Te Linde's
Operative Gynecology

Te Linde's

Operative Gynecology
Seventh Edition

John D. Thompson, M.D.

Professor
Department of Gynecology and Obstetrics
Emory University School of Medicine
Atlanta, Georgia

John A. Rock, M.D.

Chairman
Department of Gynecology and Obstetrics
The Union Memorial Hospital
Professor
Gynecology/Obstetrics and Pediatrics
The Johns Hopkins University School of Medicine
Baltimore, Maryland

46 Contributors

J. B. Lippincott Company

Philadelphia New York London Hagerstown

Acquisitions Editor: Lisa McAllister
Sponsoring Editor: Paula Callaghan
Project Editor: Virginia Barishek
Indexer: Alexandra Nickerson
Design Coordinator: Kathy Kelley-Luedtke
Designer: Terri Siegel
Production Manager: Caren Erlichman
Production Coordinator: Sharon McCarthy
Compositor: Circle Graphics
Printer/Binder: R. R. Donnelley & Sons Company

Seventh Edition

6   5   4   3   2   1

Library of Congress Cataloging-in-Publication Data

Te Linde's operative gynecology / [edited by] John D. Thompson, John
   A. Rock. — 7th ed.
      p.   cm.
   Includes bibliographical references.
   Includes index.
   Rev. ed. of: Te Linde's operative gynecology / Richard F.
Mattingly, John D. Thompson. 6th ed. © 1985.
   ISBN 0-397-50835-2
   1. Generative organs, Female—Surgery. I. Te Linde, Richard W.
(Richard Wesley), date. Te Linde's operative gynecology.
II. Thompson, John D. (John Daniel), date.   III. Rock, John A.
IV. Mattingly, Richard F. (Richard Francis), date. Te Linde's
operative gynecology.   V. Operative gynecology.
   [DNLM: 1. Genital Diseases, Female—surgery. WP 660 T2721]
RG104.T4 1992
618.1'45—dc20
DNLM/DLC
for Library of Congress   90-13389
                                                                                CIP

The authors and publisher have exerted every effort to ensure that drug selection and
dosage set forth in this text are in accord with current recommendations and practice at
the time of publication. However, in view of ongoing research, changes in government
regulations, and the constant flow of information relating to drug therapy and drug
reactions, the reader is urged to check the package insert for each drug for any change
in indications and dosage and for added warnings and precautions. This is particularly
important when the recommended agent is a new or infrequently employed drug.

Contributors

MICHAEL S. BAGGISH, M.D.
Professor and Chairman
Department of Obstetrics/Gynecology
State University of New York
Health Science Center
Chief, Crouse-Irving Memorial Hospital
Syracuse, New York

JOSEPH BUSCEMA, M.D.
Assistant Professor
Department of Gynecology and Obstetrics
The Johns Hopkins University School of Medicine
Baltimore, Maryland

WILLIAM J. BUTLER, M.D.
Associate Professor and Chief
Division of Reproductive Endocrinology, Infertility, and
    Reproductive Genetics
Department of Obstetrics and Gynecology
Albany Medical College
Assistant Attending
Obstetrics and Gynecology
Albany Medical Center Hospital
Albany, New York

LARRY C. CAREY, M.D.
Chairman, Department of Surgery
University of South Florida
Harbourside Medical Tower
Tampa General Hospital
James Haley Veterans Administration Hospital
H. Lee Moffitt Cancer Research Center
Tampa, Florida

CARMEL J. COHEN, M.D.
Professor
Department of Obstetrics, Gynecology, and
    Reproductive Science
Director
Division of Gynecologic Oncology
Mount Sinai School of Medicine of The City University
    of New York
New York, New York

JOHN L. CURRIE, M.D.
Assistant Professor
Department of Gynecology and Obstetrics
The Johns Hopkins University School of Medicine
Assistant Clinical Professor
Department of Obstetrics and Gynecology
University of Maryland School of Medicine

Vice Chairman
Department of Obstetrics and Gynecology
Director of Gynecologic Oncology and Gynecology
St. Agnes Hospital
Attending Gynecologist
The Johns Hopkins Hospital
Baltimore, Maryland

JOHN O. L. DE LANCEY, M.D.
Assistant Professor
Department of Obstetrics and Gynecology
University of Michigan Medical School
University of Michigan Medical Center
Ann Arbor, Michigan

JAMES H. DORSEY, M.D.
Chairman
Department of Gynecology
Greater Baltimore Medical Center
Assistant Professor
Department of Gynecology and Obstetrics
The Johns Hopkins University School of Medicine
Clinical Associate Professor
Department of Obstetrics and Gynecology
University of Maryland School of Medicine
Baltimore, Maryland

A. GATEWOOD DUDLEY, M.D.
Associate Clinical Professor
Department of Gynecology and Obstetrics
Emory University School of Medicine
Atlanta, Georgia

MICHELLE R. DUDZINSKI, M.D.
Assistant Professor
Division of Gynecologic Oncology
Department of Obstetrics and Gynecology
The Johns Hopkins University
Attending Physician
The Johns Hopkins Hospital
Baltimore, Maryland

PETER J. FABRI, M.D.
Professor and Vice Chairman
Department of Surgery
University of South Florida
Chief of Surgery
James A. Haley Veterans Administration Medical Center
Tampa, Florida

MALCOLM G. FREEMAN, M.D.
Professor of Gynecology and Obstetrics
Associate Professor of Pediatrics, Pathology, and
   Psychiatry
Emory University School of Medicine
Emory University Hospital
Grady Memorial Hospital
Atlanta, Georgia

CLAIRE M. FRITSCHE, M.D.
Assistant Professor of Medicine
Nephrology Division
Medical College of Wisconsin
Froedtert Memorial Lutheran Hospital
Milwaukee, Wisconsin

DAVID A. GRIMES, M.D.
Professor
Department of Obstetrics and Gynecology
University of Southern California School of Medicine
Women's Hospital
Los Angeles, California

WILLIAM A. GROWDON, M.D.
Clinical Associate Professor
Obstetrics and Gynecology
University of California, Los Angeles
UCLA Medical Center
Los Angeles, California

LEE A. HEBERT, M.D.
Division of Nephrology
Department of Internal Medicine
The Ohio State University
The Ohio State University Hospitals
Columbus, Ohio

ARMAND E. HENDEE, M.D.
Professor
Department of Gynecology and Obstetrics
Emory University School of Medicine
Atlanta, Georgia

MICHAEL P. HOPKINS, M.D.
Associate Professor
Department of Obstetrics and Gynecology
Northeastern Ohio Universities College of Medicine
Akron, Ohio

IRA R. HOROWITZ, M.D.
Assistant Professor
Department of Gynecology and Obstetrics
The Johns Hopkins University School of Medicine
Director
Department of Gynecologic Oncology
The Union Memorial Hospital
Baltimore, Maryland

JOHN H. ISAACS, M.D.
The Mary Isabelle Caestecker Professor of Obstetrics
   and Gynecology
Stritch School of Medicine
Loyola University
Chicago, Illinois

HOWARD W. JONES, JR., M.D.
Professor of Obstetrics and Gynecology
Eastern Virginia Medical School
Professor Emeritus, Gynecology and Obstetrics
The Johns Hopkins University School of Medicine
Gynecologists-Sentara Norfolk General Hospital
Norfolk, Virginia

MICHAEL H. KEELAN, JR., M.D.
Professor of Cardiology
Medical College of Wisconsin
Milwaukee, Wisconsin

JACOB LEMANN, JR., M.D.
Professor of Medicine
Chief, Nephrology Section
Medical College of Wisconsin
Froedtert Memorial Lutheran Hospital
Milwaukee, Wisconsin

SHIRLEY McCARTHY, M.D., Ph.D.
Associate Professor
Yale University School of Medicine
Director, Magnetic Resonance Imaging
Yale-New Haven Hospital
New Haven, Connecticut

PHILIP B. MEAD, M.D.
Clinical Professor of Obstetrics and Gynecology
University of Vermont College of Medicine
Hospital Epidemiologist
Medical Center Hospital of Vermont
Burlington, Vermont

GEORGE W. MITCHELL, M.D.
Professor of Obstetrics and Gynecology
University of Texas at San Antonio
Medical Center Hospital, San Antonio
San Antonio, Texas

GEORGE W. MORLEY, M.D.
Norman F. Miller Professor of Gynecology
   and Associate Professor
Department of Obstetrics and Gynecology
University of Michigan Medical School
Ann Arbor, Michigan

ANA ALVAREZ MURPHY, M.D.
Assistant Professor
University of California, San Diego
UCSD Medical Center
San Diego, California

DAVID H. NICHOLS, M.D.
Director of Gynecologic Pelvic Surgery
Massachusetts General Hospital
Boston, Massachusetts

ELVOY RAINES, J.D., M.P.H.
Vice President
Powell Adams and Rinehart
Washington, D.C.

JOHN H. RIDLEY, M.D.
Clinical Professor Emeritus
Department of Gynecology and Obstetrics
Emory University School of Medicine
Atlanta, Georgia

JOHN A. ROCK, M.D.
Chairman
Department of Gynecology and Obstetrics
The Union Memorial Hospital
Professor
Gynecology/Obstetrics and Pediatrics
The Johns Hopkins University School of Medicine
Baltimore, Maryland

WILLIAM A. ROCK, JR., M.D.
Professor of Pathology
University of Mississippi Medical Center
Director, Division of Laboratory Medicine
University Medical Center Hospitals and Clinics
Jackson, Mississippi

FELIX N. RUTLEDGE, M.D.
Professor of Gynecology
University of Texas
M.D. Anderson Cancer Center
Houston, Texas

DONALD P. SCHLEUTER, M.D.
Professor of Medicine
Pulmonary and Critical Care Medicine
Medical College of Wisconsin
Milwaukee, Wisconsin

MICHAEL R. SPENCE, M.D., M.P.H.
Professor and Chairman
Department of Obstetrics and Gynecology
Hahnemann University School of Medicine
Hahnemann University Hospital
Philadelphia, Pennsylvania

ADOLF STAFL, M.D., Ph.D.
Professor
Department of Obstetrics and Gynecology
Medical College of Wisconsin
Milwaukee, Wisconsin

DONALD P. SWARTZ, M.D., M.Sc., F.R.C.S.(C)
Professor
Department of Obstetrics and Gynecology
Albany Medical College
Chief, Division of General Gynecology
Attending in Obstetrics and Gynecology
Albany Medical Center
Consultant in Obstetrics and Gynecology
St. Peter's Hospital
Albany, New York

JOHN D. THOMPSON, M.D.
Professor
Department of Gynecology and Obstetrics
Emory University School of Medicine
Atlanta, Georgia

L. LEWIS WALL, M.D., D.Phil.
Assistant Professor
Department of Gynecology and Obstetrics
Emory University School of Medicine
Atlanta, Georgia

EDWARD E. WALLACH, M.D.
Dorothy Edward Professor of Gynecology
Director, Department of Gynecology and Obstetrics
The Johns Hopkins University School of Medicine
Director, Department of Gynecology and Obstetrics
The Johns Hopkins Hospital
Baltimore, Maryland

CLIFFORD R. WHEELESS, JR., M.D.
Professor, Gynecology and Obstetrics
Director, Gynecologic Oncology
Emory University School of Medicine
Atlanta, Georgia

TIFFANY J. WILLIAMS, M.D.
Professor, Obstetrics and Gynecology
Mayo Medical School
Consultant, Gynecologic Surgery
Mayo Medical Center
Rochester, Minnesota

ANNE WISKIND, M.D.
Assistant Professor
Department of Obstetrics and Gynecology
Emory University School of Medicine
Atlanta, Georgia

J. DONALD WOODRUFF, M.D.
Richard W. Te Linde Professor Emeritus
Gynecologic Pathology
Professor Emeritus, Obstetrics and Gynecology
The Johns Hopkins Hospital
Baltimore, Maryland

HOWARD A. ZACUR, M.D., Ph.D.
Associate Professor
Deputy Director
Department of Gynecology and Obstetrics
The Johns Hopkins University School of Medicine
Baltimore, Maryland

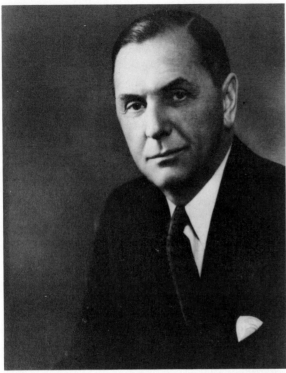

Richard W. Te Linde (1894–1989)

This is truly my last foreword to the text, *Operative Gynecology*. Howard Kelly first published his two-volume text in 1897. As the Johns Hopkins University celebrates its 100th anniversary it is truly appropriate to publish the seventh edition of *Operative Gynecology* in 1992. There has been steady advancement in operative technique with the development of the concepts of asepsis, antibiotics, and various methods to limit or prevent complications. Gynecologic surgery is in most instances safe and effective in improving women's health.

During this past century this textbook has deleted procedures which have been replaced by more effective and safer procedures. This edition is no exception. With the rapid development of operative endoscopy and the documentation of the usefulness of laser, both have had a positive impact in our specialty. These procedures have been introduced in this textbook. Other less valuable techniques have been deleted.

My colleagues have told me that more practicing physicians in our specialty have restricted their practice to gynecology. I am hopeful that the specialty will return to its surgical roots as proposed by Kelly and Cullen. The gynecologic surgeon should be trained to handle all disease in the abdomen.

I am 95 years old and have been privileged to see this specialty grow and prosper through the years. I wish to thank the present editors, John D. Thompson and John A. Rock, for carrying on the work so ably. I also wish to thank the gynecologists of this country and abroad for the acceptance of this work. It is my hope that I have made a contribution to *Operative Gynecology* and that this text will continue to serve the intellectual and technical needs of gynecologists who are interested in pelvic surgery. I leave this book in good hands and wish my colleagues Godspeed.

Richard W. Te Linde, M.D.
April 1, 1989

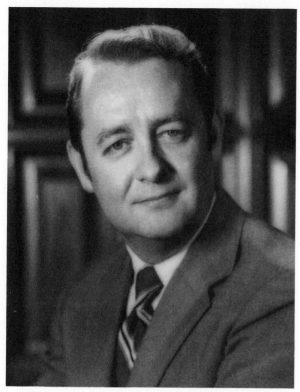

Richard F. Mattingly (1925–1986)

In their professional careers, Dr. Te Linde and Dr. Mattingly profoundly and favorably influenced the quality of contemporary gynecologic surgery through their scholarship, experience, personality, hard work, research and writing—especially their authorship and editorship of *Te Linde's Operative Gynecology* through the first six editions. We are all grateful for their dedication to professional excellence.

J.D.T.
J.A.R.

Preface

Since the publication of the first edition in 1946, *Te Linde's Operative Gynecology* has become the major textbook of gynecologic surgery for physicians in training and in practice, and the influence of this textbook has extended to many parts of the world. During the latter half of the 20th century, the dynamic changes in gynecologic surgery have been recorded in every chapter of every edition, and by the addition of new chapters and new authors. The editors of this seventh edition acknowledge their responsibility to maintain the standards of excellence firmly established in previous editions.

New to this edition is coeditor John A. Rock, M.D. Both Dr. Rock and John D. Thompson, M.D., are members of the Hopkins School of pelvic surgery. Dr. Rock is also an expert in reproductive endocrinology and infertility surgery.

The word *gynecology* comes from the Greek word *gynaios* for woman and *logia* for science. The word *surgery* comes from the Greek words for hand and work: *cheir* and *ergon*. Such a broad derivation of *gynecologic surgery* allows, indeed requires, a broad definition of the subject. Although the central focus of gynecologic surgery is clear (pathology of the reproductive system and core operative procedures), the boundaries are broad and indistinct and should include consideration of the many factors and functions that affect the general health and health care of women.

Those who are or aspire to be gynecologic surgeons have accepted an important responsibility and challenge to maintain standards of excellence in their work. To be the best gynecologic surgeon possible requires a blending of surgical sciences and technical skills.

The application of basic surgical science in the everyday practice of gynecologic surgery cannot be overemphasized. Gynecologic surgery is a beautiful and fascinating subject to study and attempt to master in technical detail. An adequate level of technical skill is important but cannot be emphasized to the exclusion of all else. In addition to technique, surgical judgment and perioperative care must also be learned. Truly great surgeons are noted not for their technical skills but for their great surgical judgment before, during, and after the operation. The intricacies of the decision-making process as applied to gynecologic surgery are often more difficult than teaching and learning the technical skills.

It should be emphasized that the ability to perform gynecologic operations with a low mortality and morbidity rate is not *ipso facto* evidence that gynecologic surgery is being practiced correctly. In addition to a low mortality and morbidity rate, one must be concerned that only patients with proper indications are chosen for surgical treatment. The knowledge needed to formulate the proper "indications for surgery" includes, first, a thorough understanding of the physiology and pathology of the female reproductive organs, as well as an understanding of the clinical manifestations of the disease process and the normal and abnormal development of psychosocial-sexual behavior. This basic knowledge is the absolute foundation of gynecologic surgery. On the basis of this knowledge, one must decide whether a patient should be offered surgical therapy, remembering that only the occasional gynecologic patient requires surgery for relief.

After the right patient has been selected for operation, the right operation must be selected for the patient. The practice of gynecologic surgery includes proper preparation of the patient for operation, proper technical performance of the operation, and proper postoperative care, follow-up, and rehabilitation. In the practice of gynecologic surgery, mistakes may be made in the course of operation by the use of improper technique. Perhaps even more mistakes may be made by using improper indications for surgery.

Proper surgical practice is not possible without including humanistic concerns. Individual human beings who suffer from disease, deformity, or malfunction are influenced by unique personal, social, and ethical concerns. Gynecologic surgery may seem to have a narrow focus, but a narrow focus in any branch of medicine or surgery is acceptable so long as recognition is given to the personal concerns of individual patients as they relate to function and care.

As the science of gynecologic surgery evolves, new wisdom and conduct will be needed. Pellegrino has said that "medicine is the most humane of the sciences, the most empiric of the arts, and the most scientific of the humanities." So it is with gynecologic surgery. After all, gynecologic surgeons are physicians first. They are members of a profession dedicated to the well-being of womankind and mankind. The gynecologic surgeon who brings the greatest amount of ability, energy, and kindly feeling to the work is the one who will best serve the patient and best exemplify the standards of the profession.

Those who practice or aspire to practice gynecologic surgery should continue to concentrate on quality in their work. Such concentration is needed to balance the increasing numbers of gynecologic surgeons and patients, the increasing complexity and detail of knowledge of reproductive and related organ physiology and pathology, and the greater technical skills required to master operative procedures. Throughout one's lifetime, education and training must always continue. High standards of quality assurance must be maintained. The incidence of immediate complications and long-term poor results must be kept to a minimum.

In spite of conscientious effort, errors in the practice of gynecologic surgery are inevitable. Osler once said, "Errors in judgment must occur in the practice of an art which consists largely in balance probabilities." The gynecologic surgeon who is conscientious and well trained and who operates with proper indications in the best interests of the patient, will serve this surgical specialty and its patients well. Just as in business and industry, quality in service, performance, and results will bring forth a competitive edge.

Socioeconomic and demographic factors will to some extent influence the environment in which gynecologic surgery is practiced in the future. A larger number of gynecologic patients will be older, requiring greater emphasis on geriatric gynecology. At the same time, more younger women will seek assistance with reproductive health problems. Nonsurgical or more conservative surgical methods will be used more often. Previously standard methods of surgical treatment will be challenged and perhaps replaced by advances in medical and surgical technology. New laparoscopy techniques will increasingly replace "open" surgery. As a result of developing technology, fewer operations will be performed in smaller hospitals and the technical skills needed to perform certain operations will be difficult to acquire and maintain. More patients will be referred to specialized facilities to obtain good cost-effective results. Concern for professional liability and cost containment will influence the choice of procedure, the indications for surgery, and the choice of surgeon. New surgical techniques will be evaluated more carefully for safety and effectiveness before they are adopted as appropriate and standard care. Standard indications for existing surgical procedures will undergo evaluation and scrutiny.

The patients we serve will expect to have a more active role in recommendations and decisions regarding the choice of surgical procedures. The surgeon must respect the patient's autonomy in all phases of medical care, especially as the role of women in society changes.

Many leaders in gynecologic surgery believe that improvements in the training of surgical residents are needed, especially if the skill of the surgeon is to equal or surpass that of his or her predecessor. Pelvic surgeons must be well versed in the general principles of surgery. They must be experienced in techniques of anatomical dissection of advanced pelvic disease; be capable of managing complications such as fistulas and other defects involving adjacent organ systems; have a broad base of operative experience; have an understanding of pathology and basic science of reproductive medicine; and have an awareness of the clinical manifestations and psychological aspects of pelvic disease. A pelvic surgeon must be able to manage the usual and straightforward, as well as the difficult, complicated, unusual, and unexpected.

If current training programs are to accomplish these aims, it will be necessary to extend the period of training. For those interested in more than the basic gynecology-obstetric residency training, formal subspecialty recognition of special competence in gynecologic surgery is needed and should be encouraged.

The reader will find many new contributions to the seventh edition that update this work and broaden the knowledge of the pelvic surgeon. We especially wish to thank Michael Baggish, Joseph Buscema, William Butler, Larry Carey, Carmel Cohen, John Currie, John De Lancey, James Dorsey, Gatewood Dudley, Michelle Dudzinski, Peter Fabri, Malcolm Freeman, Claire Fritsche, David Grimes, William Growdon, Lee Hebert, Armand Hendee, Michael Hopkins, Ira Horowitz, John Isaacs, Howard Jones, Jr., Michael Keelan, Jacob Lemann, Shirley McCarthy, Philip Mead, George Mitchell, George Morley, Ana Alvarez Murphy, David Nichols, Elvoy Raines, John Ridley, William Rock, Felix Rutledge, Donald Schleuter, Michael Spence, Adolf Stafl, Donald Swartz, Lewis Wall, Edward Wallach, Clifford Wheeless, Jr., Tiffany Williams, Anne Wiskind, Donald Woodruff, and Howard Zacur for their contributions to this expanded edition. The editors gratefully acknowledge the assistance of Glenda Smith, Claire Hackworth, Anne Terry, Patricia Poor, and the staff of the J.B. Lippincott Company in the preparation of the text.

Gynecologic surgery is a dynamic field, always in

transition. This will not cease with publication of this edition of *Te Linde's Operative Gynecology*. Therefore, this book cannot and does not pretend to define the standards of care in pelvic surgery. It does present generally recognized and accepted methods and techniques in gynecologic surgery. Methods and techniques not mentioned here may also be appropriate when special circumstances are taken into consideration. It is our hope that the information in this seventh edition of *Te Linde's Operative Gynecology* will be beneficial to those young men and women engaged in the process of learning gynecologic surgery as well as to those experienced gynecologic surgeons interested in bringing their knowledge up to date. Gynecologic surgeons who

perform the most common operative procedures will find new and useful information in the text. The surgeon whose practice is composed of the most complicated, unusual, and difficult problems will also find much useful discussion of specialized operative techniques.

Finally, the seventh edition is dedicated to the two previous editors, Dr. Richard W. Te Linde and Dr. Richard F. Mattingly, both scholars in pelvic surgery. Without their work in previous editions, the seventh edition would not exist.

John D. Thompson, M.D.
John A. Rock, M.D.

Contents

8   Control of Pelvic Hemorrhage: Blood Component Therapy and Hemorrhagic Shock   151

JOHN D. THOMPSON, WILLIAM A. ROCK, Jr., AND ANNE WISKIND

9   Postoperative Infections   195

PHILIP B. MEAD

10   Wound Healing, Surgical Instrumentation, and Suture Material   209

MICHELLE R. DUDZINSKI

20   Endometriosis   463
TIFFANY J. WILLIAMS

21   Application of Laser in Gynecology   499
JAMES H. DORSEY

22   Surgery for Benign Disease of the Ovary   525
JOHN A. ROCK

28 Evolving Aspects of Reparative Surgery   739
HOWARD W. JONES, JR.

29 Operative Injuries to the Ureter: Prevention, Recognition, and Management   749
JOHN D. THOMPSON

30 Vesicovaginal Fistulas   785
JOHN D. THOMPSON

43 Malignant Tumors of the Uterine Corpus   1253
JOHN L. CURRIE

44 Surgical Treatment of Ovarian Cancer   1303
FELIX N. RUTLEDGE

45 Pelvic Exenteration   1329
GEORGE W. MORLEY AND MICHAEL P. HOPKINS

Historical Development of Pelvic Surgery

JOHN A. ROCK

*No group should ever neglect to honor the work
of forebears upon which their contributions are
based. Great is the loss to anyone who neglects
to study the lives of those he follows.*

Howard A. Kelly

All specialties in medicine have evolved gradually. Subspecialties continue to emerge as new knowledge is developed within each field. In retrospect, isolated surgical events, especially in the 19th and 20th centuries, served as the foundation of gynecologic surgery as a distinct entity. These historical masterworks highlight the progress in the discipline and, if studied carefully, can have practical value in improving the practice of modern pelvic surgery.

In the early days of medicine in the United States, it was customary for one person to hold a combined chair of anatomy and surgery; thus, the discipline of obstetrics and gynecology was included with surgery. John Collins Warren, later to become the founder of the Massachusetts General Hospital, was the first Professor of Anatomy and Surgery at that institution. Phillip Syng Physick, often considered the father of American surgery, held the first chair of surgery divorced from anatomy in the United States at the University of Pennsylvania in 1805. Gynecology was first recognized in this country as a distinct medical discipline in 1813, when

The authors wish to express their sincere appreciation to Gert H. Brieger, M.D., William H. Welch Professor and Director of the Institute of the History of Medicine, the Johns Hopkins University School of Medicine, Baltimore, Maryland, for his suggestions for the revision of this chapter on the history of gynecologic surgery.

Theodore Woodward was appointed Lecturer in Gynecology at the Medical School of Castleton, Vermont. By the late 19th century, many medical schools had appointed professors of gynecology and obstetrics separate from surgery, although diseases of women and children continued to be taught together as a single course in many schools. Obstetrics was divorced from the chair of surgery during the first part of the 19th century. Gynecology began to be identified as a specialty during this period and its separation from general surgery was more gradual. By the beginning of the 20th century, pediatrics was separated from gynecology and obstetrics, largely through the efforts of Abraham Jacobi, a pioneer pediatrician of New York. Today gynecology is divorced almost completely from general surgery in practice, and in all medical schools in the United States it is combined with obstetrics. The final combination of gynecology and obstetrics as a distinct and major medical specialty in the United States is largely the result of the establishment of the American Board of Obstetrics and Gynecology in 1930 and of the development of residency training programs that combined gynecologic and obstetric education and training. However, attempts continue today to give pelvic surgery the status of a distinct surgical discipline separate from obstetrics.

Important advances in pelvic surgery have been made by many gynecologic surgeons in other countries, particularly those in Britain and Europe. Therefore, the history of pelvic surgery in the United States must be viewed as a conjoining of surgical concepts and experience from abroad with the rapidly growing technology and science in North America during the 19th and 20th centuries.

OOPHORECTOMY

Pelvic surgery may be said to have begun in the backwoods of Kentucky when Ephraim McDowell (Fig. 1-1) successfully removed a large ovarian tumor from Jane Todd Crawford. He had studied under John Bell of Edinburgh, who suggested the operation to McDowell. The operation, performed on Christmas morning in 1809, was done without the benefit of anesthesia or asepsis. McDowell considered the operation an experiment, as it truly was, and frankly told the patient so. She agreed to accept the risk and demonstrated her faith in her doctor and the Lord by singing hymns during the operation. While McDowell was performing the operation, his house was surrounded by a crowd of the patient's friends, who intended to shoot or hang him if the patient died. Fortunately, she made a rapid recovery and lived for 32 years, to die at the mature age of 78. McDowell's publication of his first three successful cases of ovariotomy (oophorectomy) marks the beginning of abdominal surgery. The operation fell into disrepute shortly thereafter because of misuse. The brothers Atlee of Lancaster, Pennsylvania, were among those who performed the procedure during the middle of the 19th century for a wide range of nonsurgical indications. At the tenth annual meeting of the American Gynecological Society in 1885, William T. Howard reported that Washington Lee Atlee had performed 255 operations for removal of the ovary.

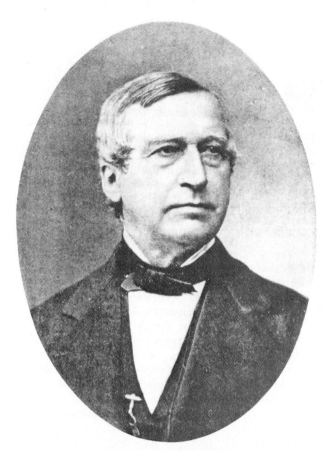

Figure 1–2. Washington Lee Atlee (1808–1878).

MYOMECTOMY

In 1840, Amussat of France performed the first recorded myomectomy. In the United States, the operation was done shortly thereafter, in 1844, by Washington Atlee (Fig.1-2). In 1850, Professor Mussey wrote: "Of all the achievements of modern surgery we meet with, none [is] more striking or extraordinary than the operation performed by Professor Atlee for the removal of fibrous tumors." A generation later, J. Marion Sims wrote: "The name of Atlee stands without a rival in connection with uterine fibroids. His operations were so heroic that no man has as yet dared to imitate him." In more modern times, Victor Bonney in England and Isadore Rubin in this country were the greatest advocates of myomectomy. Their enthusiasm exceeded that of more recent gynecologists, but myomectomy has found a definite place in today's pelvic surgery.

HYSTERECTOMY

It was not until many years after "ovariotomy" was being done rather frequently and with some favorable results that an abdominal hysterectomy was suc-

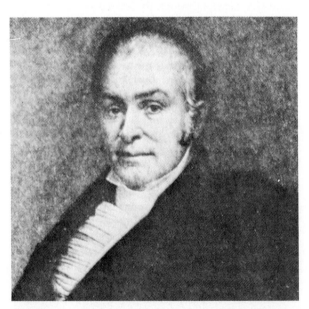

Figure 1–1. Ephraim McDowell (1771–1830), "father of abdominal surgery."

cessfully performed. Myomectomy was done before hysterectomy was attempted. In 1843, Charles Clay of Manchester performed abdominal removal of a leiomyomatous uterus, but the patient fell on the floor violently and died on the morning of the 15th day after operation. The first completely successful removal of a leiomyomatous uterus took place in Massachusetts in 1853. Dr. Walter Burnham of Lowell opened the abdomen to remove what was thought to be an ovarian cyst. Lacking adequate anesthesia, the patient suddenly vomited and extruded the large uterus through the incision. The operator could not replace it and was forced to remove it. The patient survived, and Burnham was encouraged to attempt further hysterectomies. Of his next 15 cases, only 3 survived. Sir James Young Simpson, considered a daring surgeon at the middle of the 19th century, said that the idea of removing uterine leiomyomas should be rejected "as an utterly unjustifiable operation in surgery." Lawson Tait attempted to solve the problem of leiomyomas by castration, by means of bilateral oophorectomy. At the fifth annual meeting of the American Gynecological Society in 1880, C. D. Palmer reviewed a total of 119 hysterectomies collected from the literature by Pozzi in 1875. Palmer reported a surgical mortality of 64% and estimated that if the unreported cases were included, the mortality rate at that time would have exceeded 75%.

Vaginal hysterectomy was performed in 1813 by Langenbeck in Germany and in 1829 by John Collins Warren in Boston. Both operations were unsuccessful. Fenger described the modern operation of vaginal hysterectomy in 1881. Proponents of the vaginal approach and proponents of the abdominal approach began their arguments in the late 19th century; the argument continues to some extent today. Kelly was an early proponent of vaginal hysterectomy but later changed to a preference for the abdominal approach.

TREATMENT OF VESICOVAGINAL FISTULAS

Vesicovaginal fistulas existed in ancient Egypt, which is proved by the discovery of a large fistula in the mummy of Queen Henhenit, one of the wives of King Menuhotep, who reigned about 2050 B.C. Avicenna, an Arabo-Persian physician who died in 1037, is said to have been the first to recognize that incontinence of urine in women may be due to a fistula resulting from difficult labor. He considered the condition incurable and advocated contraception in the very young as a preventative. Until the work of J. Marion Sims in the mid-19th-century United States, attempts at cure had extremely limited success. Van Roonhuyse of Holland was one of the most ardent experimenters, and de

Lamelle of France reported some successes; but failures were much more frequent. J. T. Mettauer of Virginia also struggled with the problem during this time and was the first to use metallic sutures. In 1838, he performed the first successful closure of a vesicovaginal fistula in this country, but he did not report it until 1840. In 1847, he reported six such successful cases, and in 1855 he reported a total of 27 cures.

During these preanesthesia and preasepsis days, J. Marion Sims, a Southerner, began his experiments on the cure of vesicovaginal fistulas (Fig. 1-3). The term *experiments* is appropriate, since four years of experimentation elapsed before his first success. Sims had a successful career in surgery as practiced then in Montgomery, Alabama. He had no experience in pelvic surgery; in fact, he disliked it. It was his custom to turn away patients with pelvic disorders, referring them to doctors whom he considered more competent in this field. His slave-holding planter friends owned female slaves who had been delivered by midwives, and some of these slaves suffered from large vesicovaginal fistulas, then considered incurable. With this disturbing condition the slaves were unacceptable as house servants. One of Sims's planter friends pleaded with him to attempt to cure the women. At first Sims declined the task, believing it to be hopeless; but finally his compassion for the unfortunate women persuaded him to undertake it. He worked on a group of these black women from 1845 to 1849 before achieving his first cure. During these years he housed and boarded the patients at his own expense in a small building that he constructed

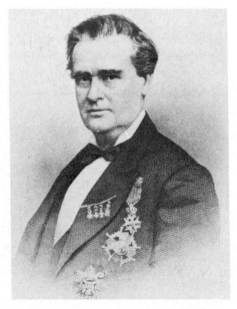

Figure 1–3. James Marion Sims (1813–1883).

for this purpose on his own property. His many failures only stimulated his determination and efforts. The colleagues who at first assisted him at the operations abandoned him, and his friends begged him to give up what appeared to be a hopeless effort; so he trained other slave patients to assist him in the operations. In his 29th operation on one patient, he was finally successful in closing her vesicovaginal fistula. He attributed his ultimate success to the use of the lateral position (now known as Sims's position); the use of silver-wire sutures, which had initially been described by Mettauer; and the use of special instruments that he devised. The most important and lasting of these instruments was Sims's speculum, which evolved from a pewter spoon he used in earlier cases. However, an almost identical instrument of polished silver had been described by von Metzler in Prague in 1846. Sims's success in his small private hospital in Montgomery, Alabama, soon became known and took him to New York City, where he became one of the founders of the Woman's Hospital. From there his fame spread to the capitals of Europe, where he was received with the greatest esteem and where he demonstrated his operative technique on several women with fistulas that had been considered incurable. All his operations were done without asepsis and without anesthesia. In the late 1920s, Mahfouz of Egypt reported on his vast experience with the repair of vesicovaginal fistulas utilizing the principles of Sims, with the great advantage of general anesthesia.

Although Sims made one of the important surgical contributions of the 19th century, he overlooked the original canine experiments by Levert (1829) with silver wire and the first successful silver-wire closure of a vesicovaginal fistula by Gosset (1834). To Sims must be accorded the recognition for perfecting and popularizing the technique of vesicovaginal fistula repair from previously developed surgical concepts. Credit for the original pioneering work and initial surgical success with silver wire must go to others.

ANESTHESIA

Anesthesia and asepsis were the two major developments of the 19th century that advanced the field of gynecologic surgery. Soporifics had long been used to lessen the pain of surgery, but none was very successful. The discovery of general anesthesia by chloroform and ether is one of the most fascinating stories in medicine. It introduced a new era in surgery, and progress thereafter was rapid.

There is much discussion as to who first used chloroform (discovered by the great German chemist Justus von Liebig in 1831) as an anesthetic, but it is certain that after a number of personal experiments with it, Simpson administered its beneficent fumes to a woman in the pangs of labor on November 4, 1847. He was the first to apply it in just this way and probably the first to use it for the relief of pain.

The discovery of ether as a general anesthetic was undoubtedly America's greatest contribution to medicine up to that time. A detailed account of the struggle for priority in this great discovery is beyond this short review, but a few salient points may be of interest.

There is little doubt that Crawford Long, a practitioner in a rural community in Georgia, first used ether as an anesthetic in surgery. He was a modest practitioner who did only such surgery and obstetrics as came his way in his general practice; the discovery was somewhat accidental. It was the custom in Long's rural community to hold "ether frolics." The participants would inhale the fumes and become quite intoxicated. During the cavorting about, the merrymakers often fell and bruised themselves. On questioning them, Long was surprised to learn that they had no recollection of falling and suffered no pain at the time of injury. From this experience he conceived the idea that surgery might be made painless by the use of this drug. He first used it in 1842, although he did not publish his results until 1849.

While Long was using ether as a surgical anesthetic, Horace Wells, a dentist, was experimenting with nitrous oxide ("laughing gas") and had some of his own teeth extracted using it. After an untoward result, however, he abandoned its use. A chemist suggested to William Thomas Green Morton, who was Wells's partner, that he use ether. Morton persuaded John Collins Warren to use it in surgery at the Massachusetts General Hospital, which he did successfully in 1846. A month later, this was reported by an observer of the operation, H. J. Bigelow. Thus, the Massachusetts group was the first to publicize the use of ether anesthesia, although Crawford Long was the first to use it. Long would probably never have received recognition had it not been for J. Marion Sims, who brought it to the attention of the medical public in an article published in 1877. As a result of this, Long's statue now stands in the Hall of Fame in New York and in the Capitol Rotunda in Washington, D.C. It is of interest to note that the name *anesthesia,* derived from the Greek word meaning "insensibility," was suggested by Oliver Wendell Holmes.

ASEPSIS, ANTISEPSIS

At the time of the development of gynecologic surgery in the mid- and late 19th century, death from sepsis was the major surgical complication. In the mid-19th century, the development of ether anesthesia extended the surgical treatment of pelvic disease and, at the same time, increased the postoperative mortality from sepsis. Hand washing was sporadic; surgeons operated in their street clothes; ligatures were attached to the outer clothing of the surgical assistant; sea sponges were used, washed, and reused many times without sterilization; and the observers of an operation were frequently invited to examine the operative field with their unwashed fingers. The success of an operative procedure was related principally to the patient's ability to mount sufficient host defenses to prevent the spread of the local tissue infection that invariably occurred.

The discovery of general anesthesia opened the door to rapid progress in pelvic surgery, but other discoveries also stimulated its development. One of these was the proof by Ignaz Semmelweis of the contagiousness of puerperal fever in the Vienna Frauenklinik. His work was published from Budapest, where he became professor in 1845. His insistence on asepsis in the delivery room was responsible for a new era in obstetrics, but his principles were also adopted for surgery. Like many revolutionary discoveries, his ideas were rejected by his colleagues, who ridiculed and persecuted him, eventually forcing him to an insane asylum, where he died at the age of 47—ironically, from septicemia.

Another event that had a profound effect on the development of surgery was the work of Baron Joseph Lister, who performed the first successful antiseptic treatment of a surgical wound at the Royal Infirmary in Glasgow in 1865, on the day preceding the death of Semmelweis. His method of sterilization included the use of carbolic acid spray, not only in the operative field to prevent the growth of pathologic bacteria, but also in the operating room. His results were published two years later, and his ideas were slowly but widely accepted. It is noteworthy that whereas Lister's was the principle of antisepsis, Semmelweis's principle was one of asepsis by thorough scrubbing to sterilize the hands of the operator. So not only did Semmelweis's work precede Lister's by 20 years, but his ideas were more advanced than those of Lister and corresponded more nearly to the customs of modern surgery. Lister also freely acknowledged his contribution to surgical asepsis as an extension of the original bacteriologic studies of Louis Pasteur. Pasteur also advanced the principles of surgical asepsis by advocating that a scalpel blade be passed through a flame before use. In the latter part of 1864, the year before Lister began to use carbolic acid on wounds, Sir Thomas Spencer Wells, the eminent British surgeon, published a paper in the *British Medical Journal* entitled "Some Causes of Excessive Mortality After Surgical Operations." Wells suggested that pus may result from germs finding their way into an appropriate medium in wounds, subsequently resulting in septicemia. Wells's concept of infection was not accepted by the academic community. Nonetheless, Lister may have been stimulated by his thought.

The use of rubber gloves was a great step in aseptic surgery. Although William S. Halsted of Johns Hopkins is generally credited with the introduction of boiled rubber gloves in surgery, the idea was not solely his. In 1939, Halsted wrote:

The operating in gloves was an evolution rather than an inspiration or happy thought. In the winter of 1889 and 1890, I cannot recall the month, the nurse in charge of my operating room (later Mrs. Halsted) complained that the solutions of mercuric chloride produced a dermatitis of her arms and hands. As she was an unusually efficient woman, I gave the matter my consideration and one day in New York requested the Goodyear Rubber Company to make as an experiment two pair of thin rubber gloves with gauntlets. In the report that I made of the first year's work at the hospital, written in November and December, 1890, and published in March, 1891, I stated that the assistant who passed instruments wore rubber gloves to protect his hands from the solution of phenol—in which the instruments were submerged—rather than to eliminate him as a source of infection. I do not recall having referred again, in my publications, to the employment of rubber gloves. Dr. Hunter Robb in 1894, in his book on aseptic technique, recommended that the operator wear rubber gloves. Dr. Robb was at that time resident gynecologist of the Johns Hopkins Hospital.

A photograph taken in the Halsted clinic of a breast operation in 1893 shows that gloves were not being worn by him at that time. Halsted states further that it was remarkable that "we could have been so blind as not to have perceived the necessity of wearing them invariably at the operating table." So to Hunter Robb, a gynecologist, belongs the credit of recommending that the operator use rubber gloves.

Horatio Storer of Boston, credited with performing the first successful cesarean hysterectomy in the world in 1869, was actually the first surgeon to wear rubber gloves while operating.

With the adoption of general anesthesia and asepsis, the way was cleared for rapid progress in all fields of surgery. Gynecologic surgery suddenly received renewed life.

OTHER ADVANCES IN OPERATIVE GYNECOLOGY, 1850–1900

Thomas Addis Emmett, a Virginian who had moved to New York, was an illustrious pupil of Sims's at the Woman's Hospital. He devised operations for the repair of the vagina and cervix. The Emmett vaginal repair has persisted, with some modifications, though the cervical repair as done by Emmett is seldom used today. Emmett did not follow his mentor, Sims, as chief surgeon at the Woman's Hospital—not from lack of ability but because of personality clashes between him and the governing board of the hospital. Previously, Sims had clashed with the board over his insistence that women with cervical cancer be admitted to the hospital.

During this era, progress was also being made in England in operative gynecology. Sir Thomas Spencer Wells performed many "ovariotomies" and published his ideas on the subject in his book *Diseases of the Ovaries.* He was one of the first in England to insist on the greatest cleanliness of the operator's hands and instruments. A little later, a Scot, Robert Lawson Tait, transferred to London and Birmingham and made these cities centers of gynecologic surgery in England. He was a violent opponent of antisepsis and antagonistic in his personal relations to the profession, but he made landmark contributions to the surgical management of ectopic pregnancy and pelvic inflammatory disease.

In the United States, leadership in pelvic surgery was transferred from New York to Baltimore. Howard A. Kelly (Fig. 1-4) graduated from the University of Pennsylvania in 1882, the year before Sims died. He spent several years in postgraduate work in Germany when that country led the world in teaching pathology under Virchow and bacteriology under Koch. He was brought to Johns Hopkins as the head of gynecology and obstet-

rics in 1889, at the age of 31, by Welch and Osler, who had known him in Philadelphia. He was a bold and aggressive surgeon and was given carte blanche to develop his ideas at the new medical school. After several years, realizing that his real interest was in pelvic surgery, he turned the Department of Obstetrics over to J. Whitridge Williams, whose illustrious career in that specialty justified Kelly's decision. Kelly had great interest in the female urinary system, realizing that the symptomatology of urinary tract disease is often intertwined with that of the reproductive organs. As a means of investigating these symptoms, Kelly invented the air cystoscope and devised ureteral catheters. He was the first to plicate the vesical sphincter for stress incontinence of urine. Dr. Kelly wrote extensively on the organization of the gynecologic operating room (Fig. 1-5). He also devised many techniques and refinements of pelvic surgery (Fig. 1-6), which were published in his textbook *Operative Gynecology,* a classic on that subject for many years. Kelly's many textbooks were beautifully illustrated by Max Brödel (Fig. 1-7), who came to the Johns Hopkins Hospital from Germany as a very young man. Brödel's contribution to operative gynecology was tremendous in his portrayal of operative techniques, pelvic anatomy, and pathologic disease. His contribution was great not only to gynecology, but to all medicine. He set a standard for medical illustration never before attained and unsurpassed since. His school for medical illustrators supplied artists to many medical centers throughout the United States. Brödel's illustrations of Richardson's technique of total abdominal hysterectomy helped turn the tide in favor of total rather than subtotal hysterectomy.

Great as Kelly's contributions to pelvic surgery were, perhaps the most enduring result of his professorship at Johns Hopkins was his establishment of the long-term residency training program, which has been copied generally throughout the United States and to some extent in foreign countries. This plan for training pelvic surgeons, which emphasizes a strong background in and knowledge of gynecologic pathology and female urology, has done more to elevate the quality of gynecologic practice than any other factor.

TREATMENT OF CERVICAL CANCER

The earliest attempts to cure cervical cancer were made by simple amputation of the cervix. In the early part of the 19th century, Marie Anne Boivin, one of the earliest female surgeons, had amputated a cervix that showed cancerous ulceration. Many others—Osiander, Dupuytren, Recamier, and Lisfranc—had performed the same operation. England was far behind France in the diagnosis and treatment of cervical cancer, possibly

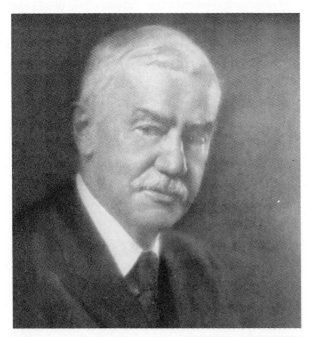

Figure 1–4. Howard A. Kelly (1858–1943). (Davis AW: Dr. Kelly of Hopkins. Baltimore: The Johns Hopkins Press, 1959.)

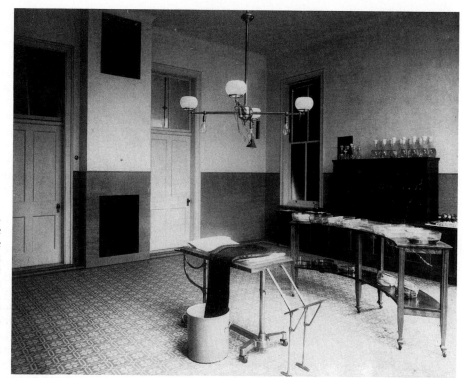

Figure 1–5. Dr. Howard A. Kelly's old operating room at the Johns Hopkins Hospital. To the left is the door to the corridor. In the center is the door to the ether room. The rubber pad was used for drainage during irrigation of the abdomen. A similar pad was developed by Dr. Kelly for drainage of blood and amniotic fluid during and after a vaginal delivery.

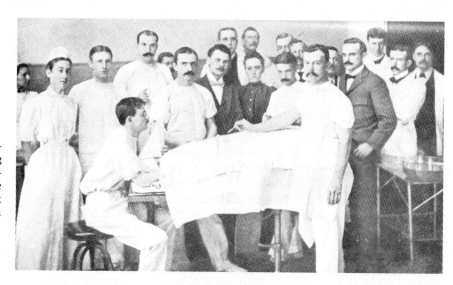

Figure 1–6. Howard Kelly operates. Grouped about the operating table, left to right, are: Emma Beckwith, head nurse; Jay Durkee (seated); Thomas S. Cullen; Max Brödel (in the center); Elisabeth Hurdon; J. E. Stokes; John G. Clark. (Davis AW: Dr. Kelly of Hopkins. Baltimore: The Johns Hopkins Press, 1959.)

because of Victorian modesty, which prevented vaginal examinations except in the most desperate cases. Sir James Young Simpson attacked the problem in England and stressed the importance of early diagnosis. He observed that cervical amputation "can be employed only in very few cases of cancroid disease of the cervix, seeing that it is only when you can catch the disease, so to speak, before it has reached the line of reflexion between the cervix and the vagina, that you can amputate with any hope or prospect of success."

Following these failures with cervical amputation, simple hysterectomy was tried. This, too, was generally unsuccessful, and it became evident that a more radical surgical approach would have to be taken if any mea-

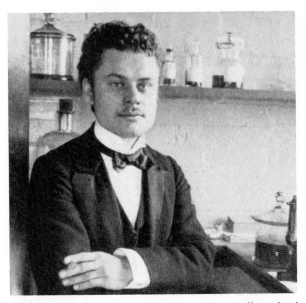

Figure 1–7. Max Brödel. (Robinson J: Tom Cullen of Baltimore. New York: Oxford University Press, 1949.)

sure of success was to be attained. In 1895, Emil Reis of Chicago attacked the problem and developed a radical abdominal operation with pelvic lymph gland dissection, which he performed on dogs and cadavers. In that same year, John Clark, a resident gynecologist at Johns Hopkins Hospital, employed this technique for the treatment of invasive cervical cancer. Three years later, Wertheim of Vienna began doing the same radical abdominal type of hysterectomy with selective pelvic lymphadenectomy and popularized it in Europe and, to a lesser extent, in the United States. His name has been associated with it since, although Clark was the first to perform the operation. Some success was attained with this radical procedure when the disease was limited to the cervix, later defined as stage I, but when the disease had progressed beyond this stage, the salvage was indeed small. Initially, the operation carried with it a 10% mortality, and ureteral, vesical, and rectal fistulas to the vagina were common. Sampson, who was later to become famous for his work on endometriosis, did special work on the blood supply of the ureter and the pathogenesis of ureteral injury in dogs while he was a resident and young faculty member at the Johns Hopkins Hospital. The intention was to preserve ureteral blood supply and thus avoid fistulas from the extensive lymph node dissection. In spite of his work, the percentage of ureteral fistulas remained high with the use of the Wertheim hysterectomy. In recent years, fistulas occur in less than 2% of such cases.

Realizing the shortcomings of operative cure of this disease, Kelly experimented with radium therapy. He and the many gynecologists who followed his early attempts attained greater success in the overall salvage of cervical cancer than had been attained by surgery. Although fistulas and other complications resulted from intravaginal radium therapy, they occurred most often in the advanced cases in which cure was impossible by surgery or irradiation.

In the 1940s, Meigs at the Massachusetts General Hospital revised and extended the Wertheim type of radical abdominal operation. He believed that with modern therapy at his disposal, such as antibiotics, blood replacement, and intravenous control of electrolytes, the procedure should be reevaluated. He proved that in expert hands the operation could be done with a mortality of not over 1%. He was unable, however, to reduce appreciably the incidence of fistulas.

Another surgical approach to the treatment of cervical cancer was made in 1908 by Schauta, who published a volume on the removal of the uterus and parametrium by the vaginal route, which he had first done in 1901. The greatest proponents of this operation were van Bouwdijk Bastiaanse of Amsterdam and Ernst Navratil of Graz, but it never obtained popularity in the United States. The greatest disadvantage of the procedure was that it did not permit the removal of pelvic lymph nodes, as does the Wertheim procedure. However, the mortality in expert hands was only 3% to 4%, in contrast to several times that percentage with the Wertheim procedure.

In a review article in 1968, Alexander Brunschwig of New York published his radical surgical method of treating advanced and recurrent cervical cancer, a procedure he first practiced 20 years previously. It consisted essentially of exenterating adjacent pelvic organs and the generative organs, with diversion of the urine and feces through the abdominal wall, depending on whether the bladder or rectum or both were removed. Initially, mortality and morbidity were high and salvage was small. The major usefulness of this procedure was in the en bloc removal of a radioresistant carcinoma of the cervix that had recurred centrally in the cervix and in which extension to the adjacent bladder and rectum could not be disproved. Current improvements in radiation techniques and dosimetry have reduced the frequency of central radiation failure in the treatment of cervical cancer as well as the clinical use of this ultraradical procedure. However, with ample blood replacement, antibiotics, and attention to electrolyte balance, these extensive procedures have found a limited place in the care of cervical cancer in carefully selected cases.

MORE MILESTONES

Thomas S. Cullen succeeded Kelly to the chair at Johns Hopkins in 1919 (Fig. 1-8). His contribution to pelvic surgery was indirect: the establishment of a gyne-

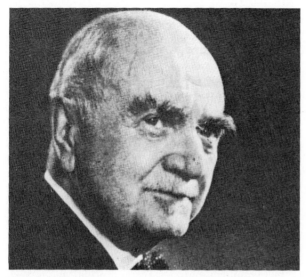

Figure 1–8. Thomas S. Cullen (1868–1953). (Robinson J: Tom Cullen of Baltimore. New York: Oxford University Press, 1949.)

cologic pathology laboratory. This was somewhat accidental. He went to Baltimore after an internship in Toronto, intending to work with Kelly in pelvic surgery, but no position was immediately available on Kelly's surgical staff. To mark time, he was sent to the Department of Pathology to work under William Welch. He established a laboratory of gynecologic pathology that remains to this day. Cullen's book *Cancer of the Uterus* (1900) was published from this laboratory and was considered the classic on the subject for many years. Cullen was succeeded in his laboratory by Emil Novak, who published extensively from it, especially in the field of ovarian tumors. Thus, indirectly, with an understanding of the pathology of the pelvic organs, pelvic surgery was placed on a scientific rather than a purely technical level.

Endometriosis, one of the most common conditions requiring pelvic surgery, was first described by Russell in Cullen's laboratory in 1899. The disease was publicized by extensive studies of its histology by Sampson, who had been one of Kelly's early residents. His publications began in the early 1920s and extended to 1940. His theory of retrograde menstruation was the subject of the great controversy during this period. It was greatly strengthened by the experimental work of Te Linde and Scott, who in 1950 created endometriosis artificially in monkeys by permitting them to menstruate into the peritoneal cavity, thus demonstrating the ability of the cast-off endometrium to grow on the serosal surfaces. The effect of hormones on this artificially created endometriosis was studied by Scott and Wharton, and Kistner of Boston proposed the therapeutic use of progesterone to produce a sustained pseu-

dopregnancy. However, surgery, augmented by the use of the carbon dioxide laser, remains the backbone of therapy.

In the realm of vesicovaginal fistulas, the surgical tenets of Sims still hold. Also, Latzko's contribution in 1914 of partial colpocleisis for closure of a high post-hysterectomy fistula was a major step in the curability of fistulas of this type. Silver-wire sutures in the vagina have now been superseded by delayed-absorbable suture material.

Because of three important advances, rectovaginal fistulas and third-degree perineal tears are curable today in a much higher percentage of cases than before. The first of these dates from 1882, when Warren described his method of turning down a flap of vaginal mucosa to replace the defect in the terminal end of the anterior wall of the rectum. A better technique was described in 1902 by Nobel. A second advance was the use of Sulfasuxidine and neomycin for bowel sterilization. Finally, the cutting of the anal sphincter, as described by Norman Miller in 1939, was considered to be a major step in anal sphincter repair at that time. It made possible the release of pressure from gas and feces, thus preventing the impaction of fecal material in the bowel for several days after the operation. This procedure has been abandoned in modern surgery because it led to weakening of the anal sphincter and persistence of anal incontinence of intestinal gas.

In 1912, Antoine Basset of Paris reported his study of 147 cases of primary carcinoma of the clitoris and described an operation for extensive removal of the malignant tumor and the regional lymph nodes. The Basset operation, which was popularized in the United States by Taussig, was a major contribution to reducing the mortality from cancer of the vulva. This procedure, now individualized for each patient, remains the standardbearer for the treatment of vulvar carcinoma.

CYTOLOGY AND CARCINOMA IN SITU

One of the greatest advances in gynecology in the 20th century may be the improvement in the cure rate for cervical cancer that has resulted from the development of cytology and the recognition of carcinoma in situ. In conjunction, these two discoveries have permitted the detection of cervical cancer in the microscopic, hence curable, stage. Without cytology, very few microscopic carcinomas would be discovered. Without the recognition and proper interpretation of the microscopic picture known as carcinoma in situ, cytology would be of little value. The first publication of Papanicolaou and Traut appeared in 1943. Subsequent publications by them and others, notably Ruth Graham, demonstrated beyond doubt that cytologic studies could almost infallibly detect cervical cancer. First in

1927 and subsequently in many articles in the 1930s, Walter Schiller of Vienna described a lesion in the surface epithelium of the cervix that we now recognize as carcinoma in situ. The same microscopic picture had been noted by Cullen, Rubin, and Schottlander and Kermauner shortly after the turn of the century, but its relation to invasive cancer was not understood. This relationship was proposed by Galvin and Te Linde in an article published in 1944, and in several subsequent reports. Since then the relationship has been amply confirmed, and early cervical cancer has become a detectable and curable disease.

As emphasized in this text, the development of colposcopy in Germany by Hinselmann in 1925 and the introduction of this technique into the United States in the 1960s have provided a new dimension to the assessment of the abnormal cervix as detected by cytology. Colposcopy has also improved the accuracy of diagnosis of early cervical carcinoma. When used by an experienced colposcopist, the stereoscopic magnification provided by colposcopy makes unnecessary blind random cervical biopsies or the routine use of conization for the diagnosis of localized lesions, which can be completely visualized.

TREATMENT OF UTERINE PROLAPSE

The surgical cure of uterine prolapse was first attempted after the advent of anesthesia and asepsis. Up to that time, pessaries of all types had been the vogue. Some of the first surgical attempts were made by ventrofixation, but this proved unsatisfactory, the results often being temporary. Vaginal operations that rarely succeeded included amputation of the elongated cervix, constriction of the vaginal outlet and reconstruction of the perineum, and operations for diminishing the caliber of the vagina, usually by removing a strip or triangle of mucosa and suturing the edges together. The almost complete union of the labia majora was tried in Germany. Then, in 1888, A. Donald of Manchester and his assistant, Fothergill, devised what became known as the Manchester operation. Although infrequently used in the United States today, this operation, with various minor modifications, merits a prominent place in the history of attempts to cure uterine prolapse.

The best method of treating uterine prolapse and allied conditions is still in dispute. Vaginal hysterectomy with suitable plastic vaginal repair has gained wide acceptance in the United States. Among the contributors to our present knowledge are Watkins of Chicago (the interposition operation), Spalding of San Francisco and Richardson of Baltimore (the composite operation), Heaney of Chicago (the vaginal hysterectomy), and LeFort of France. Heaney's greatest contribution

was the development of a meticulous technique for the vaginal removal of the uterus, applicable in the removal of the benign uterus even when no prolapse exists.

TREATMENT OF URINARY INCONTINENCE

Great progress has been made in the surgical cure of urinary incontinence in the present century. Simple plication of the sphincter with or without cysto-urethrocele repair, as advocated by Kelly in 1913, and later by Kennedy and others, fails to cure the condition in some cases. In 1910, Rudolf Goebell of Germany first used the pyramidalis muscles to give continence to a child with congenital incontinence (possibly caused by spina bifida occulta). Frangenheim modified the original procedure by using a strip of rectus sheath attached to the pyramidalis muscles. Further modifications were made by Stoeckel in Germany and Aldridge in the United States, and out of this work there has evolved the so-called sling operation in its various modifications. In 1949, Victor Marshall and Andrew Marchetti of New York and Kermit Krantz, now of Kansas City, published their first results on the retropubic technique of vesicourethral suspension, a procedure that has gained considerable popularity in the United States.

During the past three quarters of a century, more than 100 abdominal, vaginal, or combined operative procedures have been developed for the control of genuine stress urinary incontinence. These operations are variations of the original Kelly technique of vaginal plication of the urethrovesical sphincter mechanism and the abdominal approach for the retropubic suspension of the urethra as initially described by Marshall, Marchetti, and Krantz.

In recent years, due in part perhaps to previous editions of this text, there has been a resurgence of interest in female urology in many gynecologic clinics in this country and abroad. This interest has been heightened by the development of high-technology methods for the advanced study of the urodynamic mechanisms that act as causative factors of urinary incontinence. These sophisticated urodynamic studies, particularly useful for the patient with a previous operative failure, have significantly improved the long-term surgical cure of this socially disabling condition.

TREATMENT OF CONGENITAL MALFORMATIONS

Significant progress has been made within the last 40 years in reconstructive procedures for congenital malformations of the female generative tract. Many ingenious operations have been devised for forming a vagina when it is congenitally absent. Among the originators of procedures, now only of historical interest, are Baldwin, Frank, Wharton, Graves, and Shirodkar. In 1938, McIndoe devised a simple method of lining the newly formed vaginal cavity with a split-thickness skin graft. The operation has been extremely successful in most hands and has made obsolete other methods, many of which are more complicated and more dangerous.

In 1907, Paul Strassmann of Berlin was the first to unify a double uterus. His operation was done through a transverse incision in the uterine fundus and merely bisected, without removing, the septum. More recently, an operation characterized by excision of the septum or the inner aspects of the two horns has been very successfully done. The procedure was described in 1953 by Jones and Jones of Johns Hopkins.

In the 1940s, the epochal work of Lawson Wilkins, a pediatrician, on intersexuality opened the door for surgical work on reconstruction of the genitalia according to the child's physical and emotional instincts. This surgery was initiated chiefly by Howard Jones.

LAPAROSCOPY

The introduction and general acceptance of laparoscopy marks a real milestone in the history of pelvic surgery. The idea of viewing the intra-abdominal organs for diagnosis, however, is not new.

In 1911, Bertram M. Bernheim, an assistant surgeon at the Johns Hopkins Hospital, described two cases in which a proctoscope was passed through a small abdominal incision. He observed the abdominal organs using a reflected light. The next year, Jacobaes in Stockholm reported 115 examinations, of which 42 were abdominal and 27 thoracic. Interest was aroused internationally, and Meirelles of South America, Renon and Rosenthal in France, Roccoivilla in Italy, and Ordoff in Chicago all described original techniques and ideas of laparoscopy.

In 1929, Kalk, an outstanding German surgeon, was an avid exponent and promoter of peritoneoscopy. He designed and constructed numerous lens systems and various endoscopes, and described 100 laparoscopy examinations with significant detail. It is probably through Kalk's influence that modern laparoscopy acquired credibility. In 1930, Ruddock from the United States became an avid proponent of peritoneoscopy and published reports on over 2500 cases in which local anesthesia and room air were used for the procedure. A significant advance was made by Fourestier, Gladu, and Valmiere, who developed a cool method for transmitting intense light in 1947. In the same year, Hopkins and Kampany introduced fiber optics.

In spite of the general use of peritoneoscopy abroad, it was not generally accepted as a diagnostic tool in the United States until Decker published extensively from 1949 to 1967 on visualization of the pelvic organs using the culdoscope. He introduced the culdoscope into the cul-de-sac after puncturing it through the posterior fornix. The patients were placed in the knee/chest position, allowing air to rush in by suction. Culdoscopy has been almost completely replaced by laparoscopy in most clinics.

The rebirth and modernization of laparoscopy can be traced to the early work of Palmer in Paris in 1940. His careful experiments on creation of a pneumoperitoneum and the control of intra-abdominal pressure were valuable contributions to the science of laparoscopy. He used the term *gynecologic celioscopy* rather than *laparoscopy* and preferred this procedure to culdoscopy because it reduced the risk of pelvic infection. He believed that surgical techniques could be better applied through the laparoscope than through the culdoscope.

In 1974 Semm of Germany reported the performance of gynecologic surgery through the laparoscope. Gomel in 1977 reported sharp dissection and neosalpingostomies in nine patients, eight with previous tuboplasties.

In recent years, many operative procedures formerly requiring a major pelvic operation have been successfully performed through the laparoscope. Among these are tubal sterilization, lysis of pelvic adhesions, evaluation of chronic pelvic pain and infertility, evaluation of treated pelvic malignancies, and, more recently, use of the carbon dioxide laser for vaporization of endometriosis implants throughout the pelvis.

MICROSURGERY

Gynecologic microsurgery was pioneered by Kurt Swolin of Sweden. In 1966, he reported the advantage of magnification in placing fine sutures for tubal reconstruction. In a subsequent year, he reported the results of microsurgical reconstruction in 50 women. Gomel and Winston, among others, demonstrated the advantage of microsurgical technique in tubal and ovarian reconstruction. Over the past two decades, studies have revealed that the principles of microsurgical techniques should be employed in tubal and ovarian reconstruction procedures, that is, a gentle technique using fine needles and nonreactive suture material, delicate instruments, magnification, constant irrigation, and precise hemostasis. This philosophy of gentle technique has been shown to limit iatrogenic postoperative adhesion formation following gynecologic surgery.

Bibliography

Barnes AC. A comment on historical "truth." Prospec Biol Med 1977; Autumn:131.

Bernheim BM. Organoscopy. Ann Surg 1911;53:764.

Bonney V. Technique and results of myomectomy. Lancet 1931;220:171.

Brunschwig A. Whither gynecology? Am J Obstet Gynecol 1968;100:122.

Castiglioni A. A history of medicine. New York: AA Knopf, 1941.

Clark JG. A more radical method of performing hysterectomy for cancer of the uterus. Bull Johns Hopkins Hosp 1895;6:120.

Cognat MA, Dessapt B. The history of microsurgery. In: Phillips J, ed. Microsurgery in gynecology. Downey, Calif.: American Association of Gynecologic Laparoscopists, 1977.

Cullen TS. Cancer of the uterus: its pathology, symptomatology, diagnosis, and treatment. New York: Appleton, 1900.

Davis AW. Dr. Kelly of Hopkins. Baltimore: The Johns Hopkins Press, 1959.

Decker A. Culdoscopy: its diagnostic value in pelvic disease. JAMA 1949;140:378.

Decker A. Culdoscopy. Am J Obstet Gynecol 1952;63:654.

Decker A. Culdoscopy. Philadelphia: FA Davis, 1967.

de Lamelle J. Traite des Fistulas Vesicouterines et Vesicouterine-Vaginales. Paris: 1892.

Eskew PN, Watt GW. Postgraduate medical education in obstetrics and gynecology. Obstet Gynecol 1981;58:642.

Fourestier N, Gladu A, Valmiere J. Perfectionnements a l'endoscopie medicale. Realisation bronchoscopique. Presse Med 1952; 60:1291.

Galvin GA, Te Linde RW. The minimal histological changes in biopsies to justify a diagnosis of cervical cancer. Am J Obstet Gynecol 1944;48:774.

Goebell R. Zur operativen beseitegung der angeborenen incontinentia vesical. Z Cynäk Urol 1910;2:187.

Gomel V. Salpingostomy by laparoscopy. J Reprod Med 1977;18:265.

Gosset M. Calculus in the bladder: incontinence of urine—vesicovaginal fistula. Advantages of gilt-wire suture. Lancet 1834;1:345.

Halsted WS. An account of the introduction of gloves etc. Menasha, Wis.: George Banta Publishing, 1939.

Harris S. Woman's Surgeon. New York: Macmillan, 1950.

Heaney NS. Report of 565 vaginal hysterectomies performed for benign pelvic disease. Am J Obstet Gynecol 1934;28:751.

Jones HW, Jones GS. Double uterus as an etiological factor in repeated abortion: indications for surgical repair. Am J Obstet Gynecol 1953;65:325.

Kalk H. Erfahrungen mit der laparoskopie. Z Klin Med 1929;111:303.

Kelly HA. Operative gynecology. New York: Appleton, 1898.

Kennedy WT. Incontinence of urine in the female: some functional observations of the urethra illustrated by roentgenograms. Am J Obstet Gynecol 1937;33:19.

Latzko W. Behandlung hochsitzender blasen und mastdarm scheiden fistlen noch uterus exterpetion mit hohen scheidenverschluss. Zbl Gynaek 1914;38:906.

LeFort L. Nouveau procede pour la guerison du prolapsus uterin. Bull Gen Ther 1877; 92:337.

Levert HS. Experiments on the use of metallic sutures, as applied to arteries. Am J Med Sci 1829;4:17.

Mahfouz Bey NJ. Urinary and recto-vaginal fistulae in woman. J Obstet Gynaec Brit Empire 1929;36:581.

Mettauer JT. Vesico-vaginal fistula. Boston Med Surg J 1840;22:154.

Miller NF, Brown W. The surgical treatment of complete perineal tears in the female. Am J Obstet Gynecol 1937;34:196.

Noble GH. A new technique for complete laceration of the perineum designed for the purpose of eliminating infection from the rectum. Trans Am Gynecol Soc 1902; 27:357.

Palmer R. Instrumentation et technique de la coelioscopie gynecologique. Gynecol Obstet (Paris) 1947;46:420.

Papanicolaou GN, Traut HF. Diagnosis of uterine cancer by the vaginal smear. New York: Commonwealth Fund, 1943.

Richardson EH. A simplified technique for abdominal pan-hysterectomy. Surg Gynecol Obstet 1929;48:248.

Richardson EH. An efficient composite operation for uterine prolapse and associated pathology. Am J Obstet Gynecol 1937;34:814.

Robb H. Aseptic surgical technique. Philadelphia: JB Lippincott, 1904.

Robinson J. Tom Cullen of Baltimore. New York: Oxford University Press, 1949.

Rubin IC. Progress in myomectomy. Am J Obstet Gynecol 1942;44:197.

Ruddock JC. Peritoneoscopy. West J Surg 1934;42:392.

Ruddock JC. Application and evaluation of peritoneoscopy. Calif Med 1949;71:110.

Ruddock JC. Peritoneoscopy: a critical clinical review. Surg Clin N Am 1957;37:1249.

Schiller W. Untersuchen zur entstehung der geschulste, collumearzinom des uterus. Virchow Arch Path Anat 1927; 263:279.

Schottlander J, Kermauner F. Zur kenntnis des uterus karzinoms. Berlin: Karger, 1912.

Semm K. Endocoagulator: new possibilities for tubal surgery via pelviscopy. Excerpta Medica 1974;370:242.

Sims M. On the treatment of vesico-vaginal fistulas. Am J Med Sci 1852;23:59.

Sims M. The story of my life. New York: Appleton, 1884.

Spalding AB. A study of frozen sections of the pelvis with description of an operation for pelvic prolapse. Surg Gynecol Obstet 1919;29:529.

Speert H. Obstetrics and gynecologic milestones, essays in eponymy. New York: Macmillan, 1958.

Speert H. Obstetrics and gynecology in America, a history. Baltimore: Waverly Press, 1980.

Swolin K. Experimental studies on the prophylaxis of post-operative intra-abdominal adhesions. Acta Obstet Gynecol Scand 1966;43:473.

Swolin K. Fertilitat superationen literatur und methodik. Acta Obstet Gynecol Scand 1967;46:234.

Taylor PJ, Gomel V. Introduction. In Gomel V, Taylor PJ, Yuzpe AA, Rioux J, eds. Laparoscopy and hysteroscopy in gynecologic practice. Chicago: Yearbook Medical Publisher, 1986.

Te Linde RW, Scott RB. Experimental endometriosis. Am J Obstet Gynecol 1950;60:1147.

Warren JC. A new method of operation for relief of rupture of the perineum through the sphincter and rectum. Trans Am Gynecol Soc 1882;7:322.

Watkins TJ. The treatment of cystocele and uterine prolapse after the menopause. Am J Obstet Gynecol 1899;15:420.

Wells TS. Some causes of excessive mortality after surgical operations. Br Med J 1864;2:284.

Wertheim E. Zur frage der radical operation beim uterus krebs. Arch Gynak 1900;61:627.

Wilkins L. The diagnosis and treatment of endocrine disorders in childhood and adolescence. Springfield, Ill.: Charles C Thomas, 1950.

Psychological Aspects of Pelvic Surgery

MALCOLM G. FREEMAN

It is not enough for a surgeon to be trained and proficient in gynecologic diagnosis and the technical skills of surgery. He or she must also be prepared to predict, recognize, and at least begin treatment of the psychological (including emotional, sexual, psychosomatic, and other behavioral) consequences of gynecologic disease and its treatment. These include preoperative and postoperative evaluation and supportive therapy of patients, and often of their immediate family members as well.

Gynecologists deal with surgical procedures so regularly and often so routinely that there is a considerable risk of losing perspective about the impact of surgery on the life of the individual woman who is subjected to this stress. For the surgeon the gynecologic operation is an ordinary and frequent event of usually simple dimension. For the patient each procedure is a unique experience that may immediately threaten her sense of health and well-being, her control over her own body, and her security; sometimes it can even threaten or destroy the central core of her sexual identity. Even though the ultimate purpose of surgical treatment is to enhance the patient's health, the process of accomplishing that goal may be acutely threatening. It is appropriate for surgeons to remind themselves of the psychological stresses that are often precipitated by the removal of body parts that are emotionally synonymous with a woman's feminine nature, and of the stresses that are an inherent part of the hospital/surgical treatment. It is also important to be aware of and comfortable with the usual psychological mechanisms by which patients react to surgical stress.

Much of the information in this chapter will doubt-less be familiar to every experienced surgeon. The chapter is intended to create some organization and system within which fragmented knowledge can be seen in a clear and recognizable pattern; a pattern that can be remembered and utilized to facilitate the patient care process and ease the anxiety and emotional stress of the surgical subject. Much of what is said about the impact of gynecologic surgery on women's lives is equally applicable to breast surgery, since the breast has most of the same real and symbolic sexual and identity meanings as do genitalia.

The patient who experiences ablative genital (or breast) surgery is influenced by many emotional factors. These vary in degree from subject to subject but are usually additive in nature. The patient, as she passes through the presurgical, surgical, and postsurgical experience, is stressed; often feels beset on every hand; and may, in fact, be inundated beyond her capacity to compensate. If help is not available to facilitate emotional healing and rehabilitation as well as physical healing and rehabilitation, then permanent emotional damage may result. Most of us have seen the postsurgical emotional cripple, the woman who

feels desexed and damaged
complains of continuing pelvic pain without obvious structural cause
no longer has desire
has a dry vagina and whose sexual excitement has vanished
has lost her ability to trust and lives in rage and bitterness
feels old before her time

is abandoned by her lover or drives her lover away terminates her sexual identity and begins to draw in the edges of her life

These women have been emotionally stressed beyond their ability to compensate and heal.

Most women, of course, do heal and take up their lives, raise their children, work at their jobs, and relate to their husbands or lovers. For some the healing is quick and the stress is modest. For others the healing is harder and the struggle to be well and whole leaves tender scars that slowly fade as time passes. Whether the healing process is slow or rapid, the same problems and processes occur and must be understood if recovery is to be facilitated.

EMOTIONAL RESPONSE TO SURGERY

Massler and Devansan have said there is an emotional response to any physical assault on the body. The magnitude of the response is expected to be proportional to the degree of emotional investment one has in the part of the body being assaulted. Among women, the parts of the body that are most vulnerable to this emotional reaction to assault are the face, hair, breasts, genitalia, and abdominal wall (scars, colostomy, ileostomy). Barnes and Tinkham have said that on the whole patients tend to react to current stress in much the same way as they have reacted to past crises and personal losses. Well-established patterns of behavior repeat themselves at such critical moments. This gives an opportunity to predict some of the patient's reactions by taking a history of her reactions to stress in the past.

The list below gives Roeske's 13 factors related to

FACTORS RELATED TO POOR PROGNOSIS FOR MENTAL HEALTH AFTER HYSTERECTOMY (3 MONTHS TO 3 YEARS POST-OP)

Gender identity (the intimate sense of herself as a woman)—the hyperfeminine cope less well
Previous adverse reactions to stress
Previous depressive episodes
Depression or other mental illness in her family of origin
A history of multiple physical complaints (especially low back pain)
Numerous hospitalizations and surgeries
Age less than 35 years at time of hysterectomy
A wish for a child or more children
Anticipation that the surgery will produce a loss of interest in and satisfaction from coitus
Husband's or other significant person's negative attitude toward hysterectomy
Marital dissatisfaction and instability
Disapproving cultural and religious attitudes
Lack of vocational or avocational involvement

---

poor prognosis for mental health after hysterectomy. These factors begin to define the patient whose emotional stability in response to genital surgical stress is apt to be less certain. I would add to Roeske's list the woman who has a hysteric (histrionic) personality, since patients of this kind often require additional emotional support to handle life stresses.

By actively inquiring about such events in the past and about the patient's reaction to them, the surgeon can be forewarned about which patients are likely to have the most difficulty handling the stress of gynecologic surgery. Equipped with this forewarning the surgeon can be prepared to offer extra support, counsel, information, or even additional psychotherapeutic consultation services when necessary.

COMMON EMOTIONAL RESPONSES TO SURGERY

A. Insecurity and vulnerability
   1. Surrender of control
   2. Sense of being manipulated
   3. Depersonalization (hospital)
   4. Helplessness
   5. Feelings of being attacked
B. Anxiety
   1. Fear of dying (may be expressed as anesthesia fear)
   2. Fear of pain
   3. Fear of loss of identity (role, independence, attractiveness, etc.)
   4. Fear of adverse effect on sexual life
C. Emotional lability, sadness, tearfulness, irritability
D. Regression and dependency
E. A feeling of illness—a state of nonhealth ("sick" role)
F. Grief

Common emotional responses to surgery in general are listed above. These responses are not unique to gynecologic surgical patients and are likely to be found in both men and women.

Insecurity

Feelings of insecurity and vulnerability are often a realistic appraisal of the patient's own situation. Giving up control of one's own body (and life) to others is terrifying for many people and most likely to be terrifying to those patients who are most insecure, since one of the common defenses against feelings of insecurity is the institution of rigid controls over all aspects of life, including self. Patients feel manipulated in a hospital setting because, in fact, they are manipulated shamelessly by staff, who tell them when to awake, take medicine, eat, bathe, walk, have visitors, have blood removed, and so on. When this manipulation is accompanied by a staff attitude that depersonalizes the patient, it adds to the feelings of helplessness. Anger results from being in a situation that the patient cannot handle successfully. As a consequence, this insecurity commonly causes patients to experience both anxiety and anger while they are confined to the hospital. Closely allied to feelings of loss of control are feelings of being attacked or assaulted. This is akin to the feelings of rape victims that have been described as feelings of loss of control of one's own space—a violation of territory. Such feelings are greatly diminished by the patient's belief that surgery will accomplish something positive (relief of pain, removal of cancer, restoration of fertility, etc.) and by feelings of trust and confidence in and liking of her surgeon. When the surgeon is cool, aloof, impersonal, or distracted, the patient's feelings of being assaulted increase.

Anxiety

Anxiety or fear associated with surgery is essentially universal. Most such fear involves fear of the unknown or of what the patient imagines she will be forced to endure during hospitalization. Fear is diminished by trust, emotional support by hospital staff, and factual information about the surgical and recovery process. According to Lalinec-Michaud and Engelsmann, spouse, siblings, and friends are most important (in that order) among nonmedical sources of support. Fear of anesthesia is often thinly disguised fear of dying as well as fear of loss of control. It may be appropriate to confront fear of dying directly so that the patient can ventilate those fears openly.

Some of the diseases with which we deal, cancer in particular, have special stresses. Schain has described fairly universal concerns among cancer patients, no matter where in the body the cancer may be located. The fear of death is, of course, common. Cancer treatments are associated with fear of morbidity. Patients sometimes fear that the treatment will be as severe as the disease. In irradiation for carcinoma of the cervix, for example, the vagina may be totally destroyed as a functional sexual organ. There may also be fear of cancer recurrence. Even if the patient has been told that she has reason to expect a cure, she may feel as though she is carrying a time bomb in her abdomen. We speak of 5-year cure rates, which says that we are never quite sure that malignancy is gone forever. There is often fear of abandonment. The patient often feels that having cancer is like having leprosy; she becomes untouchable and unclean in some way. There is a small but real risk (and a major anxiety) that the partner of the woman who has cancer might abandon her. The loss of functional ability, of social value, and of self-esteem are major concerns.

Patients fear the loss of economic competence. A woman who has worked hard every day of her life fears that she will be partially or totally disabled, so that she can no longer work. The loss of familiar role behavior is important. All of us define part of our identities by the way we carry out our expected tasks or responsibilities. If the patient cannot do these tasks, she may lose her sense of identity because she has lost her usual role.

There are also site-specific function problems. The man who has had a leg amputated because of disease has a different function problem than the woman who has had a pelvic exenteration. Breast and gynecologic diseases are unique in that they attack sexual identity directly, as well as body image and self-esteem. Genital organs are one of the important ways in which we define our sexual identity.

Regression and Dependency

Regression to a less self-sufficient and less emotionally mature state is commonly observed in most people who are ill or undergo surgery. It is also one of the most difficult behaviors with which family and friends deal. Women usually fulfill multiple roles as wage earner, wife and/or mother, cook, housekeeper, chauffeur, seamstress, confidant, advisor, shopper, and so on. Family members who are used to depending on the patient to satisfy part of their needs are often angry and confused when illness and physical incapacity interfere with her capacity to perform her usual functions. They often apply overt or subtle pressure (including guilt) on the patient to exert herself to fulfill her usual roles.

All these factors, as well as a feeling of nonhealth, contribute to an emotional fragility that shows itself as extremely labile emotions, including feelings of sadness, depression, tearfulness, and irritability. Usual emotional defense mechanisms are often temporarily weakened or destroyed.

Grief

Medical staff often do not appreciate the important role of grief when considering a patient's reaction to her illness. Grief is a normal and natural emotional response to loss of any kind and can be considered essential to emotional healing. The stages of grief are well enough defined to make understandable behavior that may otherwise seem incomprehensible.

The first and most primitive emotional response to loss is *denial*. Denial takes many forms. The patient may demonstrate denial, for instance, by not going to see the physician if she has abnormal bleeding or by simply pretending that it is not there. Not remembering things she has been told by the physician may be denial. The patient, on returning home, may say, "Well, I don't really remember what he said." She may forget the important things or deny the seriousness of the problem. Denial is a very primitive response but one that allows people to function temporarily and survive emotional stresses that they might be unable to handle otherwise.

The second stage of grief is *bargaining with God.* The patient has the opportunity to bargain with God only when anticipating a loss. The surgical patient may say to herself: "I promise to be a good person if only I don't have to die." "I will be kind to my children and I will not complain to my husband and I will go to church regularly."

The next stage of grief is *guilt.* Feelings of guilt occur whether the grief reaction is before or after the loss. Most of the guilty feelings are completely inappropriate, in that the "guilty" act rarely is directly related to the cause of loss. Many people feel that any bad event is likely to be a punishment from God. Therefore, if something bad happens, the patient may feel as though she did wrong and is guilty. This gives rise to a series of "if onlys": "If only I had had my annual Pap smear. If only I had gone to the doctor regularly." When a mother has died: "If only I had gone to see my mother more often," or " . . . taken her out to dinner" or " . . . I had paid her rent instead of letting her do it on her Social Security." The guilt feelings come from a belief in magical or supernatural cause and effect. Guilt feelings may sometimes be devastating and incapacitating but are more often transitory.

Along with guilt, people who go through grief usually have some degree of *depression.* Depression is often characterized by feelings of helplessness, hopelessness, and/or worthlessness. Other symptoms include middle-of-the-night insomnia, nightmares, loss of appetite or excessive eating, lethargy, difficulty making decisions, psychosomatic symptoms, and so on. To get a history of depression we ask the patient if she has these feelings. Depressed patients usually agree that those feelings characterize their day-to-day responses. Postsurgical depression is very common. When prolonged, it indicates that the patient has been unable to work through the grief process and find resolution. Depression as a part of grief is often rage turned inward (ie, suppressed), and when the patient is able to identify her rage and ventilate it, the depression usually begins to lift. When the patient takes charge of her life again and makes decisions, even small ones, she begins to feel better and feelings of helplessness, hopelessness, and worthlessness abate. The stage during which the patient ventilates *anger* can be difficult for those providing care, but it should be accepted as healthy. During the stage of anger, the patient may go to the extreme of writing letters to the newspaper or of suing her physi-

cian. She may complain bitterly about the nursing staff, the doctors, or the size of the bill, or she may read all the literature on unnecessary surgery. Such actions are a form of protest at the stress that has been dealt to her body and mind. In the great majority of instances, this behavior means that the depression is lifting and the patient is beginning to move toward the resolution of her grief. Ventilation by talking is very helpful for depressed patients; so are physical exercise and taking actions to take charge of her own life.

Finally, *resolution* and *integration* occur. The stressful experience of loss eventually becomes an accepted part of one's life, the memory of which causes sadness and regret but no longer causes the devastating immobilization that is found in the earlier stages of grief. The integration of this experience does not mean that it is forgotten, only that it has less affect (feeling) tied to it.

When a woman is dealing with grief, she may have worked through the majority of the process and still, for a period of several years, have flashes of grief. There will be a word, an image, something that happens on television, that brings all the acute grief feelings back severely for a few moments and then passes. It is important to note that the stages of grief do not always follow in the orderly sequence described earlier. For many people, they are intermingled. The patient may feel fragments of anger, depression, or guilt at the same time. Grief is common, and whenever the behavior of a patient seems excessive, bizarre, or out of the realm of what would usually be anticipated, it is useful to look for the role that grief may be playing.

Symbolic Value of the Uterus

Specific emotional issues are related to hysterectomy. Physicians tend to deal directly with the anatomic, physiologic, and pathologic situations that justify uterine removal. We spend little time considering the unconscious or symbolic value of the uterus. To the patient, the symbolic value of the uterus is often of great importance and must be dealt with in some manner by the patient before uterine removal can be reconciled. Roeske points out that most premenopausal women express some form of ambivalence about giving up this valued part of themselves. When hysterectomy offers relief from fear of pregnancy, relief from pain, from continuous or excessive bleeding, from disability, from incontinence, or from cancer, it is apt to be viewed as a positive and appropriate procedure. This is particularly true for women over 35 years of age who have had children.

Even when hysterectomy offers relief from distress, however, the loss of the uterus often stirs up conscious or unconscious ambivalent feelings related to its symbolic value. One symbolic significance of the uterus is related to menstruation. The onset of menstruation is a rite of passage into feminine adulthood. When a girl has her first period, she often feels that she has become a woman. Many women do not regard menstruation as simply a bother; they consider it a sign of their femininity, and its presence confirms that femininity. Some women feel that menstruation is a cyclic cleansing, that during the month poisons accumulate in the body and cause edema, premenstrual tension, grumpiness, or other change in emotional status; with the beginning of menstrual flow, these unpleasant emotions and physical feelings fade away. Some women use the rhythmicity of the menstrual cycle as a means of timing and ordering their lives. Like the phases of the moon, the menstrual cycle gives them a sense of routine, of regularity, of predictability that has emotional significance. The loss of that rhythmicity leaves them feeling empty.

For many women the uterus has symbolic significance as a sexual organ. If the patient believes that the uterus is essential to sexual response, then, in fact, it often becomes so. Such women may become sexually dysfunctional when the uterus is removed. Women may also believe that the uterus is closely tied to feelings of attractiveness and sexual desirability. Removal of it constitutes a desexing, a destruction of their identity and function as women. Many women who have all the children they want and who do not want to get pregnant again are still disturbed that sterilization or hysterectomy removes the possibility of pregnancy. This possibility in their lives has a symbolic feminine meaning that they regret losing. The uterine presence means completeness and wholeness, and its removal leaves an emptiness in them.

Some women regard the uterus as a source of youth, strength, energy, and well-being, and as the regulator of general body health. Such a woman may believe that she has lost her youth because she has lost her uterus.

Many women think that a partner will be able to tell that she has no uterus and that, because of its absence, her partner will experience sex differently and see her as less of a woman, as old or defective. Such women fear that the partner will despise or abandon them for a woman who is complete—either complete in the sense of being able to offer him a child or complete in the sense of not having been desexed, damaged, or made worthless. All these terms are commonly used by women in describing their reaction to loss of their uterus.

Lamont, who studied rehabilitation among exenterative surgery patients, says that sexual happiness is not a question of anatomy or endocrinology, especially in the woman who previously has been sexually well adjusted. Loss of sexual function is more likely to be related to a patient's feeling of unattractiveness. Lamont's view may be slightly one-sided, but only slightly. There are certainly surgical procedures that damage a woman's ability to be sexually responsive and happy. The woman who has a scarred irradiated vagina, for instance, may lose that ability. However, most women who have learned how can continue to be sexually responsive even with the loss of breasts, vulva, vagina, uterus, tubes, ovaries, or rectum so long as their brain is intact and so long as they feel like sexually attractive people.

Sexual Dysfunction

Derogatis has said that "sexual dysfunction is attendant upon gynecologic surgery even . . . when it does not involve dramatic procedures or a malignancy. In cases where threat to life and external disfiguration are added, the incidence of dysfunction is considerably higher." The incidence of sexual dysfunction among postoperative hysterectomy patients has been the subject of several studies. Table 2-1 is from Derogatis's paper describing hysterectomy patients who report postoperative sexual dysfunction. The percentage of women reporting dysfunction increases as these studies become more recent. In 1950, with Huffman's study, the frequency was believed to be about 10%. In the last two studies, from 1974 and 1977, the frequency was up to 38% and 37%. Studies of other types of gynecologic surgery also point out high rates of postoperative sexual dysfunction (see Campion and colleagues, Andersen and Hacker, Andersen and colleagues).

Andersen and Hacker have proposed a useful research model for the study of psychosexual adjustment in gynecologic oncology patients.

Direct and Indirect Sexual Disorders

Gynecologic patients (and sometimes their partners) have direct and indirect sexual disorders that result from surgery or disease. The direct physiologic effects cause dyspareunia and have to do with estrogen loss (with subsequent vaginal atrophy, pain, scarring), with

TABLE 2–1
Proportion of Hysterectomy Patients Reporting Postoperative Sexual Dysfunction

STUDY, YEAR	SEXUAL DYSFUNCTION, %
Huffman, 1950	10
Dodds et al, 1961	15
Patterson and Craig, 1963	18
Munday and Cox, 1967	28
Richards, 1974	38
Dennerstein et al, 1977	37

loss of lubrication secondary to atrophy or to autonomic nerve fiber disruption, and with vaginal shortening (when it is extreme). There may be loss of vulva, clitoris, or vagina, depending on the type of surgery, and there may be loss of strength and health. The indirect effects result from the loss of self-esteem, the change in body image, and the loss or change in the patient's sense of sexual identity. These changes may cause loss of desire, loss of excitement (which includes loss of lubrication and dyspareunia), and loss of orgasm (anorgasmy). Sexual dysfunctions may lead to deterioration of a relationship or to the loss of a partner as an indirect effect.

Direct effects on the male partner sometimes have to do with the loss of the female partner's physical attractiveness. A response of this type seems to be much less common than most women suppose. A woman's physical attractiveness to her partner is usually less important than she fears it might be. In most instances in which one partner complains of the other's physical appearance, the complaint is a mask for deeper interpersonal issues. Among most men, the importance of "prettiness" in a beloved partner rapidly declines when men reach their mid-30s, and other factors, such as compatibility and mutual caring, become more important. Even though men continue to appreciate physical attractiveness in women, it seldom is a crucial factor in a valued relationship. Women tend to be very critical of their own appearance and quite realistic about their own physical faults, as they are about those of their husbands'. Men often have a romantic fantasy about their wives' appearance that changes relatively little as the years pass, providing the relationship continues to be gratifying in other ways.

There is also a "fantasy" identity. People relate to their own perception of their partner's identity rather than to the person himself or herself. This perception may be quite different from the partner's own self-perception. When a woman has had a surgical procedure and extirpation of reproductive organs, it is rare but possible for her partner to begin to perceive her differently, and this change may change the relationship for better or worse.

There is sometimes a fear of contagion. One of the reasons that male partners sometimes leave women who have had gynecologic cancer is a subtle or unconscious belief, even though this seems unrealistic, that the cancer may be contagious.

A loss or change in the female partner's sexual availability may have an impact on her male partner. The fear of causing pain or injury to the female partner has a major inhibiting effect on many men. Emotional isolation and loss of nurturing occur in men as a result of the physical disability of the wife.

The male partner may also experience indirect effects because of such things as a change in the patient's assertive role. The woman's usual assertive sexual role may be temporarily or permanently lost as a result of the surgical experience. Her sexual response may change. Her dependency and insecurity, particularly during the healing phases, may lead to a major change in response from the male partner. All these changes may result in temporary loss of desire, excitement, or orgasm in the male partner.

THE SURGEON'S INFLUENCE ON EMOTIONAL RESPONSE TO SURGERY

How does the surgeon help or hinder the patient's emotional response to surgery? Barnes and Tinkham have said:

Surgeons tend to be activists rather than empathetic listeners and many of them need to distance themselves from the patient's feelings and fears as a kind of protective insulation against the things they see every day. Some do not hear the patient and instead relate to a uterus or a breast or an appendix, and not a human being in distress. At times one observes a kind of cut and run syndrome in some surgeon-patient relationships. There are also doctors with a tendency to react to their patient's problems in terms of their own personal and moral value systems.

In other words, not all of us are as supportive or empathetic as we might be. Even though we see ourselves as pragmatic problem solvers who do all that is reasonable and logical to contribute to our patient's health, our patients sometimes see us in quite another and less flattering way.

To be satisfied, the patient needs two assurances from her surgeon, besides technical competence and professional efficiency. The patient needs to know that she has the surgeon's complete attention during the patient/physician interaction, and she needs to believe that the surgeon is willing and able to accept and help her to cope with her feelings as well as her physical dysfunction. Actually, neither of these requirements is difficult. It is not hard for the surgeon to give the patient the impression that she has his or her full attention if, in fact, that is the case. When the surgeon pushes other things out of mind, looks directly at the patient continuously, and listens carefully, the patient is apt to think she has her listener's attention. When the surgeon responds appropriately to what she is saying, she is sure of it. Dealing with the patient's feelings is usually not difficult if the surgeon accepts the viewpoint that the patient's feelings are a part of the gynecologic disorder. Most of the feelings surgical patients have are predictable and familiar to the surgeon but not to the patient. The surgeon's application of common sense will be enormously helpful to the patient. It is important for the surgeon to avoid being defensive about the patient's complaints and comments, particularly when she is ventilating anger. It is important to hear her anger and accept it whether or not the surgeon agrees.

The surgeon should begin by finding out what the patient's expectations may be about what will be done to her body and what the consequences of surgery will be on her life. As she tells the surgeon these things, her knowledge, fears, and biases emerge fairly quickly. The surgeon is then able to cope with them by supplementing her knowledge with appropriate explanations of anatomy and physiology and by describing in detail the usual preoperative, operative, and postoperative routines and experiences. The patient should be told in detail exactly what she and her family can expect. Physical sensations, bandages, incisions, catheters, tubing, medications, and so on should all be described. The anticipated amount of discomfort and techniques to handle discomfort should be outlined. The patient's own role in convalescence and recovery should be defined. The nature of common complications should be described, although a true "informed consent" may be nearly impossible. A timetable for discomfort, medication, ambulation, bowel movements, and discharge from the hospital should be given. Factors that determine when sexual intercourse can resume should be described. The patient's questions and fears should be heard and answered.

This interaction should never be assigned to anyone other than the surgeon. A physician's assistant, resident, or nurse is not a satisfactory substitute, although each may reinforce this training process. When preparation for surgery is properly carried out, the patient's anxiety is greatly allayed, her postoperative care is simplified, and her need for pain medication is apt to be greatly reduced. Instead of feeling like a powerless victim, she is likely to feel like an important partner in a cooperative enterprise—which she is.

It is important to remember that whatever the patient's feelings may be, they must be accepted. Information, reassurance, and support will usually quickly modify many dysfunctional feelings and lead to a more healthy attitude and understanding of the surgical process. The surgeon also needs to remember that not all the patient's feelings must be changed. It is enormously helpful for most patients to be able to talk about fears and ventilate their anxiety even if nothing definitive can be done about them at that moment.

The surgeon also needs to remember that a patient's family is an important part of her support system and can be a potent ally or a bitter enemy to the health care team. The family's need for information, reassurance, support, and attention cannot be neglected.

It is important that the surgeon be available to patients. Too often, receptionists or secretaries seem to think that their role is to shield the physician from patients rather than to facilitate that contact. Often the physician is unaware of this staff behavior or covertly may encourage it. Few dissatisfactions make patients more angry than being unable to reach their physician within a reasonable length of time.

Touching

The art of touching—the therapeutic laying on of hands—is important. Human beings need to be and enjoy being touched, providing the toucher is a person they trust and accept. The touch itself is soothing, supportive, reassuring, and accepting, particularly to the sick and emotionally vulnerable patient. Physicians should be taught not to paw the patient but to *touch* her when they have some reason to do so. Being lonely, frightened, and sick is a reason for the patient to be touched by her physician. To hold the patient's hand while talking to her, or to touch her shoulder is therapeutic. In the old days before fetal monitoring, we evaluated the quality of labor by sitting at the patient's bedside with our hand on her abdomen feeling uterine contractions. It was interesting to see how often the presence of the physician and a warm hand on her abdomen made the patient relax, rest, and become more comfortable even during active labor. It is important to recognize how powerful and positive touching is when it is done in a therapeutic way, that is, for the patient's benefit rather than the surgeon's. Often a gentle touch can say things that words do not.

PSYCHOSEXUAL REHABILITATION

Psychosexual rehabilitation after gynecologic or breast surgery has as its goal the restoration of sexual function, sexual identity, body image, and self-esteem. Most of this rehabilitation is a gradual process that the patient does for herself, but it can be facilitated by the health care team.

As healing takes place, there is a gradual loss of dependency. The patient's strength increases and she starts to resume her usual roles, which helps her feel more like her old self. Gradually she begins to lose the sick role and to see herself again as a well person.

Every patient who undergoes surgery will go through the grief process to some extent. Though grief is inevitable and normal, it is also uncomfortable. The grief process can be speeded by encouraging the patient to ventilate, to talk about her feelings rather than repressing them or brooding unnecessarily. Everyone needs support systems, particularly when under stress. Support systems are people who are able to supply emotional support when stress is heavy and the need for ventilation and encouragement is great. The physician and other health care workers can and do function as part of a patient's support system, but most of the support is given by spouse, family, and friends. A good friendship offers mutual but often not simultaneous support. Rarely is a spouse alone sufficient support; usually others are necessary to share the load. Sometimes the patient's spouse may seem to her to be part of the problem rather than part of the solution.

Part of the rehabilitation comes from validation of the patient's sexual identity from herself, from others, and from her roles. As she begins to see herself as a sexual person and as her sexual partner, family, and friends indicate their continuing acceptance of her as an important, powerful, sexual person, that mantle rests more and more comfortably on her shoulders. The woman who has had a mastectomy, for example, needs the affirmation of knowing that her partner sees her as attractive and sexually desires her; without that affirmation she may have trouble seeing herself as a sexual person.

Cosmetics, dress, and grooming are an important part of rehabilitation. We live in a culture that places great emphasis on women's physical appearance. When a postoperative patient combs her hair, puts on lipstick, and demands her own nightgown instead of a hospital gown, she has begun to heal. When the patient feels that surgery has been disfiguring in some way, she needs to find a way to compensate with dress or grooming in order to feel whole and complete again. This need cannot be neglected.

THE FOUR PLEASURES

When sexual functional loss has occurred, real compensation is needed. The patient's surgical treatment cannot be said to be complete until she has been returned to a level of sexual functioning that she judges to be gratifying and satisfactory. Patients who talk about their sexual lives regularly describe four different pleasures associated with sexuality. They describe these same four pleasures so regularly that we can assume they are universal in our culture. Understanding the four pleasures offers the key to sexual rehabilitation of men or women who have lost some portion of their usual sexual function.

The Pleasure of Touching

The pleasure of touching—of being held, caressed, cuddled, stroked, kissed, and hugged and of feeling warm skin—is not necessarily sexual; it derives from a basic human need. In our society it is difficult for adults to have their touching needs met in any way outside of sexual interaction. For many women who have never experienced an orgasm, sexual interaction is nevertheless profoundly enjoyable because of the touching and concentrated attention they receive during the experience. Women who have orgasm easily and regularly often complain about their sexual interactions if insufficient time is devoted to "foreplay" and "afterplay"—in other words, when insufficient touching has taken place to gratify their needs. Often when something has happened to interfere with genital sexual expression, all physical contact abruptly stops, so that touching and affection needs are no longer met. The couple's relationship actually may suffer more from loss of touching and simple affection than from loss of intercourse. When touching has ceased and needs for simple affection and nurturing are no longer met, the partners begin to feel alienated and needy. Encouraging the couple to resume and emphasize touching usually brings them closer together and decreases tension, and good feelings increase. Simple touching can be carried out even when a patient is postoperative or in early convalescence. Touching also helps affirm feelings of being accepted, wanted, needed, and sexually desirable.

The Pleasure of Genital Caressing

Genitalia (including breasts and nipples in both sexes) are extremely sensitive to touch. Genital and breast play is a regular part of courtship and intensely gratifying to most people, whether it is followed by orgasm or not. Orgasm itself is a brief sensation, whereas genital caressing can and sometimes does continue for hours with a relatively low expenditure of energy. During premarital courtship whole body touching and genital caressing is a major focus, and both male and female partners go to great lengths to make sure it can take place without outside interruption.

When a patient is recovering from surgery or has had surgical loss of coital function, genital caressing as a giver or receiver is often possible and intensely gratifying. Although excessive sexual excitement in women who are in their first few weeks after pelvic surgery is not advisable, the pleasure of breast caressing may be comforting to the patient.

Women who have lost the ability to have vaginal intercourse because of vaginal loss may substitute interfemoral or anal intercourse if either is acceptable to them. Women who have lost their vulva from surgery or disease may still be able to have vaginal intercourse or may receive intense sexual pleasure from abdominal, inguinal, perianal, or inner thigh caressing. A sexual gratification substitute can usually be found for any genital loss unless the inhibitions or ethical code of the couple prohibit alternatives or experimentation.

The Pleasure of Orgasm

An orgasmic response tends to be pleasurable and relieve sexual tension. An orgasm may be painful, but that is rare. In general, men and women enjoy orgasms whether produced by dreams, fantasy, caressing, a stream of water, masturbation, a vibrator, oral contact, vaginal intercourse, anal intercourse, or any other means. Most people tend to value one means of producing orgasms more than another, but this is a matter of personal preference. Although all orgasms may be physiologically identical, people perceive and value orgasm very differently.

When a woman has previously learned to be orgasmic with genitalia intact, she can often learn to be orgasmic again in spite of major genital loss, including loss of the clitoris. When the ability to have orgasm by one favorite means is temporarily or permanently impossible following pelvic surgery, the patient can be encouraged to try alternative ways to achieve orgasmic relief, so long as the alternatives do not violate her value system. Sometimes the patient needs help reconsidering her value system, where it came from, and what it means to her.

The Pleasure of Giving Pleasure to a Partner

Most people value their ability to be a source of pleasure for a beloved partner. To give pleasure and have a role in creating excitement and gratification gives a person a sense of identity and of being needed and valued. Men often carry this feeling to an extreme, so that they may feel responsible for their partner's pleasure. This attitude can become a performance trap and should be avoided. Each person ultimately is responsible for his or her own pleasure.

Women who lose their ability to engage in vaginal intercourse may still feel they fulfill their feminine role if they can be a source of pleasure for a sexual partner. When a patient has functional sexual loss, her ability to compensate may be evaluated by reviewing the "four pleasures" and defining alternative ways of feminine response.

OFFERING HELP

The surgeon cannot offer help in psychological rehabilitation to patients without taking a psychological and sexual history covering both her preoperative life and the postoperative recovery period. As defined earlier in this chapter, psychological factors that may be related to subsequent emotional distress are not difficult to determine historically. Similarly, sexual history is not difficult to obtain from patients (see Freeman) providing the surgeon is willing to ask the questions. The limiting factor in sexual history taking is rarely patient reticence. More often it is physician awkwardness and discomfort (anxiety). In survey after survey (Bernal, Gould, Moth et al, Webb and Wilson-Barnett) patients describe the desirability of more sexual information from their physicians. Physicians must become comfortable asking for sexual information and providing needed sexual information to their patients.

Whenever a patient's psychosexual rehabilitation after surgery seems to have become impaired and she fails to make steady progress toward resumption of her usual role, with appropriate self-esteem, energy, identity, and ability to handle life stresses, she should be offered help. Help should be offered early (after a period measured in days or weeks) rather than late (months to years), since intervention, if early, is often easy and brief. Otherwise, long-term psychotherapy can be required if confirmed patterns of emotional dysfunction must be dealt with. Help should be given first by the surgeon and then, if more help is needed, by a psychotherapist who is interested in and familiar with these problems.

Some gynecologists suggest that the time to do a hysterectomy is when a patient begs for it. It is not necessary for a patient to beg for surgery before the surgeon decides to do it, but when she believes the procedure will be of enormous benefit, wants it done, and chooses it without any coercion, she is very likely to be pleased by the procedure and gratified by having had it. She is also apt to recover from it quite well and to resume her life after a reasonable period of convalescence. When she goes into the procedure with reluctance and anxiety and a fear that she will come out as a different and damaged person, her recovery may well be delayed and stormy.

The pelvic surgeon's responsibility transcends the performance of the surgical procedure, no matter how technically demanding that may be. The appropriate decisions about whether to operate, when to operate, and what procedure to do and the considerate management of the patient's return to health are the hallmarks of an accomplished surgeon. They distinguish the specialist from the surgical technician. The informed gynecologic surgeon possesses the knowledge and ability to do a better job of helping the patient return to health.

Bibliography

Andersen BL, Hacker NF. Psychosexual adjustment following pelvic exenteration. Obstet Gynecol 1983;61:331.

Andersen BL, Hacker NF. Psychosexual adjustment of gynecologic oncology patients: a proposed model for future investigation. Gynecol Oncol 1983;15:214.

Andersen BL, Hacker NF. Psychosexual adjustment after vulvar surgery. Obstet Gynecol 1983;62:457.

Andersen BL, Turnquist D, La Polla J, Turner D. Sexual functioning after treatment of in situ vulvar cancer: preliminary report. Obstet Gynecol 1988;71:15.

Barnes AB, Tinkham CG. Surgical gynecology. In: Notman MT, Nadelson CC, eds. The woman patient: medical and psychological interfaces. New York: Plenum Press, 1978.

Bernal EW. Hysterectomy and autonomy. Theor Med 1988;9:73.

Campion MJ, Brown JR, McCance DJ, Atia W, Edwards R, Cuzick J, Singer A. Psychosexual trauma of an abnormal cervical smear. Br J Obstet Gynecol 1988;95:175.

Cutler WB, Garcia CR. The medical management of menopause and premenopause. Philadelphia: JB Lippincott, 1984.

Derogatis LR. Breast and gynecologic cancers: their unique impact on body image and sexual identity in women. In: Vaeth JM, Blomberg RC, Adler L, eds. Body image, self-esteem, and sexuality in cancer patients. New York: S Karger, 1980.

Freeman MG. Introduction to the sexual history. In: Walker HK, Hall WD, Hurst JW, eds. Clinical methods. 2nd ed. Boston: Butterworth, 1980.

Gould D. Hidden problems after a hysterectomy. Nursing Times 1986 June 4:43.

Lalinec-Michaud M, Engelsmann F. Depression and hysterectomy: a prospective study. Psychosomatics 1984;25:550.

Lamont JA, DePetrillo AD, Sargeant EJ. Psychosexual rehabilitative and exenterative surgery. Gynecol Oncol 1978;6:236.

Massler DJ, Devansan MM. Sexual consequences of gynecologic operations. In: Comfort A, ed. Sexual consequences of disability. Philadelphia: George F Stickley, 1978.

Moth I, Andreasson B, Jensen SB, Bock JE. Sexual function and somatopsychic reactions after vulvectomy. Dan Med Bull 1983; 30(suppl 2):27.

Roeske NCA. Hysterectomy and other gynecological surgeries: a psychological view. In: Notman MT, Nadelson CC, eds. The woman patient: medical and psychological interfaces. New York: Plenum Press, 1978.

Schain WS. Sexual functioning, self-esteem and cancer care. In: Vaeth JM, Blomberg RC, Adler L, eds. Body image, self-esteem, and sexuality in cancer patients. New York: S Karger, 1980.

Webb C, Wilson-Barnett J. Hysterectomy: a study in coping with recovery. J Adv Nurs 1983;8:311.

Professional Liability of the Gynecologic Surgeon

ELVOY RAINES

The gynecologic surgeon shares the company of a growing number of medical and surgical specialists who practice their profession under a cloud of professional liability risk. The threat of litigation has never been greater, and this threat is reflected in the sizable insurance premiums they must pay and the ever-more-stringent protocols imposed by hospitals. It is also apparent in the evolution of the physician/patient relationship, as well as adjustments to the content and method of surgical practice not necessarily dictated by medical or scientific considerations.

There are important practical and professional considerations that should be understood by the gynecologic surgeon to prevent injury and unjustified exposure to a legal claim, as well as to preserve the scientific integrity of the decision-making process. The final outcome of these protective actions should be one in which the surgeon can practice without the fear of a lawsuit affecting his or her judgment.

This chapter is not a substitute for appropriate legal counsel, nor is it an exhaustive explanation of tort, or personal injury, law. Physicians interested in a fuller treatment of the subjects and legal theories raised here are referred to the bibliography for further reading.

THE PHYSICIAN/PATIENT RELATIONSHIP

Establishment of the Relationship

There are circumstances when the liability of the physician is nonexistent or limited (as in emergencies), but this discussion will focus upon the common physician/patient relationship where a duty of some sort is owed by the physician to the patient: a duty to perform as agreed between the parties and a duty not to injure the patient.

In general, the physician/patient relationship is contractual: one party is paid for services provided by another. But there is also a personal, physical aspect, since the physician (and especially the surgeon) actually touches the patient, either topically or invasively. Legal consequences attach in either instance, and lawsuits against physicians may be based upon contract or tort law. For this reason, the relationship of the parties may determine, first, whether a basis for a claim ever arises and then how the claim is resolved.

The manner in which the physician/patient relationship is established and maintained may be as important

23

to professional liability risk management as the quality of care actually provided. For instance, the physician should be careful to take on patients carefully selected for their compatibility with the practice and professional services offered; he must be diligent in the initial stages of the relationship to make certain that he is the proper provider for the emerging and apparent health care needs of the patient. This is made easier when the surgeon limits his practice to a manageable number of patients within a defined scope of services for which his training and skills are appropriate.

The patient shares responsibility for understanding the respective roles of the physician and patient in the pursuit of a mutually satisfactory outcome; therefore, accurate perception of patient expectations is essential to avoid later surprise or disappointment that can lead to litigation.

The patient should be involved—actually encouraged to participate—in her care, including activities of compliance with a therapeutic plan and monitoring of symptoms. The physician should make time available to talk about shared responsibilities and the critical role of patient participation and cooperation. Involvement of the patient improves the likelihood that communication will be free and effective, that potential misunderstandings will be avoided, and that any actual incidents will be managed in a more efficient and timely manner.

Informed Consent

A developing body of law (and much confusion and concern in some parts of the medical community) surrounds the concept of informed consent—that process by which the patient acquires an understanding of the contemplated surgical procedure and gives the physician permission to act. If the physician acts without permission, or beyond the limits or scope of permission, he or she may violate the agreement (contract) that is the basis of the physician/patient relationship or may be liable, under tort law, for personal injury, however slight.

It should be emphasized—and integrated into a surgeon's practice habits—that informed consent is a process. Although it is evidenced generally by a form signed by the patient stating that she understands the recommended procedure, risks, alternatives, and so on, the form is only representative of the process: it simply serves to show in writing that the process did occur. The process is the key, essential to appropriate professional practice, and one that should occur with any procedure or treatment.

The patient is the final decision maker. Of course there are exceptions due to age and mental or legal competence, but in general dealings with patients, the surgeon should acknowledge—and emphasize to the patient—that there are shared and respective responsibilities between physician and patient, and the decision to accept a physician's recommendation of surgery ultimately is the patient's alone.

If permission is given, and if the act is to be legally defensible, it must be based upon all elements *material* to the patient. Generally, courts will expect the patient to act on the value system of the fictional "reasonable man," that creation of the law that approximates the average person in terms of education and intellectual capacity. Material elements will almost always include a description of the procedure and why it is recommended; the risk of complication, side-effect, or injury associated with the procedure; alternatives to the procedure, including taking no action; the projected outcome and relative chances of success for the procedure; and information about costs for both the procedure and aftercare. Those risks that are known to exist and occur with some frequency should be explained, even if slight in terms of impact; rare but severe complications (those that cause permanent impairment or death) should also be explained.

Communication Between Physician and Patient

The patient and the physician both have obvious reasons for striving to maximize the quality of their communications. It might be argued that the physician has the added incentive of knowing that if a failure of communication leads to a lawsuit, he or she is the one who will suffer most, legally, for that failure.

The most effective means of reducing exposure to professional liability is effective communication: it prevents mistakes, misunderstandings, and inaccurate expectations; it also prevents lawsuits. The surgeon may improve the quality of communication by attending to details that may require extra time initially but that ultimately save time and energy for the physician, and consequences and costs for the patient: allow time for uninterrupted discussions with the patient, encourage the patient to ask questions, see that the patient follows directions and is a participant in her care, and reference and record all conversations (including telephone conversations) in the patient's file.

Special Duties of the Specialist

The existence of a duty owed the patient by the physician is necessary for liability. Also necessary is a breach of that duty, and an injury that is caused by that breach of duty. The gynecologic surgeon, like other specialists, will be held to a higher standard of care in a court's analysis of the duty and the breach than would a generalist, perhaps even one performing the same procedure. In the past, a "locality rule" was in effect, even for specialists, that set the standard as that which a similarly trained physician in that locality would be expected to meet; today, except in a very few jurisdictions, specialists are held to a nationally applied standard of care, rigidly enforced by courts and easily established by a plethora of expert witnesses.

Liability for the Acts of Others

The surgeon is responsible for his own actions, but he may also bear the legal responsibility for acts of those providing care and services to the patient under his direction. Courts explain this transference of liability in terms of "vicarious liability" or *respondeat superior.* Simply stated, the primary physician may be liable for the acts of another person, even another physician, where the second person causes injury to the patient during the course and scope of his or her employment and there is some relationship between the providers that would give the primary physician control or right of control over the second person's actions.

A second, and less easily applied, rule of liability for the actions of others is established under the legal theory of *res ipsa loquitur.* This concept means roughly "the thing speaks for itself" and is a form of strict liability, wherein by circumstantial proof negligence may be inferred from the fact that an injury occurred that does not normally occur in the absence of negligence. This inference shifts the burden of proof to the defendant physician. Requisite elements, in addition to the presumption of negligence, are that the injury is caused by an instrumentality within the exclusive control of the physician and that there is no contributing action by the patient.

The surgeon must be aware that the theory of *respondeat superior* may apply in the operating room as well as in the office: employees may place him or her in positions of liability, but members of the health care team providing surgical assistance, laboratory and record interpretation, and follow-up care also may cause injury for which he or she is liable. For that reason, adequate, effective communication between the surgeon and colleagues, other providers, and staff is essential to meaningful risk management.

The competence of other physicians and assistants must be assured, and the gynecologic surgeon should not involve them in patient care if their abilities are not known. More specifically, nonphysician assistants should be adequately trained and experienced for the assignments delegated to them, and supervised in their performance. It is unwise to delegate care to medical students and residents without adequate supervision, and the surgeon should be especially sensitive to signs that the patient feels slighted when others provide care in the attending physician's stead.

Termination of the Physician/Patient Relationship

Just as the physician/patient relationship is a product of agreement between the parties, so too should be the termination of the relationship. Unless treatment is no longer required or the patient terminates the relationship, the physician wishing to terminate his or her obligation to provide professional services should give adequate and timely notice to the patient, refer the case if necessary and advisable, and provide all records and information necessary to a proper response by the replacing physician. Failure to ensure continuous coverage may result in a lawsuit for abandonment and negligence. If the physician wishes to limit the relationship from the outset, that should be made clear in the initial information of the relationship; the surgeon, for instance, may wish to explain that his or her services will be provided with the understanding that the patient will return to her referring physician, who provides her routine gynecologic care.

Documentation of the circumstances and process of termination of the relationship is critical. Notice to the patient might require certified mail to guarantee receipt, and acknowledgement by the referral physician of acceptance of the case demonstrates a continuum of care. Hospitalized patients require extremely careful referral if the relationship terminates while they are inpatients, including details of date and time of case management transfer.

PRACTICE MANAGEMENT

Recordkeeping

After effective communication, the single most important aspect of liability risk management is the maintenance of good records. As a determinant of the defensibility of a case, it may be the most important element. There is no substitute for an articulate, fully informative record as a mechanism for communication among members of the health care team, and as a permanent written record of treatment decisions and effects. In the absence of a record or elements of a record, only the memories of the parties are available, and that places the allegations of the plaintiff on a par with the defenses of the defendant.

Gynecologic surgeons must devote considerable attention to recordkeeping, since their exposure to a lawsuit is so high. For 1980, statistics indicate that six of the eight most frequently performed operative procedures were among those commonly performed by gynecologists. (The eight most frequently performed procedures, in order of frequency, are biopsy, diagnostic dilatation and curettage, excision of lesion of skin or tissue, hysterectomy, ligation and division of fallopian tubes, cesarean section, repair of inguinal hernia, and oophorectomy.) In simple numbers, gynecologic surgeons have a greater degree of exposure to lawsuit because they have a greater number of patient/surgical encounters. Therefore, prompt, accurate recording of information is essential.

Completeness, accuracy, and adequacy are critical elements in recordkeeping. For completeness, the physician should pay special attention to the medical history, and the record should include progress notes (as well as information regarding a patient's failure to comply with therapeutic plans), consent forms, lab reports, consultant reports, correspondence, and notes of conversations, both in person and on the telephone. Questions asked should have answers in the record; lab tests ordered should be followed by a reading and interpretation in writing. Flat, unqualified predictions (". . . is not a threat to her general health") should not appear in the record, and self-deprecating humor or other irrelevant asides should not appear. To ensure an up-to-date record, timely writing or dictation of the operative record is essential; dictated records should be reviewed for typographical errors or other mistakes. Written remarks must be legible. The chart is a clinical record of care rendered, and remarks should be precise, professional, complete, and accurate. Finally, completeness includes making sure that the record is internally consistent; inconsistencies in the physician's comments or in those added by others should be explained in the record.

Any blank spaces or alterations in the record can be especially damaging to the defensibility of a physician's actions. Unanswered questions or absence of comments suggests that important matters went unattended, and alterations suggest inconclusiveness or an attempt at subterfuge. Something should be written at *every* patient visit, and the surgeon should never delay in completing essential information. There should be no obliteration of already recorded information, and if a mistake is made or a change is necessary for any reason, the incorrect statement should be lined through once (so the original may be still legible) and the correction made, dated, and initialed with an explanation for the change. When sharing records, surgeons should provide copies, retaining the originals in their files at all times.

Consultation, Second Opinion, or Referral

The surgeon should resort readily to consultation, or referral if necessary, rather than relying upon "hopes" or "odds" for achieving a positive outcome; no surgeon should expect that his or her knowledge is complete and superior in all instances, for a court will quickly demonstrate that theirs is the final judgment of appropriate medical practice. Information should be explained to the patient in a correct, timely, and responsible manner, with bad news conveyed in a serious and professional manner rather than jokingly or casually.

Too frequently, physicians decide that they can perform a given procedure as well as anyone or that they do not wish to risk losing a patient to a competing physician; such short-sightedness leads only to lawsuits. Timely consultation suggests prudence on the part of the physician, and recorded opinions of two physicians make the defensibility of the primary physician much greater.

Consultations should be obtained any time the patient or a member of the family makes a request, when a poor outcome is expected, or when some uncertainty remains about the diagnosis or treatment.

Awareness of Current Literature and Procedural Specifications

The surgeon is expected to be current to the date of the procedure on readings related to all relevant professional practice considerations. Any lapse reflects badly on the competence of the physician and reduces the defensibility of his or her actions. State-of-the-art opinions and guidelines should be followed closely, and technical information and standards must be a functional part of the surgeon's knowledge. Expert witnesses need only display the professional literature to establish a failure in professional performance.

Office Staff Appreciation of Liability Issues

As explained in relation to vicarious liability, the actions of others may cause the physician to acquire an unnecessary liability risk. This is true also of behavioral considerations for the physician's staff. Inappropriate behavior or antagonistic remarks by nurses, clerks, and secretaries can sour the best physician/patient relationship. Therefore, all staff members should be involved in risk management. Among the basic considerations are the following: retain copies of all telephone messages and conversations with patients, record all missed appointments or variances in compliance with therapy, note inconsistencies in patient statements about history or progress, and keep all financial and billing records separate from medical and surgical records.

At this point, special mention should be made of appropriate use of the telephone. The physician should avoid as much as possible the practice of diagnosing, prescribing, or instructing over the telephone. As an instrument of communication, it has considerable limitations because the conversants cannot see one another and may not hear each other's statements correctly. If instructions are given by telephone, very careful records and follow-up should be part of the process.

Communication with the Insurance Carrier

Surgeons who do not communicate freely and regularly with their insurance carrier may find it difficult to understand the true role of an insurer. It is important to understand that the risk of the physician is the risk of the insurer, at least to a degree, and that the physician has no greater ally in risk management efforts. A basic yet thorough understanding of the policy is essential. In addition, it is essential to know the names and locations of claims managers and the criteria for reporting incidents to the insurer.

Early reporting of incidents is critical to maintaining a defensible practice. For the surgeon, this is an even more important habit, and one that will be fairly commonly practiced, since surgery naturally involves a core percentage of unanticipated outcomes or incidents. It is impossible to perform as a surgeon for any considerable period without committing an act or being identified with an outcome that could become the basis for a lawsuit. Therefore, perception of the occurrence of incidents, and a prompt reporting to the insurer, allow time and perspective for insurer and insured to anticipate and prepare a defense against claims of potential plaintiffs. If no case arises, the exercise of incident management (described in more detail later) will permit the physician to examine critically his or her own performance.

Communication with Other Physicians, Nurses, and Staff

"Physicians get physicians sued" is a statement that the surgeon will hear repeatedly. And it is true. Moreover, nurses get physicians sued, and residents, and other hospital staff members. The failure of these providers to confine their observations to clinical facts and objective analysis of patient care is the primary cause of lawsuits generated from the medical community. The solution is not a conspiracy of silence but a more professional pattern of behavior within the confines of the hospital and in the physician's office. A basic rule is never to write or say anything that you would be reluctant to repeat on a witness stand.

The quality of communication is critical as well. Studies have shown a significant variance in the understanding of terminology, especially quantifying terms such as *sometimes* and *always,* with variations from region to region and between professions. Specificity, opportunities for questions, and periodic review of the effectiveness of communication aid the surgeon in ensuring that correct understandings occur.

ZONES OF RISK

The gynecologic surgeon will find the majority of his or her practice related to diseases of the female genital tract. However, aspects of other specialties find application in good gynecologic practice: endocrinology, internal medicine, and obstetrics, for example. Therefore, the gynecologic surgeon must have a thorough knowledge of female reproductive physiology and of the concurrent mental and emotional factors that are so integral to reproductive ability and sexual function. Furthermore, the interaction and interdependence of the gynecologic surgeon with other specialists mandates an ability to coordinate efforts and cooperate toward a positive outcome.

Common gynecologic conditions may not necessarily require surgery, and the surgeon should exercise prudence in selecting and recommending treatment modalities.

The initial examination of the patient, and all preoperative evaluations, should be comprehensive and detailed. This early and preliminary investigation is critical to correct management of care thereafter.

Accurate diagnosis is essential prior to any elective operative procedure. Especially important is the identification of pregnancy, and any suggestion of pregnancy should forestall elective procedures until all factors are known.

Gynecologic surgery generally involves fewer complications than some other surgical encounters, and therefore potential liability is somewhat reduced; however, there is no special immunity from error or injury in gynecologic surgery, and the surgeon must direct special attention to a variety of zones of risk inherent in such surgical encounters.

Diagnosis and Treatment

Diagnostic issues account for about 18.4% of claims. Treatment issues are the basis for legal claims in over half of all cases. For the gynecologic surgeon, these factors present a formidable risk that must be translated into a manner of practice that will minimize the risk of delay in diagnosis, misdiagnosis, or failure to diagnose.

For example, for gynecologists fully 51% of diagnostic failure claims involve cancer; 73% of allegations of failure to diagnose are for breast cancer. It would seem, therefore, that gynecologists should have an extremely high index of suspicion for examination of the patient's breast in a rigorous practice of screening. Other special areas of risk involve surgical injury and infection, and problems related to contraception, abortion, and sterilization (6.8% of claims are abortion-related and 9.5% are for failure of sterilization).

Adequate training in the techniques and procedures for breast examination, diagnosis, and follow-up is essential. Moreover, the appropriate referral of patients, or consultation, is basic to a defensible practice.

Surgical injury, particularly bowel and urinary tract injuries, is also common enough to merit special consideration and anticipation; postoperative infection is the most common complication. When such an injury occurs (nicked ureters, perforations of the uterus, and so on) the appropriate steps in incident management must be taken.

Problems related to contraception and sterilization account for many of the claims against gynecologists. Incomplete abortion, failure to diagnose or mismanagement of ectopic pregnancy, and failed sterilization procedures are common areas of risk.

Injuries from Medication or Equipment and Facilities

Medication issues account for about 7% of claims, and equipment or facilities-related injuries account for about 3%. Both percentages are small; nevertheless, both areas contribute to the liability exposure of the surgeon. The administration of drugs and the care and maintenance of office and hospital equipment are matters that require the surgeon's awareness and understanding. No drug or item of equipment should ever be used without a full knowledge of its function and of possible complications.

Special Areas of Risk for the Gynecologic Surgeon

Besides the preceding issues, the gynecologic surgeon has a unique level of liability exposure in the performance of laparoscopy, laparotomy, cancer screening, hysterectomy, oophorectomy, abortion, and conception control. Professional services related to these special areas of risk should incorporate the highest degree and quality of communication, informed consent, and attention to detail in recordkeeping and case follow-up. The surgeon who knows the areas of legal risk is forearmed and able to anticipate the occasional poor outcome or small error and deal more effectively with it.

Fistulas

Pelvic surgery—particularly total abdominal hysterectomy or vaginal hysterectomy and repair—may lead to the development of vesicovaginal or ureteral fistulas. Rectovaginal fistulas are likely to occur with vaginal repair, abdominal hysterectomy, incision and drainage of a Bartholin abscess, sigmoid resection, and hemorrhoidectomy.

When injury is recognized while an operation is in progress, it should be repaired at once. However, some fistulas will be recognized in the first days after a surgical procedure; in such instances, the surgeon may wish to delay repair until inflammation, local swelling, and identified infection have diminished.

Hysterectomy

Total hysterectomy is the second most frequently performed surgical procedure in the United States. Today, many hysterectomies are performed for conditions that are potentially dangerous, partially disabling, or simply uncomfortable. Therefore, because of the relatively elective nature of the procedure in some instances, and because of the risk of infection or injury to the urinary tract and other organs, special attention to medical and legal concerns such as informed consent is appropriate.

Dilatation and Curettage

Dilatation and curettage ranks third in frequency among surgical procedures. Although most physicians consider it a minor operative procedure, there is a risk of complication, such as perforation of the uterus, and the surgeon should be fully prepared to deal with any complications arising during or after the procedure.

Abortion

Another procedure considered relatively routine, abortion is a zone of risk for the gynecologist who is less than experienced or who is providing services to women at high risk, in the later stages of pregnancy, or in inadequately equipped facilities. Complications and injuries that often lead to lawsuits include uterine perforation, cervical laceration, hemorrhage, incomplete removal of the fetus and placenta, and anesthetic problems.

Sterilization and Contraception

Two emerging zones of risk for the gynecologist in terms of professional liability are contraception and sterilization procedures. Inappropriate prescription of contraceptive methods or insertion of devices, disregard of or failure to identify contraindications, and failure to manage complications adequately all expose the physician to lawsuits.

Surgical laparoscopy for sterilization may lead to electrosurgical injuries or hemorrhage, but more commonly the gynecologist is sued on the basis of failures of informed consent or of negligence in the performance of the procedure: the patient expects to be sterile and then becomes pregnant. Such cases lead to claims of "wrongful birth" or "wrongful conception." There may be recovery even if the fetus is aborted. Therefore, it is imperative that the gynecologist explain in detail and to the patient's full understanding the possibility of a sterilization procedure's being unsuccessful and the consequent risk, however remote, of a pregnancy. Since most states now recognize the right of action of wrongful birth, this is one area of professional liability risk that must be effectively managed. It can be, with a careful discussion of the procedure with the patient.

INCIDENT MANAGEMENT

Every physician encounters unexpected problems, unanticipated complications, and actual errors of skill or judgment. The management of these events is critical to whether a lawsuit results. The techniques of incident management have been mentioned in previous sections of this chapter, but a full treatment follows.

The occurrence of an incident involving injury to the patient, however insignificant to the physician, should be treated professionally and diligently. At the first opportunity, a full report of the incident should be shared with the insurer; in a hospital, the incident should be reported to the risk management team or the legal counsel, as well as to the chief of service or department head. But attention must first be paid to the patient and her problem must be resolved.

The first and most important step is to avoid concealment, subterfuge, lying, or minimization of the injury in communicating with the patient and her family. Honesty is the best protection from a legal viewpoint and the most effective medical course to follow. A calm, uninterrupted conversation should be conducted with the patient, explaining precisely what occurred and

what will be necessary to mitigate the damage. A full disclosure of what occurred is absolutely essential, but the surgeon should avoid embellishing the facts with details that will create anxiety or apprehension beyond the scope of the actual problem. Certain terms should be avoided in conversation: the surgeon should not mention negligence or malpractice; similarly, he or she should not confess to fault but rather explain that complications occur and, referring back to the properly conducted process of informed consent, remind the patient that such an event was discussed as a possibility.

For the repair of injuries caused in the course of surgery, a second process of informed consent may be necessary, unless the error is corrected during the course of the original procedure. In either case, the explanation of the repair procedure must be quite detailed, and the risk and complications that relate to that procedure must be fully explained. The scope of permission granted in the process of informed consent will weigh heavily in a court's consideration of whether the additional surgery was necessary and whether the patient was appropriately prepared with information and explanations.

INFORMED CONSENT: SURGERY BY RESIDENTS AND SUBSTITUTES

Hospitals affiliated with institutions for health care education and training are faced with the special problem of consent to surgery extending to physicians other than the attending physician who is known to the patient. Although the hospital and medical staff may understand the routine and necessary involvement of surgeons-in-training and the performance of surgery by physicians other than those to whom the patient has specifically granted consent, it is unwise to presume that the patient gives "implied consent" by entering a teaching hospital.

Consent forms for the teaching hospital should include a reference to the fact that residents and substitute physicians may either perform the surgery in its entirety or assist in the surgery to which the patient has been asked to consent (Fig. 3-1). Additionally, the attending physician should explain to the patient that such participation or substitution may occur. If the patient objects, the objection should be noted in the record and every effort made to prevent violation of the objection. If the institution cannot ensure compliance, then, except in an emergency, the patient should be encouraged to utilize a different institution.

Emergencies provide the only defensible exception to consent to substitutes, and they should be thoroughly documented as such.

[NAME OF HOSPITAL]
CONSENT TO HOSPITAL ADMISSION AND
MEDICAL TREATMENT

Name of Patient: _____

Name of Attending Physician(s): _____

Date of Admission: _____ Time: _____ (AM) (PM)

1. I, (or [NAME OF AUTHORIZED REPRESENTATIVE] acting on behalf of) [NAME OF PATIENT], suffering from a condition requiring hospital care, hereby consent to the rendering of such care, which may include routine diagnostic procedures and such medical treatment as the named attending physician(s) or others of the hospital's medical staff consider to be necessary.

2. I understand that the practice of medicine and surgery is not an exact science and that diagnosis and treatment may involve risks of injury, or even death. I acknowledge that no guarantees have been made to me as to the result of examination or treatment in this hospital.

3. I understand that:
   (A) It is customary, absent emergency or extraordinary circumstances, that no substantial procedures are performed upon a patient unless and until he or she has had an opportunity to discuss them with the physician or other health professional to the patient's satisfaction;
   (B) Each patient has the right to consent, or to refuse consent, to any proposed procedure or therapeutic course; and
   (C) No patient will be involved in any research or experimental procedure without his or her full knowledge and consent.

4. I understand that many of the physicians on the staff of this hospital, including the attending physician(s) named above, are not employees or agents of the hospital but, rather, are independent contractors who have been granted the privilege of using its facilities for the care and treatment of their patients. Further, I realize that among those who attend patients at this hospital are medical, nursing, and other health care personnel in training who, unless requested otherwise, may be present during patient care, as a part of their education. Still or motion pictures and closed circuit television monitoring of patient care also may be used for education purposes, unless a patient expressly requests otherwise.

5. This form has been fully explained to me, and I am satisfied that I understand its content and significance.

Date of Execution: _____

_____   _____
[SIGNATURE OF PATIENT]   [SIGNATURE OF WITNESS]

(If patient is unable to consent or is a minor, complete the following:) Patient [is a minor _____ years of age] (is unable to consent because]:

_____

_____

_____   _____
[SIGNATURE OF LEGAL GUARDIAN OR CLOSEST AVAILABLE RELATIVE]   [SIGNATURE OF WITNESS]

Figure 3–1. Consent form.

CONCLUSION

Gynecologic surgeons have several opportunities to manage and control their legal risk, and several corresponding periods of special exposure. Diligence in practice, both in the office and in the hospital, and attention to those occasions and the procedures that carry heightened risk for the physician, will permit the most effective risk and incident management and the diminution of liability problems. Surgeons should create and maintain a strong, complete presurgical record; they should personally perform the functions involved in the process of obtaining informed consent; they should respond to complications in a timely and responsible manner, involving the patient when possible; and they should give equal attention to the postoperative relationship with the patient.

The law offers protection and privilege for the gynecologic surgeon, and careful practitioners will familiarize themselves with local rules and regulations, as well as general concepts such as those explained here. In this way, they may not only function as surgeons but also be comfortable with the liability that is a basic element of their position of trust and their professional relationship with patients.

Bibliography

Alton W. Malpractice: a trial lawyer's advice for physicians. Boston: Little, Brown & Co, 1977.

American College of Obstetricians and Gynecologists. Professional liability and its effects: report of a 1987 survey of ACOG's membership. Washington, D.C.: ACOG, 1988.

Andrews LB. Informed consent statutes and the decision-making process. J Legal Med 1984;5(2):163.

Chayet NL, Reardon TM. Trouble in the medical staff: a practical guide to hospital initiated quality assurance. Am J Law Med 1981; 7(3):301.

Curran WJ, Shapiro ED. Law, medicine and forensic science. Boston: Little, Brown & Co, 1981.

Danner D. Medical malpractice: a primer for physicians. New York: The Lawyers Co-operative, 1988.

Danzon PM. Medical malpractice: theory, evidence and public policy. Cambridge, Mass.: Harvard University Press, 1985.

Fineberg KS, Peters JD, Willson JR, Kroll DL. Obstetrics/gynecology and the law. Ann Arbor, Mich.: Health Administration Press, 1984.

Fiscina SF. Medical law for the attending physician: a case-oriented analysis. Carbondale, Ill.: Southern Illinois University Press, 1982.

Holder AR. Medical malpractice law. 2nd ed. New York: John Wiley & Sons, 1978.

King JH, Jr. The law of medical malpractice in a nutshell. St. Paul: West, 1977.

Kramer C. Medical Malpractice. New York: Practising Law Institute, 1976.

Levine M. Surgical malpractice. La Mesa, Calif.: Trans-Media, 1970.

Pegalis S, Wachsman H. American law of medical malpractice. 3 vols. Rochester: New York Lawyers Co-operative Publishing Company, 1980.

Pollack R. Clinical aspects of malpractice. Oradel, N.J.: Medical Economics Books, 1980.

Prosser WL. Handbook of the law of torts. St. Paul: West, 1971.

Richards EP III, Rathbun KC. Medical risk management: preventive legal strategies for health care providers. Rockville, Md.: Aspen Publications, 1983.

Roberts DK, Shane JA, Roberts ML. Confronting the malpractice crisis: guidelines for the obstetrician-gynecologist. Kansas City: Eagle Press, 1985.

Rosoff AJ. Informed consent. Rockville, Md.: Aspen Publications, 1981.

Rozovsky FA. Consent to treatment. Boston: Little, Brown & Co, 1984.

United States Department of Health and Human Services. Report of the task force on medical liability and malpractice. Washington, D.C.: U.S. Government Printing Office, 1987:190–412/70133.

4

Anatomy of the Female Pelvis

JOHN O. L. DE LANCEY

VULVA AND ERECTILE STRUCTURES

The bony pelvic outlet is bordered by the ischiopubic rami anteriorly, and the coccyx and sacrotuberous ligaments posteriorly. It can be divided into anterior and posterior triangles, which share a common base along a line between the ischial tuberosities. The tissues filling the anterior triangle have a layered structure similar to that of the abdominal wall (Table 4-1). There is a skin and adipose layer (vulva) overlying a fascial layer (perineal membrane) that lies superficial to a muscular layer (levator ani muscles).

Subcutaneous Tissues of the Vulva

The structures of the vulva lie on the pubic bones and extend caudally under its arch (Fig. 4-1). They consist of the mons, labia, clitoris, vestibule, and associated erectile structures and their muscles. The mons is comprised of hair-bearing skin over a cushion of adipose tissue that lies on the pubic bones. Extending posteriorly from the mons, the labia majora are composed of similar hair-bearing skin and adipose tissue, which contain the termination of the round ligaments of the uterus and the obliterated processus vaginalis (canal of Nuck). The round ligament may give rise to leiomyomas in this region, and the obliterated processus vaginalis can be a dilated embryonic remnant in the adult.

The labia minora, vestibule, and glans clitoris can be seen between the two labia majora. The labia minora are hairless skin folds, each of which splits anteriorly to run over, and under, the glans of the clitoris. The more anterior folds unite to form the hood-shaped prepuce of the clitoris, while the posterior folds insert into the under side of the glans as the frenulum.

Unlike the skin of the labia majora, the cutaneous structures of the labia minora and vestibule do not lie on an adipose layer but upon a connective-tissue stratum that is loosely organized and permits mobility of the skin during intercourse. This loose attachment of the skin to underlying tissues allows the skin to be easily dissected off the underlying fascia during skinning vulvectomy in the area of the labia minora and vestibule.

In the posterior lateral aspect of the vestibule, the duct of the major vestibular gland can be seen 3–4 mm outside of the hymenal ring. The minor vestibular gland openings are found along a line extending anteriorly from this point, parallel to the hymenal ring and extending toward the urethral orifice. The urethra protrudes slightly through the vestibular skin anterior to the vagina and posterior to the clitoris. Its orifice is flanked on either side by two small labia. Skene's ducts open into the inner aspect of these labia and can be seen as small, punctate openings, when the urethral labia are separated.

Within the skin of the vulva are specialized glands that can become enlarged and thereby require surgical removal. The holocrine sebaceous glands in the labia majora are associated with hair shafts, and in the labia minora they are free-standing. They lie close to the surface, which explains their easy recognition with minimal enlargement. In addition, lateral to the introitus and anus, there are high densities of apocrine sweat glands, along with the normal eccrine sweat glands. The former structures undergo change with the menstrual cycle, having increased secretory activity in the premenstrual period. They can become chronically infected, as in hidradenitis suppurativa, or neoplastically enlarged, as in hidradenomas, both of which may require surgical therapy. The eccrine sweat glands present in the vulvar skin rarely present abnormalities, but on occasion they can form palpable masses as syringomas.

TABLE 4–1
Layers of the Anterior Triangle of the Perineum

Skin
Subcutaneous tissue
  Camper's fascia
  Colles's fascia
Superficial space
  Clitoris and its crura
  Ischiocavernosus muscle
  Vestibular bulb
  Bulbocavernosus muscle
  Greater vestibular gland
  Superficial transverse perineal muscle
Deep space–perineal membrane
  Compressor urethrae
  Urethrovaginal sphincter

The subcutaneous tissue of the labia majora is similar in composition to the skin of the abdominal wall. It consists of lobules of fat interlaced with connective tissue septa. Although there are no well-defined layers in the subcutaneous tissue, regional variations in the relative quantity of fat and fibrous tissue exist. The superficial region of this tissue, where fat predominates, has been called Camper's fascia, as it is on the abdomen. In this region there is a continuation of fat from the anterior abdominal wall, called the digital process of fat, that is easily separated from the surrounding tissues and that is employed as a Martius fat pad graft to cover vaginal fistulas.

In the deeper layers of the vulva there is less fat, and the interlacing fibrous connective tissue septa are much more evident than those in Camper's fascia. This more

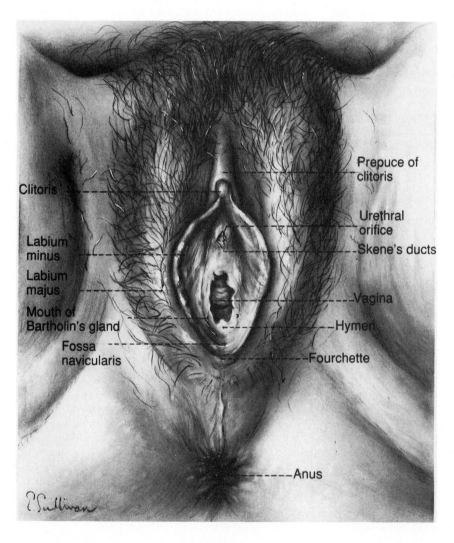

Figure 4–1. External genitalia.

fibrous layer is called Colles' fascia and is similar to Scarpa's fascia on the abdomen. Its interlacing fibrous septa of the subcutaneous tissue attach laterally to the ischiopubic rami and fuse posteriorly with the posterior edge of the perineal membrane (ie, urogenital diaphragm). Anteriorly, however, there is no connection to the pubic rami, and this permits communication between the area deep to this layer and the abdominal wall. These fibrous attachments to the ischiopubic rami and to the posterior aspect of the perineal membrane limit the spread of hematomas or infection in this compartment posterolaterally but allow spread into the abdomen. This clinical observation has led to considering Colles' fascia as a separate entity from the superficial Camper's fascia, which lacks these connections.

Superficial Compartment

The space between the subcutaneous tissues and the perineal membrane, which contains the clitoris, crura, vestibule bulbs, and the ischiocavernosus and bulbocavernosus muscles, is called the superficial compartment of the perineum (Fig. 4-2). The deep compartment is the region just above the perineal membrane; it is discussed later.

The erectile bodies and their associated muscles within the superficial compartment are applied to the caudal surface of the perineal membrane. The clitoris is composed of a midline shaft (body) capped with the glans. This shaft lies on, and is suspended from, the pubic bones by a subcutaneous suspensory ligament. The paired crura of the clitoris bend downward from

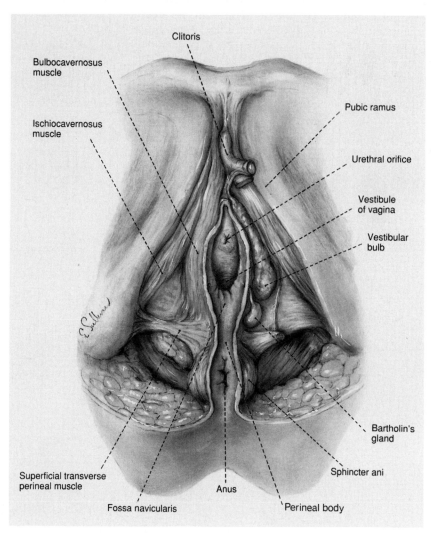

Figure 4–2. Superficial compartment and perineal membrane.

the shaft and are firmly attached to the pubic bones, continuing dorsally to lie on the inferior aspects of the pubic rami. The ischiocavernosus muscles originate at the ischial tuberosities and the free surfaces of the crura, to insert on the upper crura and body of the clitoris. A few muscle fibers, called the superficial transverse perineal muscles, originate in common with the ischiocavernosus muscle from the ischial tuberosity and lie medial to the perineal body.

The paired vestibular bulbs lie immediately under the vestibular skin and are composed of erectile tissue. They are covered by the bulbocavernosus muscles, which originate in the perineal body and lie over their lateral surfaces. These muscles, along with the ischiocavernosus muscles, insert into the body of the clitoris and act to pull it downward.

Bartholin's greater vestibular gland is found at the tail end of the bulb of the vestibule and is connected to the vestibular mucosa by a duct lined with squamous epithelium. The gland lies on the perineal membrane and beneath the bulbocavernosus muscle. The intimate relationship between the enormously vascular erectile tissue of the vestibular bulb and Bartholin's gland is responsible for the hemorrhage associated with removal of this latter structure.

The perineal membrane and perineal body are important to the support of the pelvic organs. They are discussed in the section on the pelvic floor.

Pudendal Nerve and Vessels

The pudendal nerve is the sensory and motor nerve of the perineum. Its course and distribution in the perineum parallel the pudendal artery and veins that connect with the internal iliac vessels (Fig. 4-3). We describe the course and division of the nerve with the understanding that the vascular channels parallel them.

The pudendal nerve arises from the sacral plexus (S2–S4), and the vessels originate from the anterior division of the internal iliac artery. They leave the pelvis through the greater sciatic foramen by hooking around the ischial spine and sacrospinous ligament to enter the pudendal (Alcock's) canal through the lesser sciatic foramen.

The nerve and vessels have three branches: the clitoral, perineal, and inferior hemorrhoidal. The clitoral branch insinuates itself into the perineal membrane along its path to supply the clitoris. The perineal branch (the largest of the three branches), enters the sub-

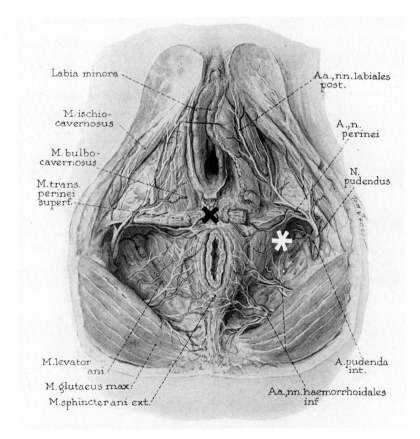

Figure 4–3. Pudendal nerve and vessels, with the position of the ischiorectal fossa (*) and the perineal body (X) indicated.

cutaneous tissues of the vulva behind the perineal membrane. Here it supplies the bulbocavernosus, ischiocavernosus, and transverse perineal muscles. It also supplies the skin of the inner portions of the labia majora, the labia minora, and the vestibule. The inferior hemorrhoidal branch goes to the external anal sphincter and perianal skin.

Lymphatic Drainage

The pattern of the vulvar lymphatic vessels and of drainage into the superficial inguinal group of lymph nodes has been established by both injection studies and clinical observation. It is important to the treatment of vulvar malignancies; an overview of this system is provided here. This area is described and illustrated in more detail in Chapter 39.

Tissues external to the hymenal ring are supplied by an anastomotic series of vessels in the superficial tissues that coalesce to a few trunks lateral to the clitoris and proceed laterally to the superficial inguinal nodes (Fig. 4-4). The vessels draining the labia majora also run in an anterior direction, lateral to those of the labia minora and vestibule. These lymphatic channels lie medial to the labiocrural fold, establishing it as the lateral border of surgical resection.

Injection studies of the urethral lymphatics have shown that lymphatic drainage of this region terminates in either the right or left inguinal nodes. The clitoris has been said to have some direct drainage to deep pelvic lymph nodes, bypassing the usual superficial nodes, but the clinical significance of this appears to be minimal.

The inguinal lymph nodes are divided into two groups, the superficial and the deep nodes. The superficial nodes are 12–20 in number and lie in a T-shaped distribution parallel to and 1 cm below the inguinal ligament, with the stem extending down along the saphenous vein. The nodes are frequently divided into four quadrants with the center of the division at the saphenous opening. The vulvar drainage goes primarily to the medial nodes of the upper quadrant. These nodes lie deep in the adipose layer of the subcutaneous tissues, in the membranous layer, just superficial to the fascia lata.

The large saphenous vein joins the femoral vein through the saphenous opening. Within 2 cm of the inguinal ligament several superficial blood vessels branch from the saphenous vein and the femoral artery. They include the superficial epigastric vessels that supply the subcutaneous tissues of the lower abdomen, the superficial circumflex iliac vessels that course laterally to the region of the iliac crest, and the superficial external pudendal that supply the mons, labia majora, and clitoral hood.

Lymphatics from the superficial nodes enter the fossa ovalis and drain into the deep inguinal nodes, which number one to three and lie in the femoral canal of the femoral triangle. They pass through the fossa ovalis (saphenous opening) in the fascia lata that lies approximately 3 cm below the inguinal ligament, lateral to the pubic tubercle, along with the saphenous vein on its way to the femoral vein. The membranous layer of the subcutaneous tissues spans this opening as a trabeculate layer called a fascia cribrosa, pierced by lymphatics. The deep nodes are found under this fascia in the femoral triangle.

The femoral triangle is the subfascial space of the upper one third of the thigh. It is bounded by the inguinal ligament, sartorius muscle, and adductor

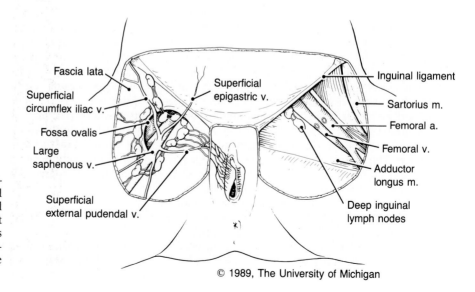

Figure 4–4. Lymphatic drainage of the vulva and femoral triangle. Superficial inguinal nodes are shown in the right thigh, and deep inguinal nodes are shown on the left thigh. Fascia lata has been removed on the left.

Fascia lata

Superficial circumflex iliac v.

Fossa ovalis

Large saphenous v.

Superficial external pudendal v.

Superficial epigastric v.

Inguinal ligament

Sartorius m.

Femoral a.

Femoral v.

Adductor longus m.

Deep inguinal lymph nodes

© 1989, The University of Michigan

longus muscle. Its floor is formed by the pectineus, adductor longus, and the iliopsoas muscles. The femoral artery bisects it vertically between the anterior superior iliac spine and the pubic tubercle. The femoral vein lies medial to the artery; the femoral nerve is lateral to it.

As these vessels pass under the inguinal ligament, they carry with them an extension of the transversalis fascia, which is the extraperitoneal connective tissue deep to the rectus abdominis muscle called the femoral sheath. These sheaths are prolonged for approximately 2–3 cm below the inguinal ligament before fusing with the vascular adventitia. Besides the two parts of the femoral sheath that accompany these vessels, a third portion—the femoral canal—can be found in the space medial to the vein. The abdominal opening of this is the femoral ring. The femoral canal contains the deep inguinal lymph nodes. Lymph channels from these nodes pierce the membrane filling the femoral ring to communicate with the external iliac nodes. Also within this region, the femoral vessels give rise to the deep external pudendal vessels. These pudendal branches run deep to the femoral vein over the pectineus to pierce the fascia lata. Here they become subcutaneous and there are anastomoses with the branch of the internal pudendal branches as well as the deep femoral and lateral circumflex femoral.

THE PELVIC FLOOR

With assumption of the upright posture by humans, the opening within the bony pelvis has come to lie at the bottom of the abdominopelvic cavity. This required the evolution of a supportive system to prevent the pelvic organs from being pushed downward through this opening. In the female, this system must withstand these downward forces but allow for the passage of the large and cranially dominant human fetus. The supportive system that has evolved to meet these needs consists of a fibromuscular floor that forms a shelf spanning the pelvic outlet and that contains a cleft for the birth canal and excretory drainage. A series of visceral ligaments and fasciae tethers the organs and maintains their position over the closed portions of the floor. The floor consists of the levator ani muscles and the perineal membrane. The openings in these structures for parturition and elimination have required the development of ancillary fibrous elements that are concentrated over open areas in the muscular floor to support the viscera in these weak areas. This section discusses the structures of the pelvic floor; the fibrous supportive system is described in the section on the pelvic viscera and cleavage planes and fascia.

Perineal Membrane (Urogenital Diaphragm)

The perineal membrane forms the inferior portion of the pelvic floor. It is a triangular sheet of dense, fibromuscular tissue that spans the anterior half of the pelvic outlet (see Fig. 4-2). It has previously been called the urogenital diaphragm, and this change in name reflects the appreciation that it is not a two-layered structure with muscle in between, as had previously been thought. It is a membrane, with the skeletal muscle of the striated urogenital sphincter (formerly the deep transverse perineal muscle) above. Because of the presence of the vagina, the perineal membrane cannot form a continuous sheet to close off the anterior pelvis in the female, as it does in the male. It does provide support by attaching the vagina and perineal body to the ischiopubic rami, thereby limiting their downward descent. This layer of the floor arises from the inner aspect of the inferior ischiopubic rami above the ischiocavernosus muscles and the crura of the clitoris. The medial attachments of the perineal membrane are to the urethra, the walls of the vagina, and the perineal body.

Just cephalad to the perineal membrane lie two arch-shaped muscles that begin posteriorly to arch over the urethra. These are the compressor urethrae and the urethrovaginal sphincter. They are a part of the striated urogenital sphincter muscle in the female and are continuous with the sphincter urethrae muscle (Fig. 4-5). They act to compress the distal urethra. Posteriorly, intermingled within the membrane are skeletal muscle fibers of the transverse vaginal muscle and some smooth muscle fibers. The dorsal and deep nerve and vessels of the clitoris are also found within this membrane and are described later.

The primary function of the perineal membrane is related to its attachment to the vagina and perineal body. By attaching these structures to the bony pelvic outlet, the perineal membrane supports the pelvic floor against the effects of increases in intra-abdominal pressure, and against gravity. The amount of downward descent that is permitted by this mechanism can be assessed by placing a finger in the rectum, hooking it forward, and pulling the perineal body downward. If the perineal membrane has been torn during parturition, then an abnormal amount of descent is detectable, and the pelvic floor sags and the introitus gapes.

Perineal Body

Within the area bounded by the lower vagina, the perineal skin, and the anus is a mass of connective tissue

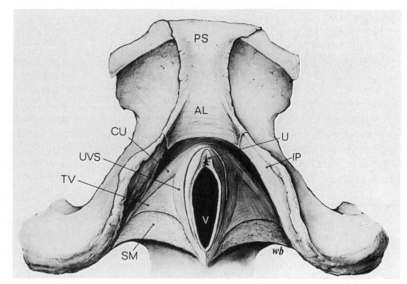

Figure 4–5. Structures visible after removal of the perineal membrane and superficial genital structures: AL, arcuate pubic ligament; CU, compressor urethrae; IP, ischiopubic ramus; PS, pubic symphysis; SM, smooth muscle; TV, transverse vaginae muscle; U, urethra; UVS, urethrovaginal sphincter; V, Vagina. (Used with permission, Alan R. Liss.)

called the perineal body (see Fig. 4-3). The term *central tendon of the perineum* has also been applied to this structure and is descriptive, suggesting its role as a central point into which many muscles insert.

The perineal body is attached to the inferior pubic rami and ischial tuberosities through the perineal membrane and superficial transverse perineal muscles. Anterolaterally, it receives the insertion of the bulbocavernosus muscles. On its lateral margins, the upper portions of the perineal body are connected with some fibers of the pelvic diaphragm. Posteriorly, the perineal body is attached to the coccyx by the external anal sphincter that is embedded in the perineal body anteriorly; it is attached at its other end to the coccyx. These connections anchor the perineal body and its surrounding structures to the bony pelvis and help to keep it in place.

Posterior Triangle–Ischiorectal Fossa

In the posterior triangle of the pelvis, the ischiorectal fossa lies between the pelvic walls and the levator ani muscles (see Fig. 4-3). It has an anterior recess that lies above the perineal membrane. It is bounded medially by the levator ani muscles and anterolaterally by the obturator internus muscle. The main portion of the fossa is lateral to the levator ani and external anal sphincter, and it has a posterior portion that extends above the gluteus maximus. Traversing this region is the pudendal neurovascular trunk.

Anal Sphincters

The external sphincter lies in the posterior triangle of the perineum (see Fig. 4-3). It is a single mass of muscle, which has traditionally been divided into superficial and deep portions. The superficial part attaches to the coccyx posteriorly and sends a few fibers into the perineal body anteriorly. The fibers of the deep part generally encircle the rectum and blend indistinguishably with the puborectalis (see later), which forms a loop under the dorsal surface of the anorectum and which is attached anteriorly to the pubic bone.

The internal anal sphincter is a thickening in the circular muscle of the anal wall. It lies just inside the external anal sphincter and is separated from it by a visible intersphincteric groove. It can be identified just beneath to the anal submucosa in repair of a chronic fourth-degree laceration of the perineum. The longitudinal layer of the bowel, along with some fibers of the levator ani, separates the external and internal sphincters.

Levator Ani

Unfortunately, the extreme intra-abdominal pressures generated during embalming greatly distort the levator ani muscles by forcing them downward. Most anatomy atlases therefore fail to give a true picture of the horizontal nature of this strong supportive shelf of muscle. Examination of the normal standing patient is the best way to appreciate the nature of this closure mechanism, for the lithotomy position causes some relaxation of the musculature. During routine pelvic examination of the nullipara, the effectiveness of this closure can be appreciated, as it is often difficult to insert a speculum if the muscles are contracted and not relaxed.

To understand the lateral attachments of the levator ani, it is necessary to discuss two muscles that act on the hip, the obturator internus and the piriformis, which cover the inner surfaces of the pelvic wall (Fig. 4-6). The fascia overlying the obturator internus provides a part of the origin of the levator ani muscles, and the cardinal ligament has significant attachments to the fascia overlying the piriformis. The obturator internus arises from the inner surface of the obturator foramen and membrane and leaves the pelvis through the lesser sciatic foramen to insert into the medial surface of the greater trochanter. The piriformis takes its origin from the anterior aspect of the sacrum and passes through the greater sciatic foramen to insert into the upper border of the greater trochanter. This latter muscle is important to the gynecologist as a cause of deep-seated pain in the piriformis syndrome. Palpating the tender muscle posterior and superior to the ischial spine and sacro-

spinous ligament assists in making this diagnosis. Both pelvic wall muscles are lateral rotators and abductors of the thigh.

The opening between the bones and muscles of the pelvic wall is spanned by the muscles of the pelvic diaphragm: the pubococcygeus, the iliococcygeus, puborectalis, and the coccygeus muscles. The most medial of these muscles is the puborectalis/pubococcygeus complex. The pubococcygeus portion of these muscles has an insertion into the anococcygeal raphe and the superior surface of the coccyx, while the puborectalis represents those inferior fibers that pass behind and insert into the rectum. Both portions arise from the inner surface of the pubic bones and pass the urethra without attaching to it. Some fibers attach to the lateral vaginal wall and external anal sphincter and form a sling around the rectum before returning to a similar course on the other side. The pubococcygeus portion passes posteriorly from its origin lying above the iliococcygeus muscle, where its fibers insert into the anococcygeal raphe and the coccyx.

The iliococcygeus muscle arises from a fibrous thickening in the fascia overlying the obturator internus called the arcus tendineus levatoris ani. From these broad origins the fibers of the iliococcygeus pass be-

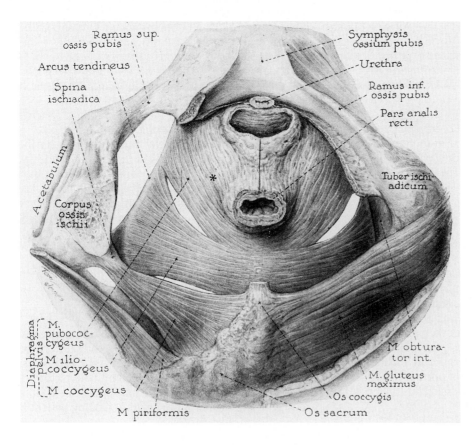

Figure 4–6. Anatomy of the pelvic floor. (* marks the puborectalis portion of the pubococcygeus muscle.)

hind the rectum and insert into the midline anococcygeal raphe and the coccyx. The coccygeus arises from the ischial spine and the sacrospinous ligament to insert into the borders of the coccyx and the lowest segment of the sacrum.

These muscles are covered on their superior and inferior surfaces by superior and inferior fasciae. When the levator ani muscles and their fasciae are considered together, they are called the pelvic diaphragm, not to be confused with the urogenital diaphragm (perineal membrane).

The muscle fibers of the pelvic diaphragm form a broad U-shaped layer of muscle with the open end of the U directed anteriorly. The open area within the U through which the urethra, vagina, and rectum pass is called the urogenital hiatus. The normal tone of the muscles of the pelvic diaphragm keep the base of the U pressed against the backs of the pubic bones, keeping the vagina and rectum closed. The region of the levator ani between the anus and coccyx formed by the anococcygeal raphe (see the earlier discussion) is clinically called the levator plate. It forms a supportive shelf upon which the rectum, upper vagina, and uterus can rest. The relatively horizontal position of this shelf is determined by the anterior traction on the fibrous levator plane of the pubococcygeus and puborectalis muscles and is important to vaginal and uterine support.

The iliococcygeus and coccygeus muscles receive their innervation from an anterior branch of the ventral ramus of the third and fourth sacral nerves, whereas the medial portions of the puborectalis and pubococcygeus are supplied by the pudendal nerve.

THE PELVIC VISCERA

This section on the pelvic viscera discusses the structure of the individual pelvic organs and considers specific aspects of their interrelationships (Fig. 4-7). Those aspects of blood supply, innervation, and lymphatic drainage that are idiosyncratic to the specific pelvic viscera are covered here. However, the section on the retroperitoneum, where the overall description of these systems is given, provides the general consideration of these latter three topics.

Genital Structures

Vagina

The vagina is a pliable hollow viscus whose shape is determined by the structures that surround it and by its attachments to the pelvic wall. These attachments are to the lateral margins of the vagina, so that its lumen is a transverse slit, with the anterior and posterior walls in contact with one another. The lower portion of the vagina is constricted as it passes through the urogenital hiatus in the levator ani. The upper part is much more capacious. The vagina is bent at an angle of 120° by the anterior traction of the levators at the junction of the lower one third and upper two thirds of the vagina (Fig. 4-8). The cervix lies within the anterior vaginal wall, making it shorter than the posterior wall by approximately 3 cm, with the former being approximately 7–9 cm in length, although there is great variability in this dimension.

When the lumen of the vagina is inspected through the introitus, many landmarks can be seen. The anterior and posterior walls have a midline ridge, called the anterior and posterior columns, respectively. These are caused by the impression of the urethra and bladder and the rectum on the vaginal lumen. The caudal portion of the anterior column is distinct and is called the urethral carina. The recesses in front of and behind the cervix are commonly called the anterior and posterior fornices of the vagina, and the creases along the side of the vagina, where the anterior and posterior walls meet, are called the lateral vaginal sulci.

The relationships of the vagina can be understood by dividing it into thirds. In the lower third, anteriorly the vagina is fused with the urethra, posteriorly with the perineal body, and laterally to each levator ani by the "fibers of Luschka." In the middle third are the vesical neck and trigone anteriorly, the rectum posteriorly, and the levators laterally. In the upper third, the anterior vagina is adjacent to the bladder and ureters (which allow these latter structures to be palpated on pelvic exam), posterior to the cul-de-sac, and lateral to the cardinal ligaments of the vagina.

The vaginal wall contains the same layers as all hollow viscera, that is, a mucosa, submucosa, muscularis, and adventitia. Except for the area covered by the cul-de-sac, it has no serosal covering. The mucosa is of the nonkeratinized stratified squamous type and lies on a dense, dermislike submucosa. The similarity of these layers to dermis and epidermis has resulted in their being called the "vaginal skin."

The vaginal muscularis is adherent to the submucosa, and the pattern of the muscularis is a bihelical arrangement. Outside the muscularis there is an adventitia that has varying degrees of development in different areas of the vagina. This layer is a portion of the connective tissue in the pelvis called the endopelvic fascia and has been given a separate name because of its unusual development. When it is dissected in the operating room, the muscularis is usually adherent to it, and this combination of specialized adventitia and muscularis is the surgeon's "fascia," which might better be called the fibromuscular layer of the vagina, as Nichols suggested in *Vaginal Surgery*.

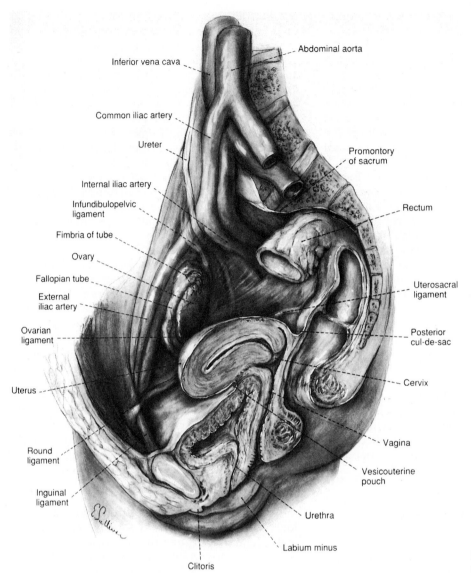

Figure 4–7. The pelvic viscera.

Uterus

The uterus is a fibromuscular organ whose shape, weight, and dimensions vary considerably, depending on both estrogenic stimulation and previous parturition. It has two portions, an upper muscular corpus and a lower fibrous cervix. In the reproductive-age woman, the corpus is considerably larger than the cervix, but before menarche, and after the menopause, their sizes are similar. Within the corpus, there is a triangularly shaped endometrial cavity surrounded by a thick muscular wall. That portion of the corpus that extends above the top of the endometrial cavity (ie, above the insertions of the fallopian tubes) is called the fundus.

The muscle fibers that make up most of the uterine corpus are not arranged in a simple layered manner, as is true in the gastrointestinal tract, but are arranged in a more complex pattern. This pattern reflects the origin of the uterus from paired paramesonephric primordia, with the fibers from each half crisscrossing diagonally with those of the opposite side.

The uterus is lined by a unique mucosa, the endometrium. It has both a columnar epithelium that forms glands and a specialized stroma. The superficial portion of this layer undergoes cyclic change with the menstrual cycle. Spasm of hormonally sensitive spiral arterioles that lie within the endometrium causes shedding of this layer after each cycle, but a deeper basal layer of

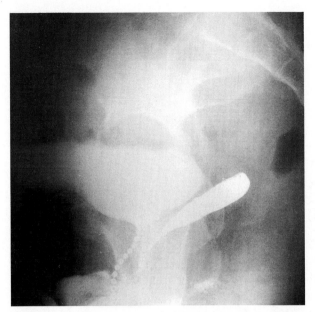

Figure 4–8. Bead chain cystourethrogram with barium in the vagina showing normal vaginal axis in the standing position.

the endometrium remains to regenerate a new lining. Separate arteries supply the basal endometrium, explaining its preservation at the time of menses.

The cervix is divided into two portions: the portio vaginalis, which is that part protruding into the vagina, and the portio supravaginalis, which lies above the vagina and below the corpus.

The substance of the cervical wall is made up of dense fibrous connective tissue with only a small (approximately 10%) amount of smooth muscle. What smooth muscle there is lies on the periphery of the cervix, connecting the myometrium with the muscle of the vaginal wall. This smooth muscle and accompanying fibrous tissue are easily dissected off the fibrous cervix and form the layer reflected during intrafascial hysterectomy. It is circularly arranged around the fibrous cervix and is the tissue into which the cardinal and uterosacral ligaments and pubocervical fascia insert.

The portio vaginalis is covered by nonkeratinizing squamous epithelium. Its canal is lined by a columnar mucous secreting epithelium that is thrown into a series of V-shaped folds that appear like the leaves of a palm and are therefore called plicae palmatae. These form compound clefts in the endocervical canal, not tubular racemose glands, as formerly thought.

The upper border of the cervical canal is marked by the internal os, where the narrow cervical canal widens out into the endometrial cavity. The lower border of the canal, the external os, contains the transition from squamous epithelium of the portio vaginalis to the columnar epithelium of the endocervical canal. This occurs at a variable level relative to the os and changes with hormonal variations that occur during the woman's life. It is in this active area of cellular transition that the cervix is most susceptible to malignant transformation.

There is little adventitia in the uterus with the peritoneal serosa being directly attached to most of the corpus (Fig. 4-9). The anterior portion of the uterine cervix is covered by the bladder, and therefore has no serosa. Similarly, as will be discussed later, the broad ligament invests the lateral aspects of the cervix and corpus and therefore has no serosal covering there. The posterior cervix does have a serosal covering.

Adnexal Structures and Broad Ligament

The fallopian tubes are paired tubular structures, 7–12 cm in length. Each has four recognizable portions. At the uterus, the tube passes through the cornu as an interstitial portion. Upon emerging from the corpus, a narrow isthmic portion begins with a narrow lumen and thick muscular wall. Proceeding toward the abdominal end, next is the ampulla, which has an expanding lumen and more convoluted mucosa. The fimbriated end of the tube has many frondlike projections to provide a wide surface for ovum pickup. The distal end of the fallopian tube is attached to the ovary by the fimbria ovarica, which is a smooth muscle band responsible for bringing the fimbria and ovary close to one another at the time of ovulation. The outer layer of the tube's muscularis is composed of longitudinal fibers; the inner layer has a circular orientation.

The lateral pole of the ovary is attached to the pelvic wall, by the infundibulopelvic ligament and the ovarian artery and vein contained therein. Medially, it is connected to the uterus through the utero-ovarian ligament. During reproductive life it measures approximately 2.5–5 cm long, 1.5–3 cm thick, and 0.7–1.5 cm wide, varying with its state of activity or suppression, as with oral contraceptive medications. Its surface is mostly free, but has an attachment to the broad ligament through the mesovarium, as will be discussed later.

The ovary has a cuboidal to columnar covering and consists of a cortex and medulla. The medullary portion is primarily fibromuscular, with many blood vessels and much connective tissue. The cortex is composed of a more specialized stroma, punctuated with follicles, corpora lutea, and corpora albicantia.

The round ligaments are extensions of the uterine musculature and represent the homologue of the gu-

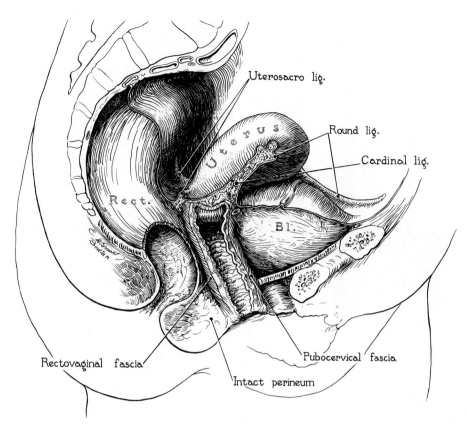

Figure 4–9. Ligamentous supports of the uterus.

bernaculum testis. They begin as broad bands that arise on each lateral aspect of the anterior corpus. They assume a more rounded shape before they enter the retroperitoneal tissue, where they pass lateral to the deep inferior epigastric vessels and enter each internal inguinal ring. After traversing the inguinal canal, they exit the external ring and enter the subcutaneous tissue of the labia majora. They have little to do with uterine support.

The ovaries and tubes comprise the uterine adnexa. They are covered by a specialized series of peritoneal folds called the broad ligament. During embryonic development the paired müllerian ducts and ovaries arise from the lateral abdominopelvic walls. As they migrate toward the midline, a mesentery of peritoneum is pulled out from the pelvic wall from the cervix on up. This leaves the midline uterus connected on either side to the pelvic wall by a double layer of peritoneum.

Within the upper layers of these two folds, called the broad ligaments, lie the fallopian tubes, round ligaments, and ovaries (Fig. 4-10). The cardinal and uterosacral ligaments (see Fig. 4-9) are at its lower margin. These structures are *visceral* ligaments and are therefore comprised of varying amounts of smooth muscle, vessels, connective tissue, and other structures. They

are not the pure ligaments associated with joints in the skeleton.

The ovary, tube, and round ligament each have their own separate mesentery, called the mesovarium, mesosalpinx, and mesoteres, respectively. These are arranged in a constant relationship, with the round ligament placed ventrally, where it exits the pelvis through the inguinal ligament, and the ovary placed dorsally. The tube is in the middle and is the most cephalic of the three structures. At the lateral end of the fallopian tube and ovary, the broad ligament ends where the infundibulopelvic ligament blends with the pelvic wall. The cardinal ligaments lie at the base of the broad ligament and will be described under the section on supportive tissues and cleavage planes.

Blood Supply and Lymphatics of the Genital Tract

The blood supply to the genital organs comes from the ovarian arteries and uterine and vaginal branches of the internal iliac. A continuous arterial arcade connects these vessels on the lateral border of the adnexa, uterus, and vagina (Fig. 4-11).

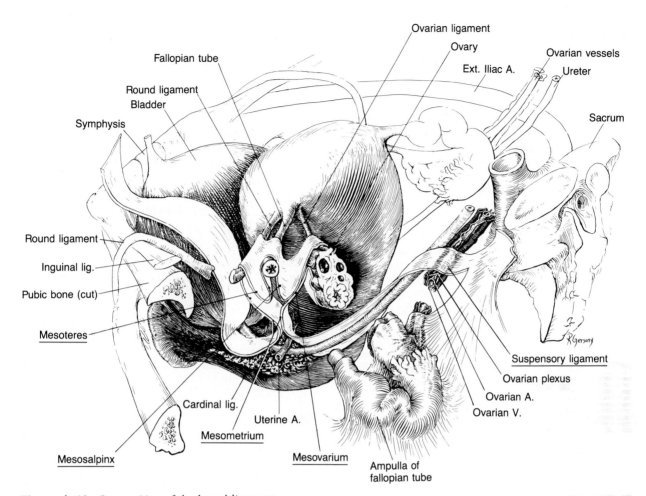

Figure 4–10. Composition of the broad ligament.

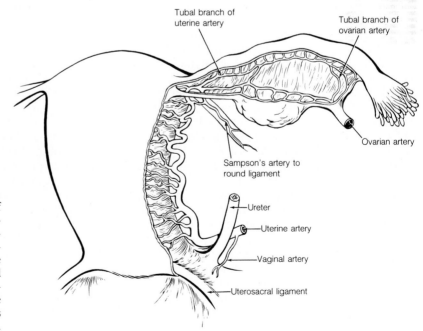

Figure 4–11. Collateral circulation of uterine and ovarian arteries. Uterine artery crosses over the ureter in the cardinal ligament, gives off cervical and vaginal branches before ascending in the wall and serosal surface of uterus and anastomosing with medial end of ovarian artery. Note the small branch of the uterine or ovarian artery that nourishes the round ligament (Sampson's artery).

45

The blood supply of the upper adnexal structures comes from the ovarian arteries that arise from the anterior surface of the aorta just below the level of the renal arteries. The accompanying plexus of veins drains into the vena cava on the right and the renal vein on the left. The arteries and veins follow a long, retroperitoneal course before reaching the cephalic end of the ovary. They pass along the mesenteric surface of the ovary to connect with the upper end of the marginal artery of the uterus. As the ovarian artery runs along the hilum of the ovary, it not only supplies the gonad, but sends many small vessels through the mesosalpinx to supply the fallopian tube, including a prominent fimbrial branch at the lateral end of the tube.

The uterine artery originates from the internal iliac artery. It usually arises independently from this source but may have a common origin with either the internal pudendal or vaginal artery. It joins the uterus at approximately the junction of the corpus and cervix, but this position varies considerably both with the individual and with the amount of upward or downward traction placed on the uterus. Accompanying each uterine artery are several large uterine veins that drain the corpus and cervix.

On arriving at the lateral border of the uterus (after passing over the ureter and giving off a small branch to this structure), the uterine artery flows into the side of the marginal artery that runs along the side of the uterus. Through this connection it sends blood both upward toward the corpus and downward to the cervix. As the marginal artery continues along the lateral aspect of the cervix, it eventually crosses over the cervicovaginal junction and lies on the side of the vagina.

The vagina receives its blood supply from a downward extension of the uterine artery along the lateral sulci of the vagina and from a vaginal branch of the internal iliac artery. These form an anastomotic arcade along the lateral aspect of the vagina at 3:00 and 9:00 o'clock. Branches from these vessels also merge along the anterior and posterior vaginal walls. The distal vagina also receives supply from the pudendal vessels, and the posterior wall has a contribution from the middle and inferior hemorrhoidal vessels.

Lymphatic drainage of the upper two thirds of the vagina and uterus is primarily to the obturator and internal and external iliac nodes, and the distal-most vagina drains with the vulvar lymphatics to the inguinal nodes. In addition, some lymphatic channels from the uterine corpus extend along the round ligament to the superficial inguinal nodes, and some nodes extend posteriorly along the uterosacral ligaments to the lateral sacral nodes. These routes of drainage are discussed more fully in the discussion of the retroperitoneal space.

The lymphatic drainage of the ovary follows the ovarian vessels to the region of the lower abdominal aorta, where they drain into the lumbar chain of nodes (paraaortic nodes).

The uterus receives its nerve supply from the uterovaginal plexus (Frankenhauser's ganglion) that lies in the connective tissue of the cardinal ligament. Details of the organization of the pelvic innervation are contained in the section on retroperitoneal structures.

Lower Urinary Tract

Ureter

The ureter is a tubular viscus approximately 25 cm long, divided into abdominal and pelvic portions of equal length. Its small lumen is surrounded by an inner longitudinal and outer circular muscle layer. In the abdomen, it lies in the extraperitoneal connective tissue on the posterior abdominal wall, crossed anteriorly by the left and right colic vessels (see Fig. 4-7). Its course and blood supply are described in the section on the retroperitoneum.

Bladder

The bladder can be divided into two portions, the dome and the base. The musculature of the spherical bladder does not lie in simple layers, as do the muscular walls of tubular viscera such as the gut and ureter. It is best described as a meshwork of intertwining muscle bundles. The musculature of the dome is relatively thin when the bladder is distended. The base of the bladder, which is thicker and varies less with distention of the dome, consists of the urinary trigone and a thickening of the detrusor, called the detrusor loop. This is a U-shaped band of musculature, open posteriorly, that forms the bladder base anterior to the intramural portion of the ureter. The trigone is made of smooth muscle that arises from the ureters that occupy two of its three corners. It continues as the muscle of the vesical neck and urethra. There it rests upon the upper vagina. The shape of the bladder depends upon its state of filling. When empty, it is a somewhat flattened disk, slightly concave upward (see Fig. 4-7). As it fills, the dome rises off the base, eventually assuming a more spherical shape.

The distinction between the base and dome has functional importance, because they have differing innervations. The bladder base has alpha-adrenergic receptors that contract when stimulated and thereby favor continence. The dome is responsive to beta stimulation, or cholinergic stimulation, with contraction that causes bladder emptying.

Anteriorly, the bladder lies against the lower abdominal wall. It lies against the pubic bones laterally and inferiorly, and abuts against the obturator internus and levator ani. Posteriorly, it rests against the vagina and cervix. These relationships are discussed further in consideration of the pelvic planes and spaces.

The blood supply of the bladder comes from the superior vesical artery, which comes off the obliterated umbilical, and the inferior vesical, which is either an independent branch of the internal pudendal artery or arises from the vaginal artery.

Urethra

The urethral lumen begins at the internal urinary meatus and has a series of regional differences in its structure. It passes through the bladder base in an intramural portion for a little less than a centimeter. This region of the bladder, where the urethral lumen traverses the bladder base, is called the vesical neck.

The urethra itself begins outside the bladder wall. In its distal two thirds it is fused with the vagina (see Fig. 4-7), with which it shares a common embryologic derivation. From the vesical neck to the perineal membrane, which starts at the junction of the middle and distal thirds of the bladder, the urethra has several layers. An outer, circularly oriented skeletal muscle layer (urogenital sphincter) mingles with some circularly oriented smooth muscle fibers. Inside this layer is a longitudinal layer of smooth muscle that surrounds a remarkably vascular submucosa and nonkeratinized squamous epithelium that responds to estrogenic stimulation.

Within the submucosa is a group of tubular glands that lie on the vaginal surface of the urethra. These paraurethral (or Skene's) glands empty into the lumen at several points on the dorsal surface of the urethra, but two prominent openings on the inner aspects of the external urethral orifice can be seen when the orifice is opened. Chronic infection of these glands can lead to urethral diverticula, and obstruction of their terminal duct can result in cyst formation. Their location on the dorsal surface of the urethra reflects the distribution of the structures from which they arise.

At the level of the perineal membrane, the distal portion of the urogenital sphincter begins. Here the skeletal muscle of the urethra leaves the urethral wall to form the urethrovaginal sphincter (see Fig. 4-5) and compressor urethrae (formerly called the deep transverse perineal muscle). Distal to this portion, the urethral wall is fibrous, and forms a nozzle for aiming the urinary stream. The mechanical support of the vesical neck and urethra, which are so important to urinary continence, are discussed in the section of this chapter devoted to the supportive tissues of the urogenital system.

The urethra receives its blood supply both from an inferior extension of the vesical vessels and from the pudendal vessels.

Sigmoid Colon and Rectum

The sigmoid colon begins its S-shaped curve at the pelvic brim. It has the characteristic structure of the colon, with three tenia coli lying over a circular smooth muscle layer. Unlike much of the colon, which is retroperitoneal, the sigmoid has a definite mesentery in its midportion. The length of the mesentery and the pattern of the sigmoid's curvature vary considerably. It receives its blood supply from the lower-most portion of the inferior mesenteric artery, the branches called the sigmoid arteries.

As it enters the pelvis, the colon straightens its course and becomes the rectum. This portion extends from the pelvic brim until it loses its final anterior peritoneal investment below the cul-de-sac. It has two bands of smooth muscle (anterior and posterior). Its lumen has three transverse rectal folds that contain the mucosa, submucosa, and circular layers of the bowel wall. The most prominent fold, the middle one, lies anteriorly on the right about 8 cm above the anus, and it must be negotiated during high rectal examination or sigmoidoscopy.

As the rectum passes posterior to the vagina, it expands into the rectal ampulla. This portion of the bowel begins under the cul-de-sac peritoneum and fills the posterior pelvis from the side. At the distal end of the rectum, the anorectal junction is bent at an angle of 90° where it is pulled ventrally by the puborectalis fibers' attachment to the pubes and posteriorly by the external anal sphincter's attachment dorsally to the coccyx.

Below this level the gut is called the anus. It has many distinguishing features. There is a thickening of the circular involuntary muscle called the internal sphincter. The canal has a series of anal valves to assist in closure, and at their lower border the mucosa of the colon gives way to a transitional layer of non-hair-bearing squamous epithelium before becoming the hair-bearing perineal skin.

The relationships of the rectum and anus can be inferred from their course. They lie against the sacrum and levator plate posteriorly and against the vagina anteriorly. Inferiorly, each half of the levator ani abuts against its lateral wall and sends fibers to mingle with the longitudinal involuntary fibers between the internal and external sphincters. Its distal terminus is surrounded by the external anal sphincter.

The anorectum receives blood supply from a number of sources (Fig. 4-12). From above, the superior rectal (hemorrhoidal) branch of the inferior mesenteric artery lies within the layers of the sigmoid mesocolon. As it reaches the beginning of the rectum it divides into two branches and ends in the wall of the gut. A direct branch from the internal iliac artery arises from the pelvic wall on either side and supplies the

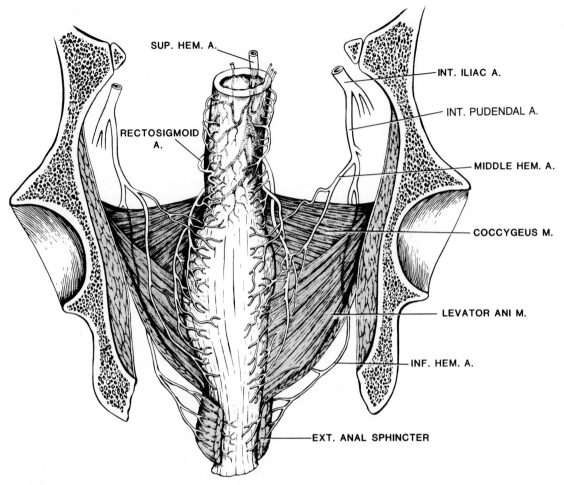

Figure 4–12. Rectosigmoid colon and anal canal, showing collateral arterial circulation from superior hemorrhoidal (inferior mesenteric), middle hemorrhoidal (hypogastric or internal iliac), and inferior hemorrhoidal (internal pudendal) arteries.

rectum and ampulla above the pelvic floor. The anus and external sphincter receive their blood supply from the inferior rectal (hemorrhoidal) branch of the internal pudendal artery, which reaches the terminus of the gastrointestinal tract through the ischiorectal fossa.

PELVIC CONNECTIVE TISSUE AND CLEAVAGE PLANES

The pelvic viscera are connected to the lateral pelvic wall by their adventitial layers and thickenings of the connective tissue that lie over the pelvic wall muscles (Fig. 4-13). These attachments, as well as the attachments of one organ to another, separate the different surgical cleavage planes from one another. These condensations of the adventitial layers of the pelvic organs have assumed supportive roles, connecting the viscera to the pelvic walls, besides their usual role in transmitting the organs' neurovascular supply from the pelvic wall. An understanding of their disposition is important to both vaginal and abdominal surgery.

Because of the prominent development of this adventitial connective tissue, it has been given the special designation of endopelvic fascia. It is not a layer similar to the layer encountered during abdominal incisions (rectus abdominus "fascia"). It is a meshwork of collagen and elastin, which are the fused adventitial layers of the visceral structures and pelvic wall muscles. In some areas there is considerable smooth muscle within this tissue, as is true in the area of the pubocervical fascia. Although surgical texts often speak of this fascia as a specific structure separate from the viscera, this is not strictly true. These layers can be separated from the

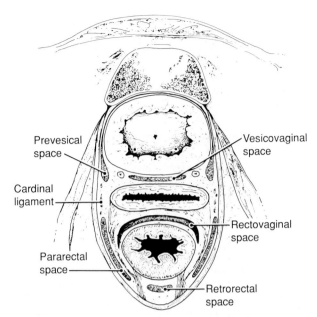

Figure 4–13. Cross section of the pelvis showing cleavage planes.

viscera, just as the superficial layers of the bowel wall can be separated from the deeper layers, although they are not themselves separate structures.

Pelvic Connective Tissue

The term *ligament* is most familiar when it describes a dense connective tissue band that links two bones, but it also describes ridges in the peritoneum or thickenings of the endopelvic fascia. The ligaments of the genital tract are very diverse. Although they share a common designation (ie, ligament), they are composed of many types of tissue and have different functions.

Uterine Ligaments

The broad ligaments are peritoneal folds that extend laterally from the uterus and cover the adnexal structures. They have no supportive function and were discussed in the section on the pelvic viscera.

At the lower end of the uterus, somewhat above the external os, are two fibromuscular bands called the uterosacral ligaments (see Fig. 4-9). They lie on either side of the pouch of Douglas and are composed of smooth muscle, nerves, and connective tissue. Near the cervix, they are discrete, but they fan out in the retroperitoneal layer to have a broad, if somewhat ill defined, area of attachment over the second, third, and fourth segments of the sacrum. These ligaments hold the cer-

vix posteriorly in the pelvis over the levator plate of the pelvic diaphragm.

The cardinal ligaments lie at the lower edge of the broad ligaments, between their peritoneal leaves. They attach to the cervix below the isthmus and fan out to attach to the pelvic walls over the piriformis muscle in the area of the greater sciatic foramen. Although when placed under tension they feel like ligamentous bands, they are composed simply of perivascular connective tissue and nerves that surround the uterine artery and veins. Nevertheless, these structures have considerable strength, and the lack of a separate "ligamentous band" in this area does not detract from their supportive role. They provide support not only to the cervix and uterus, but also to the upper portion of the vagina to keep these structures positioned posteriorly over the levator plate of the pelvic diaphragm and away from the urogenital hiatus.

Vaginal Fasciae and Attachments

The upper one third of the vagina is suspended within the pelvis by the downward extension of the cardinal ligaments (see Fig. 4-9). Anterior to the vagina in this area is the vesicovaginal space; posterior to it is the cul-de-sac. In its middle third, the vagina develops significant lateral and posterior attachments to the pelvic wall at the arcus tendineus fasciae pelvis, separate from the cardinal ligaments. The arcus tendineus is a thickening of the obturator and levator fasciae and represents the lateral attachment of the vaginal adventitia. These lateral attachments, the upper attachments to the cervix and cardinal ligament, and the lower attachment through the perineal membrane to the pubic bones suspend the anterior vaginal wall across the pelvis. The connective tissue of the anterior wall's adventitia and these attachments form a sheet of tissue in this area called the pubocervical fascia. Whether it should be considered as a separate, surgically useful structure has been somewhat controversial.

Posterolaterally, the vagina is attached to the parietal endopelvic fascia over the pelvic diaphragm and sacrum through the rectovaginal septum (fascia of Denonvilliers). This latter structure is connected cephalically to the depth of the cul-de-sac peritoneum and caudally to the perineal body. It is thought to be a fusion fascia left when the peritoneal pouch that extends to the perineal body in the fetus progressively closes from below, upward to the level of the cul-de-sac in the adult. Its distal attachment to the perineal body serves to suspend this structure, thereby playing a role in introital support. It is adherent to the posterior vaginal wall and lies anterior to the rectovaginal space.

The lower one third of the vagina is firmly attached to its surrounding structures. Anteriorly, it is attached to the pubic bones by the perineal membrane. Posteriorly, it fuses with the perineal body; laterally, it adheres to the medial borders of the levator ani. These are the strongest of the vagina's connections, and they are usually preserved even in cases of complete vaginal prolapse.

Urethral Supports

The support of the proximal urethra is important in the maintenance of urinary continence during times of increased abdominal pressure. The distal portion of the urethra is inseparable from the vagina, because of their common embryologic derivation, so that the support of these two viscera, in this area cannot be separated from one another. These tissues are fixed firmly in position by connections of the periurethral tissues and vagina to the pubic bones through perineal membrane. These supports of the distal urethra have extensions covering both anterior (ventral) and posterior (dorsal) aspects of the pubic bones and have been called the anterior and posterior pubourethral ligaments. The posterior ligament attaches 1 cm above the inferior border of the pubic symphysis, just lateral to the midline.

The proximal urethra, however, is normally a mobile structure, and women can control its position. This control depends upon a combination of the attachments of the paraurethral tissues to the arcus tendineus fasciae pelvis and to the medial portion of the levator ani muscle (pubococcygeus/puborectalis portion) (Figs. 4-14 and 4-15). Besides these supportive structures, a separate extension of the detrusor musculature runs from the vesical neck anteriorly to the arcus tendineus fasciae pelvis. Properly called the pubovesical muscle or ligament, it has no role in urethral support.

Cleavage Planes and Spaces

Each of the pelvic viscera can expand somewhat independently of its neighboring organs. The ability to do this comes from their relatively loose attachment to one another, which permits the bladder, for example, to expand without equally elongating the adjacent cervix. This allows the viscera to be easily separated from one another along these lines of cleavage. These surgical cleavage planes are called spaces, although they are not strictly empty but are filled with fatty or areolar connective tissue. The pelvic spaces are separated from one another by the connections of the viscera to one another and to the pelvic walls.

Prevesical Space

The prevesical space of Retzius (see Figs. 4-14 and 4-19) is separated from the undersurface of the rectus abdominis muscles by the transversalis fascia and can be entered by perforating this layer. Ventrolaterally, it is

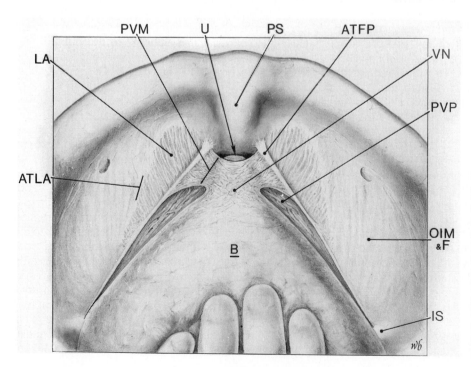

Figure 4–14. Space of Retzius. Abbreviations: ATFP, arcus tendineus fasciae pelvis; ATLA, arcus tendineus levatoris ani; B, bladder; IS, ischial spine; LA, levator ani; OIM&F, obturator internus muscle and fascia; PS, pubic symphysis; PVM, pubovesical muscle; PVP, paraurethral vascular plexus; U, urethra; VN, vesical neck. (Copyright Alan R. Liss, with permission, Neurourol Urodynam 1989;8:53.)

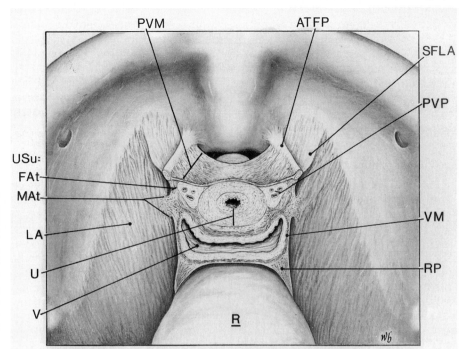

Figure 4–15. Urethral supports. Additional abbreviations: RP, rectal pillar; USu, urethral supports; FAt, fascial attachment of the urethral supports; MAt, muscular attachments of the urethral supports; SFLA, superior fascia of the levator ani; V, vagina; VM, vaginal muscularis. (Copyright Alan R. Liss, with permission, Neurourol Urodynam 1989; 8:53.)

bounded by the bony pelvis and muscles of the pelvic wall; cranially, it is bounded by the abdominal wall. The proximal urethra and bladder lie in a dorsal position. The dorsolateral limit to this space is the attachment of the bladder to the cardinal ligament and the attachment of the pubocervical fascia to the arcus tendineus fasciae pelvis. These separate this space from the vesico-vagino-cervical space. This lateral attachment is to the arcus tendineus fasciae pelvis, which lies on the inner surface of the obturator internus and pubococcygeus/puborectalis muscles.

Important structures lying within this space include the dorsal clitoral vessels under the symphysis at its lower border and the obturator nerve and vessels as they enter the obturator canal. A branch to the obturator canal often comes off the external iliac and lies on the pubic bone, so that dissection in this area should be done with care. Lateral to the bladder and vesical neck is a dense plexus of vessels that lie at the border of the lower urinary tract. They are deep to the pubovesical muscle, and although they bleed when sutures are placed here, this venous ooze usually stops when the sutures are tied. Also within this tissue, lateral to the bladder and urethra, lie the nerves of the lower urinary tract. The upper border of the pubic bones that form the anterior surface of this region has a ridgelike fold of periosteum called the iliopectineal line. This is sometimes used to anchor sutures during urethral suspension operations.

Vesicovaginal and Vesicocervical Space

The space between the lower urinary tract and the genital tract is separated into the vesicovaginal and vesicocervical spaces by a thin septum, the supravaginal septum (see Fig. 4-13). The lower extent of the space is the junction of the proximal one third and distal two thirds of the urethra, where it fuses with the vagina, and it extends to lie under the peritoneum at the vesicocervical peritoneal reflection. It extends laterally to the pelvic side walls, separating the vesical and genital aspects of the cardinal ligaments.

Rectovaginal Space

On the dorsal surface of the vagina lies the rectovaginal space (see Fig. 4-13). It begins at the apex of the perineal body, some 2–3 cm above the hymenal ring. It extends upward to the cul-de-sac and laterally around the sides of the rectum to the attachment of the rectovaginal septum to the parietal endopelvic fascia. It contains loose areolar tissue and is easily opened with finger dissection.

At the level of the cervix, some fibers of the cardinal/uterosacral ligament complex extend downward behind the vagina, connecting it to the lateral walls of the rectum and then to the sacrum. These are called the rectal pillars and separate the midline rectovaginal space in this region from the lateral pararectal spaces. These pararectal spaces allow access to the sacrospinous ligaments (mentioned later). They also form the lateral boundaries of the retrorectal space between the rectum and sacrum.

Region of the Sacrospinous Ligament

The sacrospinous ligament is another region that has become more important to the gynecologist operating for problems of vaginal support. The sacrospinous ligament lies on the dorsal aspect of the coccygeus muscle. The rectal pillar separates it from the rectovaginal space.

As its name implies, the sacrospinous ligament courses from the ischial spine to the lateral aspect of the sacrum. In its medial portion it fuses with the sacrotuberous ligament and is a distinct structure only laterally. It can be reached from the rectovaginal space by perforation of the rectal pillar to enter the pararectal space or by dissection directly under the enterocele peritoneum. This area is covered in more detail in Chapter 32.

Many structures are near the sacrospinous ligament, and their location must be remembered during surgery in this region. The sacral plexus lies immediately next to the ligament on its cephalic border and comes to lie on its lateral surface as the nerve passes through the greater sciatic foramen. Just before its exit, the plexus gives off the pudendal nerve, which, with its accompanying vessels, passes lateral to the sacrospinous ligament at its attachment to the ischial spine. The nerve to the levator ani muscles lies on the inner surface of the coccygeus muscle in its midportion. In developing this space, the tissues that are reflected medially and cranially to gain access contain the pelvic venous plexus of the internal iliac vein, as well as the middle rectal vessels. If they are mobilized too vigorously, they can cause a considerable hemorrhage.

RETROPERITONEAL SPACES AND LATERAL PELVIC WALL

The retroperitoneal space of the posterior abdomen, the presacral space, and the pelvic retroperitoneum contain the major neural, vascular, and lymphatic supply to the pelvic viscera. These areas are explored during operations to identify the ureter, interrupt the pelvic nerve supply, arrest serious pelvic hemorrhage, and remove potentially malignant lymph nodes. Because this area is free of the adhesions from serious pelvic infection or endometriosis, it can be used as a plane of dissection when the peritoneal cavity has become obliterated. The structures found in these spaces are discussed in a regional context, because that is the way they are usually approached in the operating room.

Retroperitoneal Structures of the Lower Abdomen

The aorta lies on the lumbar spine slightly to the left of the vena cava, which it overlies. The portion of this vessel below the renal vessels is encountered during retroperitoneal dissection to identify the para-aortic lymph nodes. The renal blood vessels arise at the second lumbar vertebra. The ovarian vessels also arise from the anterior surface of the aorta in this region. In general, the branches of the vena cava follow those of the aorta, except for the vessels of the intestine, which flow into the portal vein, and the left ovarian vein, which empties into the renal vein on that side.

Below the level of the renal vessels and just below the third portion of the duodenum, the inferior mesenteric artery arises from the anterior aorta. It gives off ascending branches of the left colic artery and continues caudally to supply the sigmoid through the three or four sigmoid arteries that lie in the sigmoid mesentery. These vessels follow the bowel as it is pulled from side to side, so that their position may vary, depending on retraction.

Inferiorly, a continuation of the inferior mesenteric artery forms the superior rectal artery. This vessel crosses over the external iliac vessels to lie on the dorsum of the lower sigmoid. It supplies the rectum, as will be described in the section concerning that viscus.

The aorta and vena cava have segmental branches that arise at each lumbar level and are called the lumbar arteries and veins. They are situated somewhat posteriorly to the aorta and vena cava and are not visible from the front. When the vessels are mobilized, as is done in excising the lymphatic tissue in this area, they come into view.

At the level of the fourth lumbar vertebra (just below the umbilicus) the aorta bifurcates into the left and right common iliac arteries. After about 5 cm, the common iliac arteries (and the medially placed veins) give off the internal iliac vessels from their medial side and continue toward the inguinal ligament as the external iliacs. These internal iliac vessels lie within the pelvic retroperitoneal region and are discussed later.

The aorta and vena cava in this region are surrounded by lymph nodes on all sides. Surgeons usually refer to this lumbar chain of nodes as the para-aortic nodes, reflecting their position. They receive the drainage from the common iliac nodes and are the final drainage of the pelvic viscera. In addition, they collect the lymphatic drainage from the ovaries that follows the ovarian vessels and does not pass through the iliac nodes. The nodes of the lumbar chain extend from the right side of the vena cava to the left of the aorta and can be found both anterior and posterior to the vessels.

The ureters are attached loosely to the posterior abdominal wall in this region, and when the overlying colon is mobilized, they remain on the body wall. They are crossed anteriorly by the ovarian vessels, which contribute a branch to supply the ureter. Additional blood supply to the abdominal portion comes from the renal vessels at the kidney, and the common iliac.

This region can be exposed either by a midline peritoneal incision to the left of the small bowel mesentery or, retroperitoneally, by reflection of the colon. During embryonic development, the colon and its embryonic mesentery fuse with the abdominal wall. A cleavage plane exists here that allows the colon and its vessels to be elevated to expose the structures of the posterior abdominal wall. Because the ureter and ovarian vessels originally arise in this area, they are not elevated with the colon.

Presacral Space

The presacral space begins below the bifurcation of the aorta and is bounded laterally by the internal iliac arteries (Figs. 4-16 and 4-17). Lying directly on the sacrum are the middle sacral artery and vein, which originate from the dorsal aspect of the aorta and vena cava (and not from the point of bifurcation, as sometimes shown). Caudal and lateral to this are the lateral sacral vessels. The venous plexus of these vessels can be extensive, and bleeding from it can be considerable.

Within this area lies the most familiar part of the pelvic autonomic nervous system, the presacral nerve (superior hypogastric plexus). The autonomic nerves of the pelvic viscera can be divided into a sympathetic (thoracolumbar) system and a parasympathetic (craniosacral) system. The former is also called the adrenergic system, and the latter is called the cholinergic system, according to their neurotransmitters. Alpha-adrenergic stimulation causes increased urethral and vesical neck tone, and cholinergic stimulation increases contractility

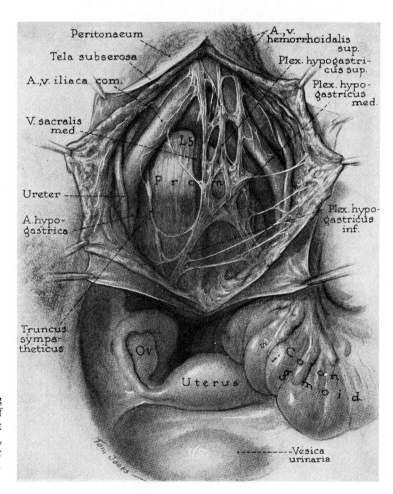

Figure 4–16. Presacral nerve plexus, showing passage of sympathetic trunk over bifurcation of aorta. Note division of trunk into left and right presacral nerves. (Curtis AH, Anson BJ, Ashley FL, et al: The anatomy of the pelvic autonomic nerves in relation to gynecology. Surg Gynecol Obstet 1942; 75:743.)

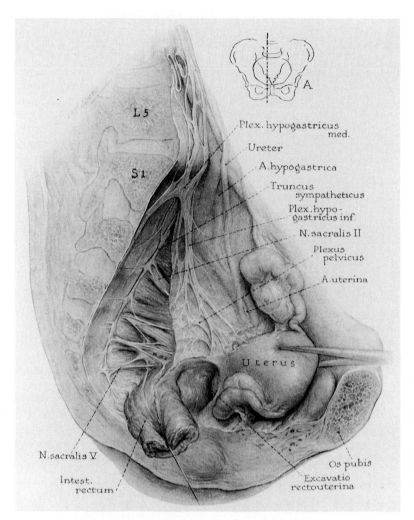

Labels on figure:
L 5
S 1
N.sacralis V
Intest. rectum
Plex. hypogastricus med.
Ureter
A. hypogastrica
Truncus sympatheticus
Plex. hypo-gastricus inf.
N. sacralis II
Plexus pelvicus
A. uterina
Uterus
Os pubis
Excavatio rectouterina
A

Figure 4–17. Nerves of the female pelvis. Current terminology refers to the plex. hypogastricus inf. as the hypogastric nerve, and the plexus pelvicus and the inferior hypogastric plexus. (Anson BJ: An atlas of human anatomy. Philadelphia: WB Saunders, 1950; with permission of WB Saunders.)

of the detrusor muscle. Similarly, adrenergic stimulation in the colon and rectum favors storage, and cholinergic stimulation favors evacuation. Adrenergic agonists, which are used for tocolysis, suggest that these influence contractility of the uterus. As is true in the male, damage to the autonomic nerves during pelvic lymphadenectomy may have a significant influence on orgasmic function in the female.

How these autonomic nerves reach the organs that they innervate has surgical importance. The terminology of this area is somewhat confusing, because many authors use idiosyncratic terms. The structure, however, is simple: a single ganglionic midline plexus overlying the lower aorta (superior hypogastric plexus) that splits into two trunks without ganglia (hypogastric nerves), each of which connects with a plexus of nerves and ganglia lateral to the pelvic viscera (inferior hypo-

gastric plexus). We shall follow the terms outlined in the *Nomina Anatomica.*

The superior hypogastric plexus lies in the retroperitoneal connective tissue on the ventral surface of the lower aorta and receives input from the sympathetic chain ganglia through the thoracic and lumbar splanchnic nerves. It also contains important afferent pain fibers from the pelvic viscera, which makes its transection effective in primary dysmenorrhea. It passes over the bifurcation of the aorta and extends over the proximal sacrum before splitting into two hypogastric nerves that descend into the pelvis in the region of the internal iliac vessels. The hypogastric nerves end in the inferior hypogastric plexus, which are broad expansions of the hypogastric nerves. Their sympathetic fibers come from the downward extensions of the superior hypogastric plexus and pelvic splanchnic nerves from the continuation of the sympathetic chain into the pelvis. Parasympathetic fibers come from sacral segments 2–4 via the pelvic splanchnic nerves (nervi erigentes) to join these ganglia. They lie in the pelvic connective tissue of the lateral pelvic wall, lateral to the uterus and vagina.

The inferior hypogastric plexus (formerly called the pelvic plexus) is divided into three portions: the vesical plexus anteriorly, the uterovaginal plexus (Frankenhauser's ganglion), and the middle rectal plexus. The uterovaginal plexus contains fibers that derive from two sources. It receives sympathetic and sensory fibers from the tenth thoracic through the first lumbar spinal cord segments. The second input comes from the second, third, and fourth sacral segments and consists primarily of parasympathetic nerves that reach the pelvic plexus through the pelvic splanchnic nerves. The uterovaginal plexus lies on the dorsal (medial) surface of the uterine vessels, lateral to the sacrouterine ligaments' insertion into the uterus. It has continuations cranially along the uterus and caudally along the vagina. This latter extension contains the fibers that innervate the vestibular bulbs and clitoris. These nerves lie in the tissue just lateral to the area where the uterine artery, cardinal ligament, and uterosacral ligament pedicles are made during a hysterectomy for benign disease, and within the tissue removed during a radical hysterectomy.

The location of the sensory fibers from the uterus in the superior hypogastric nerve (the presacral nerve) allows the surgeon to alleviate visceral pain from the uterine corpus by transecting this structure. It does not provide sensory innervation to the adnexal structures or, for that matter, to the peritoneum and is therefore not useful for alleviating pain in those sites. Another important way in which the autonomic nervous system is involved is through damage to the inferior hypogastric plexus during radical hysterectomy. The extension of the surgical field lateral to the viscera interrupts the connection of the bladder and sometimes the rectum to their central attachments.

The ovary and uterine tube receive their neural supply from the plexus of nerves that accompany the ovarian vessels and that originate in the renal plexus. These fibers come from the 10th thoracic segment, and the parasympathetic fibers from extensions of the vagus.

As the lumbar and sacral nerves exit from the intervertebral and sacral foramina, they form the lumbar and sacral plexuses. The lumbar nerves and plexus lie deep within the psoas muscle on either side of the spine. The sacral plexus lies on the piriformis muscle, and its major branch, the sciatic nerve, leaves the pelvis through the lower part of the greater sciatic foramen. The sacral plexus supplies nerves to the muscles of the hip, pelvic diaphragm, and perineum, as well as to the lower leg (through the sciatic nerve). The femoral nerve from the lumbar plexus is primarily involved in supplying the muscles of the thigh.

Pelvic Retroperitoneal Space

Division of the internal and external iliac vessels occurs in the area of the sacroiliac joint. Just before passing under the inguinal ligament to become the femoral vessels, the external iliac vessels contribute the deep inferior epigastric and deep circumflex iliac. There are no other major branches of the external iliac in this region.

Internal Iliac Vessels

Unlike the external iliac artery, which is constant and relatively simple in its morphology, the branching pattern of the internal iliac arteries and veins is extremely variable (Figs. 4-18 and 4-19). A description of a common variant will be included here. The internal iliac artery supplies the viscera of the pelvis and many muscles of the pelvic wall and gluteal region. It usually divides into an anterior and posterior division about 3–4 cm after leaving the common iliac artery (Table 4-2). The vessels of the posterior division (the iliolumbar, lateral sacral, and superior gluteal) leave the internal iliac artery from its lateral surface to provide some of the blood supply to the pelvic wall and gluteal muscles. Trauma to these hidden vessels should be avoided during internal iliac artery ligation as the suture is passed around behind vessels.

The anterior division has both parietal and visceral branches. The obturator, internal pudendal, and inferior gluteal vessels primarily supply muscles, whereas the uterine, superior vesical, vaginal (inferior vesical), and middle rectal vessels supply the pelvic organs. The internal iliac veins begin lateral and posterior to the arteries. These veins form a large and complex plexus within the pelvis, rather than having single branches, as do the arteries. They tend to be deeper in this area than the arteries, and their pattern is highly variable.

Ligation of the internal iliac artery has proven to be helpful in the management of postpartum hemorrhage. Burchell's arteriographic studies have shown that physiologically active anastomoses between the systemic and pelvic arterial supplies were immediately patent following ligation of the internal iliac artery (Fig. 4-20) These anastomoses, shown in Table 4-2, connected the arteries of the internal iliac system with systemic blood vessels either directly from the aorta, as is true for the lumbar and middle sacral, or indirectly through the

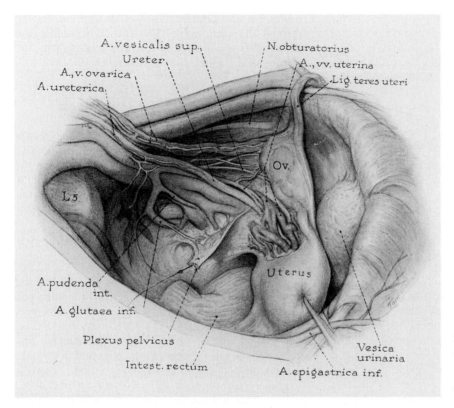

Figure 4–18. Arteries and veins of the pelvis. (Anson BJ: An atlas of human anatomy. Philadelphia: WB Saunders, 1950; with permission of WB Saunders.)

inferior mesenteric artery in the case of the superior hemorrhoidal vessels. These in vivo pathways were quite different from the anastomoses that had previously been hypothesized on purely anatomic grounds.

Pelvic Ureter

The course of the pelvic ureter within the pelvis is important to gynecologic surgeons and is fully considered in Chapter 29. A few of the important anatomic landmarks are considered here (see Fig. 4-18). After passing over the bifurcation of the internal and external iliac arteries, just medial to the ovarian vessels, the ureter descends within the pelvis. Here it lies in a special connective tissue sheath that is attached to the peritoneum of the lateral pelvic wall and medial leaf of the broad ligament. This fact is responsible for the observation that when the retroperitoneal space is entered, the ureter still adheres to the peritoneum and does not remain laterally with the vessels.

The ureter crosses under the uterine artery ("water flows under the bridge") in its course through the cardinal ligament. There is a loose areolar plane around it to allow for its peristalsis here, creating a tunnel through the denser fibrous tissue. At this point it lies along the anterolateral surface of the cervix, usually about 1 cm from it. From there it comes to lie on the anterior vaginal wall and then to proceed for a distance of about 1.5 cm through the wall of the bladder.

During its pelvic course, the ureter receives blood from the vessels that it passes, specifically the common iliac, internal iliac, uterine, and vesical arteries. Within the wall of the ureter, these vessels are connected to one another by a convoluted vessel that can be seen running longitudinally along its outer surface.

Lymphatics

The lymph nodes and lymphatic vessels that drain the pelvic viscera vary in their number and distribution, but they can be organized into coherent groups. Because of the extensive interconnection of the lymph nodes, spread of lymph flow, and therefore malignancy, is somewhat unpredictable. Recognizing this, some important generalizations about the distribution and drainage of these tissues are still helpful. Distribution of the pelvic lymph nodes is discussed further in Chapter 42 on invasive carcinoma of the cervix. Figures 42-25 to 42-28 show this anatomy.

The nodes of the pelvis can be divided into the external iliac, internal iliac, common iliac, medial sacral, and pararectal nodes. The medial sacral nodes are few and follow the middle sacral artery. The pararectal

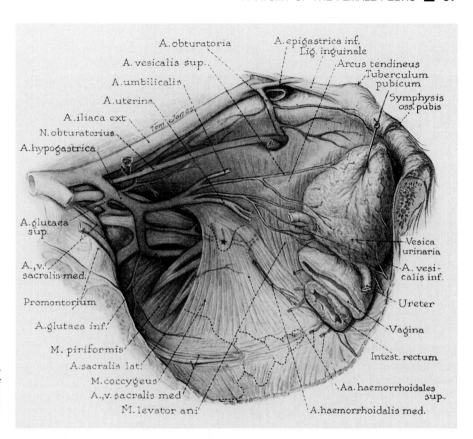

Figure 4–19. Structures of the pelvic wall. (Anson BJ: An atlas of human anatomy. Philadelphia: WB Saunders, 1950; with permission of WB Saunders.)

nodes drain that part of the rectosigmoid above the peritoneal reflection, the part supplied by the superior hemorrhoidal artery. The medial and pararectal nodes are seldom involved in gynecologic disease.

The internal and external iliac nodes lie next to their respective blood vessels, and both end in the common iliac chain of nodes, which then drain into the nodes along the aorta. The external iliac nodes receive the drainage from the leg through the inguinal nodes. Nodes in the external iliac group can be found lateral to the artery, between the artery and vein, and on the medial aspect of the vein. These groups are called the anterosuperior, intermediate, and posteromedial groups, respectively. They can be separated from the underlying muscular fascia and periosteum of the pelvic wall along with the vessels, thereby defining their lateral extent. Some nodes at the distal end of this chain lie in direct relation to the deep inferior epigastric vessels and are named according to these adjacent vessels. Similarly, nodes that lie at the point where the obturator nerve and vessels enter the obturator canal are called obturator nodes.

The internal iliac nodes drain the pelvic viscera and receive some drainage from the gluteal region along the posterior division of the internal iliac vessels as well.

TABLE 4–2
Collateral Circulation Following Internal Iliac Artery Ligation

INTERNAL ILIAC	SYSTEMIC
Iliolumbar	Lumbar
Lateral sacral	Middle sacral
Middle hemorrhoidal	Superior hemorrhoidal

These nodes lie within the adipose tissue that is interspersed among the many branches of the vessels. The largest and most numerous nodes lie on the lateral pelvic wall, but many smaller nodes lie next to the viscera themselves. These nodes are named for the organ by which they are found (eg, parauterine).

Not only is it difficult in the operating room to make some of the fine distinctions mentioned in this anatomic discussion, but there is little clinical importance in doing so. Surgeons generally refer to those nodes that are adjacent to the external iliac artery as the external iliac group of nodes and to those next to the internal iliac artery as the internal iliac nodes. This leaves those nodes that lie between the external iliac

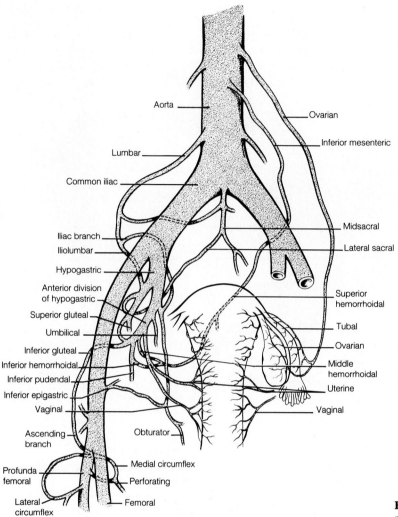

Aorta

Ovarian

Inferior mesenteric

Lumbar

Common iliac

Midsacral

Iliac branch

Iliolumbar

Lateral sacral

Hypogastric

Anterior division
of hypogastric

Superior
hemorrhoidal

Superior gluteal

Tubal

Umbilical

Ovarian

Inferior gluteal

Middle
hemorrhoidal

Inferior hemorrhoidal

Inferior pudendal

Uterine

Inferior epigastric

Vaginal

Vaginal

Ascending
branch

Obturator

Profunda
femoral

Medial circumflex

Perforating

Lateral
circumflex

Femoral

Figure 4–20. Collateral circulation of pelvis.

vein and internal artery, which are called interiliac nodes.

The lines of lymph flow from the uterus tend to follow its attachments, draining along the cardinal, uterosacral, and even round ligaments. This latter connection can lead to metastasis from the uterus to the superficial inguinal nodes, whereas the former connections are to the internal iliac nodes, with free communication to the external iliac nodes and sometimes to the lateral sacral nodes. The anastomotic connection of the uterine and ovarian vessels makes lymphatic connections between these two drainage systems likely, and metastasis in this direction possible.

The vagina and lower urinary tract have a divided drainage. Superiorly (upper two thirds of the vagina and the bladder), drainage occurs along with the uterine lymphatics to the internal iliac nodes, whereas the

lower one third of the vagina and distal urethra drain to the inguinal nodes. This demarcation, however, is far from precise.

The common iliac nodes can be found from the medial to the lateral border of the vessels of the same name. They continue above the pelvic vessels and occur around the aorta and the vena cava. These nodes can lie anterior, lateral, or posterior to the vessels.

THE ABDOMINAL WALL

Knowledge of the layered structure of the abdominal wall will permit the surgeon to enter the abdominal cavity with maximum efficiency and safety. A general summary of these layers is provided in Table 4-3. The abdomen's superior border is the lower edge of the rib

TABLE 4–3
Table of Abdominal Wall Layers

Skin
Subcutaneous layer
  Camper's fascia
  Scarpa's fascia
Musculoaponeurotic layer
  Rectus sheath—formed by conjoined aponeuroses of the
    External oblique muscle
    Internal oblique muscle }
                { fused in lower abdomen
    Transversus abdominis muscle }
Transversalis fascia
Peritoneum

cage (r7–12). Inferiorly, it ends at the iliac crests, inguinal ligaments, and pubic bones. It ends posterolaterally at the lumbar spine and its adjacent muscles.

Skin and Subcutaneous Tissue

The fibers in the dermal layer of the abdominal skin are oriented in a predominantly transverse direction following a gently curving concave upward line. This predominance of transversely oriented fibers results in more tension on the skin of a vertical incision and in a wider scar.

Between the skin and the musculoaponeurotic layer of the abdominal wall lies the subcutaneum. It is made of globules of fat held in place and supported by a series of branching fibrous septa. In the more superficial portion of the subcutaneous layer, called Camper's fascia, the fat predominates, and the fibrous tissue is less apparent. Closer to the rectus sheath, the fibrous tissue predominates relative to the fat in the region known as Scarpa's fascia. Camper's and Scarpa's fasciae are not discrete or well-defined layers but represent regions of the subcutaneum. Scarpa's fascia is best developed laterally and is not seen as a well-defined layer during vertical incisions.

Musculoaponeurotic Layer

Deep to the subcutaneous tissue is a layer of muscle and fibrous tissue that holds the abdominal viscera in place and controls movement of the lower torso (Figs. 4-21 and 4-22). Within this area are two groups of muscles: vertical muscles in the anterior abdominal wall and oblique flank muscles. The rectus abdominis muscle is found on either side of the midline, and the pyramidalis muscle is located just above the pubes. Lateral to these are the flank muscles: the external oblique, internal oblique, and transversus abdominis. The broad, sheetlike tendons of these muscles form aponeuroses that unite with their corresponding member of the other side, forming a dense white covering of the rectus abdominis muscle properly called the rectus sheath (rectus "fascia").

Rectus Abdominis and Pyramidalis Muscles

Each paired rectus abdominis muscle originates from the sternum, and cartilages of ribs 5–7, and inserts into the anterior surface of the pubic bone. Each muscle has three tendinous inscriptions. These are fibrous interruptions within the muscle that firmly attach it to the rectus abdominis sheath. In general, they are confined to the region above the umbilicus, but they can be found below it. When this happens, the rectus sheath is attached to the rectus muscle there, and these two structures become difficult to separate during a Pfannenstiel incision.

The pyramidalis muscles arise from the pubic bones and insert into the linea alba in an area several centimeters above the symphysis. Their development varies considerably among individuals. Their strong attachment to the midline makes separation of their attachment here difficult by blunt dissection.

Flank Muscles

Lateral to the rectus abdominis muscles lie the broad, flat muscles of the flank. The aponeurotic insertions of these muscles join to form the conjoined tendon, or rectus sheath, which covers the rectus abdominis. Because of its importance, it is covered separately later.

The most superficial of these muscles is the external oblique. Its fibers run obliquely anteriorly and inferiorly from their origin on the lower eight ribs and iliac crest. Unlike the external oblique's fibers, which run obliquely downward, the fibers of the internal oblique fan out from their origin from the anterior two thirds of the iliac crest, the lateral part of the inguinal ligament, and the thoracolumbar fascia in the lower posterior flank. In most areas, they are perpendicular to the fibers of the external oblique, but in the lower abdomen, their fibers arch somewhat more caudally and run in a direction similar to those of the external oblique.

As the name *transversus abdominis* implies, the fibers of the deepest of the three layers run in a primarily transverse orientation. They arise from the lower six costal cartilages, the thoracolumbar fascia, the anterior three fourths of the iliac crest, and the lateral inguinal ligament. The caudal portion of the transversus abdominis muscle is fused with the internal oblique muscle. This explains why, during transverse incisions of the

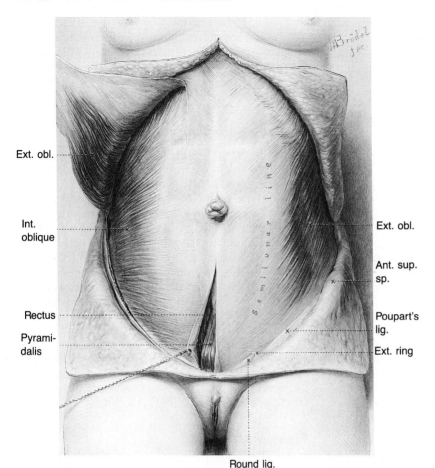

Ext. obl.

Int. oblique

Rectus

Pyrami- dalis

Round lig.

Ext. obl.

Ant. sup. sp.

Poupart's lig.

Ext. ring

Figure 4–21. External oblique, internal oblique, and pyramidalis muscles. (Kelly HA: Gynecology. New York: Appleton, 1928.)

lower abdomen, only two layers are discernible at the lateral portion of the incision. Although these fibers are not strictly parallel, their primarily transverse orientation and the transverse pull of their attached muscular fibers place vertical suture lines in the rectus sheath under more tension than transverse ones. For this reason, vertical incisions are more prone to dehiscence.

Rectus Sheath (Conjoined Tendon)

The line of demarcation between the muscular and aponeurotic portions of the external oblique in the lower abdomen occurs along a vertical line through the anterior superior iliac spine (Fig. 4-23). The internal oblique and transversus extend farther toward the midline, coming closest at their inferior margin, at the pubic tubercle. Because of this, muscular fibers of the internal oblique are found underneath the aponeurotic portion of the external oblique during transverse incision. In addition, it is between the internal oblique and transversus that the nerves and blood vessels of the flank are to be found and their injury avoided.

In forming the rectus sheath, the conjoined aponeuroses of the flank are separable lateral to the rectus muscles, but fuse near the midline. As they reach the midline, these layers lose their separate directions and fuse. Many specialized aspects of the rectus sheath are important to the surgeon. In the lower one fourth of the sheath, it lies entirely anterior to the rectus muscle. Above that point, it splits to lie both ventral and dorsal to it. The transition between these two arrangements occurs midway between the umbilicus and the pubes and is called the arcuate line. Cranial to this line, the midline ridge of the rectus sheath, the linea alba, unites these two layers. Sharp dissection is usually required to separate these layers during a Pfannenstiel incision. A vertical peritoneal incision cuts the posterior sheath.

The lateral border of the rectus muscle is marked by the semilunar line of the rectus sheath. Above the arcuate line, this is the level at which the anterior and posterior layers of the sheath split. Below it the transversalis fascia fuses with the sheath. The semilunar line is not always where the three layers of flank muscles join. During a transverse lower abdominal incision, the ex-

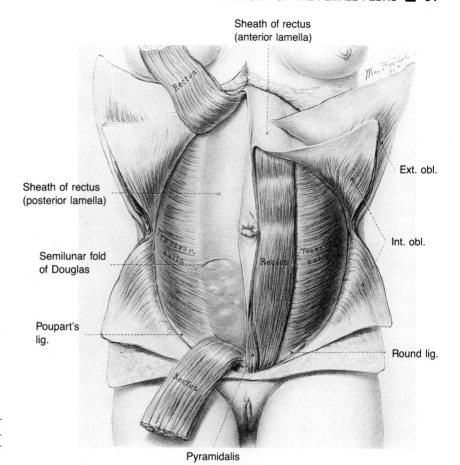

Figure 4–22. Transversus abdominis and rectus abdominis muscles. (Kelly HA: Gynecology. New York: Appleton, 1928.)

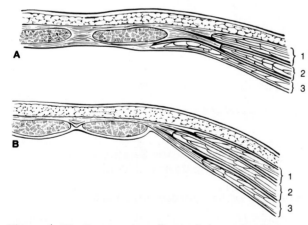

Figure 4–23. Cross section of lower abdominal wall. *A,* The anterior fascial sheath of the rectus muscle from external oblique (*1*) and split aponeurosis of internal oblique muscles (*2*). The posterior sheath is formed by aponeurosis of transversalis muscle (*3*) and split aponeurosis of internal oblique. *B,* Lower portion of abdominal wall below arcuate line (*linea semicircularis*) with absence of a posterior fascial sheath of the rectus muscle and all of the fascial aponeuroses (*1, 2, 3*) forming the anterior rectus sheath.

ternal and internal oblique aponeuroses are frequently separable near the midline.

The inguinal canal lies at the lower edge of the musculofascial layer of the abdominal wall. Through the inguinal canal, in the female, the round ligament extends to its termination in the labium majus. In addition, the ilioinguinal nerve and the genital branch of the genitofemoral nerve pass through the canal.

Transversalis Fascia, Peritoneum, and Bladder Reflection

Inside the muscular layers, and outside the peritoneum, lies the transversalis fascia, a layer of fibrous tissue that lines the abdominopelvic cavity. It is visible during abdominal incisions as the layer just underneath the rectus abdominis muscles suprapubically. It is separated from the peritoneum by a variable layer of adipose tissue. It is frequently incised or bluntly dissected off the bladder to take the tissues in this region "down by layers."

The peritoneum is a single layer of serosa. It is thrown into five vertical folds by underlying ligaments

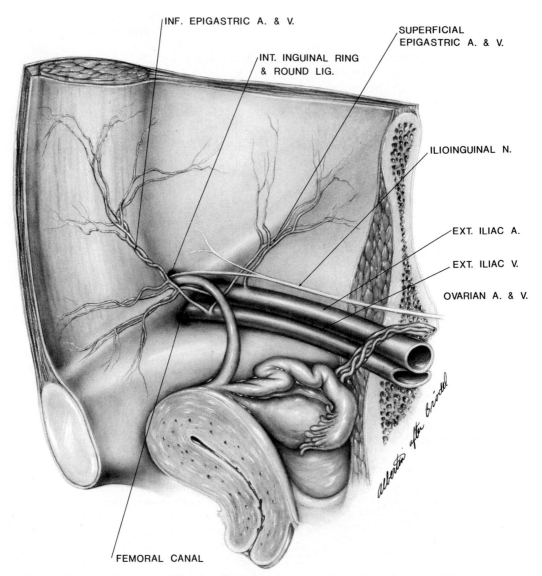

INF. EPIGASTRIC A. & V.

INT. INGUINAL RING & ROUND LIG.

SUPERFICIAL EPIGASTRIC A. & V.

ILIOINGUINAL N.

EXT. ILIAC A.

EXT. ILIAC V.

OVARIAN A. & V.

FEMORAL CANAL

Figure 4–24. Sagittal view of female pelvis, showing inguinal and femoral anatomy.

or vessels that converge toward the umbilicus. The single median umbilical fold is caused by the presence of the urachus (median umbilical ligament). Lateral to this are paired medial umbilical folds that are raised by the obliterated umbilical arteries that connected the internal iliac vessels to the umbilical cord in fetal life, and the corresponding lateral umbilical folds caused by the inferior epigastric arteries and veins.

The reflection of the bladder onto the abdominal wall is triangular in shape, with its apex blending into the medial umbilical ligament. Because the apex is highest in the midline, incision in the peritoneum lateral to the midline is less likely to result in bladder injury.

Neurovascular Supply of the Abdominal Wall

Vessels of the Abdominal Wall

The blood vessels that supply the abdominal wall can be separated into those that supply the skin and subcutaneous tissues and those that supply the musculofascial layer. Although there is only one set of epigastric vessels in the subcutaneous tissues (superficial epigastric), there are both superior and inferior epigastric vessels in the musculofascial layer, so care must be taken in using these terms to avoid confusion.

The superficial epigastric vessels run a diagonal

course in the subcutaneum from the femoral vessels toward the umbilicus, beginning as a single artery that branches extensively as it nears the umbilicus. Its position can be anticipated midway between the skin and musculofascial layer, in a line between the palpable femoral pulse and the umbilicus. The external pudendal artery runs a diagonal course from the femoral artery medially to supply the region of the mons pubis. It has many midline branches, and bleeding in its territory of distribution is heavier than that from the abdominal subcutaneous tissues. The superficial circumflex iliac vessels proceed laterally from the femoral vessels toward the flank.

The blood supply to the musculofascial layer of the lower abdominal wall follows lines similar to the subcutaneous vessels. Besides having a supply derived from the external iliac, near the femoral origin of the superficial vessels, this layer receives vessels from the abdominal extensions of the intercostal and subcostal vessels.

The branches of the external iliac, the inferior epigastric and the deep circumflex iliac, parallel their superficial counterparts (Fig. 4-24). The circumflex iliac lies between the internal oblique and transversus abdominis muscle. The inferior epigastric artery and its two veins originate lateral to the rectus muscle. They run diagonally toward the umbilicus and intersect the muscle's lateral border midway between the pubis and

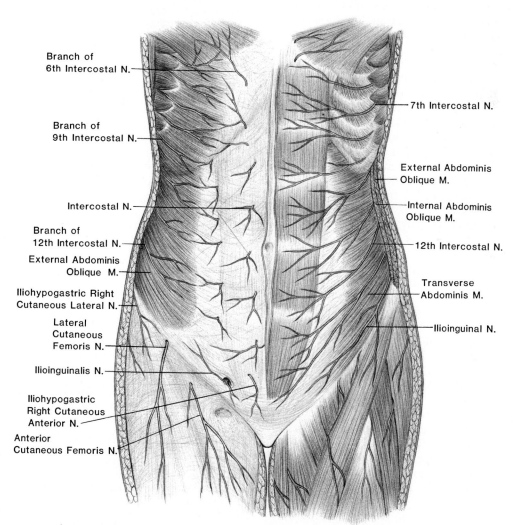

Figure 4–25. Nerve supply to the abdomen. (*Right*) Deep innervation of T6–T12 to the transversalis, internal oblique, and rectus muscles. (*Left*) Superficial distribution, including cutaneous nerves, after penetration and innervation of the external oblique muscle and fascia. Innervation of the groin and thigh is also shown.

the umbilicus. Below the point at which the vessels pass under the rectus, they are found lateral to the muscle deep to the transversalis fascia. After crossing the lateral border of the muscle, they lie on the muscle's dorsal surface, between it and the posterior rectus sheath. As the vessels enter the rectus sheath, they branch extensively, so that they no longer represent a single trunk. The angle between the vessel and the border of the rectus muscle forms the apex of Hesselbach's triangle (inguinal triangle), whose base is the inguinal ligament.

Nerves of the Abdominal Wall

The innervation of the abdominal wall (Fig. 4-25) comes from the abdominal extension of intercostal nerves 7–11, the subcostal nerves (T12), and ilio-hypogastric nerves (T12 and L1), and the ilioinguinal (L1) nerves. Dermatome T10 lies at the umbilicus.

After giving off a lateral cutaneous branch, each intercostal nerve pierces the lateral border of the rectus sheath. There it provides a lateral branch that ends in the rectus muscle. The anterior branch then passes through the muscle and perforates the rectus sheath to supply the subcutaneous tissues and skin as the anterior cutaneous branches. Incisions along the lateral border of the rectus lead to denervation of the muscle, which may render it atrophic and weaken the abdominal wall. Elevation of the rectus sheath off the muscle during Pfannenstiel incision stretches the perforating nerve, which is sometimes ligated to provide hemostasis from the accompanying artery. This may leave an area of cutaneous anesthesia.

The iliohypogastric and ilioinguinal nerves pass medial to the anterior superior iliac spine in the abdominal wall. The former supplies the skin of the suprapubic area. The latter supplies the lower abdominal wall, and by sending a branch through the inguinal canal, it supplies the upper portions of the labia majora and the medial portions of the thigh. These nerves can be entrapped in the lateral closure of a transverse incision.

The genitofemoral (L1 and L2) and femoral cutaneous (L2 and L3) nerves can be injured during gynecologic surgery. The genitofemoral nerve lies on the psoas muscle (see Fig. 4-24), where pressure from a retractor can damage it and lead to anesthesia in the medial thigh and lateral labia. The femoral cutaneous nerve can be compressed either by a retractor blade lateral to the psoas or by too much flexion of the hip in lithotomy position, causing anesthesia over the anterior thigh.

Bibliography

Anson, Barry J. An atlas of human anatomy. Philadelphia: WB Saunders, 1950:241.

Burchell RC. Arterial physiology of the human female pelvis. Obstet Gynecol 1968;31:855.

Campbell RM. The anatomy and histology of the sacrouterine ligaments. Am J Obstet Gynecol 1950;59:1.

Cox HT. The cleavage lines of the skin. Br J Surg 1941;29:234.

Curry SL, Wharton JT, and Rutledge F. Positive lymph nodes in vulvar squamous carcinoma. Gynecol Oncol 1980;9:63.

Dalley AF. The riddle of the sphincters. Am Surg 1987;53:298

Daseler EH, Anson BJ, Reimann AF. Radical excision of the inguinal and iliac lymph glands. Surg Gynecol Obstet 1948;87:679.

DeLancey JOL. Correlative study of paraurethral anatomy. Obstet Gynecol 1986;68:91.

DeLancey JOL. Structural aspects of the extrinsic continence mechanism. Obstet Gynecol 1988;72:296.

Fernstrom I. Arteriography of the uterine artery. Acta Radiologica Stockholm (Suppl) 1955;122:21.

Fluhmann CF, Dickmann Z. The basic pattern of the glandular structures of the cervix uteri. Obstet Gynecol 1958;11:543.

Forster DS. A note on Scarpa's fascia. J Anat 1937;72:130.

Funt MI, Thompson JD, Birch H. Normal vaginal axis. So Med J 1978;71:1534.

Goerttler K. Die architektur der muskelwand des menschlichen uterus und ihre funktionelle bedeutung. Morph Jarb 1930;65:45.

Goff BH. The surgical anatomy of cystocele and urethrocele with special reference to the pubocervical fascia. Surg Gynecol Obstet 1948;87:725.

Hudson CN. Lymphatics of the pelvis. In: Philipp EE, Barnes J, Newton M, eds. Scientific foundations of obstetrics and gynecology. 3rd ed. London: William Heinemann, 1986:1

Huffman J. Detailed anatomy of the paraurethral ducts in the adult human female. Am J Obstet Gynecol, 1948;55:86.

Hughesdon PE. The fibromuscular structure of the cervix and its changes during pregnancy and labour. J Obstet Gynaecol Br Commononw 1952;59:763.

Huisman AB. Aspects on the anatomy of the female urethra with special relation to urinary continence. Contrib Gynecol Obstet 1983;10:1.

Hutch JA. Anatomy and physiology of the bladder, trigone and urethra. New York: Appleton-Century-Crofts, 1972.

Klink EW. Perineal nerve block: an anatomic and clinical study in the female. Obstet Gynecol 1953;1:137.

Krantz KE. The anatomy of the urethra and anterior vaginal wall. Am J Obstet Gynecol 1951;62:374.

Krantz KE. Innervation of the human uterus. NY Acad Sci (Annals) 1959;75:770.

Kuhn RJ, Hollyock VE. Observations on the anatomy of the rectovaginal pouch and septum. Obstet Gynecol 1982;59:445.

Lawson JON. Pelvic anatomy. I Pelvic floor muscles. Ann R Coll Surg Engl 1974;54:244.

Lawson JON. Pelvic anatomy. II Anal canal and associated sphincters. Ann R Coll Surg Engl 1974;54:288.

Milley PS, Nichols DH. The relationship between the pubo-urethral ligaments and the urogenital diaphragm in the human female. Anat Rec 1971;170:281.

Milley PS, Nichols, DH. A correlative investigation of the human rectovaginal septum. Anat Rec 1969;163:443.

Milloy FJ, Anson BJ, McAfee DK. The rectus abdominis muscle and the epigastric arteries. Surg Gynecol Obstet 1960;110:293.

Morley GW, DeLancey JOL. Sacrospinous ligament fixation for eversion of the vagina. Am J Obstet Gynecol 1988;158:872.

Muellner SR. Physiology of micturition. J Urol 1951;65:805.

Nesselrod JP. An anatomic restudy of the pelvic lymphatics. Ann Surg 1936;104:905.

Nichols DH. Sacrospinous fixation for massive eversion of the vagina. Am J Obstet Gynecol 1982;142:901.

Nichols DH. Vaginal surgery. 2nd ed. Baltimore: Williams & Wilkins, 1983:219.

Oelrich TM. The striated urogenital sphincter muscle in the female. Anat Rec 1983;205:223.

Nichols DH, Milley PS, Randall CL. Significance of restoration of normal vaginal depth and axis. Obstet Gynecol 1970;36:251.

Oh C, Kark AE. Anatomy of the perineal body. Dis Col Rect 1973;16:444.

Parry-Jones, E. Lymphatics of the vulva. J Obstet Gynecol Br Emp 1963;70:751.

Plentl AA, Friedman EA. Lymphatic system of the female genitalia. Philadelphia: WB Saunders, 1971:15.

Ramsey, EM. Vascular anatomy. In: Wynn, RM, ed. Biology of the uterus. New York: Plenum Press, 1977:60.

Range RL, Woodburne RT. The gross and microscopic anatomy of the transverse cervical ligaments. Am J Obstet Gynecol 1964;90:460.

Reiffenstuhl G. The clinical significance of the connective tissue planes and spaces. Clin Obstet Gynecol 1982;25:811.

Ricci JV, Lisa JR, Thom CH, Kron WL. The relationship of the vagina to adjacent organs in reconstructive surgery. Am J Surg 1947;74:387.

Ricci JV, Thom CH. The myth of a surgically useful fascia in vaginal plastic reconstructions. Quart Rev Surg Ob Gyn 1954;2:253.

Richardson AC, Edmonds PB, Williams NL. Treatment of stress urinary incontinence due to paravaginal fascial defect. Obstet Gynecol 1981;57:357.

Roberts WH, Habenicht J, Krishingner G. The pelvic and perineal fasciae and their neural and vascular relationships. Anat Rec 1964;149:707.

Roberts WH, Krishingner GL. Comparative study of human internal iliac artery based on Adachi classification. Anat Rec 1967;158:191.

Sampson JA. Ureteral fistulae as sequelae of pelvic operations. Surg Gynecol Obstet 1909;8:479.

Schreiber H. Konstruktionsmorphologische Betrachtungen uber den Wandungsbau der menschlichen Vagina. Arkiv fur Gynaekologie 1942−43;174:222.

Skandalakis JE, Gray SW, Rowe JS. Anatomical complications in general surgery. New York: McGraw-Hill, 1983:297.

Stulz P, Pfeiffer, KM. Peripheral nerve injuries resulting from common surgical procedures in the lower portion of the abdomen. Arch Surg 1982;117:324.

Tobin CE, Benjamin JA. Anatomic and clinical re-evaluation of Camper's, Scarpa's and Colles' fasciae. Surg Gynecol Obstet 1949;88:545.

Uhlenhuth E, Nolley GW. Vaginal fascia, a myth? Obstet Gynecol 1957;10:349.

Zaccharin RF. The anatomic supports of the female urethra. Obstet Gynecol 1968;21:754.

Preoperative Care

5

JOHN A. ROCK

The hallmark of a competent surgeon is embodied in the type of patient that he or she selects for a specific operative procedure. As part of this selection process, a succinct but inclusive history and physical examination are necessary to clarify the severity of the patient's symptoms, identify the disease process or anatomic defect, and verify the need for the recommended surgery. At a moment in medical history when such judgments are commonly being challenged by second surgical opinions and medical and legal scrutiny, the gynecologic surgeon is well advised to give the highest priority to this patient selection process. Reports of second surgical opinions may exaggerate in suggesting that over 50% of the gynecologic symptoms used as indications for major pelvic surgery could be alleviated by more conservative nonoperative treatment (McCarthy, Finkel). Nevertheless, there is a growing consumer concern that the indications for pelvic surgery may in recent years have become too lax for the patient's welfare. For example, is it in the patient's best interest when a 45-year-old female has a hysterectomy for no other symptoms or clinical findings than a history of menometrorrhea when neither a dilatation and curettage nor medical management has been utilized? We disagree with a popular tendency to consider the uterus at the completion of childbearing to be a superfluous organ that should be removed. The view that the retained uterus is merely a potential site for cancer is at odds with a rational understanding of the true risk of modern medical management of cervical and endometrial malignancy as compared with the risks of major surgery, including the potential psychological sequelae.

No longer does a patient seek a surgeon solely on the basis of his or her technical skill. Of equal importance are a reputation for the exercise of proper clinical judgment and choice of appropriate indications for surgery. Although it is a delight to observe an operation by a technically adept surgeon, if the operation is done on poor indications, the patient may suffer a loss, not a gain. Too often a patient is subjected to an unnecessary major operation when a minor procedure would have sufficed. Not infrequently, the surgeon operates with-

out knowledge of the basic pathologic lesion and without having conducted a proper diagnostic investigation.

Surgery may be indicated on solid grounds, or it may be done without defensible indications. It may be adequate or inadequate. It may be excessive and only add to the patient's misery. Before performing surgery, the surgeon would do well to consider one of three basic indications. As students, we frequently heard them and they are worth repeating: the indications for surgery are (1) to save life, (2) to relieve suffering, and (3) to correct deformity. If a contemplated surgery cannot be justified on the basis of one or more of these indications, the surgeon should take another long look at the problem.

This chapter will review the preoperative evaluation, which includes taking a thorough history and performing a complete gynecologic examination. The evaluation of the pulmonary, cardiovascular, gastrointestinal, and urinary systems is stressed. Finally, appropriate laboratory examinations and preoperative procedures are discussed.

HISTORY TAKING

The preoperative care of the patient begins in the office or outpatient department with the careful taking of a complete history. Good history taking, careful preoperative examination, and the preparation of the patient, physically and mentally, are essential to good surgical results. No matter how busy the gynecologist may be, it is essential that he or she take the history personally. When the patient comes for gynecologic advice, the personal talk with the physician may be extremely beneficial to her. Personal contact is also of the greatest value to the physician, since the evaluation of the case can be guided by an overall clinical impression of the patient's symptoms rather than by a complete reliance on findings on the pelvic examination. Too often the busy surgeon disregards the maxim that "the patient will tell you what is wrong with her, if you will only give her time." Good history taking requires time and patience, and neither of these is found easily by the gynecologist, and in particular by a gynecologist/obstetrician who has a large obstetrics practice in addition to a heavy surgical schedule. However, the reward for following such a course is the avoidance of unnecessary surgery. Unindicated operations, particularly when performed upon those mentally troubled by some difficult problem of life, not only may prove to be unsuccessful in relieving the patient's symptoms but may concentrate her attention on the pelvic organs and aggravate invalidism. It is our practice not to make a rapid decision regarding the recommendation for major pelvic surgery on the first consultation if the condition is not urgent. Preferably, the patient should be counseled on the need for surgery after all aspects of her physical and emotional makeup are thoroughly evaluated. The surgeon who is quick with the knife and short on words of explanation is usually the one who has the poorest doctor/patient relationship and the greatest malpractice experience.

The history should be concise, but accuracy should not be sacrificed for the sake of brevity. For several years it has been our custom to use a form in obtaining the history. There are objections to any form, for no one has ever devised a perfect form for every case. However, if one uses records for clinical research, important omissions are far more infrequent when information is compiled on a form. There should be no restriction in recording the present illness, and the greatest freedom is permitted the physician in documenting the details of the patient's present condition. Often events in the patient's history do not fit into any medical form but may have an important bearing on the present illness. These too should be recorded properly and completely in the present illness.

A few points should be stressed in taking a gynecologic history. The menstrual history must be accurate and detailed, since the clue to a correct diagnosis of the gynecologic condition for which surgery is being considered often appears in the pattern of the menstrual irregularity. This holds true whether the menstrual disturbance results from an organic lesion or has a dysfunctional cause. In fact, differentiation between dysfunctional and early organic disease is one of the most common and difficult clinical distinctions that must be made. Of major importance are the accurate dates of the last and the previous menstrual period. When there is great discrepancy between menstrual dates and pelvic findings in a patient with a suspected pregnancy, the sensitive radioimmunoassay tests for hCG are invaluable for the diagnosis. In women under the age of 30, a history of maternal use of intrauterine diethylstilbestrol (DES) during the first trimester of pregnancy is important in alerting the gynecologist to the potential presence of various anatomic abnormalities, such as vaginal

adenosis, an anatomic (cockscomb) alteration of the cervix, or a T-shaped deformity of the uterus. A documented history of herpes (type 2) viral infection of the lower genital tract has long-term implications for future recurrences and symptomatology.

The reproductive history is of great importance to the gynecologist, particularly the history of previous pregnancies and their complications—such as dystocia, postpartum infection, abortions, urinary tract infections, excessive-size infants, vaginal tears, or pulmonary embolism, to list but a few. A well-taken marital history may reveal dyspareunia and unsatisfactory sexual relations, which may, in turn, explain symptoms that resemble organic pelvic disease.

The symptomatology of urinary tract disease is so closely related to that of disease of the reproductive tract that it is important to obtain a complete urologic history and, on occasion, an investigation of the urinary tract before making a final diagnosis and a decision about treatment. All too commonly, women have a vaginal repair with plication of the bladder neck for symptoms of urinary frequency, urgency, and dysuria, while the real problem lies undiagnosed as a chronic infection or a neurogenic dysfunction of the bladder. It is well to remember that a disorder of the lower urinary tract may produce symptoms suggestive of reproductive tract disease, and vice versa. For this reason, we have advocated basic urologic training for every gynecologist. The gynecologist who is adept at using the cystoscope is better prepared to evaluate the case than one who must depend completely on the urologist's report.

GYNECOLOGIC EXAMINATION

It is incumbent upon the gynecologist to assess the patient's general health completely as well as to perform a gynecologic examination. As the primary physician for women, the gynecologist/obstetrician frequently is the only physician who has seen the patient, particularly if her initial physician consultation concerns a problem involving the reproductive tract. It is important therefore to perform a complete physical examination, which must include a blood pressure assessment, weight measurement, examination of the thyroid, auscultation of the heart and lungs, and examination of the breasts, abdomen, and pelvis. Particular attention must be placed on any evidence of abnormal sexual development, including ambiguity of the external and internal female genitalia and abnormal hair growth on the extremities, chest, abdomen, and pubic regions. A critical evaluation of cardiac and pulmonary function before any proposed surgical procedure is carried out must be the responsibility of the gynecologist. Whether additional medical consultation is required must be determined before a general anesthetic is administered. A meticulously collected, midstream, clean-catch or catheterized urine specimen should be examined and a urine culture obtained in all cases in which the symptoms even remotely suggest the possibility of urinary tract disease. Although there is a reported 2% to 3% incidence of urinary tract infection or significant bacteriuria (Kass) following a single catheterization, recent evidence suggests that such complications occur more frequently among patients in whom urinary tract infection or abnormal bladder function existed prior to the catheterization. Hence, we still believe that transurethral catheterization, if properly performed, is not a hazard to the normal bladder and may provide valuable information in the total assessment of the patient's gynecologic symptoms.

Breasts

The breasts are first inspected for symmetry, size, condition of the nipples, and presence of a gross lesion. Normal breast tissue, which feels rather shotty to the fingertips, is often erroneously considered to be tumorous by the patient and even by physicians who are unfamiliar with the proper method of breast palpation. The breasts should be examined with the patient in both the upright and the supine positions for symmetry, contour, and a palpable mass. In the supine position, the patient's shoulder should be raised slightly with a towel to bring the lateral aspect of the breast tissue level with the remaining portion of the breast. The arm should be raised above the head to flatten the breast against the thoracic cage, which will permit easy examination of the full thickness of the breast tissue. The examination should be done with the flat surface of the physician's fingers and palm; a significant lesion will almost always be detected in this manner. Any suspicious lesion should be evaluated by mammography (xeroradiography), needle aspiration, or biopsy to confirm or discount the existence of a significant breast lesion (see Ch. 35). The nipples and adjacent areolar tissue are then gently compressed, and the presence and character of any secretions are noted. Cytologic (Papanicolaou) examination of breast secretions has been reported by Masukawa and associates and others to diagnose very early cases of breast carcinoma prior to the clinical discovery of a gross lesion. The finding of secretions often gives valuable information when pregnancy is suspected, but minimal galactorrhea is not uncommon in parous women many years after the last child, and occasionally it is found in women who have never been pregnant.

Abdomen

Examination of the abdomen includes both inspection and palpation; percussion and auscultation are also useful. Bulging of the flanks suggests free abdominal fluid, but thin-walled ovarian cysts and irregularly shaped uterine leiomyomas may give a similar clinical picture. Although large ovarian cysts and leiomyomas most commonly cause protrusion of the anterior abdominal wall, there are many confusing exceptions. Palpation for a fluid wave through the lateral quadrants of the abdomen is also useful. Percussion for areas of flatness or tympany and for shifting dullness may aid in determining whether the distention is due to intraperitoneal fluid or to intestinal gas. Auscultation is especially useful in differentiating among a large tumor, a distended bowel, or an advanced pregnancy as the cause of abdominal enlargement.

Pelvis and Rectum

An accurate evaluation of the female reproductive tract is essential in establishing the underlying cause of the patient's gynecologic symptoms. Although a detailed description of a pelvic examination is not given here, it is important to stress some of the steps in evaluating the female pelvis. The bladder should be emptied by voiding prior to an adequate pelvic examination. If the patient has urinary tract symptoms, a clean-catch or catheterized urine specimen should be obtained for complete urinalysis and for culture and antibiotic sensitivity studies. Should the patient complain of urinary incontinence, she should be examined with a full bladder in the lithotomy and erect positions to demonstrate stress incontinence of the urethral sphincter. On inspecting the vulva for gross lesions, the Bartholin and Skene glands should be examined for evidence of cyst formation and for purulent exudate as sources of gynecologic infection. Particular attention should be given to the mons pubis and the labia majora and minora for subtle changes in skin pigment, for vesicle formation, or for small, raised lesions that may represent evidence of viral infection or early neoplasia. The outlet should be closely inspected for relaxation of the anterior and posterior vaginal walls, and the vaginal mucosa should be observed for infection and estrogen effect. The patient should be encouraged to bear down and to cough in order to demonstrate the degree of relaxation of the anterior and posterior vaginal walls and the extent of uterine descensus, without the use of a tenaculum. The urethra should be compressed along its entire length to test for a possible suburethral diverticulum, often manifested by the expression of purulent material from the urethral meatus or by a tender suburethral mass. The cervix should be evaluated for abnormal gross pathology, particularly ulceration, neoplastic growths, and abnormal discharge. A Papanicolaou smear should be taken, combining a sample of posterior vaginal pool material with cells scraped from the entire circumference of the external os and adjacent endocervical canal. This type of combined cytologic smear is extremely valuable in detecting cervical and endometrial lesions and should always be included in a complete gynecologic examination. A remote history of a negative Papanicolaou smear does not exclude the possibility of a cervical or endometrial neoplasm, because of the frequency (10%–20%) of false-negative cervical-vaginal smears. A patient should not undergo pelvic surgery without having had a recent cytologic study of the cervix performed by the gynecologist. Because 80% to 90% of all preclinical malignancies of the cervix demonstrate no significant gross lesion, it is impossible to be certain of the condition of the cervix without a Papanicolaou smear or a colposcopically directed cervical biopsy (see Ch. 41). The uterus is examined bimanually by the abdominal–vaginal route for position, size, mobility, irregularity, and tenderness to motion. Both adnexal regions are evaluated vaginally and by rectovaginal examination.

Rectal examination should never be neglected in the routine pelvic examination. Besides giving information about the competence of the anal sphincter and about lesions in the anal canal and lower rectum, it is an effective method of detecting pelvic pathology and especially of evaluating the broad and uterosacral ligaments, the cul-de-sac of Douglas, the uterus, and the adnexa. In this procedure, the index finger is inserted into the vagina and the middle finger is inserted into the rectum (Fig. 5-1). This technique permits examination of the rectum to a higher level than does examination with the index finger, as well as an opportunity to evaluate the ovaries, the cul-de-sac, and the posterior aspect of the broad ligament. When the pelvic findings are doubtful or inconclusive, a more adequate examination should be done under general anesthesia before a final decision for or against surgery is made. In fact, pelvic examination under anesthesia should always precede any gynecologic procedure, whether major or minor. Frequently, suspected pelvic pathology is completely ruled out by thorough preoperative pelvic examination and a needless laparotomy is avoided. The most common area of clinical confusion is in establishing the presence of an ovarian cyst, which may be confused with bowel, bladder, or uterine leiomyomas. If a normal ovary can be palpated and a cyst is not identified under anesthesia, the patient has been spared a needless operative procedure. All patients having a dilatation and curettage should have a pelvic examination under anesthesia, and the pelvic organs should be described in detail for future reference.

LABORATORY EXAMINATIONS

A determination of hemoglobin level, a hematocrit, a white blood count and differential count, and a complete urinalysis should be a part of every preoperative workup of a gynecologic patient. Symptoms suggestive

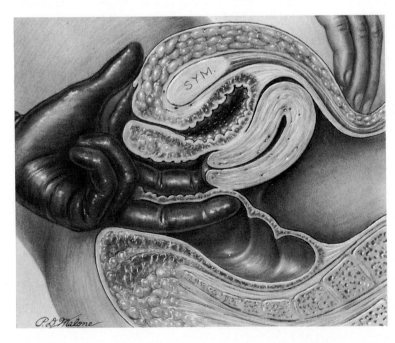

Figure 5–1. Rectovaginal-abdominal examination.

of hepatic, renal, or metabolic disease should be thoroughly investigated by specifically related laboratory studies, such as liver function studies, assessments of fasting or 2-hour postprandial blood glucose levels, enzyme determinations, and assessments of total protein with albumin/globulin ratio and of thymol turbidity, cephalin flocculation, prothrombin time, and total bilirubin levels. A history of renal disease requires evaluation with an excretory urogram, blood urea nitrogen, serum creatinine, and possibly creatinine clearance studies, along with complete urinalysis and urine culture. When masculinizing or feminizing ovarian tumors are suspected, determinations of plasma androgen and estrogen levels are frequently helpful. For all patients having extensive pelvic surgery, a baseline electrolyte panel is important as a basis for postoperative fluid and electrolyte replacement therapy. An excretory urogram may be obtained in the differential diagnosis of a pelvic mass. Chest x-ray examination with anteroposterior and lateral views is a routine hospital admission procedure. Patients over 40 years of age should have an electrocardiogram (ECG) prior to major pelvic surgery. Ultrasonography may be a useful diagnostic tool in separating uterine from adnexal disease, in diagnosing an intrauterine from an extrauterine pregnancy, and in measuring the growth of uterine myomas (see Ch. 26). However, it should never be considered as exceeding the diagnostic accuracy of a thorough pelvic examination; to do so may subject the patient to unnecessary diagnostic studies and the risk of unnecessary surgery.

PREOPERATIVE EVALUATION

The outcome of pelvic surgery is related to four major factors: (1) the severity and reversibility of the organic disease, (2) the presence of a surgically resectable disease process, (3) the pelvic surgeon's knowledge of the disease process, and (4) the skill and judgment of the surgeon. Diminished cardiac, pulmonary, or renal reserve produces an unstable physiologic background for extensive or emergency surgery. Arteriosclerosis, with its ischemic and compromising effects on the heart, produces myocardial changes detectable by ECG in more than 75% of patients with this condition. Full cardiac stabilization and digitalization should be afforded all patients in whom there is a significant dysfunction as evidenced by diminished cardiac reserve.

Dehydration and hypovolemia are serious and frequently critical factors in the development of postoperative complications. Without adequate interstitial fluid and vascular volume replacement prior to surgery, the patient's cardiac reserve may fail to maintain a normal circulation, and vasomotor collapse or acute renal tubular necrosis may result. In an effort to maintain an ideal urinary output of approximately 50–60 ml/hr, dehydration must be avoided for any prolonged period of time preoperatively, during surgery, and postoperatively. Proper hydration is assured if approximately 250–300 ml/hr of intravenous fluids are given during surgery. This rate, which is approximately twice the average fluid replacement rate given in the postoperative state, compensates for the insensible fluid loss from the exposed peritoneal surfaces. Because the cardiovascular tree in elderly patients lacks resilience, adequate blood and fluid replacement during surgery is essential to avoid the devitalizing effects of hypovolemia, shock, and hypoxia.

Chronic pulmonary disease is a frequent respiratory complication, although less so in women than in men. Such obstructive changes in the bronchial tree and alveoli, including bronchiectasis and emphysema, produce an excellent environment for respiratory infection, impair oxygen exchange, and result in respiratory acidosis. Atelectasis, pneumonia, and the Adult Respiratory Distress Syndrome (ARDS) are difficult to control in such a setting, to the degree that ARDS is one of the major postoperative complications that may result in death.

Particular attention must be given to the elderly patient, whose cardiac, pulmonary, or renal reserve requires meticulous evaluation and preoperative correction of any physiologic and functional abnormality. In a survey at the Milwaukee County Medical Complex of 500 male and female surgical patients 80 years of age or older, the following preoperative complications were noted: (1) nearly one third were malnourished (below 100 lb); (2) anemia was present in 15% of the patients, and among these, one in four required preoperative blood transfusions; (3) hypertension, cardiomegaly, or arteriosclerotic heart disease was present in more than 50% of the patients, and the ECG was abnormal in 80%; and (4) acute or chronic lung disease was present in over 25%. Of paramount importance was that the mortality rate among such patients was four to five times higher than the expected rate when emergency surgery prevented their proper evaluation and preparation.

AGE AS A FACTOR IN PELVIC SURGERY

Having defined the potential medical complications and operative risks that pertain to elderly women, it is important to state that chronologic age, by itself, is no longer an accurate indicator of organ function. Atheromatous changes in the cardiovascular system are uncommon in women until well past the climacteric. This biologic phenomenon is but one of the many factors that promote increasing female longevity. The average female lifespan in the United States has increased to 78 years. As a consequence, more women are entering the period of their life where gynecologic disease is more prevalent and surgery is necessary.

The predictable life expectancy at various ages in the elderly has likewise changed. According to actuarial life tables, an 80-year-old woman has an additional life expectancy of 6.5 years; at 85 there is a 5-year life expectancy; and at 90 years, a 3.5-year expectancy. It is a fact that such changes in longevity have influenced the need for surgery in the aging female. Many clinics show the current incidence of major surgery to be highest in the 60- to 69-year-old age group. However, when excellent surgical skill is combined with meticulous medical control of concurrent disease and physiologic and pharmacologic competence in the field of anesthesiology, there is only a minimal increase in surgical risks for the elderly female (ie, over the age of 65) above those for the premenopausal patient.

PULMONARY EVALUATION

DONALD P. SCHLUETER

Despite continuing advances in anesthesia, surgical techniques, pharmacology, and our understanding of the physiologic events during the postoperative period, pulmonary complications associated with abdominal surgery remain a major problem. Preexisting pulmonary disease, especially chronic obstructive lung disease, is one of the most significant factors predisposing to operative and postoperative respiratory complications. Overall, pulmonary complications have been reported in 5% to 56% of patients having lower abdominal surgery. Stein and associates have shown that 70% of patients with chronic bronchitis and emphysema develop atelectasis and pneumonia postoperatively, whereas only 3% of patients with normal preoperative lung function encounter similar difficulties. Gold and Helvich reported a 24% incidence of operative and postoperative complications in an asthmatic population as compared with 14% in the control group. Although respiratory complications occur most frequently with obstructive lung disease, factors that alter lung elasticity (such as fibrosis or thoracic mechanics and, particularly, obesity) will also lead to an increased incidence of postoperative problems. The importance of age as a factor in all types of postoperative complications, especially those involving the respiratory system, increases sharply after age 50. With aging there are changes in air flow rates, lung volumes, lung elasticity, physiologic dead space, arterial oxygen tension (Pao_2), and alveolar–arterial oxygen gradient, all of which result in less efficient respiratory function. Tissue hypoxia is more likely to occur in this group, since circulatory responses to hypoxia are diminished.

Few data are available dealing specifically with the effects of smoking on the incidence of postoperative complications. However, ample evidence implicates smoking as a significant factor in the production of respiratory symptoms and in the etiology of obstructive lung disease. Physiologic alterations, including increased airway resistance, decreased flow rates, impaired ventilation distribution, increased carboxyhemoglobin levels, and decreased Pao_2 levels have been reported in smokers. Even smoking a single cigarette has been shown to result in a significant increase in airway resistance. Tobacco smoke can lead to a decrease in surfactant activity and thus promote alveolar instability and microatelectasis. Defense against infection is altered because of depression of mucociliary function and alveolar macrophage activity. All these factors combined place the smoker at a higher risk for anesthesia and surgery. Shapiro has estimated that patients who smoke quadruple their risk of pulmonary complications; those over 65 have three times the risk; and those with a body weight more than 20% above the ideal have twice the normal rate of complications.

An often-neglected factor in pulmonary evaluations is chronic alcoholism. Alcoholics have more respiratory symptoms and an increased incidence of pulmonary infections because of altered host defenses. Physiologic changes resulting in a decreased diffusing capacity, increased shunting, and decreased surfactant production are frequently found.

The operative site and type of procedure will have a significant effect on the incidence of postoperative respiratory complications following abdominal surgery. The incidence following lower abdominal surgery is somewhat lower than that for upper abdominal procedures. With these procedures, pain and associated abdominal distention are frequent causes of respiratory complications, because of their limiting effects on ventilatory capacity.

Preoperative Pulmonary Evaluation

The question of who should have a preoperative pulmonary evaluation beyond the usual routine history and physical exam is frequently raised. Certain observations that the physician can make to alert him or her to potential respiratory complications are summarized later. These high-risk patients should undergo a more extensive pulmonary evaluation. However, any patient in whom a history of respiratory symptoms has been elicited is a candidate. She should be questioned specifically about the frequency, volume of sputum, and productivity of a cough. An attempt should be made to quantitate the degree of dyspnea by determining if it is present at rest or is worse in certain positions, what level of exercise causes symptoms, and what particular activity is most aggravating. The presence or absence of wheezing and precipitating factors should also be noted. A careful smoking history is extremely important. The past medical history should elicit any prior illnesses involving the lungs or thorax, and it is helpful to determine from surgical history whether the patient had experienced any postoperative respiratory complications.

The preoperative assessment of the patient with pulmonary impairment actually begins with the physician's first impression, that is, with the patient's general appearance. The robust, energetic individual with a trim figure and good musculature certainly is more likely to handle the stress of the postoperative period satisfactorily than is the sedentary person with poor posture, flabby musculature, and obesity. Inspection of the thorax for deformities, mobility limitations, and muscle weakness and atrophy is vital, since any one of these abnormalities may interfere with adequate ventilation. Such simple tests as having the patient blow out a match at arm's length will demonstrate the presence of obstruction. This can be further substantiated by timing her forced expiration, which should be complete in 3 seconds, and listening with a stethoscope for the presence of wheezes. Respiratory excursions can be determined by percussion in the full inspiratory position (normally 4–6 cm). Thorough auscultation of the chest should be carried out, both with quiet breathing and with forced expiration, to detect rales, rhonchi, or wheezes that may be indicative of the presence of secretions or airway obstruction. Differences in the intensity of breath sounds should be noted, since they may indicate the presence of pleural disease or of decreased ventilation. The abnormalities can then be verified by percussion. Obviously, a chest roentgenogram should be routine in all candidates for surgical procedures. Pulmonary function studies provide an objective measurement of the degree of respiratory impairment. A wide variety of test procedures is available; carefully selected, they can provide information about a specific physiologic abnormality without unnecessary stress to the patient.

Physiologic Evaluation

In general, pulmonary function tests should be performed in all patients in whom respiratory symptoms are elicited or in whom significant abnormalities have been demonstrated on chest examination, as well as in heavy smokers and those at increased risk of postoperative respiratory complications, as previously described.

The basic screening test of pulmonary function is spirometry. This test requires a maximum forced expiration by the patient from full inspiration while the change in volume with time is traced on a recording spirometer. From this tracing, measurements of forced vital capacity (FVC), 1-second forced expired volume $(FEV_{1.0})$/FVC ratio, forced expiratory flow from 200 ml to 1200 ml $(FEF_{200-1200})$, and forced expiratory flow from 25% to 75% of the forced vital capacity (FEF_{25-75}) are obtained. In many laboratories a flow/volume curve is generated simultaneously during the forced expiration. This test can detect obstruction in the small airways. The latter finding is important, since obstruction in the small airways is not usually detected on auscultation of the chest but can lead to significant disturbances in ventilation/perfusion relationships and to hypoxemia.

Since these tests are effort dependent, adequate cooperation from the patient is necessary for meaningful results. It is obvious that in a patient who is seriously ill or incapable of understanding instructions, the results are not reliable in quantitating the impairment. The two major kinds of defects that will be demonstrated by spirometry are restrictive defects and obstructive ones. *Restrictive pulmonary disease* includes those conditions in which there is actual reduction in the volume of air-containing tissue, and it affects primarily the volume of air that can be inspired. In these conditions, the FVC and the $FEV_{1.0}$ are reduced, whereas the $FEV_{1.0}$/FVC ratio and expiratory flow rates are normal. *Obstructive disease* includes those conditions in which there is reduction and prolongation of air flow during expiration. This results in a normal or low FVC and a reduction in $FEV_{1.0}$, $FEV_{1.0}$/FVC ratio, and expiratory flow rates. A determination of lung volume is necessary to quantitate the changes in lung volume and to determine if the reduction in FVC is secondary to airway obstruction or restriction. This can be accomplished by a gas dilution technique using helium. With this method the functional residual capacity (FRC) is measured and the total lung capacity (TLC) and residual volume (RV) are derived. In restrictive disease all lung volumes are decreased, and in obstructive disease they are elevated. The degree of air trapping can be estimated from the RV/TLC ratio (Fig. 5-2). In addition, the time required for equilibration of the marker gas will give some indication of the distribution of inspired gas, being prolonged when distribution is abnormal. Problems in oxygen transfer due either to disturbance in ventilation/perfusion relationships or to alveolar capillary membrane abnormalities can be evaluated by measuring the carbon monoxide diffusing capacity. Regional ventilation/perfusion disturbances can be visually demon-

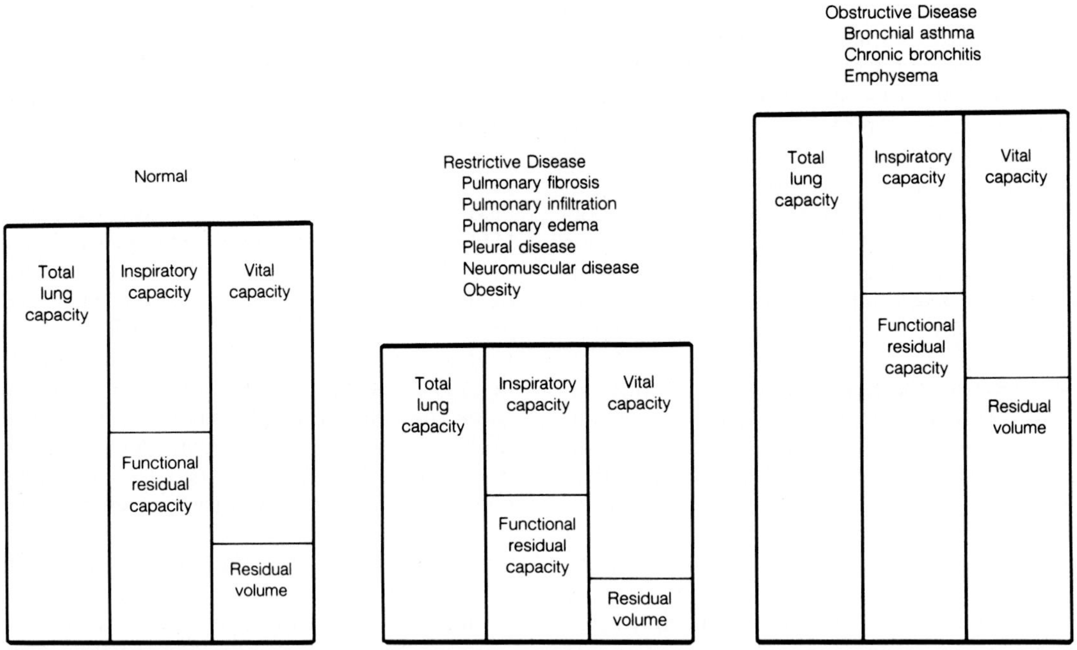

Obstructive Disease
Bronchial asthma
Chronic bronchitis
Emphysema

Restrictive Disease
Pulmonary fibrosis
Pulmonary infiltration
Pulmonary edema
Pleural disease
Neuromuscular disease
Obesity

Normal

Figure 5–2. Normal lung compartments and changes that are found in restrictive and obstructive lung disease.

strated by radioactive scanning techniques using xenon.

Arterial blood gas studies should be performed preoperatively in all patients with evidence of pulmonary disease. An elevated arterial carbon dioxide tension ($Paco_2$) is indicative of inadequate ventilation, whereas a low Pao_2 is most frequently associated with ventilation/perfusion mismatching, diffusion defect, or anatomic shunting. Shunting can be verified by the inability to raise the Pao_2 above 550 mm Hg after breathing 100% oxygen for 30 minutes. Hemoglobin concentration should also be measured, since this determines the oxygen-carrying capacity of the blood. The laboratory indicators of potential postoperative respiratory complications are summarized below.

LABORATORY INDICATORS OF POTENTIAL POSTOPERATIVE RESPIRATORY COMPLICATIONS

COPD on chest x-ray
Severe thoracic deformity on chest x-ray
FVC less than 50% of predicted
$FEV_{1.0}$ less than 2 liters or less than 50% of predicted
MVV less than 50% of predicted
FEF_{25-75} less than 1.0 liter/sec
Pao_2 less than 65 mm Hg
$Paco_2$ greater than 45 mm Hg

FVC = forced vital capacity; $FEV_{1.0}$ = 1-second forced expired volume; MVV = maximum voluntary ventilation; FEF_{25-75} = forced expiratory flow from 25% to 75% of FVC; COPD = chronic obstructive pulmonary disease.

Problems Associated with Obstructive Lung Disease

The three most common obstructive pulmonary diseases are chronic bronchitis, emphysema, and asthma. Although bronchitis and emphysema frequently occur together and the discussion is facilitated by considering them in one section, significant differences alter the approach to therapy and the expected response. The following definitions have been proposed by the World Health Organization and are generally accepted. Chronic bronchitis is a clinical disorder characterized by excessive mucus secretion in the bronchial tree. Chronic cough is present on most days for a minimum of 3 months in the year and for not less than 2 successive years. Emphysema is an anatomic alteration of the lung characterized by an abnormal enlargement of the air spaces distal to the terminal nonrespiratory bronchiole, accompanied by destructive changes of the alveolar walls. Table 5-1 lists some of the distinguishing clinical and laboratory features of these two diseases. Obviously, with combined disease these differences become less distinct. It is important to consider the mechanisms of obstruction in these two diseases, since they provide some idea of what to expect from the various therapeutic modalities employed. Bronchitis is essentially an intrinsic airway disease, with the obstruction resulting from bronchoconstriction, mucosal edema, and accumulation of secretions. The bronchoconstriction can be reversed with a variety of bronchodilators,

TABLE 5–1
Differential Characteristics in Chronic Obstructive Lung Disease

CHARACTERISTIC	BRONCHITIC TYPE	EMPHYSEMATOUS TYPE
Body build	Stocky, obese	Thin, wasted
Age	40–60 years	Usually > 50 years
Dyspnea	Sustained, progressive	Variable
Cough	Major symptom	Minor problem
Sputum	Often profuse	Scanty
Wheezing	Episodic	Uncommon
Cyanosis	Common	Uncommon
Pao_2	Frequently low	Normal or slightly low
$Paco_2$	Frequently elevated	Usually normal
Heart failure	Common	None
Respiratory failure	Frequent	Infrequent
Response to therapy	Good	Poor

the mucosal edema can be reduced with decongestants, and the secretions can be mobilized with humidification, expectorants, and mucolytic agents. In emphysema, although the preceding mechanisms may play a role, the major cause of obstruction is the loss of the normal tractional support of the airways provided by the connective-tissue structure of the lung. It is a destructive process in the lung and is therefore irreversible. For this reason, response to therapy is usually not dramatic. With these facts in mind, the preoperative preparation of the patient will be considered.

Patients with obstructive lung disease should be admitted to the hospital several days prior to surgery. The first step in preparation is the cessation of exposure to inhaled irritants; that is, the patient must stop smoking. This will probably do more to prevent postoperative complication than any other measure. An air-conditioned room will be helpful when the weather is hot and humid. In addition, fellow patients and visitors will not be allowed to smoke in the room.

Bronchial infection may be present, particularly if the cough is very productive or symptoms severe. Therefore, a sputum smear and culture should be obtained. If the sputum is purulent, even if a specific pathogen is not isolated, the patient should receive a course of antibiotics. Ampicillin or tetracycline in a dosage of 2.0 g/day is preferred, since both are effective against the most common pathogens involved, *Streptococcus pneumoniae* and *Haemophilus influenzae*. With isolation of a specific organism, other antibiotics may be indicated. In some cases it may be advisable to postpone surgery to a later date.

Bronchodilators should be used on a round-the-clock basis when bronchospasm is present. An adrenergic agent such as terbutaline, metaproterenol, or albuterol is indicated. Theophylline should form the basis of bronchodilator therapy. Many slow-release preparations are available that can be given orally at 12-hour intervals. With this dosage schedule, relatively uniform theophylline blood levels can be obtained in the therapeutic range of 10–20 mg/ml. Determination of the serum concentration of theophylline, which can be done in most hospitals, facilitates maintaining therapeutic levels and avoiding toxicity. For patients unable to take medications orally, a continuous intravenous infusion of aminophylline at a rate of 0.5–0.7 mg/kg/min usually provides therapeutic levels. Aerosolized bronchodilators such as isoproterenol (Isuprel), isoetharine (Bronkosol), or metaproterenol (Alupent) with saline given by nebulizer or intermittent positive pressure breathing (IPPB) every 4–6 hours is often very effective in reversing bronchospasm and stimulating cough and clearing secretion. Metaproterenol may have some advantages because of its longer action. The nebulizer usually provides better distribution of aerosol, although some patients are able to coordinate their inspiration better with the IPPB treatment. Controlled studies have failed to show any statistically significant differences between these two methods of administration in the incidence of postoperative respiratory complications. If IPPB is to be used postoperatively in these patients, they should be introduced to its use preoperatively when they are alert and free of pain and can cooperate completely. Since this type of therapy is most frequently employed in the immediate postoperative period in patients with airway obstruction, the patient is already experienced; consequently, therapy is more effective. When the patient has recovered enough to use a nebulizer effectively for delivering the bronchodilator, IPPB can be discontinued. The use of a metered dose inhaler is discouraged because of difficulties with coordination during this period and potential overuse.

Bronchial secretions should be reduced by the foregoing medical measures. Remaining secretions can be removed by reducing their viscosity with mist therapy, which can be provided by a heated aerosol, a pressure nebulizer, or an ultrasonic generator and administered with a face mask. It may be somewhat more effective if given after the IPPB treatment. Thick mucus secretions may be thinned by nebulizing N-acetylcysteine (Mucomyst). A bronchodilator should be added to this agent, since the mucolytic agent may cause bronchospasm. Expectorants have been in use for many years, but there is little evidence that they are more effective than water. Adequate hydration is extremely important, and patients should be encouraged to drink at least eight glasses of water daily.

Physical therapy is very helpful in teaching the patient with obstructive lung disease to breathe more efficiently, and instruction in postural drainage and effective coughing will improve her ability to mobilize secretions.

Bronchial asthma, in general, involves a younger age group. It is an episodic disease with symptoms occurring during certain seasons of the year, allowing some selectivity for surgical procedures; and the physiologic disturbances are usually almost completely reversible. Asthma is defined as a disease characterized by an increased responsiveness of the trachea and bronchi to various stimuli and is manifested by a general narrowing of the airways that changes in severity either spontaneously or as the result of therapy. The preoperative preparation of the asthmatic patient is much the same as that for the patient with chronic bronchitis or emphysema. She should be removed from all irritants, not only cigarette smoke but pollen, dust, fumes, and any other materials known to trigger an acute attack in the patient. Emotional stress is an important precipitating factor in this disease, and the period of preoperative preparation can be used to lessen tension and anxiety through reassurance and sympathetic discussion of the problem. A mild tranquilizer may be helpful. The therapeutic program should include regular oral and aerosolized bronchodilators, humidification, hydration, and antibiotics if the sputum is purulent. If the sputum is very viscid and difficult to raise, N-acetylcysteine (Mucomyst) can be helpful but must be used with caution and with a bronchodilator, since it may cause severe bronchospasm. It is extremely important to question the patient thoroughly regarding medications to determine if she is receiving corticosteroids or has taken them within the previous 6 months. They should be continued orally until surgery and then given parenterally. If steroids have been used during the previous 12 months, adrenal response to the stress of surgery may be diminished. Acute adrenal insufficiency can be prevented by administration of hydrocortisone preoperatively in a dose of 100 mg IM the night before

surgery and 100 mg IM the morning of surgery. If the surgery is particularly prolonged or complicated, it may be necessary to give additional hydrocortisone during and after surgery.

Because of their ventilatory depressant potential, preanesthetic agents must be used cautiously in all patients with obstructive lung disease. Morphine and meperidine are particularly prone to reduce the ventilatory response to hypercapnia, and this effect may be potentiated by promethazine. Atropine and scopolamine tend to decrease liquid secretions, which may result in the formation of mucus plugs and contribute to postoperative atelectasis and pneumonia.

Inhalation anesthesia by way of an endotracheal tube is preferred when moderate to severe obstructive lung disease is present, since it provides complete control of ventilation during surgery and the postoperative period. It also provides a ready access to the bronchial tree for removal of secretions during the period when the cough mechanism is depressed. Halothane has proven to be a very satisfactory agent because it relaxes bronchial smooth muscle, is nonirritating to the airways, does not stimulate tracheobronchial secretions, and is associated with rapid induction of and recovery from anesthesia.

Much discussion has focused on the preoperative preparation of the patient with obstructive lung disease; however, this is important because a program such as that outlined, if assiduously applied, can significantly reduce respiratory complication and hence the postoperative recovery period.

Problems Associated with Restrictive Lung Disease

The incidence of postoperative respiratory complications tends to be lower in patients with restrictive lung disease, particularly when it is limited to the lung, than in patients with obstructive disease. This is probably because patients with restrictive lung disease are usually able to compensate for the increased work of breathing and maintain adequate ventilation. In addition, hypercapnia is infrequent in these patients, and oxygen can be administered without fear of depressing ventilation. Because of the increased retractive force of the respiratory system, the cough mechanism remains effective in removing secretions. The major exceptions to these statements involve markedly obese patients and patients with neuromuscular disease involving the thorax. Figure 5-2 lists the predominantly restrictive diseases that result in a reduction in the volume of air-containing tissue. Physiologically, this reduction results in a decrease in vital capacity and lung volumes without airway obstruction except when the disease is very severe. Oxygen transfer is usually impaired, as shown by a low diffusion lung carbon monoxide (low D_LCO) level, and hypoxemia without hypercapnia is the rule.

Hypoxemia can be corrected in most cases of restrictive pulmonary disease by increasing the inspired oxygen concentration. However, in some patients with primarily thoracic cage disease or with extreme obesity, hypercapnia may accompany the hypoxemia, and suppression of ventilation may occur with high inspired oxygen concentration.

The patient with restrictive disease limited to the lungs requires only brief preoperative preparation, including instruction in the use of IPPB, deep breathing, and coughing. More recently, incentive spirometers and similar devices have been used to achieve a maximum sustained inspiration that appears effective in preventing and reexpanding the atelectatic lung. However, a recent study by Jung and associates (1980) of patients undergoing abdominal surgery failed to show any advantage of one method over the other in reducing postoperative respiratory complications.

Since patients with restrictive disease may be taking corticosteroids or may have taken them in the recent past, they should be questioned specifically about this, and therapy should be instituted as previously described. Special attention should be given to patients with evidence of impaired ventilation as indicated by the presence of hypercapnia. IPPB or incentive spirometry and measures directed at liquefying secretions should be instituted several days prior to surgery, along with chest physiotherapy and instruction in coughing. Oxygen should be administered carefully, particularly to obese patients with hypercapnia, since correction of the hypoxemia may significantly depress ventilation. Measurement of the ventilatory response to carbon dioxide preoperatively is helpful in determining which individuals are likely to experience depression of ventilation with oxygen. Weight reduction will usually decrease or eliminate this type of response. Retention of fluid and congestive heart failure occur relatively frequently in patients with restrictive disease, so diuresis and cautious digitalization, if indicated, should be done prior to surgery. Olgivie cautions that preoperative evaluation by an experienced chest physician may be indicated in patients with severely impaired respiratory function.

CARDIOVASCULAR EVALUATION

MICHAEL H. KEELAN, JR.

Advances in medical and surgical therapy have been responsible for prolongation of productive life in a significant number of patients with cardiovascular disease. Antibiotics and surgical procedures have altered the natural history of congenital and rheumatic heart diseases. Coronary artery disease continues to be the major cause of death in this country, but mortality has declined in recent years. Aggressive management of this disease now includes transluminal angioplasty and direct intracoronary thrombolysis in addition to surgical revascularization. Recognition and treatment of hypertension have resulted in a decreased incidence of malignant progression of this disease. In summary, the likelihood of facing problems of unrelated medical and surgical illnesses in the cardiac patient continues to increase.

Patients with severe preoperative cardiac disease, including ECG evidence of severe ischemia, heart block, or congestive heart failure, are most likely to experience postoperative cardiac problems. The evaluation and management of these patients presents a challenge to surgeon, anesthesiologist, and cardiologist alike. Cadanelli and associates reported a 13.5% incidence of heart disease in 1664 patients presenting for gynecologic surgery. Twelve percent of the cardiac patients demonstrated clinical or ECG deterioration, and overall mortality among these was less than 1%. The anticipation of potential problems depends on the preoperative recognition and understanding of the fundamental cardiac disease process.

The clinical history will readily identify the patient with overt cardiorespiratory symptoms. Interpretation of atypical symptoms tests the skill of the most experienced clinician. This is particularly evident in the evaluation of chest pain syndromes. The classic description of ischemic chest pain is well known and easily recognized. Angina pectoris should also be suspected, if discomfort of any qualitative description is localized between the waist and the jaw and is predictably evoked by effort or emotion. Coronary risk factors must be carefully weighed in any patient whose history suggests possible angina pectoris. Anginal pain that occurs at rest, particularly in the early morning, suggests the diagnosis of vasospastic disease. The association of other vasoregulatory disorders, such as migraine or Raynaud's phenomenon, enhances the probability of coronary artery spasm as a diagnosis. A prominent heart murmur, pulmonary rales, or peripheral edema direct immediate attention to the cardiovascular system. Vascular bruits, gallop sounds, or abnormal venous pulsations are more subtle findings but are equally important signs of cardiac or vascular disease.

Routine laboratory studies in the preoperative patient often fail to reveal the extent of underlying cardiac pathology. The resting ECG is helpful if it is abnormal, but a normal tracing is no reassurance in a patient with classic symptoms of progressive angina pectoris. Furthermore, the ECG reverts to normal in approximately

25% of patients with proven myocardial infarction. The exercise ECG is frequently used to assess patients with suspected angina pectoris. The test is not sufficiently sensitive to be helpful if the patient has a typical history of ischemic pain. The history alone is 90% predictive of coronary disease, whereas the stress test has only 75% to 80% sensitivity. In recent years, nuclear scanning has assumed a prominent role in the diagnosis of coronary artery disease by noninvasive testing. Stress tests are performed using either thallium-201 (^{201}Tl) or technetium-99M (^{99M}Tc). ^{201}Tl is an analogue of potassium and is distributed to and taken up by the myocardium in proportion to blood flow. It is injected intravenously at peak exercise, and scanning is performed in at least three projections within 15 minutes of the completion of exercise. The scan is repeated 3–4 hours later using similar projections. Failure of uptake in a region of myocardium suggests stenosis or occlusion of the artery to the corresponding region. If the delayed scan shows reperfusion of the previously underperfused area, the test is considered positive for ischemia. Failure to reperfuse identifies severe ischemia or old infarction. The ^{201}Tl perfusion scan enhances the sensitivity of stress testing in both males and females, but it is worth noting that false-positive scans are more frequent in females. The ^{99M}Tc blood pool scan is combined with a computerized program that permits analysis of left or right ventricular wall motion. Radioisotope angiocardiography can be performed before and during graded exercise. This study yields valuable information concerning cardiac reserve. It is a less reliable predictor of coronary disease than is the ^{201}Tl perfusion scan because of the low specificity of the test.

The standard chest x-ray provides adequate evaluation of the cardiac silhouette and lung fields in most patients. Accurate determination of individual chamber size and thickness is best provided by ultrasonic (echo) cardiography. The sector scan (2D) echo is a useful technique for evaluation of ventricular wall motion, valve orifice size, and intracardiac masses such as thrombus or myxoma.

Preoperative attention to electrolyte concentrations and renal function help to avoid "surprise" arrhythmias during the perioperative period. All medications must be reviewed, since many patients will be taking one or more cardiac drugs. Serum drug level determinations are available for digitalis and a variety of antiarrhythmic agents. Routine assessment of serum digoxin level is not recommended. The test should be obtained if there is a question of drug intoxication or a lack of patient compliance with the prescribed regimen. Blood volume measurements may be useful in patients whose total volumes are often contracted (eg, the elderly or those with extensive malignancies).

Coronary Artery Disease

Coronary artery disease rarely afflicts premenopausal women without major risk factors such as hyperlipidemia, hypertension, diabetes mellitus, or smoking. Use of an anovulatory drug appears to increase the risk of coronary disease in patients over 40 years of age. Realistically, ischemic heart disease is a disease of men and postmenopausal women. The diagnosis is made by history (angina pectoris or prior documented myocardial infarction) or by ECG evidence of infarction. Various electrocardiographic changes, including left bundle branch block and ST–T changes, suggest the diagnosis of ischemic disease, but they are not definitive. Even significant Q waves, the hallmark of transmural myocardial infarction, are not always diagnostic. Hypertrophic cardiomyopathy and mitral valve prolapse are noncoronary diseases in which the cardiogram may demonstrate a pseudoinfarction pattern. A preoperative diagnosis of coronary artery disease increases the surgical risk for complications, but multiple factors influence the overall prognosis. Unstable coronary disease is a major risk factor. Patients with recent onset of angina, progressive angina, or rest angina should be fully evaluated by a cardiac consultant prior to elective surgery. Surgery should be deferred until the patient has stabilized with appropriate pharmacologic or surgical therapy. Myocardial infarction within the previous 6 months should also be considered a potentially unstable condition. Surgery performed within this interval is accompanied by an unacceptably high incidence of both reinfarction and fatality. Emergency surgery is occasionally necessary in patients with unstable coronary syndromes. Most patients will have been treated with combinations of vasodilators, including nitrates, calcium channel blockers, or β-adrenergic blocking agents. Whenever possible, these drugs should be continued through the perioperative course or tapered off gradually if they must be discontinued. The availability of direct invasive monitoring of left ventricular filling pressure using the balloon-tipped floating pulmonary artery catheter has made it possible to monitor hemodynamic parameters throughout the critical perioperative period. Filling pressures and systemic arterial pressure are optimized, thereby avoiding inadvertent fluid overload and unnecessary increase in myocardial oxygen demand. Of course, ECG monitoring is also used. In patients with exceptionally unstable disease, the preoperative insertion of the intraaortic counterpulsation balloon catheter has provided stabilization during the operative procedure. This device augments the central aortic diastolic pressure, thereby increasing coronary perfusion. The balloon deflates rapidly, producing a dramatic fall in end-diastolic aortic pressure. The impedance to ejection is reduced and systolic cardiac emptying is enhanced.

Congestive heart failure, overt or covert, is the single most important predictor of cardiac complications in the surgical patient. Because of its overall frequency, coronary disease is the likely cause for heart failure in most patients presenting for surgery. Elective surgery should not be done in patients whose signs and symptoms are overt. Patients with gross cardiomegaly or gallop rhythm should be carefully assessed with either echocardiography or nuclear ventriculography. Invasive hemodynamic monitoring is indicated for patients with a severe reduction in resting left ventricular function who may urgently require surgery. Similar monitoring should be considered for any patient with a recent history of heart failure regardless of the current findings. Cardiac rhythm disturbances, particularly ventricular premature beats, are also associated with increased surgical risk. This risk is most prominent, however, when the ectopic beats are associated with a decrease in left ventricular function. In the absence of defined cardiovascular disease, premature ventricular beats are not harbingers of sudden death or symptomatic ventricular tachycardia and need not be treated at all. Commonly used antiarrhythmics such as quinidine, procainamide, and, particularly, disopyramide are cardiac depressants, and routine use of these drugs preoperatively is not recommended. Patients with known coronary artery disease and frequent ventricular ectopic beats, especially couplets or salvos, should be treated instead with intravenous lidocaine. Infusion is begun prior to induction. An initial bolus injection of 1–1.5 mg/kg is followed 15–20 minutes later by a similar dose. After the first bolus an infusion of 1–4 mg/min is begun. The doses should be reduced by half in elderly patients or those with liver disease. Atrial ectopic beats are often predictors of more complex atrial arrhythmias, such as atrial flutter or fibrillation. They may be the first sign of impending cardiac failure. Digitalis is recommended for this reason. Routine preoperative administration of digitalis is *not* recommended for all patients with coronary disease. This drug may be detrimental to some patients with reduced coronary reserve, because of the increased oxygen demand associated with the augmented contractile state. Its use should be restricted to (1) patients with clinical congestive heart failure; (2) patients with objective evidence of poor left ventricular function without decompensation; or (3) patients with atrial arrhythmias. Rapid "eleventh-hour digitalization" should be avoided to reduce the incidence of toxicity.

Contrary to popular belief, the greatest risk for myocardial infarction is not necessarily within the immediate intraoperative period. High rates of perioperative myocardial infarction are noted on the third and the fourth postoperative days. Surveillance with daily ECGs during this time is recommended. When indicated, creatine phosphokinase (CPK) enzymes should be obtained with myocardial brain fraction analysis. The enzymes are not obtained routinely unless there is a change in the cardiogram or the patient's clinical status suggests a cardiac event.

In summary, elective surgery should be deferred in patients with unstable syndromes. Following myocardial infarction, a 6-month delay is advised. Patients with unstable angina should be stabilized by appropriate pharmacologic and/or surgical therapy. Optimal perioperative assessment should include hemodynamic as well as electrocardiographic monitoring for unstable patients in need of urgent surgery.

Valvular Heart Disease

The incidence of rheumatic fever has declined dramatically in recent years. Mitral valve prolapse is now widely recognized as perhaps the most common of all valvular abnormalities. Its predilection for the female is also well known. The etiology is diverse, but in most patients it is not well known. The disease may be familial, and it is often accompanied by a variety of poorly explained symptoms including chest pain and fatigue. Multiple arrhythmias have been described. These include ventricular ectopic beats, atrial tachyarrhythmias, bradycardiac rhythms, and, rarely, sudden death. Autonomic dysfunction involving abnormalities of both sympathetic and parasympathetic tone has also been identified in many patients. This syndrome has often been described as being a nuisance rather than a threat.

Innovative advances in valvular repair may defer or delay valve replacement in some patients, but in most patients with advanced valvular disease, defective valves still require replacement with a prosthetic device. Bioprostheses are available and are used primarily in elderly patients or others in whom the risk of long-term anticoagulation is excessive. Because of the relatively poor durability of these valves, they have not displaced the synthetic prosthesis as the valve of choice for most young or middle-aged patients. Improved long-term results following valve replacement mean that more patients with prosthetic valves survive to endure the trials of other medical and surgical disorders.

Patients with valvular disease generally exhibit more predictable courses than do patients with coronary disease. Those in functional classes III to IV (New York Heart Association classification) have symptoms that limit their daily activities either moderately or severely. The surgical risk is greatest for these patients. Most of these patients will be taking digitalis, a diuretic, and perhaps a vasodilator. Surgery should be deferred until overt heart failure has improved and the patient is clinically stable. Invasive monitoring is also recommended during the operative procedure. All patients with valvular disease should be treated with antibiotic prophylaxis against endocarditis. Patients with severe aortic stenosis have an increased risk for surgery, and this group is not always symptomatic. Echocardiographic evaluation is recommended for all patients with harsh ejection murmurs.

The anticoagulated patient poses a special challenge. It had been recommended that Coumadin be stopped several days before surgery, allowing the prothrombin time to decline to approximately 15 seconds, at which time surgery would be done. Postoperatively, the Coumadin was resumed as soon as it was deemed safe to do so. This protocol has been successful in a number of patients, but both clotting and hemorrhagic complications have been reported. The risk for thromboembolism is greater in patients with mitral prostheses. For this group we prefer to administer fresh frozen plasma (*not* vitamin K) immediately before surgery, and begin IV heparin as soon as possible postoperatively. The regular Coumadin dose is reinstituted at the same time. This regimen has proven to be both effective and safe.

Patients with valvular disease are at risk according to their functional status. Those with critical aortic stenosis are exceptions, and ultrasonic cardiac examination is helpful in the evaluation of these patients. Special attention to endocarditis prophylaxis is necessary in all patients with valvular disease. Anticoagulation poses a minimal problem in the performance of routine surgical procedure if proper protocol is employed.

Congenital Heart Disease

The natural history of most forms of serious congenital heart disease dictates that surgical correction be performed early in life. If surgery is not possible, mortality is high and the patients do not survive to adulthood. Exceptions to this rule include patients with cyanotic heart disease such as Eisenmenger's complex and tetralogy of Fallot, who may live well into the adult years without cardiac surgical intervention. Patients with acyanotic disorders such as congenital aortic stenosis, atrial septal defect, and small ventricular septal defects often survive into adulthood without major complications. Functional classification may be misleading, particularly in patients with cyanotic disease, who may seem to be surprisingly free of symptoms despite marked erythrocytosis, hypoxemia, and cyanosis. Low-level stress tests combined with arterial oximetry give a better assessment of the true cardiac reserve in these patients. Increased blood viscosity may lead to problems of thrombosis, and decreased platelets frequently are associated with a bleeding tendency. In general, patients with congenital heart disease should be treated prophylactically for endocarditis, although those with atrial septal defect need not be.

Women with acquired or congenital valvular heart disease should receive antibiotic coverage. Additionally, women with high-pressure cardiac shunts, valvular prostheses, and/or previous episodes of endocarditis should receive endocarditis prophylaxis. Mitral valve prolapse is the main indication for antibiotic prophylaxis prior to instrumentation. A recommended antibiotic regimen is ampicillin (2 g IM or IV) and gentamicin (1.5 mg/kg IM) approximately 1 hour prior to surgery. The same dosage is repeated 8 hours later. Vancomycin (1 g given slowly IV) may be given to patients allergic to ampicillin.

Hypertension

In the absence of cardiac or renal complications, hypertension of itself adds little risk to surgical procedures. Since various antihypertensive medications are currently available, it is imperative to review drugs carefully and to do it well in advance of anticipated surgery. Agents commonly used in the management of mild to moderate hypertension include diuretics, rauwolfia, and beta blockers. Other currently available drugs capable of inducing significant cardiovascular effects include monoamine-oxidase inhibitors, guanethidine, hydralazine, prazosin, and captopril. In patients with mild hypertension, medications can generally be discontinued completely during the preoperative period without ill effect. If severe diastolic hypertension exists (diastolic pressures in excess of 115 mm Hg), it is best to continue antihypertensives to the time of surgery and reinitiate them in the early postoperative period. Rarely, it may be necessary to continue antihypertensives by the intravenous route. Nitroprusside and hydralazine are suitable drugs. With evidence of cardiomegaly or past congestive heart failure, the patient should receive digitalis in anticipation of surgery.

The approach to the surgical patient with cardiac disease should include a cooperative effort on the part of the gynecologist, anesthesiologist, and the internist-cardiologist. Although the risk of mortality and morbidity understandably is greater in this patient, the risks, as summarized in Table 5-2, can be minimized by careful preoperative, intraoperative, and postoperative management.

TABLE 5–2
Risks in Surgical Patients with Cardiovascular Disorders

DISORDER	RISK FACTORS	PRECAUTIONS
Atherosclerotic heart disease	Unstable angina Recent myocardial infarction Arrhythmias* Congestive heart failure*	Delay elective surgery 6 months ECG and hemodynamic monitoring Nuclear or echoencephalogram (ECHO) evaluation of left ventricular function
Valvular heart disease	Endocarditis Congestive heart failure Critical aortic stenosis Anticoagulants†	Antibiotic prophylaxis ECHO Hemodynamic monitoring
Congenital heart disease	Endocarditis (endarteritis) Thrombosis, hemorrhage	Antibiotic prophylaxis Evaluation of clotting factors
Hypertension	Drug interactions	Maintenance of therapy for severe hypertension only
Cardiomyopathy	Arrhythmias Congestive heart failure Anticoagulants	As for arteriosclerotic heart disease and valvular heart disease

* Arrhythmias and reduced functional capacity are potentially serious risk factors to patients regardless of etiology of heart disease. They require careful consideration of renal status, electrolyte balance, and drug therapy during the preoperative period. Monitoring central venous pressure and daily weights will help to maintain optimal fluid balance.
† See text discussion under "Valvular Heart Disease."

Thromboembolism

Virchow noted a triad of factors that contributed to the occurrence of deep venous thrombosis: hypercoagulability, stasis, and vessel wall injury. Prior to surgery the patient should be evaluated for factors that place her at increased risk for thromboembolic disease. High-risk factors include malignant disease, previous radiation therapy, obesity, severe venous varicosities, acute and chronic pelvic infection, leg edema, and oral contraceptive use prior to surgery. Other risk factors include surgical procedures with excessive blood loss, prolonged anesthesia, a past history of thromboembol-

ism, or a family history of hypercoagulability. An assessment of risk may be determined as defined by Bonnar (Table 5-3).

Prophylactic measures to prevent stasis include elastic stockings and early ambulation. Additional prophylactic measures include miniheparin, intraoperative dextran, and/or pneumatic inflated sleeve devices. Miniheparin is indicated for patients with a high risk for developing thrombosis during or after surgery. Subcutaneous heparin (5000 units) is given 2 hours prior to operative procedure and every 8 hours thereafter for 7 days postoperatively (see Ch. 6).

External pneumatic calf compression is delivered in

TABLE 5–3
Assessment of Risk of Venous Thromboembolism in Gynecologic Patients

THROMBOEMBOLIC COMPLICATIONS	LOW RISK*	MODERATE RISK†	HIGH RISK‡
Calf vein thrombosis	<3%	10%–30%	30%–60%
Proximal vein thrombosis	<1%	2%–8%	6%–12%
Pulmonary embolism	<0.01%	0.1%–0.7%	1%–2%

* Under 40 years; operative procedures less than 30 minutes; no immobilization.
† Over 40 years; estrogen therapy; operative procedures more than 30 minutes; obesity; postoperative infection.
‡ Previous thromboembolism; abdominal or pelvic operation for malignant disease; immobilization.
(After Bonnar J. Venous thromboembolism and gynecologic surgery. Clin Obstet Gynecol 1985; 28(2):435.)

a pulsatile fashion so as to reduce venous pooling in calf veins of the leg and augment venous flow at the level of the femoral veins as well as the vena cava. Clarke-Pearson and associates have noted a reduction in postoperative venous thromboembolism when external pneumatic calf compression was maintained intraoperatively for at least the first 5 postoperative days. Duration of compression was 12 seconds every minute. The prophylactic measures outlined earlier should be considered for patients at significant risk for deep venous thrombosis.

GASTROINTESTINAL SYSTEM

Gastrointestinal symptoms may be noted in women presenting for elective gynecologic surgery. Patients with bowel symptoms should receive appropriate consultation. In general, a barium enema and upper gastrointestinal series are reserved for patients with severe symptoms and/or gastrointestinal bleeding. Barium enema and endoscopy are usually necessary when a patient is noted to have a positive stool guaiac.

Symptoms must be evaluated with each individual in mind. Nevertheless, a high index of suspicion of bowel involvement in gynecologic disease process may alert the surgeon to suggest a complete evaluation. After appropriate studies, the surgeon may be rewarded with a clear appreciation of the technical requirements needed for surgery and perhaps further preoperative measures needed to prepare the patient for surgery.

Proper mechanical cleansing of the large intestine should be accomplished prior to elective surgery. Cleansing enemas should be given early in the evening so that sufficient time is allowed to evacuate the large bowel before surgery in the morning. Enemas help to reduce the incidence of fecal impaction and promote the return of normal bowel function after surgery.

If it is anticipated that the operation may result in an entry into the large intestine or may necessitate removal of a section of the colon, a complete bowel prep should be performed. Mechanical preparation usually includes a single day of oral gut lavage solution (Golytely). This solution should be ingested at a rate of 1.5 liters per hour until the diarrheal effluent is clear. Beck and coauthors noted quantitative stool cultures obtained before and following preparation of the bowel. Intraoperative cultures also were taken. Stool cultures were similar using Golytely as compared with the traditional 3 days of liquid diet, cathartics, and enemas. Patients were noted to have less weight loss, and an excellent cleansing effect on the bowel was noted at surgery.

Antibiotic coverage to reduce the high bacterial count inside the lumen should include neomycin (1 g PO) and erythromycin base (1 g PO), each given three or four times the day prior to surgery. Antibiotic prophylaxis should be used in conjunction with the mechanical and antibiotic bowel preparation.

URINARY SYSTEM

Gynecologic disease may produce anatomic distortion of the urinary tract. Complete or partial obstruction of the ureter with secondary hydronephrosis may result. A preoperative evaluation may include both radiologic and blood chemistry studies. An excretory urogram in the past was considered an integral part of the preoperative evaluation. However, a recent report by Piscitelli and coauthors addresses the use of an excretory urogram before hysterectomy for benign disease. The authors suggest that the clinical findings may be used to select a preoperative excretory urogram for those patients who are likely to have abnormalities of importance to the pelvic surgeon. Interestingly, endometriosis, pelvic inflammatory disease, pelvic relaxation, and previous intra-abdominal surgery were associated with an increased prevalence of abnormal findings. Factors likely to be associated with an abnormality of the urinary tract include a uterine size of 12 weeks or larger or an adnexal mass of 4 cm or larger.

Insufficient renal function is a major risk factor in elective operations. Abnormalities in renal function may alter the metabolism of drugs administered to the patient. Patients with azotemia have a three-fold greater risk of adverse drug reactions than women with normal renal function. All patients should receive an assessment of renal function as determined by a serum creatinine and blood urea nitrogen study prior to major surgery.

PREPARATION OF THE PATIENT FOR THE OPERATION

In most instances the patient is seen by the anesthesiologist prior to surgery. At that time, the anesthesia risks will be assessed.

Anesthesiologists classify surgical procedures according to the patient's risk of mortality (Table 5-4). An emergency operation doubles the mortality risks for classes 1, 2, and 3; produces a slightly increased risk in class 4; and does not change the risk in class 5. A dialogue between surgeon and anesthesiologist often results in the best form of anesthesia for the patient, taking into consideration the technical requirements of the operation.

A povidone-iodine (Betadine) douche and a vaginal

TABLE 5–4
Dripps–American Society of Anesthesiologists'
Classification of Physical Status

CLASS	DESCRIPTION
1	A normal healthy patient
2	A patient with mild-to-moderate systemic disease
3	A patient with severe systemic disease with limited activity but not incapacitated
4	A patient with incapacitating, constantly life-threatening systemic disease
5	A moribund patient not expected to survive 24 hours with or without operation

(Jewell ER, Persson AV. Preoperative evaluation of the high-risk patient. Surg Clin North Am 1985; 675:4. Adapted from new classification of physical status. Anesthesiology 24:111, 1963.)

suppository of nitrofurazone (Furacin), inserted high in the vagina the night preceding surgery, have been useful in decreasing the frequency of cuff cellulitis postoperatively. Many gynecologists routinely prepare the atrophic vagina of the postmenopausal patient with estrogen vaginal suppositories or cream for 4–6 weeks preoperatively. This has been particularly useful for patients undergoing vaginal surgery, since thickening the vaginal mucosa makes the tissues easier to dissect. There is no clinical evidence, however, that the vaginal flora are significantly altered or reduced by an increase of intracellular glycogen in the vaginal epithelium or by a drop in the vaginal pH—changes that are produced by estrogen preparations and the lactobacillus organisms.

The meal on the evening before an operation should be light and easily digestible. Overloading the alimentary tract shortly before the operation is particularly hazardous, not only as an anesthetic risk but also because it increases postoperative discomfort from nausea and gas formation. It is important that the patient have an adequate night's rest prior to the operation. Since the hospital environment usually causes apprehension, a mild sedative is advisable to ensure a good night's sleep.

The patient should be in the fasting state overnight, with nothing by mouth from midnight, unless the operation is scheduled for late in the day. In such cases, a light breakfast of a liquid diet is permissible, not later than 6 hours preoperatively. The lower colon should be cleansed by a preoperative enema on the evening prior to surgery and again before the operation is performed. Adequate time should be scheduled to permit complete evacuation of the enema. If necessary, repeat enemas should be given until the colon is completely empty of fecal material. A patient should not be awakened at dawn by an attendant to be given an enema when the operation is posted at noon. Not only is such a procedure a discourtesy to the patient, but the lower bowel may become refilled with fecal material because of increased intestinal peristalsis from the anxiety of awaiting the operative procedure. Preoperative sedation is usually requested by the anesthesiologist when he or she examines the patient on the night before surgery.

The use of prophylactic broad-spectrum antibiotics has become commonplace in recent years for certain patients undergoing vaginal and abdominal surgery. Although this practice has as many opponents as it has advocates, certain types of pelvic surgery have shown specific benefit. Patients undergoing vaginal hysterectomy, for example, have a high incidence of cuff cellulitis, particularly patients who are premenopausal and have a highly vascular reproductive tract. In these cases, postoperative collections of serum and blood from venous sinusoids in the vaginal cuff provide an excellent nutrient in which vaginal flora can grow and multiply. Postoperative cuff cellulitis occurs in as many as 30% to 50% of these cases. Here a broad-spectrum, single antibiotic agent has proven useful in producing a significant reduction in the incidence of febrile morbidity to no more than 5% to 10%. When given as intraoperative treatment (2 hours before surgery and every 6 hours, for a total of three doses), one of the new-generation cephalosporins, semisynthetic penicillins, or semisynthetic broad-spectrum β-lactamase antibiotics is a highly effective agent.

The infections that occur following surgery on the female reproductive tract arise from the introduction of the normal vaginal flora into the surgical field. Pelvic surgery provides ideal conditions for the development of both aerobic and anaerobic infections, principally those that are polymicrobial rather than monomicrobial in origin. When surgery is performed on the reproductive tract through a bacteriologically contaminated field, such as the vagina, bacteria are seeded into the pedicles and surgical margins of pelvic tissues. This provides an excellent nidus for infection in the devitalized tissue bed. The destruction of tissue by clamps and sutures lowers the tissue oxidation-reduction potential, frequently referred to as the redox potential. This process of lowering tissue oxygen levels enhances the growth of facultative anaerobes that normally inhabit the vagina. As the tissue hypoxia progresses, strict anaerobes are the primary bacteria that survive and proliferate. Therefore, the usual postoperative infection in the vaginal vault, although initially polymicrobial, can be prevented if an adequate tissue level of a broad-spectrum antibiotic is present at the time of the operative contamination. The short-term (24-hour) intraoperative use of a broad-spectrum antibiotic has proven to be as effective as long-term (5–7 days) use in preventing postoperative infectious morbidity. Therefore, a preoperative, intraoperative, and postoperative dose of a broad-spectrum antibiotic that has particular sensitivity to gram-negative organisms, given at 6-hour intervals, will inhibit the growth of aerobic organisms. The reduced utilization of oxygen, by inhibiting the growth of aerobic organisms, will interrupt the oxidative-reductive cycle and prevent lowering of the redox potential. The secondary benefit of maintaining a high tissue oxygen level is the suppression of the growth of anaerobic bacteria. This simple technique of controlling the microbiologic environment of bacteria has proven effective in controlling the growth of both aerobic and anaerobic bacteria in a potentially contaminated operative field such as the vaginal vault (see Ch. 27).

In 1973, Ledger, Sweet, and Headington were among the first to demonstrate the effectiveness of short-term prophylactic antibiotic therapy. Since that time, innumerable studies have demonstrated that the various aminoglycoside or cephalosporin antibiotics have predictable effects in suppressing the growth of gram-negative aerobic bacteria, which are the most common type of bacterial infective agents in the operative site following vaginal or abdominal hysterectomy. Because the most common complication associated with vaginal hysterectomy is infection, the available data clearly indicate that with the intraoperative use of short-term antibiotics, the incidence of postoperative pelvic infection can be reduced dramatically. Although originally this benefit from prophylactic antibiotics was considered to be effective principally for the premenopausal patient, a decrease in infectious morbidity has also been demonstrated in the postmenopausal patient, particularly when a vaginal repair has been undertaken in conjunction with a vaginal hysterectomy. Recent reviews of this subject by Duff and Park and by Polk and associates provide clear evidence of the clinical benefit of this technique of controlling pelvic infection that has resulted from gynecologic surgery.

By reducing infection, postoperative short-term antibiotic prophylaxis results in a shortened hospital stay and a decrease in medical expense for the majority of patients. A prophylactic antibiotic should be a drug that is *not* used as a treatment of choice for overt pelvic infection. Further, the antibiotic should have a low incidence of toxic side-effects and should be capable of achieving an effective tissue concentration at the operative site within a short period following administration. Several agents have been shown to be effective in reducing pelvic infection following vaginal and abdominal hysterectomy, including ampicillin, cephaloridine (Loridine), cephalothin (Keflin), cephradine (Anspor), cefazolin (Ancef), and doxycycline (Vibramycin), to list but a few.

Prophylactic antibiotics may be effective in reducing the incidence of postoperative infectious morbidity, but they should never be used as a substitute for time-honored principles of adequate hemostasis and gentle handling of tissues. Although Wangensteen has made the uncomplimentary statement that "antibiotics will turn a third-class surgeon into a second-class surgeon, but will never turn a second-class surgeon into a first-class surgeon," there is a changing attitude regarding the effectiveness of the short-term, intraoperative use of broad-spectrum antibiotics in modern pelvic surgery. (Prophylactic antimicrobials are also discussed in Chapter 9.)

PREOPERATIVE PROCEDURES IN THE OPERATING SUITE

The patient is brought to the operating room area and is transferred to the operating table in the anesthesia room adjoining the surgical suite. A Kelly pad is placed on the foot of the operating table so that liquids used for the vaginal cleanup will drain into a floor basin. Most operations can be done without shaving the patient. If necessary, however, the patient's lower abdomen or vulva or both may be shaved in the anesthesia room prior to surgery. Since several minutes are required to attain a surgical plane of anesthesia, no time is lost as a result of shaving while the patient is unconscious. Removing excess hair with scissors may be more comfortable to the patient.

After shaving and catheterization, the patient is usually sufficiently anesthetized for a careful bimanual pelvic examination. In this examination, the operator can obtain very valuable information that may not be obtainable when the patient is awake. Following the pelvic examination, the perineum and the vagina are cleansed before all pelvic surgery. There is always the possibility that the findings at operation may make a total abdominal hysterectomy advisable, even when the preoperative plan in the operator's mind did not include such an extensive procedure. It is extremely disconcerting to find that a total hysterectomy must be performed at the time of a laparotomy if the vagina is not properly prepared. To prevent this circumstance, we have made the preoperative vaginal cleanup a routine procedure. To clean the perineum and the vagina, the nurse or surgical assistant first scrubs the vulva and the perineum with a sponge that is soaked with surgical soap or povidone-iodine solution and held in the gloved hand. Then the vagina is scrubbed with a soapy sponge held in the fingers. Following the vaginal scrub, the operator's fingers are spread to enlarge the outlet and the perineum is depressed to permit the soapy water or iodine solution to run out of the vagina. The solution is flushed away with sterile water that is poured into the vagina by the nurse. From this point on, the cleanup is done with a sterile sponge on a sponge forceps. This is used several times to clean the vagina with the appropriate antiseptic solution.

Next, an unfolded sterile sponge is inserted into the vagina. The end of the vaginal sponge is left protruding from the outlet, and the sponge forceps is left attached to facilitate its removal during the operation. The sponge absorbs any secretions that may come from the cervical canal as the result of operative manipulation. At operation, the sponge is removed by a nurse who pulls on the sponge forceps just before the vagina is opened at the time of total hysterectomy. If a hysterectomy is not done, the vaginal sponge is removed at the completion of the laparotomy.

After the vaginal cleanup, the abdomen is washed with chlorhexidine (Hibiclens). Particular attention is paid to cleansing the umbilicus with a Q-tip sponge. The abdomen is prepared by the nurse or surgical assistant with a 5-minute scrub using a povidone-iodine (Betadine) or similar antiseptic solution. The surgically prepared area should extend from the inferior rib cage, superiorly, to the mid-thigh, inferiorly. The lateral margins of the skin preparation should extend to the anterior iliac crest and anterior axillary line. In recent years, many clinics have used Viodrape placed over the skin to protect the incision from contamination by skin bacteria.

UNIVERSAL PRECAUTIONS FOR THE PREVENTION OF SEROPOSITIVITY FOR ACQUIRED IMMUNODEFICIENCY SYNDROME

As surgeons are at risk for acquiring seropositivity for acquired immunodeficiency syndrome (AIDS) through contamination from fluids and blood products, certain precautions should be taken at the time of surgery. In 1987 the Centers for Disease Control published a document that recommended that blood and other body fluid precautions be consistently used for all patients regardless of their blood-borne infectious status. This extension of blood and other body fluid precautions to all patients is referred to as "Universal Blood and Fluid Precautions" or "Universal Precautions." Under Universal Precautions, blood and certain body fluids of all patients are considered potentially infectious for human immunodeficiency virus (HIV), hepatitis B virus (HBV), and other blood-borne pathogens.

Universal Precautions are intended to prevent parenteral, mucous membrane, and nonintact skin exposure of the surgeon to blood-borne pathogens. In addition, immunization with HBV (hepatitis B virus) vaccine is recommended as an important adjunct to the Universal Precautions for surgeons who are exposed to blood products.

Protective barriers reduce the risk of exposure of the surgeon's skin or mucous membranes to potentially infectious materials. In the operating room protective barriers include gloves, gowns, masks, and protective eyeware. Gloves should reduce the incidence of contamination of the hands, but they cannot prevent penetrating injuries due to needles and other sharp instruments. Masks and protective eyeware, or face shields, should reduce the incidence of contamination of mucous membranes of the mouth, nose, and eyes. Special care should be taken to prevent injuries with needles, scalpels, or other sharp instruments or devices. Care should be taken to wash immediately and thoroughly hands and other skin surfaces that are contaminated with blood, body fluids containing visible blood, or other body fluids to which Universal Precautions apply.

Bibliography

Alexander S. Surgery in the cardiac patient. Surg Clin North Am 1970;50:567.

American Heart Association Committee Report. Prevention of bacterial endocarditis. Circulation 1977;56(1):139A.

Anderson DO, Ferris BC. Role of tobacco smoking in the causation of chronic respiratory disease. N Engl J Med 1962;267:787.

Antman EM, Stone PH, Muller JE, et al. Calcium channel blocking agents in the treatment of cardiovascular disorders. Part I: Basic and clinical electrophysiologic effects. Ann Intern Med 1980;93:875.

Appel GB, Neu HC. The nephrotoxicity of antimicrobial agents. N Engl J Med 296;663:1977. First of three parts.

Appel GB, Neu HC. The nephrotoxicity of antimicrobial agents. N Engl J Med 1977;296:722. Second of three parts.

Appel GB, Neu HC. The nephrotoxicity of antimicrobial agents. N Engl J Med 1977;296:784. Third of three parts.

Arkins R, Smessaert AA, Hicks RG. Mortality and morbidity in surgical patients with coronary artery disease. JAMA 1964;190:485.

Beck DE, Harford FJ, DiPalma JA. Comparison of cleansing methods in preparation for colonic surgery. Dis Col Rect 1985;28(7):491.

Behrendt DM, Morrow AG. General operative procedures after cardiac valve replacement—results and methods of management of 33 patients. Arch Surg 1968;96:824.

Berger SA, Nagar H, Gordon M. Antimicrobial prophylaxis in obstetric and gynecologic surgery: a critical review. J Reprod Med 1980;24:185.

Beta-Blocker Heart Attack Study Group. The beta-blocker heart attack trial. JAMA 1981;246:2073.

Bomalski JS, Phair JG. Alcohol, immunosuppression, and the lung. Arch Int Med 1982;142:2073.

Bonnar J. Venous thromboembolism and gynecologic surgery. Clin Obstet Gynecol 1985;28(2):432.

Cadanelli GP, Cavatorta E, Verrilli D. Chirurgia gynecologia e cardiopatie. Quad Clin Obstet Gynec 1967;22:911.

Centers for Disease Control. Universal precautions for prevention of transmission of human immunodeficiency virus, hepatitis B virus, and other bloodborne pathogens in health-care settings. MMWR 1988;37(24):377.

Clarke-Pearson DL, Creasman WT, Coleman ER, Synan IS, Hinshaw WM. Perioperative external pneumatic calf compression as thromboembolism prophylaxis in gynecologic oncology: report of a randomized clinical trial. Gynecol Oncol 1984;18:226.

Clarke-Pearson DL, Synan IS, Hinshaw WM, Coleman E, Creasman WT. Prevention of postoperative venous thromboembolism by external pneumatic calf compression in patients with gynecologic malignancy. Obstet Gynecol 1984;63(1):93.

Cohn JN, Franciosa JA. Vasodilator therapy in cardiac failure. N Engl J Med 1977;297:27.

Criteria Committee of the New York Heart Association. Diseases of the heart and blood vessels: nomenclature and criteria for diagnosis. 6th ed. Boston: Little, Brown, 1964.

Cunningham FG, Hamsell DL, DePalma RT, et al. Moxalactam for obstetric and gynecologic infections: in vitro and dose-finding studies. Am J Obstet Gynecol 1981;139:915.

Dana JB, Ohler RL. Influence of heart disease on surgical risk. JAMA 1956;162:878.

Devereaux RB, et al. Mitral valve prolapse. Circulation 1976;54:3.

Dodek A. The serum digoxin test: a clinical perspective. Cardiol Dig 1979;14:19.

Dreifus LS, Rabbino MD, Watanabe Y, Tabesh E. Arrhythmias in the postoperative period. Am J Cardiol 1963;12:431.

Duff P, Park RC. Antibiotic prophylaxis in vaginal hysterectomy: a review. Obstet Gynecol (suppl) 1980;55:193.

Eidenmiller LR, Awe C, Hodam RP, et al. General surgical procedures in valve replacement patients. Am Surg 1969;35:559.

Gazes PC. Non-cardiac surgery in cardiac patients—preoperative and operative management. Postgrad Med 1971;49:171.

German PM, Stackpole DA, Levenson DK, et al. Second opinion for elective surgery. N Engl J Med 1980;302:1169.

Gold MJ, Helvich M. A study of the complications related to anesthesia in asthmatic patients. Anesth Analg (Cleve) 1963;42:283.

Goldman L, Caldera DL, Southwick FS, et al. Cardiac risk factors and complications in noncardiac surgery. Medicine (Baltimore) 1978;57:357.

Greene HG. Cephalosporin therapy of soft tissue infections: an overview. J Int Med Res 1980;8(suppl 1):53.

Hoeprich PD. Current principles of antibiotic therapy. Obstet Gynecol 1980;55(suppl):121.

Horan LG, Flowers NC, Johnson JC. Significance of the diagnostic Q wave of myocardial infarction. Circulation 1971;43:428.

Jarkuberm JS, Braunwald E. Present status of digitalis treatment of acute myocardial infarction. Circulation 1972;45:891.

Journal of the American Medical Association. Recommendations for prevention of HIV transmission in health-care settings: leads from the MMWR. JAMA 1987;258(Supplement 2S):1441.

Jung R, et al. Comparison of three methods of respiratory care following upper abdominal surgery. Chest 1980;78:31.

Kannel WB, Feinlieb M. The natural history of angina pectoris in the Framingham Study—prognosis and survival. Am J Cardiol 1972;29:154.

Kass EH. The role of asymptomatic bacteriuria in the pathogenesis of pyelonephritis. In: Quinn EL, Kass EH, eds. Biology of pyelonephritis. Boston: Little Brown & Co, 1960:399.

Katholi RE, Nolan SP, McGuire B. Living with prosthetic heart valves, subsequent noncardiac operations and the risk of thromboembolism or hemorrhage. Am Heart J 1976;92:162.

Keelan MH, Jr. Evaluation of the gynecological patient with heart disease. Clin Obstet Gynecol 1973;16:80.

Ledger WJ. Prevention, diagnosis and treatment of postoperative infections. Obstet Gynecol 1980;55(suppl):203.

Ledger WJ, Sweet RL, Headington JT. Prophylactic cephaloridine in the prevention of postoperative pelvic infections in premenopausal women undergoing vaginal surgery. Am J Obstet Gynecol 1973;115:766.

Masukawa T, Levinson EF, Forst JK. The cytologic examination of breast secretions. Acta Cytol (Baltimore) 1966;10:261.

Mattingly RF. Surgery in the aging female. Clin Obstet Gynecol 1964;7:573.

Mattingly RF. The prophylactic use of antibiotics in pelvic surgery: a discussion. Obstet Gynecol 1980;55(suppl):267.

Mattingly TW. Patients with coronary disease as a surgical risk. Am J Cardiol 1963;12:279.

McCarthy EG, Finkel ML. Second consultant opinion for elective gynecologic surgery. Obstet Gynecol 1980;56:403.

Mills P, Rose J, Hollingsworth J, et al. Long term prognosis of mitral valve prolapse. N Engl J Med 1977;297:13.

Norwegian Multicenter Study Group. Timolol-induced reduction in mortality and reinfarction in patients surviving acute myocardial infarction. N Engl J Med 1981;304:801.

Okada RD, Boucher CA, Strauss HW, et al. Exercise radionuclide imaging approaches to coronary artery disease. Am J Cardiol 1980;46:1188.

Olgivie C. Physician among surgeons: thoughts on preoperative assessment. Thorax 1980;35:881.

Peterman TA, Cates W, Curran JW. The challenge of human immunodeficiency virus (HIV) and acquired immunodeficiency syndrome (AIDS) in women and children. Fertil Steril 1988;48(4):571.

Piscitelli JT, Simel DL, Addison WA. Who should have intravenous pyelograms before hysterectomy for benign disease? Obstet Gynecol 1987;69(4):541.

Polk BF, Shapiro M, Goldstein P, et al. Randomised clinical trial of perioperative cefazolin in preventing infection after hysterectomy. Lancet 1980;8166:437.

Savino JA, Del Guercio LRM: Preoperative assessment of high-risk surgical patients. Surg Clin N Am 1985;65(4):763.

Schlueter DP. Pulmonary risks. Clin Obstet Gynecol 16:91, 1973.

Selzer A, Cohn KE. Some thoughts concerning prophylactic use of digitalis. Am J Cardiol 1970;26:214.

Shapiro B. Evaluation of respiratory function in the perioperative period. ASA Refresher Courses 1979;221:1.

Skinner JF, Pearce ML. Surgical risk in the cardiac patient. J Chronic Dis 1964;17:57.

Stahlgren LH. An analysis of factors which influence mortality following extensive abdominal operations upon geriatric patients. Surg Gynecol Obstet 1961;113:283.

Stein M, Koota GM, Simon M, et al. Pulmonary evaluation of surgical patients. JAMA 1962;181:765.

Stone PH, Antman EM, Muller JE, et al. Calcium channel blocking agents in the treatment of cardiovascular disorders. Part II: Hemodynamic effects and clinical applications. Ann Int Med 1980;93:886.

Swartz WH. Prophylaxis of minor febrile and major infectious morbidity following hysterectomy. Obstet Gynecol 1979;54:285.

Swartz WH, Teichholz LE, Donoso F. Mitral valve prolapse—a review of associated arrhythmias. Am J Med 1977;62:377.

Tarhan S, Moffitt EA, Taylor WF, et al. Myocardial infarction after general anesthesia. JAMA 1972;220:1451.

Tinker JH, Tarhan S. Discontinuing anticoagulant therapy in surgical patients with cardiac valve prostheses: observations in 180 operations. JAMA 1978;239:738.

U.S. Department of Health and Human Services, National Center for Health Statistics. Monthly vital statistics report. 1981;29(13). (Published and unpublished data.)

Virchow R. Die Cellular pathologie in Ihre Begrundung auf physiologische und pathologische bewebelehre. Berlin: A. Hirschwald, 1858.

Wann LS, Dillon JC. Echocardiography of the aortic valve. In: DeVlieger M, ed. Handbook of clinical ultrasound. New York: John Wiley & Sons, 1978:453.

Wightman JA. A prospective survey of the incidence of postoperative pulmonary complications. Br J Surg 1968;55:85.

Postanesthesia and Postoperative Care

6

IRA R. HOROWITZ
JOHN A. ROCK

The most critical period of a patient's postoperative course occurs within the first 72 hours following surgery. Precise monitoring of the cardiovascular, renal, and respiratory systems provides the most valuable information about the patient's postoperative condition. Postoperative morbidity can be decreased with an appropriate preoperative evaluation of the surgical candidate. It is important to identify those patients at risk for developing venous thrombosis and to administer appropriate prophylaxis. Improved nutritional status in the preoperative and postoperative periods also improves wound healing and decreases the postoperative recovery time.

VASCULAR COMPLICATIONS

Incidence of Venous Thrombosis

Approximately half a million patients hospitalized every year have a deep venous thrombosis or pulmonary embolism. Of this number, 50,000 die. Fifteen percent of gynecology patients experience venous thrombosis, with a range of 5% to 45%, depending on the procedure performed and associated risk factors. Pulmonary embolism is responsible for 40% of the postoperative deaths in the gynecology patient. The sudden occurrence in a postoperative patient of respiratory distress that is followed by hypotension, chest pain, and cardiac arrhythmias signals a complication that can convert a successful operative procedure into a postoperative mortality. Recently, diagnostic studies have provided more accurate information on the frequency of this vascular complication and have identi-

fied those patients with deep venous thrombosis who are at risk to shed emboli. Preoperative and postoperative prophylaxis using heparin, dextran, antiembolic stockings, and intermittent pneumatic compression devices for moderate- and high-risk patients has reduced the incidence of pulmonary emboli. Clarke-Pearson and coauthors, using univariate and regression analysis, have designed a prognostic model to evaluate the risks of postoperative deep venous thrombosis for an individual patient. Preoperative prognostic factors identified in a prospective study of 411 gynecology patients were type of surgery, age, leg edema, nonwhite patient, severity of venous varicosities, prior radiation therapy, and prior history of deep venous thrombosis.

Essentially all the major factors contributing to postoperative venous thrombosis were described by Virchow more than 125 years ago, including (1) an increase in blood coagulability, (2) venous stasis, and (3) trauma to the vessel wall. Tissue injury activates blood coagulation by the extrinsic and intrinsic pathways (Fig. 6-1) by exposing the blood either to increased levels of tissue thromboplastin (extrinsic) or to subendothelial collagen in the vessel wall, which activates factor XII (intrinsic). Venous damage is particularly prevalent in patients undergoing radical surgery where skeletonization of the pelvic vasculature is performed. When postoperative infection and pelvic cellulitis occur, there is an acceleration of the clotting mechanism due to the release of tissue thromboplastin (extrinsic) and the activation of factor VII (extrinsic) by collagen. The activation of both extrinsic and intrinsic pathways results in the conversion of factor X to an active form that, in turn, interacts with factor V, calcium, and phospholipid from platelet factor 3 to convert prothrombin to thrombin

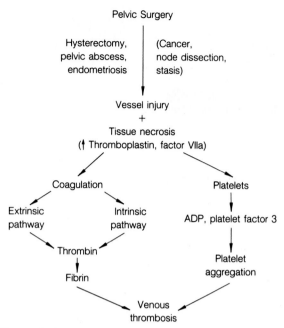

Figure 6–1. Formation of venous thrombus following various surgical procedures with the activation of clotting factors and aggregation of platelets.

dynamics occur in the preoperative, operative, and postoperative periods. Many investigators have found it advisable to perform the preoperative studies on high-risk patients on an ambulatory basis or, if the patient has been hospitalized for a significant time, to discharge her home for several weeks to increase her physical activity prior to elective surgery. Doran and others have shown that venous return from the lower extremities is decreased to one half its normal rate during the operative procedure. The decrease results from the loss of muscle tone that is caused by muscle relaxation from anesthetic agents. Iodine-125 (^{125}I)-labeled fibrinogen-scanning studies have demonstrated that venous clotting is initiated during the operative procedure in 50% of the patients who develop thrombosis in the postoperative period. Blood flow from the lower extremities is further reduced to approximately 75% the normal drainage flow immediately following surgery. This reduced flow rate persists for 10–14 days, because of the loss of pump action of the leg muscles. The major site of clot formation is in the soleal venous sinuses of the calf, a portion of the venous arcade that joins the posterior tibial and peroneal veins that drain the soleus muscle. Thrombi from these sinuses occur frequently

(Fig. 6-2). Thrombin is the rate-regulating proteolytic enzyme that controls the conversion of fibrinogen to fibrin, the basic component of a venous thrombus. Other coagulation factors that are known to be increased following surgery are, principally, factors VIII, IX, and XI, which increase as a result of activating the intrinsic pathway, and factor XII, which is activated by tissue collagen. There is also an increase in circulating platelets, platelet adhesiveness, and aggregation within 72–96 hours following surgery. In addition, fibrinogen and circulating fibrinolysin inhibitors increase. Normally, the fibrinolytic system, which is composed principally of plasmin formed from its inactive precursor, plasminogen, balances the clotting mechanism by digesting fibrin and fibrinogen and inactivating factors V and VIII. An acceleration of the clotting mechanism leads to a thrombus in either the venous or the arterial system. An excess of fibrinolytic activity causes blood to fail to clot and can produce serious hemorrhage. A proper balance of both is required for normal circulation.

Venous stasis is the cornerstone of postoperative thrombus formation. In the lower extremities and pelvis, it results in platelet aggregation and the adhesion of platelets to the vein wall with the release of a thromboplastin-like substance that forms a platelet–fibrin–red cell network that results in thrombus formation. These physiologic changes in venous hemo-

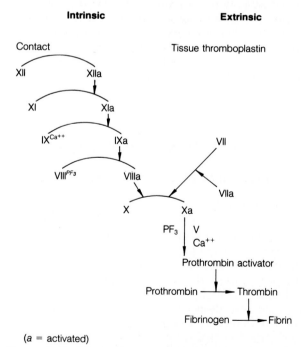

(*a* = activated)

Figure 6–2. Schematic representation of the cascade clotting mechanism, illustrating the role of extrinsic and intrinsic factors. Increases in tissue thromboplastin-like substance and collagen-activated factor XII initiate the formation of fibrin through the extrinsic and intrinsic pathways, principally by the activation of factor X.

behind the valves that are located at the point at which the sinuses drain into the collecting veins. Thrombi form frequently in these large sinuses or valve cusps in bedridden patients.

Another factor leading to venous stasis is prolonged surgery with tight packing of the intestines in the upper abdomen and obstruction of the underlying vena cava. The type and length of operation are directly related to the incidence of postoperative venous thrombosis, as outlined in Table 6-1.

Diagnosis of Venous Thrombosis

The traditional clinical methods used to diagnose venous thrombosis of the lower extremities are of limited value. Such methods may be in error in 50% of the cases and provide both false-positive and false-negative information. This diagnostic problem is due to the silent and insidious nature of the venous thrombus formation process, which occurs principally in the deep soleal veins in the lower extremities. Because the clinical diagnosis of this vascular complication is so inaccurate, more objective methods of diagnosis are required. In recent years, venography, ^{125}I-labeled fibrinogen scanning, Doppler ultrasound, and serial impedance plethysmography have been used along with a variety of other imaging techniques. Venography is regarded as the most definitive method for the diagnosis of venous thrombosis and has been used as the reference source against which other techniques are measured.

Venography

The venogram has had the widest clinical use of all available techniques in the study of venous thrombosis, with the most extensive clinical correlation in cases involving the large veins of the lower extremities. Venography is generally reserved for cases where there is clinical suspicion of venous thrombosis or a pulmonary embolus. Because it is an invasive technique, venography has limited usefulness as a screening procedure.

[125]I-Labeled Fibrinogen Scanning

Recent studies have used scintillation counterscanning of the lower extremities following the administration of ^{125}I-labeled fibrinogen. The incorporation of iodinated fibrinogen into a developing thrombus was first tested by Hobbs and Davies in 1960. The British study of Kakkar and coauthors in 1975 was one of the first to give clear evidence of the clinical accuracy of this technique in a collaborative, randomized study of more than 4000 patients. This study demonstrated a 93% correlation of the fibrinogen-scanning technique with venography in identifying a developing venous thrombus in the lower extremities. Preoperative monitoring is initiated 24 hours after the intravenous injection of 100 μc of ^{125}I-labeled fibrinogen; subsequently, monitoring is performed in the immediate postoperative period and daily thereafter. An iodine preparation is administered to prevent ^{125}I uptake by the thyroid. Scintillation readings taken at 2-in. intervals along the

TABLE 6–1
Risk Categories of Thromboembolism in Gynecologic Surgery

FACTOR	RISK CATEGORY		
	Low Risk	*Medium Risk*	*High Risk*
Age	Under 40 years	40 years and over	40 years and over
Contributing factors			
Surgery	Uncomplicated or minor	Major abdominal or pelvic	Major, extensive malignant disease involved
			Prior radiation treatment
Weight	Normal	Moderately obese (75–90 kg or >20% above ideal weight)	Mobidly obese (≥115 kg or >30% above ideal weight)
Medical diseases			Previous venous thrombosis
			Varicose veins (severe)
			Diabetes (insulin dependent)
Thromboembolism			
Calf vein thrombosis	2%	10–35%	30–60%
Iliofemoral vein thrombosis	0.4%	2–8%	5–10%
Fatal pulmonary embolism	0.2%	0.1–0.5%	1%
Recommended prophylaxis	Early ambulation and graduated-compression stockings	Low-dose heparin or dextran or intermittent pneumatic compression	Dextran or low-dose heparin and/or intermittent pneumatic compression

lower leg that monitor the venous flow in the deep veins of the calf are compared with precordial readings, and a percentage of the heart count is plotted graphically for each leg. Venous thrombosis is suspected when the level of radioactivity at any point in the leg is 20% greater than either the reading taken 24 hours earlier at the same point or the reading taken at the same point in the other leg. A diagnosis of venous thrombosis can be made if the scan remains abnormal for more than 24 hours. However, the test has specific limitations. It is unreliable in the upper thigh, because of the close proximity of the bladder, where the iodine is excreted in the urine, and because of the large veins and arteries in the pelvis, which increase the background noise. It is relatively insensitive in the diagnosis of established venous thrombosis, being positive in only 70% of the cases. Further, as long as 72 hours may be required before enough iodinated fibrinogen to give a positive result is deposited in the formed thrombus. Its major use, therefore, is in the prophylactic screening of high-risk patients to detect the earliest stage of deep venous thrombus formation.

Impedance Plethysmography

Impedance plethysmography is based on the measurement of the electrical resistance in a specific area of the body, such as the lower extremities. When blood flow has been reduced by venous outflow obstruction, such as with venous thrombosis, there is a marked reduction in the electrical resistance over the involved vessel. This technique is most specific in venous occlusion in the larger veins of the thigh—namely, the lower iliac, femoral, and popliteal. Its overall accuracy is 95% that of venography, but it is much less useful than venography for the detection of small calf vein thrombi. This is due to the caliber of the small soleus sinuses and the subtle changes in blood flow through these vessels. The ability of impedance plethysmography to detect asymptomatic venous thrombi in the calf veins has been found to be less than 50% that of venography.

Huisman and coauthors evaluated 471 outpatients clinically suspected of having acute deep venous thrombosis. Four sequential impedance plethysmograms were obtained on days 1, 2, 5, and 10 of the study. Of the 137 patients with abnormal results, 117 (85%) had abnormal results on day 1; the remaining 20 patients turned positive on subsequent days. Compared with the venogram, serial impedance plethysmography had a specificity of 92% and a sensitivity of 100%. By performing serial studies, the authors were able to improve their ability to diagnose deep venous thrombosis. In a similar study involving 252 patients, Vaccaro and coworkers reported a sensitivity of 84.2% and a specificity of 78.2% when attempting to diagnose deep venous thrombosis with a single study.

Doppler Ultrasound

The use of Doppler ultrasound, a noninvasive technique, has become more prevalent during the past decade for the diagnosis of venous thrombosis. In its major physiologic use, in the measurement of the velocity of blood flow in large vessels, a reflected signal is converted to the audible range and directed through a loudspeaker. No signal is heard when venous thrombosis is present, because of the obstruction of the vein. When used in the upper thigh, the technique is highly sensitive to venous thrombosis in the lower iliac, femoral, or popliteal vessels. However, sensitivity decreases rapidly in smaller vessels, particularly in the soleal sinuses of the calf, where the accuracy rate, in most series, is less than 60%. The technique is of limited value as a routine screening test for high-risk patients.

Real-Time Ultrasound

Real-time ultrasound diagnosis of deep venous thrombosis has recently been compared to venography. Aitken and Godden demonstrated a sensitivity of 94% and a specificity of 100% in evaluating a group of 46 patients with real-time ultrasound. In a similar study evaluating 121 patients, Appelman and coauthors found real-time ultrasound to have a sensitivity of 96% and a specificity of 97%.

Duplex Doppler Imaging

Recently, real-time ultrasound and Doppler examination have been combined in a procedure known as duplex B-mode imaging or duplex Doppler imaging, which enables the radiologist to visualize the thrombus and measure blood flow through the vessels. Langsfeld and associates examined 431 patients and diagnosed thrombi in 86. They reported a sensitivity of 100% and observed two false-positives, which resulted in a specificity of 78%. Upon further evaluation, it was found that, early in the protocol, the duplex B-mode imaging of one patient had been read incorrectly. The second patient had a term pregnancy and the observed decreased blood flow was a result of aortocaval compression from the pregnant uterus. An accurate study could have been obtained by positioning the patient on her side. Duplex B-mode imaging is a noninvasive procedure and will probably replace venography as the gold standard to diagnose deep venous thrombosis.

Indium-111 Platelet Imaging

[125]I-labeled fibrinogen is of limited value in detecting thrombi in the proximal femoral vein and in diagnosing pelvic thrombosis or pulmonary emboli. Clarke-Pearson and coauthors advocated using indium-111 (^{111}In) platelet imaging to diagnose deep venous thrombosis

and pulmonary emboli. When compared with diagnostic tests such as pulmonary angiography, lung scans, venograms, and ^{125}I fibrinogen counting, ^{111}In platelet imaging was found to have a sensitivity of 100% and a specificity of 90%. In recent animal studies, Oster and coauthors suggested using [111]In- or iodine-123–radiolabeled monoclonal antiplatelet antibodies for thrombus identification with radioimmunoscintigraphy. Peters and coauthors used ^{111}In-radiolabeled monoclonal antibodies in platelets in six patients, three of whom had thrombus formation. Two patients were positive and the third, with a chronic deep venous thrombosis (DVT), was radioimmunoscintigraphy-negative. Radiolabeled monoclonal antibodies are easier to produce than ^{111}In-radiolabeled platelets and do not have the risk of hepatitis and human T-cell lymphotrophic virus III (HTLV III) transmission that donor ^{125}I fibrinogen and ^{111}In platelets have. Additional trials in humans are needed.

Magnetic Resonance Imaging

Magnetic resonance imaging (MRI), in the past 3 years, has been used to evaluate venous clots. Rapoport and coauthors demonstrated in in vitro studies that acute clot when compared with stagnant blood resulted in a marked reduction in relaxation time of both T1 and T2 measurements. The relaxation time was also reduced as the clot aged. Spritzer and coauthors prospectively evaluated 16 patients and 17 extremities to compare limited-flip-angle, gradient-refocused MRI with venography. By pulsing, flowing blood is excited while the adjacent tissue becomes saturated and therefore produces a signal of lower intensity. Stasis of blood flow would act in a manner similar to that in the adjacent tissues with decreased intensity. In a study of 16 of 17 lower extremities, the authors were able to locate the thrombus correctly. The 17th extremity was correctly diagnosed to have iliac and femoral vein clots; however, MRI had also suggested the presence of calf and popliteal thrombi that were not confirmed on venography. Using the GRASS images (gradient-recalled acquisition in a steady state), Mintz and coauthors reported MRI diagnosis of puerperal ovarian vein thrombosis. MRI thrombus diagnosis is in its infancy. As our understanding of this technique increases and technology improves, MRI will prove to be a valuable noninvasive tool to diagnose thrombus formation. The advantage MRI has over computed tomography (CT) is that it does not require the use of intravenous contrast.

Risk Factors for Vascular Complications

Several factors have been observed that present a clinical profile of the patient who is prone to venous thrombosis and pulmonary embolism (see Table 6-1).

Among the many clinical factors that predispose to venous thrombosis in women, the following are the most prevalent: age greater than 40, obesity greater than 20% above ideal weight, prolonged surgery, and immobility in the preoperative, intraoperative, and postoperative periods. Pelvic malignancy, previous thromboembolism, severe diabetes, heart failure, previous radiation therapy, and chronic pulmonary disease also increase the risk of vascular thrombi.

Age

In autopsy studies by Sevitt and Gallagher, the incidence of deep venous thrombosis was greatest in patients over 60 years of age. Many additional studies have demonstrated a linear increase in fatal pulmonary emboli as patient age increases. The major correlation in such patients relates to degenerative changes in the vascular tree. The incidence of pulmonary embolism following major surgery increases sharply in women over 40 years of age.

Obesity

The risk of thromboembolism is decidedly increased in the obese patient. Breneman recognized obesity as one of the most significant factors in thromboembolic disease in the operative patient. His study of patients with thromboembolic disease demonstrated that they were 21.6% above their ideal weight. Obesity increases the likelihood of thrombus formation largely because of increased venous stasis, which is aggravated by postoperative immobility.

Immobility

Prolonged inactivity in the preoperative patient causes an impairment in the venous circulation of the lower extremities. Preoperative immobilization, such as that required for prolonged diagnostic evaluation, produces a decrease in muscle tone of the lower extremities with diminished venous flow. These hemodynamic changes result in sludging of the platelets and red cells and set the stage for venous thrombosis during the operative period. Flanc and associates and Kemble have clearly demonstrated this, using ^{125}I-labeled fibrinogen scanning before and immediately after surgery. They observed that in 50% of patients who ultimately developed postoperative thrombosis, the clot formation began during the operative procedure. Similarly, the patient who has undergone prolonged anesthesia with generalized muscle relaxation has more venous stagnation of the lower extremities and a higher incidence of postoperative thromboembolism. It is important to reemphasize that the nidus for venous thrombosis frequently occurs before or, more commonly, during the operative procedure. Consequently, prophylactic treatment for the high-risk patient should be initiated prior to surgery and should be continued until the patient is fully ambulatory.

Postoperative immobilization provides an added physiologic insult to preexisting venous stasis. As many as 66% of patients who develop postoperative venous thrombosis have thrombosis, as detected by ^{125}I-labeled fibrinogen scanning, within 48 hours of surgery. Such anatomic positions as sitting with the legs crossed, sitting with the legs dangling from the bed, and sitting in an exaggerated Fowler's position impair venous return from the lower extremities. The high-risk patient (Table 6-2) in particular should be ambulated vigorously and, when confined to bed, should have the legs and trunk elevated approximately 15° above the horizontal. Immobilization in bed can be more hazardous than the physiologic impact of advancing age.

Other Factors

Other factors that lead to increased risk of thrombosis and pulmonary embolism include varicose veins, previous thromboembolism, severe diabetes, cardiac failure, and chronic pulmonary disease—all of which impair circulation, resulting in stasis and an increased frequency of venous thrombosis. Malignancy is also a factor in venous thrombosis, although the exact mechanism is not fully understood. Many tumors undergoing tissue breakdown are known to elaborate a thromboplastinlike substance that may predispose to increased thrombosis. In addition, previous radiation therapy increases the cancer patient's risk of developing venous thrombosis.

It is evident that a clinical profile can be developed for the high-risk patient. The paradigmatic high-risk patient is a woman who is more than 40 years of age, is 30% above her ideal weight, is diabetic, has varicose veins and/or heart disease, has been in the hospital for a prolonged period for medical evaluation or treatment, and has a malignant tumor. Regardless of the nature of the pelvic disease, the greater the number of risk factors, the longer the operation, and the more difficult the surgical procedure, the more frequent is the occurrence of venous thrombosis and pulmonary embolus. Patients who embody one or more of these surgical risks should have intensive monitoring and prophylactic treatment for venous thrombosis.

Treatment of Venous Thrombosis

Prophylaxis

The most effective treatment of venous thrombosis is prevention. Because between 5% and 45% of patients undergoing major gynecologic surgery develop venous thrombosis of the lower extremity, a prophylactic method of preventing this complication should be considered prior to surgery. In about 20% of cases, venous thrombi in the calf veins extend to the popliteal or femoral vessels, and in an estimated 40% of these, the patient will develop pulmonary emboli. These facts are sufficient to warrant the prophylactic treatment of the high-risk patient in an effort to avoid this life-threatening sequence of events.

Low-Dose Heparin. Many randomized prospective studies document the reduction of deep venous thrombosis from an incidence of 35% to 45% in untreated high-risk patients to approximately 7% in similar patients treated prophylactically with low-dose heparin. These studies have been conducted during the past three decades and were verified in 1975 by Kakkar and coauthors in a multicenter study of more than 4000 surgical patients over 40 years of age (Table 6-3). This study evaluated the effectiveness of low-dose heparin given prophylactically at doses of 5000 IU of calcium heparin, subcutaneously, 2 hours before surgery and every 8 hours after for the subsequent 7 postoperative days. The study demonstrated the benefit of low-dose heparin by reducing the incidence of thrombi from 25% in the untreated control group to 8% in the low-

TABLE 6–2
Profile of Patient at High Risk
for Venous Thrombosis

FACTOR	CONDITION
Age	>40 years
Obesity	
Moderate	75–90 kg or >20% above ideal weight
Morbid	≥115 kg or >30% above ideal weight with reduced fibrinolysin and immobility
Immobility	
Preoperative	Prolonged hospitalization; venous stasis
Intraoperative	Prolonged operative time; loss of pump action of calf muscles; compression of vena cava
Postoperative	Prolonged bed confinement; venous stasis
Trauma	Damage of wall of pelvic veins
	Radical pelvic surgery
Malignancy	Release of tissue thromboplastin
	Activation of factor X; reduced fibrinolysin
Radiation	Prior radiation therapy
Medical diseases	Diabetes mellitus
	Cardiac disease; heart failure
	Severe varicose veins
	Previous venous thrombosis with or without embolization
	Chronic pulmonary disease

TABLE 6–3
Pulmonary Embolism and Deep Venous Thrombosis in Patients on Low-Dose Heparin and in Controls

	LOW-DOSE HEPARIN	CONTROL
No. of patients	2045	2076
No. of deaths from all causes	80	100
Deaths caused by pulmonary embolism (verified at autopsy)	2	16
Deep venous thrombosis	8%	25%

Adapted from Kakkar et al, 1975.

dose-heparin-treated group. The most significant observation from this study was that 16 patients in the control, untreated group and only two patients in the heparin-treated group died of acute massive pulmonary embolism as revealed on autopsy.

Of interest is the fact that in the prophylactic use of low-dose heparin, there is no significant alteration of clotting time and, as a consequence, there is no increase in operative or postoperative bleeding. This phenomenon is attributed to the mechanism of action of heparin, which binds to antithrombin III and exerts its major anticoagulant effect in combination with this naturally occurring inhibitor. Together they inhibit the activated coagulation factors XIIa, XIa, Xa, and thrombin. Low doses of heparin interfere with the early stages of coagulation before thrombin is formed, thereby preventing thrombus formation without significantly altering the clotting factors in the plasma. These results as well as those of other studies recorded in Table 6-4 indicate that this method of prophylactic heparin therapy has been eminently successful in reducing the incidence of deep venous thrombosis in the surgical patient. Low-dose subcutaneous heparin, administered at a reduced dose of 5000 IU 2 hours preoperatively and every 12 hours postoperatively for 5 days, has proven efficacious in preventing thromboembolism.

Dihydroergotamine/Low-Dose Heparin. Nine years after Kakkar's landmark study, Sasahara and co-authors evaluated dihydroergotamine (DHE)/heparin prophylaxis in the prevention of deep venous thrombosis (Table 6-5). Dihydroergotamine mesylate, 0.5 mg, exerts a selective constrictive effect on the veins and venules and has a minimal effect on arteries and arterioles. By combining heparin with DHE, it is possible to alter the coagulability of blood with heparin and to decrease venous stasis and accelerate peripheral venous return with DHE. The incidence of deep venous thrombosis was significantly decreased in patients treated with 5000 IU of DHE/heparin sodium every 12 hours until postoperative day 5 as compared with patients who received other treatments (see Table 6-5). DHE mesylate is contraindicated in patients with severe vascular disease, severe hypertension, sepsis, or impaired liver or kidney function. The results of collaborative studies of prophylactic doses of DHE/heparin (5000 IU twice daily) are comparable to studies mentioned in this chapter in which prophylactic doses of heparin (5000 IU three times daily) are administered or intermittent pneumatic compression devices are employed.

Dextran 70/Dextran 40. In 1972, Bonnar and Walsh suggested using dextran 70 to prevent thrombo-

TABLE 6–4
Results of Prophylactic Treatment of Venous Thrombosis Following Gynecologic Surgery*

STUDY	DATE	TYPE OF SURGERY	NO. OF PATIENTS	VENOUS THROMBOSIS (%)				
				Control	*Heparin*	*Dextran*	*Oral AC[†]*	*Pneumatic Calf Compression*
Bonnar et al	1973	Simple hysterectomy	260	15.0	—	0.1	—	—
		Radical malignant	62	33.0	—	5.0	—	—
Ballard et al	1973	Major gynecol age 40	110	29.0	3.6	—	—	—
McCarthy et al	1974	Major gynecol	130	—	10.9	16.2	—	—
Baetschi et al	1975	Major gynecol	458	—	2.3	—	4.7	—
Gjonnaess and Abildgaard	1976	Major gynecol age 50	95	8.0	2.0	—	—	—
Adolf et al	1978	Major gynecol	454	29.3	7.0	—	—	—
Taberner et al	1978	Major gynecol	146	23.0	6.0	—	6.0	—
Clarke-Pearson et al	1983	Gynecol malignant	185	12.4	14.8	—	—	—
Clarke-Pearson et al	1984	Gynecol malignant	107	34.6	—	—	—	12.7

*Detected by ^{125}I-labeled fibrinogen scan.
†AC = anticoagulants.

TABLE 6–5
Thrombosis Prevention with Dihydroergotamine Mesylate Prophylaxis

TREATMENT AND DOSE*	NO. OF PATIENTS TREATED	PATIENTS WITH DVT Frequency (%)	PATIENTS WITHOUT DVT Frequency (%)	P†
DHE/heparin sodium, 5000 IU	214	18 (8.4)	196 (91.6)	—
DHE/heparin sodium, 2500 IU	226	32 (14.2)	194 (85.8)	0.0396
Heparin sodium, 5000 IU	222	32 (14.4)	190 (85.6)	0.0341
DHE mesylate, 0.5 mg	110	18 (16.4)	92 (83.6)	0.0263
Placebo	108	22 (20.4)	86 (79.6)	0.0024

Adapted from Sasahara et al, 1984.
*All treatment modalities administered 2 hours prior to surgery and every 12 hours postoperatively for 5 days.
†P level compares with DHE/heparin sodium, 5000 IU.

sis after pelvic surgery. Bernstein and coauthors decreased the incidence of leg vein thrombosis from 33% to 5% in patients undergoing radical hysterectomies who received dextran 70 prophylaxis. Dextran's mechanism in preventing thrombosis is through an effect on decreasing platelet function, coagulation factors V and VII, and fibrinolysis. To obtain adequate prophylaxis, dextran 70 is initiated during the operative procedure or immediately at its conclusion. Infusion of 1 L of dextran 70 over 6–8 hours should provide protection for 5 days. Dextran 40, however, is cleared rapidly and should be administered at a continuous infusion rate of 20 cc/hr. Alternatively, 500 cc of dextran 40 may be transfused over a period of 4–6 hours daily. Dextran 70 has been found to be as efficacious as low-dose heparin in preventing thromboembolism in patients undergoing major surgical procedures. In 1986 the NIH Consensus Development Conference on Prevention of Venous Thrombosis and Pulmonary Embolism advocated the use of dextran prophylaxis in patients at moderate and high risk for developing venous thrombosis.

Low-Molecular-Weight Heparin. Low-molecular-weight heparin (LMWH) is not available in the United States at the time of this writing. Several clinical trials, however, are presently being performed in Europe. LMWH fragment potentiates the inhibition of factor Xa and should have less of an effect than heparin in prolonging the partial thromboplastin time. Bergqvist and coauthors compared low-dose heparin, 5000 IU twice daily, with LMWH (kabi 2165), 5000 IU once daily, in a randomized, prospective, double-blind multicenter trial. Thrombus formation was observed in 4.3% of the patients receiving low-dose heparin and in 6.4% of those receiving LMWH. Hemorrhagic complications were much more prevalent in the group treated with LMWH, 11.6% versus 4.7% of those treated with heparin. These results were recently supported by a large multicenter study in France (Samama and co-authors) comparing subcutaneous heparin, 5000 IU three times daily, with LMWH (Enoxaparine) at doses of 20 mg, 40 mg, or 60 mg, once daily. The researchers did not find any of the preceding regimens to be significantly superior. Twenty milligrams per day of Enoxaparine was found to be as safe and efficacious as unfractionated heparin, 5000 IU subcutaneously t.i.d., in preventing postoperative thrombus formation. Sasahara and coauthors evaluated LMWH and heparin sodium with the addition of DHE mesylate, 0.5 mg, to each. No significant difference was observed when comparing the ability of LMWH/DHE and H/DHE to prevent postoperative deep venous thrombosis. In addition, hemorrhagic complications of LMWH/DHE q.d. and H/DHE b.i.d. were comparable. The authors believe that the once-daily regimen of LMWH/DHE will gain greater patient and nursing staff acceptance and prove cost effective.

Compression Modalities. Initial studies in 1944 by Stanton and coauthors used static compression to decrease venous stasis. By decreasing the luminal diameter, blood flow velocity was increased. Sigel and coauthors showed an increase in blood velocity of 20% in patients using graduated elastic compression stockings versus 200% with intermittent sequential pneumatic compression. When comparing intermittent sequential pneumatic compression with uniform intermittent calf compression, Mittleman and coauthors found the former to be more effective in increasing blood flow in the thigh region. It is accepted that compression modalities decrease at least one component of Virchow's triad, stasis. Several investigators believe compression modalities may have a marked effect on a second component in Virchow's triad, coagulability. Several authors (Allenby and associates, Tarnay and associates, Caprini and associates) have shown that intermittent pneumatic compression (IPC) stimulates fibrinolysis. The role of IPC in increasing prostaglandin production has been suggested in two recent studies. Guyton and coauthors identified an increased production of 6-ketoprostaglandin F1 in patients undergoing IPC when compared with controls. Frangos and coauthors illustrated in human endothelial cell cultures a 16-fold increase in prostacyclin production in cells under conditions of pulsatile shear stress versus a twofold increase with constant shear stress when compared with controls.

Graduated Compression Stockings

Initial studies evaluating antiembolic stockings were inconclusive and relied on several different methods to diagnose thrombosis (clinical DVT and pulmonary embolism [PE] versus ^{125}I fibrinogen uptake). In 1975, Sigel and coauthors designed a graduated compression thromboembolism-deterrent (TED) stocking with pressures of 18, 14, 8, 10, and 8 mm Hg from the ankle to upper thigh. Scurr and coauthors evaluated the efficiency of TED Hose in 75 patients over 40 years of age undergoing major abdominal surgery with only one leg covered by the TED Hose. During clinical evaluation or ^{125}I fibrinogen testing, 19 patients developed a DVT in the control leg and only one in the stockinged leg. An additional 110 patients were evaluated by Inada and coauthors, with each patient wearing TED Hose on one leg. Deep venous thrombosis was found in 14.5% of the controls and 3.6% of the legs with stockings. Malignancy has been shown to predispose patients to the formation of deep venous thrombosis, secondary to stasis and plasminogen production by the tumor. Allan and coauthors demonstrated the efficacy of graduated compression stockings in preventing DVT formation in patients undergoing major abdominal surgery for benign and malignant diseases. The presence of a DVT was demonstrated by ^{125}I fibrinogen testing, with the following results: in patients with benign disease, DVT was present in 24.5% of the control limbs and 6.1% of the stockinged limbs, whereas in patients with malignancy, the figures were 27.9% of the control limbs versus 11.5% of the stockinged limbs. The NIH Consensus Development Conference on Prevention of Venous Thrombosis and Pulmonary Embolism in March, 1986, suggested that graduated compression stockings with early ambulation would provide sufficient prophylaxis in the low-risk gynecology and obstetrics operative candidate.

External Intermittent Pneumatic Compression

External compression of the lower extremities decreases stasis and improves fibrinolysis. Nicolaides and coauthors (1980) compared intermittent sequential pneumatic compression, nonsequential (one-chamber)

pneumatic compression, and heparin in preventing postoperative deep venous thrombosis. Using pressures of 35, 30, and 20 mm Hg sequentially for 12 seconds at the ankle, calf, and thigh, Nicolaides and associates observed a 240% increase in the peak blood velocity. When using a single chamber inflated at 35 mm Hg for 12 seconds, the peak blood velocity increased 180%. Using the ^{125}I fibrinogen test, the authors demonstrated that the intermittent sequential pneumatic compression device was as effective as heparin, 5000 units/12 hours, in preventing deep vein thrombosis. The sequential device was also found to be more effective than the single chamber in preventing thrombosis of the lower extremities. In addition, intermittent sequential pneumatic compression increased the time interval for clot formation proximal to the calf when compared with heparin. In another study, Nicolaides and coauthors (1983) compared electrical calf stimulation, low-dose subcutaneous heparin, and intermittent sequential compression and the use of TED stockings in 150 patients over the age of 30 undergoing major abdominal surgery. The incidence of ^{125}I-fibrinogen-detected DVT was 18%, 9%, and 4%, respectively. In a prospective study, Clarke-Pearson and coauthors demonstrated the efficacy of external pneumatic calf compression in preventing postoperative venous thromboembolism in patients undergoing surgery for a gynecologic malignancy. All 107 patients were prospectively screened for deep venous thrombosis with impedance plethysmography and ^{125}I fibrinogen testing. The control group did not receive thromboembolic prophylaxis, whereas nonsequential external pneumatic pressure cuffs with pressures of 40–45 mm Hg every 12 seconds were placed on the lower extremities of the remaining patients. Deep venous thrombosis or pulmonary embolism was present in 34.6% of the controls compared with 12.7% of those who received external pneumatic calf compression devices intraoperatively and for 5 postoperative days ($P < .005$). The NIH Consensus Development Conference on Prevention of Venous Thrombosis and Pulmonary Embolism recommended external pneumatic compression as a prophylactic measure in patients at moderate and high risk. Patients with a malignancy were felt to benefit from a combination of low-dose heparin and external pneumatic compression.

Thrombosis in Malignancies

Since its initial description in 1868, Trousseau's syndrome of migratory thrombotic disease in neoplasias has been described in conjunction with a multitude of primary tumors. The predominant histology is an adenocarcinoma. In a comprehensive review of the literature in 1977, Sach and coauthors at the Johns Hopkins Hospital identified 123 cases with Trousseau's syndrome. The patients presented with thrombus formation in several locations: venous, arterial, and cardiac. Nusbacher, in a series of 68 patients presenting with carcinoma, noted that 75% initially presented with migratory thrombophlebitis prior to the diagnosis of a neoplasia and 50% had a pulmonary embolism. In 128 patients who had pulmonary embolism documented by angiography, Gore and coauthors showed an increased incidence in diagnosing malignancies after a pulmonary embolism. The increased hypercoagulable state of a malignancy predisposes the patient to embolic processes, including pulmonary embolism.

Treatment of patients with Trousseau's syndrome consists of identification of the malignancy and appropriate treatment. Anticoagulation with IV heparin followed by oral Coumadin compounds is required to decrease the thrombosis and consumption of platelets and clotting factors. Several patients have been found to be resistant to Coumadin and require daily maintenance with heparin. Sach and coauthors noted that all patients not responding to heparin were not sensitive to Coumadin compounds. However, a majority resistant to Coumadin responded to heparin. Proponents of Coumadin therapy suggest that Coumadin is a small nonpolar molecule that can diffuse out of the vascular space and act directly at the tumor site or intravascularly as an anticoagulant. Heparin is a large, charged compound unable to diffuse out of the vascular compartment and as such may not have a direct effect on the third-spaced tumor cells that produce a procoagulant. Heparin should be used as first-line therapy in patients with migratory thrombophlebitis. When the patient is fully anticoagulated, attempts should be made to administer an oral agent such as Coumadin. Patients resistant to Coumadin should be treated with subcutaneous or intravenous heparin on an outpatient basis.

After identification of a primary malignancy, patients with Trousseau's syndrome are treated by decreasing fibrin degradation, decreasing platelet consumption, and decreasing clot migration and embolization. Physical examination findings consistent with thrombophlebitis, arterial emboli, and bleeding may herald the presence of a malignancy. In addition to treating patients' coagulopathy, identifying its etiology should include evaluating for a malignancy. As previously mentioned, an embolus is frequently the result of the hypercoagulable state of a malignancy that may be present. Hematologic changes, including increased fibrinopeptide A (FPA), increased fibrin split products (FSP), increased turnover rate of fibrinogen, prolonged prothrombin time (PT), and microangiopathic hemolytic anemia, frequently present as a result of intravascular coagulation and fibrinolysis in patients with neoplasias.

Trousseau's syndrome in patients with gynecologic malignancies has not been addressed extensively in the gynecologic literature. Intravascular coagulation and fibrinolysis and migratory thrombosis in the form of venous and arterial emboli as well as pulmonary embolism continue to present the gynecologist with a clinical dilemma.

Anticoagulant Therapy

There is general agreement that deep venous thrombosis should be treated initially with intravenous heparin, using 5000 to 10,000 IU as an intravenous bolus. This produces therapeutic levels for anticoagulation in most patients. Since the major effect of an intravenous bolus of heparin will be cleared from the plasma within 4 hours, maintenance doses of heparin should be either by intermittent intravenous injections at intervals of 4–6 hours or, preferably, by continuous intravenous infusion at a rate of 1000–1200 IU per hour. We prefer to use a constant-infusion intravenous pump that is reliable in delivering small continuous doses of heparin, because when heparin is administered by intermittent intravenous bolus, 15% to 25% of patients will receive either an inadequate or an excessive dosage. Continuous heparinization by the intravenous route prevents the rise and fall of the heparin level and avoids recurrent thrombosis during the period of inadequate anticoagulation and potential bleeding complications when heparin levels are increased.

The level of anticoagulation should be carefully monitored 30 minutes prior to each scheduled intermittent bolus. In patients receiving continuous intravenous infusion, the level of anticoagulation may be assessed at any time. An anticoagulation level equivalent to a Lee-White clotting time that is two to three times the control level is considered adequate. Alternatively, an activated partial thromboplastin time of 1.5–2 times the control levels indicates adequate anticoagulation. Obviously, the monitoring method should be in accordance with the local preference of the clinical laboratory being used. Once optimal levels are established, clotting studies may be done at 24-hour intervals to determine proper maintenance doses of heparin. The duration of intravenous treatment is difficult to specify, but treatment should be continued for at least 5–7 days, until there has been resolution of the thrombus in the leg veins or until thrombi have become firmly organized and attached to the vessel wall. If clinical signs of improvement are not clearly demonstrated, more than 7 days of treatment may be required.

The symptomatic patient with acute thrombophlebitis should also be maintained at bed rest until the symptoms of pain and fever have subsided. The patient's leg should be maintained in an elevated position until the edema has completely subsided, at which time progressive ambulation is permitted. It is our policy to restrict ambulation until the leg edema has subsided. After 5–7 days of heparin therapy, oral anticoagulation is initiated. The combined medication of oral Coumadin and tapered doses of heparin is used for approximately 48–72 hours, after which Coumadin therapy is continued alone. Proper Coumadin therapy is aimed at maintaining a prothrombin time approximately 2.5 times the normal control. The Coumadin therapy is usually continued for 4–6 weeks.

The rationale for the treatment of asymptomatic deep venous thrombosis of the lower extremity has been questioned by many surgeons. In brief, some simply ignore this subclinical diagnosis and consider this vascular phenomenon to be an innocuous sequela of pelvic surgery. However, if patients with established venous thrombosis are not treated, the risk of serious morbidity or, possibly, mortality must be considered. The major risk is the extension of the venous thrombus into the popliteal and proximal veins of the thigh, which reportedly occurs in approximately 20% of cases. A Doppler scan, plethysmogram, or venogram is required to identify a proximal thrombosis. It is estimated that 40% of these patients, or 8% of the group with thrombosis of the calf veins, will have pulmonary emboli and, more important, recurrent embolization. On the conservative side, one might question the advisability of treating the 80% of patients who do not have proximal migration of the venous clot into the thigh to protect the 20% who do. If the 8% risk of pulmonary embolization is not sufficient reason for treatment, one should consider that once extension of the thrombosis into the proximal vessels has occurred, nearly two thirds of the patients will have residual disease in the venous system of the leg, with loss of valve function and impairment of venous return. This complication will frequently lead to the postphlebitic syndrome of chronic pain and lymphedema of the lower extremity. Because of these unhappy consequences, the prudent surgeon should consider the brief treatment of documented deep venous thrombosis to be a relatively cost-efficient method of managing this vascular complication of pelvic surgery.

Acute iliofemoral thrombosis is one of the most serious and hazardous complications of venous thrombosis of the lower extremity. An estimated 40% of patients with this condition develop pulmonary emboli. This condition is difficult to misdiagnose because in the acute stage, commonly called phlegmasia cerulea dolens, the leg becomes exquisitely tender, edematous, and cyanotic. During the acute stage there may be high morbidity from gangrene as well as high mortality from pulmonary embolism. This condition also results in a high incidence of chronic postphlebitic venous obstruction with chronic pain and peripheral edema. Effective ther-

apy requires immediate anticoagulation as outlined. If complete occlusion occurs, surgical treatment is usually required. Unless the clot is removed from the iliofemoral vessels, propagation into the vena cava and pulmonary embolization may occur in as many as 50% of cases, according to Mavor.

Venography is useful in confirming the diagnosis of iliofemoral thrombosis and is essential in evaluating the extent of involvement of the contiguous deep veins. When a pulmonary embolus has occurred, venography is also helpful in determining the presence of nonocclusive contralateral thrombosis from the opposite leg, which may be the site of origin of the embolus. Most cases of iliofemoral thrombosis are insidious in origin and can be treated medically with heparin therapy if diagnosed early, thereby avoiding complete vascular occlusion leading to massive swelling of the leg with pooling of blood, which may produce hypovolemia. Although the risk of mobilization of an embolus is always present, when gangrene has set in it is urgent that immediate thrombectomy be performed, with clearance of the iliofemoral segments. With the use of intravenous heparin therapy and early thrombectomy, the incidence of pulmonary emboli has been extremely low. In these acutely ill patients, intravenous heparin must be maintained continuously until there is complete resolution of the leg edema, inflammation, and pain in the calf and thigh. Only then can the patient be ambulated and the process of oral anticoagulation be initiated. These patients require not only early and aggressive management, both medical and surgical, but continuation of the anticoagulation therapy for 6–9 months for complete vascular canalization and prevention of recurrent thrombosis.

PULMONARY COMPLICATIONS

DONALD P. SCHLUETER

Hypoventilation

Hypoventilation is one of the most frequent and dangerous complications in the immediate postoperative period, even in patients with normal lungs. To assess ventilation, the expired gas can be collected and the volume expired per minute (minute volume = V_E) can be determined. However, a portion of this gas ventilates non-gas-exchanging areas of the lung, namely, conducting airways referred to as dead space. This ventilation is wasted, since it does not participate in gas exchange. The normal dead space volume is approximately equal in pulmonary milliliters to the person's ideal weight in pounds (ie, a 150-lb female has a dead space volume of 150 ml). To calculate the effective or alveolar ventilation, the dead space must be subtracted from the tidal volume and the difference multiplied by the respiratory rate. Gross errors in the estimation of ventilation can be made if only V_E is considered. If tidal volume decreases from 500 to 250 ml but respiratory rate doubles from 14 to 28 respirations per minute (rpm), minute volume remains at 7.0 l. However, assuming a dead space of 150 ml, the alveolar ventilation under these conditions decreases from 4.9 to 2.8 l, resulting in significant alteration in blood gases. This type of respiratory pattern is common in the patient with abdominal surgery, who tends to decrease tidal volume to avoid pain. Hypoventilation is defined as a level of alveolar ventilation that is insufficient to prevent accumulation of carbon dioxide. The causes include depression of central respiratory control from obesity, neuromuscular disease, pain, restrictive dressings, immobility, hypomobility, and increased carbon dioxide production. Obviously, patients with obstructive and restrictive respiratory impairment are much more likely to develop hypoventilation during this critical early postoperative period.

Inadequate ventilation may not be clinically obvious unless an estimate of alveolar ventilation is made. Ultimately, arterial blood gas studies are the most accurate measure of alveolar ventilation. Table 6-6 shows the effect of decreasing alveolar ventilation on the arterial blood gases. From these data, it can be seen that although the arterial carbon dioxide tension ($Paco_2$) rises almost linearly as alveolar ventilation decreases, changes in oxygenation (Sao_2 = arterial oxygen saturation) are modest until respiratory acidosis is severe. Thus, the best indicator of adequate ventilation is the $Paco_2$. A normal arterial oxygen tension (Pao_2) in the presence of a severe respiratory acidosis (elevated $Paco_2$) would implicate the administration of oxygen as a causative factor in the hypoventilation.

Acute Ventilatory Failure

The treatment of acute ventilatory failure manifested by hypoventilation and a $Paco_2$ greater than 50 mm Hg is mechanical ventilatory support until the causative fac-

TABLE 6–6
Effect of Decreasing Alveolar Ventilation on Arterial Blood Gases

ALVEOLAR VENTILATION (l/min)	ARTERIAL BLOOD GASES			
	Pao_2 (mm Hg)	Sao_2 (%)	$Paco_2$ (mm Hg)	pH
5.0	100	96	40	7.40
4.0	82	94	50	7.32
3.0	68	87	75	7.20
2.0	30	40	105	7.05

tors can be alleviated. This may require several hours to several days. It is important, therefore, to leave the endotracheal tube in place following surgery until adequate spontaneous ventilation and arterial blood gas levels have been demonstrated. The adequacy of respiratory mechanics can be determined by measuring tidal volume and inspiratory effort. The tidal volume should exceed 10 ml/kg, and inspiratory pressure should be greater than − 20 cm H_2O. The tidal volume alone is not a reliable indicator of respiratory adequacy in a patient with abnormal lungs because of changes in physiologic dead space. Under these circumstances, $Paco_2$ is used as a guide, since an elevated or rising $Paco_2$ is the best clinical indicator of inadequate alveolar ventilation and progressive respiratory acidosis. Weaning is accomplished either by taking the patient off the ventilator with supplemental oxygen and periodic monitoring of arterial blood gas levels or by intermittent mandatory ventilation. The latter technique allows the gradual reduction of ventilator support with the advantage of providing a known minimum minute ventilation and the security of the monitoring systems of the ventilator. This method is particularly helpful in patients who have poor ventilatory reserve or who have been intubated for prolonged periods. After extubation, treatment can be continued with supplemental oxygen and intermittent positive pressure breathing (IPPB) until the patient's respiratory status is stabilized.

Acute Respiratory Failure

Acute respiratory failure can be defined as a disturbance in respiratory function that results in a Pao_2 of less than 50 mm Hg with or without carbon dioxide retention. Although a number of conditions can result in this finding (notably, a large pulmonary embolus), this discussion will be limited to Adult Respiratory Distress Syndrome (ARDS). In 1967, Ashbaugh and coworkers described sudden respiratory failure in 12 adult patients who had dyspnea, hypoxemia, reduced respiratory compliance, and diffuse alveolar infiltrates that resembled pulmonary edema without evidence of prior lung disease or congestive failure. This syndrome is a form of nonhydrostatic pulmonary edema that represents the final pathways of the response of the lungs to acute diffuse alveolar injury from a variety of causes. A broad spectrum of disorders has been associated with ARDS. These disorders are listed in Disorders Associated with Adult Respiratory Distress Syndrome.

ARDS is relatively common, affecting about 150,000 persons per year, with a mortality rate approaching 50%, despite current supportive measures. The hallmark of ARDS is progressive hypoxemia that is refractory to conventional oxygen therapy. Suggested criteria are listed in Criteria for the Diagnosis of Adult Respira-

DISORDERS ASSOCIATED WITH ADULT RESPIRATORY DISTRESS SYNDROME
Shock of any etiology Infections and sepsis Trauma Liquid aspiration Fat and amniotic fluid embolism Drug overdose Inhaled toxins, including oxygen Intravascular coagulation Pancreatitis Eclampsia

CRITERIA FOR THE DIAGNOSIS OF ADULT RESPIRATORY DISTRESS SYNDROME

1. Clinical history of predisposing condition
2. Clinical respiratory distress
   a. Tachypnea greater than 20 breaths per minute
   b. Labored breathing
3. Chest x-ray showing diffuse pulmonary infiltrates
4. Pa_{O_2} less than 50 mm Hg or F_iO_2* greater than 0.6
5. Increased shunt fraction
6. Increased dead space ventilation
7. Decreased total respiratory compliance

*F_iO_2 = Forced inspiratory oxygen concentration.
Adapted from Petty TL, Fowler AH, 1982.

tory Distress Syndrome. Initially, it may be difficult to distinguish ARDS from cardiac failure and pulmonary edema. Using the Swan-Ganz catheter to monitor pulmonary capillary wedge pressure is extremely helpful in making this distinction and helps to determine cardiac output and tissue oxygen delivery.

The pathogenesis of ARDS is complex; a summary of potential mechanisms is shown in Figure 6-3. A recent review by Divertie found that damage to the alveolar capillary membrane resulting in increased capillary permeability is precipitated by complement activation, subsequent aggregation of granulocytes, and liberation of proteases and superoxide radicals. Obviously, therapy must be directed at reversing the primary physi-

ologic abnormality, which is, basically, progressive hypoxemia. The cornerstone of therapy is ventilatory support with positive end-expiratory pressure (PEEP) until repair of the capillary damage can occur. PEEP improves ventilation-perfusion relationships, and consequently oxygenation, by increasing functional residual capacity and stabilizing the alveoli at low levels of inflation. Particularly at high levels, PEEP may have an adverse effect on tissue oxygen delivery (cardiac output × Pa_{O_2}); therefore, careful monitoring of this product is necessary as the PEEP level is increased. The use of corticosteroids in ARDS has been controversial. However, steroids have been shown to inhibit complement-induced granulocyte aggregation, to cause disaggrega-

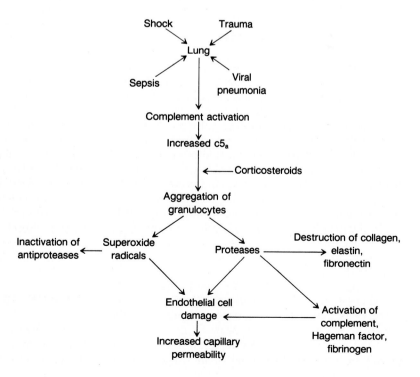

Figure 6–3. Summary of the mechanisms involved in the pathogenesis of ARDS.

tion of neutrophils, and to block the increase in sheep lung vascular permeability after endotoxemia. Sibbald and coauthors demonstrated decreased passage of radiolabeled albumin from serum into pulmonary edema fluid in patients with ARDS after methylprednisolone had been administered. Steroids (methylprednisolone sodium succinate [Solu-Medrol]) may be beneficial if given early in the emergency of ARDS in a dosage of 1–2 g/d but should be discontinued after 48 hours to avoid the possible complications of sepsis.

Judicious management of fluid intake is essential in maintaining adequate perfusion of vital organs and avoiding further complications. Since one of the major determinants of fluid flux in the lung is the hydrostatic pressure in the pulmonary capillaries, this pressure assumes greater than normal importance in the presence of increased capillary permeability. Measurement of pulmonary capillary wedge pressure is the only reliable method of monitoring fluid administration. If adequate perfusion cannot be maintained when the pulmonary wedge pressure is within the upper limits of the normal range (10–12 mm Hg), pressor agents should be considered. Colloid should be administered only if the serum protein level is low, because rapid equilibration of protein concentrations between the capillary and interstitial spaces occurs.

With an increasing understanding of the mechanisms of ARDS, early recognition, and aggressive intervention, the prognosis in ARDS has improved. The long-term outlook is variable, but most patients who survive are left with surprisingly few pulmonary sequelae.

Atelectasis

That airway obstruction can lead to atelectasis is well known and is readily recognized clinically and roentgenographically. The cause may be mucus plugs or inappropriate endotracheal tube placement. A more common and less obvious postoperative problem is so-called microatelectasis, which results from failure to inspire deeply or from constant volume ventilation of the lung. It appears that occasional large inflations are necessary to replenish surfactant and prevent alveolar collapse. Secretions accumulating during anesthesia may result in obstruction of small airways and contribute to the problem. Specifically, during inhalation of a high concentration of oxygen, atelectasis may develop rapidly in areas of the lung where small airways have become obstructed.

Microatelectasis is difficult to detect clinically and roentgenographically. The earliest indication of its occurrence is a fall in Pao_2 and oxygen saturation in the presence of a normal to low $Paco_2$.

In the early stages of development, the Pao_2 can usually be returned to normal by increasing the inspired oxygen concentration. Chest physiotherapy, deep breathing, coughing, incentive spirometry, and IPPB are helpful in resolving the problem. As atelectasis becomes more widespread, positive pressure ventilation and hyperinflation may be necessary to reverse the process. For extensive atelectasis, bronchoscopy to remove mucus plugs may be necessary.

Pneumonia

Postoperative pneumonia has become less frequent with the introduction of early ambulation and intensive respiratory therapy in the immediate postoperative period. Since pneumonia is frequently associated with atelectasis and hypoventilation, prevention or prompt reversal of these conditions is the best prophylactic measure. Animal studies have shown that even with instillation of infected material directly into the lower respiratory tract, pneumonia could not result without such additional factors as atelectasis and hypoventilation. A decrease in the activity of cilia caused by drugs or altered humidity may interfere significantly with bacterial clearing. This is particularly true in patients with obstructive lung disease. In patients with an endotracheal tube in place, the normal protective mechanisms of the upper respiratory system are abolished. Infection is much more likely to develop in this group and is directly related to the duration of intubation. Gram-negative organisms, usually *Proteus* or *Pseudomonas,* are most frequently encountered under these circumstances. Deep tracheal secretions should be aspirated into a sterile sputum trap for culture and antibiotic susceptibility studies. Pathogenic organisms are invariably isolated, but it must be emphasized that a positive sputum culture cannot be equated with pulmonary infection requiring antibiotic therapy. Treatment must be based on such additional criteria as fever, persistence of purulent sputum, leukocytosis, positive blood culture, and physical and roentgenographic signs of pneumonia. Prophylactic antibiotic therapy rarely has a place in the treatment of patients on assisted ventilation except in emergency situations, such as acute aspiration or fulminating infection, in which the gram-stained sputum smear should be used as a guide for initial therapy. Meticulous aseptic technique must be used in suctioning to prevent the introduction of infection. Adequate humidification is essential to facilitate the removal of secretions.

CARE OF THE URINARY BLADDER

The most common postoperative problem of the female bladder is atony caused by overdistention and the reluctance of the patient to initiate the voluntary phase of voiding. Following abdominal surgery, the patient is frequently unwilling to contract the abdominal muscles to produce sufficient intra-abdominal pressure against the dome of the bladder to initiate the voiding reflex. Following anterior colporrhaphy, spasm, edema, and tenderness of the pubococcygeus muscles may obstruct the process of voiding. The operative trauma from plication of the pubovesicocervical fascia causes edema of the urethral wall and submucosa, especially at the urethrovesical junction, thus contributing to the urinary obstruction.

For spontaneous voiding to occur, the parasympathetic function of the bladder detrusor must be coordinated with the voluntary motor function of the abdominal wall and the levator muscles. In the past, it has been customary to insert an indwelling urethral catheter for 5 or more days following vaginal plastic surgery. Although this technique is still used in many clinics, a suprapubic catheter has proven to be very effective in urinary drainage. The suprapubic technique was developed and introduced to the gynecologic literature in 1964. When inserted at the time of surgery, the suprapubic Silastic tube eliminates the necessity for repeated bladder catheterization until spontaneous voiding occurs. Although used preferentially following anterior vaginal colporrhaphy, suprapubic bladder catheterization is also useful when the need for prolonged bladder drainage is anticipated, such as after radical Wertheim hysterectomy. A suprapubic catheter may also be inserted when a Marshall-Marchetti-Krantz urethral suspension is performed.

The procedure for suprapubic bladder drainage is performed either before or after the operative procedure. Catheter placement consists of the insertion of a No. 12 French gauge Silastic (silicone) catheter into the bladder through a needle trocar (Fig. 6-4). A No. 12

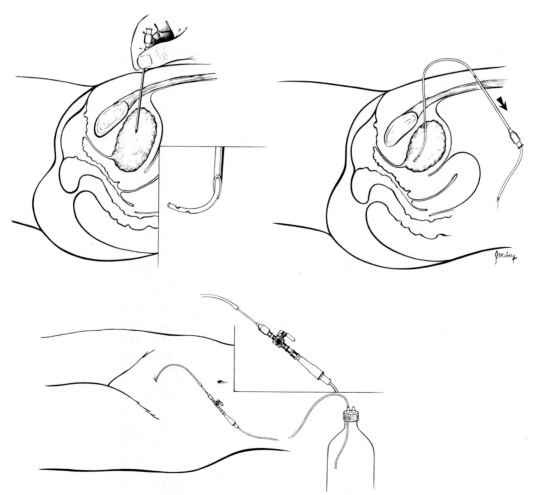

Figure 6–4. Method of inserting suprapubic tube through needle and drainage into bottle. Suprapubic catheterization avoids the trauma to the urethra caused by repeated catheterization or an indwelling catheter.

French gauge pigtail (Bonano) Teflon catheter and other modifications have also been used by many surgeons. The bladder is filled with 300 ml of sterile water and the needle trocar is inserted through the surgically cleaned anterior abdominal wall, approximately 2 cm above the symphysis pubis. When the stylet is removed from the trocar, clear fluid should pass from the bladder under pressure. Approximately 10 cm of the suprapubic catheter is threaded through the trocar, following which the trocar is removed by sliding it over the indwelling tube. The opposite end of the Silastic catheter is connected to a sterile 1-l drainage bottle or to a sterile closed drainage urinometer bag. The tubing should be filled with fluid at all times and should be anchored to the skin with silicone paste or sutured to the skin to avoid accidental removal. A two-way stopcock is inserted between the catheter and drainage tubing for easy opening and closing of the system. The system is not irrigated unless there is plugging of the bladder catheter and failure of drainage.

Alternatively, at the Johns Hopkins Hospital, a Foley catheter is placed through the abdominal wall. After placing a Kelly clamp through the urethra and elevating the dome of the bladder, an incision is made on the abdominal wall superior to the Kelly clamp. A No. 14 French gauge Foley catheter is then pulled through into the bladder and connected to gravity drainage. If a suprapubic urethropexy is performed, a 2–3-cm opening is made in the dome of the bladder and the bladder is inspected to ensure that no sutures penetrated through the mucosa. The Foley catheter is placed into the bladder and sutured in place with a 2.0 absorbable purse-string suture. Using the preceding techniques for insertion of a suprapubic Foley catheter, we have decreased the frequency of catheter obstruction.

Suprapubic catheters at the Johns Hopkins Hospital are frequently used after vaginal reconstruction for ambiguous genitalia and suprapubic urethropexies. Transurethral Foley catheters, however, have replaced suprapubic catheters in the majority of patients undergoing abdominal or vaginal hysterectomy and anterior colporrhaphy with a Kelly urethral plication. Seven to 10 days postoperatively the catheters are removed and postvoid residuals are evaluated. Patients with more than 100 ml of residual urine after spontaneous voiding require an extended period of transurethral catheterization or suprapubic catheterization. The gynecologic oncologists at our institution advocate the use of transurethral Foley catheters in patients undergoing radical hysterectomy. The catheter is routinely removed 14–21 days postoperatively and residuals are evaluated as previously mentioned.

It is our opinion, as well as that of others, that prophylactic antibiotics, when given with the use of an indwelling bladder catheter, are ineffective in preventing urinary tract infection. Although urinary tract symptoms may be delayed with the use of prophylactic antibiotics, it is our experience that the incidence of infection is unchanged but that a subsequent urinary tract infection may result from resistant organisms that are more difficult to treat later. Therefore, we prefer to treat only patients who have significant bacteriuria and pyuria, which includes approximately 10% to 15% of the patients with suprapubic drainage. This incidence of bladder infection is a significant improvement from the common rate of 70% to 90% (Kass and Sossen) when a urethral catheter is retained for more than 72 hours.

GASTROINTESTINAL TRACT MANAGEMENT

Dysfunction of the gastrointestinal tract remains a challenge in postoperative management. Each patient should be treated as an individual and not placed on a standard protocol for advancing diets. Patients who have had uncomplicated surgery may be given clear liquids on the first postoperative day if bowel sounds are present, if abdominal examination reveals no distention, and if the patient is no longer nauseated from her anesthesia. After flatus is passed, the diet should be accelerated as tolerated to a regular diet. Seriously ill or malnourished patients or patients requiring extensive bowel surgery would benefit from preoperative and postoperative parenteral nutrition.

Patients requiring extensive bowel manipulation, dissection, and excision will undoubtedly experience a delay in the return of bowel function and require the placement of a nasogastric tube at the time of surgery. Nasogastric tubes may have a single or double lumen. Single-lumen tubes such as Levin-type tubes or Cantor tubes are connected to a source of low intermittent suction. Although either tube is acceptable in a patient with a small-bowel obstruction, some surgeons prefer the long Cantor tube, which passes through the small intestines with the assistance of a mercury-filled balloon attached to its distal port. Double-lumen tubes, such as the Salem Sump, have a second lumen that functions as a pressure valve. This tube can be connected to a source of low constant suction or high intermittent suction. If the second port is occluded, it should be managed as a single-lumen tube. It is imperative that all gastric contents be replaced equally with normal saline or half normal saline containing 20–40 mEq KCl/L. Patients on nasogastric suction should also have an electrolyte panel obtained daily to ensure adequate replacement.

It is important to differentiate between postoperative ileus and postoperative obstruction (Table 6-7) if

TABLE 6–7
Differential Diagnosis Between Postoperative Ileus and Postoperative Obstruction

CLINICAL FEATURE	POSTOPERATIVE ILEUS	POSTOPERATIVE OBSTRUCTION
Abdominal pain	Discomfort from distention but not cramping pains	Cramping progressively severe
Relationship to previous surgery	Usually within 48–72 hours of surgery	Usually delayed, may be 5–7 days for remote onset
Nausea and vomiting	Present	Present
Distention	Present	Present
Bowel sounds	Absent or hypoactive	Borborygmi with peristaltic rushes and high-pitched tinkles
Fever	Only if related to associated peritonitis	Rarely present unless bowel becomes gangrenous
Abdominal x-rays	Distended loops of small and large bowels; gas usually present in colon	Single or multiple loops of distended bowel, usually small bowel with air fluid levels
Treatment	Conservative with nasogastric suction, enemas, cholinergic stimulation	Partial conservative with nasogastric decompression; or Complete surgical

proper therapy is to be initiated promptly with beneficial results. The distinction may be difficult. This is because partial bowel obstruction is frequently accompanied by a secondary ileus as part of the clinical picture. Only by close clinical monitoring of the bowel sounds, serial abdominal x-ray studies, and frequent white blood cell counts can one clearly separate these two postoperative complications. Obviously, adynamic ileus is the more frequent clinical entity, a fact that may mislead the surgeon into a false sense of security unless he or she remains acutely aware of the distinguishing features of intestinal obstruction. Serial monitoring of the white blood cell count and differential count is an important method for differentiating between bowel obstruction and paralytic ileus. A key feature of advancing bowel obstruction is necrosis of the bowel wall, which will cause a progressive leukocytosis, along with distention and peritonitis. The most common gynecologic disease process associated with both ileus and intestinal obstruction is severe pelvic inflammatory disease. Notoriously, acute exacerbation of pelvic inflammatory disease or rupture of a pelvic abscess is associated with prolonged ileus. Occasionally, fibrous adhesions form and secondary bowel obstruction occurs. Postoperative pelvic peritonitis from any cause, including cellulitis resulting from hematoma formation and secondary infection of the vaginal cuff, is frequently associated with ileus, whereas intestinal obstruction only rarely results from such a complication.

In contrast to pelvic surgery for benign disease, any cancer surgery, including pelvic exenteration for cervical carcinoma, is frequently complicated either by postoperative adynamic ileus or by intestinal obstruction. When radical surgery is preceded by preoperative irradiation, the small bowel is frequently compromised by a protracted ileus.

TOTAL PARENTERAL NUTRITION

Nutritional support has been proven efficacious in patients undergoing major surgery, with impaired bowel function, with inadequate oral intake, and with cancer. A few patients require total parenteral nutrition (TPN) for prolonged periods secondary to their inability to obtain adequate calories orally. Parenteral nutrition may be administered through a peripheral or central access, depending on the patient's initial nutritional status and the time required on TPN.

Hospitalized patients may require TPN for disease processes such as gastrointestinal tract obstruction, prolonged ileus, short-bowel syndrome, radiation enteritis, intra-abdominal abscess, pancreatitis, regional enteritis, or enterocutaneous fistula. A patient with any condition that will prevent oral intake of adequate amounts of food for more than 7–10 days will probably require central parenteral nutrition. Since it is much easier to maintain an adequate nutritional state than to improve a poor one, the decision to use TPN should not be delayed.

Peripheral alimentation is used in patients who are not in a catabolic state and who require nutritional support for less than 7 days. At the Johns Hopkins Hospital, peripheral total hyperalimentation solution (THAS) has an osmolality of 800 mOsm versus 1850 mOsm for standard THAS and 2050 mOsm for concentrated THAS (Table 6-8). Alternatively, central THAS is used in patients requiring prolonged nutritional sup-

TABLE 6–8
Parenteral Nutrition Formulas at the Johns Hopkins Hospital

FORMULA	Unit Volume (ml)	Amino Acids (g)	Nitrogen (g)	Dextrose (g)	Total Kcal	Na (mEq)	K (mEq)	Mg (mEq)	Ca (mEq)	Phos* (mM)	Cl (mEq)	Acetate (mEq)	mOsm	P Cal %	Calories to Nitrogen
Standard THAS	1000	41 (4.25%)	6.5	250 (25%)	1020	30	20	5	5	5	30	67	1850	16.7	157:1
Concentrated THAS	1000	58 (6%)	9.2	280 (28%)	1190	6	—	—	—	6	—	53	2050	20	130:1
Hi-Pro THAS	1000	72 (7.5%)	11.5	175 (17.5%)	885	7.5	—	—	—	7.5	2	67	1700	32.6	77:1
Hi-Cal THAS	1000	41 (4.25%)	6.5	350 (35%)	1360	5	—	—	—	5	—	37	2200	12.5	209:1
Peripheral THAS†	1000	29 (3%)	4.6	70 (7%)	360	35	24.5	5	4	3.5	40	44	800	33	78:1
Low-nitrogen THAS	1000	29 (3%)	4.6	50 (5%)	290	3	—	—	—	3	—	27	600	40.6	63:1
Fat emulsion 10%	500				550					7.5			280		
Fat emulsion 20%	500				1000					7.5			330		

* 1 mM phosphate = 2 mEq phosphate.
† Peripheral PN is always coinfused with 1000 cc 10% fat emulsion.

port for more than 1 week and/or the promotion of anabolism.

Starvation and Stress

The starvation seen in severely ill, hospitalized patients is different from simple starvation in the way it affects the metabolic benefits of infused nutrients. Most patients can tolerate a weight loss of 5% to 10%. But a 40% loss of body weight is uniformly fatal. In addition to the fat supplies and skeletal muscle, vital body proteins are depleted, affecting the liver, spleen, and pancreas.

Even though a human weighing 70 kg stores approximately 100,000/Kcal as fat for energy, the enzymes required to convert fat to glucose are not intrinsic; consequently, the body must make glucose from protein. This protein degradation is then used for gluconeogenesis to form glucose, which serves as a principal energy source in several vital organs, including the central nervous system, and in red and white blood cells.

An adaptive process to conserve vital body proteins must take over. After 3 weeks of starvation, nitrogen output in the urine will fall to 3 g/d from the normal level of 10–15 g/d, indicating a lesser rate of protein breakdown and conservation of body cell mass. Physical activity will decrease, and the basal metabolic rate will fall by approximately 12% to 20%.

The body's adaptation to starvation involves many parts of the metabolic process. The central nervous system converts to using ketones and ketoacid substrates for energy, which allows the breakdown rate of protein to drop by about 70%. Another adaptive process decreases the use of glucose by muscle tissue; when insulin levels fall, muscle uses an energy substrate of fatty acids and, therefore, less glucose. Later in the starvation process the elevated levels of ketoacids and ketones directly depress gluconeogenesis further.

Most of the endocrine systems are involved in the response to starvation. The insulin level falls rapidly, but levels of glucagon, growth hormone, and catecholamines increase, generating more glucose from protein substrate, which depletes the body cell mass rapidly. Later in the starvation process, glucagon returns to normal, growth hormone levels remain elevated, catecholamines decrease, and gluconeogenesis is slowed.

The kinds of changes that allow for conservation of body cell mass during simple starvation do not operate after injury, trauma, or infection. Afferent information, such as pain and other nerve responses to injury, along with hypovolemia and hypotension, is integrated in the central nervous system and hypothalamus, causing efferent responses that adjust the body to the stress condition. Levels of catecholamines and glucocorticoids become elevated, accentuating gluconeogenesis and preventing decreases in basal metabolic rates. Antidiuretic hormone levels are increased and the renin/angiotensin system is activated, allowing fluid retention, which prevents early detection of the degree of weight loss.

During stress, urinary nitrogen levels may increase to 20 g or more per 24 hours, corresponding to a loss of 600 g of hydrated body protein. Body weight decreases, since proteins, carbohydrates, and fats are all being degraded for energy, but the adaptive responses seen in simple starvation do not operate in the different hormonal milieu created by the stress condition.

Provision of nutrients can offset some of this nitrogen loss and even produce positive nitrogen balance. During starvation, the provision of 150 g of glucose (the amount in 3 l of 5% dextrose IV solution) will reduce nitrogen loss even further than the maximum physiologic adaptive mechanisms, because glucose prevents much of the obligatory gluconeogenesis, creating a protein-sparing effect. As Moore explained in his concise review, if high levels of glucose are supplied (up to 750 g/d), protein sparing can be optimized and nitrogen output decreased to 1.8 $g/m^2/d$.

During periods of injury and stress, patients must receive energy intake at least equal to energy expenditure; and to attain positive nitrogen balance, they must receive amino acid nitrogen in excess of urinary losses. Although fat alone cannot provide this energy intake, a combination of glucose and fat is effective.

Initiating Total Parenteral Nutrition

Safe venous access is required for initiating TPN. A reliable intravenous catheter should be placed into a large central vein with the catheter tip located so that blood flow will dilute the highly concentrated nutritional fluids. The insertion site should also allow easy fixation of the catheter at the entrance site, minimum catheter movement during body movements, and easy dressing changes. A subclavian vein approach satisfies the requirements for safe catheter placement, but neither internal jugular vein nor antecubital fossa placement is optimal. The internal jugular vein should be used only if the subclavian approach has failed. Movement of the head and neck results in an increased incidence of occluding venous access when the internal jugular vein has been cannulated.

Use of the Subclavian Vein for Intravenous Infusions

In 1952, Aubaniac, a French physician, was among the first to advocate the use of the subclavian vein for intravenous infusions. J. N. Wilson cannulated the superior vena cava through a percutaneous puncture of the subclavian vein. He reported a high percentage of successful cannulations and a low incidence of complications.

Anatomy of Infraclavicular Subclavian Vein. As Figure 6-5 shows, the subclavian vein is located within the costoclavicular-scalene triangle, which is bounded anteriorly by the medial end of the clavicle, posteriorly by the upper surface of the first rib, and laterally by the anterior scalene muscle. The anterior scalene muscle separates the subclavian vein from the subclavian artery, which lies beneath and along the lateral aspect of the muscle. The subclavian vein is covered by 5 cm of the clavicle medially and joins the internal jugular vein near the medial border of the anterior scalene muscle to form the innominate vein. The innominate vein descends behind the sternum and joins with the opposite innominate vein to form the superior vena cava. The

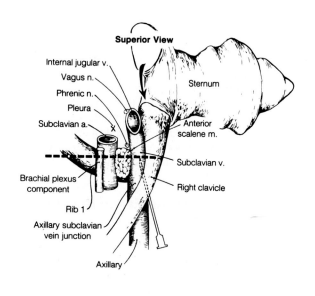

Superior View

Internal jugular v.
Vagus n.
Phrenic n.
Pleura
Subclavian a.
Sternum
Anterior scalene m.
Subclavian v.
Right clavicle
Brachial plexus component
Rib 1
Axillary subclavian vein junction
Axillary

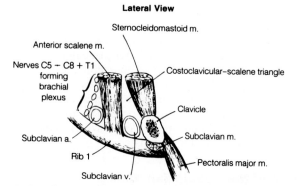

Lateral View

Sternocleidomastoid m.
Anterior scalene m.
Nerves C5 – C8 + T1 forming brachial plexus
Costoclavicular–scalene triangle
Clavicle
Subclavian a.
Rib 1
Subclavian m.
Subclavian v.
Pectoralis major m.

Figure 6–5. Anatomical relationships of subclavian vein. *Dotted line* represents the location of transverse section for lateral view. (Adapted from Moosman DA: The anatomy of infraclavicular subclavian vein catheterization and its complications. Surg Gynecol Obstet 1973; 136:71.)

subclavian vein, which is approximately 3 or 4 cm long, continues as the axillary vein below the clavicle, en route to the axilla. Several other significant structures occupy this region. The phrenic nerve courses across the anterior surface of the anterior scalene muscle near its attachment to the first rib and courses medially to lie posterior to the subclavian vein. It can be injured if the posterior wall of the vessel is penetrated. The internal thoracic nerve and the apical pleura are in contact with the posterior surface of the subclavian vein at its junction with the internal jugular vein. The roots of the brachial plexus formed by the fifth, sixth, seventh, and eighth cervical and the first thoracic nerves lie lateral to the anterior scalene muscle on the lateral side of the subclavian artery. If a cannulating needle is directed too far laterally, the brachial nerve plexus could be injured or the subclavian artery could be punctured. The thoracic duct on the left side and the lymphatic duct on the right cross the anterior scalene muscle on either side of the thorax to enter the superior aspect of each subclavian vein near its junction with the internal jugular vein. These lymphatic vessels are rarely encroached upon during subclavian catheterization.

Subclavian Catheter Placement. The subclavian catheter is inserted with the patient in the supine position, with the foot of the bed elevated 6–12 in. to increase the pressure in the subclavian vein and produce venous distention. After meticulous aseptic preparation of the skin with povidone-iodine (Betadine), the skin and subcutaneous tissues are infiltrated with a 1% solution of lidocaine (Xylocaine) if the patient is awake. The point of needle insertion is approximately 1 cm below the junction of the inner and middle third of the clavicle (Fig. 6-6A). Most central venous catheter units include an external introducer catheter (Teflon) and an internal infusion catheter (silicone). The outer, Teflon sheath accommodates a No. 12 needle, which fits snugly into and protrudes beyond the end of the Teflon catheter.

The needle and sheath are introduced into the skin with the shaft of the needle held almost parallel with the anterior chest wall (see Fig. 6-6A). The needle is directed medially and advanced along the undersurface of the clavicle. It is not necessary to scrape the posterior surface of the clavicle to ensure that the pleura are protected from puncture. By applying suction constantly, the needle passes beneath the skin and immediately aspirates dark red blood, which confirms entry into the vein. If the vein is not entered, the needle is withdrawn and readvanced in a similar manner but in a slightly more cranial or caudal direction. As soon as a free flow of blood is obtained, the introduced Teflon sheath is advanced far enough to be certain that it is securely placed within the vein. The sheath is held in place by the connector, the finger is placed over the end

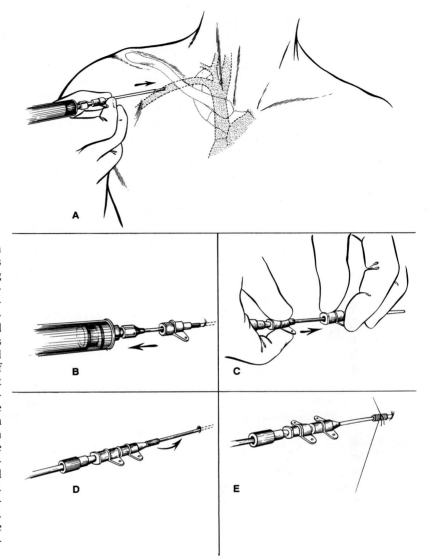

Figure 6–6. Insertion of subclavian catheter for monitoring central venous pressure. *A,* After locally anesthetizing the puncture site, the needle with overlying introducer catheter is directed medially between the first rib and the clavicle at the junction of the middle and inner third of the clavicle. The needle is held parallel to the anterior chest wall and advanced along the undersurface of the clavicle. Entry into the vein is evident with aspiration of blood in attached syringe. *B,* The needle and syringe are removed from the Teflon sheath and a finger is held over the end of the open catheter to prevent entry of air. *C,* The silicone infusion catheter is now inserted through introducer catheter until the two connectors meet and lock firmly. *D,* The intravenous fluid line is connected to the silicone infusion catheter. *E,* The suture sleeve is advanced to the skin surface, where the catheter is sutured firmly to the skin.

of the needle to prevent air embolism, and the internal needle is replaced (see Fig. 6-6*B*) by the silicone infusion catheter that accompanies the central venous pressure (CVP) kit (see Fig. 6-6*C*). A thin wire stylet inside the infusion catheter allows the catheter to be advanced easily; occasionally, the stylet must be withdrawn slightly in order to advance the catheter as far as possible into the innominate vein and superior vena cava. The silicone infusion catheter is advanced until the attached connector can be securely wedged into the connector of the Teflon sheath (see Fig. 6-6*C*).

After the infusion catheter is connected to an intravenous fluid line, the Teflon sheath is carefully withdrawn from the vein, remaining partially in the subcutaneous tissue while leaving an ample length of the infusion catheter in the vena cava (see Fig. 6-6*D*). A suture sleeve on the introducer sheath is slid down to the puncture site and sutured to the skin (see Fig. 6-6*E*). The tip of the catheter is preferably positioned in the superior vena cava and should not be advanced into the right atrium or ventricle, where it could cause accidental trauma to the heart wall or cardiac arrhythmias. To ensure its continued sterility and proper function, the subclavian vein catheter should not be used to replace fluids or withdraw blood for laboratory studies, if it is at all possible to avoid these uses. A central venous line for hyperalimentation is an exception to this rule. The dressing should be changed daily and the catheterization site cleaned with povidone-iodine or a similar antimicrobial solution.

Patient Evaluation

A complete medical history and physical examination must be obtained prior to initiating parenteral nutrition. Particular attention should be paid to identifying patients with cardiovascular or renal disease, hyperlipidemia, diabetes, and thyroid disease. THAS modification can include decreasing or eliminating fat emulsion in patients with severe cardiovascular disease or hyperlipidemia, administering low-nitrogen THAS to patients with renal failure (see Table 6-8), and increasing the insulin dosage in patients with diabetes mellitus.

The patient's degree of malnutrition should be assessed by taking measurements of several physical indicators, such as actual body weight (ABW) and ideal body weight (IBW), usual body weight (UBW) (preillness), creatinine/height index, triceps skin fold thickness (TSFT), and arm circumference (AC). At the Johns Hopkins Hospital, the AMC (arm muscle circumference) is calculated and used as an index of nutritional status:

$$AMC = AC - (TSFT \times 3.14)$$

Fat stores are reflected in the triceps skin fold measurement; somatic proteins are evaluated by measuring muscle mass such as the AMC. The Frisancho standards are used to interpret body weight (kg), triceps (mm), and bone-free arm muscle area (cm^2).

Patients found to be in the fifth to 10th percentiles are severely malnourished and require an anabolic environment. Weight loss is considered significant when the (UBW − ABW)/UBW × 100 is greater than 10%. Weight loss during starvation occurs at a rate of 0.4 kg/d. Survival is also compromised when the ABW falls below the 70th percentile of the IBW. In addition to the preceding physical measurements, a thorough evaluation of chemical indicators is required (Table 6-9) prior to initiating total parenteral nutrition. Extensive monitoring is required while the patient is receiving TPN (Table 6-10).

The physical and chemical measurements of malnutrition are subject to many influences during illness and should be treated as confounding variables. For example, albumin values less than 3.2 g/dl are frequently used to indicate malnutrition. Starker and coauthors observed that in hospitalized patients, albumin values in conjunction with body weight measurements provided a better indication of sodium balance and extracellular fluid volume than albumin values alone. In addition, albumin serum levels are required for the maintenance of the intravascular colloid oncotic pressure and as a carrier protein.

The half-life of albumin is 20 days and thus reflects a depletion of visceral proteins of at least 3 weeks' duration. Transferring with a half-life of 8−9 days provides the clinician with a measurement of recent protein status changes. Since transferrin is required to bind Fe^{2+}, its level is affected by intravascular iron status and can increase during pregnancy, in patients with hepatitis, and in patients receiving estrogen supplementation. Serum protein content can be reduced in protein-losing enteropathy, nephropathy, chronic infections, and uremia and during catabolism. Transferrin reflects recent losses and therefore remains a better indicator of protein status and change than albumin. Total lymphocyte counts of less than 1500 mm^3 are indicative of an immunocompromised patient. Immunologic skin testing for recall antigens and total lymphocyte counts has been correlated to both nutritional status and morbidity and mortality. Its usefulness in the assessment of nutritional status is limited to confounding variables such as cancer, side-effects of cancer treatment protocols, stress of trauma or surgery, and infection. Phosphorus and the trace elements are thoroughly evaluated prior to initiating and during total parenteral nutrition because they are frequently depleted with many disease states and are required when alimenting (Tables 6-11 and 6-12).

TABLE 6–9
Pretreatment Screening at the Johns Hopkins Hospital

LABORATORY EVALUATION
Complete blood count (CBC) with differential
Prothrombin time/partial thromboplastin time (PT/PTT)
Electrolyte panel
Chemistry panel
Albumin
Transferrin (?)
Total lymphocyte count
Triglycerides
Magnesium
Phosphorus
Copper
Zinc
Selenium

TABLE 6–10
Treatment Monitoring

TEST	FREQUENCY
Electrolyte panel	Twice weekly
Chemistry panel	Weekly
Magnesium	Weekly
Transferrin	Weekly
Triglycerides	Monthly/as needed
Zn, Cu, Se	Monthly/as needed

TABLE 6–11
Standard Trace Minerals at the Johns Hopkins Hospital Compared to AMA/FDA Guidelines

MINERAL	DAILY DOSAGE	AMA/FDA GUIDELINES
Zinc	3 mg	2.5–4.0 mg
Copper	1.2 mg	0.5–1.5 mg
Manganese	0.3 mg	0.15–0.8 mg
Chromium	12 mcg	10–15 mcg
Selenium	60 mcg	50–60 mcg*

*No firm AMA/FDA recommendations

Nutritional Requirements

Total parenteral nutrition consists of six components: carbohydrates, fat, protein, electrolytes, vitamins, and trace elements. The Harris-Benedict Basal Energy Expenditure (BEE) accounts for two thirds of the total daily energy requirements, with the remaining one third obtained from protein. Daily requirements for protein are between 1.5 and 2.5 g/kg/d. Patients receiving TPN who are severely malnourished and stressed will require larger amounts of protein daily. The BEE is calculated as follows:

TABLE 6–12
Trace Minerals

MINERALS AND LEVELS	DEFICIENCY Symptoms	DEFICIENCY Etiology	TOXICITY Symptoms	TOXICITY Etiology
Zinc, 55–150 mg/dl	Diarrhea, mental depression, alopecia, night blindness, dermatosis, impaired taste, hypogonadism, impaired wound healing	Gastrointestinal (failure of ingestion, absorption, retention) Large wounds Protein-energy malnutrition Cancer	Vomiting Diarrhea Neurologic damage ("zinc shakes")	Increased ingestion from galvanized containers Metal fume fever
Selenium, 90–150 μg/dl (synergism with vitamin E)	Myositis with muscle weakness Cardiomyopathy with arrhythmias and congestive heart failure	Unsupplemented TPN	Liver cirrhosis Alopecia Pathologic loss of nails Dermatitis	Increased ingestion (rare)
Chromium, 50–200 μg/d	Neuropathy Encephalopathy New insulin-dependent diabetes mellitus	Unsupplemented TPN Increased renal loss secondary to injury Gastrointestinal losses	Respiratory Lung cancer	Workers' manufacturing products containing hexavalent chromium
Phosphorus, 3.0–4.5 mg/dl	Nausea, vomiting, anorexia, dysarthria, paresthesia, hemolytic anemia, peripheral neuropathy, respiratory depression, congestive heart failure, renal glycosuria	Gastrointestinal (failure of ingestion, absorption, retention) Cellular anabolism Respiratory/metabolic alkalosis Al(OH)$_3$ antacids Alcoholism	Neurotoxicity secondary to compensatory hypocalcemia	Renal failure Hypoparathyroidism
Magnesium, 136–145 mEq/l	Nausea, vomiting, muscle weakness, lethargy, tetany, muscle tremor, personality changes	Gastrointestinal (failure of ingestion, absorption, retention) Cellular catabolism, acidosis, K$^+$ depletion Glomerular dysfunction	Hyporeflexia, lethargy, respiratory depression, cardiac arrest	Magnesium supplementation in patients with renal compromise
Copper, 70–155 μg/dl	Hypochromic anemia not responsive to iron, neutropenia	THAS without copper or high amino acids Gastrointestinal (failure of ingestion, absorption, retention) Pregnancy, lactation (increased requirements) Renal losses	Jaundice–hepatic necrosis Intravascular hemolysis Gastric hemorrhage Tremors, choreoathetoid movements, dementia, rigidity, dysarthria	Iatrogenic Wilson's disease Absorption of copper nitrate salves in burn patients

$$\text{cal/d} = 655.0955 + 9.5634\,(\text{wt}) + 1.8496\,(\text{ht}) \\ \times 4.6756\,(\text{A})$$

where wt = weight (in kg), ht = height (in cm), and A = age (in years).

Once the patient has reached the estimated daily calorie goal, a 24-hour nitrogen balance study is performed by obtaining a 24-hour urine collection and an A.M. electrolyte panel. If a large quantity of fluid from the nasogastric tube, ileostomy, fistula, or wound is present, this should also be collected and sent for nitrogen measurements.

$$N_2(g) \text{ balance} = N_2(g) \text{ in} \times N_2(g) \text{ out}$$

At the Johns Hopkins Hospital, we add 4 to the N_2 out, which accounts for nitrogenous losses in the stool and skin. This does not include an estimate of the losses from the gastrointestinal tract and wound, as previously described.

$$N_2(g) \text{ balance} = N_2(g) \text{ in} \times [N_2(g) \text{ out} + 4] \\ N_2(g) \text{ out} = \text{urine vol (ml)} \\ \times \text{ urine urea } N_2 \text{ (mg/dl)} \\ N_2(g) \text{ in} = \text{amino acids/d/6.24} \\ 6.24 = \text{g protein/g nitrogen}$$

Patients with normal renal and liver function at the Johns Hopkins Hospital are started on standard THAS (see Table 6-8). Each liter provides a total of 1020 Kcal, including 41 g of amino acids and 250 g of dextrose. The osmolality of this solution is 1850 mOsm, which therefore necessitates a central venous access. The calories-to-nitrogen ratio of this solution is 157:1 and is optimal in nonstressed patients. The addition of lipids is also effective in promoting a positive nitrogen balance. The total daily sodium concentration should be equivalent to normal saline (150 mEq/l). This can be altered to accommodate patients who require sodium restriction or loading. Table 6-13 outlines the recommendation for daily electrolyte requirements. It should be noted that acetate serves as a precursor to bicarbonate, since the latter is not compatible in the THAS solution. Multivitamins are added daily to 1 l of THAS (Table 6-14), whereas trace elements are divided equally in the volume to be infused during a 24-hour period.

Blood glucose levels in patients receiving PN should be between 100 and 200 mg%. A minimum of 10 units should be added to each liter when required. This permits approximately 50% to adhere to the plastic tubing. This can be supplemented with subcutaneous doses of regular insulin to obtain the desired blood glucose level. Approximately one half to two thirds of the previous day's requirements are added in divided doses to the THAS solutions.

TABLE 6–13
Daily Electrolyte Requirements for Parenteral Nutrition

	DOSAGE
ELECTROLYTE	*mEq/day*
Sodium	60–150
Potassium	60–240
Phosphate	30–45
Calcium	10–15
Magnesium	8–26
Acetate	80–120
Chloride	60–150

TABLE 6–14
Standard Multivitamins at the Johns Hopkins Hospital (AMA/FDA Formula)*

VITAMIN	DAILY DOSAGE	VITAMIN	DAILY DOSAGE
A	3300 IU	Niacin	40 mg
D	200 IU	Pyridoxine	4 mg
E	10 IU	Pantothenic acid	15 mg
C	100 mg	B_{12}	5 mcg
Thiamine	3 mg	Folic acid	0.4 mg
Riboflavin	3.6 mg	Biotin	60 mg

*Vitamin K is ordered separately (see Fig. 6-7).

Intravenous lipids provide a nonprotein source of energy and serve as a source of essential fatty acids. Ten percent fat emulsions (550 Kcal/500 cc) and 20% fat emulsions (1000 Kcal/500 cc) are commercially available. In patients receiving standard THAS, 500 cc of 10% fat emulsion are infused twice weekly at a rate of 42 cc/hr. However, when fat emulsion is used with peripheral THAS, the patient requires 2 l of peripheral THAS and 1 l of 10% fat emulsion daily. Twenty percent fat emulsions can also be used for calories in patients with glucose intolerance or patients who require a decreased protein calorie percentage. Patients deficient in fatty acids present with dermatitis, hemolytic anemia, thrombocytopenia, elevated liver enzymes, and poor wound healing.

In an attempt to improve glucose tolerance, the first liter should be started at a rate of 42 cc/hr. The second day, the solution can be increased to 84 cc/hr, and on day 3 it can be increased to 124 cc/hr. If the patient is unable to tolerate this schedule, increments can be decreased to 21 cc/hr each day (Fig. 6-7). Treatment monitoring is outlined in Table 6-10. Total nitrogen balance should be recalculated if there is a marked change in the patient's condition or the parenteral nu-

Page No. _____ | Patient's Name and History No. _____

ALL PN ORDERS TO BE WRITTEN BY 12 NOON TO BEGIN AFTER 2100 HRS. (9 PM)				

Figure 6–7. Sample parenteral nutrition order form used at the Johns Hopkins Hospital.

The order form contains the following sections:

ORDERED (DATE / TIME) | PARENTERAL NUTRITION (PN) ORDERS (24 HOUR SUPPLY) | NOTED BY | ORDER COMPLETED (DATE / TIME) | INITIALS

1 Infuse D10W at 20ml/hr via PN line until X-Ray confirms position.

2 Urine S & A's q6 hr. notify H.O. if ≥ 3+ Glucosuria.

3 Daily I & O's / Daily Weights.

4 Alimentation Solutions
Standard ☐; Concentrated ☐; Hi-Pro ☐; Hi-Cal ☐; Peripheral ☐; Low Nitrogen ☐
a) Bottle # ___ @ ___ ml/hr to start at ___ hrs.
b) Bottle # ___ @ ___ ml/hr
c) Bottle # ___ @ ___ ml/hr

5 MODIFICATIONS TO EACH LITER
a) Sodium (20-140 mEq)   as acetate _____ mEq
                         as chloride _____ mEq
b) Potassium (10-80 mEq) as acetate _____ mEq
                         as chloride _____ mEq
c) Phosphate (0-15 mM)   as sodium _____ mM
                         as potassium _____ mM
d) Calcium Chloride (0-5 mEq)   _____ mEq
e) Magnesium Sulfate (0-12 mEq)   _____ mEq
f) Regular Insulin (5-70 units)   _____ units

6 Daily Multivitamins ☐; Daily Trace Minerals ☐

7 Vitamin K 1 mg/liter ☐

8 Fat Emulsion 10% ☐; Fat Emulsion 20% ☐; ___ ml @ 42 ml/hr

9 Other additives:

SIGNATURE _____ M.D. # _____

---

trition administered. Table 6-15 lists the essential and nonessential amino acids.

Cardiac and Respiratory Insufficiency

Patients with congestive heart failure require decreased sodium and decreased total fluid volume. The best solution can be prepared from the most concentrated solutions of glucose, amino acid, and fat available. Fluid-restricted solutions may also be beneficial for patients with respiratory failure, who should receive less total glucose in favor of more fat, since the respiratory quotient (CO_2/O_2) of glucose (1.00) is greater than that of fat (0.70), and excess glucose will increase the

TABLE 6–15
Amino Acids

ESSENTIAL	NONESSENTIAL
Arginine	Alanine
Histidine	Aspartic acid
Isoleucine	Glutamic acid
Leucine	Glutamine
Lysine	Glycine
Methionine	Serine
Phenylalanine	Tyrosine
Threonine	
Tryptophan	
Valine	

load of CO_2 the lungs must excrete. Excessive total caloric intake resulting in fat synthesis from glucose substrate may severely compromise respiratory function, since large amounts of CO_2 are released (respiratory quotient 8.0).

Discontinuing Total Parenteral Nutrition

Prior to discontinuation of TPN, the patient should tolerate an enteral diet that provides adequate calories. It is permissible to aliment patients with an enteral diet prior to decreasing the THAS solution. An abrupt discontinuation of central parenteral nutrition results in a rebound hypoglycemia. Our recommendation is to decrease the THAS step-wise to 42 cc/hr prior to discontinuation. Some institutions recommend that the patient receive 10% dextrose for an additional 12 hours once central parenteral nutrition has been discontinued.

The Team Approach to Total Parenteral Nutrition

TPN can now be safely administered to patients in many hospitals because of the existence of a team of physicians, nurses, and health care professionals. Although the composition and exact function of the team members vary between hospitals, most teams consist of a physician, a nurse, a pharmacist, and a nutritionist. The role of the team varies in each institution from consultation to complete management of the patient's nutritional needs. The team approach by either method is highly beneficial, providing a high concentration of personnel with knowledge, expertise, and interdisciplinary communication at the patient's bedside. Team members can provide continuing education on nutrition therapy, can continuously audit and collect quality control data, and can investigate ways to improve the safety and efficacy of TPN as a treatment modality. Most teams operate with a standardized protocol that covers patient assessment, catheter insertion techniques, solutions used, and monitoring functions performed.

ROUTINE ORDERS

When the patient has fully recovered from the anesthetic and is ready for return to the nursing floor and routine postoperative care, we have found the basic postoperative orders shown in Figure 6-8 to be useful. They are only a general outline. This list should be expanded to include the special needs of each postoperative patient.

It is imperative that each patient be evaluated prior to being transferred from the recovery room. If the patient is not ready for transfer, additional efforts are made to stabilize the patient or transfer her to an intensive care bed. Upon transferring, the frequency of rounding should be based on the severity of the patient's condition. All patients should be evaluated on the evening of surgery and appropriate documentation made in the chart. A thorough evaluation of the vital signs, catheter drainage (nasogastric, peritoneal, and Foley), and pulmonary status is required, and abdominal examination is performed. Each physician has a desired protocol for postoperative management. The routine orders outlined in this chapter provide the clinician with a framework to design patient care plans that address the individual patient's requirements. Laboratory and radiographic evaluation of the postoperative patient is also tailored to the individual patient. Unfortunately, many physicians are predominantly concerned with quantitative test values. It is, however, just as important to develop a close rapport with your patient, the patient's family, and the nursing staff. Only through good communication can the gynecologic surgeon deliver optimum medical care.

ESTROGEN REPLACEMENT THERAPY

During the past decade, few subjects in medicine have engendered greater controversy than has the use of estrogen by postmenopausal women. In the postoperative patient who has undergone bilateral oophorectomy at the time of pelvic surgery, important metabolic changes occur as a result of estrogen deficiency. The most significant effects include vasomotor symptoms, genitourinary atrophy, and osteoporosis. In counseling the patient about the advisability or the necessity of oophorectomy and surgical castration at the time of surgery, it is important that the surgeon take the time to explain all the benefits and risks of post-oophorectomy estrogen replacement.

Prophylactic oophorectomy is reasonable if the patient is approaching menopause, since ovarian cancer is the major cause of death from gynecologic malignancy and its cure rate has remained unchanged for the past three decades. These facts have encouraged many gynecologists to remove the ovaries at the time of hysterectomy in patients who are 45 years of age or older and approaching menopause. The ease of oral estrogen replacement has made this surgical approach quite acceptable.

Among the most important sequelae of castration or of natural menopause is bone demineralization or osteoporosis. With the sudden decrease in plasma estrogen following oophorectomy, there is bone reabsorp-

---

BASIC POSTOPERATIVE ORDERS

Patient's Name: _____.

1. Admit to Unit #_____.
2. Diagnosis:
3. Allergies:
4. Condition:
5a. Vital signs:
   _____ q 15 minutes until stable
   _____ q 2 hours for 24 hours
   _____ q 8 hours, if stable
5b. Notify House Officer (H.O.) if
   BP < 90/60, > 160/100
   Pulse <60, >120
   Temp >38.0°C
6. Activity:
   _____ Bed rest
   _____ Ambulate
   _____ Other (specify)
7. Diet:
   _____ NPO
   _____ Other (specify)
8. Intravenous fluids:
9. Incentive inspirometer q 2 hours while awake
10. Encourage deep breathing.
11. Drains:

Type	Location	Drainage
_____ Nasogastric	_____ Stomach	_____ Low/intermittent suction
_____ Peritoneal	_____ Pelvis	_____ Bulb suction
_____ Foley catheter	_____ Bladder	_____ Gravity

12a. Fluid intake and output chart.
12b. Notify H.O. if urine output <30 cc/h.
13. Pain medication: Specify
   (a) route of administration
   (b) dosage
14. Antiemetic medication: Specify
   (a) route of administration
   (b) dosage
15. Antibiotics
16. Venous thrombosis prophylaxis
17. Other medications
18. Catheterize q 6 hours, or sooner, if bladder is full and patient unable to void.

Figure 6–8. Sample of basic postoperative orders.

---

tion without change in the chemical composition of the bone. This reabsorption involves the entire skeleton, although the soft cancellous bone undergoes the demineralization process before the hard cortical bone. For this reason earliest effects of advancing osteoporosis are seen in spontaneous fracture of the distal radius, the weight-bearing vertebral bodies, and the neck of the femur.

In 1979, more than 125,000 women in the United States suffered a fracture of the proximal femur, and 12% died as a direct result. Of white women over 60 years of age, 25% have radiographic or clinical evidence of vertebral crush injuries. Although bone loss is a normal aging process for both men and women, the most significant physiologic event associated with skeletal fractures in women is the loss of ovarian function, whether due to oophorectomy or to spontaneous menopause. While there are apparently no estrogen receptors in bone, estrogen plays an important role in calcium metabolism. Osteoporosis is perhaps the most significant abnormality resulting from estrogen deficiency and is a major cause of morbidity and mortality.

Several theories have been proposed to explain the mechanism of action of estrogen in retarding bone reabsorption. Estrogen is known to suppress the action of parathyroid hormone at the osteoclastic cellular level and thereby suppress the effect of parathormone on bone reabsorption. A diminished plasma level of estrogen results in an increased sensitivity in these cells to parathyroid hormone stimulation, which in turn results in an acceleration of bone reabsorption. As a result of the estrogen deficiency, bone demineralization causes an increase in serum calcium. This, in turn, suppresses parathyroid hormone secretion. Consequently, the beneficial effect of parathyroid hormone on renal tubular reabsorption of calcium and the formation of the active, dihydroxy form of vitamin D is diminished. The low level of 1,25-dihydroxy vitamin D results in an increased renal excretion of calcium and a diminished calcium absorption from the gastrointestinal tract. If low-dose estrogen is provided on a continued basis, the action of the parathyroid hormone on bone reabsorption is decreased. This, in turn, lowers the serum calcium level. The lowered serum calcium level enhances parathyroid hormone release, which has a positive effect on calcium metabolism by increasing renal tubular reabsorption of calcium. Calcium absorption from the gastrointestinal tract is also increased because activated vitamin D levels are higher.

Although the foregoing may be a plausible explanation of the role of estrogen in bone reabsorption, the exact mechanism is by no means fully understood. Many investigators believe that estrogen does not affect osteoclast activity directly, since estrogen receptors have not been shown to be present in bone. There is some evidence that the effect of estrogen on bone metabolism is mediated by its control of calcitonin secretion. Calcitonin, a peptide hormone synthesized by the C cells of the thyroid gland, is decreased in the postmenopausal patient; calcitonin is known to reduce both the number of osteoclasts and their physiologic activity. The administration of estrogen not only prevents bone loss but also raises the plasma level of calcitonin to premenopausal levels. Therefore, another possible explanation of the pathogenesis of postmenopausal osteoporosis is the accelerated decline in calcitonin secretion that is associated with loss of ovarian function.

Photon absorptiometry studies have made it eminently clear that premature castration and the cessation of ovarian function at menopause are both associated with a dramatic and continued decline in bone density. Lindsay and coauthors demonstrated that when oophorectomized, perimenopausal patients were treated with estrogen for periods of up to 8 years, significant bone loss did not occur. When estrogen was withdrawn, bone mineral content fell at a normal postmenopausal rate, demonstrating the long-term prevention of bone loss by estrogen. This group also demonstrated a significant reduction in height loss among postoophorectomized women who were treated prophylactically with small doses of mestranol (mean dosage was 20 μg/d). It seems evident, therefore, that bone demineralization can be delayed with estrogen replacement ther-

apy. Although no therapy now available can restore bone mass in a patient with osteoporosis, women who have premature ovarian failure or bilateral oophorectomy before 50 years of age would benefit if treated prophylactically with estrogen. At particular risk of osteoporosis are slender white or Asian women who smoke, have early menopause, have a low calcium intake, drink alcohol excessively, and are physically inactive. Kriska and coauthors recently identified an association between historical physical activity and bone density.

There are many orally active estrogen compounds. Conjugated equine estrogen in the dosage of 0.625 mg/d for 25 days of each month is one of the more common agents used. Medroxyprogesterone acetate in a dosage of 10 mg/d is administered on days 16–25 when cycling is desired. Ethinyl estradiol in a dosage of 0.02 mg/d or mestranol in a dose of 25–30 μg/d will produce similar biologic effects. The prophylactic use of estrogen must be decided on an individual basis and should not be discontinued unless contraindications develop. Creasman and coauthors have suggested that estrogen supplementation in patients after treatment for stage I endometrial carcinoma is not contraindicated.

Patients receiving sequential or continuous therapy with estrogen and progesterone have demonstrated decreased vertebral bone loss. According to Savvas and coauthors, patients receiving estradiol, 50 mg, and testosterone, 100 mg, in subcutaneous implants were less likely to develop osteoporosis when compared with those receiving sequential estrogen and progesterone therapy. Calcitonin and fluoride have also been shown to be efficacious in decreasing bone loss. Pak and coauthors demonstrated an increase in mineralized bone, increased vertebral bone mass, and reduced frequency of vertebral fractures when using intermittent sodium fluoride treatment without 1,25-dihydroxy vitamin D. Future estrogen supplementation protocols to decrease osteoporosis may include agents such as calcitonin and fluoride.

The remaining major physiologic changes associated with loss of estrogen—namely, vasomotor symptoms and genitourinary atrophy—may or may not be clinically symptomatic. Although the hot flush appears to occur in synchrony with a pulsatile surge of luteinizing hormone, the change in hormone level is not the major causative factor. The major defect is in the heat regulatory mechanism in the intact hypothalamus. It has been postulated that gonadotropin-releasing hormone and the heat regulatory center are affected concomitantly by α-adrenergic stimulation. This stimulation produces a secondary autonomic response that causes a hot flush. Although the precise stimulatory mechanism is as yet incompletely explained, estrogen replacement has a dampening effect on both the pulsatile gonadotropin release mechanism and the thermogenic center. The treatment for vasomotor symptoms and genitourinary atrophy, however, may be given on a very temporary basis until the patient has adjusted to the change in circulating estrogen level. Genitourinary symptoms are less frequent and have a delayed onset. A troublesome clinical problem of estrogen deprivation is the urethral syndrome. This is a recurrent sterile urethritis that causes dysuria, nocturia, and urinary frequency and urgency. The syndrome is usually well controlled with estrogen replacement therapy, with the most immediate response being produced by local vaginal estrogen.

The atrophic changes of the vagina are late sequelae of the diminished plasma estrogen level and do not occur for many months or years following the removal of the ovaries. Such changes as vaginal dryness, dyspareunia, irritation, and, occasionally, postcoital bleeding are associated with atrophy of the vaginal epithelium. Although vasomotor and genitourinary symptoms are troublesome, they produce no serious long-term health hazards to the patient.

Postmenopausal women receiving estrogen supplements have a marked reduction in cardiovascular disease and mortality. Estrogen supplementation partially exerts this protective effect through increasing serum levels of high-density lipoproteins (HDL). Low-density lipoproteins (LDL), which are atherogenic and increase the risk of cardiac morbidity and death, are also decreased in patients receiving postmenopausal estrogen supplementation. Exercise, in addition to estrogen therapy, will result in increased HDL and bone density. Some studies have suggested that norethindrone, megestrol acetate, medroxyprogesterone acetate, and levonorgestrel decrease HDL levels. Wren and Garrett demonstrated that low-dose levonorgestrel (30 mg) and low-dose estrogen therapy in postmenopausal women do not affect HDL levels. Additional studies by Ravnikar and coauthors evaluating medroxyprogesterone acetate sequentially administered with estrogen did not result in a decrease of HDL serum levels. Although several prospective studies are in progress, it appears that postmenopausal estrogen and progesterone supplementation diminishes the risk of cardiovascular disease and death in addition to preventing bone demineralization with resultant osteoporosis. (Estrogen replacement therapy is also discussed in Chapters 27 and 43.)

Bibliography

Adam S, Williams V, Vessey MP. Cardiovascular disease and hormone replacement treatment: a pilot case-control study. Br Med J 1981;282:1277.

Adar R, Papa MZ, Amsterdam E, et al. Antithrombosis routines and hemorrhagic complications: a seven year survey comparing vascular and general surgical operations. J Cardiovasc Surg 1985;26:275.

Adolf J, Buttermann G, Weidenbach A, et al. Optimization of postoperative prophylaxis of thrombosis in gynecology. Geburtsh Frauenheilk 1978;38:98.

Aitken AGF, Godden OJ. Real-time ultrasound diagnosis of deep vein thrombosis: a comparison with venography. Clin Rad 1987;38:309.

Allan A, Williams JT, Bolton JP, et al. The use of graduated compression stockings in the prevention of postoperative deep vein thrombosis. Br J Surg 1983;70:172.

Allenby F, Pflugg JJ, Boardman L, et al. Effects of external pneumatic intermittent compression on fibrinolysis in man. Lancet 1973;2:1412.

Almond DJ, Guillou PJ, McMahon MJ. Effect of intravenous fat emulsion on natural killer cellular function and antibody-dependent cell cytotoxicity. Hum Nutr Clin Nutr 1985;39:227.

Aloia JF, Vaswani A, Yeh JK, et al. Calcitriol in the treatment of postmenopausal osteoporosis. Am J Med 1988;84:401.

AMA Department of Foods and Nutrition. Guidelines for essential trace element preparation for parenteral use. JAMA 1979;241:2051.

Anderson S. Thermography and plethysmography in the diagnosis of deep venous thrombosis—a comparison with phlebography. Acta Med Scand 1986;219:359.

Angus RM, Eisman JA. Osteoporosis: the role of calcium intake and supplementation. Med J Aust 1988;148:63.

Apelgren KN. Triple lumen catheters: technological advance or setback? Am Surg 1987;53:113.

Appelman PT, DeJong TE, Lampmann LE. Deep venous thrombosis of the leg: US findings. Radiology 1987;163:743.

Aronen HJ, Pamilo M, Suoranta HT, Suramo I. Sonography in differential diagnosis of deep venous thrombosis of the leg. Acta Radiol 1987;28:457.

Ashbaugh DG, Bigelow DB, Petty TL, et al. Acute respiratory distress in adults. Lancet 1967;2:319.

Askanazi J, Carpentier YA, Elwyn DH, et al. Influence of total parenteral nutrition of fuel utilization in injury and sepsis. Ann Surg 1980;191:40.

Askanazi J, Elwyn DH, Silverberg PA, et al. Respiratory distress secondary to a high carbohydrate load. Surgery 1980;87:596.

Athanasoulis CA. Therapeutic applications of angiography. Part 1. N Engl J Med 1980;302:1117.

Aubaniac R. L'injection intraveineuse sousclaviculaire: advantages et technique. Presse Med 1952;60:1456.

Ausman RK, Quebbeman EJ, Altmann CL. Liver malfunction associated with parenteral nutrition. In: Johnston IDA, ed. Advances in clinical nutrition. Boston: MTP Press, 1983.

Baertschi U, Schaer A, Bader P, et al. A comparison of low dose heparin and oral anticoagulants in the prevention of thrombophlebitis following gynaecological operations. Geburtsh Frauenheilk 1975;35:754.

Bain C, Willett W, Hennekens CH, et al. Use of postmenopausal hormones and risk of myocardial infarction. Circulation 1981;64:42.

Baker JP, Detsky AS, Wesson DE, et al. Nutritional assessment: a comparison of clinical judgment and objective measurements. N Engl J Med 1982;306:969.

Baker WH, Mahler DK, Foldes MS, et al. Pneumatic compression devices for prophylaxis of deep venous thrombosis (DVT). Am Surg 1986;52:371.

Baker WL. Hypophosphatemia. Am J Nurs 1985;85:998.

Ballard RM, Bradley-Watson PJ, Johnstone FD, et al. Low doses of subcutaneous heparin in the prevention of deep vein thrombosis after gynaecological surgery. J Obstet Gynaecol Br Commonw 1973;80:469.

Baran GW, Frisch KM. Duplex Doppler evaluation of puerperal ovarian vein thrombosis. Am J Radiol 1987;149:321.

Barbul A, Fishel RS, Shimazu S, et al. Intravenous hyperalimentation with high arginine levels improves wound healing and immune function. J Surg Res 1985;38:328.

Bates GW. On the nature of hot flash. Clin Obstet Gynecol 1981;24:231.

Becker DM. Venous thromboembolism. Epidemiology, diagnosis, prevention. J Gen Int Med 1986;1:402.

Bell WR, Starksen NF, Tong S, et al. Trousseau's syndrome: devastating coagulopathy in the absence of heparin. Am J Med 1985;79:423.

Bellantani MF, Blackman MR. Osteoporosis: diagnostic screening and its place in current care (clinical conference). Geriatrics 1988;43:63.

Bergqvist D. Dextran in the prophylaxis of deep-vein thrombosis, Letter. JAMA 1987;258:324.

Bergqvist D, Burmark US, Frisell J, et al. Low molecular weight heparin once daily compared with conventional low-dose heparin twice daily. A prospective double-blind multicentre trial on prevention of postoperative thrombosis. Br J Surg 1986; 73:204.

Bernstein K, Ulmsten U, Astedt B, et al. Incidence of thrombosis after gynecologic surgery evaluated by an improved ^{125}I-fibrinogen uptake test. Angiology 1980;3:606.

Bistrian BR, Blackburn GL, Hallowell E, et al. Protein status of general surgical patients. JAMA 1974;230:858.

Bjornson HS, Colley R, Bower RH, et al. Association between microorganism growth at the catheter site and colonization of the catheter in patients receiving total parenteral nutrition. Surgery 1982;92:720.

Black P MCL, Crowell RM, Abbott WM. External pneumatic calf compression reduces deep venous thrombosis in patients with ruptured intracranial aneurysms. Neurosurgery 1986;18:25.

Blackburn GL, Bistrian BR, Maini BS, et al. Nutritional and metabolic assessment of the hospitalized patient. J Parenter Enter Nutr 1977;1:11.

Blackburn GL, Etter G, Mackenzie T. Criteria for choosing amino acid therapy in acute renal failure. Am J Clin Nutr 1978;31:1841.

Body JJ, Borkowski A. Nutrition and quality of life in cancer patients. Eur J Cancer Clin Oncol 1987;23:127.

Bonnar J. Venous thromboembolism and gynecologic surgery. Clin Obstet Gynecol 1985;28:432.

Bonnar J, Walsh J. Prevention of thrombosis after pelvic surgery by British Dextran 70. Lancet 1972;1:614.

Bonnar J, Walsh J, Haddon M, et al. Coagulation system changes induced by pelvic surgery and the effect of dextran 70. Bibl Anat 1973;12:351.

Breneman JC. Postoperative thromboembolic disease: computer analysis leading to statistical prediction. JAMA 1965;193:576.

Brenner DA. Total parenteral nutrition at home. Outpatient Ther Med 1987;2:1.

Brismar B, Hardstedt C, Jacobson S. Diagnosis of thrombosis by catheter phlebography after prolonged central venous catheterization. Ann Surg 1981;194:779.

Brown CE, Battocletti JH, Sprinivasan R, et al. In vivo 31P nuclear magnetic resonance spectroscopy of bone mineral for evaluation of osteoporosis. Clin Chem 1988;34:1431.

Brown JG, Ward PE, Wilkinson AJ, Mollan RAB. Impedance plethysmography: a screening procedure to detect deep-vein thrombosis. J Bone Joint Surg Br 1987;69(2):264.

Brown R, Bancewicz J, Hamid J, et al. Delayed hypersensitivity skin testing does not influence the management of surgical patients. Ann Surg 1982;196:672.

Burch JC, Byrd BF, Vaughn WK. The effects of long-term estrogen on hysterectomized women. Am J Obstet Gynecol 1974;118:778.

Bush TL, Barrett-Connor E, Cowan DK, et al. Cardiovascular mortality and noncontraceptive use of estrogen in women: results from Lipid Research Clinics Program Follow-up Study. Circulation 1987;75:1102.

Buzby GP, Mullen JL, Mathews DC, et al. Prognostic nutritional index in gastrointestinal surgery. Am J Surg 1980;139:160.

Caprini JA, Chuckler JL, Zuckerman L, et al. Thrombosis prophylaxis using external compression. Surg Gynecol Obstet 1983;156:599.

Carpentier YA. Indications for nutritional support. Gut 1986;27:14.

Cauley JA, La Porte RE, Sandler RB, et al. The relationship of physical activity to high density lipoprotein cholesterol in postmenopausal women. J Chron Dis 1986;39:687.

Chory ET, Mullen JL. Nutritional support of the cancer patient: delivery systems and formulations. Surg Clin N Am 1986;66:1105.

Chow R, Harrison JE, Notarius C. Effect of two randomised exercise programmes on bone mass of healthy postmenopausal women. Br Med J 1987;295:6611.

Clarke-Pearson DL, Coleman RE, Siegel R, et al. Indium 111 platelet imaging for the detection of deep venous thrombosis and pulmonary embolism in patients without symptoms after surgery. Surgery 1985;98:98.

Clarke-Pearson DL, Coleman RE, Synan IS, et al. Venous thromboembolism prophylaxis in gynecologic oncology: a prospective controlled trial of low-dose heparin. Am J Obstet Gynecol 1983;145:606.

Clarke-Pearson DL, Creasman WT. Diagnosis of deep venous thrombosis in ob-gyn by impedance phlebography. Obstet Gynecol 1981;58:52.

Clarke-Pearson DL, DeLong ER, Synan IS, Creasman WT. Complications of low-dose heparin prophylaxis in gynecologic oncology surgery. Obstet Gynecol 1984;64:689.

Clarke-Pearson, DL, DeLong, ER, Synan, IS, et al. Variables associated with postoperative deep venous thrombosis: a prospective study of 411 gynecology patients and creation of a prognostic model. Obstet Gynecol 1987;69:146.

Clarke-Pearson DL, Jelovsek FR, Creasman WT. Thromboembolism complicating surgery for cervical and uterine malignancy: incidence, risk factors, and prophylaxis. Obstet Gynecol 1983;61:87.

Clayton JK, Anderson JA, McNicol GP. Effect of cigarette smoking on subsequent postoperative thromboembolic disease in gynecological patients. Br Med J 1978;2:402.

Clinical Nutrition Cases. Is chromium essential for humans? Nutr Rev 1988;46:17.

Colditz GA, Taden RL, Oster G. Rates of venous thrombosis after general surgery: combined results of randomised clinical trials. Lancet 1986;2:143.

Colditz GA, Willett WC, Stampfer MJ, et al. Menopause and the risk of coronary heart disease in women. N Eng J Med 1987;316:1105.

Colley R, Wilson J, Kapusta E, et al. Fever and catheter-related sepsis in total parenteral nutrition. J Parenter Enter Nutr 1979;3:32.

Collins CG. Suppurative pelvic thrombophlebitis. Am J Obstet Gynecol 1970;108:681.

Comerota AJ, Katz M, Grossi RJ, et al. The comparative value of noninvasive testing for diagnosis and surveillance of deep vein thrombosis. J Vasc Surg 1988;7:40.

Common HH, Seaman AJ, Rosch J, et al. Deep vein thrombosis treated with streptokinase or heparin. Follow-up of a randomized study. Angiology 1976;27:645.

Cooper HA, Bowie EJW, Owen CA. Evaluation of patients with increased fibrinolytic split products (FSP) in their serum. Mayo Clin Proc 1974;49:654.

Cranley JJ, Canos AJ, Sull WJ. The diagnosis of deep vein thrombosis. Arch Surg 1976;111:34.

Creasman WT, Henderson D, Hinshaw W, et al. Estrogen replacement therapy in the patient treated for endometrial cancer. Obstet Gynecol 1986;67:326.

Czer LSC, Appel P, Shoemaker WC. Pathogenesis of respiratory failure (ARDS) after hemorrhage and trauma. II. Cardiorespiratory patterns after development of ARDS. Crit Care Med 1980;8:513.

Dalen N, Lamke B, Wallgren A. Bone-mineral losses in oophorectomized women. J Bone Joint Surg 1974;56:1235.

D'Alonzo WA, Alavi A. Detection of deep venous thrombosis by Indium-111 leukocyte scintigraphy. J Nuc Med 1986;27:631.

Dalsky GP, Stocke KS, Ehsani AA, et al. Weight-bearing exercise training and lumbar bone mineral content in postmenopausal women. Ann Int Med 1988;108:824.

Dark DS, Pingleton SK, Kerby GR. Hypercapnia during weaning: a complication of nutritional support. Chest 1985;88:141.

Davis RB, Theologides A, Kennedy BJ. Comparative studies of blood coagulation and platelet aggregation in patients with cancer and nonmalignant diseases. Ann Int Med 1969;71:69.

Delafosse B, Bouffard Y, Viale JP, et al. Respiratory changes induced by parenteral nutrition in postoperative patients undergoing inspiratory pressure support ventilation. Anesthesiology 1987;66:393.

Dempsey DT, Mullen JL, Buzby GP. The link between nutritional status and clinical outcome: can nutritional intervention modify it? Am J Clin Nutr 1988;47:352.

Dihydroergotamine-heparin to prevent postoperative deep vein thrombosis. Med Lett Drugs Ther 1985;27:688:45.

Dillon JD, Schaffner W, Van Way CW, et al. Septicemia and total parenteral nutrition: distinguishing catheter-related from other septic episodes. JAMA 1973;223:1341.

Dinsmore RE, Wedeen V, Rosen B, et al. Phase-offset technique to distinguish slow blood flow and thrombus on MR images. Am J Roent 1987;148:634.

Divertie MB. Adult respiratory distress syndrome. Mayo Clin Proc 1982;57:371.

Doran FSA. Prevention of deep vein thrombosis. Br J Hosp Med 1971;6:773.

Duxbury B McD. Therapeutic quality control leading to further clinical assessment of oral anticoagulation. Acta Haemat 1986;76:65.

Elwyn DH. Nutritional requirements of adult surgical patients. Crit Care Med 1980;8:9.

Endl VJ, Auinger W. Early detection of postoperative deep-vein thrombosis in gynecological patients by the ^{125}I-fibrinogen test. Wien Klin Wochenschr 1977;89:304.

Everett HS, Ridley JH. Female urology. New York: Harper-Hoeber, 1968.

Felmlee JP, Ehman RL. Spatial presuturation: a method for suppressing flow artifacts and improving depiction of vascular anatomy in MR imaging. Radiology 1987;164:559.

Fischer JE. Surgical nutrition. Boston: Little, Brown, 1983.

Flanc C, Kakkar VW, Clarke MB. The detection of venous thrombosis of the legs using ^{125}I-labeled fibrinogen. Br J Surg 1958;55:742.

Fletcher JP, Little JM. A comparison of parenteral nutrition and early postoperative enteral feeding on the nitrogen balance after major surgery. Surgery 1986;100:21.

Francis DMA, Shenton BK. Fat emulsion adversely affects lymphocyte reactivity. Aust N Z J Surg 1987;57:323.

Francis RM, Peacock M. Local action of oral 1.25-dihydroxycholecalciferol on calcium absorption in osteoporosis. Am J Clin Nutr 1987;46:315.

Frangos JA, Eskin SG, McIntire, LV. Flow effects on prostacyclin production by cultured human endothelial cells. Science 1985;227:1477.

Frisancho AR. New standards of weight and body composition by frame size and height for assessment of nutritional status. Am J Clin Nutr 1984;40:808.

Frisancho AR. Nutrition anthropometry. J Am Diet Assoc 1988;88:553.

Furman RH. Coronary heart disease and the menopause. In: Ryan KJ, Gibson DC, eds. Menopause and aging. 1971; DHEW publication no. (NIH) 73-319.

Gallagher JC, Nordin BEC. Estrogens and calcium metabolism. In: Van Keep PA, Lauritzen C, eds. Frontiers of hormone research. Vol. 2. Aging and estrogens. Basel: S Karger, 1973.

Gallagher JC, Nordin BEC. Calcium metabolism and the menopause.

In: Curry AS, ed. Biochemistry of women. Cleveland: CRC Press, 1974.

Gazzaniga AB, Day AT, Sankary H. The efficacy of a 20 per cent fat emulsion as a peripherally administered substrate. Surg Obstet Gynecol 1985;160:387.

Genton E. Pulmonary embolism and infarction. In: Chung ED, ed. Cardiac emergency care. Philadelphia: Lea & Febiger, 1979.

Genton E, Turpie AGG. Venous thromboembolism associated with gynecologic surgery. Clin Obstet Gynecol 1980;23:209.

Gever LN. Embolex: to prevent a double postop danger. Nursing 1986;16:73.

Gjonnaess H, Abildgaard U. Bleeding in gynecological surgery: influence of low dose heparin. Int J Gynaecol Obstet 1976;14:9.

Goldberg RJ, Seneff M, Gore JM, et al. Occult malignant neoplasm in patients with deep venous thrombosis. Arch Intern Med 1987;147:251.

Goodnight SH Jr. Bleeding and intravascular clotting in malignancy: a review. Ann NY Acad Sci 1974;230:271.

Gordon GS. Postmenopausal osteoporosis: cause, prevention and treatment. Clin Obstet Gynecol 1977;4:169.

Gordon SG, Franks JJ, Lewis B. Cancer procoagulant A: a factor X activating procoagulant from malignant tissue. Thromb Res 1975;6:127.

Gordon T, Kannel WB, Hjortland MC, McNamara PM. Menopause and coronary heart disease: The Framingham Study. Ann Int Med 1978;89:157.

Gore JM, Appelbaum JS, Greene HL, et al. Occult cancer in patients with acute pulmonary embolism. Ann Intern Med 1982;96:556.

Gray LA, Christopherson WM, Hoover RN. Estrogens and endometrial carcinoma. Obstet Gynecol 1977;49:385.

Griffin MR, Stanson AW, Brown ML, et al. Deep venous thrombosis and pulmonary embolism: risk of subsequent malignant neoplasms. Arch Intern Med 1987;147:1907.

Gruber UF, Saldeen T, Brokopt T, Ekolf B. Incidences of fatal postoperative pulmonary embolism after prophylaxis with dextran 70 and low dose heparin. An international multicentre study. Br Med J 1980;280:69.

Guyton DP, Khayat A, Schreiber H. Pneumatic compression stockings and prostaglandin synthesis: a pathway to fibrinolysis? Crit Care Med 1985;13:266.

Guyton DP, Khayat A, Schreiber H, Husni EA. Endogenous plasminogen activator and venous flow: therapeutic implications. Crit Care Med 1987;15:122.

Hammond CB, Jelovsek FR, Lee KL, et al. Effects of long-term estrogen replacement therapy: I. metabolic effects. Am J Obstet Gynecol 1979;133:525.

Hammond CB, Ory SJ. Endocrine problems in the menopause. Clin Obstet Gynecol 1982;25:19.

Hands LJ, Royle GT, Kettlewell MGW. Vitamin K requirements in patients receiving total parenteral nutrition. Br J Surg 1985;72:665.

Hart DM, Farish E, Fletcher DC, et al. Ten years postmenopausal hormone replacement therapy-effect on lipoproteins. Maturitas 1984;5:271.

Hauser CJ, Shoemaker WC, Turpin I, et al. Oxygen transport responses to colloids and crystalloids in critically ill surgical patients. Surg Gynecol Obstet 1980;150:811.

Haydock DA, Hill GL. Improved wound healing response in surgical patients receiving intravenous nutrition. Br J Surg 1987;74:320.

Heird WC, Grundy SM, Hubbard VS. Structured lipids and their use in clinical nutrition. Am J Clin Nutr 1986;43:320.

Helgason S. Estrogen replacement therapy after the menopause. Acta Obstet Gynecol Scand 1982;107(suppl):1.

Hilgard P. Experimental vitamin K deficiency and spontaneous metastases. Br J Cancer 1975;35:391.

Hirsh J, Deykin D, Poller L: "Therapeutic range" for oral anticoagulant therapy. Chest 1986;89:11S.

Hirsh J, Genton E, Hull R. Venous thromboembolism. New York: Grune & Stratton, 1981.

Hirsh J, Hull RD, Raskob GE. Clinical features and diagnosis of venous thrombosis. J Am Coll Cardiol 114B, 1986.

Hirvonen E, Malkonen M, Manninen V. Effects of different progestogens on lipoproteins during postmenopausal therapy. N Engl J Med 1981;304:560.

Hoak JC, Connor WE, Warner ED. The antithrombotic effects of sodium heparin and sodium warfarin. Arch Intern Med 1966;117:25.

Hobbs JT, Davies JW. Detection of venous thrombosis with ^{131}I-labeled fibrinogen in the rabbit. Lancet 1960;2:134.

Hodgkinson CP, Hodari AA. Trocar suprapubic cystostomy for postoperative bladder drainage in the female. Am J Obstet Gynecol 1966;96:773.

Hoshal VL. Total intravenous nutrition with peripherally inserted silicone elastomer central venous catheters. Arch Surg 1975;110:644.

Huisman MV, Buller HR, Ten Cate JW, et al. Serial impedance plethysmography for suspected deep venous thrombosis in outpatients. The Amsterdam General Practitioner Study. N Engl J Med 1986;314:823.

Hull RD, Raskob GE, Hirsh J. Prophylaxis of venous thromboembolism: an overview. Chest 1986;89:3745.

Inada K, Koike S, Shirai N, et al. Effects of intermittent pneumatic leg compression for prevention of postoperative deep venous thrombosis with special reference to fibrinolytic activity. Am J Surg 1988;155:602.

Ireton-Jones CS, Turner WW, Jr. The use of respiratory quotient to determine the efficacy of nutrition support regimens. J Am Diet Assoc 1987;87:180.

Irving M. ABC of nutrition. Br Med J 1985;291:1403.

Jeffcoate TNA, Tindall VR. Venous thrombosis and embolism in obstetrics and gynecology. Aust N Z J Obstet Gynaecol 1965;5:119.

Joist JH, Sherman LA, eds. Venous and arterial thrombosis: pathogenesis, diagnosis, prevention and therapy. New York: Grune & Stratton, 1979.

Joseph RR, Day HJ, Sherwin RM, et al. Microangiopathic haemolytic anaemia associated with consumption coagulopathy in a patient with disseminated carcinoma. Scand J Haematol 1967;4:271.

Judd HL, Cleary RE, Creasman WT, et al. Estrogen replacement therapy. Obstet Gynecol 1981;58:267.

Kakkar VV, Corrigan TP, Fossard DP. Prevention of postoperative pulmonary embolism by low dose heparin. Lancet 1975;2:45.

Kass EH, Sossen HS. Prevention of infection of urinary tract in presence of indwelling catheters. JAMA 1959;169:1181.

Kemble JVH. Incidence of deep vein thrombosis. Br J Hosp Med 1971;6:721.

King CR, Daly JW. The prevention of postoperative pulmonary emboli with low-molecular-weight dextran. Am J Obstet Gynecol 1975;123:46.

Kline A, Hughes LE, Campbell H, et al. Dextran 70 in prophylaxis of thromboembolic disease after surgery: a clinically oriented randomized double-blind trial. Br Med J 1975;2:109.

Knight LC, Maurer AH, Ammar IA, et al. Evaluation of indium: 111-labeled anti-fibrin antibody for imaging vascular thrombi. J Nucl Med 1988;29:494.

Kotz KL, Geelhoed GW. Lethal thromboembolism and its prevention in pelvic surgery: a review. Gynecol Oncol 1981;12:271.

Kriska AM, Sandler RB, Cawley JA, et al. The assessment of historical physical activity and its relation to adult bone parameters. Am J Epidemiol 1988;12:1053.

Langsfeld M, Hershey FB, Thorpe L, et al. Duplex B-mode imaging for the diagnosis of deep venous thrombosis. Arch Surg 1987;122:587.

Leiter LA, Marliss EB. Survival during fasting may depend on fat as well as protein stores. JAMA 1982;248:2306.

Lieberman JS, Borrero J, Urdaneta E, et al. Thrombophlebitis and cancer. JAMA 1961;177:542.

Lindhagen A, Bergqvist A, Bergqvist D, Hallbook T. Late venous function in the leg after deep venous thrombosis occurring in relation to pregnancy. Br J Obstet Gynaecol 1986;93:348.

Lindquist O. Relationship between menstrual status and development of osteoporosis. Acta Obstet Gynecol Scand [Suppl] 1982;110:22.

Lindsay R. Prevention of osteoporosis. Clin Orthopaed Relat Res 1987;222:44.

Lindsay R, Aitken JM, Anderson JB, et al. Long-term prevention of postmenopausal osteoporosis by oestrogen. Lancet 1976;1:1038.

Lindsey R, Hart DM, Forrest C, et al. Prevention of spinal osteoporosis in oophorectomised women. Lancet 1980;2:1151.

Lindsey R, Hart DM, MacLean A, et al. Bone response to termination of estrogen treatment. Lancet 1978;1:1325.

Longerbeam JK, Vannix R, Wagner W, et al. Central venous pressure monitoring. Am J Surg 1965;110:220.

Lueg MC. Postmenopausal osteoporosis: treatment with low-dose sodium fluoride and estrogen. S Med J 1988;81:597.

MacIntyre I, Stevenson JC, Whitehead MI, et al. Calcitonin for prevention of postmenopausal bone loss. Lancet 1988;1:900.

Maki DG, Weise CE, Sarafin HW. A semiquantitative culture method for identifying intravenous-catheter-related infection. N Engl J Med 1977;296:1305.

Malluche HH, Faugere MC, Friedler RM, et al. 1,25-dihydroxy vitamin D3 corrects bone loss but suppresses bone remodeling in ovariohysterectomized beagle dogs. Endocrinol 1988;125:1998.

Mamelle N, Meunier PJ, Dusan R, et al. Risk-benefit ratio of sodium fluoride treatment in primary vertebral osteoporosis. Lancet 1988;2:361.

Mammer EF, ed. Venous thromboembolism. Semin Thromb Hemost 2:4, April 1976.

Markwardt F. Pharmacological approaches to thrombin regulation. Ann NY Acad Sci 1986;485:204.

Marshall DH, Horsman A, Nordin BEC. The prevention and management of post-menopausal osteoporosis. Acta Obstet Gynecol Scand [Suppl] 1977;65:49.

Mattingly RF, Moore DE, Clark DO. Bacteriologic study of suprapubic bladder drainage. Am J Obstet Gynecol 1972;114:732.

Mavor GE. Surgery of deep vein thrombosis. Br J Hosp Med 1971;6:755.

McCarthy TG, McQueen J, Johnstone FD, et al. A comparison of low dose subcutaneous heparin and intravenous dextran 70 in the prophylaxis of deep venous thrombosis after gynaecological surgery. J Obstet Gynaecol Br Commonw 1974;81:486.

McDevitt E. Thromboembolic complications following gyneologic operations: role of prophylactic anticoagulant therapy. In: Sherry S, Brinkhous KM, Genton E, et al, eds. Thrombosis. Washington, D.C., National Academy of Sciences, 1969.

McGee CD, Ostro MJ, Kurran R, Jeejeebhoy KN. Vitamin E and selenium status of patients receiving short-term total parenteral nutrition. Am J Clin Nutr 1985;42:432.

Meema HE, Bunker ML, Meema S. Loss of compact bone due to menopause. Obstet Gynecol 1965;26:333.

Miller SP, Sanchez-Avalos J, Stefanski T, et al. Coagulation disorders in cancer: I. clinical and laboratory studies. Cancer 1967;20:1452.

Mintz MC, Levy DW, Axel A, et al. Puerperal ovarian vein thrombosis: MR diagnosis. Am J Radiol 1987;149:1273.

Mirtallo JM, Schneider PT, Mauko K, et al. A comparison of essential and general amino acid infusions in the nutritional support of patients with compromised renal function. J Parenter Enter Nutr 1982;6:109.

Mittleman JS, Edwards WS, McDonald JB. Effectiveness of leg compression in preventing venous stasis. Am J Surg 1982;144:611.

Mobin-Uddin K, Callard GM, Bolooki H, et al. Transcaval interruption with umbrella filter. N Engl J Med 1972;286:55.

Mohr DN, Ryu JH, Litin SC, Rosenow EC, III. Recent advances in the management of venous thromboembolism. Mayo Clin Proc 1988;63:281.

Moore FD. Energy and the maintenance of the body cell mass. J Parenter Enter Nutr 1980;4:228.

Moosman DA. The anatomy of infraclavicular subclavian vein catheterization and its complications. Surg Gynecol Obstet 1973;136:71.

Moser KM, LeMoine JR. Is embolic risk conditioned by location of deep venous thrombosis? Ann Int Med 1981;94:439.

Mullin TJ, Kirkpatrick JR. The effect of nutritional support on immune competency in patients suffering from trauma, sepsis, and malignant disease. Surgery 1981;90:610.

Munk-Jensen N, Pors Nielsen S, Obel EB, et al. Reversal of postmenopausal vertebral bone loss by oestrogen and progesterone: a double-blind placebo controlled study. Br Med J 1988; 296:1150.

Need AG, Horowitz M, Morris HA, et al. Effects of nandrolane therapy on forearm bone mineral content in osteoporosis. Clin Orthop 1987;225:273.

Nicolaides AN, Fernandes JF, Pollock AV. Intermittent sequential compression of the legs in the prevention of venous stasis and postoperative deep venous thrombosis. Surgery 1980;87:69.

Nicolaides AN, Miles C, Hoare M, et al. Intermittent sequential pneumatic compression of the legs and thromboembolism-deterrent stockings in the prevention of postoperative deep venous thrombosis. Surgery 1983;94:21.

Nordenstrom J, Carpentier YA, Askanazi J, et al. Metabolic utilization of intravenous fat emulsion during total parenteral nutrition. Ann Surg 1982;196:221.

Notelovitz M, Johnston M, Smith S, et al. Metabolic and hormonal effects of 25-mg and 50-mg 17 beta-estradiol implants in surgically menopausal women. Obstet Gynecol 1987;70:749.

Nusbacher J. Migratory venous thrombosis and cancer. NY J Med 1964;64:2166.

O'Keefe SJD, Bean E, Symmonds K, et al. Clinical evaluation of a "3-in-1" intravenous nutrient solution. S Afr Med J 1985;68:82.

Oster G, Tuden RL, Colditz GA. Prevention of venous thromboembolism after general surgery: cost-effectiveness analysis of alternative approaches to prophylaxis. Am J Med 1987;82:889.

Oster MW. Thrombophlebitis and cancer: a review. Angiology 1976; 27:557.

Oster ZH, Srivastava SC, Som P, et al. Thrombus radioimmunoscintigraphy: an approach using monoclonal antiplatelet antibody. Proc Natl Acad Sci USA 1985;82:3465.

Ottosson UB, Johansson BG, von Schoultz B. Subfractions of high-density lipoprotein cholesterol during estrogen replacement therapy: a comparison between progestogens and natural progesterone. Am J Obstet Gynecol 1985;151:746.

Pacifici R, McMurty C, Vered I, et al. Coherence therapy does not prevent axial bone loss in osteoporotic women: a preliminary comparative study. J Clin Endocrinol Metab 1988;66:747.

Padberg FT, Ruggiero J, Blackburn GL, et al. Central venous catheterization for parenteral nutrition. Ann Surg 1981;193:264.

Pak CYC, Sakhaee K, Zerwekh JE, et al. Safe and effective treatment of osteoporosis with intermittent slow release sodium fluoride augmentation of vertebral bone mass and inhibition of fractures. J Clin Endocrinol Metab 1989;68:150.

Pangrazzi J, Abbadini M, Zametta M, et al. Antithrombotic and bleeding effects of a low molecular weight heparin fraction. Biol Pharmacol 1985;34:3305.

Peters AM, Lavender JP, Needham SG, et al. Imaging thrombus with radiolabelled monoclonal antibody to platelets. Br Med J 1986;293:1525.

Peterson CE, Kwaan HC. Current concepts of warfarin therapy. Arch Intern Med 1986;146:581.

Petitti DB, Wingard J, Pellegrin F, Ramcharan S. Risk of vascular

disease in women: smoking, oral contraceptives, non-contraceptive estrogens, and other factors. JAMA 1979;242:1150.

Petty TL, Fowler AA. Another look at ARDS. Chest 1982;82:98.

Peuscher FW, Cleton FJ, Armstrong L, et al. Signifance of plasma fibrinopeptide A (FPA) in patients with malignancy. J Lab Clin Med 1980;96:5.

Poller L, McKernan A, Thomson JM, et al. Fixed minidose warfarin: a new approach to prophylaxis against venous thrombosis after major surgery. Br Med J 1987;295:1309.

Polley KJ, Nordin BE, Baghurst PA, et al. Effect of calcium supplementation on forearm bone mineral content in postmenopausal women: a prospective sequential controlled trial. J Nutr 1987;117:1929.

Poulose KP, Kapcar AJ, Reba RC. False positive ^{125}I fibrinogen test. Angiology 1976;27:258.

Prevention of venous thrombosis and pulmonary embolism. N.I.H. consensus development conference on prevention of venous thrombosis and pulmonary embolism. JAMA 1986;256:744.

Proudfit CM. Estrogens and menopause. JAMA 1976;236:939.

Quebbeman EJ. Estimating energy requirements in patients receiving parenteral nutrition. Arch Surg 1982;117:1281.

Quebbeman EJ. A re-evaluation of energy expenditure during parenteral nutrition. Ann Surg 1982;195:282.

Quick AJ. Modern concepts of venous thrombosis. Practitioner 1951;166:213.

Quigley MM, Hammon CB. Estrogen replacement therapy: help or hazard? N Engl J Med 1979;301:646.

Ramchandani P, Soulen RL, Fedullo LM, Garnes VD. Deep vein thrombosis: significant limitation of noninvasive tests. Radiology 1985;156:47.

Rapoport S, Sostman HD, Pope C, et al. Venous clots: evaluation with MR imaging. Radiology 1987;162:527.

Ravnikar V, Murin V, Nutkik J, et al. Blood lipid levels in post-menopausal women on hormone replacement therapy. 35th Annual Meeting, Soc Gynecol Invest 1988; Abstract no. 422.

Rayburn W, Wolk R, Mercer N, Roberts J. Parenteral nutrition in obstetrics and gynecology. Obstet Gynecol 1986;41:200.

Reginster JY, Denis D, Albert A, et al. 1-year controlled randomised trial of prevention of early postmenopausal bone loss by intra-nasal calcitonin. Lancet 1987;2:1481.

Rickles FR, Edwards RL. Activation of blood coagulation in cancer: Trousseau's syndrome revisited. Blood 1983;62:14.

Rickles FR, Edwards RL, Barb C, et al. Abnormalities of blood coagulation in patients with cancer: fibrinopeptide A generation and tumor growth. Cancer 1983;51:301.

Riis BJ, Christiansen C. Measurement of spinal or peripheral bone mass to estimate early postmenopausal bone loss? Am J Med 1988;84:646.

Rinaldo JE, Rogers RM. Adult Respiratory Distress Syndrome. N Engl J Med 1982;306:900.

Rivlin RS. Osteoporosis: nutrition. Public Health Reports Jul-Aug, 1987;(suppl):131.

Rose D, Yarborough MF, Canizaro PC, Lowry SF. One hundred and fourteen fistulas of the gastrointestinal tract treated with total parenteral nutrition. Surg Gynecol Obstet 1986;163:345.

Rosner NH, Doris PE. Diagnosis of femoropopliteal venous thrombosis: comparison of duplex sonography and plethysmography. Am J Roentgenol 1988;150:623.

Ross RK, Paganini-Hill A, Mack TM, et al. Menopausal oestrogen therapy and protection from death from ischaemic heart disease. Lancet 1981;1(8225):858.

Rudman D, Williams PJ. Nutrient deficiencies during total parenteral nutrition. Nutr Rev 1985;43:1.

Ryan DA. Hazard associated with the use of a common pathway for infusion and vascular monitoring. Anaesthesia 1985;40:1134.

Sach GH, Levin J, Bell WR. Trousseau's syndrome and other manifestations of chronic disseminated coagulopathy in patients with neoplasms: clinical pathophysiologic and therapeutic features. Medicine 1977;S6:1.

Salvian AJ, Baker JD. Effects of intermittent pneumatic calf compression in normal and postphlebitic legs. J Cardiovasc Surg 1988;29:37.

Samama M, Bernard P, Bonnardot JP, et al. Low molecular weight heparin compared with unfractionated heparin in prevention of postoperative thrombosis. Br J Surg 1988;75:128.

Sanders RA, Sheldon GF. Septic complications of total parenteral nutrition: a five year experience. Am J Surg 1976;132:214.

Sandler DA, Martin JF. Liquid crystal thermography as a screening test for deep-vein thrombosis. Lancet 1985;1:665.

Sandstedt S, Lennmarken C, Symreng T, et al. The effect of preoperative total parenteral nutrition on energy-rich phosphates, electrolytes and free amino acids in skeletal muscle of malnourished patients with gastric carcinoma. Br J Surg 1985;72:920.

Sasahara AA, DiSerio FJ, et al. Dihydroergotamine-heparin prophylaxis of postoperative deep vein thrombosis: a multicenter trial. JAMA 1984;251:2960.

Sasahara AA, Koppenhagen K, Haring R, et al. Low molecular weight heparin plus dihydroergotamine for prophylaxis of postoperative deep vein thrombosis. Br J Surg 1986;73:697.

Savvas M, Studd JW, Fogelman I, et al. Skeletal effects of oral oestrogen compared with subcutaneous oestrogen and testosterone in postmenopausal women. Br Med J 1988;297:331.

Schiff MJ, Feinberg AW, Naidich JB. Noninvasive venous examinations as a screening test for pulmonary embolism. Arch Intern Med 1987;147:505.

Schlueter DP. High-risk gynecology: pulmonary risks. Clin Obstet Gynecol 1973;16:91.

Scurr JH, Ibrahim SZ, Faber RG, LeQuesne LP. The efficacy of graduated compression stockings in the prevention of deep vein thrombosis. Br J Surg 1977;64:371.

Seem E, Stranden E, Stiris MG. Computed tomography in deep venous thrombosis with limb oedema. Acta Radiol Diag 1985;26:727.

Seiden AM, Pensak ML. Postoperative deep venous thrombosis and pulmonary embolism: diagnosis, management and prevention. Am J Otol 1986;7:377.

Semmens JP, Wagner G. Effects of estrogen therapy on vaginal physiology during menopause. Obstet Gynecol 1985;66:15.

Sevitt S, Gallagher NG. Venous thrombosis and pulmonary embolism: a clinical pathological study in injured and burned patients. Br J Surg, 1961;48:475.

Shils ME, Young VR, eds. Modern nutrition in health and disease. 7th ed. Philadelphia: Lea and Febiger, 1988.

Shoemaker WC, Appel P, Czer LSC, et al. Pathogenesis of respiratory failure (ARDS) after hemorrhage and trauma: I. cardiorespiratory patterns preceding the development of ARDS. Crit Care Med 1980;8:504.

Sibbald WJ, Anderson RR, Reid B, et al. Alveolo-capillary permeability in human septic ARDS: effect of high dose corticosteroid. Ther Chest 1981;79:133.

Sigel B, Edelstein AL, Felix WR, et al. Compression of deep venous system of the lower leg during inactive recumbency. Arch Surg 1973;106:38.

Sigel B, Edelstein AL, Savitch L, et al. Type of compression for reducing venous stasis: a study of lower extremities during inactive recumbency. Arch Surg 1975;110:171.

Sitges-Serra A, Puig P, Jaurrieta E, et al. Catheter sepsis due to Staphylococcus epidermidis during parenteral nutrition. Surg Gynecol Obstet 1980;151:481.

Smith DC, Prentice R, Thompson DJ, et al. Association of exogenous estrogen and endometrial carcinoma. N Engl J Med 1975; 293:1164.

Sobel S. Osteoporosis: regulatory view. Public Health Reports Jul—Aug, 1987;(suppl):136.

Soong BCF, Miller SP. Coagulation disorders in cancer: III. fibrinolysis and inhibitors. Cancer 1970;25:867.

Speroff L, Glass RH, Kase NG. Clinical gynecologic endocrinology and infertility. 4th ed. Baltimore: Williams and Wilkins, 1989.

Spritzer CE, Sussman SK, Blinder RA, et al. Deep venous thrombosis evaluation with limited-flip-angle, gradient-refocused MR imaging: preliminary experience. Radiology 1988;166:371.

Sproul EE. Carcinoma and venous thrombosis: the frequency of association of carcinoma in the body or tail of the pancreas with multiple venous thrombosis. Am J Cancer 1938;34:566.

Stamp TC, Jenkins MV, Loveridge N, et al. Fluoride therapy in osteoporosis: acute effects on parathyroid and mineral homeostasis. Clin Sci 1988;75:143.

Stampfer MJ, Willett WC, Colditz GA, et al. A prospective study of postmenopausal estrogen therapy and coronary heart disease. N Engl J Med 1985;313:1044.

Stanton JR, Freis ED, Wilkins RW. Acceleration of linear flow in deep veins with local compression. J Clin Inves 1944;28:553.

Starker PM, Gump FE, Askanazi J, et al. Serum albumin levels as an index of nutritional support. Surgery 1982;91:194.

Starker PM, LaSala PA, Askanazi J, et al. The influence of preoperative total parenteral nutrition upon morbidity and mortality. Surg Gynecol Obstet 1986;162:569.

Stevenson JC, Whitehead MI, Padwick M, et al. Dietary intake of calcium and postmenopausal bone loss. Br Med J 1988; 297:6640:15.

Stewart RD, Sanislow CA. Silastic intravenous catheter. N Engl J Med 1961;265:1283.

Sturdee DW, Wilson KA, Pipili E, et al. Physiological aspects of menopausal hot flush. Br Med J 1978;2:79.

Sue-Ling HM, Johnston D, McMahon MJ, et al. Pre-operative identification of patients at high risk of deep venous thrombosis after elective major abdominal surgery. Lancet 1986;1:1173.

Sugimura K, Yamasaki K, Kitagaki H, et al. Bone marrow diseases of the spine: differentiation with T1 and T2 relaxation times in MR imaging. Radiology 1987;165:541.

Summaria L, Caprini JA, McMillan R, et al. Relationship between postsurgical fibrinolytic parameters and deep vein thrombosis in surgical patients treated with compression devices. Am Surg 1988;54:156.

Sun NCJ, Bowie EJW, Kazmier FJ, et al. Blood coagulation studies in patients with cancer. Mayo Clin Proc 1974;49:636.

Sun NCJ, McAfee WM, Hum GJ, et al. Hemostatic abnormalities in malignancy, a prospective study of one hundred eight patients. Am Soc Clin Path 1979;7:10.

Sy WM, Seo IS. Radionuclide venography: imaging monitor in deep-vein thrombosis of the pelvis and lower extremities. Br J Rad 1986;59:325.

Szklo M, Tonascia J, Gordis L, Bloom I. Estrogen use and myocardial infarction risk: a case-control study. Prevent Med 1984;13:510.

Taberner DA, Poller L, Burslem RW, et al. Oral anticoagulants controlled by the British comparative thromboplastin versus low-dose heparin in prophylaxis of deep vein thrombosis. Br Med J 1978;1:272.

Tarnay TJ, Rohr PR, Davidson AG, et al: Pneumatic calf compression, fibrinolysis and the prevention of deep venous thrombosis. Surgery 1980;88:489.

Taussig FJ. Bladder function after confinement and after gynecological operations. Trans Am Gynecol Soc 1915;40:351.

Thomas D, ed. Thrombosis. Br Med Bull 1978;2:34.

Tice DA. Low dosage of heparin. Surg Gynecol Obstet 1976;143:970.

Torosian MH, Daly JM. Nutritional support in the cancer-bearing host: effects on host and tumor. Cancer 1986;58:8(suppl):1915.

Tracey KJ, Legaspi A, Albert JD, et al. Protein and substrate metabolism during starvation and parenteral refeeding. Clin Sci 1988;74:123.

Trousseau A. Phlegmasia alba doleng: Clinique Medicale de l'Hotel-Dieu de Paris. London: New Sydenham Society 1868;3:695.

Turner GM, Cole SE, Brooks JH. The efficacy of graduated compression stockings in the deep vein thrombosis after major gynaecological surgery. Br J Obstet Gynacol 1984;91:588.

Turpie AGG, Hirsh J, Jay RM, et al. Double-blind randomised trial of Org 10172 low-molecular weight heparinoid in prevention of deep-vein thrombosis in thrombotic stroke. Lancet 1987;1: 8532:523.

Twombly GH. Hemorrhage in gynecologic surgery. Clin Obstet Gynecol 1973;16:135.

Underwood SR, Firmin DN, Klipstein RH, et al. Magnetic resonance velocity mapping: clinical application of a new technique. Br Heart J 1987;57:404.

Utian WH. Menopause in modern perspective. New York: Appleton-Century-Crofts, 1980.

Vaccaro P, Van Aman M, Miller S, et al. Shortcomings of physical examination and impedance plethysmography in the diagnosis of lower extremity deep venous thrombosis. Angiology 1987; 38:232.

Valerio D, Hussey JK, Smith FW. Central vein thrombosis associated with intravenous feeding: a prospective study. J Parenter Enter Nutr 1981;5:240.

Van den Brande PM. The efficacy of dextan 40 in preventing early postoperative thrombosis following difficult lower extremity bypass. J Vasc Surg 1985;2:643.

Van Ooijen, B. Subcutaneous heparin and postoperative wound hematomas: a prospective, double-blind, randomized study. Arch Surg 1986;121:937.

Vernet O, Christin L, Schutz Y, et al. Enteral versus parenteral nutrition: comparison of energy metabolism in lean and moderately obese women. Am J Clin Nutr 1986;43:194.

Vinton NE, Laidlaw SA, Ament ME, et al. Taurine concentrations in plasma and blood cells of patients undergoing long-term parenteral nutrition. Am J Clin Nutr 1986;44:398.

Virchow R. Handbuch der speciellen Pathologie and Therapie. Vol II. Erlangen and Stuttgart: F Enke, 1854.

Von Schulthess GK, Augustiny N. Calculation of T2 values versus phase imaging in the distinction between flow and thrombus in MR imaging. Radiology 1987;164:549.

Walsh JJ, Bonnar J, Wright FW. A study of pulmonary embolism and deep leg vein thrombosis after major gynaecological surgery using labelled fibrinogen-phlebography and lung scanning. J Obstet Gynaecol Br Commonw 1974;81:311.

Wardlaw G. The effects of diet and life-style on bone mass in women. J Am Diet Assoc 1988;88:17.

Weinstein MC. Estrogen use in post-menopausal women: costs, risks, and benefits. N Engl J Med 1980;303:308.

Weiss NS, Szekely DR, Austin DF. Increasing incidence of endometrial cancer in the United States. N Engl J Med 1976;294:1259.

Welch GW, McKeel DW, Silverstein P, et al. The role of the catheter composition in the development of thrombophlebitis. Surg Gynecol Obstet 1974;138:421.

Willatts SM. Nutrition. Br J Anaesthiol 1986;58:2:201.

Williams TJ, Julian CG. Tidal drainage in the postoperative bladder. Am J Obstet Gynecol 1962;83:1313.

Wilson JE. Diagnostic methods for deep venous thrombosis (editorial). Arch Int Med 1980;140:893.

Wilson JN, Grow JB, Demony CV, et al. Central venous pressure in optimal blood volume maintenance. Arch Surg 1962;85:563.

Wilson PWF, Garrison RJ, Castelli WP. Postmenopausal estrogen use, cigarette smoking, and cardiovascular morbidity in women over 50: The Framingham Study. N Engl J Med 1985;313:1038.

Wren B, Garrett D. The effect of low-dose piperazine oestrogen sulphate and low-dose levonorgestrel on blood lipid levels in postmenopausal women. Maturitas 1985;7:141.

Yoda Y, Abe T. Fibrinopeptide A (FPA) level and fibrinogen kinetics in patients with malignant disease. Thromb Haemostas 1981;46:706.

Young GP, Thomas RJS, Bourne DWF, Russell D McR. Parenteral nutrition. Med J Aust 1985;143:597.

Zacharski LR, Rickles FR, Henderson WG, et al. Platelets and malignancy: rationale and experimental design for the VA cooperative study of RA-233 in the treatment of cancer. Am J Clin Oncol 1982;5:593.

Ziel HK, Finkle WD. Increased risk of endometrial carcinoma among users of conjugated estrogens. N Engl J Med 1975;293:1167.

7

Water, Electrolyte, and Acid–Base Metabolism

CLAIRE M. FRITSCHE
LEE A. HEBERT
JACOB LEMANN, JR.

In the normal adult, about 50% to 70% of body weight is water. Fatty tissue contains little water; therefore, with increasing degrees of obesity, the percentage of body weight that is water approaches 50%. With increasing degrees of leanness, the percentage of body weight that is water approaches 70%. The approximate distribution of body water in health is shown in Table 7-1. Osmotic and oncotic forces are important determinants of water distribution; thus we must begin with a review of these concepts.

OSMOTIC FORCES (OSMOLALITY, OSMOTIC PRESSURE)

If a solute is added to pure water, the presence of the second molecular species interferes with the normal "activity" of water molecules. As a result, water diffuses more slowly through the solution, and the solution must be raised to a higher temperature before boiling will occur and lowered to a cooler temperature before freezing will occur. These effects of solute on the colligative properties of water are principally related to the number of molecules present per unit volume rather than to the specific kind of molecule or to the total weight of solute present. The determination of osmolality is a measure of the number of molecules in the solution that are effective in reducing the concentration and, therefore, the chemical properties of water. The slower rate of diffusion of water caused by the solute accounts for the fact that water diffuses from zones of low osmolality (high water concentration) to zones of high osmolality (low water concentration). The hydrostatic pressure that must be applied to the zone of high osmolality to oppose exactly osmotic pressure is equal to the osmotic pressure between the zones of high and low osmolality. The effect of solute concentration on the freezing point vapor pressure of water is the basis for the clinical measurement of osmolality in body fluids.

The osmolality of normal extracellular fluid (ECF) is determined almost entirely by sodium and its accompanying anions. Under certain conditions, other substances, such as glucose, mannitol, alcohol, and urea, can accumulate and contribute importantly to plasma osmolality. The contribution of each of these solutes to plasma osmolality can be directly determined in the clinical laboratory by measuring freezing point depression or by calculation. Calculation of plasma osmolality (P_{osm}) from the known concentration of solutes is as follows:

$$P_{osm} = 2 \times [Na] \text{ mEq/L} + \text{glucose millimoles/L} \\ + \text{urea millimoles/L} \\ + \text{osmolar concentration of other solutes.}$$

For normal plasma,

$$P_{osm} = 2 \times 140 \text{ mEq/L} + (900 \text{ mg glucose/L})/ \\ (180 \text{ mg glucose/mOsm}) \\ + (140 \text{ mg urea nitrogen/L})/ \\ (28 \text{ mg urea nitrogen/mOsm}) \\ + \text{other solutes (negligible in normal plasma)} \\ = 290 \text{ mOsm/L}$$

(mOsm = milliosmoles)

Most laboratories use different units, and the formula can be shortened to:

$$P_{osm} = 2 \times Na^+ \, (mEq/L)$$

$$+ \frac{glu \, (mg/dL)}{18} + \frac{BUN \, (mg/dL)}{2.8} = \frac{mOsm}{L}$$

The osmolalities of intracellular fluid (ICF) and ECF are equal because cell walls (except for the collecting duct of the kidney) are always freely permeable to water. Potassium is the major intracellular cation, and is found in concentrations of approximately 150 mEq/L of cell water. Thus potassium and its accompanying anions—principally phosphate and protein—account for almost all of the osmolality of ICF. In health, Na^+ is excluded from cells and K^+ is maintained in cells in most cases because of cellular $Na^+ - K^+$ adenosine-triphosphatase.

ONCOTIC FORCES (ONCOTIC PRESSURE, COLLOID OSMOTIC PRESSURE)

Just as crystalloids in solution, such as Na^+, Cl^-, and urea, reduce the concentration of water, so also do colloids, such as albumin and globulins. In biologic solutions, however, the contribution of proteins in lowering the effective concentration of water is far less than that of crystalloids, since there are far fewer protein molecules than crystalloid molecules. One gram of albumin (mol wt 68,000) theoretically yields 0.015 mOsm ($[1,000 \, mg/68,000 \, mg/mM] \times 1 \, mOsm/mM$), whereas 1 g of sodium chloride theoretically yields 34.3 mOsm ($[1,000 \, mg/58.5 \, mg/mM] \times 2 \, mOsm/mM$). Thus, gram for gram, sodium chloride is theoretically 2300 times more effective in increasing the osmolality of a solution than albumin. The oncotic pressure of solutions is expressed in millimeters of mercury for the same reason that osmotic forces are expressed in units of hydrostatic pressure.

Even though oncotic forces are small relative to osmotic forces, they are important in biologic systems because plasma proteins are selectively retained in the intravascular space. Thus the effective concentration of water and electrolytes is selectively reduced in the intravascular compared with the interstitial space. All other things being equal, this will result in diffusion of water and electrolytes from the interstitial to the intravascular space. At the capillary level, however, where these oncotic forces are at work, the capillary blood hydrostatic pressure opposes an inward diffusion of water and electrolytes. At the arterial end of the capillary, the effect of capillary blood oncotic pressure (about 35 mm Hg) pushing fluid outward is greater than the effect of capillary blood hydrostatic pressure (equivalent to 25 mm Hg) causing inward diffusion of fluid. Therefore, net outward movement of water and electrolytes occurs. At the venous end of the capillary, the capillary blood oncotic pressure (equivalent to about 25 mm Hg) exceeds capillary blood hydrostatic pressure (now about 15 mm Hg) and, therefore, net inward movement of water and electrolytes occurs. In health, the rate of fluid outflow from the arterial end of the capillary equals the rate of uptake at the venous end of the capillary.

REGULATION OF WATER AND ELECTROLYTE DISTRIBUTION BETWEEN INTRACELLULAR AND EXTRACELLULAR COMPARTMENTS

Osmotic forces regulate the distribution of water between ECF and ICF, and under all steady-state conditions, ECF osmolality equals ICF osmolality. The implications of these principles when water or solute is added to body fluids are as follows.

Effect of Addition of Water on ECF and ICF Volume and Osmolality

The ingestion of water or the intravenous infusion of water, as 5% solution of glucose in water, results in expansion of all body fluid compartments. Because the osmolality of all body compartments is the same, the water is distributed in the body water compartments in proportion to their size. For example, 1000 mL of a 5% solution of dextrose in water is infused into a normal 60-kg person with plasma osmolality = 290 mOsm/L and serum sodium = 140 mEq/L. Assuming that there is no excretion of the water, the change in volume of the body water compartments (see Table 7-1) when complete mixing has occurred is as follows: The ICF is increased by about 666 mL and the ECF is increased by about 333 mL. The intravascular water, which is one-fourth of the ECF, is increased by only about 83 mL. Plasma osmolality decreases by about 2%. This is sufficient to completely suppress antidiuretic hormone (ADH) release and cause a maximum water diuresis in a normal person.

Effect of Addition of Solute on ECF and ICF Volume and Osmolality

If solutes are ingested or infused that penetrate cells slowly (e.g., glucose), or are actively excluded from cells (e.g., Na^+), water is obligated to remain with these

TABLE 7–1
Body Water Compartments in Health

PARAMETER	TOTAL BODY WATER	INTRACELLULAR WATER	EXTRACELLULAR WATER*
Percentage of total body water	100%	67%	33%
Percentage of body weight	60%	40%	20%
Actual volume (liters) in a 60-kg person	36	24	12
Osmolality (mOsm/kg of water)	290	290	290

*The intravascular water space is about one-fourth of the extracellular water space. The intravascular volume is substantially larger than the intravascular water space because of the additional space occupied by blood cell and plasma proteins. The intravascular volume (blood volume) is about 7% of body weight or slightly more than 4 liters in a 60-kg person.

solutes in the ECF so that conditions of osmotic equilibrium between ICF and ECF are met. If these solutes are given in isotonic solutions (i.e., if the osmolality of the solution equals that of body fluids), conditions of osmotic equilibrium are met without shifts of water between ICF and ECF. Thus the ECF is selectively expanded. On the other hand, if these solutes are ingested without water or given as hypertonic solutions, ECF osmolality will rise as these solutes move into the ECF, and water will diffuse from ICF to ECF until osmolality in the two compartments is equal. Thus the ECF is expanded as the ICF is contracted.

Although certain other solutes, such as urea and ethyl alcohol, increase plasma osmolality, they do not affect the steady-state distribution of water between ECF and ICF because these solutes readily penetrate cells and rapidly distribute throughout the body water space. Nevertheless, in non-steady states, such as rapid removal of urea by hemodialysis, transient redistribution of water between ECF and ICF does occur. Such shifts of fluid in brain tissue can lead to significant changes in brain function.

REGULATION OF WATER AND ELECTROLYTE DISTRIBUTION BETWEEN THE INTRAVASCULAR AND INTERSTITIAL COMPARTMENTS

As discussed above, the regulation of fluid and electrolyte transfer at the capillary level is determined by the balance among oncotic forces, hydrostatic forces, and capillary permeability to plasma proteins. These forces can be perturbed in the following ways.

Hypoalbuminemia results in a fall in plasma oncotic pressure, a rise in the effective concentration of water and electrolytes in the intravascular space, and, all other things being equal, net movement of water and electrolytes in the interstitial space. As a consequence, intravascular volume decreases, and the kidney responds by retaining sodium and water in an attempt to restore intravascular volume to normal. If the hypoalbuminemia is sufficiently pronounced (less than 2.5 g/dL), and the expected renal retention of sodium and water occurs, edema will develop before a new equilibrium between outflux and influx of fluid at the capillary level is achieved.

The sequence of events that leads to edema formation is depicted in Figure 7-1. Note that the stimulus to renal sodium and water retention in hypoalbuminemia is a decrease in intravascular volume. In many hypoalbuminemic patients, the retention of sodium and water does not completely restore intravascular volume to normal. In fact, in some patients with marked hypoalbuminemia, massive edema (expansion of the interstitial volume) may be present, yet the intravascular volume may be dangerously low, even to the point of shock.

Marked edema also can develop in the presence of extensive lymphatic obstruction, distal to a venous obstruction, or because of ischemic injury. In these situations, the edema seldom accumulates at such a rate that a serious decrease in intravascular volume becomes

Decrease in plasma albumin
↓
Decrease in plasma oncotic pressure
↓
Capillary outflux exceeds influx
↓
Intravascular volume decreases, interstitial volume increases
↓
Renal sodium and water retention develops
↓
Edema develops when a large interstitial fluid volume is needed to raise interstitial pressure enough to prevent the excessive capillary outflux caused by hypoalbuminemia

Figure 7–1. Sequence of events leading to edema formation in hypoalbuminemia.

clinically evident. Once the edema in such patients is established, the intravascular volume and the renal, endocrine, and hemodynamic factors regulating the intravascular volume usually return to normal. Thus, if diuretic therapy is used to reduce the lymphedema, it can do so, but intravascular volume will be decreased below normal, possibly adversely affecting hemodynamics.

REGULATION OF WATER AND SODIUM EXCHANGES WITH THE EXTERNAL ENVIRONMENT

The following discussion focuses on the normal response of the kidney to perturbations of sodium or water balance because an examination of the state of renal sodium and water excretion often is key to the understanding of the pathogenesis of a disorder of fluid and electrolyte balance and usually provides the basis for planning appropriate fluid and electrolyte therapy.

Water Balance

Water balance equals water intake minus water output. Sometimes it is assumed that the measurement of fluid intake and output, as it is performed clinically, is a measure of water balance. The difficulty in assessing the state of water balance from the measurement of intake and output is indicated in Table 7-2, which lists all the sources of intake and output of water from the body. It is evident from this table that only a few of the important components of water balance are included in the measurement of intake and output. For this reason, some serious disturbances of water balance may not be reflected in the intake and output record. Fortunately the accurate measurement of water balance does not require that special techniques be used to measure the various sources of intake and output of water from the body. Instead, in most clinical situations, changes in water balance can be assessed simply by following changes in body weight.

In the great majority of clinical situations, changes in water balance occur secondarily to changes in sodium balance. For example, in the pathogenesis of fluid retention in congestive heart failure, the primary event is positive sodium balance because of a decreased renal capacity to excrete sodium. The ingested water that is retained is retained as a secondary event to maintain plasma osmolality at some level set by the thirst mechanism. If sodium had not been retained, water would not have been retained. For this reason, the key to preventing fluid retention in such patients is the regulation of sodium intake and output, not water intake.

Less commonly, a change in water balance is the primary event, and changes in sodium balance are secondary to the change in water balance. To recognize such situations, it is necessary to understand the normal renal response to primary changes in water balance. Because the capacity of the kidneys to concentrate and dilute the urine is commonly evaluated by measurement of urine specific gravity, it is first necessary to consider the relation between urine osmolality (U_{osm}) and specific gravity (sp gr).

$$sp\ gr = W_s / W_{H2O}$$

where

W_s = weight of the solution
W_{H_2O} = weight of an equal volume of water.

In normal urine, there is, on the average, a linear relation between urine osmolality and specific gravity, as shown in Figure 7-2. This relation is disturbed when molecules that have molecular weights much higher than the predominant normal urinary solutes are excreted in large amounts. Thus, in the presence of large numbers of molecules with high molecular weight, specific gravity is no longer a reliable index of osmolality. The normal, predominant urinary solutes are sodium, potassium, and chloride ions, and urea, which have molecular weights of 23, 39, 35, and 60, respectively. The commonly encountered urinary solutes that cause large increases in specific gravity but small increases in urine osmolality are glucose (mol wt 180), mannitol (mol wt 181), dextran (mol wt 20,000–40,000), iodine-containing radiographic contrast (mol wt 600–800), and protein (but only with

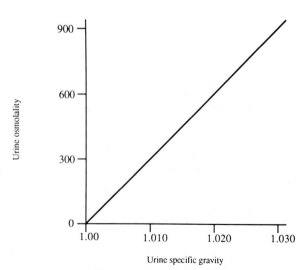

Figure 7–2. Approximate relation between specific gravity and osmolality in normal urine.

TABLE 7–2
Components of Water Balance*

SOURCES	MEASURED CLINICALLY	COMMENTS
Water Intake		
Oral intake of liquids, intravenous fluids	Yes	
Water in solid food	Rarely	Water content of solid food in diet of normal adult averages 800–1000 mL/d
Metabolic water	No	The average adult forms about 200–300 mL of water daily by oxidation of carbohydrate and fat to water and CO_2
Water absorbed by way of respiratory tract during use of gases hydrated by ultrasonic nebulizer	No	Up to 350 mL of water can be absorbed daily at respiratory volumes of 10 L/min
Water Output		
Sensible losses		
Urine	Yes	Output variable in health, depends on water intake. Usual range is 600–2500 mL/d. With renal insufficiency and loss of renal concentrating capacity, urine flow rate depends principally on rate of solute excretion.
Sweat	No	In hot environments, several liters of water can be lost daily.
Stool	Rarely	A normally formed stool contains 80–100 mL of water. Diarrheal stools are principally water: diarrheal losses can be quantitated by collecting and weighing the feces.
Other sensible losses		
Gastric drainage, transudation from skin, etc.	Variable	
Insensible losses		
Evaporation from skin	No	Normally 450 mL lost daily. In the average-sized adult, with fever, losses increase about 10% per degree F.
Evaporation from lung surfaces	No	Normally 450 mL lost daily. Losses increase by 50% with doubling of ventilatory rate.

*Water balance = Water intake − water output.

heavy proteinuria). If these substances are absent, urine specific gravity can be relied on to reflect urine osmolality. If these substances are present, urine osmolality must be measured directly to determine the true extent to which the kidneys have concentrated or diluted the urine.

Normal Renal Response to Water Deprivation

The permeability of the collecting duct to water is markedly increased when ADH is released. Thus, as the tubular fluid enters the collecting duct, water diffuses from the collecting duct into the hypertonic medullary interstitium. This results in a marked reduction in urine volume and a marked increase in urine osmolality. In health, the osmolality of the medullary interstitium is 900 to 1200 mOsm/L. Thus, in states of maximum water conservation, the urine osmolality approaches 900 to 1200 mOsm/L. In such circumstances, urine flow rates approximate 0.5% or less of the normal glomerular filtration rate, resulting in urine flow rates of about 20 mL/h, or 500 mL/d when kidneys function normally. The elderly are unable to concentrate their urine, with maximum osmolalities among the aged often less than 800 mOsm/L.

Normal Response to Water Loading

The administration of water or hypotonic solutions results in a reduction in the osmolality of body fluids. A 2% reduction in plasma osmolality (e.g., P_{osm} 290→284 mOsm/L, serum sodium 140→137 mEq/L) is sufficient to result in a complete suppression of ADH secretion. In an average, healthy adult, the ingestion of 1000 mL of water is more than enough to elicit such a response and the formation of a maximally dilute urine. When ADH secretion is inhibited and renal function is normal, urine specific gravity usually is less than 1.005, urine osmolality is less than 100 mOsm/kg, and urine flow rates approach 15% to 20% of the glomerular filtration rate (i.e., 10–15 mL/min, 600–900 mL/h). Elderly patients also cannot dilute their urine as well as the young, the minimum osmolality being 200 mOsm/L or slightly higher.

Sodium Balance

Sodium balance equals sodium intake minus sodium output. The components of sodium balance are shown in Table 7-3. From this table, it is evident that the kidneys play the central role in the regulation of sodium balance by adjusting sodium excretion to match sodium intake. Unless there are abnormal losses of sodium through the skin or gut, sodium balance can thus be assessed simply by determining dietary sodium intake and measuring the urinary excretion of sodium. These measurements usually are not necessary because if the patient has free access to water and an intact thirst mechanism, water will be ingested and retained in proportion to the level of sodium retention. Thus changes in sodium balance are reflected by changes in body weight. Occasionally the measurement of urine sodium excretion is useful. For example, when body weight and serum sodium concentration are stable, and there are no abnormal extrarenal sodium losses, the measurement of the 24-hour urinary excretion of sodium accurately reflects sodium intake.

Normal Renal Response to Sodium Restriction and Sodium Loading

When sodium intake is abruptly reduced from a normal (e.g., 170 mEq/24 h) to a very low level (e.g., 10 mEq/24 h), approximately 3 to 4 days are required until

TABLE 7–3
Components of Sodium Balance*

SOURCES	COMMENTS
Sodium Intake	
Dietary	Normal adult intake of salt is about 10 g NaCl daily (~170 mEq Na^+ and Cl^- or 4 g Na^+). Restricted dietary salt intake usually is 2 g sodium (87 mEq NaCl) daily.
Parenteral	1000 mL normal saline (0.9% saline) = 9 g NaCl = 155 mEq Na^+ + 155 mEq Cl^-
Sodium Output	
Urine	Variable. In health, reflects intake, since virtually all ingested NaCl is excreted in urine
Skin	Negligible except with sweating. Sweat contains 50–60 mEq Na^+/L and several liters of sweat may be lost each day in hot environments.
Gastrointestinal secretion	
Normally formed stool	Na^+ ~ 1 mEq/24 h
Diarrheal stool	
Secretory (infectious)	Na^+ ~ 130 mEq/L
Fermentative (malabsorption)	Na^+ ~ 50 mEq/L
Vomitus or gastric aspirate	
Normally acid gastric juice	Na^+ ~ 40 mEq/L
Achlorhydria	Na^+ ~ 130 mEq/L
All other GI secretions (bile, pancreatic juice, small-bowel secretions)	Na^+ ~ 130 mEq/L

*Sodium balance = Sodium intake − sodium output

maximum renal sodium conservation occurs. During this period of adjustment, renal sodium output exceeds intake, and water is lost with sodium in isosmotic proportion from the ECF. One to 2 liters of ECF usually are lost in the change from a normal to a very low sodium intake. Thus normal people come into balance on a low sodium intake, but the ECF volume may then be regulated at a suboptimal level. The potential danger to such a patient lies in the fact that the person is then more vulnerable to the potential hypotensive effects of anesthesia or additional volume losses that may occur during surgery.

The normal renal response to salt loading is analogous to that of salt restriction, in that it takes several days for the renal excretion of sodium to increase in response to the higher level of sodium intake. Thus, when balance is finally achieved, ECF volume is being regulated at an expanded level. This can be undesirable. For example, the patient with underlying heart disease who comes into sodium balance on a high sodium chloride intake will be more vulnerable to the development of congestive heart failure if additional fluids are administered.

CLINICAL ASSESSMENT OF DISORDERS OF WATER AND ELECTROLYTE METABOLISM

Disorders of ECF electrolyte composition may be detected by measurement of the serum electrolyte concentrations. Identification of the process (or processes) behind the disturbance of electrolyte composition and the planning of subsequent therapy are critically dependent on one's being able to accurately assess whether the disturbance in ECF electrolyte composition is associated with volume expansion, volume contraction, or a normal volume.

In the evaluation of a patient's ECF volume status, it must be kept clearly in mind that the critical volume is that portion of the intravascular volume that is effective in determining the filling pressure of the ventricles and, hence, the cardiac output. Hereafter, this theoretical volume will be referred to as the effective intravascular volume (IVV).

In light of the above definition, an optimum effective IVV is that intravascular volume that maintains an optimum cardiac output and thus optimizes tissue perfusion. Although in many clinical situations the actual intravascular volume and the effective IVV are the same and can be expected to change in direct proportion, in a number of important clinical states the actual intravascular volume is different from the effective IVV. For example, in acute metabolic acidosis, increased venoconstriction can develop, resulting in an abnormal increase in central venous pressure (CVP) and cardiac output. Under this circumstance, the actual intravascular volume could be less than normal while the effective IVV is greater than normal. That is, because of the increase in venous tone, a lower than normal intravascular volume can maintain a normal effective IVV.

Acute changes in venous tone induced by drugs (e.g., morphine, furosemide, norepinephrine), changes in acid–base status, or the presence of bacterial endotoxin also can disrupt the normal relation between the actual intravascular volume and the effective IVV.

The most reliable clinical means for assessing the status of the effective IVV currently is the measurement of the pulmonary capillary wedge pressure. This measurement is an estimate of the pulmonary capillary pressure, which, in turn, is a measure of the filling pressure of the left ventricle. Factors that increase pulmonary capillary wedge pressure tend to increase cardiac output by increasing capillary outflux. When effective IVV is considered within these constraints, it becomes clear that under virtually any physiologic or pathophysiologic circumstance, an optimum effective IVV is that intravascular volume which results in a pulmonary capillary wedge pressure that is high enough to promote optimal cardiac output and yet low enough to prevent pulmonary edema.

Fortunately, in the great majority of clinical situations, it is not necessary to resort to measuring pulmonary wedge pressure to assess whether a disturbance of ECF composition is associated with an effective IVV that is abnormally high, abnormally low, or normal. Instead, an accurate assessment of the effective IVV usually can be made by a careful clinical assessment using the criteria listed in Table 7-4. This table lists the bedside and laboratory means to assess volume status according to whether the findings are consistent with an effective IVV that is less than normal, or an effective IVV that is nearly normal or expanded.

Also shown in Table 7-4 are the conditions under which the given means for evaluating the intravascular volume must be qualified (i.e., the conditions that may render the meaning of the finding indeterminant with respect to the evaluation of intravascular volume). For example, the relation between an increase in weight and a change in intravascular volume is rendered indeterminant if, at the same time, the patient has developed a third space, as in bowel obstruction. In this instance, the entire weight gain could be caused by the accumulation of fluid outside the intravascular volume. Thus the finding of weight gain in this setting cannot be used as evidence of an increase in effective IVV.

We suggest that the evaluation of effective IVV, using the criteria in Table 7-4, be approached in the following manner: First, whenever a finding can be significantly qualified, it should not be used in arriving at a final

TABLE 7–4
Assessment of Effective Intravascular Volume (IVV)

SUGGESTIVE EVIDENCE	QUALIFYING CONDITIONS*
Significantly Decreased Effective IVV	
History of fluid and electrolyte deprivation or loss (e.g., vomiting, diarrhea)	Difficulty in establishing by history whether the magnitude of loss or deprivation is sufficient to result in negative balance of water and electrolytes
Decrease in body weight below normal not explained by inadequate calorie intake.	None
Blood pressure less than usual for patient or orthostatic hypotension	(a) Patient receiving methyldopa (Aldomet), prazosin (Minipress), minoxidil (Loniten), or other drugs that interfere with vascular α-receptors; (b) autonomic insufficiency as in diabetics, quadraplegics, and after prolonged bed rest.
Elevated serum creatinine associated with concentrated urine ($U_{osm}/P_{osm} > 1.5$), and Na^+ conservation: ($U_{Na} < 20$ mEq/L) or % $E/F_{Na} < 1\%$†	Decreased renal perfusion owing to: (a) severe hepatic failure (hepatorenal syndrome); (b) severe cardiac failure. Acute, high-grade urinary tract obstruction. (see text)
Low central venous pressure (CVP) or pulmonary capillary wedge pressure	(See text)
Decreased tissue turgor	(See text)
Hematocrit above normal	Presence of conditions that may cause erythrocytosis
Nearly Normal or Expanded Effective IVV (i.e., Absence of Significant Intravascular Volume Depletion)	
Hypertension with patient in sitting or standing position and no orthostatic fall in blood pressure	None
Presence of cardiac failure: Left ventricular failure: audible third heart sound (S_3), or pulmonary edema	Patients with markedly reduced cardiac output and very large left ventricles may have decreased effective IVV despite an audible S_3.
Right ventricular failure: peripheral edema with increased venous pressure (neck vein distention, increased IVP)	Right ventricular failure but normal left ventricular function (see text)
Increase in weight above normal not explained by increased caloric intake	(a) Significant hypoalbuminemia; (b) development of "third spaces" (e.g., ascites, bowel obstruction)
Increased CVP	(See text)
Increased pulmonary capillary wedge pressure	(See text)
Edema, ascites, or pleural effusion	(See text)
Hematocrit less than normal	Presence of conditions that may cause loss, destruction, or decreased production of red blood cells

*Qualifying conditions are circumstances that may render the meaning of the finding indeterminant with respect to the evaluation of the effective IVV.

†%E/F_{Na} = percentage of excretion of filtered sodium (see text).

decision. Second, as many independent means as practical should be used to assess the effective IVV to minimize the effect of possible error on the final decision. The greater the number of independent, unqualified findings that can be marshalled in favor of a given clinical decision, the more likely it is that the decision is correct. If such a systematic approach to clinical decision making is used, it should be possible to arrive at an accurate evaluation of volume status in most circumstances.

DATA BASE FOR ASSESSMENT OF EFFECTIVE INTRAVASCULAR VOLUME

Body Weight

All patients should be weighed on admission to the hospital and then periodically during their hospital stay. In patients undergoing surgery, or in whom problems in fluid and electrolyte balance are anticipated, weight must be measured daily.

Alterations in body weight are the result of changes in body water content plus solid tissue content (fat, protein, bone). Gains or losses of solid tissue are almost always related to changes in caloric intake and seldom exceed 0.25 kg/24 h. For example, a patient who takes no calories for 24 hours is forced to consume her endogenous stores of fat and protein to meet the energy requirements for continued life. The complete oxidation of fat yields 9 calories per gram, and protein yields 4 calories per gram. It can be readily calculated that the complete oxidation of 0.25 kg of solid tissue (in starvation, a mixture of about 87% fat, 13% protein) will yield enough calories to meet basal daily energy needs. Thus changes in weight exceeding 0.25 kg/24 h are almost always attributable to changes in water balance. Although the relation between body weight and effective IVV can be variable, usually the relation between changes in body weight and intravascular volume can be correctly assessed by the application of the following guidelines: (1) A decrease in body weight below normal (for the patient), and not explainable on the basis of inadequate caloric intake, can be assumed to be accompanied by a decrease in intravascular volume. (2) An increase in body weight above normal not explainable by increased nutrition can be assumed to be accompanied by an increase in intravascular volume except when the weight gain develops in association with the following conditions: (a) significant hypoalbuminemia: serum albumin less than 2.5 g/dL; (b) venous obstruction; or (c) development of third spaces (e.g., obstructed or ischemic bowel). Under these three general conditions, an increase in body weight may not reflect an increase in the effective IVV.

Renal Function

Creatinine, a by-product of muscle energy metabolism, is produced at a constant rate that is related to muscle mass. Normal men produce 20 to 25 mg/kg (ideal body weight)/24 h, whereas women produce 15 to 20 mg/kg (ideal body weight)/24 h. Nearly all of the creatinine produced is excreted by glomerular filtration. Therefore, changes in the concentration of serum creatinine reflect changes in the glomerular filtration rate (GFR), and the clearance of creatinine (C_{cr}) is an index of the GFR:

$$C_{cr} = U_{cr}V/S_{cr} \sim GFR$$

where

U_{cr} = urinary creatinine concentration;
V = urine volume per unit time; and
S_{cr} = serum creatinine.

Thus, by rearranging the above equation:

$$S_{cr} \sim U_{cr}V/GFR.$$

Normally, as muscle mass (which is proportional to $U_{cr}V$) increases, the GFR increases proportionately less. Therefore, on the average, children have lower serum creatinine values than adults, and large adults have higher serum creatinine levels than small adults. Because of these considerations, a single range of serum creatinine values cannot be applied to everyone. The suggested normal ranges of serum creatinine for adults, according to ideal body weight, are shown in Table 7-5. Creatinine clearance, expressed as milliliters per minute, can be estimated, using the formula derived by Cockcroft and Gault, from the patient's age, body weight, and serum creatinine level as follows for men:

$$C_{cr}, mL/min = \frac{(140\text{-age}) \times (\text{weight, kg})}{(72) \times (S_{cr}, mg/dL)}$$

This result multiplied by 0.85 provides a better estimate for women because of their relatively smaller muscle mass. Azotemia is arbitrarily defined here as a serum creatinine level greater than the upper limit of normal for body size, as shown in Table 7-5. The blood urea nitrogen level is influenced by dietary protein intake, tissue metabolism, and urine flow rate, in addition to the GFR, and should not be relied on to assess changes in the GFR.

The following guidelines are suggested for the eval-

TABLE 7–5
Normal Relation Between Body Size and Serum Creatinine Level

IDEAL BODY WEIGHT	EXPECTED RANGE OF SERUM CREATININE LEVEL*
<55 kg (120 lb)	0.6–1.0 mg/dL
55–80 kg (120–175 lb)	0.8–1.2 mg/dL
>80 kg (175 lb)	1.0–1.4 mg/dL

*Autoanalyzer picric acid method.

uation of the intravascular volume in light of the state of renal function. The azotemia can be assumed to be due to decreased renal perfusion if the serum creatinine level is elevated, the urine is concentrated ($U_{osm}/P_{osm} > 1.5$; sp gr > 1.015), and renal sodium conservation is present ($U_{Na} < 20$ mEq/L) on a random and untimed urine sample or % E/F_{Na} less than 1%, where

$$
\begin{aligned}
\%E/F_{Na} &= \text{percent fractional excretion of filtered Na}^+ \\
&= (\text{Excreted Na}^+) \times 100/(\text{Filtered Na}^+) \\
&\quad (U_{Na} \times S_{cr} \times 100/ \\
&\quad (S_{Na} \times U_{cr})
\end{aligned}
$$

where

U_{Na} = urinary Na$^+$ concentration, mEq/L;
S_{cr} = serum creatinine concentration, mg/dL;
S_{Na} = serum Na$^+$ concentration, mEq/L;
U_{cr} = urine creatinine concentration, mg/dL.

If severe cardiac failure and severe liver failure (hepatorenal syndrome) can be excluded, the decreased renal perfusion can be assumed to be due to a decreased effective IVV.

Edema, Ascites, or Pleural Effusion

Guidelines for interpreting the status of intravascular volume in the presence of edema, ascites, or pleural effusion are as follows: (1) Effective IVV is increased when edema, pleural effusion, or ascites occurs in the setting of congestive heart failure. (2) Increased effective IVV cannot be assumed in the presence of edema, ascites, or pleural effusion if there is significant hypoalbuminemia or venous obstruction, or if the accumulation of fluid is in a relatively small area of capillary injury (e.g., pleural effusion caused by pulmonary infarction).

Tissue Turgor

Tissue turgor is a function of the elasticity of the solid components of tissue and the degree of distention of the tissues by interstitial fluid. If tissue becomes depleted of interstitial fluid, it is less elastic (i.e., it less readily returns to its original shape after being deformed). Skin turgor is best assessed on the forehead and anterior chest. In patients under 50 years of age, the turgor of the dorsum of the hand also can be used. In older patients, the elasticity of the solid components of tissue is decreased, and the turgor of the skin becomes unreliable in interpreting changes in interstitial volume.

Central Venous Pressure

The measurement of CVP is a relatively simple but useful means for monitoring cardiac function and cardiovascular status. For the valid measurement of CVP, the catheter must be placed in the large intrathoracic veins near the right atrium (as assessed by chest radiograph) and the catheter must be patent (as assessed by the cyclic variation of CVP with ventilatory movements: decreased CVP during inspiration, increased CVP during expiration). In the normal adult, CVP is about 5 to 12 cm H_2O.

A CVP of less than 3 cm H_2O is commonly seen in children and young adults who have no evidence of a decreased effective IVV. In older adults and the elderly, a CVP of less than 3 cm H_2O can be assumed to reflect a significant decrease in effective IVV.

The CVP is an index of the filling pressure of the right atrium, which, in turn, is an index of the filling pressure of the right ventricle. In uncomplicated circumstances, expansion of the intravascular volume results in an increased CVP, whereas contraction of the intravascular volume results in a decreased CVP. It must be emphasized that the CVP cannot be used to assess the adequacy of left ventricular function in patients in whom left ventricular function may be impaired relative to right ventricular function. The CVP also is unreliable when lung disease is present, since CVP measurements are commonly falsely elevated. In such patients, left ventricular function can be monitored by observing for signs and symptoms of left ventricular failure (dyspnea, development of an audible third heart sound [S_3], or pulmonary edema), or by direct measurement of pulmonary capillary wedge pressure. Under normal circumstances, the pulmonary capillary wedge pressure is approximately equal to the CVP $+$ 6 mm Hg.

Pulmonary Capillary Wedge Pressure

Technical refinements of the Swan-Ganz catheter make it possible to measure pulmonary artery systolic and diastolic pressure, CVP, pulmonary wedge pressure, and cardiac output using the thermodilution technique with the same catheter. This permits a definitive assessment of the volume status of the patient, since it can be determined whether the cardiac output is appropriate for a given pulmonary wedge pressure. Specific guidelines for the interpretation of the relation between pulmonary wedge pressure and cardiac output are as follows.

The Patient with Normal Volume Status. Pulmonary wedge pressure can be expected to be between 8 and 12 mm Hg in patients with a normal cardiopulmonary system and a normal effective IVV. Cardiac output will be normal. Pulmonary wedge pressure can be less than 8 mm Hg without indicating volume contraction; in that circumstance, the cardiac output will be normal, despite the unusually low pulmonary wedge pressure.

The Patient Who Is Volume Contracted. Patients who have a normal cardiopulmonary system but who are significantly volume depleted usually have a pulmonary wedge pressure of less than 8 mm Hg and their cardiac output is less than normal. In patients with chronic pulmonary hypertension—for example, those with chronic left ventricular failure—a higher than normal pulmonary wedge pressure is needed to drive a satisfactory cardiac output. Thus, in such patients, pulmonary wedge pressure can be above the normal range but be inappropriately low for the patient. This situation can be identified by showing that (a) cardiac output is less than normal, despite the elevated pulmonary wedge pressure; (b) volume infusion causes an increase in cardiac output toward a more favorable range; and (c) despite further increase in pulmonary wedge pressure with volume expansion, pulmonary function does not deteriorate (Pao$_2$ does not decrease, Paco$_2$ does not increase, pulmonary compliance does not worsen).

The Patient Who Is Volume Expanded. In patients with a normal cardiopulmonary system, pulmonary wedge pressure usually is above 18 mm Hg when volume expansion is substantial. Cardiac output is above normal. If cardiac function is impaired, cardiac output will be inappropriately low for the level of pulmonary wedge pressure.

When a given pulmonary wedge pressure is being interpreted, the serum albumin level also should be taken into consideration, since it is the serum albumin level that opposes the effect of capillary hydrostatic pressure, to cause migration of fluid from the capillary lumen to the interstitial space. Thus, at any given elevated pulmonary wedge pressure, pulmonary edema will develop more rapidly in the patient who is hypoalbuminemic compared with a patient who has a normal serum albumin concentration.

In some patients, it is not possible to obtain a reliable pulmonary wedge pressure. In most of these patients, the pulmonary artery diastolic pressure is a good estimate of the pulmonary wedge pressure. If pulmonary hypertension is present, pulmonary vascular resistance is increased; thus pulmonary artery diastolic pressure may not be a good index of the pulmonary wedge pressure. In such patients, it is important to be able to obtain a wedge pressure. Finally, in patients who are being ventilated with high levels of positive end-expiratory pressure, pulmonary wedge pressure may become an unreliable index of left atrial filling pressure because the high intrapulmonary pressures may cause obstruction of the catheter orifice. Patients must be

briefly taken off the ventilator for accurate measurements. Other circumstances in which pulmonary artery wedge pressure measurements may be inaccurate include the presence of mitral stenosis or pulmonary venous obstruction.

Blood Pressure

The following guidelines are suggested for the evaluation of the effective IVV from measurement of blood pressure: (a) a nearly normal or expanded effective IVV can be assumed in patients with hypertension that is demonstrated in the sitting or standing position; (2) effective IVV may be decreased in patients who previously were hypertensive but who have become normotensive; and (c) effective IVV may be decreased in patients who develop orthostatic hypotension (a drop in systolic pressure greater than 10 mm Hg in changing from the supine to the sitting or standing position). Orthostatic hypotension also can be present, in the absence of volume contraction, as a result of prolonged bed rest, during the use of such antihypertensive agents as methyldopa (Aldomet) or of vasodilators (prazosin, minoxidil). If the pulse rate does not rise as blood pressure falls when a patient stands, autonomic neuropathy should be considered as a cause for postural hypotension.

Systemic Vascular Resistance

Other measurements of hemodynamic importance derived from Swan-Ganz readings include calculations of resistance across the pulmonary and systemic vascular beds. The calculations are as follows:

$$PVR = \frac{P_{\overline{PA}} - P_{\overline{PAW}} \times 80}{\dot{Q}T}$$

$$SVR = \frac{P_{\overline{SA}} - P_{\overline{RA}} \times 80}{\dot{Q}T}$$

PVR = pulmonary vascular resistance
SVR = systemic vascular resistance
P$_{\overline{PAW}}$ = mean pulmonary artery wedge pressure
P$_{\overline{PA}}$ = mean right atrial pressure
P$_{\overline{SA}}$ = mean systolic arterial pressure
$\dot{Q}T$ = cardiac output in liters per minute

Normal values for PVR are 50 to 150 dyne-sec/cm and for SVR, 800 to 1200 dyne-sec/cm. PVR is elevated in hypovolemic shock, cardiogenic shock, pulmonary embolism, or airway obstruction and diminished in septic shock. SVR is elevated in hypovolemic shock, cardiogenic shock, and pulmonary embolism and sometimes elevated in right ventricular infarct and cardiac tamponade; it is decreased in end-stage liver disease and septic shock.

CLINICAL ASSESSMENT OF DISORDERS OF EXTRACELLULAR FLUID COMPOSITION (SODIUM AND WATER)

The schema for the evaluation of the hyponatremic patient depends on the assessment of volume status. That is, a determination must first be made of whether the patient's hyponatremia is associated with a decreased, a normal, or an increased effective IVV. Once this initial separation is made, based on the assessment of intravascular volume, a further separation, based only on the state of renal sodium and water excretion, is made. Each of the final categories contains relatively few diagnostic possibilities, and in most instances, the presence or absence of each of these conditions in a given patient can be readily determined. The schema for the evaluation of the hypernatremic patient is analogous, except that it depends on the assessment of the state of renal water excretion.

Clinical Assessment of Hyponatremia

In the discussion that follows, only patients with "true" hyponatremia are considered (i.e., hyponatremia in which serum osmolality is decreased in proportion to the reduction in serum sodium concentration, after appropriate correction for any elevation in the plasma urea nitrogen). By making this distinction, hyponatremia caused by accumulation of ECF solutes such as glucose or mannitol can be excluded. In this type of hyponatremia, the decreased concentration of ECF sodium is the result of the shift of water from cells to the ECF in response to the osmotic gradient caused by the accumulation of the solute. As a consequence, the hyponatremia is associated with an increased plasma osmolality. These patients also can be readily identified by the presence of hyperglycemia sufficient to explain the decrease in serum sodium concentration, or by a history of administration of large amounts of mannitol— for example, in adults, more than 100 g—usually in the presence of a decreased capacity to excrete mannitol (decreased GFR).

We also exclude spurious hyponatremia resulting from the abnormal accumulation of plasma lipids or proteins. In such circumstances, the concentration of sodium in plasma water is normal; however, the concentration of sodium expressed per liter of whole plasma is reduced because an abnormally large volume of whole plasma is occupied by the lipids or proteins, which do not contain plasma water and electrolytes. Thus, when aliquots of hyperlipemic or hyperproteinemic plasma are analyzed, a lesser amount of sodium is determined to be present in a given volume of whole plasma. Plasma osmolality, however, is normal because lipids and proteins do not contribute importantly to plasma osmolality (see Osmotic Forces above). These patients can be readily identified by the presence of markedly elevated total serum protein levels (e.g., multiple myeloma) or grossly lipemic serum. The distinction can be readily made if lipemic serum is centrifuged and the lipoprotein layer removed before evaluation, if flame photometry is being used for measurement of serum Na^+. Spurious hyponatremia is not a consideration in most laboratories today, since serum Na^+ concentration is determined by ion-specific electrodes, and increased levels are not affected by lipemic serum.

Hyponatremia and Volume Depletion Associated with Renal Sodium Wasting

The normal renal response to volume depletion and hyponatremia is the virtual elimination of sodium from the urine (see Sodium Balance above and Fig. 7-3). Thus the presence of an excessive amount of urinary sodium under these conditions indicates that renal sodium loss is the cause or a major contributing factor to the state of sodium depletion. A spot urine sodium concentration greater than 40 mEq/L, a $\%E/F_{Na}$ greater than 1%, or a urinary sodium excretion rate greater than intake indicates such renal sodium wasting. The following conditions are associated with hyponatremia, intravascular volume depletion, and renal sodium wasting:

Chronic Renal Disease. All types of renal disease can be associated with renal salt wasting. In adults with such a disorder, the serum creatinine level is virtually always higher than 2 mg, and usually much higher before a significant salt leak develops. These azotemic patients usually require 85 to 170 mEq of sodium daily (5–10 g of sodium chloride) to maintain salt balance at a normal effective IVV. Thus, if sodium intake is decreased in azotemic patients by anorexia or vomiting, or if additional sodium losses occur (e.g., diarrhea or diuretic therapy), the inability of the diseased kidneys to conserve sodium and water normally may rapidly lead to the development of significant sodium and water deficits. Water intake usually continues, and thus sodium balance is more adversely affected than water balance. As a consequence, the patient becomes volume-contracted with hyponatremia. With the onset of

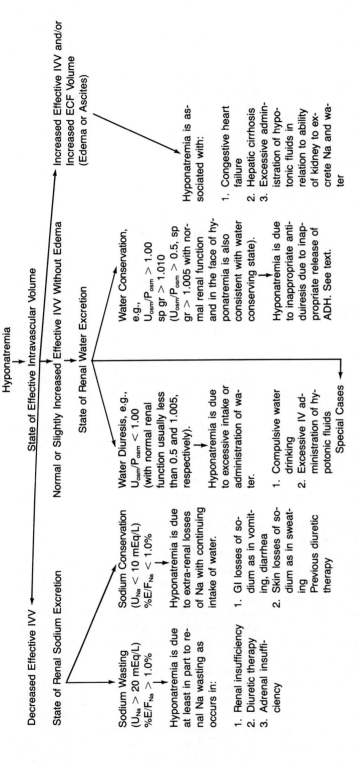

Hyponatremia

State of Effective Intravascular Volume

Decreased Effective IVV

Normal or Slightly Increased Effective IVV Without Edema

Increased Effective IVV and/or Increased ECF Volume (Edema or Ascites)

State of Renal Sodium Excretion

State of Renal Water Excretion

Sodium Wasting
($U_{Na} > 20$ mEq/L)
%E/F$_{Na} > 1.0$%

Hyponatremia is due at least in part to renal Na wasting as occurs in:

1. Renal insufficiency
2. Diuretic therapy
3. Adrenal insufficiency

Sodium Conservation
($U_{Na} < 10$ mEq/L)
%E/F$_{Na} < 1.0$%

Hyponatremia is due to extra-renal losses of Na with continuing intake of water.

1. GI losses of sodium as in vomiting, diarrhea
2. Skin losses of sodium as in sweating
   Previous diuretic therapy

Water Diuresis, e.g.,
$U_{osm}/P_{osm} < 1.00$
(with normal renal function usually less than 0.5 and 1.005, respectively).

Hyponatremia is due to excessive intake or administration of water.

1. Compulsive water drinking
2. Excessive IV administration of hypotonic fluids

Special Cases

Water Conservation, e.g.,
$U_{osm}/P_{osm} > 1.00$
sp gr > 1.010
($U_{osm}/P_{osm} > 0.5$, sp gr > 1.005 with normal renal function and in the face of hyponatremia is also consistent with water conserving state).

Hyponatremia is due to inappropriate antidiuresis due to inappropriate release of ADH. See text.

Hyponatremia is associated with:

1. Congestive heart failure
2. Hepatic cirrhosis
3. Excessive administration of hypotonic fluids in relation to ability of kidney to excrete Na and water

(Hyponatremia with essentially normal effective IVV but water diuresis occurs with water loading, and water conservation occurs with water restriction.)

1. Severe K$^+$ depletion associated with water depletion. Identifying features: history of diuretic administration, presence of hypokalemic metabolic alkalosis.
2. Resetting of "osmostat." Probably a rare complication of chronic disease. See text.
3. Polydipsic vomiting. Identifying features: protracted vomiting but continued large oral intake of water, metabolic alkalosis.

Figure 7–3. An approach to the assessment of the hyponatremic patient. This approach considers only patients with true hyponatremia (i.e., in nonazotemic patients, serum osmolality is reduced in proportion to the decrease in serum sodium). Thus patients are excluded who have lowered concentrations of serum sodium because of hyperlipidemia, hyperproteinemia, or the abnormal accumulations of solutes in the ECF, such as glucose or mannitol. %E/F$_{Na}$ = Fractional excretion of sodium.

congestive heart failure or the nephrotic syndrome, the salt leak of chronic renal failure usually disappears, and salt intake must be restricted.

Diuretic Therapy (Thiazides or Loop Diuretics Such as Furosemide, Bumetanide, and Ethacrynic Acid). Diuretics induce a renal salt-wasting state, and if the urinary output of sodium exceeds intake, sodium depletion ensues. Rarely diuretics may cause hyponatremia without evidence of volume depletion if severe potassium depletion has been a result of their use (see Fig. 7-3).

Adrenal Insufficiency (Addison's Disease). Destruction of the adrenal gland or sudden withdrawal of chronic, daily glucocorticoid therapy results in inadequate adrenal function. The lack of mineralocorticoid causes renal salt wasting, but renal potassium retention, and leads to sodium depletion. The lack of glucocorticoid results in a decreased capacity to excrete a water load and leads to hyponatremia, but not to volume depletion or hyperkalemia.

Hyponatremia and Volume Depletion Associated with Renal Sodium Conservation

A spot urine sodium concentration of less than 20 mEq/L or %E/F_{Na} less than 1% in a hyponatremic, volume-contracted patient is evidence of normal renal sodium conservation, and indicates that the cause of the sodium depletion is nonrenal in origin or that it occurred during prior diuretic therapy. The fact that the serum sodium concentration is lower than normal indicates that water balance is less negative than sodium balance. The following conditions may result in volume depletion and hyponatremia as a result of extrarenal losses of sodium.

Gastrointestinal Losses. If losses of fluid from the upper gastrointestinal tract (e.g., vomiting, gastric aspiration) cause the hyponatremia, and if the gastric juice is normally acid, metabolic alkalosis will be present. If diarrheal losses cause the hyponatremia, metabolic acidosis may be present. In patients with gastric achlorhydria, upper gastrointestinal losses also can lead to metabolic acidosis.

Losses of Sodium from the Skin. Sweat contains about 50 mEq/L of sodium and is a hypotonic fluid. Thus the effect of sweat losses that are not replaced is the development of hypernatremia. In most situations, the water losses from the skin are replaced more adequately than the sodium losses. Thus most patients who develop significant sodium losses from sweating become hyponatremic. Skin losses of fluid and electrolytes also can occur after burns or other skin injuries. These are isotonic losses of sodium, and will lead to hyponatremia if the water losses are more adequately replaced than the sodium losses.

Losses of Sodium Because of Prior Diuretic Therapy. The natriuretic action of most diuretics is less than 24 hours. Hyponatremia is made worse if water intake is excessive.

Hyponatremia and Normal Volume Status Associated with Water Diuresis

In a patient with normal renal function who has become hyponatremic from the administration or ingestion of excessive amounts of water, intravascular and ECF volume are normal to slightly expanded, and one can expect to find high rates of urine flow in association with maximally, or nearly maximally, dilute urine (see Water Balance above). In a patient with preexisting renal functional impairment, water loading also results in increases in urine flow rate and dilution of the urine; however, maximally dilute urine cannot be formed. Hyponatremia secondary to water loading may be seen in compulsive water drinkers, who usually are severely neurotic or psychotic, or after excessive intravenous administration of hypotonic fluids. Many of these patients additionally have high levels of ADH for various reasons (e.g., drugs, psychosis). Without this elevation of ADH, presuming normal renal function, consumption of 20 L of water would be necessary for development of frank hyponatremia.

Hyponatremia and Normal to Slightly Elevated Volume Status Associated with Water Conservation

As discussed above, in a patient with normal renal function who is hyponatremic and has evidence of normal or slightly elevated intravascular volume without edema, it is appropriate to observe a brisk water diuresis. When high flow rates of hypotonic urine are not observed, the patient is exhibiting an inappropriate antidiuresis. This may be due to the inappropriate release of ADH, although other mechanisms also can be involved (e.g., decreased renal blood flow, certain drugs). An additional characteristic of such patients is that administered sodium is promptly excreted in the urine perhaps because of the effect of atrial natriuretic factors. On the other hand, when sodium intake is curtailed, renal sodium conservation is observed. These patients also exhibit normal adrenal and renal function, and are not edematous. The syndrome of inappropriate antidiuresis has been associated with various clinical states, including malignant tumors (e.g., in the lung or pancreas), central nervous system disorders (e.g., head trauma, meningitis), infections (e.g., tuberculosis, bacterial pneumonias), the postoperative state, hypopituitarism, and myxedema, and with many drugs (Table 7-6). Infusion of oxytocin to induce uter-

TABLE 7–6
Antidiuretic Drugs

Sulfonylureas (chlorpropamide, tolbutamide)
Cytotoxic agents (vincristine, cyclophosphamide)
Nicotine
Morphine
Barbiturates
Carbamazepine
Psychotropics (tricyclics)
Clofibrate
Isoproterenol
Nonsteroidals
Salicylates
Acetaminophen
Vasopressin
Oxytocin

ine contraction also can cause hyponatremia because of the antidiuretic effects of oxytocin.

Under the category of hyponatremia associated with normal intravascular volume are three special categories. The feature that sets these apart is that patients in these categories may exhibit evidence of water conservation when water is withdrawn, or an appropriate or nearly appropriate water diuresis when water is administered. That is, it appears that osmoregulation has been reset to "defend" a lowered plasma osmolality. The first special case is an unusual response to diuretic therapy, characterized by hyponatremia, severe potassium depletion, and metabolic alkalosis. Despite the hyponatremia and normal intravascular volume, exchangeable sodium is near normal, suggesting intracellular movement of sodium. Potassium replacement must be accomplished before specific treatment of hyponatremia. The second case is an unusual manifestation of chronic illness, such as pulmonary tuberculosis, resetting the osmostat. The third case involves patients with sodium depletion from any cause in whom the decrease in effective IVV is minimized by excessive water intake and water retention. This effect of excessive water intake can occur in any of the causes of sodium depletion.

Hyponatremia Associated with Increased Effective IVV or Increased ECF Volume (Edema or Ascites)

Congestive Heart Failure. When hyponatremia develops spontaneously in the course of chronic congestive heart failure (i.e., is not the result of excessive water administration or diuretic therapy), it usually is indicative of severe cardiac insufficiency, and a poor prognosis. The cause of the hyponatremia in such patients has been ascribed to a decreased capacity to increase renal free water clearance perhaps because of

(a) increased fractional reabsorption of glomerular filtrate proximal to the renal diluting sites of the distal nephron and (b) an elevated ADH level.

Cirrhosis of the Liver. Patients with cirrhosis and ascites have a decreased capacity to excrete a water load, possibly because of the same mechanisms operative in patients with congestive heart failure.

Excessive Administration of Hypotonic Fluids. This usually is an iatrogenic situation, and must be especially guarded against in postoperative patients whose ADH levels are elevated because of pain or drugs, and in elderly patients who are unable to maximally dilute their urine.

Clinical Assessment of Hypernatremia

All patients with hypernatremia are volume-contracted, except those in whom hypernatremia develops as a result of excessive administration of hypertonic saline or sodium bicarbonate, or in those rare examples of essential hypernatremia (Fig. 7-4). The following discussion considers only the first group of patients; the section on treatment (see below) considers all forms of hypernatremia.

Hypernatremia Associated with Formation of Concentrated Urine

The normal renal response to decreased intake of water or increased extrarenal losses of water is the formation of maximally concentrated urine (see Water Balance above). In most clinical situations in which hypernatremia is the result of water depletion, the expected renal response is $U_{osm}/P_{osm} > 1.5$, and sp gr > 1.015. Thus the finding of hypernatremia with evidence of renal conservation of water indicates that the hypernatremia is due to excessive nonrenal losses of water or to solute diuresis.

Excessive Nonrenal Water Loss. Hypernatremia typically develops in patients with accelerated rates of nonrenal water loss because of a hot environment, fever, or hyperventilation in whom water losses are not replaced because the patient cannot perceive or communicate thirst. Despite the hypernatremia, sodium deficits also usually are present because initially, as water deficits develop, renal sodium excretion increases to maintain normal plasma osmolality and serum sodium concentration. When more than about 15% of ECF volume is lost, renal conservation of sodium occurs and, if the water losses continue, hypernatremia develops. The presence of volume deficits is indicated by the signs of intravascular volume depletion, as previously described. Urine flow rate usually is less than 35 mL/h.

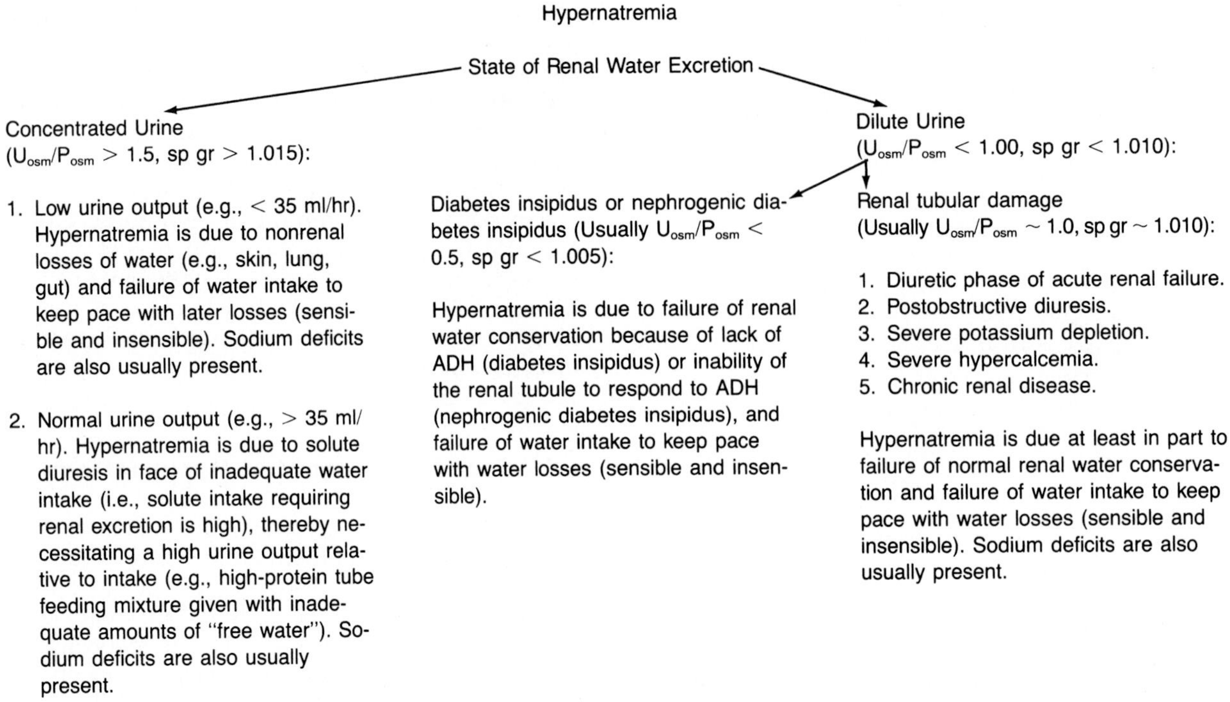

Hypernatremia

State of Renal Water Excretion

Concentrated Urine
($U_{osm}/P_{osm} > 1.5$, sp gr > 1.015):

1. Low urine output (e.g., < 35 ml/hr). Hypernatremia is due to nonrenal losses of water (e.g., skin, lung, gut) and failure of water intake to keep pace with later losses (sensible and insensible). Sodium deficits are also usually present.

2. Normal urine output (e.g., > 35 ml/hr). Hypernatremia is due to solute diuresis in face of inadequate water intake (i.e., solute intake requiring renal excretion is high), thereby necessitating a high urine output relative to intake (e.g., high-protein tube feeding mixture given with inadequate amounts of "free water"). Sodium deficits are also usually present.

Diabetes insipidus or nephrogenic diabetes insipidus (Usually $U_{osm}/P_{osm} < 0.5$, sp gr < 1.005):

Hypernatremia is due to failure of renal water conservation because of lack of ADH (diabetes insipidus) or inability of the renal tubule to respond to ADH (nephrogenic diabetes insipidus), and failure of water intake to keep pace with water losses (sensible and insensible).

Dilute Urine
($U_{osm}/P_{osm} < 1.00$, sp gr < 1.010):

Renal tubular damage
(Usually $U_{osm}/P_{osm} \sim 1.0$, sp gr ~ 1.010):

1. Diuretic phase of acute renal failure.
2. Postobstructive diuresis.
3. Severe potassium depletion.
4. Severe hypercalcemia.
5. Chronic renal disease.

Hypernatremia is due at least in part to failure of normal renal water conservation and failure of water intake to keep pace with water losses (sensible and insensible). Sodium deficits are also usually present.

Figure 7–4. An approach to the assessment of the hypernatremic patient. This approach does not consider patients with hypernatremia secondary to excessive administration of hypertonic saline.

Solute Diuresis. The amount of water that must accompany the excretion of a given amount of solute in the urine is determined by the osmolality of the renal medullary interstitial fluid (with which the collecting duct fluid must equilibrate) and the plasma level of ADH activity (which determines the permeability of the collecting duct to water and, therefore, the rate at which water will move from the collecting duct to medullary interstitial fluid to achieve osmotic equilibrium). Hypernatremia will result if water intake does not keep pace with renal water losses because although renal sodium excretion also is increased in solute diuresis, renal sodium reabsorption is affected proportionately less than water reabsorption. Large amounts of mannitol infused intravenously or high-protein mixtures fed by nasogastric tube (each gram of protein yields 8 mOsm, as urea, phosphate, and potassium) can cause a solute diuresis sufficient to cause hypernatremia if water intake is inadequate. In solute diuresis, urine volume usually is greater than 35 mL/h.

Hypernatremia Associated with Formation of Dilute Urine

The finding of an isotonic or hypotonic urine in the face of hypernatremia indicates that, at least in part, the hypernatremia is due to failure of normal renal conservation of water. Failure to concentrate the urine under these conditions may be due to lack of ADH (hypothalamic-pituitary diabetes insipidus) or to impaired renal tubular function that interferes with the development of a hypertonic medullary interstitium (renal tubular damage).

Central diabetes insipidus or nephrogenic diabetes insipidus should be suspected immediately in a patient with hypernatremia when the urine is very dilute (i.e., $U_{osm}/P_{osm} < 0.5$, or sp gr < 1.005).

In patients with renal tubular damage, the ability to concentrate and dilute the urine is decreased. As a result, under all conditions, the urine is isotonic or nearly isotonic with plasma. Hypernatremia can supervene when water losses exceed sodium losses and water intake does not keep pace with water losses. Despite the hypernatremia, significant sodium deficits usually are present because renal sodium wasting also usually is a feature of these disorders. The following are examples of clinical situations in which renal tubular damage can be associated with hypernatremia.

The Diuretic Phase of Acute Renal Failure. Occasionally, in a patient recovering from acute renal injury, tubular function is more severely affected than glomerular function. Thus an inordinately large fraction of the glomerular filtrate escapes reabsorption, resulting in high urine flow rates. The period of inappropriate diuresis can persist for a period lasting from a few days to several weeks.

Postobstructive Diuresis. The sudden release of chronic urinary tract obstruction often is followed by a period of several days or weeks in which urine flow rates are abnormally high. Some patients develop short-lived nephrogenic diabetes insipidus.

MANAGEMENT OF WATER AND ELECTROLYTE BALANCE

The approach to the management of water and electrolyte balance has two parts. First, a plan must be formulated to correct the patient's existing deficits or excesses of sodium or water. This plan must take into consideration the magnitude of the imbalances, the rate at which correction should be attempted, and the criterion that must be applied to assess the adequacy of correction. Second, a plan must be formulated to provide replacement of normal and abnormal ongoing losses of water and electrolyte. General guidelines are presented in Tables 7-7 and 7-8 and are discussed below.

Correction of Volume Deficits

Estimating the Magnitude of Sodium or Water Deficits

If the patient has been weighed daily, the magnitude of the water deficit owing to external losses of water can be estimated from the decrease in body weight. The coexisting sodium deficits can be estimated by examining the weight deficits in light of the serum sodium concentration. For example, if the patient has acutely lost 3 kg in weight and the serum sodium concentration is within ±10% of normal serum sodium concentration (i.e., 126–154 mEq/L), little error is incurred by assuming that the patient has lost 3 L of ECF (i.e., isotonic saline) and, therefore, replacement therapy should be about 3 L of 0.9% saline (155 mEq/L). There is no advantage in using an equivalent amount of Ringer's lactate, since the kidneys will adjust electrolyte excretion to make up for small differences between the composition of the ECF and the isotonic saline.

In patients in whom sodium and water deficits cannot be documented by changes in body weight, or in whom the losses are from the intravascular volume into internal "third spaces," approximate but useful guidelines are available to estimate the magnitude of the intravascular volume deficit. These guidelines are as follows: A loss equivalent to 15% of ECF volume (about 2–3 L in the average adult) results in a decrease in tissue turgor, but blood pressure and renal function, as judged by serum creatinine level, usually are normal. Losses of sodium and water in excess of 15% of ECF volume usually are accompanied by decreased tissue turgor, orthostatic or frank hypotension, and significant elevation of serum creatinine level.

Correction Rates for Volume Deficits and Criteria for Assessment

Sodium and water losses great enough to result in hypotension represent a medical emergency, and rapid intravenous administration of isotonic saline is indicated until the hypotension is reversed. Thereafter, the rate of intravenous therapy is guided by the adequacy of the intravascular volume as assessed by other criteria, particularly the measurement of blood pressure and pulse in the supine and sitting positions, urine flow rate, and CVP or pulmonary wedge pressure. In patients with less severe degrees of volume depletion, salt and water deficits often can be corrected by increasing oral intake. Salt can be added to food (the salt packets commonly present on hospital trays provide slightly more than 1 g of sodium chloride), or plain sodium chloride tablets can be given, with water ad libitum, letting the patient's thirst mechanism dictate water intake. As a guide to the amount of sodium chloride that should be added to the diet to restore the deficits, it should be recalled that 1 L of ECF contains 140 mEq of sodium, or about 9 g of sodium chloride. The adequacy of replacement therapy can be assessed over the ensuing days by measurement of change in body weight and blood pressure and by the decrease in serum creatinine level.

Correction of Volume Excess

Expansion of effective IVV sufficient to precipitate pulmonary edema is a medical emergency and requires the usual treatment of pulmonary edema, including placing the patient in the sitting position or elevating the head of the bed, as well as the administration of oxygen, vasodilators such as nitrates, hydralazine or angiotensin converting enzyme inhibitors (e.g., captopril, enalapril, lisinopril), digitalis, and loop diuretics, as needed. If the pulmonary edema does not improve, phlebotomy may be needed to relieve the vascular congestion. If the volume excess is less severe (e.g., simple edema), the problem usually can be controlled by decreasing salt intake or adding a diuretic drug, or both. The effectiveness of treatment can be guided by the decrease in body weight and periodic measurement of serum electrolyte and creatinine levels.

TABLE 7–7
General Guidelines for Planning Fluid and Electrolyte Therapy
in Complicated Cases

Volume-Contracted Patients (From Water and Electrolyte Loss)

Replace deficits:

Moderate volume contraction (e.g., decreased effective IVV causing azotemia but not hypotension). Plan to replace deficits in about 24 h (e.g., 0.9% saline at 200–250 mL/h). If patient is hypernatremic, 0.9% and 0.45% saline may be alternated.

Severe volume contraction (e.g., decreased effective IVV causing hypotension). Give 0.9% saline as rapidly as practicable until the hypotension is corrected.

Estimate maintenance needs and add this amount to the fluids used to correct the preexisting water and electrolyte deficits.

For patients with normal renal function and no abnormal losses:

Maintenance	*Equivalent Intravenous Fluid Orders*
Water: 2500–3000 mL/24 h	Alternate: 5% dextrose in 0.45% saline with 5% dextrose in 0.25% saline
Sodium: 150 mEq/24 h	Each day add:
Potassium: 40 mEq/24 h	Multivitamins to 1st liter Potassium chloride 20 mEq to 1st and 2nd liters Infuse at 100–125 mL/hr
Nutrition (Short-term)	At least 400 carbohydrate calories/24 h

For patients with acute renal failure with no urine output and no abnormal losses:

Maintenance	*Equivalent Intravenous Fluid Orders*
Water: 600 mL/24 h	600 mL 20% glucose in water and multivitamins per 24 h
Sodium: 0	
Potassium: 0	
Nutrition:	At least 400 carbohydrate calories/24 h

See Table 7-8 if patients have abnormal losses of water and electrolytes.

Monitor patient frequently:

Weight daily

Measure serum creatinine and electrolyte levels daily or more frequently if necessary.

Measure CVP or pulmonary wedge pressure in complicated cases. If patient has normal cardiopulmonary function, CVP is sufficient. If cardiac disease or pulmonary hypertension is suspected, pulmonary wedge pressure measurement is preferred.

Evaluate water and electrolyte needs daily or more frequently in patients with high rates of abnormal losses.

Volume-Expanded Patient (Increased Effective IVV)

Correct volume excess:

Mild (e.g, simple edema): Decrease NaCl intake.

Moderate (e.g., mild pulmonary vascular congestion): Induce diuresis with diuretic and allow the sodium and water losses to go unreplaced.

Severe volume excess (e.g., severe pulmonary edema): Steps 1 and 2 and phlebotomy or ultrafiltration (if the patient is anemic) and/or digitalis, vasodilators, if heart disease is present.

Estimate ongoing losses (as above) and begin replacing when volume excesses have been corrected.

Monitor patient frequently.

Correction of Hyponatremia

The approach to the correction of hyponatremia depends on (a) whether the patient has significant central nervous system symptoms as a result of the hyponatremia (coma or seizures) and (b) the cause of the hyponatremia. If the patient has coma or seizures as a result of hyponatremia, the serum sodium level is commonly less than 125 mEq/L, and usually the reduction has occurred rapidly, over a few hours to days. In these situations, regardless of the cause of the hyponatremia, the serum sodium level should be rapidly raised toward normal by the intravenous administration of 3% saline. The serum sodium level should be raised to 125 mEq/L at a rate of 1 to 2 mEq/h. The rate of replacement can be slowed once the serum sodium level reaches 125

TABLE 7–8
Major Sources, Loss Rates, and Replacement Fluids in Abnormal Water and Electrolyte Loss

SOURCES	RATE OF LOSS	REPLACEMENT FLUID
Fever	Insensible water losses (normally 450 mL/24 h from skin and 450 mL/24 h from lung) increase by about 10% per degree F or 20% per degree C for each degree of temperature above normal	Replace with 5% dextrose in water
Hyperventilation	Doubling alveolar ventilation (i.e., 50% reduction in $Paco_2$) increases insensible water losses from lung by 50%. Thus the increase in alveolar ventilation required to reduce $Paco_2$ from 40 to 20 mm Hg increases insensible loss from lung from 450 to 675 mL/24 h.	Replace with 5% dextrose in water
Gastric fluid	Rates of loss from nasogastric suction usually are 1 to 2 L/24 h but can be much greater. Normal composition of gastric juice is approximately H^+ 100 mEq/L; sodium 40 mEq/L; potassium 10 mEq/L; and chloride 150 mEq/L.	Replace with 0.45 normal saline and potassium chloride (usually 20 to 40 mEq/L) as needed*
Diarrheal fluid	Losses can vary from trivial to several liters daily. In adults, diarrheal fluid usually resembles ECF except that the bicarbonate concentration is higher (about 30–50 mEq/L) and chloride concentration is lower (about 80 mEq/L). Potassium concentration is variable (10–40 mEq/liter)	Replace with 0.45 normal saline and 50 mEq of sodium bicarbonate/L and potassium chloride (usually 20 mEq/L), as needed*
Urine in acute renal failure	Because of tubular injury, urine sodium concentration usually is between 40 and 80 mEq/L and is largely independent of urine flow rate.	Replace with 0.45 normal saline and potassium chloride, as needed*

* The rate of potassium replacement usually is determined by the serum potassium concentration rather than the rates of potassium loss. For example, even though a patient in acute renal failure may be losing 30 mEq/24 h potassium in the urine, it may not be necessary to replace this amount, since potassium may be entering the ECF at an even faster rate because of catabolism of cellular proteins. On the other hand, the potassium losses in gastric fluid may amount to only 10 to 20 mEq/24 h, yet far greater amounts of potassium may have to be administered to maintain a normal serum potassium level, since gastric aspiration may lead to metabolic alkalosis, causing renal potassium wasting and extensive diffusion of potassium into ICF.

mEq/L, since neurologic symptoms are rare above this concentration. Rapid elevation of the serum sodium concentration to normal or hypernatremic levels must be avoided, since such rapid correction may cause central pontine myelinolysis. The correction using 3% saline (513 mEq/L) can be calculated as follows:

$$\text{volume TBW} = 0.6 \times \text{total body weight in kg}$$
$$\text{volume TBW} \times (\text{desired } [Na^+] - \text{actual } [Na^+])$$
$$= \text{total } Na^+ \text{ (mEq)}$$
$$[Na^+] \text{ is expressed in mEq/L}$$

The total amount of sodium required can then be replaced at a rate of 2 mEq/h using hypertonic saline. For example, if a 71-kg woman with neurologic symptoms has a serum sodium level of 113 mEq/L, correction to a serum sodium level of 125 mEq/L can be managed as follows:

$$\text{Volume TBW} = 0.6 \times 71 = 42.6$$
$$42.6 \times (125 - 113) = 511 \text{ mEq } Na^+$$

Therefore, this patient requires 1 L of 3% saline to raise her serum sodium level by 12 mEq. The liter of hypertonic saline is administered over 6 to 12 hours. Serum electrolyte levels should be checked every few hours and rates of replacement readjusted as necessary. The infusion of hypertonic saline results in diffusion of water from ICF to ECF until isosmotic conditions are restored. This results in reduction of cell volume and an increase of ICF osmolality toward normal as well as in an expansion of ECF volume. The expansion of the ECF by the hypertonic saline may precipitate or worsen congestive heart failure. Therefore, patients receiving hypertonic saline should be carefully observed for signs of pulmonary edema and, if present, vigorously treated with a loop diuretic.

Hyponatremia Associated with Volume Depletion

The administration of isotonic saline in amounts sufficient to replace existing sodium deficits usually result in complete correction of the hyponatremia, as discussed, in connection with the treatment of volume depletion, since restoration of effective IVV toward normal allows a water diuresis. If specific disease states, such as adrenal insufficiency or diarrhea, are associated with the development of the hyponatremia and volume depletion, these also require treatment.

Hyponatremia Associated with Normal Intravascular Volume

If the hyponatremia is associated with excessive intake of water, restricting water intake to normal will correct the hyponatremia. If the hyponatremia is due to an inappropriate antidiuresis, water intake must be restricted below normal—for example, to about 800 mL of measured liquid intake daily in an average-sized adult (see Table 7-2). This usually results in negative water balance, a fall in body weight, and a rise in serum sodium concentration toward normal. Excess total body water (TBW) can be calculated as follows:

$$\text{actual TBW} = 0.6 \times \text{total body weight in kg.}$$
$$(\text{actual serum } [Na^+]/\text{desired serum } [Na^+])$$
$$\times \text{actual TBW} = \text{desired TBW}$$
$$\text{actual TBW} - \text{desired TBW} = \text{excess TBW (L)}$$
$$[Na^+] \text{ is expressed in mEq/L}$$

If a specific cause for the inappropriate antidiuresis can be identified, it should be eliminated (see Table 7-6).

Hyponatremia Associated with Expanded Intravascular Volume and Extracellular Fluid

The spontaneous development of hyponatremia in the course of severe congestive heart failure or liver failure is an ominous sign. The hyponatremia usually does not cause any clinical symptoms, and although it can be successfully treated by water restriction, clinical improvement usually does not follow. Furthermore, during such treatment, patients complain bitterly of thirst. Thus water restriction sufficient to raise serum sodium concentration to normal is not indicated. It does seem prudent, however, to restrict water to prevent the serum sodium concentration from decreasing to less than 120 mEq/L in an effort to prevent possible central nervous system symptoms of hyponatremia.

Correction of Hypernatremia

Hypernatremia Secondary to Water Depletion

The amount of water needed to correct the serum sodium concentration toward normal is given in the following equation:

$$\text{actual TBW} = 0.6 \times \text{total body weight in kg}$$
$$(\text{actual serum } [Na^+]/\text{desired serum } [Na^+])$$
$$\times \text{actual TBW} = \text{desired TBW}$$
$$\text{desired TBW} - \text{actual TBW} = \text{amount water}$$
$$\text{necessary to lower serum } [Na^+]$$
$$[Na^+] \text{ is expressed in mEq/L}$$

The rate of correction usually is 1 to 2 mEq/h. This deficit usually would be corrected with hypotonic fluid given over 24 to 48 hours along with the water and electrolytes needed to maintain day-to-day water and electrolyte balance. The underlying cause of the hypernatremia also must be corrected if possible.

Hypernatremia Secondary to Excessive Administration of Hypertonic Saline

In this circumstance, which rarely does occur when intra-amniotic infusion of hypertonic saline is used to induce abortion, hypernatremia is due solely to positive sodium chloride balance. Therefore, treatment consists simply in inducing a state of negative sodium chloride balance while maintaining a slightly positive water balance. If the hypernatremia is associated with impairment of central nervous system function (usually $Na^+ > 160$ mEq/L), 2 to 3 L of 5% solution of glucose in water should rapidly be given intravenously, together with sufficient furosemide to induce a urine flow rate of about 10 to 20 mL/min. About 100 mg of furosemide intravenously is an appropriate initial dose. This will result in the excretion of urine containing about 140 mEq/L of sodium and chloride and 10 mEq/L of potassium. If, at the same time, only the water and potassium are replaced (e.g., replacement of each 1000 mL of urine with 1000 mL of 5% solution of glucose in water plus 10–20 mEq of potassium chloride, given intravenously), the patient will be selectively depleted of sodium chloride, and within several hours plasma electrolytes can be restored to normal. During this period of correction, serum and urine electrolyte levels must be frequently monitored to assess the adequacy of intravenous replacement therapy, particularly the rate of potassium administration.

POTASSIUM METABOLISM

Disorders of potassium metabolism frequently coexist with disorders of sodium and water balance. When, for example, there are gastrointestinal losses of water and electrolytes, sodium and potassium losses often go hand in hand. The recognition and management of potassium depletion under these circumstances are discussed above in connection with the management of disorders of sodium and water balance. It also is important to recognize those disorders in which disturbances of potassium balance are the primary abnormality or the major feature of the electrolyte disturbances.

Hyperkalemia

Hyperkalemia is defined as a serum potassium level greater than 5 mEq/L. Serum potassium levels between 5 and 6 mEq/L usually cause little or no functional abnormality, but such levels indicate that an abnormality of potassium regulation is present. This sign should be heeded and its cause investigated, since further small elevations in serum potassium concentration can seriously impair cardiac and skeletal muscle function. At a serum potassium level of 6 or 7 mEq/L, the electrocardiogram (ECG) begins to show tall, peaked T waves and skeletal muscle weakness may be present. At a serum potassium level greater than 7 mEq/L, severe ECG abnormalities may be present, including complete suppression of atrial activity and an idioventricular rhythm that can then lead to ventricular tachycardia and fibrillation. Profound skeletal muscle weakness leading to respiratory arrest also can develop. If serious hyperkalemia is suspected, an ECG should be obtained immediately along with a blood specimen for potassium measurement. The ECG findings will establish whether life-threatening hyperkalemia is present. Table 7-9 lists the principal clinical conditions associated with hyperkalemia.

Pseudohyperkalemia can result from hemolysis of red cells as a result of the mechanical trauma of venipuncture. Such pseudohyperkalemia can be readily recognized, since both potassium and hemoglobin are released by the damaged cells. If the serum potassium level has been significantly raised by in vitro hemolysis, the serum will be visibly pink owing to the presence of free hemoglobin. Patients with extraordinarily high white blood cell counts or platelet counts also can exhibit pseudohyperkalemia from excessive traumatic in vitro lysis of these cells.

Pseudohyperkalemia can be avoided by drawing venous blood samples under low pressure into a heparinized syringe.

Treatment of Hyperkalemia

Life-Threatening Hyperkalemia. (ECG shows sine waves or loss of atrial activity and a broad QRS complex. Serum potassium level usually is greater than 7.0 mEq/L)

1. Infuse intravenously, 10 mL of 10% calcium gluconate over a few minutes with ECG monitoring to observe for reversal of ECG changes toward nor-

mal. The same infusion of 10 mL of 10% calcium gluconate can be repeated once. Calcium ion directly antagonizes the effects of potassium on myocardial metabolism. The onset of action is a few minutes.

2. Infuse 50 g of glucose, 10 units of regular insulin, and 50 mEq of sodium bicarbonate. The onset of action is approximately 15 minutes. Additionally, an intravenous infusion of glucose, insulin, and sodium bicarbonate (e.g., 500 mL of 10% dextrose in water plus 15 units of regular insulin plus 50 mEq of sodium bicarbonate) may be started. Infuse over several hours. This maneuver causes potassium to move intracellularly. The amount of glucose infused must be altered or omitted in the hyperglycemic diabetic patient.

3. As soon as practical, give cation exchange resin (Kayexalate) by mouth, nasogastric tube, or retention enema (e.g., 20–50 g of Kayexalate every 2 to 4 hours). An equal number of grams of sorbitol should be given if the Kayexalate is given into the upper gastrointestinal tract. Sorbitol, a sugar that is poorly absorbed from the intestine, causes an osmotic diarrhea and prevents concretions of Kayexalate from forming within the gut. Kayexalate is an ion-exchange resin. It removes potassium by binding potassium and releasing sodium into body fluids.

Moderate Hyperkalemia. (ECG shows only peaked T waves; serum potassium level usually is less than 7.0 mEq/L)

1. Reduce potassium intake (normal potassium intake is 60–100 mEq/24 h). Reducing dietary potassium to 50 to 60 mEq/24 h usually is sufficient to correct mild hyperkalemia.

2. Kayexalate may be needed periodically to control serum potassium level.

3. Correct metabolic acidosis, if present.

Hypokalemia

Hypokalemia is defined as a serum potassium level less than 3.5 mEq/L (Table 7-10). Significant symptoms usually do not result from hypokalemia unless the serum potassium level is less than 3 mEq/L. An important exception is the patient receiving digitalis preparations. In such patients, hypokalemia, or even low normal serum potassium levels, can increase myocardial irritability and lead to serious arrhythmias. In addition to increasing myocardial irritability, hypokalemia can cause profound muscle weakness and ileus. Chronic

(text continues on page 146)

TABLE 7–9
Causes of Hyperkalemia

CAUSE	EFFECT
Excessive intake of potassium Transfusion of blood stored for prolonged periods	Shortened life span of stored RBCs after transfusion leads to excessive release of RBC potassium to ECF. Plasma potassium of stored blood also is increased (30 mEq/L) after 14 days of storage.
Excessive oral or intravenous intake of potassium	Acute ingestion of 500 mEq potassium chloride can cause fatal hyperkalemia with normal renal function. If renal function is impaired, even normal potassium intake can cause severe hyperkalemia.

Excessive release of intracellular stores of potassium
    Chemotherapy of malignancies
    Catabolism of hematomas
    Rhabdomyolysis
    Succinylcholine action on muscle
    Sepsis with excessive catabolism of muscle protein
    Acute digitalis poisoning
    Familial hyperkalemic periodic paralysis
    Intravenous hypertonic glucose or mannitol
    Intravenous arginine
    Metabolic acidosis
	The potential for any of these conditions to cause serious hyperkalemia is greatly increased when they coexist with impaired renal function.
	
	H^+ displaces K^+ from intracellular sites, causing increased diffusion of K^+ into ECF.

Impaired renal capacity to excrete potassium Grossly reduced glomerular filtration rate	Almost all of filtered potassium is reabsorbed. Excreted potassium represents almost exclusively potassium secreted by the tubules. Nevertheless, grossly reduced glomerular filtration rate is associated with grossly reduced tubular function and hence the tendency to hyperkalemia.
Impaired tubular function Hyperkalemic renal tubular acidosis	Some patients with normal or mildly reduced glomerular filtration rate can have substantial impairment of potassium secretion (e.g., lupus patients with interstitial nephritis, mild obstructive uropathy)

Decreased aldosterone secretion
    Addison's disease
    Primary hypoaldosteronism
    Hyporeninemic hypoaldosteronism
	Aldosterone is necessary for normal potassium and H^+ secretion and normal Na^+ absorption in the distal renal tubule.
	Common in patients with diabetes mellitus or obstructive uropathy.

Drugs that suppress angiotension formation (β-blocking agents, e.g., propranolol; prostaglandin synthetase inhibitors, e.g., indomethacin, ibuprofen; angiotensin converting enzyme inhibitors, e.g., captopril, enalapril, lisinopril)	Angiotensin II causes aldosterone secretion; β-blockers and nonsteroidal anti-inflammatory agents directly suppress angiotensin formation by suppressing renin production. Captopril prevents angiotensin II formation by blocking conversion of angiotensin I.
Drugs that interfere with renal potassium secretion	Spironolactone competitively inhibits the action of aldosterone. Triamterene and amiloride block potassium secretion even in the absence of aldosterone.
Ureteral implantation into jejunal loop	Increased reabsorption of potassium from jejunum causes predisposition to hyperkalemia.

TABLE 7–10
Causes of Hypokalemia

CAUSE	COMMENTS ON PATHOGENESIS
Decreased potassium intake	With 0 mEq potassium intake, stool potassium is about 10 mEq/2 h, urinary potassium is <30 mEq/24 h or is <20 mEq/L
Excessive renal losses of potassium	Urinary potassium usually greater than 30 mEq/24 h or 20 mEq/L
Diuretic therapy	All diuretics except for spironolactone, triamterene, and amiloride cause renal potassium wasting. Mechanism: Diuretics cause increased sodium delivery to distal tubular sites where sodium is reabsorbed in exchange for potassium or hydrogen ion.
Diuretic phase of acute tubular necrosis and other causes of osmotic diuresis	Mechanism: Same as above
Metabolic alkalosis	Mechanism: Renal tubular cell potassium concentration increased resulting in enhanced potassium secretion.
Gentamicin or amphotericin B nephrotoxicity	Renal tubular damage presumably causes increased back flux of potassium into renal tubules in the case of amphotericin.
Increased renal mineralocortocoid effects	Increased activity of distal tubular site, which reabsorbs sodium in exchange for potassium or H^+
Mineralocorticoid therapy (DOCA, 9 α-fluodrocortisone)	
Primary aldosteronism	
Secondary aldosteronism (e.g., cirrhosis of the liver, renal artery stenosis, malignant hypertension)	
Cushing's syndrome	
Excessive licorice or chewing tobacco (glycyrrhizic acid)	
Bartter's syndrome	
Renal tubular acidosis (RTA)	Mechanism:
	Distal RTA: ? increased renal potassium secretion in exchange for sodium at the distal tubular site because of decreased availability of H^+ for secretion
	Proximal RTA: Increased bicarbonate excretion leads to increased renal potassium excretion.
Excessive gastrointestinal losses of potassium	
Vomiting, gastric drainage, diarrhea, laxative abuse	Renal potassium excretion also increased in the case of vomiting or gastric drainage
Villous adenoma of rectum	Loss of potassium-rich mucus per rectum
Shift of potassium from the extracellular to the intracellular fluid	
Correction of metabolic acidosis	H^+ leave cells, K^+ enter cells during correction of metabolic acidosis.
Correction of hyperglycemia	K^+ enter cells with glucose to provide cation to balance anion that forms during metabolism of glucose.
Hypokalemic periodic paralysis	Unexplained familial disorder
Miscellaneous	
Ureterosigmoidostomy	Colonic secretion of HCO_3^- and K^+ with absorption of Na^+ and Cl^- results in hypokalemic metabolic acidosis.

severe hypokalemia also can cause metabolic alkalosis and decreased capacity to concentrate the urine. The ECG in hypokalemia often shows U waves, although this finding is not diagnostic of hypokalemia.

Treatment of Hypokalemia

Mild asymptomatic hypokalemia usually can be corrected simply by eliminating the cause of the potassium wasting or by increasing potassium intake. If the hypokalemia is due to diuretic therapy, potassium depletion usually can be avoided by adding spironolactone or triamterene. Potassium supplementation also can be used, but if the patient is on a low sodium chloride intake, the potassium supplement must be given as potassium chloride. The use of the other, more palatable potassium salts, such as gluconate, citrate, or acetate, and all forms of potassium in food is much less effective in correcting hypokalemia, and this treatment is used primarily in patients on a normal sodium chloride intake.

Severe or symptomatic hypokalemia usually requires intravenous administration of potassium chloride. In general, the use of intravenous solutions that contain greater than 40 mEq/L of potassium should be avoided, since infusing high concentrations of potassium could cause hyperkalemia. In correcting even severe potassium deficits, it is seldom necessary to infuse more than 120 to 160 mEq/24 h of potassium chloride. When higher rates are used, it is essential to frequently monitor the patient's ECG and serum potassium level.

DISORDERS OF ACID–BASE METABOLISM

The major acid–base buffer system of the ECF is the carbonic acid–bicarbonate system. Thus it has been traditional to define acid–base disturbances in terms of alterations of this buffer system:

$$H^+ + HCO_3^- \underset{R_2}{\overset{R_1}{\rightleftarrows}} H_2CO_3 \underset{R_4}{\overset{R_3}{\rightleftarrows}} CO_2 + H_2O$$

In the steady state, according to the law of mass action, the H^+ concentration of body fluids is determined by the following relations:

$$H^+ = \frac{K \cdot H_2CO_3}{HCO_3^-}$$

H_2CO_3 is not measured clinically. However, H_2CO_3 = P_{CO_2}, and P_{CO_2} can be measured clinically (a is the solubility coefficient of carbon dioxide).

$$H^+ = \frac{K \cdot a \cdot pCO_2}{HCO_3^-} = \frac{K'pCO_2}{HCO_3^-}$$

This is the Henderson equation. It states that, in the steady state, the H^+ concentration in body fluids is determined by the ratio of the P_{aCO_2} (the respiratory component of acid–base regulation) to HCO_3^- (the metabolic component of acid–base regulation). From these considerations, the basic nomenclature of acid–base disorders follows. The Henderson-Hasselbach equation is the logarithmic form of the Henderson equation. In the logarithmic form, the equation is more difficult to analyze. Thus, for the purposes of the present discussion, we prefer to analyze acid–base disturbances in terms of the Henderson equation. Table 7-11 shows the directional changes in acid–base parameters for the primary acid–base disorders. Figure 7-5 shows the expected range of arterial blood pH, P_{aCO_2}, and bicarbonate concentrations for the primary acid–base disturbances.

The Primary Acid–Base Disorders

Metabolic Acidosis

Metabolic acidosis begins as a reduction in plasma HCO_3^- and a rise in H^+. In response to these changes, alveolar ventilation is increased, resulting in a decrease in P_{CO_2} and restoration of H^+ toward normal (see Fig. 7–5 for appropriate decrease in P_{CO_2} for given HCO_3^- reduction in metabolic acidosis). The decrease in plasma HCO_3^- can be the result of the following:

1. An excessive rate of production of nonvolatile acids requiring buffering by HCO_3^- (e.g., diabetic ketoacidosis, lactic acidosis, methanol ingestion)
2. A normal rate of production of nonvolatile acids, but a decreased ability of the kidney to regenerate the HCO_3^- consumed in the buffering reaction (e.g., chronic azotemic renal disease, distal renal tubular acidosis)
3. Excessive losses of HCO_3^- (e.g., gastrointestinal losses from diarrhea, renal losses in proximal renal tubular acidosis)
4. Combinations of the above

Causes of Metabolic Acidosis

Increase in Unmeasured Anions—
"Anion Gap Acidosis"

Mechanism: Increased nonvolatile acid production
　　Diabetic ketoacidosis
　　Alcoholic ketoacidosis
　　Lactic acidosis
　　Salicylate poisoning
　　Ethylene glycol poisoning
　　Paraldehyde poisoning
　　Methanol poisoning

TABLE 7–11
Primary Disorders of Acid–Base Regulation

ACID–BASE DISTURBANCE	PRIMARY (INITIATING) EVENT	SECONDARY (COMPENSATORY) EVENT	RESULTANT CHANGE IN BLOOD H^+ AND pH
Metabolic acidosis	$\downarrow HCO_3^-$	$\downarrow P_{CO_2}$	$H^+ \uparrow$, pH $\downarrow$
Metabolic alkalosis	$\uparrow HCO_3^-$	$\uparrow P_{CO_2}$ (Minimal and only with severe increase in HCO_3^-)	$H^+ \downarrow$, pH $\uparrow$
Respiratory acidosis			
Acute (24 h)	$\uparrow Pa_{CO_2}$	Negligible $\uparrow HCO_3^-$	$H^+ \uparrow$, pH $\downarrow$
Chronic (3–7 days or longer)	$\uparrow Pa_{CO_2}$	Important $\uparrow HCO_3^-$	
Respiratory alkalosis	$\downarrow Pa_{CO_2}$	$\downarrow HCO_3^-$	$H^+ \downarrow$, pH $\uparrow$

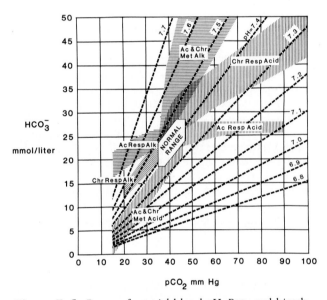

Figure 7–5. Range of arterial blood pH, P_{CO_2} and bicarbonate concentrations in the primary acid–base disturbances. The width of the bands indicates the 95% confidence limits of the range of variables. (From Arbus GS. Can Med Assoc J 1973; 109:291, redrawn and expanded to include chronic respiratory alkalosis)

Mechanism: No increase in nonvolatile acid production
  Renal failure

No Increase in Unmeasured Anions— "Nonanion Gap Acidosis" (Hyperchloremic Metabolic Acidosis)

Mechanism: Excessive HCO_3^- loss
  Diarrhea

Drainage of pancreatic juice
Ureterosigmoidostomy
Proximal renal tubular acidosis
Carbonic anhydrase inhibiting diuretics
Mechanism: Excessive HCl production
  Ammonium chloride, arginine HCl or lysine HCl administration
  Intravenous hyperalimentation solution containing cationic amino acids
Mechanism: Decreased renal HCO_3^- production
  Distal renal tubular acidosis (classic and hyperkalemic)

Although classification based on rates of acid production and excretion is useful for teaching acid–base pathophysiology, it is not satisfactory as a diagnostic approach to the individual patient with metabolic acidosis because there are no readily available means to measure acid production or excretion. Instead, the diagnostic approach should be to determine whether the decrease in plasma HCO_3^- is associated with a normal or an increased concentration of unmeasured anion in the plasma, which is calculated as follows:

Unmeasured anion = Na^+ mEq/L − (Cl^- + HCO_3^-) mEq/L.

Normal unmeasured anion concentration is from 8 to 12 mEq/L. In health, the unmeasured anions are mostly protein anions along with small quantities of sulfate, phosphate, and organic acids. In metabolic acidosis associated with increased unmeasured anions, the increase in unmeasured anions can be due to accumulation of sulfate and phosphate (as in renal failure) or nonvolatile organic acids (such as ketoacids, as in diabetic ketoacidosis).

In patients with metabolic acidosis, increased unmeasured anions, and increased acid production, the fall in serum bicarbonate level is a result of the rise in unmeasured anion. For example, in lactic acidosis, each lactic acid anion produced reacts with body buffers as follows:

$$H \text{ lactate} + NaHCO_3 \rightarrow Na \text{ lactate} + H_2CO_3$$
$$\downarrow$$
$$H_2O + CO_2 \uparrow$$

Thus the rise in blood lactate level is accompanied by a fall in blood bicarbonate level.

In metabolic acidosis with increased unmeasured anion and no increase in acid production (renal failure), the fall in bicarbonate level is due to inadequate renal acid excretion (renal bicarbonate production). The rise in unmeasured anion in renal failure is principally due to retention of sulfate and phosphate anions because of the reduced renal capacity to excrete these ions by glomerular filtration.

Treatment of Metabolic Acidosis. Moderate degrees of metabolic acidosis (plasma bicarbonate level greater than 15–18 mEq/L) usually are well tolerated for short periods. If metabolic acidosis is acute and severe (plasma bicarbonate level less than 10 mEq/L), dyspnea, depressed cardiac function, and obtundation can result. In such a setting, it often is necessary to infuse sodium bicarbonate intravenously to correct the acidosis. The effective space of distribution of bicarbonate is approximately equal to body water (about 50% of body weight). Thus, for a 60-kg woman with severe metabolic acidosis in whom it is desired to acutely raise plasma bicarbonate level from 6 to 10 mEq, approximately 120 mEq of sodium bicarbonate is required (4 mEq/L × 30 L = 120 mEq). This normally would be infused over 1 to 2 hours. Bicarbonate could then be given at a slower rate until the acidosis was corrected. In general, the serum bicarbonate concentration should not be acutely raised to levels greater than 15 to 18 mEq/L. Too-rapid correction requires infusion of large amounts of sodium bicarbonate, and this may cause overexpansion of the ECF and congestive heart failure. Finally, rapidly restoring the plasma bicarbonate level to normal may produce alkalosis because of persistence of a low P_{CO_2}. That is, if plasma bicarbonate is rapidly restored to normal or above in the treatment of metabolic acidosis, alveolar ventilation frequently persists at elevated levels for an additional 24 to 48 hours. Thus the low P_{CO_2} with normal plasma bicarbonate level can result in severe alkalosis, which, in turn, can cause cardiac arrhythmias, tetany, and seizures.

Metabolic Alkalosis

Causes of Metabolic Alkalosis

Mechanism: Chloride depletion and possibly ECF volume depletion (responds to sodium chloride and potassium chloride repletion)

Vomiting
Gastric drainage
Certain diuretics
Abrupt relief of hypercapnia
Congenital chloride diarrhea
Cystic fibrosis
Mechanism: mineralocorticoid excess (responds to removal of mineralocorticoid or mineralocorticoid inhibition)
Hyperaldosteronism
Bartter's syndrome
Cushing's syndrome
Licorice ingestion
Mechanism: Increased renal acid excretion (responds to removal of offending mechanism)
"Milk alkali" syndrome
Hypercalcemia
Mechanism: Massive alkali administration
Massive blood or plasma transfusions
Massive $NaHCO_3$ ingestion

A detailed discussion of metabolic alkalosis is beyond the scope of this review. Instead, attention is focused on the metabolic alkalosis that can follow gastric drainage because it is the form of metabolic alkalosis most commonly encountered in surgical patients.

Figure 7-6 depicts the normal handling of HCl and $NaHCO_3$ produced by the gastric mucosa. Note that the initial reactants ($NaCl + H_2CO_3$, step 1) are the same as the final products ($NaCl + H_2CO_3$, step 4). Thus gastric acid secretion normally has no net effect on acid–base regulation. If the gastric HCl is lost from the body and the chloride loss is not replaced, metabolic alkalosis will ensue, as shown in Figure 7-7.

Step 1 HCl is formed and enters gastric fluid
Step 2 $NaHCO_3$ is formed and enters body fluids
Step 3 HCl moves to duodenum and reacts with $NaHCO_3$ (from bile or pancreatic fluid)
Step 4 $NaCl$ and H_2CO_3 are formed

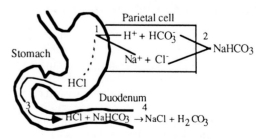

Summation: No net effect on acid-base balance since:
One H^+ and one HCO_3^- are formed in Steps 1 and 2.
One H^+ and one HCO_3^- are destroyed in Step 4.

Figure 7–6. Normal disposal of hydrochloric acid and sodium bicarbonate formed by gastric mucosa.

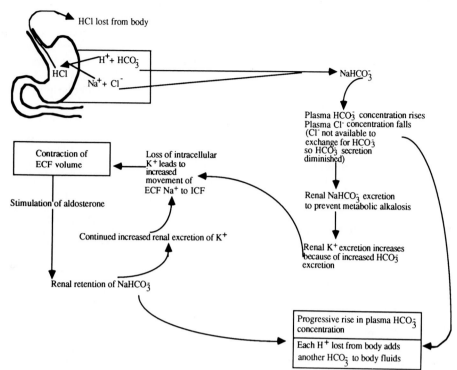

Figure 7–7. Pathogenesis of metabolic alkalosis from loss of gastric hydrochloric acid.

Severe potassium depletion alone also can cause metabolic alkalosis. Although the mechanism is not clearly established, apparently severe potassium depletion causes intracellular acidosis, which, at the renal tubular cell level, results in increased renal acid excretion (renal bicarbonate production) and an increased renal threshold for bicarbonate, so that the high filtered loads of bicarbonate can be retained by the kidney.

Treatment of Metabolic Alkalosis. Metabolic alkalosis can have serious consequences, such as tetany, major motor seizures, production of hypokalemia and cardiac arrhythmias (particularly in patients receiving digitalis), suppression of alveolar ventilation, and decrease in cerebral blood flow. Furthermore, the presence of metabolic alkalosis often is a sign that the patient is significantly volume-contracted. For these reasons, it is important to treat metabolic alkalosis and its underlying causes. Effective treatment consists in replacing sodium, potassium, and chloride deficits as they occur, as discussed above. Rarely it is necessary to treat metabolic alkalosis with intravenous infusion of hydrochloric acid, ammonium chloride, or arginine hydrochloride or with a carbonic anhydrase inhibitor (acetazolamide). This form of treatment is necessary in a patient who cannot undergo the sodium bicarbonate diuresis necessary to correct the metabolic alkalosis. This inability usually is the result of severely impaired renal or cardiac function.

Respiratory Acidosis

Respiratory acidosis results from decreased alveolar ventilation. This causes decreased CO_2 excretion by the lungs and an increase in blood $Paco_2$. With acute rises in $Paco_2$, H^+ rises linearly with increasing $Paco_2$ because there is little change in plasma HCO_3^- concentration. However, after 24 hours of hypercapnia, there is a significant increase in renal acid excretion (bicarbonate production), which results in a rise in plasma HCO_3^- concentration and a fall in plasma H^+. These plasma concentrations usually reach a steady state by 3 to 7 days. (See Fig. 7-5 for HCO_3^- elevation appropriate for acute and chronic $Paco_2$ elevations.)

Causes of Respiratory Acidosis

Mechanism: Any condition that decreases alveolar ventilation
  "Bellows" failure (e.g., respiratory muscle paralysis, fractured ribs)
  Obstructive pulmonary disease (e.g., asthma, pulmonary emphysema, foreign body in the trachea)
  Decrease in respiratory center drive (e.g., sedative drugs, O_2 therapy in chronic hypercapnia, Pickwickian syndrome)

Treatment of Respiratory Acidosis. The only treatment for respiratory acidosis is to increase alveolar ventilation (by such means as endotracheal tube, mechanical ventilators, or bronchodilators). Within minutes, severe respiratory acidosis can be reversed with adequate ventilation. In patients with chronic respiratory acidosis, severe posthypercapneic alkalosis will develop if $Paco_2$ is rapidly restored to normal and the patient is unable to initiate and sustain a bicarbonate diuresis. This inability usually is because of sodium chloride or potassium chloride deficits. If sodium chloride or potassium chloride is provided to correct volume contraction and intracellular potassium deficits, a bicarbonate diuresis will ensue and correction of metabolic alkalosis will be achieved.

Respiratory Alkalosis

Respiratory alkalosis results from an increase in alveolar ventilation. This causes an increase in CO_2 excretion along with a fall in blood $Paco_2$. Concomitantly, plasma HCO_3 is reduced primarily as a result of the action of intracellular buffers (see Fig. 7–5 for HCO_3^- concentrations appropriate for acute $Paco_2$ reductions).

Causes of Respiratory Alkalosis

Mechanism: Any condition that increases alveolar ventilation

Hyperventilation syndrome—a manifestation of an anxiety reaction

Hepatic failure

Fever

Aspirin intoxication

Central nervous system disorders (e.g., tumors, cerebrovascular accident, infection, trauma)

Early sepsis

Hypoxemia (heart failure, pulmonary emboli, restrictive lung disease, altitude, severe anemia)

Iatrogenic (excessive ventilator therapy)

Treatment of Respiratory Alkalosis. The symptoms of acute respiratory alkalosis (e.g., paresthesias, light-headedness, tetany) can be rapidly controlled by raising $Paco_2$ to normal (e.g., by rebreathing into a paper bag). If the patient is being supported on the respirator, the dead space may be increased or tidal volume and respiratory rate decreased while maintaining oxygenation. Definite treatment consists in removing the cause of hyperventilation. Respiratory alkalosis also can cause tetany and seizures, and predispose to cardiac arrhythmias (by causing an intracellular shift of K^+), particularly in patients receiving digitalis.

Bibliography

Arbus GS. An in vivo acid-base nomogram for clinical use. Can Med Assoc J 1973;109:291.

Arieff AI, deFronzo RA. Fluid, electrolyte and acid-base disorders. 1st ed. New York: Churchill Livingstone, 1985.

Arieff AI. Hyponatremia, convulsions, respiratory arrest, and permanent brain damage after elective surgery in healthy women. N Engl J Med 1986;314:1529.

Ayus JC, Krothapalli RK, Arieff AI. Treatment of symptomatic hyponatremia and its relation to brain damage: a prospective study. N Engl J Med 1987;317:1190.

Cockcroft DW, Gault MH. Prediction of creatinine clearance from serum creatinine. Nephron 1976;16:31.

Cohen JJ, Kassirer JP. Acid base. Boston: Little, Brown, 1982.

Harrington JL. Metabolic alkalosis. Kidney Int 1984;26:88.

Klahr S. The kidney and body fluids in health and disease. New York: Plenum, 1984.

Knochel JP. Neuromuscular manifestation of electrolyte disorder. Am J Med 1982;72:521.

Lennon EJ, Lemann J Jr. Fluid and electrolyte balance. In: TeLinde RW, Mattingly RF, eds. Operative gynecology. 6th ed. Philadelphia: JB Lippincott, 1985.

Matthay MA. Invasive hemodynamic monitoring in critically ill patients. Clin Chest Med 1983;4:233.

Maxwell MH, Kleeman CR, Narins RG. Clinical disorders of fluid and electrolyte metabolism. 4th ed. New York: McGraw-Hill, 1987.

Narins RG. Therapy of hyponatremia. Does haste make waste? N Engl J Med 1986;314:1573.

Narins RG, Emmett M. Simple and mixed acid-base disorders: a practical approach. Medicine 1980;59:161.

Ponce SP, Jennings AE, Madias NE, Harrington JT. Drug induced hyperkalemia. Medicine 1985; 64:357.

Robertson G, Aycinesa P, Zerbe R. Neurogenic disorders of osmoregulation. Am J Med 1986;2:339.

Schrier RW. Pathogenesis of sodium and water retention in high-output and low-output cardiac failure, nephrotic syndrome, cirrhosis and pregnancy. N Engl J Med 1988;319:1065.

Schrier RW, ed. Renal and electrolyte disorders. 2nd ed. Boston: Little, Brown, 1980.

Steiner RW. Interpreting the fractional excretion of sodium. Am J Med 1984;77:699.

Williams SE. Hydrogen ion infusion for treating severe metabolic alkalosis. Br Med J 1976;2:1189.

Control of Pelvic Hemorrhage: Blood Component Therapy and Hemorrhagic Shock

JOHN D. THOMPSON
WILLIAM A. ROCK, JR.
ANNE WISKIND

The performance of any surgical procedure involves control of pain, control of infection, and control of bleeding; control of bleeding is the subject of this chapter. Recognition and correction of an abnormal hemostatic mechanism and the prevention and control of bleeding are fundamental to the success of any operation. Preoperative, intraoperative, and postoperative hemorrhage are potential complications in every patient undergoing gynecologic surgery. Preoperative hemorrhage may be encountered in a variety of circumstances, such as in patients with intraperitoneal bleeding from a ruptured tubal pregnancy or in patients taking heparin who have a massive intraperitoneal hemorrhage with ovulation. Intraoperative and postoperative hemorrhage may result from vascular injury and failure to control bleeding during surgery. In all settings (preoperative, intraoperative, and postoperative) the bleeding may be caused or aggravated by a systemic bleeding diathesis that may or may not be related to the patient's other reason for hemorrhage.

In any case, satisfactory outcome in gynecologic surgery depends primarily on the competence of the pa-

tient's hemostatic mechanisms and the technical skills of the surgical team, and secondarily on the availability of measures to compensate for deficiencies in either if the need should arise. Fortunately, in modern gynecologic surgery practice, death from hemorrhage is rare and almost always preventable. This is testimony to the technical skill of gynecologic surgeons and the attention they give to details in caring for their patients in the preoperative, intraoperative, and postoperative periods.

Many benign and malignant gynecologic conditions are associated with an increase in menstrual blood loss (menorrhagia), an increase in the duration of menstrual flow (metrorrhagia), an increase in the frequency of menstrual periods (polymenorrhea), or combinations of all three. Repeated small menstrual hemorrhages, such as occur with menorrhagia, will reduce the iron stores in the body over time. The daily dietary intake of iron usually is sufficient to replace the iron lost with normal menstruation, but it is inadequate to replace the increased loss of iron associated with heavy menstruation. In contrast, a severe hemorrhage over a few hours does not deplete the body's iron reserves; a considerable reserve will remain to reform hemoglobin and restore a normal hematocrit, although this process may be hastened by the administration of iron.

A patient with a history of heavy, prolonged, or frequent menstruation who is scheduled for elective gynecologic surgery should be given iron supplementation, even if the hematocrit and hemoglobin values are relatively normal. The hemoglobin and hematocrit values usually do not drop until the bone marrow iron reserves are depleted over an extended period.

Iron supplementation is wise in any patient with a history of increased menstrual blood loss, especially before elective surgery. A blood transfusion is seldom necessary to correct iron deficiency or iron deficiency anemia in a gynecologic patient. Blood transfusion should be reserved for patients in hypovolemic shock and patients with aregenerative forms of anemia. Occasionally it is necessary to transfuse a patient who cannot tolerate or will not take iron; a patient whose anemia is associated with pelvic cancer and who should not wait several weeks to be operated on; a patient whose anemia is associated with a pelvic infection and who probably will not respond to iron supplementation; and a patient whose bleeding is too heavy and too continuous. Most patients who have an iron deficiency anemia, however, can correct the anemia by taking ferrous sulfate or ferrous gluconate. It may be necessary to administer iron intramuscularly in patients who cannot tolerate or will not take iron orally. After the hemoglobin and hematocrit values return to normal, even major gynecologic surgery can usually be accomplished without the additional risk of blood transfusions. As pointed out by Thompson, the liberal use of oral iron to correct anemia caused by gynecologic disease significantly reduced the need for blood transfusion on the gynecology service at the Johns Hopkins Hospital. Patients should be admitted to the hospital for elective gynecologic surgery with the highest possible hemoglobin and hematocrit values. This is the first and perhaps the most important rule in reducing the risks of surgical bleeding.

In the preoperative preparation of patients sometimes a faster method is substituted for a safer one without justification. This is especially true of the gynecologic surgeon who chooses to transfuse an anemic patient, regardless of her individual situation and regardless of the risks of transfusion. The practice of routinely transfusing anemic patients preoperatively is observed on busy gynecologic surgery services, where unfortunately the question too often is not whether to transfuse, but how fast to transfuse. The establishment of modern blood banks and the ready availability of blood have saved countless lives but undoubtedly have increased the tendency to use blood unnecessarily. In an editorial appropriately titled "One Pint of Blood"

Crisp emphasized these points, and said: "The anemias should be studied with more care and blood transfusions reserved for the aregenerative forms of anemia. Oral therapy takes longer but in an elective procedure it is much safer." There is no need to routinely transfuse patients arbitrarily before operation just to bring a hematocrit level back to 30% or a hemoglobin back to 10 g. Mild anemia is not associated with an increase in preoperative morbidity or delayed wound healing as long as intravascular volume and tissue perfusion remain normal. There is no evidence that transfusion will help to combat infection. Mild anemia is associated with normovolemia and adequate tissue perfusion and oxygen tension, and healing, therefore, is not compromised. Cardiovascular function also is not adversely affected unless the anemia is profound.

FUNDAMENTAL CONCEPTS OF NORMAL COAGULATION

A surgeon who accepts the responsibility for performing a surgical procedure must understand at least the basic mechanisms of normal hemostasis that can be relied on when surgical injury to tissue is inflicted, and must be able to recognize when normal hemostasis is interdicted, so that available remedies to protect against excessive bleeding may be found. Hemostasis is a complex, intricate, integrated, complementary, and countervailing system that maintains a delicate balance between normal coagulation and hypocoagulation or hypercoagulation. Gynecologic surgery, as a form of intra-abdominal surgery, demands an understanding of excessive bleeding or clotting and its treatment. Bleeding may be anticipated or unexpected, but in any case it is a serious complication to be dealt with in an organized and expeditious manner. Unusual clinical situations may arise that require hematologic consultation for resolution. A specialist in coagulation disorders can provide invaluable assistance in the diagnosis and treatment of many rare disorders of coagulation.

The following is a discussion of the principles and concepts of normal hemostasis, abnormal hemostasis (congenital and acquired), and management techniques.

Effective hemostasis is the result of all aspects of the coagulation system functioning together to stop bleeding. Coagulation is the working interrelationship of five aspects of a complex biochemical and vascular system that causes the formation and dissolution of the fibrin platelet plug. These five components are (1) vasculature, (2) platelets, (3) plasma clotting proteins, (4) fibrinolysis and clot inhibition, and (5) the hypercoagulable response. How these five components interrelate in the normal setting must be understood before one can appreciate how the five relate to bleeding or abnormal clotting in disease states.

Vasculature

The vasculature presents an endothelial-lined flexible conduit through which red cells, white cells, platelets, and all of the plasma proteins flow. At the interface between the flowing blood and vessel wall are several inhibitory biochemical systems that prevent the generation of the platelet-thrombin clot. The antiplatelet substance prostacyclin, produced deep in the vessel wall, inhibits platelet adhesion to the vessel wall. The surface antithrombin III–heparin sulfate complex inhibits deposition of thrombin and fibrin.

A tear in the vessel wall removes the endothelial cell layer, exposing the basement membrane, smooth muscle, collagen, and supporting adventitia. These substances are biochemical activators of platelets and have their own thromboplastic activity, which initiates fibrin generation and deposition. Therefore, the disruption in the vessel wall removes the protective covering of the endothelial cells, exposing platelet clumping and clot-initiating substances that produce a platelet-fibrin mass that will plug the tear in the vessel wall. A disease or medication that interferes or intensifies this process can cause bleeding or inappropriate clotting. The vessel wall is diagrammed in Figure 8-1.

Congenital diseases associated with inadequate connective tissue and vascular dysfunction associated with bleeding are rare. The more frequently seen conditions are hereditary hemorrhagic telangiectasia, Ehlers-Danlos syndrome, and Marfan syndrome, which are characterized by defects in the quality of collagen. Defective collagen is responsible for poor clot formation and platelet activation when needed at the injured site. No disease is known to be associated with excessive inappropriate clotting related to the vasculature as a structure. The congenital disease closest to that definition is predisposition to atherosclerosis owing to abnormalities in lipid metabolism, such as hypercholesterolemia.

Acquired diseases of the vessel associated with bleeding include deficiencies in vitamin C, Cushing's syndrome, acute and chronic inflammatory diseases such as infectious vasculitis and immune vasculitis, pyrogenic purpura, emboli purpura, and anaphylactoid reactions from drugs. Myeloproliferative disorders, such as multiple myeloma and Waldenström's macroglobulinemia, produce abnormal proteins that interfere with vascular function and therefore permit bleeding.

Routine laboratory assessment of vascular function is extremely primitive. The capillary fragility test, the only routinely available test used to assess vascular function, has limited value. It is sensitive to only the severest vascular structure abnormalities. More in-depth studies include vascular biopsies and skin window testing procedures, which are research procedures. There are no routinely available methods for assessing increased vascular activity in the area of inappropriate clotting.

Platelet Function

Platelets are disk-shaped fragments of the large multinucleated megakaryocytes released from the bone marrow on a daily basis (normal count is 150,000 to 400,000/mm^3) (Fig. 8-2). Their life span is 8 to 10 days. These microscopic fragments have a well-defined substructure that can be directly correlated with platelet function.

The surface activation of the receptor sites on the platelet causes it to change first to a sphere and finally to a spiderlike structure with pseudopods in all directions. This release reaction is the summation of biochemical and structural changes in the platelet, which are characterized as follows. The surface receptor sets up a biochemical chain reaction, resulting in the generation of thromboxane A$_2$. This causes contraction of the protein thrombasthenin, which causes the ejection of the platelet contents. Of great importance are the dense granules with nonmetabolic adenosine diphosphate (ADP). ADP is a potent platelet-aggregating agent that, in a dominolike sequence, stimulates more platelets, generating a large platelet plug.

The congenital diseases associated with poor platelet

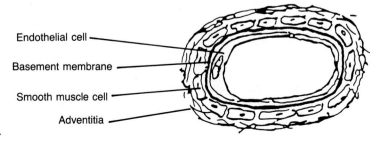

Endothelial cell

Basement membrane

Smooth muscle cell

Adventitia

Figure 8–1. Vessel cross section.

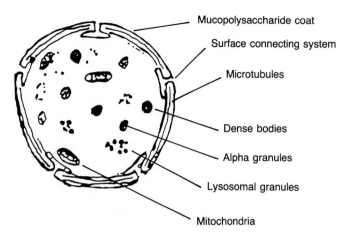

Mucopolysaccharide coat

Surface connecting system

Microtubules

Dense bodies

Alpha granules

Lysosomal granules

Mitochondria

Figure 8–2. Platelet cross section.

function are divided into four types of dysfunction: (1) adhesion to collagen, (2) adhesion to subendothelium, (3) release reaction defects, and (4) ADP aggregation defects. With the exception of von Willebrand's disease, a defect in the adhesion to subendothelium, all the congenital defects are rare and not essential to this discussion. Von Willebrand's disease (Table 8-1) is a classically autosomal, dominantly inherited disorder resulting from absence, decreased production, or abnormal function of a large multimeric protein synthesized by megakaryocytes and vascular endothelium. This protein is responsible for the proper binding and activation of platelets to the collagen surface exposed in vascular trauma. Its absence results in the failure of platelets to bind normally to disruptions in the vasculature, preventing formation of the platelet plug necessary for normal hemostasis. The condition remains undetected in the vast majority of the patients until some form of vascular trauma occurs or surgery is performed. In addition, such patients are particularly sensitive to aspirin or other antiplatelet medication, and bleed excessively in surgery while taking this kind of medication. Von Willebrand's disease is the most common congenital platelet disorder, and is the disease

most likely to go undetected until surgery. This disorder is particularly treacherous because in its milder forms history of bleeding in surgery is negative and the preoperative coagulation screen is normal (ie, a normal bleeding time). Acquired defects in platelet function are much more common, and can be classified into two groups: (1) those that are a result or consequence of a disease such as renal failure, myeloproliferative disorders (polycythemia vera, chronic myelogenous leukemia), and increased fibrin split products in consumptive coagulopathies, and (2) those that are iatrogenic, such as those caused by medications (aspirin, nonsteroidal antiinflammatory drugs, antibiotics, antihistamines, tricyclic antidepressants, dextran) and cardiopulmonary bypass surgery.

Congenitally increased platelet function has not been described. Acquired disorders associated with increased platelet function, however, are common. The stress of routine surgery or trauma (fractured hip, femur, or pelvis) may create a hypercoagulable state with thrombocytosis and increased platelet activity.

The laboratory assessment of platelet function has been expanded from the research laboratory and is more readily available to the surgeon. The routine anal-

TABLE 8–1
More Commonly Seen Rare Congenital Clotting Disorders

NAME	INCIDENCE	TREATMENT
Factor VIII (classic hemophilia A, sex-linked)	60–80/million	FVIII concentrate
Factor IX (classic hemophilia B, sex-linked)	15–20/million	FIX concentrate
Von Willebrand's disease (dominant; autosomal)	5–10/million	Cryoprecipitate (DDAVP)*

*DDAVP—Deamino-D-arginine vasopressin.

The remainder of the known congenital clotting factors are very rare, and occur with such low frequency that their discussion, diagnosis, and management can be found elsewhere. (See Harker LA. Hemostasis manual. 2d ed. Philadelphia, FA Davis, 1974; Corriveau DM, Fritsma GA. Hemostasis and thrombosis. Philadelphia: JB Lippincott, 1988; Triplett DA, ed. Laboratory evaluation of coagulation. Chicago: ASCP Press, 1982.)

ysis of platelet function should begin with a platelet count and template bleeding time. In special cases platelet adhesion and platelet aggregation are useful in identifying the inadequate or overstimulated platelet. In addition, biochemical markers for increased platelet utilization or turnover can be demonstrated with platelet factor 4 and beta-thromboglobulin assays.

Plasma-clotting Proteins

Plasma-clotting proteins are a group of serine proteases and cofactors that interact in a synergistic system to generate fibrin. The activation of the clotting system can be initiated in two ways: either by contact activation with factor XII or through thromboplastin activation of factor VII. The clotting cascade is diagrammed in Figure 8-3. As we will see later in the discussion of fibrinolysis and antithrombin systems, anticoagulation forces are initiated at the inception of clotting. The tear in the vessel wall, described earlier, begins the orderly activation of the plasma-clotting system. The fibrin contribution to the platelet-fibrin plug is initiated with the activation of factor XII by collagen and factor VII with tissue juice (thromboplastin). Any congenital or acquired disorder of the clotting factors may lead to inadequate or no generation of fibrin. Each clotting factor has a different role and significance in the overall generation of fibrin. This also is true with abnormal increases in some clotting factors that are associated with inappropriate clotting.

The congenital factor deficiencies associated with bleeding can be divided into the two groups: those that are relatively common and those that are rare. The relatively common group includes hemophilia A (factor VIII deficiency) and hemophilia B (factor IX deficiency). Both are seen in the male and rarely in the female as disorders with sex-linked inheritance patterns. The rare group includes all the remaining factors that have an autosomal recessive inheritance pattern or a dominant pattern with variable penetrance (see Table 8-1).

The acquired factor deficiencies are common and usually multiple in clinical appearance. A frequently seen hospital-acquired multiple deficiency is due to iatrogenic vitamin K deficiency with loss of factors II, VII, IX, and X. This deficiency often is the result of multiple antibiotic therapy that kills the vitamin K−producing bacterial flora in the intestine, and the nothing-by-mouth status of many critically ill patients, resulting in the loss of food sources of vitamin K. Other common acquired multifactor deficiencies are seen in acute and chronic liver disease, as in viral hepatitis and alcoholic cirrhosis; consumptive coagulopathies, seen in sepsis and placenta abruptio; washout coagulopa-

thies, seen in multiple-transfusion patients after severe blood loss, as in ruptured abdominal aneurysms; and major trauma, as from automobile accidents or gunshot wounds.

The laboratory assessment of the plasma clotting factors has traditionally begun with the prothrombin time (PT; factors V, VII, and X, prothrombin, and fibrinogen) and the activated partial thromboplastin time (APTT; factors VIII, IX, XI and XII). Specific factor assays also can identify the exact deficiencies. Remember that a factor deficiency as low as 30% may generate a normal prothrombin time and activated partial thromboplastin time. This relation is important in investigating minimal prolongations of the PT or APTT, which appear insignificant but could be hiding a moderately severe deficiency. The extrinsic pathway inhibitor modulates activated X but is not apparently significant in disease.

The sensitivity of the PT and APTT reagents are essential to the appreciation of the proper use of these tests as preoperative screening tests, or in monitoring warfarin and heparin anticoagulant therapy. Recent publications from Europe and the United States stress the importance of and need for a standardized prothrombin reagent system in the United States. The lack of sensitivity of the rabbit brain thromboplastin used in the United States has led to the overcoumarinization of some patients. The original 2.0 to 2.5 times the control value was based on the more sensitive human thromboplastin. Current recommendations have lower ratios (Table 8-2). These ratios are applicable only in stable, coumarinized patients. Studies of different APTT reagents have revealed a similar variability of sensitivity to heparin.

Fibrinolysis

The activation of the fibrinolytic system begins with the activation of the plasma substrate plasminogen. This substrate is converted by naturally occurring activators such as urine urokinase, kallikrein, and clot-activated proteases to the active enzyme plasmin. Plasmin is the active enzyme that, if free or clot-bound, lyses fibrin clots and destroys fibrinogen. This enzyme is modulated by α_2-antiplasmin and antitrypsin, which destroy the active enzyme plasmin.

This enzymatic conversion of fibrinolysis normally is initiated by clot formation, or primarily by a direct activator such as urokinase, or tissue plasminogen activator (tPA). tPA released from the endothelium activates tissue plasminogen, and is neutralized by tPA inhibitor. Sometimes direct activation is seen in liver disease and during extracorporeal bypass. This activation also may be secondary to disease, as in a consumptive coagulo-

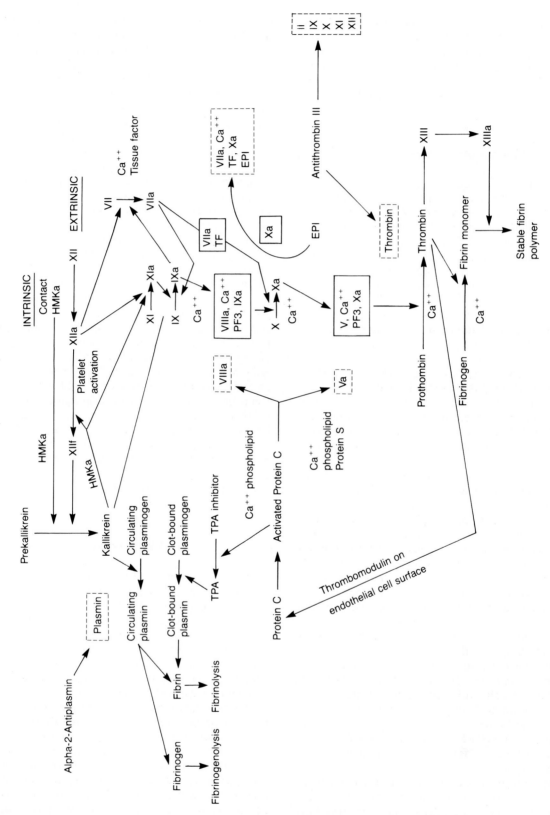

Figure 8–3. Clotting cascade. *Dotted line* indicates destruction of factor(s). (*HMKa*, high-molecular-weight kininogen.)

TABLE 8–2
Therapeutic Prothrombin Time Ratios

INTERNATIONAL NORMALIZED RATIO [INR] WITH *WHO* STANDARD "1"		PROTHROMBIN TIME RATIOS USING LESS RESPONSIVE THROMBOPLASTIN (HIGHER ISI VALUES)*		
		2.0	2.3	2.6
1. Prophylaxis for high-risk surgery	2.0–2.5	1.4–1.6	1.4–1.5	1.3–1.4
2. Prophylaxis for hip surgery Treatment of deep vein thrombosis and pulmonary embolism Prevention of embolism in atrial fibrillation, valvular heart disease, myocardial infection	2.0–3.0	1.4–1.7	1.4–1.6	1.3–1.5
3. Prevention of embolism in prosthetic heart valves and recurrent systemic thromboembolism	3.0–4.5	1.7–2.1	1.6–1.9	1.5–1.8

*ISI, International Sensitivity Index.
(Modified from Hirsh J, Levine M. Review article: confusion over the therapeutic range for monitoring oral anticoagulant therapy in North America. Throm Haemost 1988; 59:129.)

pathy such as bacterial sepsis, or a large abdominal aneurysm.

Hypercoagulable State

With physiologic stress of many kinds, such as emotional stress and surgical stress, there is a response of fright or flight. This response to stress also is evident in the coagulation system. The plasma-clotting proteins, such as fibrinogen and factor VIII, increase; the platelet count and stickiness may increase as well. This normal response is important in ensuring hemostasis at the time of increased need. When this process is exaggerated, uncontrolled, or unmodulated, inappropriate clotting may occur, which produces venous and arterial clots and all their sequelae. In gynecologic surgery the normal physical hypercoagulable state as well as the inappropriate state must be understood to appreciate the diagnosis, intervention, and management of postoperative vascular occlusive complications. Virchow, in 1845, was the first to conceptualize the triad of blood flow, vessel wall, and the content of blood itself as a basis for inappropriate clotting. An understanding of the relation of the three parts is essential to understanding what has occurred in the problem patient.

CONGENITAL CAUSES OF INAPPROPRIATE CLOTTING

The congenital etiology of inappropriate clotting has long been an ill-defined group, and has only recently been more completely elucidated by laboratory pro-

cedures (Table 8-3). Procoagulants, when increased on a congenital basis, have been associated with a propensity to generate clots. These include factor V and factor VIII. Their occurrence, however, is extremely rare, and they would not be present frequently enough to warrant testing every suspect case. Naturally occurring inhibitors of clotting are defined as those factors that actively destroy clotting factors or substrates as they are formed. The more frequently seen of these rare deficiencies include antithrombin III, protein C, and protein S.

Antithrombin III

Antithrombin III was described by Brinkhous and coworkers in 1939, and named by Seegers and Marciniak in 1962. The role of antithrombin III as a surface inhibitor of clotting was described by Buonassisi in 1973 as a cofactor with naturally occurring heparin sulfate on the endothelial cell surface. Antithrombin III is a protease inhibitor made by the hepatocyte with a normal activity of 80% to 120%. This serine protease inhibitor has a neutralizing affinity for thrombin as well as factors XII, IX, X, and XI. It is heparin-activated antithrombin III that produces the anticoagulant effect of heparin. The heparin–antithrombin III complex binds with thrombin irreversibly, removing the thrombin from any clotting activity. The heparin is later released from the antithrombin III to initiate the binding process to antithrombin III and thrombin again.

In 1965 Egeberg first described congenital deficiency of antithrombin III. As a congenital deficiency, it occurs with a frequency of 0.02% to 0.05% in the general

TABLE 8–3
Congenital Causes for Inappropriate Clotting

PROCOAGULANTS	MECHANISM
Factor V	More rapid or efficient generation of fibrin
Factor VIII	More rapid or efficient generation of thrombi
Inhibitors of Clotting	
Antithrombin III	With naturally occurring heparin sulfate has antithrombin activity, as well as neutralizing factors
Protein C	On the endothelial surface with thrombomodulin is activated to inhibit a tissue plasminogen activator inhibitor, as well as with protein S cofactor neutralizes Factors Va and VIIIa.
Protein S	A cofactor for protein C that neutralizes Factors Va and VIIIa
Impaired Fibrinolysis	
Plasminogen	Decreased absolute or functional levels result in persistent clots
Fletcher factor (prekallikrein)	Plasma deficiency results in persistent clots
Factor XII	Same as Fletcher factor
Tissue plasminogen activator	Activates plasminogen on thrombosis which if decreased does not initiate fibrinolysis
Plasminogen activator inhibitor (PAI-1)	Blocks activation of plasminogen
Dysfibrinogenemia	Produces nonlysable clots
Vascular Component	
Ineffective release of activator from vessel wall	Failure to lyse clots
Homocystinuria	

population and in 2% to 3% of those patients with deep vein thrombosis in Scandanavia. Three classes of such congenital deficiency have been characterized: type I, the more common type, with a parallel decrease in functional activity (progressive antithrombin III activity, and heparin cofactor assay and antigen); type II, the rare type, with a decrease in functional activity (as above) and a normal antigen quantitation; and type III, with normal antigen, normal progressive antithrombin III assay, and decreased heparin cofactor assay.

An antithrombin III deficiency that causes clinical symptoms is the result of the autosomal dominant transmission of the defect. The disease worsens with age but with a variable expression. An activity level of only 50% to 60% of normal in affected patients underscores its critical importance in the (normal) control and prevention of spontaneous thrombosis. Affected patients usually are made apparent clinically by some insult such as surgery or pregnancy.

It is therefore possible for such a patient being seen for the first time to be either a young or an older woman, depending on the occurrence of the initiating or challenging event. When investigating a patient with a deep vein thrombosis or other thrombotic event, caution must be taken in interpreting the results. Patients on intravenous heparin therapy, for instance, may have levels of 60% to 80%; levels below 50% in such patients are suspicious of an antithrombin III deficiency. Studies should be repeated when heparin therapy is discontinued.

Once a diagnosis of antithrombin III deficiency is made, a change to lifelong coumarin therapy is indicated. An increase in antithrombin III is seen after coumarin therapy.

Acquired deficiencies in antithrombin III are seen most frequently in liver cirrhosis, consumptive coagulopathy in liver disease, and earlier studies of oral birth control medication with estrogen. A deficiency also is seen in protein-losing enteropathies such as ulcerative colitis, and nephrotic syndrome by way of the kidney.

Protein C

Protein C is a naturally occurring serine protease that functions to neutralize factors Va and VIIIa as well as to permit the activation of tPA by blocking the tPA inhibitor with cofactor protein S.

This protease was described by Seegers and Marchiniak as an anticoagulant in 1962 and characterized by Stenflow in 1976 as a protease that requires vitamin K for gamma carboxylation. Esmon and Owen, Kisiel and colleagues, and Malar and associates further elucidated the anticoagulant activity of protein C with the inactivation of factors Va and VIIIa. Esmon and others and Comp and coworkers further demonstrated that the activation by thrombin as well as an endothelial substance, thrombomodulin, was needed for the orderly and rapid activation of protein C. The normal plasma concentration of protein C is with activity usually expressed from 80% to 120% of normal. Levels below 40% are associated with inappropriate clotting. Again, caution must be used in making the diagnosis of protein C deficiency because coumarin therapy normally will decrease the protein C level. A ratio of the activities of factors II, VII, and X to their antigens can be used to diagnose protein C deficiency while the patient is on coumarin therapy.

Another vitamin K–dependent substance, protein S, was isolated by DiScipio and colleagues in 1977 as a cofactor for the activation of protein C in its inactivation of factor Va. Protein S is a regulator of protein C.

Because activated protein C also is a blocker of an inhibitor of tPA, it also allows the orderly dissolution of clots by permitting tPA to activate plasminogen.

Congenital absences of protein C and protein S are well documented with inappropriate venous and arterial thrombosis. The incidence of this congenital defect is estimated to be 1 : 16,000 (?) and 1 : 160,000 to 360,000 live births in the United States. The estimated heterozygote rate is 100 to 200 to 300 births. The age range of presentation also varies as in antithrombin III.

IMPAIRED FIBRINOLYSIS

A congenital decrease in the plasma substrate plasminogen results in inadequate fibrinolysis of thrombi. This deficiency may be qualitative as well as quantitative with similar effect.

A congenital decrease in tPA that normally is released from the vascular endothelium is associated with impaired fibrinolysis. An abnormal increase in plasminogen activator inhibitor also will reduce the level of tPA, resulting in inappropriate clotting.

The decrease or absence of Fletcher factor (prekallikrein) and factor XII also may result in impaired fibrinolysis because of a decrease in activation of circulating plasminogen at the time of clot activation.

ACQUIRED CAUSES OF INAPPROPRIATE CLOTTING

The number of acquired causes of inappropriate clotting is much greater than the number of congenital causes and is expanding every day because the same chemistry of the congenital mechanism may be identified as a deficiency in an ongoing disease process.

Factor VIII has been shown to determine the rate of thrombin production and is a cause for thrombogenesis and coronary artery disease. Increases in dietary fat also increase factor VIII:C levels, resulting in an increased aggregability of platelets, which causes platelet thrombi to increase. Also of note is that smoking as a cause of coronary artery disease may in fact be mediated through a rise in fibrinogen.

Natural physiologic states also may increase the levels of plasma-clotting factors. Rather than a single factor being the cause of inappropriate clotting, in these cases it is most likely that the complementary activity of all factors working synergistically produces inappropriate clotting. In pregnancy, factor VIII:C and fibrinogen are increased. A frequent reaction to trauma such as leg fracture or surgery is an increase in factor VIII:C and fibrinogen levels and in the platelet count.

Disease states associated with inappropriate clotting include both acute and chronic forms. The acute forms are seen in diseases such as thrombotic thrombocytopenic purpura (absence of unknown platelet inhibitor) and nephrotic syndrome with loss of antithrombin III in the urine along with other plasma proteins. The chronic forms are seen in such diseases as diabetes mellitus (endothelial hyperplasia of smaller arterioles, reduced prostaglandin I_2 production, and hypersensitivity of platelets), heavy cigarette smoking, and diets high in fat and cholesterol. Neoplastic diseases such as carcinoma of the lung, colon, and prostate are associated with severe thromboembolic complications. Myeloproliferative diseases, including polycythemia vera, chronic myelogenous leukemia, and essential thrombocythemia, are associated with inappropriate clotting. The lupus-like inhibitor seen in lupus patients as well as in infectious diseases and other autoimmune diseases is associated with inappropriate clotting as well as spontaneous abortions.

Iatrogenic causes for inappropriate clotting are common findings in the hospital setting, and generate great concern. Such causes are the (1) postsurgical state, (2) medication, (3) prosthetic devices, and (4) immobilization for any reason.

As a physiologic acute phase response to surgical stress, an exaggerated outpouring of clotting factors and platelets in combination with a decrease in physiologic inhibitors may result in clot formation. This frequently occurs in deep leg veins, particularly in association with venous stasis.

Prosthetic devices such as grafts, shunts, and artificial heart valves can provide a clottable surface that will form a nidus for initial thrombosis quickly followed by further clot formation, resulting in obstruction or embolization.

The vascular component of acquired thrombotic disease has only recently been described in detail. It appears that decreased blood flow through a vein may decrease the contact of thrombin to thrombomodulin, diminishing the contact with protein C and predisposing the vein for thrombosis. On the other hand the arterial side with high blood flow rates has a rich capillary bed with greater contact with protein C, lysing clots more efficiently. Local thrombus formation may be generated by other direct mechanical disruption to the vascular endothelium, traumatic damage to vessel wall, infectious or chemical damage to the vessel wall, and vasculitis.

PREOPERATIVE COAGULATION SCREENING

For the preoperative evaluation, gynecologic patients must of necessity be divided into two categories: those having routine or elective surgery and those having emergency surgery.

Elective Surgery

The elective gynecologic surgical patient must be evaluated from two aspects: general medical history and specific nature of the surgery. The medical history taken at the bedside, with review of the medical chart when available, is an excellent place to begin. Table 8-4 highlights the most important positive and negative findings to be identified.

Preoperative coagulation screening is of limited value without complete knowledge of the patient's past and current history. It does not replace a good history and physical examination. Such screening should not be expected to reveal the estimated blood loss in the routine surgical procedure. It is essential, however, to resolving and eliminating risk factors that can affect postoperative bleeding (Tables 8-5 and 8-6).

Risk factors such as (a) unknown history, or known history in an emergency surgical procedure, (b) positive personal or family history for bleeding or bleeding with or without surgery, and (c) known history of taking medications that may affect coagulation, such as antiplatelet medication, vitamin K deficiency (nothing-by-mouth status with long use of antibiotics), and fibrinolytic therapy (decreased fibrinogen) are assessed by preoperative screening (see Table 8-4).

Preoperative coagulation screening also is useful in assessing the degree of change in the coagulation status

TABLE 8-4
Pertinent Medical History to Screen for Coagulation Problems

History of spontaneous bruising or bleeding
History of unusual bruising or excessive bleeding after surgery
Family history of bruising or bleeding after surgery
Medication associated with bruising or bleeding
Current medication within past week
Previous coagulation testing
Current coagulation testing

TABLE 8-5
Tests to Indicate Coagulation Status

TEST	NORMAL RANGE	LEVEL OF ALARM	SIGNIFICANCE
Hematocrit	37%–47%	25%	Tissue anoxia
White cell count	4,000–12,000	3000	Susceptibility to infection, infection, leukemia
		25,000	
Platelet count	140,000–400,000	100,000–700,000	Bleeding, myeloproliferative disorder
Fibrinogen	150–400 mg/dL	100 mg/dL	Bleeding, liver disease, intravascular consumption
Prothrombin time	10–13 s	14 s	Bleeding factor deficiency
Activated partial thromboplastin time	28–38 s	40 s	Bleeding, factor deficiency, inhibitor
Clot retraction	Complete clot 60 min; retraction complete 120 min	No clot	Low platelets or fibrinogen
		Clot lysis	Fibrinolysis
Bleeding time	1–9 min	9 min	Bleeding

TABLE 8-6
Coagulation Profiles

BRIEF COAGULATION PROFILE	COMPLETE COAGULATION PROFILE
CBC (includes WBC differential)	CBC (includes WBC differential)
Platelet count	Platelet count
Prothrombin time	Prothrombin time
Partial activated thromboplastin time	Partial activated thromboplastin time
	Fibrinogen
	Bleeding time

of the patient after a high-risk or difficult surgical procedure. A degree of change may not be significant when compared with the preoperative value, but alone, with no comparison, may be interpreted as an ominous sign of bleeding or change in the patient's coagulation status.

In the elective surgical case a diagnosed congenital or acquired bleeding disorder necessitates a coordinated approach that involves surgeon, blood bank, laboratory, and consulting clinical pathologist or hematologist to achieve success. The kind of bleeding disorder identified dictates the kinds of replacement blood components, medication, preoperative and intraoperative therapy, and laboratory monitoring. The cost of the required support must be reviewed not only in terms of initial costs, but also in terms of managing complications.

The decision to transfuse blood and blood components must be made with all the current knowledge on the patient's status. The surgeon must actively seek the patient's past history, hematology and coagulation test results, and chemistry results as appropriate (Fig. 8-4). The surgeon must be aware of the patient's hematologic and coagulation status throughout the case. Then, and only then, does the proper selection of blood components solve problems. The surgeon's surgical dictations and progress notes also should reflect the observations, test results, and course of action taken.

The risk of blood-borne infections and adverse reactions is always present, but the documented need for blood as a lifesaving substance will validate the decision. When blood is transfused when indicated but is not justified in writing, this lifesaving substance becomes a liability to all who use it. The routine preoperative orders for blood require a knowledge of the specific needs of the patient and the surgeon's usual transfusion requirements for a specific surgical procedure. For the routine gynecologic procedure, such as simple hysterectomy in an otherwise healthy woman, a

type and antibody screen are appropriate. With the type and antibody screen the patient's blood is screened for unexpected antibodies. No specific blood units are set aside, but blood is available from the general inventory in an emergency. If an unexpected antibody is identified, the blood bank should notify the ordering physician and set aside 2 units of antigen-negative crossmatched compatible blood for use in an emergency situation.

In an emergency the blood bank may release blood immediately, with a type and match to follow, with a 99.99% safety factor when the previous screen for unexpected antibodies was negative. Additionally, when the surgeon can wait 10 to 15 minutes, an immediate spin crossmatch may be performed to further verify ABO compatibility between donor and recipient. The value of the type and antibody screen is in monetary savings for the patient without undue or unnecessary risk to the patient.

In the more complex procedure, such as pelvic exenteration for cancer, where there usually is significant blood loss, a type and crossmatch for the average number of units used is appropriate. With extremely difficult procedures or other complicating diseases, additional blood, fresh frozen plasma, and platelets may be required during the procedure and should be requested preoperatively.

Ideal or time-proven guidelines are difficult to establish for every operative case. The surgeon will gain with his or her surgical experience, and over time establish his or her usual transfusion requirements for both type and antibody screen, as well as type and crossmatch. The hospital quality assurance program in planning with the transfusion service or blood bank and transfusion committee should establish guidelines to assist the surgeon in identifying the usual blood transfusion needs.

Emergency Surgery

As the emergency procedure is begun, decisions regarding blood replacement must be made. A direct approach to blood replacement therapy and the complications of such therapy depends on a clear understanding of the following concepts.

As bank blood replacement corrects the blood volume problem, it may create an acquired bleeding disorder, "thrombocytopenic hemophilia."

The patient's bleeding potential is dynamic and will change rapidly and frequently with the loss of blood and replacement therapy.

Direct monitoring before, during, and after surgery offers the best chance to diagnose and manage the

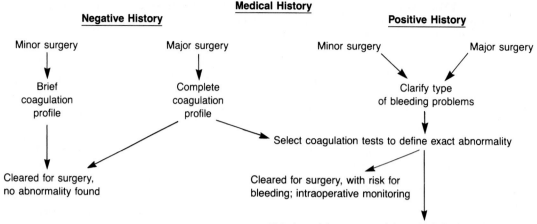

Figure 8–4. Evaluation of candidate for elective surgery.

bleeding. Direct monitoring also allows formulation of plans and adjustment of the replacement therapy program.

Surgery for emergency situations proceeds, even if the patient's medical history is unknown (Fig. 8-5). The fact that an underlying cause for potential bleeding may exist presents a complicated situation requiring ongoing testing and management decisions. Although such problems may not be immediately identified or verified, the surgeon must be prepared to request support from appropriate specialists if a congenital or acquired defect is suspected. If the patient is lucid or a relative is present, answers to such questions as the following should be obtained:

Has the patient been admitted to a hospital in the past? Where? Are medical records available?

Does the patient have a bleeding tendency, liver disease, or renal disease? Has there been previous surgery or other medical problems?

What medications is the patient currently taking or has she taken in the past (aspirin or *other non-steroidal* antiinflammatory drugs that may affect platelet function)?

Does the patient have surgery scars, and if so, where and how large are they? Such scars may suggest previous blood transfusions and the possible presence of platelet antibodies, as well as testimony to successful surgery. After this history has been obtained, the patient's current coagulation status should be evaluated. If test results are initially abnormal, surgery may proceed, but if possible, an additional freshly drawn blood sample should be tested before extensive replacement therapy is begun. (See Table 8-5 for standard coagulation profile.)

COMPONENT THERAPY FOR REPLACEMENT BEFORE SURGERY

With surgery planned, the preoperative data can be evaluated. Assuming the patient does not have *hemophilia, severe liver disease, or liver failure,* a prolonged PT and APTT may suggest an acquired or congenital bleeding disorder. (The blood sample must be properly drawn and mixed well, and must not be taken from an A-line containing heparin or from an infusion site.) Assistance from a clinical pathologist or hematologist should be requested if an intrinsic bleeding disorder is suspected.

If the patient is bleeding before surgery, packed red blood cells should be given. If bleeding is severe, fresh frozen plasma, cryoprecipitate, or platelets should be given as indicated. Whole blood (8 days old) is deficient in coagulation factor V and factor VIII in the plasma portion as well as in platelets. Although the levels of these factors may produce normal PT and APTT readings, they are insufficient for a patient undergoing surgery and blood loss. (Mild hemophilia also may produce a normal APTT reading.) When packed red blood cells and fresh frozen plasma are not available, whole blood may be used, although it may create a greater coagulation deficit when given in large amounts, making intraoperative monitoring even more critical.

The goals of emergency preoperative screening are as follows:

To determine whether a coagulation defect exists before surgery is begun and possibly to identify the cause

To establish a baseline for assessing the changes owing to massive blood replacement and the success of specific component therapy

To establish immediate component therapy needs

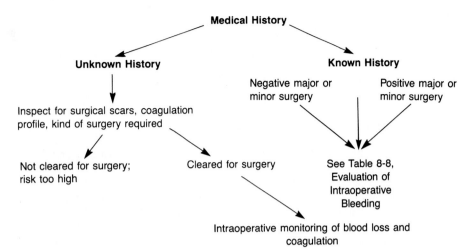

Figure 8–5. Evaluation of candidate for emergency surgery.

Minimum preferred values to be achieved before surgery are listed in Table 8-7.

Packed red cells are given as needed, and 2 units of fresh frozen plasma should be given in excess of 6 units of packed red blood cells to begin normalizing the PT and APTT. Platelet transfusions should not be given routinely until a deficiency is documented during surgery and when the surgical procedure is nearly completed. Correcting the fibrinogen level should be delayed until after the intraoperative monitoring results are seen. The transfusion of plasma in whole blood or in fresh frozen plasma may correct the fibrinogen deficiency. Poor clot retraction may be due to deficient platelets and fibrinogen, and the presence of clot lysis suggests intravascular coagulation. Additional investigative procedures (with specialty input) are suggested for further evaluating and managing the complex case.

COMPONENT THERAPY FOR REPLACEMENT DURING SURGERY

According to Schifman and Steinbrown, when intraoperative blood loss exceeds 15% of the patient's estimated blood volume, red blood cell transfusion is appropriate to replace the acute blood loss. As a general

rule, 15% of an adult's blood volume = patient's weight (in kilograms) × 10. For example: for a 50-kg woman (110 lb.), 15% of blood volume = 50 × 10 = 500 mL; for a 75-kg woman (165 lb.), 15% of blood volume = 75 × 10 = 750 mL; for a 100-kg woman (220 lb.), 15% of blood volume = 100 × 10 = 1000 mL. The patient's estimated blood volume, the estimated intraoperative blood loss, the presence of preoperative anemia, and the risk of hypoxic complications must all be taken into consideration when deciding whether or not to transfuse (Table 8-8).

When *massive blood replacement* therapy is under way, intraoperative monitoring of coagulation at 2-hour intervals, or after every 10 units of blood transfused, usually is sufficient. Remember that a patient bleeding during a surgical procedure has a higher demand for clotting factors and platelets than a patient at bed rest. In many oncology cases in which the patient is undergoing chemotherapy a platelet count of 50,000/mm^3 is ade-

TABLE 8–7
Minimum Preferred Values Before Surgery

Hematocrit	>25%
Platelet count	>150,000/mm^3
Fibrinogen	>150 mg/dL
Prothrombin time	<13 s
Activated partial thromboplastin time	<39 s
Clot reaction	Clot at one hour, no lysis

TABLE 8–8
Evaluation of Intraoperative Bleeding

I. Known medical history
  A. Positive
    Manage according to preoperative plan
  B. Negative
    1. Intraoperative coagulation profile: Assess amount of blood loss, transfuse up to 6 units packed red blood cells. After 6th unit repeat coagulation profile and prepare to transfuse components.
    2. Evaluate as to whether cause of bleeding is surgical or nonsurgical.
II. Unknown medical history
  A. Attempt to acquire history.
  B. Intraoperative coagulation profile: Assess amount of blood loss, transfuse up to 6 units packed red blood cells. After 6th unit repeat coagulation screen and prepare to transfuse components.

quate; in a surgical case in which the patient is bleeding a 50,000/mm^3 platelet count is not adequate to achieve a good platelet plug. The use of blood and blood components in the management of massive bleeding because of a major vessel rupture has the following three main objectives:

1. To maintain sufficient blood volume and circulating red cells to sustain life
2. Assuming extensive loss of plasma-clotting factors and platelets, to replace sufficiently to achieve adequate coagulation and hemostasis
3. To avoid falling so far behind in replacement that management involves not only bleeding from a vascular tear, but also bleeding at the microvascular level because of insufficient clotting factors and platelets

Each of these objectives requires repeated assessment of the patient throughout the surgical procedure. Careful monitoring by established routine ordering policies often is the best way to assure monitoring in a crisis situation created by massive bleeding.

Formulas for blood transfusion that are applied ritualistically without the benefit of laboratory data may resolve the need to treat but do not answer the needs of the patient. The formulas described below are designed to initiate the marshaling of blood bank resources, and do not replace the thoughtful analysis of laboratory data coupled with the selection of a specific blood component to correct a specific deficit. The following guidelines are recommended for component therapy in clinical situations with massive blood replacement to maintain normal hemostasis.

1. For every 6 to 8 units of red blood cells (packed red blood cells or whole blood), give 2 units (500 mL) of fresh frozen plasma. The size and age of the patient affect blood replacement. If the patient's blood volume can accommodate an additional 500 mL of fresh frozen plasma, this amount should be transfused and the PT and APTT monitored.
2. Platelets should be given as the platelet count falls below 100,000/mm^3 in massive hemorrhage. (Measurement error of a platelet count may be high as ± 20,000/mm^3 in a bleeding patient.) When a long surgical procedure is anticipated, or when more than 10 units of blood are given, 10 units of platelets in a volume of 500 mL should be given toward the end of the surgical procedure. This amount should be administered at least once to provide a maximum bolus effect. Unless their use is reserved until near the end of the procedure, platelets, which often are difficult to obtain, may be lost and unavailable when needed

because of continued blood loss and replacement during extensive surgical repair. Because pooling and transporting the platelets may take up to an hour, the blood bank should be given sufficient notice to have them available in surgery when needed. In assessing the patient's coagulation status, it should be remembered that clotting factors will be constantly changing. Ten units of platelets will not only achieve maximum bolus effect in an average patient (5 units in a child or small adult), but also enable evaluation of platelet utilization. A platelet count of 70,000 should be expected in a 70-kg person after transfusion of 10 units of platelets. Monitoring the platelet count after transfusion and for the next several hours will reveal the success of replacement, utilization, and life of the platelets. If fewer than 10 units of platelets are given, it often is not possible to determine whether a therapeutic level has been reached, or whether bleeding has continued because of other causes.

3. When the PT and APTT are prolonged (more than 14 seconds and 40 seconds, respectively) after replacement therapy, intrinsic disease must be considered initially, if only to be ruled out later. A borderline hemophiliac or patient with liver disease may manifest excessive bleeding after stress, trauma, or blood replacement, because of the increased coagulation needs. A mild hemophilia or liver disease is rare as an unknown, but it is possible (the recovery room values of a PT and an APTT near normal usually goes against those conditions). Therefore, administration of fresh frozen plasma in these 2-unit (500 mL) doses should begin to correct the deficiencies caused by massive red blood cell replacement. If oozing continues despite the rapid transfusion of 6 units of fresh frozen plasma, a clotting problem or other ongoing bleeding disorder should be suspected and additional support sought.
4. When the fibrinogen level falls below 100 mg/dL, transfusion of 20 units of cryoprecipitate will provide about 150 mg/dL in a 70-kg person. A low fibrinogen level is rare because fibrinogen is stable and present in whole blood and fresh frozen plasma. Liver disease or intravascular consumption must be suspected if the fibrinogen level is initially less than 100 mg/dL and remains low throughout surgery and recovery. The 20 units of cryoprecipitate will achieve therapeutic levels quickly and permit monitoring over several hours.

The goals of intraoperative monitoring are as follows:

To assess changes in the coagulation mechanism resulting from blood loss and replacement therapy

To identify the coagulation components affected, and determine the correct components to initiate therapy

To assess the success of replacement component therapy in an extensive operative procedure

To enable selection of components to achieve the following values: PT less than 14 seconds; APTT less than 40 seconds; fibrinogen more than 100 mg/dL; and platelets more than 80,000/mm^3. If surgical hemostasis appears to have been achieved from a technical viewpoint and bleeding is present but mild, one can "wait to see" for 2 hours. If bleeding is profuse and worsening, first 2 to 4 units of fresh frozen plasma and a 10 unit-dose of platelets are given and then packed red cells as needed. The patient is monitored when the transfusion is completed. Laboratory monitoring is repeated after 1 to 2 hours, whether the patient is bleeding or not, to determine the success of replacement.

COMPONENT THERAPY FOR POSTOPERATIVE REPLACEMENT

The presurgical and intrasurgical alarm levels for hematocrit, platelet count, PT, APTT, fibrinogen, and clot retraction also apply postoperatively, and a comparison of these values provides an accurate assessment of the bleeding patient. Significant clinical bleeding with good postoperative coagulation values suggests surgical bleeding. When laboratory values are abnormal, however, further surgery may be delayed until an attempt at aggressive specific component therapy is made. We have found that when abnormal coagulation studies exist, the following causes predominate, in order of frequency (most frequent first):

1. Low platelet count, owing to transfusion of only whole blood or blood bank plasma
2. Prolonged PT and APTT, owing to factor V and factor VIII deficiencies from whole blood or blood bank plasma. In administering aggressive replacement therapy, it should be remembered that some patients have a meager blood volume. Careful monitoring of venous and arterial pressure, as well as cardiac output, should be considered in blood component therapy. Often a slower rate of administration may achieve hemostasis without cardiovascular overload. In rare cases phlebotomy may be required to create needed space for transfusion. If nearly normal coagulation values are achieved but bleeding continues, surgical causes for bleeding should be considered.
3. Low fibrinogen level, owing to dilution with

plasma expanders, or concurrent development of a disseminated intravascular coagulation

The goals of postoperative monitoring are as follows:

To determine whether a coagulopathy was created by blood replacement, and to determine current status

To assess the success of specific component therapy and identify the need for additional components

To enable the surgeon to distinguish surgical from nonsurgical bleeding

The routine use of postoperative monitoring, whether the patient is bleeding or not, will achieve these goals. As the surgeon reviews the results of every case, he or she will develop a valuable assessment of his or her patients' usual postoperative coagulation states. With this knowledge the unexpected is recognized and resolved in a more timely manner.

RISKS OF BLOOD TRANSFUSION

Transfusions of whole blood were given sporadically before 1900, but usually to treat specific diseases rather than to replace lost blood volume. Indeed, heavy bleeding was thought to be beneficial and therapeutic for many diseases. Even as late as World War I the importance of blood loss and replacement was not recognized, since shock was thought to be due to toxins released from traumatized tissue. It was the work of Cannon and Bayliss in 1919 and Blalock in 1930 that brought proof that the important factors in shock were the loss of circulating blood volume and the decreased return of venous blood to the right heart.

Landsteiner discovered the four major blood groups in 1900. Banking and storage of donated blood became possible with refrigeration and the addition of sugar and later sodium citrate as an anticoagulant. In World War II a remarkable program was organized to collect and store large quantities of type O (so-called universal donor) blood for shipment to U.S. military hospitals throughout the world. Many lives were saved by the use of this banked blood to treat the shock associated with battle casualties. This experience firmly established the need for blood banks and the importance of blood transfusions in combatting hypovolemic shock from hemorrhage before, during, or after surgery.

To be safe, homologous blood must be collected from carefully selected volunteer donors and properly matched to the potential recipient. Although many lives have been saved by properly administered transfusions, gynecologic surgeons must be aware of the potential hazards of perioperative transfusions. The risks of red blood cell transfusion were recently reviewed by a National Institutes of Health and Food and Drug Administration Consensus Development Conference on Perioperative Red Cell Transfusion and published in 1988. The following excerpt is taken directly from their report.

In deciding whether to use red blood cell transfusion in the perioperative period, the need for possibly improved oxygenation must be weighed against the risks of adverse consequences, both short-term and long-term. The disadvantages are of two general types: transmission of infection and adverse effects attributable to immune mechanisms.

Any infectious agent that is present in the blood of a donor at the time of donation is potentially transmissible to a susceptible recipient. The consequence may be seen as clinical morbidity and mortality after an incubation period characteristic of the agent or recognized only by serological or other types of laboratory testing. If the agent produces chronic infection, clinical mortality may not be seen until years after the transfusion.

In modern blood banking practice, bacterial contamination of red blood cell units is rare. For practical purposes, the transmissible agents of greatest concern are viruses.

Human hepatitis viruses are the most frequently transmitted infectious agents. The incidence of Non-A, non-B infection after recent changes in criteria for donor acceptance and the introduction of nonspecific laboratory tests (antibody to hepatitis B core antigen and alanine aminotransferase) is not precisely known, but it may be 1 : 100 or less per unit. Hepatitis B virus infection, for which a specific screening procedure has been in use since 1971, still occurs, and prior to recent changes in donor populations was in the range 1 : 200 to 1 : 300 per unit.

Human immunodeficiency virus(es), about which there is the greatest public concern, presently poses only a remote hazard because of donor selection and laboratory screening procedures. It is variously estimated that the risk of HIV transmission by transfusion is 1 : 40,000 to 1 : 1,000,000. That level of risk is unlikely to be appreciably decreased in the foreseeable future even if additional screening tests are added. The consequences of HIV infection are rarely seen until two or many more years have elapsed, but ultimately morbidity and mortality are extremely high.

Cytomegalovirus infection occurs with moderate frequency among those recipients without prior infection. Most of these infections are asymptomatic, except among immunocompromised people.

Human T-cell lymphotropic viruses occur with low but not negligible frequency among donor populations in the United States. It is not known whether transfusion-transmitted infection with these viruses among adults results in T-cell leukemia/lymphoma and/or neurological disease several to many years later.

On rare occasions, other microbial agents, including parvoviruses, plasmodia, Epstein-Barr virus, and Babesia, cause infection and disease.

It is known for the human hepatitis viruses that the incidence of infection in recipients increases with the number of donor exposures. This relationship is probably true for other transfusion-transmitted infections. If homologous transfusion is to be used, therefore, the number of units administered should be kept to a minimum.

Immunologic consequences also complicate homologous red blood cell transfusion. Hemolytic and nonhemolytic reactions are largely caused by alloimmunization to red blood cell and leukocyte antigens. Compatibility testing virtually has eliminated immediate hemolytic transfusion reactions; when they occur, they are largely due to human error. Nonhemolytic febrile reactions occur in 1% to 2% of recipients due to sensitization to leukocyte antigens. This may be minimized by the use of leukocyte-poor blood products.

The incidence of fever, chills, and urticaria is 1 : 100; of hemolytic transfusion reactions is 1 : 6000; and of fatal hemolytic transfusion reactions is 1 : 100,000. Components of red blood cell transfusions, possibly leukocytes, may induce immunosuppression. The clinical significance of the phenomenon is unclear and presently is under investigation in a number of areas.

Although blood transfusions are and will remain an essential component of perioperative gynecologic care, an awareness of their associated risks should require careful consideration in every patient before electing their use. Certainly, there is every reason to carefully consider the risk-benefit ratio of giving "just one bottle of blood." Indeed, it is the rare clinical situation in which this action can be justified.

The growing public concern about transfusion-associated infections should make gynecologic surgeons aware of the importance of being selective in using transfusion therapy. The public has been greatly sensitized by transfusion-associated transfer of acquired immunodeficiency syndrome. The most common transfusion-related viral infection, however, is non-A, non-B hepatitis, accounting for 90% to 95% of cases of transfusion-acquired hepatitis and possibly as many as 3000 deaths per year in the United States. Ultimately, on further testing, many of these cases will be found to have hepatitis C. Certainly, when mortality or significant morbidity occurs with blood transfusion, the gynecologic surgeon must be able to show that the transfusion was indicated.

According to Friedman and associates, in every age range the mean hematocrit of men is higher than that of women. Women adapt to this relative state of "anemia" physiologically by a variety of mechanisms. Their red blood cells have a greater capacity than those of men to release oxygen. The erythrocyte oxygen dissociation curve of women is right-shifted when compared with that of men. Levels of 2,3,-disphosphoglycerate, adenosine triphosphate, and glucose-6-phosphate are higher in the red blood cells of women than in those of men. Because of these physiologic adaptations, Friedman and colleagues suggest that a lower hematocrit support level to govern the blood transfusion of female surgical patients be considered.

There are a variety of methods to support circulating volume, but there is no available material to support oxygen transport. Future research may be successful in developing modified hemoglobin solutions and perfluorochemical emulsions for oxygen transport, but there currently is no substitute for red blood cells for this purpose.

AUTOLOGOUS BLOOD TRANSFUSION

Blood collected from a patient for retransfusion at a later time into the same patient is called autologous blood. Autologous blood transfusions have been endorsed by the Council on Scientific Affairs of the American Medical Association and by the Committee on Hospital Transfusion Practice of the American Association of Blood Banks. If established guidelines are followed, autologous blood is the safest type of blood for transfusion. It does not eliminate all risks associated with red blood cell transfusion, since there is still the possibility of a hemolytic reaction caused by the rare clerical error. It does eliminate the risk of alloimmunization and the risk of transferring such infections as hepatitis, malaria, cytomegalovirus, and acquired immunodeficiency syndrome. In patients with rare blood types who have antibodies to common blood antigens, it may be the only blood available for transfusion. Autologous blood transfusion is acceptable to most Jehovah's Witnesses who have a religious objection to transfusion with homologous blood or blood products. The use of auto-

logous blood decreases the need for banked blood, which may then be reserved for other purposes. Depending on a variety of circumstances, the use of autologous blood for transfusion may reduce the general cost of blood transfusion therapy. About 65% to 80% of predeposited autologous blood donations are reinfused during or immediately after surgery. Blood that is not used by the donor can be used for other patients, thus reducing the demands on the nation's blood supply.

Intraoperative Autologous Transfusion

The frequency of autologous transfusion has increased appreciably in the past decade, especially for cardiovascular operations. Keeling and associates reported on the use of the Haemonetic Cell Saver for autologous intraoperative transfusion in 725 consecutive general hospital patients. Seventy-five percent were cardiovascular patients, but a variety of other patients, including gynecology-obstetric patients, were represented.

A general subject review of intraoperative autologous transfusion was published by Popovsky and associates in 1985. These authors point out that although the technology of the earlier experiences was comparatively crude and associated with technical problems and complications, better methods have been developed in recent years to eliminate problems in the operation and maintenance of the machinery and to make intraoperative autologous transfusion safe. Our experience in gynecologic surgery reported by Shapiro, although limited at this point to a series of 25 myomectomy operations, has demonstrated to our satisfaction that it is convenient to use and does not in any way interfere with the performance of the procedure.

The Haemonetic Cell Saver operates by retrieving blood from the operative site by suctioning into a double-lumen catheter, in which it is immediately anticoagulated with heparin. It is then collected in a cardiotomy reservoir where a filter removes gross debris. The blood is then pumped to a spinning centrifuge bowl where the red blood cells are separated, washed with normal saline solution, and then concentrated to a hematocrit of about 50%. The supernatant waste that is subsequently collected contains saline, anticoagulant, activated coagulation factors, platelets, leukocytes, free hemoglobin, and other small debris. The washed packed red blood cells are pumped into a reinfusion bag. The blood is then directly transfused to the patient through a filter. The reagents and the collecting system are sterile and disposable. The entire process takes 8 to 10 minutes to process about 250 mL of packed cells. The machine is maintained and operated by a trained technician.

At least until additional data is available to the contrary, intraoperative autologous transfusion should be considered contraindicated in patients with malignant disease and in patients with bacterial contamination of blood in the operative field. Although the addition of antibiotic agents to the cell-washing system may reduce or eliminate contaminating bacteria, some bacteria with the potential of causing systemic infection if retransfused may remain. There is a theoretical concern that malignant cells contained in retransfused blood may be responsible for generalized seeding of the malignant process. Although there is no data to support or deny this position—for medicolegal reasons at least—intraoperative autologous transfusion should be considered contraindicated in a patient with cancer unless the need is desperate. It is difficult to distinguish the hematologic changes induced by intraoperative autologous transfusion from the changes induced by hemorrhage and massive transfusion with homologous blood. The guidelines for use of component therapy are the same for both groups.

Merrill and associates reported the use of intraoperative autotransfusion in 38 patients with ruptured ectopic pregnancy. Transfusion-related morbidity occurred in six patients; two patients developed clinical coagulopathy, two patients developed pulmonary edema, and two patients developed minor transfusion reactions from concomitantly used bank blood. The total amount of retransfused blood was 49,475 mL, or 59% of the total amount of blood administered, a saving of about 90 units of banked blood.

It must be remembered that both autologous (intraoperative) and homologous blood are essentially packed red blood cells. A risk for autologous blood transfusions is in forgetting that only the patient's packed cells are transfused. The patient still will need fresh frozen plasma and platelets when massive transfusion of autologous blood is used.

Predeposit Autologous Blood Transfusion

With increasing frequency, gynecologic patients scheduled for elective surgery are asking to predeposit their own blood in the blood bank just in case a blood transfusion is needed. Indeed, experience has shown that such autologous blood can be collected and stored as whole blood, red blood cells, plasma, or platelets for retransfusion into the same patient during surgery if needed or at some other time. Donation may be scheduled at weekly intervals up to 3 days before surgery. Oral iron therapy is administered, and the hematocrit

and hemoglobin levels must not be low. The American Association of Blood Banks' standards for elective preoperative autologous blood donation include the following guidelines: (a) a hemoglobin of no less than 11 g/dL or a packed cell volume of no less than 34% and (b) phlebotomy no more frequently than every 3 days and not within 72 hours of surgery. If a patient's condition is stable enough to allow elective surgery, then preoperative donation for autologous transfusion is not contraindicated. Mann and associates studied the safety of autologous blood donation before elective surgery for a variety of potentially high-risk patients. Of 300 patients in the study, 46 were at least 70 years old. Four percent of patients experienced minor reaction to blood donation. This method of providing autologous blood should have applicability in gynecologic surgery. Experience suggests that it should be encouraged when practical.

The number of centers providing autologous blood transfusion programs will probably continue to increase, especially after the outbreak of the acquired immunodeficiency syndrome epidemic and the public knowledge of the possibility of spread by homologous blood transfusion, even though rare. Programs to encourage selected patients to donate their own blood before surgery are becoming increasingly popular despite the numerous logistical problems that must be solved. Only 2% of the blood currently collected in the United States is for predeposit autologous transfusion.

Much of gynecologic surgery is elective, and many patients are comparatively healthy. Elective gynecologic surgery often is scheduled 3 to 4 weeks in the future. During this time many patients can have blood predeposited for use during operation. Axelrod and associates suggest that 2 units of predeposited blood is sufficient for patients scheduled for hysterectomy. Only 10% to 20% of patients undergoing elective hysterectomy require blood transfusion, depending on the skill of the operator and the extent and nature of the gynecologic pathology.

Goodnough and associates have found that the administration of recombinant human erythropoietin increases the amount of autologous blood that can be collected before surgery. The volume of red cells donated by patients treated with erythropoietin during the study was 41% greater than that donated by patients given placebo.

BASIC SURGICAL PRINCIPLES TO AVOID EXCESSIVE BLEEDING IN PELVIC SURGERY

Bleeding caused by coagulation disorders is at the microvascular level. All the blood components used in replacement therapy cannot plug up holes in arteries and veins. Techniques of avoiding or controlling bleeding from pelvic vessels are most essential in efforts to reduce the risk of pelvic hemorrhage.

The following discussion will be of little importance to the seasoned pelvic surgeon, but it may be helpful to those who are learning basic techniques of gynecologic surgery. Assuming that the patient has been properly evaluated and prepared for surgery, the judgment and skill of the surgeon will determine, to a great extent, the amount of blood that will be lost during the operation. A good medical history and physical examination are still good screening tools to assess the patient's risk for bleeding. Regardless of the thoroughness of the preoperative evaluation, visual inspection of the first and any subsequent incisions alerts the surgeon to the possibility of excessive bleeding. There should be no hesitation to seek specialty support if clinically indicated.

The speed with which the dissection is performed should be varied from one phase of the operation to the other, but should progress deliberately without fiddling. For example, the incision can be fashioned with some alacrity, but dissection around deep pelvic veins must be done with great caution to avoid injury and bleeding. It is impossible to place too much emphasis on the need for optimum exposure to limit blood loss. When operating vaginally a contracted pelvic outlet will limit exposure for vaginal hysterectomy. A leiomyomatous uterus may require morcellation to allow exposure sufficient for safe vaginal removal. A Schuchardt incision may be required to improve exposure when operating vaginally. If exposure is inadequate, bleeding from vessels in the upper broad ligament may not be controllable from below, and an abdominal incision will be necessary to achieve final hemostasis from above. When operating abdominally the exposure achieved will depend on the choice of incision, the method of retracting, the placement and intensity of the lights, and the presence of willing and skilled assistants. Suction should be available to keep the field as free of blood as possible, and is preferred over sponges for two reasons. First, sponges are more traumatic to delicate serosal surfaces. And second, a determination of the amount of blood lost can be more accurate if the largest percentage has actually been suctioned into a calibrated bottle and measured. One may then add to this exact amount an estimate of the amount of blood lost on the drapes, sponges, and lap packs. A record of the amount of blood lost should be as accurate as possible and can be of great value in making correct decisions subsequently about the patient's care, especially regarding the need for blood replacement in case there is a suspicion of hypovolemia.

For pelvic laparotomy the patient usually is placed in modest Trendelenburg position. In this position the packs required to keep the intestines displaced in the upper abdomen tend to stay in place better, thereby enhancing exposure. An anesthetic for muscle relaxation is needed to keep the patient from pushing her bowels into the operative field, especially at times when the dissection is tedious and exposure of the field is mandatory to safely perform dissection. If a hypotensive anesthetic technique is used, the amount of blood lost will be decreased. The effect of the hypotensive anesthesia on reduction of blood loss will be enhanced if the operative field is elevated above the level of the heart, as in the Trendelenburg position. Hypotensive anesthesia, although useful in extensive operations, usually is not needed for routine major gynecologic surgery and should never be used as a substitute for hemostasis.

It usually is possible, and always desirable, to keep the number of clamps in the operative field to an absolute minimum. If the field is cluttered with clamps, the operators cannot see as well to operate. The length of the instruments must vary, depending on the thickness of the abdominal wall, the depth of the pelvis, and other variables. Pedicle clamps, tissue forceps, dissecting scissors, needle holders, and all other instruments must be longer when operating on obese patients and when doing extensive operations in a deep pelvis. The handles of the instruments must come all the way out and above the level of the incision so as not to interfere with the operator's view of the pelvis. There is an unfortunate tendency for gynecologic surgeons to use instruments that are too short. The operator must stand high enough to see down into the pelvis rather than barely looking over the edge of the incision. The patient's incision should be at the level of the operator's waist, not at the level of the operator's chest.

Vessel clamps used in surgery today are descendants of the original instruments developed by Ambrose Paré, a French military surgeon who began in 1537 to treat amputation wounds by clamping and ligation of vessels and by applying clean dressings rather than using hot cautery and boiling oil. Gynecologic surgeons of today may select from a variety of instruments to clamp vessels. Hemostats, Kelly clamps, Kocher clamps, and Adson clamps have been most popular. Other clamps developed for hysterectomy and said to be less traumatic include the Masterson and Rogers clamps. Haney clamps are heavier and designed to be used as a single clamp in vaginal hysterectomy. Double clamps are used on the top of the broad ligament for security. In abdominal hysterectomy a double clamp technique is used on the uterine arteries and the infundibulopelvic ligaments.

Cushing, a neurosurgeon, introduced the hemostatic silver metal clip in 1908 to occlude cranial vessels inaccessible to ligation. More recently clips have been made of stainless steel, tentalum, and the new synthetic absorbable nonopaque polydioxane polymer. The latter has the advantage of not causing the streaked artifact of metal clips when subsequent computed tomography of the pelvis is performed. Clips cause little tissue reaction, usually are easily and rapidly applied, and provide secure control of bleeding vessels in relatively inaccessible places in the pelvis where ligation would be more difficult. A small vessel can be quickly occluded with a clip even before the vessel is cut, thus keeping the field dry and the tissues to be dissected free of blood staining. Clips are especially useful in retroperitoneal dissections. They are available in several sizes. The applicator may be loaded with multiple clips, obviating the need for reloading and facilitating rapid use, and may be straight or obliquely angled. If appropriately used, clips can reduce blood loss, facilitate dissection, and reduce operating time.

Working with Bovie, Cushing also pioneered the use of the electrocautery for surgical hemostasis. Modern electrosurgical units are radiofrequency generators that supply 500,000 to 2 million Hz of alternating current to the tip of the electrode. The amount of current is preselected by the surgeon. It rapidly dissipates throughout the body and returns to the unit through the ground plate, which provides a large surface area of contact over a heavy muscle mass, usually the anterior surface of the thigh. Failure to properly secure the ground plate may cause burns at the other sites as the current seeks to discover alternate pathways to leave the body.

The surgeon may use the electrocautery for dissection of tissues set on the "cutting" current and for the hemostasis set on the "coagulation" current. The needle point electrode can be used for precise monopolar cautery of small vessels. The tissue surrounding the site of monopolar cautery, however, is damaged to a greater extent than necessary. If the vessel is grasped with a fine-pointed clamp or forceps, hemostasis is achieved by a low-current bipolar cautery and excess tissue necrosis is avoided, since the current will pass between the two points of the forceps or clamp grasping the vessel. This method of hemostasis is quick and convenient. Used properly, it can cause less tissue necrosis than ligatures. Experience in its use will result in maximum efficiency with minimum tissue damage, and a shorter operating time.

Among the many contributions to surgery made by William S. Halsted, first chief of surgery at Johns Hopkins Hospital, was the teaching of a surgical technique that emphasized meticulousness in dissection, gentleness in the handling of tissues, accuracy in hemostasis, precision in wound approximation, and absolute asepsis. Such a meticulous technique has become widely known in the United States as the Halstedean technique. It promotes good tissue healing by reducing tissue damage and wound infection. The accuracy of dissection, hemostasis, and tissue approximation is emphasized over speed, but wasting time with unnecessary hesitation, indefiniteness, and indecision can increase blood loss and infection. The experienced surgeon will be able to finish procedures in a deliberate, purposeful, timely, and precise manner.

On the basis of a thorough knowledge of pelvic anatomy, the dissection should emphasize the development of pelvic planes and spaces. This will avoid unnecessary bleeding and allow more accurate placement of clamps on vessels. Certain parts of the dissection can be delayed until later, especially if not needed now and blood loss is likely to be increased. For example, in performing abdominal hysterectomy the dissection of the bladder away from the cervix and vagina may be associated with blood loss and should not be done at the beginning of the operation. To avoid unnecessary blood loss, it should be done later.

Even simple maneuvers can reduce blood loss. For the same reasons, in doing a cervical conization, the cervical stroma should be injected with sterile saline solution. If a quantity sufficient to actually distend and blanch the cervix is used, an internal tourniquet is created, compressing small vessels and reducing the amount of blood loss. The posterior cervical cone should be taken first. If the specimen is taken from the anterior cervical lip first and bleeding is profuse, it will be difficult to see the posterior cervical lip and it will not be possible to perform the operation expeditiously to keep blood loss to a minimum. In doing vaginal hysterectomy saline can be injected beneath the posterior vaginal mucosa to act as an internal tourniquet and to help identify the correct plane for dissection. A needle point attachment to the electrosurgical unit can be used to make the incision and to precisely coagulate small bleeding vessels as they are encountered, thus reducing blood loss. When the incision in the posterior vagina is finished, the same technique can be used to incise the anterior vaginal mucosa behind the anterior cervical lip. The same technique also will reduce the amount of blood loss in anterior colporrhaphy. With this operation, however, as with some others, the amount of blood lost will depend, to some extent, on the time required to complete the procedure, since bleeding from paravesicle veins cannot always be controlled with sutures or coagulation. In this situation one is encouraged and allowed to finish the operation quickly and to control the continued venous oozing with a pack placed tightly in the vagina against the anterior wall. The pack should be removed in 24 hours.

In the early days of abdominal pelvic surgery, in the

19th century, postoperative hemorrhage was common because an effective technique of hemostasis was not known. In these earliest years the usual method of performing abdominal hysterectomy used a *ligature en masse* around the lower uterus. This mass ligature saved time and was used to occlude both uterine and ovarian vessels simultaneously. The uterine corpus with adnexa attached was simply amputated above the ligature. The stump thus formed was such a large mass of tissue that it could not be safely returned to the peritoneal cavity because of the danger of intraperitoneal bleeding. Therefore, sometimes the stump was fixed extraperitoneally in the incision, so that it was available for hemostatic clamping if the need arose. It was not until 1889 that Stimson published a technique for secure individual ligation of the uterine and ovarian vessels that was responsible for significantly reducing the incidence of postoperative hemorrhage. Kelly published a similar technique with illustrations in 1891.

Today in abdominal operations all major vascular pedicles should be individually ligated doubly and securely. Delayed absorbable sutures should be used and the knots firmly tied. Catgut suture knots tend to swell and come apart in tissue fluid. If vessels can be skeletonized (as with uterine vessels), ligation will be securer. Unfortunately the ovarian arteries cannot be easily skeletonized, and must be securely ligated in the infundibulopelvic ligament tissue about them according to the technique shown in Figures 27-7 and 27-8. A vascular pedicle such as the infundibulopelvic ligament should always be ligated first with a free tie around its base to occlude the vessels. Hemostasis is then secured with a transfixion suture ligature placed distally. This technique will avoid hematoma formation as well as the rare occurrence of a traumatic arteriovenous fistula. If a suture ligature is to be held long for traction or later identification, there is a danger that it will be pulled off, with immediate bleeding the result. Sutures used to ligate uterine vessels should be cut and never held for traction for that reason. During vaginal hysterectomy the upper broad ligament containing the utero-ovarian ligament and the fallopian tube must be doubly clamped. The lateralmost clamp is replaced with a free tie completely around the pedicle. Tied tightly, this ligature will compress the vessels in the pedicle so that the most medial clamp (the one closest to the uterus) can then be replaced with a suture ligature placed through the pedicle and then tied tightly around both sides of the pedicle. This ligature may be held long for identification and traction without fear of bleeding (see Fig. 27-45).

Gynecologic surgeons usually do not have the luxury of using tourniquets to control bleeding. There are, however, two special procedures in which tourniquets have been used to advantage. These are myomectomy and uterine unification operations. The tourniquet is fashioned in the manner of a Rummel tape tourniquet. It is used by vascular, thoracic, and trauma surgeons to occlude major vessels. A medium-sized soft plastic tube or rubber tape is used and threaded through a 4-in length of a No. 22F or No. 24F soft red rubber catheter. A tourniquet loop can be placed around the uterine isthmus through a small hole made in the broad ligament just lateral to the uterine vessels. Loops also can be placed around both infundibulopelvic ligaments through the same hole in the broad ligament. When these are snugged down tightly and held with a clamp, the entire circulation to the uterus can be occluded. The sterile doptone should be used, to be certain that arterial pulsations have disappeared completely. This technique can reduce blood loss to a minimum in these two procedures especially when hypotensive anesthesia is used. (Fig. 8-6). Similarly, vessel loops also can be used when repairing defects in the walls of large pelvic vessels.

Unnecessary bleeding in the area of dissection stains tissues, obscures visibility, restricts technical freedom, and gradually adds up to a significant amount of blood loss that may require replacement. Reducing the circulation to the operative field by *deliberate induction of hypotension* is a safe and effective anesthetic technique in properly selected patients, but requires planning and cooperation between the surgeon and the anesthesiologist. A reduction in arteriolar resistance will lower blood pressure and reduce, to a certain degree, bleeding in the operative field. The main mechanism for control of operative field bleeding with hypotensive anesthesia lies in reduction of venous tone, which reduces ventricular filling and cardiac output, the major determinant of blood pressure. The desired reduction in venous tone is achieved by one or more of the following anesthetic techniques: ganglionic blockade; spinal or epidural anesthesia; specific venodilating agents, such as sodium nitroprusside or glyceryl trinitrate; and the effect of some anesthetic agents. The use of induced hypotension is more effective if the operative field is raised above the level of the heart to encourage local venous emptying by gravity. For this purpose a modest Trendelenburg position should be used.

Deliberate hypotension is now an established practice, although some anesthesiologists are more enthusiastic about its use than others, and must be trained in the technique to use it safely. It has been most effective in operations on the head, face, neck, and upper thorax. Our experience with its use in extensive pelvic dissections for malignant disease has been uniformly favorable. The blood loss in extensive hysterectomy can be reduced 50% or more and the need for blood replace-

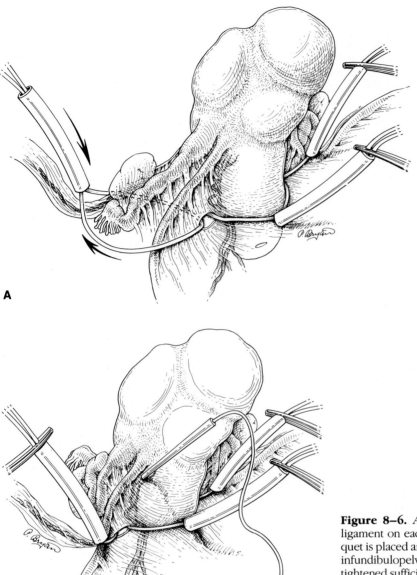

A

B

Figure 8–6. *A,* Through a small hole in the broad ligament on each side of the uterus, a Rummel tourniquet is placed around the lower uterus and around each infundibulopelvic ligament. *B,* When the tourniquets are tightened sufficiently, the blood flow to the uterus stops. The absence of arterial pulsations can be determined with the sterile doptone.

ment reduced by a corresponding amount. In a report by Powell and coworkers a deliberate hypotensive technique utilizing nitroglycerin and general anesthesia decreased the blood loss in extensive hysterectomy and pelvic lymphadenectomy by 70% when compared with a control group. The percentage of patients requiring blood transfusion was reduced from 81% to 11.5%. There is no doubt that deliberate hypotension is a valuable technique, but it cannot be a substitute for careful surgical hemostasis. "Reactionary hemorrhage," bleeding that occurs after the blood pressure

returns to normal, will present problems unless hemostasis is meticulous.

INTRAOPERATIVE MEASURES TO CONTROL PELVIC HEMORRHAGE

A survey by Bergqvist and Bergqvist published in 1987 gave information about the incidence of vascular injuries during gynecologic surgery in Sweden. Interestingly, the incidence of major vascular injuries was highest with laparoscopy, a procedure that usually is not associated with life-threatening hemorrhage. In 1975 Loffer and Pent reported that the total incidence of vascular injuries with laparoscopies was 6.4 : 1000 procedures. Most vascular injuries involved vessels in the abdominal wall and mesosalpinx. Life-threatening injuries to the major vessels (aorta, common iliac artery, and external iliac artery) also occur, however, and require immediate laparotomy for control. Small lacerations can be repaired with No. 5-0 monofilament nylon arterial suture after placing arterial or bulldog clamps or vessel loops above and below the bleeding site. More extensive injuries may require synthetic grafts. Experts in vascular surgery may be needed, but the operation to stop the bleeding must not be delayed until their arrival. Failure to take immediate action can result in death from exsanguination. Death after aortic puncture during laparoscopic sterilization was reported by Peterson and associates. Most of the major vascular injuries that occurred with pelvic laparotomy involved the external and internal iliac vein, according to Bergqvist and Bergqvist.

Despite adequate technical skills and careful dissection, serious hemorrhage may suddenly appear, especially during retroperitoneal dissections on the lateral pelvic sidewalls and around the sacrum. When it happens, it is hoped that the field will not be cluttered with unnecessary clamps, exposure will be adequate, the patient's condition will be stable, and anesthesia will be sufficient to maintain good relaxation. If the bleeding vessel cannot be quickly clamped, the simplest and most effective method of controlling the bleeding is provided by the index finger of the gloved hand. Pressure applied in this way will tamponade the lacerated vessel. With cessation of bleeding, the operative site can be cleared of accumulated blood by suctioning, exposure of the area can be improved, and the surgeon can gain a few moments to evaluate the situation and choose the best possible course of action. Arterial bleeding in the pelvis usually is easily controlled. The vessels are thick-walled and not easily torn further. Blood spurting from the vessel leads to its easy identification. If the artery can be clamped, it usually can be ligated or a clip can be applied, or both. If a vessel has mostly retracted from view with only one small edge still visible, that edge may be grasped with a clamp and gently twisted, thus decreasing the amount of bleeding sufficient to allow clipping or ligation. The difficult problem with hemorrhage in the pelvis stems from lacerations of deep pelvic veins, and can vary in magnitude from trivial to life-threatening. Pelvic veins may be fragile, tortuous, hidden from view, and distended. Blood returning through the lacerated vein may come from multiple deeper sources that are unavailable for ligation. Placing clamps and sutures blindly is dangerous and may even make the problem worse. Electrocoagulation of a laceration in a large vein should not be attempted, since it will inevitably result in a larger hole that will be even more difficult to secure. Sometimes the best procedure is to hold the finger against the bleeding site for a minimum of 7 minutes, after which the bleeding may stop or be easily controlled in other ways. Digital pressure to control venous bleeding takes advantage of the fact that the pressure in pelvic veins is very low. The initial use of digital pressure also is less likely to cause further tearing and trauma to the vein. Sometimes additional careful dissection in the area is required to free the vessel above and below, to allow more precise ligation or clipping. A long, finely pointed instrument can be used to clamp the vessel, and clips can be placed on each side. If the vessel can be sufficiently liberated, another instrument can be gently slipped beneath the first one so that its point is free. Then a fine free tie can be placed around the clamp. If necessary, clips also may be placed on each side of the tie. Temporary placement of packs in the pelvis in the vain hope of controlling the bleeding usually only delays the more definitive measures that will be required. A pack usually does not cause precise pressure against the bleeding point and hides bleeding beneath it. It may be allowed, however, as a temporary expedient to prepare for definitive action.

When dissecting in the pelvis one should avoid making a deep hole the bottom of which cannot be exposed in case a vein there might be lacerated. For example, development of the pararectal space must be done carefully because of the danger of injuring deep veins. The space is developed between the ureter and the hypogastric artery. The dissection is directed posteriorly at first, but soon changes to a more caudal direction. Failure to make this directional change will result in laceration and bleeding from veins in the bottom of the space. If development of the pararectal space is difficult, it should not be forced.

There are several other places in the pelvis and abdomen that deserve special mention. The removal of lymph nodes around the aorta and vena cava can result in serious hemorrhage from either vessel if not done carefully and with adequate exposure. An incision that provides sufficient exposure for the routine pelvic operation is not ordinarily sufficient for dissection around the aorta and vena cava unless it can be extended. A laceration in the aorta must be repaired. The aorta cannot be ligated without serious consequences. Although the vena cava usually can be ligated without serious consequence, a laceration in the vena cava should be repaired by placing a finger over it and gaining the necessary exposure by retraction and suctioning. Then continuous No. 5-0 Prolene suture should be used to close the laceration from side to side as the finger is slowly withdrawn. The same technique can be used to repair lacerations in other large veins, such as the common and external iliac veins. These two veins usually can be ligated without serious consequences, but we prefer to repair the laceration if possible, and it usually is possible. Lacerations of the common and external iliac arteries must always be repaired. These vessels cannot be ligated without serious consequences, including gangrene in the lower extremities. If the laceration is not repairable, the artery must be replaced.

One of the most dangerous places in the pelvis to dissect is in the region of the bifurcation of the common iliac artery and vein. This is the "axilla" of the pelvis, where many lymph nodes that drain the cervix are found. The hypogastric vein and its branches are at risk of injury when dissecting between the distal common iliac artery and the psoas muscle and deeper in the area of lumbosacral nerve trunks. When pulling on surrounding areolar tissue a relatively loose and thin-walled vein may inadvertently be pulled into the scissor dissection. The vein wall may not be distinct, especially when the tissue is blood-stained. One is wise to proceed cautiously. Furious hemorrhage threatening exsanguination may result from laceration of either the external iliac vein or the hypogastric vein where they join together, or from their major branches in the area. On the medial side of these veins the lateral sacral veins disappear into the sacral foramina. Fatal hemorrhage can result from laceration of these vessels. They cannot be clamped and ligated. They cannot be clipped. They are kept open by their attachment to the walls of the foramina. Extreme measures usually are needed to control the bleeding. One may try to pack the foramen with bone wax, but this usually is not successful. Alternatively, multiple layers (sandwiches) of absorbable gelatin sponge (Gelfoam) and microfibrillar collagen (Avitene) may be tightly sewn over the foramen. This area deserves its reputation as the "corona mortis" in the pelvis.

In the presacral region bleeding usually can be avoided by choosing a plane of dissection that is superficial to the anterior sacral artery and vein. Indeed, the retrorectal space is easily entered and developed inferiorly to the tip and lateral margins of the sacrum without appreciable bleeding, provided the dissection is carefully made with the hand and in the correct plane superficial to the presacral fascia and the vessels that overlie the periosteum of the sacrum. Kahn and Fang have recommended using metal thumbtacks to control presacral hemorrhage when the usual methods fail. Sterilized metal thumbtacks are placed directly over the bleeding point in the presacral fascia and pushed all the way into the sacrum with the thumb. An intercom-

municating network of presacral veins is protected by a covering layer of presacral fascia. Bleeding from the veins may be aggravated by clips, ligatures, or cautery. Packs, hemostatic agents, and thumbtacks are more effective in controlling the bleeding in this area.

Numerous variations in the branches of the hypogastric artery and vein will be encountered in dissecting the obturator fossa, especially in the floor of the fossa. The "web" of paracervical tissue separating the paravesicle and pararectal spaces contains branches of the hypogastric artery and vein. These vessels must be carefully ligated with clips or sutures in doing an extensive hysterectomy. With care, the dissection can be carried to the depths of the paravesicle space and pararectal space by carefully ligating or clipping each vessel encountered. The obturator artery and vein can be found adjacent to the obturator nerve. These vessels should be carefully ligated or clipped before they exit the fossa through the obturator foramen. If these vessels are allowed to retract into the upper thigh without being ligated, bleeding into the thigh may be a significant problem. The circumflex iliac vein will be seen emptying into the external iliac vein just above the inguinal ligament. Careful dissection around it usually avoids injury or the need for ligation.

In rare cases major bleeding points deep in the pelvis cannot be controlled by ligating or clipping vessels. Under these circumstances, if the bleeding has been controlled with a long clamp, it is permissible to leave the clamp on the vessel and close the incision around it as far as possible. Two days later the patient may be returned to the operating room for removal of the clamp. Rather than leave in a clamp, it may be more appropriate to use 2-in gauze packing to compress the vessel as tightly as possible against the pelvic wall. The pack should be removed 2 days later in the operating room, at which time careful additional debridement of devitalized tissue, irrigation, and placement of clean drains may be done.

Whenever an extensive pelvic dissection is anticipated, preparations should be made in advance in case pelvic hemorrhage is suddenly encountered. Adequate quantities of blood should be available to replace lost volume. More blood should be requested in advance of its need. A responsible member of the operating team or anesthesia team should be asked to monitor blood loss, blood replacement, and urine output. In the excitement of the moment it is possible to lose count of the number of units of whole blood, blood components, crystalloids, and other fluids that have been given, and how much blood has been lost. A dependable route for administering blood must be maintained. Without it, blood replacement is not possible. All other physiologic functions (eg, blood pressure, pulse, central venous pressure, blood gases, hematocrit values) should be carefully monitored. If massive hemorrhage occurs, or even if a possibility of its occurrence exists, a Swan-Ganz catheter should be placed for better control of volume replacement. In extreme cases where no other vessels are available intraoperatively, transfusions may be given under pressure directly into the common iliac artery with the needle pointed toward the heart.

Finally, as stated well by Breen and associates, "few gynecologists have not had a routine procedure abruptly transformed into a life-threatening drama. Under these circumstances the attitude of the surgeon may be the deciding factor in the outcome of the situation. Though a degree of alarm is a normal reaction, the surgeon must keep a clear head, even in the presence of massive hemorrhage. One important factor is the surgeon's realistic appraisal of his or her personal limitations; it is a wise individual who accepts these limitations and seeks assistance."

POSTOPERATIVE BLEEDING

Fortunately, with normal hemostasis and proper surgical technique, postoperative hemorrhage should be a rare occurrence. Every patient, however, should be carefully monitored for the first 24 hours after operation. Routinely, blood pressure, pulse rate, and respiratory rates are checked every 15 minutes for the first 2 hours after a major gynecologic operation. Thereafter, these vital signs are checked every 30 minutes until stable and then every 2 hours during the first 24 hours. This schedule may be altered, depending on the circumstances. Also, the abdominal incision and the perineum should be inspected for bleeding. Any sign of restlessness in the patient may be an indication of blood loss. A hematocrit usually is done about 6 hours after the operation is completed and again on the first postoperative morning. It may be done at any other time there is a suspicion of postoperative bleeding or anemia.

Occult intraperitoneal bleeding is one of the most serious postoperative complications after abdominal or vaginal surgery. It usually does not develop suddenly in the recovery room. More commonly a small artery begins bleeding into the peritoneal cavity. The vital signs in the recovery room may remain stable. Indeed, the vital signs may be stable for 12 to 18 hours after the operation is completed, and then suddenly severe hypotension, tachycardia, tachypnea, restlessness, and abdominal distention lead to a diagnosis of intraperitoneal hemorrhage. The diagnosis of intraperitoneal bleeding in the postoperative patient may be difficult. Peritoneal signs are subtle and may be masked by incisional pain and analgesic medications. Unfortunately the initial examination of the abdomen may be quite benign. The peritoneal cavity has an enormous capacity for occult blood loss without appreciable abdominal distention. As much as 3000 mL of blood (about 65% of the total blood volume of a 70-kg person) may be hidden in the peritoneal cavity with only 1 cm increase in the radius of the abdomen. Occult intraperitoneal hemorrhage is even more serious when one considers that the postoperative patient may not have had replacement of all the blood that was lost at the initial operation and may already have a slight hypovolemia when sent to the recovery room. Peritoneal lavage, described by Root and associates in 1965, is a valuable diagnostic tool in patients suspected of having occult postoperative intraperitoneal bleeding. It is not necessary when the diagnosis is unequivocal and associated with definite evidence of hypovolemia. It may be especially valuable, however, when the diagnosis is not certain in a patient whose vital signs are stable. It may be done with a blunt Touhey needle placed through the abdominal wall in a lower abdominal quadrant. It also may be done with a semiopen method, utilizing a small incision to insert a catheter. A nasogastric tube and Foley catheter should be placed before lavage to avoid injury to a distended stomach or bladder. If initial aspiration yields more than 10 mL of blood, reexploration is indicated. If lavage with normal saline solution (15 mL/kg) yields a red blood cell count of 100,000/mm^3, occult intraperitoneal bleeding is likely to be found at reexploration. A white blood cell count greater than 500/mm^3 suggests significant intestinal injury and is an indication for reexploration.

Immediate return to the operating room for reexploration while at the same time lost blood volume is rapidly replaced is indicated without delay. Sometimes it is difficult for the surgeon who did the original operation to conclude that reoperation is needed without hesitation. The results of watchful expectancy and procrastination, however, can be devastating in this situation. The experienced surgeon knows that the most common reason for postoperative shock is improper surgical hemostasis. A vessel has become disligated. There may be a temptation to blame the coagulation system and look for some defect in clotting factors. An established routine coagulation profile, ordered at the first suspicion, often eliminates this option. There also may be a temptation to try some nonoperative means of controlling the bleeding, like the MAST trousers (medical antishock trousers) or intra-arterial embolization of the bleeding vessels. Although these procedures may be valuable in unusual situations, the good surgeon quickly realizes that the best solution is immediate reexploration and ligation of the offending vessel while lost blood volume is simultaneously replaced. After reexploration such patients are at increased risk for developing postoperative complications, such as pulmonary atelectasis, abdominal distention from ileus, postoperative infection, incisional complications, and coagulation disorders from multiple transfusions. The anticipation of these complications allows the adoption of measures to prevent or manage them correctly if they should occur.

Postoperative hemorrhage from the vaginal vault usually comes from the vaginal artery in the lateral vaginal fornix, or from one of its branches. Most often the lateral vaginal angle, including the vaginal artery, is not properly secured or becomes disligated. To prevent such bleeding, the lateral vaginal angle stitch should be anchored in tissue lateral to the angle so that the angle cannot slip out. This stitch should not be held for traction because it may become loose.

Excessive vaginal bleeding may be noted in the recovery room or after the patient has returned to her room. Every attempt should be made to establish an objective measurement of the amount of blood lost, and to follow vital signs and changes in hematocrit values. One must realize that the vagina is a distensible organ. If a clot occludes the vaginal introitus, a large amount of blood—sometimes several hundred milliliters—can distend the vagina behind it and not be evident on a perineal pad. When significant bleeding is present the patient should be returned to the operating room. Sometimes adequate examination can be done with analgesia, but anesthesia should be used if necessary. The vaginal apex should be inspected. If the bleeding point can be seen, it should be ligated from below. Figure-of-eight No. 0 or 00 delayed absorbable transfixion sutures should be placed to include the vaginal mucosa and underlying paravaginal tissue. Care must be taken to avoid the inadvertent placement of a suture into the musculature of the bladder wall, the ureter, or the underlying rectum. If bleeding is not controlled by this technique, it is unwise to continue to add suture on suture in a frantic effort to control the vaginal bleeding. In such cases it is probable that the bleeding vessels have retracted well above the vaginal apex and cannot be reached by this approach.

If surgical hemostasis cannot be achieved transvaginally, laparotomy may be necessary. A vaginal pack seldom will control significant bleeding from the vaginal vault. One may apply pressure against a well-placed vaginal pack while the patient is being prepared for laparotomy. Our experience suggests that postoperative vaginal vault hemorrhage is more frequent when catgut sutures are used for hemostasis. Indeed, in some patients the hemorrhage will be delayed until 10 to 14 days after surgery, when the catgut loses its tensile strength. Posthysterectomy disruption of the vaginal vault with hemorrhage also may result from coitus, as reported by Hacker and associates. Their two cases occurred 2 and 8 weeks after total abdominal hysterectomy. In one case the blood loss was 2500 mL, and ligation of the hypogastric, ovarian, and uterine vessels was required to control the hemorrhage.

Bleeding from anterior and posterior colporrhaphy usually is from veins that have not been secured. A fairly tight vaginal pack will effectively compress these vessels and control the bleeding. The patient will feel an uncomfortable sensation of urgency of urination that will be relieved when the pack is removed in 24 to 48 hours. It seldom is necessary to reexplore an anterior or posterior colporrhaphy to locate and ligate a specific bleeding vessel.

A *postoperative pelvic hematoma* can cause serious morbidity, especially if it is large and becomes infected. Hematomas can develop above the vaginal vault, along the pelvic sidewall, in the paravesicle space, in the abdominal wall, and in the ischiorectal fossa and vulva. A hematoma in the ischiorectal fossa and on the vulva may be obvious on examination when the patient complains of discomfort in the area. If below the puborectalis muscle attachment to the vagina, it will not dissect into the pelvis above, but will be limited to the perineum and buttocks. A pelvic hematoma may finally be recognized in a patient whose postoperative discomfort and anemia exceed what is normally expected, whose temperature is progressively increasing, and whose postoperative abdominal distention is slow to resolve. If a patient is on anticoagulant therapy, even simple coughing can spontaneously result in a tremendous postoperative pelvic hematoma. Abdominal and pelvic examinations reveal a mass. Ultrasonography is helpful in delineating its exact size and location. An extended, morbid, and complicated postoperative course can be alleviated if the hematoma can be drained. Sometimes simple drainage through the vaginal vault can be accomplished by probing with a uterine dressing forceps. A small Penrose drain may be inserted through the drainage tract and left in place for a day or so. If drainage cannot be achieved in this simple way, drainage with guidance of computed tomography or through an abdominal incision may be necessary. In our experience, if the hematoma can be drained, the patient's recovery will be more prompt. In exceptional cases where drainage may be difficult or contraindicated and infection is not a serious problem, the hematoma may be allowed to gradually resolve over a few months. Unfortunately sometimes a hematoma will not resolve completely, but persist and continue to cause pain. We occasionally have removed large pieces of an organizing hematoma as long as 1 year later. For these reasons we prefer to drain pelvic hematomas initially whenever possible.

A few *other special circumstances* may be mentioned. Hemorrhage after uterine curettage is extremely rare, even with perforation of the uterus. The perforation usually is with the uterine sound and through the corpus. The curettage should be stopped and the patient's vital signs checked for several hours. If she is not already in the hospital, she may be admitted for overnight observation. It is extremely unlikely that any problem will develop, and hospital admission as a precautionary measure may be unnecessary. On the other hand, if the perforation has occurred with a wide blunt instrument, such as a curette or a suction device, if the patient is pregnant, or if fatty tissue appears in the curettage specimen, the patient must be hospitalized and closely observed for intraperitoneal bleeding. Laparoscopy also may be done in high-risk cases to assess the damage and find out if active bleeding is present. A misdirected cervical dilator can lacerate the uterine artery and vein, with subsequent intraperitoneal bleeding or broad ligament hematoma formation. Laparotomy is required to control the bleeding and evacuate the hematoma. A hysterectomy may or may not be necessary, depending on assessment of the damage to the uterus.

Hemorrhage from cervical conization may occur in the first 24 hours or 7 to 14 days later, when cervical sutures lose their tensile strength. In our experience delayed hemorrhage after conization of the cervix is more common if catgut is used to suture the cervix. It also is more common if one cuts deeply into the cervical stroma or if the patient is pregnant. If the patient is bleeding heavily at any time after conization, the cervix should be inspected. Measures to control the bleeding include resuturing, hot cautery, silver nitrate, and Monsel's solution. If bleeding is not profuse, a pack may be tried. In taking the conization specimen one must be certain that the apex of the cone intersects the endocervical canal. If the cervical incision is misdirected to one side or the other, the uterine vessels are in danger of laceration. Serious hemorrhage or broad ligament hematoma will result. To prevent this problem, the cervix should first be sounded to ascertain the direction of the endocervical canal and the incision planned accordingly.

UNUSUAL METHODS OF CONTROLLING PELVIC HEMORRHAGE

Hypogastric Artery Ligation

One of the most effective and rapid methods of controlling severe pelvic hemorrhage is by ligation of both hypogastric arteries. In 1893 at the Johns Hopkins Hospital, Howard Kelly performed bilateral hypogastric artery ligation to control hemorrhage during hysterectomy for uterine cancer. Hypogastric artery ligation was later introduced by Mengert and then extensively investigated by Burchell.

Because of the major collateral circulation with the aorta and femoral artery, including the lumbar, iliolumbar, middle sacral, lateral sacral, superior and middle hemorrhoidal, and gluteal arteries, it is important to ligate the anterior division of the hypogastric artery distal to the posterior parietal branch, as demonstrated in Figure 8-7. When the hypogastric artery is ligated *proximal* to the posterior division, flow may still occur distal to the point of ligation by reversed flow through the iliolumbar and lateral sacral collateral arteries. When the hypogastric artery is ligated *distal* to the posterior division, flow may still occur distal to the point of ligation, but only by reversed flow in middle hemorrhoidal arteries, and flow in the iliolumbar and lateral sacral arteries above the point of ligation will continue to be normal.

In ligating the hypogastric artery the peritoneum is opened on the lateral side of the common iliac artery near its bifurcation, with the ureter left attached to the medial peritoneal reflection to avoid disturbing its blood supply. The posterior branch of the hypogastric artery must be clearly identified before the selection of the point of dissection and double ligation of the anterior division. The artery is dissected and carefully mobilized free from the underlying hypogastric vein. Nonabsorbable suture (No. 0 silk) is passed around the

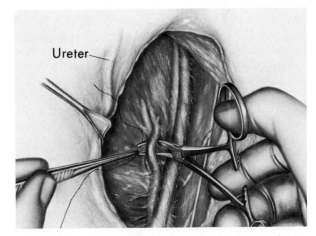

Figure 8–7. Ligation of right hypogastric artery, showing peritoneal reflection with attached ureter from bifurcation of iliac artery, and silk ligature placed around anterior division of hypogastric artery.

artery with an Adson or right-angle clamp, and tied. A second free-tie is placed distal to the initial ligature to avoid recanalization. Transfixion of the vessel is not essential or desirable in this procedure. The major advantages of ligating the anterior division of the hypogastric artery are in isolating the collateral arterial circulation from the pelvis and in reducing the pulse pressure in the bleeding artery, as demonstrated by Burchell. This reduction in pulse pressure permits thrombosis of the bleeding vessel to occur. When possible, we believe that the arterial branch closest to the bleeding point should be ligated. Because the uterine artery is the first visceral branch of the hypogastric artery, it may be feasible to identify this artery and ligate it separately, if this vessel should be the origin of the pelvic bleeding. This is a much more difficult procedure than ligating the entire anterior division of the hypogastric artery, and should not be attempted in the face of massive pelvic bleeding, distorted pelvic anatomy, and shock.

In the presence of massive bleeding when the uterus has not been removed (as may occur in certain obstetric operations) it is important to separately identify and ligate each ovarian artery after each hypogastric artery has been ligated because of the important collateral communication of the aorta with the ovarian and uterine arteries. This procedure is easily accomplished by extending the peritoneal incision above the pelvic brim and the bifurcation of the common iliac artery, being careful to remain lateral to the ureter and to avoid traumatizing the ovarian vessels. If there is difficulty in distinguishing the artery from the ovarian vein, ligation of both the ovarian artery and vein within the infundibulopelvic ligament is acceptable. Even though ligating both the arterial and venous circulation to the ovary leads to a high incidence of postoperative cystic enlargement of the ovary, this complication is preferable to the risk of recurrent pelvic bleeding when the ovarian arteries are not ligated. Each ovarian artery should be dissected free from its retroperitoneal position at or above the pelvic brim and free-tied with No. 0 silk suture. Only one ligature is necessary for each. The artery should not be cut, to avoid the need for multiple ligatures and the risk of retraction and retroperitoneal bleeding of the vessel. A single hemoclip also can be placed on each ovarian artery as a quicker and easier method of occlusion. Care must be taken to avoid injury to the ovarian vein when the artery is being freed for ligation. If injury occurs, control of bleeding may be troublesome. The left ovarian vein can be particularly troublesome; if it should retract beneath the peritoneum, its drainage into the left renal vein makes it difficult to trace.

Rather than ligating the ovarian artery in the infundibulopelvic ligament, Cruikshank and Stoelk have described a technique of ligating this artery at the point of its anastomosis with the uterine artery in the medial mesosalpinx. This point of ligation allows maintenance of the blood flow to the tube and ovary but occludes the ovarian artery blood flow to the uterus.

In cases of life-threatening uterine hemorrhage Fehrman prefers bilateral ligation of the uterine arteries as primary treatment. When this method was used in 66 patients with post–cesarean delivery hemorrhage, emergency hysterectomy to achieve final hemostasis was necessary in 6 patients. If bilateral uterine ligation is not effective in controlling the uterine bleeding, the author recommends supplementary ligation of the round ligaments and the ovarian ligaments at their junction with the uterine corpus. He also believes that bilateral uterine artery ligation is more effective treatment for life-threatening uterine hemorrhage than bilateral hypogastric artery ligation.

Intra-arterial balloon tamponade, a technique described by Fogarty and coworkers in 1963, could be useful in pelvic surgery for temporary control of bleeding while more definitive hemostatic procedures are carried out.

The vaginal artery may originate as a separate branch from the hypogastric artery. Uncontrollable bleeding from the vagina will not be stopped by hysterectomy or by ligation of the uterine arteries. Hypogastric artery ligation is required.

Amazingly, there are many reports of full-term deliveries after bilateral hypogastric artery ligation with and without bilateral ovarian artery ligation. This is ample testimony to the abundant collateral blood supply to the uterus that can develop over time. According to Burchell, the blood flow to the pelvis is reduced by as much as 50% and yet there remains an adequate reserve to nourish a term pregnancy. Ischemic necrosis of pelvic tissues never occurs unless additional collateral pathways are destroyed.

The collateral circulation of the female pelvis is extensive, and provides a variety of intercommunicating sources of arterial blood from various sites along the arterial tree. These collateral vessels anastomose with the hypogastric artery and the blood supply to the uterus through a number of circuitous arterial pathways in the pelvis. During a difficult hysterectomy the collateral circulation may create problems in achieving adequate hemostasis. Therefore, it is important to have a clear understanding of the various extrapelvic arteries that communicate with the pelvic circulation.

The collateral circulation of the pelvis may be divided into three main arterial groups: (1) those vessels that communicate with branches from the aorta, (2) those that communicate with branches from the external iliac artery, and (3) those that communicate with branches from the femoral artery (Fig. 8-8).

Intra-arterial Embolization

Although hypogastric artery ligation is an effective and direct method of controlling postoperative hemorrhage in the female pelvis, some patients are poor surgical risks for additional major surgery while in the hypotensive state. In particular, patients with cardiopulmonary compromise or debilitating disease or patients who are of an advanced age may develop more serious complications if another major surgery should be undertaken when they are in a precarious hemodynamic state. Transcatheter arterial embolization by angiography has been added to the various methods of controlling pelvic hemorrhage. In 1969 Nusbaum and coworkers described this method to control bleeding from esophageal varices by selectively cannulating the superior mesenteric artery and infusing small doses of vasopressin into terminal vessels. The subsequent use of particulate matter to achieve hemostasis within bleeding viscera developed rapidly. Its use in the control of pelvic and postoperative bleeding was popularized by Athanasoulis and associates. Numerous embolic materials have been used, one of the more effective being Gelfoam pledgets of various sizes mixed with a small amount of saline solution to facilitate injection through an arterial catheter. Although many other compounds are used for transcatheter embolization, including autologous clot, subcutaneous tissue, small Silastic spheres, and metal coils, Gelfoam is one of the most practical and easily injected materials. It is sterile, nonantigenic, remains in the vessels for 20 to 50 days, and forms a fibrin mesh framework on which blood clot may develop. Its immediate effect is to obstruct the distal artery or arteriole and reduce the pulse pressure in the bleeding vessel, thereby permitting clot formation and cessation of bleeding. Although initially developed for use in the gastrointestinal tract, this method has wide application for the control of bleeding in many areas of the body, including the central nervous system, kidney, head, and neck, as well as the control of hemorrhage from genitourinary organs. One of its earliest uses in the field of gynecology was for the control of massive vaginal hemorrhage in patients with advanced carcinoma of the cervix.

The method of intravascular injection is quite simple, although it requires the expertise of a person skilled in angiography. Percutaneous catheterization of the femoral artery under local anesthesia provides direct access in a retrograde manner to the hypogastric artery. If prior hypogastric artery ligation has obstructed this pathway, arteriography of the pelvic vasculature through one of the collateral arteries usually localizes the specific bleeding vessel. When the site of the bleeding is identified by angiography, either the hypogastric artery or the specific collateral vessel is cannulated and small pieces of Gelfoam, small metal coils, or other hemostatic materials are injected into the peripheral vessel under direct angiographic observation. When it becomes evident by repeat angiography that the vessel has been occluded, the catheter is removed and the patient is carefully monitored for evidence of further bleeding. This technique is quick, safe, and effective, and may remove the need for additional surgery. No procedure, however, is without risk of complication, and this angiographic procedure is no exception. Pelvic pain and fever can occur as a result of localized ischemia and secondary cellulitis, but these symptoms and signs usually are transient. Cases of bladder ischemia and vesicovaginal fistula have been reported after vascular embolization, usually after occlusion of the hypogastric artery in patients who also have received prior megavoltage pelvic irradiation.

Selective angiographic arterial embolization has been used to control postoperative hemorrhage after abdominal and vaginal hysterectomy and other gynecologic operations, hemorrhage from cervical cancer and gestational trophoblastic disease, postpartum hemorrhage, hemorrhage from abdominal pregnancy, and retroperitoneal hemorrhage. In 1989 O'Hanlan and associates reported the results of embolotherapy in six patients whose postoperative hemorrhage was associated with pelvic surgery. The arterial embolization achieved hemostasis in three patients. The remaining three patients required reoperation for final hemostasis. The authors point out that in each of the cases that required reoperation, the information obtained by arteriography directed the surgeon immediately to the site of bleeding, thus expeditiously facilitating the control of bleeding. Posttreatment fever with positive blood cultures in two patients suggested the advisability of prophylactic antibiotics.

Life-threatening pelvic hemorrhage from multiple sites and uncontrollable by standard means may be promptly controlled by direct intraoperative embolization of the hypogastric artery on one side, or on both sides if the bleeding is bilateral, as reported by Saveracker and associates.

Antishock Trousers

The principle of external counterpressure was originally described by Crile in 1903. He used an inflatable rubber suit to counter the postural hypotension that developed in patients who were operated on in the semirecumbent or sitting position. The idea was picked up in World War II and used to combat the centrifugal forces experienced by fighter pilots during aerial maneuvers. It was subsequently used in the Korean War to (text continues on page 182)

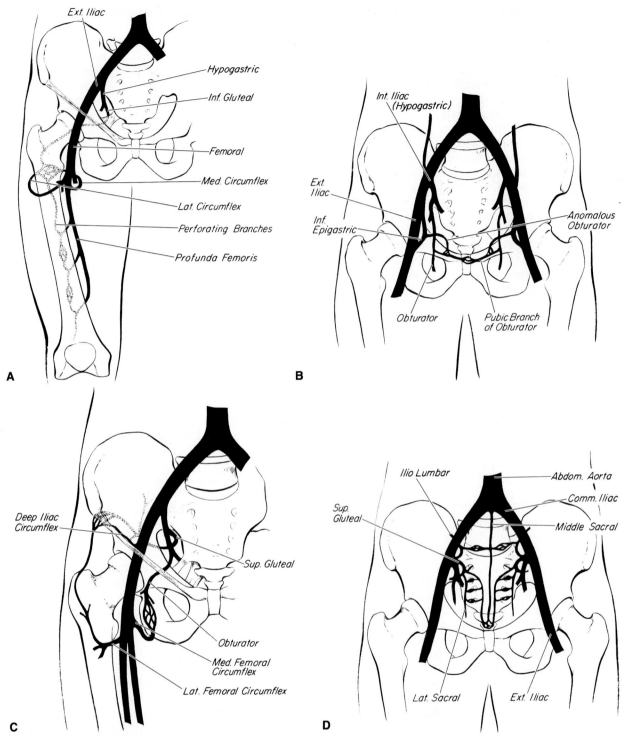

Figure 8–8. *A,* Anastomoses of deep medial and lateral femoral circumflex arteries around hip joint to posterior division (inferior gluteal) of hypogastric artery. *B,* Anastomosis of external iliac and hypogastric arteries through obturator originating anomalously from inferior epigastric artery. *C,* Collateral arterial circulation between external iliac and hypogastric arteries through anastomoses with iliolumbar and superior gluteal arteries. Note anastomoses from medial and lateral femoral circumflex vessels with obturator and superior gluteal branches of hypogastric artery. *D,* Anastomosis of middle sacral artery from aorta with hypogastric branches, including lateral sacral and iliolumbar arteries. (*Figure continues.*)

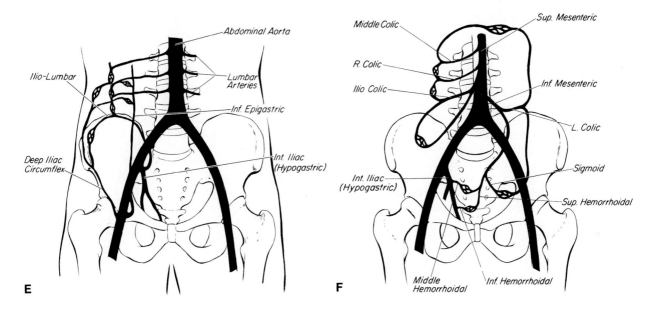

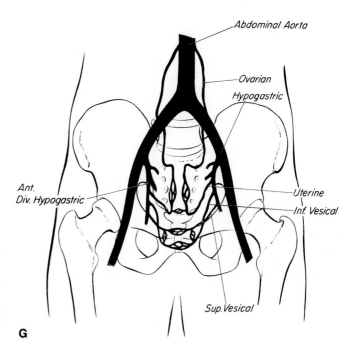

Figure 8–8. (*continued*) *E,* Collateral circulation of aorta and hypogastric arteries through lumbar and iliolumbar anastomoses. *F,* Collateral circulation of inferior mesenteric artery to branches of hypogastric artery, from superior hemorrhoidal to middle and inferior hemorrhoidal arteries. *G,* Arterial arcade and anastomosis between ovarian and uterine arteries.

transport casualties from the battlefield to the hospital. According to Gardner, its usefulness in patients with intra-abdominal bleeding was discovered serendipitously.

External counterpressure by means of an inflatable garment wrapped around the legs and abdomen (sometimes called the MAST suit or G suit, or pneumatic antishock garment) has been used for the temporary control of acute, profuse intra-abdominal hemorrhage while the patient is being prepared for surgery. In some cases the bleeding can be controlled and surgery can be avoided. This technique has been used in more than 175 cases of surgically uncontrollable hemorrhage, as reported in the literature, with temporary or complete control of the hemorrhage. Its use has been described by Pelligra and Sandberg, by Pearse and associates, and by others.

The suit is made of polyvinyl, wraps around the patient, and secures with Velcro fasteners. It contains an abdominal pneumatic bladder that extends from the xiphoid to the pubis, and has two separate leg bladders. It is inflated to a pressure between 25 mm Hg and 40 mm Hg (some clinics have used pressures of 100 mm Hg or higher). When applied for periods of from 2 to 48 hours results usually have been satisfactory in increasing intra-abdominal pressure to a level that controls the source of arterial or venous bleeding. We have found this technique to be most effective in cases where all previous surgical attempts to identify and control the source of intra-abdominal bleeding after pelvic surgery were unsuccessful. We also have used it for the patient in profound shock from intra-abdominal hemorrhage, such as that caused by a ruptured tubal pregnancy, while the blood volume is being rapidly replaced before surgery. It has been used to control the intra-abdominal hemorrhage caused by multiple sites of placental separation in patients with abdominal pregnancy.

There are definite disadvantages and dangers to the use of external counterpressure by means of an inflatable garment. Absolute contraindications to the use of the garment include pulmonary edema, known rupture of the diaphragm, and left ventricular dysfunction. Abdominal examination is not possible unless the garment is removed. Likewise, pelvic examination is impossible. If pressures are not carefully monitored, circulation to the lower extremities can be impaired sufficient to cause progressive muscle necrosis, crush syndrome, and death. Pressures of more than 40 mm Hg should be applied only in extreme circumstances and then for only brief periods. All inflatable garments should be equipped with pressure-monitoring devices. A study by Bicknell and associates has cast some doubt on the usefulness of inflatable garments for trauma patients. In an urban setting rapid transport and other resuscitation measures appear to be effective without wasting precious minutes to fit the patient into an inflatable garment.

Logothetopulos Pack

Some surgeons, such as Parente and associates, have found the Logothetopulos pack to be of assistance in compressing the retracted, bleeding vessels in the pelvis. This technique includes the formation of a large pack of loose gauze within an outstretched, opened piece of gauze or plastic sheet. This can be used in an umbrella manner within the pelvic cavity by tying the four corners of the opened gauze together, creating a ball or bag, and placing traction on the free end of the pack when it is pulled through the vaginal vault. This approach attempts to compress the bleeding vessels against the pelvic floor by the downward traction and pressure exerted with the pack. It may be used at the time of either abdominal or vaginal surgery for compression of bleeding vessels that cannot be controlled by other means. The pack can be left in place with perineal traction for 24 to 48 hours until the bleeding has ceased. It is removed vaginally by first withdrawing the internal gauze and then the outside bag (Fig. 8-9).

Absorbable Hemostatic Agents

The use of microfibrillar collagen for the local control of intraoperative bleeding was mentioned previously. This bovine collagen material can be applied directly and compressed against an area of a small bleeding vessel. It acts as a fibrin nidus to accelerate thrombus formation on the surface of the vessel. It will not control bleeding from a small arteriole or venule. Caution must be exercised in the use of this material because it may produce secondary fibrosis in the pelvis and even a persistent palpable mass. There have been reports of retroperitoneal fibrosis and ureteral obstruction secondary to the use of this material. These sequelae have cautioned the pelvic surgeon against applying this agent near the ureter. When used in other sites we have found fewer adverse reactions. If a localized hemostatic agent is considered necessary, the use of Gelfoam or topical thrombin may prove to be more efficacious with less fibrosis. More important, the surgeon should not rely on any agent for control of a significant amount of arterial or venous bleeding. Instead, every effort should be made to identify the bleeding vessel and to occlude it with either a hemoclip or a ligature.

In one case of severe bleeding from deep pelvic veins we were successful in finally controlling the bleeding

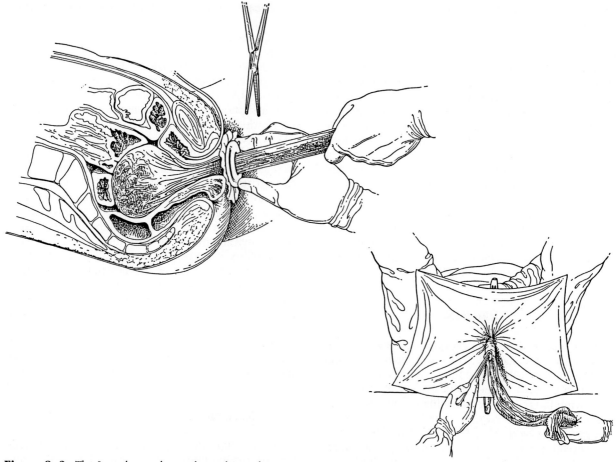

Figure 8–9. The Logothetopulos pack used in pelvic surgery.

with multiple layers ("sandwiches") of Gelfoam and Avitene cut to appropriate size from sheets and stacked one on top of the other. If coagulation factors have been depleted with multiple transfusions, the Gelfoam should be soaked in thrombin. As the material is applied, the field should be as dry as possible. Some constant pressure may be applied by placement of sutures that can be tied over top of the sandwiches.

Malviya and Deppe have reported the successful use of fibrin glue, a biodegradable tissue adhesive and sealant and topical hemostatic agent, to control life-threatening hemorrhage in one obstetric and two gynecologic patients. The fibrin glue is prepared from equal amounts of cryoprecipitate (highly concentrated human fibrinogen) and bovine thrombin. It imitates the last stages of physiologic coagulation at the local site. Equal volumes are drawn into separate syringes and applied directly to the bleeding site in a field as dry as possible. A firm rubbery clot is formed in 2 minutes.

This technique has been used successfully in microvascular, cardiovascular, and thoracic surgical procedures, and has recently been effective in controlling hemorrhage in liver transplantation. It should be helpful in extensive pelvic dissections for gynecologic cancer, especially to control low-pressure pelvic vein bleeding that is not controllable by other standard measures.

Aortic Compressor

An instrument such as the one described by Conn and associates to temporarily compress and stop circulation through the aorta to the pelvis may be useful in special cases to control pelvic hemorrhage. It is used by vascular surgeons in operations for aortic aneurysms and by trauma surgeons to control traumatic hemorrhage from the aorta or large pelvic vessels. When massive arterial bleeding in the pelvis is difficult to control, temporarily occluding the aorta by compressing it against the lumbar vertebrae may be helpful. It is less effective in hemorrhage from pelvic veins. Indeed, because the vena cava also is compressed, pelvic veins temporarily may become distended. The aortic compressor may be helpful when excessive blood loss from extensive myomectomy is anticipated, especially if a tourniquet cannot be fitted around the lower uterus. It also is useful in removing large pelvic tumors whose blood supply is difficult to isolate or control. It is a temporary expedient to control an urgent problem. The operator can simply compress the aorta with his or her hand until the aortic compressor arrives.

When the aorta is occluded for more than a few minutes, clots may form in vessels at distal sites. This may be avoided by injecting heparin distal to the point of occlusion and by releasing the compressor periodically to allow the blood to flow.

SHOCK

Shock may be defined in various ways, but in practical terms it is the state of inadequate tissue perfusion characterized by cardiac output inadequate to provide normal circulation in the major organs. Whether the underlying factor is myocardial failure, obstruction of arterial pathways (pulmonary embolus or coronary occlusion), increased peripheral capillary resistance, widespread peripheral vascular pooling, or direct blood loss, the end result is the same: insufficient circulating blood volume to ensure adequate tissue perfusion. Historically, Blalock, at the Johns Hopkins Hospital, was one of the earlier investigators to propose a classification of shock according to various causative mechanisms, and the general categories in use today are similar to those proposed by him. They include hemorrhagic shock, septic shock, neurogenic shock, cardiogenic shock, and various combinations of these.

Although each type of shock is related to a particular pathophysiologic pattern, in practice a combination of these interrelated factors usually is involved in the more serious forms of circulatory collapse. Sepsis, with its adverse effect on cellular metabolism, is a frequent complication in patients with acute blood loss. Irrespective of whether shock is initiated by a single factor or a combination of factors, the end stage of shock is the same: a decreased cardiac output, diminished circulating blood volume with progressive hemoconcentration, alterations in cell metabolism, hypoxia and acidosis, peripheral capillary dilatation, and, finally, failure of return of blood to the heart, resulting in cardiac standstill.

Pathophysiology of Hemorrhagic Shock

The basic pathophysiologic problem in all types of shock is tissue hypoxia, which produces cellular metabolic disarrangements that revolve around anaerobic glucose metabolism. This anaerobic process produces increased blood levels of lactic acid, amino acids, fatty acids, and phosphoric acids, which lower the blood pH and produce systemic acidosis.

Decreased oxygen delivery to tissues results in the decline in aerobic glycolysis by cells and a consequent decrease in the production of adenosine triphosphate (ATP), which governs the exchange of extracellular sodium and intracellular potassium and limits the production of proteins and enzymes. A decrease in ATP synthesis causes a loss of the sodium pump mechanism and permits an influx of sodium and water into the cell and an efflux of potassium from the cell. The net metabolic effect of these changes is an increased serum level of blood pyruvate and lactate, an increase in serum potassium (hyperkalemia), an intracellular shift of sodium and water with a depletion of serum sodium, and gradual hemoconcentration—all changes that are characteristic of metabolic acidosis. The ionic changes caused by the loss of the sodium pump mechanism causes hypopolarization of the cell membrane, opening voltage-sensitive calcium channels. This results in an influx of extracellular calcium, causing an increase in cellular metabolism and a further depletion of cellular ATP stores. The opening of the calcium channels also allows an efflux of intracellular magnesium. Because the ATP–magnesium complex is the biologically active form of ATP in the cell, the loss of magnesium hinders the utilization of the remaining intracellular ATP. The continued increase of intracellular calcium concentration results in the swelling of mitochondrial cristae and a disruption of the Krebs cycle with an uncoupling of oxidative phosphorylation. At this point, on the cellular level, the effects of shock become irreversible. Concomitantly, there is intracellular release of lysosomal enzymes, which causes both lysis of the cell membrane and degradation of proteins, carbohydrate, and fat. Together these peptide fragments, cellular debris, and lysosomal enzymes pass into the circulation and may produce adverse effects in more distant parts of the body.

The effects of tissue hypoxia on the cellular level are reflected systemically by altered organ functions. In the gastrointestinal tract, ischemia has the most marked effect on the mucosal layer. The integrity of the mucosal barrier is lost, and the circulatory system is invaded by intestinal bacteria and their toxins. Mucosal damage is most marked in the stomach, where superficial erosions and petechial bleeding may contribute to further blood loss. Decreased oxygen delivery to the liver results in failure of the hepatic reticuloendothelial system, which allows bacteria absorbed from the gastrointestinal tract to gain access to the circulation. The bacterial toxins adversely affect cell function and vascular tone and activate the coagulation and complement cascades. Pancreatic lysosomes seem particularly susceptible to hypoxic damage, and their disruption also may impair reticuloendothelial function. Decreased kidney perfusion may result in acute renal failure owing to tubular necrosis. The lung often responds to prolonged uncorrected hypovolemia with the development of the adult respiratory distress syndrome, which is discussed in more detail later in this chapter. Myocardial function may be impaired by lactic acidosis and by circulating myocardial depressants such as kinins and myocardial depressant factor, which is released from the pancreas. Myocardial oxygenation may be compromised by progressive tachycardia, rising ventricular end-diastolic pressure, and falling arterial systolic pressure.

To prevent the effects of shock from becoming irreversible, it is essential that the patient be maintained in appropriate hemodynamic balance. This balance depends on three interrelated factors: (1) an adequate cardiac output—an effective pump; (2) a reasonably normal blood volume—an effective circulatory fluid; and (3) a normal vascular tone. Alterations in any one of these basic hemodynamic prerequisites will produce compensatory changes in the remaining two. Early compensatory changes in acute blood loss include tachycardia and an increase in peripheral vascular resistance owing to elevated levels of circulating catecholamines triggered by peripheral chemoreceptors. The result of these compensatory mechanisms is an adequate circulation to provide tissue oxygenation with the maintenance of a normal systolic blood pressure. These early autonomic changes temporarily mask the symptoms and clinical signs of an altered circulating blood volume. The pulse pressure (the difference between the systolic blood pressure and diastolic blood pressure), however, is narrowed because of an increase in the diastolic blood pressure, which results from the increased vascular tone. This narrowed pulse pressure is one of the early changes in hypovolemic shock, and differentiates it from septic shock, which is characterized by vasodilation from the bacterial endotoxin surge, resulting in a widened pulse pressure. When blood volume loss reaches 30% or more these adaptive changes fail to support a normal cardiac output and an adequate peripheral circulation, resulting in a fall in systemic blood pressure. As the hypovolemia progresses, the cell becomes anoxic, sodium and water enter the cell, and potassium and lactate are forced into the serum. The clinical effect of this metabolic shift is the accumulation of an increasing amount of lactate in the serum, reflected by progressive acidosis.

The barometer of hemorrhagic shock is at the capillary level, where increased peripheral vascular constriction, caused by the release of sympathomimetic amines, produces arteriovenous shunting and accelerates the process of cellular anoxia, anaerobic metabolism, and lactic acidosis. As calcium enters the cell, magnesium leaves the cell, mitochondria swell, lysosomes rupture and the cell is destroyed. The anoxic process becomes irreversible. This cycle is complicated by the fact that the arterial precapillary sphincter mechanism is apparently more sensitive to a low pH than the distal venous sphincter. As acidosis advances and the precapillary sphincter decompensates, the venous sphincter maintains its tone and an increase in capillary pooling is produced. Consequently blood is pooled in the peripheral capillary bed, which is estimated to be capable of accommodating a blood volume 500 times greater than normal. The subsequent effect is further reduction of the circulating volume, increased tissue hypoxia, and decreased clearance of metabolites. Once this stage is reached, no therapy can be effective.

Clinically, hemorrhagic shock may be divided into three phases: early, intermediate, and late or irreversible. A dramatic example of early hemorrhagic shock is seen in the gradual intraperitoneal accumulation of blood from a ruptured ectopic pregnancy. Such cases clearly demonstrate the early stage of shock by a temporary decrease in cardiac output and arterial blood pressure. This is followed by compensatory changes of the sympathetic nervous system and decreased vagal nerve activity. In effect, these adaptive measures tend to temporarily increase the heart rate and restore cardiac output and arterial pressure. These changes are augmented by an increase in peripheral arterial resistance and an inotropic effect on the cardiac muscle, producing more forceful myocardial contractions. At this stage the patient with an ectopic pregnancy experiences increasing symptoms of abdominal and pelvic pain, but the magnitude of the intraperitoneal blood loss may be masked by these adaptive hemodynamic responses. If the patient is seen at this time, her blood pressure will be relatively normal when she is in the supine position, owing to the compensatory mechanisms of early shock. This process can be unmasked by having the patient sit or stand, which will demonstrate orthostatic hypotension. The pulse rate will be rapid, and the patient will be hypovolemic from intraperitoneal hemorrhage. This form of early, "warm" shock is reversible, and is not associated with prolonged cellular acidosis. If it is not promptly treated, the hemodynamic compensatory changes may fail. When patients are delayed in obtaining prompt medical care, the blood loss may progress to a more critical and frequently irreversible phase.

There are several physiologic defense mechanisms aimed at maintaining adequate plasma volume in the face of hemorrhage. Plasma refill is an important early compensatory mechanism in hemorrhagic shock. It was previously thought that the fastest rate at which humans could refill plasma volume by the intravascular absorption of interstitial water was 90 mL/h. Recent studies have demonstrated that interstitial fluid can re-enter the vascular space to compensate for severe hypovolemia at about 10 times this rate, or about 900 mL/h. Hemorrhagic shock, then, is a phenomenon that is related to intravascular volume, the rate of blood loss, and the rate of plasma refill. Over a long period one can slowly lose an enormous amount of blood without clinical evidence of hypotension or shock. On the other hand, a rapid loss of a small amount of blood can result in clinical shock. One of the major differences between these two hemodynamic conditions is related to plasma refill. The continuous refill of the intravascular compartment by interstitial fluid will prevent shock in cases of insidious and slow blood loss. This physiologic mechanism will not compensate for rapid blood loss, even though the total amount lost is smaller.

Another important adaptive mechanism is provided through the kidneys. A decrease in renal blood flow is immediately sensed by the juxtaglomerular apparatus of the afferent renal arterioles, leading to the release of renin into the plasma and the subsequent conversion of renin to an inactive polypeptide, angiotensin I, which is metabolized in the liver to angiotensin II, a potent arteriolar constrictor. Angiotensin II also induces the secretion of catecholamines from the adrenal medulla and aldosterone from the adrenal cortex. The release of aldosterone as well as of antidiuretic hormone from the pituitary promotes the conservation of water and sodium by the kidneys. High doses of antidiuretic hormone also increase splanchnic vasoconstriction induced by the sympathetic stimulation, circulating catecholamines, and angiotensin. Hemorrhage also induces the release of adrenocorticotropic hormone, causing a rise in plasma cortisol, which may be necessary for a normal hemostatic response to hemorrhage. Increased levels of circulating catecholamines also stimulate glucagon secretions, which stimulate hepatic gluconeogenesis, resulting in hyperglycemia. An adequate level of glucose is essential, as it serves as an energy substrate critical for maintenance of homeostasis. Declining plasma glucose levels have been associated with poor outcomes. When the limits of these physiologic adaptations have been exceeded, the patient will enter a phase of hypovolemia, impairment of venous return, and cardiac output inadequate to sustain normal tissue perfusion.

The intermediate stage of shock is the pivotal stage in terms of reversibility (Fig. 8-10), since compensatory mechanisms alone are no longer effective in maintaining adequate circulation. During the intermediate phase cardiac output may be decreased more than can be counterbalanced by the reflex inotropic mechanisms and, as a consequence, many vital organs will have inadequate circulation. There is a preferential distribution of blood to the heart and brain from less vital organs. Prolonged impairment of oxygen supply to the kidneys will produce progressive renal shutdown and will accelerate the metabolic acidosis by changes in cellular function of the distal renal tubules. Peripheral ischemia, associated with sympathetic stimulation of the sweat glands, produces cold, clammy extremities and the early signs of advanced, or "cold," shock. If the intermediate phase of shock goes untreated, it will progress to the terminal phase. Diminished cardiac output and impaired cerebral perfusion are manifested by progressive mental confusion and later by coma.

The final, irreversible phase of hemorrhagic shock produces the clinical picture of progressive cerebral and cardiovascular ischemia (Fig. 8-11), owing to intense peripheral vasoconstriction. The patient becomes unresponsive to external stimuli, appears ashen-gray, and is anuric. Cardiac arrhythmia develops, and the patient finally expires in cardiac arrest. Most heroic attempts to reverse this stage of the metabolic process are unsuccessful because the myocardium and central nervous system have undergone cellular death and are unable to respond to any kind of stimulation or aggressive therapy.

Treatment

Each patient must have an accurate hemodynamic evaluation before beginning any type of treatment. The basic goals of all types of treatment are similar: (a) to improve the effective circulating blood volume and (b) to improve cellular perfusion and oxygenation. The major effect of this therapy is to increase the effective blood flow to organs and tissues, regardless of the causative factors. The control of hemorrhage, or the prevention of further hemorrhage, frequently prompts surgical intervention. The general objectives in the treatment of shock are outlined in Table 8-9.

Oxygenation

Tissue hypoxia is the essential problem in the shock patient. Hypoxia may result from inadequate ventilation, intrapulmonary shunting, low hematocrit, circulatory insufficiency, or a combination of these factors. All

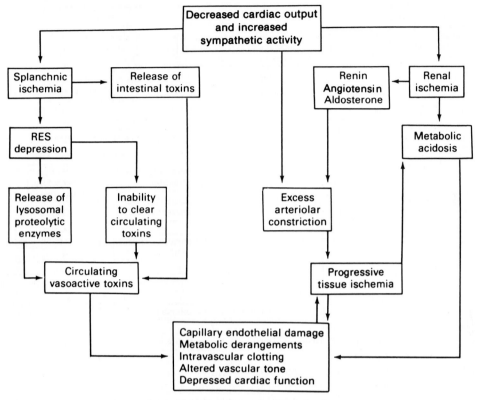

Figure 8–10. Pathophysiologic changes in intermediate shock.

patients in shock should receive supplemental oxygen. If the airway is clear and the respiratory rate and tidal volume are adequate, 100% oxygen should be administered by a closed mask or a nasal cannula at the rate of 12 L/min. If there is any doubt about the ability of the patient to maintain adequate, spontaneous ventilation or protect her airway, endotracheal intubation should be performed and mechanical ventilation initiated. Re-

spiratory failure is a common cause of death in patients in acute shock.

Fluid Replacement

Restoration of the circulating volume is a fundamental concern in the patient with hemorrhagic shock. As an initial step, the patient's legs should be elevated

TABLE 8–9
General Objectives in Treating Shock

INDICATION	OBJECTIVE
Systolic blood pressure	$\geq$90 mm Hg
Urine output	>40 ml/hr
Central venous pressure	12–15 cm H_2O
Pulmonary capillary wedge pressure	12–15 mm Hg
Skin	Warm, no cyanosis
Sensorium	Oriented
Blood gases	
Pao_2	80–100 mm Hg
$Paco_2$	30–35 mm Hg
pH	7.35–7.50
Hemoglobin	12–14 g%

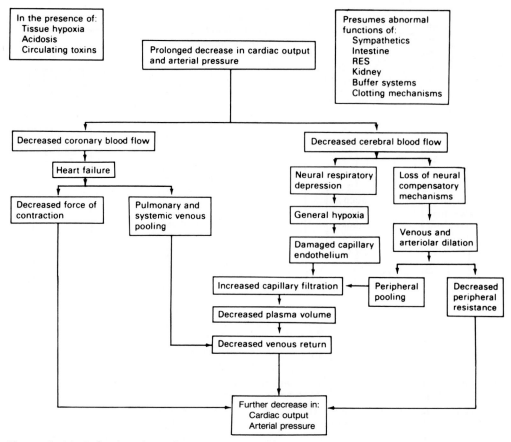

Figure 8–11. Pathophysiologic changes in irreversible shock.

about 30 degrees to facilitate venous return. The Trendelenburg position has the potential to compromise both respiration and cerebral blood flow, and its use should be discouraged.

An organized approach to fluid replacement in the patient in hemorrhagic shock may be facilitated by an understanding of the physiologic and clinical manifestations that accompany the percentage of acute blood volume loss. A class I hemorrhage includes an acute blood loss up to 15%, which results in a mild resting tachycardia with normal blood pressure, pulse pressure, respiratory rate, skin color, and temperature. A class II hemorrhage represents a 15% to 30% blood volume loss. These patients may appear slightly anxious with more pronounced tachycardia and tachypnea and a narrowed pulse pressure. The systolic pressure usually is maintained. A capillary refill test may be positive (> 2 seconds). Urine output usually is only mildly affected. The majority of these patients eventually may require blood transfusion, but initially can be stabilized

with crystalloids. A class III hemorrhage represents 30% to 40% of blood volume loss. These patients are confused and markedly anxious with classic signs of inadequate tissue perfusion, including marked tachycardia, tachypnea, and a measurable fall in systolic pressure. They usually have a measurable fall in urine output, and the capillary refill test is always positive. These patients almost always require transfusion; however, this decision is based on the patient's response to the initial crystalloid infusion as described later. Class IV hemorrhage involves greater than 40% of blood volume loss and is immediately life-threatening. These patients usually have a markedly depressed mental status. The skin is cold and pale. There is a significant depression in systolic blood pressure with a very narrow pulse pressure or unobtainable diastolic pressure. Tachycardia is marked. Anuria usually is present. Loss of more than 50% of the patient's blood volume results in loss of consciousness, pulse, and blood pressure (Fig. 8-12).

Increased pulse rate
Increased respiratory rate
Peripheral venous constriction (progressive)
Decreased pulse pressure
Poor capillary filling
Thirst
Hypotension
Agitation
Oliguria
Peripheral cooling
Pallor
Trunk cooling
Anuria
Diminished pain sensation
Loss of deep reflexes
Acidotic breathing
Deep pallor
Loss of consciousness
DEATH

Figure 8–12. Clinical signs of progressive hypovolemia.

Loss of less than 15% of the blood volume usually can be managed with volume replacement with crystalloid alone; this may be amended, based on clinical symptoms. Losses of more than 15% of blood volume may require transfusion, depending on the initial patient response to crystalloid infusion. The initial management for fluid resuscitation in patients in hemorrhagic shock consists of placing two large-bore intravenous catheters, usually 14 or 16 gauge, in peripheral veins. These may be hard to place in a patient in shock, and a surgical cutdown of a peripheral vein may be necessary. The placement of a central venous catheter also is an option; however, a complication such as a pneumothorax may prove fatal in an already compromised patient and peripheral access should be established when possible. At the time of insertion of the intravenous line, blood should be drawn for type and crossmatching and complete blood count with platelet count, coagulation profile, and complete biochemical profile. The establishment of adequate vascular volume is more important than the specific type of fluid administered, although whole blood has no equal in the treatment of hemorrhagic shock.

Isotonic electrolyte solutions are used for initial fluid resuscitation. This type of fluid provides transient intravascular expansion and further stabilizes the vascular volume by replacing accompanying fluid losses. Ringer's lactate solution is the initial fluid of choice, with normal saline solution being the second choice. Although normal saline is satisfactory, it has the potential to cause hypochloremic acidosis, especially if renal function is impaired. The usual initial dose is 1 to 2 L for an adult (or 10 to 25 mL/kg of body weight) with further therapy depending on the response. Patients usually fall into three groups based on the initial fluid therapy. The first group of patients respond rapidly to the initial fluid bolus and remain stable when the initial fluid bolus has been completed and their fluids are slowed. Such patients usually will have lost less than 20% of their blood volume. No further fluid boluses or immediate blood administration is indicated for this small group of patients.

The second group of patients, which is the largest group, are transient responders. These patients respond to the initial fluid bolus; however, as these fluids are slowed, their circulatory perfusion indices begin to show deterioration. Most of these patients will have lost 20% to 40% of their blood volume and still may be bleeding. Continued fluid administration and initiation of blood are indicated. These patients may require type-specific blood rather than fully crossmatched blood, depending on their hemodynamic status.

The third group of patients demonstrate no response to the initial fluid administration. Most require immediate blood transfusion and surgical intervention to control exsanguinating hemorrhage. On rare occasions the failure to respond to the fluid challenge may be due to cardiac failure. Central venous pressure monitoring may help to differentiate between these two groups of patients. As a rule of thumb, at least three times as much crystalloid solution is required to replace a specific amount of blood loss.

Instead of crystalloids, some physicians prefer fluid repletion with intravascular colloids, including the use of plasma, albumin, and hypertonic solutions such as high or low molecular weight dextran and polyethyl starches. These molecules are large enough to stay within the vascular tree and do not easily permeate the capillary wall, resulting in an oncotic plasma expansion. There is little in the literature to establish the superiority of crystalloids or colloids in the management of hypovolemia. The ready availability of crystalloid solutions, their ease of storage, and their low cost are arguments in favor of their use. Some reports claim an increased survival with the administration of colloid solution, but this has not been clearly established. Plasma and albumin are associated with hepatitis risks. Low molecular weight dextran is rapidly eliminated from the circulation and offers little advantage over simple crystalloid solutions. High molecular weight dextran has been associated with thromboplastin-like properties and may interfere with platelet function, resulting in further bleeding from disseminated intravascular coagulation. Also, it may cause an anaphylactic reaction. Caution should be used to avoid replacing more than 20% of the total blood volume with colloids.

Hypertonic saline solutions have been used in animal studies for the treatment of controlled hemorrhagic shock and initially showed beneficial effects, resulting in increased systemic blood pressure, cardiac output, and peripheral blood flow. When hypertonic saline was used in cases of uncontrolled hemorrhage it was found to significantly increase blood loss and early mortality. In addition, the use of hypertonic saline has been associated with the occurrence of an acute hyperosmolality state, which is associated with a high mortality and neurologic damage, that may be partially explained by the adverse effect of the hyperosmolar load on cerebral hemodynamics. Thus the use of hypertonic saline has no clinical role in the treatment of hypovolemic shock.

Blood is ideal substance for volume resuscitation in the patient with hemorrhagic shock. Its use, however, is associated with certain risks, including the minimal risk of transfusion reaction and the transmission of infectious diseases such as the hepatitis virus and the human immunodeficiency virus. The use of blood and blood component therapy is described in detail elsewhere in this chapter. Because of the problems associated with blood transfusion as well as the scarcity of blood products, many attempts have been made to find a blood substitute. The use of fluorocarbon solutions, specifically Fluosol DA, has recently met with some success. This compound carries oxygen in a simple solution, with 40 cc of oxygen/100 mL at an oxygen pressure of 100 torr in vitro. The half life is 24 hours. The use of these solutions, however, has been associated with pulmonary, hepatic, respiratory, reticuloendothelial system, and renal toxicity, and there is little clinical data available to judge the efficacy of these compounds.

For many years there has been interest in the development of hemoglobin solutions as volume-expanding, oxygen-carrying resuscitation fluids. The development of a pyridoxalated, polymerized, stroma-free human hemoglobin has shown some promise in animal models. Stroma-free hemoglobin is not associated with the transmission of hepatitis or with transfusion reactions. It has the ability to function as an oxygen carrier with an oxygen hemoglobin dissociation curve that is the same as for red blood cells. In addition, the solution is oncotically active and acts as a plasma expander. Unfortunately it has a very short plasma half life, as it is rapidly excreted in the urine. It also has been found to elicit an immune response when injected into animals in hemorrhagic shock. The clinical significance of this finding is unknown.

Careful monitoring of the response to volume replacement in patients with hemorrhagic shock is essential both to ensure that adequate volume is given and to avoid giving too much volume. An important laboratory method of monitoring colloid and crystalloid fluid replacement is through the use of serum osmolality (normal = 290 mOsm/L). Regardless of the type of fluids given—whole blood, albumin, crystalloids, or other colloids—adequate intravascular volume replacement therapy may require several times the normal blood volume in fluid replacement before there is evidence of clinical improvement, since the amount of peripheral pooling is unpredictable. With the infusion of such large amounts of intravenous fluids it is essential that the fluid volume be carefully monitored with frequent assessment of central venous pressure or pulmonary artery occlusive pressure readings, to avoid the complication of cardiac overload and pulmonary edema. This may be especially important in the patient who has had a slow or insidious bleed, and who may have a low hemoglobin but a relatively normal intravascular volume through the reabsorption of interstitial fluid. Nonetheless, until low central venous pressure or pulmonary wedge pressure levels return to normal, aggressive replacement of intravascular volume is the key to improvement in tissue perfusion and the patient's clinical response.

Patient volume status should be monitored by accurate recording of urine output. In general, urine output is an excellent clinical indicator of tissue perfusion. If the kidneys produce at least 30 to 40 mL/h of urine, it is probable that all other organs are adequately perfused. Urine specific gravity is an excellent index of the extent of hydration (normal specific gravity is 1.010–1.015).

Meticulous control of fluid and electrolyte balance is essential in altering peripheral cellular metabolism. Correction of tissue oxygenation is important in the prevention and treatment of potentially fatal hyperkalemia caused by shock. The extracellular release of potassium into the serum is a frequent complication of shock that may develop with alarming rapidity. The clinical signs of hyperkalemia include decreased deep tendon reflexes, muscle weakness, acroparesthesias, and cardiac arrhythmias. The use of the following agents is beneficial in the management of hyperkalemia: calcium gluconate (10 mL of 10% solution given slowly, intravenously); sodium bicarbonate (1 ampule [45 mEq] given slowly, intravenously); or insulin and glucose (30 units of crystalline insulin in 500 mL of 20% dextrose over 30 to 60 minutes, intravenously). These agents either counteract the physiologic effect of extracellular potassium or produce a temporary shift of potassium into the cell and rapidly lower the serum potassium level. This effect also may be achieved by cation exchange, whereby 1 g of polystyrene sulfonate (Kayexalate) removes 1 mEq of serum potassium by exchanging 3 mEq of sodium. This may be given rectally (15 g of Kayexalate and 60 mL of 70% sorbitol in 200 mL of water) as an enema, which should be retained for 30 to 60 minutes; it may be repeated every 6 to 12 hours as needed or given orally (15 g of Kayexalate in 60 mL of 70% sorbitol solution in water every 6 to 12 hours as needed).

Hyperglycemia is a normal physiologic response to shock resulting from catecholamine-induced hepatic gluconeogenesis. During fluid resuscitation it is important to maintain a relative plasma hyperglycemia, as glucose plays a key role as an energy substrate for the heart, brain, and vascular smooth muscle, which are critical to maintain hemostasis. Declining plasma glucose levels have been associated with hemodynamic decompensation.

Vasoactive Drugs

The role of vasoactive drugs in the management of hypovolemic shock is extremely limited. Because the hemodynamic changes after shock have produced a marked increase in peripheral vascular constriction owing to the increased level of circulating catecholamines, the use of potent vasoconstrictive agents may cause further impairment of peripheral tissue perfusion. The effect of this treatment would be further production of tissue anoxia and perpetuation of metabolic acidosis. In patients with profound shock and anuria the use of chronotropic or inotropic drugs to augment cardiac output by increasing heart rate or alternating contractility by stimulation of cardiac beta receptors may play a small role. Dopamine is one of the most widely used agents in the treatment of shock. It stimulates both alpha$_1$ and beta receptors; however, at low doses the beta activity is predominant. This has an inotropic effect on the heart, resulting in increased cardiac output, but without a significant incidence of arrhythmias. Myocardial oxygen consumption is only moderately increased. A particularly important effect of dopamine in the shock patient is the improvement of renal blood flow, glomerular filtration rate, sodium excretion, and urine output. The effects are dose-dependent. Dopamine doses in the range of 2 to 5 μg/kg/min are considered "renal doses," and usually increase renal blood flow and urine output with little effect on cardiac output or systemic vascular resistance. At doses of 5 to 10 μg/kg/min the beneficial effects of renal blood flow and urine output are somewhat maintained, and cardiac output is increased. At doses over 15 μg/kg/min the alpha adrenergic effect dominates, leading to peripheral vasoconstriction and reduced renal blood flow and urine output (Fig. 8-13). Dobutamine, a synthetic catecholamine, acts as an inotropic agent by the stimulation of beta receptors in the myocardium. It can be used in conjunction with renal doses of dopamine for an inotropic effect when indicated.

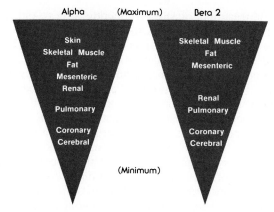

Figure 8–13. Graded receptor response of various organs to α and β-2 adrenergic stimulation.

Pulmonary Complications in Hemorrhagic Shock

The adult respiratory distress syndrome (ARDS) may result as a latent sequela to the hemodynamic changes of shock. The patient may show signs of tachypnea and develop rales throughout the lungs within 24 hours after the restoration of the blood pressure to normal values. The clinical picture of respiratory distress is associated with a Pao$_2$ as low as 40 to 60 mm Hg along with an elevated Paco$_2$. Administration of 100% oxygen may not improve the situation, and may give clinical evidence of pulmonary shunting from areas of the lung that are partially perfused but not ventilated. Endotracheal intubation with controlled mechanical ventilation should be instituted expeditiously when indicated, to compensate for respiratory acidosis that may develop. The respiratory distress appears to be a result of changes in the integrity of the alveolar capillary membrane that produce diffuse pulmonary interstitial edema without cardiomegaly. A characteristic ground-glass appearance of the lung fields with normal cardiac silhouette is visible on chest x-ray films. The apparent loss of alveolar surfactant leads to atelectasis and exaggeration of the right-to-left pulmonary shunt of unoxygenated blood. The physiologic mechanism that is responsible for this pulmonary insult appears to be the initial damage to the alveoli and pulmonary capillaries from the transient or prolonged state of hypotension and hypoxemia. As a result, severe hypoxemia is difficult to correct, despite use of 100% oxygen and mechanical ventilation. The interstitial edema seen with ARDS can be differentiated from cardiogenic pulmonary edema by the presence of a normal pulmonary artery occlusion pressure or central venous pressure with central hemodynamic monitoring.

The treatment of ARDS frequently is more difficult than cardiac and hemodynamic resuscitation in patients with hypovolemic shock. It is essential that meticulous fluid and electrolyte balance be maintained to avoid further insult to the damaged lung. The use of oxygen is obligatory for the hypoxemic state. Many cases require oxygen delivery through an endotracheal tube by a volume-cycled mechanical ventilator. It is important to institute positive end-expiratory pressure (PEEP) to improve the inflation of the pulmonary alveoli and to enhance oxygen exchange. Many patients require high deliveries of inspired oxygen and high positive-pressure ventilation to maintain adequate oxygenation. It is desirable to keep the forced inspiratory oxygen less than 50% to avoid the risk of oxygen toxicity. If a PEEP of 15 cm H_2O or greater is required to maintain adequate oxygenation, a Swan-Ganz catheter should be used to evaluate cardiac output, as increasing levels of PEEP decrease the venous return to the heart and may compromise the cardiac output and decrease the effective circulating volume.

Treatment of Acidosis

The effect of progressive metabolic acidosis due to hypoxemia and anaerobic glycolysis is cytotoxic, with the release of lysosomal enzymes and cell death. Acidosis also increases the tone of both afferent arteriolar and efferent venous sphincters—the efferent more than the afferent vessels—with progression of peripheral pooling and cellular anoxia. The only effective treatment of metabolic acidosis in patients with hemorrhagic shock is the reestablishment of an adequate vascular volume to restore cellular and organ perfusion with adequately oxygenated blood. Thus the goal of therapy is to restore the circulating volume and reverse the anaerobic metabolism with volume resuscitation and not bicarbonate infusion. With a serum pH of less than 7.2 after restoration of adequate volume, however, sometimes the infusion of sodium bicarbonate is necessary.

Antibiotics

Infection remains the leading cause of late morbidity and mortality after hemorrhagic shock. Proposed mechanisms include bacterial invasion from the ischemic gastrointestinal mucosa, failure of the hepatic reticuloendothelial system because of liver hypoxia, and increased cellular toxins from cell breakdown. Thus patients with hemorrhagic shock should be covered with broad-spectrum antibiotic therapy, especially those effective against intestinal flora.

Bibliography

Al-Mondhiry H. Disseminated intravascular coagulation: experience in a major cancer center. Thrombos Diathes Haemorrh 1975;34:181.

Amrein PC, Ellman L, Harris WH. Aspirin-induced prolongation of bleeding time and perioperative blood loss. JAMA 1981;245:1825.

Bennet B, Towler HMA. Haemostatic response to trauma. Br Med Bull 1985;67:274.

Benson RE, Isbister JP. Massive blood transfusion. Anaesth Intensive Care 1980;8:152.

Beris P, Miescher PA. Hematological complications of antiinfective agents. Semin Hematol 1988;25:123.

Better OS, Stein JH. Early management of shock and prophylaxis of acute renal failure in traumatic rhabdomyolysis. N Engl J Med 1990;322:825.

Boral LI, Dannemiller FJ, Stanford W, et al. A guideline for anticipated blood usage during elective surgical procedures. Am J Clin Pathol 1979;71:680.

Boral LI, Henry JB. The type and screen: a safe alternative and supplement in selected surgical procedures. Transfusion 1977;17:163.

Bowie EJ, Owen CA. Hemostatic failure in clinical medicine. Semin Hematol 1977;14:341.

Bowie EJW, Owen CA. The significance of abnormal preoperative hemostatic tests. In: Spaet TH, ed. Progress in hemostasis and thrombosis. Vol 5. New York: Grune & Stratton, 1980:170.

Brinkhous K, Smith H, Warner E, et al. Inhibition of blood clotting; an unidentified substance which acts in conjunction with heparin to prevent the conversion of prothrombin to thrombin. Am J Physiol 1939;125:683.

Brockman AW, van der Linden IK, Velt Kamp JJ, et al. Prevalence of isolated protein C deficiency in patients with venus thrombotic disease and in the population [Abstract]. Thromb Haemost 1983;50:350.

Buonassisi V. Sulfated mycopolysaccharide synthesis and secretion in endothelial cell cultures. Exp Cell Res 1973;76:363.

Burns ER, Billet HH, Frater RWM, et al. The preoperative bleeding time as predictor of postoperative hemorrhage after cardiopulmonary bypass. J Thorac Cardiovasc Surg 1986;92:310.

Ciavarella S, Reed RL, Counts RB, et al. Clotting factor levels and the risk of diffuse microvascular bleeding in the massively transfused patient. Br J Haematol 1987;67:365.

Collins JA, Murawski K, Shafer AW. Massive transfusion in surgery and trauma. Prog Clin Biol Res 1982;108:1–319.

Comp P, Nixon R, Esmon C. A functional assay for protein C, and antithrombotic protein, using a thrombomodulin complex. Blood 1984;63:15.

Conard J, Brosstad F, LieLarson M, et al. Molar antithrombin III concentration in normal human plasma. Haemostasis 1983;13:363.

Consensus Conference. Fresh frozen plasma indications and risks. JAMA 1985;253:551.

Consensus Conference. Platelet transfusion therapy. JAMA 1987;257:1777.

Consensus Conference. Perioperative red blood cell transfusion. JAMA 1988;260:2700.

Corriveau DM, Fritsma GA. Hemostasis and thrombosis: in the clinical laboratory. Philadelphia: JB Lippincott, 1988.

Cowley RA, Trump BF, eds. Pathophysiology of shock, anoxia, and ischemia. Baltimore: Williams & Wilkins, 1982.

DiScipio R, Hermodson M, Yates S, et al. A comparison of human prothrombin, Factor IX (Christmas Factor), Factor X (Stuart factor), and protein S. Biochemistry 1977;16:698.

Edmunds LH, Addonizio VP. Massive transfusion. In: Colman RW, Hirsh J, Marder VJ, et al, eds. Hemostasis and thrombosis: basic principles and clinical practice. 2nd ed. Philadelphia: JB Lippincott, 1987:913.

Egeberg O. Inherited antithrombin III deficiency causing thrombophilia. Thrombo Diathes Haemorrh 1965;13:513.

Esmon CT, Owen W. Identification of an endothelial cell cofactor for thrombosis catalyzed activation of protein C. Proc Natl Acad Sci USA 1981;78:2249.

Esmon NL, Owen W, Esmon C. Isolation of a membrane bound cofactor for thrombin catalyzed activation of protein C. J Biol Chem 1982;257:859.

Halal F, Quenneville G, Laurin S, et al. Clinical and genetic aspects of antithrombin III deficiency. Am J Med Gen 1983;14:737.

Harker LA. Hemostasis manual. 2nd ed. Philadelphia: FA Davis, 1974.

Hirsh J, Deykin D, Poller L. "Therapeutic range" for oral anticoagulant therapy. Chest 1986;89(suppl):11.

Hirsh J, Levine M. Review article: confusion over the therapeutic range for monitoring oral anticoagulant therapy in North America. Thromb Haemost 1988;59:129.

Iberti TJ. Thrombocytopenia following peritonitis in surgical patients. Ann Surg 1986;204:341.

Jespersen J, Munkvad, Gram J. Induction of coagulant activity and increase of t-PA and PAI-1 in plasma after thrombolysis in patients with myocardial infarction [Abstract]. Fibrinolysis 1990;4(suppl 3):95.

Johnson H, Knee-Ioli S, Butler TA, et al. Are routine preoperative laboratory screening tests necessary to evaluate ambulatory surgical patients? Surgery 1988;104:639.

Kisiel W, Canfield W, Ericsson L, et al. Anticoagulant properties of bovine plasma protein C following activation by thrombin. Biochemistry 1977;16:5824.

Kitchens CS. Concept of hypercoagulability: a review of its development, clinical application, and recent progress. Semin Thromb Hemost 1985;11:293.

Krieger JN, Hilgartner MW, Redo SF. Surgery in patients with congenital disorders of blood coagulation. Ann Surg 1977;185:290.

Lee VS, Tarassenko L, Bellhouse BJ. Platelet transfusion therapy: platelet concentrate preparation and storage. J Lab Clin Med 1988;111:371.

Malar R, Kleiss A, Griffin J. Human Protein C: inactivation by Factor V and VIII in plasma by the activated molecule. Ann NY Acad Sci 1981;370:303.

Malar RA, Kleiss AJ, Griffin JH. An alternative extrinsic pathway of human blood coagulation. Blood 1982;60:1352.

Mannucci PM, Tripodi A. Laboratory screening of inherited thrombotic syndromes. Thromb Haemost 1987;57:247.

Meade TW. The epidemiology of hemostatic and other variables in coronary artery disease. In: Verstraete, Vermylen, Liynen, Arnout, eds. Thrombosis and hemostasis 1987. International Society on Thrombosis and Haemostasis. Leuven University Press, 1987:37.

Miletich J, Sherman L, Broze G. Absence of thrombosis in subjects with heterozygous protein C deficiency. N Engl J Med 1987;317:991.

Miller N, Hultin MB, Gounder M, et al. Hereditary antithrombin III deficiency: case report and review of recent therapeutic advances. Am J Hematol 1986;21:215.

Morgan CH, Penner JA. Bleeding complications during surgery: part I. Defects of primary hemostasis and congenital coagulation. Lab Med 1986;17:207.

Morgan CH, Penner JA. Bleeding complications during surgery: part II. Acquired hemorrhagic disorders. Lab Med 1986;17:262.

Nagy I, Losonczy H. Three types of hereditary antithrombin III deficiency. Thromb Haemost 1979;42:187.

National Committee for Clinical Laboratory Standards (NCCLS) Document H21-A, vol 6, no 26. Collection, transport, and preparation of blood specimens for coagulation testing and performance of coagulation assays.

Pineo GF, Regoeczi E, Hatton MW, et al. The activation of coagulation by extracts of mucus: a possible pathway of intravascular coagulation accompanying adenocarcinomas. J Lab Clin Med 1973;82:255.

Poller L, Hirsh J. Special report: a simple system for the derivation of international normalized ratios for the reporting of prothrombin time results with North American thromboplastin reagents. Am J Clin Pathol 1989;92:124.

Rabkin B, Rabkin MS. Individual and institutional liability for transfusion-acquired diseases. JAMA 1986;256:2242.

Rao LM, Rapaport SI. Studies of a mechanism inhibiting the initiation of the extrinsic pathway of coagulation. Blood 1987;69:645.

Rao LM, Rapaport SI. Factor VIIa catalyzed activation of Factor X independent of tissue factor: its possible significance for control of hemophilic bleeding by infused Factor VIIa. Blood 1990;75:1069.

Rapaort SI. Preoperative hemostatic evaluation: which tests, if any? Blood 1983;61:229.

Reich NE, Hoffman CG, de Wolfe VG, et al. Recurrent thrombophlebitis and pulmonary emboli in congenital Factor 5 deficiency. Chest 1976;69:113.

Rickles FR, Edwards R. Activation of blood coagulation in cancer: Trousseau's syndrome revisited. Blood 1983;62:14.

Rodgers CRP, ed. A critical reappraisal of the bleeding time. Semin Thromb Hemost 1990;16:1.

Rodgers GM, Shuman MA. Congenital thrombotic disorders. Am J Hematol 1986;21:419.

Rohrer MJ, Michelotti MC, Nahrwold DL. A prospective evaluation of the efficacy of preoperative coagulation testing. Ann Surg 1988;208:554.

Salzman EW. Hemostatic problems in surgical patients. In: Colman RW, Hirsh J, Marder VJ, et al, eds. Hemostasis and thrombosis: basic principles and clinical practice. 2nd ed. Philadelphia: JB Lippincott, 1987:920.

Sas G, Peto I, Banhegyi D, et al. Heterogeneity of the "classical" antithrombin III deficiency. Thromb Haemost 1980;43:133.

Seegers W, Marciniak E. Inhibition of autoprothrombin C activity in plasma. Nature 1962;193:1188.

Seyer AE, Seaber AV, Dombrose FA. Coagulation changes in elective surgery and trauma. Ann Surg 1981;193:210.

Siegal T, Seligsohn U, Aghai E, et al. Clinical and laboratory aspects of disseminated intravascular coagulation (DIC): a study of 118 cases. Thromb Haemost 1978;39:122.

Stead NW, Bauer KA, Kinny TR, et al. Venous thrombosis in a family with defective release of vascular plasminogen activator, and elevated F VIII/von Willebrand Factor. Am J Med 1983;74:33.

Stenflow J. A new vitamin K dependent protein: purification from bovine plasma, and preliminary characterization. J Biol Chem 1976;251:355.

Stirling Y, Woolf WRS, North MJ, et al. Haemostasis in normal pregnancy. Thromb Haemost 1984;51:176.

Thaler E, Lechner K. Antithrombin III deficiency and thrombolism. Clin Haematol 1981;10:369.

Triplett DA, ed. Laboratory evaluation of coagulation. Chicago: ASCP Press, 1982.

Triplett DA, Brandt JT. Lupus anticoagulants: misnomer, paradox, riddle, epiphenomenon. Hematol Pathol 1988;2:121.

Walker F. The regulation of activated protein C by a new protein: a possible function for bovine protein S. J Biol Chem 1980;255:5521.

Walker F. Regulation of activated protein C by protein by protein S. The role of protein C in Factor Va inactivation. J Biol Chem 1981;256:11128.

Winman B. Altered fibrinolysis as a risk factor in cardiovascular disease [Abstract]. Fibrinolysis 1990;4(suppl 3):111.

9

Postoperative Infections

PHILIP B. MEAD

A broad-based knowledge of infectious diseases will enable the gynecologic surgeon to minimize the occurrence of postoperative infections and skillfully manage those patients who become infected despite optimal surgical care. Prevention requires knowledge of risk factors for infection after gynecologic surgery, and familiarity with specific techniques that reduce the incidence of or avoid infection-related morbidity, including use of antimicrobial prophylaxis. Effective management of the infected postoperative patient demands various skills. The surgeon must anticipate the likely presence of certain pathogens and understand how to isolate these pathogens in culture. The clinical syndromes that may be encountered postoperatively must be appreciated, so that a strategy to deal with each may be developed. In particular, an aptitude for evaluating the causes of postoperative fever must be developed and facility with the choice and use of antimicrobials must be mastered. In addition to possessing these necessary skills, the surgeon must take an active part in protecting all surgical personnel from the small, but finite risk of surgically acquired blood-borne infection. This chapter reviews each of these facets of gynecologic infectious disease.

PATHOGENS

Vaginal Flora

The bacteriology of the female genital tract is considerably more complex than is implied by the usual textbook description of a sparse flora mainly consisting of lactobacilli. Mean total bacterial counts in vaginal secretions actually approximate 10^8 to 10^9 bacteria per milliliter. The predominant facultative organisms are lactobacilli, various species of streptococci, *Gardnerella vaginalis, Staphylococcus epidermidis, Corynebacterium* species, and strains of Enterobacteriaceae (especially *Escherichia coli*). Anaerobes are numerically dominant (10 : 1); anaerobic gram-positive cocci, gram-positive bacilli, and gram-negative bacilli are all present in counts greater than 10^5 mL. These observations are relevant to gynecologic surgery because the normal flora also mirror the major pathogens in nonvenereal infections of the female pelvis (Table 9-1). This supports an endogenous route of infection, which was postulated by Schottmueller more than 80 years ago and has subsequently become a cornerstone of gynecologic infectious disease theory. An unexplained exception to this association is *Bacteroides fragilis,* which is commonly isolated from pelvic abscesses, despite its relative infrequency in the normal vaginal flora.

Various influences can modify the cervicovaginal flora: Bartlett and coworkers have found relatively consistent mean levels of anaerobes and a significant decrease in concentrations of aerobes in premenstrual specimens, whereas Neary and others have found greater colonization with *Bacteroides* species during the first week of the cycle. Recommendations for timing of gynecologic surgery in relation to the menstrual cycle based on such observations have never been verified by randomized trials.

Mead has reported that patients with invasive cervical cancer have an increased frequency of vaginal colonization with *E. coli* and *Bacteroides* species.

Ohm and Galask have shown that after abdominal or vaginal hysterectomy, facultative gram-negative rods (*E. coli, Klebsiella, Proteus, Enterobacter*), *B. fragilis,* and enterococci are more common in 5-day postoperative cultures than in preoperative cultures from the same patients. Although numerous studies have documented increased enterococcal colonization after perioperative cephalosporin prophylaxis, this state cannot be reliably predicted simply on the basis of the antibiotic used. Other factors are involved, as shown by increased enterococcal colonization in the placebo groups. Hospi-

TABLE 9–1.
Pathogens Responsible for Infections Following Gynecologic Surgery

Aerobic Gram-positive Cocci

  Staphylococcus aureus
  Streptococcus viridans group
  Group B streptococcus
  Enterococcus

Aerobic Gram-negative Bacilli

  Escherichia coli
  Proteus mirabilis
  Klebsiella species
  Gardnerella vaginalis

Anaerobes

  Peptostreptococcus species
  Peptococcus species
  Bacteroides bivius
  Bacteroides disiens
  Bacteroides melangiogenicus
  Bacteroides capillosis
  Bacteroides fragilis group
    B. fragilis
    B. ovatus
    B. thetaiotaomicron
    B. distasonis
    B. vulgatus
  Clostridium perfringens
  Fusobacterium species

talization on an obstetrics or gynecology ward exerts a profound effect on the vaginal flora, regardless of surgery, antibiotic prophylaxis, or therapy, and this change tends to be in the direction of more virulent organisms, including enterococci, *B. fragilis,* and resistant Enterobacteriaceae.

Bacterial Vaginosis

Bacterial vaginosis (homogeneous vaginal discharge, pH higher than 4.5, amine odor when mixed with potassium hydroxide, presence of clue cells) is characterized bacteriologically by vaginal overgrowth of *G. vaginalis,* anaerobic bacteria (*Bacteroides* species, *Mobiluncus* species, and anaerobic cocci), and *Mycoplasma hominis.* Postpartum endometritis and the intra-amniotic infection syndrome have been associated with bacterial vaginosis. It also is probable that the high concentration of potentially virulent organisms in bacterial vaginosis is an important inoculation source for posthysterectomy or other pelvic infection. If such an association can be confirmed, as seems likely, preoperative testing and treatment should offer a simple means of decreasing postoperative pelvic infections.

Natural History

The animal model of intra-abdominal infection devised by Weinstein and colleagues has clarified our understanding of the distinctive roles of different bacteria in the natural history of pelvic infection. These investigators documented a biphasic response to infection: an early-onset phase with high rates of sepsis and death in which gram-negative aerobic bacteria predominate (peritonitis stage) and a late-onset phase with abscess formation in which anaerobes predominate (abscess stage). Although there are differences between the animal model and human infections, the timing of symptoms, the pathologic picture seen, and the microorganisms involved are amazingly similar.

COLLECTION OF MICROBIOLOGIC SPECIMENS

Specimens for culture must be appropriate to the clinical setting, correctly collected, and properly transported if meaningful results are to be achieved. Adherence to the following guidelines is essential.

Urine

Acceptable specimens for urine culture may be clean-voided, obtained by urethral catheterization, or aspirated from an indwelling catheter with a sterile needle. The disinfected distal end of the catheter or, preferably, the sampling port should be used. Unless refrigerated during storage and transport, no urine arriving in the laboratory more than 2 hours after its collection should be cultured.

Blood

The recovery of organisms from bloodstream infections is probably most closely related to the volume of blood cultured, with about 30 mL the optimal volume. An aerobic and an anaerobic bottle should be inoculated from each venipuncture. Two or three sets of cultures are adequate for each septic episode, depending on the volume of blood accommodated by each bottle. Conversely, it is inappropriate to collect only a single set of blood cultures because it is more difficult to assess the clinical significance of such organisms as *S. epidermidis, Propionibacterium acnes, Bacillus* species, and *Corynebacterium* species, which are ordinarily considered contaminants, but which may cause disease in certain patients.

Pus

Pus is an excellent specimen from which responsible pathogens can be isolated. It should be aspirated in a sterile syringe and submitted either in a transport vial (a diaphragm-stoppered bottle with an anaerobic atmosphere that contains prereduced agar and a redox indicator) or directly in the syringe itself after the needle is inserted into a sterile rubber stopper. Pus from abdominal wounds also can be submitted on a prereduced, anaerobically sterilized swab gently plunged into Cary-Blair transport medium.

Infected Tissue

Tissue such as the wall of an abscess provides an excellent specimen for culture. It may be submitted in an anaerobic transport tube, but if it is kept moist on saline-dampened sterile gauze and transported promptly, special anaerobic transport techniques are probably unnecessary. All specimens of pus or tissue should be Gram-stained. This procedure provides invaluable, immediate data and, in the case of certain fastidious organisms, may yield information not available from cultures.

Infected Operative Sites

Consensus is lacking concerning the optimal method, or even the wisdom, of culturing infected pelvic sites when pus or tissue cannot be obtained (eg, pelvic cellulitis). Culture of needle aspirates or fine needle aspiration biopsies has been suggested, but documentation of the validity of such specimens is largely anecdotal. It is difficult, if not impossible, to avoid contamination with normal flora in any specimen obtained transvaginally. Such cultures are hard to interpret and in fact are susceptible to misinterpretation. A rational approach to this problem is to consult a clinical microbiologist when the need for a culture or choice of specimen to be obtained is uncertain. After reviewing the case and discussing possible options, the need for culture or technique necessary for obtaining an interpretable specimen usually can be defined.

Grossman and colleagues have demonstrated that routine culture of the vaginal cuff at the time of hysterectomy is not predictive of the subsequent development of pelvic or abdominal wound infection. Their findings do not justify routine culture of the vaginal cuff at the time of surgery in an attempt to predict or more specifically treat subsequent pelvic infection.

It cannot be overemphasized that the value of the information gained from the microbiology laboratory is in direct proportion to the day-to-day rapport established between the gynecologic surgeon and the clinical microbiologist. It also is prudent to treat a culture specimen and report from a febrile patient with the same personal concern accorded a biopsy specimen and report from a patient with suspected cancer.

RISK FACTORS

A multiplicity of factors, many beyond the surgeon's control, influence the likelihood of the development of a postoperative infection.

A recent study documents a higher febrile morbidity rate for abdominal as compared with vaginal hysterectomy. The difference is almost certainly attributable to the greater efficacy of prophylactic antibiotics for vaginal operations.

The incidence of postoperative infection is higher in patients of lower socioeconomic status than in patients of higher socioeconomic status, irrespective of the surgical approach to hysterectomy. Although the reasons for this higher incidence have never been elucidated, it is a consistent finding.

Age has inconsistently been shown to be a risk factor for infection after hysterectomy. Premenopausal women are at increased risk in some studies, especially after vaginal hysterectomy. It is not known whether this increased infection risk in younger women is due to differences in the bacterial flora of the cervix and vagina or to greater difficulty in obtaining hemostasis.

Duration of surgery is directly correlated with postoperative infection rates in most studies. For infections of the operative site (ie, "deep" infections), duration of surgery probably reflects the degree of technical difficulty of a procedure or the skill of the surgeon, or both. For abdominal incisions, increased duration of surgery allows greater contamination of the wound.

Obesity is associated with a markedly increased risk of postoperative infection, reflecting an interplay of factors, including prolonged operative time, decreased tissue oxygenation, and altered nutritional and metabolic status. Comorbidities (eg, diabetes, cirrhosis, steroid therapy) that affect the host's immune competence also predispose to postoperative infection.

Perioperative anemia appears not to play a role. There is no support for transfusion to a certain hemoglobin level or hematocrit to promote wound healing. Likewise, there is no clear evidence that anemia increases the frequency or severity of postoperative infections. There also are no data to suggest that transfusion of red cells has a salvage effect on infection.

Patients with cancer are more likely to develop postoperative infection, an effect explained by multiple host factors, radical surgical procedures, factors inherent in the tumor itself, and irradiation and chemotherapy.

England and coworkers have shown that the use of epinephrine as a vasoconstrictor in vaginal hysterectomy does not significantly reduce blood loss and results in a higher incidence of postoperative vaginal cuff infection.

The following risk factors for incisional wound infections have been identified by Cruse and others: increased duration of surgery, age less than 1 year or more than 50 years, prolonged preoperative hospitalization, shaving of the skin site, and use of passive wound drains.

CLINICAL SYNDROMES: DEFINITIONS AND MANAGEMENT STRATEGIES

A helpful approach to management of the patient with a presumed postoperative pelvic infection is to classify the infection into one of the following categories.

Vaginal Cuff Abscess

Vaginal cuff abscesses present with fever early in the postoperative period and occasionally with rectal pressure or pelvic pain. There are few other systemic symptoms; a purulent discharge or palpable collection at the vaginal cuff, often an infected hematoma, are the only significant findings. Response to simple drainage by digital palpation or needle aspiration of the vaginal vault is rapid. Although perhaps unnecessary, we treat these patients with antimicrobials in addition to drainage.

Pelvic Cellulitis

The most common pelvic infection after hysterectomy, pelvic cellulitis presents with fever later in the postoperative course (2nd to 5th day), lower abdominal tenderness, and, occasionally, peritoneal signs or ileus. Pelvic examination reveals marked induration but no fluctuant mass. Treatment consists of systemic antimicrobial agents.

Septic Pelvic Thrombophlebitis

Septic pelvic thrombophlebitis is almost always diagnosed by exclusion in a patient who has been febrile but has not responded to antimicrobial therapy. A hectic fever curve and a constant tachycardia are typical. Abdominal and pelvic findings are minimal, and there is no evidence of a pelvic or incisional abscess by pelvic examination, ultrasonography, or computed tomogra-

phy (CT) scanning. A PO_2 of less than 80 mm Hg in a nonsmoker supports the diagnosis. Treatment consists of full heparin anticoagulation for 7 to 10 days. Patients usually respond dramatically, becoming afebrile within 24 to 48 hours. Additional long-term anticoagulation therapy with warfarin sodium (Coumadin) is considered only for patients with associated pulmonary embolism. We also treat patients who have septic pelvic thrombophlebitis with antimicrobials that are effective against heparinase-producing *Bacteroides* species (eg, clindamycin, metronidazole, cefoxitin).

Postoperative Adnexal Abscess

Fever and abdominal pain late in the postoperative period, together with a tender palpable adnexal mass, suggest adnexal abscess. Occasionally ultrasonography or CT scanning is necessary to demonstrate the mass. These infections occur almost exclusively in premenopausal patients. Initial antimicrobial therapy must include agents that are effective against *B. fragilis* (eg, clindamycin, metronidazole). Failure to respond, as evidenced by continued fever after 48 to 72 hours or increase in the size of the mass, mandates laparotomy for removal of the abscess. A pelvic abscess may be drained by means of colpotomy if the following absolute prerequisites are met: the mass is fluctuant, it adheres to the parietal pelvic peritoneum, and it dissects into the midline of the upper one-third of the rectovaginal septum.

Osteomyelitis Pubis

Osteomyelitis of the pubis is a rare infection that results from either bacteremic seeding or extension of a contiguous focus of infection. Most cases in women occur after urethral suspension, radical vulvectomy, or pelvic exenteration. In the study conducted by Hoyme and colleagues, symptoms (pubic bone pain and tenderness, avoidance of ambulation, and pain on abduction) did not appear until more than 8 weeks after the initial operation. Wound drainage, low-grade fever, moderate leukocytosis, and an elevated erythrocyte sedimentation rate or alkaline phosphatase level may be present. Blood and bone biopsy specimens or aspirated material should be cultured. Radiography and various radioactive scanning techniques are useful diagnostic methods. Antimicrobial therapy must be prolonged, and capable of covering both *Staphylococcus aureus* and aerobic gram-negative bacteria, the usual pathogens, unless a specific organism is isolated. Although untested for this indication, the new quinolone group of antimicrobials have the proper antimicrobial spectrum and can be administered orally. Surgical debridement may be necessary as well.

Ligneous Pelvic Cellulitis

Campbell has described a pelvic cellulitis that is characterized by unremitting fever and widespread tender induration in the pelvis. The firmness of the affected areas is so great that the description of "a frozen pelvis" often is given. In the past patients with this diffuse "woody" induration have responded to corticosteroids after antimicrobial therapy produced no response. Most infectious disease specialists have not seen this syndrome during the past decade, suggesting that the use of effective anti-anaerobic antimicrobials has relegated ligneous pelvic cellulitis to a place of historical interest only.

Incisional Wound Infections

At least three varieties of wound infection should be recognized by the gynecologic surgeon.

Early-Onset Wound Infection. Early-onset wound infection caused by group A β-hemolytic streptococci develops during the first 24 to 48 hours after surgery. This rare infection is a cellulitis that responds to high-dose parenteral penicillin. Patients should be isolated for the first 24 hours of therapy and an attempt made to determine the source of infection; often the source is a colonized caregiver. Group B β-hemolytic streptococci may cause a similar early-onset infection.

Late-Onset Wound Infection. Most wound infections become apparent 5 to 7 days after surgery when low-grade fever and wound drainage develop. A fever curve typical of an abscess—a single high spike in the late afternoon or early evening—also is a common presentation. The wound should be opened down to the fascia over the entire extent of the infection, material for culture and Gram stain obtained, and the fascia examined for its integrity. Treatment consists of irrigations and wet-to-dry dressings, so that the wound granulates in from the base. Although drainage of a wound abscess is the definitive therapy, many surgeons administer a brief course of systemic antimicrobials until the wound is clean and granulating well. About 25% of wound infections are caused by *S. aureus,* often from an exogenous source; the remaining 75% are caused by vaginal organisms introduced at the time of surgery. In selected situations (eg, obese patients) one may consider secondary closure of an infected wound when it appears clean clinically and a quantitative wound culture obtained after the manner of Magee and coworkers and Robson and coworkers predicts success.

The use of delayed primary closure in contaminated cases usually obviates the complication of wound infection.

Necrotizing Fasciitis. A third variety of wound infection has been described under a plethora of names, including necrotizing fasciitis, clostridial cellulitis, non-clostridial anaerobic cellulitis, anaerobic cutaneous gangrene, Fournier gangrene, synergistic necrotizing cellulitis, gangrenous erysipelas, hospital gangrene, acute dermal gangrene, and necrotizing erysipelas. All of these conditions have a similar pathogenesis, treatment, and prognosis. Each is essentially an infection of the subcutaneous tissues (ie, the superficial fascia) that spreads in the fascial clefts overlying the deep fascia (Fig. 9-1). The deep fascia usually, but not always, is spared; skin involvement results only secondarily after the vessels to the skin thrombose. Necrotizing fasciitis is a synergistic infection caused by groups of aerobic and anaerobic bacteria. Presenting complaints are local pain and edema. Because the skin is not primarily involved, the wound may appear normal, making early clinical recognition difficult and causing fatal delay in appropriate treatment. Despite the minimal local findings, patients may appear severely ill. Definitive diagnosis is made at surgery when the operator discovers extensive undermining of surrounding tissues and lack of resistance in the superficial fascial plane (ie, the subcutaneous tissue or "fat") to probing with a blunt instrument. Treatment includes broad-spectrum antibiotic therapy (eg, clindamycin plus ampicillin plus gentamicin) and radical debridement to include removal of all necrotic and pale tissue. Acceptable margins are reached when the subcutaneous tissue cannot be separated from the underlying normal deep fascia or from normal skin. The reported mortality rate from necrotizing fasciitis, an infection that occurs most often in diabetics, ranges from 21% to 76%.

EVALUATION OF POSTOPERATIVE FEVER

Although fever and infection are not synonymous, fever is the physical sign that alerts physicians to the possible presence of infection and that initiates diagnostic action. The efficient and precise evaluation of fever is a skill essential for the management of postoperative patients. Ledger has offered the useful insight that clues to the cause of fever usually are based on the interval between surgery and the onset of fever.

Onset Within 48 Hours of Surgery

Garibaldi and associates suggest that most cases of early postoperative fever are noninfectious in origin. Most patients who develop fever without an identifiable source become febrile within the first 2 postoperative days, a pattern significantly different from the timing of postoperative wound and urinary tract infections (Fig. 9-2). The cause of early, unexplained fever remains ill-

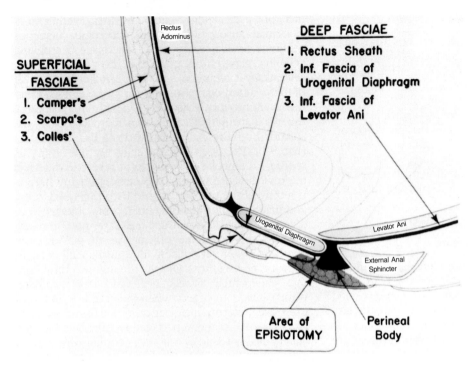

Figure 9–1. Diagrammatic representation of the fascial layers of the lower abdomen and perineum in paramedian sagittal section. (Shy KK, Eschenbach DA. Obstet Gynecol 1979; 54:296. Reprinted with permission from The American College of Obstetricians and Gynecologists.)

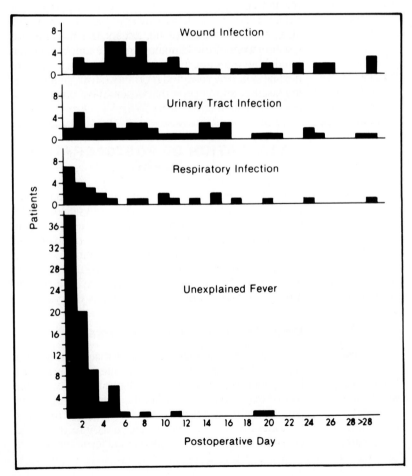

Figure 9–2. Days of onset for postoperative infections and unexplained fever. (Garibaldi RA, Brodine S, Matsumiya S, Coleman M. Infect Control 1985; 6:274. Reprinted with permission from SLACK, Inc.)

defined. Possible noninfectious causes include hypersensitivity reactions to anesthetics or other medications, and pulmonary atelectasis. Physiologic responses to intraoperative tissue trauma or hematoma formation include the release of pyrogenic substances into the circulation. Patients with early postoperative fever must be properly evaluated to rule out obvious infection, but empiric antibiotic therapy should be withheld if no source of infection is identified.

Extravasation of urine after unrecognized ureteral damage at surgery may result in a high-spiking fever early in the postoperative period.

Spitzer and coworkers have reported three patients who developed high fevers within 5 hours after laser surgery of the vagina. All defervesced promptly, one without treatment.

Infectious causes of early postoperative fever include pneumonia, contaminated intravenous infusions (extremely rare), group A β-hemolytic streptococcal wound infections, pelvic infections after intrauterine manipulation (eg, radium implantation), operative manipulation that exacerbates an unrecognized established infection (eg, pelvic inflammatory disease), and early-onset sepsis.

Onset More Than 48 Hours After Surgery

Urinary tract infections, infections of the operative site, and abdominal wound infections become evident 48 or more hours after surgery. Noninfectious fevers also can appear at this time but are less common.

Late Manifestations of Postoperative Infections

Fever with onset late in the postoperative course, usually after discharge from the hospital, suggests an adnexal abscess, wound infection, or, rarely, osteomyelitis pubis.

When fever develops very late in the postoperative course of a patient who was transfused with any blood product, one must consider transfusion-associated infection (eg, hepatitis B; non-A, non-B hepatitis including hepatitis C; malaria; brucellosis; babesiosis; infection caused by human immunodeficiency virus, cytomegalovirus, or Epstein-Barr virus).

ANTIMICROBIAL THERAPY

Postoperative pelvic infections are polymicrobic; isolates occur in the rough proportions of 20% aerobic gram-positive cocci, 20% gram-negative rods, and 60% anaerobes. The aerobic gram-positive cocci are predominantly streptococci and less frequently *S. aureus;* enterococci are believed to be synergistic partners with other organisms and not primary pathogens. The gram-negative rods are common Enterobacteriaceae: *E. coli, Klebsiella,* and *Proteus mirabilis.* Anaerobes are numerically dominant. With these simple facts in mind it is not difficult to design effective antimicrobial regimens and to anticipate the deficiencies of any given regimen. It makes little sense to be dogmatic about the initial choice of antibiotics, since there are almost always multiple appropriate regimens and acceptable alternatives (Table 9-2).

A regimen of clindamycin, 900 mg, plus gentamicin, 2 mg/kg loading dose followed by 1.5 mg/kg maintenance dose (assuming normal renal function), each given intravenously every 8 hours, provides excellent coverage of *S. aureus,* aerobic streptococci, aerobic gram-negative rods, and anaerobes. This regimen has proved significantly more effective than penicillin and gentamicin in controlled clinical trials and is currently the standard against which other regimens should be compared. This combination is ineffective against enterococci, however, and it has the potential for nephrotoxicity and ototoxicity (gentamicin) or for diarrhea and pseudomembranous enterocolitis (clindamycin). The addition of ampicillin or high-dose penicillin extends the spectrum of the clindamycin–gentamicin regimen to include enterococci. This "triple therapy" has the broadest spectrum but has never been systematically studied in a controlled trial. It should be used initially only in the most seriously ill patients, such as those with necrotizing fasciitis or those who are in septic shock.

Metronidazole is extremely active against *B. fragilis* and other obligate anaerobes; it is not effective against *Actinomyces* and has no activity against aerobic bacteria. It has been effective for pelvic infections, including abscesses, when combined with another antimicrobial, usually gentamicin.

Various cephalosporins and extended-spectrum penicillins have been used successfully to treat mild to moderately severe postoperative pelvic infections (eg, cefoxitin, ceftizoxime, cefotetan, ticarcillin/clavulanic acid, ampicillin/sulbactam, piperacillin, mezlocillin). These agents offer the advantage of single-agent therapy and avoid problems associated with gentamicin (ie, inadequate dosing, measuring peak and trough levels, ototoxicity, and nephrotoxicity).

All of these regimens should be continued intravenously for at least 4 days, and until 24 to 48 hours after the patient becomes afebrile and asymptomatic and the white blood cell count returns to normal. Treatment of pelvic cellulitis usually can be completed in 4 or 5 days. Controlled trials have documented the safety of this short-course antibiotic therapy.

Although it is common clinical practice to discharge

TABLE 9–2.
Treatment Choices for Gynecologic Infections

TYPE OF INFECTION	TREATMENT CHOICES		
	Recommended Regimen	*Failures*	*Penicillin Allergy*
Postoperative			
Mild to moderate	Extended-spectrum cephalosporins or extended-spectrum penicillins	Clindamycin + gentamicin	Clindamycin + gentamicin
Severe	Clindamycin + gentamicin	Clindamycin + gentamicin + ampicillin or imipenem	Clindamycin + gentamicin
Pelvic abscess	Clindamycin + gentamicin or metronidazole + gentamicin	Reevaluate need for surgical drainage	Clindamycin + gentamicin or metronidazole + gentamicin
Staphylococcal infections (eg, toxic shock syndrome or severe staphylococcal wound infection)	Nafcillin or oxacillin	Consultation indicated	Vancomycin

(American Collge of Obstericians and Gynecologists: Antimicrobial Therapy for Gynecologic Patients [ACOG Technical Bulletin 97]. Washington DC, ACOG, 1986, p 3. Reprinted with permission from The American College of Obstetricians and Gynecologists.)

patients on regimens of oral tetracycline, ampicillin, or cephalexin with instructions to complete 10 days of treatment, most infectious disease authorities have doubted the value of such a policy, and two studies have provided evidence that oral antibiotics after parenteral antibiotics are not necessary.

Failure of properly chosen initial antimicrobial therapy should prompt a careful search for an undrained soft-tissue collection (ie, wound infection or pelvic abscess), septic pelvic thrombophlebitis, or one of the rarer syndromes previously described. Failure because of inadequate antimicrobial coverage per se is uncommon but may occur, usually when highly resistant anaerobes are present or superinfection with enterococci has occurred. Resistant anaerobes are treated by the addition of clindamycin or metronidazole to the regimen. Enterococcal superinfection is suggested when patients do not respond to regimens that are not effective against enterococci (eg, cephalosporins; less commonly after clindamycin plus gentamicin), particularly when this organism is isolated in pure culture or heavy growth from the infected site. Beyond these two possibilities it usually is more productive to look for an undrained abscess, septic pelvic thrombophlebitis, or a noninfectious fever than to juggle the antimicrobial regimen.

PREVENTIVE MEASURES

Haley has shown that nearly two thirds of all hospital-acquired infections can be prevented, including one-quarter to one-half of all wound infections. In addition to an effective hospitalwide infection control program, the following specific actions will help to keep postoperative infections to the irreducible minimum.

Prevention of Urinary Tract Infections

Correct and appropriate use of indwelling urinary catheters offers the greatest opportunity for lowering the incidence of urinary tract infections. Urinary catheters should be inserted only when necessary and never solely for the convenience of patient care personnel; they should be left in place only as long as absolutely necessary. Only staff who are skilled in the correct techniques of aseptic insertion and maintenance should handle catheters. A sterile, continuously closed drainage system should be maintained, and the catheter should be properly secured to prevent movement and urethral traction. Handwashing before manipulation of the catheter should be emphasized.

An indwelling catheter should never be "covered" with antimicrobials; as long as the catheter is in place, one should use antimicrobials only to treat symptomatic infection. It is far more important to maintain a daily fluid intake that will produce at least 2500 mL of urine each day. Urinary tract infection is unlikely to occur when urine output is adequate, even with a catheter in place. Some surgeons recommend a short course of oral antibiotics to be started when the catheter is removed from postoperative patients who are at high risk for asymptomatic bacteriuria.

Prevention of Postoperative Pneumonia

Patients who will receive anesthesia for an abdominal operation or who have substantial pulmonary dysfunction (eg, chronic obstructive lung disease, abnormal pulmonary function tests, musculoskeletal abnormality of the chest) should receive preoperative and postoperative respiratory therapy and instruction designed to prevent postoperative pulmonary complications. Preoperative therapy should include treatment of pulmonary infections, efforts to facilitate removal of respiratory secretions, and, especially, discontinuance of smoking. Preoperative instruction should include discussion of the importance of frequent coughing, deep breathing, and ambulation in the postoperative period. Postoperatively, pain that interferes with coughing and deep breathing should be controlled, and the patient should be encouraged and assisted in coughing, deep breathing, and early ambulation.

Prevention of Operative Site and Incisional Wound Infections

Strategies to minimize deep and superficial wound infections derive directly from knowledge of those risk factors discussed earlier.

If the operation is elective, all identifiable bacterial infections, excluding those for which the operation is performed, should be treated and controlled before the operation. Of particular importance in gynecologic surgery is the preoperative identification and treatment of bacterial vaginosis. The current therapy for bacterial vaginosis is metronidazole, 500 mg by mouth twice a day for 7 days.

Although not proved in controlled trials, the following interventions to alter host factors seem worthwhile: tight control of blood glucose in diabetics; oral, enteral, or parenteral nutrition in malnourished patients; and discontinuance or reduction of doses of adrenal steroids when possible.

A shorter period of preoperative hospitalization has been associated with lower wound infection rates in at least five studies. All other things being equal, day-of-surgery admissions are probably ideal.

Unless hair near the operative site is so thick that it will interfere with the surgical procedure, it should not be removed. Clipping hair or using a depilatory has been suggested if hair must be removed. If shaving is necessary, it should be performed immediately before the operation.

Bathing the patient preoperatively with an antimicrobial-containing detergent has been suggested as a preventive measure because it reduces colonization with typical pathogens such as *S. aureus.* Although there is no evidence that such bathing reduces infection rates, it is easy, safe, and inexpensive. We favor the use of a chlorhexidine shower of the entire body, including the scalp, on two separate occasions before surgery.

A preoperative povidone-iodine douche should be administered to patients whose vaginas will be entered during surgery.

The most important measure to prevent wound infections is good operative technique. Speed, gentle tissue handling, meticulous hemostasis, eradication of dead space, and minimization of devitalized tissue, tension on tissue, and foreign materials in the wound will all reduce postoperative infection. The surgeon must balance the need to operate quickly with the need for atraumatic handling of tissue and precise dissection.

At least eight studies have demonstrated that reporting surgeon-specific wound infection rates is an effective way of lowering these rates by as much as 55%. All hospitals should tabulate surgeon-specific, procedure-specific wound infection rates and provide these rates to surgeons confidentially on a regular basis.

There is preliminary evidence that enteral elemental feeding in the postoperative period is more advantageous than total parenteral nutrition in protecting the gut barrier, reducing metabolic stress, maintaining normal hepatic function, and thus decreasing the risk of sepsis. An intact gut barrier blocks translocation of bacteria and endotoxins that otherwise activate complement and stimulate macrophages and neutrophils to elaborate inflammatory mediators. Studies are urgently needed to define the value of early enteral feeding in postoperative gynecologic surgical patients who are unlikely to tolerate oral feedings for 3 or more days after surgery.

Prophylactic Antimicrobials

For some gynecologic operations prophylactic antimicrobials are effective in reducing the risk of wound or operative site infections. In classic studies performed more than 30 years ago, Miles and colleagues showed that there is a well-defined short period, beginning with the incision and lasting for about 3 hours, when developing wound infection can be suppressed by antibiotics. Antibiotics cause maximum suppression of infection if given before bacteria gain entrance to the tissue, and are ineffective if bacteria have been in the tissue more than 3 hours before the antibiotics are given. It is not surprising that a multitude of clinical trials have demonstrated that a single dose of a parenteral antibiotic given just before an operation provides optimal antimicrobial prophylaxis for procedures lasting up to 2 hours; earlier administration is unnecessary and undesirable. When surgery is delayed or prolonged, a second dose may be advisable. Fundamental goals include minimizing the number of bacteria present and maximizing the amount of available antibiotic at the site of the potential contamination for the duration of that contamination. Once the skin or mucous membrane incision is closed and the period of contamination is over, there is little theoretical justification for giving additional doses. In numerous studies longer courses of therapy have seldom shown any additional benefit, and may be harmful.

First-generation cephalosporins have been widely used for prophylaxis in gynecologic surgery. They have not been shown to be less effective than second- or third-generation agents, have a narrower range of activity, are less likely to induce bacterial production of β-lactamase, and are less expensive. Cefazolin, because it has a longer half-life than other first-generation cephalosporins, is viewed as the cephalosporin of choice for prophylaxis. We use the following regimen: cefazolin, 1 g, by intravenous push (over less than 5 minutes) given immediately before incision and repeated if the procedure lasts more than 3 hours.

PROPHYLACTIC ANTIMICROBIALS FOR SEPTIC PROCEDURES

Vaginal hysterectomy: Effective; use in all premenopausal patients; some authorities recommend use in all patients.

Abdominal hysterectomy: Effective, but less consistently so than with vaginal hysterectomy. Some authorities recommend if the combined operative site infection plus abdominal wound infection rate is greater than 10%.

Radical hysterectomy: Several studies support the use of prophylaxis in radical hysterectomy. There is an urgent need for studies comparing short-course (intraoperative) cefazolin prophylaxis with more prolonged, broader-spectrum coverage. Unlike simple abdominal or vaginal hysterectomy, in which the addition of suction drainage to antibiotics does not further reduce morbidity, in radical hysterectomy prophylactic antibiotics plus suction drainage significantly decrease infectious morbidity.

Tuboplasty: Use is common, but studies to document efficacy are unavailable.

Repair of cystocele and rectocele: Prophylactic antibiotics have not been effective.

Antibiotics for Dirty or Contaminated Surgery

Antimicrobials given during dirty or contaminated surgery should be considered as treatment of an established infection rather than as prophylaxis. In these cases the antibiotic regimen should be continued after the immediate postsurgical period for the usual therapeutic course.

Summary

It should be stressed that antibiotic prophylaxis is only one component of care of the gynecologic patient, and certainly not the most important one. The goal should be the performance of necessary surgery, skillfully carried out in the operating room, in patients whose preoperative and postoperative courses are managed by knowledgeable, conscientious, compassionate gynecologic surgeons. In certain situations antibiotic prophylaxis may complement such care, but it can never replace any portion of it.

PROTECTION OF THE SURGICAL TEAM

Current emphasis on protecting the surgical team, admittedly galvanized by fear of acquired immunodeficiency syndrome, is returning needed, but neglected, procedures to their proper place in the practice of surgery. Blood-transmissible infections acquired by parenteral injury (needlestick, scapel cut) or mucosal splash (eye, mouth) or through nonintact skin (dermatitis) provide the only appreciable risk to the surgeon. The risk of hepatitis B infection after a contaminated needlestick ranges from 6% to 30%; the risk of human immunodeficiency virus (HIV) infection under similar circumstances is less than 0.5%. Hagen and associates have calculated the surgeon's risk of HIV infection when operating on an HIV-infected patient as between 1:4,500 and 1:130,000. The risk when operating on an untested patient from a low-prevalence area for HIV was similarly calculated as between 1/450,000 and 1/1.3 billion.

The Centers for Disease Control has issued guidelines for preventing transmission of HIV and hepatitis B virus during invasive procedures. Of particular importance to surgeons are the use of eye coverings if splashes are likely to occur, impervious gowns if blood exposure to arms or thorax is expected, and avoidance of direct patient care by surgeons with exudative skin lesions or weeping dermatitis. Needles and sharp instruments represent the greatest risk to the surgeon, with needlesticks accounting for 95% of intraoperative injuries. Hand-to-hand passing of sharp instruments should be avoided by designating an area of the Mayo stand where they can be placed by the scrub nurse and picked up by the surgeon. No completely satisfactory alternative to palpation of the needletip when suturing "blindly" deep in the pelvis has been devised; studies documenting the left index finger as the most common site of needlestick injury in surgeons highlight the potential risk of this technique.

Despite enormous concern over HIV, hepatitis B still represents the greatest threat to surgeons; seroprevalence rates among surgeons are five to eight times greater than among the general public. Hepatitis B vaccine is safe and immunogenic. Clearly all susceptible surgeons should receive hepatitis B immunization, not only for their personal health protection, but also to prevent the remote but real possibility of transmission of hepatitis B infection to their patients.

Several studies have demonstrated that most hospitalized patients who harbor blood-borne diseases are not identified as infected. Accordingly, the Centers for Disease Control strongly recommend the use of universal precautions, under which the blood and certain body fluids of *all* patients are considered potentially infectious. If special techniques to reduce the likelihood of intraoperative exposure to blood-borne pathogens are developed, preoperative testing for HIV and hepatitis B virus might be considered a desirable supplement to universal precautions in the future. No such techniques have been identified to date, and in any event preprocedure testing would have no utility for emergency procedures.

Bibliography

Altemeier WA, McDonough JJ, Fullen WD. Third day surgical fever. Arch Surg 1971;103:158.

Anonymous. Antimicrobial prophylaxis for surgery. Med Lett Drugs Ther 1983;25:113.

Anonymous. The choice of antimicrobial drugs. Med Lett Drugs Ther 1988;30:33.

Bartlett JG. Recent developments in the management of anaerobic infections. Rev Infect Dis 1983;5:235.

Bartlett JG, Moon NE, Goldstein PR, et al. Cervical and vaginal bacterial flora: ecologic niches in the female lower genital tract. Am J Obstet Gynecol 1978;130:658.

Bartlett JG, Onderdonk AB, Drude E, et al. Quantitative bacteriology of the vaginal flora. J Infect Dis 1977;136:271.

Bartlett JG, Onderdonk AB, Louie T, et al. Lessons from an animal model of intraabdominal sepsis. Arch Surg 1978;113:853.

Berkelman RL, Martin D, Graham DR, et al. Streptococcal wound infections caused by a vaginal carrier. JAMA 1982;247:2680.

Brooker DC, Savage JE, Twiggs LB, et al. Infectious morbidity in gynecologic cancer. Am J Obstet Gynecol 1987;156:513.

Brough SJ, Hunt TM, Barrier WW. Surgical glove perforations. Br J Surg 1988;75:317.

Brown SE, Allen HH, Robins RN. The use of delayed primary wound closure in preventing wound infections. Am J Obstet Gynecol 1977;127:713.

Burke JF. The effective period of preventive antibiotic action in experimental incisions and dermal lesions. Surgery 1961;50:161.

Cabbad M, Sijin O, Minkoff H. Short course of antibiotics for postcesarean section endometritis. Am J Obstet Gynecol 1987; 157:908.

Campbell C. Two unusual uses of steroid hormones in pelvic infection. Clin Obstet Gynecol 1969;12:247.

Centers for Disease Control. Nosocomial infection surveillance, 1984. MMWR 1986;35:1755.

Centers for Disease Control. Recommendations for preventing transmission of infection with HTLVIII/LAV during invasive procedures. MMWR 1986;35:221.

Centers for Disease Control. Recommendations for prevention of HIV transmission in health-care settings. MMWR 1987;36:25.

Centers for Disease Control. Update: acquired immunodeficiency syndrome and human immunodeficiency virus infection among health-care workers. MMWR 1988;37:229.

Centers for Disease Control. Update: universal precautions for prevention of transmission of human immunodeficiency virus, hepatitis B virus, and other bloodborne pathogens in health-care settings. MMWR 1988;37:377.

Cruse PJE, Foord R. The epidemiology of wound infection. A ten-year prospective study of 62,939 wounds. Surg Clin North Am 1980;60:27.

Cuchural GJ, Tally FP, Jacobus NV, et al. Susceptibility of the *Bacteroides fragilis* group in the United States: analysis by site of isolation. Antimicrob Agents Chemother 1988;32:717.

Dicker RC, Greenspan JR, Strauss LT, et al. Complications of abdominal and vaginal hysterectomy among women of reproductive age in the United States. Am J Obstet Gynecol 1982;144:841.

DiPiro JT, Bowder TA, Hooks VH. Prophylactic parenteral cephalosporins in surgery. JAMA 1984;252:3277.

Donowitz GR, Mandell GL. Beta-lactam antibiotics. N Engl J Med 1988;318:490.

Dudley HAF, Sim A. AIDS: a bill of rights for the surgical team? Br Med J 1988;296:1449.

Duff P. Antibiotic prophylaxis for abdominal hysterectomy. Obstet Gynecol 1982;60:25.

Duff P, Park RC. Antibiotic prophylaxis in vaginal hysterectomy: a review. Obstet Gynecol 1980;55:1935.

Edlich RF, Rodeheaver GT, Thacker JG. Technical factors in the prevention of wound infections. In: Simmons RL, Howard RJ, eds. Surgical infectious diseases. New York: Appleton-Century-Crofts, 1982:chap 22.

Emmons SL, Krohn M, Jackson M, et al. Development of wound infections among women undergoing cesarean section. Obstet Gynecol 1988;72:559.

England GT, Randall HW, Graves WL. Impairment of tissue defenses by vasoconstrictors in vaginal hysterectomies. Obstet Gynecol 1983;61:271.

Eschenbach DA, Hillier S, Critchlow C, et al. Diagnosis and clinical manifestations of bacterial vaginosis. Am J Obstet Gynecol 1988;158:819.

Filker R, Monif GRG. The significance of temperature during the first 24 hours postpartum. Obstet Gynecol 1979;53:358.

Garibaldi RA, Brodine S, Matsumiya S, et al. Evidence for the non-infectious etiology of early postoperative fever. Infect Control 1985;6:273.

Garner JS. CDC guideline for prevention of surgical wound infections, 1985. Am J Infect Control 1986;14:71.

Gerberding JL, Henderson DK. Design of rational infection control policies for human immunodeficiency virus infection. J Infect Dis 1987;156:861.

Greenwalt TJ, Buckwalter JA, Desforges J, et al. Perioperative red blood cell transfusion. JAMA 1988;260:2700.

Grossman JH III, Adams RL, Hierholzer WJ, et al. Endometrial and vaginal cuff bacteria recovered at elective hysterectomy during a trial of antibiotic prophylaxis. Am J Obstet Gynecol 1978;130:312.

Hagen MD, Meyer KB, Pauker SG. Routine preoperative screening for HIV. JAMA 1988;259:1357.

Hager WD. Ob-gyn infections: bacterial causes and antibiotic choices. Contemp OB/GYN 1987;29:121.

Hager WD, Vernon M, Pascuzzi M. Efficacy of oral antibiotics following parenteral antibiotics for serious infections in obstetrics and gynecology. Abstr. #14. Snowmass, CO: Infectious Disease Society for Obstetrics-Gynecology, Aug 4, 1988.

Haley RW: Managing hospital infection control for cost-effectiveness. Chicago: American Hospital Publishing, 1986.

Hamod KA, Spence MR, Rosenshien NB, et al. Single-dose and multi-dose prophylaxis in vaginal hysterectomy: a comparison of sodium cephalothin and metronidazole. Am J Obstet Gynecol 1980;136:976.

Hemsell DL, Bawdon RE, Hemsell PG, et al. Single-dose cephalosporin for prevention of major pelvic infection after vaginal hysterectomy: cefazolin versus cefoxitin versus cefotaxime. Am J Obstet Gynecol 1987;156:1201.

Hemsell DL, Heard ML, Nobles BJ, et al. Single dose cefoxitin prophylaxis for premenopausal women undergoing vaginal hysterectomy. Obstet Gynecol 1984;63:285.

Hemsell DL, Hemsell PG, Heard ML, et al. Preoperative cefoxitin prophylaxis for elective abdominal hysterectomy. Am J Obstet Gynecol 1985;153:225.

Hemsell DL, Nobles B, Heard MC. Recognition and treatment of posthysterectomy pelvic infections. Infect Surg 1988;7:47.

Hemsell DL, Reisch J, Nobles B, et al. Prevention of major infection after elective abdominal hysterectomy: individual determination required. Am J Obstet Gynecol 1983;147:520.

Ho JL, Barza M. Role of aminoglycoside antibiotics in the treatment of intra-abdominal infections. Antimicrob Agents Chemother 1987;31:485.

Hoyme UB, Tamimi HK, Eschenbach DA, et al. Osteomyelitis pubis after radical gynecologic operations. Obstet Gynecol 1984;63:475.

Hussain SA, Latif AB, Choudhary AA. Risk to surgeons: a survey of accidental injuries during operations. Br J Surg 1988;75:314.

Iffy L, Kaminetzky HA, Maidman JE, et al. Control of perinatal infection by traditional preventive measures. Obstet Gynecol 1979;54:403.

John JF. What price success? The continuing saga of the toxic therapeutic ratio in the use of aminoglycoside antibiotics. J Infect Dis 1988;158:1.

Josey WE, Staggers SR. Heparin therapy in septic pelvic vein thrombophlebitis: a study of 46 cases. Am J Obstet Gynecol 1974;120:228.

Kaiser AB. Antimicrobial prophylaxis in surgery. N Engl J Med 1986;315:1129.

Kelen GD, Fritz S, Qaqish B, et al. Unrecognized human immunodeficiency virus infection in emergency department patients. N Engl J Med 1988;318:1645.

Klimek JJ, Ajemian ER, Gracewski J, et al. A prospective analysis of hospital-acquired fever in obstetric and gynecologic patients. JAMA 1982;247:3340.

Ledger WJ. Infections following gynecologic operations. In: Faro S, ed. Diagnosis and management of female pelvic infections in primary care medicine. Baltimore: Williams & Wilkins, 1985:chap 8.

Ledger WJ. Infection in the female. 2nd ed. Philadelphia: Lea & Febiger, 1986.

Ledger WJ, Campbell C, Wilson JR. Postoperative adnexal infection. Obstet Gynecol 1968;31:83.

Lett WJ, Ansbacher R, Davidson BL, et al. Prophylactic antibiotics for women undergoing vaginal hysterectomy. J Reprod Med 1977;19:51.

Lettau LA, Smith JD, Williams D, et al. Transmission of hepatitis B with resultant restriction of surgical practice. JAMA 1986;255:934.

McNamara MT, Mead PB. Diagnosis and management of the pelvic abscess. J Reprod Med 1976;17:299.

Magee C, Haury B, Rodeheaver G, et al. A rapid technique for quantitating wound bacterial count. Am J Surg 1977;133:760.

Marcus R. Surveillance of health care workers exposed to blood from patients infected with the human immunodeficiency virus. N Engl J Med 1988;319:1118.

Marsden DE, Cavanagh D, Wisniewski BJ, et al. Factors affecting the incidence of infectious morbidity after radical hysterectomy. Am J Obstet Gynecol 1985;152:817.

Mead PB. Cervical-vaginal flora of women with invasive cervical cancer. Obstet Gynecol 1978;52:601.

Mead PB. Prophylactic antibiotics in gynecology. In: Ledger WJ, ed. Antibiotics in obstetrics and gynecology. Boston: Martinus Nijhoff, 1982:3.

Mead PB. Antimicrobial therapy for gynecologic infections. ACOG Techn Bull 1986; No. 97 (Oct).

Mead PB. Enterococcus in obstetrics and gynecology. Infect Surg 1986;5(suppl):6.

Mead PB, Pories SE, Hall P, et al. Decreasing the incidence of surgical wound infections. Arch Surg 1986;121:458.

Mendelson J, Portnoy J, Victor JRDS, et al. Effect of single and multidose cephradine prophylaxis on infectious morbidity of vaginal hysterectomy. Obstet Gynecol 1979;53:31.

Micha JP, Jucera PR, Birkett JP, et al. Prophylactic mezlocillin in radical hysterectomy. Obstet Gynecol 1987;69:251.

Miles AA, Miles EM, Burke J. The value and duration of defense reactions of the skin to the primary lodgement of bacteria. Br J Exp Pathol 1957;38:79.

Moore EE. Early postinjury enteral feeding: attenuated stress response and reduced sepsis. Contemp Surg 1988;31:1.

Morrow CP, Hernandez WL, Townsend DE, et al. Pelvic celiotomy in the obese patient. Am J Obstet Gynecol 1977;127:335.

Neary MP, Allen J, Okubadejo OA, et al. Preoperative vaginal bacteria and postoperative infections in gynaecological patients. Lancet 1973;2:1291.

Nev HC. Clinical use of the quinolones. Lancet 1987;2:1319.

Ohm J, Galask RP. The effect of antibiotic prophylaxis on patients undergoing vaginal operations. Am J Obstet Gynecol 1975;123:597.

Ohm MJ, Galask RP. The effect of antibiotic prophylaxis on patients undergoing total abdominal hysterectomy. Am J Obstet Gynecol 1976;125:448.

Orr JW, Taylor PT. Avoiding postoperative infection in the patient with gynecologic cancer. Infect Surg 1987;6:666.

Roberts DB. Necrotizing fasciitis of the vulva. Am J Obstet Gynecol 1987;157:568.

Robson MC, Lea CE, Dalton JB, et al. Quantitative bacteriology and delayed wound closure. Surg Forum 1968;19:501.

Rosene K, Eschenbach DA, Tempkins LS, et al. Polymicrobial early postpartum endometritis with facultative and anaerobic bacteria, genital mycoplasmas and chlamydia trachomatis. J Infect Dis 1986;153:1028.

Rotter ML, Larsen SO, Cooke EM, et al. A comparison of the effects of preoperative whole body bathing with detergent alone and with detergent containing chlorhexidine gluconate on the frequency of wound infections after colon surgery. J Hosp Infect 1988;11:310.

Schottmueller H. Significance of several anaerobes in pathology, especially in puerperal illnesses. Mitt Grenzt der Med und Chir 1910;21:450.

Scott JR. Pelvic infections following vaginal hysterectomy. Hosp Pract 1973;8(Dec):101.

Sevin B-U, Ramos R, Lichtinger M, et al. Antibiotic prevention of infection complicating radical abdominal hysterectomy. Obstet Gynecol 1984;64:539.

Shy KK, Eschenbach DA. Fatal perineal cellulitis from an episiotomy site. Obstet Gynecol 1979;54:292.

Simmons BP. CDC guidelines for the prevention and control of nosocomial infections: guideline for prevention of intravascular infections. Am J Infect Control 1983;11:183.

Soper DE, Kemmer CT, Conover WB. Abbreviated antibiotic therapy for the treatment of postpartum endometritis. Obstet Gynecol 1987;69;127.

Spitzer M, Krumholz BA, Seltzer VL. Fevers in patients undergoing vaginal laser surgery. Obstet Gynecol 1988;71:480.

Stamenkovic I, Lew PD. Early recognition of potentially fatal necrotizing fasciitis. N Engl J Med 1984;310:1689.

Stovall TG, Ambrose SE, Ling FW, et al. Short-course antibiotic therapy for the treatment of chorioamnionitis and postpartum endomyometritis. Am J Obstet Gynecol 1988;159:404.

Strand CL, Shulman JA, eds. Bloodstream infections. Chicago: ASCP Press, 1988.

Swartz WH. Prophylaxis of minor febrile and major infectious morbidity following hysterectomy. Obstet Gynecol 1979;54:284.

Weinstein WM, Onderdonk AB, Bartlett JG, Gorbach Sl. Experimental intra-abdominal abscesses in rats. Development of an experimental model. Infect Immunol 1974;10:1250.

10

Wound Healing, Surgical Instrumentation, and Suture Material

MICHELLE R. DUDZINSKI

WOUND HEALING

The healing process is fundamental to all of surgery; without the ability to heal, no surgical trauma would be tolerated. This process, which is present in all tissues, allows for the repair of minor scrapes and bruises as well as major operative insults. Wound healing is identical, regardless of tissue type or degree of injury. The resultant scar formation, however, depends on the amount of tissue trauma and the foreign substances used to repair the wound. This chapter focuses on wound healing and its interaction with surgical technique, instrument choice, and suture selection.

Biologic Basis of Wound Healing

The wound healing process can be divided into four stages: inflammation, epithelialization, fibroplasia, and maturation (Fig. 10-1). Although these four phases afford an organized discussion of particular events during the healing process, they often occur simultaneously and in concert.

Inflammation

The initial response to injury is inflammation. This event can be divided into two separate processes, the vascular and the cellular response, which are initiated simultaneously. Immediately after injury there is a vaso-constriction of the local microvasculature that lasts for about 5 to 10 minutes and results in hemostasis and the accumulation of cellular elements within these vessels. Platelets accumulate in the wound and interact with thrombin to initiate clotting. The release of histamine from mast cells promotes subsequent vasodilation and an increase in vascular permeability, which results in the leakage of plasma and cellular elements into the area of injury. This is noted clinically as edema, or swelling.

Simultaneously the cellular response of the inflammatory process begins. Migration, margination, and diapedesis of leukocytes occur. Chemotaxis promotes the migration and concentration of polymorphonuclear leukocytes into the area of injury. These cells, which phagocytize and digest bacteria as well as foreign and necrotic debris by way of lysosomal enzymes, predominate for the first 2 to 3 days after injury. The activity of the polymorphonuclear leukocyte is completed by the 3rd postinjury day unless infection is present. Mononuclear leukocytes are transformed into macrophages, which migrate to the wound and become the predominant cells by the 3rd day, as described by Willoughby. These cells continue the work of phagocytizing bacteria and debris and are the characteristic cell of the chronic inflammatory response. As noted by Leibovich and Ross, they also play a critical role in attracting fibroblasts to the wound and initiating their maturation and proliferation. These fibroblasts may appear in the wound area as early as 24 hours after injury.

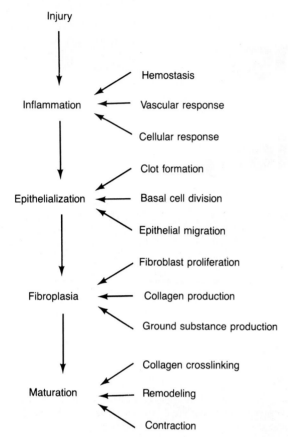

Figure 10–1. Stages of wound healing.

Epithelialization

The second phase of wound healing, epithelialization, as described by Odland and Ross, initially results in the formation of a superficial layer of cells across the wound. This layer serves as a protective barrier against bacteria and foreign substances. After injury basal cells surrounding the wound edge enlarge and proliferate. The formation of clot in the tissue defect creates an underlying fibrin bridgework on which the epithelial cells migrate across the wound (Fig. 10-2). This migration occurs from the wound edges toward the center and is governed by contact inhibition. Cessation of cell movement occurs when the epithelial cell comes into circumferential contact with similar cells. Within 48 hours the approximated wound edges may be completely covered with an epithelial layer. This layer is thin and poorly attached, which makes it highly susceptible to trauma. Proliferation and differentiation of epithelial cells continue until the epithelial layer is rejuvenated. Even this layer affords little structural integrity to the wound until an underlying fibrous scar forms. Failure of epithelialization to achieve coverage of injured tissue results in continued proliferation of basal cells, which may lead to malignant transformation. This potential is of particular importance in wounds associated with radiation injury.

Fibroplasia

Fibroplasia results in the formation of the fibrous scar that will ultimately afford tensile strength to the wound. The tensile strength of a wound is the load per cross-sectional area of tissue that can be supported by that wound; it is the most important feature of wound integrity. The process of gain in tensile strength by wounds has been well described by Howes and associates. Essential to fibroplasia is the differentiation of fibroblasts from local mesenchymal cells, which migrate into the wound as early as 24 hours after injury, as shown by Ross and coworkers. These cells attach to the fibrin scaffolding in the wound deposited during initial clot formation and undergo proliferation. Within 3 to 4 days these cells manufacture glycoproteins and mucopolysaccharides, which compose the essential elements of ground substance. This substance forms the milieu in which fibroplasia will occur. The fibroblasts then begin the production of collagen. They are the predominant cells in the wound by 10 days after injury, and may continue collagen production for up to 6 weeks. Collagen is a complex protein structure. There are five recognized, distinct collagen types that can be formed by various combinations of seven collagen chains (Table 10-1). Initially the fibroblast secretes triple-helical protein chains called tropocollagen. Each is composed of two identical α_1-chains and one distinct α_2-chain. Every third amino acid in each chain is a glycine. The molecular weight of the collagen molecule is about 300,000 daltons. These tropocollagen units bond into chains to form collagen filaments. These filaments form bundles that ultimately constitute strong collagen fibers (Fig. 10-3). The tensile strength of the wound is directly proportional to the production of these collagen fibers, and increases most rapidly during fibroplasia. Collagen provides the framework for new capillary formation, which in turn provides nutrients and oxygen to the healing wound. This complex of collagen and capillaries forms what is known as granulation tissue. By the end of 4 weeks the rate of collagen synthesis declines and the number of fibroblasts in the wound area decreases.

Maturation

Maturation, which includes collagen cross-linking, remodeling, and wound contraction, results in the final tensile strength of the wound and its ultimate appearance. The collagen scar formed during fibroplasia is characterized by a disorganized array of collagen fibers. Some of these fibers subsequently undergo degradation and are replaced by new fibers that are laid down in a more organized manner. These organized collagen fibers then

A. Cell migration
   with contact inhibition
B. Mitosis
C. Hemostatis/Vasoconstriction
D. Vasodilation/increased permeability
E. Endothelial buds
F. Fibroblast migration
G. Mononuclear leukocytes
H. Fibrin strands

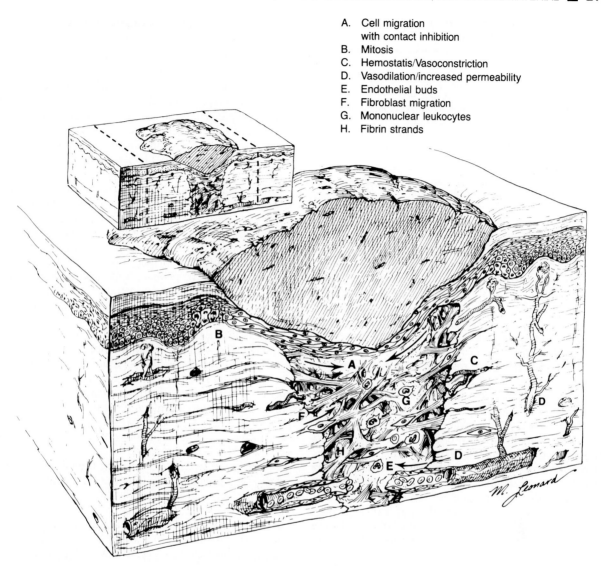

Figure 10–2. The wound healing process. (Adapted from Wound Healing. Ciba Clin Symp 1977; 29:11)

undergo covalent cross-linking to further increase the tensile strength of the wound. The balanced process of collagen degradation and production that allows organized cross-linking of the collagen fibers is known as remodeling. This process, which results in increased tensile strength, may continue for years. Skin wounds gain only 5% of maximum strength in the 1st week. Furthermore, the maximum tensile strength achieved in any wound usually is less than that of the unwounded tissue. Fortunately, in most circumstances, only 15% to 20% of unwounded strength is necessary to resist the stresses of daily life, and this is achieved by the 21st day post wounding (Fig. 10-4). The final appearance of the scar formation depends on the balance of collagen synthesis and break-down during remodeling. If collagen synthesis exceeds breakdown, exuberant scar tissue forms, resulting in hypertrophic scars or keloid formation. The predilection for keloid formation is familial.

Wound contraction may begin as early as 5 days after injury, and is characterized by the movement of the wound margins toward the center of the defect. During this process myofibroblasts actively use contractile proteins to reduce the separation of the wound margins, resulting in wound closure. The success of wound contraction in achieving this result is limited by the mobility of the surrounding tissue. Progression of wound contraction may result in debilitating deformity of the tissue surrounding the wound, known as contracture.

TABLE 10–1
Collagen Types

TYPE	TISSUE DISTRIBUTION
I	Skin, bone, ligament, tendon, fascia
II	Hyaline cartilage, intervertebral disk
III	Uterus, muscular arteries, intestine, adult and fetal skin
IV	All basement membrane structures
V	Amnion, chorion, synovium, cartilage, skeletal muscle, smooth muscle

(Adapted from Cuono CB. Physiology of wound healing. In: Dagher FJ, ed. Cutaneous wounds. Mount Kisco, NY: Futura Publishing Co, 1985:7.)

All tissues, including skin and viscera, heal by the same basic process described above. In most cases this healing process results in scar formation, as the ability to regenerate specialized tissues does not exist except in the liver and in simple epithelial surfaces such as gastrointestinal mucosa, respiratory epithelium, and epidermis. The formation of a fibrous scar in many tissues may be detrimental and result in pathologic processes. This is commonly seen after intra-abdominal operative procedures, with peritoneal scarring and resultant adhesion formation leading to visceral obstruction. Although there currently are no known methods to accelerate the healing process, scar formation can be reduced in certain circumstances by decreasing the inflammatory response. Minimization of tissue trauma by the use of meticulous surgical technique, proper instrumentation, and appropriate suture material may aid in this goal. The intraperitoneal instillation or systemic administration of various agents, including steroids, antihistamines, anticoagulants, antibiotics, antiprostaglandins, and dextran and other high-molecular-weight solutions, to prevent adhesion formation has been investigated, and continues to be an area of active research.

Wound Classification

Operative and traumatic wounds are classified according to the degree of bacterial contamination that is present at the time of injury. Classifications include clean, clean-contaminated, contaminated, dirty, and infected. These classifications can be used as indicators of the risk of subsequent wound infection, and may influence the method of wound closure. A clean wound is a nontraumatic, uninfected incision made under aseptic conditions that does not enter the respiratory, alimentary, oropharyngeal, or genitourinary tract. It is closed by primary approximation. The infection rate with this type of wound usually is less than 5%. A clean-contaminated wound is an operative wound that involves entrance into an uninfected respiratory, alimentary, oropharyngeal, or genitourinary tract. This type of wound usually is closed by primary approximation. The infection rate for a clean-contaminated wound is about 10%. Many gynecologic procedures, including hysterectomy and vaginal repairs, fall into this category. Included in this classification are clean wounds that have been contaminated by a minor break in aseptic technique. Contaminated wounds include operative procedures that involve gross soilage or fresh traumatic wounds. Procedures with spillage from the lower gastrointestinal tract or entry into an infected genitourinary or biliary tract are included in this category, as are operations with a major break in aseptic technique. The infection rate with this type of wound is about 15%. Closure of a contaminated wound depends on the clinical circumstance and the clinical judgment of the surgeon. Dirty and infected wounds are clinically infected before operation, heavily contaminated, or traumatic wounds more than 6 hours old. Procedures for existing infections or abscesses are included in this category. The infection rate with this type of wound approaches 30%.

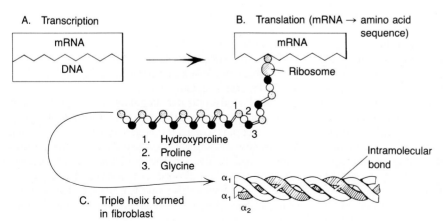

Figure 10–3. Formation of collagen. (Adapted from Wound Healing. Ciba Clin Symp 1977; 29:11)

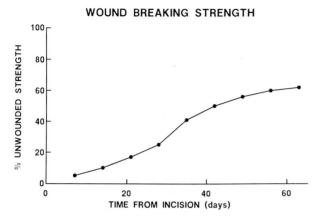

Figure 10–4. Percentage of unwounded strength achieved in the healing wound from time of incision.

Closure usually is by secondary intention or delayed primary closure.

Types of Wound Healing

The healing of surgical incisions or traumatic wounds is subdivided into three types, depending on the tissue injury and the nature of the wound closure. These types of wound healing are described as primary intention, secondary intention, and delayed primary closure.

Primary Intention

Healing by primary intention occurs when a surgical incision made with aseptic technique is reapproximated in a layered manner. The apposition of the tissue layers allows healing to occur promptly with minimal scar formation. This technique is appropriate for clean and clean-contaminated wounds as well as for some fresh traumatic lacerations.

Secondary Intention

Healing by secondary intention occurs when the skin and the subcutaneous tissues of a surgical or traumatic wound are allowed to heal by spontaneous closure. This is achieved by contraction and granulation. The wound usually is treated by frequent dressing changes, debridement, and irrigation to reduce the risk of infection and to promote healing. The wound heals from the wound surfaces gradually filling in the defect. With this technique healing time is prolonged and scar formation is excessive. It is appropriate for contaminated and dirty wounds.

Delayed Primary Closure

Healing by delayed primary closure occurs when tissues that had been allowed to granulate are subsequently approximated. These wounds are initially allowed to heal by secondary intention. The sutures for closure often are placed intraoperatively and left untied for subsequent use. Wound management should be aggressive in these patients, with daily debridement and more frequent wound dressing changes. As noted by Edlich and coworkers, once the open wound gains sufficient resistance to infection by the formation of granulation tissue, an uncomplicated closure can be performed. Optimal time for closure is variable, depending on the amount of tissue necrosis, initial risk of wound infection, and rate of granulation. Closure time usually is 3 to 6 days postinjury. In closing the wound the tissues should be carefully reapproximated as in a primary closure. According to Hugo and associates, delayed primary closure does not delay the development of wound tensile strength. Compared with healing by secondary intention, delayed primary closure lessens the total time required for wound healing and results in less scar formation.

Factors That Affect Wound Healing

There are a myriad of factors that may delay or interrupt the physiologic processes involved in wound healing. Some of the most important factors are local microvasculature and tissue oxygenation, the patient's age and underlying disease processes, the patient's nutritional status, and therapeutic and pharmacologic interventions. Although each of these factors is discussed separately, it should be kept in mind that several of these factors may coexist in the same patient and have cumulative detrimental effects on the wound healing process. Therefore, these factors must be identified and evaluated before decisions are made regarding the method of closure and subsequent wound management in an individual patient.

Microcirculation and Local Tissue Oxygenation

Local tissue perfusion and adequate tissue oxygenation are vital to the wound healing process. Any pathologic condition that interrupts or reduces local perfusion of injured tissue will severely compromise the healing wound. This may result from reduced perfusion pressure secondary to shock of cardiogenic, neurogenic, hypovolemic, or infectious origin. Furthermore, there may be compromise or interruption of the vessels that supply the injured tissues secondary to trauma, vasoconstriction, strangulating sutures, electrocautery coagulation, local external pressure, thrombotic or embolic occlusion, or underlying vascular disease. Local tissue perfusion also may be compromised by reduced environmental temperature leading to vasoconstriction in the injured tissue. In addition, elevated blood viscosity or an elevated hematocrit may lead to reduced flow secondary to sludging in the microvasculature. Abnormalities in coagulation may compromise tissue perfusion through embolic or thrombotic events. Bleeding disorders and platelet dysfunctions often lead to difficulties acquiring hemostasis in injured tissue, with subsequent seroma or hematoma formation. Such fluid collections may result in separation of the healing tissues as well as provide a medium for subsequent bacterial growth and infection. Therefore, sustaining local perfusion, correcting underlying coagulation disorders, and acquiring meticulous hemostasis are essential for adequate wound healing.

As well documented by Stevens, prolonged reduced oxygen tension has detrimental effects on healing tissues. Molecular oxygen is necessary for collagen synthesis, and as shown by Uitto and Prockop, formation of collagen under anoxic conditions may result in less stable collagen with fibers of low mechanical strength. Anemia reduces the oxygen-carrying capacity of the blood and can interfere with oxygen delivery to injured tissue. Anemia alone, however, may not result in decreased oxygen tension in the tissues. Therefore, although the correction of anemia may be important in many circumstances, maintenance of adequate local perfusion to injured tissues is essential for the normal wound healing process.

Patient's Age and Underlying Diseases

Both medical condition and age influence the patient's ability to heal surgical and traumatic wounds. There is evidence by Prockop and colleagues indicating that advanced age is associated with a delayed rate of wound healing. It is still uncertain whether this is due to more efficient healing mechanisms in younger patients or a consequence of frequent underlying disease processes in the elderly that interfere with wound healing. The optimal management of underlying disease before surgical intervention is therefore important in elderly patients.

Diabetes mellitus is one of the most frequently encountered disease processes that has a direct effect on wound healing. The diabetic patient's propensity toward atherosclerosis, small-vessel disease, impaired inflammatory response, and infection results in deficient wound healing and a higher incidence of wound complications. In atherosclerosis the blood flow to peripheral tissues is reduced, causing tissue hypoxia and malnutrition. Further compromise of tissue oxygenation may be caused by small-vessel disease. Insulin deficiency has been shown to impair the inflammatory response as well as cell proliferation. Insulin-deficient states adversely affect leukocyte phagocytosis, chemotaxis, and intracellular killing of bacteria. These defects in the inflammatory phase of healing result in impaired fibroblast proliferation and collagen synthesis, as shown by Leibovich and Ross. Diabetics also are more susceptible to infection because of their hyperglycemic state, poor vascular perfusion, and impaired leukocyte function. Cruse and Foord demonstrated a 10.7% rate of wound infection in diabetics, which was five times greater than that in nondiabetics. Obese patients also are at increased risk for wound infection. This may result from glucose intolerance in response to surgical stress. Control of diabetes in the perioperative period is imperative for adequate wound healing. This requires close monitoring of blood glucose levels with therapy by insulin, diet, or oral hypoglycemics, as required. Some diabetic patients must be admitted several days preoperatively to achieve maximum control of their diabetes before the surgical procedure. Postoperatively, during the wound healing process, continued surveillance and control of blood glucose levels are mandatory.

Patients with collagen vascular diseases or autoimmune diseases also are at risk for impaired wound healing. These patients may have compromise of the inflammatory response, deficits in collagen synthesis or aggregation, or reduced integrity of the microvasculature as a direct result of their disease process.

Patients with underlying malignancies may be compromised by nutritional deficits, metabolic derangements, immunosuppression, and hypercoagulability. Therapeutic measures such as chemotherapy and radiation therapy, which also may have detrimental effects on wound healing, are described separately. Likewise, any patient who is immunocompromised secondary to an infectious process or inborn deficiencies has a reduced inflammatory response and, consequently, an impairment in wound healing.

Nutrition

The patient's nutritional status plays an integral part in wound healing. Malnutrition leading to deficiencies of proteins, vitamins, or minerals significantly compromises the biologic processes involved in wound healing. Therefore, particular attention must be paid to these factors in patients with surgical and traumatic wounds.

Protein deficiency may impair wound healing. Rhoads and coworkers have demonstrated that protein depletion may prolong the inflammatory phase and impair fibroplasia. Peacock also has shown that the rate of gain of tensile strength is significantly reduced in protein-depleted animals. The mechanisms by which protein deficiencies affect healing tissues are largely unknown. The addition of the D- and L-form of methionine, or cystine to the diet of laboratory animals will reverse the effects of protein depletion. Cystine, a sulfur-containing amino acid, may be important in the healing process, since the development of disulfide bonds is necessary for the formation of tropocollagen.

Vitamins are essential to the healing process. The relation of vitamin C (ascorbic acid) to wound healing is well established. This vitamin is known to play a critical role in the hydroxylation of proline and lysine, which is essential for the cross-linking of collagen fibers during fibroplasia and remodeling. Consequently, a deficiency of vitamin C (scurvy) leads to a significant impairment in collagen aggregation, resulting in reduced tensile strength of healing or remodeling wounds. Repleting deficiencies of vitamin C is advantageous to the healing process; however, administering excessive amounts of this vitamin is not beneficial. The role of vitamin A in the healing process is unknown, but deficiencies may lead to abnormalities in wound healing. Ehrlich and Hunt have demonstrated that vitamin A is an antagonist to the inhibitory effects of steroid agents on wound healing. Specifically, vitamin A is thought to counteract the stabilization of lysosomal membranes produced by steroids. Vitamin E has been shown by Ehrlich and associates to interfere with collagen synthesis and wound repair. Its clinical use to prevent hypertrophic scar formation, however, is only theoretical.

The role of minerals in the healing process is well recognized. Ferrous iron is an essential mineral cofactor for the hydroxylation of proline and lysine during collagen synthesis. Copper is a critical cofactor for the polymerization of collagen molecules. Zinc is an essential cofactor for cellular proliferation; deficiencies of this mineral result in delayed epithelialization and decreased wound strength. Proliferation of inflammatory cells, fibroblasts, and epithelial cells are all facilitated by the presence of zinc. Magnesium also has been shown to play a role in the synthesis of collagen. Further research is needed to elucidate the role of other minerals in the healing process.

Pharmacologic Agents

Steroids, nonsteroidal anti-inflammatory agents, and chemotherapeutic agents may have significant effects on the healing process. It is essential, therefore, to identify which medications a patient has been exposed to before making decisions about wound closure and wound management.

The increasing use of steroids in the treatment of various disorders makes this type of medication a concern in surgical patients. Steroids have a myriad of effects on the wound healing process, including stabilization of lysosomal membranes, with resultant decreased inflammatory response; inhibition of fibroblast proliferation; reduction of the rate of protein synthesis, epithelialization, and neovascularization; reduction of tensile strength; and inhibition of contraction. Steroids cause the greatest impairment of wound healing when administered during the first 3 days after injury. Subsequent administration also may slow healing but to a lesser degree. Wound contraction is inhibited regardless of time of administration. The administration of vitamin A has been shown to reverse the effects of steroids on wound healing by counteracting the stabilization of lysosomal membranes, thereby allowing the inflammatory response to occur. The inhibition of wound contraction is not reversed, however.

Although a history of chronic steroid use is not a contraindication to surgical intervention, special care must to taken ensure wound integrity during the delayed healing process. The fascial wound layer should be closed with permanent suture, and the removal of skin sutures should be delayed. Consideration should be given to the use of internal retention sutures or stay sutures for added strength.

Steroids also are known to reduce the production of scar tissue and can be used to diminish keloid formation by intralesional injection. The resultant increase in collagenase activity with decreased collagen synthesis and inhibition of fibroblast proliferation results in keloid regression.

The use of nonsteroidal anti-inflammatory drugs for treating conditions associated with pain and inflammation is ubiquitous in today's society. In pharmacologic doses these medications reduce the inflammatory response, but they do not have a significant effect on wound healing. Consequently, no special closure techniques are required for wounds of patients who are taking these medications.

Patients who are receiving chemotherapy often require surgical intervention. The effects of chemotherapy on wound healing are not well defined. Although studies in laboratory animals demonstrate a detrimental effect of chemotherapy on wound healing, most clinical studies in humans have not demonstrated a significant increase in wound complications. Clinical studies involving nitrogen mustard, cyclophosphamide, thiotepa, vincristine, mitomycin, and doxorubicin (Adriamycin) demonstrate no significant increase in wound complications at therapeutic doses. Little data are available on 6-mercaptopurine, dactinomycin, bleomycin, cisplatin, and dacarbazine. The effect of methotrexate on wound healing can be diminished by the administration of folinic acid, and is of little clinical significance. Wound complications may be increased in patients receiving 5-fluorouracil in the first 2 weeks after surgery, and chronic topical application may totally prevent wound healing. The administration of chemotherapy alone, therefore, is not a contraindication to surgical intervention in most cases.

The systemic effects of chemotherapy, including neutropenia, thrombocytopenia, and malnutrition, may have a profound influence on the healing process. Neutropenia predisposes to wound infection, with resultant tissue necrosis and wound breakdown. Thrombocytopenia may result in hematoma formation and lack of apposition of the healing wound edges. Surgical intervention should be avoided in these patients until the bone marrow recovers. Malnutrition as a result of the malignant process or the emesis caused by chemotherapy also may significantly impair wound healing. The administration of parenteral nutrition may be necessary to replete protein, vitamin, and mineral stores before surgical therapy if adequate wound healing is to be expected.

Radiation

Radiation therapy, which frequently is used to treat gynecologic malignancies, can have profound detrimental effects on wound healing and indeed also can cause chronic nonhealing wounds in the radiation field. The prime cause of poor wound healing after radiation is the decrease in blood supply to the tissues, owing to an obliterative endarteritis of the microvasculature, as demonstrated by Telok and coworkers. Subintimal fibrosis ultimately results, with a decrease or total occlusion of the vascular lumen. The acute reaction of skin to radiation is erythema and desquamation. The skin normally heals by reepithelialization from remaining viable germinal cells. Chronically radiated skin may develop abnormal pigmentation and woody induration with fibrosis of the subcutaneous tissue and dermal thinning.

Chronic nonhealing wounds can result in the radiation field acutely if a sufficient dose is administered to prevent repopulation of the epithelial cells, or they can result years after radiation treatment by either spontaneous or traumatic breakdown of previously damaged tissues. These wounds are painful and extremely difficult to treat. They appear as necrotic ulcers with a raised edge. Such wounds can be difficult to differentiate from recurrent tumor, and show no tendency toward spontaneous healing. Unlike surgical wounds in healthy tissue, which heal with time, the necrosis of tissue caused by radiation tends to be progressive over time as the obliterative endarteritis leads to further fibrosis and ischemia. Although the newer, high-energy radiotherapy techniques are relatively skin-sparing, necrosis can still occur under intact skin with resultant ulcer formation; deeper tissues, such as the vaginal apex, also are at risk.

The therapy for radiation-induced ulcers begins with optimization of local and systemic factors. Nutritional support is important in malnourished patients. Local debridement, with the removal of necrotic tissue, and the implementation of antibiotic therapy may be necessary to eliminate any infectious process. No attempt should be made to debride until bleeding tissue is reached, as this may lead to an increase in the size of the wound. Occasionally, successful closure can slowly be achieved by vigorous wound care and the use of topical debriding agents. Hyperbaric oxygen therapy also has been used in the treatment of radiation ulcers. This technique may increase the oxygen tension in ishemic tissue and, therefore, promote wound healing.

The definitive treatment of radiation ulcers is wound closure. This requires total excision of all radiation-damaged tissues. Both the ulcer and the surrounding tissues should be excised until healthy, nonirradiated tissue is reached. If the area of damage is small, the wound may be closed primarily. To achieve a satisfactory closure without tension, a skin graft or myocutaneous flap often is required. A well-vascularized bed, which is necessary for the survival of a skin graft, is not always easily obtained after radiation therapy. If a skin graft is chosen as the method of closure, split-thickness grafts, which require less blood supply, have a greater chance of successful closure than full-thickness grafts. As noted by Robinson, the myocutaneous flap is ideal for closure of radiation defects, as it receives its blood supply from outside the radiation field, therefore obtaining oxygenation and nutrients independently of the radiated wound and also providing supplementation to the damaged bed.

When choosing the location of a surgical incision in a previously irradiated patient, the area of radiation should be avoided, especially if radiation-induced skin changes are present. When an incision must be made through previously irradiated tissue, there often is thin skin overlying densely fibrotic subcutaneous tissue, with little vascularity. Wound healing in such tissue is definitely compromised, and the type of closure to be used should be given serious consideration. Primary closure may be successful in wounds with minimal fibrosis, especially if care is taken to avoid bacterial contamination or seroma or hematoma formation. Secondary or delayed primary closure may be a wise choice in severely damaged tissues, as the risk of wound breakdown is high. Excision of the radiated tissues with subsequent closure of healthy tissue is ideal, but usually cannot be accomplished because of the extensiveness of the radiation damage.

Wound Infections

Wound infection is a possible complication whenever an incision in made; it also is dealt with in Chapter 9. The risk factors for wound infection are well known (Table 10-2). These include both surgical factors and patient-related systemic factors. The effects of tissue oxygenation, underlying disease, nutrition, pharmacologic agents, and radiation on wound healing have already been discussed.

Most wound infections are caused by bacterial contamination at the time of the surgical procedure. Wounds that contain more than 10^5 bacterial organisms per gram of tissue are at high risk for infection and breakdown. Patients who have undergone a surgical procedure for an intra-abdominal infection or who have had spillage of large-bowel contents during the procedure are at greater risk for significant wound contamination by bacteria.

Bacterial contamination may be prevented by adherence to strict aseptic technique. The skin should be prepared with a bactericidal solution, and the operative team should wash their hands and forearms thoroughly with a bactericidal preparation before making the skin incision. Gloves should be changed immediately if they are punctured or torn. An attempt should be made to clear an infection at a distant site in a patient about to undergo a surgical procedure, to prevent blood-borne contamination of the wound. Bacterial contamination during bowel surgery can be reduced by isolating the operative site from the remainder of the operative field, using laparotomy packs, and by using a separate set of instruments until the bowel is closed. All instruments and sponges used in the procedure should then be removed from the operative field.

Copious irrigation of the wound at the time of closure will decrease the number of bacteria present, and thus lower the risk of infection. Likewise, in patients who are at high risk for wound contamination, perioperative prophylactic antibiotics are useful to reduce the likelihood of infection. As demonstrated by Burke, antibiotics are most effective in preventing wound infection when given 1 hour before incision, thus ensuring that tissue levels of the antibiotic are present at the time of bacterial contamination.

Wound healing may be impaired and the number of bacteria necessary to produce infection reduced by several other surgical factors. Suture material acts as a foreign body in the wound, and may promote wound infection. De Holl and others demonstrated that the presence of suture material in a contaminated wound potentiates the development of wound infection. The use of suture material in the subcutaneous tissues should, therefore, be avoided, and is unnecessary if meticulous hemostasis has been obtained. If sutures must be used, a small-caliber, synthetic absorbable suture that is not highly inflammatory, such as polyglycolic acid (Dexon) or polyglactin 910 (Vicryl), should be chosen.

Drains placed in the subcutaneous tissue also act as a foreign body, and may potentiate infection, as demonstrated by Magee and associates. If meticulous hemostasis has been obtained and dead space will not be present in the subcutaneous tissue, drainage is unnecessary. The presence of dead space in the wound has been shown by de Holl and coworkers to potentiate infection. Occasionally, therefore, in the very obese patient on whom an extensive operative procedure has been performed, or when significant dead space is present, a subcutaneous drain may be indicated and should always be of the closed-suction type. Such drains should be brought through the skin by way of a separate stab incision, and should be removed as soon as possible.

Devitalization of tissue also promotes wound infection. Tissue in the wound may be devitalized by excessive use of cautery, excessive placement of sutures, or excessive mechanical trauma. Gentle handling of tissues and the use of electrocautery only as necessary to produce hemostasis are recommended. As previously stated, the use of sutures should be avoided except as needed to obtain hemostasis in larger blood vessels.

In 1982 the Centers for Disease Control gathered a group of physicians to develop guidelines for the prevention of surgical wound infection (Polk and coworkers). All gynecologists should be well versed in these guidelines and should apply them to their surgical practices (see box, pp. 218–219).

TABLE 10–2
Risk Factors in Wound Infection

Surgical Factors

Contamination
Devitalization of tissue
Presence of foreign bodies
Long operative time
Extensive wound dissection
Presence of dead space

Systemic Factors

Anemia
Past history of radiation
Underlying disease
Immunocompromised state
Malnutrition
Previous wound infection at same site
Infection at distant site

GUIDELINES FOR PREVENTION OF SURGICAL WOUND INFECTION

CATEGORIZATION

A categorization scheme has been used to rank each of the recommendations in the guidelines. A summary of the ranking scheme follows.

Category I (Strongly Recommended).—Measures in category I are strongly supported by well-designed and controlled clinical studies that show effectiveness in reducing the risk of nosocomial infections or are viewed as useful by the majority of experts in the field. Measures in this category are judged to be applicable to the majority of hospitals, regardless of size, patient population, or endemic nosocomial infection rate, and are considered practical to implement.

Category II (Moderately Recommended).—Measures in category II are supported by highly suggestive clinical studies or by definitive studies in institutions that might not be representative of other hospitals. Included in this category are measures that have not been adequately studied but have a strong theoretical rationale. Category II measures are judged to be practical to implement. They are *not* to be considered a standard of practice for every hospital.

Category III (Weakly Recommended).—Measures in category III have been proposed by some investigators, authorities, or organizations, but, to date, they lack both supportive data and a strong theoretical rationale. Thus, they might be considered important issues that merit further evaluation, and they might be implemented in some hospitals, especially those that have specific nosocomial infection problems or sufficient resources.

1. SURVEILLANCE AND CLASSIFICATION

1. *a.* At the time of operation or shortly after, all operations should be classified as clean, clean-contaminated, contaminated, or dirty and infected (category I).
   b. The classification should be recorded as such in the medical record (category II).
2. The person in charge of surveillance of surgical patients should gather information necessary to compute the classification-specific wound infection rates for all operations in the hospital. These rates should be computed at least every six to 12 months, entered into the records of the infection control committee, and made available to the department of surgery (category I).
3. Every six to 12 months, procedure-specific clean-wound infection rates should be computed for the hospital and all active surgeons. These rates should be given to all surgeons so that they can compare their own rates with those of others; the rates can be coded so that names do not appear (category II).
4. An effort should be made to contact discharged patients to determine the infection rate for the 30 days after operation (category III).

2. PREPARATION OF THE PATIENT

1. If the operation is elective, all bacterial infections that are identified, excluding ones for which the operation is performed, should be treated and controlled before the operation (category I).
2. The preoperative hospital stay should be as short as possible. In particular, tests and therapeutic measures that would prolong the stay beyond one day should be performed as outpatient services if possible (category III).
3. If the operation is elective and the patient is grossly malnourished, the patient should receive preoperative oral or parenteral hyperalimentation (category II).
4. If the operation is elective, the patient should bathe (or be bathed) the night before with an antiseptic soap (category III).
5. *a.* Unless hair near the operative site is thick enough to interfere with the surgical procedure, it should not be removed (category II).
   b. If hair removal is necessary, it should be done as near the time of operation as possible, preferably immediately before (category II).
6. *a.* The area around and including the operative site should be scrubbed with a detergent solution and then covered with an antiseptic solution. This area should include the entire incision and an adjacent area large enough for the surgeon to work during the operation without contacting unprepared skin (category I).
   b. Tincture of chlorhexidine, iodophors, and tincture of iodine are the recommended antiseptic products for preparing a patient's operative site. Plain soap, alcohol, or hexachlorophene is not recommended as a single agent for operative site preparation, unless the patient's skin is sensitive to the recommended antiseptic products. Aqueous quaternary ammonium compounds should not be used (category I).
7. For major operations involving an incision and requiring use of the operating room (OR), the patient should be covered with sterile drapes in such a manner that no part of the patient is uncovered except the operative field and those body parts necessary for the administration of anesthesia (category I).

3. PREPARATION OF THE SURGICAL TEAM

1. Everyone who enters the OR should wear at all times (1) a high-efficiency mask that fully covers the mouth and nose, (2) a cap or hood that fully covers the head hair, and (3) shoe covers. A beard should be fully covered by the mask and hood (category I).
2. *a.* The surgical team (those who will touch the sterile surgical field, sterile instruments, or an incisional wound) should scrub their hands and arms to the elbows with an antiseptic before each operation. Scrubbing should be done before every procedure and for at least five minutes before the first procedure of the day (category I).
   b. Between consecutive operations, scrubbing for two to five minutes may be acceptable (category III).
   c. Chlorhexidine, iodophors, and hexachlorophene are the recommended active antimicrobial ingredients for the surgical hand scrub. Aqueous quaternary ammonium compounds (eg, benzalkonium chloride) should not be used (category I).
   d. Hexachlorophene should not be used by pregnant women (category II).
3. *a.* After the hands are scrubbed with an antiseptic and dried with a sterile towel, the surgical team should don sterile gowns (category I).
   b. Gowns used in the OR should be made of reusable or disposable fabrics that have been shown to be nearly impermeable to bacteria, even when wet (category II).
4. *a.* The surgical team should wear sterile gloves. If a glove is punctured during the operation, it should be promptly changed (category I).
   b. For open bone operations and orthopedic implant operations, two pairs of sterile gloves should be worn (category II).

4. VENTILATION AND AIR QUALITY IN THE OR

1. All OR doors should be kept closed except as needed for passage of equipment, personnel, and the patient; personnel allowed to enter the OR, especially after an operation has started, should be kept to a minimum (category I).
2. For new construction, OR ventilation should include at least 25 air changes per hour. All inlets for outside air should be located as high above ground as possible and remote from exhaust outlets of

(continued)

all types. All air, recirculated or fresh, should be filtered before entering the OR (category I).

5. CLEANING AND CULTURING

1. The OR should be cleaned between surgical operations, daily, and weekly, according to established procedures for each scheduled cleaning (category I).
2. *Routine* culturing of the OR environment or personnel should *not* be done (category I).
3. Use of tacky or antiseptic mats at the entrance to the OR is *not* recommended for infection control (category I).

6. OPERATIVE TECHNIQUE

The surgical team should work as efficiently as possible in order to handle tissues gently, prevent bleeding, eradicate dead space, and minimize devitalized tissue and foreign material in the wound (category I).

7. WOUND CARE

1. Incisional wounds that are classified as dirty and infected should not ordinarily have skin closed over them at the end of an operation, that is, they should not be closed primarily (category I). (However, when an operation is performed to treat a low-grade infection involving an implanted device, it is sometimes better to close the wound after operation to prevent superinfection with microorganisms more virulent than those already causing infection.)
2. If drainage is necessary for an uninfected wound, a closed suction drainage system should be used and placed in an adjacent stab wound rather than the main incisional wound (category I).
3. Personnel should wash their hands before and after taking care of a surgical wound (category I).
4. Personnel should not touch an open or fresh wound directly unless they are wearing sterile gloves. When the wound is sealed, dressings may be changed without gloves (category I).
5. Dressings over closed wounds should be removed if they are wet or if the patient has signs or symptoms suggestive of infection, eg, fever or unusual wound pain. When the dressing is removed, the

wound should be inspected for signs of infection. Any drainage from a wound that is suspected of being infected should be cultured and smeared for a Gram stain (category I).

8. PROPHYLACTIC ANTIBIOTICS (GENERAL PRINCIPLES)

1. Parenteral antibiotic prophylaxis is recommended for operations that (1) are associated with a high risk of infection (eg, most alimentary tract operations, cesarean sections, hysterectomies, and selected biliary tract operations) or (2) are not frequently associated with infection but are associated with life-threatening consequences if infection occurs (eg, cardiovascular, neurosurgical, and orthopedic operations involving implantable devices) (category I).
2. Except in cesarean sections, parenteral antibiotic prophylaxis should be started within two hours before the operation. These antibiotics should not be continued for more than 48 hours, and a 12-hour limit is desirable for most types of wounds and operations (category I). (For cesarean sections, prophylaxis is usually given intraoperatively after the umbilical cord is clamped.)
3. Oral, absorbable prophylactic antibiotics should not be used to supplement or extend parenteral prophylaxis (category I).
4. If oral antibiotics are used as prophylaxis with colorectal operations, their use should be limited to the 24 hours before the operation (category I).
5. Antibiotics selected for use as prophylaxis should have been proved effective for prophylaxis of operative wound infections in randomized, prospective, and controlled trials whose results have been published (category II).
6. Antibiotics given to patients whose wounds are classified as dirty and infected should be considered therapeutic rather than prophylactic. The antibiotic and its duration of use should be determined by clinical factors, for example, the pathogens likely to be involved, the site and severity of infection, and clinical response (category I).

9. TOPICAL ANTIMICROBIAL PRODUCTS

If used in the wound, topical antimicrobial products, whether antibiotics or antiseptics, should be free of serious local or systemic side effects (category I).

(Polk HC, Simpson CJ, Simmons BP, et al. Guidelines for prevention of surgical wound infection. Arch Surg 1983; 118:1213.)

Wound Management

After closure of the wound, a sterile dressing should be applied. This dressing not only protects the suture line, but also immobilizes the skin around the wound. The dressing should be changed as necessary to keep the wound dry. The dressing may be removed after 48 to 72 hours.

Skin sutures or staples usually are removed by the 5th to 7th postoperative day to avoid the development of inflammation and epithelialized tracts around them. Further splinting of the skin should be provided by adhesive strips for about 21 days after suture removal, to prevent widening of the scar during collagen formation.

An infected wound should be opened to allow drain-

age of purulent material, and debrided of all necrotic tissue and foreign bodies. The wound should be packed open with sterile gauze. A debriding, cleansing, and packing regimen may then be used several times daily until healing is accomplished by secondary intention or until delayed primary closure is performed. Although many wound care regimens exist, sharp debridement followed by wet-to-dry dressing is commonly used. After removal of large necrotic tissue fragments with fine scissors and forceps, the wound should be irrigated with saline solution. A fine layer of saline-moistened gauze should be placed directly against the wound edges and then be covered by a dry dressing of sterile gauze. The entire dressing will dry over several hours and, when changed, will remove small pieces of necrotic material that will be adherent to the gauze. This regimen, when performed three to four times daily, allows the formation of healthy granulation tissue and secondary wound healing. Wounds left open at the time of the surgical procedure because of excessive contamination should be cared for in a similar manner. Once granulation tissue has formed, delayed primary closure may be performed.

Antibiotics are seldom necessary in the management of wound infection. Once drainage has been performed, local care usually is sufficient to result in the healing process. Occasionally a subcutaneous cellulitis may occur, and should be treated with aggressive systemic antibiotic therapy. Necrotizing fasciitis occurs rarely and can be life-threatening. Leukocytosis, fever, extensive erythema, soft-tissue swelling, and bullae formation are indications of this serious infection. Treatment consists of aggressive, wide surgical incision and drainage, with extensive debridement of all infected tissue. Broad-sprectrum systemic antibiotic therapy is necessary, including anaerobic coverage.

SURGICAL INSTRUMENTATION

Meticulous atraumatic surgical technique is necessary to avoid hindering the wound healing process by tissue devitalization. The gynecologic surgeon should be thoroughly familiar with the instruments available and their proper use. Excessively large pedicles and undue compression of tissues should be avoided.

Standard Surgical Instruments

Scalpels

Scalpel handles and surgical blades come in various sizes (Fig. 10-5). A standard No. 3 handle with a No. 10 blade is most commonly used to incise the skin. The correct method of holding the scalpel is shown in Figure 10-6. The blade should be held perpendicular to the skin when making the incision, to avoid beveling the skin edges. The belly of the blade, not the point, should be used. A No. 15 blade should be selected when making small incisions. For fine dissection the scalpel should be held like a pencil (Fig. 10-7), and the portion of the blade closer to the tip should be used. This technique permits greater precision and control. The No. 11 blade is most appropriate when performing a cold-knife conization, making a stab incision for drain placement, or draining abscesses. Longer knife handles are available for dissecting deeper tissues.

The scalpel is the instrument of choice for skin incisions. As demonstrated by Hambley and colleagues, it produces the least epidermal destruction and collagen denaturation compared with an ultrasonic knife, electrosurgery, or a carbon dioxide laser (Fig. 10-8). Faster healing also is evident. Madden and others have shown that wounds made with a steel scalpel are more resistant to infection than those made with a laser or an electrosurgical device. The use of separate scalpels for the skin incision and the incision of subcutaneous and deeper tissues is unnecessary and does not decrease the wound infection rate, as shown by Hasselgren and associates.

The scalpel also is a useful tool for intra-abdominal dissection. It may be used for the incision of uterine pedicles at hysterectomy and can be used with much precision in the lyses of bowel adhesions.

Scissors

There are a myriad of scissor types and sizes available for surgical dissection, some of which are shown in Figure 10-9. Mayo scissors are designed for cutting

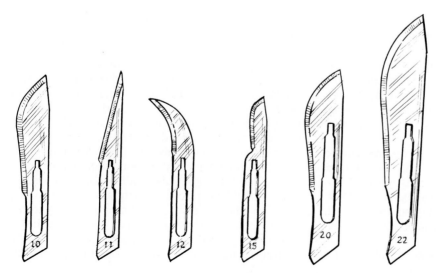

Figure 10–5. Surgical scalpel blades.

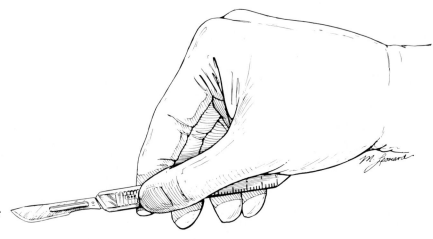

Figure 10–6. Proper technique for holding scalpel.

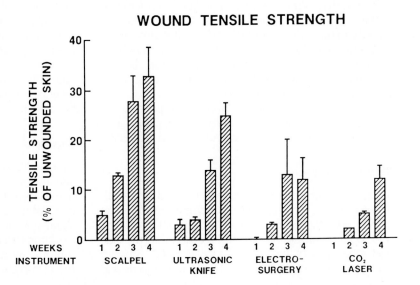

Figure 10–7. Scalpel technique for fine dissection.

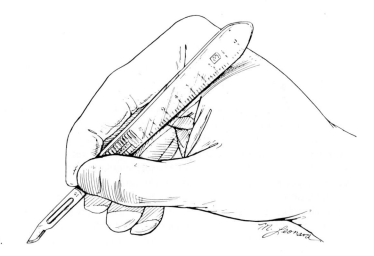

Figure 10–8. Wound tensile strength as percentage of unwounded pig skin for various instruments at weekly intervals. (From Hambley R, Hebda PA, Abell E, et al. J Dermatol Surg Oncol 1988; 14:1213)

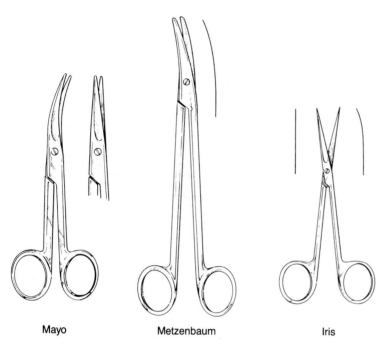

Mayo   Metzenbaum   Iris   **Figure 10–9.** Surgical scissors.

tough structures, such as fascia. They are available with either curved or straight blades. In gynecology Mayo scissors are most commonly used when entering the abdominal wall fascia; for dividing the round ligaments, infundibulopelvic ligaments, and parametrial and paracervical pedicles; and for incising the vaginal cuff.

Metzenbaum scissors are a much finer dissecting tool. They are lighter, with finer curved blades, and are used for both cutting and dissecting tissue. Metzenbaum scissors are used most commonly in gynecologic surgery for incising peritoneum, dissecting and incising intra-abdominal adhesions, and performing careful dissection, as in the retroperitoneal space. These scissors, as well as Mayo scissors, come in various lengths.

Mayo and Metzenbaum scissors that are used for incising tissue should not be used to cut suture material, as this may damage their blades. Instead, straight or curved suture scissors should be used. These also are available in various lengths, which can be chosen according to the depth of dissection.

Iris scissors are delicate instruments for precise dissection of small structures. They are most appropriately used in gynecology for vulvar and perineal surgery.

Tissue Forceps

Tissue forceps, both smooth and toothed, are available in varying lengths to grasp and immobilize tissue during dissection (Fig. 10-10). The size of the forceps and its teeth should be selected according to the size and toughness of the tissue to be grasped. Smooth forceps are most commonly used to stabilize tissue and to hold gauze sponges when packing or cleaning wounds. They are not used to grasp skin, as excessive pressure is required for adequate stabilization. The presence of teeth allows stabilization of tissue with minimal pressure. Toothed forceps should not be used on tissues that may be perforated. Thumb forceps with teeth and Russian forceps are commonly used when grasping fascial structures. The Adson forceps is useful in approximating the skin for staple or suture placement. Intra-abdominally, the DeBakey forceps is most useful when manipulating the peritoneum and when grasping fine bleeding points. The ring forceps can be used in the retroperitoneal space, as it has no teeth and, therefore, will not damage the pelvic vasculature.

When using forceps the tissue should be grasped only with enough force to manipulate and stabilize the tissue. Needles should never be grasped with tissue forceps, as this may destroy the forceps' fine teeth. Rather, in suturing, the tissue around the needle should be grasped and held in place until the needle driver can be used to complete the suture placement.

Clamps

Selection of the correct instrument can greatly facilitate the surgical procedure. Although the common names used for surgical clamps are not standard from one institution to another, a working knowledge of the clamps available is necessary.

Clamps used for hemostasis include the Halsted mosquito, Kelly, and Crile clamps (Fig. 10-11). The size of the clamp chosen should be governed by the size and

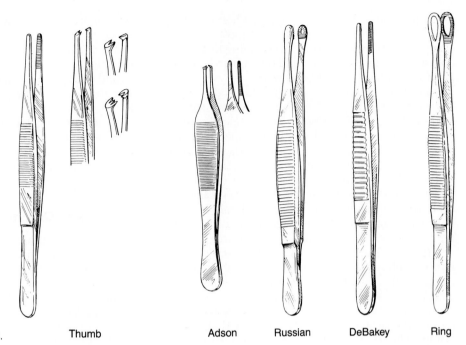

Figure 10–10. Tissue forceps.

Thumb   Adson   Russian   DeBakey   Ring

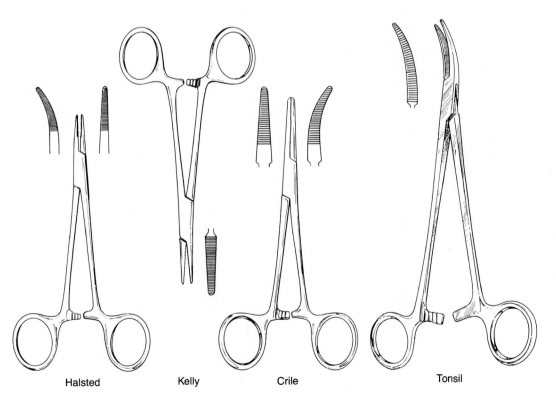

Halsted   Kelly   Crile   Tonsil

Figure 10–11. Hemostatic clamps.

location of the vessel to be clamped. When operating deep in the pelvis, the tonsil clamp is most useful for clamping small blood vessels. In obtaining hemostasis only the tips of the clamp should be used and only the point of bleeding should be grasped.

Many other specialized clamps are used in gynecologic surgery (Fig. 10-12). The Allis clamp has fine teeth, and is useful for grasping fascia, vaginal mucosa, and tissue to be removed as a biopsy specimen. The Kocher clamp has larger teeth and exerts much pressure. It is useful for grasping tough tissue, such as fascia, when strong traction is required. Kocher clamps also have been used to clamp the parametrial and paracervical tissues during hysterectomy. Care should be taken to avoid traumatization of the uterine vasculature with the teeth when using Kocher clamps in this manner.

The Babcock clamp has no teeth and is atraumatic. It is extremely useful for grasping and stabilizing the fallopian tube, round ligament, bladder, or bowel when atraumatic manipulation is required.

The most commonly used clamps for hysterectomy include the Heaney, Heaney-Ballantine, and Masterson clamps (Fig. 10-13), and the Kocher clamp. All are used to clamp the parametrial and paracervical tissue, with the Masterson clamp being the least traumatic (Fig. 10-14). Hysterectomy clamps are available with curved or straight blades. The curved instruments usually are used when clamping the infundibulopelvic ligaments, the uterine arteries, and the vaginal angles. The straight

varieties are useful when clamping the parametrial and paracervical tissues.

The right-angle clamp is extremely useful both as a dissecting tool and when passing suture material around pedicles. It often is used to develop the tunnel over the ureter during radical hysterectomy and to develop the avascular space under the infundibulopelvic ligament during simple hysterectomy. It also is appropriately used in developing the avascular space between the pelvic vasculature and the lymph node-bearing tissue during pelvic or para-aortic node sampling.

Hemostatic Clip Applicators

Hemostatic clip applicators, available in short and long lengths, are invaluable in obtaining hemostasis during radical pelvic surgery. They allow rapid ligation under direct vision of vessels in deep spaces that often are difficult to reach. Clips are available in small, medium, and large sizes, and should be chosen according to the size of the vessel or pedicle to be ligated. The metal clips are made of stainless steel, tantalum, or titanium, and are nonreactive in tissues and nonmagnetic. Titanium offers the advantage of producing less artifact on a computed tomography scan. All clips are radiopaque, which makes them useful in marking the location of intra-abdominal structures for postoperative identification.

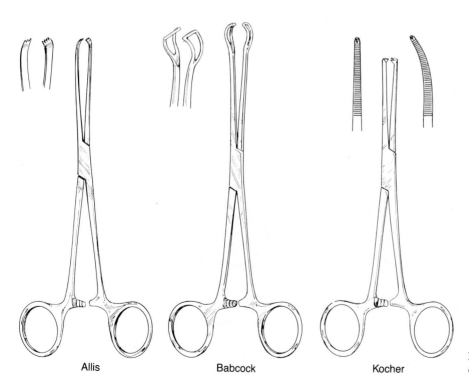

Allis   Babcock   Kocher

Figure   10–12. Specialized clamps.

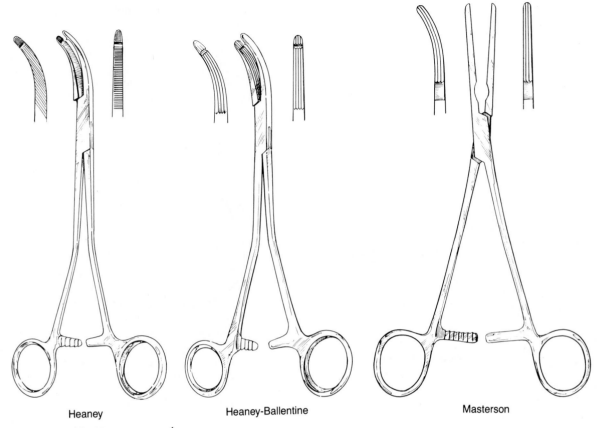

Figure 10–13. Hysterectomy clamps.

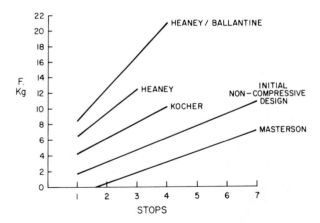

Figure 10–14. Forces exerted at a 2-mm opening and 1 cm from the tip by various gynecologic clamps. (From Masterson BJ, Sullivan TG. Am J Obstet Gynecol 1978; 132:113)

Automatic clip applicators, some with titanium clips, also are available, and can substantially lessen surgical procedure time and nurse workload. They are efficient and easy to use, and avoid the difficulty of premature closure of the clip applicator, with resultant loss of the

clip before application on the tissue. Some varieties of automatic applicators have somewhat larger heads, which can be difficult to use when delicate dissection is required.

Retractors

Both manual and self-retaining retractors are regularly used to obtain proper exposure, which is the key to success in pelvic surgery. The most commonly used self-retaining abdominal wall retractors are the Balfour and the O'Connor-Sullivan (Fig. 10-15). When using these retractors care must be taken to select the blade length that will provide adequate exposure without undue compression of underlying pelvic sidewall structures. Self-retaining ring retractors, such as the Bookwalter (see Fig. 10-15) and the Turner-Warwick, also are extremely useful in gynecologic surgery, especially in an obese patient. They offer a variety of blades of variable width and length that can be placed at any location around the ring, thus providing excellent exposure and often eliminating the need for additional hand-held retractors.

Manual retractors that are useful for skin and sub-

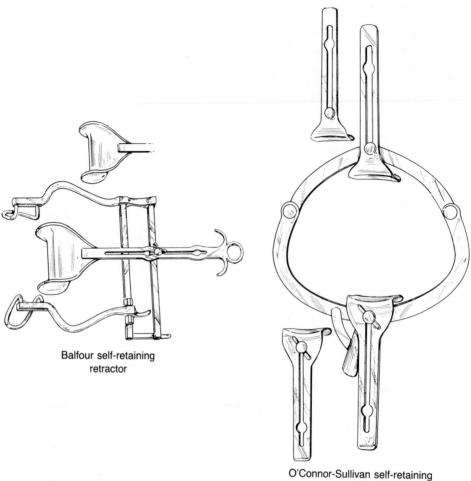

Balfour self-retaining
retractor

O'Connor-Sullivan self-retaining
retractor

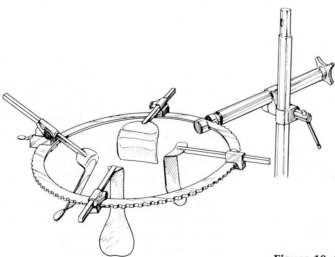

Bookwalter retractor

Figure 10–15. Self-retaining abdominal
wall retractors.

cutaneous tissue include the Army-Navy, Parker, small Richardson, and Weitlander retractors and various skin rakes and hooks. The larger Richardson and the Deaver retractor provide exposure intra-abdominally (Fig. 10-16).

Specialized retracting instruments, such as vein retractors and vessel loops, often are used for radical pelvic surgery. Specialized longer instruments and retractors also may be necessary when operating on an extremely obese patient. Availability of these should be assured before beginning the surgical procedure.

Electrosurgical Instrument

The electrocautery device was developed by William Bovie, an electrical engineer working with Harvey Cushing. Although the modern electrosurgical instrument is much more versatile than the original device,

the term "Bovie" is still routinely used when referring to all instruments of this class.

The Bovie can be used both to obtain hemostasis by coagulation of tissue and to cut tissue. In the coagulation mode short bursts of high-frequency electric current are generated, which allow cooling of the tissue between bursts and result in coagulation. When the Bovie is used on the cutting setting the energy output is continuous, resulting in vaporization of tissue with a cutting effect. Instruments also may blend the current for combined coagulation and cutting. This offers the advantage of obtaining hemostasis while incising the tissue. Twenty to 80 W are most commonly used.

The electrosurgical instrument is shaped like a pencil, and should be held as such (Fig. 10-17). The switches designating cutting or coagulation are easily operated by the index finger. In older models a foot pedal is utilized. Use of the electrosurgical device as a cutting instrument usually is begun after the skin incision has been made with a traditional scalpel. The

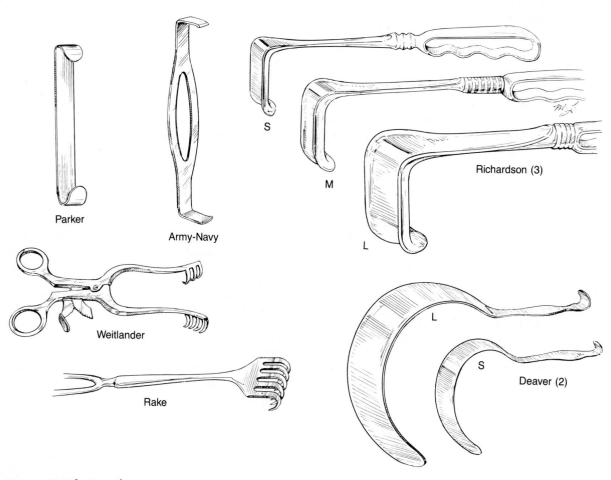

Figure 10–16. Manual retractors.

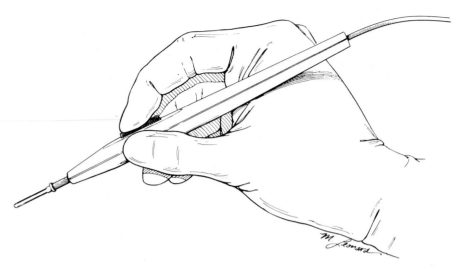

Figure 10–17. Technique of utilization of Bovie handpiece.

technique of handling the instrument is similar to that used to make an incision with a scalpel, and the tissues should separate quickly and easily. Care should be taken to avoid inadvertent incision of intra-abdominal structures that are adherent to the parietal peritoneum when using the electrocautery to make an abdominal incision. Carbon buildup on the blade should be removed regularly on a specialized scratch pad.

In using the Bovie for coagulation, the site of bleeding may be grasped with a fine clamp or tissue forceps and electric current applied to the clamp. The site of bleeding also may be coagulated by application of the Bovie tip directly on the tissues.

Surgical Stapling Instruments

Surgical stapling instruments are discussed in detail in relation to the specific procedures in which they are used. The discussion here is, therefore, limited to their relation to the wound healing process. Surgical stapling instruments that contain wire staples are widely used in bowel resections and anastomosis, and offer some advantages over conventional suturing techniques. The stapling instruments place a double row of B-shaped staggered staples that allow the microvasculature to course through the staple line (Fig. 10-18). This permits improved healing of the tissues, owing to greater vascularity. This is of utmost importance, especially in a patient who has undergone radiation. As demonstrated by Wheeless and Smith and shown in Figure 10-19, a stapled anastomosis has greater blood flow than a two-layer standard or Gambee anastomosis.

Healing of the stapled anastomosis is enhanced by the nonreactive nature of the wire staples, the uniformity of the anastomosis formed, and the increased speed

with which the procedure can be performed. There is little trauma to the tissues involved in the anastomosis; consequently there is relatively little fibrosis or adhesion formation around it.

Surgical stapling instruments also have been used in closing the vaginal cuff at the time of hysterectomy. The theoretical advantages of this technique are a shorter operating time and less contamination of the abdomen by vaginal bacteria. Wire staples initially were used. This method did not gain wide acceptance, as staples often would be visible at the vaginal cuff, sometimes caused dyspareunia or penile lacerations, and often had to be removed postoperatively.

A copolymer absorbable staple is available in a TA 55–type instrument with a rotating head for use on the vagina. The copolymer degenerates by hydrolysis, and maintains more than 50% tensile strength for longer than 2 months. Although the copolymer is relatively nonreactive, the staple size is quite large. McNeeley and colleagues demonstrated in rabbits that the copolymer-stapled cuff resulted in increased adhesion formation at the vaginal apex and greater tissue necrosis compared with chromic suture. There also was no decrease in bacterial contamination when utilizing the stapling technique. Many physicians routinely use vaginal cuff staplers, but others continue to close the vaginal cuff in the conventional manner with synthetic absorbable sutures. Lesser acceptance of the vaginal cuff staples, compared with the intestinal staples, may be due to increased tissue necrosis, difficulty of placement of the stapling instrument into some pelves, expense of the instrument, and the relative quickness and ease with which the cuff can be closed in the conventional manner. Analysis of further use will be necessary to determine if there is any advantage of the absorbable vaginal cuff staples over the conventional suture closure.

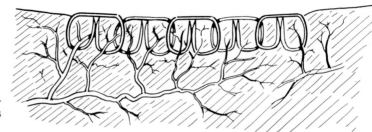

Figure 10–18. Microvasculature remains intact owing to staggered nature of surgical staples in double B formation.

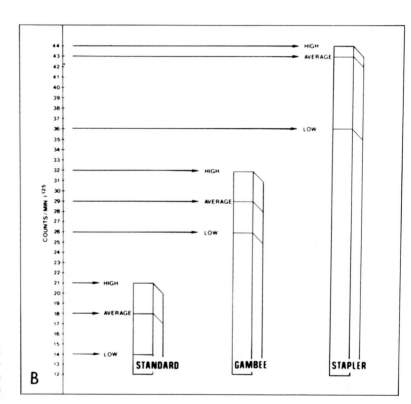

Figure 10–19. Counts per minute of ^{125}I flowing through three anastomoses: standard, Gambee, and stapler. (From Wheeless CR, Smith JJ. Obstet Gynecol 1983; 62:513)

Cavitron Ultrasonic Surgical Aspirator

The Cavitron Ultrasonic Surgical Aspirator (CUSA) has come into widespread use for tumor debulking in gynecologic oncology. The instrument consists of the main control console, which regulates power, and the handpiece, which is gas sterilizable. The handpiece, which is held like a pencil (Fig. 10-20), is available straight or angled, and consists of a titanium hollow tip with a 2-mm opening, a protective plastic flue that exposes only the last 4 mm of the titanium amplifier, and an electric coil and transducer. As described by Chopp and coworkers, alternating the electromagnetic field 23,000 times per second results in expansion and contraction of the transducer, which is amplified by the connecting body and tip. When in use the interchange-able tip has a longitudinal excursion of 150 μm around the resting position, with a resultant 300-μm total stroke. This fragments tissue in a 1- to 2-mm radius around the tip.

The vibration produces considerable heat, and cooling is provided by saline irrigation over the tip at a rate of 3 to 10 ml/min. This solution mixes with the fragmented tissue and is removed by way of the suction device. The tissue is collected in a cannister in the control console, and can be pathologically evaluated by histologic or cytologic techniques. As demonstrated by Chopp and others, the tissue cell damage produced by the CUSA is 25 to 30 μm, and is similar to that produced by a cold scalpel. This is in contrast to the 75 to 100 μm of tissue cell damage produced by electrocautery.

Fragmentation of tissue with the CUSA depends on

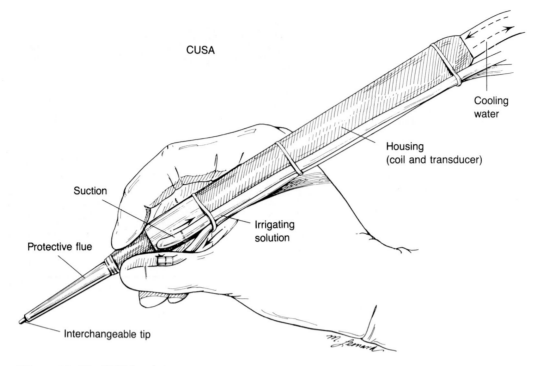

CUSA

Cooling
water

Housing
(coil and transducer)

Suction

Irrigating
solution

Protective flue

Interchangeable tip

Figure 10–20. CUSA handpiece.

tissue water content. The higher the water content, the less power required to fragment tissue. Fibrous tissue is much more resistant to fragmentation, and requires more power. Because blood vessels usually are more fibrous than surrounding tissues, proper use of the CUSA can result in removal of tissue with isolation of the blood vessels, which can then be ligated for hemostasis. When the CUSA is used at a higher power setting, fragmentation is more rapid and blood vessels may be punctured.

The CUSA is most commonly used in gynecologic surgery for ovarian carcinoma debulking. Although its use can be time-consuming, it allows removal of tumor tissue from the diaphragm, bowel serosa, stomach, and spleen that might otherwise not be resectable, and does so without damage to underlying structures. It can, therefore, aid in optimal debulking without major organ resection. Although many ovarian carcinoma tumor implants can easily be removed using the CUSA, those that are densely fibrotic or calcified may present some difficulty.

Reports of the use of this instrument in ovarian carcinoma debulking by Adelson and colleagues and Deppe and colleagues suggest that a combination of standard surgical resection and CUSA aspiration may be best for maximal tumor removal with acceptable operating time. Further investigation will be necessary to determine if the added tumor removal possible with the CUSA results in a survival advantage for patients.

SUTURE MATERIALS

Modern suture materials have been designed to combine the qualities of low tissue reaction, resistance to infection, knot security, maintenance of tensile strength, and ease of handling. Sutures can be divided into categories of absorbable and nonabsorbable and further subdivided into natural or synthetic, monofilament or polyfilament. In this section, characteristics of the available suture materials, surgical knots, surgical needles, and needle drivers are examined.

General Characteristics of Suture Material

The general characteristics of suture material are well described in the *Wound Closure Manual* distributed by Ethicon, Inc. Because all suture materials are foreign substances, the smallest-caliber suture material of sufficient strength to hold the tissues should be used. Suture sizes are derived from thread sizes, as simple thread was used as the first suture material. The largest nonsteel suture size available is No. 5, and the caliber of the suture decreases as size decreases to No. 0. Smaller suture is designated as 00, 000, 4-0, and downward, with the smallest size available being 11-0. As depicted by Stone, the diameter allowable for each suture size is a range; therefore, not all suture materials of the same

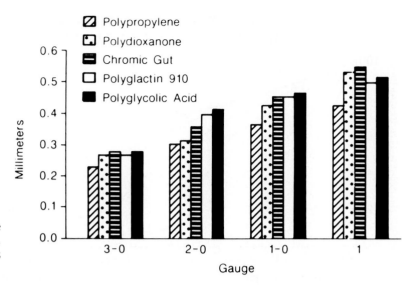

Figure 10–21. Suture diameters of five commonly used materials in four gauges. (From Stone IK. Clin Obstet Gynecol 1988; 31:712)

size are identical in diameter (Fig. 10-21). The degree of adhesion formation around suture material correlates with the suture size, as demonstrated by Holtz. Therefore, especially for intra-abdominal sutures, the smallest possible size of appropriate tensile strength should be chosen.

The knot-pull tensile strength of different sutures varies widely; data for each type are available from the manufacturer. In general, the tensile strength of the suture chosen should be governed by the strength of the tissues into which the suture is placed. The pull-out strength (in pounds) in tissues, as determined by van Winkle and Hastings, are as follows: fascia, 8.3; muscle, 2.8; peritoneum, 1.9; and fat, 0.44. The knot-pull tensile strength (in pounds) for various sutures has been determined by Ethicon (Table 10-3). As can be seen, a smaller-diameter synthetic absorbable suture has about the same tensile strength as surgical gut that is one size larger. The use of a synthetic absorbable suture will, therefore, allow the surgeon to choose a suture of smaller diameter, which causes less tissue reaction.

As the synthetic suture materials are absorbed, they gradually lose tensile strength. The tensile strength of various sutures in vivo after 1 to 6 weeks is shown in Figure 10-22 (data from Ethicon). As can be seen, absorbable braided sutures (Vicryl, Dexon) lose about 35% to 40% of their tensile strength by 2 weeks, and by 5 weeks they have little remaining strength. Of the monofilament absorbable sutures (polyglyconate [Maxon] and polydioxanone [PDS II]), PDS II retains its tensile strength longest, with about 50% remaining at 6 weeks.

Although all suture materials cause some degree of tissue reaction, some are more inert than others. As discussed by Sanz and colleagues, all suture materials produce some degree of inflammation for the first 5

TABLE 10–3
Knot-Pull Tensile Strength (in Pounds)

SIZE	ABSORBABLE SUTURES		NONABSORBABLE SUTURES	
	Gut	*Vicryl*	*Silk*	*Prolene*
1	11.1	14.8	8.8	11.0
0	8.4	10.8	6.8	7.8
00	5.7	7.9	5.0	5.7
000	3.9	5.0	3.1	3.8

(Adapted from Ethicon. Wound closure manual. Somerville, NJ: Ethicon, 1985:96.)

days after placement. The reaction consists of both acute and chronic inflammatory cells. After this initial period the inflammation is predominantly chronic, and the degree of inflammatory response varies with suture type (Fig. 10-23). Absorbable synthetic materials in general are degraded by hydrolysis, and elicit less inflammatory response than naturally occurring materials, which are degraded by phagocytosis. The maintenance of tensile strength of surgical gut may be markedly decreased in the presence of infection. Nonabsorbable synthetic sutures demonstrate very low tissue reactivity. They do not undergo hydrolysis or phagocytosis, but become permanently encapsulated within the surrounding tissues.

Both absorbable and nonabsorbable sutures may be monofilament or polyfilament. In general, multifilament sutures exhibit better handling characteristics and ease of tying than the monofilament. The monofilament sutures also are more easily damaged in handling, which may result in loss of tensile strength. The braided sutures, however, may be more easily contaminated by

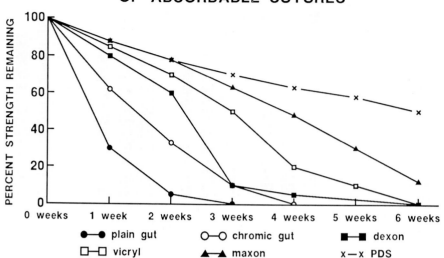

IN VIVO TENSILE STRENGTH OF ABSORBABLE SUTURES

Figure 10–22. The tensile strength of various suture materials after 1 to 6 weeks in vivo. (Data on file, Ethicon Research Foundation)

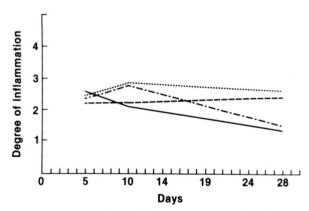

Figure 10–23. Inflammatory response at 5, 10, and 28 days after surgery by type of suture used: chromic catgut (dotted line), Vicryl (dashed line), Maxon (dot-dashed line), and PDS (solid line) sutures. (From Sanz LE, Patterson JA, Kamath R, et al. Obstet Gynecol 1988; 71:418)

bacteria. This may result in chronic suture infection, as bacteria between the braids may not be accessible to the leukocytes of the normal inflammatory response. Braided suture should, therefore, be used with caution in the presence of infection.

Absorbable Sutures

Table 10-4 lists various absorbable sutures and their characteristics. Loss of tensile strength of several absorbable sutures is shown in Figure 10-22. The rate of absorption is independent of loss of tensile strength, and varies with the suture material. Sutures may retain

tensile strength for prolonged periods and then absorb rapidly, or they may lose tensile strength rapidly and absorb slowly.

For many years catgut was the main suture material used by gynecologists for pelvic surgery. The synthetic absorbable sutures now available offer many advantages over catgut, and the use of catgut in gynecology is appropriately decreasing.

Natural Absorbable Suture. Surgical plain and chromic catgut are manufactured from the submucosa of sheep intestine or the serosa of beef intestine, treated with formaldehyde to increase tensile strength, and twisted into strands to make various caliber threads. Treating plain catgut with chromium salts causes intramolecular cross-linking, which results in stronger tensile strength and slower absorption. The advantages of catgut include excellent knot-holding properties and ease of handling. The disadvantages include the intense inflammatory reaction, with resultant scarring produced by the foreign protein, and rapid loss of tensile strength, especially when infection is present. Tensile strength of plain catgut is maintained for only 7 to 10 days, and phagocytosis of the suture is complete by 70 days. Chromic catgut maintains tensile strength for 14 to 28 days and is absorbed by 90 days.

Most surgeons choose the synthetic absorbable sutures over catgut for the majority of surgical procedures, to avoid the intense tissue reaction. Catgut should not be routinely used in gynecologic surgery. Indeed, there remains little indication for the use of catgut in any gynecologic surgical procedure.

Synthetic Absorbable Sutures. The introduction of polyglycolic acid (Dexon) and polyglactin 910

TABLE 10–4
Characteristics of Absorbable Suture Materials

TYPE	BASIC MATERIAL	TIME TO COMPLETE ABSORPTION	TISSUE REACTIVITY
Plain catgut	Sheep or cattle intestine	70 days	Moderate
Chromic catgut	Catgut treated with chromium salt	90 days	Moderate
Vicryl	Polyglactin 910	56–72 days	Mild
Dexon	Polyglycolic acid	40–90 days	Mild
PDS II	Polydioxanone		Slight
Maxon	Polyglyconate	180 days	Slight

(Vicryl) in the early 1970s has revolutionized surgical sutures, and most surgeons use these materials. Dexon is composed of thin filaments of a linear copolymer of glycolic acid that are braided into various sizes of polyfilament suture. Vicryl is composed of a copolymer of lactic and glycolic acid that is melted, stretched into filaments, and braided. Both cause minimal tissue reaction and hold their tensile strength well, retaining 60% to 65% of tensile strength at 2 weeks. Dexon and Vicryl are degraded by slow hydrolysis. Absorption is minimal until 30 to 40 days and is complete by 90 to 120 days. Vicryl is absorbed slightly faster than Dexon.

Dexon and Vicryl maintain good knot security. Their ease of handling is improved by coating the fibers. A compulsive square knot-tying technique should be used with these materials, as incorrectly tied knots tend to slip. Using a surgeons' knot as the first throw will offer additional security, as will adding two additional hitches and a longer cut end of 8 to 10 mm.

Another advantage of these sutures is their resistance to breakage. Because of this, it is possible to use a much smaller caliber material than would be necessary for catgut. Thus, almost all pelvic surgery can be accomplished with 2-0 or smaller ligatures and sutures. Larger pedicles may require 0 caliber to allow cinching down without cutting, but seldom is No. 1 suture required. Except in special circumstances, virtually all visceral suturing can be accomplished with these materials.

Maxon and PDS II are synthetic absorbable monofilament sutures with high tensile strength that is maintained for extended periods. About 70% to 80% of their tensile strength is maintained at 2 weeks and 50% to 60%, at 4 weeks. They cause only slight tissue reaction. Like Dexon and Vicryl, they are absorbed by slow hydrolysis. Absorption is minimal until about the 90th day and is not complete until about 180 days. The absorption rate for PDS II has recently been improved, and the new data are not yet available.

Maxon and PDS are extremely useful when tensile strength is required for prolonged periods, such as in fascial closure, and in most circumstances can be used in place of nonabsorbable sutures. Because of their monofilament construction, they may be used in the presence of infection. The main disadvantage of these materials is the poor handling qualities found with most monofilament suture. Multiple knots are required for adequate knot security.

Nonabsorbable Sutures

A suture that maintains its tensile strength for more than 60 days may be considered nonabsorbable (Table 10-5). Such sutures must be removed when placed in exposed tissues and will become encapsulated when surrounded by tissues. Although most nonabsorbable sutures remain permanently encapsulated in the body tissues, silk is gradually absorbed over about 2 years, and nylon degrades at 15% to 20% per year. Since the introduction of the delayed absorbable synthetic sutures, the frequency of use of nonabsorbable sutures in gynecologic surgery has been decreasing.

Natural Nonabsorbable Suture. Silk and cotton have been used as suture material for decades. Indeed, surgical silk's superb ease of handling and knot control are the standards by which other suture materials are judged. Silk, however, causes more tissue reaction than any other nonabsorbable suture. This intense inflammatory reaction can lead to sinus formation, expulsion, and frank infection. To form silk suture, silk filaments are braided or twisted together. For this reason silk suture should not be used in contaminated tissues.

The use of silk has been supplanted somewhat by absorbable synthetic sutures. Because of its good handling characteristics, however, it is still used by many surgeons, especially for gastrointestinal surgery.

Surgical cotton is seldom used in gynecologic surgery. It is the weakest of nonabsorbable materials, but may have increased tensile strength when wet. It loses 50% of tensile strength in 6 months and 60% to 70% by 2 years. Cotton has poor handling qualities when wet and is now seldom used.

Metal Suture. The use of metal as a suture material

TABLE 10–5
Characteristics of Nonabsorbable Suture Materials

GENERIC NAME	TRADE NAME	BASIC MATERIAL	TISSUE REACTIVITY
Surgical cotton		Natural cotton fibers	Moderate
Surgical silk		Raw silk	Moderate
Nylon	Dermalon	Monofilament	Low
	Ethilon	Monofilament	
	Neurolon	Multifilament	
	Surgilon	Multifilament	
Polypropylene	Prolene	Monofilament	Minimal
Polyester	Mersilene	Braided–plain	Minimal
	Ethibond	Braided–coated	Minimal
	Tevdek	Braided	Mild
Surgical steel	Flexon	Monofilament	Low
		Multifilament	

has strong historical significance. James Marion Sims used silver wire in his landmark repairs of fistulas, and generations of pelvic surgeons used stainless steel wire in the fascial closure of contaminated wounds and the reclosure of abdominal evisceration. Stainless steel wire is the strongest available suture material with the greatest knot security. It has little tissue reactivity. Its major drawbacks are its extremely poor handling characteristics. It tends to kink and can fracture at points of deformity. It is difficult to tie, and when larger sizes are used, it is twisted and not tied. Surgical steel also can puncture gloves, and injure operating room personnel. The wide variety of synthetic nonabsorbable sutures have made the use of wire almost obsolete.

Synthetic Nonabsorbable Suture. Nylon suture is available in both monofilament and multifilament form. It is nonreactive in tissues, has a very high tensile strength, and degrades slowly by hydrolysis at 15% to 20% per year. Monofilament nylon sutures offer relatively poor handling and knot security. The initial throw should be a surgeons' knot followed by a minimum of five additional throws for adequate knot security. This suture should not be used for fascial closure in slender patients, as the voluminous knot may be palpable through the skin. The technique of burying the knot beneath the fascia when using a running closure should be used. Braided nylon offers improved handling properties but should not be used if infection is present. Polypropylene suture is similar in characteristics to nylon, offering minimal tissue reaction and indefinite high tensile strength. This monofilament suture is totally nonabsorbable.

Polyester, the strongest of the synthetic nonabsorbable sutures, has a tensile strength slightly greater than nylon and polypropylene. It elicits minimal tissue reaction and maintains its tensile strength indefinitely. All polyester sutures are braided and should not be used in the presence of infection or contamination. Some manufacturers have produced coated polyester sutures with improved handling characteristics but poorer knot security. A minimum of five knot throws should be used for adequate knot security.

Suture Selection

Suture selection should be based on the strength of the tissues being sutured, the rapidity of healing of these tissues, the need for nonreactivity (presence or absence of infection), and the handling characteristics and knot security of the suture material. The variety of suture materials currently available and their outstanding characteristics frequently make the choice of suture a matter of personal preference, institutional tradition, training bias, and availability. Suture length should be determined by the depth of dissection. The length should be sufficient to facilitate the tying of a secure knot. Cost may mandate the suture used, as manufacturers attempt to enter into exclusive contracts with hospitals to keep costs down.

Surgical Needles and Needle Holders

There are a myriad of needles available, of which most surgeons use relatively few. Needles are available as free needles, which have an eye and must be threaded with the suture material, or as swaged needles, which have the suture material already attached. Swaged needles offer the advantage of being a continuous unit without the added bulk of eye and threaded suture material and, therefore, lessen tissue trauma. Swaged needles are always new and sharp, and are discarded after use. There also is a decreased probability of inadvertent glove puncture, as the needles do not require threading, which minimizes handling. The swaged needle eliminates the frustration of the suture unthreading inadvertently, which occurs with rethreadable needles, and also makes misplaced needles easier to locate because of the attached suture material. Most surgeons currently use swaged needles for gynecologic procedures.

Swaged needles are available with suture and needle either permanently affixed or with the ability for controlled release. With controlled-release sutures (pop-offs) the suture can be quickly removed from the needle with a slight tug of the needle driver. The use of these needles greatly increases the speed with which interrupted sutures can be placed.

Needles used in gynecologic surgery are, for the most part, straight or curved and of an atraumatic tapered or cutting variety (Fig. 10-24). Straight needles, such as the Keith cutting needle, are most commonly used in suturing skin and are used by hand. Curved needles are available as 1/4, 3/8, 1/2, and 5/8 circles. The choice of needle size and curvature depends on the tissue to be sutured and the depth of dissection. The most commonly used needles are the 3/8 and 1/2 circles. The greater the curvature of the needle, the more easily it can be manipulated in deep, confined spaces.

Tapered needles are designed to be atraumatic, and are used for most gynecologic surgery. They produce the smallest hole possible in the tissue being sutured and the least tissue trauma. They are used for all aspects of gynecologic surgery except skin closure. The CT needle is most commonly used in the ligation of the pedicles during hysterectomy and in the closure of the abdominal wall. The SH needle is smaller and tapered, which is extremely useful for suture ligature of small pedicles and blood vessels. The MO needle, which is somewhat heavier and tapered, is useful in denser tissues.

Cutting needles have at least two honed edges that will cut through tough tissue and are, therefore, most useful in closing skin. A conventional cutting needle has its third cutting edge on the inside, concave surface of the needle and easily cuts tissue in the direction of the pull of the needle. The reverse cutting needle has its third cutting edge on the outside, convex surface of the needle, which reduces the possibility of inadvertently cutting through tissue at the edges of the incision. Retention needles are of the reverse cutting variety. Cutting needles produce a larger hole than tapered needles, and great care must be taken in their use to avoid unnecessary laceration of the tissues being sutured. They are never used intra-abdominally, as there would be a possibility of lacerating blood vessels and other delicate tissues.

Tapercut needles, which combine a reverse cutting edge for the first 1/32 in with a tapered body, and blunt needles with a tapered body and a rounded blunt point also are available.

All curved needles are designed to be used with a needle holder. The ease of suturing with a curved needle depends on the duplication of the needle's curve by the needle driver as the suture is placed. This is accomplished by exaggerated supination of the wrist, usually starting from a pronated position. This also may be facilitated by slight rotation of the clamp holding the pedicle after placement of the needle point.

The Heaney needle holder, with its angled head, automatically angulates the needle so that the curved arc can be more easily performed. This is useful in vaginal surgery. A similar effect can be obtained by angulating the needle about 45 degrees at the tip of the

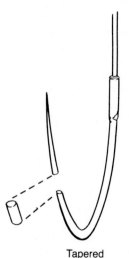 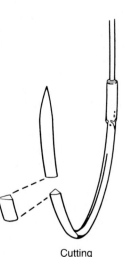

Figure 10–24. Curved surgical needles.

Tapered   Cutting   Reverse cutting

needle holder. This technique is especially useful in the very large patient or deep in the pelvis, where longer instruments must be used.

Needle holders are available in various lengths to facilitate suture placement regardless of the depth of dissection. The jaws of the needle holder are variable, and may be smooth or diamond-cut. Some have a tungsten carbide insert, which increases the hardness of the jaws. In selecting the needle holder the surgeon should choose one that matches the needle size. Larger, heavier needles require needle holders with heavier jaws to prevent movement of the needle in the needle holder during placement of the suture. Likewise, needles of small caliber should be driven with smaller, more delicate needle holders.

Needles should be grasped by the needle holder one-quarter to one-half the distance from the swaged end to the point. The suture itself should never be grasped by the needle holder, as this may damage the suture and decrease its breaking strength, as demonstrated by Stamp and associates. This is especially important when monofilament synthetic sutures are being used.

Surgical Knots

The integrity of any suture depends on the placement of a secure knot. Careful learning of the correct technique and many hours of practice with a knot-tying handbook are required. The two-handed tie, which is more reliable and precise, should be mastered before the one-handed tie. The instrument tie should be learned for certain skin closures and for the occasional situation in which a very short suture must be tied.

The square knot and the surgeons' knot provide the greatest knot security (Fig. 10-25). Indeed, a square knot can maintain up to 90% of the tensile strength of the uninterrupted strand. In tying a proper square knot the two sides should be mirror images of each other and the knot should be tied flat. The knot may be tied by a two-handed, one-handed, or instrument tie technique. The number of throws after the initial two depends on the type of suture material being used. Sawing of the suture during tying should be avoided, as this may weaken the suture material with resultant breakage.

Knots may be formed by using a tension or a nontension technique. In using a tension tie both ends of the suture must be held taut at all times while the second throw is placed. Failure to maintain tension will result in loosening of the knot. When using a nontension tie the first throw must be placed flat. There must then be no tension or jerking on the suture ends until the second throw is completed. The placement of a surgeons' knot, in which the first throw is doubled, facili-

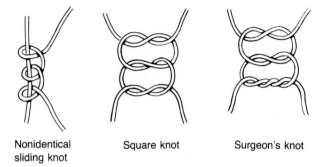

Nonidentical sliding knot   Square knot   Surgeon's knot

Figure 10–25. Commonly used surgical knots.

tates the nontension tie, and is extremely useful when operating deep in the pelvis.

As described by Trimbos, although the symmetric flat square knot is thought to be the securest surgical knot, asymmetric sliding knots are most commonly used by gynecologic surgeons. A sliding knot is produced when one end of the suture is held taut as the knot is tied. They are most easily tied, especially in deep, confined areas of the pelvis. Trimbos found identical sliding knots to be the most unreliable. Nonidentical and parallel sliding knots did not differ in reliability.

Recent studies by van Rijssel and associates confirm the value of the traditional square knot in knot security and strength. In comparing square knots and sliding knots of equal throws, the square knot is superior for all suture materials. The three-throw sliding knot (granny knot) performs the poorest, both in security and in strength. The placement of a surgeons' knot initially helps to hold the knot on the tissue but does not result in greater knot security. Interestingly, van Rijssel and others found that when the caliber of the suture is smaller, there is little difference in security between square knots and nonidentical sliding knots that contain one extra throw.

Van Rijssel and coworkers also have demonstrated that tissue reaction surrounding surgical knots is more a function of suture material and suture size than the number of knots placed in the suture material. Knot strength can be increased by using a larger size suture; knot reliability can be increased by placing a greater number of throws. This should be kept in mind when choosing suture materials.

CONCLUSION

Although wound healing cannot be accelerated, it can be hindered. The medical condition of the patient should, therefore, be optimized before any surgical procedure. The use of meticulous technique, correct surgical instrumentation, and knowledgeable suture selection will result in decreased patient morbidity and optimum wound healing.

Bibliography

Adelson MD, Baggish MS, Seifer DB, et al. Cytoreduction of ovarian cancer with the cavitron ultrasonic surgical aspirator. Obstet Gynecol 1988;72:140.

Alexander JW. Surgical infections and choice of antibiotics. In: Sabiston DC, ed. Textbook of surgery. 13th ed. Philadelphia: WB Saunders, 1986:chap 14.

Altemeier WA, Burke JF, Pruit BA, Sandusky WR, eds. Manual on control of infection in surgical patients. American College of Surgeons. Philadelphia: JB Lippincott, 1976:29.

Baker BL, Whitaker WL. Interference with wound healing by the local action of adrenocortical steroids. Endocrinology 1950;46:544.

Beresford JM. Automatic stapling techniques in abdominal hysterectomy. Surg Clin North Am 1984;64:609.

Blomstedt B, Osterberg B, Bergstand A. Suture material and bacterial transport. Acta Chir Scand 1977;143:71.

Bourne RB, Bitar H, Andreae PR, et al. In-vivo comparison of four absorbable sutures: Vicryl, Dexon plus, Maxon and PDS. Can J Surg 1988;31:43.

Bryant WM. Wound healing. Ciba Clin Symp 1977;29:2.

Burke JFP. The effective period of preventive antibiotic action in experimental incisions and dermal lesions. Surgery 1961;50:161.

Carrico TJ, Mehrhog AI, Cohen IK. Biology of wound healing. Surg Clin North Am 1984;64:721.

Chopp RT, Shah BB, Addonizio JC. Use of ultrasonic surgical aspirator in renal surgery. Urol 1983;22:157.

Cox CE. Principles of operative surgery: antisepsis, technique, sutures and drains. In: Sabiston DC, ed. Textbook of surgery. 13th ed. Philadelphia: WB Saunders, 1986:chap 13.

Cruse PJE, Foord R. A prospective study of 23,649 surgical wounds. Arch Surg 1973;107:206.

Cuono CB. Physiology of wound healing. In: Dagher FJ, ed. Cutaneous wounds. Mount Kisco, NY: Futura Publishing Co, 1985:1.

De Holl D, Rodeheaver G, Edgerton M, et al. Potentiation of infection by suture closure of dead space. Am J Surg 1974;127:716.

Deppe G, Malviya VK, Malone JM. Debulking surgery for ovarian cancer with the cavitron ultrasonic surgical aspirator (CUSA)—a preliminary report. Gynecol Oncol 1988;31:223.

Dudrick SJ, Baue AE, Eiseman B, et al, eds. Manual of preoperative and postoperative care. American College of Surgeons. 3rd ed. Philadelphia: WB Saunders, 1983.

Edlich RF, Rodeheaver GT, Thacker JG, Edgerton MT. Fundamentals of wound management in surgery: technical factors in wound management. Plainfield, NJ: Chirurgecom, 1977:67.

Ehrlich HP, Hunt JK. Effects of cortisone and vitamin A on wound healing. Ann Surg 1968;167:324.

Ehrlich HP, Hunt TK. The effect of cortisone and anabolic steroids on the tensile strength of healing wounds. Ann Surg 1969;170:203.

Ehrlich HP, Tarver H, Hunt TK. Inhibitory effects of vitamin E on collagen synthesis and wound repair. Ann Surg 1972;175:235.

Ethicon. Wound closure manual. Somerville, NJ: Ethicon, Inc. 1985.

Falcone RE, Nappi JF. Chemotherapy and wound healing. Surg Clin North Am 1984;64:779.

Ferguson MK. The effect of antineoplastic agents on wound healing. Surg Gynecol Obstet 1982;154:421.

Goodson WH, Hunt TK. Wound healing and the diabetic patient. Surg Gynecol Obstet 1979;149:600.

Goodson WH, Hunt TK. Wound healing in experimental diabetes mellitus: importance of early insulin therapy. Surg Forum 1978;29:95.

Gottrup F. Delayed primary closure of wounds. Infect Surg 1985; 4:171.

Hambley R, Hebda PA, Abell E, et al. Wound healing of skin incisions produced by ultrasonically vibrating knife, scalpel, electrosurgery, and carbon dioxide laser. J Dermatol Surg Oncol 1988;14:11.

Hasselgren PO, Hagberg E, Malmer H, et al. One instead of two knives for surgical incision. Arch Surg 1984;119:917.

Herrman JB. Tensile strength and knot security of surgical suture materials. Am Surg 1971;37:209.

Holtz C. Adhesion induction by suture of varying tissue reactivity and caliber. Int J Fertil 1982;27:134.

Howes EL, Harvey SC, Hewitt WJ. Rate of fibroplasia and differentiation in the healing of cutaneous wounds in different species of animals. Arch Surg 1939;38:934.

Howes EL, Plotz CM, Blunt JW, et al. Retardation of wound healing by cortisone. Surgery 1950;28:177.

Howes EL, Sooy JW, Harvey SC. The healing of wounds as determined by their tensile strength. JAMA 1929;92:242.

Hugo NE, Epstein L, Cone A, et al. The effect of primary wounding on the tensile strength of secondary wounds. Surg Gynecol Obstet 1970;131:516.

Hunt JK. Control of wound healing with cortisone and vitamin A. In: Longacre JJ, ed. The ultrastructure of collagen. Springfield, IL: Charles C Thomas, 1976:497.

Leibovich SJ, Ross R. The role of the macrophage in wound repair. Am J Pathol 1975;78:71.

Luce EA. The irradiated wound. Surg Clin North Am 1984;64:821.

McMurry JF. Wound healing with diabetes mellitus. Surg Clin North Am 1984;64:769.

Madden JW, Arem AJ. Wound healing: biologic and clinical features. In: Sabiston DC, ed. Textbook of surgery. 13th ed. Philadelphia: WB Saunders, 1986:chap 11.

Madden JE, Edlich RF, Custer JR, et al. Studies in the management of the contaminated wound. Am J Surg 1970;119:222.

Magee C, Rodeheaver GT, Golden GT, et al. Potentiation of wound infection by surgical drains. Am J Surg 1976;131:547.

Masterson BJ, Sullivan TG. Development of a noncrushing vascular clamp for pelvic surgery. Am J Obstet Gynecol 1978;132:113.

McNeeley SG, Elkins T, Portz DM, et al. Comparison of copolymer staple versus chromic suture during hysterectomy: gross, histologic, and microbiologic findings. Obstet Gynecol 1988;72:862.

Odland G, Ross R. Human wound repair. I. Epidermal regeneration. J Cell Biol 1968;39:135.

Orgill D, Demling R. Current concepts and approaches to wound healing. Crit Care Med 1988;16:899.

Peacock EE. Effects of dietary proline and hydroxyproline on tensile strength of healing wounds. Proc Soc Exp Biol Med 1960;105:380.

Peacock EE. Wound healing and wound care. In: Schwartz SI, ed. Principles of surgery. 5th ed. New York: McGraw-Hill, 1989:chap 8.

Peacock EE. Wound repair. 3rd ed. Philadelphia: WB Saunders, 1984.

Polk HC, Simpson CJ, Simmons BP, et al. Guidelines for prevention of surgical wound infection. Arch Surg 1983;118:1213.

Prockop DJ, Kivirikko KI, Tuderman L, et al. The biosynthesis of collagen and its disorders. Part II. N Engl J Med 1979;301(2 Pt 2) :77.

Reinisch JT, Puckett CL. Management of radiation wounds. Surg Clin North Am 1984;64:795.

Rhoads JE, Fliegelman MT, Panzer LM. The mechanism of delayed wound healing in the presence of hypoproteinemia. JAMA 1942;118:121.

Robinson DW. Surgical problems in the excision and repair of irradiated tissue. Plast Reconstr Surg 1982;70:179.

Robson MC, Heggers JP. Delayed wound closures based on bacterial counts. J Surg Oncol 1970;2:379.

Robson MC, Duke WF, Krizek TJ. Rapid bacterial screening in the treatment of civilian wounds. J Surg Res 1973;14:426.

Ross R, Everett NB, Tyler R. Wound healing and collagen formation. VI. The origin of the wound fibroblast studies in parabiosis. J Cell Biol 1970;44:645.

Ruberg RL. Role of nutrition in wound healing. Surg Clin North Am 1984;64:705.

Rudolph R, Arganese T, Woodward M, et al. The ultrastructure and etiology of chronic radiotherapy damage in human skin. Ann Plast Surg 1982;9:282.

Rudolph R, Utley J, Woodward M, et al. The ultrastructure of chronic radiation damage in rat skin. Surg Gynecol Obstet 1981;152:171.

Sanz LE. Wound management—matching materials and methods for best results. Contemp Obstet Gynecol 1987;30:86.

Sanz LE, Patterson JA, Kamath R, et al. Comparison of Maxon suture with Vicryl, chromic catgut, and PDS sutures in fascial closure in rats. Obstet Gynecol 1988;71:418.

Sowa DE, Masterson BJ, Nealon N, et al. Effects of thermal knives on wound healing. Obstet Gynecol 1985;66:436.

Stamp CV, McGregor W, Rodeheaver GT, et al. Surgical needle holder damage to sutures. Am Surg 1988;54:300.

Steichen F, Ravitch MM. Stapling in surgery. Chicago: Year Book Medical Publishers, 1984.

Stein TA, Vaughn RW, Wise L. Glucose tolerance in the obese surgical patient. Surg Gynecol Obstet 1979;148:380.

Stephens FU, Dunphy JE, Hunt TK. The effect of delayed administration of corticosteroids on wound contraction. Ann Surg 1971;173:214.

Stevens FO. Effects of changes in inspired oxygen and carbon dioxide tensions on wound tensile strength: an experimental study. Ann Surg 1971;173:515.

Stone IK. Suture materials. Clin Obstet Gynecol 1988;31:712.

Telok Ha, Mason ML, Wheelock MD. Histopathologic study of radiation injuries of the skin. Surg Gynecol Obstet 1950;90:335.

Tobin GR. Closure of contaminated wounds: biologic and technical considerations. Surg Clin North Am 1984;64:639.

Trimbos JB. Security of various knots commonly used in surgical practice. Obstet Gynecol 1984;64:274.

Trimbos JB, van Rijssel EJC, Klopper PJ. Performance of sliding knots in monofilament and multifilament suture material. Obstet Gynecol 1986;68:425.

Uitto J, Prockop DJ. Synthesis and secretion of underhydroxylated procollagen at various temperatures by cells subject to temporary anoxia. Biochem Biophys Res Commun 1974;60:414.

Van Rijssel EJC, Brand R, Admiraal C, et al. Tissue reaction and surgical knots: the effect of suture size, knot configuration, and knot volume. Obstet Gynecol 1989;74:64.

Van Rijssel EJC, Trimbos JB, Booster MH. Mechanical performance of square knots and sliding knots in surgery: a comparative study. Am J Obstet Gynecol 1990;162:93.

Van Way CW, Buerk CA, eds. Basic surgical skills. St Louis: CV Mosby, 1986.

Van Winkle W, Hastings JC. Considerations in the choice of suture material for various tissues. Surg Gynecol Obstet 1972;135:114.

Von Fraunhofer JA, Storey RS, Stone IK, et al. Tensile strength of suture materials. J Biomed Mater Res 1985;19:596.

Wheeless CR. Stapling techniques in operations for malignant disease of the female genital tract. Surg Clin North Am 1984;64:591.

Wheeless CR, Smith JJ. A comparison of the flow of iodine 125 through three different intestinal anastomoses: standard, Gambee, and stapler. Obstet Gynecol 1983;62:513.

Williamson MB, Fromm HJ. Effect of cystine and methionine on healing experimental wounds. Proc Soc Exp Bio Med 1957;80:523.

Willoughby DA. Some views on the pathogenesis of inflammation. In: Montagna W, Bentley JP, Dobson R, eds. The dermis. Vol 10. Advances in biology of skin. New York: Appleton-Century-Crofts, 1970:221.

Incisions for Gynecologic Surgery

JOHN D. THOMPSON

It is the responsibility of the gynecologic surgeon to decide, before each operation begins, which one among several abdominal incisions available is most suited to the successful performance of the procedure planned. A careful consideration of a variety of circumstances presented by each patient is required before the decision can be finalized. Mistakes can result in a bad outcome. The success of any operation depends on the length of the incision, the correct placement of the incision, the choice of sutures, and the method of closure. The incision influences the relative ease with which the pelvic dissection can be accomplished by providing limited or optimal exposure and access. Limited exposure through small incisions is dangerous, and makes identification of contiguous structures and organs at risk of injury difficult. The time spent fashioning the incision may exceed the time spent removing or correcting the gynecologic and other intra-abdominal pathology. Indeed, performing the abdominal incision is in itself a major surgical procedure. An abdominal incision that is correctly placed, properly fashioned, and closed with perfect healing that preserves the integrity of the abdominal wall strength and function is a source of pride for the gynecologic surgeon and satisfaction for the patient.

ANATOMY OF THE ANTERIOR ABDOMINAL WALL

The surgeon must be completely familiar with the anatomy of the anterior abdominal wall before an intelligent decision can be made on a particular type of incision. The abdominal wall is a functional unit composed of beautifully integrated component parts. It protects the visceral organs and vasculature contained within the abdominal cavity. The abdominal muscles assist in respiration; aid in defecation, urination, coughing, and childbirth by increasing intra-abdominal pressure; and work synergistically with the muscles of the back to flex, extend, and rotate the trunk and the pelvis. The principal anatomic structures of the abdominal wall include muscles, their fascial sheaths and aponeuroses, nerves, arteries, veins, lymphatics, and fat. Considerable individual variation in the contour of the abdominal wall occurs, depending on age, muscle mass and tone, obesity, intra-abdominal pathology, previous pregnancies, posture, and other factors. Such variations in contour affect abdominal wall topography and may present major problems in the correct placement of incisions.

As Figure 11-1 shows, the anatomy of the abdominal wall includes two lateral striated muscles coursing obliquely between the lower margin of the rib cage and the brim of the pelvis on each side. These are the external and internal oblique muscles. Beneath these are the transversalis muscles, which lie directly on the peritoneum. These three paired muscles fuse in the midline at the linea alba by means of their fasical aponeuroses. The central portion of the abdominal wall receives its major support from the paired rectus abdominis muscles, which lie on either side of the linea alba; these muscles originate from the costal margins of the fifth, sixth, seventh, and eighth ribs and insert into the superior pubic rami. The paired pyramidalis muscles arise from the crest of the pubic symphysis and

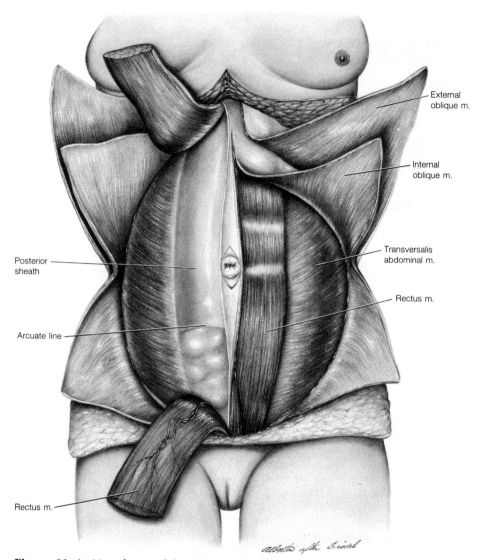

Figure 11–1. Musculature of the abdominal wall showing (*left*) reflection of external and internal oblique muscles along with anterior division of rectus sheath, which exposes the transversalis and rectus muscles. Note tendinous inscriptions in rectus sheath above the umbilicus. The rectus muscle has been reflected (*right*) to demonstrate the posterior rectus sheath and the abrupt cessation of the posterior lamella of the internal oblique at the linea semicircularis (*arcuate line*). Below the arcuate line the intestines are separated from the abdominal wall by the peritoneum and the attenuated fascia of the transversalis muscle.

insert into the lower linea alba. Their function is minor, but they may supply some support to the lower abdominal wall. In making abdominal incisions, preservation of the pyramidalis muscles is not essential.

A cross section of the lower abdominal wall shows that the fascia of the abdominal muscles envelop the anterior and posterior surface of the rectus muscles and anchor the external oblique, the internal oblique, and the transversalis muscles to the vertical (rectus) mus-

cles (Fig. 11-2). There is excellent fascial support anteriorly and posteriorly to the rectus muscles above the arcuate (semicircular) line. Here the fascial aponeurosis of the external oblique and the split fascial aponeurosis of the internal oblique fuse together anterior to the rectus muscle and insert in the midline (linea alba). Above the arcuate line the posterior lamella of the internal oblique aponeurosis fuses with the aponeurosis of the transversalis muscle, passes posterior to

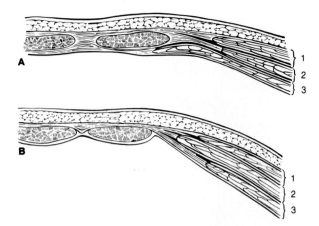

Figure 11–2. Cross section of lower abdominal wall. *A,* The anterior fascial sheath of the rectus muscle from external oblique (*1*) and split sponeurosis of internal oblique muscles (*2*). The posterior sheath is formed by aponeurosis of transversalis muscle (*3*) and split aponeurosis of internal oblique. *B,* Lower portion of abdominal wall below arcuate line (*linea semicircularis*) with absence of a posterior fascial sheath of the rectus muscle and all of the fascial aponeuroses (*1, 2, 3*) forming the anterior rectus sheath.

the rectus muscle, and inserts in the midline. The lower half of the lower abdominal wall is weakened below the arcuate line, at a level about horizontal to the anterior superior iliac spine, where the posterior division of the rectus sheath disappears. Here the divided lamella of the internal oblique muscle combines and passes anterior to the rectus muscle. From this lower portion of the lower abdominal wall to the pubic rami only the attenuated transversalis fascia and the peritoneum lie adjacent to the posterior surface of the muscle. It is in this weakened section of the lower abdomen that most of the incisional hernias occur after pelvic surgery through lower midline incisions (see Fig. 11-1). The distribution and course of the nerves and blood vessels of the abdominal wall bear directly on the postoperative healing and function of the abdominal wall. The quality of the tissues, including the abdominal fascia and muscles, the lines of elasticity, and the direction of muscle contractility influence healing and affect the strength of the resultant scar.

There is a distinct difference in the function of the four main paired muscles of the anterior abdominal wall. The rectus abdominis muscles are primarily muscles of locomotion. Although they do participate to a minor degree in increasing intra-abdominal pressure, their primary function is to approximate the xiphoid process to the symphysis pubis (as in doing sit-ups). The three paired flat muscles on each side of the abdominal wall (the external oblique, the internal oblique, and the transversus abdominis muscles) have a

minor function in locomotion by assisting in rotation of the trunk. Their major functions are to assist with respiration and to assist in increasing intra-abdominal pressure. Each time they contract they pull at the linea alba. In other words, the linea alba represents the point of insertion of six (three on each side) of the eight major muscles of the anterior abdominal wall. Therefore, cutting the linea alba, as in a lower midline incision, actually cuts a major part of the insertion of these six muscles. Contraction of these muscles in the postoperative period causes considerable tension on a suture line in the linea alba as well as considerable discomfort.

The blood supply to the abdominal wall comes from several sources. Laterally, the abdominal wall is supplied by the lower intercostal and lumbar arteries (T8-12 and L1) and the superficial and deep circumflex iliac arteries, which course along the inguinal ligament and along the iliac crest. The main blood supply of the midabdomen and the rectus muscles comes from two vascular systems: from above, from the superior epigastric artery and vein, which are terminal branches of the internal mammary vessels; from below, from the inferior epigastric artery and vein, which arise from the external iliac vessels beneath Poupart's ligament (Fig. 11-3). This freely anastomosing vascular system provides one continuous arterial and venous channel on both sides of the anterior abdominal wall, extending from the subclavian artery and vein above to the external iliac vessels below. This system also anastomoses with the intercostal and lumbar vessels, which supply branches to the external and internal oblique and transversus abdominis muscles. The anterior abdominal wall has an excellent blood supply except at the linea alba. The limited vascularity of this central line of fascial fusion is just one factor to be considered in choosing a secure method of closure of lower midline incisions that will, one hopes, avoid a high incidence of impaired healing, incisional hernias, and eviscerations.

The inferior epigastric vessels ascend from beneath the inguinal ligament, medial to the inguinal ring and superficial to the transversalis fascia (see Fig. 11-3 and Fig. 4-24, which shows blood supply of lower abdominal wall from the inside). At this lowest point they form the lateral margin of Hesselbach's triangle, the base of which is the inguinal ligament and the medial border of which is the lateral border of the rectus muscle. The vessels continue their cranial course between the peritoneum and the undersurface of the rectus muscle to finally enter the posterior rectus sheath at the arcuate line. Along its course the rectus muscle is attached to the anterior rectus sheath at its several transverse tendinous inscriptions, but posteriorly it is free of attachments. Transverse inscriptions are more numerous above the umbilicus and may be absent below the umbilicus. Bleeding from branches of the inferior epi-

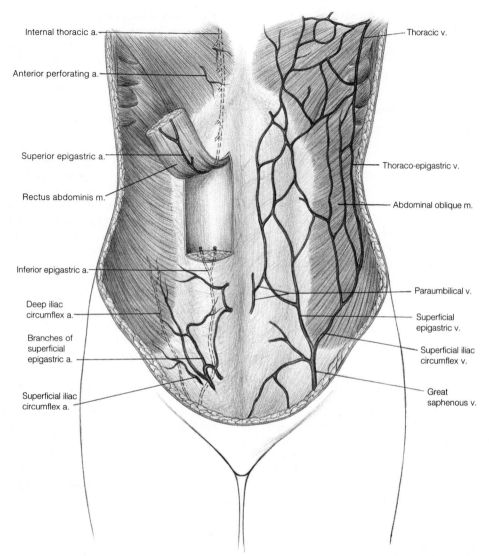

Figure 11–3. Arterial and venous circulation of abdominal wall. The superior and inferior epigastric arteries provide a rich arcade for the rectus muscles, arising superiorly from the internal thoracic artery and inferiorly from the external iliac artery. The venous system has a similar origin, with the exception that the superficial inferior epigastric vein communicates with the saphenous vein of the leg.

gastric vessels beneath the rectus muscle may dissect superiorly and inferiorly the entire length of the posterior sheath, and below the arcuate line the bleeding may dissect laterally and inferiorly along the retroperitoneal pelvic planes and spaces, causing extensive hematomas of the abdominal wall and pelvis. Large quantities of blood may be lost in these loose tissues. Such bleeding into the rectus abdominis muscle and sheath can produce confusing acute abdominal symptoms and signs, especially in a postoperative patient. This problem was discussed by Cullen and Brodel in a classic description of the anatomy of the rectus muscle and more recently by Fletcher and Joseph. The entity usually results from trauma to the unprotected portion of the inferior epigastric artery below the arcuate line (linea semicircularis), where the protection of the vessels is limited to the attenuated fascia of the transversus abdominis muscle and the peritoneum. A thoughtful discussion of the blood supply of the abdominal wall was published by Nahai and associates.

The venous drainage of the abdominal wall accompanies the arteries. The veins of the abdominal wall may be dilated in patients with obstruction of blood flow through the liver and porta hepatus.

The nerve supply to the abdominal wall is easily damaged by incisions, some more than others. The intercostal and lumbar nerves run parallel to the ribs, and enter the abdominal wall laterally between the transversus abdominis and internal oblique muscles. They continue in an oblique and downward course to innervate each segment of the rectus abdominis muscle along its lateral border. This is a most important anatomic point in planning abdominal incisions. A long vertical incision placed lateral to the rectus abdominis muscle will effectively denervate the muscle and render it essentially useless. However, a midline incision in the linea alba or a transverse incision through the rectus muscle will not interfere with innervation of abdominal musculature.

After entering the rectus sheath and rectus muscles laterally, the terminal branches of the thoracic nerve pass through the anterior rectus sheath and supply the skin as cutaneous nerves. The 12th thoracic nerve is joined by L1 and forms the iliohypogastric nerve that supplies motor fibers to the internal and external oblique and transversus abdominis muscles, along with sensory fibers to the skin of the upper and lateral aspects of the thigh. It passes medially, where it communicates with the ilioinguinal nerve and carries sensory fibers to the subcutaneous tissues and skin of the external inguinal ring and the skin over the symphysis pubis. The umbilicus is innervated by the T10 dermatome. The umbilicus is an important landmark on the abdominal wall and in gynecology. In an abdomen with normal tone and contour it is a reference point for the fourth lumbar vertebra and the bifurcation of the aorta.

A minimal loss of skin sensation can result from abdominal incisions. Although unavoidable in most cases, it can be annoying to the patient. Numbness of the skin below a transverse abdominal incision is a frequent occurrence. If the transverse incision is extended laterally, numbness of the skin of the upper anterior thigh also may be noted (see Fig. 4-25, nerve supply of abdominal wall).

The lymphatic drainage of the upper abdominal wall passes directly to the axillary lymph nodes. The lymphatic drainage of the lower abdomen passes to the inguinal nodes and then to the iliac nodes. Some lymphatics around the umbilicus drain toward the liver through the falciform ligament. When an incision is placed transversely in the lower abdomen, lymphatic drainage of the abdominal wall above the incision site will be interrupted. Some tissue swelling may develop temporarily until collateral lymphatic drainage can be established.

An important anatomic point about the skin of the abdominal wall should be mentioned. In 1861, Langer, an Austrian physician, punctured the skin of cadavers in multiple places and found that an elliptical hole was made. The distance between the sides of the ellipse varied in different regions of the body. On this basis he described cleavage lines of the skin that pull the skin edge apart when cut across. These have become known as Langer's lines. Langer's lines usually run horizontally across the abdomen. A vertical midline incision in the skin of the abdomen cuts perpendicular to Langer's lines. A horizontal incision cuts parallel to Langer's lines. Therefore, horizontal (transverse) incisions heal with a very fine scar. Vertical (longitudinal) incisions heal with a broad scar, especially in the lower abdomen. Langer's lines are important in considering the cosmetic result of abdominal incisions (Fig. 11-4).

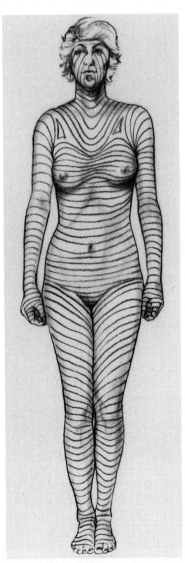

Figure 11–4. Langer's lines run horizontally across the lower abdomen. A transverse incision cuts parallel to Langer's lines and heals with a fine scar.

ABDOMINAL INCISIONS FOR GYNECOLOGIC SURGERY

The history of abdominal incisions is fascinating. Almost every conceivable vertical, horizontal, and oblique incision with many modifications and even combinations has been described in the past century. The abdomen originally was routinely opened with a longitudinal incision through the linea alba. In many of these early cases the patient was in desperate condition, the diagnosis was obscure, and the anesthesia was suboptimal. An incision that could be made rapidly and extended if necessary was needed. An incision in the linea alba involved cutting only one almost avascular layer. The abdominal cavity could be opened and closed simply and rapidly. These were important considerations in the early days of abdominal surgery. Ephram McDowell, the "father of abdominal surgery," chose a midline incision to do the first successful abdominal operation in 1809. He removed a large ovarian tumor from Mary Todd Crawford with a total operating time of 25 minutes.

In the early days of abdominal surgery there was a reluctance to do transverse incisions because they could not be done as rapidly. There also was genuine concern that cutting the abdominal muscles would interfere with their function. It was known, for example, that if the bicep muscle in the upper arm were transected across its belly, the distal half would atrophy because the nerve supply of the biceps is axial. It was thought that the rectus abdominis muscle would suffer a similar fate. As pointed out earlier, however, the innervation of the rectus muscle is segmental, and therefore it will not atrophy if transected transversely. The fear that the rectus would retract and leave a defect in the abdominal wall also was unfounded. The transected ends of the rectus muscle cannot retract, since the entire muscle is firmly attached to the anterior rectus sheath with several transverse inscriptions. The transected rectus muscle heals securely by simply forming another transverse inscription. After these points were realized and confirmed, and as speed became less essential in performing most elective operations, transverse incisions for abdominal surgery became more popular.

Baudelocque was the first to describe a lower abdominal transverse incision in 1823. Subsequently the most popular transverse incisions used in gynecologic surgery were described by Kustner in 1896, by Pfannenstiel in 1896, by Maylard in 1907, and by Cherney in 1941. In 1901 MacKenrodt described a lower abdominal transverse incision similar to the one described by Maylard. Actually, Maylard first used the transverse incision dividing the rectus muscles in the upper abdomen in 1899. In 1894 McBurney described an oblique muscle-splitting incision to be used in operating for appendicitis. It is of some interest that most transverse incisions are identified by the name of the surgeon who first described the incision. Few longitudinal abdominal incisions are known by a person's name.

General Principles and Requirements

The choice of which incision to use is always a compromise between several relative advantages and disadvantages of each incision with the circumstances presented by each patient always in mind. Sometimes the gynecologic surgeon unconsciously chooses the incision he or she is most comfortable with rather than the one that is best suited for the patient. The surgeon should be able to use all of the incisions described herein, rather than to use one approach or technique routinely or reflexively in all patients, regardless of the circumstances.

There are no hard and fast rules in choosing an incision. The following discussion is an attempt to guide the gynecologic surgeon in making the right decision. One should consider the following points.

Anticipated Pathology. A small, benign ovarian cyst can be easily removed through a limited incision, such as a Pfannenstiel or Kustner incision. Operations for bilateral tubo-ovarian abscesses or a leiomyomatous uterus require a transverse Maylard or a lower midline incision for removal. A leiomyomatous uterus pulled upward through a Pfannenstiel incision may completely fill the incision and leave no room around the tumor to operate. Unless the decision can be made with certainty at an earlier time, the best time to decide which incision to make is during the pelvic examination under anesthesia just before the operation begins. The abdominal wall is relaxed and the pelvic pathology is most easily felt at this time.

Type of Operation Planned. If an abdominal hysterectomy is to be done, an incision that allows identification of all contiguous structures in the operative field will be needed. It is doubtful if this can be achieved with the limited exposure provided by a Pfannenstiel or Kustner incision. A simple myomectomy can be done through a Pfannenstiel or Kustner incision. An extensive myomectomy requires greater exposure through a Maylard or lower midline incision.

Desired Exposure. Even when the pelvic dissection is confined to a small area, the pathology may be strategically located in a place that is difficult to visualize through a limited incision (eg, resection of endometriosis in the cul-de-sac). Only an ample incision allows the exposure required for careful and complete dissection. Satisfactory exposure of the operative field is obtained not only by means of a proper incision, but also by means of retractors, packs, correct positioning of the patient on the operating table, good lighting, and relaxation provided by a well-administered anesthetic.

Extensibility of the Incision. The incision with the greatest potential for extensibility is the lower midline incision. It can be extended superiorly around the left side of the umbilicus all the way to the xiphoid process if necessary. When operating for ovarian cancer, sampling para-aortic nodes, removing extremely large tumors of the uterus or ovaries, or diagnosing or correcting incidental pathology in the upper abdomen, the possibility of extending an incision in the lower abdomen superiorly into the upper abdomen is important. The transverse Maylard incision is limited in extensibility to the upper abdomen, although this can be accomplished to a degree by carrying the incision laterally and obliquely upward along Poupart's ligament and through the lateral flat muscles to the level of the anterior superior iliac spine, or even higher if necessary. If a Pfannenstiel incision has been done and the exposure is inadequate, the incision should not be converted to a Maylard incision by cutting the rectus muscles because the anterior rectus sheath has already been widely separated from the rectus muscles. The ends of the muscles will retract and will not come together when the edges of the aponeurosis are later reapproximated. The Pfannenstiel incision, however, can be converted into a Cherney incision to great advantage when additional exposure is required. Thus, although not as suitable as vertical incisions for exploratory procedures, transverse incisions are of great usefulness for elective operations in which the site and extent of the pelvic and abdominal pathology are known with reasonable certainty.

Configuration of the Abdominal Wall. The body build of the patient, especially if obese, can be an important determinant in choosing an incision. In my view, a large panniculus over the lower abdomen should not contraindicate a transverse incision. Indeed, a transverse incision that allows simultaneous removal of the panniculus may be the optimum incision unless circumstances dictate otherwise. A longitudinal midline incision also may be done with satisfactory results, as indicated by the experience of Morrow and associates.

Presence of Previous Surgical Scars. If a previous pelvic laparotomy has been done and the procedure planned can be done satisfactorily through the same incision, the scar should be excised and the repeat laparotomy done through the same site to avoid making a separate incision. If the planned procedure cannot be done correctly in the same site by excising the old scar, then a new incision should be made without hesitation. Some patients who had the first operation for limited pathology through a Pfannenstiel incision will need a

Maylard, Cherney, or midline incision if a second operation is required for more extensive pathology. In performing repeated abdominal surgeries, care should be taken to avoid "tram lines" (making another incision alongside a previous one), since there is a slight but real risk of skin necrosis between the two incisions. Oblique confluence of two incisions also should be avoided.

Necessity for Speed in Entering the Abdomen. The abdominal cavity can be entered much more quickly through a lower midline incision. Indeed, the entry can be made in only a few seconds if the patient's condition is desperate. In gynecology it is a most unusual situation in which such speed is required to make a difference in the outcome of the operation.

Security of the Closure. Many gynecologic surgeons have the impression that transverse incisions heal more securely than longitudinal incisions, have a lower incidence of wound disruption, and a lower incidence of postoperative hernia. This impression goes back many years. In 1916 Moschcowitz discussed the principles of anatomy and physiology of abdominal muscles and their application to the transverse incisions, and stated that not one single postoperative hernia had occurred in any of his patients with a transverse incision. As reported by Tollefson and Russell, Farris accumulated data comparing 1060 transverse incisions with 603 vertical incisions for similar operations on the same service, and concluded that wound disruption was five times more frequent with vertical incisions. Incisional hernia was two and one-half times more common. Thompson and associates, Whitaker, and others report similar findings. Ellis, however, points out in his defense of the midline abdominal incision that most studies of this subject have not been well controlled and that midline incisions are more likely to be done in "cases of great urgency"—hemorrhage, trauma, and sepsis—or in patients who require reoperation through the same incision. Indeed, the poor reputation for disruption accorded to the midline incision may be a reflection of inadequate methods of closure, especially in high-risk cases. The security of the wound comes mostly from the method of closure. More modern methods of incision closure and recent improvements in suture material may help to reduce the incidence of poor healing in all incisions. Until recently there was a preference for meticulously closing incisions in layers, sometimes with catgut sutures. Now, to provide a securer closure, incisions are more likely to be closed with synthetic nonabsorbable or delayed absorbable sutures, taking wide bites a minimum of 1 cm from the wound edge and placed at intervals of 1 cm or less using the Smead-Jones technique. Most surgeons would agree that the Pfannenstiel incision provides the best wound security of all gynecologic incisions. Unfortunately, because of this, sometimes it is used inappropriately when an incision that provides better exposure should be used instead.

Cosmetic Appearance of the Abdomen. This matter is more important to some women than to others. The question, "Doctor, what kind of incision will I have?" is certainly an indication of her concern for the cosmetic appearance of her abdomen. The skin incision is the only part of the operation she will see, and how it looks will determine, to some extent, how she feels about her surgery. Gynecologic surgeons also take pride in the appearance of their incisions. For this and possibly other reasons, and whenever possible, the gynecologic laparotomy should be performed through a transverse lower abdominal incision about 3 finger-breadths above the symphysis pubis. Made in a direction parallel to Langer's lines, the skin incision will heal as a very fine line that will be almost invisible after the initial erythema has disappeared (see Fig. 11-4). The gynecologic surgeon takes pride in all other aspects of the operation as well, and will certainly not allow preservation of the cosmetic appearance of the abdominal wall to be a primary consideration in choosing an incision. The transverse Maylard incision is rapidly becoming the most popular incision for gynecologic surgery, and especially for those operations that are done for benign disease. It satisfies most of the essential requirements of an incision to provide accessibility, extensibility, and security, and at the same time protects the cosmetic appearance of the abdominal wall.

Other Considerations. The scalpel is the preferred instrument for fashioning incisions. According to the experimental work of Sowa and associates, wounds made with the standard steel scalpel are stronger compared with wounds made with other types of incisional instruments. The scalpel's use also may be associated with a lower incidence of incisional infections. Bleeders in the incision are clamped with small clamps and ligated with fine suture. An incision can be made with an electrosurgical unit with a low incidence of infection if a needle point rather than a blade is used, if the correct cutting technique and current are used, and if small bleeders are coagulated precisely without unnecessary charring. A steel scalpel is used first to incise the superficial skin and then the needle point Bovie is substituted to fashion the remainder of the incision. This technique also saves a little time and avoids leaving unnecessary suture material in the wound.

If possible, one should avoid extending an incision by making a "T" in the fascia or skin. One also should avoid developing complicated flaps that involve the aponeurosis of the abdominal wall unless necessary for plastic procedures. A long vertical incision along the lateral border of the rectus muscle should be avoided, since it would effectively denervate the rectus muscle on the same side and lead to weakness in the abdominal wall. All of these procedures are associated with a high incidence of postoperative incisional hernia.

The influence of abdominal incisions on postoperative pulmonary function and complications was discussed by Greenall and associates. Although previous authors had reported fewer postoperative pulmonary complications with transverse incisions, these authors found no significant difference. Incisions in the lower abdominal wall are much less likely to interfere with pulmonary function than incisions in the upper abdomen anyway. The gynecologic surgeon can choose an incision that will allow the best possible exposure.

A discussion of the technique of fashioning abdominal incisions for gynecologic operations is divided into longitudinal, transverse, and other incisions.

Longitudinal Incisions

Median Incisions

Many abdominal operations on the female reproductive tract are performed through a low midline incision. The incision can be made rapidly and easily, and can be extended above the umbilicus when necessary. Consequently it has the greatest advantage of adequate operative exposure with the least time requirement. The length of the incision is important in the healing process, even though it is frequently stated that "the incision heals from side to side, and not from end to end." As measured by Sloan, tension on a midline incision is roughly proportional to the square of the length of the incision; that is, a 30-lb force is necessary to approximate the edges of a 3-in incision, whereas an 80-lb force is necessary to approximate a 5-in incision. The skin incision is continued through the fat to the linea alba, traditionally using a clean knife other than the one used on the skin, although this may not be necessary (Fig. 11-5A). Bleeders are occluded with Halsted clamps and tied with No. 4-0 delayed absorbable suture.

Using the flat end of the scalpel, the adherent fat is dissected laterally from the midline of the aponeurosis for about 1 cm to permit adequate exposure, easy identification of the midline, and accurate placement of sutures when the aponeurosis is closed.

The aponeurosis is incised at the linea alba for the full length of the incision (Fig. 11-5B). In parous women there usually is no difficulty in finding the midline because the underlying rectus muscles normally are separated from previous stretching of the abdominal wall (diastasis recti). In nulliparous women the midline may not be immediately evident. In such cases the pyramidalis muscles, which arise from the symphysis pubis, are the most useful landmarks in directing the surgeon to the midline. The medial border of each

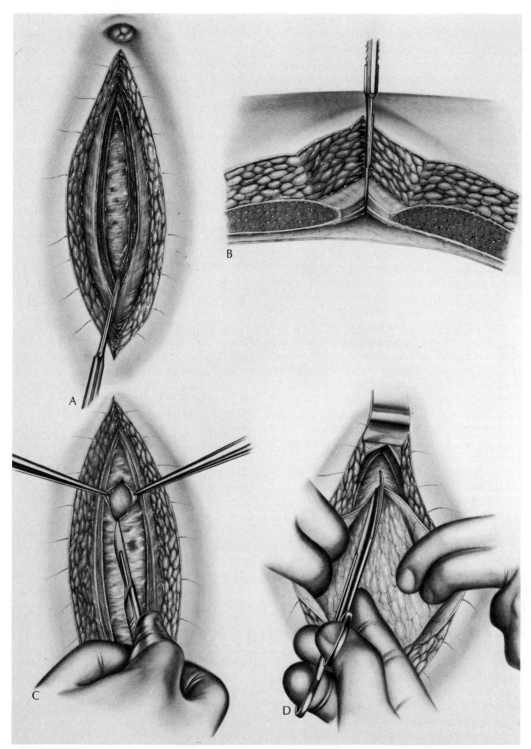

Figure 11–5. *A*, Cutting of linea alba in low midline incision with scalpel. *B*, Cross section of abdominal wall showing skin, subcutaneous fat, anterior and posterior rectus sheaths, and underlying peritoneum. *C*, Opening of peritoneum with knife and demonstration of small bowel protruding into peritoneal opening. *D*, Enlargement of peritoneal opening to the region of the umbilicus with Mayo scissors.

muscle passes upward and inward, and inserts into the lower one third of the linea alba. To provide optimum exposure, the incision in the anterior rectus sheath and between the tendinous portion of the rectus muscles must extend inferiorly all the way to the symphysis pubis. Near the umbilicus the rectus muscles can be further separated by using the handle of the scalpel. Hemostasis should be final and complete before the peritoneal cavity is entered.

The peritoneal fat is incised, and the peritoneum becomes visible beneath. The urachus, the embryologic remnant of the allantois, is frequently seen as it courses from the dome of the bladder to the umbilicus; it also identifies the midline of the lower abdomen. Above the arcuate line the posterior rectus sheath may be incised as a separate layer, revealing a varying amount of preperitoneal fat beneath. After this is cleared away the peritoneum in the upper incision is picked up with mouse-tooth forceps by the operator and the assistant. It is carefully incised to avoid accidental laceration of the underlying bowel, which may be adherent beneath the peritoneum (Fig. 11-5C). Pushing the fat away with the knife handle before incising the peritoneum allows good visualization of the underlying bowel, and is an excellent surgical precaution. The cut edges of the peritoneum are grasped with Kelly clamps, and the peritoneal incision is enlarged with the knife and scissors while the assistant and the operator elevate the abdominal wall (Fig. 11-5D). Enlargement of the peritoneal incision toward the symphysis is done under direct vision, with care being exercised to avoid injury to the dome of the bladder.

Special care must be taken in entering the peritoneal cavity, particularly when there has been a previous laparotomy; when the bladder is distended or possibly displaced upward by a tumor; when there is a large tumor, such as a uterine leiomyoma or an ovarian tumor, pressing tightly against the parietal peritoneum; and when the history and clinical findings suggest the presence of extensive pelvic inflammatory disease. In entering the abdomen through a previous scar, it is advisable to incise the peritoneum at the highest level to avoid possible injury to an adherent bladder. When a large tumor presses against the parietal peritoneum, it is best to attempt entrance above the tumor by nicking the peritoneum slightly and listening for the rush of air into the peritoneal cavity. Injury to the bladder occurs more frequently at the time of entry into the peritoneal cavity, in the experience of Everett and Mattingly, than at any other time during pelvic surgery. It is therefore important for the gynecologist to observe the thickness of tissues that he or she is incising. If the tissues appear muscular or vascular, it is well to abandon entrance at that point and attempt an opening at a higher level,

perhaps even above the umbilicus if necessary. Adherent bowel from previous surgery or pelvic inflammatory disease must be identified by gently opening the thin layer of peritoneum, if there is not another available site of entry, and removing the adherent bowel from the peritoneum with careful scissor or digital dissection under direct vision.

After the peritoneal cavity has been entered, the abdominal walls are retracted with either self-retaining or wide-bladed retractors. It is advisable to protect the abdominal muscles with moist laparotomy packs placed beneath the retractor blades, particularly when prolonged surgery is anticipated. Although the Trendelenburg position is helpful in displacing the intestines in the upper abdomen, a steep position is neither necessary nor desirable with the use of modern methods of anesthesia and muscle relaxants. In particular, any patient with limited cardiac reserve should not be subjected to steep Trendelenburg's position, as this may compromise the adequacy of pulmonary ventilation during surgery.

A routine and careful exploration and palpation of the upper abdomen are carried out at this point and before the bowel is packed off. Pelvic surgeons develop their own routine for doing this examination. It may be done by feeling the gallbladder, the liver, and the right kidney, in that order. The pancreas and the stomach are palpated as the hand sweeps across to the opposite side of the upper abdominal cavity. After feeling the left kidney and the spleen (if possible), the operator feels along the aorta and vena cava and also notes any enlargement or firm consistency of lymph nodes along these vessels. The small and large bowel and the appendix also must be examined. The idea is to discover pathology in the upper abdomen that might be related to the pathology in the pelvis and may alter the plan of operation. One also may discover incidental pathology that might need further diagnostic tests or treatment at a later time.

After first releasing all bowel adhesions in the pelvis, the intestines may be held gently in the upper abdomen with two or three moist laparotomy packs; too many packs may place undue pressure on the bowel and restrict diaphragmatic excursions. If the bowel does not remain out of the operative field with two laparotomy packs carefully placed over the small intestines and pushed into the lateral spaces in the abdomen, it is probable that the anesthesia is inadequate and that the abdominal muscles need to be further relaxed. It also is well to remember that the average moist laparotomy pack, when formed into a sphere, occupies about 240 cc of available intra-abdominal space; consequently excessive packs will crowd the upper abdomen and restrict movement of the diaphragm. In addition, excessive compression of the small bowel between laparotomy packs will temporarily damage the terminal motor nerve endings and may contribute to postoperative adynamic ileus.

Laparotomy packs may cause microscopic damage to the delicate serosal surface of the intestine. This damage can be visible even as small subserosal petechial hemorrhages, and will predispose to the development of postoperative adhesions. The bowel should always be handled gently. Placing laparotomy packs in plastic bags may help to prevent this serosal damage with subsequent adhesion formation.

Paramedian Incision

In making a paramedian rectus incision, a longitudinal incision of desired length is placed in the skin between the umbilicus and the symphysis 1 to 2 cm either to the right or to the left of the midline. This choice depends on the operation planned and the side of the pelvis where one expects to find the pathology. The anterior rectus sheath also is incised longitudinally 1 to 2 cm from the midline, and freed from the underlying rectus muscle. At this point the operator may choose to retract the rectus muscle laterally, in which case the inferior epigastric vessels beneath the muscle usually are gently retracted uninjured with the muscle. Alternatively, the rectus muscle may be split longitudinally 1 to 2 cm from its medial border, ligating the inferior epigastric vessels if necessary to avoid or stop troublesome bleeding. The peritoneum beneath the rectus muscle is then incised longitudinally 1 to 2 cm from the midline.

A paramedian incision has good extensibility; good exposure, especially on the side of the pelvis over which it is made; good muscle cover; and good healing and strength when closed. Exposure deep in the cul-de-sac and on the opposite side of the pelvis may be limited. If a transrectus technique is used, the medial fibers of the muscle will be weakened by denervation. This is of little consequence in limited incisions, but extending the incision may result in noticeable weakness and atrophy. Some gynecologic surgeons prefer a paramedian incision over a median incision when a longitudinal incision is made. A paramedian incision is thought to be stronger, since it avoids cutting directly through the linea alba. Cox and associates reported a prospective randomized controlled clinical trial comparing the incidence of postoperative incisional hernias after median and paramedian incisions. Twenty-two incisional hernias were found within 1 year: 20 in the median group and 2 in the paramedian group. A left paramedian incision is especially useful when operating for disease that involves the sigmoid colon and left pelvic sidewall. If a paramedian incision is placed parallel to a previous median incision, or vice versa, the blood supply between the two incisions may be inadequate, causing slough or delayed healing.

Transverse Incisions

There are four principal transverse lower abdominal incisions used for pelvic surgery: (1) the Maylard, or true transverse rectus muscle–cutting, incision; (2) the Cherney incision, in which the rectus muscle is detached from the pubic symphysis; (3) the Pfannenstiel incision, in which the rectus aponeurosis is incised transversely; and (4) the Kustner incision (sometimes called the modified Pfannenstiel), in which a median incision is made in the linea alba.

The Pfannenstiel incision has been championed by a number of gynecologic surgeons but has not been as popular in the United States as the lower midline incision. Critics of the Pfannenstiel incision emphasize the longer time required for opening and closing the abdomen as well as the increased amount of bleeding caused by dissecting the aponeurosis from the rectus muscles. In addition, exposure is limited when compared with a midline incision or true transverse Maylard incision, with no opportunity for enlargement of the incision, if the disease process should be found to extend above the pelvic brim, unless it is converted to a Cherney incision. In the event that bowel surgery is contemplated, any transverse incision may limit access to the upper abdomen and interfere with the location of a colostomy site in the lower abdomen. The transverse techniques are not advised for large pelvic tumors or when any surgical procedure is contemplated in the upper abdomen.

According to Speert, prevention of incisional hernia was Pfannenstiel's principal objective. Originally he also wrote that his incision provided a better view of the operative field than even the longitudinal incision. Later, after additional experience, even Pfannenstiel recognized the limitations of exposure provided by his incision. In recanting, he suggested that his incision was appropriate only in cases where "a smaller opening of the abdomen suffices for carrying out all the procedures in a thorough and conservative manner and is indicated principally for procedures on the internal genitalia which permit conservation of the uterus." In other words, Pfannenstiel did not believe that his incision provided sufficient exposure to perform an abdominal hysterectomy.

The advantages cited for the transverse incision include the well-known fact that incisional hernias are infrequent with these methods, whereas they are more common after vertical incisions. This is undoubtedly one of the strongest points in favor of transverse incisions. Griffiths has reported an increased incidence of postoperative inguinal hernias among men who have retropubic prostatectomy performed through a Pfannenstiel incision. This has not been confirmed in women. The incisions also have a cosmetic advantage, since the scar is located in the lower abdomen or hidden near the margin of the pubic hairline. These incisions also are reported to entail less postoperative discomfort.

As discussed in Chapter 4, the transverse type of incision, especially the Maylard, is associated with a higher frequency of femoral nerve injury, as emphasized by Hudson and colleagues. This complication occurs more commonly in thin patients in whom the lateral margins of the incision extend into the lateral abdominal wall and in whom a self-retaining retractor with lateral blades is used. The lateral blades of the retractor may rest on the psoas muscles and press downward on the femoral nerve in its location just superior to the inguinal ligament. A self-retaining retractor with deep lateral blades should not be used with a Maylard or Cherney incision. If a self-retaining retractor is used, the lateral blades should be only deep enough to fit under the edges of the incision or, preferably, should be removed. The ilioinguinal and iliohypogastric nerves that innervate the mons pubis and labia also may be damaged by retractor entrapment, excision, suture ligation, or electrocoagulation with the possibility of causing postoperative discomfort.

Maylard Incision

The Maylard incision is a true transverse rectus muscle−cutting incision in which all layers of the lower abdominal wall are incised transversely. The limitation of operative exposure encountered with the Kustner or Pfannenstiel incision is avoided. By cutting the rectus and lateral abdominal muscle transversely, excellent exposure for almost any type of pelvic procedure is obtained, especially on the lateral sides of the pelvis.

There are many enthusiastic advocates of the Maylard incision, including Russell, Morley, McDuff, and others. The advantages of this incision have been discussed in detail by Tollefson and Russell and by Daversa and Landers. In addition to the advantages of improved exposure of the operative site and stronger healing, these authors mention a lower incidence of adhesions, fewer postoperative pulmonary complications, earlier and better postoperative ambulation, less postoperative incisional pain, reduced requirement for postoperative pain medication, and better recovery of intestinal peristalsis when compared with longitudinal incisions. The Maylard incision is only slightly more time-consuming

to make but has some limitation of extensibility to deal with problems in the upper abdomen.

Additional exposure may be achieved by extending the incision further laterally and above the anterior superior iliac spine. When this is done, the exposure may be adequate to remove fairly large pelvic tumors and to do extensive abdominal hysterectomy and pelvic lymphadenectomy. Even the lower para-aortic lymph nodes may be safely removed through this incision.

The Maylard incision is shown in Figure 11-6. Before the skin incision is made, a series of three or four markings are made perpendicular across the planned line of the incision. Markings with a sterile pencil are preferable to scratches made with a scalpel. These markings will be helpful later in approximating the skin margins. The skin incision is straight across or curved slightly upward 3 to 5 cm above the superior border of the pubic symphysis. This usually is at the superior border of the pubic hairline or slightly below (see Fig. 11-6A). The skin incision should not be made in a deep skin crease or beneath a large panniculus of fat. The superficial branches of the inferior epigastric artery and vein will be encountered, as the fat and aponeurosis are incised transversely in the same line. The aponeurosis should not be separated from the underlying muscle. The rectus muscles are transected transversely with a scalpel or preferably with a needle point Bovie using a zig-zag motion, coagulating small vessels inside the muscle as they are encountered. The inferior epigastric vessels will be identified at the lateral border of each rectus muscle usually lying within a pad of preperitoneal fat (see Fig. 11-6B). The fat pad can be picked up between the thumb and index finger. A clamp can be passed beneath the fat pad, and the vessels divided between clamps and both ends ligated with No. 2-0 delayed absorbable suture. The incision can be extended laterally for several centimeters to provide optimum exposure. Hemostasis should be final and complete before the peritoneum is opened. The peritoneum is opened laterally at its thinnest part. The incision is then extended across to the opposite side just above the bladder (see Fig. 11-6C). The urachus is transected in the midline just above the apex of the bladder. The obliterated hypogastric arteries (lateral umbilical ligaments) are transected laterally. An indwelling transurethral Foley catheter is placed before the operation begins, to ensure that the bladder is empty. It is our custom to sew laparotomy pads to the edges of the peritoneum to protect the incision, assist in retraction, and aid in closure of the peritoneum. Abdominal exploration and lysis of adhesions are done as previously described. A suitable self-retaining retractor is put in place, taking care that the lateral blades do not rest on the femoral nerves. Our current preference is to

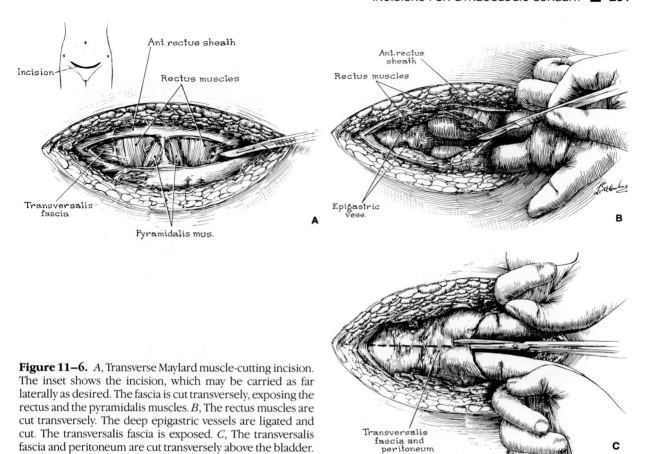

Figure 11–6. *A,* Transverse Maylard muscle-cutting incision. The inset shows the incision, which may be carried as far laterally as desired. The fascia is cut transversely, exposing the rectus and the pyramidalis muscles. *B,* The rectus muscles are cut transversely. The deep epigastric vessels are ligated and cut. The transversalis fascia is exposed. *C,* The transversalis fascia and peritoneum are cut transversely above the bladder.

use the Bookwalter retractor with very shallow lateral blades. The bowel is placed in the upper abdomen with the hand and held there with laparotomy packs and the upper blade of the retractor. When using the Bookwalter retractor with the Maylard incision, the lateral blades may be removed after the upper and lower blades have been positioned. Then the operation can proceed with optimum exposure.

Krupski and associates have described a rare complication of transverse abdominal incisions in which the inferior epigastric artery is ligated. In patients with impaired arterial circulation to the leg because of an obstruction at the terminal aorta and common iliac arteries, the blood flow in the inferior epigastric artery may be reversed from its normal cranial direction to a caudal direction to provide additional collateral circulation to the lower extremity. In this situation, ligation of the inferior epigastric artery could result in lower-extremity ischemia. In a gynecologic patient with clinical evidence of impaired circulation in the lower extremities, a midline incision should be used. If a transverse Maylard incision is used, every attempt should be

made to avoid ligation of the inferior epigastric arteries, especially if directional Doppler flow studies show a reversal of flow, as demonstrated by Kwaan and Connolly.

Cherney Incision

The only difference between the transverse Maylard incision and the Cherney incision is in the manner of dividing the rectus muscles. In the Maylard incision the rectus muscles are transected across about 3 to 5 cm above their insertion into the symphysis pubis. On the other hand, Cherney advocated freeing the rectus muscles at their tendinous attachments to the symphysis pubis and retracting them upward for exposure. Breen and others who have used this incision extensively report excellent exposure, few technical problems, and secure healing. Indeed, it is one of the strongest transverse incisions. There seems to be an almost psychological inhibition to cutting the tendinous insertion of any muscle, especially the rectus muscle. However, its reattachment to the undersurface of the rectus sheath

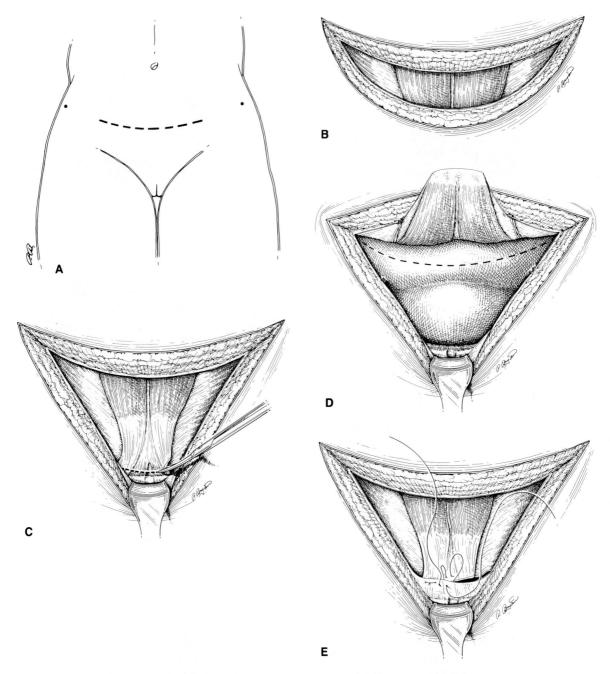

Figure 11–7. *A,* The Cherney incision begins with a transverse elliptical skin incision 2 to 3 cm above the symphysis pubis. *B,* The incision is carried transversely through the skin, subcutaneous fat, and fascia. The rectus muscles are exposed. *C,* After separating the fascia from the muscles inferiorly, the tendinous portions of the rectus muscles are exposed and dissected from the periosteum of the superior border of the symphysis pubis. *D,* The tendinous portions of the muscles are retracted superiorly and the peritoneum is incised transversely above the bladder. *E,* When the operation is completed, the tendinous portions of the rectus muscles are sutured beneath the fascia of the anterior abdominal wall just above the pubic symphysis. Permanent synthetic suture material should be used.

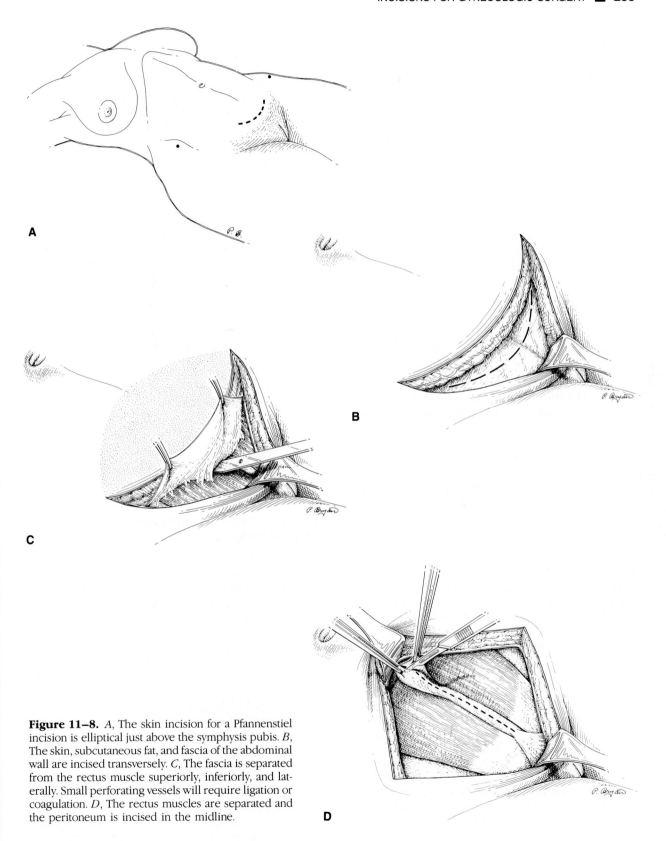

Figure 11–8. *A*, The skin incision for a Pfannenstiel incision is elliptical just above the symphysis pubis. *B*, The skin, subcutaneous fat, and fascia of the abdominal wall are incised transversely. *C*, The fascia is separated from the rectus muscle superiorly, inferiorly, and laterally. Small perforating vessels will require ligation or coagulation. *D*, The rectus muscles are separated and the peritoneum is incised in the midline.

just above the symphysis usually is easy and secure, but involves an extra step when compared with the Maylard incision (Fig. 11-7).

Although the Cherney incision has not achieved the same level of popularity as the Maylard, it is reported to have definite advantages for gaining access to the retro-pubic space of Retzius for urethropexy procedures and for gaining access to the lateral retroperitoneal spaces for extraperitoneal pelvic lymphadenectomy.

Pfannenstiel Incision

The original, true Pfannenstiel incision is described as a transverse incision that is slightly curved (concavity upward) and may be made at any level suitable to the surgeon (Fig. 11-8A). It usually is 10 to 15 cm long, and extends through the skin and subcutaneous fat to the level of the rectus fascia. The rectus fascia is incised transversely on either side of the linea alba, which is cut separately, joining the two lateral incisions but leaving the rectus fascia intact across the midline (Fig. 11-8B). The rectus sheath is separated from the underlying muscle by inserting the fingers on either side of the cut edge of the sheath and pulling the fascia in opposite directions, with one hand toward the head and the other hand toward the feet. This maneuver will free the fascia from the anterior surface of the rectus muscle as far as desired between the symphysis and the umbilicus (Fig. 11-8C). The rectus muscles are then separated in the midline, and the peritoneum is opened vertically (see Fig. 11-8D). This procedure avoids the necessity of dissecting the subcutaneous fat away from the anterior rectus fascia, as is done in the Kustner incision. How-ever, it separates the perforating nerves and small blood vessels that enter the fascia from the underlying mus-cles and nourish the fascia, and may weaken the inci-sion.

If greater exposure is required, the Pfannenstiel inci-sion should be converted to a Cherney incision by separating the tendinous portion of the rectus muscles from the symphysis. A Pfannenstiel incision should not be converted to a Maylard.

If the Pfannenstiel incision is extended laterally be-yond the edge of the rectus muscles and into the sub-stance of the external and internal oblique muscles, injury to the iliohypogastric and ilioinguinal nerves may occur, as reported by Sippo and associates. The nerves may be incised or excised, in which case a neuroma may form. The nerve may be caught in a suture or in the surrounding scar tissue in the incision. This also is a danger when a Maylard or Cherney inci-sion is extended laterally. When closing these lateral extensions, sutures should be placed only in the exter-nal oblique fascia. Deep sutures in the substance of the muscles may entrap these nerves and cause postopera-tive pain.

Kustner Incision

The Kustner incision, also incorrectly called the mod-ified Pfannenstiel incision, is shown in Figure 11-9. The slightly curved transverse skin incision begins below the level of the anterior superior iliac spine and extends just below the pubic hairline, through subcutaneous fat, down to the aponeurosis of the external oblique muscle and the anterior sheath of the recti in the same manner as all other transverse incisions (see Fig. 11-9A). The superficial branches of the inferior epigastric artery and vein may be encountered in the subcutaneous fat at the lateral margin of the incision. When encountered, they are ligated. The fascia is cleaned superiorly and inferiorly until a sufficient area is exposed from the region of the umbilicus to the symphysis to permit an adequate vertical incision in the linea alba. Excessive separation of the fat from the fascia in the lateral mar-gins of the incision is unnecessary and may provide sites for a small postoperative hematoma. Separation of the rectus muscles and entrance into the peritoneum are as in the ordinary midline incision (see Fig. 11-9B). Because of the importance of obtaining adequate he-mostasis in the subcutaneous fat of the skin flaps, this incision is definitely more time-consuming than the low midline incision or the Pfannenstiel incision. It offers little or no advantage. Its extensibility is severely limited.

Oblique Incisions

Gridiron (Muscle-Splitting) Incision of McBurney

The McBurney incision is a good choice for an un-complicated appendectomy and also may be used for the extraperitoneal drainage of an abscess from pelvic inflammatory disease. In pelvic inflammatory disease, when drainage becomes necessary for an indolent broad ligament abscess that does not respond to antibi-otics and does not point into the cul-de-sac for drainage, drainage through a gridiron incision is most effective. The incision is made as for an appendectomy, except that it is made a little lower and the peritoneal cavity is not entered. Similarly, if drainage of the pelvis should be required during a pelvic laparotomy, avoid draining the abscess through a midline incision, and use a small gridiron (stab wound) incision for placing drains in the pelvis. In treating a large tubo-ovarian abscess that extends out of the pelvis and does not respond to antibiotic therapy, extraperitoneal drainage through a McBurney incision also is possible by approaching the abscess laterally. This permits entrance into the site of infection without soiling the peritoneal cavity.

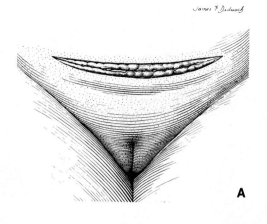

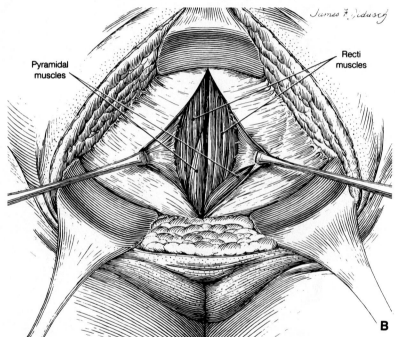

Figure 11–9. Kustner incision. *A,* Skin incision just below hairline. *B,* Midline incision through fascia, exposing rectus and pyramidalis muscles. The rectus muscles are retracted laterally and the peritoneum is incised in the midline.

The gridiron incision is made obliquely downward and inward over McBurney's point (Fig. 11-10*A*). The location may be varied when the incision is done for appendectomy during pregnancy or when it is used for abscess drainage, as mentioned. As described by Delany, the incision in the skin may be made at a lower level to preserve the cosmetic appearance of the abdominal wall. The incision is carried through the skin and subcutaneous fat to the external oblique muscle. The fibers of the muscle are separated in the direction in which they run (Fig. 11-10*B*). The internal oblique and the transversus abdominis are separated in the line of their fibers (Fig. 11-10*C*). At this point the internal oblique and the transversus abdominis course in the same direction and are closely fused. Retractors are placed to widen the divided muscle fibers, and the preperitoneal fat is exposed. The peritoneum is incised and the peritoneal cavity entered. The cecum lies close to the peritoneum at this point, and care must be taken to avoid injury to the bowel. The appendix usually can be found without difficulty, although in suppurative appendicitis the exposure may not be adequate. If additional exposure is needed, the incision may be extended upward and laterally. If more room is needed medially, the incision may be extended through the lateral border rectus muscles. The inferior epigastric vessels may require ligation if encountered.

When using the McBurney incision to drain a pelvic abscess, entrance into the peritoneal cavity should be

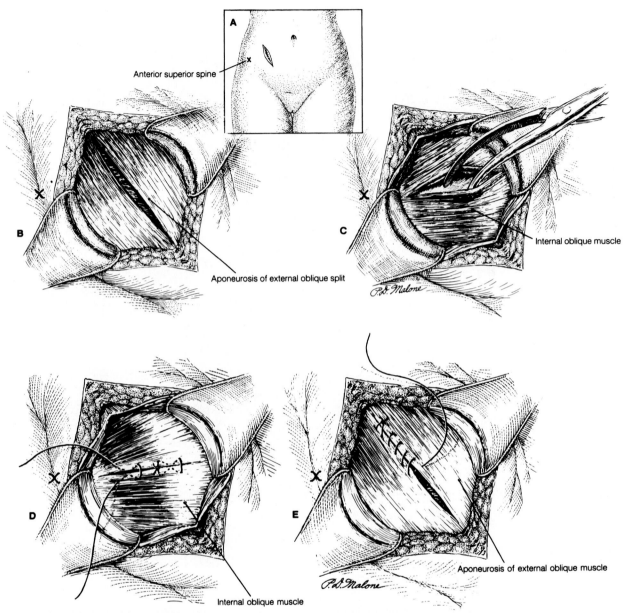

Figure 11–10. Gridiron incision. *A*, Position of incision. *B*, Fibers of external oblique have been split. *C*, Internal oblique muscle being split with Kelly clamp. *D*, Gridiron incision closing: internal oblique fibers approximated with figure-of-eight of No. 0 delayed absorbable sutures. *E*, Aponeurosis of external oblique is closed with continuous or interrupted No. 0 delayed absorbable sutures.

avoided, if possible. Instead, the peritoneum should be gently reflected way from the abdominal wall inferiorly and the abscess entered beneath the round ligament for extraperitoneal drainage. Thickened, indurated tissue may make this difficult. If the parietal peritoneum is adherent to the peritoneal surface of the abscess, drainage still may be possible without transversing free space in the peritoneal cavity. One should avoid contaminating the general peritoneal cavity with pus, if possible.

The gridiron incision may be used in the left lower quadrant to drain an abscess on the left side of the pelvis. It also can be used to perform sigmoid colostomy.

Rockey-Davis Incision

An alternative to the McBurney incision is the Rockey-Davis (or Elliot) incision. It is a transverse incision placed at the junction of the lower and middle thirds of a line extending from the anterior superior iliac spine to the umbilicus. Medially, the incision extends to the border of the rectus muscle. The aponeurosis of the external oblique muscle is split in the line of its fibers. The internal oblique and transversus muscle fibers can be separated by blunt finger dissection. The peritoneum is incised transversely. This incision has provided satisfactory exposure to pathology in either lower abdominal quadrant. A similar incision made lower on the abdomen will preserve the cosmetic appearance of the abdominal wall.

Closing the Abdomen

After completion of the pelvic operation, all laparotomy packs are removed and the sigmoid is placed over the operative field to prevent the small intestines from becoming adherent in the cul-de-sac. The omentum is drawn down over the viscera, and closure of the abdominal incision begins.

The many variables that must be considered and decisions that must be made in wound closure are discussed by Martyak and Curtis.

The closure techniques described below are standard techniques. Most gynecologic surgeons establish standard techniques for closing standard incisions made for standard operations done in standard patients. Certainly, this is convenient and time-saving and usually acceptable. It is unacceptable, however, if the routine closure will not hold when an unanticipated postoperative complication occurs or if the routine becomes so routine that exceptions are not made when indicated. There are many factors that place patients at high risk for developing incisional problems. Healing can be impaired and delayed for many reasons. A discussion of factors that influence wound healing can be found in Chapter 10. In each patient these factors must be taken into account so that the routine incision closure may be altered when indicated.

One of the greatest advances in surgery, including gynecologic surgery, in recent years has been the introduction of improved suture materials for wound closure. Chemical technology has produced synthetic alternatives to silk and catgut that have been shown to be superior by extensive laboratory and clinical testing. Synthetic delayed absorbable sutures provide more uniform and predictable absorption, greater tensile strength for longer periods, better knot security in tissue fluids, and less tissue reaction. These synthetic

sutures include Ethicon's Vicryl (polyglactin 910) and Davis and Geck's Dexon (polyglycolic acid). Even newer suture materials, such as Ethicon's PDS II (polydioxanone monofilament) and Davis and Geck's Maxon (polyglyconate monofilament), are now available, and provide even longer strength retention than Vicryl or Dexon. All are superior to chromic catgut, as shown by the experimental work of Sanz and associates and many others. Goligher, for example, showed that catgut had insufficient strength for use in abdominal wound closure and was associated with dehiscence in 11% of patients. Synthetic nonabsorbable sutures also are available, and are being used in place of silk sutures (Ethicon's Ethibon, DeKnatel's Tevdek II, Ethicon's Ethilon and Prolene). These newer synthetic sutures are an excellent addition to the armamentarium of the gynecologic surgeon. They should be used for wound closure in place of catgut and silk. Catgut has almost no place in gynecologic surgery, and its use has declined in recent years. A discussion of the characteristics of suture materials, proper methods of obtaining knot security, and suture technique also can be found in Chapter 10.

Median or Paramedian Incision

In closing the median or paramedian incision the margins of the peritoneum are approximated, beginning at the upper end; both the peritoneum and the posterior rectus sheath are sutured together with a continuous No. 2-0 delayed absorbable suture. A three-point stitch is used to evert the cut peritoneal edges and make the intraperitoneal suture line as smooth as possible (Fig. 11-11). To improve the exposure of the peritoneal edge, the peritoneum is grasped with Kelly clamps, which exteriorize the margins for the operator to suture. If the intestines should interfere with the closure, they may be retracted with a malleable spatula or, if great difficulty is experienced, a laparotomy pad may be inserted over the intestines and withdrawn just before completion of the closure. In high-risk patients two to four retention sutures of No. 2 nylon or polypropylene are placed in the abdominal wall (Fig. 11-12A). These sutures pass through the skin, fat, and anterior rectus sheath, but to prevent bleeding, pain, and partial muscle necrosis from a distended abdomen, they avoid the muscles (Fig. 11-12B). In cases where additional support to the abdominal incision is required, such as with secondary closure after evisceration, the rectus muscle is encircled, making certain that the sutures remain outside the peritoneal cavity. Small pieces of fine rubber tubing are placed on each suture to ensure that, when tied, the sutures do not cause pressure necrosis of the skin over the incision (Fig. 11-12C).

If retention sutures are used, they are tied loosely

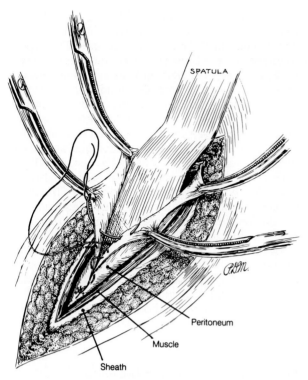

Figure 11–11. Method of closure of the peritoneum that results in everted peritoneal three-point edges. No. 2-0 delayed absorbable suture is used.

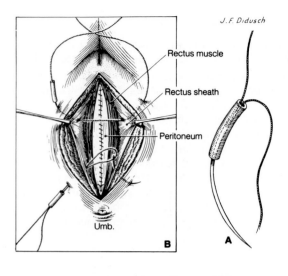

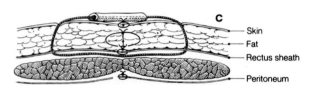

Figure 11–12. Method of placing tension sutures. *A*, Long cutting needle threaded with No. 2 nylon and shod with rubber tubing. *B*, Method of placing sutures through skin, fat, and fascia. *C*, Layer-for-layer closure of the abdomen and position of tension suture through skin and subcutaneous fat, and beneath anterior rectus fascia.

enough across the incision to permit two fingers to pass between the suture and the skin. They are used primarily to hold the incision together in the event of abdominal distention. Constricting retention sutures can impair circulation to the incision and produce local ischemia, which may result in poor healing. Healing of the incision is more effective when the skin edges fall together without tension and without undue pressure from deep sutures. If retention sutures are too tight with abdominal distention, they should be loosened to avoid cutting through the skin. In high-risk patients they may be left in place for several weeks.

As in all aspects of incisions and closures, there is difference of opinion regarding the value of retention sutures. In a well-controlled study Hubbard and Rever compared 203 midline incisions closed with and 209 midline incisions closed without retention sutures. Three cases of wound dehiscence occurred when retention sutures were used, and none occurred when they were not used. Because modern suture materials and suture techniques provide better wound security, we are not likely to use retention sutures except in very high-risk patients.

The rectus muscles are not sutured together in the

median incision unless there is sufficient diastasis to cause symptoms. In that case a special closure resembling a ventral hernia repair is used. In the routine closure the fascial edges are approximated with interrupted, figure-of-eight sutures of No. 0 delayed absorbable suture (Vicryl or Dexon) or synthetic braided non-absorbable suture (Ethibond or Tevdek II), taking generous bites on each side. These stitches are shown in Figure 11-13*A*. A stronger fascial closure is the Smead-Jones technique, in which a far-near, near-far modification of the horizontal mattress stitch is used. This technique offers the advantage of a wider fascial anchor of the suture and avoids the problem of suture pull-through along the fascial edge (Fig. 11-14).

It is no longer considered appropriate to close abdominal incisions in layers with fine sutures placed close to the edge of the aponeurosis and tied tightly. Experiments on wound healing by Jenkins demonstrate clear superiority of the placement of musculofascial sutures in the abdominal wall at 1- to 2-cm intervals, allowing a generous 2-cm or greater margin of fascia, including the medial border of the underlying muscle,

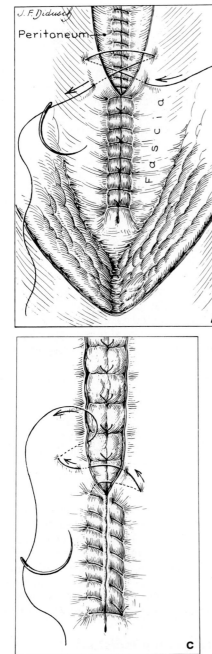

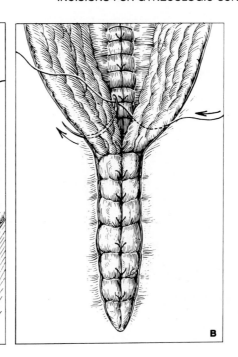

Figure 11–13. Layer-for-layer closure of the lower midline incision. *A*, The peritoneum has been closed with a continuous No. 2-0 delayed absorbable suture. The fascia is being closed with figure-of-eight No. 0 delayed absorbable sutures. *B*, The fat is approximated with interrupted No. 3-0 or 4-0 delayed absorbable sutures. *C*, The skin is closed with staples or with a No. 3-0 silk suture, interrupted or continuous.

especially in patients who are high-risk for poor wound healing. A continuous mass suture of monofilament plastic or continuous double-stranded nylon gives results equal to or better than interrupted sutures and is faster. Maxon (No. 0 or No. 1) also gives good results used in the same way. Schoetz and associates used a continuous No. 1 PDS II suture to close 172 midline incisions, many of which had been performed on pa-

tients who had risk factors for impaired wound healing. There were no eviscerations or dehiscences; five incisional hernias occurred. Wasiljew and Winchester reported satisfactory results with a continuous no. 1 Vicryl suture for midline incisions. A wide purchase of aponeurotic tissue gives increased holding power to the closure, since it increases the total amount of collagen included in the suture. The musculofascial margins

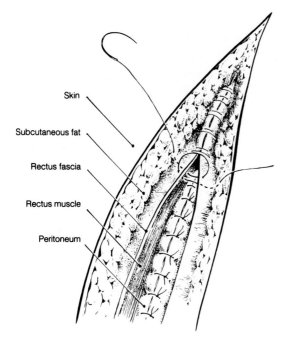

Skin

Subcutaneous fat

Rectus fascia

Rectus muscle

Peritoneum

Figure 11–14. Modification of far-near, near-far suture (Smead-Jones). Suture passes deeply through lateral side of anterior rectus fascia and adjacent fat, crosses the midline of the incision to pick up the medial edge of the rectus fascia, then catches the near side of the opposite rectus sheath, and finally returns to the far margin of the opposite rectus sheath and subcutaneous fat. (Adapted from Baggish MS, Lee WK. Abdominal wound disruption. Obstet Gynecol 1975; 46:533)

should not be approximated snugly, as formerly taught, but should be approximated loosely enough to permit 2- to 3-cm distention of the abdominal wall postoperatively. The analogy is to the technique for bowel closure, in which tight, necrosing sutures in the mucosal margins of a bowel anastomosis are avoided to prevent ischemia and suture pull-through or knot failure. In many cases of incisional hernia or evisceration the surgeon frequently finds free loops of suture material which have been tied too tightly and have cut through the fascial edges. It should be pointed out that the knot in the suture should be tied tightly and securely. However, the force applied to the tissue for approximation should not be too great. The less force applied to the tissue, the less chance that necrosis will occur, allowing the suture to pull through the tissue. But the knot should be tied tightly.

A continuous suture technique leaves less suture material in the wound when compared with placing multiple interrupted sutures, all of which must be tied several times. A continuous suture will not strangulate tissue as long as it approximates tissue with firm, rather than tight, tension.

After closure of the fascia the subcutaneous fat is approximated with interrupted No. 3-0 or No. 4-0 delayed absorbable suture (Fig. 11-13*B*). This step is omitted by some surgeons. The skin is closed with silk by the preferred stitch of the operator, or with skin staples. Figures 11-13*C* and 11-15*A* demonstrate skin closure with a continuous on-end mattress suture. This skin suture requires a little more time than the simple continuous suture, but it makes an excellent closure. It is particularly useful when one is dealing with the lax skin of a parous woman, since it prevents inversion of skin margins. Figure 11-15*B* shows a horizontal mattress stitch. We prefer a lock stitch (Fig. 11-15*C*) when hemostasis is desired and the skin bleeders are too superficial to ligate; these usually are controlled by pressure on the skin margins. Figure 11-15*D* demonstrates a continuous suture, which is quite satisfactory when the skin is firm. Figure 11-15*E* demonstrates a simple interrupted stitch. Interrupted stitches, particularly the vertical mattress (Fig. 11-15*F*), are placed with a straight Keith needle instead of the usual curved skin needle. This interrupted technique makes an ideal skin closure, although it is more time-consuming than the continuous suture. We have found the use of disposable skin staples to be a more rapid method of skin closure that has less foreign body reaction and stitch abscess from skin bacteria than various other suture techniques. The staples are ordinarily removed on the 5th or 6th postoperative day, and sterile adhesive strips are applied across the incision to hold the edges of the skin together. In special circumstances the skin staples may be left in place for a longer time, but there is a risk of leaving permanent staple scars.

Closing the skin edges with silk suture is not recommended for clean-contaminated or contaminated incisions. The large quantity of suture required for continuous skin closure potentiates the spread of bacteria along suture tracts in the subcutaneous fat, with the possibility of involving the entire length of the incision. The skin edges of a clean-contaminated or contaminated incision should be closed with disposable skin staples or packed open and closed later.

Transverse Incisions

When the Pfannenstiel incision is being closed, the peritoneum and rectus fascia are closed separately, as in the midline incision. Retention sutures are not used. When the Kustner incision is being closed, special attention must be directed to obliterating all dead space by anchoring the subcutaneous fat to the underlying fascia with No. 3-0 delayed absorbable sutures. Additional sutures are used to approximate the opposing margins of subcutaneous fat. The skin margins may be closed with a continuous subcuticular No. 4-0 delayed

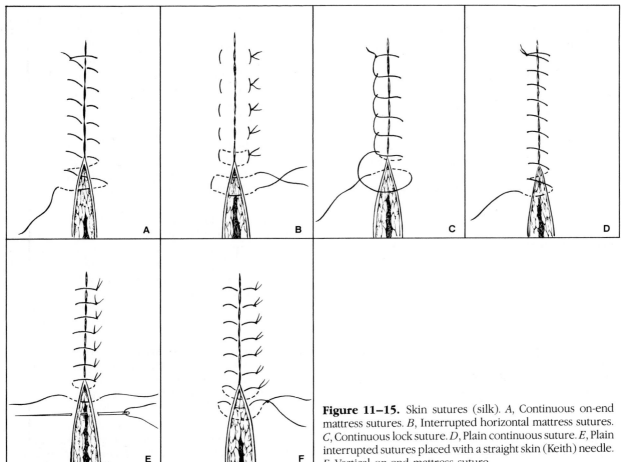

Figure 11–15. Skin sutures (silk). *A*, Continuous on-end mattress sutures. *B*, Interrupted horizontal mattress sutures. *C*, Continuous lock suture. *D*, Plain continuous suture. *E*, Plain interrupted sutures placed with a straight skin (Keith) needle. *F*, Vertical on-end mattress suture.

absorbable suture. Alternatively, skin staples may be used.

The transverse Maylard incision is closed by suturing the peritoneum transversely with a continuous No. 2-0 delayed absorbable suture. The edges of the peritoneum should be everted. The cut ends of the rectus muscles will be drawn together when the abdominal wall aponeurosis is approximated. No attempt should be made to bring the rectus muscles together separately. The edges of the aponeurosis should be approximated with a continuous No. 0 Maxon or PDS II suture. Contraction of the oblique muscles of the abdomen or strain of the incision tends to draw the muscles and the edges of aponeurosis tighter together and strengthens the closure. The edges of the subcutaneous fat are approximated with No. 4-0 delayed absorbable suture, bringing the hatch marks on the skin as close together as possible. The skin is closed according to the preference of the surgeon, usually with a continuous subcuticular No. 4-0 delayed absorbable suture or with

disposable skin staples. A subcuticular continuous closure with fine delayed absorbable suture is excellent for immediate closure of a clean or clean-contaminated transverse incision.

The value of closing the peritoneum in Pfannenstiel and lower midline incisions has been questioned. Tulandi and associates have reported fewer postoperative adhesions when the peritoneum is not closed. Although we might be willing (reluctantly) to omit peritoneal closure with the Pfannenstiel and lower midline incisions, we would insist on peritoneal closure with a Maylard incision. Leaving the peritoneum open with a Maylard incision would leave the ends of the rectus muscles exposed in the peritoneal cavity—an undesirable result.

McBurney's Gridiron Incision

The gridiron incision is closed with sutures similar to those used for the midline incision, although there is less strain on the suture line. As is true for the transverse incision, tension on the gridiron incision from contraction of the abdominal muscles draws the edges of the muscle and fascia closer together. The peritoneum is closed with a continuous suture of No. 2-0 delayed absorbable suture. The internal oblique and the transversus abdominis are closed as a single layer with figure-of-eight sutures of No. 0 delayed absorbable suture (see Fig. 11-10*D*). The margins of the external oblique are closed with interrupted or figure-of-eight sutures (see Fig. 11-10*E*). The fat and skin are closed as described. The skin of this incision is closed with interrupted sutures of fine silk, by which a firm approximation can be obtained, or by using skin staples.

Special Circumstances

Contaminated Wounds

The presence or absence of infection may be the major determinant of the final integrity of the incision. Depending on the type of operation done, the pathology for which the operation is performed, and other factors, varying degrees of bacterial contamination of the incision may result. Wounds may be classified as clean, clean-contaminated, contaminated, and dirty and infected wounds. For example, a clean-contaminated incision results from a total abdominal hysterectomy because the operation involves entrance into the vagina and possible contamination of the operative site with vaginal bacteria. If an accidental entry into the unprepared bowel occurs during a gynecologic laparotomy, the wound should be classified as contaminated. When the operation is done for a pelvic abscess and pus is spilled in the operative field, the wound is classified as dirty and infected. It is important for the gynecologic surgeon to think about this classification because the amount of bacterial contamination of the wound affects the choice of the method of closure of the incision. Patients will have a high probability of wound infection when the bacterial contamination is sufficient to overwhelm the host resistance to infection and to interfere with the local processes of wound repair, such as fibroblast activity and the production and organization of collagen, as shown by Bucknall. Patients who also may have one or more diseases (eg, diabetes, cancer, malnutrition) that interfere with one or more of the natural defense mechanisms of host resistance to infection are at even greater risks when the incision is contaminated with bacteria. So the gynecologic surgeon must not only evaluate the magnitude of wound contamination, but also estimate the extent to which the patient's defense against infection may be impaired.

The choice of sutures for incisional closure may be different when an incision is contaminated. Because natural healing is not as efficient when wound infection is present, a stronger suture material is needed to retain tensile strength for a longer time until the wound is healed. Bacteria in the wound accelerates the degradation of absorbable sutures and their usual loss of tensile strength. This is especially true of catgut suture. Synthetic absorbable sutures are better able to maintain their tensile strength and knot security when infection is present in the wound. This is in contrast to catgut suture, which loses strength and disintegrates more rapidly in the presence of bacterial contamination of wounds. Bacterial growth is inhibited in the presence of delayed absorbable sutures. Bacteria can hide in braided sutures and continue to contaminate the wound. Monofilament sutures are cleaner and less reactive in tissue. According to Bucknall, a monofilament nylon suture provides better wound security than delayed absorbable sutures in the presence of bacterial contamination. Neither catgut nor silk would be appropriate to use in a contaminated wound.

When the fascia of a contaminated wound is closed correctly, healing usually is secure. The subcutaneous fat, which has a poor blood supply, is a more likely site for wound infection. The vast majority of wound infections develop in the subcutaneous fat, especially when it is thick. When a grossly contaminated wound is closed primarily, the incidence of wound infection is very high, sometimes as much as 50%. With this in mind, many gynecologic surgeons have used a delayed type of closure of the contaminated abdominal incision, especially when the host defense mechanisms against infection also are impaired. The fascia is closed as indicated, usually with a Smead-Jones or mass continuous suture of monofilament nylon. The wound is irrigated with a copious amount of saline solution and packed lightly with a dry dressing. Interrupted mattress sutures are placed in the skin but not tied. Twice each day the wound is inspected and irrigated, and a fresh dry dressing is applied. On the 4th postoperative day, if the wound is clean with fresh granulation tissue, the skin sutures are tied and the skin edges brought closer together with sterile adhesive strips. Such a method of secondary closure is almost uniformly successful, and is associated with a very low incidence of wound complications.

Drains

Sometimes drainage of the abdominal cavity is deemed appropriate. For example, retroperitoneal drains are needed after pelvic lymphadenectomy to avoid lymphocele and ureteral fistula. Intraperitoneal drains may be needed when an operation for active tubo-ovarian abscesses results in oozing of peritoneal surfaces in the pelvis and incomplete removal of necrotic and infected tags of tissue. If their use is indicated, drains should be placed through separate stab wounds several centimeters from the skin incision without exception. We have almost completely discontinued using drains made of soft, collapsible rubber tubing, such as the Penrose or "cigarette" drain. Plastic tubes connected to a closed system for suction are preferable.

Drainage of the wound itself is best provided by a Jackson-Pratt closed-suction drain inserted through a separate stab wound. If it is determined that the wound may need drainage, one might also consider leaving it open for delayed closure. We do not recommend routine drainage of transverse Maylard incisions or routine drainage of the space of Retzius after suprapubic urethropexy procedures.

High-Risk Patients

In addition to bacterial contamination of the wound, a number of other special circumstances presented by the patient may interfere with wound healing. These must be taken into consideration when choosing the incision and planning the closure. Obesity, especially when the condition is morbid, presents challenges in incision placement and closure. One should avoid placing an incision through a heavily irradiated part of the abdominal wall. If this cannot be avoided, then the securest closure is needed to keep the wound from bursting until healing is secure. Patients with chronic pulmonary disease and a chronic cough need an incision and closure that will withstand the effect of repeated, incessant, and sudden increases in intra-abdominal pressure and strain on the suture line associated with constant coughing. Malnutrition, anemia, and weight loss are associated with many chronic diseases, including liver disease, kidney disease, chronic infection, and aging. These problems direct their attention not only to using a secure wound closure technique, but also to the possible use of various techniques of hyperalimentation preoperatively and postoperatively to improve nutrition and wound healing. Advanced age and diabetes have their own special adverse effects on wound repair that must be considered in advance. The experience of Morrow and associates and of Pitkin confirm the high incidence of wound infections among obese diabetic patients. And this is only a partial list. Especially dreaded is a combination of several of these factors in the same patient.

Morrow and associates, recognizing the special challenges of gynecologic surgery in the obese patient, suggest promoting it to an area of special interest. They prefer a midline incision in obese patients, citing less blood loss, a shorter operating time, and adequate exposure as advantages. Suction drains are placed above the fascia. The wound is irrigated with copious amounts of warm saline solution to remove fat and tissue debris. A primary Smead-Jones closure with No. 1 or No. 0 nylon is preferred. In their experience with 39 patients weighing from 200 to 325 pounds, there were five wound infections (all in diabetics) and no wound dehiscences. This method also was used by Gallup, who reported a wound complication rate of 3.1%.

We agree that a midline incision can be the correct incision in some obese patients. We also have used a transverse Maylard incision to advantage. It allows excellent exposure. A large panniculus of the lower abdomen may be removed at the same time. The incision should not be made in the unhealthy skin crease beneath the panniculus, where the warm, moist, sometimes macerated skin provides an excellent environment for anaerobic bacterial growth. The peritoneum is closed with a continuous No. 0 delayed absorbable suture, the aponeurosis is closed with a continuous no. 1 Maxon or PDS suture, the wound is irrigated copiously, Jackson-Pratt drains are inserted through separate incisions at each end, and the skin is approximated with metal clips, which may be left in place for a bit longer than usual. Delayed closure of the skin and fat also may be appropriate.

COMPLICATIONS OF ABDOMINAL INCISIONS

The important complications of abdominal wall incisions can be characterized, among other things, by their time of occurrence after surgery. Wound infection and dehiscence or evisceration occur early in the postoperative period. Sutures sinuses and incisional hernias are late manifestations of impairment of primary wound healing.

Wound Infections

Wound infections have been reviewed by Cruse and by Edlich and associates, and also are discussed in Chapter 9.

The frequency of postoperative wound infections varies from one clinic to another, and is related to many factors, including the experience of the surgeon, the type of procedure performed, the clinic population operated on, and the surgical condition of the patient. The usual rate of significant wound infections is 5% or less for all major abdominal operations. The incidence is somewhat higher in patients with pelvic inflammatory disease.

One of the most frequent causes of wound infection is the direct implantation of bacteria at the operating table. An inoculum of bacteria may reach the incision from either the skin of the patient or the skin of the operator. A study at Duke University by Moylan and Kennedy demonstrated the importance of gown and drape barriers in the prevention of wound infection. In 2253 consecutive general surgical operations the use of the disposable gown and drape system rather than reusable cotton cloth material reduced the incidence of postoperative infection from 6.4% to 2.3%. Earlier work by Beck and Collett demonstrated conclusively that cotton materials, when wet, actually wick bacteria through the fabric and cause contamination of the wound. Of interest in the Duke study was the fact that the disposable gown and drape system resulted in a lowered infection rate in both clean and clean-contaminated operations. Further, their study showed that there was no difference in the infection rate between clean and clean-contaminated procedures when prophylactic antibiotics were given preoperatively, intraoperatively, and postoperatively. Operative procedures that exceeded 90 minutes in length had a much higher infection rate than did shorter-length operations. It is a well-known fact that elderly patients, especially those over age 60, are more prone to wound infection complications than younger patients. This may be the result of poor nutrition, decreased immune response, or other aging factors. It also was shown in the Duke study and in other investigations that women have a statistically higher wound infection rate than men. This phenomenon may be related to wound seeding from subclinical infections in the vaginal tract. Cole and Bernard determined that 20% to 40% of all surgical gloves are punctured during the course of an average operation, and that such puncture sites could contaminate the wound with 4,000 to 18,000 staphylococci within 20 minutes.

Newer antiseptic scrub techniques have been developed, including povidone-iodine (Betadine), 4% chlorhexidine gluconate (Hibiclens), and the standard 3% hexaclorophene (pHisoHex). A study by Peterson and coworkers evaluating these compounds as surgical scrub preparations showed that of the three, chlorhexidine gluconate in detergent solution produced the best immediate and persistent reduction in normal hand flora. Preoperative baths and scrubbing the patient's abdomen the night before surgery with an antiseptic solution, such as povidone-iodine, have reduced the frequency of postoperative wound infection in many clinics where surgical patients are primarily from low socioeconomic groups. The patient's abdomen should not be shaved until immediately before surgery, to avoid superficial skin lacerations that would permit bacterial invasion. The deep recesses of the umbilicus should receive special attention by vigorous cleaning with a cotton-tipped applicator. During most operations the patient's skin is inadequately isolated from the inci-

sion with skin towels or adherent plastic drapes, although the latter are considered to be more effective than loose skin towels. Studies suggest that the use of disposable drapes and towels, and adherent skin drapes may contribute to a reduction in wound infections.

Whenever a bacteria-containing organ is opened—mainly the bowel, gallbladder, or urinary tract—there is a marked increase in the infection rate of the abdominal incision. Small areas of infection often occur in low midline incisions, particularly at the lower end of the incision, where the hair follicles may harbor bacteria that are not sterilized by the surgical scrub. As mentioned, these cases are benefited by scrubbing the abdomen for 20 minutes the evening before surgery. The number of wound infections also correlates with the obesity of the patient. Beneath a large panniculus is a favorite place for anaerobes and aerobes to multiply. The fact that folds in the skin, moistened by perspiration, harbor more bacteria than dry skin is the rationale on which many surgeons leave the incision exposed for delayed closure postoperatively in a very obese patient. The incision should be thoroughly irrigated with saline before closure of the subcutaneous tissues to make certain that a hematoma is not overlooked in the operative site, particularly when the patient is obese. Prophylactic antibiotics and subcutaneous drains are useful in controlling wound infections when infection has been encountered in the pelvis, particularly when a stab wound is required for drainage. For the antibiotic to prove effective in reducing incisional infections—that is, for it to result in a therapeutic tissue level at the time of surgery—it must be given in sufficient time preoperatively to be absorbed. Many effective perioperative antibiotic regimens have been published. Cephalosporins have been the most popular antibiotics used for this purpose.

Coliform bacilli, particularly *Escherichia coli* and *Aerobacter aerogenes,* are the most common contaminants of the incision in postoperative patients, along with *Staphylococcus aureus.* In most cases the wound infection develops to the stage of clinical recognition within 5 to 6 days postoperatively. The temperature usually remains slightly elevated, and the patient may complain of tenderness in the incisional area, although this symptom is not consistently present. In most instances the wound infection is discovered in a routine search for the cause of a temperature elevation and is noted by the presence of reddening of the skin with fluctuation or induration of the subcutaneous tissues.

The wound should be cultured and opened, and bacterial sensitivity studies should be obtained, so that the patient can be treated with the appropriate antibiotics. The wound is cleaned daily with hydrogen peroxide and povidone-iodine solution. Hot compresses are used if there is considerable induration of the adjacent tissue, as moist heat is superior to dry heat in aiding drainage of the infected tissue. The area of the incisional infection should be stimulated to granulate from the base upward by the use of an iodoform wick, urea crystals, and the like. After healing has been initiated the skin edges may be debrided and drawn together by narrow strips of sterile adhesive tape (Steri-strips) or, if necessary, by secondary closure.

Although a rare complication of gynecologic surgery, the fulminating course of necrotizing fasciitis caused by hemolytic *Streptococcus* and *Staphylococcus,* as well as a variety of virulent gram-negative bacteria, deserves early diagnosis, vigorous antibiotic treatment, and prompt, aggressive, and extensive debridement. The wound harboring this necrotizing process is excruciatingly painful initially, and demonstrates dark vesicles, dusky discoloration, and widespread ecchymosis. There is rapid progression of subcutaneous and fascial necrosis, and septicemia, and death occurs in 20% to 30% of the patients. This condition, which has been reviewed by Borkowf, must be differentiated from gas gangrene (*Clostridium*) and progressive synergistic bacterial gangrene for proper management.

Wound Dehiscence and Evisceration

In the broadest sense, the term *dehiscence* includes the separation of any of the suture layers of the abdominal wall, although it usually is used synonymously with the terms *evisceration, wound disruption,* and *burst abdomen.* In the latter definitions the disruption includes all layers of the abdominal wall and protrusion of the intestines through the incision.

Reports of the frequency of actual dehiscence and evisceration vary considerably in the surgical literature, between 0.3% and 3% of all cases of pelvic surgery. Pratt reports the occurrence of eight dehiscences in about 2500 gynecologic laparotomies (0.3%) at the Mayo Clinic, and all eight cases had vertical incisions and extensive operations. Keill and coworkers reported an incidence of wound dehiscence of 0.68% in cases with transverse incisions compared with 2% in cases with vertical incisions. Mowat and Bonnar observed a decrease in the incidence of wound dehiscence from 2.9% to 0.3% when the transverse incision was used for cesarean section. As noted by Rollins, about 50% of patients with a serious wound complication have had prior abdominal or pelvic surgery. Complete disruption and evisceration is one of the most serious of all wound complications. A 10-year study by Helmcamp at the New York Hospital found a mortality rate of 2.9%, or 2 deaths among 70 cases.

Causative Factors

The various reported factors associated with wound dehiscence may be summarized in four general categories: (1) the type and location of the incision, (2) the specific type of suture, (3) the inherent strength of the tissues (wound healing), and (4) mechanical factors.

The importance of the type of incision has been previously discussed. Low midline incisions have a higher rate of wound dehiscence than transverse or gridiron incisions. In addition, the strength of the incision is inversely proportional to its length.

The choice of a permanent or absorbable suture in the closure of an incision has been long debated as a factor in wound healing. Previous reports failed to document a difference between the frequency of wound disruption in cases in which the fascial closure was accomplished by nonabsorbable suture and those in which absorbable catgut was used. Recent evidence has established that a difference does exist. In a study of more than 1000 major abdominal procedures Baggish and Lee demonstrated a reduction in the incidence of wound disruption from 0.4% when catgut was used for incisional closure to 0.1% when polyglycolic delayed absorbable suture material and the Smead-Jones fascial closure techniques was used. In an important study on wound healing Jenkins showed that when a tightly sewn laparotomy wound becomes elongated by abdominal distention, the sutures come under undue tension, with a significant risk of breakage, pull-through, or knot failure. All of these complications were demonstrated to be preventable by placing stitches 1 cm apart with sufficient generosity of suture material that the total suture used equals at least four times the wound length. Of equal importance was the inclusion of a wide (2 cm) margin of fascia and the medial border of the muscle layer in the suture closure. This study and others suggest that the tissues should be approximated loosely to permit as much as 30% increase in the length of the incision owing to abdominal distention during the postoperative period. Therefore, large, loose sutures are preferable to tight, forceful, strangulating sutures that cause ischemia of the margins of the incision, and that may result in suture pull-through, breakage, or knot failure. Although the tissue is approximated without undue tension, the knots should be securely tied.

The inherent strength of the tissue has been related to various factors, including vitamin C deficiency, protein deficiency, anemia, wound infection, and the patient's age. Unquestionably, major surgical wounds have a higher disruption rate in the elderly patient than in the young patient, a finding that has been observed by many surgeons. In addition, inflammation disrupts collagen deposition in a wound, with separation of tissue by the accumulation of purulent exudate. Such inflammatory response weakens the fascial suture line, produces premature fragmentation of absorbable suture, and allows permanent suture to pull through the fascial edge of the incision. Patients with a chronic disease, notably an advanced neoplasm, are known to have poor wound healing owing to limitation of collagen deposition and fibroblastic activity. Surgery through a previous operative site is known to produce a weaker scar because of limitation of blood supply and diminished fibroblastic activity. Obesity is a common feature in most reports of wound disruption, and is related to the amount of tension on the suture line. Frequency of wound infection also is increased in such patients. The thickness of the subcutaneous fat layer has a direct bearing on wound infection and failure of healing. Pitkin reported the incidence of abdominal wound infection or separation to be increased sevenfold in 300 obese women in comparison with a matched control group of normal-weight subjects. Hematoma formation in the incision is a frequent cause of poor healing and produces an excellent nidus for sepsis. It frequently is associated with wound disruption and evisceration and is one of the preventable factors in such complications.

One of the most striking findings in most large series of wound dehiscence is the association of infection and mechanical factors, including pulmonary complications and abdominal distention. In the study by Guiney and associates 87% of their cases experienced one or more such complications in contrast to a 15% occurrence in a control group. Excessive vomiting and coughing, abdominal distention, and hiccups have been implicated as causative factors in increasing tension on the suture line. Many surgeons have championed the use of tension (stay) sutures to support the suture line in such cases, particularly when tension and strain are increased. Although many believe that retention sutures help to prevent dehiscence, there are those who either are uncertain about the merits of retention sutures or consider the retention suture merely as a safeguard against evisceration. We prefer to use the stay suture in high-risk patients as a method of avoiding expulsion of the bowel through the completely separated abdominal wound if an evisceration should occur. By this method the wound edges are firmly held together, but with the stay sutures anchored through the anterior rectus fascia and without producing ischemia to the suture line. When used, the stay sutures should be left in place for 10 to 14 days in high-risk patients.

Diagnosis

Evisceration must be recognized early and treated promptly, since the mortality rate has been reported to be as high as 15% to 20%. Some cases of evisceration occur entirely without symptoms, and are discovered on routine inspection of the incision. Most cases, however, present symptoms and signs that at least call for investigation. Dehiscence usually occurs within the 5th to 8th postoperative day, and is associated with infection in more than half of the cases. The patient frequently is conscious of something "giving way." One of the most common signs is the presence of a watery, serosanguineous drainage from the incision, which should alert the astute clinician to the possibility of an impending evisceration. When such drainage occurs in the presence of discomfort in the region of the incision, disruption should be strongly suspected. The incision may be gently probed with a sterile instrument or with a sterile gloved finger, looking for defects in the fascia and peritoneum. When the evisceration is discovered, or suspected, a sterile towel should be placed over the incision and a tight adhesive bandage applied for temporary control of the protrusion of the bowel through the incisional site, and the patient should be transferred to the operating room for a more complete examination under anesthesia.

Treatment

Immediate closure of the disrupted incision is indicated. Because this complication may be life-threatening, delay in secondary closure is not recommended, since the patient's condition will not improve until the incision is reapproximated. Secondary closure after evisceration is best accomplished by through-and-through sutures of an inert material, preferably no. 2 nylon sutures (Fig. 11-16A). Before closure the wound should be thoroughly cleansed at the operating table, under general anesthesia, and gentle debridement should be accomplished where needed. The intestines should be manipulated as little as possible when being replaced in the peritoneal cavity. The wound is cultured for aerobic and anaerobic bacteria, and antibiotic sensitivities are obtained. The sutures are placed through the entire thickness of the abdominal wall, including the peritoneum, as demonstrated in Figure 11-16B. Current statistics show that the incidence of secondary incisional hernia is decreased by closure of the fascial margins, loosely, with interrupted sutures of a delayed absorbable suture material that include a wide margin of fascia and the inner border of the abdominal musculature. In recent years we have found through-and-through nylon sutures to be as effective and inert as silver wire sutures and less discomforting and traumatic to the wound. After being inserted the sutures are held with clamps but are not tied until all are placed. This procedure pulls the abdominal wall away from the viscera and guards against injury to the bowel. The stay sutures are placed about 2 cm apart. When the sutures are closed by tying, the skin and abdominal muscles are

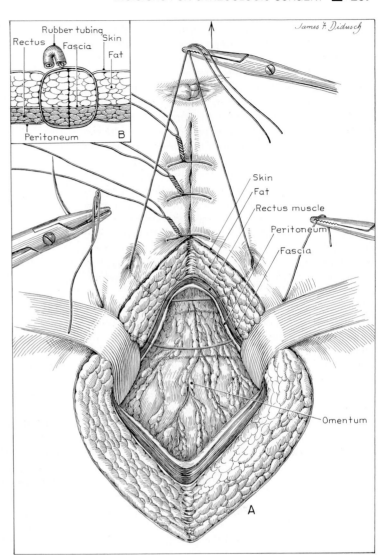

Figure 11–16. Secondary closure of disrupted wound with through-and-through silver-wire or preferably, No. 2 nylon sutures. *A*, Method of closure. *B*, Suture twisted tight and approximating the wound edges.

well approximated; if more careful approximation is desirable, interrupted sutures or disposable skin staples may be placed between the stay sutures.

A broad-spectrum antibiotic is initiated and modified according to the bacteriology and antibiotic sensitivity. Postoperatively, the patient is treated with a nasogastric tube for decompression of the bowel, and intravenous fluid replacement is maintained until bowel function returns to normal and oral feedings are well tolerated. The sutures are left in place until healing appears to be complete, which usually requires about 14 to 21 days. We frequently discharge the patient to her home and remove the sutures sometime later, when healing is complete.

Incisional Hernia

An incisional hernia is caused by incomplete healing of the operative wound in which the peritoneum remains intact while the fascial margins and adjacent muscles separate, leaving a defect beneath the subcutaneous fat into which the bowel may herniate.

Causative Factors

The causative factors related to poor healing and hernia formation are similar to those for wound dehiscence. Instead of complete dehiscence and evisceration of the wound, hernia formation results from incomplete dehiscence in which the peritoneum, subcutaneous fat, and skin remain intact. Most cases of ventral hernia follow an incisional infection, with impairment of both fibroblastic activity and the synthesis of collagen during the active phase of wound healing. Increased intra-abdominal pressure from coughing and vomiting, along with necrosis of the fascial margins, permits the sutures to pull through the edge of the fascia. These changes result in separation of the wound edges and failure of fibroblastic bridging of the fascia. This complication occurs more frequently in the lower abdominal incision because of the anatomic deficit of a posterior fascial sheath beneath the rectus in the area inferior to the semicircular line. Ventral hernias occur after low midline incisions in about 0.5% to 1% of all gynecologic surgery; the incidence increases to about 10% after a wound infection, whereas after dehiscence and reclosure the chance of hernia formation increases to 25%.

Although the initial fascial defect may be small, the size of the resultant hernia may assume varying proportions and involve the entire length of the lower abdominal wall. The size of the hernia depends on the mobility of the bowel and omentum and the final aperture in the ventral defect. A large amount of small bowel and omentum can escape from a very small fascial defect into an easily expandable subcutaneous space. The smaller the fascial defect through which small bowel has herniated, the greater the frequency of incarceration, obstruction, and infarction.

Diagnosis

The diagnosis of a ventral hernia is not difficult in view of the fact that the abdominal wall is distended in such cases (Fig. 11-17) and the patient complains of lower abdominal discomfort. The patient may observe peristalsis of the bowel beneath the skin, and may not note the regression of the mass while in the recumbent position with recurrence of the abdominal distention while erect. The hernia is more noticeable on coughing and straining, and may increase in size with time because of either enlargement of the hernial ring or incorporation of additional segments of bowel in the hernial sac. It is rare that a ventral hernia produces acute symptoms of visceral torsion and infarction, and therefore the repair of the hernia usually is on an elective basis.

Treatment

The principles of ventral hernia repair include (1) dissection of the hernial sac from the subcutaneous fat, rectus fascia, and peritoneal margin; (2) excision of the redundant hernial (peritoneal) sac; and (3) closure of

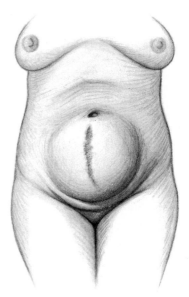

Figure 11–17. Ventral hernia in a low midline incision.

the abdominal wound, using a layer-for-layer closure, an overlap repair of the rectus fascia, or the placement of a synthetic mesh prosthesis (Prolene).

The low midline incisional scar is excised, and the underlying subcutaneous fat is mobilized free from the adjacent hernial sac. Sharp dissection is used to separate the skin and underlying fat widely from the margins of the hernial sac (Fig. 11-18A). It is important to defer opening the sac until the boundaries of the hernia have been delineated and dissected, as this aids in identifying the various tissue planes. To identify the margins of the fascial ring, it is advisable to open the sac and separate any underlying bowel from the peritoneal surface of the sac (Fig. 11-18B). Loops of small bowel and adherent omentum frequently obscure the true identity of the sac, and many pockets of the peritoneal lining are formed by fibrous bands that anchor the bowel to the peritoneum. After releasing the omentum and bowel, with particular attention given to hemostasis, it is important to determine if the hernial defect can be adequately closed with the adjacent fascia before excising the lining of the sac. If there is adequate fascial tissue remaining after the dissection, either a layer-for-layer or an "overlap" fascial closure should be done. If there is inadequate fascia available to close, the defect must be bridged with Prolene mesh. Most incisional hernias can be closed without the use of a mesh support. When there has been failure of an initial hernial repair, when the hernial defect is so large that the edges cannot be adequately approximated, or when the tissues of the abdominal wall are quite attenuated, the use of synthetic mesh is strongly advised.

The layer-for-layer closure is accomplished after closure of the peritoneum as the initial layer. The fascial margins of the anterior rectus sheath are then sutured with either a nonabsorbable No. 0 (silk, Tevdek, Ethibon) suture (Fig. 11-18C). Interrupted far-near, near-far pulley sutures (modified Smead-Jones) that include the inner margin of the abdominal musculature are placed to avoid subsequent pull-through of the suture from the edge of the incision. These sutures serve as internal stay sutures and increase the tensile strength of the wound while healing occurs.

If there is adequate fascial margin of good strength, a "vest-over-pants" closure will give extra support to the defect and produce a double-layer closure of the fascia (Fig. 11-18D). It is necessary to separate the peritoneum and posterior rectus sheath from the hernial margins to permit an overlap of the anterior fascia. The peritoneum is closed separately with a continuous suture of No. 2-0 delayed absorbable suture of polyglactin material. The anterior rectus sheath of the hernial margins is separated widely on each side of the wound. Horizontal mattress sutures of a permanent suture material are placed 3 to 4 cm distant from the fascial edge, and pass through only the free margin of the opposite fascia before returning to the distal portion of the anterior fascia. The sutures are held untied until all have been placed. When the sutures are tied, the free fascial margin is drawn firmly beneath the opposite fascial layer, producing a double support to the hernial closure. The remaining free fascial margin is sutured to the fascial surface (Fig. 11-18E) to complete the double-layer closure.

When closure of the fascial margins is complete, perforated drainage tubes may be inserted beneath the skin flaps and sutured to the anterior rectus fascia with fine catgut, for subsequent drainage (see Fig. 11-18E). Penrose drains do not provide a satisfactory method for wound drainage. Perforated plastic tubes or rubber catheters give a better conduit for removal of serum by negative suction pressure in a potentially infected site. Jackson-Pratt drains are ideal. The drains should exit through the skin several centimeters away from the primary incision.

Large Hernias

In repairing a ventral hernia with a large fascial defect and poor abdominal tissue, it may be necessary to reinforce the hernial defect with a polypropylene prosthetic mesh such as Prolene. In using mesh it is important to dissect the hernial sac as previously described and to carefully define the layers of the abdominal wall (Fig. 11-19A). Because of the placement of a foreign body in the abdominal incision, meticulous hemostasis and aseptic technique are essential. The implanted mesh must completely bridge the entire defect, with adequate margins for suturing to the adjacent rectus muscles.

After the hernial sac is removed and the margins of the fascial defect are freed, the rectus muscle is freed from the underlying posterior fascial sheath and peritoneum (see Fig. 11-19A). The fascia and peritoneum beneath the rectus muscle should be dissected widely around the margins of the defect to permit closure of the peritoneum without tension. A large piece of mesh is then inserted between the rectus muscle and the closed peritoneum (Fig. 11-19B). The mesh should be maintained under slight tension; therefore, the lateral sutures that anchor the mesh to the fascia should be strategically placed so that the mesh does not buckle when the overlying rectus muscles are approximated in the midline. Nonabsorbable No. 0 Tevdek or Ethibon sutures are used to anchor the mesh to the rectus abdominis muscle. Closure of the rectus fascia over the mesh is then attempted as far as possible, using the far-near, near-far closure technique (Fig. 11-19C). If the rectus muscles or fascia cannot be approximated in the midline, the attenuated hernial sac is used to bridge the gap and cover the underlying mesh. In this case the margins of the hernial sac are preserved, so that they can be sutured to the lateral margins of the anterior rectus fascia. Alternatively, when the peritoneum and posterior fascia cannot be separated from the margins of the hernia, the mesh may be placed on the anterior surface of the rectus and abdominal muscles and beneath the anterior fascia, rather than posteriorly. Although it is preferable to place the mesh beneath the abdominal muscles to prevent infection from the incision, placement beneath the anterior fascia has proved to be much easier and anatomically quite satisfactory.

Drainage tubes or catheters are placed longitudinally on either side of the fascial incision, and the subcutaneous fat and skin are closed separately. Suction is applied to the drainage tubes to give negative pressure beneath the skin and prevent elevation of the skin flaps by serum or blood. The drains may be removed by the 5th day but must be left in place until there has been complete cessation of incisional drainage.

Postoperatively, the patient is ambulated on the day after surgery, without prolonged bed rest. It is advisable, however, that the abdominal incision be protected from excessive stress and strain of coughing, vomiting, and retching. An elastic binder is helpful. If the bowel becomes distended, it should be decompressed immediately with a nasogastric tube until normal bowel function has returned. Prophylactic antibiotics often are used perioperatively to prevent secondary infection in the operative site. Antibiotics are particularly indicated for patients in whom mesh has been used for closure of a large hernial defect.

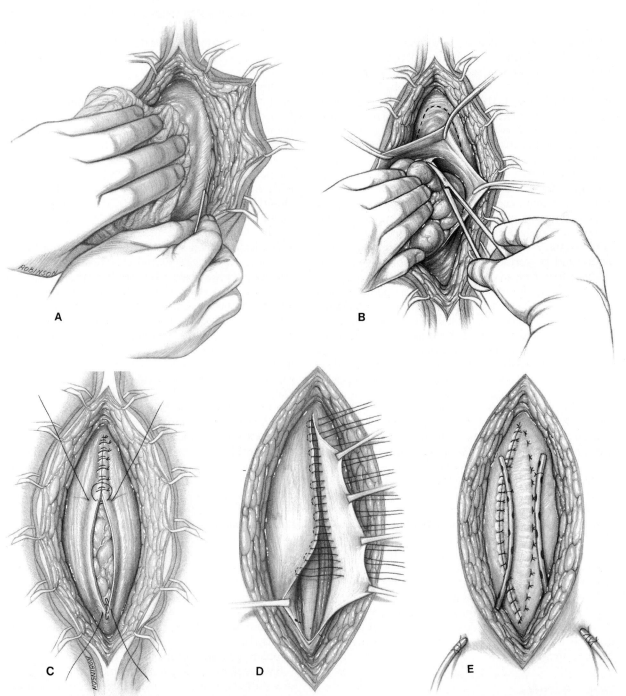

Figure 11–18. Repair of ventral hernia. *A,* Wide dissection of subcutaneous fat from lateral boundaries of ventral hernia. *B,* Hernial sac opened and adherent bowel and omentum released from the peritoneal surface. Note the superior margin of the fascial defect (*dotted line*). *C,* Layer-for-layer closure of midline ventral hernia. Redundant hernial sac has been excised and fascial margins are sutured by far-near, near-far technique. Crown stitch is demonstrated at lower pole, showing anchoring of apex of defect to lateral fascial margins. When possible, the peritoneum is closed as a separate layer. *D,* Vest-over-pants technique of midline hernia repair. The peritoneum is separated from hernia and closed. Anterior rectus fascia dissected widely; horizontal mattress sutures are placed distant from fascial edge and passed through the opposite fascial margin. When the sutures are tied, fascial margins are drawn firmly beneath opposite layer, producing a double fascial layer closure of hernia. *E,* Completion of vest-over-pants closure of midline ventral hernia showing suture of free margin of the fascial flap to the underlying fascial surface. Perforated plastic closed suction drainage tubes are sutured to the fascia to permit adequate drainage.

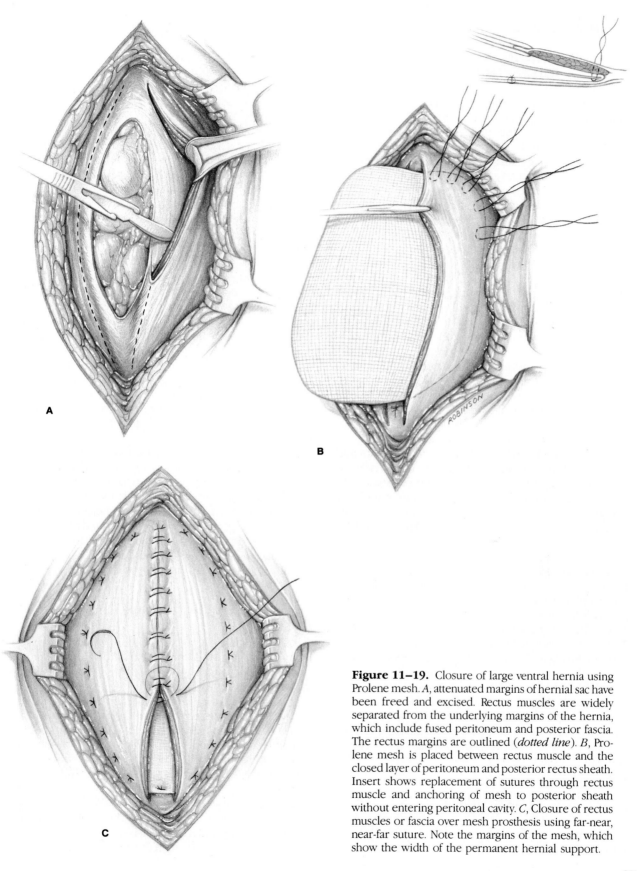

Figure 11–19. Closure of large ventral hernia using Prolene mesh. *A,* attenuated margins of hernial sac have been freed and excised. Rectus muscles are widely separated from the underlying margins of the hernia, which include fused peritoneum and posterior fascia. The rectus margins are outlined (*dotted line*). *B,* Prolene mesh is placed between rectus muscle and the closed layer of peritoneum and posterior rectus sheath. Insert shows replacement of sutures through rectus muscle and anchoring of mesh to posterior sheath without entering peritoneal cavity. *C,* Closure of rectus muscles or fascia over mesh prosthesis using far-near, near-far suture. Note the margins of the mesh, which show the width of the permanent hernial support.

PANNICULECTOMY AND ABDOMINOPLASTY

The morbidly obese patient with a large, protruding panniculus of the lower abdominal wall presents a major technical problem and a surgical risk for pelvic surgery. Not only is the operative procedure technically difficult because exposure of the surgical field is limited when operating through a large panniculus, but wound healing also is seriously compromised. The increased incidence of wound infection and hematoma formation and the potential for development of a ventral hernia put the obese patient in the high-risk category for both significant complications after pelvic surgery. In the past, surgical treatment of symptomatic pelvic disease was not often undertaken in such patients, and alternative methods, frequently less effective, were adopted.

With the current sophistication of anesthesia techniques, the intensive care monitoring of the postoperative patient, and the medical control of cardiopulmonary reserve, the obese patient has become a less serious risk and a more frequent surgical candidate. To alleviate the anatomic problem of surgical exposure and to reduce the frequency of postoperative wound complications, panniculectomy and abdominoplasty have become more common procedures when performed as a part of major abdominal surgery.

Panniculectomy was first described by Demars and Marx in 1890, as reported by Elbax and Falguel. Howard Kelly (1910) was among the first of a list of surgeons to recommend removal of a large panniculus at the time of pelvic surgery, remarking that, for cosmetic purposes alone, the procedure was warranted. The procedure then fell into oblivion for the next 50 years, until a resurgence of interest developed in the field of plastic and reconstructive surgery. During the 1970s and 1980s there were many descriptions and reports on abdominal panniculectomy, but few have emerged from the gynecologic literature until the experience from the Mayo Clinic was reviewed by Pratt and Irons in 1978. This large series included 126 panniculectomies performed during a 20-year period, of which 85 were done specifically to facilitate exposure to the surgical field. A modified transverse elliptic incision was used for most cases, and V-shaped wedges of tissue were removed from the angles of the incision to reduce the redundant skin. Although 34.5% of the patients had some degree of postoperative morbidity, the average hospital stay was only 14 days.

Indications

The major indication for panniculectomy is abdominal obesity with an accumulation of fat that produces an abdominal wall that protrudes over the symphysis pubis and the upper thighs. The degree of abdominal obesity may be accentuated by short stature and loss of subcutaneous tissue support from advanced age. Although there are no absolute indications for this procedure based on weight alone, morbid obesity usually is defined as a weight of more than twice the ideal body weight as derived from the Metropolitan Life Insurance tables on desirable weight. Such patients usually weigh more than 115 kg. Most women in this weight category have a large abdominal panniculus when examined in the erect position. Excision is recommended for this group of patients when pelvic surgery by the abdominal route is indicated, particularly in those who are physically inconvenienced by the weight and size of the abdominal fat pad. The patient also must be counseled and must become strongly motivated to a weight reduction program, as it is impractical to perform an extensive abdominoplastic procedure in a patient who makes no change in her nutritional habits. If the surgical procedure is not urgent, it should be deferred until there is clinical evidence of a weight loss of about 40% to 50% of the optimal weight loss that is planned. Although the panniculectomy may remove as much as 35.5 kg, the purpose of the preoperative weight loss is to establish a normal eating pattern before the operation.

Patients who have a large diastasis recti in association with the panniculus also are candidates for this procedure, at which time plication of the rectus fascia should be done, either directly or using a vest-over-pants, layered technique. In many instances the rectus abdominoplasty is of as much cosmetic and therapeutic benefit to the patient as is the panniculectomy. When both anatomic conditions coexist, the panniculectomy alone will not give a satisfactory surgical result.

Technique

Of the various operative techniques available for panniculectomy and abdominoplasty, the elliptical transverse incision, originally described by Kelly, has proved to be the procedure of choice. We have found two modifications of the transverse panniculectomy to be useful. The most common procedure includes an elliptical "watermelon" incision (Fig. 11-20A) extending from the lateral aspect of the lumbar regions to about 3 to 4 cm above the umbilicus. If the patient requests the preservation of the umbilicus, it can be excised and transplanted to the upper pedicle of skin. Inferiorly, the transverse incision follows the concave skin fold that separates the overhanging panniculus from the suprapubic skin. The underlying fat is excised deeply in a slightly wedged manner, with the deep portion of the fat

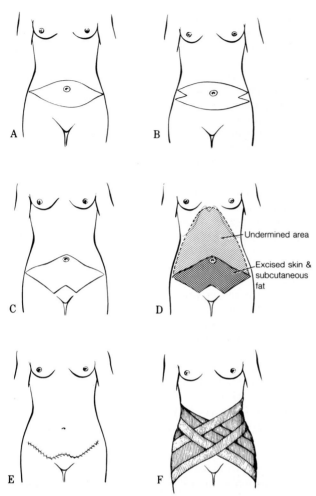

Figure 11–20. Panniculectomy incisions. *A,* Elliptical transverse incision extending from region of iliac crest extends above and below umbilicus. *B,* V-shaped incision in lateral angles eliminates folds of skin in abdominal wall. *C,* W-shaped incision over the mons pubis extends along the inguinal ligament to the iliac crest. *D,* The upper incision passes above the umbilicus. Wide mobilization of the upper skin flap is carried to the sternum and rib margins. *E,* After removal of panniculus and skin, the upper skin flap is sutured without tension to the lower skin margin. *F,* A firm elastic dressing is criss-crossed over the abdominal wall for abdominal support and to prevent seroma formation.

extending outward and slightly beyond the skin margin to avoid ischemia of the incision. Meticulous attention must be given to absolute hemostasis, a time-consuming procedure, to avoid postoperative hematoma formation and infection. The excessive use of cautery, which produces a favorable environment for bacterial growth in devitalized tissue, should be avoided. The lateral angles of the incision may require separate "V"

incisions to avoid the unsightly folds of redundant fat (Fig. 11-20*B*). When these V-shaped wedges are closed, the angle of the incision is converted into a Y-shaped configuration, which eliminates the excessive skin in the lateral aspects of the abdominal wall. After the removal of the large panniculus the abdomen may be opened either transversely or vertically. If an abdominoplasty is required to approximate the widely separated rectus muscles, a midline incision is necessary. In this way a tight closure of the rectus fascia or a vest-over-pants repair, as shown in Figure 11-18*D* and *E,* will give additional strength to the abdominal wall. If the rectus fascia is of poor quality and will not provide adequate support to the abdominal wall, a mesh graft may be inserted at the completion of the procedure, either above or below the rectus muscle (see Fig. 11-19). Alternatively, if the fascia of the rectus sheath can be plicated in the midline, wide plication and anchor of the medial margins of the rectus muscle at the closure of the procedure will close the diastasis and give a firm abdominal wall.

A second type of transverse panniculectomy is a "W" technique, initially described by Regnault in 1972 and shown in Figure 11-20*C*. The incision is outlined before the operative procedure in the form of a W over the symphysis pubis, inside the hairline. The incision is started in the center of the mons pubis and extended laterally and downward on each side to the inguinal fold near the external inguinal ring. The line then follows above the inguinal ligament in the panniculus skin crease to the region of the iliac crest on each side of the pelvis. The upper margin of the incision is drawn above the umbilicus to the upper margin of the redundant fat. If the umbilicus is to be relocated, the new umbilical site is drawn in the upper skin flap before the incision is made, and is transposed to the upper skin flap after the incision is closed. The panniculus is excised before the pelvic operation in the manner described.

At the completion of the panniculectomy, the abdomen is opened either vertically or transversely in accordance with the surgeon's preference, as wide exposure of the anterior abdominal wall is produced. A vertical incision through the linea alba is preferred, since this provides an opportunity to plicate the rectus fascia or to perform a layered, vest-over-pants closure of the abdominal wall. In closing the W-shaped incision of Regnault after the abdominal or pelvic operation is completed, the upper flap of the abdominal skin is mobilized superficial to the fascia as far as necessary to the region of the xiphoid process and to the inferior margin of the costochondral junctions of the rib cage (Fig. 11-20*D*). Here it is particularly important to reemphasize the necessity for meticulous ligation and control of all small bleeding vessels. A thin layer of fat is left attached to the fascia to facilitate the postoperative absorption of serous fluid. As shown in Figure 11-20*E,* the upper skin flap is sutured to the W-shaped, pubic skin margins, using interrupted sutures of no. 2-0 delayed absorbable suture for the subcutaneous fat. Multiple fine sutures are used to anchor the skin flap to the abdominal wall to prevent seroma formation and loculation. Suction drainage is always used beneath the upper skin flap, using a small Silastic or a polyethylene catheter that is brought out through separate lateral stab wounds above the suture line. If the upper skin flap will not reach the pubic skin without excessive tension, the patient is placed in a slightly jackknife position on the operating table by having the back elevated and the legs maintained in a straight horizontal position. When the skin margins have been approximated over the pubis and along the inguinal ligament, additional V-shaped incisions can be taken from the lateral angles of the incision if there is redundant skin present.

The skin is closed after either procedure with interrupted vertical mattress sutures of No. 3-0 silk. Alternatively, we have used inert skin staples or a removable fine subcuticular suture to approximate the skin margins. Skin staples can be left in place without the risk of infection until the skin incision has shown adequate healing. Rather than being removed all at once, they can be removed over a period of several days and replaced with sterile strips of adhesive. The new umbilicus is placed in the skin flap by making a 2-cm horizontal incision in the center flap, about 2 cm below the waistline. Fine interrupted No. 2-0 or No. 3-0 subcuticular sutures are used to anchor the fat of the incision to the transplanted umbilicus, and the skin is approximated with No. 3-0 silk vertical mattress sutures. A firm Elastoplast tape dressing is applied under tension over the abdominal wall in a crisscross manner, beginning at the rib cage and extending to the thighs (Fig. 11-20*F*). This abdominal support will relieve tension on the suture line and also prevent seroma and hematoma formation beneath the skin flaps.

PERINEOTOMY INCISIONS

Adequate exposure is just as important with vaginal surgery as it is with abdominal surgery. When exposure is not adequate with abdominal operations, the incision is extended or some other measure used to improve exposure. There also are measures that one can use to improve exposure with vaginal operations. A tight vaginal introitus may restrict exposure of the upper vagina. It may be enlarged at the beginning of the operation by simply making a midline or mediolateral episiotomy incision. A mediolateral incision can be made on one or both sides of the vaginal introitus. If a midline episiotomy is made and closed transversely, the vaginal

introitus may be made larger than before, if that is deemed advisable. These incisions may be closed with No. 2-0 or No. 3-0 delayed absorbable suture. They almost always heal per primum, and can be a real advantage in facilitating the performance of operations in the upper vagina when exposure is limited by a tight vaginal introitus.

Sometimes the entire vagina is small in caliber because of virginity or nulliparity, atrophic shrunken vaginal mucosa, previous colporrhaphy, or previous radiation or disease in the vagina. The vaginal vault may be fixed in a relatively high position with relatively little descensus. These circumstances may be so severe as to require that the operation be done abdominally because adequate exposure through the vagina is impossible to achieve. On the other hand, sometimes the exposure required can be obtained by making a Schuchardt incision. The entire vagina may be enlarged with this incision with a remarkable improvement in exposure of the upper vagina. Sometimes a patient whose problem might otherwise have necessitated an abdominal approach can have the advantage of a perfectly satisfactory vaginal operation if a Schuchardt incision is made.

According to Speert, Langenbeck made a deep relaxing incision into the perineal body in attempting vaginal hysterectomy for uterine cancer in 1828. Similar incisions were used by Olshausen in 1881 and Duhrssen in 1891. Karl Schuchardt described his incision in 1893:

> in order to make more accessible from below a uterus whose mobility is limited. . . . With the patient in the lithotomy position and her buttocks elevated, a large, essentially sagittal incision is made, somewhat convex externally, beginning between the middle and posterior third of the labium majus, . . . extending posterior toward the sacrum, and stopping two fingerbreadths [*sic*] from the anus. The wound is deepened only in the fatty tissue of the ischiorectal fossa, leaving the funnel of the levator ani muscle, the rectum behind it, and the sacral ligaments intact. Internally, the sidewall of the vagina is opened into the ischiorectal fossa and the vagina divided in its lateral aspect by a long incision extending up to the cervix. There thus results a surprisingly free view of all the structures under consideration.

This incision has since become known as the Schuchardt incision.

The incision ordinarily is made on the patient's left side by a right-handed operator (Fig. 11-21*A*). A left-handed operator may find it technically easier to make the incision on the patient's right side. Bilateral inci-

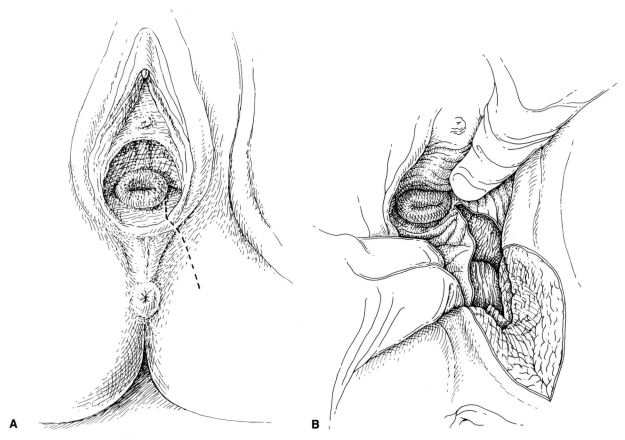

Figure 11–21. *A*, The Schuchardt incision begins at the 4 o'clock position at the vaginal introitus and extends into the buttock and up the posterolateral wall of the vagina to the cervix. *B*, The ischiorectal fossa fat is exposed. The puborectalis muscle is divided. The left paravesical and pararectal can be exposed through the incision.

sions have been advocated in extreme cases. The side on which the incision is made might be dictated by the location of the pathology to be removed. Injection of the tissues to be incised with sterile saline solution may be helpful, especially beneath the vaginal mucosa in the line of the incision. The assistant pulls upward to the left with the index finger placed as deep as possible in the vagina just to the left of the urethra. The operator makes countertraction by placing two fingers in the vagina and pulling downward to the right. This pull and counter-pull in opposite directions stretches the left vaginal wall. The incision is made with the electrosurgical unit beginning at the four o'clock position at the introitus and extending downward in the skin of the buttock to the level of the anus. The incision is then carried upward through the vaginal mucosa into the upper one-third of the vagina. As the incision is deepened, the fingers of the operator's left hand are used to displace the rectum medially to protect it from injury. The isch-

iorectal fossa fat will be visible below the puborectalis muscle. The muscle is incised with the electrosurgical knife (Fig. 11-21*B*). If necessary, the left paravesical space can be developed. For the best possible exposure the apex of the vaginal incision should intersect any incision made around the cervix. Bleeders are coagulated or ligated and a laparotomy pack is sutured to the edges of the vaginal incision to help retain a posterior retractor in place.

At the end of the operation the Schuchardt incision is closed with No. 2-0 and No. 3-0 delayed absorbable sutures, attempting to approximate the puborectalis muscle edges and to obliterate the dead space in the ischiorectal fossa. It usually is not necessary to drain the incision.

A Schuchardt incision most often is used for extensive vaginal hysterectomy for early invasive cervical cancer. We also have used it when doing extensive dissections to remove endometriosis in the vaginal vault, to gain better exposure for difficult vaginal hysterectomy or vesicovaginal fistula repair, to repair injuries to the lower ureter, to remove organized hematomata just above the puborectalis muscle, to drain lymphocysts vaginally, and to remove benign cystic teratomata in the lower presacral area behind the rectum. It can convert a technically difficult, complicated, and dangerous vaginal operation into one that is simple, easy, and safe. It is extremely helpful whenever increased exposure of the vaginal vault is required. It is difficult to understand why perineotomy incisions are so quickly done for obstetric operations and so reluctantly done for gynecologic operations.

Bibliography

Baggish MS, Lee WK. Abdominal wound disruption. Obstet Gynecol 1975;46:530.

Baudelocque A. Nouveau procede pour practiquer l'operation Cesarienne, Thesis No. 132. Paris, 1823.

Beck, WC, Collett TS. False faith in the surgeon's gown and drape. Am J Surg 1952;83:152.

Breen, JL. Transverse incisions and the total abdominal hysterectomy. Gynecol Surg Film Festival, New York, September, 1987.

Brokowf HI. Bacterial gangrene associated with pelvic surgery. Clin Obstet Gynecol 1973;16:40.

Bucknall TE. Factors influencing wound complications: a clinical and experimental study. Ann R Coll Surg Engl 1983;65:72.

Cherney LS. A modified transverse incision for low abdominal operations. Surg Gynecol Obstet 1941;72:92.

Cole WR, Bernard HR. Inadequacies of present methods of surgical skin preparation. Arch Surg 1964;89:215.

Cox CE. Principles of operative surgery: antisepsis, technique, sutures, and drains. In: Sabistan DC Jr, ed. Textbook of surgery. 13th ed. Philadelphia: WB Saunders, 1986.

Cox PJ, Ausobsky JR, Ellis H, Pollock AV. Towards no incisional hernias: lateral paramedian versus midline incisions. J R Soc Med 1986;79:711.

Cruse PJE, Foord R. The epidemiology of wound infection. A 10-year prospective study of 62,939 wounds. Surg Clin North Am 1980;60:27.

Cullen TS, Brodel M. Lesions of the rectus abdominis muscle simulating an acute intra-abdominal condition. Bull J Hopkins Hosp 1937;61:295.

Daversa B, Landers D. Physiological advantages of the transverse incision in gynecology. Obstet Gynecol 1961;17:305.

Delany HM, Carnevale NJ. A "bikini" incision for appendectomy. Am J Surg 1976;132:126.

Elbaz JS, Flageul G. Plastic surgery of the abdomen. New York: Masson, 1979:42.

Ellis H. Commentary on midline abdominal incisions. Br J Obstet Gynaceol 1984;91:1.

Everett HS, Mattingly RF. Urinary tract injuries resulting from pelvic surgery. Am J Obstet Gynecol 1956;71:502.

Fletcher HS, Joseph WL. Bleeding into the rectus abdominis muscle. Int Surg 1973;58:97.

Funt MI, Thompson JD, McDuff HC Jr. Abdominal incisions and closures. Obstet Gynecol Update Tapes 1981.

Gallup DG. Modifications of celiotomy techniques to decrease morbidity in obese gynecologic patients. Am J Obstet Gynecol 1984;150:171.

Goldman JA, Feldberg D, Dicker D, et al. Femoral neuropathy subsequent to abdominal hysterectomy: a comparative study. Eur J Obstet Gynecol Reprod Biol 1985;20:385.

Goligher JC. Visceral and parietal sutures in abdominal surgery. Am J Surg 1976;131:130.

Goligher JC, Irvin TT, Johnston D, et al. A controlled clinical trial of three methods of closure of laparotomy wounds. Br J Surg 1975;62:823.

Greenall MJ, Evans M, Pollock AV. Midline or transverse laparotomy? A random controlled clinical trial. Part II: Influence on postoperative pulmonary complications. Br J Surg 1980;67:191.

Guillou PJ, Hall TJ, Donaldson DR, et al. Vertical abdominal incisions: a choice? Br J Surg 1980;67:395.

Guiney EJ, Morris PJ, Donaldson GA. Wound dehiscence. Arch Surg 1966;92:47.

Halpern SL. Quick reference to clinical nutrition. Philadelphia: JB Lippincott, 1979.

Haxton H, Clegg J, Lord M. A comparison of catgut and polyglycolic acid sutures in human abdominal wounds. Abdom Surg 1974;16:239.

Helmkamp BF. Abdominal wound dehiscence. Am J Obstet Gynecol 1977;128:803.

Howard RJ, Simmons RL, eds: Surgical infectious diseases. 2nd ed. East Norwalk, CT: Appleton and Lange, 1988:chap 18 and 19.

Hubbard TB Jr, Rever WB Jr. Retention sutures in the closure of abdominal incisions. Am J Surg 1972;124:378.

Hudson AR, Hunter GA, Waddell JP. Iatrogenic femoral nerve injuries. Can J Surg 1979;22:62.

Hunt TK. Physiology of repair. In: Gibson T, ed. Wound healing. First International Symposium on Wound Healing. Rotterdam, April 1974. Montreux: Foundation for International Cooperation in the Medical Sciences, 1975.

Irvin TT, Koffman CG, Duthie HL. Layer closure of laparotomy wounds with absorbable and nonabsorbable suture materials. Br J Surg 1976;63:793.

Jenkins TPN. The burst abdomen: a mechanical approach. Br J Surg 1976;63:873.

Jones TE, Newell ET, Brubaker RE. The use of alloy steel wire in the closure of abdominal wounds. Surg Gynecol Obstet 1941;72:1056.

Keill RH, Keitzer WF, Nichols WK, et al. Abdominal wound dehiscence. Arch Surg 1973;106:573.

Kelly HA. Excision of the fat of the abdominal wall: lipectomy. Surg Gynecol Obstet 1910;10:229.

Kirk RM. Effect of method of opening and closing the abdomen on incidence of wound bursting. Lancet 1972;2:352.

Krupski WC, Sumchai A, Effeney DJ, et al. The importance of abdominal wall collateral blood vessels. Arch Surg 1984;119:854.

Kustner O. Der suprasymphysare kreuzschnitt, eine methode der coeliotomie bei wenig umfanglichen affektioen der weiblichen beckenorgane. Monatsschr Geburtsh Gynakol 1896;4:197.

Kwaan JH, Connelly JE. Doppler assessment of the inferior epigastric artery flow patterns as a screening test for aortoiliac obstruction. Am J Surg 1979;138:117.

Langer K. Cleavage of the cutis (the anatomy and physiology of the skin). Presented at the Meeting of the Royal Academy of Sciences, April 25, 1861. Clin Orthop 1973;91:3.

Mackenrodt A. Die radikaloperation des gebarmutterscheidenkrebes mit ausravmung des beckens. Verh Dtsch Gynakol 1901;9:139.

Martyak SN, Curtis LE. Abdominal incisions and closure. A systems approach. Am J Surg 1976;131:476.

Masterwon BJ. Wound healing in gynecologic surgery. In: Masterson BJ, ed. Manual of gynecologic surgery. New York: Springer-Verlag, 1979.

Mayerowitz BR, Gruber RP, Laub DR. Massive abdominal panniculectomy. JAMA 1973;225:408.

Maylard AE. Direction of abdominal incisions. Br Med J 1907;2:895.

McBurney C. The incision made in the abdominal wall in cases of appendicitis, with a description of a new method of operating. Ann Surg 1894;20:38.

McDowell E. Three cases of extirpation of diseased ovaria. Electic Repertory Anal Rev 1817;7:242.

Morrow CP, Hernandez WL, Towsend DE, et al. Pelvic celiotomy in the obese patient. Am J Obstet Gynecol 1977;127:335.

Moschcowitz AV. Transverse incisions in the upper abdomen. An Surg 1916;64:268.

Mowat J, Bonnar J. Abdominal wound dehiscence after cesarean section. Br Med J 1971;2:256.

Moylan JA, Kennedy BV. The importance of gown and drape barriers in the prevention of wound infection. Surg Gynecol Obstet 1980;151:465.

Nahai F, Brown RG, Vasconez LO. Blood supply to the abdominal wall as related to planning abdominal incisions. Am Surg 1976;42:691.

Peterson AF, Rosenberg A, Alatary SO. Comparative evaluation of surgical scrub preparations. Surg Gynecol Obstet 1978;146:63.

Pfannenstiel JH. Uber die vortheile des suprasymphysaren fascienguerschnitt fur die gynaekologischen koeliotomien. Samml Klin Vortr Gynaekol (Leipzig) Nr 268, 1900;97:1735.

Pitkin RM. Abdominal hysterectomy in obese women. Surg Gynecol Obstet 1976;142:532.

Pratt JH. Wound healing: evisceration. Clin Obstet Gynecol 1973;16:126.

Pratt JH, Irons GB. Panniculectomy and abdominoplasty. Am J Obstet Gynecol 1978;132:165.

Regnault P. Abdominal lipectomy, a low W incision. Int J Aesthetic Plast Surg 1972.

Regnault P. Abdominoplasty by the W technique. Plast Reconstr Surg 1975;55:265.

Rollins RA, Corcoran JJ, Gibbs CE. Treatment of gynecologic wound complications. Obstet Gynecol 1966;28:268.

Sanz Patterson JA, Kamath R, Willett G, et al. Comparison of Maxon suture with Vicryl, Chromic catgut, and PDS sutures in fascial closure in rats. Obstet Gynecol 1988;71:418.

Savage RC. Abdominoplasty combined with other surgical procedures. Plast Reconstr Surg 1982;70:437.

Schoetz DJ, Coller JA, Veidenheimer MC. Closure of abdominal wounds with polydioxanone. Arch Surg 1988;123:72.

Schuchardt K. Eine neue methode der gebarmutterexstirpation. Zentralbl Chir 1893;20:1121.

Sippo WC, Burghardt A, Gomez AC. Nerve entrapment after Pfannenstiel incision. Am J Obstet Gynecol 1987;157:420.

Sloan GA. A new upper abdominal incision. Surg Gynecol Obstet 1927;45:678.

Sowa DE, Masterson BJ, Nealon N, et al. Effects of thermal knives on wound healing. Obstet Gynecol 1985;66:436.

Speert H. Obstetric and gynecologic milestones. New York: Macmillan, 1958:630–636, 665–671.

Tera H, Aberg C. The strength of suture knots after one week in vitro. Acta Chir Scand 1976;142:301.

Tera H, Aberg C. Tissue strength of sutures involved in musculoaponeurotic layer sutures in laparotomy incision. Acta Chir Scand 1976;142:349.

Thompson JB, MacLean KF, Collier FA. Role of the transverse abdominal incision and early ambulation in the reduction of postoperative complications. Arch Surg 1949;59:1267.

Tollefson DG, Russell KP. The transverse incision in pelvic surgery. Am J Obstet Gynecol 1954;68:410.

Tulandi T, Hum HS, Gelfand MM. Closure of laparotomy incisions with or without peritoneal suturing and second-look laparotomy. Am J Obstet Gynecol 1988;158:536.

Usher FS. The repair of incisional and inguinal hernias. Surg Gynecol Obstet 1970;131:525.

Van Winkle W Jr, Hastings JC, Barker E, et al. Effect of suture materials on healing skin wounds. Surg Gynecol Obstet 1975;140:7.

Wallace D, Hernandez W, Schlaerth JB, et al. Prevention of abdominal wound disruption utilizing the Smead-Jones closure technique. Obstet Gynecol 1980;56:226.

Wasiljew BK, Winchester DP. Experience with continuous absorbable suture in the closure of abdominal incisions. Surg Gynecol Obstet 1982;154:378.

Whitaker WG Jr. Transverse abdominal incisions. Southern Surg 1948;14:143.

12

New Imaging Techniques in Gynecology

SHIRLEY McCARTHY

The advances in cross-sectional imaging have dramatically changed the practice of radiology and gynecology. Ultrasonography, computed tomography (CT), and magnetic resonance imaging (MRI) are tomographic techniques that enable visualization of organs and tissues previously unseen with standard plain film radiography.

These cross-sectional techniques each depend on different physical properties to generate tomographic images of the anatomy. Ultrasonography depends primarily on differences in acoustic impedance, especially the rigidity of tissues. It is, therefore, particularly accurate in the differentiation of solid versus cystic structures. CT depends on tissue differences in x-ray attenuation. Calcium, water, fat, and air, having quite different attenuation coefficients, are thus clearly separated. Soft tissues, however, usually have only subtle density differences, hence intravenous contrast often is necessary to improve the separation of normal and abnormal by means of differences in vascularity or vascular permeability. MRI relies on four tissue parameters: hydrogen content (in fat or water), T1 and T2 (tissue magnetic relaxation times), and blood flow. The way hydrogen nuclei (protons) behave in a magnetic field depends on their local physical and chemical environment. The relaxation times (T1 and T2) determine the rates at which protons emit their signal after excitation with radiowaves. Because these differences are far greater than differences in radiographic contrast (electron density), there is inherently more contrast with MRI. A wide range of contrast differences (T1-, T2-, or proton density–weighted images) are available to identify a certain tissue or disease. Furthermore, because rapidly flowing blood does not generate a signal, vessels stand out from adjacent structures, obviating the need for intravenous contrast administration to identify them. MRI is biologically safe because the energies involved are so small (ie, are nonionizing, unlike standard x-ray techniques). An x-ray photon interacting with tissue is at least 10 billion times more energetic than an electromagnetic photon. Hazards exist, however, since the magnetic field used is many times that of earth's gravity. Patients with pacemakers, implanted electronic devices, and certain types of cerebral aneurysm clips cannot undergo MRI.

UTERUS

Normal

The normal uterus can be identified by any cross-sectional imaging technique: ultrasonography, CT, or MRI. Because the contrast resolution of CT is insufficient to demonstrate the tissue structure within the uterus and CT entails ionizing radiation, there is no reason to use this technique in a premenopausal woman unless uterine malignancy is being staged. Internal uterine anatomy can be visualized on both ultrasonography and MRI. The myometrium on sonography (Fig. 12-1) normally demonstrates a homogenous low to moderate level of echogenicity in contradistinction to the endometrial stripe, which is seen as a moderate to high amplitude thin echogenic line. With transabdominal ultrasonography, depending on bladder distention, the uterus may be seen in varying degrees of version. In women with retrodisplaced uteri the central linear echo complex that identifies the uterine cavity may be seen in only 20% of patients. Because the fundus of the uterus is situated farther from the transducer and

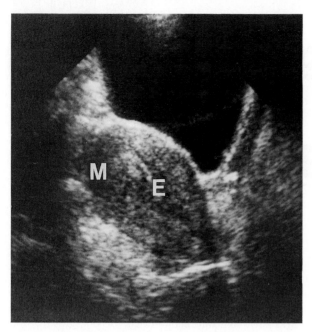

Figure 12–1. Transabdominal ultrasound demonstrating normal, moderate echogenic myometrium (*M*) and the echogenic endometrial stripe (*E*).

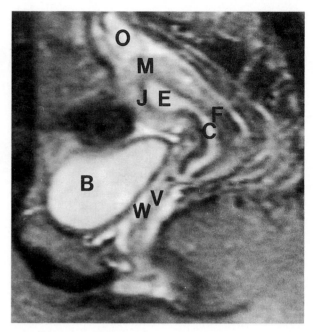

Figure 12–2. Sagittal MR scan showing the corpus, cervix, and vagina in one plane. Note the endometrium (*E*), junctional zone (*J*), myometrium (*M*), endocervical canal (*C*), fibrous stroma (*F*), vaginal canal (*V*), vaginal wall (*W*), bladder (*B*), and ovary (*O*).

may be partially shadowed by the rest of the uterus, the fundus can simulate a leiomyoma. Leiomyomas may distort the uterus such that a retroverted uterus is simulated; these tumors also can obliterate the central echo complex, thereby prohibiting confident identification of the uterus. Transvaginal sonography offers an alternative view that can obviate some of these pitfalls.

With MRI the uterus can always be identified because of a characteristic zonal anatomy apparent with this modality. Bowel, bone, body habitus, uterine position, or masses contiguous with the uterus do not impede reliable identification of this zonal anatomy. On T2-weighted scans the endometrium appears as a bright (high-signal) zone contiguous with the equally bright endocervical canal (Fig. 12-2). Also seen is a surrounding dark (low-signal) band, the junctional zone, which is continuous with the fibrous stroma of the cervix. The origin of this zone is as yet unknown, but it may be part of the myometrium, which appears as a moderate-signal structure. Despite numerous histologic studies, no discrete tissue layer has been identified. Nonetheless, a decrease in magnetic relaxation times (T1 and T2) and in water content compared with the endometrium and myometrium have been documented.

The hormonal milieu can be appreciated by visualization of the relative tissue thicknesses of these uterine layers as well as by the corpus–cervix ratio. The zonal anatomy of the uterus is visualized in premenarchal, reproductive-age, and postmenopausal women; however, as one might expect, the endometrium and myometrium are both smaller in the nonreproductive-age groups. In women who are taking oral contraceptives (Fig. 12-3), a significant decrease in endometrial width has been noted, as well as an increase in myometrial signal intensity. The latter has been attributed to myometrial edema, which accompanies oral contraceptive use. With gonadotropin-releasing hormone analog there is a statistically significant decrease in both endometrial and myometrial size.

Developmental Variants

Uterine malformations are classically evaluated with hysterosalpingography. Anomalies of the nongravid uterus occasionally are detected on ultrasonography, but sonography usually serves as an adjunct to hysterosalpingography. Hysterosalpingography does have limitations, particularly in the differentiation of septate from bicornuate uteri. Although the cornua of the septate uterus typically demonstrate a more acute angle than that seen with the bicornuate uterus, there is overlap. Ultrasonography or MRI can demonstrate the presence of myometrial tissue between the endometrial cavities. Because the zonal anatomy is so reliably demonstrated with MRI, it can be used to quantify the amount of interposed myometrium and demonstrate the external contour of the uterus (Fig. 12-4). A direct coronal view through the corpus can be obtained even in severely retrodisplaced uteri. Identification of the external contour of the uterus may not always be possible with ultrasonography, owing to position or the presence of myoma or adnexal masses, which may look like the second uterine horn. The relative accuracy of transvaginal sonography is unknown. The diagnosis of uterus didelphys requires injection of both cervices during hysterosalpingography, whereas both cornua and cervices can be readily shown with MRI (Fig. 12-5). The identification of two cervices on sonography is not reliable. Although the cervix and the vagina are always visualized with MRI, it is not known whether a thin vaginal septum, for example, can be visualized, since insufficient studies exist to date. Uterine hypoplasia can be diagnosed by hysterosalpingography, sonography, or MRI. In the same study, ultrasonography or MRI also can be used to demonstrate the urinary tract without added cost or risk to the patient.

Benign Diseases

Although ultrasonography can be used to screen for the presence of leiomyomas, MRI is the procedure of choice in the evaluation of these tumors in patients when therapeutic decisions need to be made—for example, in infertility patients. Although a leiomyomatous uterus can be identified with ultrasonography, discrete localization of individual leiomyomas usually is not possible. The most common sonographic finding is an abnormal uterine contour. Uterine enlargement and an inhomogeneous echo texture are frequent findings as well. These tumors demonstrate a wide variety of appearances but typically are hypoechoic with poor sound transmission. The sonogram can be falsely normal. In contrast, MRI can depict the number, size, location, and presence of degeneration (Figs. 12-6 and 12-7). Large feeding vessels also are demonstrated (Fig. 12-8). MRI is more accurate than ultrasonography or hysterosalpingography in localizing these tumors in infertile patients before myomectomy. Although submucosal lesions can be localized with hysterosalpingography, intramural lesions can only be inferred if large. Subserosal lesions are not seen, whereas they are clearly depicted with MRI and distinguished from adnexal masses. MRI is particularly useful in discerning whether a mass is ovarian or uterine in origin. Subserosal fibroids may simulate ovarian masses on pelvic examination and sonography. In a study of 30 patients who had undergone ultrasonography or CT, MRI provided additional information or increased diagnostic confidence in 25 of these 30 patients (Fig. 12-9).

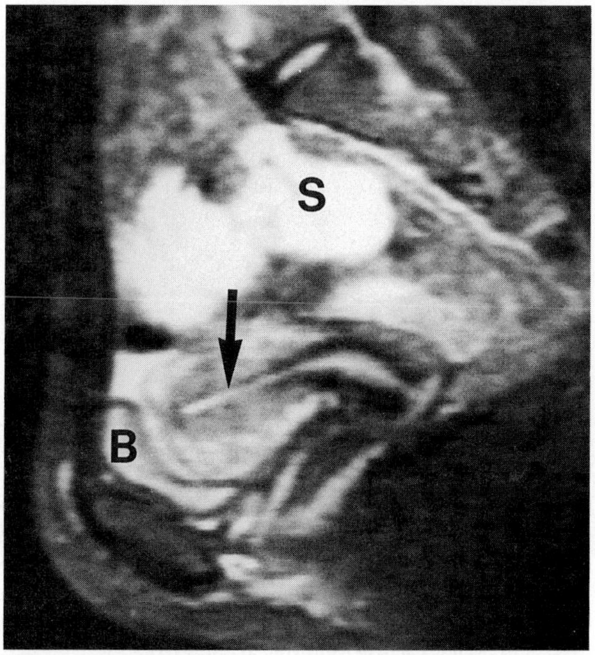

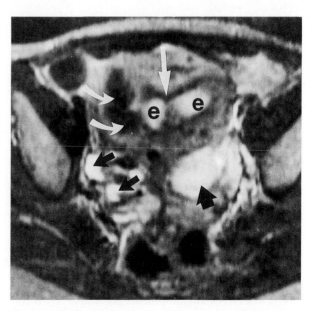

Figure 12–3. Sagittal MR scan showing the thin endometrium (*arrow*) seen in women who are taking oral contraceptives. Note bladder (*B*) and small bowel (*S*).

Figure 12–4. Axial MR scan of a patient with a septate uterus. Note septum (*white arrow*) between two endometrial cavities (*e*). Also note two intramural fibroids (*curved arrows*) and extensive endometriosis in the cul-de-sac (*black arrows*).

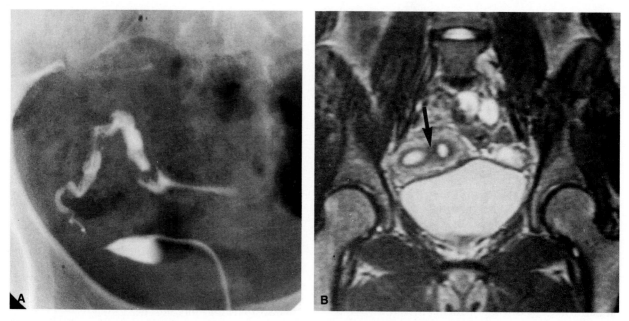

Figure 12–5. *A*, Hysterosalpingogram (in a patient with two cervices discovered on routine pelvic examination) shows one uterine horn. The other cervical os could not be canulated. *B*, MR scan shows two separate endometrial cavities separated by a small amount of myometrium (*arrow*).

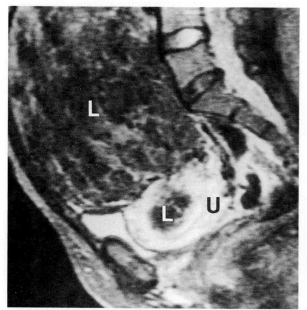

Figure 12–6. Sagittal MR scan showing a large subserosal and a small intramural leiomyoma (*L*). Uterus (*U*) is compressed inferiorly.

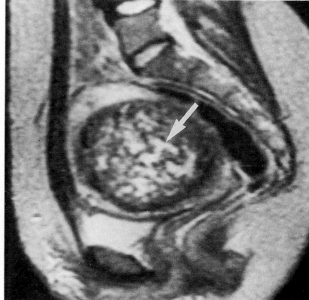

Figure 12–7. Sagittal MR scan showing a large intramural leiomyoma that has undergone degeneration, manifested by the high signal (*arrow*) internal component.

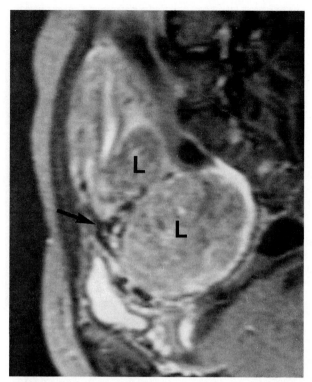

Figure 12–8. Sagittal MR scan showing one intramural leiomyoma (*L*) and a large subserosal leiomyoma (*L*). Note numerous vessels (*arrow*) feeding these benign tumors.

Dooms, Hricak, and Tscholakoff were able to depict adnexal masses as separate from the uterus in 23 of 23 cases. Leiomyomas can obscure the deep pelvis and displace the ovaries into the false pelvis, where transvaginal sonography cannot reach and transabdominal sonography has no acoustic window secondary to overlying bowel. In 23 cases of leiomyomatous disease, Zawin and coworkers identified 44 of 46 ovaries, in contrast to 21 of 46 ovaries with ultrasonography. Additionally, determination of uterine volume with MRI was possible in all patients, but with sonography it was not possible with volumes greater than 140 ml (Fig. 12-10).

Response to drug therapy can be monitored with MRI, since total intrauterine volume and individual leiomyoma volumes can be quantitated to assess therapeutic efficacy. The response of an individual leiomyoma also can be documented. Zawin and associates noted a statistically significant decrease in the size of individual leiomyomas and the number of vessels visualized in women using gonadotropin-releasing hormone analog. Gross vascularity of the leiomyoma can be assessed, thus enabling better timing of myomectomy after medical therapy. The precise anatomic local-

ization of these tumors also permits better choice of treatment options (eg, vaginal hysteroscopy versus myomectomy) (Fig. 12-11).

Adenomyosis, another cause of uterine enlargement, can be identified with MRI and distinguished from leiomyomatous disease. An often neglected diagnosis, adenomyosis appears as a focal or diffuse thickening of the junctional zone with or without bright foci, which represent the heterotopic endometrium (Fig. 12-12). This disease can be separated from leiomyomas, since the latter are typically well circumscribed owing to a pseudocapsule, whereas adenomyosis interdigitates with the myometrium. Adenomyosis usually is not diagnosable with sonography, since the findings are nonspecific. Walsh, Taylor, and Rosenfield described a honeycomb sonographic appearance of the myometrium in four cases, whereas Bohlman and coworkers described uterine enlargement with a decreased echogenicity in seven cases. In a study by Togashi, Ozasa, Konishi, and associates the cause of uterine enlargement was prospectively diagnosed with MRI in 92 of 93 cases of women with adenomyosis, leiomyomas, or coexistent disease.

Tumors

Imaging is primarily used for the staging of endometrial carcinoma diagnosed with dilatation and curettage. Ultrasonography is of limited use in staging endometrial carcinoma. Although it may show enlargement of the uterus with abnormal echogenicity, these findings are nonspecific, and can be due simply to uterine fibroids. An intact endometrial halo can be seen with superficial invasion, whereas an absent halo may indicate deep invasion. The major utility of CT in the staging of uterine carcinoma is in the assessment of extrauterine spread, particularly spread to the pelvic sidewall, lymph nodes (Fig. 12-13), and distant metastases (eg, liver). Hricak, Stern, Fisher, and others have demonstrated an overall accuracy of MRI in staging endometrial cancer of 92%, with an accuracy of 82% in evaluating depth of myometrial invasion. The superior contrast resolution of MRI compared with CT enables detection of tumor spread within the uterus, thereby enabling more accurate staging of early, curable disease (Fig. 12-14). Long and associates demonstrated an MRI accuracy of 92% in separating deep invasion (>50%) from superficial invasion (<50%) and focal disease (Fig. 12-15). Early carcinoma limited to the endometrium may appear simply as an expansion of the central high signal zone not distinguishable from adenomatous hyperplasia. In postmenopausal women who are not receiving estrogen replacement, this zone

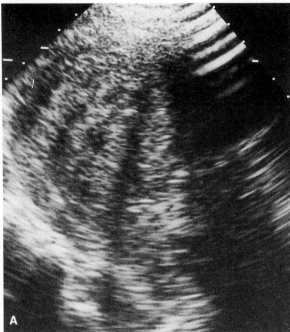

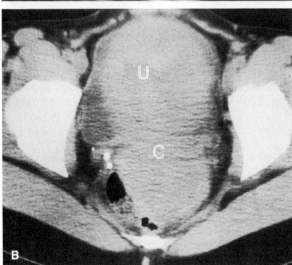

Figure 12–9. Febrile postpartum patient with a large bulky uterus. *A*, Ultrasound showing echogenic uterus. *B*, CT scan conducted to rule out infection does not have the contrast resolution to display internal gynecologic anatomy. Corpus uterus (*U*) and cervix (*C*) appear similar. *C*, Axial MR scan shows that a large leiomyoma (*L*) has prolapsed into the upper endocervical canal (*arrow*). This submucosal fibroid had obstructed uterine contents. Once removed, adequate drainage occurred.

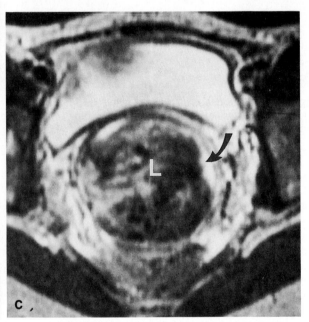

should be about 3 mm or less. Gross tumor limited to the endometrium can be measured. Complete integrity of the junctional zone is the main criterion for the absence of myometrial invasion (Fig. 12-16).

Gestational Trophoblastic Disease

The sonographic appearance of gestational trophoblastic disease (GTN) is nonspecific, and is seen in complete or partial hydatidiform mole, hydropic de-

generation, degenerating fibroids, endometrial carcinoma, and adenomyosis. Doppler ultrasonography can facilitate the diagnosis of this disease because of the high vascularity typical of this tumor. Taylor and colleagues, in recording the signal from the uterine arteries with Doppler ultrasonography, have shown higher systolic and diastolic shifts in GTN compared with those in postabortal, gravid, and nongravid women. On MRI, GTN typically obliterates the zonal architecture. The presence of numerous enlarged vessels can be directly visualized (Fig. 12-17); however, MRI is not particularly

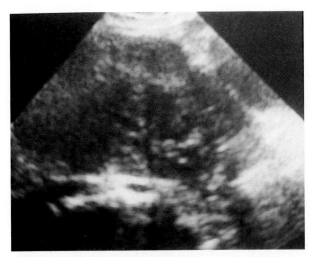

Figure 12–10. Sonogram showing leiomyomatous uterus. Note that the field of view is restricted such that an accurate total intrauterine volume cannot be obtained.

useful or practical for total body staging of choriocarcinoma because of the long scan times and inability to demonstrate lung micrometastases. CT is the imaging modality of choice in the exclusion of metastases because of its capability to efficiently scan almost the entire body (ie, brain, chest, abdomen, and pelvis) (Fig. 12-18). CT is superior to MRI in the evaluation of the chest, since both the mediastinum and lung parenchyma are well depicted, whereas only the mediastinum can be examined with MRI.

CERVIX

Imaging of the cervix primarily concerns the staging of malignancy. Ultrasonography is of limited use in staging cervical carcinoma, since it does not always permit visualization of the entire cervix and extracervical spread (specifically lymphadenopathy) usually is not detected. As with endometrial cancer, CT is not particularly valuable in the evaluation of early disease, since the contrast resolution does not permit routine separation of the tumor from normal cervical tissue. Extracervical organ planes are not well separated by CT. For example, the urethra and the vagina usually appear as one structure on CT, whereas MRI routinely delineates these structures separately (Fig. 12-19) as well as differentiating the bladder wall from the cervix. A large necrotic tumor may be identifiable with CT because of the low density of fluid, and larger tumors may be appreciated owing to distortion or enlargement of the cervix (Fig. 12-20). Unfortunately, the normal shape of the cervix is quite variable. CT is not accurate in differ-

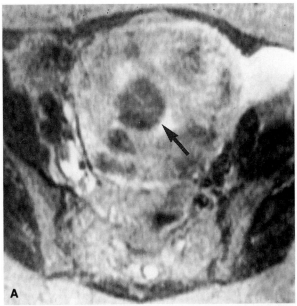

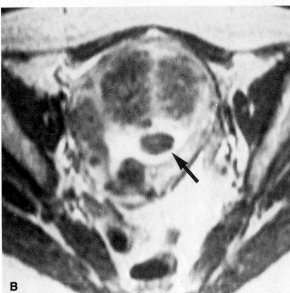

Figure 12–11. *A,* Note large submucosal leiomyoma (*arrow*). *B,* On gonadotropin-releasing hormone analogue therapy, it has significantly decreased. Also note that four intramural leiomyomas (not shown in *A* because on higher section) have decreased along with size of uterus. This study also is technically better because of less bowel peristalsis on the second examination.

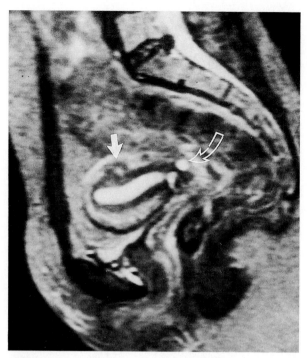

Figure 12–12. Sagittal MR scan through uterus showing adenomyosis (*straight arrow*) and an incidental nabothian cyst (*curved arrow*).

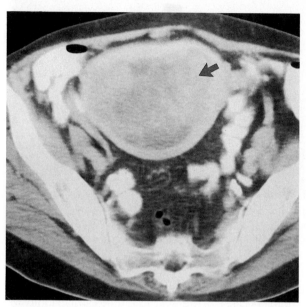

Figure 12–14. CT scan showing a uterine sarcoma (*arrow*). It cannot be ascertained whether or not there is myometrial invasion.

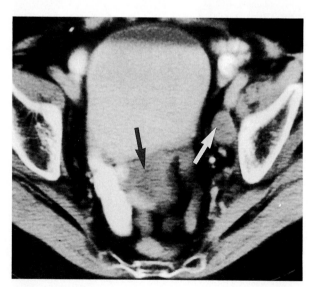

Figure 12–13. CT showing endometrial cancer (*black arrow*). Although extent in the uterus is difficult to ascertain, there is clearly a large obturator lymph node (*white arrow*).

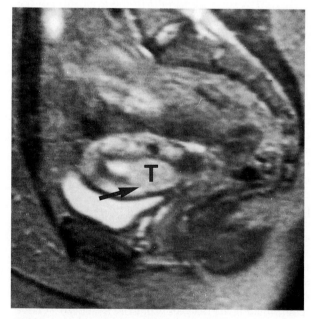

Figure 12–15. Sagittal MR scan showing an endometrial cancer (*T*) with more than 50% invasion of the myometrium (*arrow*).

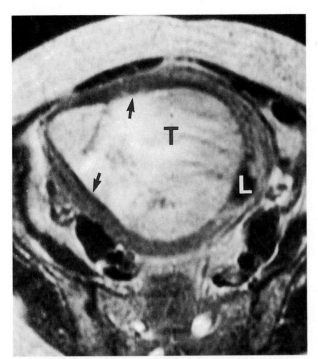

Figure 12–16. Axial MR scan of a patient with a mixed müllerian tumor (*T*). Note that this tumor has not invaded the myometrium because the junctional zone is intact (*arrow*). There also is an incidental leiomyoma (*L*).

entiating IB from IIB lesions; however, it is useful in the evaluation of clinical stages 3B to 4 disease, with a reported success rate of 92%. Tumor extension into the parametrium can be detected, but not routinely (Fig. 12-21). Extension to the pelvic sidewall is more consistently identified. Detection of enlarged pelvic or periaortic lymph nodes is the major value of CT in this disease. If CT is conducted, there is no reason to obtain an intravenous urogram in these patients, since CT reliably documents renal excretion, the course and size of the ureters, and the presence and location of an obstruction. Urography is quite insensitive for the demonstration of extension of any tumor.

MRI does not reliably detect carcinoma in situ; however, gross tumor size and extent are much better seen with MRI than with CT. Togashi, Nishimura, Sagoh, and others have reported an overall accuracy of MRI in staging cervical cancer of 76%, a 95% accuracy in demonstrating invasive disease (stage IB or higher), and an 89% accuracy in specifically assessing parametrial status. MRI can depict the location and extent of tumor invasion of the cervical stroma and depict tumor beneath relatively normal epithelium or within the endocervical canal that is not detectable by colposcopic examination (Fig. 12-22).

MRI and CT are equally accurate in detecting lymphadenopathy. Both techniques rely on size criteria for the diagnosis of lymph node involvement: a lymph node size equal to or greater than 1.5 cm. Clearly, early microscopic involvement will be missed; however, the convention of a minimum size of 1.5 cm prevents too many false-positive diagnoses.

Recurrent tumor can be screened with CT. Nevertheless, a fibrotic mass that is postoperative or secondary to radiation therapy cannot be distinguished from recurrence unless interval scans show an increase in size. Percutaneous biopsy specimens of suspicious masses can be obtained by CT (Fig. 12-23). MRI can be used noninvasively to differentiate fibrosis from recurrence. Ebner and coworkers showed a highly significant difference in the signal intensity of recurrent tumors versus fibrotic masses in 22 patients who had had gynecologic tumors and were at least 1 year post radiation therapy.

OVARY

Although the normal ovaries are well visualized with MRI (Fig. 12-24), ultrasonography remains the standard screening technique for evaluation of the ovaries. Particularly in the evaluation and treatment of infertility, sonography can establish that anatomically normal ovaries are present, that normal follicular development occurs during the menstrual cycle, and that there is a response to pharmacologic induction of ovulation. In the last case, when ovaries become greater than 5 cm in length with replacement of normal echogenic tissue by multiple septated cysts, ovarian hyperstimulation has occurred.

Polycystic ovarian disease usually is diagnosed by hormonal means; nonetheless, the sonographic findings of enlarged ovaries that contain multiple tiny cysts are suggestive of the disease. In about 30% of such patients with this disease, ovarian size is within normal limits. Mitchell and associates have shown that MRI can demonstrate the characteristic gross pathologic findings of polycystic ovarian disease (ie, numerous subcapsular cysts surrounding an abundant central stroma) (Fig. 12-25). Because MRI entails no ionizing radiation, it can be used to examine both the ovaries and the adrenals to exclude an adrenal or an ovarian tumor as a cause for elevated androgen levels.

Ovarian Masses

Most ovarian masses are initially assessed with ultrasonography. Once the mass has been identified with sonography, the differential, although large, can be narrowed by assessing the echogenicity and architecture

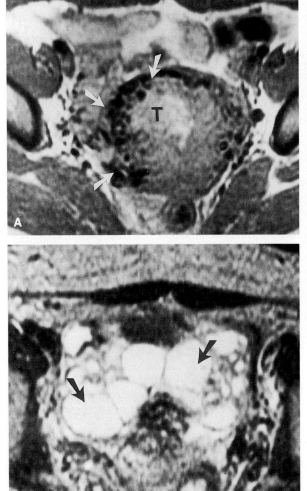

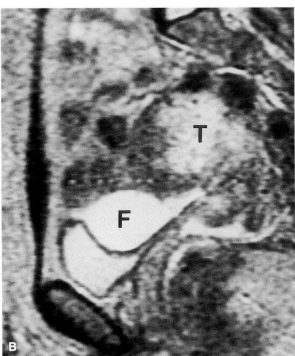

Figure 12–17. *A*, Axial MR scan showing numerous vessels (*arrows*) feeding a focus of tumor (*T*) in a patient with gestational trophoblastic disease. *B*, Sagittal MR scan showing obliteration of the uterine zonal architecture by tumor (*T*). Note fluid (*F*) in the pelvis. *C*, There are numerous theca lutean cysts (*arrows*).

of the lesion. Functional or physiologic cysts constitute the majority of lesions, and these appear completely cystic. Cystadenomas, cystic teratomas, and ovarian abscesses can be completely cystic but often have a complex nature because of debris or septations. Lesions that appear to be predominantly solid on sonography include granulosa cell tumor, adenocarcinoma, solid teratoma, arrhenoblastoma, fibroma, and metastases to the ovaries. Ectopic pregnancies, endometriomas, and ovarian torsion have a variable appearance. Unfortunately, fluid- or feces-filled loops of intestine can simulate cystic adnexal masses. In the case of suspected ectopic pregnancy, transvaginal sonography can provide an earlier, more definitive diagnosis by confirming

an empty uterus or small fluid collections. An intrauterine pregnancy can be confirmed by 5 weeks.

MRI is not used as a screening technique for the presence of an ovarian mass, since it is more expensive than sonography. However, MRI is the procedure of choice after an indeterminate ultrasonography (ie, a study in which the origin or nature of the mass is uncertain). MRI is superior to sonography or CT in localizing a mass to the ovary or uterus and in providing a more limited differential diagnosis (Fig. 12-26). Specific diagnoses possible with MRI include simple or hemorrhagic cysts, dermoids, endometriomas, and subserosal fibroids. Commonly, a complex lesion seen with ultrasonography can be specifically identified as a

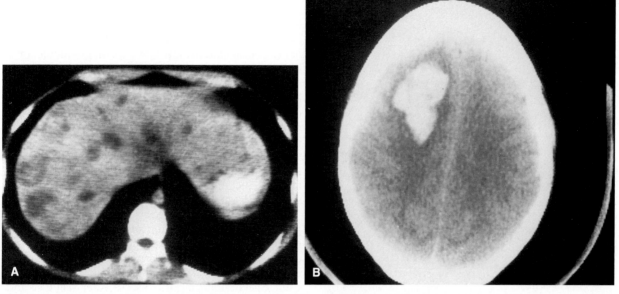

Figure 12–18. Patient with metastatic choriocarcinoma. *A,* CT scan of the liver shows numerous hepatic metastases. *B,* CT scan of the head shows a hemorrhagic metastasis to the right hemisphere.

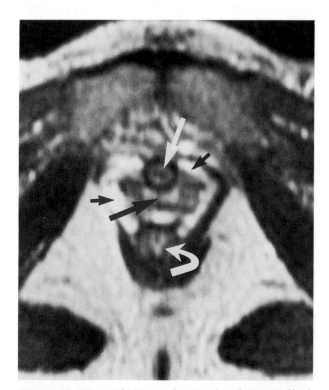

Figure 12–19. Axial MR scan showing the advantage of high contrast resolution. Note separation of the urethra (*white arrow*) from vagina (*black arrow*) and rectum (*curved arrow*). The surrounding bright area represents the perivaginal venous plexus (*small black arrows*).

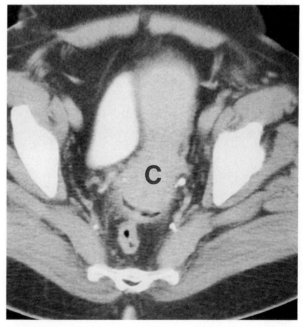

Figure 12–20. CT scan of a patient with cervical carcinoma. Note that the cervix (*C*) is prominent; however, there is no density change to enable localization of the actual tumor site.

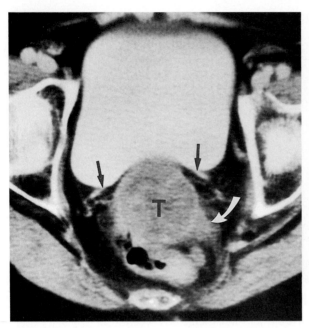

Figure 12–21. CT scan of a patient with a large necrotic cervical cancer (*T*). Note the ureters (*arrows*) are clearly identified and unaffected. There is parametrial invasion on the left (*curved arrow*).

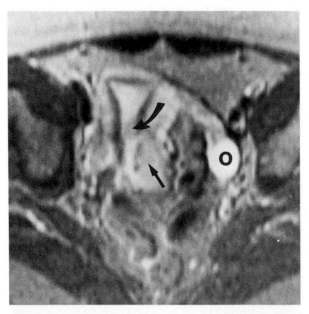

Figure 12–22. Axial MR scan showing tumor infiltration of the cervical stroma (*arrows*) with a small polypoid focus of tumor in the endocervical canal at the level of the internal os (*curved arrow*). Note incidental dominant follicle on left ovary (*O*).

dermoid or an endometrioma with MRI, since fat and blood have a characteristic appearance on MRI. Fatty lesions are bright on both the T1- and T2-weighted sequences (Fig. 12-27), and can demonstrate an internal chemical shift artifact that is pathognomonic for a lesion containing a fat–fluid interface. This artifact is due to the 3 parts-per-million difference in resonance frequency of hydrogen nuclei bonded in water versus hydrogen nuclei bonded in fat. Endometriomas, because of the paramagnetic behavior of iron in hemoglobin, exhibit a characteristic signal behavior (Fig. 12-28). Dermoids or malignant teratomas can be unmistakably diagnosed with CT owing to their contained fat and calcium; however, CT should not serve as a simple screening technique.

Endometriosis, a disease in which imaging has not proved particularly useful, can be followed with MRI once the diagnosis is established by laparoscopy. Implants smaller than 5 mm and adhesions are not currently visible with this technique; thus, MRI cannot be used to accurately stage the disease. After diagnosis and staging by laparoscopy, MRI can be used to follow the response of endometriomas to treatment (eg, gonadotropin-releasing hormone analog therapy). In women with adhesions that impair laparoscopic visualization, MRI can demonstrate disease not visible to any technique. In a study of 88 endometriotic lesions, comparison to concurrent laparoscopy demonstrated an MRI sensitivity of 71% and specificity of 82% for the identification of endometriomas. In a study by Friedman and colleagues, ultrasonography detected endometriosis in only 4 of 37 patients (10.8%). Even with direct correlation between known areas of disease, there were 33 false-negative sonograms. CT is of little value in this disorder, since it uses ionizing radiation in reproductive-age women and the contrast resolution is insufficient to distinguish endometriosis from even normal adnexa. There is no typical CT density for endometriosis.

Although MRI is more specific (ie, offers a more limited differential diagnosis than sonography in the routine evaluation of ovarian masses), it uses the same morphologic criteria for the identification of malignant lesions as used for CT and ultrasonography: septations, mural nodules, and ascites (Fig. 12-29). Because the imaging times with MRI are relatively long and thus motion artifact from peristalsis obscures the bowel wall as well as peritoneal surfaces, MRI is not particularly useful in staging the spread of ovarian cancer to the peritoneum. In the detection of hepatic metastases (from any primary tumor), MRI is equivalent or better than CT. However, CT remains the procedure of choice in the routine staging of ovarian cancer, since it can

(*text continues on page 295*)

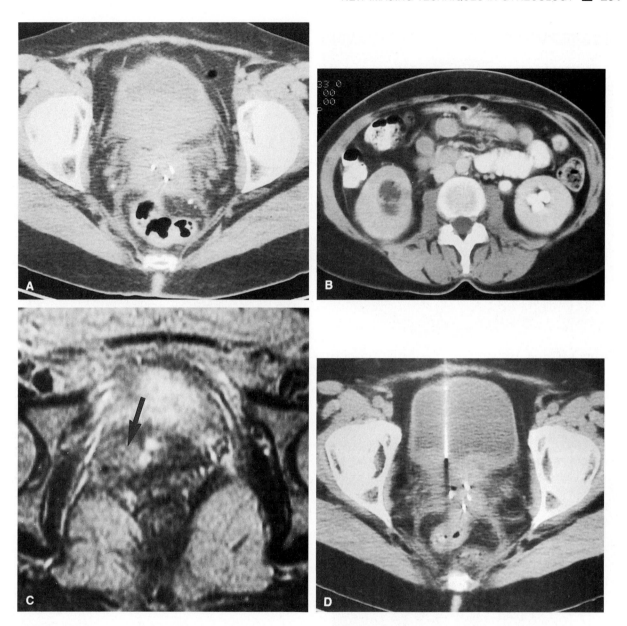

Figure 12–23. Patient with recurrent cervical cancer. *A,* CT scan through pelvis shows prominent cervix (*C*) and bilateral ureteric obstruction (*arrows*). *B,* CT at level of kidneys shows bilateral hydronephrosis with delayed excretion on right. *C,* Axial MR scan (at a lower section than CT section) shows one area of increased signal intensity (*arrow*) compatible with recurrent tumor. *D,* CT-guided biopsy of that specific area shows recurrent tumor.

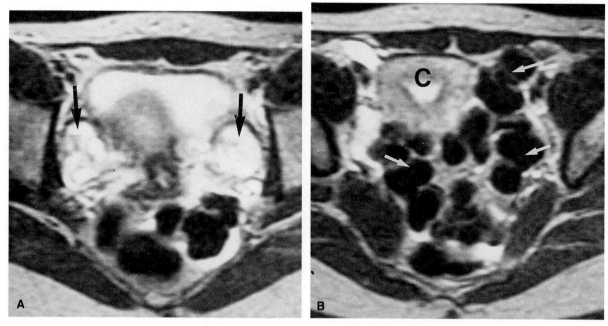

Figure 12–24. *A,* Axial MR section showing both ovaries containing multiple cysts (*arrows*). *B,* Higher axial section demonstrates a normal corpus (*C*) and numerous loops of air-filled bowel (*arrows*) that appear black (*signal void*). Because air does not contain hydrogen nuclei, there is no signal on MRI.

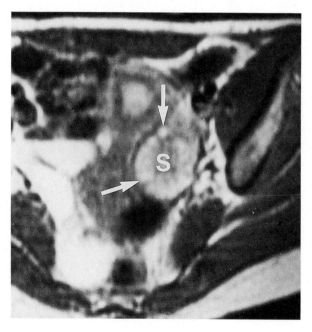

Figure 12–25. Axial MR scan showing polycystic ovarian disease. Note numerous subcapsular cysts (*arrows*) and abundant stroma (*S*).

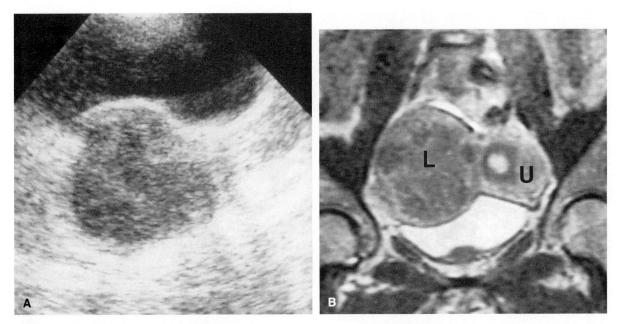

Figure 12–26. *A*, Sonogram shows fibroid uterus; however, adnexal mass cannot be excluded. *B*, MR demonstrates that the leiomyoma (*L*) is clearly subserosal and not an adnexal mass. Note that it is continuous with myometrium of the corpus uterus (*U*).

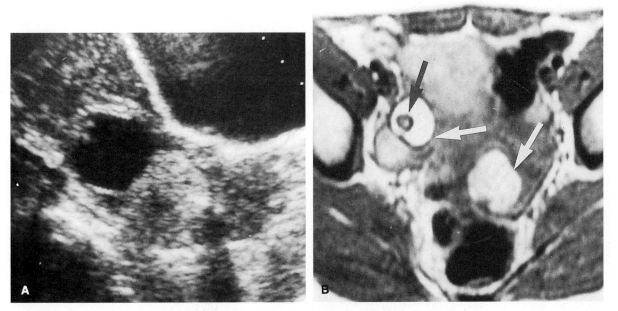

Figure 12–27. *A*, Sonogram showing echogenic and cystic adnexal lesions. *B*, MR scan showing these lesions (*white arrows*) to be isointense with fat (on all pulse sequences), representative of dermoids. Note that right one contains an area of signal void (*black arrow*), which is calcium.

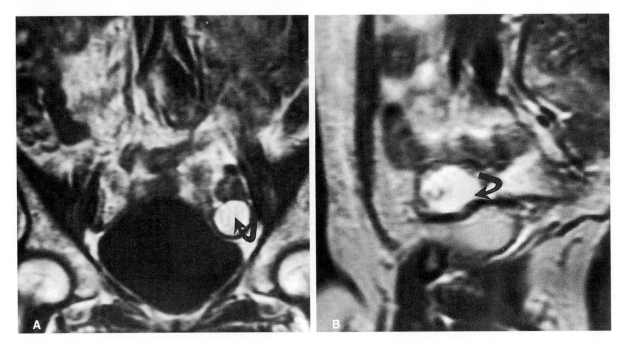

Figure 12–28. *A,* Coronal section showing endometrioma on the left ovary (*curved arrow*). *B,* Sagittal section with a different pulse sequence (*contrast*) showing the lesion also to be high signal (brighter than fat), compatible with an endometrioma.

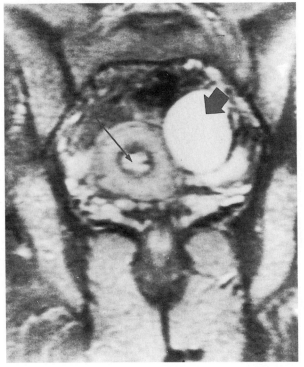

Figure 12–29. Coronal MR scan showing a septated cystic lesion of the left ovary (*short arrow*) that was shown to be a cystadenoma at surgery. Note intrauterine device within uterine cavity (*long arrow*).

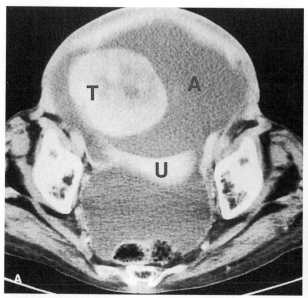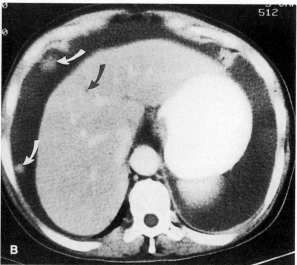

Figure 12–30. *A*, CT scan through the pelvis showing a large ovarian tumor (*T*) that is clearly malignant, since extensive ascites (*A*) is present. Note uterus (*U*). *B*, CT scan more cephalad showing peritoneal metastases (*white arrows*) and a small liver metastasis (*black arrows*).

demonstrate the primary tumor, small peritoneal metastases, and hepatic metastases in a single time-efficient study (Fig. 12-30).

Bibliography

Arrive L, Hricak H, Martin MC. Pelvic endometriosis: MR imaging. Radiology 1989;171:687.

Bohlman ME, Ensor RE, Sanders RE. Sonographic findings in adenomyosis of the uterus. AJR 1987;148:765.

Buy J, Ghossain MA, Moss AA, et al. Cystic teratoma of the ovary: CT detection. Radiology 1989;171:697.

Callen P, DeMartini W, Filly R. Central uterine cavity echo: a useful anatomic sign in the ultrasonographic evaluation of the female pelvis. Radiology 1979;131:187.

Cooperberg PL, Kidney MR. Ultrasound evaluation of the ovary. In: Callen PW, ed. Ultrasonography in obstetrics and gynecology. Philadelphia: WB Saunders, 1988;423.

Cooperberg PL, Kidney MR. Ultrasound evaluation of the uterus. In: Callen PW, ed. Ultrasonography in obstetrics and gynecology. Philadelphia: WB Saunders, 1988;396, 403.

Davis WK, McCarthy S, Moss AA, Braga C. Computed tomography of gestational trophoblastic disease. J Comput Assist Tomogr 1984;8:1136.

Demas BE, Hricak H, Jaffe RB. Uterine MR imaging: effects of hormonal stimulation. Radiology 1986;159:123.

Dooms GC, Hricak H, Crooks LE, Higgins CB. Magnetic resonance imaging of the lymph nodes: comparison with CT. Radiology 1984;153: 719.

Dooms GE, Hricak H, Tscholakoff D. Adnexal structures: MR imaging. Radiology 1986;158:639.

Dore R, Moro G, D'Andrea F, et al. CT evaluation of myometrium invasion in endometrial carcinoma. J Comput Assist Tomogr 1987;11:282.

Dudiak CM, Turner DA, Patel SK, et al. Uterine leiomyomas in the infertile patient: preoperative localization with MR imaging versus US and hysterosalpingography. Radiology 1988;167:627.

Ebner F, Kressel HY, Mintz MC, et al. Tumor recurrence versus fibrosis in the female pelvis: differentiation with MR imaging at 1.5T. Radiology 1988;166:333.

Feldberg MAM, van Waes P, Hendriks MJ. Direct multiplanar CT findings in cystic teratoma of the ovary. J Comput Assist Tomogr 1984;8:1131.

Fishman EK, Scatarige JC, Saksouk FA, et al. Computed tomography of endometriosis. J Comput Assist Tomogr 1983;7:257.

Fleischer AC, Dudley BS, Entman SS, et al. Myometrial invasion by endometrial carcinoma: sonographic assessment. Radiology 1987;162:307.

Friedman H, Vogelzang RL, Mendelson EB, et al. Endometriosis detection by US with laparoscopic correlation. Radiology 1985; 157:217.

Hamlin DJ, Burgener FA, Beecham JB. CT of intramural endometrial carcinoma: contrast enhancement is essential. AJR 1981;137:551.

Hamlin JD, Pettersson H, Fitzsimmons J, Morgan LS. MR imaging of uterine leiomyomas and their complications. J Comput Assist Tomogr 1985;9:902.

Haynor DR, Mack LA, Soules MR, et al. Changing appearance of the normal uterus during the menstrual cycle: MR studies. Radiology 1986;161:459.

Hillman BJ, Clark RL, Babbitt G. Efficacy of the excretory urogram in the staging of gynecologic malignancies. AJR 1984;143:997.

Hricak H, Alpers C, Crooks L, Sheldon P. Magnetic resonance imaging of the female pelvis: initial experience. AJR 1983;141:1119.

Hricak H, Demas BE, Graga CA, et al. Gestational trophoblastic neoplasm of the uterus: MR assessment. Radiology 1986;161:11.

Hricak H, Stern JL, Fisher MR, et al. Endometrial carcinoma staging by MR imaging. Radiology 1987;162:297.

Hricak H, Tscholakoff D, Heinrichs L, et al. Uterine leiomyomas: correlation of MR, histopathologic findings and symptoms. Radiology 1986;158:385.

Johnson RJ, Blackledge G, Eddleston B, Crowther K. Abdomino-pelvis computed tomography in the management of ovarian carcinoma. Radiology 1983;146:447.

Lee JKT, Gersell DJ, Balfe DM, et al. The uterus: in vitro MR-anatomic correlation of normal and abnormal specimens. Radiology 1985;157:175.

Lee JKT, Heiken JP, Ling D, et al. Magnetic resonance imaging of abdominal and pelvic lymphadenopathy. Radiology 1984;153:181.

Long F, Scoutt L, McCarthy S, et al. MRI and synthetic imaging of endometrial carcinoma. Magn Reson Imaging 1988;6:62.

McCarthy S, Scott G, Majumdar S, et al. Uterine junctional zone: MR study of water content and relaxation properties. Radiology 1989;171:241.

McCarthy S, Tauber C, Gore J. Female pelvic anatomy: MR assessment of variations during the menstrual cycle and with use of oral contraceptives. Radiology 1986;160:119.

Mark AS, Hricak H, Heinrichs LW, et al. Adenomyosis and leiomyoma: differential diagnosis with MR imaging. Radiology 1987;163:527.

Megibow AJ, Hulnick DH, Bosniak MA, Balthazar EJ. Ovarian metastases: computed tomographic appearances. Radiology 1985;156:161.

Mendelson EB, Bohm-Velez M, Neiman HL, Russo J. Transvaginal sonography in gynecologic imaging. Semin Ultrasound CT MR 1988;9:102.

Mintz MC, Grumbach K. Imaging of congenital uterine anomalies. Semin Ultrasound CT MR 1988;9:167.

Mintz MC, Thickman DI, Gussman D, Kressel HY: MR evaluation of uterine anomalies. AJR 1987;148:287.

Mitchell DG, Hill MC, Hill S, Zaloudek C. Serous carcinoma of the ovary: CT identification of metastatic calcified implants. Radiology 1986;158:649.

Mitchell DG, Mintz MC, Spritzer CE, et al. Adnexal masses: MR imaging observations at 1.5T, with US and CT correlation. Radiology 1987;12:319.

Mitchell KG, Gefter WB, Spritzer CE, et al. Polycystic ovaries: MR imaging. Radiology 1986;160:425.

Miyasaka Y, Hachiya J, Furuya Y, et al. CT evaluation of invasive trophoblastic disease. J Comput Assist Tomogr 1985;9:459.

Nishimura K, Togashi K, Itoh K, et al. Endometrial cysts of the ovary: MR imaging. Radiology 1987;162:315.

Sanders C, Rubin E. Malignant gestational trophoblastic disease: CT findings. AJR 1987;148:165.

Scoutt L, McCarthy S, Lange R, Bourque A, Schqartz P. MR imaging: utility in the evaluation of ovarian masses. Radiology 1990;177:242.

Stark DD, Wittenberg J, Butch RJ, Ferrucci JT. Hepatic metastases: randomized, controlled comparison of detection with MR imaging and CT. Radiology 1987;165:399.

Taylor KJW, Schwartz P, Kohorn E. Gestational trophoblastic neoplasia: diagnosis with Doppler US. Radiology 1987;165:445.

Togashi K, Nishimura K, Itoh K, et al. Ovarian cystic teratomas: MR imaging. Radiology 1987;162:669.

Togashi K, Nishimura K, Sagoh T, et al. Carcinoma of the cervix: staging with MR imaging. Radiology 1989;171:245.

Togashi K, Ozasa H, Konishi I, et al. Enlarged uterus: differentiation between adenomyosis and leiomyoma with MR imaging. Radiology 1989;171:531.

Vick CW, Walsh JW, Wheelock JB, Brewer WH. CT of the normal and abnormal parametria in cervical cancer. AJR 1984;143:597.

Walsh JW, Amendola MA, Hall DJ, et al. Recurrent carcinoma of the cervix: CT diagnosis. AJR 1981;136:117.

Walsh JW, Goplerud DR. Computed tomography of primary, persistent and recurrent endometrial malignancy. AJR 1982;139:1149.

Walsh JW, Goplerud DR. Prospective comparison between clinical and CT staging in primary cervical carcinoma. AJR 1981;137:997.

Walsh JW, Taylor KJW, Rosenfield AT. Gray-scale sonography in the diagnosis of endometriosis and adenomyosis. AJR 1979;132:87.

Whitley NO, Brenner DE, Francis A, et al. Computed tomographic evaluation of carcinoma of the cervix. Radiology 1982;142:439.

Worthington JL, Balfe DM, Lee JKT, et al. Uterine neoplasms: MR imaging. Radiology 1986;159:725.

Yeh H, Futterweit W, Thornton JC. Polycystic ovarian disease: US features in 104 patients. Radiology 1987;163:111.

Zawin M, McCarthy S, Scoutt L, Comite F. Endometriosis: appearance and detection at MR imaging. Radiology 1989;171:693.

Zawin M, McCarthy S, Scoutt L, et al. Monitoring therapy with a gonadotropin-releasing hormone analog: utility of MRI imaging. Radiology 1990;175:503.

Zawin M, McCarthy S, Scoutt L, Comite F. High-field MRI and US evaluation of the pelvis in women with leiomyomas. Magn Reson Imaging 1990;8:371.

13

Normal and Abnormal Uterine Bleeding

DONALD P. SWARTZ
WILLIAM J. BUTLER

Cyclic uterine bleeding, which begins in the anatomically and physiologically normal female, marks an important stage of reproductive maturation. Accurate informational and empathetic psychologic preparation of the young woman *before* the onset of this potentially disturbing function is important to her early reaction to menstruation—and almost certainly also to her long-term view of it.

Although clinical experience has led to empiric definitions of variations in menstrual pattern that are described as abnormal uterine bleeding or dysfunctional uterine bleeding, many women, perhaps appropriately, tend to conclude that any departure from prior personal menstrual experience is abnormal. Conversely, some women accept or ignore significant variation in their menstrual function to the extent that serious health impairment occurs (eg, severe iron deficiency anemia).

Some terms are generally used to facilitate description and record keeping regarding patterns of uterine bleeding. Those used in this discussion are defined as follows:

Polymenorrhea—menstrual cycle interval less than 21 days

Oligomenorrhea—menstrual cycle interval more than 37 days

Metrorrhagia—menstrual bleeding longer than 7 days or interval bleeding

Menorrhagia—excessive or prolonged menstrual bleeding

Postmenopausal bleeding—uterine bleeding occurring more than 12 months after the last menstrual period of a menopausal woman

Breakthrough bleeding—intermenstrual bleeding in a menstrual cycle that is the result of exogenous hormones

Current medical therapy is effective in the management of most disturbances of menstrual function that occur in the absence of infection, gestation, or uterine tumor. Successful therapy depends on a complete understanding of normal menstrual physiology and of the available agents. New surgical diagnostic and therapeutic technologies are available with which to manage patients who fail to respond to conventional endocrine manipulation.

NORMAL MENSTRUAL PHYSIOLOGY

Menstruation is the physiologic shedding of the endometrium associated with uterine bleeding, occurring at monthly intervals from menarche to menopause. Between these two physiologic landmarks, menstruation may occur 400 to 500 times. According to classical theory, the superficial functional layer of the endometrium is shed during menstruation, with regeneration proceeding from the remaining intact basalis. It is surprising that this process of monthly shedding and regeneration can occur so often without producing permanent tissue damage. A new concept that may explain this paradox holds that most of the functional endometrium is conserved during menses and that dynamic physiologic processes control the metamorphosis between proliferative and secretory endometria. An interruption of these normal cyclic processes can lead to irregular endometrial breakdown and dysfunctional uterine bleeding.

The endometrium is an endocrine organ that responds to circulating blood levels of estrogen and progesterone. In the unstimulated resting phase, the glands are narrow and lined by low cuboidal cells with few mitoses. The stromal cells are small and spindly with little cytoplasm or mitotic activity. Protein synthesis and secretory activity are minimal. Estradiol production by the developing follicle stimulates metabolic activity in the endometrium. The estradiol has multiple effects. Deoxyribonucleic acid (DNA) synthesis is activated and, subsequently, ribonucleic acid (RNA) synthesis and mitochondrial enlargement signify induction of the metabolic machinery necessary for protein synthesis and mitosis. These actions are mediated by estrogen receptors. A well-documented effect of estrogen in multiple tissues is the induction of receptors, both for itself and other hormones. Steroid hormones have a relatively low molecular weight and probably enter cells by passive diffusion where they are bound by cellular receptors. The classical concept described binding of the steroid by a cytoplasmic receptor with subsequent translocation of the steroid-receptor complex into the nucleus where it transformed, bound to DNA, and exerted its biologic effect. New experimental evidence has shown that data demonstrating cytoplasmic steroid receptors were experimental artifact. The receptors are nuclear proteins that undergo transformation after hormone binding. Estrogen increases endometrial responsiveness by increasing the concentration of its own receptor (replenishment) as well as inducing progesterone receptors. These estrogen receptors reach a maximal concentration in the middle to late proliferative phase of the menstrual cycle. Progesterone receptors are also induced and their concentration peaks in the late proliferative phase.

With development and elongation of the glands, secretory granules appear in the cytoplasm and glycogen collects in basal vacuoles of the glandular cells. Arteriolar vessels grow up into the endometrium as part of the general proliferative response. Several enzymes such as alkaline phosphatase, 5α-reductase, and possibly phospholipase A_2 are induced by estradiol. Phospholipase A_2, which releases arachidonic acid from phospholipid esters, controls the rate-limiting step in prostaglandin synthesis. Estradiol also stimulates cyclooxygenase synthesis of prostaglandin $F_{2\alpha}$ and prostaglandin E_2, both of which have a role in menstrual function. $PGF_{2\alpha}$ has vasoconstrictive and muscle contraction effects, and PGE_2 is generally a vasodilator but also causes contraction in uterine smooth muscle. Alterations in the relative levels of $PGF_{2\alpha}$ and PGE_2 may alter menstrual bleeding patterns. Progesterone also has multiple biologic effects that are mediated through its estrogen-induced receptors. These basic functions are to induce secre-

tory change in the proliferative endometrium as a prelude to implantation of the embryo and to inhibit synthesis of both estrogen and progesterone receptors to limit the biologic activity of estrogen and progesterone. This process primarily has a suppressive effect on DNA synthesis in endometrial cells and results in dynamic inhibition of cell mitosis. Accompanying this process is the development of RNA-filled channels between the nucleoli and nuclear membranes responsible for the active synthesis of cytoplasmic enzymes during the secretory phase of the cycle. The enzymes 17β- and 20α-hydroxysteroid dehydrogenase (HSD) are induced and modulate steroid activity. 17β-HSD catalyses the conversion of estradiol to the relatively weaker estrogen estrone, which, when sulfated by the enzyme estrogen sulfotransferase, can no longer bind to estrogen receptors. 20α-HSD alters progesterone receptor binding and activity. Lytic enzymes such as acid phosphatase are also induced but kept inactive within Golgi-derived lysosomes, the membranes of which are stabilized by progesterone.

Several investigators have described increased levels of protease inhibitors such as α_1-antitrypsin and antithrombin III in secretory phase uterine fluid. They may be involved in the mechanism of menstrual bleeding. A specific protein, progestogen-associated endometrial protein, has been identified with levels that correlate to the intensity of secretory change. The function is as yet undetermined, but it may play a role in prostaglandin metabolism as well as serve as a marker for progesterone response in the endometrium. Morphologically, progesterone causes coiling of the spiral arterioles and endometrial glands. Glandular cells expel apical glycogen vacuoles and subsequently flatten into a low cuboidal form. Differentiation of stromal cells from reticular spindle-shaped cells into plump predecidual cells and phagocytic granulated cells containing another protein, relaxin, which may be important in implantation, defines two layers in the functional endometrium, the superficial compactum and deeper spongiosum. The endometrium reaches its greatest thickness, 5 to 6 mm, at this time. The stage is set for menstruation.

Menstruation is controlled by many complex, interrelated, and incompletely understood factors. Normal menstruation results from progesterone withdrawal from an estrogen-primed endometrium. The changes in the endometrium that occur with menstruation were described by Markee, who observed endometrial tissue transplanted to the anterior chamber of the eye of the rhesus monkey. He described the cyclic changes in the endometrial vascularity and the development of coiled vessels supplying the superficial two thirds of the endometrium. The estrogen-primed endometrium of the follicular phase is compact with relatively underdeveloped vasculature. Progesterone converts this endometrium into a thick, edematous, secretory lining that is glycogen enriched and prepares the metabolically active stroma and glands with an increased vasculature to receive and nourish a fertilized ovum. If implantation does not occur, estrogen and progesterone levels fall and prostaglandin synthesis and lysosomal membrane rupture occur, causing constriction of the spiral arterioles, ischemic necrosis, and sloughing of the endometrium superficial to the basalis layer. This process begins in the premenstrual phase of the cycle with cessation and inspissation of ground substance and supporting tissues by lytic enzymes released from lysosomes, tonic contractions of spiral arterioles with reduction of blood flow to the tissues, loss of stromal edema, and kinking of the coiled spiral arterioles caused by a reduction in endometrial thickness. A generalized state of ischemia develops in the superficial layers of endometrium and bleeding into the stroma begins, acid phosphatase and prostaglandin substances released from autolyzed cells cause more intense vasoconstriction of spiral arterioles, and the devitalized tissue sloughs as small hemorrhages in the stroma coalesce. According to Beller, coagulation factors are decreased in normal menstrual discharge. Fibrinogen is absent and plasminogen and plasmin inhibitor are decreased in amount. Menstrual blood does not clot, but as it collects in the vagina, it may form red blood cell aggregates with mucoid substances, mucoproteins, and glycogen. These red cell aggregates may appear to be blood clots but contain no fibrin.

According to classical theory, during menstruation the superficial compacta and the intermediate stratum spongiosum layers of the endometrium are shed, leaving the basalis layer intact. New endometrium is regenerated from the basalis. In Markee's studies, regeneration of new capillaries from the basalis could be seen. Restoration of the endometrial circulation was correlated with the cessation of menstrual bleeding. The loss of blood from the process of normal menstruation is limited by recovery of tone in the myometrium and in endometrial vasculature, cessation of cellular autolysis, eventual clotting over the endometrial surface, and active regeneration of glands, stroma, and vessels in the basalis layer in response to rising estrogen levels in the new cycle. Another theory holds that endometrium is relatively protected from the destructive lytic activity of lysosomal enzymes by a mucinous carbohydrate coat that covers the free surfaces of endometrial cells. This coat allows retention of most of the endometrium during menstruation and may explain the lack of permanent damage.

Endometrial regression during menstruation is then described as the result of four processes: (1) autophagy, (2) heterophagy, (3) extrusion of secretory products, and (4) elimination of fluids without extensive shedding of tissue. Autophagy and heterophagy describe the processes of lytic digestion of intracellular debris in vacuoles and extracellular debris ingested in phagosomes. Both serve to eliminate damaged tissue and allow regeneration of normal endometrial cells. With fluid loss and secretion, the functionalis regresses to a resting state, ready to regenerate in the next cycle. This theory also can partially explain the observation that initial endometrial regeneration occurs in the absence of estrogen. The lack of estrogen dependence could be secondary to the lesser proliferative response required after regression compared with complete endometrial shedding. Much work still needs to be done to define the complex processes involved in menstruation.

It is not surprising that a variety of alterations in the systems that control menstruation may occur and produce abnormal uterine bleeding, even in the absence of obvious disease. Prolonged estrogen stimulation can result in endometrium that outgrows its blood supply and has asynchronous development of endometrial glands, stroma, and blood vessels. Similarly, a failure of progesterone production also may have profound effects on endometrial glands, stroma, and blood vessels. Abnormal synthesis of acid mucopolysaccharides may result in the release of excessive amounts of hydrolytic enzymes into the stroma. Lysosome release from endometrial glands, influenced by plasma progesterone levels, may affect menstrual flow. Patients with menorrhagia produce altered types of prostaglandins from their endometrium and myometrium. Smith and associates have shown that the amount of menstrual flow is influenced by a change in the endometrial conversion of prostaglandin endoperoxide from PGF_2 to PGE_2. In their studies, women with menorrhagia synthesized mainly the vasodilator PGE_2 in the endometrium.

Menstruation has three clinical characteristics: (1) the menstrual interval or cycle length, (2) the duration of flow, and (3) the amount of flow. Although the mean cycle length is 28 to 29 days, a menstrual interval of 21 to 37 days may be considered normal. A patient with a menstrual interval shorter than 21 days is said to have polymenorrhea. A patient with a menstrual interval longer than 37 days is said to have oligomenorrhea. When menses have been absent for 6 months or longer, the patient is said to have amenorrhea. The menstrual interval may vary from month to month by several days. Regularity of the menstrual cycle is more important than exact approximation to the 28-day mean menstrual interval. Variation in the length of the menstrual interval in regular ovulatory cycles usually occurs in the preovulatory (proliferative) phase of the cycle and is more frequent among postmenarchal teenagers and in women approaching menopause.

A duration of flow of 7 days or less is considered to be normal. Beyond 7 days, the patient is bleeding into the intermenstrual phase of the cycle, which is defined as metrorrhagia. Regardless of the length of the menstrual flow, 70% of the blood loss will usually occur by the second day and 90% by the third day. A total blood loss of 20 to 80 mL, representing 10 to 35 mg iron, is considered within normal limits. The mean menstrual blood loss for a normal period is approximately 40 mL. Signs of iron deficiency are present, however, in a significant proportion of women who lose more than 60 mL blood with each menstrual flow. Hallberg and associates found that iron deficiency is common among women who lose more than 80 mL menstrual blood. Unfortunately, objective measurement of menstrual blood loss is rarely made in women complaining of heavy menstruation or women with unexplained iron deficiency anemia. The patient's history of normal or heavy menstrual blood loss is an inaccurate indicator of the amount of flow. It is also difficult to estimate the amount of blood loss by counting the number of days of menstrual flow or the number of pads and tampons used, as emphasized by Grimes. Iron deficiency anemia is a late manifestation of excessive menstruation. Serum iron (ferritin) levels are more sensitive than hematocrit and hemoglobin levels in detecting depletion of iron stores before anemia develops, as shown in the study by Guilebaud and associates. The availability of a convenient, standardized, objective method of measuring menstrual blood loss would improve the clinical practice of gynecology significantly, especially because 20% of women will have a problem with excessive menstrual blood loss during the reproductive years. The method of Hallberg and Nilsson is based on the simultaneous use of tampons and pads for the collection of menstrual blood. These are extracted with 5% sodium hydroxide, thus converting hemoglobin to alkaline hematin. The concentration is then determined spectrophotometrically. The method is simple and gives accurate results but is not widely used.

DYSFUNCTIONAL UTERINE BLEEDING

Dysfunctional uterine bleeding (DUB) is a symptom complex that includes any abnormal uterine bleeding in the absence of a pregnancy, neoplasm, infection, or other intrauterine lesion. Such bleeding is most often the result of endocrinologic dysfunction that inhibits normal ovulation. The state of chronic anovulation results in unopposed estrogen stimulation of the endometrium with irregular breakdown and bleeding. Hyper- and hypothyroidism, hyperprolactinemia, hormone-producing ovarian tumors, and Cushing's disease are endocrine syndromes that can all induce anovulation, but the primary etiology is recycling failure, commonly described as the polycystic ovary or Stein-

Leventhal syndrome. An imbalance in hypothalamic pulsatile release of gonadotropin releasing hormone (GnRH), pituitary synthesis or release of follicle-stimulating hormone (FSH) or luteinizing hormone (LH), or ovarian follicular production of estradiol, androgens, or progesterone can all upset the delicate balance that induces cyclic ovulation and menstrual function. Exogenous androgen production in the adrenal glands or estrone production in adipose tissue will give an identical clinical picture. Recycling failure and chronic anovulation syndrome therefore serve as "waste basket" diagnoses for these multiple endocrine etiologies. DUB in the presence of ovulatory cycles calls for further investigation to rule out a bleeding diathesis or other pathology.

DUB is partially a diagnosis of exclusion. The major diagnostic value of endometrial curettage is to rule out other pathologic conditions that can produce similar clinical symptoms. The immediate effect of a curettage is to control bleeding by removal of incompletely shed and possibly hyperplastic endometrium with thrombosis of arterioles and venous sinuses. Although possibly therapeutic, more commonly there is continuation of the abnormal bleeding pattern secondary to a failure to correct the underlying endocrine dysfunction. An understanding of the diverse etiologies that can result in DUB will provide an easier and more practical diagnostic scheme and more effective therapeutic intervention.

Pathophysiology

The most common etiology for DUB is estrogen withdrawal or estrogen breakthrough bleeding from an anovulatory patient. In the absence of progesterone exposure with its growth-limiting inhibition of DNA synthesis and mitosis, the estrogenic proliferative response exceeds the structural integrity of its stromal matrix and the endometrium breaks down with irregular bleeding. The amount of bleeding correlates directly to the level of estrogen stimulation, with chronic high estrogen milieus as seen in obesity, chronic anovulation syndrome, and perimenarchal and perimenopausal patients having the greatest amount of blood loss. Unopposed estrogen results in vascular endometrial tissue with relatively scant stroma, giving glands a back-to-back appearance. This endometrium is fragile and undergoes repetitive spontaneous breakdown with bleeding. In the absence of the normal control mechanisms that limit menstrual blood loss, this bleeding can be prolonged and excessive. Unopposed estrogen stimulation, over time, can induce a hyperplastic response in the proliferating endometrium (Fig. 13-1A). Eventually, such hyperplasia may develop the cytologic changes associated with neoplasia—atypical adeno-

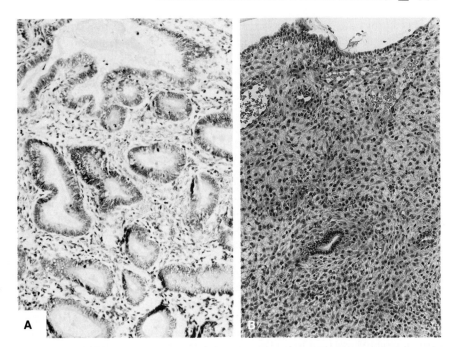

Figure 13–1. *A*, Endometrial hyperplasia before treatment showing hyperplastic cellular changes of glands. *B*, Hyperplastic endometrium after continuous progestin treatment.

matous hyperplasia or even low-grade adenocarcinoma. As such cellular transformation takes time, probably 10 to 20 years, the young patient with DUB has a low risk of hyperplasia/neoplasia and, in most cases, probably does not require endometrial sampling; however, the perimenopausal patient is certainly at higher risk and sampling is mandated.

Jones and associates studied the endometria from patients with dysfunctional bleeding and found hyperplasia present in 63% of the cases. Secretory endometrium was noted in 17% and nonsecretory endometrium of the interval, postmenstrual, or atrophic type in the remaining 20%. Thus, in at least 17% of this series, normal cyclic hormonal function and ovulation had occurred before the endometrium was examined. It is possible that many cases that showed the postmenstrual type of endometrium would have shown secretory changes had the curettage been done later. The exact percentage of DUB cases associated with ovulatory cycles has not been determined, but is a minority. Prospective hormonal studies using daily serum estrogen and progesterone levels are more accurate in defining anovulation than the historic studies of endometrial histology, which may be misleading because of previous hormonal therapy. Prospective studies provide clear evidence that the major cause of irregular shedding of the endometrium that produces clinical symptoms is failure of regular ovulation. DUB must be considered to be an endocrine problem that is best treated with hormonal therapy initially, with more invasive treatment reserved for resistant cases.

Symptoms and Diagnosis

DUB occurs frequently at the extremes of menstrual life, but also may develop at any intervening time. The type of bleeding is variable, from infrequent heavy flow (oligomenorrhea) to almost continuous bleeding or spotting. The age of onset and duration of irregularity can provide important clues to etiology. In the perimenarchal girl, anovulation is common, with more than 50% of cycles being anovulatory in the first 2 years after menarche. Complications of pregnancy are also frequent in this age group and must be ruled out before initiation of treatment for DUB. The new sensitive radioimmunoassays for the β subunit of human chorionic gonadotropin (HCG) are an accurate method for evaluating the possibility of pregnancy without obtaining an invasive tissue diagnosis. Although relatively rare, endocrinologically active ovarian neoplasms do occur, and should be particularly excluded in prepubertal vaginal bleeding. Other causes of irregular bleeding in the adolescent include genital trauma and blood dyscrasias such as idiopathic thrombocytopenic purpura, von Willebrand's disease, or leukemia.

The adult woman with DUB may have either an acute or chronic history of menstrual irregularity. Onset at menarche and persistence into adulthood is a classic history for chronic anovulation syndrome, but adult onset congenital adrenal hyperplasia (CAH) must be differentiated in the patient with coexistent androgen excess. A more acute history requires differential diagnosis of other endocrinologic causes of anovulation such as thyroid and prolactin disorders, as well as complications of pregnancy, neoplastic processes such as fibroids or hormone-producing ovarian tumors, intrauterine lesions such as polyps and synechiae, and blood dyscrasias. Women over age 30 with a history consistent with chronic anovulation should undergo endometrial sampling because of a risk of hyperplasia.

The perimenopausal woman with DUB has a much higher risk of hyperplasia/neoplasia and should always undergo a dilation and curettage (D & C). Several years before menopause, the menstrual cycles usually shorten secondary to a decreased proliferative phase with moderate elevation of FSH and subsequent frequent anovulatory cycles. This unopposed estrogen environment is therefore conducive to development of both DUB and hyperplasia. Postmenopausal bleeding is discussed later in the chapter.

DUB is, to some extent, a diagnosis of exclusion. Problems of pregnancy, such as incomplete or missed abortion, subinvolution of the placental site, placental polyp, trophoblastic disease, and extrauterine pregnancy must be ruled out. All gynecologic malignancies may cause abnormal bleeding. Even common epithelial tumors of the ovary may produce estrogen and cause uterine bleeding. Submucous leiomyoma and endometrial polyps may be present in older women but are not a problem in differential diagnosis in teenagers. Excessive anovulatory bleeding is common with polycystic ovarian disease, with luteal phase defects and with functional cysts of the ovary. Blood dyscrasias are associated with increased menstrual blood loss.

The workup should include a complete history and physical examination. Pelvic examination may disclose an adnexal mass, vaginal laceration, or fibroid uterus. Laboratory studies should include HCG, FSH, LH, thyroid function tests, prolactin, and serum androgens if indicated. A marked increase in dehydroepiandrosterone sulfate calls for an adrenocorticotropic hormone stimulation test to rule out adult onset CAH. Endometrial biopsy or D & C is necessary in the older patient or when there is clinical suspicion of an abnormal pregnancy, but is otherwise contraindicated in the adolescent. Blood clotting studies are particularly important in the presence of ovulatory DUB. Ultrasonography is useful in the evaluation of pelvic masses, with vaginal ultrasound particularly informative in early pregnancies. Hysterosalpingography or hysteroscopy are most effective aids in the diagnosis of intrauterine pathology.

Treatment of Dysfunctional Uterine Bleeding

Because most patients with DUB have an underlying etiology of anovulation with unopposed estrogen stim-

ulation of the endometrium, medical treatment with progestational compounds is the mainstay of therapy. Although the precise management may differ depending on the patient's age, adequate progestin stimulation will decrease DNA synthesis and cell proliferation, deplete estrogen receptors, and increase the conversion of estradiol to the less potent estrone sulfate. These effects will induce maturation of the endometrium, healing of superficial breaks, enhancement of the stromal matrix with increased structural stability, and cessation of bleeding. Withdrawal of the progestin after adequate exposure results in orderly and uniform shedding of the endometrium with a finite, self-limited bleed.

The progestin dosage and duration of therapy must induce a complete secretory transformation or it will fail to inhibit all estrogenic effects, and islands of proliferative endometrium will remain. Whitehead has shown in patients on postmenopausal estrogen replacement, which mimics the unopposed estrogen environment of chronic anovulation, that 4% develop endometrial hyperplasia with only 7 days of progestin exposure, 2% with 10 days exposure, and 0 with 12 days of progestin. He recommends 12 days of progestin every month to counteract estrogen's proliferative effects. Medroxyprogesterone acetate 10 mg or norethindrone acetate 5 mg/qd may be prescribed, and after initial control of the dysfunctional bleeding, the 12-day course can be repeated at monthly intervals to prevent the development of hyperplasia. It is convenient to start each new course on the first day of each month. A regular withdrawal may be expected to start either during the last 2 days of progestin or within several days after the last pill. Failure to withdraw could signify pregnancy, development of hypoestrogenemia, or, rarely, induction of ovulation by progestin stimulation of the estrogen-primed patient, in which case, because of endogenous progesterone production, the menses may be delayed 2 weeks. As a word of caution, this regimen is not contraceptive.

Chronic unopposed estrogen can produce a lush endometrium that may bleed heavily during progestin withdrawal. Speroff, Glass, and Kase recommend treatment using combination oral contraceptives in a "step-down" regimen. Four pills are given daily for 5 to 7 days for acute control of bleeding. Withdrawal of medication will result in a heavy bleed, on the fifth day of which a low dose cyclic oral contraceptive is started and repeated for three cycles to allow orderly regression of the excessive proliferative endometrium. Combination oral contraceptives induce atrophy of the endometrium because the chronic estrogen–progestin exposure suppresses pituitary gonadotropins and inhibits endogenous steroidogenesis. They are useful for long-term management of DUB in patients without contraindications, and have the added benefit of pregnancy prevention. Particularly in perimenarchal patients, heavy prolonged bleeding can denude the basal endometrium, making it unresponsive to progestins. Curettage for control of hemorrhage is contraindicated because of a high risk of development of intrauterine synechiae (Asherman's syndrome) if the basalis is curetted. High dose intravenous estrogen (conjugated estrogens 25 mg/q4h until bleeding abates) will give acute control by proliferative repair of the endometrium, after which oral conjugated estrogens in combination with a progestin or the progestin alone can be used to induce orderly withdrawal bleeding.

In patients who fail to respond to hormonal therapy, hysteroscopy may reveal previously missed pathology such as a submucous myoma or polyp. These diagnoses are particularly frequent in patients with ovulatory dysfunctional bleeding. If a diagnostic curettage has not been performed previously, one can be done in conjunction with the hysteroscopy for both diagnosis and temporary therapy. If atypical hyperplasia has been identified and preservation of fertility is desired, more aggressive progestin therapy is recommended. Medroxyprogesterone acetate 30 mg or megestrol 20 mg daily for 3 months should be followed by repeat endometrial sampling to assess the efficiency of the medical treatment (see Fig. 13-1B). If atypical hyperplasia persists, high dose progestin protocols may be tried but hysterectomy must be considered.

Menorrhagia can be reduced when prostaglandin E_2 and prostacyclin synthesis is decreased by flufenamic and mefenamic acid medication. Both of these drugs inhibit the cyclooxygenase enzyme necessary for endometrial production of prostaglandin under estrogen stimulation. These compounds are most effective when given in therapeutic dosage for 7 to 10 days before the expected onset of the next menstrual period in ovulatory DUB patients as shown by Fraser, Pearse, and Shearman.

Two new treatment modalities show promise in DUB refractory to other therapy. Long-acting derivatives of GnRH, GnRH agonists, downregulate pituitary synthesis of FSH and LH and induce a "medical castration." Withdrawal of endogenous steroid stimulation will result in endometrial atrophy. Anecdotal reports have described excellent short-term control of DUB during a 6-month therapeutic trial, with possible prolonged control of bleeding during the period of endometrial regeneration after withdrawal of the drug. Currently, the only available analog must be administered parenterally, either by subcutaneous or intramuscular injection. Endometrial ablation by hysteroscopic application of the Nd-YAG laser fiber provides good control of menorrhagia in patients who have failed with medical therapy and are not candidates for more definitive surgical intervention. This fiberoptically guided laser causes deep tissue coagulation, but with limited pene-

tration, giving it the capability to destroy the endometrium without myometrial penetration. Appropriate indications for surgery and the incidence of complications such as postoperative bleeding and pulmonary edema from intravascular absorption of the uterine distending medium have not yet been defined, but the procedure may offer an alternative to conventional surgical treatment (see Ch. 17).

Should the patient fail to respond to repeated curettage or endocrine therapy, more definitive therapy, primarily hysterectomy, should be considered in relation to the age of the patient and her desire for future childbearing. Although a hysterectomy may be considered an admission of therapeutic defeat, it is frequently an expeditious method of resolving a refractory and recurrent type of DUB. In general, the ovulatory type of bleeding has the poorest response to replacement hormonal therapy and the highest incidence of recurrence. When bleeding persists after repeated curettage and cyclic hormonal therapy, hysterectomy may be required. If other conditions are present that should be corrected surgically, such as a relaxed vaginal outlet, rectocele, cystocele, or uterine descensus, the authors recommend vaginal hysterectomy with support of the vaginal vault and repair of the vaginal wall relaxation. When hysterectomy is indicated in premenopausal women under age 50 years, normal ovarian tissue is conserved. In a patient under age 30 years, radical surgical treatment must be avoided because one can almost always control the uterine bleeding by repeated curettage or by increasing amounts of cyclic hormone therapy. Today, the availability and use of estrogen and progesterone has changed the need for hysterectomy. Hysterectomy is not indicated in young women to treat DUB. Hysterectomy may be indicated in older women when hormonal therapy has failed and curettage has been performed at least twice.

Blood transfusions are seldom required when DUB is associated with anemia, but may be given if the anemia is so severe that symptoms are present. Oral iron therapy should be started at the first sign of heavy menstruation to prevent depletion of iron stores, and should be given for 3 to 6 months after normal hemoglobin and hematocrit levels have been restored in patients with iron deficiency anemia.

POSTMENOPAUSAL BLEEDING

When uterine bleeding occurs more than 12 months after the last regular menstrual periods, it is defined as postmenopausal bleeding. The first diagnostic consideration is to ensure that the origin of the bleeding is from the uterus. In the elderly woman, bleeding from the urethra or the rectum may be reported as vaginal bleeding. Vaginal or cervical lesions causing the bleeding symptom should be diagnosed readily on careful inspection or biopsy. Cancers of the vagina or cervix or cervical polyps require diagnosis and appropriate treatment.

When the source of the bleeding is believed to be the uterine cavity, diagnostic D & C continues to be the most commonly performed diagnostic and therapeutic procedure. Office endometrial biopsy, if positive for endometrial carcinoma or sarcoma, can often expedite appropriate comprehensive evaluation and therapy. However, an endometrial biopsy that reveals benign endometrium histology does not exclude absolutely the presence of a malignant process elsewhere within the endometrium. For that reason, advocacy of office hysteroscopy is growing—proponents claim the ability to selectively biopsy the area of the visualized endometrium most likely to contain a neoplastic process, if present. Another major use for the hysteroscope is to exclude the endometrial polyp as a source of the bleeding—a source that may not always be removed by conventional curettage. Suction curettage, as utilized for pregnancy termination, may be a more efficient diagnostic and therapeutic procedure, especially in the postmenopausal patient. The conventional suction curettage procedure is now used for all curettages.

Hormone-induced postmenopausal uterine bleeding may be the result of endogenous or exogenous hormonal effects. The proliferation of endometrium in the uterus of a patient who is not receiving exogenous hormonal therapy is generally attributed to the endogenous production of estrone. Estrone is the peripheral conversion product of the weak androgenic precursor androstenedione (85% from adrenal, 15% from ovary), and its synthesis occurs primarily in adipose tissue. The usually prescribed replacement hormonal therapy is some sequential program of at least 12 days of progestin, with exogenous estrogen added when failure of withdrawal bleeding to occur indicates hypoestrogenemia. However, many regimens of postmenopausal hormonal replacement therapy have been introduced in recent years including programs that utilize continuous estrogen accompanied by continuous low dose progestin.

In any patient with postmenopausal uterine bleeding, the recommended diagnostic procedures may produce a tissue sample of endometrium or no tissue may be obtained. That no tissue is obtained is not uncommon in some patients with marked hypertension and in patients undergoing chronic anticoagulant therapy.

When endometrial tissue is present in the postmenopausal bleeding patient, a wide range of histology may be noted. Occasionally, simple proliferative endometrium is found. The endometrium may exhibit simple hyperplasia, more marked adenomatous hyperplasia, or hyperplasia with atypia cells that results in a diagnosis of atypical endometrial hyperplasia. Later in the menopausal years, it is not uncommon to obtain endometrium that has the characteristics of cystic hyperplasia, often referred to in the older literature as "Swiss cheese hyperplasia."

The management of postmenopausal uterine bleeding not associated with exogenous hormonal therapy must include the exclusion of an estrogen-producing ovarian tumor (eg granulosa cell tumor). When that is not present, management of the several types of endometrial hyperplasia other than that of atypical adenomatous hyperplasia can generally be accomplished by monthly administration of a progestin such as medroxyprogesterone acetate 10 mg/day for 12 days or norethindrone acetate 5 mg/day for 12 days monthly until two or three monthly administrations have failed to produce any evidence of uterine withdrawal bleeding. Endometrial biopsy is then repeated in approximately 6 months, and if no further bleeding occurs and if no endometrial tissue is obtained on biopsy attempts, then the problem is generally resolved for a considerable time, if not permanently. More aggressive hormonal therapy may consist of continuous high dose progestin for 3 to 6 months (ie, Megestrol 20 mg–160 mg/day). Atypical adenomatous endometrial hyperplasia is considered by most to be the equivalent of an intraepithelial malignancy, and hysterectomy is generally advised.

The woman who is receiving any one of the regimens currently in use as postmenopausal hormonal replacement therapy may have uterine bleeding. Unopposed estrogen is no longer recommended for postmenopausal hormone replacement in the woman who has an intact uterus because it may result in the development of hyperplasia in between 18% and 32% of patients. Use of sequential estrogen-progestin regimens have been shown to significantly decrease this risk with 12 days of progestin reducing the risk to less than 1%. The bleeding that accompanies the more commonly utilized sequential estrogen-progestin regimens should occur predictably at the conclusion of the progestin phase of the cyclic administration. Most students of this subject now agree that such predictable and appropriately timed withdrawal bleeding does not indicate any need to sample the endometrial histology. Just as intermenstrual bleeding during the regular menstruating years dictates investigation and management, so patterns of bleeding that do not follow the anticipated schedule of bleeding require investigation and management. Regimens of continuous estrogen and low dose progestin replacement therapy are commonly accompanied by quite irregular bleeding patterns for at least 4 to 8 months of the regimen. They are utilized in anticipation that as the months of use increase, the proportion of women becoming completely amenorrheic will increase so that the majority of women using the program will be happier in the long run with the regimen than with the conventional sequential regimen in which the majority of women bleed regularly at the conclusion of the progestin phase of the cycle—at least for 6 to 24 months.

The most important point about the significance of postmenopausal bleeding is its frequent association with a gynecologic malignancy, especially endometrial adenocarcinoma. Although the incidence of malignancy to explain postmenopausal bleeding has decreased in recent decades, diagnostic efforts must continue to emphasize the discovery of a malignancy by appropriate diagnostic procedures, especially careful pelvic examination and uterine curettage. When endometrial carcinoma is suspected, an endometrial biopsy is helpful only if positive. The definitive test is D & C.

DILATATION OF THE CERVIX

Recamier invented the curette in 1843. Since that time, dilatation of the cervix and curettage of the endometrial cavity is the second most frequent gynecologic procedure performed in the United States. It is used to diagnose uterine malignancy, to complete an incomplete or missed abortion, to evaluate the causes of infertility, to control DUB, and to relieve dysmenorrhea. Because medical therapy for DUB and dysmenorrhea has become more effective, dilatation of the cervix and curettage of the uterus is needed less often for these two problems, especially in young women.

Dilatation of the cervix is carried out as a preliminary step to curettage of the uterine cavity. As a therapeutic measure, it is done for acquired or congenital cervical stenosis, for dysmenorrhea, for introduction of intracervical and intrauterine radium or cesium, occasionally for insertion of an intrauterine contraceptive device, to allow drainage of the uterine cavity in the presence of pyometra, for sterility, or as a part of other operations on the cervix.

Most indications for cervical dilatation are obvious. However, in connection with primary dysmenorrhea and sterility, there is room for controversy. It is a recognized fact that many cases of primary dysmenorrhea are not cured by cervical dilatation. Because of frequent failures, some gynecologists have almost abandoned it as a therapeutic technique. We do not subscribe totally to this pessimistic point of view. Unfortunately, in most instances, it is impossible to detect those cases of dysmenorrhea that will be relieved by cervical dilatation. Often the operation must be done as a therapeutic test, but fortunately it is such a minor procedure that one is justified in performing it on that basis. In nulliparous women in whom pain is greatest just before or during the early part of the menstrual flow, there is a possibility of relief from cervical dilatation. However, this result is unpredictable. Before proceeding with the operation, it is advisable to permit the patient to decide whether her menstrual pain is sufficiently severe to justify an operation that may be of limited or no benefit.

Ibuprofen, sodium naproxen, and mefenamic acid have proven to be so effective in the management of dysmenorrhea that a thorough trial of these agents is indicated first. Because it has become evident that endometriosis can occur much earlier than once considered true, the woman with dysmenorrhea unrelieved by these nonsteroidal anti-inflammatory drugs should be considered for laparoscopy.

In a postmenopausal patient with cervical stenosis, a pyometra may be discovered when the uterus is sounded. The pus should be cultured for anaerobic and aerobic organisms and the cervix should be dilated. A short, soft, rubber or plastic tube may be sutured in place to keep the cervical canal open while the uterine cavity is draining. Although antibiotics may not be strictly necessary in all cases, fever and pelvic pain and tenderness herald the onset of spreading pelvic infection.

Curetting a pyometra may produce parametritis or wider pelvic cellulitis. Because the risk of perforation during curettage is increased, resulting in the potential for development of serious peritonitis, curettage should be delayed until adequate drainage has occurred (3 to 10 days depending on magnitude) and antibiotic therapy should be used. Curettage is mandatory to exclude endocervical or endometrial malignancy that are associated frequently with pyometra.

Technique of Cervical Dilatation

The patient is placed on the table in the lithotomy position. A careful pelvic examination is done to locate the position of the uterine corpus. The vagina and the perineum are cleaned with the usual vaginal preparation of povidone-iodine (Betadine). The cervix is grasped with a four-pronged tenaculum (Fig. 13-2, *left*) and gently drawn toward the vaginal outlet. We favor the straight Jacobs clamp, especially when difficult dilatation is either anticipated or encountered. Its use is much less likely to result in cervical laceration than is the use of the single tooth tenaculum. A sound (Fig. 13-2, *right*) is passed through the cervical canal into the uterine cavity carefully to avoid creating a false passage. Resistance is greatest at the internal cervical os. Occasionally, a fine silver probe is needed to find the proper passage if the canal is stenotic. Passing the uterine sound gives one confirmatory information on the position of the uterus, the length of the uterine cavity, and

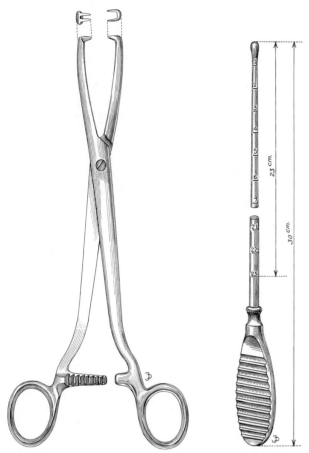

Figure 13–2. *Left*, Straight Jacobs clamp, used for pulling down cervix when performing curettage. *Right*, Uterine sound.

the angulation between the cervical canal and the uterine cavity. The degree of stenosis of the cervical canal can be detected in this manner.

The cervical canal is dilated with a small Hegar's dilator (Fig. 13-3). The uterine wall may be perforated by improper passage of the dilator; usually this is due to a lack of knowledge or to disregard of the position of the uterus. When acute anteflexion is present, the dilator may perforate posteriorly (Fig. 13-4). When retrodisplacement exists, the perforation usually occurs anteriorly (Fig. 13-5). This complication may be avoided by sounding the uterine cavity before dilating the cervix and following the direction of the endocervical canal and uterine cavity indicated by the sound. The dilator rarely perforates the fundus except when there is an atrophic postmenopausal uterus or when an invasive tumor or pregnancy has produced softening of the uterine wall. After the 3 mm or 4 mm Hegar's dilator is passed, successively larger ones are used. For ordinary

curettage, dilatation to 8 mm or 9 mm suffices. When dilatation is done for dysmenorrhea or sterility, we prefer to carry the dilatation up to 10 mm. There is concern that excessive dilatation may be associated with an incompetent cervix in a subsequent pregnancy. If cervical dilatation is difficult, "half-size" Hegar's dilators with incremental diameters of 0.5 mm are useful (see Fig. 13-3).

The Hank-Bradley dilator has the same shape and contour as the Hegar's dilator, but has a more tapered shank (Fig. 13-6). It also has the added advantage of a hollow center, which prevents a piston effect in which air is forced into the uterine cavity during progressive dilatation of the cervix. Because of the positive pressure created within the uterine cavity by passing a Hegar's dilator, blood, endometrium, fragments of neoplastic tissue, or infected material could be forced into the fallopian tubes or peritoneal cavity. Beyth and associates have demonstrated that, in a significant number of patients, endometrial tissue will be found in peritoneal

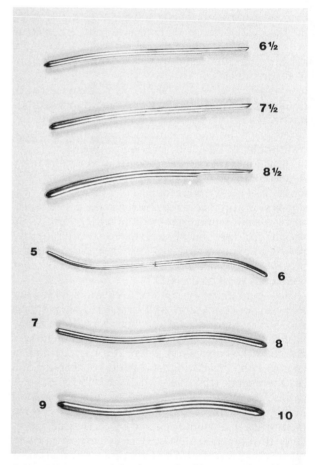

Figure 13–3. Graduated Hegar's dilators and "half-size" Hegar's dilators.

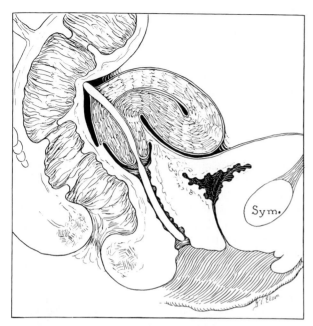

Figure 13–4. Perforation of the acutely anteflexed uterus. The uterus was thought to be in retroposition, and the Hegar's dilator was erroneously directed posteriorly.

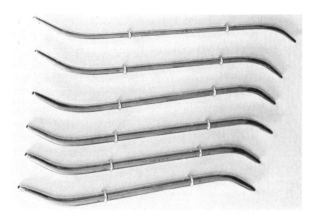

Figure 13–6. Hank-Bradley dilators in graduated sizes. Note central canal that extends through length of dilator.

fluid after curettage. Concern has been voiced about the possibility of reflux of endometrial carcinoma cells into the peritoneal cavity with forceful dilatation of a postmenopausal cervix in a patient found to harbor endometrial carcinoma. On the other hand, in the small postmenopausal uterus, it is quite easy to perforate the fundus of the uterus with the tip of the Hank-Bradley dilator while attempting to achieve the maximum dilating effect from the widest portion of the instrument. The Hank-Bradley dilator is used more commonly when curettage is being performed for an incomplete abortion because it permits the release of blood through the dilator while the cervix is being dilated. When dilatation is for removal of placental tissue, dilatation up to No. 19 or No. 20 Hank-Bradley (equivalent to a 9 mm or 10 mm Hegar's) is often necessary to permit the introduction of a large blunt curette and placental forceps.

Cervical injury is a potential problem when the cervix is forcefully dilated in preparation for removal of products of conception. The cervical tenaculum may lacerate the cervix. The internal cervical os may be damaged. The cervix is most resistant to dilatation at about 8 mm. Tapered Pratt dilators require less force than blunt Hegar's dilators. The incidence of cervical incompetence may be related to the degree of cervical dilatation. Insertion of laminaria into the cervical canal several hours before cervical dilatation may make the procedure less difficult and traumatic, as suggested by Manabe and Manabe.

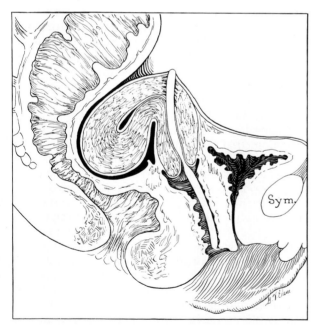

Figure 13–5. Perforation of the retroflexed uterus. The uterus was thought to be in anteposition, and the Hegar's dilator was erroneously directed anteriorly.

CURETTAGE OF THE UTERUS

Indications and Contraindications

It is important that D & C be done for a proper indication, be done correctly so the most useful information is obtained, and be done safely. A curettage done properly and with aseptic technique involves little risk, but if precautions are disregarded, complications and even death may result.

The chief purpose of curettage of the uterus is the removal of endometrial or endocervical tissue for histologic study in cases in which there has been abnormal uterine bleeding. Although classical curettage of the uterus continues to be a useful procedure, new practices and instrumentation permit the procurement of endometrium as a screening diagnostic test under many circumstances. Appropriate use of such procedures can reduce significantly the need for operating room curettage. Previously, careful pelvic examination under relaxation anesthesia was an important adjunctive diagnostic aid during conventional D & C. Improvement in precision and availability of ultrasound and other imaging techniques has diminished that aspect to some degree.

During the past 50 years, many instruments have been devised for the sampling of endometrial tissue and evaluation of the endometrial cavity. One of the most useful instruments for outpatient use is the Novak curette. Although this curette was initially devised to obtain a sample of the endometrium by suction and aspiration, it is more commonly used as a miniature curette that contains a serrated edge surrounding its biopsy aperture. The curette is approximately 5 mm in diameter and can usually be passed through a small cervical canal, even in nulliparous women. However, the postmenopausal cervical canal is frequently stenotic and is difficult to penetrate without minimal dilatation. The Novak curette has been used with increasing effectiveness in providing an adequate sample for dating the endometrium in infertility cases, as well as for the initial screening evaluation of a patient with abnormal bleeding. Its principal value is in avoiding a formal D & C under anesthesia if the tissue removed contains adenocarcinoma. However, if the cause of postmenopausal bleeding is not identified in a screening endometrial biopsy by the Novak curette, then a standard curettage is obligatory. In office biopsy of the endometrium in more than 20,000 patients of all ages, Hofmeister detected 273 cases of endometrial carcinoma, of which 32 (14.28%) were totally asymptomatic. The endometrial carcinoma detection rate was 1.76% of the total group of 23,202 patients. Hofmeister's routine use of the office endometrial biopsy, using a modification of the Novak and Randall curette, provides one of the largest clinical experiences to date for this instrument. Unfortunately, only patients who had continued uterine bleeding or who demonstrated an atypical endometrial pattern in the office biopsy were subjected to a complete curettage. Therefore, the true false–negative rate for the Novak-type curette in the

detection of endometrial cancer has not been determined accurately. In other studies, the accuracy with which endometrial cancer is detected by the Novak curette varied from 76% to 92%, as summarized by Cohen, Gusberg, and Koffier. However, a thorough endometrial curettage under anesthesia is not infallible in the detection of endometrial cancer.

More recently, the use of vacuum suction curettage has gained popularity as an office procedure not requiring general anesthesia. This technique consists of using a small metal or plastic cannula with an outside diameter of 3 mm that has a slightly curved tip and an opening on the concave surface for easy insertion through a small endocervical canal. The cannula is connected to a plastic tubular chamber containing a cylindrical plastic filter. At the opposite end of the chamber, there is a plastic spout that is connected to a negative pressure source. The apparatus is prepackaged in a sterile disposable container and the vacuum source can be either a commercial pump or a faucet in which approximately 60 cm of negative water pressure is developed for proper suction through the curette. Several improvements have been made in the technology. This Vabra aspirator instrument has the advantage and the convenience of being completely prepared and disposable but the disadvantage of a high price, which must be borne by the patient. Several studies have compared the results of suction curettage with those of a regular curettage under anesthesia in the same patient. Cohen and associates studied 98 patients by this technique and found that identical histologic patterns resulted from both methods. In only five patients there was no correlation between the results of the two techniques, and none of these had cancer. At the Medical University of South Carolina, Lutz and associates found the suction curettage to be 98% accurate in evaluating high-risk women with abnormal bleeding for endometrial malignant disease.

Many other devices have been developed to apply the suction aspiration principle to obtain an endometrial sample. Some use specially designed syringes that develop effective vacuum pressures (Fig. 13-7). The vacuum pumps produced for suction abortion can be utilized to perform a thorough endometrial aspiration.

A remarkably simple device has been distributed that does not require syringe or pump. It is a disposable 3.1 mm O.D. hollow plastic tube with an aspiration port at its tip and a solid plastic obturator. The obturator fits the tube so closely that when the obturator is slowly withdrawn while the device is in the uterine cavity, sufficient suction results to obtain excellent endometrial specimens (Fig. 13-8).

These new tools permit almost painless endometrial sampling providing little or no cervical dilatation is required. A quick acting nonsteroidal anti-inflamma-

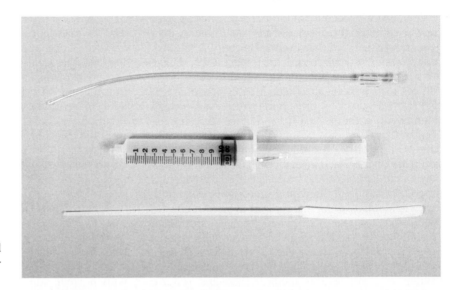

Figure 13–7. An endometrial suction sampling (UTER CYTE) instrument with syringe vacuum.

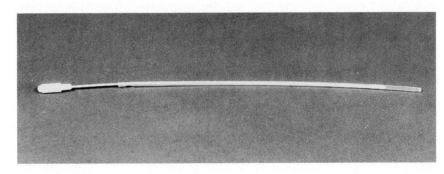

Figure 13–8. A useful suction endometrial sampling Pipelle instrument—3.1 mm OD and no pump or syringe required.

tory drug (eg, 550 mg sodium naproxen) administered 15 to 30 minutes before the procedure has provided satisfactory analgesia for the majority of patients. If dilatation of the cervix is required, paracervical block anesthesia is also initiated by injecting 4 or 5.0 cc of 1% lidocaine at both 3 o'clock and 9 o'clock, exercising care to avoid intravascular injection.

Although this method may be an easy outpatient technique for evaluating the histology of the endometrium in patients with abnormal bleeding, it does not fulfill the requirements for a thorough curettage, should the cause of the uterine bleeding fail to be determined. Only if an endometrial biopsy or a suction curettage shows frank adenocarcinoma should one have total confidence in these findings. Even in the most experienced hands, endometrial carcinoma can be quite elusive. None of the office methods can assure the removal of an endometrial polyp. Therefore, endometrial carcinoma could be missed in a polyp, as could the source of benign bleeding. Office curettage should be used only as a screening procedure; and, if the office procedure is negative, then it should not be accepted as a substitute for a more thorough D & C under anesthesia. For the same reasons, hysteroscopy should be utilized before concluding that no intrauterine pathology is present.

Indications for obtaining endometrial histology by one or more of the aforementioned methods include

Abnormal bleeding at any premenopausal age
 Especially when it is not corrected promptly by medical management
 Especially in women over age 35 years
 Especially if a submucous myoma is suspected, and include hysteroscopy or hysterosalpingography
Postmenopausal bleeding
 Of any amount
 Regardless of finding atrophic vaginitis, polyp, or urethral caruncle
Prehysterectomy
 In the postmenopausal woman to exclude endocervical or endometrial carcinoma
Postmenopausal vaginal surgery without hysterectomy

When office procedures have been deemed to have failed to establish the diagnosis, it is preferable to use a general anesthetic during D & C. Not only is the procedure easier to perform with the patient fully relaxed, but it is more comfortable for the patient. Most patients will opt for a general anesthetic for this procedure. It also provides an ideal opportunity to do a thorough examination of the pelvic organs. Before the examination, the bladder should be empty and an enema should have been given and expelled. When the anterior abdominal wall is relaxed from the anesthesia, a thorough pelvic examination should be done before the patient is draped. Occasionally, new and important pelvic findings will be discovered. In a study of 2666 women who required a curettage, McElin and coworkers found an unanticipated adnexal mass in 30 patients at the time of pelvic examination under anesthesia before D & C. Twenty-eight were benign and two were malignant. In women who are serious medical risks and require curettage for postmenopausal bleeding, the operation is performed without anesthetic other than hypodermic or intravenous administration of a sedative combined with paracervical nerve block.

However, a single curettage will not remove all of the surface endometrium completely from the uterine cavity. Repeated studies have demonstrated the inability of a thorough curettage to remove more than 50% to 60% of the endometrium when the procedure has been done by experienced gynecologists immediately before a planned hysterectomy. Stock and Kanbour, from the McGee Hospital in Pittsburgh, observed that in 60% of hysterectomy specimens studied, less than 50% of the endometrial surface had been curetted by a prehysterectomy curettage. They also found that in 26 cases, endometrial carcinoma had been classified as clinically normal-appearing tissue on prehysterectomy curettage; six of these carcinomas were reported as benign on frozen section. These facts and other similar experiences indicate that it is difficult to be certain of the histology of the endometrium by gross examination of the curettings. If the symptoms warrant a curettage, then the endometrium deserves a histologic diagnosis.

Curettage is also done when bleeding occurs from a cervical stump. It is frequently performed as a part of a cervical conization to rule out extension of cervical carcinoma into the endometrium. Helmkamp and associates found no evidence of endometrial abnormality in any of 114 curettage specimens removed at the time of 114 cervical conizations. These authors recommend that curettage at the time of cervical conization should not be done routinely but should be done selectively in postmenopausal and perimenopausal patients, when the cytology smear shows abnormal glandular cells and when an intrauterine abnormality is suspected.

The chief contraindication to curettage is infection.

Acute endometritis and salpingitis constitute conditions under which curettage should be avoided. At times, however, curettage must be done for the removal of infected placental tissue, in which case it should be preceded by an adequate period of parenteral antibiotic therapy to achieve a therapeutic tissue level of antibiotics. Patients with endometritis associated with retained products of conception will remain unwell until the infected, necrotic material is cast off spontaneously or is removed by the curette. Curettage is also contraindicated when pyometra is present.

Technique of Curettage of the Uterus

We have increasingly used the abortion suction apparatus to perform diagnostic and therapeutic endometrial evacuation. The connecting tubing is flushed with normal saline to ensure recovery of all tissue fragments. Overall, the use of suction should result in less trauma to the uterine wall and should provide a more complete sample of the endometrium. The perineum need not be shaved before uterine curettage. However, before the patient comes to the operating room, an enema is given and expelled so that hard stool in the rectum and sigmoid will not interfere with the accuracy of the pelvic examination under anesthesia. After the patient is anesthetized, she is placed in the lithotomy position and the bladder is emptied with a catheter. The pelvic organs are examined thoroughly before the patient is prepped and draped. The procedure includes a bimanual rectovaginal–abdominal exam. The examination under anesthesia is one of the most informative features of this operation because it can provide anatomical details of the reproductive tract that are unrecognizable without anesthesia. The vagina and perineum are cleaned with the usual technique.

Fractional curettage is an attempt to remove tissue samples from the endocervical canal differentially from tissue removed from the endometrial cavity. The cervical canal should be curetted before dilatation of the cervical canal and curettage of the endometrial cavity. The Gusberg curette is a small, specially shaped instrument that is particularly useful in curetting the endocervix. A differential curettage of the endocervix, separate from the endometrium, is important in the diagnosis of endometrial carcinoma that may have extended to the endocervix (see Ch. 43). All patients with perimenopausal bleeding should have a fractional curettage, a procedure that is frequently neglected. If the endocervical curettage is not done, a second fractional curettage is required to determine the anatomical boundaries of endometrial carcinoma.

The value of fractional curettage has been questioned, but Chen and Lee and others have emphasized the importance of cervical stromal invasion, rather than the mere finding of tumor tissue in the endocervical curettings, as the crucial criterion affecting staging and prognosis. The uterine cavity is always sounded to determine its size and to confirm the position determined from examination under anesthesia. The cervical canal is dilated with Hegar's or Hank-Bradley dilators. A dilatation to an 8 mm or 9 mm Hegar's is sufficient for the usual diagnostic curettage. A gauze is placed in the posterior vaginal fornix along the posterior retractor so that the blood and the endometrium removed from the uterus may fall on it (Fig. 13-9). The uterine cavity is explored initially in search of an endometrial polyp before the curettage is performed, using a narrow stone forceps (Fig. 13-10 *A* and *B*). This forceps can be opened and closed as the tip of the forceps is moved systematically across the dome of the uterus and the anterior and posterior walls. An endometrial polyp can easily be missed with an ordinary curette. As a result, unnecessary hysterectomies have been done because of supposed persistent or recurrent dysfunctional bleeding following a curettage (Fig. 13-11). If polyp forceps are routinely used, such operations may be avoided. It is

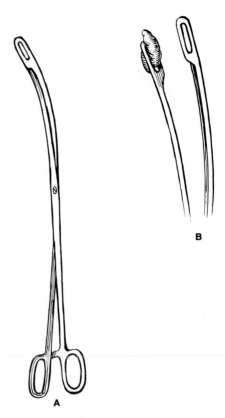

Figure 13–10. *A*, Ureteral stone forceps, an excellent instrument for removing endometrial polyps. *B*, A polyp grasped in forceps that was missed at curettage.

easier to identify and remove an endometrial polyp if the uterine cavity is explored with the stone forceps before the uterus is curetted. In a 28-month period, during which time the forceps were used routinely at the Johns Hopkins Hospital, Josey found that the diagnosis of endometrial polyp was made 130 times. In 83 of these cases, the polyp was removed by forceps. Although the sessile form of a submucous myoma is diagnosed easily by noting an irregularity of the uterine wall with the curette, the pedunculated variety, like the endometrial polyp, may escape detection because of its narrow stalk. Often such a leiomyoma may be grasped with the polyp forceps. A uterine septum may also be detected with the forceps.

A small or medium-sized, malleable, bluntly serrated curette (Fig. 13-12) is then introduced into the uterus and, in a systematic manner, the entire uterine cavity is curetted. The anterior, lateral, and posterior walls are scraped gently but firmly and finally the top of the cavity is scraped with a side-to-side movement (Fig. 13-13).The handle of the curette should never be held against the palm of the hand. Instead, it should be held gently as one would hold a pencil. The instrument is

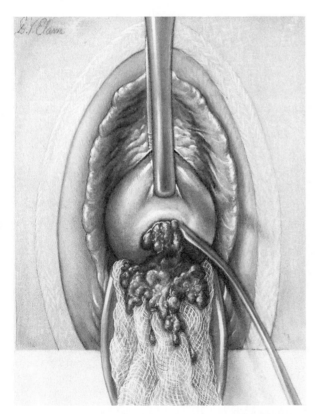

Figure 13–9. Method of collecting curettings and blood on gauze.

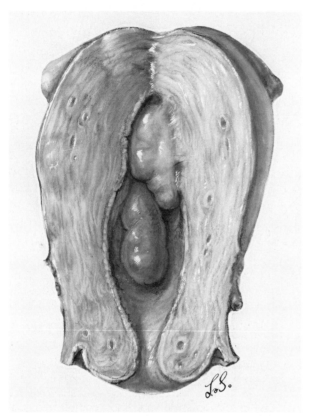

Figure 13–11. Opened uterus, showing two separate endometrial polyps.

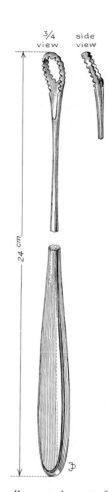

Figure 13–12. Small serrated curette for routine curettage.

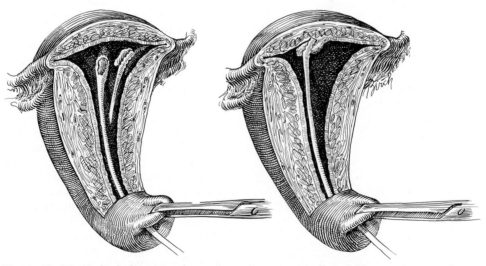

Figure 13–13. Method of curetting the uterine cavity systematically. *Left*, The anterior posterior, and lateral walls of cavity are curetted systematically. *Right*, The top of cavity is then curetted thoroughly.

held loosely as it is inserted for the full distance. Pressure is then exerted against the uterine wall as the curette is drawn in an outward direction. Because the instrument is malleable, its curvature may be changed to conform to the contour of the uterine cavity.

The unclotted blood is absorbed quickly by the gauze sponge, leaving the relatively clean endometrium to be placed in a prepared container with appropriate fixative. The curettings should never be mashed or scraped but should be picked carefully from the sponge with a smooth tip forceps and placed immediately in the fixative. In so doing, the curettings are examined carefully to be certain that no fatty tissue or other unusual tissue is present. Fragments of hyperplastic endometrium may sometimes appear tan or yellow.

When curettage is done as a curative measure for removal of placental tissue, a large, blunt, smooth curette is used to lessen the chances of perforation and endometrial sclerosis. The larger and softer the uterus, the larger the curette used should be and the more careful one should be to avoid these complications. When large masses of placental tissue are present, the ovum forceps are most useful when used in conjunction with the curette. High vacuum suction is now utilized almost routinely for the removal of placental tissue.

Routine blind biopsy of the cervix is usually unrewarding if a negative cytologic smear has been obtained and there is no suspicious cervical lesion. We no longer do a blind biopsy of the cervix at the time of curettage unless an abnormal lesion is present. If a patient has recent negative cytology and has a profuse, recurrent, mucous discharge associated with cervicitis and Nabothian cysts, cervical cauterization or laser vaporization may be done at the time of curettage, but biopsy confirmation to exclude occult malignancy should be obtained.

Complications of Cervical Dilatation and Uterine Curettage

If the position and the consistency of the uterus are carefully noted on bimanual examination under anesthesia before the curettage is undertaken, perforation will rarely occur. When the position of the uterus is not known to the operator, perforation may occur with remarkable ease. Special care should be exercised in patients who have a uterus that is acutely anteflexed or retroflexed. In the presence of cervical stenosis, pregnancy, or intrauterine malignancy, perforation is more likely. The postmenopausal atrophic uterus may be perforated with only slight force applied to the uterine sound or the curette. Perforation is discovered when the sound or the curette fails to encounter resistance at the point where it normally should, as judged by the palpated size of the uterus.

Perforation by the uterine sound or cervical dilator causes less damage than perforation by the sharp curette or suction cannula. Sharp curettage for legally induced abortion has a major complication rate two to three times higher than suction curettage, according to Grimes and Cates. The two principal dangers of uterine perforation are bleeding and trauma to the abdominal viscera. Lateral perforation through the uterine vessels is especially dangerous from the standpoint of intraperitoneal hemorrhage and broad ligament hematoma formation. Damage can occur to bowel, omentum, mesentery, ureter, and fallopian tube. Perforation of the anterior or posterior wall of the uterus by a small curette in performing a diagnostic curettage is usually not a serious accident. However, it is usually necessary to discontinue the curettage. The patient should be watched carefully for signs of hemorrhage or infection. If signs of hemorrhage develop, the abdomen should be opened and the uterine wound sutured. If signs of infection occur, broad-spectrum antibiotics should be given. If a pelvic abscess develops, then the abscess should be drained if possible. Serious hemorrhage or infection occur only rarely. When serious damage from perforation is suspected, laparoscopy may be done to assess the extent of the damage and the repair needed. According to MacKenzie and Bibby, complications occurred in 1.7% of patients undergoing D & C. McElin and associates reported that 0.5% of patients had postoperative febrile morbidity following D & C. Uterine perforation occurred in 0.63% of cases.

One should be absolutely certain that the endometrial cavity has been entered when D & C is done for postmenopausal bleeding. A relatively stenotic internal cervical os and a fear of uterine perforation may prevent entry into the uterine cavity above the internal cervical os, resulting in a failure to curette the uterine cavity and a failure to diagnose the cause of the bleeding.

Perforation of the uterus during legally induced abortion (or of any pregnant uterus) is a more serious complication than perforation of the nonpregnant uterus. First, there is the requirement to complete the removal of all remaining pregnancy tissue to prevent sepsis. To do that blindly with a defect in the uterine wall is unsafe. Second, the pregnant uterus is a much more vascular organ than is the nonpregnant uterus and intraperitoneal bleeding may be profuse without significant external bleeding. Third, it is often difficult to be certain when the perforation occurred. If a high vacuum suction vacurette has passed through the myometrium and the vacuum has been activated, major bowel injury may be present.

These considerations have resulted in the following protocol:

1. *Never* activate the vacuum suction if there is *any question* regarding the safe location of the vacurette within the uterine cavity.
2. Laparoscope all patients with a pregnant uterus in whom perforation is believed to have occurred. With the laparoscope in place, a second operator can evacuate remaining placental tissue while the laparoscopist monitors safety. Many perforations in which no other visceral damage has occurred are fundal. Laparoscopic observation will confirm that bleeding is minimal following which the patient can be managed conservatively. We administer antibiotics and follow hematocrit values for 24–48 hours. If there is no evidence of continued bleeding or developing infection, then the patient is discharged.
3. At laparoscopy, if there is any evidence of intestinal injury or any suspicion of such injury, or if bleeding is significant, then laparotomy is mandatory. Unfortunately, bowel injury by high vacuum suction may require bowel resection and anastomosis.

Fig 13-14 shows a uterus removed immediately after a perforation. The uterus was removed because of intraperitoneal bleeding. Word analyzed 70 accidental uterine perforations. Among these, an unplanned hysterectomy was done on seven unprepared patients. In none did the intraperitoneal findings indicate the need for hysterectomy. In fact, the hysterectomy only compounded the surgical error. Fifty-five patients were treated conservatively, and only one developed a complication in the form of a pelvic abscess, which was drained by colpotomy. Forty-one of the 70 perforations occurred in postmenopausal women.

When a large, boggy, postabortion, or puerperal uterus is perforated by a large curette or placental forceps in removing placental tissue, there is more danger of hemorrhage, infection, or injury to bowel. The treatment that should be given and the procedures that should be followed are discussed in Chapter 14.

Asherman's syndrome is a pathologic condition of intrauterine adhesions that may cause secondary amenorrhea, other menstrual irregularities, infertility, or recurrent abortion. Numerous investigators have shown a strong association between puerperal D & C and the formation of synechiae that may partially or completely obliterate the endometrial cavity. No incidence figures are available as no prospective studies have been done, but other factors besides pregnancy that have been identified to increase the risk of endometrial sclerosis after D & C are infection, scant endometrium that exposes the basalis to trauma and a hypoestrogenic state. Rarely significant synechiae are seen in the absence of an antecedent curettage. Cases have been reported after severe endometritis, tuberculosis, and myomectomy or cesarean section. Diagnosis is made by clinical history, hysterosalpingography, or hysteroscopy. Therapy requires lysis of the adhesions by repeat curettage or preferably with hysteroscopic scissors or KTP (potassium-titanyl-phosphate) laser. Patency of the uterine cavity is maintained with an intrauterine device or balloon catheter and endometrial regeneration stimulated with oral estrogen therapy. The prognosis with signifi-

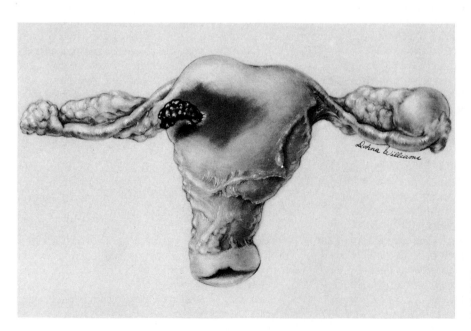

Figure 13–14. Result of uterine perforation. Specimen removed directly after perforation.

cant adhesions is poor. Only 40% of patients will become pregnant and approximately half of these will undergo spontaneous abortion or premature delivery. Consideration should be given to the risks of adhesion formation before the curettage of a pregnant or infected uterus, and possibly a less vigorous scraping performed in an attempt to minimize endometrial trauma.

Outpatient Curettage

Over the years, attempts have been made to lower the cost of D & C by making it an outpatient procedure. In 1957, Vermeeren, Chamberlain, and Te Linde presented a series of 10,000 minor gynecologic operations done on an outpatient basis on the gynecology service at the Johns Hopkins Hospital. The results were quite satisfactory. These women were usually operated on under general anesthesia and were discharged following recovery from anesthesia. D & C was the operation most frequently performed. The success and safety of such a program depends on careful selection of patients and a willingness to admit patients to the hospital for observation should complications occur. Today, D & C is often done satisfactorily on an outpatient basis or in an ambulatory surgery center. Reports by Sandmire and Austin and by Martin and Rust are among many that record favorable experience with this procedure.

Today, much endometrial sampling is performed as an office procedure. In many circumstances, a thorough office suction curettage can be accomplished with paracervical block and oral analgesic medication. Because none of the office sampling procedures may be quite as definitive as classical D & C under general anesthesia (eg an endometrial polyp may persist), it is essential to exercise keen clinical judgment with respect to whether the patient's presenting problem has been diagnosed fully—and if it has not completely resolved, then one must promptly initiate the indicated additional investigations and procedures.

Bibliography

Aksel S, Jones GS. Etiology and treatment of dysfunctional uterine bleeding. Obstet Gynecol 1974;44:1.

Anderson ABM, Haynes PJ, Guillebaud J., et al. Reduction of menstrual blood loss by prostaglandin synthesis inhibition. Lancet 1976;1:774.

Asherman J. Amenorrhea traumatica (atretica). J Obstet Gynaecol Br Emp 1948;55:23.

Barnett JM. Suction curettage on unanesthetized outpatients. Obstet Gynecol 1973;42:672.

Beller FK. Observations on the clotting of menstrual blood and clot formation. Am J Obstet Gynecol 1971;111:535.

Beyth Y, Yaffe H, Levii I, et al. Retrograde seeding of endometrium: a sequela of tubal flushing. Fertil Steril 1975;26:1094.

Chen SS, Lee L. Reappraisal of endocervical curettage in predicting cervical involvement by endometrial carcinoma. Obstet Gynecol 1986;31:50.

Chiazze L Jr, Brayer FT, Macisco JJ Jr, et al. The length and variability of the human menstrual cycle. JAMA 1968;203:377.

Cohen CJ, Gusberg SB, Koffier D. Histologic screening for endometrial cancer. Gynecol Oncol 1974;2:279.

Davies AJ, Anderson ABM, Turnbull AC. Reduction by naproxen of excessive menstrual bleeding in women using intrauterine devices. Obstet Gynecol 1981;57:74.

Denis R Jr, Barnett JM, Forbes SE. Diagnostic suction curettage. Obstet Gynecol 1973;42:301.

Fraser IS, Baird DT. Blood production and ovarian secretion rates of estradiol-17.3 and estrone in women with dysfunctional uterine bleeding. J Clin Endocrinol Metabol 1974;38:727.

Fraser IS, Pearse C, Shearman RP, et al. Efficacy of mefenamic acid in patients with a complaint of menorrhagia. Obstet Gynecol 1981;58:543.

Fraser IS, et al. Pituitary gonadotropins and ovarian function in adolescent dysfunctional uterine bleeding. J Clin Endocrinol Metabol 1973;37:407.

Fritsch N. Ein Fall von volligen Schwund der gebarmutter Hohle nach Auskratzung. Zentralbl Gumsrl 1894;18:1337.

Gregg RH. The praxiology of the office dilatation and curettage. Am J Obstet Gynecol 1981;140:179.

Grimes D. Estimating vaginal blood loss. J Reprod Med 1979;22:190.

Grimes D, Cates W Jr. Complications from legally-induced abortion: a review. Obstet Gynecol Surv 1979;34:177.

Guillebaud J, Barnett MD, Gordon YB. Plasma ferritin levels as an index of iron deficiency in women using intrauterine devices. Br J Obstet Gynaecol 1979;86:51.

Hallberg L, Hogdahl A, Nilsson L, et al. Menstrual blood loss and iron deficiency. Acta Med Scand 1966;180:639.

Hallberg L, Nilsson L. Constancy of individual menstrual blood loss. Acta Obstet Gynecol Scand 1964;43:352.

Hallberg L, Nilsson L. Determination of menstrual blood loss. Scand J Clin Lab Invest 1964;16:244.

Haynes PJ, Hodgson H, Anderson ABM, et al. Measurement of menstrual blood loss in patients complaining of menorrhagia. Br J Obstet Gynaecol 1977;84:763.

Healy DL, Hodgen GD. The endocrinology of human endometrium. Obstet Gynecol Surv 1983;38:509.

Helkamp BF, Denslow BL, Boufiglio TA, et al. Cervical conization: when is dilatation and curettage indicated? Am J Obstet Gynecol 1983;146:893.

Hofmeister FJ. Endometrial biopsy: another look. Am J Obstet Gynecol 1974;118:773.

Hofmeister FJ. Endometrial curettage. In: Symmonds CM, Zuspan FT, eds. Clinical and diagnostic procedures in obstetrics and gynecology. New York: Marcel Dekker, 1984.

Jensen JA, Jensen JG. Abragio mucosae uteri e aspiratione. Ugeskr Laeger 1968;130:2121.

Jensen JG. Vacuum curettage. Outpatient curettage without anesthesia: a report of 350 cases. Dan Med Bull 1970;17:199.

Josey WE. Routine intrauterine forceps exploration at curettage. Obstet Gynecol 1958;11:108.

Joshi SG. Progestin-regulated proteins of the human endometrium. Semin Reprod Endocrinol 1983;1:221.

Kelly HA. Curettage without anesthesia on the office table. Am J Obstet Gynecol 1925;9:78.

Klein SM, Garcia CR. Asherman's syndrome: a critique and current review. Fertil Steril 1973;24:722.

Lomano JM. Photocoagulation of the endometrium with the Nd:YAG laser for the treatment of menorrhagia: a report of ten cases. J Reprod Med 1986;31:149.

Lutz MH, Underwood PB Jr, Kreutner A, et al. Vacuum aspiration: an efficient outpatient screening technique for endometrial disease. South Med J 1977;70:393.

MacKenzie IZ, Bibby JG. Critical assessment of dilatation and curettage in 1029 women. Lancet 1978;2:566.

Manabe Y, Manabe A. Nelaton catheter for gradual and safe cervical dilatation: an ideal substitute for laminaria. Am J Obstet Gynecol 1981;140:465.

Markee JE. Menstruation in intraocular endometrial transplants in the rhesus monkey. Contr Embryol Carneg Justn 1940;28:219.

Martin PL, Rust JA. Surgical gynecology for the ambulatory patient. Clin Obstet Gynecol 1974;17:205.

McElin TW, Bird CC, Reeves BD, et al. Diagnostic dilatation and curettage. Obstet Gynecol 1969;33:807.

Mengert WF, Slate WG. Diagnostic dilatation and curettage as an outpatient procedure. Am J Obstet Gynecol 1960;79:727.

Narula RK. Endometrial histopathology in dysfunctional uterine bleeding. J Obstet Gynecol India 1967;17:614.

Novak E. Relation of hyperplasia of endometrium to so-called functional uterine hemorrhage. JAMA 1920;75:292.

Novak E. A suction curette apparatus and endometrial biopsy. JAMA 1935;104−1497.

Pacheco JC, Kempers RD. Etiology of postmenopausal bleeding. Obstet Gynecol 1968;32:40.

Reyniak JV. Dysfunctional uterine bleeding. J Reprod Med 1976;17:293.

Scandmire HF, Austin SD. Curettage as an office procedure. Am J Obstet Gynecol 1974;119:82.

Smith SK, Abel MH, Kelly RW, et al. A role for prostacyclin (PG12) in excessive menstrual bleeding. Lancet 1981;1:522.

Smith SK, Abel MH, Kelly RW, et al. Prostaglandin synthesis in the endometrium of women with ovular dysfunctional uterine bleeding. Br J Obstet Gynaecol 1981;88:434.

Southam AI, Richart RM. The prognosis for adolescents with menstrual abnormalities. Am J Obstet Gynecol 1966;94:637.

Speroff L, Glass RH, Kase NG. Clinical gynecologic endocrinology and infertility. 4th ed. Baltimore: Williams & Wilkins, 1989:276.

Stock RJ, Kanbour A. Pre-hysterectomy curettage: an evaluation. Obstet Gynecol 1975;45:537.

Swartz, DP, Jones GES. Progesterone in anovulatory uterine bleeding: clinical observations. Fertil Steril 1957;8:103.

Taylor PJ, Graham G. Is diagnostic curettage harmful in women with unexplained infertility? Br J Obstet Gynaecol 1982;89:296.

Teare AJ, Rippey JJ. Dilatation and curettage. S Afr Med J 1979;55:535.

Tseng L Gusberg SB, Gurpide E. Estradiol receptor and 17 B-dehydrogenase in normal and abnormal human endometrium. Ann NY Acad Sci 1977;286:190.

Vermeeren J, Chamberlain RR, Te Linde RU. Ten thousand minor gynecologic operations on an outpatient basis. Obstet Gynecol 1957;9:139.

Whitehead MI, Frazier D. The effects of estrogens and progestagens on the endometrium. Obstet Gynecol Clin North Am 1987;14:299.

Whitehead MI, King RJ, McQueen J, et al. Endometrial histology and biochemistry in climacteric women during estrogen and estrogen/progestogen therapy. J R Soc Med 1979;72:322.

Wilborn WH, Flowers CE Jr. Cellular mechanisms for endometrial conservation during menstrual bleeding. Semin Reprod Endocrinol 1984;2:307.

Word B. Current concepts of uterine curettage. Postgrad Med 1960;28:450.

Word B, Gravlee LC, Wideman GL. The fallacy of simple uterine curettage. Obstet Gynecol 1958;12:642.

Surgical Management of Abortion

14

DAVID A. GRIMES

Human reproduction is an inefficient enterprise. Compared with other biologic functions, such as digestion or locomotion, reproduction is characterized by false steps and frequent failures. Abortion is probably the most frequent outcome of human conception. Hormonal surveillance of early pregnancies indicates that more than half of all fertilized ova do not survive to 28 weeks' gestation (Little, 1988; Edmonds and coworkers, 1982). Moreover, of the minority of conceptions that do not terminate through spontaneous loss, approximately one in four ends in induced abortion in the United States (Centers for Disease Control, 1990). This winnowing by spontaneous and induced abortion increases the likelihood that children born are both healthy and wanted.

On a national scale, the scope of the challenge posed by spontaneous and induced abortion is broad. Several million spontaneous abortions occur annually, and approximately 1.6 million induced abortions occur annually (Centers for Disease Control, 1990). Thus, the surgical management of abortion remains a principal focus of gynecology. Induced abortion is the most frequently performed operation in gynecology in the United States.

This chapter provides an overview of the surgical management of abortion. It reviews the incidence, risk factors, and treatment of spontaneous abortion, illegal abortion, and legal abortion.

SPONTANEOUS ABORTION

Incidence

The true incidence of spontaneous abortion is uncertain because of the difficulty in recognizing early conceptions and losses. Estimates have indicated that 78% of conceptions fail to result in a live birth, and the pioneering histologic studies of Hertig suggested an embryonic mortality rate of 40% by the time of the expected menstrual period. However, as Shapiro, Levine, and Abramowicz put it, no method short of observing a cohort of women who undergo monthly pregnancy tests can provide a satisfactory assessment of early pregnancy losses. When Edmonds and associates followed this suggestion and monitored β-human chorionic gonadotropin (HCG) in the urine of a cohort of volunteers attempting to conceive, they found that 62% of conceptions were lost before 12 weeks' gestation. Most (92%) of these losses occurred subclinically, and the woman was unaware that she had been pregnant. The high incidence of spontaneous abortion of unsuspected pregnancies has been corroborated by others (Wilcox and coworkers, 1988); two thirds of such losses occurred before the pregnancy was clinically detected. These estimates did not include the unknown but presumably sizable proportion of fertilized ova lost before implantation.

Most studies of spontaneous abortion have addressed only pregnancies recognized by the woman. Overall, spontaneous abortion rates of 15% to 17% have been reported. These data support the clinical maxim that approximately one in six women who recognize they are pregnant will experience a spontaneous abortion.

Risk Factors

Several important risk factors for spontaneous abortion are known. The risk of spontaneous abortion increases with advancing maternal age, particularly for women over age 35 years. Likewise, the risk increases with advancing paternal age. Race also plays a role. At each stage of pregnancy, women of minority races have higher rates of spontaneous abortion than do white women. The racial discrepancy in rates is most marked at 12 to 19 weeks' gestation (Shapiro and coworkers, 1971).

Independent of the effect of age, the risk of spontaneous abortion increases with increasing gravidity. In addition, a history of one or more spontaneous abortions increases the risk of spontaneous abortion in subsequent pregnancies. This effect is seen at all gestational ages. The risk of spontaneous abortion increased linearly with increasing numbers of prior spontaneous abortions in one recent study (Risch and coworkers, 1988). On the other hand, the length of the interval between pregnancies appears to have little impact.

Both gestational age and the aging of sperm and egg appear to influence the likelihood of spontaneous abortion. In general, the probability of spontaneous abortion is inversely related to gestational age. Rates are presumably high in the first weeks of pregnancy, though not well quantified. Assuming a total fetal loss of 22%, Shapiro and associates estimated gestational age-specific rates of spontaneous abortion to be 8% at 4 to 7 weeks' gestation, 8% at 8 to 11 weeks; 5% at 12 to 19 weeks; and 2% at 20 or more weeks. Although spontaneous abortion occurs predominantly in the first 12 weeks of pregnancy, with the mean being 9 weeks (Wilcox and coworkers, 1988), many losses occur later in pregnancy. A study by Guerrero and Rojas has suggested that conceptions that do not occur near the time of the shift in basal-body temperature are more likely to be aborted than those that do.

Smoking also appears to increase the risk of spontaneous abortion. In one study (Kline and associates, 1977), the risk was nearly doubled, and in more recent studies (Risch and coworkers, 1988; Hemminki and coworkers, 1983), the increase in risk was slight. Because smoking is not known to be teratogenic, its effect on rates of spontaneous abortion may be mediated through an increased rate of expulsion of normal conceptuses.

Fever in early pregnancy may lead to spontaneous abortion. In one study, rates of spontaneous abortion of euploid conceptuses were increased twofold to threefold if fever had preceded the abortion (Kline and associates, 1985). External stress also may increase the likelihood of such abortions. Heavy occupational lifting and physical effort have been associated with higher rates of spontaneous abortion after controlling for the effect of other factors (Goulet and Theriault, 1987). Infection with *Chlamydia trachomatis,* mycoplasmas, or other organisms does not appear to play a role in the etiology of spontaneous abortion (Munday and colleagues, 1984).

No seasonality of spontaneous abortion rates has been identified. The number of spontaneous abortions, however, fluctuates significantly. The incidence of spontaneous abortion peaks in the spring and again in the late fall; this pattern reflects the marked seasonal variation in numbers of conceptions. However, the proportion of conceptions that end in spontaneous abortion varies little from month to month (Warren and coworkers, 1980).

The Role of Spontaneous Abortion

Spontaneous abortion serves primarily as a quality control mechanism. Only a minority of each cohort of conceptuses survives pregnancy. Human reproduction apparently tolerates a broad diversity of conceptions; much more stringent and exacting criteria determine the probability of surviving to viability.

An extensive literature supports this teleologic role for spontaneous abortion as a screening device for abnormal pregnancies (Stein and coworkers, 1975). The frequency of chromosomal abnormalities in aborted conceptus is high, ranging from 30% to 61% in surveys of different populations (Hassold and coworkers, 1980); in decreasing order of frequency, the most common abnormalities are trisomy, sex chromosome monosomy, and triploidy. The earlier the gestational age at abortion, the higher the frequency of chromosomal anomaly. Almost all anomalies, including some (such as cleft lip) that would not seem to handicap survival, increase the likelihood of spontaneous abortion.

Multiple gestations, common in other species, are atypical in humans and appear to be at high risk of fetal death. For example, in a study by Dessaive and associates of women with threatened abortions, four women with twins identified by ultrasonography at 8 weeks' gestation were followed to delivery; three delivered normal singletons, and only one delivered twins. Thus, three twins were lost without their fellow passengers in the uterus being adversely affected. Most fetuses with abnormalities are in some way identified and rejected by the body. The incidence of chromosomal or other abnormalities in fetuses that survive this selection process is low.

Prevention of Spontaneous Abortion

Although an abnormal karyotype is the most important risk factor for spontaneous abortion, a variety of other risk factors have been proposed. These include endocrine defects, infections, environmental toxins, and immunologic factors. In addition, several surgically correctable conditions have been linked with spontaneous abortion. Uterine synechiae—that is, intrauterine adhesions—have been suggested as a cause of repeated spontaneous abortion. If synechiae are identified in this clinical setting, lysis of adhesions by hysteroscopy may be advisable.

Abnormalities of müllerian fusion also have been implicated as a cause of spontaneous abortion. Although the incidence of early abortion is probably not increased, the incidence of abortion at or after 13 weeks' gestation may be in the range of 20% to 25% (Simpson, 1981). Septate and bicornuate uteri seem to have more adverse effects than uterus bicornis bicollis. Women with müllerian anomalies who experience spontaneous abortions at or after 13 weeks' gestation may be candidates for reconstructive operations, which are described elsewhere in this text (see Ch. 20).

Leiomyomas, a common condition, also have been attributed as a cause of spontaneous abortion. The evidence supporting this association, however, is limited. Submucous leiomyomas would be expected to have more effect than intramural or subserosal tumors. Women with leiomyomas who experience abortions at or after 13 weeks' gestation may be candidates for myomectomy (see Ch. 26). However, current data suggest that myomectomy, if performed only because of infertility, is of minimal benefit; the effect of myomectomy on rates of spontaneous abortion has not been adequately evaluated.

The efficacy of strategies designed to reduce the risk of spontaneous abortion has not been well established. Indeed, one small cohort study of women with a history of three or more consecutive spontaneous abortions in early pregnancy found no treatment to be as effective as conventional treatments in achieving subsequent live births (Vlaanderen and Treffers, 1987).

Management

Threatened Abortion

Threatened abortion, characterized by bleeding of intrauterine origin without cervical dilation or expulsion of tissue, has traditionally been managed by watchful waiting. The likelihood of spontaneous abortion under these circumstances appears to be about 50% (Sande and colleagues, 1980). If fetal outcome could be reliably predicted in such situations, then couples might be spared substantial emotional anguish.

Fetal well-being early in pregnancy is usually determined through monitoring maternal blood or urine levels of hormones produced by the fetoplacental unit. These hormones include HCG, human placental lactogen, estriol, estradiol, and progesterone. Like hormone assays performed to determine fetal well-being late in pregnancy, such tests have two disadvantages: (1) test results are not immediately available and (2) the validity of the tests varies widely. For example, for women with threatened abortion, the predictive value of an abnormally low plasma estradiol (percentage of women with an abnormal result who spontaneously abort) ranges from 53% (Eriksen and Philipsen, 1980) to 95% (Dessaive and coworkers, 1982). Other investigators have suggested that pregnancy associated plasma protein-A is useful in predicting abortion, although this approach is experimental (Westergaard and coworkers, 1985).

Ultrasonography has been used as a prognostic tool by a number of investigators hoping to avoid the disadvantages of hormone assays. Representative studies are listed in Table 14-1, with the validity of prediction based on ultrasonography calculated for each report. Sensitivity is the ability of ultrasonography to identify correctly those women who will spontaneously abort; specificity is the ability to identify correctly those who will not. A measure of direct interest to the clinician is the predictive value of an abnormal scan; that is, what percentage of women with an abnormal scan will, indeed, abort. To be clinically useful in predicting spontaneous abortion, a test must have very high sensitivity and predictive value of an abnormal scan. Specificity and predictive value of a normal scan are of little consequence. If ultrasonography incorrectly identifies a

TABLE 14–1
Validity of Ultrasonography in Predicting Spontaneous Abortion Among Women with Threatened Abortion

AUTHOR	ULTRASONOGRAPHIC CRITERIA	SENSITIVITY (%)	SPECIFICITY (%)	PREDICTIVE VALUE OF ABNORMAL SCAN (%)
Duff, 1975	Morphology and fetal heart motion	92	73	86
Anderson, 1980	Fetal heart motion	97	99	98
Eriksen and Philipsen, 1980	Fetal heart motion	85	95	91
Hertz, Mantoni, and Svenstrup, 1980	Fetal heart motion	69	83	74
Sande et al, 1980	Fetal heart motion	88	84	74
Stoppelli et al, 1981	Not specified	88	93	94
Dessaive, Hertogh, and Thomas, 1982	Morphology and fetal heart motion	70	89	91
Sakamoto and Okai, 1982	Morphology	88	96	94
	Fetal heart motion	97	100	100

woman as destined to have a spontaneous abortion, curettage performed on the basis of this error would abort a viable pregnancy. On the other hand, if ultrasonography incorrectly predicts a normal pregnancy outcome, no intervention ensues and no adverse effect results from the diagnostic error.

Two sonographic criteria have been shown in one study to have high specificity: (1) a gestation sac ≥ 25-mm mean diameter without an embryo and (2) distorted sac shape (Nyberg, Laing, and Filly, 1986). On the other hand, the sensitivity of these criteria was very low. Repeating the ultrasonography exam improves the diagnostic accuracy of this procedure. As shown in Table 14-1, the sensitivity of ultrasonography ranges from 69% to 97%, depending on the study population and diagnostic criteria used. The predictive value of an abnormal scan ranges from 74% to 100%. When morphologic criteria and evidence of fetal heart motion have been compared, fetal heart motion has been more accurate in predicting spontaneous abortion (Sakamoto and Okai, 1982).

The accuracy of fetal heartbeat determination increases with gestational age. Before 8 menstrual weeks' gestation, fetal heart motion cannot always been seen, and errors in assessing age can further confound interpretation of results. A woman thought to be 10 weeks' pregnant and with no visible fetal heart activity could really be 6 weeks' pregnant with normal, but imperceptible, cardiac activity. If fetal heart activity is absent at or after 8 weeks' gestation, and if the estimated gestational age is accurate, then ultrasonography may have enough predictive value to guide intervention, if so desired. Several reports concur that once fetal cardiac activity is documented by ultrasonography in the first 12 weeks of pregnancy, the likelihood of spontaneous abortion is low. Rates of 2% have been reported from Canada (Wilson and associates, 1986) and England (MacKenzie, Holmes, and Newton, 1988). Increasing use of vaginal ultrasound can be expected to improve diagnostic validity, especially at early gestational ages.

Surgical Intervention

For women with inevitable abortion (characterized by progressive cervical dilatation without expulsion of products of conception) and for those with threatened abortion in whom the pregnancy has been judged nonviable, evacuation of the uterus is appropriate management. Unless concurrent problems such as uterine infection or anemia exist, evacuation of the uterus can be handled like an elective legal abortion (described later).

Two decisions must be made: (1) where the curettage is to occur and (2) by what technique. The choice between outpatient curettage in the physician's office or curettage in an emergency room may depend on the time of day and available equipment. For uncomplicated cases, hospitalization and curettage in an operating room add to the costs, inconvenience, and emotional burden occasioned by spontaneous abortion yet offer no medical benefits over outpatient curettage (Farrell, Stonington, and Ridgeway, 1982). The choice of evacuation technique depends on the state of the cervix, gestational age, and availability of equipment. For curettage evacuations, suction curettage is preferable to sharp curettage, yet suction equipment may not be available. Suction curettage is both faster and safer than sharp curettage and may cause less damage to the basal layer of the endometrium. A flexible Karman cannula with syringe as a source of suction is portable, inexpensive, and convenient for outpatient use.

Distinguishing between an incomplete abortion, in which some but not all the products of conception have been expelled, and complete abortion is frequently difficult. The woman's description of tissue may not be helpful, and not all women are aware that they should save expelled tissue for the physician's inspection. Likewise, the aperture of the cervix, size of the uterus, and presence or absence of bleeding may not indicate whether the abortion is complete or incomplete. This distinction is important because incomplete abortion requires evacuation of the uterus; curettage after a complete abortion is discretionary. In the absence of evidence that the abortion is complete, many physicians perform a curettage, which can be both diagnostic and therapeutic. Most suction evacuations will yield products of conception. However, ultrasonography may provide information about the completeness of abortion. In one small series (Jeong and associates, 1981), a central uterine-cavity echo was associated with absence of products of conception on curettage. This technique appears to merit further investigation.

Regardless of the completeness of abortion, the physician should know the woman's rhesus factor (Rh) type. Spontaneous abortion is a potentially sensitizing event for Rh-negative women at risk. Rates of use of Rh immunoglobulin (RhIG) after spontaneous abortion are significantly lower than after induced abortion. A 50-mcg dose should be given to RhIG candidates who are at approximately 12 weeks' gestation or before, and a 300-mcg dose should be administered to those who abort later in pregnancy.

The profound grief that frequently accompanies spontaneous abortion has received little notice. Women and, to a lesser extent, men experience the usual stages of grief. Guilt may be the most difficult stage to resolve without help, and counseling plays an important role (Leppert and Pahlka, 1984).

Complications of Spontaneous Abortion

Attentive gynecologic care has reduced the risk of complications from spontaneous abortions in recent years. Nevertheless, women continue to die from such complications. From 1972 to 1980, 101 women died in the United States from spontaneous abortions unrelated to intrauterine contraceptive device (IUD) use. By 1980, the risk of death was 1.7 deaths for every million live births. Leading causes of death unrelated to IUD use were infection (48%), hemorrhage (21%), and embolism (11%). The risk of death increased with gestational age; women who were older, unmarried, and of minority races also were at increased risk of death (Berman and coworkers, 1985).

FETAL DEATH IN UTERO

Definitions

Fetal death in utero (FDIU) is the cessation of fetal life before termination of pregnancy. This diagnosis is further categorized by the gestational age at fetal death and length of retention of the dead fetus. Death before the 20th week of gestation is termed "spontaneous abortion" and death thereafter, "antepartum fetal death." If the dead fetus is retained for 8 or more weeks (or a "prolonged period"), then the term "missed abortion" is used.

From both a clinical and a nosologic point of view, the proliferation of terms related to FDIU is both unnecessary and confusing. These diagnostic categories all should be viewed as variations of a single obstetric entity.

Incidence

FDIU is uncommon. Approximately 200,000 women with FDIU were hospitalized in the United States from 1972 to 1978 (Dorfman and coworkers, 1983). During this 7-year interval, approximately 22.5 million live births occurred in the United States. Thus, the incidence of FDIU requiring hospitalization is estimated to be 9 cases per 1000 live births. By comparison, approximately one case of FDIU and 35 legal abortions occur for every 100 live births in the United States.

Management

Recent data on the natural history of FDIU are scarce. Past data have suggested that most dead fetuses are expelled spontaneously within 3 weeks of death (Dorfman and coworkers, 1983). However, the gestational age at the time of death influences the probability of expulsion within a given interval: the more remote from term, the longer the time required (Foley, 1981). Only 29% of women with fetal deaths before 34 weeks' gestation delivered within 2 weeks after death compared with 75% of women with fetal deaths occurring later in pregnancy.

Once fetal death is confirmed, the next—and perhaps most important—step is to counsel the parents (Fig. 14-1). Helping the couple to grieve appropriately can minimize psychologic sequelae from this often devastating loss. After these two initial steps, subsequent clinical management is largely discretionary. The risk of coagulation defects within 5 weeks of fetal death is minimal, as is the risk of infection, provided the membranes are intact. However, the emotional burden of carrying a dead fetus, often for weeks, can compound the misery experienced by the parents. Thus, although either watchful waiting or uterine evacuation can be chosen, most couples opt for intervention. Because there is no compelling medical indication for one course over the other, this decision generally should be left to the parents after they have been fully informed about the alternatives.

If uterine evacuation is elected, then the physician should confirm that the woman's coagulation system is intact before intervening. Two approaches to evacuation exist: (1) surgery or (2) labor induction. The choice between surgery and labor induction should reflect the skill and experience of the physician, the size of the fetus and uterus, the availability of equipment and drugs, and the preference of the woman (Hodgson and Ditmanson, 1980). If dilatation and evacuation (D & E) is planned, then accurate determination of the size of the fetus by ultrasonography is helpful.

Suction curettage is a safe and easy way to evacuate pregnancies at or before 14 weeks' gestation; thereafter, D & E can be used by those experienced in this technique. Occasionally, hysterectomy will be appropriate treatment in this setting if there is preexisting pathology such as carcinoma in situ of the cervix and the woman desires sterilization. Hysterotomy has unacceptably high morbidity, mortality, and cost; this method should not be used.

If the pregnancy is about 15 or more weeks' gestation and if the physician chooses not to perform a D & E procedure, then labor induction can be performed by administering vaginal prostaglandin E_2 suppositories, which are both effective and safe. Their use requires little surgical skill (unlike D & E), and the suppositories simultaneously stimulate contractions and promote cervical ripening. The principal disadvantages of the sup-

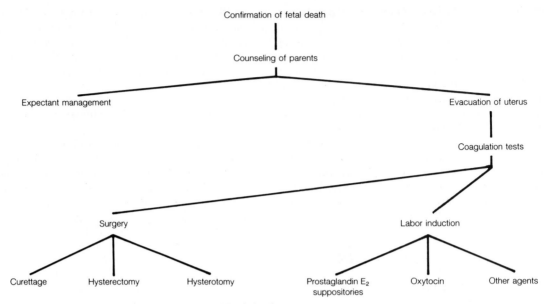

Figure 14–1. Options for management of fetal death in utero.

positories are the high incidence of vomiting and diarrhea (60% and 40%, respectively) and fever from the medication itself (50%). Hence, women should be premedicated with antiemetic and antidiarrheal drugs before administration of the suppositories; antipyretics and, occasionally, a cooling blanket may be required if the woman's temperature exceeds 39.4°C. An alternative to prostaglandin E_2 suppositories is 15-methyl prostaglandin $F_{2\alpha}$ (250 mcg), which is injected intramuscularly every 3 to 4 hours. This route of administration may be preferable when bleeding or continued leakage of amniotic fluid may dilute or wash away vaginal prostaglandin.

The traditional means of labor induction for cases of FDIU has been administration of oxytocin intravenously (IV). This treatment is familiar to all gynecologists, and the medication is inexpensive. However, oxytocin lacks the efficacy of prostaglandins because the uterus is relatively insensitive to oxytocin early in pregnancy, and the cervix is frequently unfavorable for induction of labor.

Intra-amniotic abortifacients should not be used in this setting. Instillation of hypertonic saline or hyperosmolar urea may be hazardous because of unpredictable and potentially rapid uptake into the woman's circulation due to the altered permeability of the membranes after fetal death.

A sharp-curette check of the uterine cavity to confirm complete evacuation is probably advisable after any of these evacuation techniques. As with all pregnancy terminations, RhIG candidates should be identified and given an appropriate dose of RhIG.

Complications of Fetal Death in Utero

FDIU carries risks of both morbidity and mortality for the woman. The risks of coagulation disorders and infection have received the most attention, yet recent data on their incidence are lacking. The risk of maternal death associated with FDIU is small; from 1972 to 1978, nine such deaths occurred among approximately 200,000 cases nationwide, for a death-to-case rate of 4.5 deaths per 100,000 cases (Dorfman and coworkers, 1983).

The risk of death from FDIU increases with maternal age. The risk for women aged 35 years and older was 3.6 times that for women aged 15 to 24 years. The most frequent causes of maternal death from FDIU were uterine perforation and coagulopathy. Currently, the comparative safety of available techniques for evacuating the uterus is unknown.

CERVICAL INCOMPETENCE

Incidence

Cervical incompetence is a nebulous term used to explain spontaneous abortions thought to be due to cervical factors. The term "cervical incompetence" itself is troublesome, because a woman given this diagnosis may infer that she is in some way inadequate or unworthy as a mother. Hence, the term should be used cautiously (if at all) with patients.

There is little agreement about the definition of cervical incompetence or the appropriate diagnostic criteria. Many reported cases of cervical incompetence are inconsistent with the classic picture of repetitive, acute, painless abortion in the midportion of pregnancy without associated bleeding or uterine contractions. Some physicians diagnose cervical incompetence on the basis of asymptomatic cervical dilatation observed in midpregnancy, whereas others rely on a variety of tests of unknown validity performed on nonpregnant women, for example, passage of a No. 8 (8 mm) Hegar dilator, traction on an intrauterine Foley catheter, or hysterography. In recent years, ultrasonography has been used to diagnose cervical incompetence (Westgren and Sjoberg, 1986; Michaels and associates, 1986). This technique appears to have poor validity.

Moreover, the correlation between anatomic measurements and function of the cervix in pregnancy is unknown and, currently, no valid diagnostic test of cervix incompetence exists. A history of unexplained spontaneous abortion in the middle of pregnancy may be the most useful diagnostic criterion, yet its sensitivity and specificity remain unknown. This diagnostic imprecision is reflected in reported incidence rates of cervical incompetence. Rates range from 0.05 to 1 per 100 pregnancies (Cousins, 1980). Differences in diagnosis, rather than differences in populations of women, probably account for most of this variation.

Risk Factors

The etiology of cervical incompetence is unknown but may be multifactorial. Early theories about this problem focused on cervical trauma, such as conization, laceration, or excessive mechanical dilatation. Data are lacking, however, to confirm or refute these hypothetical risk factors. The occurrence of cervical incompetence in primigravidas suggests alternative etiologies. These may include associated uterine anomalies, prenatal exposure to diethylstilbestrol, or abnormal histology of the cervix (Cousins, 1980; Hughey and McElin, 1982). In addition, cervical incompetence may be inherited.

Cervical incompetence may be but one manifestation of a spectrum of asynchronism between the uterine corpus and cervix. In normal pregnancy and delivery, biochemical and biophysical changes in the cervix in late pregnancy allow cervical dilatation and effacement to occur synchronously with labor contractions. At one extreme of asynchronism, the corpus contracts, yet cervical dilatation and effacement do not occur; this may account for the development of cervicovaginal fistulas during instillation abortions with prostaglandin $F_{2\alpha}$. At the other extreme, progressive dilatation and effacement occur prematurely and in the absence of perceptible contractions (cervical incompetence). The under-

lying pathophysiology for many cases of cervical incompetence may be biochemical; that tying a noose around the cervix is the best available treatment suggests how limited current understanding of the problem is.

Management

Three serious problems in published studies prohibit conclusions about the treatment of choice for cervical incompetence. First, without a precise and reproducible definition of cervical incompetence, comparison of success rates in published reports is impossible.

Second, some of the benefit attributed to cerclage operations may not be due to the operation itself but rather to a phenomenon termed "regression to the mean" (Cole, 1982). A variable (eg, pregnancy outcome) that is extreme or unusual when first measured (eg, fetal expulsion at 20 weeks' gestation) will tend to be nearer the mean of the population distribution at a subsequent observation (eg, another pregnancy). Although there are methods for estimating the effect of this phenomenon in studies without comparison groups, only one study of cerclage has even considered this problem (Cole, 1982).

Third, new operations frequently are adopted into clinical practice without appropriate evidence of their efficacy. Randomized clinical trials comparing two operations are rarely done when a new operation is introduced; once the operation is accepted in clinical practice, a randomized trial is frequently judged unethical. Several small and one large randomized clinical trials of cervical cerclage have been reported (MRC/RCOG Working Party, 1988). In the large trial, among 905 pregnant women with a history of early delivery or cervical surgery, the operation was found to have marginal usefulness. Important beneficial effect was found in one in every 20 to 25 cases in the trial. Because the smaller trials did not demonstrate benefits from cerclage, the role of this operation remains questionable.

A variety of approaches have been used to treat cervical incompetence. Among the more innocuous, bed rest has been suggested as primary therapy as well as adjunctive therapy after cerclage. This appears to be a reasonable approach in terms of hydraulics, although data concerning efficacy are lacking.

A Smith-Hodge pessary can be used to displace the cervix posteriorly; this technique was first described by Vitsky in 1961. Although this approach has received little attention in the United States, it does have the appeal of exerting a mechanical effect without requiring an operation. Although electrocauterization of the cervix between pregnancies has been used to treat cervical incompetence in a small number of patients, the advantages of this treatment are so few that it is not recommended.

Surgery is the principal form of therapy for cervical incompetence in the United States. Two strategies have been used: (1) primary repair of an anatomical defect and (2) reinforcement of the cervix with a circumferential suture. The repair approach, the Lash procedure, is appropriate only for nonpregnant women who have a demonstrable anatomical defect of the cervix. Moreover, the suggestion of diminished fertility after this operation is worrisome. Hence, the Lash procedure currently is used infrequently.

Several types of cerclage procedures are currently used; the McDonald and Shirodkar are the most common. Contraindications to cerclage include rupture of membranes, uterine bleeding, uterine contractions, chorioamnionitis, cervical dilatation >4 cm, polyhydramnios, or known fetal anomaly.

The McDonald procedure places a reinforcing pursestring suture around the proximal cervix. Unlike the Shirodkar procedure, however, the McDonald suture is not buried entirely (Fig. 14-2). Instead, several deep penetrations into the cervical stroma are made with a nonabsorbable suture, such as Mersilene. The advantages of this approach compared with the Shirodkar procedure are simplicity, ease of removal, and usefulness when the cervix is effaced or when fetal membranes are bulging. A notable disadvantage is the vaginal discharge associated with the exposed suture material. Because the McDonald and Shirodkar procedures have been reported to have similar efficacy, the simplicity and versatility of the McDonald operation make it preferable for most patients in need of cerclage.

The Shirodkar operation places a reinforcing band around the cervix beneath the mucosa at the level of the internal os (Figs. 14-3 and 14-4). Spinal or epidural anesthesia is recommended; Trendelenburg's position and adequate retraction facilitate placement of the suture. The original operation used aneurysm needles to place a band of fascia lata around the cervix; then the knot was tied anteriorly. In recent years, many physicians have used a wide (eg, 5 mm) Mersilene band swaged onto large atraumatic needles, with the knot tied posteriorly to avoid erosion into the bladder. The

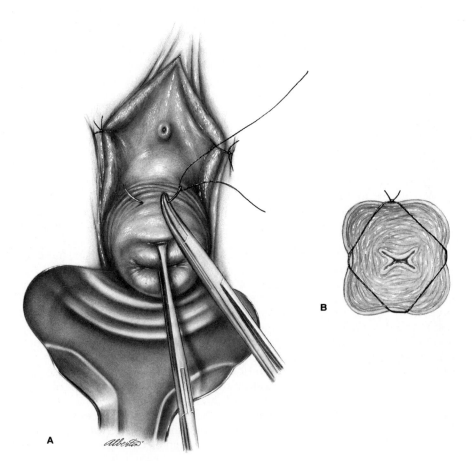

Figure 14–2. McDonald cerclage operation. *A,* Four bites are made at the junction of vaginal mucosa and cervix. *B,* A cross section of the cervix with the pursestring suture in place.

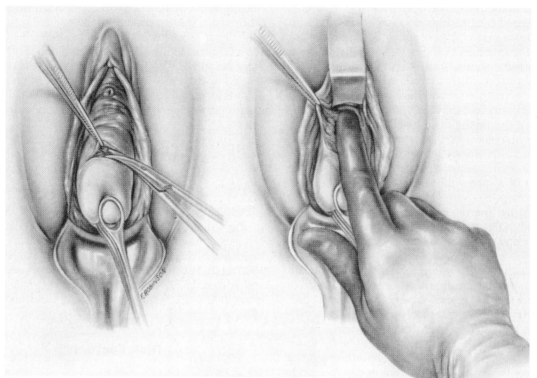

Figure 14–3. Shirodkar cerclage operation. *Left,* A transverse incision is made through the anterior vaginal mucosa at its junction with the cervix. *Right,* The bladder is pushed cephalad to enable high placement of the suture.

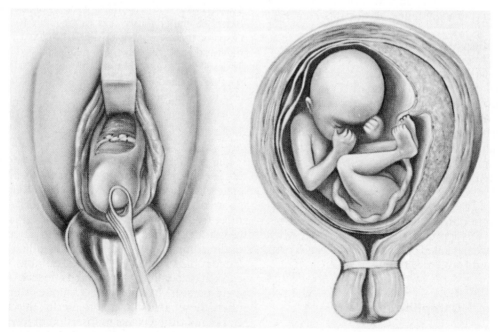

Figure 14–4. Shirodkar cerclage operation. *Left,* The encircling suture is tied to secure the cervix with an opening of 3 mm to 5 mm. The suture is anchored anteriorly with fine silk. *Right,* Correct placement of the suture.

cervical canal should remain open 3 mm to 5 mm. After the band is tied, the band and knot can be secured with several interrupted sutures of silk or other permanent material; the incisions in the mucosa are then closed with absorbable suture, thus burying the band.

Opinions are divided as to whether the cerclage procedure is best performed during or between pregnancies. Most studies (Cousins, 1980; McDonald, 1980) suggest that the timing of cerclage during pregnancy influences outcome. Cerclage at around 14 weeks' gestation appears preferable. If substantial dilatation or bulging of fetal membranes has occurred, then the likelihood of a successful cerclage is lessened. However, an attempt can be made to replace the protruding forewaters by means of a sterile Foley catheter (McDonald, 1980). Thereafter, the suture is placed and tied down, and the Foley balloon is deflated and withdrawn.

Postoperative care after cerclage for pregnant women has not been uniform. Although most authors advise bed rest for several days, and some advocate prophylactic antibiotics, tocolytic drugs, or progesterone, the usefulness of these measures has not been established. The cerclage suture can be removed at 38 weeks' gestation or when fetal pulmonary maturity has been confirmed; it should be removed immediately if membranes rupture or labor starts. Although some physicians leave a well-placed Shirodkar suture in place and deliver infants by cesarean section, the morbidity, mortality, expense, pain, and inconvenience of cesarean delivery strongly argue against this course of action.

Intraabdominal cerclage may be appropriate in rare instances. Indications include traumatic cervical laceration, congenital shortening of the cervix, previous failed vaginal cerclage, and advanced cervical effacement. This procedure places a band around the cervix at the level of the internal os in an avascular space between the branches of the uterine artery. Compared with the vaginal cerclage operations, this procedure has several important disadvantages: two abdominal operations are needed (one to place the suture, one for cesarean delivery); the surgery is performed in a highly vascular area adjacent to the ureters; and the complication rate is higher than with vaginal cerclage (Cousins, 1980). Hence, this approach should be used only when vaginal cerclage has failed or is not feasible (Novy, 1982; Wallenberg and Lotgering, 1987).

Complications

Complications of cerclage range from annoying to fatal. A partial inventory of reported complications includes hemorrhage; rupture of membranes, infection (including chorioamnionitis, abscess, and death); cervical dystocia; uterine rupture; vesicovaginal fistula; and fetal death (Charles and Edwards, 1981; McDonald, 1980; Cousins, 1980). Although the incidence of most of these complications is unknown, one report (Charles and Edwards, 1981) documented rates of chorioamnionitis ranging from 15 to 39 per 100 patients, depending on gestational age at the time of operation.

ILLEGAL ABORTION

Incidence

Despite the widespread availability of legal abortion in the United States, small numbers of illegal procedures continue to be performed. Estimates of the incidence of illegal abortion in the United States before 1970 ranged from 200,000 to 1.2 million per year (Cates and Rochat, 1976); estimates for the late 1970s ranged from 5000 to 23,000 per year (Binkin, Gold, and Cates, 1982).

Risk Factors

Little is known about characteristics of women who obtain illegal abortions. Some inferences can be drawn, however, from the characteristics of 17 women who died from illegal abortion in the United States from 1975 to 1979 (Binkin and coworkers, 1982). These women were older, of higher parity, and more likely to be black or Hispanic than women who died from legal abortion during these years. Slightly more than half lived in the South. Thus, older black or Hispanic multiparas who live in the southern United States are more likely to die from illegal abortion than are other women.

Techniques

Although a wide variety of illegal-abortion methods are used around the world, most methods in the United States can be categorized into two groups: (1) oral abortifacients and (2) intrauterine instrumentation. The most frequently used method reported in surveys in New York City in the 1960s (Polgar and Fried, 1976) was orally administered substances, including turpentine, laundry bleach, and large doses of quinine. The misconception that quinine is a safe and effective oral abortifacient persists. Intrauterine techniques were used less often; these ranged from intrauterine injection of soap or phenol disinfectants to insertion of foreign objects. As reported by the women surveyed, intrauterine techniques successfully aborted pregnancy much more often than did oral substances.

Complications of Illegal Abortion

Although intrauterine techniques have greater efficacy than oral abortifacients, the intrauterine techniques also have a higher risk of complications. For example, in a 1962 study in Chile (Liskin, 1980) 42% of women who had catheter-induced abortions were hospitalized for treatment of complications compared with 35% of those who used oral abortifacients. Similarly, transcervical administration of toxic substances carries a high risk of serious complications (Burnhill, 1985). Other important variables influencing the likelihood of morbidity include the skill of the provider, gestational age, and availability of gynecologic care. The most frequently reported complication of illegal abortion is retained products of conception, although the incidence of this and other complications is unknown.

The number of deaths from illegal abortion in the United States declined dramatically during the 1970s. For example, the rate (ie, illegal-abortion deaths per million women of reproductive age) decreased from 0.46 from 1972 to 1974 to 0.07 from 1975 to 1979, a reduction of 85% (Table 14-2). During the 1975 to 1979 interval, women in both extremes of the reproductive age span had higher death rates from illegal abortion than women of intermediate ages. However, the racial discrepancy in death rate is more striking: the mortality rate for black and Hispanic women is >10 times greater than that for white women.

As with morbidity, the likelihood of mortality is strongly related to the abortion technique. Of the 17 illegal-abortion deaths from 1975 to 1979, only one followed ingestion of an abortifacient (pennyroyal oil). The other deaths were related to intrauterine techniques, ranging from injection of cleaning solutions to insertion of foreign bodies (eg, catheters, cotton swabs, thermometers, and coat hangers). Sepsis (10 cases) and air embolism (3 cases) accounted for most of these deaths (Binkin and coworkers, 1982).

Management

Improved management of complications of illegal abortion, in addition to the decrease in such complications, has played a major role in preventing death and permanent disability. Treatment for ingestion of toxic substances is primarily medical and is not dealt with in this chapter. Incomplete abortion requires curettage.

Septic Abortion

The vast majority of women with septic abortion respond rapidly to uterine evacuation plus broad-spectrum antibiotics. Blood should not be given for the sole purpose of combating infection. Before beginning treatment, intrauterine and blood cultures should be obtained. An upright x-ray of the abdomen may identify a residual foreign body, gas bubbles in the uterus, or free air under the diaphragm; management is altered by these findings.

Antibiotics should be started IV in the emergency room. Coverage should include gram-positive, gram-negative, and anaerobic bacteria. The optimal antibiotic regimen has not been established. If the woman's condition is stable, then she can be taken directly from the emergency room to the operating room for curettage. Peak serum levels of antibiotics will be present within an hour of their administration. Further delay of uterine evacuation is unwarranted and may compromise recovery. Prompt elimination of the necrotic, infected tissue is critical. Tissue obtained during curettage should be transported quickly for microbiologic cultures. The yield of organisms, especially anaerobes, is often higher from a tissue specimen than from a swab inserted into the uterus.

Subsequent management is governed by the response of the woman and by microbiologic findings. All women with septic abortions should be closely observed after surgery, with special attention to vital signs and urine output, to detect incipient shock. Prompt aggressive therapy (see Ch. 24) is essential if septic shock develops.

Postabortal sepsis from *Clostridium perfringens* is very rare today. When this infection occurs, however, it can be catastrophic. In the absence of hemolysis, *C. perfringens* bacteremia can be managed by curettage and antibiotics. In the presence of hemolysis, hysterec-

TABLE 14–2
Annual Death Rate from Illegal Abortion by Age and Race, United States, 1972–1974 and 1975–1979

CHARACTERISTIC	RATE*	
	1972–1974	*1975–1979*
Age (yr)		
15–19	0.36	0.08
20–29	0.79	0.05
30–44	0.24	0.08
Race		
White	0.11	0.02
Hispanic	1.02	0.22
Black	2.36	0.31
Total	0.46	0.07

*Number of deaths per million women aged 15–44.
(Binkin N, Gold J, and Cates W Jr. Illegal-abortion deaths in the United States: why are they still occurring? Fam Plann Perspect 1982; 14:163. Reprinted with permission.)

tomy and more aggressive medical therapy are indicated (Green and Brenner, 1978).

LEGAL ABORTION

Incidence

Legal abortion is one of the most frequently performed operations in the United States. About 1.4 million abortions were reported to the Centers for Disease Control for 1987, and this figure is 20% less than the total number performed (Centers for Disease Control, 1990). In 1987, 356 legal abortions were reported for every 1000 live births (abortion ratio), and 24 legal abortions per 1000 women aged 15 to 44 years (abortion rate). Stated alternatively, >2% of all women of reproductive age have induced abortions each year.

Demographic Characteristics

Women who have induced abortions in the United States tend to be young, white, single, and of low parity. In 1987, 26% were teenagers; 33%, aged 20–24 years; and the remainder, 25 years and older. Most were white (66%) and unmarried (73%). Most (57%) had not had a previous birth.

Legal abortion in the United States is performed principally by curettage early in pregnancy. In 1987, 97% of all abortions were done by curettage, 1% by intrauterine instillation, and <1% by hysterotomy or hysterectomy. Approximately half (50%) of all abortions were performed at ≤8 weeks' gestation, 89% at ≤12 weeks' gestation, and about 1% at ≥21 weeks' gestation.

Techniques

All methods of abortion can be divided into two broad categories: (1) surgical evacuation and (2) labor induction. Surgical evacuation includes suction curettage (vacuum aspiration); sharp curettage; D & E (defined as transcervical evacuation at or after 13 menstrual weeks' gestation); hysterotomy; and hysterectomy. Labor induction includes administration of abortifacients either systemically (vaginal or intramuscular prostaglandins) or directly into the uterus (eg, hypertonic saline or hyperosmolar urea). In addition, several adjuncts, such as osmotic dilators or oxytocin, have an important role in abortion practice. This section reviews the principal methods of abortion in current use; detailed descriptions of these techniques have been published elsewhere (Stubblefield, 1986; Hern, 1984).

Surgical Evacuation

Suction curettage is by far the most important method of abortion in the United States; it is the most frequently used method—and the safest. The preoperative evaluation for suction curettage should include counseling, informed consent, a brief history, and a limited physical examination. The history-taking should focus only on data of relevance to the procedure, such as gynecologic problems (eg, leiomyomas) or medical problems (eg, cardiac valvular disease, asthma, or drug sensitivities) that might influence the conduct of the operation. Physical examination should include the heart, lungs, abdomen, and pelvis. Although ultrasonography is not warranted on a routine basis, it is useful if the size, shape, or position of the uterus is unclear.

Few laboratory tests are required. Determination of the hematocrit (or hemoglobin) and Rh type, in addition to a urinalysis, are appropriate. Although screening for gonorrhea, chlamydia, syphilis, and cervical neoplasia is commonly done, these tests are not obligatory unless dictated by local regulations.

Menstrual Regulation

Menstrual regulation, menstrual extraction, or minisuction are euphemisms for early suction curettage. This technique requires a flexible plastic cannula 4 mm to 6 mm in diameter, with a self-locking syringe as a source of suction (Fig. 14-5). The upper gestational-age limit for this procedure ranges from 42 to 50 days from last menstrual period. Extensive literature has documented the simplicity and safety of the technique (Laufe, 1977; Stubblefield, 1986).

Menstrual regulation differs from suction curettage in several ways. First, anesthesia is not usually required, although analgesia may ease the cramping that occurs toward the end of the evacuation. Second, dilatation is often not required for menstrual regulation. If a given cannula cannot be introduced into the uterus, then smaller flexible cannulae in the set can be used as dilators. After a cannula of appropriate size is inserted, the syringe is attached and the pinch valve released to begin the suctioning. Blood and tissue flow into the syringe. The abortion is performed by rotary and in-and-out movement of the cannula until the gritty feel of the endometrium is sensed and bubbles appear in the syringe. The cannula should not be removed while a vacuum exists in the syringe; likewise, the plunger of the syringe must never be advanced while the cannula is connected and is within the uterus, because air embolism can result. The syringe and cannula are disposable; however, with proper care and sterilization by glutaraldehyde or ethylene oxide, the equipment can be reused many times.

Two problems occur more often with menstrual reg-

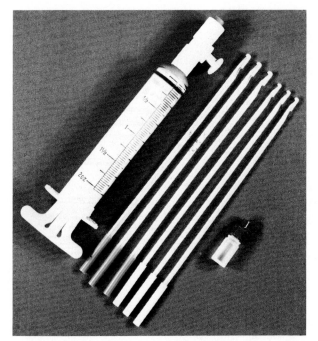

Figure 14–5. Karman cannulas, self-locking syringe with pinch valve, and bottle of silicone lubricant. (Photograph courtesy of IPAS, Carrboro, North Carolina.)

ulation than with suction curettage performed later in pregnancy: (1) the procedure may be performed on nonpregnant women and (2) the operation may fail to abort the pregnancy. Use of sensitive pregnancy tests can ensure that an unnecessary procedure will not be performed; in general, the operation should not be done in the absence of a positive test. Microscopic examination of the products of conception in addition to careful follow-up with a pregnancy test and pelvic exam can reduce the likelihood of a continuing pregnancy going unnoticed (Kaunitz and coworkers, 1985).

Suction Curettage

Suction curettage refers to dilatation of the cervix followed by vacuum aspiration of the uterine contents at 12 weeks' gestation or before. Sharp curettage, which is slower and not as safe, is analogous to diagnostic dilatation and curettage—it is not discussed further.

Preparing the patient for surgery is simple. The woman should avoid oral intake on the day of surgery, and she should bring someone with her to the facility to take her home. The woman should empty her bladder before being placed in the dorsal lithotomy position; a catheter should not be used to drain the bladder. Shaving the perineum and washing the vulva are unnecessary; the vagina is usually washed with a povidone-iodine solution, although the benefit of this practice is

not established. Likewise, routine sterile precautions (eg, drapes, caps, masks, and gowns) are unnecessary. The physician should use a "no-touch" technique: he or she wears sterile gloves and does not touch those portions of the sterile instruments to be inserted into the uterus. Although either local or general anesthesia can be used, use of local anesthesia predominates in the United States. Although local anesthesia does not completely relieve discomfort, it is less expensive and safer than general anesthesia (Peterson and coworkers, 1981).

To perform a paracervical block safely, the physician should use the smallest volume of the lowest concentration of local anesthetic. Local anesthetics vary in their toxicity; for example, chloroprocaine is substantially less toxic than lidocaine, although lidocaine is less expensive (Grimes and Cates, 1976). If lidocaine is used, a 0.5% concentration is safer than a 1% solution. The total dose of lidocaine should not exceed 2 mg/lb (lean weight) or 300 mg, whichever is less. Alternatively, use of local anesthesia with vasoconstrictor (eg, epinephrine 1 : 200,000) slows systemic absorption of anesthetic and allows a larger total dose to be used.

The site of injection of paracervical anesthesia appears to matter little; injection at almost any site adjacent to the cervix results in excellent anesthesia. Common regimens include infiltration of the cervix at the 12-o'clock position (for application of the tenaculum), then injection at four sites (at the 3-, 5-, 7-, and 9-o'clock positions) or two sites (at the 3- and 9-o'clock positions) at the junction of cervix and vagina. The injection should be submucosal to avoid inadvertent intravascular injection.

The pain of inserting the needle can be disguised by placing the tip of a 21-gauge spinal needle against the mucosa at the chosen site and having the woman cough. The Valsalva maneuver "pops" the mucosa over the needle point—frequently without any sensation of pain. This technique works better at 3-o'clock and 9-o'clock positions than at the 5-o'clock and 7-o'clock positions. Once the anesthetic has been injected, the next—and perhaps most important—step is to wait. At least 3 minutes (using a clock) should be allowed for the block to take effect; failure to wait for absorption is the usual reason for inadequate anesthesia.

Few instruments are required for suction curettage. Most physicians prefer to use a bivalve speculum. However, a speculum with standard-length blades prevents the cervix from being drawn toward the introitus during the procedure and makes the operation more difficult. The Moore modification of the Graves speculum, which has 1-in shorter blades of standard width, is well suited for this purpose and is commercially available. Two single-toothed tenaculums are helpful; one is routinely placed on the anterior cervix. If difficulty during dilatation occurs, then the other can be placed on the posterior cervix to stabilize it. Although use of a uterine sound indicates the axial depth of the uterus, sounding the uterus provides no important information and carries a risk of perforation. For this reason, many experienced physicians have abandoned its use for abortion.

If the direction of the cervical canal is in question, then the physician can gently probe with a small dilator. Pratt dilators are preferable to Hegar dilators for abortion because they require less force to dilate the cervix. A useful modification of the Pratt dilators is the Denniston dilators; these are similarly shaped but are made of plastic. Hence, they are light, slightly flexible, and inexpensive, yet they are capable of being autoclaved. Other instruments required for suction curettage include several sharp curettes of different sizes; the vacuum machine, hose, and swivel handle; and a cannula.

Traction on the cervix is important during suction curettage; it stabilizes the uterus and straightens the angle between cervix and corpus, which reduces the risk of perforation. The tenaculum should have a firm purchase on the cervix. High vertical placement at the 12-o'clock position, with one tooth in the canal and one on the anterior cervix, almost eliminates the risk of the tenaculum tearing through during dilatation, as can happen when less substantial horizontal application is made with the tenaculum. If the puncture site on the cervix bleeds when the tenaculum is removed, direct pressure for a brief time stops the bleeding. If the uterus is retroverted, some physicians prefer to place the tenaculum on the cervix at the 6-o'clock position (Fig. 14-6).

Gentleness is the key to safe cervical dilatation. The cervix should be dilated just enough to allow insertion and rotation of the desired cannula. For example, to insert an 8-mm cannula, dilatation to No. 25 French will allow free rotation. During dilatation, the dilator should be held between the thumb and index finger to limit the force applied. In addition, the other fingers should remain extended to prevent plunging forward in case resistance is suddenly lost. Dilatation need not start with the smallest dilator on the set; starting with a larger size (eg, No. 15 French instead of No. 13 French) may reduce the risk of perforating the uterus or creating a false channel.

If more than two fingers of force are required during dilation, the physician should stop and reassess the situation, rather than risk injuring the cervix. One option is to use a smaller cannula than originally planned. Alternatively, the physician can pack the cervix with one or more osmotic dilators, discontinue the procedure, then complete the operation several hours later, by which time adequate dilation will have been achieved. Performance of the procedure in two stages is far preferable to forceful dilatation.

Osmotic dilators are being used with increasing fre-

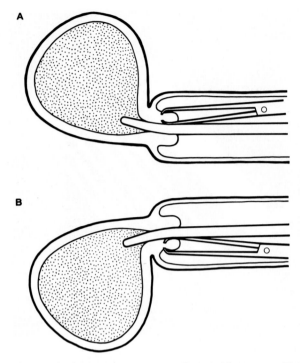

Figure 14–6. Traction on cervix during dilatation. *A*, The tenaculum is placed vertically on the anterior lip. *B*, The tenaculum is placed vertically on the posterior lip for a retroverted uterus. Note the posterior direction of the dilator.

quency for cervical dilation before curettage abortions (Fig. 14-7). Laminaria are hygroscopic sticks of seaweed that dilate the cervix over several hours. The mode of action is not well understood, but the principal mechanism appears to be desiccation of the cervix (Stubblefield, 1980). This drying may alter the ratio of collagen to ground substance, thus changing collagen cross linkages. Alternatively, laminaria may alter the elaboration, release, or degradation of uterine prostaglandins. Laminaria cause the cervix to dilate away from the laminaria; whatever the mechanism, it is more complex than mere passive stretching, as used to be thought.

Based on this concept, two synthetic osmotic dilators have been developed. The Lamicel instrument is a cylinder of polyvinyl alcohol sponge impregnated with magnesium sulfate (Grimes, Ray, and Middleton, 1987). It works within several hours and has the advantage of uniform size (either 5 mm or 3 mm diameter); assured sterility; and easy insertion and removal. Unlike laminaria, the Lamicel instrument will not assume a rigid hourglass shape that hinders removal. The other synthetic osmotic dilator, the Dilapan instrument, is made of a hydrophilic polymer of polyacrylonitrile. Its advantages are similar to those of Lamicel; on the other hand,

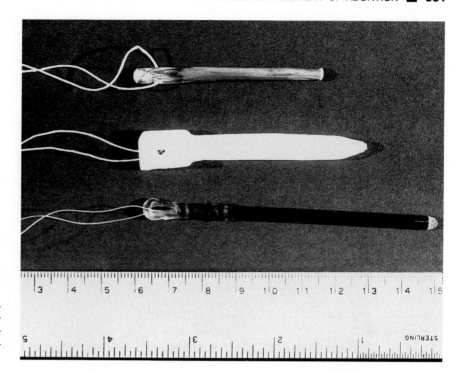

Figure 14–7. Osmotic dilators. *Top*, medium-sized laminaria. *Middle*, 5 mm diameter Lamicel instrument. *Bottom*, 4 mm diameter Dilapan instrument.

its removal can be more difficult and painful than with laminaria, and the device can fragment on removal if grasped inappropriately (Darney and Dorward, 1987). The Dilapan instrument is available in 4 mm or 3 mm diameters.

Osmotic dilators can be used conveniently in an outpatient setting. Placement of synthetic dilators for 2 hours or laminaria for 3 to 4 hours before abortion frequently dilates the cervix sufficiently for abortion. Use of laminaria has been shown to reduce fivefold the risk of cervical injury requiring suturing and of uterine perforation compared with use of metal dilators. This protection against trauma may be especially important for young teenagers with immature cervices who are at increased risk for cervical injury (Grimes and coworkers, 1984a).

After adequate dilatation has been obtained, a cannula is inserted into the uterus. In general, the diameter of the cannula in millimeters should be about one less than the weeks of gestation from last menses. For example, an 8-mm cannula is adequate for evacuating a pregnancy of 9 weeks' gestation. Some highly skilled physicians prefer to use even smaller cannulae than this guideline suggests; the advantage of needing less dilatation must be weighed against the disadvantages of longer operating time and an increased risk of incomplete abortion.

The most frequently used cannulae in the United States are clear plastic, with a slight angulation (Fig. 14-8). The cannula should be inserted only to the level of the lower uterine segment. The suction machine is turned on, and the uterine contents are then evacuated by rotation of the cannula (Fig. 14-9). In-and-out motions are unnecessary and may cause perforation of the fundus and aspiration of abdominal contents. When bubbles are seen in the cannula and the interior of the cavity feels empty, a sharp curette may be used gently to confirm the completeness of evacuation.

The operation is not finished until the aspirated tissue has been examined. The physician or another trained observer must confirm in each case that fetal tissue has been obtained to exclude the possibility of an ectopic pregnancy. Since 1972, >20 women in the United States have died from ectopic pregnancies undetected at the time of attempted suction curettage (Atrash and coworkers, 1990).

Pregnancies at or after 9 weeks' gestation should have recognizable fetal parts; earlier pregnancies may not. Identification of chorionic villi in these earlier pregnancies is essential. The bag of aspirated tissue should be rinsed under tap water to remove blood and clots. If a collection bag is not used, then the contents of the bottle can be emptied into a fine-mesh kitchen strainer (or an opened 4 × 4 gauze sponge) and rinsed.

The tissue can then be placed in a glass baking dish or a plastic basin and floated in water or white vinegar. White vinegar makes the villi appear white and facilitates their recognition. Backlighting from a horizontal x-ray viewing box is especially useful (Fig. 14-10). Villi will appear soft, fluffy, and feathery, with discernible

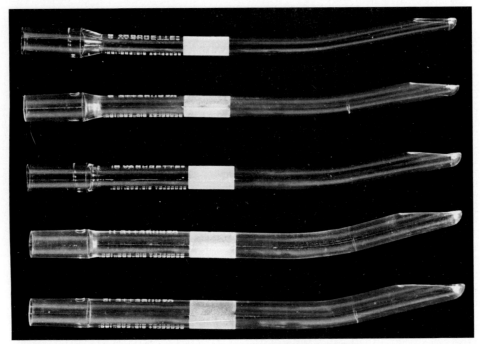

Figure 14–8. Plastic suction cannulas 8 mm to 12 mm in diameter.

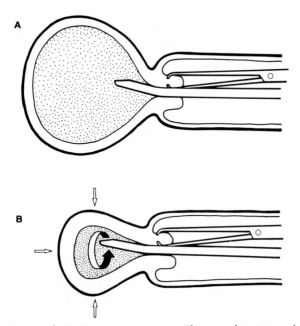

Figure 14–9. Uterine aspiration. *A*, The cannula is inserted just beyond the internal os. *B*, The products of conception are evacuated by rotary motion of the cannula.

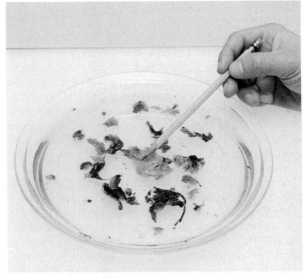

Figure 14–10. Examination of aspirated tissue. Backlighting from x-ray viewing box, in transparent dish; tissue is suspended in water or white vinegar.

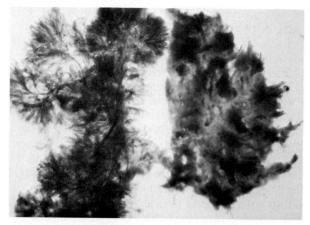

Figure 14–11. Seen immersed in water are (*left*) typical fluffy villi of placenta, and (*right*) shaggy decidua. (Reprinted from Munsick RA. Clinical test for placenta in 300 consecutive menstrual aspirations. Obstet Gynecol 1982; 60:738, with permission.)

finger-like projections; in contrast, decidua appears coarse and shaggy (Figs. 14-11 and 14-12). If villi cannot be recognized with the unaided eye, then a magnifying glass, dissecting microscope, colposcope, or standard microscope (× 100) may enable identification of villi.

If fetal tissue is not confirmed, then the woman should be reexamined, with special attention to the adnexa, and the uterus should be reevacuated. If no villi are recovered, then a sensitive pregnancy test should be done. If positive, the woman must be presumed to have an ectopic pregnancy and should be evaluated accordingly.

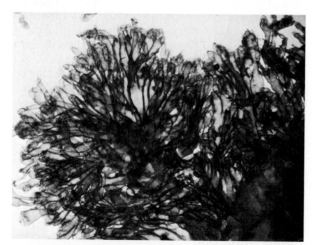

Figure 14–12. Wet-mount microscopic appearance of placental villi. (Reprinted from Munsick RA. Clinical test for placenta in 300 consecutive menstrual aspirations. Obstet Gynecol 1982; 60:738, with permission.)

Ancillary Measures

The usefulness of administering oxytocics during suction curettage is not established, although administering oxytocin or ergot derivatives reduces blood loss from suction curettage performed under general anesthesia. Although statistically significant, the reduction in blood loss is clinically unimportant. Because blood loss is less when local rather than general anesthesia is used, oxytocics probably are not warranted on a routine basis. Although ergot derivatives are commonly given by mouth for several days after suction curettage, evidence of the benefit of this practice is lacking, and the drugs cause painful uterine cramping in some women.

Prophylactic Antibiotics

Prophylactic antibiotics appear advisable for induced abortion patients. A review of the international literature on this topic suggested that routine administration of prophylaxis (usually a short course of tetracycline) was safe and cost effective (Grimes and associates, 1984b). Since that review, the world's largest cohort study of abortion complications has documented a significant reduction in febrile morbidity after suction curettage abortion when prophylaxis was given (Park and coworkers, 1985). Similarly, two randomized clinical trials with a single large preoperative dose of doxycycline have shown powerful protection against postoperative infection (Darj, Stralin, and Nilsson, 1987; Levallois and Rioux, 1988).

Because many abortion patients are not seen until the day of surgery, administration of doxycycline the evening before abortion may not be feasible. Administration of doxycyline to anxious, fasting pregnant women before surgery results in high rates of nausea and vomiting (Grimes and associates, 1984b). Hence, the most practical approach may be to begin a short-course antibiotic with food promptly after the abortion is done.

Dilatation and Evacuation

D & E is the generic term for curettage abortions at 13 or more weeks' gestation. During the 1970s, D & E emerged as the most frequently used method for abortion at ≥13 weeks' gestation. The proportion of abortions performed by curettage techniques is inversely related to gestational age: in 1987, D & E accounted for 90% of all abortions at 13 to 15 weeks' gestation, 63% at 16 to 20 weeks' gestation, and 51% of later abortions (Centers for Disease Control, 1990).

Large studies have demonstrated that D & E is clearly safer than alternative methods through 16 weeks' gestation (Grimes, 1984). At later gestational ages, the distinction blurs between D & E and labor induction methods in terms of morbidity and mortality. Hence, the choice of abortion method at this later stage may hinge on other non-medical considerations, such as cost, convenience, or compassion. Errors in estimating gestational age, especially underestimation, can have serious consequences during a D & E procedure. Hence, confirmation of gestational age by ultrasonography is strongly advised before D & E is done.

D & E differs from suction curettage in two principal ways: (1) D & E requires wider cervical dilatation and (2) forceps are needed to evacuate more advanced pregnancies. To achieve adequate dilatation, many physicians insert osmotic dilators several hours to several days before D & E (Fig. 14-13). For example, five laminaria placed overnight result in 1.5 cm to 2.0 cm dilatation with minimal or no discomfort for most women. Use of a single Lamicel instrument for approximately 4 hours produces as much dilation as do a mean of 5.5 laminaria at 14 to 16 weeks' gestation (Grimes and coworkers, 1987).

Patients must understand that once osmotic dilators have been inserted, the abortion has begun and must be completed. Rarely, a patient will change her mind about abortion after placement of an osmotic dilator. Although some women have continued their pregnancies uneventfully after removal of the devices (Van Le and Darney, 1987), other women have suffered spontaneous abortions thereafter complicated by severe chorioamnionitis.

Dilating the cervix to a large diameter over several minutes may damage the cervix. Indeed, the first large study of this question (Hogue, unpublished data) revealed a higher incidence of low birthweight infants in subsequent desired pregnancies. Hence, in the absence of evidence to the contrary, osmotic dilators

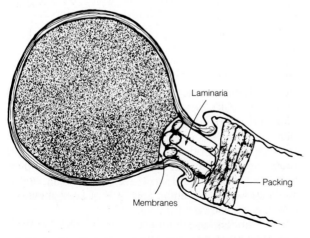

Figure 14–13. Laminaria in place after overnight placement. (Reprinted from Grimes LA, Hulka JF. Midtrimester dilatation and evacuation abortion. South Med J 1980; 73:448, with permission.)

should probably be used routinely for D & E procedures beyond approximately 14 weeks' gestation.

In the 13- to 16-week interval, D & E can be done with vacuum aspiration alone; thereafter, it is accomplished primarily with forceps extraction. A cannula 14 mm in diameter will evacuate pregnancies through approximately 16 menstrual weeks' gestation. For later pregnancies, the cannula is used principally to drain amniotic fluid at the beginning of the evacuation and to draw tissue into the lower uterus for forceps extraction. Specially designed forceps for D & E are available and are far superior to standard sponge forceps. As with suction curettage, instruments should be used only in the lower uterus to minimize the risks of perforation; the only instrument to reach the fundus should be a large sharp curette to confirm that the evacuation is complete.

Complete evacuation should then be corroborated by inspection of fetal parts before the procedure is concluded. All major fetal parts must be identified. The calvarium is the component most frequently missed during the initial evacuation. Gentle exploration of the fundal and cornual areas with a large curette or forceps will usually enable location and removal of the calvarium. Intraoperative ultrasonography may be helpful. If the retained tissue is not easily found and removed, then the physician should discontinue the operation and administer IV oxytocin to the woman for 2 to 3 hours while she is under observation in the recovery room. The woman is then returned to the operating room where the retained tissue will, almost invariably, be visible at the internal os, from which it can be removed in a few seconds.

In D & E abortions, the skill of the physician is of paramount importance. D & E abortion is an eclectic area of gynecology, analogous to radical cancer surgery or administration of chemotherapy, and physicians should not dabble in these activities. This is not to say that D & E is too difficult for most physicians to learn. On the contrary, residents can be taught to do D & E procedures skillfully. Facility with suction curettage is a prerequisite to learning to perform D & E abortions. The physician should study operative technique (Stubblefield, 1986; Hern, 1984). He or she should then observe and assist skilled physicians and then perform D & E procedures only under direct supervision. The gestational age range should be advanced cautiously as skill grows. In summary, D & E is not a trivial undertaking. Attempts by an unsupervised novice to perform a D & E abortion are dangerous.

Labor Induction

Although instillation abortions have been supplanted in part by D & E, the need for labor-induction methods for abortion continues, particularly at later gestational ages. In contrast to the proportion of abortions performed using D & E, the proportion of abortions performed by instillation techniques increases with gestational age. In 1987, 2% of abortions performed at 13 to 15 weeks' gestation were done by intrauterine instillation; at 16 to 20 weeks, the percentage was 18%; and at or after 21 weeks, 22% (Centers for Disease Control, 1990).

The abortifacients in current use can be divided into two groups: (1) hypertonic solutions (eg, saline or urea) and (2) uterotonic agents (eg, prostaglandin E_2 suppositories). The mechanism of action of hypertonic solutions is unclear, but these agents usually result in fetal death from osmotic insult; labor then usually ensues. Prostaglandins appear to act directly on the myometrium to stimulate contractions. Common doses of hypertonic solutions include 200 cc of 20% saline or 80 g of urea. Currently available prostaglandins in the United States are prostaglandin E_2 vaginal suppositories (20 mg) and 15-methyl prostaglandin $F_{2\alpha}$ (250 mcg) for intramuscular injection.

Amniocentesis is required for instillation of the abortifacient. This procedure is usually performed abdominally. Some physicians prefer a "blind" insertion in the midline, several centimeters inferior to the level of the fundus. Others mark on the woman's abdomen the location of a pocket of amniotic fluid identified at ultrasonography. Still others use real-time ultrasonography during the needle insertion.

Preparation for the amniocentesis is similar to that for diagnostic amniocentesis. The bladder should be empty. The abdomen should be cleansed with an antiseptic, and strict aseptic technique should be used. The full thickness of the abdominal wall should be infiltrated with several milliliters of local anesthetic. After needle insertion, a free flow of clear amniotic fluid should be obtained. Nitrazine paper or urine dipsticks for protein can differentiate amniotic fluid from urine if necessary. Blood-tinged fluid that clears does not present a problem; grossly bloody fluid that does not clear is a contraindication to injection of hypertonic solutions. If the uterus is small, lifting the uterus anteriorly with two fingers in the vagina can facilitate amniocentesis. Alternatively, vaginal amniocentesis posterior to the cervix can be done, but the sterility of this approach is dubious.

Withdrawal of amniotic fluid is unnecessary before the injection of abortifacient because withdrawing fluid apparently does not shorten the induction-to-abortion time. On the other hand, withdrawing several hundred milliliters of fluid (and the corresponding decrease in the size of the uterus) may displace the needle tip. Hence, only enough fluid to confirm free flow need be removed.

If hypertonic solutions are used, then they should be administered only by gravity drip. If correct needle placement is lost during the injection, the flow of solution stops. On the other hand, with syringe injection, hypertonic solutions can be injected forcibly into the myometrium in this situation.

Careful observation of the woman is required during instillation. No sedative or narcotic should be administered. The woman should be alert and watchful for any symptom (eg, burning abdominal pain, severe thirst, headache, or nausea) that might indicate faulty administration or rapid systemic uptake of the abortifacient. Any such symptom dictates immediate cessation of the infusion and close observation of the woman. If the symptom persists, the instillation should be abandoned and alternative methods or agents used for the abortion.

Administration of prostaglandins has the advantage of simplicity. An amniocentesis is not required, and inadvertent intravascular administration of hypertonic solutions cannot occur. Disadvantages of prostaglandins alone for abortion include a high frequency of nausea, vomiting, and diarrhea. Routine prophylactic use of antiemetics and antidiarrheal drugs can reduce but not eliminate these noxious side effects. Fever occurs in about one third to one half of patients given prostaglandin E_2. Another serious drawback of prostaglandins alone for abortion is that these drugs are not inherently feticidal.

Although large comparative studies are lacking, vaginal prostaglandin E_2 suppositories appear to be more effective than intramuscular 15-methyl prostaglandin $F_{2\alpha}$. With the vaginal suppositories given every 3 hours, the mean abortion time is about 13 hours, and 90% of abortions occur within 24 hours. With intramuscular 15-methyl prostaglandin $F_{2\alpha}$, mean abortion times are longer, and about 80% of abortions occur within 24 hours (Stubblefield, 1986; Rakhshani and Grimes, 1988). Hypertonic solutions can be used effectively in combination with uterotonic agents such as vaginal or parenteral prostaglandins.

Much of the morbidity (and mortality) associated with labor induction abortion is preventable. Women in labor with abortions need the same meticulous, attentive obstetric care as do women in labor with childbirth. Induction-to-abortion times of 13 to 24 hours are associated with the lowest complication rates; thus, abortion within this interval should be the goal. Serious complications increase significantly with increasing induction-to-abortion times. If labor is ineffective, then steps should be taken to stimulate labor. If the membranes rupture, then labor must conclude within a reasonable period. Similarly, active management of a retained placenta after abortion prevents morbidity. A passive approach to desultory labor in the presence of ruptured membranes exposes the woman to unnecessary risk of complications.

Ancillary Measures

Several adjuncts can expedite instillation abortions. Administering IV oxytocin shortens induction-to-abortion times with saline instillation. Intramuscular prostaglandin or vaginal prostaglandin E_2 suppositories can be used to augment labor; these agents should be considered as the pharmacologic treatment of choice for slow or failed instillation abortions.

Direct cervical dilatation is also useful. Osmotic dilators shorten induction-to-abortion times (Atienza, Burkman, and King, 1984) and protect against cervicovaginal fistulas, although this protection is not absolute. Sequential packings of dilators may be useful if adequate dilatation is not achieved with uterotonics. Alternatively, if progress is stalled, a metreurynter can be used. A sterile Foley catheter with a 30-cc to 75-cc balloon can be inserted into the uterus, the balloon inflated with a sterile solution (not air), and the catheter tied to 0.5-kg orthopedic traction at the foot of the bed. However, this method has the obvious disadvantage of placing a foreign body in the uterus.

In many cases, the preferred means of concluding a slow induction abortion is D & E. This decision should reflect gestational age, status of the cervix, skill of the physician, and the availability of equipment. Frequently, the cervix is dilated several centimeters and the evacuation proceeds quickly.

Hysterotomy and Hysterectomy

Neither hysterotomy nor hysterectomy should be considered a primary method of abortion. The morbidity, mortality, expense, and pain associated with these operations are greater than with alternative methods. Hysterotomy for abortion is an archaic operation with no contemporary uses. Hysterectomy for abortion should be restricted to cases in which preexisting pathology requires hysterectomy.

Complications of Legal Abortion

Morbidity

Legal abortion in the United States is a safe procedure. Fewer than 1 woman in 100 develops a serious complication, and fewer than 1 in 100,000 dies as a result of the operation.

Gestational age is one of two important determinants of the likelihood of morbidity. In Table 14-3, which lists serious complication rates for abortion by gestational age, the term "serious complication rates" refers to the percentage of women who had fever of 38°C or higher for 3 or more days, hemorrhage requiring transfusion, or unintended surgery (excluding curettage). These

TABLE 14–3
Serious Complication Rates for Legal Abortion by Gestational Age, United States, 1975–1978*

GESTATIONAL AGE (WK)	RATE†
≤ 6	0.4
7–8	0.2
9–10	0.1
11–12	0.3
13–14	0.6
15–16	1.3
17–20	1.9

* For women with follow-up and without concurrent sterilization or preexisting conditions; serious complications include fever of 38°C or higher for 3 days or more, hemorrhage requiring blood transfusion, and any complication requiring unintended surgery (excluding curettage).
† Per 100 abortions.

data, derived from a multicenter prospective study including 84,000 abortions, relate to those women without concurrent sterilization or preexisting medical condition and for whom follow-up information was available. Abortions performed at the 7 to 10 weeks' interval were associated with the lowest incidence of serious complications. Thereafter, complications increased progressively with advancing gestational age. The finding that serious complications are more frequent at or before 6 weeks' gestation than at later gestational ages is consistent with two previous large studies in the United States; thus, this finding appears persistent and real, although the explanation is unclear.

The method of abortion is the second principal determinant of the likelihood of complications. Table 14-4, derived from the same study as Table 14-3, demonstrates that suction curettage is the safest available abortion method. The risk of serious complications associated with D & E at or after 13 weeks' gestation is

TABLE 14–4
Serious Complication Rates for Legal Abortion by Method, United States, 1975–1978*

METHOD	RATE†
Suction curettage	0.2
D & E	0.7
Saline instillation	2.1
Prostaglandin instillation	2.5
Urea/prostaglandin instillation	1.3

* For women with follow-up and without concurrent sterilization or preexisting conditions; serious complications include fever of 38°C or higher for 3 days or more, hemorrhage requiring blood transfusion, and any complication requiring unintended surgery (excluding curettage).
† Per 100 abortions.

higher than that associated with suction curettage and lower than that associated with instillation abortion.

Abortion complications can be grouped temporally into three categories: (1) immediate, (2) delayed, and (3) late complications. Immediate complications are those that develop during or within 3 hours of the operation. Delayed complications are those that occur >3 hours and up to 28 days after the procedure. Late complications develop thereafter.

Immediate Complications

Hemorrhage

Reported rates of hemorrhage vary widely, reflecting both diverse definitions (100 ml to 1000 ml blood loss) and imprecision in estimating volumes of blood loss. Few studies have measured blood loss. Rates of hemorrhage ranging from 0.05 to 4.9 per 100 abortions have been reported in large case-series reports. However, the best index of clinically important hemorrhage is probably the rate of blood transfusion. The rate of transfusion associated with suction curettage in a large, multicenter study was 0.06 per 100 abortions. For abortions performed later in pregnancy, rates of 0.26 for D & E, 0.32 for urea–prostaglandin, and 1.72 for saline have been reported (Kafrissen and coworkers, 1984; Binkin and coworkers, 1983).

Cervical Injury

Cervical injury is one of the more frequent complications of legal abortion. A broad spectrum of trauma, however, is encompassed by this term. The most common type is a superficial laceration caused by the tenaculum tearing off during dilatation. At the other extreme are the cervicovaginal fistula and the longitudinal laceration ascending to the level of the uterine vessels. Rates of cervical injury range from 0.01 to 1.6 per 100 suction curettage abortions in large case-series reports. The incidence of cervical injury requiring sutures has been reported to be 1 per 100 suction curettage abortions (Schulz and coworkers, 1983).

Several risk factors for cervical injury during suction curettage have been identified. Among factors within the control of the physician, use of laminaria and performance of the abortion by an attending physician (rather than a resident) lower the risk significantly, whereas use of general anesthesia raises the risk significantly. Among factors beyond the control of the physician, a history of a prior abortion lowers the risk, and age of 17 years or under increases the risk. Use of laminaria and performance of the abortion under local anesthesia by an attending physician together yield a 27-fold protective effect.

Acute Hematometra

Also termed the postabortal syndrome or the "redo" syndrome, acute hematometra is an important complication of suction curettage; its etiology is unknown. The incidence of this syndrome ranges from 0.1 to 1 per 100 suction curettage abortions according to the available literature (Sands, Burnhill, and Hakim-Elahi, 1974).

Women with this condition develop severe cramping, usually within 2 hours of the abortion. Vaginal bleeding is less than expected. The woman may be weak and sweaty, and her uterus is enlarged and markedly tender. Treatment consists of prompt repeat curettage; usually neither anesthesia nor dilatation is required. Evacuation of both liquid and clotted blood leads to rapid resolution of the symptoms. The blood can be aspirated with a suction cannula, a Karman cannula and syringe, or even a catheter attached to wall suction. An oxytocic is usually given after the repeat evacuation. Whether routine use of an oxytocic would reduce the incidence of acute hematometra is unknown.

Perforation

Perforation is a potentially serious but infrequent complication of abortion. According to the most recent reports, the incidence of perforation is about 0.2 per 100 suction curettage abortions.

Several risk factors for perforation have been identified (Grimes and coworkers, 1984a). Performance of a curettage abortion by a resident rather than by an attending physician increases the risk more than fivefold; on the other hand, cervical dilatation by laminaria decreases the risk approximately fivefold. The risk of perforation increases significantly with advancing gestational age. Multiparous women have three times the risk of nulliparous women.

The two principal dangers of perforation are (1) hemorrhage and (2) damage to the abdominal contents. Lateral perforations in the cervicoisthmic region are particularly hazardous because of the proximity of the uterine vessels. Perforations of the fundus are more likely to be innocuous. Indeed, most perforations may be neither suspected nor detected.

Not all perforations require treatment. Many suspected or documented perforations require only observation. Perforation with a dilator or sound is unlikely to damage abdominal contents. On the other hand, a suction cannula or forceps in the abdominal cavity can be devastating.

If perforation is suspected, the procedure should stop immediately. If unmanageable hemorrhage, expanding hematoma, or injury to abdominal contents occurs, laparotomy should be performed promptly. Laparoscopy can be useful in documenting perforation and assessing damage; if necessary, the abortion can be completed under laparoscopic visualization.

Delayed Complications

Retained Tissue

Although retained tissue after abortion may be expelled without incident, retained tissue can lead to hemorrhage, infection, or both. This complication occurs infrequently, however. Its incidence after suction curettage abortion has been reported to be <1 per 100 abortions.

This complication usually manifests itself within several days of the abortion. Cramping and bleeding may be accompanied by fever. When women develop pain, bleeding, and low-grade fever after abortion, retained tissue must be presumed to be present. Prompt outpatient suction curettage usually resolves the symptoms, but close follow-up is advisable.

Infection

Postabortal infection is often secondary to retained tissue. The likelihood of febrile morbidity after abortion depends on the method used. The incidence of fever of 38°C or higher for 1 or more days is usually <1 per 100 abortions by suction curettage. Corresponding figures for D & E are 1.5 per 100 abortions; for urea-prostaglandin, 6.3; and for hypertonic saline, 5.0 (Kafrissen and coworkers, 1984; Binkin and coworkers, 1983) The organisms responsible for postabortal infection are similar to those responsible for other gynecologic infections (Heisterberg, 1988).

A number of risk factors for infection are known. Women are at increased risk if they have untreated endocervical gonorrhea or chlamydial infection or if their abortion is performed late in pregnancy. Likewise, use of instillation abortion instead of D & E and use of local rather than general anesthesia for suction curettage increase the risk.

Curettage and administration of broad-spectrum antibiotics are the cornerstones of therapy. Guidelines for management have been discussed previously.

Late Complications

Rh Sensitization

Legal abortion is a potentially important cause of Rh sensitization for women at risk. The likelihood of sensitization increases with advancing gestational age (and, hence, larger volumes of fetal erythrocytes). One study (Simonovits, Timar, and Bajtai, 1980) has quantified the risk of Rh sensitization from first trimester suction curettage without RhIG prophylaxis. A total of 3.1% of secundigravidas whose first pregnancy was terminated by suction curettage without RhIG prophylaxis were found to be sensitized in their second pregnancy. Subtracting 0.5% (the percentage of women estimated to have become sensitized primarily during the second pregnancy), the authors estimated the risk of sensitization from suction curettage to be 2.6%. Thus, on a nationwide basis, the clinical impact of failure to administer RhIG to candidates after abortion may be substantial. Candidates should receive 50 mcg of RhIG after abortions performed at or before 12 weeks' gestation or 300 mcg after abortions performed later in pregnancy.

Adverse Pregnancy Outcomes

A broad array of adverse reproductive outcomes, ranging from infertility to ectopic pregnancy, have been attributed to induced abortion. Most published reports, however, suffer from serious methodologic shortcomings that limit their usefulness. To examine the potential association between first-trimester–induced abortion and subsequent reproductive performance, an exhaustive review and analysis of the world literature was performed (Hogue, Cates, and Tietze, 1982). More than 150 epidemiologic studies published in 11 languages were included.

The findings of this analysis were largely reassuring. Secondary infertility and ectopic pregnancy occur so seldom that the risk of these complications is not significantly increased, even in studies with substantial power to detect differences in rates. Midtrimester spontaneous abortion is no more common among women who have had one previous abortion than among women pregnant for the first time. Similarly, the risk of premature delivery does not increase for women having undergone induced abortion.

On the other hand, low birthweight is more frequent in first births after abortion by sharp curettage performed under general anesthesia compared with first-pregnancy births. This effect is not observed after other methods of abortion such as suction curettage. The questions of the effect of repeat induced abortion and second trimester abortion have not been adequately addressed, but sharp curettage may be associated with increased risks if it is repeated. Firstborn infants of women who had one induced abortion have risks of morbidity and mortality similar to those of other firstborn children.

More recent studies have corroborated the absence of adverse effects of induced abortion on subsequent reproduction. Outcomes studied have included infertility (Stubblefield and coworkers, 1984; Daling and coworkers, 1985; MacKenzie and Fry, 1988), ectopic pregnancy (Daling, Chow, and Weiss, 1985; Burkman, Mason, and Gold, 1988), spontaneous abortion (Bracken, Bryce-Buchanan, and coworkers, 1986), and adverse obstetric outcomes (Bracken, Hellenbrand and coworkers, 1986; Frank and colleagues, 1987).

Mortality

Since 1972, when the Centers for Disease Control first began nationwide surveillance of abortion deaths, the safety of abortion has improved dramatically. As shown in Figure 14-14, the death-to-case rate has fallen from 4.1 deaths per 100,000 abortions in 1972 to 0.5 in 1985.

The causes of death from legal abortion have changed as well. From 1972 to 1978, infection and embolism were the leading causes of death (Table 14-5). However, from 1979 to 1985, complications of anesthesia (usually general anesthesia) emerged as the leading cause of death from abortion in the United States. Most of these deaths were due to hypoventilation or loss of airway resulting in hypoxia. The message from these deaths in clear: people administering general anesthesia for abortion must be skilled in airway management and observant for signs of hypoxia (Atrash, Cheek, and Hogue, 1988).

The risk of death from legal abortion is related to gestational age: the earlier the age, the safer the abor-

tion. As shown in Table 14-6, which focuses on deaths from 1979 to 1985, the death-to-case rate for abortions at ≤12 weeks' gestation was 0.5 per 100,000 abortions. The risk more than doubled in the 13- to 15-week interval. For abortions at 16 weeks and later, the risk of death was >11 times that for abortions at 12 weeks or less.

Curettage abortion (which includes suction curettage and D & E) is the safest method overall (Table 14-7). The risk of death for curettage abortions at all gestational ages was 0.6 per 100,000 abortions. Instillation abortions had a rate six times higher. Hysterotomy and hysterectomy had a rate many times higher, although this rate is based on only three deaths, and each woman had preexisting illness (Centers for Diseases Control, 1988).

CONCLUSION

Abortion is the most frequent outcome of human conception; thus, the surgical management of abortion and its complications is an important responsibility for physicians. Chromosomal anomalies are the single most important cause of spontaneous abortion. For women with threatened abortion, use of ultrasonography can help predict the outcome of the pregnancy. Evacuation of the uterus in cases of FDIU is done pri-

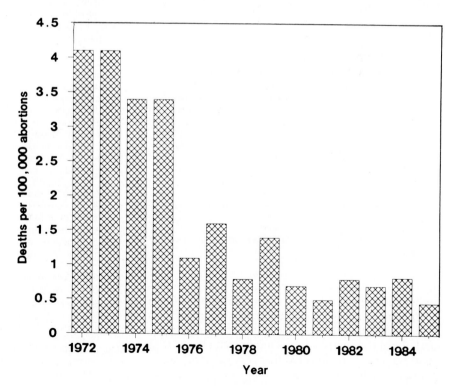

Figure 14–14. Legal abortion mortality by year, United States, 1972–1985.

TABLE 14-5
Legal Abortion-Related Deaths by Cause of Death and Interval, United States, 1972-1985

CAUSE OF DEATH	1972-1978		1979-1985	
	n	%	n	%
Hemorrhage	27	19.2	16	22.2
Infection	34	24.1	10	13.9
Embolism	34	24.1	11	15.3
Anesthesia	22	15.6	21	29.2
Other	24	17.0	14	19.4
Total	141		72	

TABLE 14-6
Death-to-Case Rates for Legal Abortion by Weeks of Gestation, United States, 1979-1985

WEEKS OF GESTATION	RATE*	RELATIVE RISK†
≤12	0.5	1.0
13-15	1.2	2.4
≥16	5.8	11.6
Total	0.7	

* Per 100,000 abortions.
† Based on an index rate for ≤12 weeks of 0.5.
(Centers for Disease Control. Unpublished data, 1988. Reprinted with permission.)

TABLE 14-7
Death-to-Case Rates for Legal Abortion by Type of Procedure, United States, 1979-1985

TYPE OF PROCEDURE	RATE*	RELATIVE RISK†
Curettage	0.6	1.0
Instillation	3.6	6.0
Hysterotomy/hysterectomy	82.9	138.2
Other	1.9	3.2
Other	0.7	

* Per 100,000 abortions.
† Based on an index rate for curettage of 0.6.
(Centers for Disease Control. Unpublished data, 1988. Reprinted with permission.)

marily for psychologic rather than medical indications; either curettage or labor induction can be used. Cervical incompetence is a poorly understood cause of spontaneous abortion. There is no uniform case definition and no valid diagnostic test. Randomized clinical trials have not clearly established that cervical cerclage improves obstetric outcomes.

Small numbers of illegal abortions continue to be done in the United States. Compared with ingestion of abortifacients, instrumentation of the uterus is both more likely to accomplish abortion and to result in complications and death. However, legally induced abortion has become one of the most frequently performed—and one of the safest—operations in the United States. Fewer than 1 per 100 of those having an abortion suffer a major complication, and fewer than 1 per 100,000 die from causes associated with the procedure. Although the rates for short-term complications of abortion are low, the potential long-term effects of abortion on subsequent fertility must be evaluated further.

Bibliography

Anderson SG. Management of threatened abortion with real-time sonography. Obstet Gynecol 1980;55:259.

Atienza MF, Burkman RT, King TM. Use of osmotic dilators to facilitate induced midtrimester abortion: clinical evaluation. Contraception 1984;30:215.

Atrash HK, Cheek TG, Hogue CJR. Legal abortion mortality and general anesthesia. Am J Obstet Gynecol 1988;158:420.

Atrash, HK, MacKay HT, Hogue CJR. Ectopic pregnancy concurrent with induced abortion: incidence and mortality. Am J Obstet Gynecol 1990;162:726.

Berman SM, MacKay HT, Grimes DA, et al. Deaths from spontaneous abortion in the United States. JAMA 1985;253:3119.

Binkin N, Gold J, Cates W Jr. Illegal-abortion deaths in the United States: why are they still occurring? Fam Plann Perspect 1982;14:163.

Binkin NJ, Schulz KF, Grimes DA, et al. Urea-prostaglandin versus hypertonic saline for instillation abortion. Am J Obstet Gynecol 1983;146:947.

Bracken MB, Bryce-Buchanan C, Srisuphan W, et al. Risk of late first and second trimester miscarriage after induced abortion. Am J Perinatol 1986;3:84.

Bracken MB, Hellenbrand KG, Holford TR, et al. Low birth weight in pregnancies following induced abortion: no evidence for an association. Am J Epidemiol 1986;123:604.

Burkman RT, Mason KJ, Gold EB. Ectopic pregnancy and prior induced abortion. Contraception 1988;37:21.

Burnhill MS. Treatment of women who have undergone chemically induced abortions. J Reprod Med 1985;30:610.

Cates W Jr, Rochat RW. Illegal abortions in the United States 1972-1974. Fam Plann Perspect 1976;8:86.

Centers for Disease Control. Unpublished data, 1988.

Charles D, Edwards WR. Infectious complications of cervical cerclage. Am J Obstet Gynecol 1981;141:1065.

Cole SK. Cervical suture in Scotland: strengths and weaknesses in the use of routine clinical summaries. Br J Obstet Gynaecol 1982;89:528.

Cousins L. Cervical incompetence, 1980: a time for reappraisal. Clin Obstet Gynecol 1980;23:467.

Daling JR, Chow WH, Weiss NS, et al. Ectopic pregnancy in relationship to previous induced abortion. JAMA 1985;253:1005.

Daling JR, Weiss NS, Voigt L, et al. Tubal infertility in relation to prior induced abortion. Fertil Steril 1985;43:389.

Darj E, Stralin E-B, Nilsson S. The prophylactic effect of doxycycline on postoperative infection rate after first-trimester abortion. Obstet Gynecol 1987;70:755.

Darney PD, Dorward K. Cervical dilation before first-trimester elective abortion: a controlled comparison of meteneprost, laminaria, and Hypan. Obstet Gynecol 1987;70:397.

Dessaive R, Hertogh R, Thomas K. Correlation between hormonal levels and ultrasound in patients with threatened abortion. Gynecol Obstet Invest 1982;14:65.

Dorfman SF, Grimes DA, Cates W Jr. Maternal deaths associated with antepartum fetal death in utero, United States, 1972–1978. South Med J 1983;76:838.

Duff GB. Prognosis in threatened abortion: a comparison between predictions made by sonar, urinary hormone assays and clinical judgement. Br J Obstet Gynaecol 1975;82:858.

Edmonds DK, Lindsay KS, Miller JF, et al. Early embryonic mortality in women. Fertil Steril 1982;38:447.

Eriksen PS, Philipsen T. Prognosis in threatened abortion evaluated by hormonal assays and ultrasound scanning. Obstet Gynecol 1980;55:435.

Farrell RG, Stonington DT, Ridgeway RA. Incomplete and inevitable abortion: treatment by suction curettage in the emergency department. Ann Emerg Med 1982;11:652.

Foley ME. The natural history of the retained dead fetus. Ir Med J 1981;74:237.

Frank PI, Kay CR, Scott LM, et al. Pregnancy following induced abortion: maternal morbidity, congenital anomalies and neonatal death. Br J Obstet Gynaecol 1987;94:836.

Goulet L, Theriault G. Association between spontaneous abortion and ergonomic factors. A literature review of the epidemiologic evidence. Scand J Work Environ Health 1987;13:399.

Green SL, Brenner WE. Clostridial sepsis after abortion with $PGF_{2\alpha}$ and intracervical laminaria tents: a case report. Int J Gynaecol Obstet 1978;15:322.

Grimes DA. Second-trimester abortion in the United States. Fam Plann Perspect 1984;16:260.

Grimes DA, Cates W Jr. Deaths from paracervical anesthesia used for first trimester abortion, 1972–1975. N Engl J Med 1976; 295:1397.

Grimes DA, Ray IG, Middleton CJ. Lamicel vs laminaria for cervical dilation before early midtrimester abortion: a randomized clinical trial. Obstet Gynecol 1987;69:887.

Grimes DA, Schulz KF, Cates W Jr: Prevention of uterine perforation during curettage abortion. JAMA 1984a;251:2108.

Grimes DA, Schulz KF, Cates W Jr. Prophylactic antibiotics for curettage abortion. Am J Obstet Gynecol 1984b;150:689.

Hassold T, Chen N, Funkhouser J, et al. A cytogenetic study of 1000 spontaneous abortions. Ann Hum Genet 1980;44:151.

Heisterberg L. Pelvic inflammatory disease following induced first-trimester abortion. Dan Med Bull 1988;35:64.

Hemminki K, Mutanen P, Saloniemi I. Smoking and the occurrence of congenital malformations and spontaneous abortions: multivariate analysis. Am J Obstet Gynecol 1983;145:61.

Hern WM. Abortion practice. Philadelphia: JB Lippincott, 1984.

Hertz JB, Mantoni M, Svenstrup B. Threatened abortion studied by estradiol-17 beta in serum and ultrasound. Obstet Gynecol 1980;55:324.

Hodgson JE, Ditmanson GM. Unsuccessful pregnancy. Minn Med 1980;63:134.

Hogue CJR, Cates W Jr, Tietze C. The effects of induced abortion on subsequent reproduction. Epidemiol Rev 1982;4:66.

Hughey MJ, McElin TW. The incompetent cervix. In: Depp R, Eschenbach DA, Sciarra JJ, eds. Gynecology and obstetrics. Vol 3. Philadelphia: Harper & Row, 1982:1.

Jeong WG, Kim CH, Bernstine RL, et al. Ultrasonic sonography in the management of incomplete abortion. J Reprod Med 1981;26:90.

Kafrissen ME, Schulz KF, Grimes DA, et al. Midtrimester abortion. JAMA 1984;215:916.

Kaunitz AM, Rovira EZ, Grimes DA, et al. Abortions that fail. Obstet Gynecol 1985;66:533.

Kline J, Stein Z, Susser M, et al. Fever during pregnancy and spontaneous abortion. Am J Epidemiol 1985;121:832.

Kline J, Stein ZA, Susser M, et al. Smoking: a risk factor for spontaneous abortion. N Engl J Med 1977;297:793.

Koonin LM, Atrash HK, Smith JC, Ramick M. Abortion surveillance, 1986–1987. In: CDC surveillance summaries, June 1990. MMWR 1990;39(no. SS-2):23.

Laufe LE. The menstrual regulation procedure. Stud Fam Plann 1977;8:253.

Leppert PC, Pahlka BS. Grieving characteristics after a spontaneous abortion: a management approach. Obstet Gynecol 1984;64:119.

Levallois P, Rioux J-E. Prophylactic antibiotics for suction curettage abortion: results of a controlled clinical trial. Am J Obstet Gynecol 1988;158:100.

Liskin L. Complications of abortion in developing countries. Population Reports 1980 Jul (series F, no 7).

Little AB. There's many a slip 'twixt implantation and the crib. N Engl J Med 1988;319:241.

MacKenzie IZ, Fry A. A prospective self-controlled study of fertility after second-trimester prostaglandin-induced abortion. Am J Obstet Gynecol 1988;158:1137.

MacKenzie WE, Holmes DS, Newton JR. Spontaneous abortion rate in ultrasonographically viable pregnancy. Obstet Gynecol 1988;71:81.

McDonald IA. Cervical cerclage. Clin Obstet Gynaecol 1980;7:461.

Michaels WH, Montgomery C, Karo J, et al. Ultrasound differentiation of the competent from the incompetent cervix: prevention of preterm delivery. Am J Obstet Gynecol 1986;154:537.

MRC/RCOG Working Party on Cervical Cerclage. Interim report of the Medical Research Council/Royal College of Obstetricians and Gynaecologists multicentre randomized trial of cervical cerclage. Br J Obstet Gynaecol 1988;95:437.

Munday PF, Porter R, Falder PF, et al. Spontaneous abortion—an infectious etiology? Br J Obstet Gynaecol 1984;91:1177.

Novy MJ. Transabdominal cervicoisthmic cerclage for the management of repetitive abortion and premature delivery. Am J Obstet Gynecol 1982;143:44.

Nyberg DA, Laing FC, Filly RA. Threatened abortion: sonographic distinction of normal and abnormal gestational sacs. Radiology 1986;158:397.

Park T-K, Flock M, Schulz KF, et al. Preventing febrile complications of suction curettage abortion. Am J Obstet Gynecol 1985;152:252.

Peterson HB, Grimes DA, Cates W Jr, et al. Comparative risk of death from induced abortion at ≤12 weeks' gestation performed with local versus general anesthesia. Am J Obstet Gynecol 1981;141:763.

Polgar S, Fried ES. The bad old days: clandestine abortions among the poor in New York City before liberalization of the abortion law. Fam Plann Perspect 1976;8:125.

Rakhshani R, Grimes DA. Prostaglandin E_2 suppositories as an abortifacient in the second trimester. J Reprod Med 1988;33:817.

Risch HA, Weiss NS, Clarke EA, et al. Risk factors for spontaneous abortion and its recurrence. Am J Epidemiol 1988;128:420.

Sakamoto S, Okai T. Ultrasonic and endocrinological aspects of first trimester miscarriage. Asia Oceania J Obstet Gynaecol 1982;8:105.

Sande HA, Reiertsen O, Fonstelien E, et al. Evaluation of threatened abortion by human chorionic gonadotropin levels and ultrasonography. Int J Gynaecol Obstet 1980;18:123.

Sands RX, Burnhill MS, Hakim-Elahi E. Postabortal uterine atony. Obstet Gynecol 1974;43:595.

Schulz KF, Grimes DA, Cates W Jr. Measures to prevent cervical injury during suction curettage abortion. Lancet 1983;1:1182.

Shapiro S, Levine HS, Abramowicz M. Factors associated with early and late fetal loss. Adv Plann Parenth 1971;6:45.

Simonovits I, Timar I, Bajtai G. Rate of Rh immunization after induced abortion. Vox Sang 1980;38:161.

Simpson JL. Repeated suboptimal pregnancy outcome. Birth Defects 1981;17:113.

Stein Z, Susser M, Warburton D, et al. Spontaneous abortion as a screening device. Am J Epidemiol 1975;102:275.

Stoppelli I, LoDico G, Milia S, et al. Prognostic value of hCG, progesterone, 17-beta estradiol and the echoscopic examination in threatened abortion during the first trimester. Clin Exp Obstet Gynecol 1981;8:6.

Stubblefield PG: Pregnancy termination. In: Gabbe SG, Niebyl JR, Simpson JL, eds. Obstetrics. Normal and problem pregnancies. New York: Churchill Livingstone, 1986:1051–1075.

Stubblefield PG. Present techniques for cervical dilatation. In: Naftolin F, Stubblefield PG, eds. Dilatation of the uterine cervix. New York: Raven Press, 1980:335.

Stubblefield PG, Monson RR, Schoenbaum SC, et al. Fertility after induced abortion: a prospective follow-up study. Obstet Gynecol 1984;63:186.

Van Le L, Darney PD. Successful pregnancy outcome after cervical dilation with multiple laminaria tents in preparation for second-trimester elective abortion: a report of two cases. Am J Obstet Gynecol 1987;156:612.

Vlaanderen W, Treffers PE. Prognosis of subsequent pregnancies after recurrent spontaneous abortion in first trimester. Br Med J 1987;295:92.

Wallenberg HC, Lotgering FK. Transabdominal cerclage for closure of the incompetent cervix. Eur J Obstet Gynecol Reprod Biol 1987;25:121.

Warren CW, Gold J, Tyler CW Jr, et al. Seasonal variation in spontaneous abortions. Am J Public Health 1980;70:1297.

Westergaard JG, Teisner B, Sinosich MJ, et al. Does ultrasound examination render biochemical tests obsolete in the prediction of early pregnancy failure? Br J Obstet Gynaecol 1985;92:77.

Westgren M, Sjoberg N-O. Surveillance of the cervix by ultrasonography at cervical incompetence. Acta Obstet Gynecol Scand 1986;65:655.

Wilcox AJ, Weinberg CR, O'Connor JF, et al. Incidence of early loss of pregnancy. N Engl J Med 1988;319:189.

Wilson RD, Kendrick V, Wittmann BK, et al. Spontaneous abortion and pregnancy outcome after normal first-trimester ultrasound examination. Obstet Gynecol 1986;67:352.

Tubal Sterilization

15

CLIFFORD R. WHEELESS, JR.

HISTORY OF STERILIZATION

Lungren is credited with performing the first tubal sterilization procedure in 1880 following a cesarean section. Since that time, more than 100 different surgical procedures have been performed on the fallopian tube for sterilization, including simple ligation, partial tubal resection, cornual resection, bilateral salpingectomy, implantation of tubal stump into the uterus or broad ligament, abdominal or vaginal fimbriectomy, and, more recently, laparoscopic procedures including coagulation, banding, clipping, laser vaporization, and cryosurgical freezing. Although many methods are available for tubal sterilization, only those techniques that are used frequently are described in this chapter.

Surgical sterilization can be done by either the vaginal or abdominal route. Boyson and McRae in 1948 recommended the vaginal operation by choice and reported a 0.6% failure rate in nonpregnant women, a level unacceptable by current standards. In 1924, Irving described an abdominal technique of burying the proximal end of the severed fallopian tube into the myometrium of the uterus. The Irving procedure was introduced as an alternative to the puerperal Pomeroy operation, which had reported failure rates up to 20% if performed during pregnancy. Husbands, Pritchard, and Pritchard in a historic report analyzed and discounted earlier reports on the Pomeroy operation; they found that in a large series of puerperal abdominal Pomeroy sterilizations the failure rate was approximately 3 per 1000. It is presumed that because of the altered anatomy and vascularity of the pregnant fallopian tube and broad ligament in pregnancy, obstetrical surgeons before the Husbands and associates report, out of concern for morbidity, were less thorough in completely ligating and excising a complete portion of the fallopian tube. Under the circumstances of incomplete ligation, transection, and resection, the risk of recanalization in pregnancy was higher. The Irving sterilization procedure had a low failure rate: <1 per 1000 cases. It is probably the procedure of choice in sterilization following cesarean section.

Interval voluntary sterilization gained popularity as the family planning movement progressed during the latter half of the 20th century. However, traditional techniques required hospital admission, a laparotomy or vaginal colpotomy under general or spinal anesthesia, and several days of hospitalization. The excessive cost and logistics made the procedure unavailable to many women of limited financial resources.

Vaginal colpotomy was reemphasized during the 1960s as a method of sterilization available to all women who desired or needed the procedure regardless of financial resources. Large numbers of these procedures were carried out in family planning camps in India by Soonawala and in Mexico by Najar on an outpatient basis under spinal or general anesthesia. Three factors prevented this approach from gaining world acceptance: (1) the need for general or spinal anesthesia with its availability and morbidity in Third World clinics; (2) surgical skill and training in vaginal operative techniques that even today make this approach available only to women who have access to surgeons with such skills; and (3) the greater incidence of postoperative pelvic infection that results from vaginal procedures compared with operating through a small abdominal incision.

The popularization of laparoscopy by Palmer and Steptoe set the stage for this procedure, which originally was introduced as a diagnostic technique, to potentially allow surgical procedures to be performed safely on an outpatient basis under local anesthesia in free-standing clinics. Outpatient female sterilization under local anesthesia was introduced into 57 countries from 1970 to 1975. Several independent studies have evaluated the results in large series in terms of cost, availability, morbidity, and failure rates. The optical physics, instruments, and operative techniques are well described in the world literature, as noted by Phillips, Hulka, and Peterson; and continued developments in instrumentation and expansion of the surgical possibilities for sterilization and pelvic surgery are summarized by Riedel and colleagues. Repetition of these descriptions is beyond the scope of this chapter.

PREOPERATIVE PREPARATION

Evaluation

A candidate for female sterilization initially should undergo a standard gynecologic history and physical examination, including a Pap smear. It is unwise to proceed with a simple tubal sterilization when the history, physical, or laboratory data indicate that significant gynecological surgery will be needed in the near future for the correction of menstrual abnormalities, neoplasia, prolapse, or urinary incontinence. The possibility of neoplasia in the female genital tract must be screened for before proceeding with a tubal sterilization procedure.

Indications for tubal sterilization in 1990 have evolved so that the procedure should be available to any adult woman who, after appropriate consideration, counseling, and informed consent, elects to have the operation. Most contemporary indications for this procedure are elective. Those medical indications that existed in earlier editions of this book are probably no longer indications. Maternal and fetal medicine has evolved so that it is possible to manage most complications of pregnancy. Medical indications for tubal sterilization are probably best described as relative contraindications versus absolute contraindications to pregnancy.

Contraindications to tubal sterilization should be those conditions that will not tolerate an anesthetic—general, local, or regional. Because of the variety of methods of tubal sterilization, massive intra-abdominal adhesions following numerous abdominal operations should not be considered a contraindication. Absolute contraindications should be gynecologic neoplasia or other gynecologic pathology that indicates the need for a major gynecologic surgical procedure in the near future. If a medical or psychiatric indication exists, then a complete consultation note should be included in the tubal sterilization records.

Informed Consent and Counseling

Although the husband is not legally required to sign a sterilization authorization, it is good practice to obtain the signature of both husband and wife. Particular care should be directed toward minors having surgical sterilization; all methods of contraception should be considered before instigating surgical sterilization of a minor. State laws vary in terms of the status of emancipated minors. Still, it is a good practice to obtain the signature of the responsible parent or guardian.

Three requirements for informed consent for surgical sterilization exist. First, it should be emphasized that the procedure is intended to be permanent. Although techniques for reversal of tubal sterilization are advanced and results are good, the patient should never enter into this procedure with the idea it can be surgically reversed—that it is a form of temporary contraception. Second, although it should be thought of as a permanent procedure, no guarantee of sterility should be implied or given. The only procedure with absolute guarantee of sterility is a total hysterectomy and bilateral salpingo-oophorectomy. Niebyl has reported pregnancies (although ectopic) after hysterectomy with retention of tubes and ovaries. In addition, pregnancies may follow total tubectomy with cornual resection. All forms of tubal sterilizations have been followed by pregnancies. Third, the patient should be informed that there are complications of tubal sterilization. Although complications are rare and the incidence is small, they may include injuries to the gastrointestinal and genitourinary tracts, infection, hemorrhage, and complications of anesthesia. These matters should be discussed before tubal sterilization and ideally confirmed in writing.

Timing of Tubal Sterilization

The occasion of a cesarean section is a common and convenient time to perform tubal sterilization. However, sterilization should not be used as an indication for abdominal delivery. Cesarean section carries greater risk of hemorrhage, shock, and postoperative complications compared with vaginal delivery followed by puerperal or interval tubal sterilization.

Puerperal sterilization is best done in the first 24 to 36 hours after delivery. The author prefers to wait at least 6 hours following delivery to reduce the likelihood of bleeding and permit the patient to rest after labor. Historically, the procedure has not been recommended later than 48 hours postpartum, because bacteria are present in the oviducts by that time and the postoperative course is more likely to be febrile. With the use of prophylactic antibiotics preoperatively, this time limitation has proven to be less rigid in recent comparative studies. If there has been premature rupture of the membranes, intrapartum fever, manual removal of the placenta, or any factor predisposing to infection and postoperative complications, then the procedure should be deferred until involution has been completed. The advantages of early puerperal sterilization include easy access to the enlarged fundus of the uterus, which may be approached by a small incision a short distance below the umbilicus, and the convenience of combining postpartum and postoperative convalescence with minimal additional hospitalization.

Interval sterilization may be done 8 weeks after delivery or at any time in the nonpregnant woman. For the patient who is not practicing contraception, interval sterilization is better carried out during the early proliferative phase of the menstrual cycle to avoid luteal phase pregnancies. Women with cardiac disease, marked hypertension, renal disease, or acute toxemia should not be subjected to sterilization in the labile early puerperium but should have an interval procedure when their medical condition has become more stable.

In patients of high parity in need of extensive vaginoplasty, the treatment of choice is a vaginal hysterectomy and repair performed no earlier than 3 months postpartum. It is illogical to perform a combined procedure of tubal ligation and vaginal repair as separate operations unless the patient is adamant in her desire to continue to menstruate or retain her uterus.

METHODS OF TUBAL STERILIZATION

Although many methods are available for tubal sterilization, only those techniques that are used frequently are discussed. These include laparoscopic techniques and the Pomeroy, Irving, Uchida, and Kroener methods. The most widely used laparoscopic sterilization techniques are electrocoagulation (unipolar or bipolar), spring-loaded clip (Hulka), and Silastic band (Yoon). Failure rates from reported studies vary widely, and the majority of such studies have had substantial methodologic limitations based on short-term and excessive loss to follow up. According to McCausland and Wheeless, there is slight variance; however, a failure rate of < 1% regardless of technique is accepted generally due to recanalization of the tube or to a tuboperitoneal fistula formed at the cornu of the uterus or the proximal stump of the tube (Fig. 15-1).

Unipolar Electrocoagulation Technique

In unipolar electrocoagulation, the operating laparoscope is introduced into the abdominal cavity and the pelvis is thoroughly inspected for abnormalities (Fig. 15-2). The electrocoagulation grasping forceps is introduced through the operative part of the laparoscope. As a safety precaution, it is important that the electric cable not be attached to the grasping forceps during its introduction but rather be attached when the surgeon is actually ready to grasp the fallopian tube.

The surgeon holds the laparoscope in one hand and manipulates the Rubin's cannula and Jacob's tenaculum with the other. The surgeon can move the uterus into the most favorable position, usually anteflexed, so that

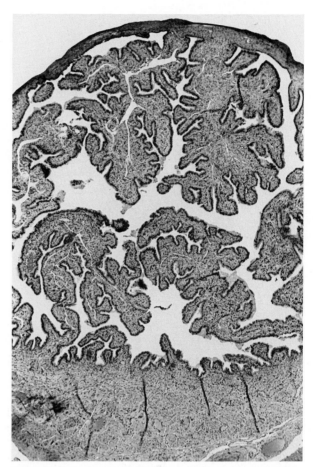

Figure 15–1. Photograph of recanalization of the tube. Note mesothelium over outer surface of the patient's tube. Muscle layers of the lower portion are left intact, indicating that the lower portion of the tube has not been transected.

the fallopian tubes, round ligaments, and ovaries are clearly visible. An assistant holds the Rubin's cannula and Jacob's tenaculum in the desired position. With the uterus fixed, the surgeon moves one hand to the operating laparoscope and the other to the grasping forceps. The fallopian tube is traced from the uterine cornu to its fimbriated end to ensure identification. The tube is grasped approximately 4 cm from the cornu with a large bite that completely encompasses it, including a portion of the mesosalpinx. The tube is moved to a safe position away from bowel and bladder. The electrocoagulation forceps is checked to be certain that its insulation is showing beyond the abdominal end of the laparoscope so that the metal of the alligator-jaw forceps is not in contact with the metal laparoscope (Fig. 15-3). By means of the foot switch, the surgeon passes electric current through the grasping forceps for approximately 5 seconds, thus thoroughly electro-

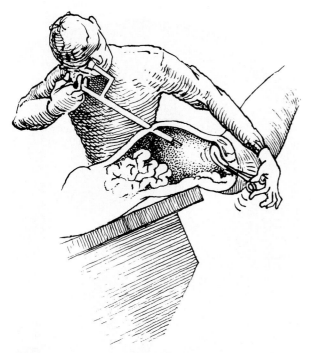

Figure 15–2. Drawing of laparoscope placed in abdominal cavity.

coagulating the tube. The tube smokes and swells, and occasionally a popping noise is heard from boiling the fluid in the tubal lumen and tissue. When the tube swells and collapses, coagulation was sufficient to permit avulsion of a segment. The electric current is turned off and only then is the grasping forceps with the coagulated segment attached drawn back into the laparoscope. It is a serious error to do this while the electric current is on because a burn of structures in contact with the trocar sleeve or laparoscope may result.

After proper electrocoagulation, the tensile strength of the coagulated portion of the tube is so weak that the forceps can easily tear it away. If electrocoagulation is complete and is only directed into the fallopian tube and not into adjacent structures, then significant hemorrhage has been rare. If hemorrhage occurs, then electrocoagulation is generally insufficient. In the rare instances of hemorrhage, bleeding points should be picked up with the electrocoagulation forceps and recoagulated. Bleeding usually can be controlled by this means.

After the "first burn" and avulsion of the tube, a "second burn" is applied to the proximal stump and not the distal stump of the tube. The stump is grasped in a nonburned area adjacent to the uterus and is electrocoagulated for 3 to 4 seconds, but not avulsed as with the first burn. If after the first burn and avulsion the tube is seen to be incompletely transected (see Fig. 15-1),

then it should be grasped again and recoagulated with a second burn until total transection is accomplished without hemorrhage. Occasionally, excessive smoke makes visualization difficult. When this occurs the laparoscope can be withdrawn from the sleeve and the trumpet valve on the sleeve opened to allow the smoke-filled carbon dioxide of the pneumoperitoneum to escape. A new pneumoperitoneum should be instituted.

After one tube has been coagulated and divided, the Jacob's tenaculum and Rubin's cannula are manipulated to expose the other tube and the process is repeated. A thorough inspection for any bleeding points should be made. The laparoscope should be withdrawn and the trumpet valve opened to evacuate the pneumoperitoneum. It is important to evacuate the carbon dioxide from the peritoneal cavity because the more carbon dioxide left behind, the more postoperative discomfort because of its irritant effect on the peritoneum. The skin incision should be closed with a single suture of No. 000 synthetic absorbable suture. There is no need to perform a closure of the peritoneum or the rectus fascia. An adhesive bandage should be applied and the patient taken to the recovery room. If local anesthesia has been used, then the patient may be discharged home in 2 hours; if general anesthesia, then after 4 hours or when stable. The patient should be instructed in daily cleansing of the incision and dressing change.

Despite following this technique, fatal intestinal burns have been reported. To reduce the risk of thermal injury, Soderstrom recommends that only low-voltage generators with a maximum peak of 600 volts and a maximum power of 100 watts be used. An isolated output system is more desirable than the ground system. When the unipolar electrode is used through an operative laparoscope, the laparoscope may act as a capacitor. The static electricity created in the scope can create a source of thermal energy if the intestine is in contact with the scope. To disperse the electricity from the scope to the abdomen and avoid a capacitor effect through the sleeve, the trocar sleeve should be made of a conductive material, that is, steel.

The site of thermal injury to the intestine is commonly the terminal ileum, although injuries to the rectosigmoid or transverse colon have been reported. Small burns of the serosa of the terminal ileum or rectosigmoid do not ordinarily require special therapy but patients who sustain them should be hospitalized for careful observation for 5 to 7 days. If signs and symptoms of peritonitis develop, then exploratory laparotomy must be performed.

The most serious gastrointestinal injuries are not recognized at the time of surgery. Patients who sustain them and who are discharged after laparoscopy reappear on the third to fifth postoperative day complaining

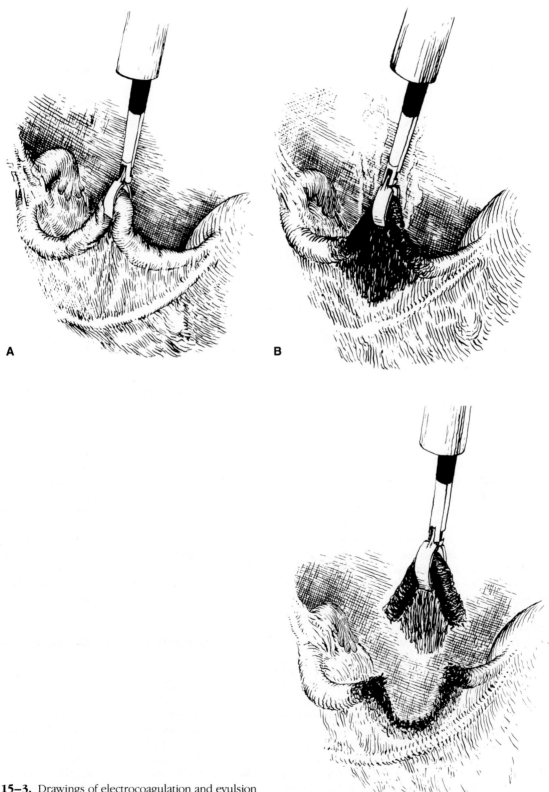

Figure 15–3. Drawings of electrocoagulation and evulsion of a segment of fallopian tube.

A

B

C

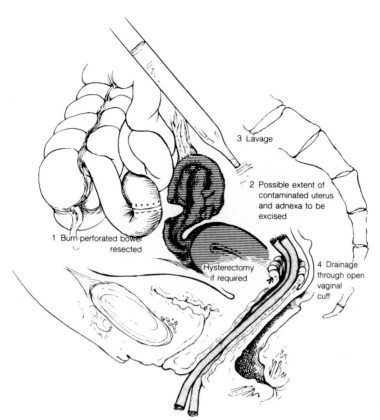

Figure 15–4. The principles of treatment of electrothermal injury to the bowel.

of bilateral lower abdominal pain. Early in the process, the necrosing bowel, before perforation, causes symptoms similar to acute appendicitis. Later, after perforation, the signs and symptoms are those of a ruptured appendix. Five principles are important in the management of this problem (Fig. 15-4). First, the damaged bowel should be resected rather than oversewn. No attempt should be made to excise the perforation site and oversew the area. The actual area of thermal bowel damage is about five times (in diameter) what it appears to be on inspection. Resection of the bowel should be made, for example, at least 5 cm away from the edge of a 1-cm burn. Second, the abdomen must be thoroughly lavaged, removing foreign matter. Third, the areas of electrocoagulation on the fallopian tubes and uterus that have been contaminated with fecal material should be completely excised even if hysterectomy is necessary. This principle is the one most frequently ignored in the management of these cases and results in postoperative pelvic abscess. Fourth, the pelvis should be drained with closed suction drains. Fifth, broad spectrum antibiotic therapy with emphasis on polymicrobial anaerobic gram-negative and enterococcus bacteria should be utilized. Thermal cellular injury greater than the observed perforation of the large

bowel may require exteriorization of the damaged segment of colon with reoperation and anastomosis after the tissue has healed. Resection and anastomosis of large bowel without proper preoperative preparation can result in serious complications. Burch and Brock reviewed a large series of colon injuries and concluded that trocar injuries secondary to a sharp instrument such as a knife wound should be sutured or stapled closed without diverting colostomy or drainage. The difference was the unrecognized extent of thermal injuries compared with sharp knife injuries.

Bipolar Electrocoagulation Technique

To reduce the chance of thermal injury to bowel and abdominal wall, the bipolar electrocoagulation technique was introduced by Rioux. Whereas unipolar systems use a small active electrode and a broad-surfaced return electrode, the grasping bipolar forceps is designed so that one jaw is the active electrode and the other is the return electrode (Fig. 15-5). The mechanism allows the electric current to heat only the tissues between the jaws. If the tissue between the jaws is only fallopian tube, then burns to adjacent structures should

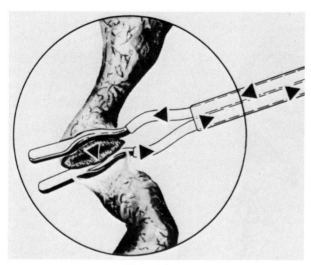

Figure 15–5. Grasping jaw of Kleppinger bipolar forceps showing the direction of electric current (*triangles*).

not occur. When the bipolar forceps is placed through an operating scope, it does not create the capacitance effect because of a "canceling act" of the wave form. Therefore, unpredictable generation of thermal energy between laparoscopic instruments and the bowel should be avoided. However, as with the unipolar technique, intestinal injuries have been reported.

The technique of laparoscopic bipolar coagulation should be similar to that of unipolar coagulation. After examination of the pelvic organs, the fallopian tube is grasped in its mobile midportion with a pair of bipolar forceps and elevated free of surrounding structure. When connecting a bipolar cord to the electrosurgery unit, the dryness of both ends of the bipolar cord should be ascertained.

If the Kleppinger bipolar forceps is used, then closing the forceps handle will compress the tube and simultaneously will bring the flat "duck-bill" portion of the tips in contact with the mesosalpinx. Activation of the electrosurgical unit will produce almost immediate coagulation in the mesosalpinx. Within a few seconds, coagulation will spread to the tube. Complete coagulation requires approximately 10 seconds longer than unipolar. When a proper bipolar generator with a proper setting is used, the cauterized segments of tube and mesosalpinx are transected with a pair of hook scissors. Transecting is important to ascertain the adequacy of electrocoagulation. If electrocoagulation has been adequate, then transection should not produce bleeding. If bleeding occurs, then repeat electrocoagulation of the vessels should be performed.

The failure rate of bipolar laparoscopic sterilization is approximately 4 per 1000 cases, which is comparable with other sterilization methods, according to Rioux and Yuzpe.

Electrosurgical complications have become less frequent since the advent of the bipolar technique. To avoid electrosurgical complications completely, mechanical methods—the band or clip techniques—should be used if possible.

Silastic Band Technique (Yoon Band)

For application of the silicone elastomer (Silastic) bands, the laparoscopic technique is the same as for the electrocoagulation procedure. The specially equipped laparoscope (Yoon band) is loaded with a Silastic band (Fig. 15-6) and inserted in the standard fashion. Each fallopian tube is identified. The tongs of the band applicator are extended and one tube is grasped at the ampullo-isthmic junction and brought into the applicator (Fig. 15-7). Spraying 2 mL of 4% lidocaine solution on the tube before application of the Silastic band reduces the patient's immediate postoperative pain secondary to ischemia. The Silastic band is pushed over a knuckle of tube. The tongs are released and the tube is dropped into the cul-de-sac. If the two-incision technique is used, then the Silastic band applicator is passed through a trocar sleeve in the second incision under observation by the viewing laparoscope, which is inserted through the first incision. The second tube is treated in the same manner as the first, and the abdominal incision (or incisions) is closed as described previously.

Occasionally, the tube is transected by the tongs and scope. If bleeding results, then it should be managed by grasping the transected bleeding stump with the tongs and applying a band on each stump to control bleeding.

Spring-Loaded Clip Technique (Hulka Clip)

The spring-loaded clip consists of two small serrated Silastic jaws held together by a metal clip and bearing

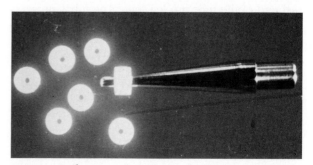

Figure 15–6. Yoon Silastic bands for tubal sterilization.

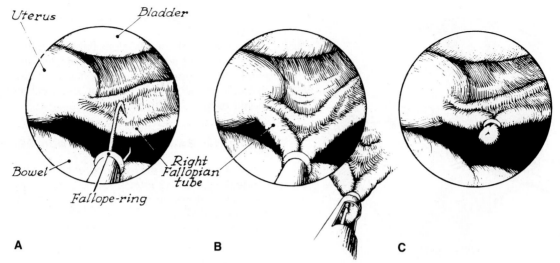

Figure 15–7. Yoon Silastic band application: *A*, tong applicator with band, fallopian tube exposed. *B*, Knuckle of tube withdrawn into band applier. *C*, The completed operation with band applied to knuckle of fallopian tube. (Reprinted from Atlas of Pelvic Surgery. 2nd ed. Philadelphia: Lea & Febiger, 1988: 279, with permission.)

teeth on the end that lock it into place (Fig. 15-8) This clip is applied perpendicular to the isthmus on the fallopian tube with an applicator. Damage to the fallopian tube with this technique has been less when compared with other techniques. Thus, the Hulka clip technique may be ideal for a young woman who might be at higher risk to later reversal of the sterilization because of changed family status.

Irving Method

The Irving sterilization has a low failure rate of <1 in 1000 cases. It has been the author's procedure of choice when accompanying a cesarean section, although it occasionally may be associated with somewhat more bleeding.

The tube should be doubly ligated with No. 00 synthetic absorbable suture about 4 cm from the uterine cornu and severed (Fig. 15-9). The sutures on the proximal end of the tube are left long. The tubal stump is mobilized by dissecting it free from the mesosalpinx. A small nick is made into the serosa on the posterior surface of the uterus near the cornu in an avascular area if possible and the musculature is penetrated with a mosquito clamp for about 2 cm to make a pocket sufficiently wide to admit the tube. The ligatures attached to the tubal stump are threaded with round needles. The needles are thrust to the bottom of the pocket, guided by a grooved director, and passed out to the uterine surface serosa several centimeters away from the pocket. The other suture attached to the tubal stump is

treated in a similar manner, bringing it to the surface of the uterus about 1 cm from the first suture. Traction is made on the sutures and the tubal stump is buried in the pocket of the uterine musculature. The sutures are tied together. A stitch of fine synthetic absorbable suture is used to close the serosal edges of the pocket.

According to Irving's original description of the operation, the ligated end of the distal portion of tube is buried between the leaves of the broad ligament. This makes a very neat appearance but adds nothing to the effectiveness of the sterilization. Occasionally, blood vessels may be nicked during this step, especially in pregnancy, and this accident has resulted in problems with control of hemorrhage. The burying of this end of the tube should be optional with the operator.

Uchida Method

The originator of the Uchida method has had extensive experience with remarkable success. Although an excellent technique, which is quite similar to Irving's original description, it has been possibly the most complex (Fig. 15-10). It is performed through a small 4-cm suprapubic minilaparotomy incision in the nonpregnant patient. Uchida used it almost exclusively as an interval sterilization procedure. The uterine fundus is maneuvered forward by a large curette or Rubin's cannula in the uterine cavity. A Babcock clamp or tubal hook is used to deliver the tube through the small incision. The mesosalpinx is dissected at its midpoint from the overlying muscular tube aided by the injection

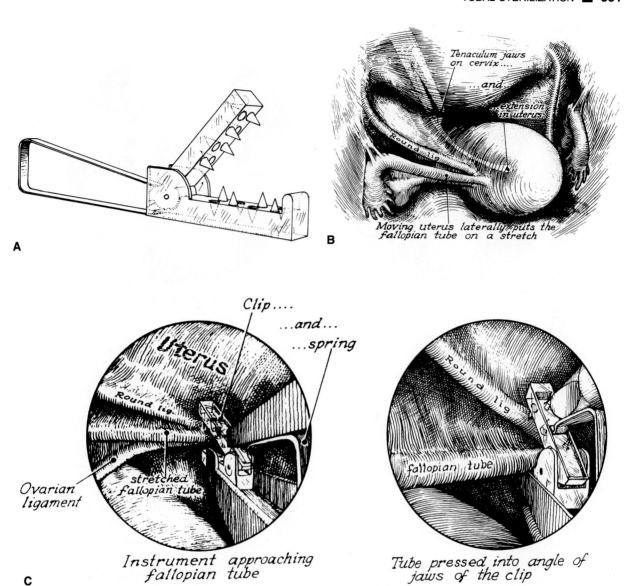

Figure 15–8. *A*, Drawing of Hulka clip with teeth in Silastic clip and locking metal spring. *B*, Drawing of technique using tenaculum in the uterus to stretch the tube. *C*, Clip in position. Stretched tube with round and ovarian ligament and clip approaching the tube. *D*, Open clip placed over tube. (*Figure continues*)

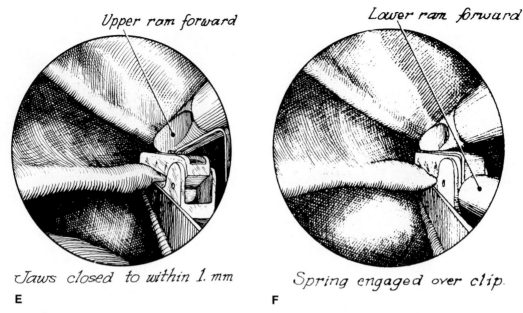

Upper ram forward

Lower ram forward

Jaws closed to within 1 mm

E

Spring engaged over clip

F

Figure 15–8. (continued) *E*, The upper ram activated forward closing jaws of clip across tube. The metal spring open and unengaged. *F*, The lower ram activated, the metal spring engaged, the clip is now locked.

of a saline-adrenalin solution at the tubal mesenteric junction in an amount sufficient to produce ballooning of the mesosalpinx. The avascular portion of the mesosalpinx is incised with scissors. The muscular tube is grasped through this incision with a clamp and delivered into a loop and the tube is divided. The serosa from the proximal end is stripped back by blunt dissection. Approximately 3 to 5 cm of tube is excised, leaving only a small stump that is ligated with synthetic permanent suture and allowed to fall back between the ballooned leaves of the broad ligament. The distal stump is ligated with a No. 000 synthetic absorbable suture that is later used to close the edges of the broad ligament and terminates with a purse-string suture around the free end of the distal tube. The suture is tied so that the distal end of the tube projects into the abdominal cavity. Alternatively, the distal tube and fimbria can be removed.

Pomeroy Method

The Pomeroy method (Fig. 15-11) can be carried out through a suprapubic 4-cm minilaparotomy incision, through a vaginal colpotomy incision as an interval procedure, or through a small subumbilical vertical incision in the immediate puerperium. One tube is delivered with a Babcock clamp that grasps the tube in the midportion. As the loop is held up, it is ligated with a No. 00 synthetic absorbable suture. The loop is cut off with scissors. At the completion of the operation, the two severed ends of the tube have a tendency to retract from one another. The process is repeated on the opposite side and the incision is closed. The tubes, several months after Pomeroy sterilization, are widely separated.

Kroener Method

The Kroener fimbriectomy can be performed through a 4-cm minilaparotomy or colpotomy incision (Fig. 15-12). When entire fimbriae are removed, the failure rate is quite low. The fimbriated end of the oviduct is drawn into the operative field with a Babcock clamp. The uterus is retracted from the field by a Heaney vaginal retractor. The mesosalpinx and outer third of the tube are clamped, doubly ligated with synthetic absorbable sutures, and excised to remove the entire fimbriated end of the tube. The initial ligature is a free tie to secure the blood vessels in the mesosalpinx while a transfixation ligature through the wall of the tube is placed between the Heaney clamp and the initial ligature to secure the collateral circula-

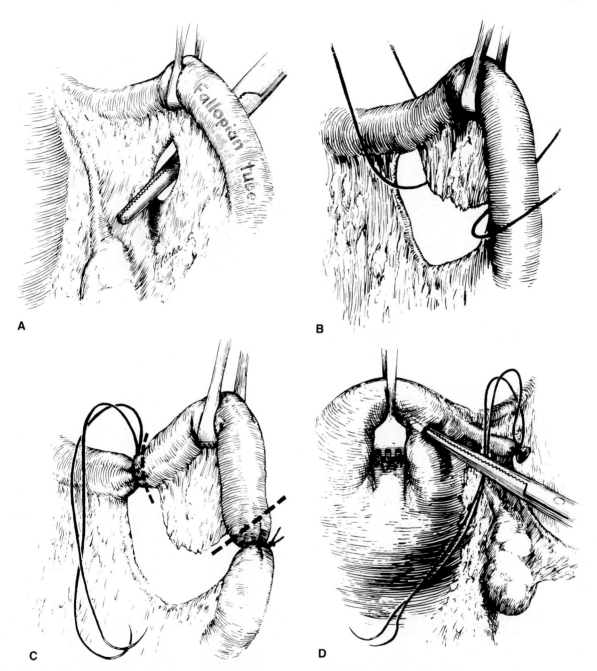

A

B

C

D

Figure 15–9. Drawing of Irving method. *A–D*, A segment of tube is isolated and tied. (*Figure continues*)

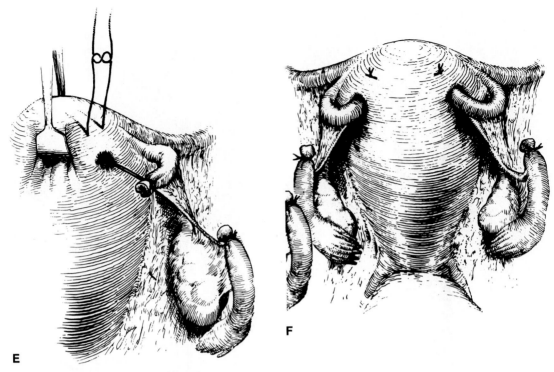

E

F

Figure 15–9. (continued) *E* and *F*, The proximal tube is clamped and used to make a pocket; the proximal tube is buried in the myometrium. (Reprinted from Atlas of Pelvic Surgery. 2nd ed. Philadelphia: Lea & Febiger, 1988: 285, with permission.)

tion and occlude the lumen of the oviduct. The fimbriated end of the tube is excised with scissors between the clamp and outer ligature. This procedure excises the fimbria and a small segment of ampullary portion of the tube to remove the functional component of the oviduct.

SEQUELAE OF TUBAL STERILIZATION

With the increasing use of a variety of surgical methods of sterilization, certain long-term sequelae of these surgical decisions should be discussed. Smibert has enumerated a wide variety of interpersonal conflicts that have evolved from elective sterilization, including regret, behavioral aberrations, and frank psychoses, although Cooper and his associates found no evidence that voluntary elective sterilization increased the risk of psychiatric disturbance in their prospective study. Peel and Potts recorded an incidence of signifi-

cant regret in fewer than 5% of sterilized patients. Akhter has found a similar incidence of 5% of patients who reported dissatisfaction with tubal sterilization. The major conflict arose in unstable marriages where subsequent fertility was desired with a new marital partner. It may be important that the marital unit be evaluated and motivations of sterilization explored preoperatively, although the final decision must rest with the adult woman. It is mandatory that the patient understands the operation is intended to be permanent before surgery is performed.

Surgical errors in the ligation and removal of a segment of adjacent anatomy (usually the round ligament or the infundibulopelvic ligament) instead of the oviduct are embarrassing complications of the procedure when performed without adequate exploration of the entire tube. Such errors are avoided with the use of the fimbriectomy technique as advocated by Kroener and Uchida, because these procedures require the identification of the fimbriated end of the tubes and result in a specimen for pathology. At the time of laparoscopic

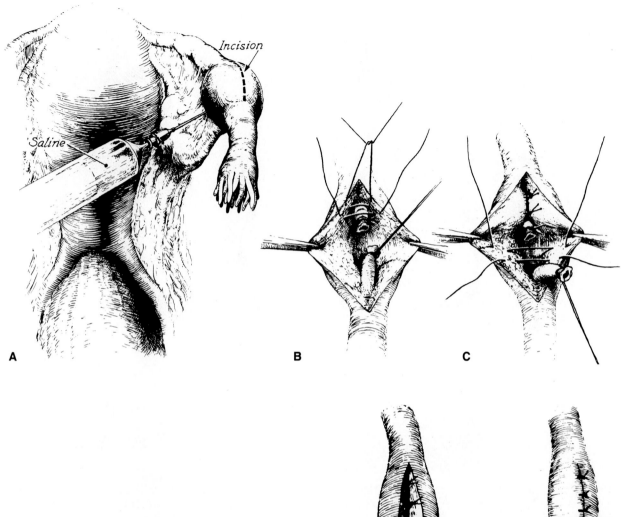

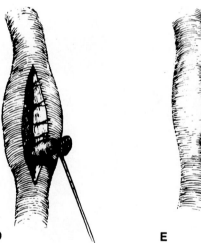

Figure 15–10. Drawings of Uchida method. *A*, The tube is injected. *B*, The serosa of the tube is retracted and a segment removed. *C*, The proximal stump of tube is buried in mesosalpinx. *D*, The distal segment is exteriorized. (Reprinted from Atlas of Pelvic Surgery. 2nd ed. Philadelphia: Lea & Febiger, 1988: 289, with permission.)

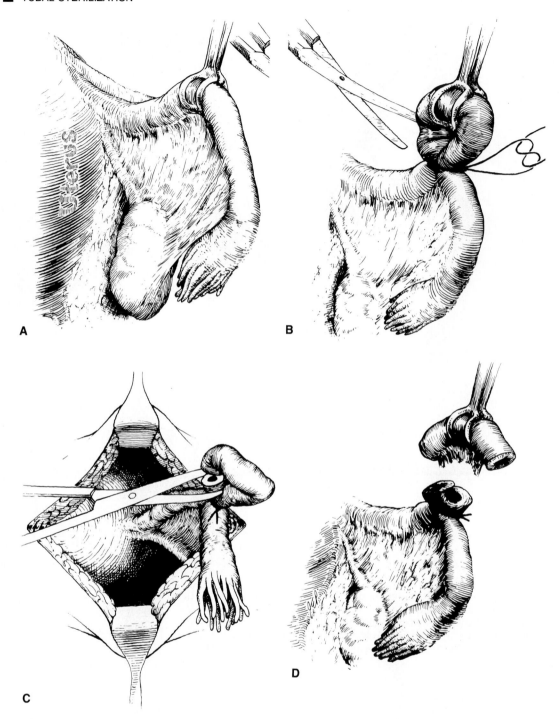

Figure 15–11. Drawings of Pomeroy operation. The tube is grasped, elevated, a knuckle tied, and the dome of the knuckle is excised. (Reprinted from Atlas of Pelvic Surgery. 2nd ed. Philadelphia: Lea & Febiger, 1988: 283, with permission.)

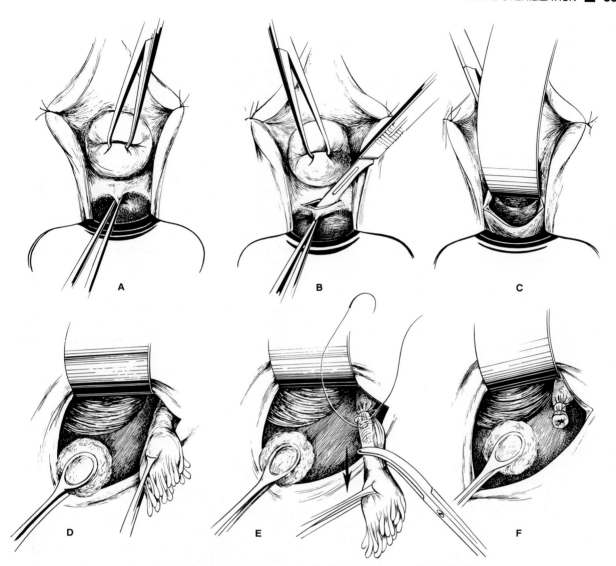

Figure 15–12. Vaginal tubal ligation—fimbriectomy. *A–C,* Colpotomy procedure. *D,* The fimbriated end of the tube is delivered into the vagina. *E* and *F,* The tube is doubly ligated, excised, and removed.

sterilization, an adequate pneumoperitoneum and positive identification of both the round ligament and the fimbriated end of the fallopian tube would minimize the danger of misidentification. Even if both tubes are properly ligated or electrocoagulated, 4 per 1000 women may conceive in the future.

Testing for failure of tubal occlusion has not been without sequelae. The hydrologic pressure generated by hysterosalpingogram may open the scar tissue sealing the fallopian tube. Hysterosalpingogram "leak rates" on x-ray may reach 25% after Pomeroy or any of the other operations, but the same series will have about 4 per 1000 pregnancies. Repeat laparoscopy and observation of the tubes will not detect microtuboperitoneal fistulae. Injection of dye under hydrologic pressure through the uterus may also open the previously occluded fallopian tube. Additional surgery on a fallopian tube found to leak dye upon injection does not guarantee permanent sterilization. The same statistics of 4 per 1000 failures applies to the repeat tubal operation as applied to the first operation. Why not utilize three, four, or five burns instead of two burns described earlier in this chapter? Likewise, why not two, three, or four Silastic bands or Hulka clips? There are simply no data to show that these heroic efforts reduce the failure rate. McCausland reported that 51% of the pregnancies following laparoscopic tubal coagulation failures are tubal gestations.

Several retrospective studies report a high prevalence of menstrual disturbances following female sterilization. However, a prospective study by Bhiwandiwala, Mumford, and Feldblum that was based on 1025 cases showed that the majority of women experienced no menstrual pattern change following sterilization. Kwak and his associates, studying sterilized women as their own controls, also found that the women had no significant menstrual irregularity following sterilization, except for previous intrauterine contraceptive device (IUD) and birth control pill users. Decreased menstrual flow was observed in women who used an IUD before sterilization and increased flow occurred in birth control pill users. Kasonde and Bonnar measured the quantity of menstrual blood loss before and after tubal sterilization and concluded that the operation made no significant difference in menstrual blood loss.

Poma reported an incidence of subsequent hysterectomy in 7% of cases with previous tubal ligation during a 7-year followup. In this regard, if there is evidence of pelvic pathology present at the time that permanent sterilization is planned, then a hysterectomy to resolve the pelvic pathology will also resolve the problem of future fertility.

Bibliography

Akhter MS. Vaginal versus abdominal tubal ligation. Am J Obstet Gynecol 1973;115:401.

Bhiwandiwala PP, Mumford SD, Feldblum PL. A comparison of different laparoscopic sterilization occlusion techniques in 24,439 procedures. Am J Obstet Gynecol 1982;144:319.

Bhiwandiwala PP, Mumford SD, Kennedy KI. Comparison of the safety of open and conventional laparoscopic sterilization. Obstet Gynecol 1985;66:391.

Boyson H, McRae LA. Tubal sterilization through the vagina. Am J Obstet Gynecol 1948;58:488.

Burch J, Brock JC. The injured colon. In: Transactions of the 97th Southern Surgical Association. Vol. 97. Philadelphia: JB Lippincott, 1985:253.

Chi I, Feldblum PL, Balogh SA. Previous abdominal surgery as a risk factor in interval laparoscopic sterilization. Am J Obstet Gynecol 1983;145:841.

Cooper, P, Gath D, Rose N, et al. Psychological sequelae to elective sterilization: a prospective study. Br Med J 1982;284:461.

Crist T, Williams P, Lee SH, et al. Laparoscopic clip sterilization in a free-stand facility: an evaluation of cost and safety. NC Med J 1983;44:546.

Dueholm S, Zingenberg HJ, Sandrgen G. Late sequelae after laparoscopic sterilization in pregnant and non-pregnant women. Acta Obstet Gynecol 1987;66:227.

Greenspang JR, Phillips JM, Rubin GL, et al. Tubal sterilizations performed in free-standing ambulatory care surgical facilities in the United States in 1980. J Reprod Med 1984;29:237.

Huggins GR, Sondheimer SJ. Comparisons of female sterilizations: immediate and delayed. Fertil Steril 1984;41:337.

Hulka JF, Omran KF. Comparative tubal occlusion: rigid and spring loaded clips. Fertil Steril 1972;23:633.

Husbands ME, Pritchard JA, Pritchard SA. Failure of tubal sterilization accompanying cesarean section. Am J Obstet Gynecol 1970;107:966.

Irving FC. A new method of insuring sterility following cesarean section. Am J Obstet Gynecol 1924;8:335.

Kjer JJ. Laparoscopy after previous abdominal surgery. Acta Obstet Gynecol Scand 1987;66:159.

Klaerke M, Bruun-Nielsen JE, Bilsgaard K. Laparoscopic sterilization with the fallope ring: technique in the puerperium. Acta Obstet Gynecol Scand 1986;65:99.

Kroener WF. Surgical sterilization by fimbriectomy. Am J Obstet Gynecol 1969;104:247.

Kwak HM, Chi I, Gardner SD, et al. Menstrual pattern change in laparoscopic sterilization patients whose last pregnancy was terminated by therapeutic abortion. J Reprod Med 1980;25:67.

Lungren SS. A case of cesarean section twice successfully performed on the same patient: with remarks on the time, indications, and details of the operation. Am J Obstet Gynecol 1881;14:76.

McCausland A. A high rate of ectopic pregnancy following laparoscopic tubal coagulation failures. Am J Obstet Gynecol 1980;136:97.

Mehta PV. Laparoscopic sterilization with fallope rings: experience with 10,100 women in rural camps. Obstet Gynecol 1981;57:345.

Najar AJG. Culdoscopy as an aid to family planning. In: Duncan GW, Falb RD, Speidel JJ, eds. Female sterilization: prognosis for simplified outpatient procedures. New York: Academic Press, 1972:41.

Niebyl J. Pregnancy following total hysterectomy. Am J Obstet Gynecol 1974;119:512.

Palmer R. Instrumentation et technique de la coelioscopie gyne-cologique. Gynecol Obstet (Paris) 1947;46:420.

Peel J, Potts M. Textbook of contraceptive practice. London: Cambridge University Press, 1969:213.

Phillips JM, Hulka JF, Peterson HB. American Association of Gynecologic Laparoscopists 1982 membership survey. J Reprod Med 1984;29:592.

Poma PA. Tubal sterilization and later hospitalization. J Reprod Med 1980;25:272.

Riedel HH, Lehmann-Willenbrock E, Conrad P, et al. German pelviscopic statistics for the years 1978–1982. Endoscopy 1986;18:219.

Rioux JE, Cloutier D. A new bipolar instrument for laparoscopic tubal sterilization. Am J Obstet Gynecol 1974;119:737.

Rioux JE, Yuzpe AA. Laparoscopic sterilization: clinical aspects. In: Sciarra JW, ed. Gynecology and obstetrics. Philadelphia: Harper & Row, 1982.

Smibert J. Pitfalls of sterilization. Med J Aust 1972;59:901.

Soderstrom RM. Electrical safety in laparoscopy. In: Phillips JM, ed. Endoscopy in gynecology.: Downey, Calif.: American Association of Gynecologic Laparoscopists, 1967:306.

Soonawala RP. Vaginal sterilization. In: Schima ME, Lubell I, Davis JE, et al, eds. Advances in voluntary sterilization. Proceedings of the Second International Conference Series No. 284, 1973. New York: American Elsevier Publishing Company, Inc., 1974:265.

Steptoe PC. Laparoscopy in gynecology. Edinburgh, Scotland: E and S Livingston, 1967:54.

Thompson BH, Wheeless CR. Gastrointestinal complications of laparoscopy sterilization. Obstet Gynecol 1973;41:669.

Uchida H. Uchida tubal sterilization. Am J Obstet Gynecol 1975;121:153.

Wheeless CR. A rapid, inexpensive and effective method of surgical sterilization by laparoscopy. J Reprod Med 1969;5:65.

Wheeless CR. Laparoscopic sterilization: review of 3,600 cases. Obstet Gynecol 1973;42:751.

Wheeless CR. Laparoscopy. Clin Obstet Gynecol 1976;19:277.

Yoon IB, Wheeless CR, King T. A preliminary report on a new laparoscopic sterilization approach: the silicone rubber band technique. Am J Obstet Gynecol 1975;120:132.

Diagnostic and Operative Laparoscopy

ANA ALVAREZ MURPHY

Laparoscopy has made a remarkable impact on gynecology in a short time. The use of the laparoscope to make safe and accurate diagnoses in a variety of settings is well recognized. The gynecologist, who is familiar with the anatomy of the female pelvis, has little difficulty in appreciating the view provided. However, acceptance of the laparoscope as an operative tool, other than for sterilization, has lagged. It is only in the 1980s that operative laparoscopy has been recognized as a powerful technique in the armamentarium of the reproductive surgeon.

Endoscopy evolved rapidly in various medical fields. The first description of endoscopy is attributed to Phillip Bozzini, who in 1805 attempted to observe the interior of the urethra with a simple tube and candlelight. Hysteroscopy was the first gynecologic endoscopic procedure to be attempted. In 1869, Pantaleoni of Ireland used a cystoscope to identify polyps in a patient complaining of irregular vaginal bleeding. It was not until 1910 that Jacobaeus of Sweden induced a pneumoperitoneum and introduced a Nitze cystoscope into the peritoneal cavity. Kalk of Germany was principally responsible for developing laparoscopy into an effective diagnostic and surgical procedure in the early 1930s. It enjoyed a modest success in Europe. In America, Ruddock introduced a biopsy forceps with diathermy coagulation and reported 500 cases with a mortality of 0.2%. Hope in 1937 emphasized its utility in the differential diagnosis of ectopic pregnancy and Anderson suggested tubal sterilization by diathermy coagulation during peritoneoscopy. Despite these reports in the late 1930s, laparoscopy did not gain much acceptance in the United States.

In 1947, Raoul Palmer of France published his first 250 cases. He used the lithotomy Trendelenburg position and created a gaseous distention. He is also credited with using a uterine cannula to elevate the uterus. Introduction of the "cold light" concept by Fourestier, Gladu, and Valmiere and fiberoptics by Kampany and Hopkins were undisputed breakthroughs for endoscopy. Before development of the cold light system in 1952, the source of light consisted of a lamp introduced into the cavities. This improvement allowed the light source to remain entirely outside the body. This immediately removed the dangers of accidents due to electrical faults and heat, and permitted intense light to be concentrated so that photographs could be taken as well as cinematographic films.

In Europe, the broad acceptance of laparoscopy in the late 1950s was due to the efforts and writing of Palmer, Fragenheim in Germany, and Albano and Cittadini in Italy. Steptoe of England, in 1967, published the first English-language monograph and Cohen published the first North American text in 1968. It was the recognition that laparoscopy could be a safe, simple, and effective means of sterilization that revived the American interest in laparoscopy. In 1962, Palmer published his initial experience with destruction by unipolar electrosurgery of the isthmic and proximal ampulla of the tube. The search for safe and effective methods of sterilization led to bipolar electrocautery, thermocoagulation, and the use of rings and clips. Semm of Germany in 1974 reported the performance of salpingectomy, myomectomy, oophorectomy, ovarian cystectomy, and salpingostomy through the laparoscope. In 1977, Gomel reported sharp dissection and neosalpingostomy in nine patients, eight with previous tuboplasties. Four of these patients subsequently achieved intrauterine pregnancies. Multiple reports have followed that attest to the successful use of laparoscopy for operative as well as diagnostic purposes.

INDICATIONS FOR LAPAROSCOPY

Diagnostic laparoscopy is an invaluable technique. It permits evaluation of tubal and peritoneal factors in the infertile patient. A thorough evaluation of the severity of pelvic adhesions or the extent of endometriosis allows selection of the appropriate treatment. It is also an important diagnostic tool in the evaluation of the patient presenting with acute and chronic pelvic pain to diagnose ectopic pregnancy, pelvic inflammatory disease, endometriosis, torsion, and other intrapelvic pathology. The evaluation of abdominal and pelvic pain may be accomplished in a more timely manner with the use of the laparoscope. A significant reduction in complications due to delay in diagnosis is apparent. A pelvic mass should be evaluated with laparoscopy in most cases. Laparotomy for some benign causes of pelvic mass can be avoided or treatment effected through the laparoscope.

Laparoscopy has a limited place in the primary diagnosis and follow-up of patients with gynecologic malignancy. In rare instances, anomalies of the müllerian or wolffian ducts may require visualization to further elucidate the defect. In addition to providing diagnostic accuracy, the laparoscope may be used to safely carry out surgical procedures. The indications for these procedures are, of course, the same as for procedures done through a laparotomy incision and are discussed later in this chapter.

CONTRAINDICATIONS TO LAPAROSCOPY

Absolute contraindications to laparoscopy include bowel obstruction, ileus, peritonitis, intraperitoneal hemorrhage, diaphragmatic hernia, and severe cardiorespiratory disease. The first three contraindications consider the unacceptably high risk of bowel perforation in patients with distended bowel. Patients with diaphragmatic hernias and severe cardiorespiratory disease may experience acute exacerbation of symptoms induced by the pneumoperitoneum raising the diaphragm, the Trendelenburg position, and decrease in venous return from gaseous compression of the large vessels. Similarly, unstable patients with brisk intraperitoneal bleeding may have further exacerbation of their already compromised cardiorespiratory status induced by the procedure.

Relative contraindications include extremes of body weight, inflammatory bowel disease, the presence of a large abdominal mass, and advanced intrauterine pregnancy. Massive obesity should be an absolute contraindication because it is nearly impossible to manipulate instruments through second punctures. Small, thin patients require a modification in technique to assure safety. The Veress needle and trocar should be inserted almost parallel to the abdominal wall because the distance between the anterior abdominal wall and the abdominal aorta is often quite small. Adhesive bowel disease and fistula formation increase the risk of bowel perforation in patients with Crohn's disease or ulcerative colitis. A large intra-abdominal mass and advanced pregnancy make visualization impossible and increase the risk of puncturing the mass. If exploration is indicated, then it should be approached through a laparotomy incision.

TECHNIQUES OF LAPAROSCOPY

Before beginning any operative procedure, an appropriate work-up is essential. Indications for the procedure and its appropriateness must be reviewed. Contraindications to endoscopic surgery must be ruled out. Informed consent should be obtained in such a manner that the patient understands the nature of the procedure, risks, complications, and alternatives, if any. The consent form for operative laparoscopy should always contain permission for possible laparotomy. It is important the patient understand what circumstances would lead to a laparotomy.

Although sterilization procedures may be performed under local anesthesia, it is imperative that general anesthesia with good muscle relaxation be used for diagnostic and operative procedures. These cases require meticulous inspection of the peritoneal cavity and may require several hours to perform. General anesthesia offers greater comfort to the patient and surgeon and increases safety. Patients should be intubated and receive assisted ventilation. The Trendelenburg position and pneumoperitoneum increase the risk of hypercarbia.

Positioning the patient appropriately can save time by facilitating the operation. The arm, corresponding to the side the surgeon stands on, should always be placed by the patient's side rather than on an extended arm support. The lithotomy position greatly facilitates manipulation of the uterine cannula as well as providing access to the vagina. The patient's buttocks should slightly protrude from the table, further facilitating uterine manipulation. Although manual manipulation may be used in specific cases, rigid cannulae are preferable, especially in long operative cases.

Laparoscopy should only be performed after assurance that the patient's stomach and bladder are empty. A nasogastric tube may be passed to assess whether the stomach may have become distended with gas during intubation. It is common practice to ensure an empty bladder by asking the patient to void before induction of anesthesia. If any doubt exists, it is safer to catheterize the patient. An indwelling Foley catheter may be inserted at the beginning of a long case and removed immediately postoperatively. A pelvic examination to assess uterine size, position, and mobility is performed before insertion of the uterine cannula. Other pelvic anomalies are noted and changes in insufflation technique made if necessary.

Pneumoperitoneum is usually achieved by insertion of the Veress or Touhy needle at the inferior rim of the umbilicus. This is a critical step in avoiding major complications. Patients with previous surgical scars, mass, or organ enlargement may require selection of an alternate site, depending on the area at risk. Alternate sites of entry include the ancillary puncture sites (Fig. 16-1), above the umbilicus in the midline, and beneath the costal margin at the edge of the lateral rectus. Insufflation through the posterior vaginal fornix should not be attempted in a patient suspected of cul-de-sac disease.

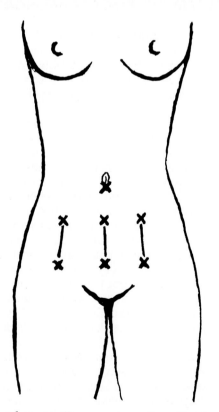

Figure 16–1. Ancillary puncture sites. (Reprinted from Murphy AA. Operative laparoscopy. Fertil Steril 1987; 47:1, with permission.)

Intraperitoneal pressures should not exceed 10 mm Hg. Appropriate position of the needle can be verified by placing a drop of water on the opening and observing its disappearance when the abdominal wall is lifted. Proper placement can also be confirmed with the syringe test. Approximately 5 cc of saline is injected through the needle and aspirated. If the needle is correctly placed, then the saline cannot be retrieved; only gas bubbles will be seen as the plunger is elevated. If fluid returns, then the surgeon may conclude that the water is contained in bowel, bladder, or preperitoneal space. The surgeon may define the limits of free space by alternately injecting and withdrawing. Loss of liver dullness after passage of 1 L of CO_2 into the abdominal cavity is also reassuring.

After insertion of the laparoscope, the surgeon should carefully examine the abdomen to assure that inadvertent damage was not caused by the Veress needle or trocar. A systematic inspection of the upper and lower abdomen should also be performed. The patient can then be placed in the Trendelenburg position to facilitate visualization of the pelvis. An ancillary puncture site is usually necessary to perform a thorough examination of the pelvis. A panoramic inspection gives a general impression of the state of the pelvis. The laparoscope is then advanced and a systematic, careful assessment is performed. The uterus is lowered and the anterior uterus as well as the uterovesical reflection are examined. Endometriotic implants can be missed if the uterus is not lowered and these areas examined. The uterus is raised and the posterior surface examined. The right adnexa is then thoroughly viewed. The medial and lateral surface of the ovary is seen. With use of the ancillary probe, the ovary can be raised to examine the lateral surface. If the procedure is not done in the early or midfollicular phase, a preovulatory follicle or corpus luteum may be encountered. Ovarian manipulation should be carefully carried out to prevent damage to these fragile vascular structures. If the ovary is adherent, then gentle pressure from the blunt probe may free the ovary from its attachment. Endometriosis should be carefully looked for on the ovary and the pelvic sidewall. Force should not be used to separate a densely adherent ovary at the time of diagnostic laparoscopy. The fallopian tube is then carefully inspected. The proximal portion is examined for nodules which may be indicative of salpingitis isthmica nodosa. The tube is viewed in its entirety for the presence of endometriosis or adhesions. The fimbriae are carefully manipulated and assessed to rule out prefimbrial phimosis or fine fimbrial adhesions that may impede ovum pickup. Posteriorly, the broad and uterosacral ligaments are examined. Fluid in the posterior cul-de-sac may obscure the view. If so, the fluid can be aspirated through the operative site on the laparoscope or the ancillary puncture site. If active infection is suspected, then the fluid may be sent for culture. The other adnexa is then similarly assessed.

Chromopertubation may be performed by injecting methylene blue or indigo carmine. It is essential that a watertight seal be achieved with the uterine cannula. Passage of dye can be observed from the fimbriated end. Lack of tubal filling may be due to obstruction, spasm, or leakage from the cervix.

In patients who have undergone prior surgical procedures, visualization may be obscured by a curtain of omentum or adhesions. To achieve adequate visualization, it may be necessary to move laterally to bypass the omentum. Alternatively, when the entire pelvic brim is covered, a thin avascular area may be found through which the surgeon may insert the laparoscope. The omentum can also be dissected sharply or bluntly to make a window through which to pass the laparoscope. Techniques of dissection are described later.

The presence of periadnexal adhesions may prevent adequate visualization. It may be necessary to insert other ancillary instruments to dissect the adhesions enough to make an adequate assessment. Extensive lysis of adhesions should not be performed at the time of diagnostic laparoscopy without adequate informed consent.

Multiple ancillary puncture sites are necessary for extensive operations. Proper placement of the second, third, and even fourth puncture site is necessary to manipulate, cut, and suture tissue. Generally, the surgeon needs at least one to two sites for stabilization and another for manipulations. The punctures are placed slightly anterior and to either side of the operative site. If the puncture site is not lateral and anterior to the area of interest, then the instruments may originate from an angle of poor visibility. These recommendations are, of course, generalizations, and the surgeon's approach should be tailored to the individual patient. Careful assessment of the operative site (anatomy) and the appropriate placement of ancillary puncture sites are critical to safe laparoscopic surgery.

The site of secondary puncture should be indented with the finger and its placement checked to ensure it provides the access required and avoids trauma to the abdominal structures. The surgeon should turn down the lights and transilluminate the anterior abdominal wall to locate large vessels before inserting an ancillary puncture site. The surgeon should keep in mind the course of the inferior epigastric artery, which comes up over the semicircular fold of Douglas and enters the rectus sheath. Hypotensive collapse of a patient from inferior epigastric vessel damage has been reported. Punctures should also be performed under visualization so that the bladder and other pelvic organs are not inadvertently punctured.

The assistant is an integral part of the operating team. The surgeon may have both hands occupied using ancillary instruments or the operating channel. It is critical that instruments be held steadily. If a video camera is available, then an experienced assistant can more actively assist the operator. Beam splitters are available that project the image while still allowing the surgeon to look through the eyepiece of the laparoscope and retain the nuances of color and depth perception, which can be lost if the surgeon operates from the screen. Operating from a screen decreases operator fatigue; however, a decrease in resolution is noted.

Assisting an experienced laparoscopic surgeon and operating under direct supervision, preferably with the aid of video, is the best way to achieve competence in laparoscopic techniques. Laparoscopic surgery should not be attempted by surgeons who have not mastered diagnostic laparoscopy and received further training. Operative laparoscopy is not for the novice, but for a well-trained gynecologic or reproductive surgeon.

EQUIPMENT FOR LAPAROSCOPY

Laparoscopes

Diagnostic laparoscopes are available with different angles of view, either straight-forward or fore-oblique (45°). The selection is the surgeon's choice, although the straight-forward view requires less adjustment for the novice laparoscopist. Diagnostic and operative laparoscopes also come in a variety of sizes from small (5–7 mm) to large (8–11 mm). Many operators prefer to begin using a smaller laparoscope and then change to the larger bore laparoscopes for better visualization and photographic documentation. Theoretically, the smaller instruments should be safer because less force is required to penetrate the abdomen. Operating laparoscopes are of greater caliber than diagnostic ones because the operating channel through which the instruments must pass varies in diameter from 3 to 5 mm. In addition, the laparoscope has a magnification system. The degree of magnification varies with the distance of the laparoscope from the object (Table 16-1), a concept that the surgeon must consider when estimating size through the laparoscope.

Many laparoscopists do not use an operating laparoscope and prefer to insert the ancillary instruments through separate incision sites. They claim improved depth perception and a wider field of vision. Proponents of the operating laparoscope, however, feel that the advantages gained from the additional angle of operation far outweigh these disadvantages.

TABLE 16–1
**Differences in Magnification in Relation to the
Distance of the Laparoscope from the Object***

WORKING DISTANCE	MAGNIFICATION		
	*Wolf**	*Olympus**	*Storz**
3 mm	—	8.2	10
5 mm	—	5.7	6
10 mm	3.19	3.2	3
15 mm	—	2.2	2
20 mm	1.71	1.7	1.5
30 mm	—	1.2	1
50 mm	0.73	0.7	0.6

* Studies were performed with a 10-mm Hopkins operating laparoscope with a 3-mm channel.
(Personal communication from Richard Wolf Medical Instruments Corp., The Olympus Co., and Karl Storz, Endoscopy-America, Inc.)

Types of Operating Laparoscopes

Three major types of operating laparoscopes are available. The most commonly used instrument is the Jacob-Palmer laparoscope, which is offset with two right angles so that the eyepiece is parallel but offset (Fig. 16-2C). This is the easiest instrument to use because the view is identical to that of the straight-forward-angle laparoscope. Its major disadvantage is that the ancillary instruments are handled close to the operator's head and can be easily contaminated. The 45°-angle operating laparoscope (Fig. 16-2D) requires more experience to use and essentially offers little advantage over the Jacob-Palmer instrument except for a small increase in the operator's field. The 90°-angle eyepiece offers a field of view that is at right angles to the operative field. This field of view can be confusing, and it takes time before

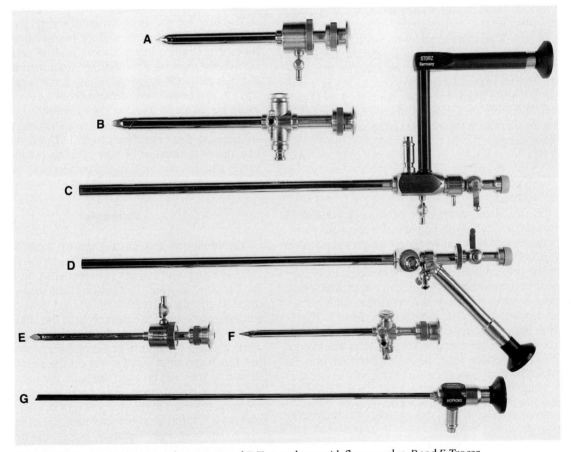

Figure 16–2. Laparoscopes and trocars. *A* and *E*, Trocar sleeve with flapper valve. *B* and *F*, Trocar sleeve with trumpet valve. *C*, Jacob-Palmer operating laparoscope. *D*, 45° angle operating laparoscope. *G*, Straight-forward diagnostic laparoscope. (Instruments made by Karl Storz Co., Tuttlingen, FRG.)

the operator adjusts to the view. However, there is less chance of contaminating the instruments.

Pneumoperitoneal Needle and Trocar

Carbon dioxide passes through the pneumoperitoneal needle after it has pierced the abdominal wall. Two needle types are available. The Touhy needle was designed for epidural anesthesia and is readily available as well as inexpensive. The Veress needle was designed to reduce the chances of accidental puncture. It has a spring that allows retraction of the blunt inner point as it traverses the abdominal wall but springs out to protect the intra-abdominal structures when it encounters the decreased pressure of the abdominal cavity.

The trocar punctures the abdominal wall after appropriate insufflation and carries with it the sleeve. The laparoscope is then inserted through the sleeve after the trocar is removed. The two basic models are (1) the flapper-valve model and (2) the trumpet-valve model. The flapper-valve model allows the laparoscope and other instruments to be inserted or withdrawn without loss of gas. The more traditional instrument is the trumpet-valve model. The trocar tip may be pyramidal or cone-shaped, but it is important that the trocar be sharp. The increased force necessary to insert a dull trocar is more likely to cause damage. Disposable trocars have the advantage of always being sharp. A spring mechanism similar to the Veress needle may also increase safety.

Gas Insufflator

A gas insufflator is used to produce a controlled pneumoperitoneum. For safety, a series of gauges monitor pressure and flow. Laparoscopic surgery is possible only if adequate pneumoperitoneum can be maintained despite multiple instrument changes. Operative procedures require multiple puncture sites, which may become sources of gas leaks. Irrigation with subsequent aspiration can also contribute to gas loss. Therefore it is imperative that a high-flow insufflator be available at least for operative procedures. Most insufflators on low flow produce approximately 0.5 to 1.0 L/min. To maintain the high flow necessary for laparoscopic surgery, a high-flow setting must be used that will produce at least 4 to 5 L/min and preferably more.

Lighting

Adequate visualization depends on the quality and power of light delivered. Xenon light is preferred, especially if the video camera is being used. Metal halide is sufficient for still photography. The beam of light is transmitted through fiberoptic cables, which must be intact to obtain optimal visualization. Broken fibers can be identified by looking at the lighted end for dark spots indicating broken cables that are not transmitting light. Liquid light cables provide superior illumination and do not have this problem.

ANCILLARY INSTRUMENTS

A myriad of ancillary instruments produced for use through a second puncture site or through the operating channel of the laparoscope provide great versatility in an endoscopy system. Broad categories of instruments are considered.

Probes

The simplest and most commonly used instrument is the blunt probe. It is essential for visualization of structures that require manipulation, such as ovaries. It is often used to stabilize structures atraumatically. Other instruments such as closed biopsy forceps or grasping forceps are often used as blunt probes. However, they must be blunt to reduce the possibility of causing trauma. Probes that are marked in centimeters are useful because the magnification of the laparoscopic lens can make estimation of size difficult—magnification varies with the distance from an object (see Table 16-1).

Forceps

The ability to stabilize a structure atraumatically is the key to many procedures. A range of forceps of different size and design is essential in an operative laparoscopy set (Fig. 16-3). Atraumatic grasping tongs and forceps are most frequently used. Small grasping forceps can be used to delicately hold the fallopian tube as the tongs gently dilate the distal fallopian tube at fimbrioplasty. Traditional grasping forceps with springs are much too injurious for use on the fallopian tube. However, they can be used safely on the utero-ovarian ligament to stabilize the ovary. Large spoon forceps are instruments used in the extraction of trophoblastic tissue from a salpingostomy site, removal of an adnexal cyst wall, and withdrawal of pieces of morcellated leiomyomata or other tissues through the trocar sleeve. Tissues that are to be removed, such as myomas or adnexa, may be grasped with large claw forceps or toothed forceps. The hinged jaws of this forceps are

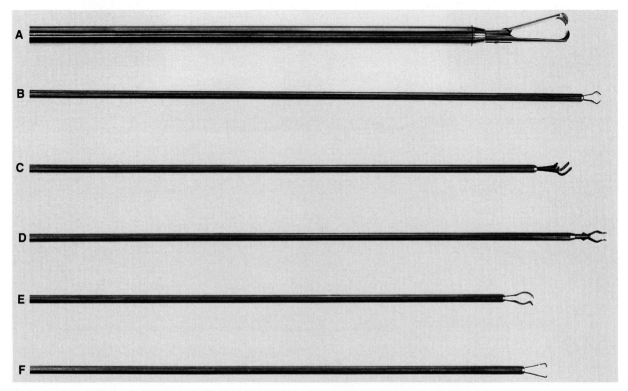

Figure 16–3. Traumatic and atraumatic grasping forceps. *A,* Traumatic claw forceps. *B,* Atraumatic grasping forceps for fixation of tissue. *C,* Atraumatic grasping forceps. *D,* Atraumatic grasping forceps or tongs. *E,* Atraumatic grasping forceps for fallopian tube. *F,* Traumatic forceps to hold sponges. (Instruments made by Karl Storz Co., Tuttlingen, FRG.)

particularly effective in stabilizing tissue while using the morcellator, or during scissors morcellation.

Punch biopsy forceps are constructed with a single sharp tooth on one or both jaws that helps keep tissues from slipping. The edges of these forceps should be kept sharp so that tissue is cut, and not avulsed, when biopsied. Hemostasis should be obtained after the tissue has been removed from the jaws so that histologic detail is not lost due to cautery damage. The Palmer drill forceps is capable of obtaining a large cylindrical core of material from the ovary. An incisional biopsy with scissors or knife is often more precise and easier to obtain.

Scissors/Scalpels

Scissors are commonly used and come in many designs that include toothed, serrated, micro, and hooked. It is essential that they be kept sharp. Scissors that avulse rather than cut can be damaging. The hook scissors (Fig 16-4*B*) are most typically used for large tissue dissection or to cut tissue after loop ligation. These should be

used cautiously because the tips overlap even when closed and may cause inadvertent damage. The microscissors (Fig 16-4*D*) are quite delicate, and are the most practical tool for fine dissection. Serrated scissors (Fig 16-4*C*) tend to "chew" through tissues and are less commonly used. They can also be used to cut suture.

Scalpels of different sizes and shapes are available for use through the operating channel of the laparoscope or an ancillary port. The unipolar cautery can be attached to some scissors as well as laparoscopy scalpels. This combines cutting with coagulation and is useful for adhesiolysis as well as linear salpingostomy.

Aspirators/Irrigators

Endoscopic aspiration of simple-appearing ovarian cysts, cul-de-sac fluid for bacteriologic and cytologic examination, and intraabdominal blood can be effected by way of endoscopic blunt and needle-tipped aspirators. Aspiration can be regulated mechanically by suction devices or manually with a large syringe. The ability to quickly evacuate a hemoperitoneum is essential, es-

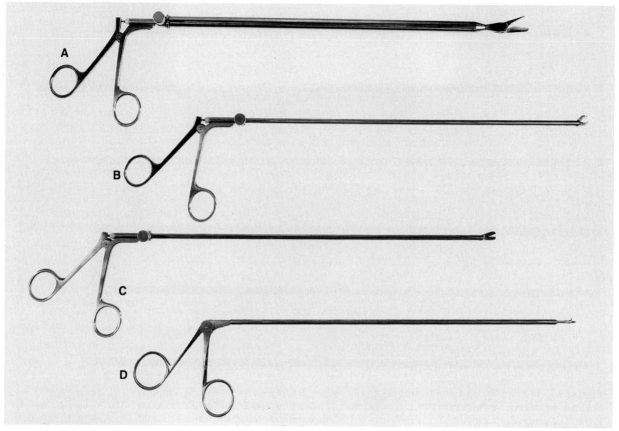

Figure 16–4. Scissors. *A*, Large. *B*, Hook. *C*, Serrated. *D*, Micro. (Instruments made by Karl Storz Co., Tuttlingen, FRG.)

pecially when doing surgery on suspected ectopic pregnancy. Combined aspiration/irrigation units are available commercially. Alternatively, one can attach the suction irrigation instrument to wall suction and to a bag of intravenous fluid. A blood pressure cuff wrapped around the solution bag helps to increase the pressure needed for rapid fluid delivery. The unit is also useful for removing char following laser use.

Morcellators

Morcellation is commonly performed during myomectomy, oophorectomy, salpingectomy, and removal of gestational tissue following conservative endoscopic surgery for ectopic pregnancy. Pieces of tissue too large to be removed intact from the pelvis may be cut into smaller pieces and removed through the laparoscopic sleeve. Alternatively, morcellation may be performed with a tissue punch device containing an automatic storage sheath that is capable of collecting numerous tissue specimens. This procedure can be time consuming and exhausting. The sheath may need to be emptied several times.

Specimens also may be removed by way of a small suprapubic incision or a colpotomy incision. Transvaginal or intra-abdominal colpotomy is performed in the standard fashion. This should be the last step of the procedure because the pneumoperitoneum will be lost and laparoscopic visualization may not be possible thereafter.

HEMOSTATIC INSTRUMENTS

The ability to achieve hemostasis is integral to any endoscopic procedure. The method selected usually depends on instrument availability, type of proposed surgical procedure, and physician preference. Physician preference usually is related to the degree of familiarity the surgeon has with a particular method.

Electrocoagulation

The majority of good, modern electrosurgical units are much safer than the early generators, which were "spark gap" units. These modern generators are low-voltage, high-frequency, solid-state units with insulated circuitry. Most offer both unipolar and bipolar modes. In a unipolar system, the current passes from the generator through the instrument to a ground plate and then back to the generator. The ground plate must be covered with a conductive jelly to obtain appropriate contact with the patient. Most units will stop automatically and emit a warning sound if the sensor part of the plate recognizes any change in the resistance of the tissue.

Cutting and coagulating current can be used in "pure" form (Fig. 16-5). Cutting current provides a constant high-energy wave form. The coagulating wave form creates an initial high-voltage peak that quickly dissipates and results in desiccation of the outer layer of the tissue and increased tissue resistance. A "blend" current consists of coagulating current blended with cutting current usually dispensed through the cut mode. The intensity of the current is regulated separately for the cutting and coagulating modes. The maximum and minimum power output may vary with each

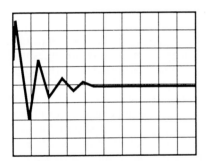

Coagulating Wave Form

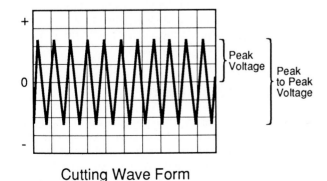

Cutting Wave Form

Figure 16–5. Coagulating and cutting wave forms.

unit. The numerical setting needed to achieve a certain power output can be determined on a graph frequently taped or welded to the top or side of the generator by the manufacturer. Current is triggered by depressing a foot pedal, one for each mode. It is essential that the current intensity be adjusted properly before usage and that only the surgeon activate the current. Proper usage demands that the tip of the instrument be kept in view of the surgeon while the current is activated. The surgeon must also be aware of the lateral spread of current, which may result in tissue necrosis at a distant site. Tissue damage can be seen 2 to 3 cm away from the area of coagulation.

Many instruments can be combined with unipolar electrocautery, most commonly scissors, point coagulators (Fig. 16-6A and C), and scalpels (Fig. 16-6B). A combination point coagulator and irrigation instrument permits irrigation of a specific site to facilitate localization and coagulation of a bleeding point (Fig. 23-6C).

The bipolar system uses the two insulated jaws of the instrument to carry the current to and from the generator. The tissue between the jaws completes the circuit and the tissue is heated (coagulated) by passage of the current. Bipolar can be dispensed in both a cutting and coagulating mode. The power density achieved is lower with coagulating current than cutting. For instance, cutting current should be used to achieve full coagulation of the fallopian tube. The total amount of energy delivered between bipolar paddles determines the adequacy of endosalpingeal destruction. By design, the power (watts) available in the coagulating mode is insufficient to drive the electrons through the already coagulated muscularis into the endosalpinx. Tubal destruction can be achieved with bipolar set at the cutting mode (25 W). Peripheral damage with bipolar is less extensive than with unipolar. Nevertheless, there is approximately 1 to 2 cm of coagulation damage around the point coagulated.

Bipolar forceps is available as a paddle-like instrument developed for sterilization (Fig. 16-6E). Its use has been generalized and it is now widely used to achieve hemostasis during operative laparoscopic procedures. Microbipolar forceps can be used for more precise coagulation (Fig. 16-6D).

The complications inherent in electrocautery are well known as are the means for preventing these accidents. With knowledge of its limitations, electrocautery can be a valuable and safe adjunct (see Ch. 15).

Thermocoagulation

For decades, high-frequency coagulation was the only means of achieving hemostasis during endoscopic

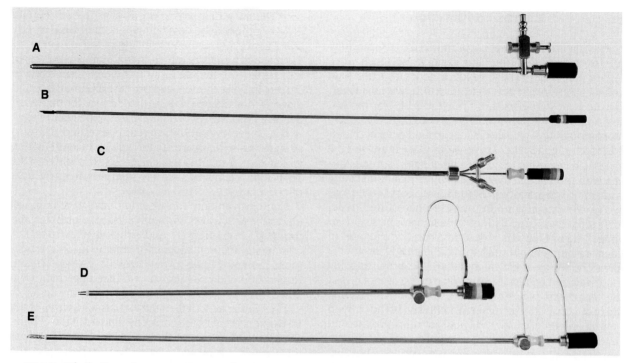

Figure 16–6. Coagulators. *A,* Point, unipolar. *B,* Unipolar scalpel. *C,* Microtip, unipolar coagulator and irrigator. *D,* Microbipolar. *E,* Bipolar paddles. (Instruments made by Karl Storz Co., Tuttlingen, FRG, and Richard Wolf Co., Rosemont, IL.)

procedures. Because of the well-documented accidents occurring from the use of high-frequency current, a "safer" method that does not use electrical current to heat the tissue was sought. This system coagulates tissue by increasing the temperature through heat convection. Electricity is used to heat the metal inside the instrument that delivers the heat. Hemostasis is achieved by heating the tissue to 100 to 120°C. As the temperature in the tissue rises slowly, a color change to white is seen. It is thought that the denaturing of proteins and desiccation cause coagulation. The desired coagulation temperature can be preselected in the range of 20 to 160°C. The temperature can be monitored visually and by a changing tone that indicates that the temperature is in the correct coagulating range. Coagulation time can also be preselected and is also coupled to the acoustic signal. Although the heated mass of metal is small, the instrument does not "cool down" immediately. If tissue is touched inadvertently, however, a penetrating injury is unlikely because the heated mass of the instrument is small and does not release much heat by convection. Nevertheless, superficial damage is possible. Careful attention to this detail is imperative.

Three instruments are available for use with the thermocoagulation unit: (1) the alligator-jaw forceps, (2) the point coagulator, and (3) the myoma enucleator. The alligator-jaw forceps, a jawed instrument, was developed for use as a means of sterilization. However, it can also be used to coagulate tissue or adhesion before sharp lysis. The most useful instrument is probably the point coagulator. Not only can it be used to obtain point hemostasis, but it is particularly helpful for endometriotic implants and for resections of endometriomas. Unfortunately, the point is fairly large and difficult to use in microsurgical work. The myoma enucleator is uniquely suited to resection of subserous and intramural myomas. It is a flat bladelike instrument approximately 3 cm in length. Hemostasis can be achieved fairly quickly and easily during a myomectomy, although color changes can be seen up to 3 cm away from the area of coagulation.

Laser

The laser is a device that produces and amplifies light, creating intense, coherent electromagnetic energy. The energy can be brought to the target site by reflection off mirrors. A lens in this path can focus the spot size and increase the power density. The beam from a fiber, however, is divergent and thus more powerful at the tip of the fiber. In general, the major types of lasers used in surgery are the CO_2, argon, 532-nm potassium-titanyl-phosphate (KTP-532), and neodymium : yttrium-aluminum-garnet (Nd : YAG) lasers.

Power density is the most important single factor in the effective operation of any laser. The power density determines the laser's ability to vaporize, excise, and coagulate various tissues. Power density is expressed in W/cm^2. The surface area of the spot size and power (watts) determine the power density. The ability of the target tissue to absorb the beam determines the area of destruction. The biologic effects depend on power density, not power in watts as read from a power meter.

The optimum power density for laser ablation or vaporization is the highest value that can be safely controlled by the surgeon. This restricts the damage to healthy tissue in the vicinity of the impact by limiting the time of exposure of the beam. The pulse or superpulse mode of the CO_2 laser is an attempt to increase power density without decreasing control and thereby decrease thermal spread and damage.

The CO_2 laser is the laser most commonly combined with laparoscopy. Special modification of the operating channel allows the focusing lens and gas to flow through the same channel (Fig. 16-7A and B). The laser energy can also be carried by an ancillary port (Fig. 16-7C and D). The need to evacuate the plume represents a drawback, and a pneumoperitoneum may be difficult to maintain. The CO_2 laser is highly absorbed by nonreflective solids and liquids, especially water. The laser energy is absorbed at a depth of 100 μm from the surface with no significant scatter from the target point. Fine focusing (high-power density) results in cutting, whereas a defocused beam (low-power density) has coagulating properties. The CO_2 has the ability to seal off blood flow in vessels up to 0.5 to 2.0 mm. Bipolar coagulation should be readily available in the event that larger vessels are encountered.

The CO_2 laser is primarily used to vaporize tissue. The argon, KTP-532, and Nd : YAG lasers have greater coagulative effect. They are of greater use in cutting through vascular tissue, such as myomas. The ability to use these lasers as cutting instruments can be increased with use of fibers or sapphire tips that convert the

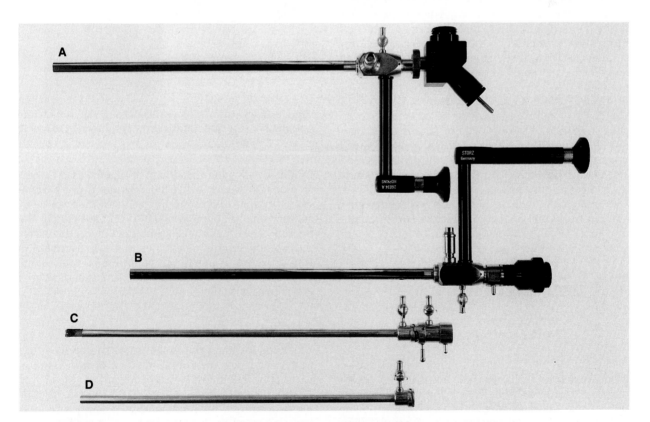

Figure 16–7. CO_2 laser laparoscopes and second puncture delivery set. *A* and *B*, CO_2 laser operating laparoscopes with coupler body. *C*, CO_2 laser laparoscopy second puncture delivery set with inner tube and outer tube with backstop. *D*, CO_2 laser laparoscopy second puncture open-end outer tube. (Instruments made by Karl Storz Co., Tuttlingen, FRG.)

properties of the laser beam to characteristics similar to those of the CO_2 laser. The depth of penetration of the argon and KTP-532 lasers is 0.4 to 0.8 mm, much deeper than that of the CO_2 laser. The depth of the Nd:YAG laser is 0.6 to 4.2 mm. The argon laser beam is preferentially absorbed by reddish pigment so its widest use has been for treatment of endometriosis. Because of its depth of penetration, the Nd:YAG laser is used for endometrial ablation, although it has been used in endometriosis. The KTP-532 laser has uses similar to those of the CO_2 laser.

Suture

Suturing can add a new dimension to operative laparoscopy. Although suturing is frequently unnecessary, certain procedures are facilitated with its use. The Roeder loop is a modification of a tonsillectomy or rectal polyp snare and is available in chromic catgut or plain. This loop can be placed around a structure and tightened, thereby ligating the tissue and blood vessels. The loop's slipknot is introduced, along with its applicator sleeve, through a 5-mm trocar. Forceps are used to position the slipknot until the suture can be tightened. In procedures such as oophorectomy, salpingectomy, and adnexectomy, three sutures are typically placed. Simple bleeding sites usually need only one suture ligature.

Suturing can also be performed with a straight needle (ST-3 and ST-4) and 2-0 plain, 2-0 chromic catgut, or 4-0 PDS (polydioxanone) suture introduced through an ancillary puncture site. A 3- or 5-mm needle holder with a spring to keep the needle in place is used. The suture is secured by either an intra-abdominal instrument tie or an extracorporeal knot (Figs. 16-8 and 16-9). The knot guide or metal push rod reintroduces the extracorporeal knot into the abdomen to tighten the knot. Greater diversity in suture material and gauges needs to be made available.

OPERATIVE PROCEDURES

Laparoscopic Procedures for Ectopic Pregnancy

The laparoscope is essential in the diagnosis of ectopic pregnancy and has recently become more widely used for therapy as well. Depending on the patient's desire for fertility and extent of disease, conservative as well as radical procedures can be performed. Refinements in technology have facilitated the early diagnosis of ectopic pregnancy, frequently in the unruptured state. Early diagnosis reduces morbidity and increases

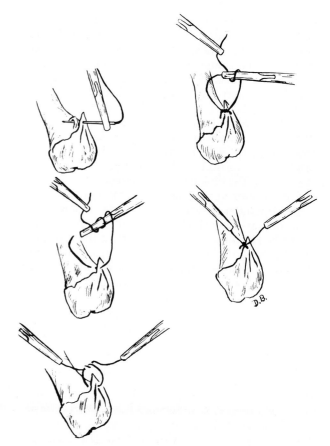

Figure 16–8. Intra-abdominal knot tying. (Reprinted from Murphy AA. Operative laparoscopy. Fertil Steril 1987; 47:1, with permission.)

fertility by allowing conservative procedures to be performed. Of course, an unstable patient is not a candidate for laparoscopic surgery. The cardiorespiratory status of an unstable patient may be exacerbated by the pneumoperitoneum raising the diaphragm, by use of the Trendelenburg position, and by a decrease in venous return from gaseous compression of the large vessels. Evidence of rupture is not a contraindication if the patient is stable.

Salpingectomy

Salpingectomy is the treatment of choice for an ectopic pregnancy when preservation of fertility is not an issue. If the fallopian tube has been markedly destroyed by rupture or severe adhesive disease, then a conservative procedure is not recommended. Many procedures for salpingectomy through the laparoscope have been described. A salpingectomy may be performed by successive electrocoagulation or thermocoagulation of the mesosalpinx and subsequent cutting with scissors or

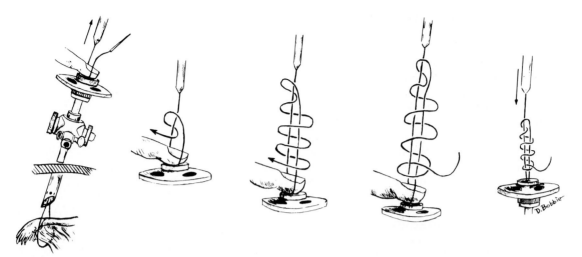

Figure 16–9. Extracorporeal knot tying. (Reprinted from Murphy AA. Operative laparoscopy. Fertil Steril 1987; 47:1, with permission.)

knife. Either unipolar or bipolar coagulation may be used. Coagulation and cutting may begin at the fimbriated end with subsequent coagulation and transection of the fallopian tube proximal to the ectopic pregnancy or vice versa (Fig. 16-10). Right-handed surgeons generally prefer to operate from right to left; thus, right fallopian tube ectopic pregnancies are resected beginning from the fimbriated end and left fallopian tube ectopic pregnancies from the proximal tube toward the fimbriated end. Unipolar cautery combined with scissors allows minimal instrument changes; however, care must be taken to avoid excessive coagulation near the ovary and its vasculature. Coagulation and cutting must be as close to the fallopian tube as possible to avoid damage to the ovary or its blood supply.

The loop or snare also may be used to perform the salpingectomy. Three loops are placed proximal to the ectopic pregnancy. The tube is then transected. The mesosalpinx usually needs to be dissected partially to allow placement of the loop in the isthmic portion. The

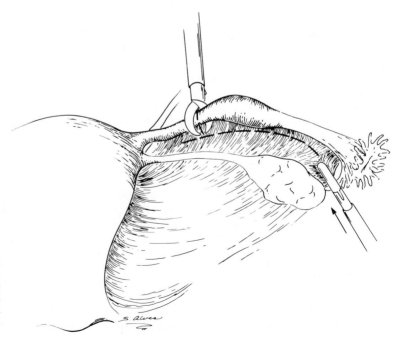

Figure 16–10. Salpingectomy by electrocoagulation or thermocoagulation. Coagulation with subsequent cutting begins at the fimbriated end. The proximal fallopian tube is thoroughly coagulated and subsequently transected.

resected fallopian tube is removed from the abdomen as discussed previously in the section on morcellators.

Conservative procedures are appropriately performed for ectopic pregnancy when the patient is desirous of future childbearing. Although earlier studies suggested that conservative procedures were not necessarily associated with improved pregnancy rates, more recent studies suggest that subsequent pregnancy rates are improved with conservative procedures when coexistent sterility factors are present. The other major argument against the conservative approach is that the risk of recurrent ectopic pregnancy is increased. This argument is unfounded because the frequency of ectopic pregnancy is the same regardless of the procedure. Obviously, the patient must be well informed of the risk of persistent trophoblast and possible need for further surgical or medical therapy. She should be followed with frequent β-HCG to monitor this potential problem.

Linear Salpingotomy

Unruptured ampullary and selected isthmic ectopic pregnancies may be treated with linear salpingostomy or salpingotomy. An incision is made along the antimesenteric border of the tubal ectopic. This can be accomplished with a unipolar needle point cautery, knife, laser (Fig. 16-11), or scissors. Before incision with the scissors, the area may be coagulated with electrocautery or thermocoagulation. To decrease blood loss, the mesosalpinx below the ectopic may be infiltrated with a dilute solution of vasopressin. Alternatively, if a vessel can be seen to be supplying the area of fallopian tube containing the ectopic, it may be selectively coagulated with bipolar to decrease blood loss.

Atraumatic forceps are used to hold the edges of the salpingotomy incision. The conceptual debris is removed with an aspirator or spoon forceps. The bed is observed closely for bleeding and to ensure that no trophoblastic tissue remains. The salpingotomy incision is usually not closed. Fistula formation at the operative site is a possible complication but does not appear to be common. If the defect is large, or marked eversion of mucosa occurs, then a 4-0 PDS suture can be used to approximate the tubal edges. The suture is tied with instruments inside the peritoneal cavity or tied outside the cavity using a slipknot as previously described. The trophoblastic tissue can usually be removed through one of the puncture sites.

Partial Salpingectomy

The conservative procedure of choice for some isthmic and interstitial pregnancies is a partial salpingectomy. It also may be performed for ruptured ectopic

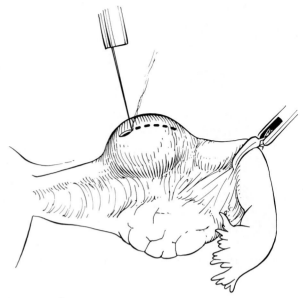

Figure 16–11. Linear salpingotomy using CO_2 laser. An incision on the antimesenteric border over the ectopic gestation is made. The contents are removed. Hemostasis is obtained and the tube is usually left to heal by secondary intention. (Reprinted from Roseff SJ, Murphy AA. Helpful techniques in laser laparoscopy. Contemp OB/GYN 1988; 32:159, with permission.)

pregnancy depending on the extent of tubal damage. A failed salpingostomy procedure may be converted to a partial salpingectomy.

Segmental resection may be accomplished with electrocautery, thermocoagulation, laser, or loop. Thorough coagulation of the tube proximal and distal to the ectopic pregnancy is achieved. The tube is incised in the area of coagulation. The tubal segment containing the ectopic pregnancy is grasped with forceps and elevated. A series of burns and cuts are placed progressively along the mesosalpinx, beneath the tubal segment being excised (Fig. 16-12). The mesosalpinx is inspected carefully and any bleeding points are recoagulated.

A variation of the Pomeroy technique for tubal sterilization can be performed with the Roeder loop or snare. The loop is placed around the ectopic gestation. The intervening tube containing the ectopic pregnancy is then resected (Fig. 16-13).

A variation of the coagulation method of sterilization consists of thoroughly coagulating the segment of fallopian tube containing the ectopic pregnancy. The tubal coagulation may be achieved with unipolar, bipolar, or thermocoagulation. Obviously, that segment of tube is destroyed and no specimen can be sent to pathology; thus, this technique is rarely used. The potential for

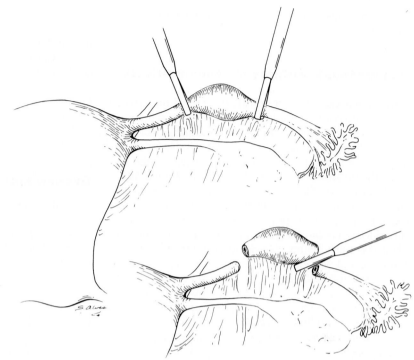

Figure 16–12. Partial salpingectomy using electrocautery or thermocoagulation. The fallopian tube proximal and distal to the ectopic gestation is coagulated and cut. The mesosalpinx below the gestation is coagulated and cut.

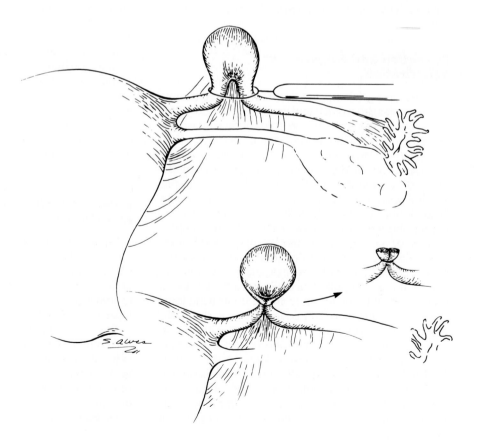

Figure 16–13. Partial salpingectomy using the sterilization technique. The loop is placed beneath the ectopic gestation. The tube above the loop containing the gestation is transected.

fertility remains, however, with tubal reanastomosis at a later time.

Laparoscopic Surgery for Endometriosis

Endometriosis is an enigmatic disease of uncertain etiology and pathophysiology. The clinical presentation of endometriosis is notoriously variable and history or physical findings alone cannot be used reliably for diagnosis. Laparoscopy has enabled the gynecologist to make the diagnosis of endometriosis with relative ease. Its importance in diagnosis and staging is unquestioned and its use as a surgical modality for treatment has become increasingly popular. Laparoscopy is ideally suited for excision, fulguration, or vaporization of implants on peritoneum. Visualization, especially of the posterior cul-de-sac, is improved. Moreover, laparoscopes magnify and can be used to facilitate identity of small proliferative or nonclassical lesions. Surgical procedures can be performed during the initial diagnostic laparoscopy with little increase in morbidity. However, the patient must be properly prepared and appropriate consent signed. This may potentially obviate further need for medical or surgical therapy. An endoscopic procedure also may be performed at a later time after options have been thoroughly discussed with the patient.

Resection and Fulguration/ Vaporization

Small superficial implants can be coagulated (unipolar or bipolar), thermocoagulated, or vaporized. When using bipolar cautery, the operator should grasp the lesion before coagulation. The accuracy of the CO_2 laser in depth of penetration and small lateral spread permits safe vaporization. The small implants are ablated. Because of its selective absorption by hemoglobin-pigmented lesions, the argon laser also has been used. Flexible-fiber lasers such as the KTP-532 are easier to master and will probably be used more frequently.

Laser or scissors can be used to excise the lesions, especially if pathologic confirmation is desired. An incision is made in a nearby normal area of peritoneum. The peritoneum is pulled medially and a blunt probe is used to separate the lesion from the underlying loose connective tissue. This technique is particularly helpful in vascular areas because sharp dissection with scissors or laser may inadvertently divide vessels. For deeper lesions, excision can be taken down to the level of healthy tissue, but this usually requires excision with laser or scissors with cautery. This technique, as described by Martin, is particularly useful for lesions suspected of being deeply penetrating. Fulguration and

vaporization techniques cause tissue distortion, which can be confusing. For example, deep lesions may be incompletely destroyed, especially with bipolar technique. Carbon can be easily confused with endometriosis at second-look laparoscopy; thus, excision may be helpful in deciding whether there is recurrence. Use of high-power density superpulse may decrease carbonization by facilitating vaporization and decreasing lateral spread. Carbon should be removed as much as possible with lavage or by use of pusher sponge.

Ovarian Endometriosis

Small surface endometriomas (< 1 cm) can be "decapitated" at the ovarian endometrioma junction and the base coagulated or vaporized. The resulting defect is not closed. Larger endometriomas (3–5 cm) are resected in a manner similar to that used at laparotomy. Endometriomas > 5 cm can be difficult to handle at laparoscopy, although resection can be accomplished. Data on the incidence of adhesion formation after laparoscopic resection of endometrioma are unavailable.

The cyst is drained and lavaged if desired. The ovarian endometrioma is opened on its axis and in the most dependent portion. The lining is inspected and a relaxing incision made. The plane of the pseudocapsule is identified. Atraumatic grasping forceps are used to hold the ovary and provide countertraction. The cyst wall lining is grasped and dissection carried out with laser, scissors, or blunt probe (Fig. 16-14). Incompletely resected areas may be further coagulated or vaporized. Extreme care must be taken when working near the hilar vessels. An alternate method involves coagulation or vaporization of the lining rather than resection. However, resection is preferable. Simple drainage of endometriomas should be avoided because the recurrence rate is high.

Endometriosis of Bladder, Bowel, and Ureter

Laparotomy has been the standard of surgical therapy for endometriosis and, for cases involving the bowel, bladder, or ureteral wall, it still is. The retroperitoneum, bowel, bladder, and ureter can be difficult to examine at laparoscopy. Palpation is more reliable at laparotomy when compared with laparoscopy.

The most common reason for laparotomy is bowel involvement with tumor in the rectovaginal septum or sidewall. If bowel involvement is suspected before surgery, then the patient should be considered for colonoscopy. The patient should also have the bowel properly prepared for possible repair or anastomosis.

Resection of endometriosis involving the bladder

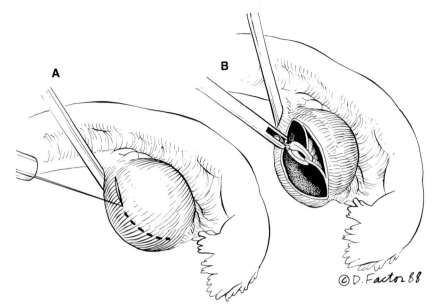

Figure 16–14. Resection of endometrioma cyst wall. *A*, The incision is made in the most dependent portion of the endometrioma in the long axis of the ovary. *B*, The cyst wall lining is stripped by blunt or sharp dissection. Any remaining cyst wall lining is coagulated or vaporized. The ovary is not sutured closed. (Reprinted from Roseff SJ, Murphy AA. Helpful techniques in laser laparoscopy. Contemp OB/GYN 1988; 32:155, with permission.)

wall requires a laparotomy. When endometriosis involves the peritoneum overlying the bladder or ureter, a laparoscopic technique similar to that used during laparotomy is utilized. An incision is made in uninvolved peritoneum away from the ureter. The peritoneum is pulled toward the midline and the ureter is bluntly dissected from the peritoneum. It should be pushed away easily with a blunt probe. Difficulty with this procedure may indicate that the ureter is infiltrated and the procedure should be abandoned laparoscopically. Alternatively, normal saline can be injected below the peritoneum to achieve separation of tissues and facilitate dissection. Electrocautery, laser, or thermocoagulation should not be used on or near the ureter. Direct injury to the ureter or injury due to spread of current or heat may follow.

Laparoscopic Surgery for Adhesive Disease

Fertility-enhancing laparoscopic surgery was reported as early as 1975 by Gomel and others with results comparable with laparotomy. Good results depend on the use of microsurgical technique. This approach represents the philosophy of gentle technique with small instruments and delicate tissue handling. Precise hemostasis should be obtained with minimum coagulation. Magnification is provided by the laparoscope.

Both laparoscopic surgery and laparotomy microsurgery can be time consuming and technically difficult. These procedures are best performed by expert laparoscopists and microsurgeons. Despite lengthy laparoscopic procedures (2–4 hours), most patients are discharged within a day of surgery, have minimal complications, and return to full activity within approximately 1 week of surgery.

Salpingo-Ovariolysis

Adhesions should be incised at both ends and removed from the cavity. Adhesiolysis is best achieved by placing the adhesion on tension by manipulating the uterus or using a probe or forceps through an ancillary site. Microscissors, knife, or laser can be introduced through the operating channel or an ancillary port. Once the adhesion is lysed on one side, the adhesion can be grasped and rolled on the forceps to provide traction.

Pelvic adhesions may differ widely, from thin and avascular to thick, multilayered, and vascular. It is preferable to lyse adhesions sharply; however, it is sometimes safer when the surgeon is dividing closely adherent structures to lyse adhesions bluntly. Multilayered adhesions should be divided one layer at a time to prevent trauma to underlying structures. It is imperative that the surgeon identify pelvic organs such as the bowel and ureter before embarking on extensive resection. Vascular adhesions can be spot-coagulated before sharp excision. It is important to consider the surrounding area of tissue damage associated with the various modalities of hemostasis and to use minimum coagulation. A dilute solution of vasopressin can be instrumental in obtaining spot hemostasis.

Fimbrioplasty/Salpingostomy

Proximal obstruction is not amenable to laparoscopic surgery at this time. Phimotic or clubbed fimbriae may be released through the laparoscope. The distal portion of the tube must be free of adhesions. The tube is distended (chromopertubation) to identify the lumen and the fallopian tube is stabilized with atraumatic forceps. Occasionally, the anterior cul-de-sac and uterus can be used to provide a platform for dissection. If the fimbriae are agglutinated, then forceps or tongs in the closed position may be introduced into the opening and then gently withdrawn. This may be repeated several times in different directions. Gentleness is necessary to avoid excessive trauma and bleeding. Occasionally, fimbrial adhesions should be sharply lysed.

Neosalpingostomy requires that the end of the tube be free of adhesions. The area of the dimple is incised sharply or with the laser (high-power density). Relaxing incisions in areas of scar are then made as is commonly done at laparotomy. This may be all that is necessary to expose the fimbriated end. Eversion also may be accomplished by grasping the luminal surface gently and using another forceps to evert the edges. Sutures of 4-0 PDS may be placed using intra-abdominal or extracorporeal technique. The CO_2 laser technique consists of applying a defocused beam of low-power density to the serosal surface (Fig. 16-15). The beam is moved continuously over the serosal area to limit damage to the tube. Absorption of water causes contraction of the serosal surface and a "flowering," exposing more muscosal area. The different techniques have not been compared.

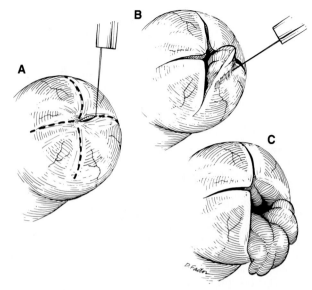

Figure 16–15. Neosalpingostomy using CO_2 laser. *A,* The initial incision is made in the area of dimple. The relaxing incisions are made along the areas of scar. This may be all that is necessary to expose the fimbriae. *B,* A defocused beam of low-power density may be "swept" along the serosal surface to effect eversion. *C,* The fimbriae are everted all the way around as the serosa contracts. (Reprinted from Roseff SJ, Murphy AA. Helpful techniques in laser laparoscopy. Contemp OB/GYN 1988; 32:164, with permission.)

Second-look Laparoscopy

Second-look laparoscopy after reconstructive surgery is frequently combined with an operative procedure. These second tuboplasties have traditionally been performed at 1 year. The results obtained with operative laparoscopy appear to be at least as successful as laparotomy with the advantage of little added morbidity to the diagnostic procedure.

Early second-look laparoscopy (1–12 weeks) after reconstructive surgery is controversial. Lysis of adhesions during this period, especially before 10 days following the procedure, is quite easy because the adhesions are filmy and avascular. No complications have been reported from early postoperative laparoscopy, although precautions should be taken not to place the ancillary probe in the previous incision. Trimbos-Kemper and associates and Jansen performed "third"-look laparoscopy to assess results of very early (8–21 days) second-look laparoscopy. Both studies found that at least 50% of adhesions lysed at second-look laparoscopy did not re-form. Moreover, they showed that adhesions would have been little improved without the postoperative laparoscopy regardless of whether adhesions were present at the first surgery. Although the evidence is suggestive, the prognostic or therapeutic benefit (increase in pregnancy rates) remains to be established.

Ovarian Biopsy/Wedge Resection

Biopsy of the ovary may be necessary to confirm or identify suspicious lesions. Two instruments are available: (1) a punch biopsy forceps and (2) drill forceps. These instruments are described in the section on ancillary instruments. Use of this technique to rule out resistant ovary syndrome in patients with premature ovarian failure is controversial. Many surgeons believe that only a true wedge resection is an adequate reflection of the true histologic features of the ovary. Because pregnancies have been documented in patients with bilateral afollicular biopsies, the indications for this procedure are few. The ovaries are usually quite small and require excision or biopsy with extreme care.

Wedge-like resections may be performed using a knife or scissors. Coagulation may be subsequently obtained with cautery or thermocoagulation.

Therapeutic multiple biopsies or wedge resection also have been recommended for patients with polycystic ovarian disease resistant to standard ovulation-induction regimens. Therapeutic multiple biopsies consist of puncturing and coagulating all visible follicles on the cortex or performing a punch biopsy.

Ovarian Cystectomy

A persistent simple cyst shown on sonography to have no external excrescences or adhesions can be aspirated. The cyst is opened and the wall is closely inspected. If the cyst wall is not suspicious, then cystectomy is performed in the same manner as that described for endometrioma. Alternatively, if the cyst wall is suspicious, then multiple biopsies of the wall may be obtained and sent for frozen section. Ovarian cysts with septa or internal echoes are not candidates for laparoscopic cystectomy. If viscid or mucinous fluid is aspirated, then the puncture should be sealed and a laparotomy should be performed. Solid tumors or tumors with a solid component should not be attempted through the laparoscope.

Adnexectomy/Oophorectomy

Two techniques for laparoscopic adnexectomy/oophorectomy have been described. The most commonly used procedure involves placement of three Roeder loops around the ovary or adnexa (Fig. 16-16). Before placement of the loops, the structures must be free of adhesions. Incisions in the mesosalpinx are sometimes necessary to facilitate placement. The adnexa is cut distal to the three loops. Small bleeding points may be coagulated on the stump but care must be taken not to coagulate the suture. However, this is rarely necessary. Alternatively, the infundibulopelvic ligament is isolated as is done at the beginning of a laparotomy oophorectomy. The "ligament" is then coagulated with bipolar forceps and transected. It is essential that the ureter be identified before coagulation. Lactated Ringer's or saline may be injected into the retroperitoneal space to help push the ureter away from the site of coagulation and increase the margin of safety. The mesosalpinx is then coagulated and cut in

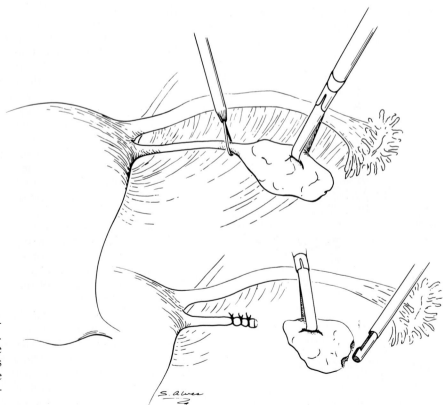

Figure 16–16. Laparoscopic oophorectomy using loop technique. Three loops are placed around the ovary encompassing the vessels and utero-ovarian ligament. The ovary is cut and morcellated if desired and appropriate.

the same manner as described for salpingectomy. The proximal fallopian tube and utero-ovarian ligament are coagulated before transection. The tissue is removed from the pelvis by any of the previously described methods.

Myomectomy

Pedunculated myomas are easily resected by coagulating the base using thermocoagulation or cautery. The myoma is transected from its base and morcellated or cut if necessary (Fig. 16-17). The defect is usually not sutured. Intramural myomas are not commonly done through the laparoscope. Instead, they are resected by first coagulating over the area to be opened if scissors are to be used. The incision is made with scissors or laser. The edges are held open with atraumatic graspers. The myoma is grasped with traumatic forceps for good traction and dissection is carried out most easily with the myoma enucleator (Fig. 16-18). This blunt bladelike instrument is attached to the thermo-coagulator. Enucleation can also be carried out with cautery or laser. If the CO_2 laser is used, then bipolar cautery should be available to obtain hemostasis when large vessels are encountered. If desired, the defect can be closed using the previously described suturing technique. Submucosal myomas should not be attempted

through the laparoscope. They are more appropriately approached through the hysteroscope. Large myomas should not be attempted when visualization is obscured due to size or location. Adhesion formation after laparoscopic myomectomy has not been studied adequately.

Uterine Suspension

Uterine suspension has become an infrequent primary operation; however, it is still occasionally used and may be performed through the laparoscope. Bilateral incisions 3 cm in length are made on the skin lateral to the inferior epigastric vessels and above the inguinal ligament. Forceps are then used to grasp the round ligament and bring it anteriorly so that it may be sutured to the anterior abdominal wall or fascia. Care must be taken not to avulse the ligament as it is brought out to the anterior abdominal wall.

COMPLICATIONS OF LAPAROSCOPY

Complications of diagnostic laparoscopy are many and well known. Meticulous adherence to proper technique is essential to prevent complications. Nevertheless, some complications such as those associated with the blind insertion of the trocar may be unavoidable.

Most major complications of laparoscopy are associated with trocar insertion or induction of pneumoperitoneum. Extraperitoneal insufflation occurs when the Veress needle fails to enter the peritoneal cavity. When the misplacement is recognized, the CO_2 is allowed to escape and the needle reinserted. The emphysema resolves spontaneously. If the preperitoneal insufflation extends to the mediastinum, then mediastinal emphysema is seen. Mediastinal emphysema is usually recognized by the anesthetist, who has difficulty ventilating the patient. As much gas as possible is allowed to escape and the patient is carefully monitored. Severe cases may require assisted ventilation. Pneumothorax is a rare complication and occurs with inadvertent insufflation of the pleural cavity when an upper abdominal site is chosen for insufflation. Emphysema of the omentum is usually a self-limited problem but may make visualization of the abdomino-pelvic structures more difficult.

The Veress needle or principal trocar may penetrate viscus or blood vessel. Meticulous attention to emptying of the bladder should make penetration of the bladder avoidable unless it is adhered. Stomach penetration usually occurs after difficult intubations, resulting in distention of the organ. If tympany is noted or doubt exists, then a nasogastric tube should be passed.

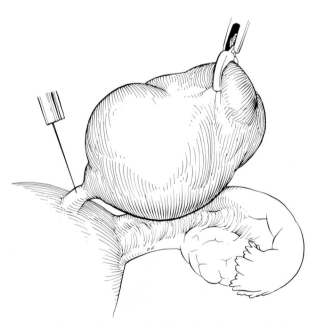

Figure 16–17. Excision of pedunculated myoma. The base is thoroughly coagulated and cut. (Reprinted from Roseff SJ, Murphy AA. Helpful techniques in laser laparoscopy. Contemp OB/GYN 1988; 32:168, with permission.)

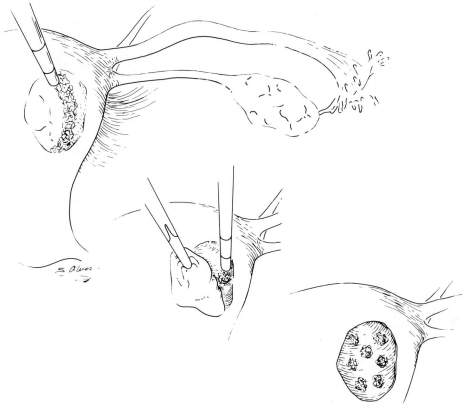

Figure 16–18. Intramural myomectomy. *Left*, The serosal surface is coagulated and cut. The pseudocapsule is identified. *Center*, The myoma is grasped and dissected using a blunt point coagulator or myoma enucleator. *Right*, The base is coagulated to achieve hemostasis. The defect may be left open or closed with suture.

The "syringe test" usually permits early recognition of stomach or bowel penetration. However, the test is not infallible. If a penetration is suspected, then the needle is withdrawn and insufflation attempted at another site. Once the laparoscope is inserted, the site of penetration is carefully examined. Through-and-through penetrations must be looked for and thoroughly evaluated because they tend to be more often associated with peritoneal soiling of bowel contents, which requires immediate corrective surgery. Most needle injuries do not require laparotomy and should be closely monitored. Trocar injury more often results in injury that must be surgically corrected. If the laparoscope enters the lumen, then it should be left in place to limit peritoneal soiling and facilitate identification of the injured site. In rare instances, the bowel is entered with the trocar only and not the sleeve. This type of injury may be easily missed because it is not suspected. Injuries to liver and spleen are unusual and associated with enlargement of the organs or upper abdominal entry site. Puncture, penetration, or laceration invariably require

surgical intervention because the organs are very vascular.

The Veress needle or trocar may traumatize omental or mesenteric blood vessels or any of the major abdominal or pelvic arteries or veins. Elevating the anterior abdominal wall and pointing the needle or trocar toward the sacrum may avoid most of these serious complications. Thin, small patients are at particular risk. Minor injuries may be observed. Injury to omental vessels may be coagulated. Major vessel injury usually requires immediate laparotomy, transfusion, and vascular repair. Injury to mesenteric vessels also may lead to compromise of a segment of bowel and bowel resection. Rarely, a penetrating injury to blood vessels is not recognized at the time of insufflation and may lead to gas embolism and death. The anesthetist should recognize the classic millwheel murmur that can be heard over the precordium.

These complications, of course, are pertinent to operative laparoscopy as well. However, operative laparoscopy has complications unique to it, including mechanical, electrical, heat, or laser-induced injury or bleeding.

All pelvic and retroperitoneal structures may be damaged during operative procedures by any of the ancillary instruments used, which include scissors, probes, and forceps. Blunt probes can cause trauma to bowel, bladder, ureter, cysts, and pelvic organs during dissection when too much force is used. Ureters may be easily damaged during dissection of ovaries adherent to the pelvic sidewall.

Sharp dissection of poorly visualized or identified structures may cause significant damage. Direct injury to bowel or ureter is much less common with dissection than injury to the vascular supply of the tissue. Most of the direct injuries occur during blind insertion of the Veress needle or trocar. Ancillary puncture sites should be placed under direct visualization to avoid these injuries. Extensive bowel dissection also may lead to postoperative ileus, which resolves in a few days.

Complications related to the use of electrosurgical instruments in laparoscopic surgery are well known. Major injuries such as skin burns, burns to intra-abdominal structures such as the bowel, and operator burns are reported; however, it is likely that minor complications are probably not reported or even suspected at times. Occult extension of tissue coagulation can cause injury to distant sites and subsequent necrosis that is not immediately evident.

Burns can be caused by direct contact of electrical or thermal energy with the organ or tissue. Some accidents occur because the field of vision is incomplete and bowel may come in contact with a charged or heated instrument without the surgeon becoming aware of it. Damage to bowel is most serious and needs to be assessed carefully. Minor injury may be observed, but frank perforation and extensive burn lead to bowel resection and colostomy in cases of damage to unprepared bowel. With electrical injury, the full extent of damage may not become immediately obvious. Occult electrical damage that may occur 2 to 3 cm distal to the burn should be remembered.

Arcs of sparks may occur in unipolar cautery as the electrons attempt to return to the dispersive electrode. As coagulation occurs, the resistance can increase, causing an interruption between the electrode and the return plate. As a consequence, arcs of sparks may occur, resulting in obvious or occult burns. The laparoscope, through which the active electrode passes, can act as a capacitor and store electrical energy. An unexpected contact with bowel or other organ may cause a burn.

Laser-induced injury to organs can result from accidental activation of the laser while aiming at the wrong target, penetrating past the actual target, and striking targets close to the true target. The surgeon may strike targets close to the true target as a result of misalign-

ment of the helium CO_2 beam, which causes the energy to hit lateral to the intended target. Accidental exposure is particularly related to repairing and aligning the equipment. In addition, safety glasses are required for the staff. The CO_2 laser will cause a surface burn to the eye. The Nd:YAG and argon lasers will penetrate to the retina. Exposure to carbon plume should be avoided because it is an irritant. It is also mutagenic in salmonella.

Bleeding accounts for approximately half of all the complications associated with laparoscopy and may include bleeding from superficial vessels to massive hemorrhage from lacerations of retroperitoneal vessels. Most of these injuries are associated with blind entry of the Veress needle or trocar. Bleeding injuries complicating a laparoscopic surgical procedure are usually related to the operator's technical skills. Tears to the oviduct, mesosalpinx, and infundibulopelvic ligament may occur from efforts to stabilize the structure or dissection. Medium vessel injury is best controlled with cautery and bipolar in particular. Minimum damage is caused if the vessel walls are grasped before coagulation. Irrigation may be necessary to pinpoint the source. Thermocoagulation may be substituted. If the bleeding site can be isolated, then a loop may be placed. The CO_2 laser, however, is not an effective coagulator of vessels >2 mm. Laparotomy to control bleeding is rarely necessary.

Abdominal wall hemorrhage is more common with operative laparoscopy because multiple ancillary sites are used, often outside the midline. Persistent bleeding can be controlled with coagulation. Rarely, the bleeding does not respond and the puncture site needs to be enlarged so that the specific cause can be located. Transillumination of the anterior abdominal wall before insertion of the puncture site should decrease trauma to large vessels such as the inferior epigastric artery and vein.

Semm reported a 0.28% overall complication rate in 8943 laparoscopies, of which 6114 were operative cases. The complications consisted of 13 cases of vessel damage, 9 cases of bowel or stomach puncture, 1 case of ureteral damage, and 2 cases of cardiac arrest. Ten laparotomies were performed because of complications (0.11%). No deaths were reported.

Operative laparoscopy is a safe technique when guidelines are observed and the surgeon is aware of the limitations of the technique. The advantages of a laparoscopic procedure are obvious. There is decreased morbidity after operative laparoscopy and the risks and complications of surgery appear to be at least equivalent to laparotomy. Additionally, the procedures appear to be as effective through the laparoscope as they are performed through a laparotomy, although conclusive data are unavailable. There is general agreement that operative laparoscopy is an important technique in the armamentarium of the gynecologic or reproductive surgeon.

Bibliography

Bahig CS. Electrosurgical burn injuries and their prevention. JAMA 1968;204:1025.

Borten M. Laparoscopic complications: prevention and management. Toronto: B.C. Decker Inc., 1986.

Bruhat MA, Manhes H, Mage G, et al. Treatment of ectopic pregnancy by means of laparoscopy. Fertil Steril 1980;33:411.

Cheng YS. Ureteral injury resulting from laparoscopic fulguration of endometriotic implant. Am J Obstet Gynecol 1976;126:1045.

Daniell JF, Herbert CM. Laparoscopic salpingostomy utilizing the CO_2 laser. Fertil Steril 1984;41:558.

Daniell JF, Meisels S, Miller W, et al. Laparoscopic use of the KTP/532 laser in nonendometriotic pelvic surgery. Colpos and Gynecol Laser Surg 1986;2:107.

Daniell JF, Pittaway DE, Maxson WS. The role of laparoscopic adhesiolysis and an in vitro fertilization program. Fertil Steril 1983;40:49.

DeCherney AH. The leader of the band is tired. Fertil Steril 1985;44:299.

DeCherney AH, Boyers SP. Isthmic ectopic pregnancy: segmental resection as the treatment of choice. Fertil Steril 1985;44:307.

DeCherney AH, Kase N. The conservative management of unruptured ectopic pregnancy. Obstet Gynecol 1979;54:451.

Doyle JB, Des Rosiers JJ. Paracervical uterine denervation for relief of pelvic pain. Clin Obstet Gynecol 1963;6:742.

Dubuisson JB, Aubriot FX. Laparoscopic salpingectomy for tubal pregnancy. Fertil Steril 1987;47:225.

Esposito JM. The laparoscopist and electro-surgery. Am J Obstet Gynecol 1976;126:633.

Fayez JA. An assessment of the role of operative laparoscopy in tuboplasty. Fertil Steril 1983;39:476.

Feste JR. CO_2 laser neurectomy for dysmenorrhea. Laser Surg Med 1984;3:327.

Feste JR. Laser laparoscopy—a new modality. J Reprod Med 1985;30:413.

Gjonnaess H. Polycystic ovarian syndrome treated by ovarian electrocautery through the laparoscope. Fertil Steril 1984;41:2.

Gomel V. Laparoscopic tubal surgery in infertility. Obstet Gynecol 1975;46:47.

Gomel V. Salpingostomy by laparoscopy. J Reprod Med 1977;18:265.

Gomel V. Salpingo-ovariolysis by laparoscopy in infertility. Fertil Steril 1983;40:607.

Gomel V, Taylor PJ. Surgical endoscopy. In: Gomel V, Taylor PJ, Yuzpe AA, et al, eds. Laparoscopy and hysteroscopy in gynecologic practice. Chicago: Year Book Medical Publishers, 1986:140.

Gomel V, Taylor PJ. The technique of endoscopy. In: Gomel V, Taylor PJ, Yuzpe AA, et al, eds. Laparoscopy and hysteroscopy in gynecologic practice. Chicago: Year Book Medical Publishers, 1986:32.

Gomel V, Taylor PJ, Yuzpe AA, et al. Indications, contraindication, complications. In: Gomel V, Taylor PH, Yuzpe AA, et al, eds. Laparoscopy and hysteroscopy in gynecologic practice. Chicago: Year Book Medical Publishers, 1986:56.

Hasson HM. Electrocoagulation of pelvic endometriotic lesions of endometriosis at laparoscopy for infertility. Am J Obstet Gynecol 1979;135:115.

Henry-Suchet J, Soler A, Loffredo V. Laparoscopic treatment of tuboovarian abscesses. J Reprod Med 1984;29:579.

Jansen RPS. Early laparoscopy after pelvic operations to prevent adhesions: safety and efficacy. Fertil Steril 1988;49(1):26.

Johns DA, Hardie RP. Management of unruptured ectopic pregnancy with laparoscopic carbon dioxide laser. Fertil Steril 1986;46(4):703.

Keye WR Jr, Dixon J. Photocoagulation of endometriosis by the argon laser through the laparoscope. Obstet Gynecol 1983;62:282.

Lauritsen JG, Pagel JD, Vangsted P, et al. Results of repeated tuboplasties. Fertil Steril 1982;37:68.

Levine RL. Economic impact of pelviscopic surgery. J Reprod Med 1985;30:655.

Lomano JM. Photocoagulation of early pelvic endometriosis with ND:YAG laser through the laparoscope. J Rep Med 1985;30:77.

Jones HW Jr, Rock JA. Reparative and constructive surgery of the female generative tract. Baltimore: Williams & Wilkins, 1983:72.

Mann WJ, Stenger VG. Uterine suspension through the laparoscope. Obstet Gynecol 1978;51:563.

Martin D. Avoid laparotomy using laser laparoscopy. Contemp Obstet Gynecol 1985;25:101.

Martin DC. CO_2 laser laparoscopy for endometriosis associated with infertility. J Reprod Med 1986;31(12):121.

Martin DC, Diamond MP. Operative laparoscopy: comparison of lasers with other techniques. Curr Prob Obstet Gynecol Fertil 1986;9:564.

McLaughlin DS. Metroplasty and myomectomy with CO_2 laser for the preservation of normal tissue and minimizing blood loss. J Rep Med 1985;30:1.

Mettler L, Giesel H, Semm K. Treatment of female infertility due to tubal obstruction by operative laparoscopy. Fertil Steril 1979;32:384.

Murphy AA. Operative laparoscopy. Fertil Steril 1987;47:6.

Murphy AA, Nager CW. Laparoscopic management of ectopic pregnancy. Contemp Obstet Gynecol 1988;32(2):102.

Olive DL, Martin DC. Treatment of endometriosis-associated infertility with CO_2 laser laparoscopy: the use of one- and two-parameter exponential models. Fertil Steril 1987;48:18.

Palmer R. Sterilisation per-coelioscopique (avec film). Presse Méd 1962;70:1106.

Patterson MEL, Jordan JA, Logan-Edwards R. A survey of 100 patients who had laparoscopic ventro suspension. Br J Obstet Gynaecol 1978;85:468.

Portuondo JA, Melchor JC, Neyro JL, et al. Periovarian adhesions following ovarian wedge resection or laparoscopic biopsy. Endoscopy 1984;16:143.

Pouly JL, Mahnes H, Mage G, et al. Conservative laparoscopic treatment of 321 ectopic pregnancies. Fertil Steril 1986;46:1093.

Pring DW. Inferior epigastric haemorrhage, an avoidable complication of laparoscopic clip sterilization. Br J Obstet Gynaecol 1983;90:480.

Raj SG, Hulka JF. Second-look laparoscopy in infertility surgery: therapeutic and prognostic value. Fertil Steril 1982;38:325.

Reich H, Johns DA, DeCaprio J, et al. Laparoscopic treatment of 109 consecutive ectopic pregnancies. J Repro Med 1988;33:885.

Reich H, McGlynn F. Laparoscopic oophorectomy and salpingo-oophorectomy in the treatment of benign tubo-ovarian disease. J Rep Med 1986;31:609.

Reich H, McGlynn F. Treatment of ovarian endometriomas using laparoscopic surgical techniques. J Reprod Med 1986;31:577.

Roseff SJ, Murphy AA. Laser laparoscopy. Contemp Obstet Gynecol 1988;32:149.

Schwartz RO, Martin JB. Laparoscopic salpingectomy for ectopic pregnancy. South Med J 1985;78:1341.

Semm K. Endocoagulator: new possibilities for tubal surgery via pelviscopy. Excerpta Medica 1974;370:242.

Semm K. Tissue-puncher and loop ligation: new aids for surgical-therapeutic pelviscopy. Endoscopy 1978;10:119.

Semm K. New methods of pelviscopy for myomectomy, ovariectomy, tubectomy and adnectomy. Endoscopy 1979;2:85.

Semm K. Endoscopic appendectomy. Endoscopy 1983;15:59.

Semm K. Endoscopic intraabdominal surgery. Kiel: Christian-Albrects-Universitat, 1984:4.

Semm K, Mettler L. Technical progress in pelvic surgery via operative laparoscopy. Am J Obstet Gynecol 1980;138:121.

Shapiro HI, Adler DH. Excision of an ectopic pregnancy through the laparoscope. Am J Obstet Gynecol 1973;117:290.

Soderstrom RM. Unusual uses of laparoscopy. J Reprod Med 1975;15:77.

Stangel JJ, Gomel V. Techniques in conservative surgery for tubal gestation. Clin Obstet Gynecol 1980;23:1221.

Steptoe PC. Laparoscopy in gynecology. Edinburgh, Scotland: E & S Livingstone, 1967:1.

Sulewski JM, Curcio FD, Bronitsky C, et al. The treatment of endometriosis at laparoscopy for infertility. Am J Obstet Gynecol 1980;138:128.

Sumioki H, Utsunomyiya T, Matsuoka K, et al. The effect of laparoscopic multiple punch resection of the ovary on hypothalamic-pituitary axis in polycystic ovary syndrome. Fertil Steril 1988;50:567.

Surrey MW, Friedman S. Second-look laparoscopy after reconstructive pelvic surgery for infertility. J Reprod Med 1982;27:658.

Tarasconi JC. Endoscopic salpingectomy. J Reprod Med 1981;26:541.

Taylor PJ, Gomel V. Introduction. In: Gomel V, Taylor PJ, Yuzpe AA, et al, eds. Laparoscopy and hysteroscopy in gynecologic practice. Chicago: Year Book Medical Publishers, 1986:1.

Trimbos-Kemper TCM, Trimbos JB, van Hall EV. Adhesion formation after tubal surgery: results of the eight-day laparoscopy in 188 patients. Fertil Steril 1985;43:395.

Yuzpe AA, Gomel V, Taylor PJ. Endoscopy in the patient with endometriosis. In: Gomel V, Taylor PJ, Yuzpe AA, et al, eds. Laparoscopy and hysteroscopy in gynecologic practice. Chicago: Year Book Medical Publishers, 1986:111.

Yuzpe AA, Gomel V, Taylor PJ, et al. Instruments for laparoscopy and hysteroscopy. In: Gomel V, Taylor PJ, Yuzpe AA, et al, eds. Laparoscopy and hysteroscopy in gynecologic practice. Chicago: Year Book Medical Publishers, 1986:7.

Operative Hysteroscopy

MICHAEL S. BAGGISH

Hysteroscopy permits direct assessment of the endocervical canal and uterine cavity. Although hysteroscopy, as described by Pantaleoni in 1869, was one of the earliest endoscopic procedures to be performed in gynecology, the technique did not incite substantial interest within the specialty until the latter part of the 1970s. Like several other techniques practiced through the years, dilatation and curettage (D & C) as a means for assessing intrauterine disease has been held in high esteem, despite its documented inaccuracies as a diagnostic tool. Similarly, few practitioners have delved into the possible risks of blind D & C, that is, the dissemination of malignant cells in cases of endometrial carcinoma as documented by Roberts, Long, and Jonasson.

During the past two decades, the thrust of modern gynecologic practice has veered to viewing abnormal tissues directly or at least localizing the pathology accurately to sample directly the site most likely to render positive results. This change in philosophy spawned procedures such as colposcopy, laparoscopy, and hysteroscopy. During the 1980s, gynecology experienced other drastic changes, with an increasing proportion of operations being done using the endoscope.

A low-risk endoscopic technique, hysteroscopy uses natural passages to enter the endometrial cavity by way of the endocervical canal. Refinement of optical and fiberoptic instrumentation, together with accessories, has elevated the hysteroscopic view to a high order of resolution and has allowed excellent visual documentation. Tremendous advances have been made in operative hysteroscopy. Procedures to treat septate uteri, such as those procedures advocated by Jones and Jones as well as Strassman, now are considered obsolete unless there is a broad septum. New techniques for ablation of the endometrium as an alternative to hysterectomy have been reported by Baggish and Baltoyannis, Goldrath, Fuller, and Segal, and Lomano. Reports by Neuwirth, Neuwirth and Amin, and DeCherney and Polan document their techniques for hysteroscopic management of removal or obliteration of submucous myoma. Other new techniques discussed in the recent literature include precise cutting of synechiae, reported by March and Israel, and office sterilization, reported by Reed and Erb. Areas of development now undergoing feasibility studies include cannulation of the tube for retrograde placement of an ovum (ie, a reverse gamete intrafallopian tube transfer procedure for women with obstructed oviducts); direct treatment of endometrial carcinoma by ablation or by photodynamic therapy before hysterectomy; and direct local injection of progesterone in cases of intractable bleeding secondary to submucous myomas.

INSTRUMENTATION

Telescopes

The best light shower and clearest optics consistent with the smallest outside diameter are most attainable when the 4-mm telescope is selected. Most commercial telescopes subtend a visual angle of 82°; however, wide-angle optics, which provide a much larger field, subtend an angle of 105°. Although 2-mm and 3-mm diameter telescopes are available, they sacrifice either lighting, optics, or both. Telescopes are usually available as 0°—straight-on view—or 30°—fore-oblique view (Fig. 17-1A). The telescope can be divided into three parts: (1) eyepiece, (2) barrel, and (3) objective lens (Fig. 17-1B). Surrounding the optics are numerous small-diameter incoherent fiberoptic bundles that provide intense, cold light to the operative field. Currently, a few manufacturers offer a choice of fixed-focus or variable-focus telescopes. The variable-focus technique exposes points < 1 mm from the objective lens to

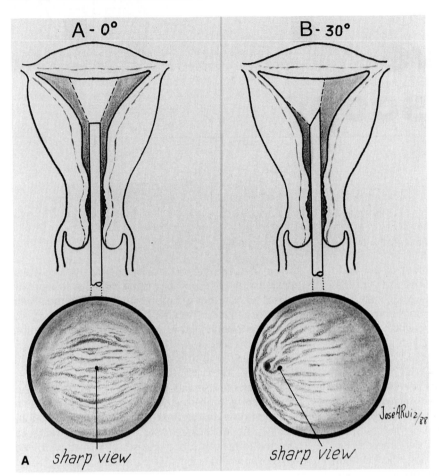

Figure 17–1. *A*, Telescopes are available with either straight-on (0°) or fore-oblique (30°) viewing objective lenses. *B*, A telescope may be conveniently subdivided into three parts: eyepiece, barrel, and objective lens. (Reprinted from Baggish MS, Barbot J, Valle RF. Diagnostic and operative hysteroscopy. Chicago: Year Book Medical Publishers, 1989, with permission.)

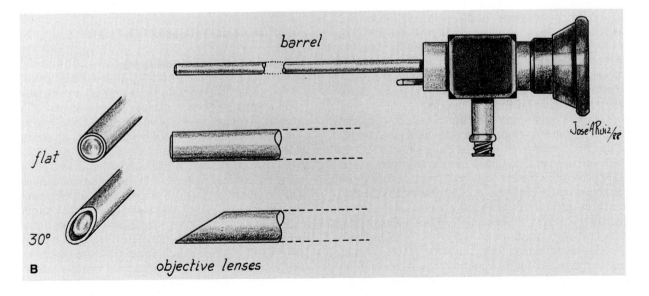

magnification and even allows light contact with the endometrium (contact hysteroscopy). The accrued benefit of the magnified or contact capability is the ability to study vascular and structural details of the tissues.

Light Generators

The quality and power of light delivered to the telescope depend on the wattage and characteristics of the remote light generator as well as the type and structural integrity of the connecting fiberoptic light cable. Three general types of light generators are available: (1) tungsten, (2) metal halide, and (3) xenon. The simplest and cheapest generator is the tungsten generator, which produces orange/yellow-tinged light; the metal halide is a powerful generator that provides sufficient light for still and television photography but casts a bluish tinge to the field. The most intense illumination is given off by the xenon light source. The xenon generator, which provides clear, white light, provides the best shower for video imaging (Fig. 17-2).

Fiberoptic light cables must be intact to convey the optimal light from the generator to the telescope. Broken fibers can be identified easily by viewing the stretched-out cable against a dark background and looking for light emitting through the sides of the cable. The liquid cable conducts light effectively and, when combined with a xenon generator, provides superior light.

Diagnostic and Operative Sheaths

To perform panoramic hysteroscopy, a sheath is required to deliver the distending medium into the uterine cavity. Types of sheaths used for hysteroscopic procedures are shown in Fig. 17-3. Sheaths are either diagnostic or operative. The 5-mm diagnostic sheath fitted with a single stopcock is all that is required for simple evaluation of the uterine cavity. The 5-mm instrument allows easy access through the narrow endocervical canal and past the point of maximal constriction, the internal os cervix. This canal can be negotiated safely under direct vision without fear of perforation. The telescope must couple securely to the hysteroscopic sheath. When the coupling is imprecise, leakage of medium will occur at the interface.

The operative sheath must necessarily be of greater diameter than the diagnostic sheath. When the sheath exceeds 6 mm, the cervix will frequently require dilatation. Most operating sheaths measure 7 mm to 8 mm in diameter. Not only the telescope but also manipulating devices and operating accessory instruments may be inserted through the operating cannula (Fig 17-4A). The operating channel must be sealed with a rubber nipple or gasket (Fig. 17-5) to prevent leakage of distending medium around the entry channel.

Recently, a new type of operating sheath has been invented, according to Baggish. This sheath is constructed with two separate operating channels, an isolated channel for the telescope, and a fourth channel for medium instillation. Isolated channels have the unique advantage of allowing the uterine cavity to be flushed of blood and other debris while maintaining the telescope in situ. The two operating channels permit an aspirating tube plus an operating instrument to be inserted into the uterine cavity simultaneously. Although dilatation is usually required for insertion of the larger operating sheaths, occasionally they may negotiate the internal os sans dilatation in multiparous women.

Accessory Instruments

A variety of operating accessories are available as rigid, semirigid, or flexible instruments. These include grasping (alligator-jaw) forceps, cup biopsy forceps, and scissors. Another handy accessory is a long, flexible needle that can be used for manipulation as well as for the injection of solutions (eg, vasopressin) into lesions. The semirigid and flexible accessories are designed to fit through the access channel(s) of the operating

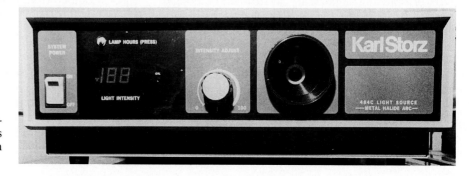

Figure 17–2. The most powerful light source that provides clear, white light is the xenon generator.

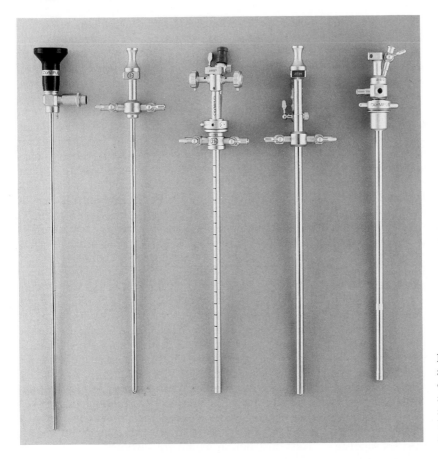

Figure 17–3. Several sheaths are available for hysteroscopic procedures. To the left from the telescope are: (1) a 5-mm diagnostic sheath; (2) an operating sheath with a deflecting bridge; (3) two views of a standard single-channel operating sheath.

sheath (Fig. 17-6). The rigid instruments are heavy duty, large devices that are themselves incorporated into the construction of and are essentially part of a specialized sheath (Fig. 17-7). Most hysteroscopists prefer the semi-rigid or flexible instruments because they permit back-and-forth movement, affording either a panoramic or a close-up view of the operative field. The rigid instruments, because of their fixed position close to the objective lens of the telescope, permit only a close-up view of the field. Although beginners seldom use them, aspirating cannulae measuring 2.0 mm in diameter are always used by experienced endoscopists. The advantages of aspirating cannulae are akin to those of sponges at the operative site and they are indispensable for clearing an otherwise cloudy field (Fig. 17-8).

The Contact Hysteroscope

Among all modern hysteroscopes only one instrument requires neither a sheath nor a distending medium. The contact hysteroscope (Fig. 17-9) is a unique instrument that is available for diagnostic purposes only, as described by Baggish and Dorsey and by Barbot and associates. The contact hysteroscope traps and transmits ambient light directed onto a special light-trapping mechanism. Because actual contact is made with the mucosa and the cavity of the endocervix and endometrium is viewed in its natural, collapsed state, bleeding will not interfere with vision when using this instrument. Unique procedures such as embryoscopy are ideally performed with the contact hysteroscope (Fig. 17-10).

The view obtained with the contact hysteroscope lies between panoramic vision and microscopy. Diagnoses are based on color, architectural pattern, contour, and touch. Compared with other hysteroscopic techniques, contact hysteroscopy is the easiest to perform but the most difficult to interpret.

The Microhysteroscope

Another specialized endoscope is the microhysteroscope. This instrument converts a panoramic hysteroscope into a high-powered microscope by switching the lens to 150 ×. Light contact is made with the mucous membrane in a fashion analogous to that of the oil-

Figure 17–4. *A*, A single-channel operating sheath consists of a single cavity that the telescope, distending medium, and operating instruments share. O.C., operating channel. (Reprinted from Baggish MS, Barbot J, Valle RF. Diagnostic and operative hysteroscopy. Chicago: Year Book Medical Publishers, 1989, with permission.) *B*, A dual-channel operating sheath is constructed with (*1*) Isolated channels for a telescope, (*2* and *3*) two operating devices, (*4*) distending medium. (Reprinted from Baggish MS, Barbot J, Valle RF. Diagnostic and operative hysteroscopy. Chicago: Year Book Medical Publishers, 1989, with permission.) *C*, Terminal portions of dual-channel operating sheaths accommodate a 0° telescope (*upper*) and a 30° telescope (*lower*).

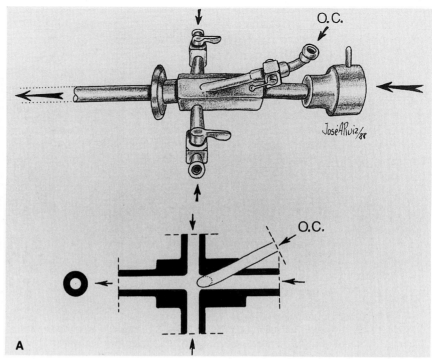

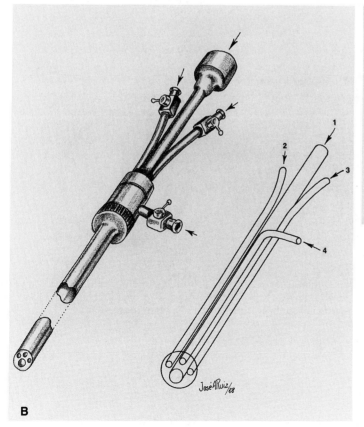

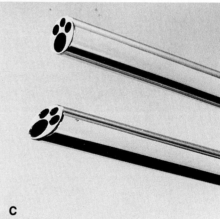

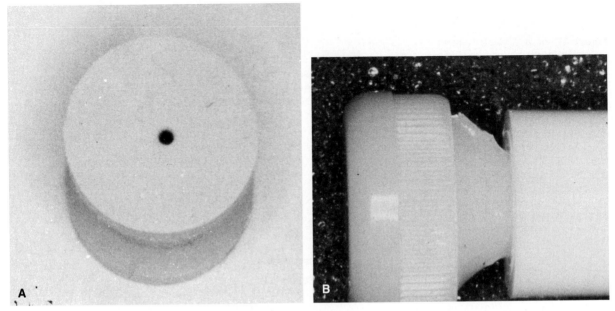

Figure 17–5. Two types of sealing nipples or gaskets fit over the entry port of the operating channel. *A*, Standard urologic nipple. *B*, A new type of Luer-lock leaf valve.

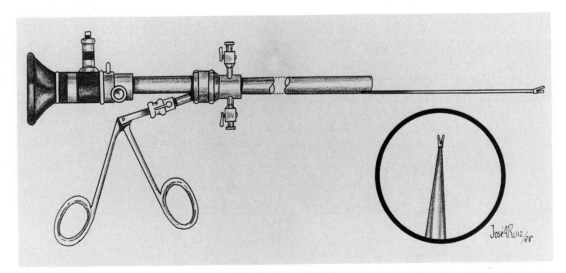

Figure 17–6. Flexible or semirigid operating instruments may be delivered to the operative site by way of the operating channel. *Inset*, Hysteroscopic view of device. (Reprinted from Baggish MS, Barbot J, Valle RF. Diagnostic and operative hysteroscopy. Chicago: Year Book Medical Publishers, 1989, with permission.)

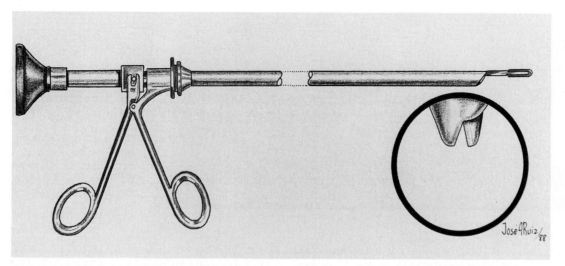

Figure 17–7. Rigid, heavy-duty operating devices form a portion of a specialized sheath. They have the disadvantage of being fixed close to the terminus of the telescope. *Inset*, Hysteroscopic view of device. (Reprinted from Baggish MS, Barbot J, Valle RF. Diagnostic and operative hysteroscopy. Chicago: Year Book Medical Publishers, 1989, with permission.)

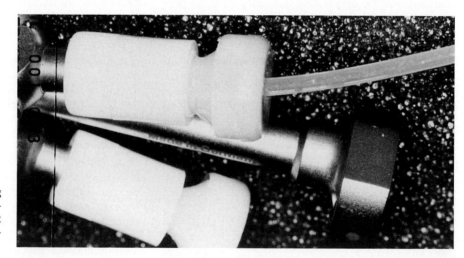

Figure 17–8. An aspirating cannula is inserted into one operating channel. The leaf gasket prevents leakage of the distending medium.

immersion lens of a microscope. A type of in vivo cytology may then be performed, as described in two reports by Hamou. The exact application of this instrument and the technique of microcolpohysteroscopy have eluded American endoscopists to date.

DISTENDING MEDIA

Hyskon (Dextran 70)

Hyskon (32% dextran 70 in dextrose) is a highly viscid solution that is optically clear. The material has the consistency of honey and does not mix with blood.

Once in the uterine cavity, particularly when there is a tight fit between the endoscopic sheath and the cervix, maintenance of distention is easy and affords the endoscopist an exceptionally good view, according to Edstrom and Fernstrom. Additionally, hyskon provides an excellent medium within which to perform operative procedures. Hyskon is generally a safe medium to use. Most diagnostic endeavors may be completed with 100 cc of hyskon or less and most operative hysteroscopic procedures can be completed with 200 cc to 500 cc of hyskon.

Hyskon can be conveniently delivered by a 50-cc syringe by way of a large-gauge plastic connecting tube (Fig. 17-11) attached to the intake port of the hyster-

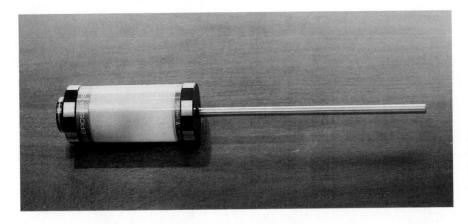

Figure 17–9. The contact hysteroscope is a specialized instrument used for diagnosis only. The cylindrical white chamber traps and transmits ambient light.

oscopic sheath. Recently, a pump has been developed to deliver the material mechanically by way of the hysteroscope into the uterine cavity.

The disadvantages of hyskon relate to its messiness, making it unsuitable for office use. The tendency for its dried residue to harden and clog hysteroscopic sheath channels may be aggravating. Clogging may be prevented by careful and thorough flushing of the instruments with hot water before storage. The most distressing side effect of this medium is the "hyskon reaction," which occurs when the hyskon macromolecules gain

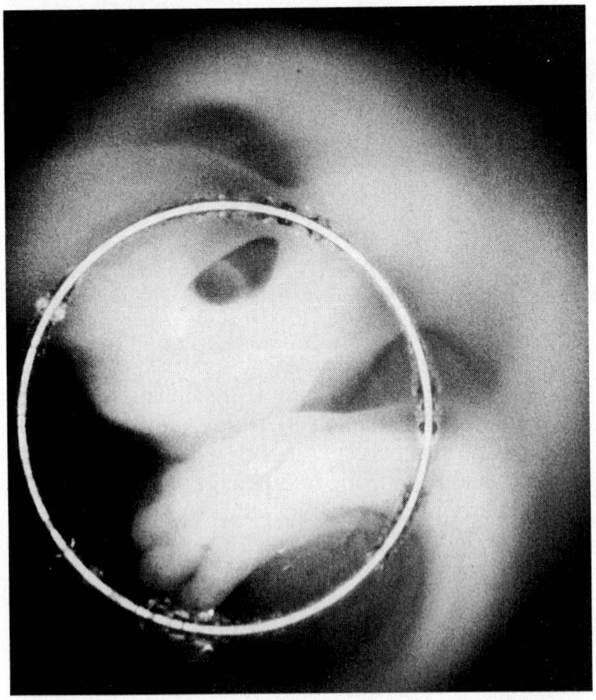

Figure 17–10. A 6-week living embryo viewed by contact hysteroscope. The diameter of the focus circle is 6 mm.

entry into the circulation and accelerate the action of thrombin-converting fibrinogen to fibrin. Plasma levels of both antihemophilic factor (factor VIII) and fibrinogen (factor I) are decreased, as reported by Mishler. The fibrinoplastic effect increases the rate of fibrin formation and polymerization. The thrombi formed are significantly more lysable than are control clots. Likewise, the hyskon is absorbed onto the surface of platelets. Platelet adhesiveness as well as aggregation is decreased. The defect mimics certain clinical features of von Willebrand's disease. Dextran 70 (hyskon) is not hydrolyzed in the bloodstream. It is metabolized following uptake into tissues. Dextran 70 will remain in the bloodstream for approximately 4 to 6 weeks, as detailed in the report by Mishler. These macromolecules also may be removed by glomerular filtration, which accounts for 70% to 80% of the total injected dose. The end result of significant absorption of hyskon is to produce an alarming bleeding diathesis. When the uterine wall is damaged (eg, endometrial ablation), hypervolemia also may occur, with resulting noncardiogenic pulmonary edema. Rarely, an idiosyncratic anaphylactoid reaction may occur. Most commonly, the aforementioned reactions happen when 700 cc or more of hyskon are instilled.

Carbon Dioxide

Carbon dioxide (CO_2) is a colorless gas that is highly soluble when mixed with blood and is a safe medium with which to distend the uterus when instilled with a proper insufflation apparatus, as described by Lindemann. This distention medium is ideal for office hysteroscopy. The hysteroscopic insufflator delivers CO_2 into the uterus at a flow rate measured in cubic centimeters per minute in contrast to the laparoscopic insufflator where CO_2 flows in at the rate of liters per minute. Obviously, the laparoscopic insufflator is both

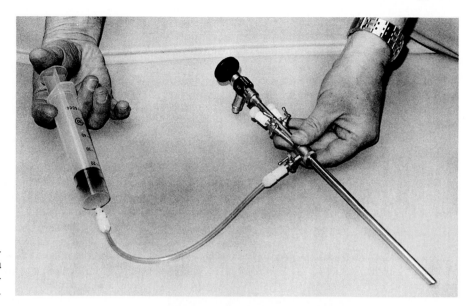

Figure 17–11. Hyskon is delivered by a 50-cc syringe and a special thick-walled (4-mm inside diameter) connecting tube.

unsuitable and unsafe for hysteroscopic insufflation. The rate of flow of CO_2 into the uterus should never exceed 100 cc/min and pressure should be adjusted below 150 mm Hg (Fig. 17-12).

When CO_2 flow is excessive, bubbles appear and obscure the field. Bleeding and CO_2 gas are incompatible; the gas and blood mix, producing an obscuring bubbling foam. CO_2 tends to flatten the endometrium and this artifact may obscure pathology. When CO_2 is improperly instilled, emboli form and can produce severe derangements in cardiovascular physiology.

The best feature in favor of CO_2 is its neatness. It does not foul instruments, it does not mess up the office or operating room, and it allows entry evaluation of the endocervical canal. CO_2 is therefore an excellent diag-

nostic medium, perhaps the best, according to Siegler and Kemmann. However, the liquid media are superior in most aspects for operative hysteroscopy. CO_2 cannot be used to flush the cavity of debris and indeed, if the pressure drops, allowing the walls of the uterus to coapt, bleeding will ensue, making this medium less than advantageous.

Normal Saline, Ringer's Lactate

Normal saline and Ringer's lactate have regained popularity with the advent of the neodymium:yttrium-aluminum-garnet (Nd:YAG) laser ablative procedures. Quinones cites that two advantages of these media are

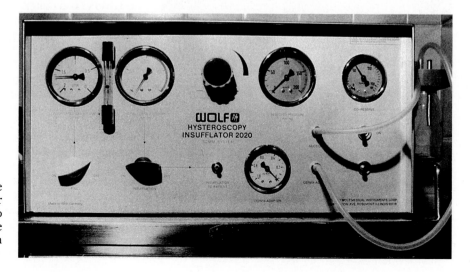

Figure 17–12. CO_2 must be infused by a special insufflator that measures flow rate (not to exceed 100 cc/min) and uterine pressure (not to exceed 150 mm Hg).

their ready and plentiful availability and cheap cost. Plastic bags containing 3 L of a solution may be mounted on an intravenous (IV) pole and enclosed in a pressure bag or wide blood pressure cuff, according to Valle (Fig. 17-13). The bag or cuff is inflated to 60 mm to 100 mm Hg pressure. The flow of medium is delivered to the intake port of the hysteroscopic sheath by standard IV tubing. The cervix must be sufficiently dilated to allow

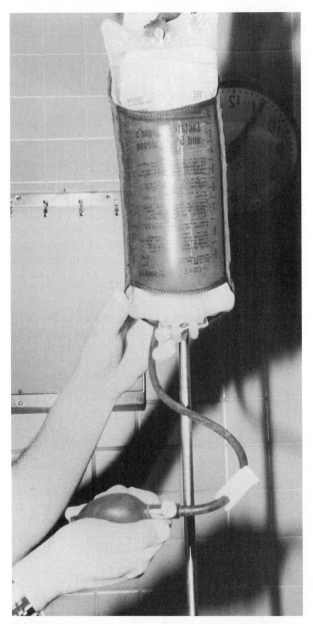

Figure 17–13. Saline, dextrose 5% in water, and Ringer's lactate are enclosed with a pressure cuff and delivered to the medium (intake) port of the hysteroscopic sheath by intravenous tubing.

continuous outflow of the medium, that is, a constant flushing of the cavity. The dual-channel operating sheath is a convenient method to deliver saline because the material may flow into the uterus and conveniently flow out through one of the operating channels. When it is desired to distend the cavity maximally, the valve on the operating channel is simply closed.

Saline and Ringer's lactate easily leak out of the uterus, and distention is difficult to maintain without large volumes of liquid flowing constantly into the cavity. The potential for fluid overload is high; thus, hypotonic material (ie, dextrose 5% in water) is hazardous because it can lead to water intoxication. These materials easily mix with blood and may obscure the operative field. Likewise, because of the large volumes required, the floor may be flooded with water, making these media unsuitable for office use. Recently, drapes have been designed with pockets to trap the overflow fluid and permit easy collection and measurement. Obviously, careful accounting of instilled and exited fluid must be done. Significant complications of saline, lactated Ringer's, or water are circulatory overload and pulmonary edema.

Electrolyte solutions are dangerous when used during operative hysteroscopy with electrical devices such as resectoscopes. In such cases, the electrical current can and will be conducted through the medium, posing risks of electrical shock to patient and endoscopist alike. When used with the Nd : YAG laser, this medium is perfectly safe and acceptable.

For operative hysteroscopy, the inexperienced hysteroscopist will be better served by dextran, which consistently provides the best view of the uterine cavity.

1.5% Glycine

Glycine is an alternative uterine distention medium that is much more commonly used for urologic electrosurgery. The material is a clear, watery liquid containing 1.5 g of glycine USP per 100 ml of solution. This sterile hypotonic solution is packaged in 2- to 4-L plastic bottles. Glycine has many of the properties of sterile water as a distending medium and is safer than electrolytic solutions when used in conjunction with the resectoscope.

When the material is absorbed into the circulation, it is metabolized to serine, then to ammonia, and finally to urea. A portion of glycine may be directly excreted by the kidneys. Because ≥20 L of glycine may be used for extensive intrauterine surgery, the risk of congestive failure and pulmonary edema must be considered. Additionally, substantial absorption of this material can lead to electrolyte and water imbalances. Women with borderline or impaired hepatic function are at risk for ammonia intoxication and those with renal damage may sustain toxic levels of plasma urea. The product circular supplied by the manufacturer also includes reports of angina-like pain, thrombophlebitis, vertigo, urticaria, transient blindness, and digitalis toxicity in digitalized patients.

TECHNIQUE OF DIAGNOSTIC HYSTEROSCOPY

The patient must be suitably prepared. A complete history and physical examination should be performed. The position of the uterus, for example, whether it is retroflexed or anteflexed, must be known. The patient should be given a thorough explanation about the hysteroscopic procedure and the possible side effects of the procedure. The surgeon and patient should decide jointly whether the procedure will be performed under local or general anesthesia. Likewise, the patient should be told about any sampling procedures that might be carried out in conjunction with the hysteroscopy.

The patient is placed in the dorsal lithotomy position. The perineum and vagina are gently swabbed with a Betadine topical anti-infective. Either a single-hinged speculum (Fig. 17-14) or Sims's retractor is placed in the vagina. A single-toothed tenaculum is attached to the anterior lip of the cervix.

A suitable telescope is selected and checked by the operator for clarity of the eyepiece and objective lens. If necessary, the lens is gently cleansed with a soft saline or water-soaked sponge. The light generator is switched on and the fiberoptic cable is attached to the telescope. The telescope is inserted into the diagnostic sheath and the selected medium flushed through the sheath, extruding air within the sheath (Fig. 17-15).

If CO_2 is the selected medium, the flow rate is adjusted to deliver 30 cc/min. The hysteroscope is engaged into the external cervical os. As the endoscope is advanced, the gas separates the walls of the endocervix, allowing an excellent view of the endocervical folds and crypts. The internal os is seen above as the endoscope is manipulated along the axis of the canal and through the os under direct vision. The isthmus is entered. Flow is adjusted to a rate of 60 cc/min (see Fig. 17-6).

Routinely, dilatation of the cervix should be avoided because even careful and gentle insertion of cervical dilators will traumatize the endocervix and endometrium. Typically, the endocervical canal shows longitudinal folds, papillae, and clefts. The vascular pattern of the normal endocervix reveals branching, treelike vessels. These are especially well observed with a focusing hysteroscope. The internal os appears as a narrow constriction at the top of the endocervical canal. The isthmus is a cylindrical extension above the os. The corpus is a capacious cavity above the isthmus (Fig. 17-16). The central point of müllerian duct fusion is seen projecting down from the fundus. The cornua occupy either side of this fused area. The tubal ostia are visible at the upper extremities of the fundal cornua and show great variation in their appearance and angle of entry into the uterine cavity. The uterine mucosa (endometrium) is smooth and pink-white in color during the proliferative phase. The gland openings appear as white-ringed elevations surrounded with netlike vessels. During the secretory phase of the cycle, the endometrium is lush and velvety; it protrudes into the cavity irregularly and can be easily mistaken for small polyps. The hue of secretory endometrium is deep pink. The interior of the cavity, particularly when liquid media are used, appears cloudy with fine debris floating in the

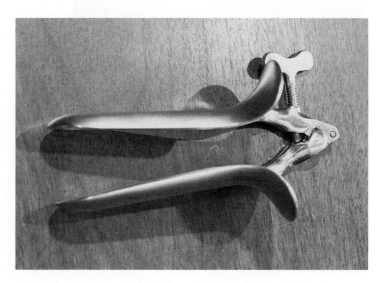

Figure 17–14. The single-hinged speculum is an excellent instrument through which to perform hysteroscopy. It may be removed after the hysteroscope is engaged into the cervix.

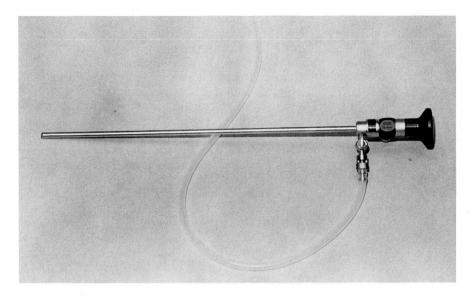

Figure 17–15. The telescope is engaged in the sheath and the medium purges air from the system.

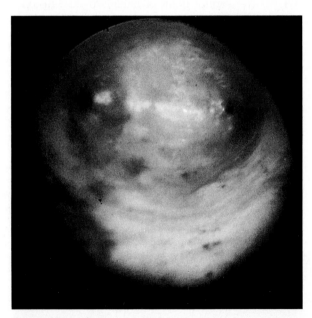

Figure 17–16. CO_2 hysteroscopy details the capacious corpus above the narrow isthmus. The tubal ostia are seen at the right and left extremes in the fundus.

medium. When CO_2 is the distending medium, the endometrium is artificially flattened. Although the cornua are easily recognized, the tubal ostia may not be seen during the latter phase of the menstrual cycle. The thickness of the endometrium can be easily appreciated by placing pressure on the telescope and pushing on the posterior wall of the uterus. This maneuver creates a groove in the endometrium.

TECHNIQUE OF OPERATIVE HYSTEROSCOPY

After completion of a diagnostic appraisal of the uterine cavity, the operator inserts the telescope into the operative sheath. A proper nipple is selected and attached to the opening of the operating channel. If a dual-channel operating sheath is available, two Luer-lock leaf-type gaskets are screwed into place (Fig. 17-17). The sheath is flushed with distending medium and a light cable is attached. Initially, an attempt should be made to insert the sheath into the cervix without resorting to dilatation. Hyskon is the recommended medium. When the internal os is viewed, a push of hyskon creates distention as simultaneous pressure is placed against the opening. Frequently, the larger sheath may negotiate the constriction and slip into the cavity. If this cannot be done, then dilatation is required. Pratt dilators are selected and lubricated with hyskon. Gentle dilatation is performed to just allow the sheath entry into the cavity with little intervening space between the sheath and the cervical mucosa, which ensures excellent distention and minimizes leakage of medium. The cavity is again scanned and the operator orients himself or herself to its landmarks. If the operator has difficulty viewing the cavity clearly, the hysteroscope has most likely been inserted too deeply and the telescope is usually in contact with the uterine wall. The recommended maneuver is to pull the instrument back while injecting a bolus of hyskon. The flow of debris within the hyskon should be followed and invariably will lead the operator to the tubal ostia.

Once a clear view is obtained, an operating instrument can be inserted into the cavity and should be

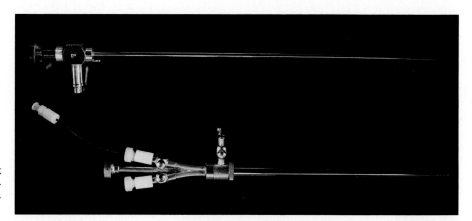

Figure 17–17. Two Luer-lock leaf valves are screwed into position (*bottom*) before performing operative hysteroscopy.

advanced so that it makes contact with the endometrium. This contact generally permits relative calibration and spatial orientation within the cavity. At this point, the knowledgeable and skilled hysteroscopist will insert an aspirating cannula and further clear the cavity of debris. If the cavity cannot be aspirated clear, or if the cavity is bloody, it must be flushed. The dual-channel hysteroscope facilitates this maneuver. Saline or Ringer's lactate is selected for this procedure. The medium channel is opened and saline is instilled under pressure. One operating channel is opened to allow the fluid to exit the cavity. After 1 L of saline has been flushed through the cavity, the operating channel is closed and hyskon is again instilled. The cavity should now appear clear. No operative procedure can ever be performed unless an absolutely unobstructed view is obtained.

Frequently, for the sake of patient safety, a simultaneous laparoscopy is also done. This procedure permits an assistant to view the serosal aspect of the uterus and provides excellent insurance against inadvertent perforation. Laparoscopy is mandatory when septa are to be cut, for adhesiotomy, and during extraction of submucous myoma.

A new and advantageous technique to master is the use of the endoscopic microchip camera coupled directly to the telescope (Fig. 17-18). The advantages of performing hysteroscopic surgery by way of the video monitor are as follows:

1. The camera, depending on the selected lens, permits magnification of the operative field. The image may fill the entire video monitor screen.
2. Use of the video camera permits the endoscopist to sit upright rather than hunched over, thus eliminating operator fatigue.
3. When the image is projected on the video screen, interest on the part of residents, nurses, and students is maintained throughout the procedure

because they are able to see the operation clearly. Therefore, they are able to learn more about the technique and can render better assistance than is possible with conventional procedures.

4. Finally, if lasers are used as operating instruments, then protective eyewear is not required because the risk of eye injury is obviated.

The endoscopic video camera should be outfitted with an appropriate lens. These lenses range in focal length from 25 to 38 mm. A 28- to 30-mm lens provides satisfactory magnification. The operator should first view the cavity by direct vision and should then attach the camera to the eyepiece of the lens. The view with the coupled camera provides magnification comparable with that obtained during microsurgery. If a video recorder is available, a tape may be inserted into the apparatus to obtain a permanent record of the procedure. A xenon light generator provides the best illumination for video techniques, although less expensive light sources may be satisfactory when newer, highly light-sensitive cameras are used.

Laser Technology

The advent of lasers has produced technological breakthroughs never before imagined for hysteroscopic surgery. Although several lasers are useful for hysteroscopic surgery, the Nd : YAG laser is preferred for a number of reasons. It is a high-output system capable of attaining powers > 100 W. The laser energy can be delivered to tissue by means of fine, flexible quartz fibers measuring 300 to 600 μm in diameter and 2 m in length. The Nd : YAG laser's major tissue action is coagulation. Most important, the laser beam's tissue interactions are exerted by front scatter, which translates into deep penetration, as described by Fisher in a work on safety in laser surgery. When a surface lesion is

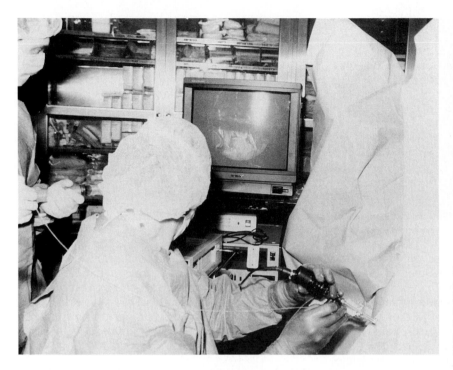

Figure 17–18. Contemporary operative hysteroscopy is performed using a microchip video camera attached to the eyepiece of the telescope. The operator and assistants all view the field by way of a high-resolution video monitor.

produced in the endometrium, the major coagulative effect actually occurs 3 to 4 mm deeper, that is, within the superficial myometrium. Additionally, the Nd : YAG laser beam traverses water and other translucent liquid media without significant loss of energy; at the same time, these liquid media exert a salutary cooling action on the laser fiber.

The transmitting quartz fiber may easily and conveniently be inserted into the operating channel(s) of the hysteroscopic sheath (Fig. 17-19). The fiber is small enough to reach any site regardless of size within the uterine cavity, including the tubal ostia and cornua. A wide variety of sapphire tips may be affixed to the end of the laser fiber. These tips act as lenses and focus the

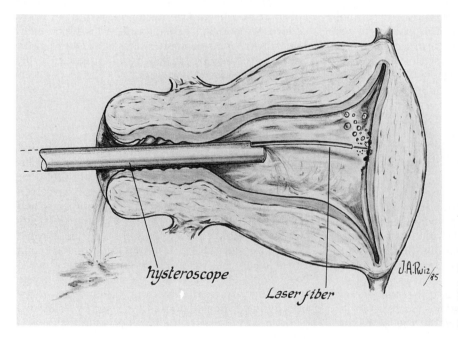

hysteroscope

Laser fiber

J.A.Ruiz/85

Figure 17–19. The Nd: YAG laser energy reaches the uterine interior by way of a fine quartz fiber introduced through the operating channel of the hysteroscope.

laser beam to a fine point suitable for focused vaporization, that is, cutting and other fine, precise maneuvers. Laser energy may be used in any distending medium without fear of electrical conduction and resultant inadvertent damage to neighboring structures (eg, bowel injury).

Urologic Resectoscope

Another important operating instrument is the resectoscope (see articles by DeCherney and associates, 1986, and by Neuwirth). This device consists of a specialized operating sheath whose terminus is designed with a mobile, small-wire loop capable of being manipulated forward and backward similar to the slide action of a trombone (Fig. 17-20). The loop is wired to an electrical generator providing suitable power to coagulate or cut tissue with which it comes into contact. The hysteroscopic telescope fits into and locks onto this specialized sheath and provides a direct view of the operative field. When this instrument is used, a non-electrolytic solution (eg, hyskon or glycine) must be instilled as the distending medium to protect the patient from potential electrical injury. Additionally, the patient should be appropriately grounded. The largest experience with this instrument has been gained in the field of urology, where it is routinely utilized for transurethral prostatectomy surgery.

SPECIFIC PROCEDURES IN HYSTEROSCOPIC SURGERY

Septate Uterus

The advent of modern hysteroscopy has rendered the correction of congenital fusion abnormalities relatively simple and straightforward by the transcervical route, according to DeCherney and associates, and March and Israel. In addition, in most instances, it has relegated transabdominal metroplasty to obsolescence. Uterine septa, contrary to popular opinion, are not associated with infertility. They are, however, a contributing factor to pregnancy wastage. During the work-up for unexplained abortion or premature delivery, timely hysterosalpingography diagnoses the fusion disorder by providing a typical picture of a Y-shaped uterus. Unfortunately, the hysterogram does not differentiate between septate and bicornuate uteri. For these defects to be accurately assessed, a diagnostic laparoscopy is required. The laparoscopic view in the case of septate uterus reveals a normal-appearing fundus. The bicornuate uterus appears typically heart shaped.

Once the correct diagnosis has been secured, the patient may be a candidate for septum resection. Large septa may necessitate a Jones (wedge) metroplasty. The Strassman procedure should be recommended for the unification of a bicornuate uterus. A simultaneous laparoscopy should always be done when hysteroscopic correction is contemplated. Obviously, the patient should be appropriately informed about the combined surgical approach. Resection may be performed by a variety of techniques (eg, scissors, laser, or resectoscope). Any one of these techniques is satisfactory.

Hysteroscopic Technique

The septum is viewed from the level of the internal cervical os. The endoscope is moved into each chamber of the divided uterine cavity and the locations of the tubal ostia are marked. The hysteroscope is again withdrawn to a level just above the internal os. The appropriate operating instrument is inserted through the sheath and the septum is cut from below upward (Fig. 17-21), as described by March. As the fundus is approached, the operator depends on the assistant to signal when the light of the hysteroscope demonstrates

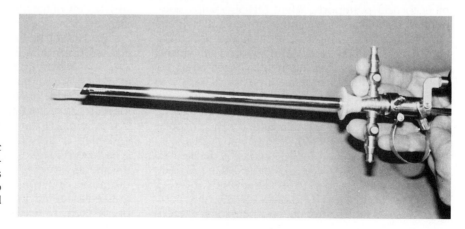

Figure 17–20. The urologic resectoscope consists of a specialized sheath whose terminus is designed with a movable loop element that slides back and forth.

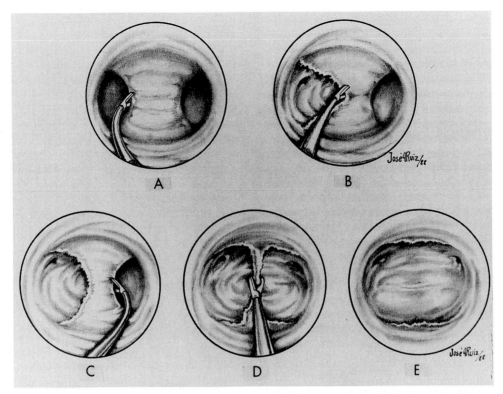

Figure 17–21. During this technique for a hysteroscopic section of a uterine septum, the operator cuts the septum from below upward (*A–D*) until a single cavity is seen (*E*). (Reprinted from Baggish MS, Barbot J, Valle RF. Diagnostic and operative hysteroscopy. Chicago: Year Book Medical Publishers, 1989, with permission.)

transmission through the intact uterine wall. The narrative between the hysteroscopist and laparoscopist will prevent perforation. It is unnecessary to excise the septum completely; that is, mere transection will eliminate the septum and unite the uterus into a single cavity. An important technical point stresses that the surgeon clip the septum squarely in the middle (Fig. 17-22). A common tendency is for the surgeon's cutting instrument to drift posteriorly. When this aberration goes unnoticed, the operating instrument will invariably cut into the myometrium, resulting in profuse bleeding. Similarly, correcting the septum too perfectly at the level of the fundus will result in deep penetration into the myometrium and subsequent hemorrhage.

If bleeding does ensue, a 30-cc Foley bag catheter is inserted into the endometrial cavity at the terminus of the operation and inflated to 15 to 18 cc. The pressure exerted by the bag on the uterine walls is sufficient to control the bleeding promptly. The bag is deflated 12 hours postoperatively and is removed if no further bleeding ensues. Patients are usually advised to take 2.5 mg of estrogen daily by mouth for 30 days postoperatively. Antibiotics are not routinely administered.

Uterine Synechiae

Adhesions form between the anterior and posterior walls of the uterus as a result of trauma or infection in a milieu of estrogen deprivation. Classically, this problem follows an abortion or postpartum hemorrhage for which a vigorous curettage has been performed to control the bleeding, as reported by March and associates. Review of the microscopic sections obtained from the curettage invariably reveals fragments of myometrium interspersed with inflamed decidua and glands. Historically, the patient does not resume menstruation; however, a minority of patients may continue to menstruate normally. Because the patient is subsequently infertile or amenorrheic, a hysterogram is performed. The radiograph reveals filling defects that vary from minimal to severe, that is, virtually obliterating the endometrial cavity. In the past, the treatment of uterine synechiae consisted of blind curettage; the results of this therapy were predictably poor. With the advent of diagnostic and contact hysteroscopy, treatment progressed to identifying the adhesions and attempting to break them by exerting pressure with the hystero-

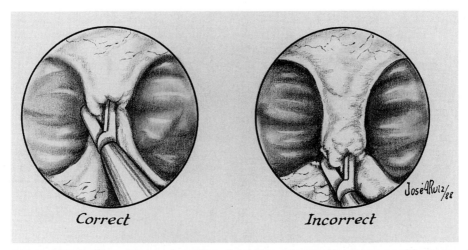

Figure 17–22. The scissors or laser fiber should be maintained in the center of the septum to avoid bleeding. (Reprinted from Baggish MS, Barbot J, Valle RF. Diagnostic and operative hysteroscopy. Chicago: Year Book Medical Publishers, 1989, with permission.)

scope. Again, this type of rugged therapy yielded poor results and a high risk of uterine perforation.

Hysteroscopic Technique

A thorough diagnostic hysteroscopy is performed to assess the degree of adhesion formation and deformity of the cavity. Small openings in the curtain of adhesions are sought out as are any normal anatomical landmarks. Here the flow pattern of tiny blood fragments and tissue debris are helpful. Either a photograph, videotape, or detailed drawing are helpful reminders in planning the strategy for cutting these adhesions.

As with septal operations, a simultaneous laparoscopy is prudently advocated to prevent perforation of the uterus. For this operation, flexible or semirigid scissors or Nd:YAG laser are the operating instruments of choice. The laser is initially set to deliver power of 25 to 30 W. Hyskon is instilled into the cavity by way of an operating sheath. Continuous maintenance of distention is one key to success. Filmy and central adhesions should be cut first, always following the hyskon flow. Marginal and dense adhesions should be attacked last, always cutting from below upward. A second hallmark to success maintains the hysteroscope in midchannel relative to the uterine walls. The cavity can usually and reasonably be restored to normal architecture. Bleeding is not uncommon during this operation, particularly when cutting marginal adhesions, because the border between adhesion and myometrium is blurred.

Upon completion of the operation, the patient is placed on conjugated estrogens 2.5 mg daily. The placement of an intrauterine device within the cavity "to keep the walls from adhering" is clearly not based on scientific fact. If immediate postoperative bleeding occurs, then a 30-cc Foley bag or specific intrauterine balloon (150 cc capacity) is placed into the uterine cavity for 12 to 24 hours. Hysterosalpingography is performed within 1 month of surgery.

Uterine Polyps

Functional and nonfunctional polyps produce intermenstrual bleeding, as reported by Barbot. Functional polyps tend to be smaller than nonfunctional polyps. If a hysterogram is performed, then a focal filling defect will be seen. The diagnosis is directly and readily made by hysteroscopy. The polyp protrudes into the endometrial cavity; in the case of a functioning polyp, the lining is identical to the surrounding endometrium. The nonfunctioning polyp presents as a white protuberance covered with branching surface vessels; within the depths of the polyp, thick-walled vessels are usually seen.

Hysteroscopic Technique

A dual-channel operating hysteroscope is inserted into the uterine cavity. An alligator-jaw forceps is inserted through one channel of the operating sheath. The polyp is grasped and pulled away from its origin on the uterine wall and stretched to expose its base. Through the other channel, scissors or an Nd:YAG laser fiber is engaged. The polyp is cut off at the base using the scissors or laser set at a power of 20 to 30 W (Fig. 17-23). The hysteroscope is withdrawn, removing with it the freed polyp, which is sent to the pathology lab for

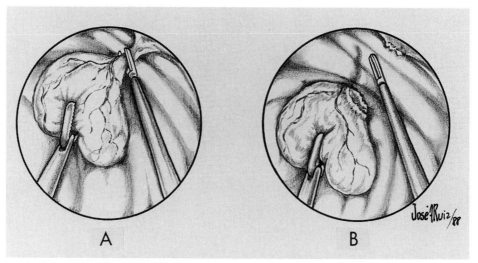

Figure 17–23. *A* and *B*, An alligator-jaw forceps stabilizes the polyp while a scissors' or laser fiber cuts the base. (Reprinted from Baggish MS, Barbot J, Valle RF. Diagnostic and operative hysteroscopy. Chicago: Year Book Medical Publishers, 1989, with permission.)

histologic evaluation. The site of removal is reinspected and the procedure terminated.

Myomata Uteri

Submucous myomas have a characteristic appearance when viewed by hysteroscopy. They appear as white, spherical masses covered with a network of fragile, thin-walled vessels. Typically, they are sessile or pedunculated. When a hysterogram is performed, the filling defect is not dissimilar to that produced by a polyp. Unfortunately, blind dilatation and curettage is an inaccurate method for diagnosing this disorder. Although subserous and intramural myomas rarely produce alarming symptoms, even when they attain relatively large size, smaller lesions in the submucous location invariably cause substantial bleeding. Additionally, because submucous myomas are commonly associated with chronic endometritis, they will interfere with implantation of the fertilized ovum and become a contributing factor to subfertility.

In the past, a diagnosis of submucous myoma was usually followed by a recommendation for hysterectomy. Today, hysteroscopic surgery offers a therapeutic option to that radical approach. Recent applications of drug therapy, for example, Danocrine and gonadotropin-releasing hormone analogs (lupron injection), provide supplementary therapy preceding surgery. The general plan is to treat symptomatic patients for 2 months before hysteroscopic surgery with either of these drugs to reduce the size and vascularity of the lesion. All patients are given a detailed informed consent that includes the recommendation for typing and holding blood as well as the possibility for hysterectomy if intractable bleeding ensues.

Hysteroscopic Technique

Two methods of treatment have been described for the hysteroscopic elimination of submucous myomas: (1) using the resectoscope (Fig. 17-24), as reported by Neuwirth and by DeCherney et al, and (2) utilizing the Nd:YAG laser (Figs. 17-25 and 17-26).

Another technique has been reported for removal of pedunculated submucous myomas. Goldrath uses laminaria tents to dilate the cervix preoperatively and then further dilate the cervix intraoperatively. Next, large grasping instruments are inserted and the pedunculated lesions are removed. Sometimes the pedicles are twisted until they snap off; then the tumor is pulled out of the uterus. Neuwirth as well as DeCherney, Cholst, and Naftolin have described a method of removing smaller (3 cm) sessile submucous myomas with the resectoscope. The lesions are excised layer by layer to the level of the base of the uterine wall. When the operation is completed, a balloon is placed into the uterine cavity for several hours to maintain hemostasis.

The Nd:YAG laser may be used in conjunction with the dual-channel operating hysteroscope. Power is set at 30 to 40 W. Through one channel, a flexible needle is inserted; the needle exerts pressure on the myoma, that is, traction. The laser cuts across the base of the myoma while the needle pushes in the same direction as the cutting fiber. The myoma may be finally cut at its base with scissors. This technique is useful for myomas 3 cm

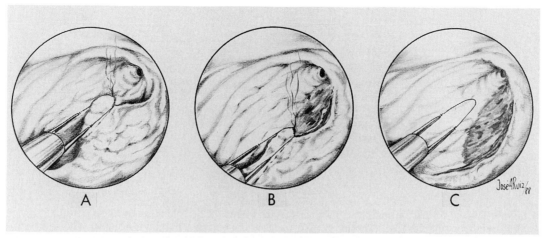

Figure 17–24. *A–C*, A submucous myoma is shaved flat by means of the resectoscope. (Reprinted from Baggish MS, Barbot J, Valle RF. Diagnostic and operative hysteroscopy. Chicago: Year Book Medical Publishers, 1989, with permission.)

in diameter. A technique similar to that used with the resectoscope also may be utilized, that is, slicing off layer upon layer of the myoma until the base is reached. For a large (≥5 cm) lesion, the laser may simply devascularize the lesion and flatten it out. This is done by running the fiber over and over the myoma, producing deep cuts into its substance until it is completely disrupted. The myoma is left to "die on the vine" and slough away. Optionally, the large myoma may be quartered with the laser and then extracted with a polyp forceps. All myomectomy operations require simultaneous laparoscopy to diminish the risk of uterine perforation or uterine wall disruption.

Endometrial Ablation

A substantial number of women undergo hysterectomy each year. According to a recent study performed by the New York State Department of Health, as re-

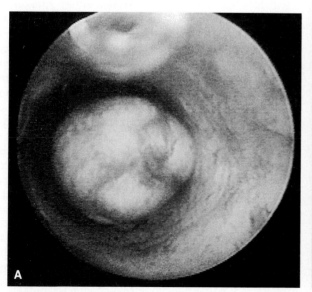
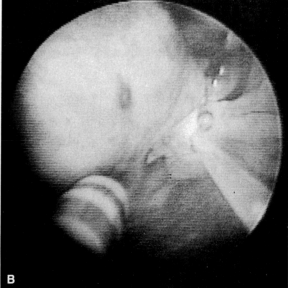

Figure 17–25. A submucous myoma. *A*, Cut with the Nd: YAG laser fiber. *B*, Then removed. The aspirating cannula (*striped*) is seen (*right*).

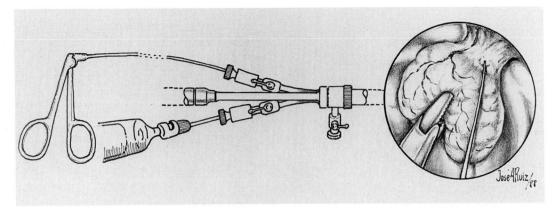

Figure 17–26. A small myoma is fixed with a grasping forceps or flexible needle while the Nd: YAG laser fiber cuts the base. (Reprinted from Baggish MS, Barbot J, Valle RF. Diagnostic and operative hysteroscopy. Chicago: Year Book Medical Publishers, 1989, with permission.)

ported by Barbot, between 650,000 and 675,000 hysterectomies are done in the United States annually and 30,065 hysterectomies were performed in New York State during 1986. Of this number, approximately 8% to 10% were done for uterine bleeding. The average length of hospital stay following hysterectomy was 8.5 days. For many women, hysterectomy may present a significant surgical risk, particularly for those individuals with bleeding disorders, with significant medical diseases, and with substantial obesity. Additionally, some women may develop psychologic problems following hysterectomy or their partners may develop sexual dysfunction.

In past years, alternative blind procedures such as cryocoagulation were implemented to control dysfunctional uterine bleeding, that is, to create a chemical or physical destruction of the endometrium without sacrificing the uterus, as described in two reports by Droegemueller and associates. Unfortunately, either the techniques themselves were associated with overwhelming noxious side-effects or the endometrium promptly regenerated. In 1981, techniques for ablating the endometrium safely under direct vision were described by Goldrath, Fuller, and Segal. In concert with growing pressures by third-party payers for less expensive treatment alternatives, practical laser and nonlaser methodologies have been described by Baggish and Baltoyannis, by Lomano, and by DeCherney, Cholst, and Naftolin. The first Nd:YAG laser methodology was described by Goldrath and associates in 1981. Most recently, Baggish and Baltoyannis reported the successful application of this technique in a group of high-risk women, attaining amenorrhea in 70% of the cases. DeCherney and Polan also reported a similar technique using the resectoscope in a high-risk group of women.

Hysteroscopic Technique

All patients selected for this surgery should undergo attempts to control uterine bleeding by hormonal therapy and curettage. If these procedures fail, then the women are candidates for endometrial ablation. Preoperatively, a diagnostic hysteroscopy should be performed together with endometrial sampling to exclude endometrial carcinoma or atypical hyperplasia. Appropriate hematologic studies and consultations should also be carried out. All patients are pretreated with Danocrine, 400 mg to 800 mg daily, for 6 to 8 weeks. Alternatively, Megace, 20 mg daily, may be prescribed. For the Nd:YAG laser technique, either hyskon or Ringer's lactate may be used as the distending medium. hyskon is always used with the resectoscope.

The operating hysteroscope is inserted into the uterine cavity. An aspirating cannula is placed into the left operating channel (Fig. 17-27A) and the cavity is aspirated until clear. The 600-μm Nd:YAG fiber is inserted next (Fig. 17-27B). Beginning in the fundus and at either the right or left tubal ostium, the fiber is dragged across the endometrium, creating a trench 1 mm to 2 mm deep (Fig. 17-28). This is repeated several times, row upon row, until the fundus is ablated and charred. Next, the posterior wall is ablated row upon row, covering the corpus and isthmus from above downward to the level of the internal cervical os. The hysteroscope is rotated 180° and the anterior wall is similarly ablated. Finally, the lateral walls are destroyed. The key to the success of this operation lies in the front scatter of the Nd:YAG laser, that is, extension two to four times beyond the visible lesion. This penetration translates into extensive superficial myometrial destruction and coagulation of the radial branches of the uterine artery.

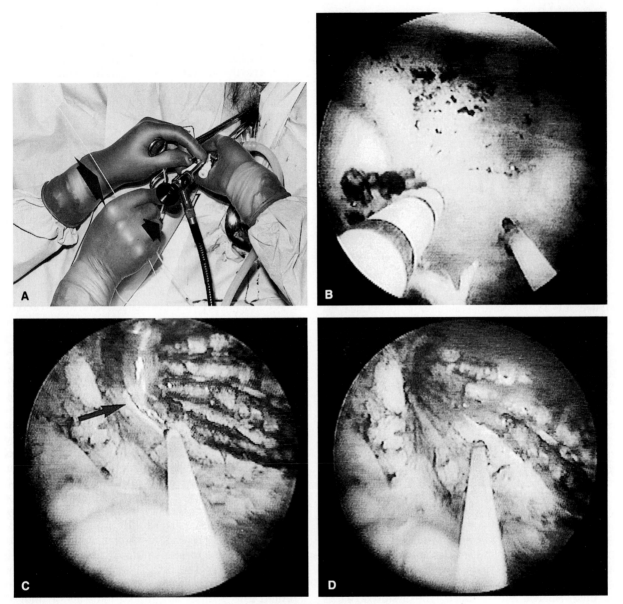

Figure 17–27. Hysteroscopic technique for endometrial ablation. *A*, An aspirating cannula is inserted through the left operating channel (*small arrow*) and the Nd: YAG laser fiber (*large arrow*) will be inserted into the right channel. *B*, The fundus and corpus are seen. The Nd: YAG laser fiber is seen (*right*) and the aspirating tube is seen (*left*). *C*, The endometrium is ablated. An escaping bubble is seen (*arrow*). *D*, Extensive damage created by the Nd: YAG laser fiber is seen in the fundus.

When the endometrium sloughs, regeneration is prevented because neither basal nor spiral arterioles survive the laser's depredations. Over a period of 6 to 8 weeks, the uterine walls scar and coapt, resulting in amenorrhea. The procedure may be carried out at a power of 30 to 40 W; a mean volume of 300 cc of hyskon is used as the distending medium. Duration of the procedure is approximately 30 minutes. Patients may be sent home on the day of surgery or the morning following surgery. The operation is usually completed without blood loss.

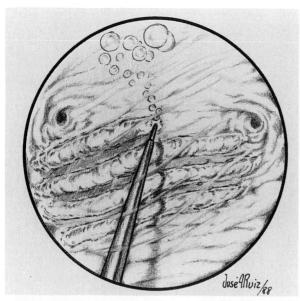

Figure 17–28. Endometrial ablation is performed by sweeping the Nd:YAG laser fiber back and forth across the endometrium, creating a series of trenches. The beam penetrates 3 mm to 4 mm beyond the endometrium into the superficial myometrium. (Reprinted from Baggish MS, Barbot J, Valle RF. Diagnostic and operative hysteroscopy. Chicago: Year Book Medical Publishers, 1989, with permission.)

Miscellaneous Procedures

IUD Removal

Although the number of intrauterine contraceptive device (IUD) insertions has diminished over recent years, the gynecologist is occasionally called upon to search for and remove a device whose indicator string is not seen in the cervix. In such circumstances, the operating hysteroscope is a vital tool with which to locate the device and to remove it under direct vision, according to Valle, Sciarra, and Freeman. The hysteroscope is inserted and the device is viewed. If a string is seen, then an alligator-jaw forceps is inserted and the string is grasped. The hysteroscope is withdrawn, pulling the device through the uterine cavity and the cervix to the exterior. If the IUD is imbedded, then a rigid grasping forceps is required. The IUD is located and the large jaws of the rigid instrument grab the extruded portion of the IUD itself. Strong pressure is exerted on the jaws as the hysteroscope's sheath is slowly withdrawn from the uterus, into the cervix, and out of the vagina.

Biopsy of Intrauterine Lesions

When a tumor is suspected, the operative hysteroscope is inserted into the cavity. A semirigid biopsy forceps is directed to the tumor site and multiple biopsies are obtained in a fashion analogous to colposcopic biopsies. A large-bore plastic cannula may be inserted by way of the operating channel and strong suction applied to the mouth of the cannula by means of a 30-cc syringe (Fig. 17-29). The cannula is removed and the contents flushed out with saline into a bottle of fixative. Alternatively, a diagnostic hysteroscope may be inserted into the uterus. The site of pathology is noted. The endoscope is withdrawn, a Novak curette is inserted into the cavity, and biopsies are taken at the previously located site. Finally, the hysteroscope may be pulled back to the level of the internal cervical os, a small Novak curette may be inserted alongside the hysteroscope, and a directed biopsy may be obtained.

Treatment of Hemangiomas and Arterio-Venous Malformations

Hemangiomas and arterio-venous malformations may be diagnosed by their characteristic hysteroscopic appearance and a history of massive, unresponsive bleeding. Historically, women with these conditions are young and of low parity. During hysteroscopic examination, the subsurface of the endometrium is covered with irregular bluish-purple vessels. These vessels form an abnormal tangle of distended channels and differ markedly from the normal fine-capillary net pattern. The abnormal channels are not dissimilar to those vessels covering the surface of submucous myomas. The Nd:YAG fiber is inserted through the operating channel and the fiber is held several millimeters above the vascular abnormality; power is turned up to 50 to 60 W. The laser is discharged without touching the vessels or the surface of the endometrium. As the laser energy impacts, the vessels collapse and coagulate. The surface blanches white. The endometrium neighboring the abnormality is also treated and coagulated. The fiber is then withdrawn. The field is aspirated clear and the hysteroscope is withdrawn. Similar treatment is repeated 2 to 3 times at 1-month intervals or until all evidence of the abnormality is obtunded.

COMPLICATIONS OF HYSTEROSCOPIC SURGERY

Intraoperative and Postoperative Bleeding

The most common complications of hysteroscopic surgery are intraoperative and postoperative bleeding. Generally speaking, intraoperative bleeding may be managed by aspirating the blood and by increasing the pressure of the distending medium so that it exceeds arterial pressure and compresses the walls of the uterus

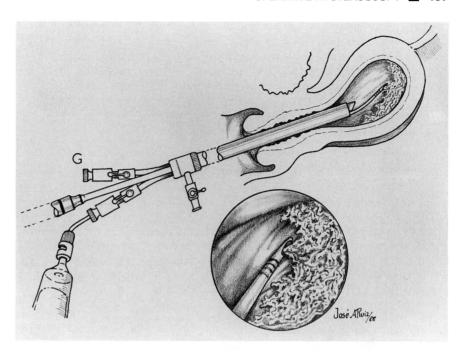

Figure 17–29. Direct sampling of an intrauterine lesion may be accomplished with a plastic cannula attached to a 30-cc syringe.

sufficiently to stop bleeding. When the counterpressure of the medium is relaxed, that is, at the termination of the procedure, bleeding may again ensue. This bleeding is best controlled by the insertion of an intrauterine balloon. Recently, a specific balloon has been marketed with 150 cc capacity. The balloon may be initially inflated to 20 to 30 cc. If this pressure does not promptly stop the bleeding, then the balloon may be distended to 50 to 60 cc until bleeding has stopped. For larger uteri, more distension to 100 to 150 cc may be required. The balloon remains in place for 6 to 8 hours, then is deflated to 20 to 30 cc for 6 hours, and then decreased to 0 cc before removal.

Fluid Overload and Pulmonary Edema

A significant and disconcerting complication of operative hysteroscopy is fluid overload with resulting pulmonary edema. This complication is most likely to happen in circumstances in which the uterine wall is damaged (eg, endometrial ablation or myomectomy). The problem may occur when either hyskon, saline, or Ringer's lactate is the distending medium. Typically, during endometrial ablation, 10 to 20 L of saline or Ringer's lactate are infused. When 500 cc of hyskon are instilled, fluid overload is possible. Intraoperatively, the anesthesiologist may note pink froth in the respirator tubing. Postoperatively, the patient typically complains of dyspnea. Auscultation of the chest reveals crackling rales over the lung fields. In such instances, the fluid

infusion should be decreased and lasix, 20 mg to 40 mg, should be administered intravenously. Obviously, the best prophylaxis to prevent fluid overload aims to limit the volume of instilled medium.

Uterine Perforation

Uterine perforation may occur during any operative hysteroscopy procedure but is most likely to happen during septum resection or myomectomy operations. The best prophylaxis against this complication is simultaneous laparoscopy. Among novice operators, perforation may even occur during insertion of the hysteroscope. With appropriate care, this perforation should not occur because the cervix and internal os should be negotiated under direct vision and the cavity should likewise be entered under direct vision. Another simple prophylactic technique, examination under anesthesia, will permit the operator to know the direction of the uterine axis. The greatest risk of perforation occurs when the septum transection is finished at the level of the uterine fundus. The operator may have difficulty determining where the septum ends and the myometrium begins. Regardless of the cutting instrument, the risk is equal.

The operator will rapidly be made aware of uterine perforation because distention becomes difficult to maintain and the flow of hyskon exits at the perforation site. An alert assistant watching through the laparoscope will warn the hysteroscopist of impending perforation by noting an increasing intensity of light transmission through the thinning uterine wall. If perforation is unnoticed and if simultaneous laparoscopy is not performed, then more serious complications will result, particularly when the laser or resectoscope is utilized. In such circumstances, the small or large intestine may be injured by conduction of electric current or by direct injury by the laser beam.

Inability to See the Operative Field

A most common, albeit minor, complication is the inability to see the operative field. Perhaps the most common cause of this problem is deep insertion of the hysteroscope so that the telescope lies directly in contact with the endometrium. The surgeon will see nothing but a red blur. The tendency is to push the hysteroscope deeper in. This is a strategic mistake because it invariably leads to perforation. An equally common mistake is overdilatation of the cervix. This error results in excessive leakage of distending medium and inability to maintain distension with resultant inability to perform the operative hysteroscopy. Blood and debris may cloud the field to such a degree that accurate operative endoscopy is impossible. The problem is a less common occurrence when hyskon is selected as the distending medium. Obviously, if the operator cannot clearly see the field, it is better to discontinue the procedure rather than press on and commit a catastrophic error. It is easy to become disoriented in the uterine cavity if normal anatomical landmarks cannot be recognized.

CO$_2$ Embolus

A rare but completely avoidable complication is CO$_2$ embolus. This occurs as a result of inappropriate CO$_2$ insufflation equipment. If a laparoscopic insufflator is used in place of a hysteroscopic insufflator, then the flow rate will be excessive in terms of liters per minute rather than milliliters per minute. This will lead to significant cardiovascular aberrations due to the excessive CO$_2$ absorption. Unbelievably, cases are on record in which CO$_2$ gas was directly infused into the uterine cavity by way of the CO$_2$ cylinder without pressure and flow-regulating devices. The predictable result of this type of CO$_2$ delivery is patient death. Signs of CO$_2$ embolus are noted on auscultation over the heart by the presence of a cogwheel murmur. Another related disaster has been reported with the use of the Nd:YAG laser in which a sheathed or gastrointestinal fiber is used for ablation rather than the recommended bare genitourinary fiber. Similarly, the identical adverse reaction

can occur when sapphire tips are mounted on the end of the gastrointestinal fiber and are cooled with nitrogen gas. In such instances, nitrogen gas or air embolism produce cardiac arrest or death of the patient. It is obvious that CO$_2$, N$_2$, or air embolism are completely avoidable complications.

Infection

Infection is an unlikely complication associated with or following hysteroscopy. Obviously, hysteroscopy should be avoided in the presence of gross cervical infection, uterine infection, or salpingitis. Following even extensive intrauterine surgery, for example, adhesiostomy or myomectomy, infection is uncommon. The endometrium seems to be peculiarly resistant to this complication. Prophylactic antibiotics should be administered only when indications exist, such as a history of rheumatic carditis or a diagnosis of prolapsed mitral valve, or with suspected chronic endometritis (submucous myoma or imbedded IUD).

Bibliography

Baggish MS. Contact hysteroscopy: a new technique to explore the uterine cavity. Obstet Gynecol 1979;54:350.

Baggish MS. A new laser hysteroscope for Nd-YAG endometrial ablation. Lasers Surg Med 1988;8:248.

Baggish MS, Baltoyannis P. New techniques for laser ablation of the endometrium in high risk patients. Am J Obstet Gynecol 1988;159:287.

Baggish MS, Barbot J, Valle RF. Diagnostic and operative hysteroscopy: a text and atlas. Chicago: Year Book Medical Publishers 1989.

Baggish MS, Dorsey JH. Contact hysteroscopic evaluation of the endocervix as an adjunct to colposcopy. Obstet Gynecol 1982;60:107.

Baggish MS, Sze EHM, Morgan G. Hysteroscopic treatment of symptomatic submucous myomata uteri with the Nd-YAG laser. J Gynecol Surg 1989;5:27.

Barbot J. Hysteroscopy for abnormal bleeding in diagnostic and operative hysteroscopy. In: Baggish MS, Barbot J, Valle RF, eds. Diagnostic and operative hysteroscopy: a text and atlas. Chicago: Year Book Medical Publishers, 1989:147–155.

Barbot J, Parent B, Doeler B. Hysteroscopie de contact et cancer de pendometre. Acta Endosc 1978;8:17.

Barbot J, Parent B, Dubuisson JB. Contact hysteroscopy: another method of endoscopic examination of the uterine cavity. Am J Obstet Gynecol 1980;136:721.

Burnett JE. Hysteroscopy-controlled curettage for endometrial polyps. Obstet Gynecol 1964;24:621–625.

DeCherney AH, Cholst I, Naftolin F. The management of intractable uterine bleeding utilizing the cystoscopic resectoscope. In: Siegler AM, Lindemann HJ, eds. Hysteroscopy: principles and practice. Philadelphia: JB Lippincott, 1984:140.

DeCherney A, Polan MI. Hysteroscopic management of intrauterine lesions and intractable uterine bleeding. Obstet Gynecol 1983;61:392.

DeCherney AH, Russell JB, Graebe RA, et al. Resectoscopic management of müllerian fusion defects. Fertil Steril 1986;45:726.

Droegemueller W, Greet BE, David JR, et al. Cryocoagulation of the endometrium at the uterine cornua. Am J Obstet Gynecol 1978;131:1.

Droegemueller W, Greet B, Makowski E. Cryosurgery in patients with dysfunctional uterine bleeding. Obstet Gynecol 1971;38:256.

Edstrom K, Fernstrom I. The diagnostic possibilities of a modified hysteroscopic technique. Acta Obstet Gynecol Scand 1970;49(4):327.

Fisher JC. Principles of safety in laser surgery and therapy. In: Baggish MS, ed. Basic and advanced laser surgery in gynecology. Norwalk, CT: Appleton-Century-Crofts, 1985:85–130.

Goldrath MH. Vaginal removal of the pedunculated submucous myoma: the use of laminaria. Obstet Gynecol 1987;70:670.

Goldrath M, Fuller T, Segal S. Laser photovaporization of endometrium for the treatment of menorrhagia. Am J Obstet Gynecol 1981;140:14.

Hamou JE. Hysteroscopic et microhysteroscopic avec un instrument nouveau: le microhysteroscope. Endosc Gynecol 1980;2:131.

Hamou JE. Microhysteroscopy: a new procedure and its original application in gynecology. J Reprod Med 1981;26:375.

Jones HW, Seegar-Jones G. Double uterus as an etiological factor in repeated abortion: indications for surgical repair. Am J Obstet Gynecol 1953;65:325.

Lindemann HJ. The use of CO_2 in the uterine cavity for hysteroscopy. Int J Fertil 1972;17:221.

Lindemann HJ, Mohr J. CO_2 hysteroscopy, diagnosis, and treatment. Am J Obstet Gynecol 1976; 124–129.

Lomano JM. Photocoagulation of the endometrium with the Nd-YAG laser for the treatment of menorrhagia: a report of 10 cases. J Reprod Med 1986;31:26.

March CM. Hysteroscopy for infertility in diagnostic and operative hysteroscopy. In: Baggish MS, Barbot J, Valle RF, eds. Diagnostic and operative hysteroscopy: a text and atlas. Chicago: Year Book Medical Publishers, 1989:136–146.

March CM, Israel R. Gestational outcome following hysteroscopic lysis of adhesions. Fertil Steril 1981;36:455.

March CM, Israel R. Hysteroscopic management of recurrent abortion caused by septate uterus. Am J Obstet Gynecol 1987;156:834.

March CM, Israel R, March AD. Hysteroscopic management of intrauterine adhesions. Am J Obstet Gynecol 1978;130:65.

Mishler JM. Synthetic plasma volume expanders—their pharmacology, safety and clinical efficacy. Clin Haematol 1984;13:75.

Neuwirth RS. A new technique for and additional experience with hysteroscopic resection of submucous fibroids. Am J Obstet Gynecol 1978;131:91.

Neuwirth RS. Hysteroscopic management of symptomatic submucous fibroids. Obstet Gynecol 1983;62:509.

Neuwirth RS. Hysteroscopic resection of submucous leiomyoma. Contemp Obstet Gynecol 1985;25:103–123.

Neuwirth RS, Amin HK. Excision of submucous fibroids with hysteroscopic control. Am J Obstet Gynecol 1976;126:95.

Pantaleoni D. On endoscopic examination of the cavity of the womb. Med Press Circ 1869;8:26–27.

Porto R, Gaujoux J. One nouvelle methode d'hysteroscopic instrumentation et technique. J Gynecol Obstet Biol Reprod 1972;7:691.

Quinones RG. Hysteroscopy with a new fluid technique. In: Siegler AM, Lindemann HJ, eds. Hysteroscopy: principles and practice. Philadelphia: JB Lippincott, 1984:41.

Reed TP, Erb RA. Hysteroscopic tubal occlusion with silicone rubber. Obstet Gynecol 1983;61:388.

Roberts S, Long L, Jonasson O. The isolation of cancer cells from the bloodstream during uterine curettage. Surg Gynecol Obstet 1960;111:3.

Siegler AM, Kemmann E. Hysteroscopic removal of occult intrauterine contraceptive device. Obstet Gynecol 1975;46:604.

Siegler AM, Kemmann EK. Hysteroscopy, a review. Obstet Gynecol Surg 1975;30:567.

Strassman EO. Plastic unification of double uterus. Am J Obstet Gynecol 1952;64:25.

Valle RF. Hysteroscopic evaluation of patients with abnormal uterine bleeding. Surg Gynecol Obstet 1981;153:521–526.

Valle RF. Hysteroscopy for gynecologic diagnosis. Clin Obstet Gynecol 1983;26:253.

Valle RF, Sciarra U. Hysteroscopy: a useful diagnostic adjunct in gynecology. Am J Obstet Gynecol 1975;122:230.

Valle RF, Sciarra JJ, Freeman DW. Hysteroscopic removal of intrauterine devices with missing filaments. Obstet Gynecol 1977;49:55–60.

Ectopic Pregnancy

JOHN A. ROCK

Ectopic pregnancy was first recognized by Busiere in 1693 on examination of the body of an executed prisoner in Paris. Gifford, in 1731 in England, made a more complete report, describing the condition in which the fertilized ovum was implanted outside the uterine cavity. This disorder has become one of the more serious complications of pregnancy. Ectopic pregnancy is now one of the leading causes of maternal morbidity and mortality in the United States, accounting for 14.7% of all maternal deaths in 1982, according to Atrash, Friede, and Hogue.

The early diagnosis of ectopic pregnancy has been made possible by the highly sensitive rapid β-human chorionic gonadotropin (β-HCG) assay and the development of abdominal and, more recently, vaginal ultrasonography. Expectant, conservative surgical and medical therapy are now possible. These conservative alternatives are usually possible when a small ectopic is present without rupture. Thus, preservation of the oviduct to preserve or enhance fertility is important. Physicians should have a high index of suspicion so they will apply advanced technology to make an early diagnosis and intervention. This chapter summarizes the contemporary methods for diagnosis and treatment of patients with an ectopic pregnancy.

EPIDEMIOLOGY OF ECTOPIC PREGNANCY

Although the total number of pregnancies has declined over the past two decades, the rate of ectopic pregnancy has increased dramatically (Table 18-1). Atrash and associates described changes in ectopic pregnancy mortality and characterized the risk of death for different groups using data on ectopic pregnancy identified by the National Vital Statistics system for the period from 1970 to 1983. The increased ratio of extrauterine to intrauterine pregnancies was related to the rising incidence of sexually transmitted disease and to the efficacy of modern antibiotic treatment in preventing inflammatory disease. The risk of death from ectopic pregnancy declined among all races and ages in all regions of the United States. However, from 1970 to 1983, women of black and other races were at significantly increased risk of death from ectopic pregnancy compared with white women.

Although the incidence of ectopic pregnancy between 1970 and 1983 increased fourfold, the risk of death from ectopic pregnancy declined by 85%. This decline may be related to improved diagnostic technology and, thus, improved management and care. With the advent of conservative surgery and the emphasis on early diagnosis, increased awareness of this condition may be an important factor in reducing the morbidity and mortality of ectopic pregnancy.

PATHOLOGY

Tubal gestation traditionally has been considered to implant and grow within the tubal lumen. Budowick and coauthors have suggested that tubal implantation actually occurs in the lumen but is soon followed by penetration into the lamina propria and muscularis to become extraluminal. Pauerstein, Hodgson, and Kramen demonstrated that trophoblastic infiltration may be predominantly intraluminal or predominantly extraluminal, or, occasionally, mixed. Currently, it is impossible to ascertain in the operating room the predominant pattern of growth of a given tubal pregnancy. In any event, fimbrial expression usually is an unacceptable method for removal of ectopic pregnancy. Not only is the method traumatic, but it does not remove all of the trophoblastic tissue. The persistence of ectopic pregnancy may require additional therapy.

411

TABLE 18–1
Numbers and Rates of Ectopic Pregnancies by Year, United States, 1970–1980

YEAR	NO. OF ECTOPIC PREGNANCIES	RATES		
		Women Aged 15–44*	Live Births †	Reported Pregnancies ††
1970	17,800	4.2	4.8	4.5
1971	19,300	4.4	5.4	4.8
1972	24,500	5.5	7.5	6.3
1973	25,600	5.6	8.2	6.8
1974	26,400	5.7	8.4	6.7
1975	30,500	6.5	9.8	7.6
1976	34,600	7.2	11.0	8.3
1977	40,700	8.3	12.3	9.2
1978	42,400	8.5	12.8	9.4
1979	49,900	9.9	14.3	10.4
1980	52,200	9.9	14.5	10.5
Total	363,900	6.9	9.9	7.7

* Rate per 10,000 females.
† Rate per 1000 live births.
†† Rate per 1000 reported pregnancies (ie, live births, legal induced abortions, and ectopic pregnancies).
(From Pregancy Epidemiology Branch, Division of Reproductive Health, Centers for Disease Control, U.S. Public Health Service, Atlanta, Georgia, 1981. Reprinted with permission.)

ETIOLOGY OF ECTOPIC PREGNANCY

Tubal Damage Secondary to Inflammation

Both the increased incidence of sexually transmitted disease resulting in salpingitis and the efficacy of antibiotic therapy in preventing total tubal occlusion following an episode of salpingitis are related to the increasing incidence of ectopic pregnancy. Levin and associates have demonstrated that the risk of ectopic pregnancy is increased in women with a primary history of pelvic inflammatory disease. Westrom compared women with pelvic inflammatory disease confirmed by laparoscopy to women matched by age and parity and found a six-times greater incidence of ectopic pregnancy for the women with pelvic inflammatory disease, an alarming rate of one ectopic pregnancy out of every 24 gestations. Similar statistics are recognized among other high-risk groups. In Jamaica, where the ectopic pregnancy rate is 1 in 28 deliveries, the frequency of pelvic inflammatory disease is proportionately high. Many of the patients in these studies had received antibiotic treatment for salpingitis.

Before the antibiotic era, salpingitis resulted in an acutely inflamed tube that usually became totally occluded, resulting in permanent sterility. Women who attempted pregnancy following a pelvic infection were successful <40% of the time. The current pregnancy rate exceeds 60% for the patients who have been adequately treated with antibiotics. After an initial infection is treated appropriately with antibiotics, agglutination of the cilia may occur and synechial bands form within the tubal lumen, resulting in partial tubal obstruction. Westrom has demonstrated by laparoscopy that occlusion occurs in approximately 12.8% of patients following treatment for a single tubal infection; after two infections, in 35%; and after three or more infections, in 75% of women. Westrom found that of the patients who achieve a subsequent pregnancy after salpingitis, 4% or 5% will have an ectopic pregnancy.

Fallopian tubes containing a gestation are frequently normal macroscopically and on gross histologic examination. Vasquez, Winston, and Brosens, using scanning electron microscopy and light microscopy studies of tubal biopsies from five groups of women, showed marked differences in the ciliated surface, which was measured planimetrically on photographs. The proportion of ciliated cells was significantly lower in biopsies taken from 25 women with tubal pregnancies compared with biopsies from seven women with intrauterine pregnancies at the same gestation. This marked deciliation also was seen in eight women biopsied during tubal surgery. Thus, the increased occurrence of sexually transmitted disease resulting in tubal epithelial damage may be a cause of the reported rise in the incidence of ectopic pregnancy. A similar mechanism may account for ectopic pregnancies reported after long-term usage of intrauterine contraceptive devices (IUDs).

Contraceptive Devices

Use of IUDs has been linked to the increased incidence of ectopic pregnancy, but a direct relationship has not been proven. In a summary of published reports on ectopic pregnancy, Tatum and Schmidt noted that 4% of the pregnancies that occurred with an IUD in place were ectopic. Ory, in a collaborative multicenter case-control study of the incidence of ectopic pregnancy in the United States from 1965 through 1977, reached a different conclusion: the IUD did not play a significant role in the increased incidence of ectopic pregnancy.

The actual number of conceptions with an IUD in place is impossible to identify. The World Health Organization task force on IUDs for fertility regulation concluded that a valid comparison of different types of IUDs regarding their association with ectopic pregnancy could not be made and, furthermore, that evidence linking IUDs and pelvic inflammatory disease has probably contributed to the presumed correlation between IUDs and ectopic pregnancy. Although the role of the IUD in the rising incidence of ectopic pregnancy cannot be proven currently, a limited cause-and-effect relationship probably does exist.

Oral Contraceptives

Studies in the United States and abroad have demonstrated that a high incidence of ectopic pregnancies involve progesterone-only oral contraceptives. It is hypothesized that progesterone-only oral contraceptives have only a minimal propulsive effect on the oviduct at the ampullary-isthmic junction and, therefore, ovum trapping may result.

Elective Abortion

Levin and coauthors demonstrated that when statistical techniques were used to control the effects of other risk factors, the history of one or more induced abortions did not significantly increase the risk of ectopic pregnancy. Nevertheless, if a woman had two or more induced abortions, the risk for tubal pregnancy doubled. A possible association between multiple induced abortions and subsequent tubal pregnancy is suggested, perhaps due to postabortal infection.

Prior Tubal Surgery

An operative procedure on the oviduct, whether a sterilization procedure or tubal reconstructive surgery, may cause an ectopic pregnancy. The incidence of ectopic pregnancies occurring after neosalpingostomy procedures for a distal tubal obstruction ranges from 2% to 18% (Table 18-2). The rate of ectopic pregnancy following a microsurgical reversal of sterilization procedure is approximately 4%, because the tubes have not been damaged by infection.

The overall incidence of ectopic pregnancy after elective tubal sterilization is approximately 16%, according to Tatum and Schmidt. Failure of sterilization may occur with the development of a tubal peritoneal fistula. These fistulas have been demonstrated radiographically by Shah, Courey, and Cunanan in 11% of

TABLE 18–2
Summary: Ectopic Pregnancy After Tubal Surgery

PROCEDURE	TECHNIQUE	% TOTAL PREGNANCY	PREGNANCY RANGE (%)	% ECTOPIC	ECTOPIC RANGE (%)
Salpingoscopy	Macr*	42	35–65	3.4	1–20
	Micr†	52	31–69	1.8	0–16
Fimbrioplasty	Macr*	42	36–50	14	10–18
	Micr	59	26–68	6	4–11
Neosalpingostomy	Macr	27	20–38	4.2	2–10
	Micr	26	17–44	7.7	0–18
Tubal anastomosis	Macr	44	25–83	9.2	0–15
	Micr	62	35–78	2.3	1–6.2
Removal of ectopic pregnancy	Salpingectomy	42	38–49	12	8–17
	Salpingostomy	57	39–73	11	0–20

* Macr, macrosurgery.
† Micr, microsurgery.
(From Levy G, Diamond MP, DeCherney AH. Ectopic pregnancy: relationship to tubal reconstructive surgery. Fertil Steril 1987; 47:543. Reproduced with permission of the publisher, The American Fertility Society.)

150 women following laparoscopic electrocoagulation. It is hypothesized that this tubal peritoneal fistula allows sperm to pass into the distal segment of the oviduct and fertilize the egg. With the increase in use of female sterilization techniques today, sterilization is becoming a more frequent cause of ectopic pregnancy. Brenner, Raj, and Mishell reported that 3% of 300 ectopic pregnancies occurring in 1976 and 1977 were due to tubal sterilization failures.

Developmental Anomalies

Intramural polyps and tubal diverticula may block or alter tubal transport of fertilized ova. Additionally, patients with congenital absence of segments of the fallopian tube with peritoneal fistulas also may be predisposed to tubal pregnancy.

Ovum Regurgitation

The fertilized egg may be regurgitated into the fallopian tube at the time of reinsertion of an embryo into the uterine fundus following in vitro fertilization. Ectopic pregnancy has been reported following embryo transfer. The National In Vitro Fertilization-Embryo Transfer Registry reported a 5% ectopic pregnancy rate in 1988. Ectopic pregnancy has been observed after gamete intrafallopian tube transfer.

Transmigration of the Ovum

Walters, Eddy, and Pauerstein reported that 16% of tubal pregnancies result from a contralateral ovulation. Transmigration of the ovum in the peritoneal cavity may occur because the oviducts and ovaries may be in close approximation in the cul-de-sac. Alternatively, this phenomenon could result from transmigration of the embryo through the endometrial cavity into the opposite oviduct.

Other Factors

Poland, Dill, and Styblo have reported morphologic and cytogenetic data from 76 embryos and fetuses obtained from pregnancies occurring in the fallopian tube. Their findings indicated that tubal implantation was associated with a high proportion of severely disorganized embryos. There also is a high incidence of maternal tubal disease. In ectopic pregnancy, the relative increase in number of embryos with severe growth disorganization may be a result of the tubal implantation site and its influence on development.

SITES OF ECTOPIC PREGNANCY

Approximately 95% of extrauterine implantations occur in the oviduct. The ampulla is the most common site, with approximately 55% of all tubal implantations; the isthmic portion has 20% to 25%; the infundibulum and fimbria have 17%; and the interstitial segment has 2% to 4%. Implantations occur less often in the ovary, the cornua, the cervix, and the peritoneal cavity (Fig. 18-1).

EFFECTS OF ECTOPIC PREGNANCY ON FUTURE REPRODUCTION

Tubal pregnancy is associated with a poor prognosis for subsequent reproduction. In most cases, an extrauterine pregnancy represents an impairment of the fertilized ovum's ability to migrate through the deep rugae of the oviduct as a result of altered tubal function. The morphologic abnormality is usually bilateral and irreversible and may produce repeated ectopic pregnancy, spontaneous abortion, or permanent sterility. In a 1975 study, Shoen and Nowak concluded that approximately 70% of the patients who have an ectopic first pregnancy are unable to produce a living child. As many as 30% of the patients who have an ectopic first pregnancy will have a repeat ectopic pregnancy, compared with the total repeat ectopic rate of between 10% and 20%. More than half of the subsequent extrauterine pregnancies will occur within a 2-year period, and 80% will occur within 4 years of the initial ectopic pregnancy. In reviewing the experience of the Kaiser Foundation hospitals, Hallatt reported a 9.2% incidence of repeat ectopic pregnancies among 1330 women who had extrauterine pregnancies. Hallatt's figure correlates well with the overall rate for repeat ectopic pregnancies. The potential reproductive capacity for a patient who has had an ectopic pregnancy depends on her reproductive history. If she is unfortunate enough to have had an ectopic pregnancy as a result of her first

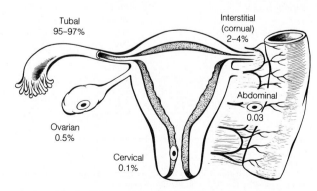

Figure 18–1. Sites and incidence of ectopic pregnancy.

reproductive effort, then the prognosis is much worse than had the complication occurred after one or more successful pregnancies.

Mueller, Daling, and Weiss have estimated that 92% percent of tubal infertility in women who have had a tubal pregnancy results from a tubal pregnancy itself or other factors that predispose to its occurrence. Approximately 20% of women who suffer tubal pregnancy will subsequently be infertile because of a tubal abnormality. Yang, Chow, and Daling noted that a history of infertility predisposes women to an increased risk of tubal pregnancy as does the use of fertility drugs. A twofold increase in the risks of tubal pregnancy exists among infertile women who were found to have no abnormality during an infertility evaluation.

TUBAL ECTOPIC PREGNANCY

The morbidity and mortality associated with extrauterine pregnancy are directly related to the length of time before diagnosis is made. In a Centers for Disease Control survey, two thirds of all patients later proven to have an ectopic pregnancy were previously seen by a physician and either the diagnosis was deferred or the condition was incorrectly assessed. The mortality rate from an ectopic pregnancy is higher in rural areas, where patients are less likely to receive early medical care.

For a successful outcome, an ectopic pregnancy must be diagnosed early. In some clinics where the complication is treated frequently, >50% of the cases are diagnosed and operated on before tubal rupture occurs. However, in approximately 85% of all cases, the symptoms that bring a patient to seek medical care are caused by a leaking or ruptured ectopic pregnancy. As many as 15% of all tubal pregnancies rupture before the first missed menstrual period, especially if a patient's periods are usually irregular.

The diagnostic record is improved somewhat in repeat ectopic pregnancies. As many as 25% to 30% of the repeat cases will be diagnosed and treated surgically before tubal rupture. Another difference is that with a repeat ectopic pregnancy, it is usually the patient herself who raises the question of an extrauterine pregnancy. Being suspicious, the patient seeks medical care earlier and provides a more specific medical history than does a patient experiencing her first ectopic pregnancy. The result is an earlier diagnosis and an improved chance for a successful outcome.

Some form of menstrual shedding occurs around the expected time of menses in more than 50% of women with an ectopic pregnancy, so most patients and their physicians are unaware that a pregnancy has occurred. The menstrual shedding may be followed by a period of amenorrhea lasting between 6 and 10 weeks, after which the clinical symptoms of ectopic pregnancy appear.

Diagnosis

Classic Symptoms: Pain, Bleeding, and Adnexal Mass

The classic presentation of pain and uterine bleeding with the finding of an adnexal mass has been the clinical hallmark of extrauterine pregnancy, but even classic presentations can be misleading, as Schwartz and DiPietro have observed. Of the patients who presented with the classic symptoms, only 14% were shown to have an ectopic pregnancy. The severity of these symptoms and signs depends on the stage of the condition, but in the early stages of an ectopic gestation, symptoms are less predictive than in the more advanced stages of the reproductive process.

A discrete, unilateral mass, separate from the adjacent ovary, has been detected in less than one third of all proven ectopic pregnancies. Locating a mass depends on many unpredictable factors, including the diagnostic skill of the examiner, the degree of pelvic peritonitis present, the presence or absence of tubal rupture, and the degree of stoicism and cooperation of the patient. Even when all factors are optimal, an adnexal mass can be felt in only half of the cases.

Diagnostic Studies

Three major improvements have made early diagnosis of extrauterine pregnancy possible: (1) the development of highly sensitive, rapid β-HCG assays; (2) the ability to use ultrasound to evaluate the uterus and the adnexa (vaginal sonography has added increased accuracy of diagnosis); and (3) the application of laparoscopy as a diagnostic tool. Culdocentesis and/or curettage may be useful under certain circumstances, eg, to help establish the presence of a hemoperitoneum or an intrauterine pregnancy, respectively.

β-HCG Assays. Urine pregnancy tests using the slide method have a β-HCG sensitivity level of 1500 to 3500 milli-international units (mIU) per milliliter (Table 18-3). The tests are frequently imprecise and have been positive in only half of the later proven cases of ectopic pregnancy, where the HCG level is often lower than the sensitivity of the urine slide test. The current availability of very sensitive and accurate serum pregnancy tests has resulted in an increased use of this method in the detection of an ectopic pregnancy. Pregnancy blood tests with a detection threshold of 200 mIU/ml are associated with an 11.9% incidence of false-negative results. A radioimmunoassay for β-HCG can detect levels of HCG as low as 5 to 10 mIU/ml of serum

TABLE 18–3
Qualitative Procedures for Detection of β-HCG

TEST	SENSITIVITY (mIU/ml)
Tube Tests	
Biocept-G (radioreceptor assay, Wampole Labs)	200
Sensitex (Roche Labs)	250
UCG-Test (Wampole Labs)	500
Accusphere (Organon, Inc.)	750
Pregnostic (Organon, Inc.)	750
Pregnosis Placentex (Roche Labs)	1000
UCG-Lyphotest (Wampole Labs)	1250
EPT (Warner-Chilcott Labs)	1250
Slide Tests	
Dri-Dot (Organon, Inc.)	1500
Pregnosis (Roche Labs)	1500
Pregnosticon (Organon, Inc.)	1500
UCG (Wampole Labs)	2000
Gravindex (Ortho Pharmaceutical Corp.)	3500

*Biocept-G also can be used as a semiquantitative test.
(From Hussa RO. Clinical utility of human chorionic gonadotropin and α-subunit measurements. Obstet Gynecol 1982; 60:1. Reprinted with permission.)

with a 0.5% incidence of false-negative results. Thus, the test is approximately 400 to 500 times more sensitive than the more conventional urinary hemagglutination tests.

The β-HCG quantitative assay requires 24 hours for desired sensitivity and reliability. A semiquantitative radioreceptor assay may be used by laboratories in which quantitative HCG assays are unavailable. The Biocept-G radioreceptor assay (Wampole Labs) can be used semiquantitatively when standardized against a qualitative method. With its lower sensitivity level of 200 mIU/ml, the radioreceptor test is positive in approximately 90% of the cases of ectopic pregnancy, compared with the β-HCG radioimmunoassay, which is positive in nearly 100% of cases.

The lower limits of increase in serum HCG for viable intrauterine pregnancy have been described in the author's laboratory using the First International Reference Preparation (First IRP). Serum quantitative HCG levels appear to increase between 30% and 50% (mean, 29.1%) for an interval of 24 hours in normal intrauterine pregnancy. A more meaningful interval determination is at 48 hours with a minimum of 66% (range, 65% to 100%) increase over baseline HCG values. Longer interval determinations are at 72 hours (range, 45% to 150%) and 96 hours (range, 75% to 200%). Interval HCG determinations interpreted within the context of several values are usually of prognostic significance with respect to normal intrauterine versus abnormal implantation sites and subsequent tro-

phoblastic development. However, Shepherd and coauthors reported that in their experience a normal rise in HCG production did not reliably differentiate an ectopic from an intrauterine pregnancy in the symptomatic patient. The authors noted that ultimately a combination of endocrine testing and ultrasonography may prove most useful.

Progesterone Assay. Matthews, Coulson, and Weld recently reported progesterone levels in 29 patients with ectopic pregnancy using a new direct radioimmunoassay that offers results within 4 hours. Patients with normal intrauterine pregnancies had serum progesterone levels >20 ng/ml and all patients with ectopic pregnancies had progesterone levels <15 ng/ml. Their results indicated that the incorporation of a progesterone assay into the work-up of a patient with suspected ectopic may be a useful clinical adjunct to standard diagnostic studies.

Ultrasound. The major use of pelvic ultrasound is to document an intrauterine pregnancy by demonstrating the gestational sac and fetus. The recent application of the imaging technique to cases with a suspected ectopic pregnancy has greatly facilitated the clinical diagnosis of the disorder.

In a normal intrauterine pregnancy, a gestational sac can be seen with abdominal ultrasonography at 5 to 6 weeks from the time of the last menstrual period, and a fetus can be identified at 6 to 7 weeks. It is not until week 7 or week 8, when the serum level of HCG reaches 13,000 to 14,000 mIU/ml or more, that a fetal heartbeat can be visualized by ultrasound. Recognition of the critical intrauterine events is sufficient for ruling out a diagnosis of extrauterine pregnancy.

Diagnosis by abdominal ultrasound can be confusing. Only a few clinics have a high ultrasound accuracy rate; the normal false-negative varies from 2% to 35%. One problem is that a "pseudogestational" sac due to a decidual cast may be mistaken for an amniotic sac. Recently, the finding of a double-sac image, representing both the decidual lining of the uterus and the amniotic sac, has been used to confirm the accuracy of a diagnosis of intrauterine pregnancy. The double-sac image can be visualized as early as 5 weeks following the last menstrual period.

Jain and associates have compared endovaginal and transabdominal ultrasound in 90 patients with a positive serum pregnancy test (Table 18-4). The specific diagnosis of ectopic pregnancy was impossible with transabdominal ultrasound before 7 weeks. Intrauterine pregnancy was detected earlier with endovaginal ultrasound because the yolk sac, fetal pole, and fetal heart motion could be seen sooner. Fetal heart motion was detected as early as 34 days after the last menstrual period in patients with fetal poles with the crown-rump length of ≥0.3 cm.

TABLE 18–4
Pregnancy Earliest Seen with Ultrasonography

EARLY INTRAUTERINE PREGNANCY	ENDOVAGINAL	TRANSABDOMINAL
Gestational Sac Seen		
Gestational sac size	0.5 cm	0.5 cm
Gestational sac age	4.3 wk	4.3 wk
Double Decidual Outline		
Gestational sac size	0.6 to 0.7 cm	1.0 cm
Gestational sac age	4.4 wk	5.0 wk
Yolk Sac Seen		
Gestational sac size	0.7 cm	1.0 cm
Gestational sac age	4.6 wk	5.0 wk
	(34 d)	(35 d)
Fetal Pole Seen		
Gestational sac size	0.7 cm	1.7 cm
Gestational sac age	4.6 wk	6.0 wk
Fetal Heart Motion Seen		
Crown-rump length	0.3 cm	0.6 cm
Gestational sac age	4.6 wk	6.5 wk
	(34 d)	(47 d)

(From Jain K, Hamper VM, Sanders RC. Comparison of transvaginal sonography in the detection of early pregnancy and its complications. Am J Radiol 1988; 151:1139. Reprinted with permission.)

Bernaschek, Rudelstorfer, and Csaicsich performed vaginosonic scans and β-HCG concentrations on 52 women with early gestational age to establish criteria for the earliest possible identification of intrauterine pregnancy. The smallest diameter of the gestational sac detected was 2 mm and the lowest β-HCG was 141 mIU/ml when an intrauterine pregnancy was correctly diagnosed. All pregnancies associated with β-HCG concentrations of >300 mIU/ml were correctly identified. No false-positive vaginoscopic findings were observed in their study.

The threshold level of HCG above which an intrauterine gestational sac is expected by abdominal sonography in a normal pregnancy (discriminatory zone) was initially characterized at a titer of ≥6500 mIU/ml using the First IRP. Others have suggested a lower threshold, 1800 mIU/ml, using the Second International Standard (Second IS). Fossum and coauthors noted that the gestational sac may be visualized 35 days from the last menstrual period, at which time the HCG was 914 ± 106 mIU/ml of the Second IS. Shapiro and coauthor reported that transvaginal ultrasound scan was able to identify the ectopic pregnancy before the expected appearance of an intrauterine sac in 92% of the patients with titers below the equivalent of 3600 mIU/ml with the First IRP. The coupling of HCG titers and ultrasound findings has greatly facilitated the diagnosis of ectopic gestation. Transvaginal sonography has enhanced the physician's ability to make the diagnosis of a tubal ectopic pregnancy by direct visualization of the ectopic in the adnexa.

In some instances, the pregnancy may be seen in the oviduct (Fig. 18-2). Thus, performance, the absence of side effects, the high rate of patient acceptance, and the clarity of images obtained with endovaginal ultrasound make this method an attractive alternative to abdominal ultrasound. The use of endovaginal ultrasound, however, is not without limitations. An overall view of the uterus and pelvis cannot be obtained. A lesion located high in the pelvis or outside the pelvis cannot be visualized, and the physician may therefore have to perform both endovaginal and transabdominal examinations. Free peritoneal fluid or hemoperitoneum secondary to a ruptured ectopic may be entirely missed with an endovaginal exam. Nevertheless, in no case in the series by Jain and associates did the endovaginal sonogram provide a false-positive finding or less information in the pelvis than did transabdominal sonography. Furthermore, Kivikoski and coauthors found that transvaginal ultrasonography was significantly more accurate in identifying an adnexal gestational sac and allowed more detailed adnexal imaging.

The use of β-HCG combined with endovaginal and abdominal sonography will assist the physician in making an early diagnosis of ectopic pregnancy. Many protocols have been suggested combining culdocentesis,

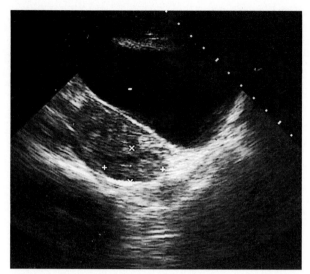

Figure 18–2. Tubal ectopic pregnancy documented by endovaginal sonography.

serum HCG, sonography, and, finally, laparoscopy. These protocols should not replace the need for a careful clinical history and examination. The protocol developed at the Johns Hopkins Hospital is changing with the development of technological advances in sonography.

Dilatation and Curettage. Although in the past, histologic changes in the endometrium accompanying an ectopic gestation were confirmed by dilatation and curettage (D&C), more accurate measurements can be achieved with newer diagnostic studies, such as the radioimmunoassay for β-HCG, ultrasonography, and laparoscopy. If there is a low plateau level of β-HCG, a D&C may be performed to establish the presence of degenerating villi. Alternatively, if a patient is bleeding excessively, a curettage may be required. In either case, the removed material may be assessed. Findings of decidua without chorionic villi, although they suggest the diagnosis of an ectopic pregnancy, do not provide absolute proof, because these findings also occur with a spontaneous abortion. Endometrial changes provide only supportive rather than diagnostic information.

The atypical epithelial changes of the gestational endometrium were first described by Polak and Wolfe in 1924, in a case of tubal pregnancy, and were expanded upon by Arias-Stella in 1954 (Fig. 18-3). The highly controversial method of identifying these changes depends on a precise definition of a definitive cell involved in the morphologic change, together with some ill-defined physiologic events that produce the changes. Arias-Stella and others remain convinced that the histologic changes represent a progressive phenomenon resulting from exaggerated proliferative and secretory

responses to the elevated hormonal levels of pregnancy. Fienberg and Lloyd disagree, maintaining that the changes are regressive and involutional and are the result of declining hormonal levels. Whatever hypothesis is proven, the endometrial changes can be associated with normal pregnancy as well as with a spontaneous abortion or an ectopic pregnancy, thus the histologic reactions have no specific value for the detection of an extrauterine pregnancy.

Recently, O'Connor and Kurman suggested that certain histologic criteria may be used to confirm the presence of an intrauterine implantation site in endometrial curettings without recognizable chorionic villi. Enlarged hyalinized spiral arteries and fibrinoid matrix were not seen in any ectopic pregnancy. These histologic criteria may be useful in determining the presence of an intrauterine implantation where no villi are recovered from D&C.

Culdocentesis. A culdocentesis is a useful diagnostic tool for identifying the presence of intraperitoneal bleeding. The simple procedure of inserting a No. 18 gauge spinal needle attached to a 50-ml aspirating syringe into the cul-de-sac between the uterosacral ligaments (Fig. 18-4) provides immediate and useful

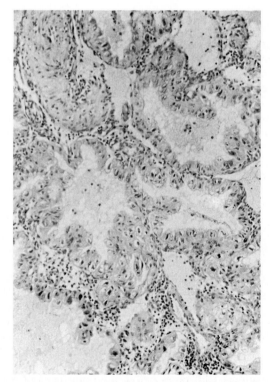

Figure 18–3. Arias-Stella reaction in endometrial cells associated with ectopic pregnancy, showing nuclear enlargement, irregularity, and hyperchromasia with cytoplasmic vacuolation.

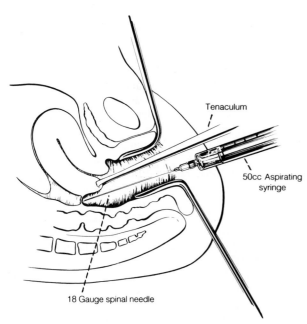

Figure 18–4. Culdocentesis. A No. 18 gauge spinal needle is inserted through the posterior fornix and enters the cul-de-sac between the uterosacral ligaments.

clinical information when unclotted blood is aspirated from the cul-de-sac. The procedure cannot be used for an absolute diagnosis, because a tubal pregnancy may not have ruptured or leaked into the peritoneal cavity. Culdocentesis can indicate the presence of free blood in the peritoneal cavity, but it cannot determine whether the blood is from an ectopic pregnancy or from some other cause of intra-abdominal bleeding. A ruptured corpus luteum hematoma or the rupture of another viscera would result in similar bleeding patterns.

Culdocentesis may be of value in patients with abdominal pain in whom one suspects early rupture. Combined with ultrasonography, culdocentesis continues to be an important diagnostic technique to assist the clinician in determining if intraperitoneal bleeding is present.

Laparoscopy. Laparoscopy is useful when an unruptured ectopic pregnancy is suspected but the patient has no signs of intraperitoneal bleeding. If a patient is in stable condition, then the examination can be deferred for 48 hours following the initial β-HCG radioimmunoassay so that a subsequent titer can be determined. Patients who have less than a 66% increase in β-HCG have a high incidence of ectopic pregnancy and should be followed closely. In such patients, laparoscopy may be indicated if a D&C does not identify products of conception. Laparoscopy (see Ch. 16) is useful for diagnosis because it allows precise visualization of

the entire female reproductive tract. Laparoscopy is a great improvement over the more cumbersome and difficult technique of culdoscopy. Once the possibility of an ectopic pregnancy has been recognized, the adnexa must be visualized to be thoroughly evaluated before the patient can be discharged from the hospital. Laparoscopy has reduced the clinical error in diagnosing an ectopic pregnancy to <4% of cases, and this simple technique has limited the need for laparotomy. When laparotomy was used to determine the presence or absence of an extrauterine pregnancy, 20% of the procedures resulted in negative findings.

Summary of Diagnostic Methods Used to Detect Tubal Ectopic Pregnancy

When a patient is seen with a clinical history suspicious for ectopic pregnancy, a careful examination is performed (Fig. 18-5). A serum β-HCG is obtained. If an intrauterine sac is visualized with fetal heart tones, then the diagnosis of intrauterine pregnancy is established. If, however, there are no fetal heart tones and there is a suboptimal elevation of β-HCG, then the asymptomatic patient may be followed with a serial quantitative β-HCG every other day. If, however, there is adnexal pain, a diagnostic laparoscopy should be performed to rule out a tubal pregnancy.

With the development of vaginal sonography, the use of a discriminatory zone is not of frequent clinical utility. The level of HCG at which a uterine sac should be visible (discriminatory zone) varies depending on the β-HCG assay. This zone also varies with the method of pelvic sonography. In the author's laboratory, the absence of an intrauterine sac with abdominal sonography and a β-HCG >10,500 signifies a probable ectopic pregnancy.

More commonly, the ectopic pregnancy will produce a low level of β-HCG from the aborting or degenerating trophoblast. The differential diagnosis should include spontaneous abortion or blighted ovum. When the diagnosis is uncertain and the patient is in an unstable condition, the patient should be evaluated immediately by laparoscopy and, if necessary, by laparotomy. If the patient is in stable condition, serial β-HCGs should be taken at 48-hour intervals and the assays should be correlated with the patient's initial serum value. If the HCG increases >66% within a 48-hour period, then the patient most probably has a normal intrauterine pregnancy and nonsurgical care is indicated. If the increase of the serial HCG level is <66% of the original value, then ectopic pregnancy should be suspected. Ultrasound can be used as a diagnostic support, showing a gestational sac in the adnexa or fluid in the cul-de-sac.

Initially, a normal increase in β-HCG may be ob-

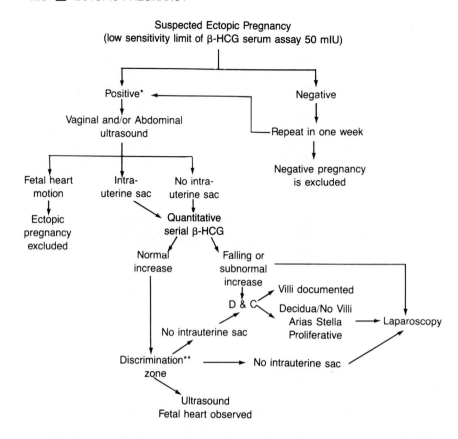

Figure 18–5. The use of sensitive and quantitative HCG. Specific radioimmunoassay and ultrasound in diagnosis of ectopic pregnancy.

served. Over time, however, the level may slowly fall, never reaching the discriminatory zone. If a possible intrauterine pregnancy is thought nonviable, a D&C may be performed. However, if there is a question of viability, then a laparoscopy is preferable to rule out an ectopic pregnancy. Once fetal heart motion is noted within the uterine cavity, the possibility of a tubal ectopic pregnancy is virtually excluded. Patients should be followed closely, especially after a superovulation regimen. In this group of patients, an increased risk of a simultaneous intrauterine and an ectopic pregnancy exists. Nevertheless, the overall risk of the two existing simultaneously is small.

A falling or subnormal increase in β-HCG in the asymptomatic patient may prompt laparoscopy if there is a question of viability of a possible intrauterine pregnancy. A falling β-HCG may occur following the death of one of several pregnancies conceived through superovulation or in vitro fertilization. Ultimately, the β-HCG level will rise if the β-HCG levels are repeated at periodic intervals. Thus, the downward trend should be dramatic or a persistent plateau should be documented with at least three β-HCG levels taken over a 1-week interval to consider a D&C before laparoscopy.

Treatment for Ectopic Pregnancy

Expectant Therapy

The early diagnosis of ectopic pregnancy by plasma HCG, ultrasound, and laparoscopy may allow the expectant treatment of tubal ectopic pregnancy. The natural history of ectopic pregnancy suggests that a majority of these tubal pregnancies may resolve without treatment. Fernandez and associates noted a spontaneous resolution of ectopic pregnancy in 64% of patients as confirmed by HCG levels of <10 mIU/ml. The mean time for resolution was 20 ± 13 days. Spontaneous resolution occurred more frequently when the initial HCG concentration was <1000 mIU/ml. The authors noted that a threshold of HCG of 1000 mIU/ml and a hemoperitoneum of <50 ml with a hematosalpinx of <2 cm appeared to be compatible with therapeutic abstention.

Garcia, Aubut, and Josiniovich suggested that expectant management of tubal pregnancies is appropriate under rigidly controlled conditions. Among 13 patients with ectopic pregnancies, titers continued to drop or could not be detected by assay (1.5 mIU/ml by 1 to 5 weeks). Seven of 10 hysterograms revealed patent tubes. A second laparoscopy in seven patients demonstrated normal tubes in all but one patient. The authors suggested that in their experience expectant management may be appropriate in asymptomatic patients with declining β-HCG who have a low risk of tubal rupture. Further investigations in larger patient groups are needed to assess the morbidity and subsequent fertility among patients so treated.

Medical Treatment

Methotrexate (MTX) may be administered to eradicate trophoblastic tissue in an ectopic pregnancy. MTX is the chemotherapy of choice in the treatment of gestational trophoblastic disease. Long-term follow-up of women who have taken MTX for gestational trophoblastic disease denotes no increase in congenital malformations, spontaneous abortions, or second tumors after chemotherapy. Toxicity may occur in 20% to 30% of patients treated with a single course of therapy but is more common in patients who receive multiple courses.

The use of high-dose short-course MTX therapy was reported by Ory and associates to resolve small unruptured ectopic pregnancies without the need for conservative surgery (Fig. 18-6). Recently, Sauer and associates reported 21 patients treated with MTX/citrovorum factor (CF). In these patients, the ectopic pregnancy was visualized and recorded to be <3 cm in diameter with intact serosa and no bleeding. Treatment with MTX administered intramuscularly with 1.0 mg/kg on postoperative days 1, 3, 5, and 7, and 0.1 mg/kg CF administered intramuscularly on postoperative days 2, 4, 6, and 8 was instituted where β-HCG levels were otherwise reaching a plateau or were slightly rising. Twenty-five of 26 ectopic pregnancies resolved without the need for laparotomy. Two patients received blood transfusions and one required a second operation for intra-abdominal bleeding. As a result of this experience, the authors suggested that MTX/CF may be safely used to treat selected cases of unruptured ectopic pregnancy and that ectopic pregnancies that form fetal elements as evidenced on ultrasound should not be managed medically. Interestingly, 18 of 21 patients responded to one course of MTX/CF, and two women required a second treatment course when the β-HCG remained elevated. For the 20 patients who responded, the median time to resolution was 27 days; the range, 5 to 60 days.

MTX has more commonly been used to treat persistent ectopic pregnancy after conservative surgery. Eight cases of persistent ectopic pregnancy were described recently by DiMarchi and associates. In these patients, persistent ectopic pregnancy resulted from proliferation of trophoblasts remaining after conservative sur-

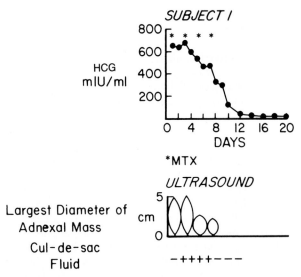

Figure 18–6. HCG levels and ultrasound findings of a patient with an unruptured tubal ectopic pregnancy less than 4 cm treated with four doses of methotrexate (0.1 mg/kg) given intramuscularly every other day. Leucovorin (10 mg/kg) was given intramuscularly on alternate days for 4 days. (Reprinted from Ory SJ, Villanueva AL, Sand PK, Tamura RK. Conservative treatment of ectopic pregnancy with methotrexate. Am J Obstet Gynecol 1986; 154:1299, with permission.)

gery. The trophoblast may be located within the muscular layer of the oviduct or between the muscularis and the serosa such that, at the time of salpingostomy, only a portion of the trophoblast within the lumen may be removed. In those patients with persistent ectopic pregnancy described in the literature, the majority were managed by a second laparotomy and salpingectomy. However, some patients recently have been treated with expectant management or MTX. It appears prudent to obtain a single follow-up β-HCG titer 2 to 3 weeks after the operation. If the titer is elevated, then serial β-HCG titers may be obtained. If the titer continues to fall, then the patient may be managed expectantly. However, if the β-HCG level remains the same or increases, then consideration should be given to a short course of MTX or perhaps an exploratory laparotomy to remove the remaining portion of the ectopic pregnancy.

MTX is an alternative that may be used for the treatment of patients with small unruptured ectopic pregnancies or if there is evidence of persistent ectopic pregnancy after conservative surgery. Because of the toxicity of this medication, patients should be carefully monitored with blood and platelet counts and liver chemistries. In most instances, ectopic pregnancy should be documented by laparoscopy before treatment with MTX.

Surgical Treatment for Ectopic Pregnancy

Conservative Surgical Treatment .The conservative management of an unruptured ectopic pregnancy usually includes one of two possible procedures: linear salpingotomy or segmental resection. A conservative surgical approach is possible when diagnosis of ectopic pregnancy is sufficiently early that rupture of the oviduct has not yet occurred.

LINEAR SALPINGOTOMY. Recent studies have found that in >50% of patients treated for ectopic pregnancy, the uninvolved tube is abnormal, usually as a result of pelvic inflammatory disease, and that 10% to 20% of patients will have a subsequent ectopic pregnancy in that tube. As many as 60% to 70% of patients who undergo salpingectomy will never have a normal pregnancy. In 1898, Howard A. Kelly was among the first to advocate conservative surgery for tubal gestation by drainage of the pregnancy per vaginam, particularly for chronic hemorrhage and formation of a pelvic hematoma. More than half a century elapsed before Stromme reported the successful use of salpingotomy to treat a patient with tubal pregnancy; the patient subsequently achieved a normal pregnancy.

In 1973, Stromme reported his more recent surgical experience with 36 cases of unruptured tubal pregnancy. Out of 21 conservative salpingotomies, five were performed on patients with only one remaining tube. Although only one term pregnancy resulted from the five single-tube procedures, Stromme's work led to the development of conservative surgical procedures during the late 1970s. Stromme's rate of 13.5% of repeat ectopic pregnancies was no higher than the rate for patients treated with radical procedures.

Since Stromme's report, much success has been achieved using the conservative salpingotomy. Even before Stromme's report, Timonen and Nieminen from Finland reported one of the largest series, 185 patients, who achieved a full-term delivery rate of 36.1% for all subsequent pregnancies. The specific benefit of this salpingotomy procedure is difficult to assess from the data, because the functional status of the opposite oviduct was not recorded. Following surgery, Timonen and Nieminen inserted a transabdominal polyethylene tube in the operated oviduct. The tube remained in place for 6 weeks and hydrotubation was utilized with 4 ml of sterile fluid containing penicillin (200,000 units) and hydrocortisone (50 mg) daily during the first postoperative week. Their repeat ectopic pregnancy rate of 16% was similar to other reports.

Järvinen, Nummi, and Pietila reported a 42% intrauterine pregnancy rate among 43 salpingotomy patients in whom both tubes were in situ. DeCherney and Kase had a 40% intrauterine pregnancy rate following salpingotomy treatment of 48 patients with an unruptured ectopic pregnancy. In a later series, 8 of 16 of DeCherney's patients (50%) had normal pregnancies, and none of the 16 patients had ectopic pregnancies. Bruhat and associates reported one of the best experiences to date with a 72% normal pregnancy rate after the salpingotomy procedure was used among a group of 25 patients. In most of the salpingotomy studies, the functional status of the uninvolved oviduct was not defined, and whether the subsequent pregnancy was achieved through the operated oviduct can only be conjectured.

Langer and associates did include a description of the uninvolved oviduct when they reported experiences with salpingotomy in 30 patients. Of the patients in whom the contralateral tube was grossly normal, 80% subsequently had normal pregnancies. When the contralateral tube was damaged or contained peritubal adhesions, only 11 patients, or 55%, achieved a viable pregnancy. In a recent report, Langer and associates reported similar findings in an update of their 15-year experience. This patient group (n = 118) experienced 142 pregnancies, 127 of which were intrauterine pregnancies following conservative surgery for unruptured ectopic pregnancy.

Among recent reports where salpingotomy was performed on a single remaining oviduct, an intrauterine pregnancy rate of approximately 50% was achieved by several investigators, but precise circumstances are difficult to define because of the incompleteness of reports. The repeat ectopic pregnancy rate in the single-tube salpingotomy patients was 20%, higher than for the series that did not report the condition of the contralateral oviduct.

In general, conservative salpingotomy is the preferred treatment for patients who desire further pregnancies. For the operation to be optimal, the oviduct should be unruptured and without serosal invasion, and the patient should be in a surgically stable condition.

TRANSABDOMINAL CONSERVATIVE PROCEDURE. A linear salpingotomy is an ideal procedure for an unruptured tubal pregnancy, because >75% of these ectopic gestations occur in the outer two thirds of the oviduct.

The procedure for linear salpingotomy starts by exposing, elevating, and stabilizing the tube. Then a linear incision is made over the distended segment of the tube (Figs. 18-7 through 18-9).

The incision is extended through the antimesenteric wall until entry is made into the lumen of the distended oviduct. When gentle pressure is exerted from the opposite side of the tube, the products of gestation are gently expressed from the lumen. Because a certain amount of separation of the trophoblast has usually occurred, the conceptus generally can be easily re-

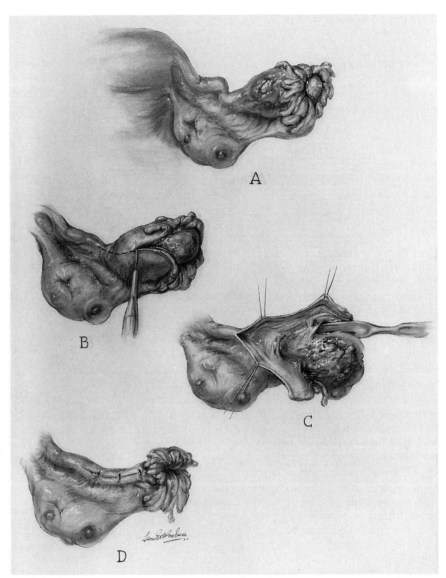

Figure 18–7. Removal of ectopic pregnancy of the distal ampulla. *A,* Distal ampulla involved with ectopic pregnancy. *B,* Initial incision on the antimesenteric border. *C,* The gestational contents are carefully removed using blunt dissection. *D,* Tubal serosa and muscularis are closed as a single layer with 5-0 nonreactive suture material.

moved from the lumen. Gentle traction by forceps without teeth or by suction may be used if necessary, but care should be taken to avoid trauma to the mucosa. Any remaining fragments of the anchoring trophoblast should be removed by profuse irrigation of the lumen with warm Ringer's lactate solution, which will prevent further damage to the mucosa.

Care must be taken to provide complete hemostasis in the tubal mucosa; failure to do so results in troublesome postoperative bleeding, which leads to the formation of intraluminal adhesions. The small tubal vessels are easily identified while the tube is being irrigated, and, if necessary, loupe magnifying glasses can be used. An operating microscope is not needed, because the

bleeding points can be easily identified with 2 × to 4 × magnification.

The mucosal margins are then closed with interrupted suture, making certain that only the serosa and muscularis are approximated and without using undue tension. Care should be taken to ensure that no suture material is retained on the mucosal surface, because even a small amount can produce a secondary inflammatory reaction with subsequent adhesion formation.

The optimum surgical approach to the isthmic ectopic pregnancy remains controversial. Conservative operations have been described: segmental resection of the involved portion of oviduct with reanastomosis at a later operation, segmental resection with primary

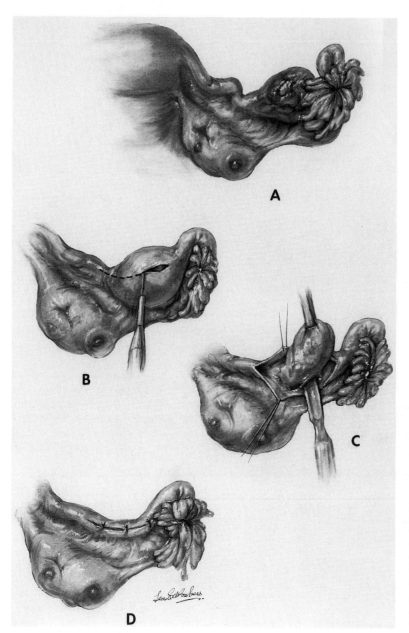

Figure 18–8. Removal of a midampullary ectopic pregnancy. *A*, Midampullary ectopic pregnancy. *B*, Antimesenteric incision with fine microdiathermy needle. *C*, The pregnancy is carefully removed by grasping the tissue and lifting while bluntly teasing the trophoblastic MAH away from the endosalpinx. *D*, The serosa muscularis are closed with interrupted 5-0 nonreactive suture material.

microsurgical anastomosis, and linear salpingostomy. In a recent report of 20 patients with isthmic ectopic pregnancies, Smith and associates compared the three surgical approaches. Their findings suggested that linear salpingostomy for isthmic ectopic pregnancy is as likely to result in later tubal pregnancy as is segmental tubal resection with primary microsurgical anastomosis. The subsequent pregnancy success rate within the three groups has not been clearly established.

Laparoscopic Procedure. A laparoscopy is performed to document the presence of ectopic preg-

nancy. Once a small unruptured ectopic has been documented, two auxiliary puncture sites are made suprapubically to allow manipulation of the fallopian tube (Fig. 18-10, *1*). The tube and mesosalpinx may be injected with a dilute solution of vasopressin. After coagulation of the antimesenteric border of the oviduct, an incision is made. (Fig. 18-10, *2A*) The contents of the tube are removed (Fig. 18-10, *2B*). The tube is left to heal by second intention (Fig. 18-10, *2C*) or is sutured. Recently, DeCherney and Diamond reported the results of 79 ampullary tubal ectopic pregnancies managed

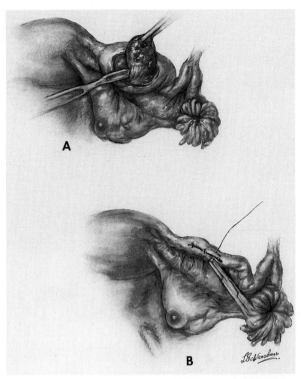

Figure 18–9. Resection of an isthmic ectopic pregnancy. *A*, The ectopic pregnancy is removed with forceps. Alternatively, one may express the pregnancy through the opening in the tube with the thumb and the forefinger. *B*, The incision is closed with 5-0 nonreactive suture material.

using laparoscopic linear salpingostomy. The incisions were allowed to heal by second intention. Two major complications, both involving continued bleeding, were recognized within 1 hour after the original procedure. There were no long-term complications. They reported a viable pregnancy rate of 38% after the procedure. The repeat ectopic pregnancy rate was 16%. The figures reported by DeCherney and by other surgeons compare favorably with pregnancy rates following conservative surgery at the time of laparotomy; that is, pregnancy rates range from 40% to 70% with a 4% to 16% repeat ectopic pregnancy rate.

PERSISTENT TUBAL ECTOPIC GESTATION. Persistent trophoblastic tissue may remain after linear salpingostomy or a segmental resection. Although there may be an initial decrease in β-HCG after surgery, the level may slowly rise, ultimately resulting in patient symptoms. The diagnosis of persistent ectopic pregnancy is confirmed by an initial measurement of serum β-HCG at 6 to 8 days postoperatively and 2-day intervals thereafter. The choice of management may include expectant therapy if the patient is asymptomatic. Alternatively, single-dose MTX may be effective. Further surgery may be required to remove the functioning trophoblastic tissue. Thus, follow-up β-HCG levels should be obtained after surgery to confirm that β-HCG has dropped to the levels associated with the nonpregnant condition.

SEGMENTAL RESECTION. Segmental resection and end-to-end reanastomosis has been proposed as an alternative treatment to salpingotomy. The procedure removes the implantation site, so it cannot be involved in a subsequent tubal pregnancy. Another objective is to restore a more normal architecture to the oviduct, a time-consuming process. The procedure requires special expertise and extensive microsurgical experience; it should not be undertaken by an inexperienced surgeon. The success of future pregnancies depends on the skill, precision, and technique used in the procedure, and once begun, the only alternative is salpingectomy. Swolin initially advocated this procedure in 1967 in Sweden. More recently, that clinic staff reported experience with 42 patients who received the segmental resection and end-to-end anastomosis. The subsequent intrauterine pregnancy rate was 23.9% and only 9.5% were able to deliver at term. A repeat ectopic pregnancy occurred in 14.3% of all pregnancies. Stangel and Gomel and DeCherney and Boyers have found segmental resection preferable to salpingotomy for patients with an isthmic pregnancy.

The resection is best performed with loupe magnification or with the operating microscope; the microsurgical techniques used are identical to those used for primary infertility surgery (see Ch. 19). Care must be taken to avoid trauma to the very vascular oviduct: only cases with minimal bleeding should be considered for the operation. The adjacent mesosalpinx also must be incised and removed with care to avoid the formation of a hematoma in the broad ligament (Fig. 18-11). The seromuscular sutures are placed using the operating microscope and No. 6-0 or 7-0 delayed-absorbable suture. The serosa is secondarily supported by interrupted sutures. Then the patency of the oviduct is tested with insufflation of the uterine cavity with indigo carmine dye.

Radical Surgical Treatment

SALPINGECTOMY. When a tubal pregnancy has ruptured, causing intraabdominal hemorrhage that must be quickly controlled, total salpingectomy must be performed. Under no circumstances should a conservative operation be attempted if a patient has extensive hematoperitoneum, because the patient is in serious cardiopulmonary jeopardy.

Many recent reports in the literature advocate the combined use of a prophylactic oophorectomy with salpingectomy, but the need for an expedient procedure does not exclude conservative management of the ovary adjacent to a ruptured tube. Theoretically, the removal of the ipsilateral ovary would cause the other

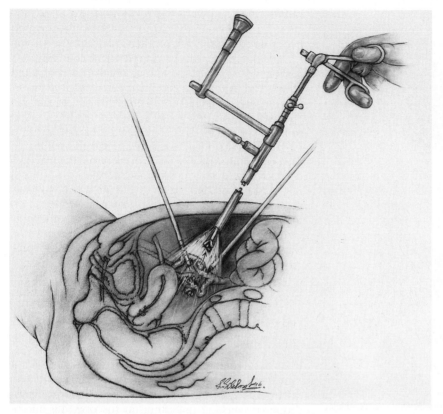

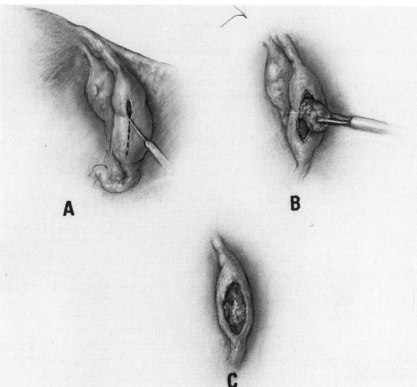

Figure 18–10. Laparoscopic salpingostomy for ectopic pregnancy. *A,* An incision is made with the fine monopolar diathermy needle along the antimesenteric border of the oviduct. *B,* The trophoblastic mass is removed with forceps. *C,* The lumen is allowed to heal by second intention.

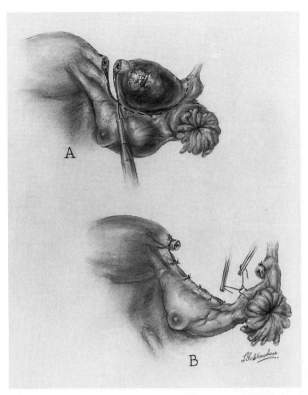

Figure 18–11. Segmental resection of midtubal ectopic pregnancy. *A,* A needle cautery is useful to resect the pregnancy. *B,* Care should be taken to approximate the mesosalpinx. Reanastomosis may be performed in 3 to 5 months.

ovary to ovulate more frequently, favoring future pregnancy. In reality, this consideration is outweighed by the fact that if the contralateral ovary were removed in a future operative procedure, then the patient would be castrated. The current high success rate of in vitro fertilization provides another reason to try to maintain functioning of both ovaries.

Total salpingectomy with partial cornual resection, the mainstay of the surgical procedures for an ectopic pregnancy, has been criticized recently for providing a residual sinus tract that allows the development of a subsequent interstitial pregnancy. The problem is not in the procedure, but in the performance. If the surgeon completely peritonealizes the cornual incision, advancing the broad and round ligaments over the uterine cornua (the modified Coffey technique of uterine suspension), then complete protection is provided from a recurrent interstitial pregnancy (Fig. 18-12). Too vigorous a cornual resection can also cause problems. A residual myometrial defect can cause uterine rupture, interstitial recanalization, or placental encroachment during a subsequent intrauterine pregnancy, and

should be avoided by making certain the interstitial section includes less than one half of the thickness of the cornual portion of the myometrium.

TECHNIQUE OF SALPINGECTOMY. A suprapubic Pfannenstiel's incision is used. The distended tube is elevated, and the mesosalpinx is clamped with a succession of Kelly clamps as close to the tube as possible (Fig. 18-12*A*). The tube is then excised by cutting a small myometrial wedge at the uterine cornu (Fig. 18-12*B*). Care should be taken to avoid a deep incision into the myometrium. A figure-of-eight mattress suture of No. 0 delayed-absorbable material is used to close the myometrium at the site of the wedge resection. The mesosalpinx is closed with interrupted ligatures of No. 0 delayed-absorbable suture. Complete hemostasis is essential to avoid hematoma of the broad ligament.

The fundus is held forward and the round and broad ligaments are sutured over the uterine cornu (Fig. 18-12*C*). The procedure, the modified Coffey suspension, accomplishes complete peritonealization. Mattress sutures anchor the broad ligament to the uterus. The No. 0 delayed-absorbable suture first penetrates the broad ligament from its anterior surface, just below the round ligament, 2 or 3 cm from the cornu. The next bite is taken into the fundus of the uterus, a little posterior and superior to the uterine incision. The suture is then placed through the posterior aspect of the broad ligament, about 1 cm lateral to the previous suture. When this suture is tied, the cornual incision and the mesosalpinx are covered with mesothelium (Fig. 18-12*D*). If there is excessive tension on this suture, or incomplete peritonealization, supporting sutures may be placed in the myometrium and the round ligament to ensure that the peritonealization suture will remain in place.

Recently there has been great interest in laparoscopic salpingectomy for a ruptured tubal pregnancy. In a recent study by Dubuisson, Aubriot, and Cardone, 100 consecutive cases of total salpingectomy by laparoscopy for the treatment of ampullary ectopic pregnancy were described. The three-puncture technique was used. Thermocoagulation and transection of the isthmus, mesosalpinx, and tubal-ovarian ligament were accomplished. The tube was subsequently removed with the use of polyp forceps through one of the suprapubic punctures. No complications were encountered at the time of surgery. Laparotomy was required for two patients who had severe pelvic adhesions and a large ectopic pregnancy. This technique should be reserved for a small ectopic pregnancy. Clearly, hospitalization time may be reduced; however, the length of time required to perform the procedure may outweigh these potential benefits. The technique of laparoscopic salpingectomy is discussed in Chapter 16.

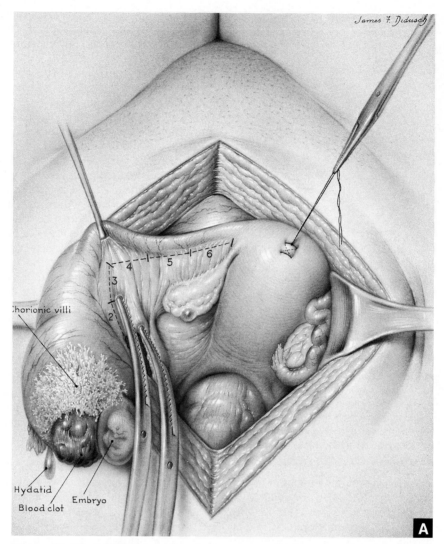

Figure 18–12. Salpingectomy for tubal pregnancy. *A,* The tube has been delivered, and the mesosalpinx is being clamped and cut using a succession of Kelly clamps. *B,* The mesosalpinx has been completely clamped and cut. The *dotted line* indicates the line of excision of the tube at the cornu. *Inset* shows the superficial wedge resection of the interstitial tube and the suture of the excised cornu. *C,* The method of placing mattress suture for peritonealization is shown with anchoring of the medial portion of the broad ligament to the uterus, a little posterior and superior to the uterine incision. *D,* Peritonealization is completed by tying mattress sutures, which brings the broad and the round ligaments over the uterine cornu.

INTERSTITIAL PREGNANCY

Interstitial pregnancy is a rare condition, accounting for no more than 2% to 4% of all tubal pregnancies. The condition occurs once for every 2500 to 5000 live births. Although many surgeons have attempted to differentiate between an interstitial pregnancy and a cornual pregnancy, the two are difficult to separate anatomically and should be classified together.

The gestational sac is protected better in the interstitial portion than in the rest of the tube, so the symptoms manifest later, and the pregnancies are more advanced when they rupture. After 2 to 3 months of amenorrhea, vaginal spotting begins. The developing chorionic villi

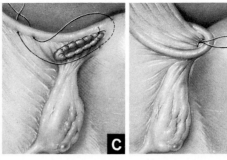

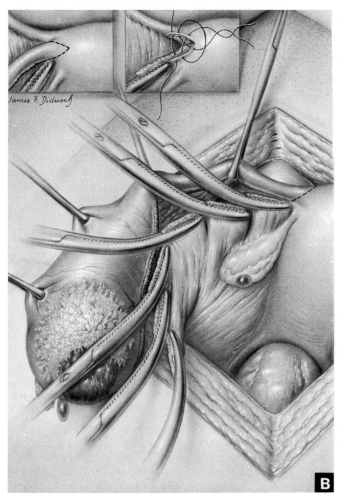

Figure 18–12. (continued)

eventually erode into the blood vessels and the uterine cornu, causing a severe hemorrhage. Because the pregnancy occurs at the most richly vascularized area of the female pelvis, the junction of the uterine and ovarian vessels, rupture usually causes profound and sudden shock.

Before 1893, the only available reports on interstitial pregnancies were from autopsies, but since then, 250 cases have been reported in the literature. Earlier diagnosis and more experience in treating this disorder have reduced the maternal mortality rate to approximately 2% to 2.5% of all interstitial and cornual pregnancies.

The diagnosis of an interstitial pregnancy is made by the critical evaluation of all the criteria used for other types of tubal pregnancy. Patients will have acute abdominal pain, intraperitoneal bleeding, a low hematocrit, and a positive serum or urine pregnancy test. Diagnostic tests include the sensitive radioimmuno-

assay or radioreceptor assay for β-HCG, culdocentesis, and ultrasonography.

Asymmetry of the uterus, often indicative of an interstitial pregnancy, may be misinterpreted as a pregnancy in a bicornuate uterus or a myoma in a pregnant uterus instead of an interstitial pregnancy. Knowledge of the previous shape of the uterus may help to confirm or exclude the existence of a bicornuate or myomatous uterus. A firm protrusion on the uterus would suggest a myoma; a soft, tender asymmetric enlargement suggests an interstitial pregnancy.

Because ultrasound cannot usually be used to identify the position of the pregnancy, laparoscopy is required to confirm the diagnosis. When the patient is experiencing massive intra-abdominal bleeding, an immediate laparotomy should be performed.

The etiologic factors for interstitial pregnancy are similar to those for the other types of tubal pregnancies; most important are pelvic inflammatory disease, operative trauma, and tumors. The management of the tubal stump at the time of salpingectomy is the subject of much controversy concerning a subsequent interstitial pregnancy.

Kalchman and Meltzer collected reports of 73 cases of interstitial pregnancy following total salpingectomy in addition to two cases resulting from their own surgery and another 24 cases occurring after partial salpingectomies. In their report, ectopic pregnancy was the original indication for 60% of the initial salpingectomies. Too vigorous a cornual resection was considered to be one of the major factors in the subsequent development of an interstitial pregnancy. Hallatt has questioned the advisability of cornual wedge resection because he feels that the technique predisposes to interstitial pregnancy and uterine rupture. Hallatt's opinion was based on four cases in a study of 123 repeat ectopic pregnancies.

When a portion of the interstitial tube is removed for the purpose of avoiding a subsequent cornual pregnancy, then surgery rarely results in interstitial pregnancy. Another problem with blaming the cornual wedge procedure for subsequent implantations is that it is impossible to determine whether a fertilized ovum entered the peritoneal side of the resected tube or if the ovum traveled to that cornu from the opposite tube.

Treatment for Interstitial Pregnancy

The choice of treatment for an interstitial cornual pregnancy depends on the extent of trauma that has occurred in the uterine wall and on the interest of the patient in preserving her childbearing function. Cornual resection and repair of the defect can be performed in >50% of the cases, and hysterectomy is required in the remainder. Hysterectomy remains the treatment of choice for patients whose pregnancy has advanced to such a stage that repair of the cornu would be technically difficult and medically hazardous.

When a small interstitial pregnancy is noted, the ectopic pregnancy may be excised and the uterus repaired while conserving the distal oviduct. Consideration then may be given to implanting the oviduct into the uterus at a second operation to preserve fertility.

When extensive resection of the myometrium is required to preserve the uterus, particularly in a patient with extensive intra-abdominal bleeding, the surgical risk is high and the risk of the uterus rupturing in a subsequent pregnancy must be considered. Efforts to conserve the uterus are therefore reserved for the patient with a stable surgical condition who is adamant about retaining the option of future childbearing.

Technique of Excision of Interstitial Pregnancy with Salpingo-Oophorectomy

Whenever possible, the ovary should be saved, but if the ovary cannot be conserved because of rupture or involvement in the ectopic pregnancy, a salpingo-oophorectomy must be performed (Fig. 18-13). As the ascending uterine vessels are approached near the cornu, they are ligated separately with a figure-of-eight suture. The interstitial pregnancy is excised in a V-shaped manner and the myometrium is approximated with a figure-of-eight closure using No. 0 delayed-absorbable suture (Fig. 18-13B). If it becomes necessary, the round ligament can be cut and resutured to the cornu and the uterine serosa using interrupted sutures (Fig. 18-13C). The round and broad ligaments are brought over the incision with mattress sutures—the modified Coffey suspension (Fig. 18-13D). Additional interrupted sutures of No. 2-0 or No. 3-0 delayed-absorbable material may be used to secure the serosa of the round ligament to the serosa of the uterus to maintain the operative site in a permanent retroperitoneal position.

OVARIAN ECTOPIC PREGNANCY

Because IUDs protect the endometrium and, to a certain degree, the proximal oviducts from implantation, future reports of extrauterine pregnancy may show an increased rate of ovarian involvement. Data from the Cooperative Statistical Program of the Population Council show an ovarian pregnancy in 1 out of every 9 ectopic pregnancies that occur among IUD users. Of pregnancies among IUD users, 4.3% are extrauterine.

There have been several reviews in the English literature on the subject of primary ovarian pregnancy. Boronow and associates summarized 62 cases in a review of the literature between 1950 and 1963. Campbell and associates added 91 cases to the list as of 1973, including three new cases of their own, and Pratt-Thomas, White, and Messer reported an additional 10 new cases in 1974. Grimes, Nosal, and Gallagher summarized the major reviews in the literature and added 18 cases of primary ovarian pregnancy from the records of six hospitals in which the reviews extended through 1980. By combining the data from their review with four other recent reports, Grimes et al determined that 34 cases of primary ovarian pregnancy occurred among 236,983 deliveries, a rate of 1 ovarian pregnancy in 7000 deliveries.

In an intrafollicular pregnancy, the second stage of meiosis, as well as ovum capacitation and fertilization,

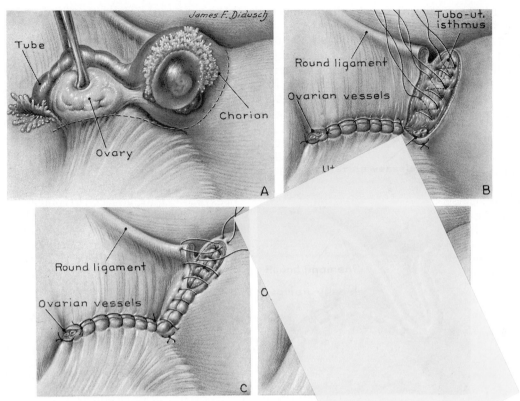

Figure 18–13. Salpingo-oophorectomy with resection of inter...tial pregnancy. *A, Dotted line* denotes line of excision. *B*, Tube, ovary, and cornual pregnancy have ...been excised. Myometrium is being approximated with figure-of-eight sutures of No. 0 delayed-abs...rbable suture. ...e that the uterine vessels have been ligated separately. *C*, The round ligame...t, which w...s cut, is being resutured to the cornu. The ovarian vessels have been ligated, and the ...road ligament has been closed with a continuous lock stitch. Serosa of the uterine wound is closed with a simple continuous stitch. *D*, The cornual wound is covered over with the round and broad ligaments.

occur within the follicle. Only 15% of cases of ovarian pregnancy are intrafollicular in origin. In an intrafollicular pregnancy, a well-preserved corpus luteum can be identified in the wall of the gestational sac. Other criteria presented by Spiegelberg for identifying an intrafollicular pregnancy are that the tube, including the fimbria ovarica, is intact and the tube is clearly separate from the ovary; the gestational sac definitely occupies the normal position of the ovary; the sac is connected with the uterus by the utero-ovarian ligament; and ovarian tissue is unquestionably demonstrated in the wall of the sac.

Diagnosis of Ovarian Pregnancy

The early diagnosis of an ovarian pregnancy is one of the most difficult of all diagnoses relating to extra-uterine gestation. Abdominal pain, amenorrhea, and bleeding are common manifestations of a tubal gestation, but chronic pelvic pain is the most frequent clinical manifestation of an ovarian gestation. Although an adnexal mass is palpable in as many as 60% of the patients, the mass is frequently confused with a leaking corpus luteum hematoma.

All of the criteria used for diagnosing a tubal pregnancy are helpful in diagnosing a primary ovarian pregnancy. In particular, the highly sensitive β-HCG radioimmunoassay is effective for identifying the presence of low HCG levels. The test can confirm the presence of a gestational process, but knowing the β-HCG level does not help determine the precise location of the gestation. One of the most common pregnancy complications to mimic an ovarian pregnancy is an incomplete spontaneous abortion with a leaking corpus luteum hematoma. In such cases, a D&C will show the remnants of trophoblastic villi that are responsible for the low level of β-HCG.

Culdocentesis is also of assistance in confirming that an extrauterine pregnancy exists, but the technique cannot differentiate between a tubal and an ovarian gestation. A tubal pregnancy can easily be ruled out with laparoscopy, but an ovarian pregnancy is still difficult to differentiate by gross appearance from a leaking corpus luteum hematoma. Ultrasonography can be used, but only when an ovarian pregnancy is advanced does the ultrasound image show a gestational sac that would raise the clinical suspicion of an ovarian pregnancy.

A critical analysis of all of the diagnostic studies, especially the sensitive radioimmunoassay for the β-HCG, must be used in making the diagnosis. When the β-HCG is positive, ultrasonography shows no intrauterine gestational sac, and culdocentesis shows free blood in the peritoneal cavity, then a laparotomy is needed to make a definite diagnosis.

Treatment for Ovarian Pregnancy

Although an ovarian pregnancy usually results in more bleeding than a leaking corpus luteum hematoma, it is still easily confused with the hematoma, and a safe approach is to proceed with surgical resection when either condition is diagnosed. Unless the diagnosis is made quite late, the ovary can be preserved by a conservative resection of the hemorrhagic portion of the gonad. Only rarely is the hemorrhage so complete that oophorectomy is required to control the bleeding. Even if the last trophoblastic villus cannot be removed in the ovarian resection, the ovary should be preserved. Any remaining trophoblastic tissue will degenerate rapidly and produce no clinical problem.

ABDOMINAL ECTOPIC PREGNANCY

An abdominal pregnancy is perhaps the rarest, as well as the most serious, type of extrauterine gestation. Reports on the frequency of abdominal pregnancy are variable, ranging from 1 in 3371 deliveries to >1 in 10,200 deliveries. Stafford and Ragan reported an incidence of 1 abdominal pregnancy in 7269 deliveries, a representative figure.

Abdominal pregnancies are classified as either primary or secondary. Most abdominal pregnancies are secondary, resulting from early tubal abortion or rupture with secondary implantation of the pregnancy into the peritoneal cavity. To be considered a primary abdominal pregnancy, the pregnancy must meet three criteria defined by Studderford in 1942: (1) both tubes and ovaries must be in normal condition with no evidence of recent or remote injury, (2) no evidence of uteroperitoneal fistula should be found, and (3) the pregnancy must be related exclusively to the peritoneal surface and must be early enough in the gestation to eliminate the possibility of secondary implantation following primary implantation in the tube.

Secondary abdominal pregnancy results when a tubal gestation attaches itself to the other viscera as the enlarging placenta spreads through the wall of the tube or is aborted through the fimbriated end. The placenta probably retains some tubal attachment, which supplies blood for the gestation to continue developing in the new peritoneal site. Rare types of secondary abdominal pregnancies have occurred following spontaneous separation of an old cesarean section scar, following uterine perforation during a therapeutic or elective abortion, and after subtotal or total hysterectomy.

Diagnosis of Abdominal Pregnancy

The early diagnosis of an abdominal pregnancy is difficult but critical, because a catastrophic hemorrhage can result from separation of the placenta. A history of recurrent abdominal discomfort, fetal movement beneath the abdominal wall, and the presence of fetal movements high in the upper abdomen should alert the clinician to the possibility of an abdominal implantation. Other clinical clues include cessation of fetal movement, vomiting late in pregnancy, fetal malposition, and closed and uneffaced cervix.

Confirmation of the diagnosis requires demonstration of the fetus outside the uterine cavity. If the uterus can be palpated separately from the fetal parts, the abdominal pregnancy can be confirmed either by hysterosalpingography or by the failure of oxytocin to stimulate the gestational mass.

The x-ray finding of fetal small parts in the lateral position overlying the maternal spine was first noted by Weinberg and Sherwin in 1956; the finding is a fairly reliable sign of an abdominal pregnancy. An x-ray examination of the abdomen, including anterior, posterior, and lateral views, is also helpful in defining malposition of the fetus, which is most commonly found in the transverse position. However, the most effective method used currently to diagnose an abdominal pregnancy is ultrasound. The ultrasound image can clearly identify the gestation as separate from the nonpregnant uterus. The use of ultrasonography should enhance the diagnostic accuracy in more than two thirds of the cases.

Maternal mortality rates have varied in the past from

4% to 29%. Rahman, Al-Suleiman, and Rahman Al-Sibai reported statistics from an Arab population of a 20% maternal mortality among 20 patients with advanced abdominal pregnancy. Recent experience has been more favorable. Clark and Jones reported maternal death estimates from 4% to 10%, and in a review of 10 cases, Delke, Veridiano, and Tancer had no case of maternal mortality, although morbidity was quite high. A high incidence of pelvic abscess, peritonitis, and sepsis results from the remnants of the placenta being retained. Fetal mortality has been notoriously high, ranging from 75% to 95% of cases.

Management of the Abdominal Pregnancy

Recent techniques of fetal monitoring have decreased the fetal mortality rate and have served as a diagnostic adjunct in the management of the abdominal pregnancy. Fetal assessment, including repeated sonography to measure biparietal diameter, nonstress testing, monitoring of fetal movements, and contraction stress tests, can provide clinical evidence of fetal maturity and fetal welfare. Despite the use of these diagnostic tools, fetal death occurred in all of the 15 cases of abdominal pregnancy reported by Martin and associates, and 3 of the 10 cases reported by Rahman and associates resulted in fetal death. Clark and Jones reported an overall fetal salvage rate of 11.4% in a study of 35 abdominal pregnancies.

One of the major factors in fetal survival is the condition of the fetal membranes. Should the membranes rupture, the fetus usually dies in the peritoneal cavity within a short time from respiratory distress. A high incidence (35%–75%) of fetal anomalies, including facial and joint deformities, torticollis, and hypoplasia of the extremities, also occur in abdominal pregnancies. These anomalies are thought to be related to the extrauterine environment of the fetus.

Management of the placenta remains a controversial issue. Most clinicians feel the best treatment is to clamp the cord, leave the placenta in situ, and close the abdomen, but allow retroperitoneal drainage if possible. The placenta can be removed after complete cessation of function, as determined by quantitative HCG titers. The placenta should be removed during laparotomy only if it is accessible and if its removal can be accomplished without excessive blood loss. When all functioning stops, the circulation has undergone fibrosis. When in doubt, leave the placenta in place and await sclerosis of its blood supply. Thompson reported leaving the placenta in the peritoneal cavity for a period of 13 years without physical harm to the patient. MTX has been used on occasion to hasten trophoblastic degeneration, which is determined by serial HCG titers.

CERVICAL ECTOPIC PREGNANCY

The cervix is a rare but hazardous site for placental implantation because the trophoblast can penetrate through the cervical wall and into the uterine blood supply. Cervical gestations have received little attention in the literature until recently, but an increased awareness of the condition has resulted in a number of recent reports. The number of reported cases now exceeds 300.

The following three criteria for the diagnosis of cervical pregnancy were established initially by Rubin in 1911: (1) there must be cervical glands opposite the placental attachment, (2) the attachment of the placenta to the cervix must be situated below the entrance of the uterine vessels or below the peritoneal reflection of the anterior and posterior surfaces of the uterus, and (3) fetal elements must not be present in the corpus uteri. A determination of whether Rubin's criteria are met is difficult without a complete study of the entire uterus, thus Paalman and McElin proposed five more practical clinical criteria for the diagnosis of this condition: (1) uterine bleeding without cramping pain following a period of amenorrhea; (2) a soft, enlarged cervix equal to or larger than the fundus—the "hourglass uterus"; (3) products of conception entirely confined within and firmly attached to the endocervix; (4) a closed internal cervical os; and (5) a partially opened external os.

The incidence of this rare entity varies; the Mayo Clinic reported 1 in 16,000 pregnancies. The highest incidence, 1 in 1000 pregnancies, was reported from Japan. The high incidence of elective abortion in Japan is probably a factor in the higher rates, and cervical pregnancy may increase in frequency in the United States with the increased use of elective abortion. Other investigators have found a high incidence of antecedent curettage.

Cervical gestations are frequently confused with a neoplastic process because of the marked vascularity and friable appearance of the cervix. Profuse bleeding may occur if the placenta is mistaken for a tumor and a biopsy taken. The gestation is also mistaken for a spontaneous abortion with the assumption that the products of conception were retained within the cervical canal (Fig. 18-14).

Treatment for Cervical Pregnancy

The treatment of a cervical pregnancy is surgical; the condition usually requires an abdominal hysterectomy. Because a true cervical pregnancy is incompatible with a viable fetus, the abnormal implantation will usually produce symptoms within the first trimester. Although

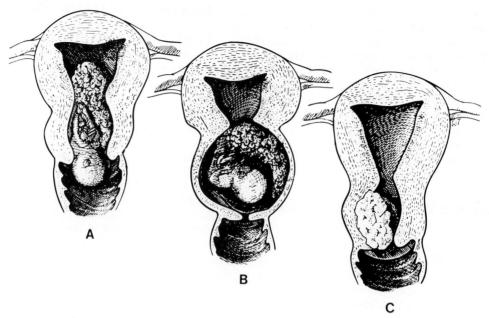

Figure 18–14. Differential diagnosis of cervical pregnancy. *A,* In the cervical phase of uterine abortion, the placenta is mainly within the expanded cervix, and the external and internal ora are dilated. *B,* In a cervical abortion (abortion into the cervix) due to stenosis of the external os, spontaneous rupture of the cervical wall may cause severe hemorrhage. *C,* Ragged, friable cervix seen in cervical pregnancy mimics that of carcinoma of the cervix. (Reprinted from Rothe DJ, Birnbaum SJ. Cervical pregnancy: diagnosis and management. Obstet Gynecol 1973; 42:65, with permission.)

conservative evacuation of an early cervical pregnancy has been accomplished by a skillful D&C, as documented by Whittle, the procedure is usually complicated by profuse hemorrhage, which generally necessitates an abdominal hysterectomy. Mortimer and Aiken have recommended that conservative measures should never be attempted if the gestation is beyond 8 weeks.

MTX therapy may be considered for the treatment of cervical pregnancy whenever uterine preservation is desirable or as an adjunct to hysterectomy. Cervical pregnancy is usually associated with implantation and development within the cervical canal but it has infrequently penetrated into the wall of the cervix. If the diagnosis of cervical pregnancy can be established, then MTX may be used to decrease vascularization of the mass, thus reducing blood loss if removal of the uterus is required.

COMBINED ECTOPIC PREGNANCY

Coexistent intrauterine and extrauterine pregnancies were described by Duverney in 1708. In 1966, Felbo and Fenger collected a total of 523 reported cases. More recently, Reece and associates reviewed the literature from 1966 to 1979 and provided 66 new cases, including five cases from the Sloane Hospital for women, bringing the total to 589 cases reported in the recent literature. In the past, combined intrauterine and extrauterine gestations have occurred in approximately 1 in 30,000 pregnancies. The increasing incidence of ectopic pregnancies may mean that the incidence of combined pregnancy is now higher, perhaps as many as 1 in 15,000 live births.

Although the precise cause of a combined pregnancy is frequently obscured, most of the factors are the same as those associated with ectopic pregnancy. Recently, the use of ovulation-inducing agents has greatly increased the incidence of multiple gestations and combined pregnancies. Berger and Taymore reported an incidence of combined pregnancy of as many as 1 in 100 stimulated patients. Still, the most common anatomical finding associated with combined pregnancies is pelvic inflammatory disease.

The combination of abdominal pain, adnexal mass, peritoneal irritation, and an enlarged uterus are the major clinical features associated with a combined pregnancy. Additional diagnostic findings include the presence of two corpora lutea found at the time of laparotomy or laparoscopy, hematoperitoneum, acute abdominal pain following the termination of an intrauterine pregnancy, or the persistence of an enlarged uterus with amenorrhea after excision of an ectopic pregnancy. Continued enlargement of the uterus and a positive pregnancy test after treatment of an ectopic pregnancy confirm the diagnosis.

Treatment for Combined Pregnancy

The major problem in the management of a combined pregnancy concerns the timing of the termination, especially if both fetuses are alive and have reached the stage of midpregnancy. In their review of the world's literature, Reece and associates found only 13 cases in which both pregnancies reached term and in which both infants were delivered and survived the neonatal period. Although fetal mortality rates have ranged from 20% to 70% for the intrauterine pregnancy, the extrauterine gestation has a mortality rate >90%. Recent experience has shown a marked improvement for the survival of the intrauterine pregnancy. Little information is available on the growth and development of infants who survive the neonatal period, but the incidence of congenital malformations and mental retardation is increased because of hypotension from the extrauterine pregnancy. Maternal mortality also has been reduced with recent aggressive medical management to a rate of 0.98%.

RH IMMUNOGLOBULIN UTILIZATION AFTER ECTOPIC PREGNANCY

Grimes has reported that Rh-negative mothers were recognized and administered Rh immunoglobulin in only 23% of cases. Fetomaternal hemorrhage associated with ectopic pregnancy can sensitize Rh-negative women at risk. A dose of 50 μg Rh immunoglobulin is usually sufficient to prevent sensitization of the patient.

Bibliography

Arias-Stella J. Atypical endometrial changes associated with the presence of chorionic tissue. Arch Pathol 1954;58:112.

Atrash HK, Friede A, Hogue CJ. Ectopic pregnancy mortality in the United States: 1970–1983. Obstet Gynecol 1987;70:817.

Beacham WD, Hernquist WC, Beacham DW, et al. Abdominal pregnancy at Charity Hospital in New Orleans. Am J Obstet Gynecol 1962;84:1257.

Berger MJ, Taymore ML. Simultaneous intrauterine and tubal pregnancies following ovulation induction. Am J Obstet Gynecol 1972;113:812.

Bernaschek G, Rudelstorfer R, Csaicsich P. Vaginal sonography versus serum human chorionic gonadotropin in early detection of pregnancy. Am J Obstet Gynecol 1988;158(part 1):608.

Boronow RC, McElin TW, West RH, et al. Ovarian pregnancy: a report of 4 cases and a 13-year survey of the English literature. Am J Obstet Gynecol 1965;91:1095.

Brenner PF, Raj S, Mishell DR Sr. Ectopic pregnancy: a study of 300 consecutive surgically treated cases. JAMA 1980;243:673.

Bruhat MA, Manhes H, Mage G, et al. Treatment of ectopic pregnancy by means of laparoscopy. Fertil Steril 1980;33:411.

Budowick M, Johnson TRB Jr, Genadry R, et al. The histopathology of the developing tubal ectopic pregnancy. Fertil Steril 1980;34:169.

Campbell JS, Hacquebard S, Mitton DM, et al. Acute hemoperitoneum, IUD, and occult ovarian pregnancy. Obstet Gynecol 1974;43:438.

Centers for Disease Control. Ectopic pregnancy surveillance, 1970–1978. Atlanta, Georgia: Centers for Disease Control, July 1982.

Clark JFJ, Jones SA. Advanced ectopic pregnancy. J Reprod Med 1975;14:30.

Cropp CS, Cowell PD, Rock JA. Failure of tubal closure following laser salpingostomy for ampullary tubal ectopic pregnancy. Fertil Steril 1987;48:887.

Cullen TS. New sign in ruptured extrauterine pregnancy. Am J Obstet Gynecol 1918;78:457.

DeCherney AH, Boyers SP. Isthmic ectopic pregnancy: segmental resection as treatment of choice. Fertil Steril 1985;44:307.

DeCherney AH, Diamond MP. Laparoscopic salpingostomy for ectopic pregnancy. Obstet Gynecol 1987;70:948.

DeCherney A, Kase N. Conservative surgical management of unruptured ectopic pregnancy. Obstet Gynecol 1979;54:451.

DeCherney AH, Romero R, Naftholin F. Surgical management of unruptured ectopic pregnancy. Fertil Steril 1981;35:21.

Delke I, Veridiano NP, Tancer ML. Abdominal pregnancy: review of current management and addition of 10 cases. Obstet Gynecol 1982;60:200.

DiMarchi JM, Kosasa TS, Kobada TY, et al. Persistent ectopic pregnancy. Obstet Gynecol 1977;20:555.

Dougherty RE, Diddle AW. Intrafollicular ovarian pregnancy: management with ovarian conservation. Obstet Gynecol 1969;3:20.

Dubuisson JB, Aubriot FX, Cardone V. Laparoscopic salpingectomy for tubal pregnancy. Fertil Steril 1987;47:225.

Felbo M, Fenger JH. Combined extra- and intrauterine pregnancy carried to term. Acta Obstet Gynecol Scand 1966;45:140.

Fernandez H, Rainhorn JD, Papiernik E, et al. Spontaneous resolution of ectopic pregnancy. Obstet Gynecol 1988;71:171.

Fienberg R, Lloyd HED. The Arias-Stella reaction in early normal pregnancy: an involutional phenomenon. Hum Pathol 1974;5:183.

Fossum GT, Kletzky OA, Davajan V, et al. Early detection of pregnancy using transvaginal ultrasound. Paper presented at the 43rd annual meeting of the American Fertility Society, September 28–30, 1987, p. 78.

Garcia AJ, Aubut JM, Sama J, Josiniovich JB. Expectant management of presumed ectopic pregnancies. Fertil Steril 1987;48:395.

Grimes DA. Rh Immunoglobulin utilization after ectopic pregnancy. Am J Obstet Gynecol 1981;140:246.

Grimes HG, Nosal RA, Gallagher JC. Ovarian pregnancy: a series of 34 cases. Obstet Gynecol 1983;61:174.

Hallatt JG. Tubal conservation in ectopic pregnancy: a study of 200 cases. AM J Obstet Gynecol 1986;54:1216.

Hussa RO. Clinical utility of human chorionic gonadotropin and α-subunit measurements. Obstet Gynecol 1982;60:1.

Jain K, Hamper VM, Sanders RC. Comparison of transvaginal sonography in the detection of early pregnancy and its complications. Am J Radiol 1988;151:1139.

Järvinen PA, Nummi S, Pietila K. Conservative operative treatment of tubal pregnancy with postoperative daily hydrotubations. Acta Obstet Gynecol Scand 1972;51:169.

Kalchman GG, Meltzer RM. Interstitial pregnancy following homolateral salpingectomy: report of 2 cases and review of literature. Am J Obstet Gynecol 1966;96:1139.

Kelly HA. Operative gynecology, vol. 2. New York, I. Appleton Co., 1898:453.

Kivikoski AI, Martin CM, Smeltzer JS. Transabdominal and transvaginal ultrasonography in the diagnosis of ectopic pregnancy: a comparative study. Am J Obstet Gynecol 1990;163(1):123.

Langer R, Bukovsky I, Herman A, et al. Conservative surgery for tubal pregnancy. Fertil Steril 1982;38:427.

Langer R, Raziel A, Ron-El R, Golan A, Bukovsky I, Caspi E. Reproductive outcome after conservative surgery for unruptured tubal pregnancy: a 15-year experience. Fertil Steril 1990;53(2):227.

Levin AA, Schoenbaum SC, Stubblefield PG, et al. Ectopic pregnancy and prior induced abortion. Am J Public Health 1982;72:253.

Levy G, Diamond MP, DeCherney AH. Ectopic pregnancy: relationship to tubal reconstructive surgery. Fertil Steril 1987;47:543.

Marchbanks PA, Annegers JF, Coulam CB, et al. Risk factors for ectopic pregnancy. JAMA 1988;269:1825.

Martin JN Jr, Sessums JK, Martin RW, et al. Abdominal pregnancy: current concepts of management. Obstet Gynecol 1988;71:549.

Matthews CP, Coulson PB, Weld RA. Serum progesterone levels as an aid in the diagnosis of ectopic pregnancy. Obstet Gynecol 1986;68:390.

Medical Research Group and AFS Special Interest Group. In vitro fertilization/embryo transfer in the United States: 1985 and 1986 results from the National IVF/ET Registry. Fertil Steril 1988;49:212.

Mitchell DE, McSwain HF, McCarthy JA, et al. Hysterosalpingographic evaluation of tubal patency after ectopic pregnancy. Am J Obstet Gynecol 1987;157:618.

Mortimer CW, Aiken DA. Cervical pregnancy. J Obstet Gynaecol Br Commonw 1968;75:741.

Mueller BA, Daling JR, Weiss NS, et al. Tubal pregnancy and the risks of subsequent infertility. Obstet Gynecol 1987;69:722.

Nylander PPS, Akande EO, Ogunbode O. Simultaneous advanced extrauterine and intrauterine pregnancy. Int J Gynecol Obstet 1971;9:102.

O'Connor DM, Kurman RJ. Intermediate trophoblast in uterine curettings in the diagnosis of ectopic pregnancy. Obstet Gynecol 1988;72:665.

Ory HW. Women's health study: ectopic pregnancy and intrauterine contraceptive devices—new perspectives. Obstet Gynecol 1981;57:137.

Ory SJ, Villanueva AL, Sand PK, et al. Conservative treatment of ectopic pregnancy with methotrexate. Am J Obstet Gynecol 1986;154:1299.

Paalman R, McElin T. Cervical pregnancy. Am J Obstet Gynecol 1959;77:1261.

Pauerstein CJ, Hodgson BJ, Kramen MA. The anatomy and physiology of the oviduct. Obstet Gynecol Annu 1974;3:137.

Polak JO, Wolfe SA. A further study of the origin of uterine bleeding in tubal pregnancy. Am Obstet Gynecol 1924;8:730.

Poland BJ, Dill FJ, Styblo C. Embryonic development in ectopic human pregnancy. Teratology 1976;14:315.

Pouly JL, Mahnes H, Mage G, et al. Conservative laparoscopic tretment of 321 pregnancies. Fertil Steril 1986;46:1093.

Pratt-Thomas HR, White L, Messer HH. Primary ovarian pregnancy: presentation of ten cases including one full-term pregnancy. South Med J 1974;67:920.

Rahman MS, Al-Suleiman SA, Rahman Al-Sibai MH. Advanced abdominal pregnancy. Obstet Gynecol 1982;59:366.

Reece EA, Petrie RH, Sirmans MF, et al. Combined intrauterine and extrauterine gestations: a review. Am J Obstet Gynecol 1983;146:323.

Rimdusit P, Kasatri N. Primary ovarian pregnancy and the intrauterine contraceptive device. Obstet Gynecol 1976;48(suppl):57.

Rock JA, Parmley TH, King TM, et al. Endometriosis and the development of tuboperitoneal fistula after tubal ligation. Fertil Steril 1981;35:16.

Rodi IA, Sauer MV, Gorrill JM, et al. The medical treatment of unruptured ectopic pregnancy with methotrexate and citrovorum rescue: preliminary experience. Fertil Steril 1986;46:811.

Romero R, Radar N. Copel JA, et al. The effect of different hCG assay sensitivity on screening for ectopic pregnancy. Am J Obstet Gynecol 1985;153:72.

Rothe DJ, Birnbaum SJ. Cervical pregnancy: diagnosis and management. Obstet Gynecol 1973;42:675.

Rubin IC. Cervical pregnancy. Surg Gynecol Obstet 1911;13:625.

Sauer MV, Gorrill MJ, Rodi IA, et al. Nonsurgical management of unruptured ectopic pregnancy: an extended clinical trial. Fertil Steril 1987;48:752.

Schwartz RO, DiPietro DL. β-hCG as a diagnostic aid for suspected ectopic pregnancy. Obstet Gynecol 1980;56:197.

Shah A, Courey NG, Cunanan RG. Pregnancy following laparoscopic tubal electrocoagulation and excision. Am J Obstet Gynecol 1977;129:459.

Shapiro BS, Cullen M, Taylor KJW, DeCherney AH. Transvaginal ultrasonography for the diagnosis of an ectopic pregnancy. Fertil Steril 1988;50(3):425.

Shepherd RW, Patton PE, Novy MJ, Burry KA. Serial β-HCG measurements in the early detection of ectopic pregnancy. Obstet Gynecol 1990;75(3):417.

Shoen JA, Nowak RJ. Repeat ectopic pregnancy: a 16-year clinical survey. Obstet Gynecol 1975;45:542.

Smith M, Vessey MP, Bounds W, et al. Progestogen-only oral contraception and ectopic gestation. Br Med J 1974;4:104.

Spiegelberg O. Zur Casuistik den Ovarial-Schwangenschaft. Arch Gynaek 1878;13:73.

Stafford JC, Ragan WD. Abdominal pregnancy: review of current management. Obstet Gynecol 1977;50:548.

Stangel JJ, Gomel V. Techniques in conservative surgery for tubal gestation. Clin Obstet Gynecol 1980;23:1221.

Stock RJ, Nelson KJ. Ectopic pregnancy subsequent to sterilization: histologic evaluation and clinical implications. Fertil Steril 1984;42:211.

Stromme WB. Salpingotomy for tubal pregnancy: report of a successful case. Obstet Gynecol 1953;1:472.

Stromme WB. Conservative surgery for ectopic pregnancy: a twenty-year review. Obstet Gynecol 1973;41:215.

Studderford WE. Primary peritoneal pregnancy. Am J Obstet Gynecol 1942;44:487.

Swolin K. Electromicrosurgery and salpingotomy: long term results. Am J Obstet Gynecol 1975;121:418.

Swolin K, Fall M. Ectopic pregnancy. Acta Eur Fertil 1972;3:147.

Tatum HJ, Schmidt FH. Contraceptive and sterilization practices and extrauterine pregnancy: a realistic perspective. Fertil Steril 1977;28:407.

Thompson LR. Abdominal pregnancy at term with later removal of placenta. Am J Surg 1966;111:272.

Timonen S, Nieminen U. Tubal pregnancy: choice of operative method of treatment. Acta Obstet Scand 1967;46:327.

Vasquez G, Winston RML, Brosens IA. Tubal mucosa and ectopic pregnancy. Br J Obstet Gynaecol 1983;90:468.

Vermesh M, Silva P, Sauer M, et al. Labor persistent tubal ectopic gestation: patterns of circulating β-human chorionic gonadotropin and progesterone and management options. Fertil Steril 1988;50:584.

Walters MD, Eddy C, Pauerstein CJ. The contralateral corpus luteum and tubal pregnancy. Obstet Gynecol 1987;70:823.

Weinberg A, Sherwin AS. A new sign in roentgen diagnosis of advanced ectopic pregnancy. Obstet Gynecol 1956;7:99.

Westrom L. Effect of acute pelvic inflammatory disease on fertility. Am J Obstet Gynecol 1975;121:707.

Whittle MJ. Cervical pregnancy management by local excision. Br Med J 1976;2:795.

Yang CP, Chow WH, Daling JR, et al. Does infertility increase the risk of tubal pregnancy? Fertil Steril 1987;48:62.

Reconstruction of the Fallopian Tube

19

JOHN A. ROCK

The major physiologic functions of the human oviduct concern the process of ovum pickup and the provision of a safe conduit for a fertilized zygote to reach the uterine cavity. Tubal surgery may be required for the control of infection, neoplasia, infertility, and fertility. Since pelvic inflammatory disease, tubal pregnancy, and tubal sterilization are discussed elsewhere in this text, this chapter discusses the remaining clinical problems that frequently require tubal surgery, concentrating on the problems associated with infertility.

In vitro fertilization has revolutionized our approach to the treatment of the infertile couple. There is now hope for the oligospermic male and the woman with severe tubal disease. Patients with distal fimbrial obstruction and severe tubal damage should be offered extracorporeal fertilization. Microsurgical tubolysis and anastomosis will continue to be useful. The contemporary microsurgical procedures presented here were developed and found useful at the Johns Hopkins Hospital.

TUBAL FACTORS IN INFERTILITY

The factors that most seriously, as well as most frequently, influence infertility are related to the anatomic and pathologic alterations of the fallopian tube. The ciliated lining of the fimbriae that embraces the surface of the ovary at the time of ovulation is responsible for ovum pickup prior to fertilization in the outer third of the fallopian tube.

The disease that most commonly alters the cilia and produces anatomic deformity of the tube is gonococcal endosalpingitis. Unless treated early, this infection will produce tubal occlusion at various locations from the uterine cornu to the fimbriae and may result in tubal obstruction, hydrosalpinx, or a tubo-ovarian inflammatory mass. The initial infection is usually the most damaging to the tubal mucosa and motility: recent evidence shows that the initial inoculum of the gonococcus may be accompanied to the tube by secondary infection from staphylococcus, streptococcus, or coliform organisms, which can result in chronic and irreversible tubal damage. Furthermore, chlamydial infection may be subclinical and equally devastating to the oviduct. Although the fallopian tube may not be completely obstructed as a result of such infections, fusion of the fimbriated appendages or impairment of ciliary activity may produce infertility by interference with ovum pickup and transport. Peritubal scarring from pelvic endometriosis or from other causes of extrapelvic infection (appendicitis or diverticulitis) may produce similar interference in tubal motility. Peritubal adhesions and impaired tubal motility explain an infertility rate of approximately 30% among patients with endometriosis even when there is demonstrable evidence of tubal patency.

Because tubal factors are among the major causes of infertility, tubal function studies should be carried out early in the investigation of the infertile couple. The remainder of the infertility evaluation should also be completed, since in approximately 15% of infertility cases two or more factors are involved. Basically, four methods of observing tubal function are currently available—tubal insufflation (Rubin's test), hysterosalpingography, pelvic endoscopy (peritoneoscopy), and salpingoscopy.

SPECIAL DIAGNOSTIC STUDIES

Tubal Insufflation

Tubal insufflation was first described by Rubin in 1920, and although there have been modifications of the original technique, this test rightfully bears his name, the Rubin's test. The procedure uses an endocervical cannula connected by rubber tubing to a mercury manometer and a source of carbon dioxide. The rate of gas flow through the system is gradually increased to approximately 30–60 ml/min. The cervix may be submerged in sterile water in the upper vagina to detect any leakage of the gas from the cervical canal. Tubal patency may be determined by (1) a direct-writing record of the rise and rapid fall of the gas pressure; (2) auscultation of the lower abdomen for the sound of gas passing from the tubes into the peritoneal cavity; and (3) direct visualization of the pressure changes on a mercury manometer. Although normal fallopian tubes demonstrate patency by the rapid escape of gas at pressures below 100 mm Hg, the test is still considered in the normal range if patency is demonstrated below 180 mm Hg. At higher pressures, however, there is a higher incidence of partial tubal obstruction. At pressures of 200 mm Hg without demonstrable patency, the test is considered negative and the tubes are either in spasm at the cornu or are pathologically obstructed. However, this test is only one of several methods of evaluating tubal patency, and a negative Rubin's test cannot be interpreted as conclusive evidence of tubal obstruction. A study by Sweeney and Gepfert documented this fact by reporting a 50% pregnancy rate ultimately in patients whose tubal insufflation tests had recorded pressures of greater than 180 mm Hg. The Rubin's test can only be interpreted as a study of gross tubal function and must be either repeated or combined with other studies for final evaluation of tubal patency. The use of a smooth muscle relaxant, such as inhaled amyl nitrite, or a mild sedative, such as Valium, 10 mg, prior to any tubal function test, may be helpful in decreasing tubal spasm.

In general, the tubal insufflation should be performed before midcycle, about the 10th day, to avoid the risk of transporting particles of endometrium through the tube, which would be possible if the test were performed during the late secretory phase.

Hysterosalpingography

Hysterosalpingography is a permanent visual record of the presence or absence of tubal patency and was first described by both Cary and Rubin in 1914. This test is always performed in the evaluation of an infertile patient, regardless of the results of the tubal insufflation study, because it serves as a permanent radiographic record that can be compared with subsequent tubal studies. If an oil-base dye is used, the study should not be performed in the latter part of the cycle because extravasation of oil into pelvic veins and lymphatics is increased when the vascularity of the endometrium and uterus is increased. Lipiodol, which made its ap-

pearance in 1922, was later abandoned by Rubin because of the occurrence of oil granuloma and lipoid salpingitis. Rubin noticed some persistence of oily media after hysterosalpingography in two thirds of the cases in one of the earliest studies he conducted. However, less than half of the cases of lipoid salpingitis reported by Elliott and associates could be attributed to oily contrast media; the remainder were thought to be caused by the ascent of oily media placed in the vagina periodically by the patient. The current use of a water-soluble opaque medium avoids such complications. Although the rapid absorption and drainage of the dye prevents the use of delayed 24-hour x-ray study of the tubes, we have not found this to be a particular disadvantage.

As is true of the tubal insufflation study, a hysterosalpingogram must be interpreted with some reservation. Not only is peritoneal spill important, but free dissemination of the dye throughout the pelvis suggests the absence of peritubal adhesions. The presence of rugal folds in the preoperative salpingogram is a favorable prognostic sign for postoperative pregnancy. Young and coworkers from the Boston Hospital for Women found a 60.7% pregnancy rate in cases with good rugal markings and a 7.3% pregnancy rate where such markings were absent.

Altemus and associates believe that the complications and shortcomings of conventional hysterography can be overcome by supplementing the study with fluoroscopic visualization of the uterus and tubes, employing image intensification. A 30-second fluoroscopic exposure is equivalent in irradiation to one conventional radiographic exposure by most modern fluoroscopic units and can avoid the necessity for multiple films when uterine or tubal filling is inadequate. This technique also avoids excessive venous or lymphatic injection when the dye is visualized in the myometrium. Fluoroscopy has been incorporated as a part of the technique of hysterosalpingography in our clinic and has been found useful.

The best evidence to date of the clinical unreliability of a negative hysterosalpingogram study is the work of Hutchins, who compared the accuracy of hysterosalpingography to that of laparoscopy with retrograde dye studies. This is one of the few current studies using general anesthesia for both procedures, which were performed at different times on the same group of infertile patients. The use of an anesthetic eliminates the complication of uterotubal spasm, which frequently produces erroneous results. The study clearly demonstrated this problem, as shown by the finding that 45 of 62 patients (73%) with proximal tubal occlusion on hysterosalpingogram had laparoscopic evidence of normal oviducts with demonstrable patency by methylene blue insufflation. Although other studies also have questioned the reliability of evidence for cornual obstruction provided by hysterosalpingography, Hutchins's study supports our view that an infertile patient should have a minimum of three separate tubal studies before the diagnosis of tubal occlusion can be established. Many comparative studies have found only a 50% to 60% agreement between laparoscopy and hysterosalpingography.

Selective transcervical fallopian tube catheterization may be accomplished with a coaxial catheter set with fluoroscopy or through the hysteroscope. Rosch and coauthors noted that ostial salpingography permitted visualization of 26% of 46 tubes found to be obstructed or poorly visualized with conventional hysterosalpingography. Recanalization was accomplished in 96% of 28 proximal tubal obstructions with the coaxial catheter set.

Peritoneoscopy

Peritoneoscopy, usually by laparoscopy, is important in the assessment of fallopian tubes in cases of prolonged infertility. It is particularly useful when there is a discrepancy between the tubal insufflation study and hysterosalpingogram.

The main information provided by a Rubin's test and hysterosalpingogram concerns tubal patency or obstruction, whereas direct visualization of the adnexa with the laparoscope provides an excellent opportunity for evaluation of tubal patency and motility, peritubal adhesions, and other pelvic disease, such as possible endometriosis or unsuspected ovarian pathology. By inserting a uterine cannula through the cervical canal, indigo carmine or methylene blue dye may be instilled into the uterine cavity with direct observation of the presence or absence of intraperitoneal spill of dye from the fimbriated end of the tubes. Of all the tubal function studies, laparoscopy is the most difficult to perform (since we prefer to conduct this procedure during anesthesia in order to evaluate the pelvis thoroughly); yet it is perhaps the most informative. Open laparoscopy allows the evaluation of patients following previous abdominal surgery. It is our policy to evaluate the pelvis by laparoscopy prior to considering definitive surgery for correction of tubal disease.

Laparoscopy provides the same information about tubal function as culdoscopy except that the approach is through the abdominal wall rather than through the cul-de-sac. It has the advantage of providing a direct view of the fallopian tubes from the anterior surface of the broad ligament and consequently provides a more complete view of the entire oviduct as well as the cul-de-sac and pelvic viscera than can be obtained through the cul-de-sac. We are convinced that the laparoscopic view of the pelvis through an infraumbilical puncture site with or without the aid of an additional probe inserted through a separate puncture site in the lower abdomen has enhanced the view of the pelvis considerably and has greatly improved our understanding of the extent of tubal abnormalities and pelvic disease. A more complete discussion of the use of laparoscopy is presented in Chapter 16.

Salpingoscopy

Salpingoscopy is an endoscopic examination of the tubal lumen. This may be accomplished with a rigid hysteroscope at laparotomy or with a flexible bronchofiberscope during laparoscopy. Adhesions, agglutination, and flattened mucosa have been described. Preliminary reports suggest that findings may correlate with subsequent pregnancy success following salpingoplasty. Additional information obtained with salpingostomy may be useful for delineating which oviducts are least likely to result in a viable pregnancy following reconstructive surgery.

MICROSURGERY

Microsurgery is usually defined as surgery requiring the use of an operating microscope; however, Gomel defines the approach broadly to include surgery performed under magnification provided by loupes (binocular lenses), hood, or microscope. In general, there is agreement that microsurgery represents the philosophy of a gentle operative technique using fine needles and sutures, delicate instruments, constant irrigation, and precise hemostasis with minimal electrodesiccation of tissue.

Magnification techniques for tubal surgery in gynecology were introduced by Swolin 1967b, who used either loupes or the operating microscope for salpingolysis and salpingostomy. Reports by Winston and by Gomel suggested improved pregnancy success following reversal of sterilization procedures in which an operating microscope was used for magnification. Similar results have been obtained with loupes or the hood.

Microsurgery is an acquired skill whose execution requires a magnification system, delicate microinstruments, and fine microsutures. Although each component may be modified to meet the operational requirements of a particular surgeon, certain general features are constant. Foremost is the execution of delicate and precise manual movements, which are governed by hand coordination and visual acuity. The small operative field and the vertical plane of vision require microinstruments. Instrument manipulation is controlled by a precise, graded pinch closure between index finger and thumb, as the instrument is supported on the first web space. Methods for knot tying and instrument handling are acquired by laboratory training. The time required to obtain these skills may vary. Several laboratory manuals outline specific training schedules, including ones by Acland, Buncke and associates, and Rock.

Magnification

Magnification of the operative field may be provided by the microscope, operating hood, or binocular lenses. Magnification may range from × 1 to × 20, depending upon the optical system. The major difficulties with the hood and the binocular lenses have been the excessive weight and short focal length required to obtain an acceptable magnification. In the past few years, however, modifications involving the use of lighter materials have obviated the weight problem. Lens adjustments have increased the focal lengths, allowing for comfortable working distances and a wider and greater depth of field of vision. At present, binocular lenses may be selected with magnifications between × 2 and × 6. Proper lighting can be provided by a fiberoptic cable covered by a sterile plastic sheath.

The operating microscope offers the advantages of a wider range of magnification and a coaxial light system. In general, the range of magnification depends on the magnification coefficient of the eyepiece and the focal length of the objective. Eyepieces of × 10 magnification and objective lengths of 250 mm provide a magnification ranging from × 3.6 to × 16.

A manual zoom system for the control of magnification and focusing, photographic attachments, and an assistance binocular observation system are available to assist the microsurgeon.

A difference of opinion about the therapeutic benefit derived by using the various systems appears to focus on the importance of the source and amount of magnification necessary for accurate control of hemostasis and the placement of fine suture. Our observations support the belief that a magnification greater than × 6 is, in most instances, unnecessary. However, there is general agreement that magnification greater than × 4 to × 6 is critical in anastomosis of the cornual-isthmic portions of the tube.

Instrumentation

Various specialized instruments are available to aid the microsurgeon; however, a basic set of microinstruments includes only jeweler's forceps, spring-handled scissors, and needle holder (Fig. 19-1). In general, instruments should facilitate though minimize hand movement; that is, the needle holders with rounded handles reduce hand movements when placing a 4 to 6-mm needle through tissue. Locks are usually cumbersome and may impede a smooth motion when tying knots.

Microelectrode monopolar or bipolar cautery is useful in obtaining hemostasis with minimal tissue trauma.

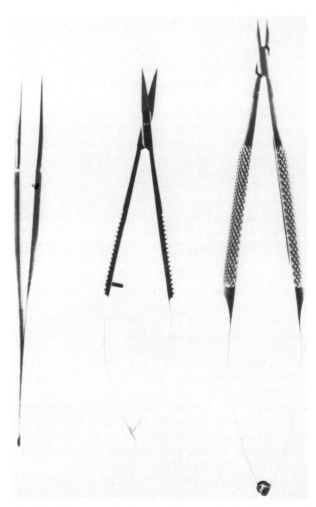

Figure 19–1. Microsurgical instruments: *Left,* jeweler's forceps (No. 4); *center,* fine straight vascular scissors; *right,* Barroquer curved needle holder. (From Jones HW Jr, Rock JA. Reparative and constructive surgery of the female generative tract. Baltimore: Williams & Wilkins, 1983.)

Constant irrigation may be provided by a bulb-tipped syringe or intravenous set to which a 16 to 18-gauge polyethylene cannula is attached. Glass or plastic rods are useful for the gentle manipulation of tubes and ovaries, as well as for elevating adhesions to facilitate their lysis and excision.

Suture Material

Suture material with minimal reactivity should be used for oviduct approximation. Winston demonstrated the superiority of No. 10-0 nylon suture as compared with No. 8-0 chromic catgut in the rabbit oviduct. Stangel and associates demonstrated that No. 9-0 polyglycolic acid suture could be used for anastomosis with minimal reactivity in the muscular layers or endosalpingeal folds. Smith reported that no inflammatory reaction was found with polyglactic acid suture as compared with the use of nylon suture, after which some tissue reaction was still present at 6 months. There have been no studies to demonstrate the correlation of a particular suture material with pregnancy success.

Good surgical technique requires the use of delicate fine suture with minimal reactivity, and the general principle does apply that the fewer sutures used, the less foreign body reaction. Use of No. 7-0 or No. 8-0 absorbable nonreactive suture with a 4 to 6-mm reverse cutting atroloc needle has proven adequate for our technique. This needle may be easily passed through serosa and muscularis with minimal tissue trauma or suture drag. This choice of suture is arbitrary, however; other surgeons have achieved similar success using various types of fine suture material.

Microsurgical Techniques

Position of the Hands

The correct positioning of the hands allows fingertip movement without fatigue. The hands, wrists, and forearms should rest on an immovable surface. In most instances, this is the patient's upper thigh and lower abdomen. Proper hand and wrist support is essential to the proper placement of suture and tying techniques.

Instruments should be held in the writing position (Fig. 19-2), which gives more stability than any other. The gynecologist is not required to touch the middle fingers together as does the vascular surgeon when performing vessel anastomosis; tying techniques are, in fact, more freehand. Vaginal packs are placed in the cul-de-sac to elevate the uterus, and a rubber pelvic diaphragm (lid) is used to support the tubes slightly below the level of the incision.

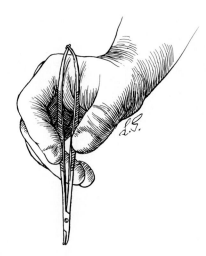

Figure 19–2. Proper hand position for grasping a microneedle holder.

Needle Handling and Placement

The suture should be grasped with the forceps in the left hand, which will stabilize the suture while the needle is positioned in the holder. Minor adjustments of the needle in the needle holder can be made by touching the needle with the left-handed forceps. The needle is in the stable position if it is set at 90° to the axis of the tips of the forceps. The needle should be grasped just behind its midpoint so that the needle tip points horizontally.

The needle should pass perpendicular to the surface of the oviductal tissue. At times, this position is difficult to achieve if the tissue edge is not everted slightly to provide the distortion that is necessary. One may elevate the edge of the tissue with left-handed forceps while simultaneously placing the needle through the tissue or simply press the tubal lumen with the forceps very gently while passing the needle (Fig. 19-3A). One should avoid grasping the thickness of the tissue with the jaws of the forceps because this is a breach of atraumatic technique. The width of the bite of tissue obtained with the needle should be between two and three times the width of the needle itself. The bite in the opposite end of the tissue, which may include muscularis or serosa, should be of equal width. Once the needle has been placed through the opposite lumen, pulling the suture in one straight movement should be avoided, as this can cause movement and visible distortion of the tissue and enlargement of the needle hole. One may avoid this with gentle, short pulls in line with the needle holes. Furthermore, using the tissue forceps

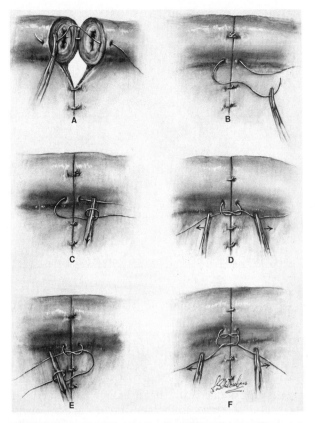

Figure 19–3. Suture placement and knot tying with micro-instruments under magnification. *A,* Needle placement. *B,* Grasping the thread with the right-handed forceps palm up. The suture is brought across as the hand is pronated. *C,* Making a loop about the tip of the left-handed forceps and grasping the short end of the suture. *D,* Tightening the first throw of the knot. *E* and *F,* A second half-knot is placed as the sequence of movements is repeated.

to keep the tail of the suture in line with the exit hole avoids damage to tissue caused by angulation of the thread at the entry hole.

Suture Placement and Knot Tying

Suture placement and knot tying with delicate instruments may be a principal source of frustration for the surgeon. However, mastering these techniques until suture placement and knot tying are second nature is essential so that the surgeon's thoughts may be directed exclusively toward the particulars of the anastomosis. A minimum of 100 hours of laboratory training is usually needed before these techniques are applied to the human oviduct.

Tying a knot consists of several maneuvers: (1) The suture is grasped with the right-handed forceps or needle holder. (2) A loop is made with the long tail of the suture. (3) The suture is wrapped over and under the pickup tips. The short end of the thread is picked up with the left-handed forceps. (4) The loop is pulled off the left-handed forceps. (5) The knot is tightened.

With a smooth motion, one should pick up the longer length of thread with the tip of the right-handed forceps, approximately 2 cm from the suture site (see Fig. 19-3*B*). The length of thread that lies between the forceps and the suture site is referred to as *loop length*. The suture is laid parallel to the oviduct. The suture should be taken with the hand (palm up); the hand is then rotated so that the suture is brought across as the hand is pronated. This first movement is critical and is often a source of error.

Once the thread has been grasped with the right hand, a single loop may be made around the tip of the left-handed forceps (Fig. 19-3*C*). This may be accomplished by winding the forceps around the thread or the thread around the forceps. An additional loop may be made if the knot is to be placed under some tension. The loop should be well onto the tip of the left-handed forceps and loose. If not, the loop will easily fall off the tip of the forceps and an additional movement will be necessary to complete the loop.

There is usually little difficulty in grasping the short end of the suture (see Fig. 19-3*C*). However, difficulty may be encountered if the end is too short, if the suture lies at an angle awkward for the forceps, or if the suture tip is hidden or is lying on a flat surface. If the short end is too short, it is usually because the loop length was too short, which was necessarily caused by some pulling of the suture with the right-handed forceps as the loop was made. The problem, therefore, may be avoided if one inspects the short end of the suture before making the loop. One may manipulate a flat or hidden suture end with the tips of the left-handed forceps, if necessary. One should not force the issue, but stop, reanalyze the position of the suture, and, if necessary, repeat the knot placement.

Once the short end of the suture has been grasped, the loop may be pulled off the left-handed forceps, drawing the knot tight (see Fig. 19-3*D*). The suture has been drawn too tightly if the tissue bunches together or the tissue edges are not approximated but overlap.

A second half-knot is placed as the sequence of movements is repeated in reverse (see Fig. 19-3 *E,F*). One should release the short tail from the left-handed pickup and take hold of the long tail next to the right-handed forceps or needle driver. One should then reverse the thread in the distal direction, creating a U-shaped opening and thereafter lift the long tail with the pickup and wrap the suture over and under the slightly opened forceps (see Fig. 19-3*E*). The short tail may then be grasped with the forceps or needle driver, pulled through the loop, and then tightened (see Fig. 19-3*F*). Each knot should be square. An additional throw may be necessary if absorbable suture is used. The number of sutures to be placed about the tubal lumen for an anastomosis varies, but the general principle applies that the fewer the knots placed about the circumference of the tube, the less the tissue reaction.

The organization of an operating room surgical team is essential. The surgical scrub nurse should be knowledgeable in microsurgical techniques and familiar with instrumentation. With careful organization of the operating theater, the best atmosphere will be provided for an efficient operation with a minimum of lost time.

Tubal Reconstruction

Historically, the field of tubal plastic surgery has had just over one century of clinical experience since the first report by Schroder in 1884 of a unilateral ampullary cuff salpingostomy. By the turn of the 20th century, most of the operative procedures in use today had been initiated by a few pioneers in infertility surgery. The historical details of this era are summarized in Table 19-1.

Pelvic laparotomy is usually deferred until two or more tubal function studies confirm the presence of tubal obstruction. Direct visualization of the tubes by laparoscopy and retrograde dye studies is always performed prior to laparotomy in order to evaluate the pelvic organs and fallopian tubes prior to committing the patient to a major operative procedure. The use of laparoscopy has greatly influenced our selection of patients for tubal surgery. Patients with far-advanced, irreversible, destructive disease of the tube are excluded as surgical candidates *before* an exploratory procedure is performed. It is our feeling that many hopeless surgical cases are operated upon simply because the surgeon has performed the exploratory laparotomy before making an adequate assessment of the extent of the tubal disease. Had the surgeon known the extent of the disease before surgery, it is unlikely that the patient would have been encouraged to have the surgical procedure. This realistic approach to the more conservative use of surgery in the treatment of irreversible tubal occlusion has greatly improved the pregnancy rates in the highly selective group of cases that are true candidates for surgery. Microsurgical tubal plastic surgery may also be performed in conjunction with a pelvic operation, primarily for relief of other symptoms, such as pelvic endometriosis or repeat ectopic pregnancy.

The carbon dioxide laser may assist the microsurgeon during tuboplasty. Opinions differ about the efficacy of the carbon dioxide laser for tuboplasty. The reported advantages include the precise vaporization of adhesions with minimal tissue damage and a consequent reduction in adhesion formation and minimal bleeding. There may be an advantage of increased ease in performing the procedure. There is, however, no evidence to suggest that the laser technique leads to an increased pregnancy success rate.

Many procedures for tubal obstruction have been described, but most of them can be included among the following procedures. In general, tubal surgery for infertility must deal with four major areas of tubal disease: (1) peritubal adhesions, for which salpingolysis is performed; (2) occlusion of the distal end of the tube, for which salpingostomy or fimbrioplasty is required; (3) segmental obstruction, for which end-to-end anastomosis has become popular in an effort to anastomose

TABLE 19–1
Historical Development of Tubal Surgery for Infertility

AUTHOR (YEAR)	OPERATIONS	CONTRIBUTION
Schroder (1884)	1	Unilateral ampullary cuff
Skutsch (1889)	1	Bilateral ampullary cuff
Martin (1891)	24	First reported postoperative pregnancy (aborted)
Polk (1894)	12	Described salpingolysis
Ries (1897)	1	First uterotubal implantation; first to use term *metrosalpingoanastomosis*
Gouillioud (1900)	1	First illustration of ampullary cuff salpingoneostomy with partial tubal resection
Burrage (1900)	17	Dorsal slit salpingoneostomy
Ferguson (1903)	6	Intraoperative tubal testing prior to tuboplasty
Turck (1909)	2	Term pregnancies following bilateral uterotubal implantations

(Siegler AM. Tubal surgery for infertility. In: Sciarra JJ, ed. Gynecology and obstetris, New York: Harper & Row, 1975.)

tubes that have been previously ligated; and (4) proximal tubal obstruction.

A major difficulty in comparing different series of surgical procedures is the lack of a universally accepted classification of tubal surgery. In an attempt to arrive at a workable classification, the Ad Hoc Committee of the International Federation of Fertility and Sterility introduced a classification that was modified by the same committee at the 10th World Congress of Fertility and Sterility in Madrid in July, 1980 (Table 19-2). This classification will create some uniformity in reporting results. However, before reliable success rates can be established, careful consideration must be given to all prognostic factors that may alter pregnancy outcome. For instance, a group of patients treated with a uniform technique may have varying pathogeneses and varying extents of adhesion formation. Therefore, all factors must be carefully delineated before surgical results can be critically evaluated.

The American Fertility Society has suggested several classifications for tubal procedures. At this time, however, no publications have classified the extent of disease based on these new systems. The usefulness of these classification systems remains to be established.

Salpingolysis

Patients with peritubular adhesions as the sole factor responsible for infertility are not common. The incidence in our institution has been approximately 4% and has remained fairly constant. Peritubular adhesions may result from postabortal or puerperal infection, residual endosalpingitis, previous appendicitis, pelvic endometriosis, or, possibly, previous gynecologic surgery. The infundibulum is by definition uninvolved. The careful excision of adhesions about the tube will restore the normal tubo-ovarian anatomic relationships. Patients with endometriosis should not be included in this series.

Tubal surgery requires careful mobilization and elevation of the adnexa so that proper hand support may allow careful excision of adhesions. If extensive adhesion formation is present, careful, painstaking removal of individual adhesions is required. Gentle, blunt dissection with the finger may allow elevation of an adnexa adhered to the pelvic sidewall onto a rubber platform after the cul-de-sac has been gently packed with a lint-free laparotomy pad. Once the adnexa are mobilized, the surgeon should carefully excise all adhesions using a fine-needle monopolar insulated microelectrode with a cutting or blended current (Fig. 19-4). Adhesions may also be removed by laser vaporization. Plastic, glass, or insulated metal rods are used to elevate adhesions so that their insertion and origin are clearly identified. All

TABLE 19–2
Classification of Tubal Procedures

1. Lysis of periadnexal adhesions (salpingolysis-ovariolysis): Classified according to adnexa with least pathology
   a. Minimal: 1 cm of tube or ovary involved
   b. Moderate: Partially surrounding tube or ovary
   c. Severe: Encapsulating peritubal and/or periovarian adhesions

2. Lysis of extra-adnexal adhesions
   a. Minimal
   b. Moderate
   c. Severe

3. Tubouterine implantation
   a. Isthmic: Implantation of isthmic segment
   b. Ampullary: Implantation of ampullary segment
   x. Combination: Different type of implantation on right and left sides

4. Tubotubal anastomosis
   a. Interstitial (intramural)–isthmic
   b. Interstitial (intramural)–ampullary
   c. Isthmic–isthmic
   d. Isthmic–ampullary
   e. Ampullary–ampullary
   f. Ampullary–infundibular (fimbrial)
   x. Combination: Different type of anastomosis on right and left tubes

5. Salpingostomy (salpingoneostomy): Surgical creation of a new tubal ostium
   a. Terminal
   b. Ampullary
   c. Isthmic
   x. Combination: Different type of salpingostomy on right and left tubes

6. Fimbrioplasty: Reconstruction of existent fimbriae
   a. By deagglutination and dilatation
   b. With serosal incision (for completely occluded tube)
   x. Combination: Different type of fimbrioplasty on right and left tubes

7. Other reconstructive tubal operations (specify)

8. Combination of different types of operations
   a. Bipolar: For occlusion at both proximal and terminal end of tube (specify)
   b. Bilateral: Different operations on the right and left sides (specify)

(From the Ad Hoc Committee of the International Federation of Fertility and Sterility. Gomel V. Classification of operations for tubal and peritoneal factors causing infertility. Clin Obstet Gynecol 1980; 23:1259.)

adhesions should be removed from the pelvis using meticulous technique, avoiding trauma to serosal surfaces. A variety of different types of adhesions to various locations may be identified. Large fibrous avascular adhesions between ovary, fallopian tube, and small bowel are particularly difficult to remove without damage to the serosal surface. An appropriately insulated manipulator prevents accidental electrocautery to surrounding tissues. Once all adhesions are removed and

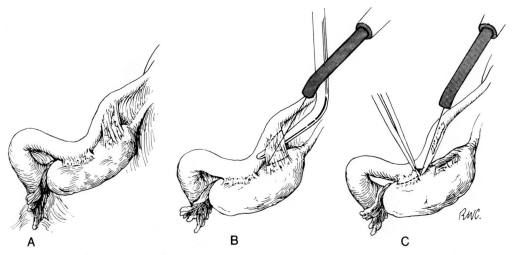

A   B   C

Figure 19–4. Salpingolysis. *A,* Peritubular adhesions may be cohesive-avascular (*left*) or filmy-vascular. *B,* Adhesions should be excised if possible. The glass rod may be inserted behind the adhesions and elevated, exposing the precise attachment to the ovary. *C,* It may not be possible to insert a rod under a densely cohesive adhesion. Careful short incisions should expose the plane of dissection. The adhesions are excised with a fine-needle monopolar-insulated microelectrode.

the anatomy is normalized, careful inspection of the fimbriae should be performed with magnification. Often, fine adhesions involving the infundibulum are missed. Careful dissection in even the best hands often results in denuded areas that must be carefully reperitonealized with fine, absorbable suture.

Postoperative pregnancy results are satisfactory following salpingolysis. Most series quote pregnancy rates ranging from 32% to 70%; our experience is similar (Table 19-3). All patients had iatrogenic or inflammatory adhesions. Patients with endometriosis were not included. Of patients with bilateral adhesions treated by salpingolysis, 68% conceived and delivered live-born

infants. Twelve ectopic pregnancies were noted among the total number of pregnancies.

Gomel has advocated salpingolysis by laparoscopy. Among 92 women, 57 (62%) achieved a term pregnancy after laparoscopic lysis of adhesions. He cautions that skilled techniques are needed to avoid trauma. In selected patients, this approach is an alternative to exploratory surgery and a microsurgical tubolysis (see Chapter 16).

Salpingoplasty

Salpingoplasty, a collective term, implies a corrective procedure involving the distal portion of the oviduct (infundibulum). It may also imply the creation of a new ostium (salpingoneostomy) or fimbrioplasty through which disagglutination or dilatation of the tubal ostium is performed.

Fimbrioplasty

The normal anatomy must be restored when the distal oviduct is being repaired. Tubo-ovarian relationships should be completely restored before patency is established. In particular, the fimbria ovarica and utero-ovarian ligament should be carefully identified.

Fimbrioplasty (Fig. 19-5) is defined as the lysis of fimbrial adhesions or dilatation of fimbrial phimosis.

TABLE 19–3
Pregnancy Success Following Salpingolysis (1961–1989)

PARAMETER	OUTCOME
No. of patients	72
No. of patients pregnant	58 (80%)
No. with living children	49 (68%)
No. of pregnancies	72
Term	49
Spontaneous abortion	11
Premature delivery	0
Ectopic pregnancy	12

(Rock JA. Pregnancy success following salpingolysis. The Johns Hopkins Hospital (Personal Series), 1989.)

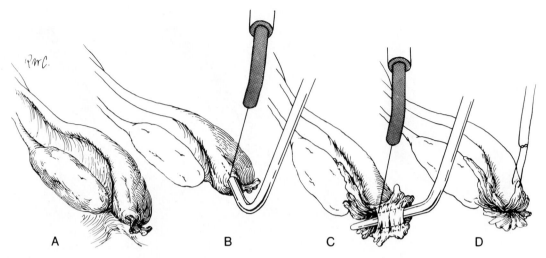

Figure 19–5. Fimbrioplasty. *A,* Incomplete tubal obstruction. *B,* Constrictive adhesive band is incised with microcautery. *C,* Fimbrial adhesions should be excised. *D,* If necessary, a minimal number of fine No. 7-0 or No. 8-0 nonreactive sutures may be placed to prevent reagglutination of the fimbriae.

On occasion, a peritoneal ring of adhesions results in a relative obstruction of the distal portion of the fallopian tube such that simple lysis of these strands will uncover normal-appearing fimbriae. In most instances, periadnexal adhesions are also present. It is important to mobilize the tube and ovary prior to attempting to establish patency by fimbriolysis.

If fimbrial agglutination is found, a fine, delicate mosquito forceps can be introduced into the phimotic opening of the tube and gently opened (see Figs. 19-5 and 19-6). The forceps are gently withdrawn in the open position, causing dilatation of the tubal ostia. By repeating this procedure in several directions, even dilatation of the fimbrial os is accomplished. In some instances, a small incision of scarred tissue may be necessary. The opening may also be aided by a few sutures of No. 8-0 polyglactic acid suture to maintain established fimbrial eversion.

Salpingoneostomy

Salpingoneostomy is the creation of a new tubal ostium where the fimbrial end is totally occluded. Terminal salpingoneostomy is the procedure of choice in establishing tubal patency. Ampullary and isthmic salpingostomy are largely historical procedures that result in dismal pregnancy success rates.

Salpingoneostomy, as performed today, avoids the removal of the distal end of the tube and emphasizes the importance of maintaining the fimbriae in as nearly normal an anatomic condition as possible (see Fig. 19-6). A successful salpingoneostomy requires a complete understanding of the normal tubo-ovarian relationships, specifically, the fimbria ovarica and the relationship of the shaft of the oviduct to the ovary. Although the fimbria ovarica may vary in length, it is always present and provides a clue to the normal axis of the oviduct. It should be clearly identified before an ostium is created.

With gentle lysis of adhesions with a monopolar insulated microelectrode, adhesions are excised and the ovaries are mobilized. The cul-de-sac may then be packed with lint-free laparotomy pads and the adnexa placed on an appropriate platform before the tubo-ovarian relationships are established. Once these relationships are established, attention is turned to the fimbria ovarica. The tubes are distended by injecting dilute methylene blue or indigo carmine dye through the fundus. Under magnification, a distinct vascular pattern that surrounds an avascular area may be easily identified. As this scar is incised (Fig. 19-7A) with cutting cautery, colored fluid will escape (Fig.19-7B). We prefer to introduce a fine forceps (Fig. 19-7C) into the tube and explore the ampullary portion of the fallopian tube. On occasion, normal-appearing fimbriae may protrude through the opening. More often than not, the fimbriae are severely damaged, agglutinated, and confined to the tubal lumen. In this case, an initial incision at 6 o'clock is performed in the direction of the fimbria ovarica (see Fig. 19-7D) and the edges are everted with No. 7-0 or No. 8-0 polyglactic acid suture (see Fig. 19-7E). The mucosa is then carefully everted with a minimal number of sutures. Bleeding capillaries may

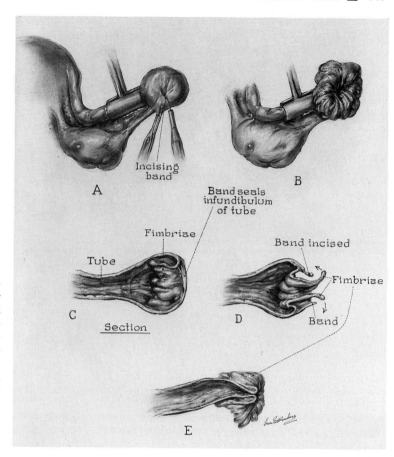

Figure 19–6. Complete distal fimbrial obstruction without significant hydrosalpinx or fimbrial destruction. *A,* Whitish scar is incised with electrocautery. *B,* Fimbrial strands are revealed. Some agglutination may be noted. Delicate fine forceps may be used to dilate the phimotic os. *C,* A cross section reveals strands sealed by a peritoneal band. *D,* When the band is incised, fimbriae are released. *E,* Fimbriae assume their normal anatomic position. (From Jones HW Jr, Rock JA. Reparative and constructive surgery of the female generative tract. Baltimore: Williams & Wilkins, 1983.)

be visualized by irrigation and coagulated with bipolar cautery at a low setting.

Prognostic Factors for Salpingoneostomy

There is a marked disparity among pregnancy success rates with different salpingoneostomy techniques. The disparity is probably a result of the inadequate description of surgical technique as well as of the lack of documentation of the degree of tubal disease and pelvic adhesion formation at the time of surgery. Furthermore, differences in classification systems have added to the confusion. Siegler has stressed the importance of uniformity in reporting results following salpingoneostomy to allow study comparison. In the classification of operations noted by the 10th World Congress of Fertility and Sterility (see Gomel's 1980 article), it was proposed that the term *salpingoneostomy* be used for those procedures designed to relieve distally obstructed fallopian tubes where no identifiable fimbriae could be recovered. Our classification differs in that not all patients who have complete distal fimbrial obstruc-

tion where salpingoneostomy is required have total destruction of the fimbriae. The condition of the fimbriae may vary once patency is established (Fig. 19-8). Thus, the condition of the fimbriae may be of prognostic value and should be taken into consideration in patients who require the creation of a new tubal ostium.

Shirodkar suggested classifying different types of hydrosalpinges on the basis of their size, the presence of peritubular adhesions, the condition of the muscular wall, the condition of the ciliary epithelium after biopsy, and the condition of the fimbriae. Pregnancy was more likely when the hydrosalpinx ranged in size between the size of the surgeon's little finger and that of the thumb, whereas pregnancy was noted to fall from 50% to 10% when the hydrosalpinx was larger than the surgeon's thumb. Young and coauthors demonstrated an increased pregnancy rate in patients noted to have rugae on preoperative hysterogram. A pregnancy rate of 61% when rugae were present decreased to 7% when rugae were not demonstrated. Garcia and Aller suggested a classification of tubal disease for patients with distal occlusion and a hydrosalpinx. This classifica-

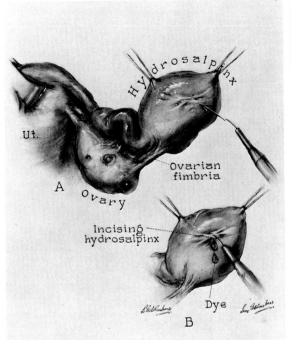

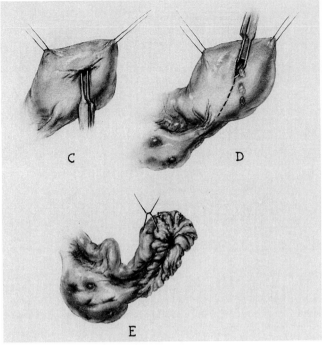

Figure 19–7. Distal fimbrial obstruction with moderate hydrosalpinx and complete fimbrial destruction. *A* and *B,* Whitish scar over the distended hydrosalpinx is incised, releasing indigo carmine dye. *C,* The ostium is first dilated with a fine forceps to release trapped fimbrial strands. *D,* If none are noted, the incision is extended down at the 6-o'clock position toward the fimbria ovarica. *E,* A cuff salpingostomy is accomplished by everting the mucosa using No. 7-0 polyglactic acid suture.

tion was based on the degree of periadnexal adhesion involvement. No correlation, however, was established between the extent of the disease and the pregnancy rate. Siegler summarized the opinion of most tubal surgeons when he stated: "The most favorable tubes for salpingostomy are those with a small hydrosalpinx, recoverable fimbriae, and minimal endosalpingeal adhesions."

A practical classification system for tubal disease was formulated (Table 19-4) using factors that have been shown to influence pregnancy, specifically the size of the hydrosalpinx, the condition of the fimbriae, the presence or absence of rugae on hysterogram, and the extent of pelvic adhesion formation. Our experience with this classification system confirms that these factors influence subsequent pregnancy success (Table 19-5). That is, the extent of tubal disease and pelvic adhesion formation are directly related to the pregnancy rate.

Boer-Meisel and coauthors also have analyzed the importance of additional factors for the prediction of subsequent conception. In addition to the diameter of the hydrosalpinx, extent of adhesions, and macroscopic

aspects of the fimbriae, the thickness of the tubal wall was analyzed. The combination of these four factors allowed the selection of three prognostic groups with regard to pregnancy outcome, that is, good, intermediate, and poor prognosis (see Table 19-5). Thus, the determination of the extent of disease will allow the selection of those patients who would have the best chances of a term pregnancy with microsurgical tubal reconstruction.

These observations were confirmed by Schlaff and coauthors in an investigation in which pregnancies occurred up to 48 months after salpingoneostomy (Fig. 19-9). This time interval has also been noted by Jansen. The delay in conception may result from a gradual regeneration of oviductal mucosal elements. This concept is supported by the work of Petrucco and Winston, who demonstrated that oviducts damaged by hydrosalpinx formation showed a highly significant decrease in both cytoplasmic and nuclear estrogen receptors compared to normal oviducts at equivalent stages of the menstrual cycle. The decrease in estrogen receptors correlated with a decrease in the percentage of ciliated cells.

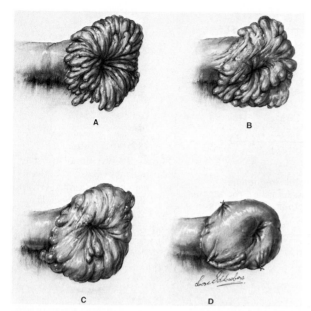

Figure 19–8. Distal fimbrial obstruction: condition of the fimbriae following salpingostomy. *A,* Normal-appearing fimbriae. *B,* Some minimal fimbrial agglutination with scarring at the 12-o'clock position. *C,* Fragmental fimbrial strands with rugal loss. *D,* Few fimbriae noted with essentially smooth flattened mucosa.

TABLE 19–4
Classification of the Extent of Tubal Disease with Distal Fimbrial Obstruction

EXTENT OF DISEASE	FINDINGS
Mild	Absent or small hydrosalpinx ≤ 15 mm diameter
	Inverted fimbriae easily recognized when patency achieved
	No significant peritubal or periovarian adhesions
	Rugal pattern on preoperative hysterogram
Moderate	Hydrosalpinx 15–30 mm diameter
	Fragments of fimbriae not readily identified
	Periovarian or peritubular adhesions without fixation, few cul-de-sac adhesions
	Absence of a rugal pattern on preoperative hysterogram
Severe	Large hydrosalpinx ≥ 30 mm diameter
	No fimbriae
	Dense pelvic or adnexal adhesions with fixation of the ovary and tube to broad ligament, pelvic sidewall, omentum, or bowel
	Obliteration of the cul-de-sac
	Frozen pelvis (adhesion formation so dense that limits of organs are difficult to define)

(Adapted from Rock JA, Katayama KP, Martin EJ, et al. Factors influencing the success of salpingostomy techniques for distal fimbrial obstruction. Obstet Gynecol 1978;52:591.)

TABLE 19–5
Pregnancy Outcome Following Salpingoneostomy with Respect to Extent of Disease

EXTENT OF DISEASE AND PROGNOSIS	SCHLAFF ET AL (1989)		BOER-MEISEL ET AL (1986)	
	Intrauterine	*Ectopic*	*Intrauterine*	*Ectopic*
Mild (good)	70%	10%	77%	4%
Moderate (intermediate)	17%	14%	21%	27%
Severe (poor)	12%	4%	3%	16%

The condition of the cilia on microscopic examination from biopsies of a hydrosalpinx has not been correlated with pregnancy rate. Crane and Woodruff found that microscopic changes offered a poor method of evaluating the physiologic disturbance produced by inflammatory disease in the oviduct. Recent scanning electron microscopy studies have demonstrated the pathologic alterations of the mucosal folds and secretion in patients with distal fimbrial obstruction. Vasquez and associates, using scanning electron microscopy, found a significant reduction in ciliated cells in a hydrosalpinx. With microbiopsy techniques,

a correlation may be established between the condition of these elements and subsequent pregnancy success.

Additional variables may further hinder the comparison of results of different series. The only adjunctive therapy found to be efficacious in the prevention of adhesion formation following tuboplasty is the intraperitoneal instillation of 32% high-molecular-weight dextran 70. The Adhesion Study Group found high-molecular-weight dextran to be effective in preventing adhesion formation in a randomized clinical trial. The mechanism of action of dextran includes the following:

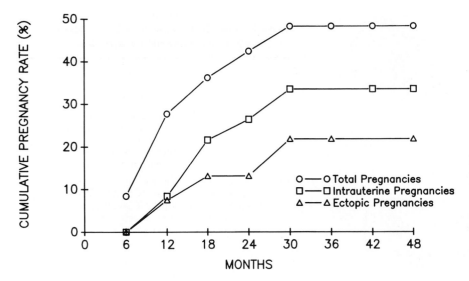

Figure 19–9. Cumulative rate of pregnancy over 48 months after salpingoneostomy. (From Schlaff WD, Hassiokos D, Damewood MD, Rock JA. Neosalpingostomy for distal tubal obstruction. Prognostic factors and impact of surgical technique. Fertil Steril (in press).

(1) The siliconizing effect of dextran is antithrombotic; that is, dextran coats raw serosal surfaces and retards peritoneal abrasions and blood clot adherence. (2) By its nonpolar properties, dextran maintains the negativity of the serosal surface and may cause repulsion of fibrinogen molecules and decrease or prevent adhesions. (3) Dextran has a mechanical effect. Tissues are held apart by a heavy fluid in the pelvis, a hydroflotation effect. Dextran establishes an osmotic gradient, increasing the volume of intraperitoneal fluid and thereby decreasing tissue apposition during the early stages of healing. (4) Dextran modifies the fiber network and renders it more susceptible to lysis. (5) Dextran does not alter the activity of thrombin but changes the kinetics of polymerization of fibrin monomers and yields a decreased clotting time. Whether this solution ultimately results in an increased pregnancy rate remains to be established.

Although many different agents have been suggested to reduce adhesion formation (Table 19-6), few have been found clearly efficacious in randomized clinical trials. At present, we suggest strict adherence to microsurgical technique and use of the following adjuncts: (1) an irrigation solution of Ringer's lactate with 5000 units of heparin and 1 g of hydrocortisone, and (2) prophylactic antibiotics.

Grant emphasized the need for postoperative hydrotubation to enhance fertility following salpingoneostomy. Contrary to his view, the efficacy of postoperative hydrotubation could not be demonstrated in our multicenter randomized clinical trial.

Swolin has suggested the use of second-look laparoscopy to lyse adhesions 8 days to 2 weeks postoperatively. Others have suggested waiting 6 months to perform a second-look laparoscopy to determine the existence of postoperative adhesions and to assess the surgical result. At that time, lysis of adhesions is possible, as well as retrograde dye insufflation.

Several studies have suggested that second-look laparoscopy may subsequently increase the term pregnancy rate. We suggest second-look laparoscopy where there are extensive periadnexal adhesions.

Overall results of salpingoneostomy, ranging from a 0% to a 31% term delivery rate, have been discouraging. Salpingoneostomy performed with magnification has resulted in intrauterine pregnancy rates similar to those following conventional techniques, although an increased ectopic pregnancy rate has been observed. The usefulness of the operating microscope in this surgery remains to be established. Our own experience, using loupe magnification, has been similar to previously reported pregnancy rates.

End-to-End Anastomoses

The role of end-to-end anastomosis is limited primarily to reconstruction of fallopian tubes in previously sterilized patients. It is used infrequently in the conservative treatment of an *unruptured* tubal pregnancy where a small segment of the tube has been destroyed by the invading trophoblast. The request for elective sterilization has become a major medical issue in recent years, with an estimated 1 million tubal sterilizations and vasectomies each performed in the United States in 1987. It is evident that the gynecologist will be called upon more frequently during the next decade to anastomose these ligated or fulgurated tubes in patients who have reversed their thinking on this matter and who desire further childbearing. Among all couples desiring no further children, sterilization is second in demand only to the contraceptive pill.

TABLE 19-6
Agents Employed for Adhesion Prophylaxis

INTENDED MECHANISM	AGENT	INTENDED MECHANISM	AGENT
Inhibit inflammatory reaction and/or fibroplasia	Corticosteroids (ACTH) Oxyphenbutazone Antihistamines Cytotoxic agents	Mechanical separation	Albumin Bladder strips Chyle Crystalloid solutions
Inhibit coagulation	Heparin Oral anticoagulants Peptone Citrates Hiruden Oxalates		Fat Gelatin Lanolin Mineral oil Oxidized cellulose Peritoneum (carp, ox, shark)
Promote fibrin lysis	Amniotic fluid Fibrinolysin Hypertonic glucose Pepsin Sodium ricinolate Steptokinase Urokinase Actase Chymotrypsin Hyaluronidase Papain Protoporphyrin Streptodornase Trypsin		Polysiloxanes Silk and rubber sheets Vitreus of calf's eye Agar Aristol Camphorated oil Collodion Dextran Fetal membranes Gum arabic Metal foils Olive oil Paraffin Pneumoperitoneum Povidine Vaseline

(From Holtz G. Prevention of postoperative adhesions. J Reprod Med 1980; 24:141. Reproduced with permission from the publisher, the Journal of Reproductive Medicine.)

Prognostic Factors for End-to-End Anastomosis

Surgical Technique. Microsurgery implies very delicate atraumatic surgical technique to minimize tissue damage. Prior to 1976, the Hellman technique using a polyethylene catheter and No. 5-0 suture material was practiced in our institution to reverse tubal ligation. At the Johns Hopkins Hospital, a comparison of Hellman's macrosurgical approach and our microsurgical technique revealed an increased pregnancy rate with the latter. There are, however, other variables that are thought to affect subsequent pregnancy success following reversal of sterilization.

Sterilization Procedure. Several types of sterilization procedures may be reversed. Depending on the extent of tubal destruction, different segments of tube are anastomosed. It is difficult to separate these variables when discussing sterilization procedures in general.

In our experience, a rather large amount of tube may be destroyed with tubal cautery procedures, especially when a triple-burn technique is employed. Of 58 women who underwent monopolar high-frequency diathermy, 39 conceived following tubal anastomosis and 30 of these delivered living children. Among ectopic pregnancies for the overall series of 246 patients with tubal reconstructive surgery, 8 of 11 occurred in patients following monopolar cautery.

The extent to which normal physiologic function returns to cauterized tubes is unknown, but the increased incidence of ectopic pregnancies suggests some interference with tubal transport. Damage to the oviduct cilia may extend 2 cm from the site of cautery. For these reasons, one should be certain that when the obliterated tube is excised and patency is established, healthy, well-vascularized tissue is present before proceeding with the anastomosis.

Others have reported good success following reversal of cauterized fallopian tubes. Winston reported that 55% of patients conceived after tubal cautery. Gomel has suggested that diathermic coagulation has one major advantage in that the pelvis is relatively clean and the tubes are free of adhesions. Although this may be true in some instances, it is by no means the rule. Associated tubal pathology has been observed in up to 30% of women after tubal cauterization using monopolar high-frequency diathermy at the Johns Hopkins Hospital.

As a result of the high variability in tubal destruction,

preoperative laparoscopy is indicated to determine the amount of distal fallopian tube available for the anastomosis. The amount of proximal tube is not an issue. That is, if destruction of the intramural portion of the fallopian tube is noted, and there is sufficient distal tube, tubocornual or tubouterine anastomosis may be performed.

Other forms of tubal sterilization may offer higher pregnancy rates following anastomosis. In particular, anastomosis following Falope ring sterilization is associated with a pregnancy rate of more than 85%. Winston has reported no failures with clip sterilization. Similar experiences have been reported by Gomel, Grunert and associates, Patterson, and Rock and associates.

Segments Anastomosed. At present, five varieties of tubal anastomoses have been identified, involving the isthmic, ampullary, and intramural portions of the fallopian tube. Recent reports record the highest pregnancy rates among isthmic-isthmic anastomosis in which there is no discrepancy in tubal lumen size.

In our experience, the site of anastomosis was not a factor in subsequent pregnancy success with Falope ring sterilization. In the cautery group, however, tubal length and site of anastomosis influenced the pregnancy rate. All women with ≤ 4 cm of oviduct in the cautery group required an ampullary-isthmic anastomosis, perhaps explaining why a reduced rate was observed.

Tubal Length. There is a direct relationship between pregnancy success and length of fallopian tube that may be reunited. Gomel has observed that fallopian tubes of less than 3 cm in total length were associated with a long interval between reconstructive surgery and occurrence of pregnancy. With oviducts of over 6 cm in length, pregnancy occurred within three to four cycles and not infrequently during the first month following surgery. A decreased pregnancy rate was noted in patients with fallopian tubes of less than 4 cm in length, and this has also been our experience. Furthermore, we have demonstrated an increased incidence of endometriosis in women whose proximal fallopian tubes are less than 4 cm in length.

We have noted a significant incidence of associated pelvic pathology in 125 patients undergoing reversal of sterilization. Thirty percent of patients, the majority of whom underwent anastomosis after tubal cautery, were noted to have associated pelvic findings. A high incidence of endometriosis and proximal hydrosalpinges was noted in the cautery group. That is, 34 of 85 (40%) oviducts sterilized by unipolar cautery had endometriosis. There were 18 (21%) fistulas.

Time Interval from Sterilization to Anastomosis. Associated tubal pathology increases with an increasing interval from previous sterilization. In particular, the condition of the cilia is significant in that decilia-

tion and tubal polyps increase 4 years after sterilization. Additionally, the pregnancy rate is less among patients who have been sterilized for 4 years or more. The pathogenesis of these intraluminal tubal polyps has not been elucidated; however, chronic inflammation has been implicated.

When shortened oviducts are less than 4 cm in length, retrograde menstruation may result in a proximal hydrosalpinx, which predisposes to the development of endometriosis and subsequent fistulization. Furthermore, the incidence of endometriosis and fistula formation increases abruptly 3 years after previous sterilization. It is probable that these associated pathologic findings are linked with a reduced pregnancy success rate.

Tubal Vascularity. Some sterilization procedures may result in a decrease in tubal vascularity, which may result in interruption of uterotubal-ovarian blood flow. Radwanska and associates noted a decrease in progesterone production in patients who underwent reversal of sterilization. These findings were supported by those of Donnez and associates; however, Meldrum was unable to demonstrate a reduction in progesterone in a similar group of patients. Unfortunately, several types of sterilization procedures were included as a group, and no particular procedure could be identified as associated with a luteal phase deficiency. Further studies in this area are needed to confirm this possible association. In principle, however, procedures that destroy a minimal amount of the fallopian tube are less likely to interfere with the vascular supply to the fallopian tube.

Magnification of the Operative Field

There has been some controversy about the efficacy of loupe lenses in providing adequate magnification for the reversal of sterilization—pregnancy success rates are comparable to those obtained with the operating microscope after anastomosis. Although the loupe lenses may provide sufficient magnification to perform an isthmic-isthmic, ampullary-ampullary, or ampullary-isthmic anastomosis, there is some question about the precision and accuracy of suture placement. There is little debate on the need for a microscope to obtain sufficient magnification to perform an isthmic-cornual anastomosis. A recent study by Rock and coauthors reported reversal of sterilization by microsurgery tubal anastomosis in 72 women using either loupe lenses ($n = 36$) or microscope ($n = 36$). The study design called for randomization of patients within tiers that were matched with the method of sterilization and the site of anastomosis. A significant difference between methods could not be demonstrated. The authors suggested that the results did not imply that any surgeon may use loupe lenses with comfort and confidence. The selection of magnification system is a personal choice and should not be influenced by concern over a difference in subsequent pregnancy success.

Technique of Tubal Anastomosis

The endosalpinx does proliferate under the influence of estrogen, as does the endometrium. For this reason, anastomosis should be performed during the proliferative phase of the cycle. Furthermore, supplemental oral estrogen given to inhibit ovulation and prolong the proliferative phase should increase tubal secretion and promote ciliogenesis. A loupe, visor, or microscope may be used to obtain magnification. Magnification with loupe lenses ranges from ×1 to ×6, whereas the microscope may provide magnification from ×3 to ×20.

Isthmic-Isthmic Anastomosis

The proximal portion of the fallopian tube is identified and its occluded tip resected (Fig. 19-10). A No. 2-0 nylon suture of 100 cm (40 in) is introduced into the lumen with fine forceps. Its passage may be facilitated by the distention of the uterine cavity and the interstitial portion of the oviduct with indigo carmine dye injected through the uterine fundus, with cervical obstruction by suitable instruments, as well as by stretching the tubal stump in a superior direction. Approximately 60 cm (25 in) of No. 2-0 nylon may be threaded through the tubal lumen and placed within the uterine cavity. The same procedure is carried out on the opposite side. There is no discrepancy in luminal size if the distal segment is truly part of the isthmus. The proximal obstructed end is resected and the No. 2-0 nylon is then passed through the oviduct and out the fimbriated end. The mesosalpinx is carefully approximated to eliminate tension at the anastomotic site. The lumina of the two ends are then approximated with No. 7-0 or No. 8-0 polyglactic acid suture on a three-eighths circle taper (BV130-4) needle. Such suture is not routinely available and must be specially ordered. No. 8-0 nylon may also be used. The needle is passed only through the muscularis of the proximal tube and through the muscularis of the distal segment (see Fig. 19-10). The sutures are tied securely, and a second layer of the three additional sutures is placed to approximate the tubal serosa. The remaining portion of the No. 2-0 nylon splint extending through the fimbriated portion of the tube is cut with approximately 1–2 cm extending beyond the fimbriae. This nylon can be easily drawn into the ampulla. The

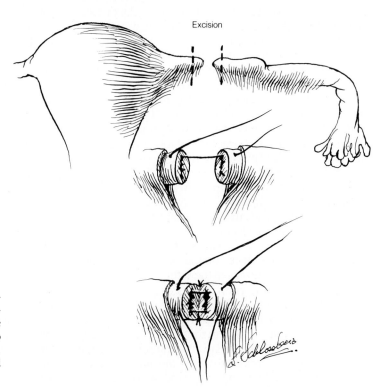

Excision

Figure 19–10. Isthmic-isthmic anastomosis. Patency of obstructed lumina is established by excision of obstructed segment. The lumina may be approximated over a No. 2-0 nylon splint in two layers after the mesosalpinx is approximated. Three sutures are placed in the muscularis, and the serosa is then approximated.

nylon splints are removed through the cervix with a Novak curette at the termination of the procedure or at the most 2–3 days after the procedure.

Isthmic-Ampullary Anastomosis

A No. 2-0 nylon splint is placed through the proximal isthmic portion of the tube into the uterus in a manner similar to that described earlier. A major difficulty is encountered in the isthmic-ampullary anastomosis, because there is a large discrepancy between the diameter of the lumen in the isthmic and the ampullary portion of the tube. This discrepancy occurs as a result of a variety of sterilization procedures. To prevent too large an opening in the ampulla, a needle technique for opening the ampulla has been described as follows: a No. 16 Teflon obturator of an intravenous catheter set is introduced through the fimbriated end of the ampullary segment of the oviduct and advanced to the obstructed site (Fig. 19-11). The needle is inserted through the obturator, and the obstructed end is perforated by the needle and the Teflon sheath (see Fig. 19-11A). After the needle is removed, the No. 2-0 nylon suture is passed in a retrograde manner through the obturator. The mesosalpinx is approximated to reduce tension at the anastomotic site. Three to five No. 7-0 or No. 8-0 polyglactic acid sutures are placed through the serosa, muscularis, and endosalpinx of the proximal (isthmic) oviduct and then through the endosalpinx, muscularis, and serosa of the distal (ampullary) tube (see Fig. 19-11B). The tip of the needle may be introduced into the ampullary lumen by being placed in the tip of the lumen of the Teflon obturator; then the tip of the obturator is withdrawn into the ampullary portion of the tube. Sutures are then tied securely (see Fig. 19-11C). In some instances, a two-layer closure is possible; in those cases, an additional, second layer of suture is placed to approximate the tubal serosa.

Alternate methods of overcoming tubal discrepancy have been described by Diamond and by Gomel. Winston prefers to circumcise the very tip of the ampulla over the bulbous end of a probe inserted through the fimbrial ostium. Before cutting across the mucosa, he suggests stripping back the peritoneal coat to facilitate subsequent two-layer closure.

In most instances, a two-layer closure is possible using this circumcision technique. A single-layer closure, however, is necessary in the rather large lumen of the distal ampullary portion of the fallopian tube. The wall of the oviduct is quite thin, and if attempts are made to circumcise the fallopian tube, extensive bleeding occurs, as well as inadvertent widening of the oviductal lumen. This is particularly frustrating when large fronds of mucosa appear through the lumen. These fronds may be troublesome when placing suture; however, using a fine metal blunt probe, they may be pushed back into the lumen as the cardinal sutures are placed.

Ampullary-Ampullary Anastomosis

The muscularis of the ampullary region is relatively delicate. Because the lumina are quite large, a suture through all layers easily approximates to the tubal lumina (Fig. 19-12). Six to eight No. 7-0 or No. 8-0 polyglactic acid sutures are placed around the circumference of the ampulla. These sutures are placed through the serosa, muscularis, and endosalpinx in each approximating lumen. No splints are used.

Intramural or Interstitial Obstruction

The length of the intramural portion of the oviduct may range from 1.5 to 2.5 cm. Its pathway is characterized by convolutions and abrupt changes in direction. The lumen follows a straight course through the uterine wall to the muscular layer and then angles sharply into the vascular layer. Thus, any attempt to pass a probe into the uterus may create a false passage.

The uterotubal junction may serve as a mechanical barrier and a site of sperm reserve in some species. The importance of intrinsic motility in sperm transport through the uterotubal junction is unclear. Motile sperm may be transported more efficiently than dead sperm. These observations suggest that contractions or fluid currents may play some role in sperm transport. Furthermore, the competence of the uterotubal junction varies with the hormonal environment in several species. Unfortunately, conflicting results in different species limit the application of these animal observations to humans.

If the uterotubal junction is removed in rabbits, the frequency of implantation of a fertilized ovum is decreased. However, in human studies Winston has reported intrauterine pregnancies in 11 of 16 patients after microsurgical tubocornual anastomosis. Thus, the uterotubal junction does not seem to be a prerequisite for intrauterine pregnancy.

Several procedures have been described to open an obstructed proximal segment. These therapies include hysteroscopic cannulization under fluoroscopy, excision of cornual polyps, and microsurgical tubocornual anastomosis (Fig. 19-13). Uterotubal implantation is no longer a primary approach, as pregnancy rates are lower than with other therapies and cesarean section is needed if a pregnancy results. It is of primary importance to preserve tubal length and as much intramural oviduct as possible. Initially, the proximal tubal obstruction may be documented by hysterosalpingogra-

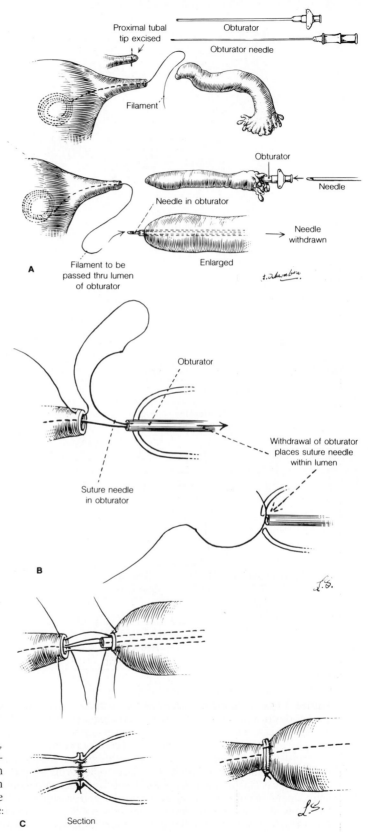

Figure 19–11. Isthmic-ampullary anastomosis. *A,* Method of performing isthmic-ampullary anastomosis. *B,* Use of obturator to place needle tip within ampullary lumen. *C,* Completed procedure. (From Jones HW Jr, Rock JA. Reparative and constructive surgery of the female generative tract. Baltimore: Williams & Wilkins, 1983.)

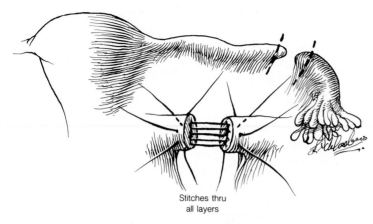

Stitches thru
all layers

Figure 19–12. Ampullary-ampullary anastomosis. Anastomosis of these lumina requires six to eight sutures of No. 7-0 or No. 8-0 absorbable sutures placed circumferentially equidistant about the oviductal lumen.

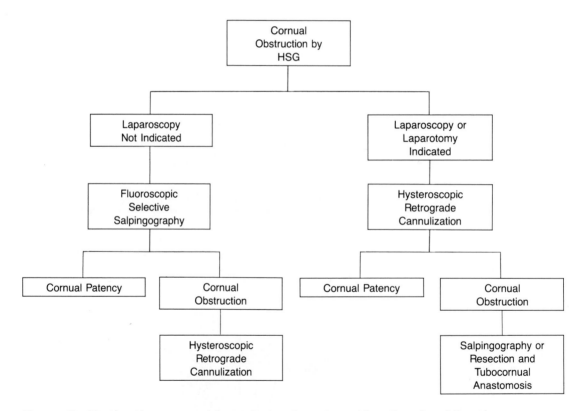

Figure 19–13. Algorithm suggested for evaluating the patient with unilateral or bilateral cornual obstruction on conventional hysterosalpingogram (HSG). If the patient is not a candidate for laparoscopy, fluoroscopic selective salpingography is performed. Hysteroscopic retrograde cannulization is a logical follow-up study if cornual patency is not demonstrated. Conversely, if abnormal pelvic findings are known or suspected to coexist, unilateral or bilateral cornual obstruction is initially investigated by hysteroscopic retrograde cannulization in conjunction with laparoscopy or laparotomy. Persistent cornual obstruction may require isthmic salpingotomy with anterograde cannulization or surgical resection and anastomosis. (Adapted from Novy MJ, et al: Diagnosis of cornual obstruction by transcervical fallopian tube cannulation. Fertil Steril 1988; 50(3):434. Reproduced with permission from the publisher, the American Fertility Society.)

phy. Transcervical fallopian tube catheterization may allow selective salpingography. If an obstruction is documented, cannulization may be attempted. If this is unsuccessful, a microsurgical tubocornual anastomosis may be performed.

Cornual-Isthmic Anastomosis

Cornual-isthmic anastomosis (Fig. 19-14), on occasion, must be performed if a small proximal portion of the interstitial oviduct is occluded. A serosal flap is developed over the proximal segment (see Fig. 19-14A). A fine knife is used to core out the obstructed portion of the fallopian tube. The obstructed segments are removed as discs (see Fig. 19-14B). The isthmic portion of the fallopian tube is then approximated to the intramural portion of the fallopian tube. This is the only procedure that requires high magnification, and in which the microscope is most useful. These procedures are usually performed at a magnification of from ×10 to ×20. Hemostasis must be achieved using high-frequency fine-needle cautery. A two-layer closure is, in most in-

stances, required. This procedure has largely replaced the need for uterotubal implantation.

Cornual-Ampullary Anastomosis

Special attention is necessary to ensure that lumen of similar size are obtained during this anastomosis. The cornual segment is prepared with a fine knife. Approximation is most difficult if the ampullary portion of the tube is transected. The catheter technique previously described for an isthmic-ampullary anastomosis or the use of a fine metal probe is essential to obtain an ampullary lumen similar in size to the cornual lumen. A two-layer closure may not be possible. Each approach should be individualized, based on the site of the ampullary or cornual segment of oviduct. A No. 2-0 nylon splint placed in the uterus as previously described is useful for manipulation of the oviduct for suture placement. We have elected to leave the splint in situ for 2–3 weeks as the healing process is completed. In our experience, anastomosis of these segments is rare. Functional success of this procedure will be maximized

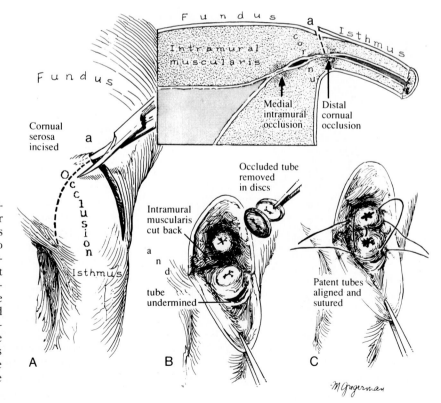

Figure 19–14. Cornual-isthmic anastomosis. Mobilization of tissues over the obstructed portion of the oviduct is required. A, A flap may be developed to allow easy access to the proximal portion of the tube. B, The distal segment of oviduct must be stabilized, especially if a large segment of tube must be removed. The tube may be separated by undermining the muscularis. Occluded portions of the tube may be removed as discs. C, The patent tubes may then be aligned and sutured. The a designates the site of the apex of the incision.

if operative techniques stress an avoidance of lumen disparity.

Transcervical Fallopian Tube Catheterization

A catheter set consists of the coaxial catheters 9 French (F), 5.5 French, and 3 French in diameter (Fig. 19-15). The catheters are introduced through a vacuum adapter under fluoroscopic guidance. Each catheter is advanced. First, the 5.5 F catheter is wedged into the cornua, the 3 F catheter with wire guide is introduced, and the wire guide for the soft tube is advanced through the obstruction. The catheter is then advanced over the wire. Alternatively, catheters may be placed into the uterotubal os via the hysteroscope. Balloon-tip catheters have also been developed to dilate the proximal portion of the oviduct once cannulation is performed.

There are no data to document pregnancy success rates after these procedures. However, patency of the proximal portion of the oviducts may be accomplished in approximately 60% of patients. These procedures are less invasive than the traditional exploratory laparotomy with anastomosis. However, the pregnancy success rates should be equivalent before the transcervical

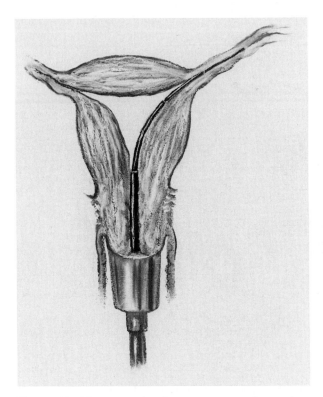

Figure 19-15. A coaxial catheter system may be used to cannulate the proximal oviduct.

fallopian tube catheterization is considered as an alternative to microsurgical tubocornual anastomosis.

Results of Anastomosis

Pregnancy success after reversal of sterilization must be considered in light of the site of the anastomosis and the sterilization procedure performed. From experience with microsurgical techniques, one may expect an overall pregnancy success rate in the range of 55% to 67% live births; the ectopic pregnancy rate approaches 3% to 4% (Tables 19-7 and 19-8).

Isthmic-isthmic anastomosis is associated with the highest pregnancy rate, whereas intramural-ampullary anastomosis has a reduced pregnancy success rate. Our own experience has noted a reduced pregnancy rate among patients requiring isthmic-ampullary anastomosis, although our procedure using a catheter technique has resulted in an improved pregnancy rate over those achieved using macrosurgical techniques. The observed reduction in pregnancy success is most likely a function of an associated reduced tubal length.

Unipolar cautery as a sterilization procedure may be reversed, although pregnancy success rates are diminished over those reported with the Falope ring and clip (see Table 19-8). Furthermore, tubal anastomosis following bilateral partial salpingectomy has a higher pregnancy rate than that following monopolar cautery. Four of our five ectopic pregnancies subsequent to anastomosis were in patients who had received monopolar cautery. Furthermore, associated pelvic pathology in the form of proximal hydrosalpinges and endometriosis is higher in patients following monopolar high-frequency diathermy. Reversal of Falope ring or clip sterilization has been associated with excellent pregnancy success rates. Larger patient series, however, are necessary to establish the superiority of these over other reversible sterilization methods.

There appear to be several variables to be considered, such as tubal polyps and endometriosis, which may only be identified after the sterilization reversal has been performed. These factors may influence subsequent pregnancy success. In particular, the tubal length and the sterilization procedures previously performed have a significant bearing on subsequent pregnancy success.

The usefulness of microsurgery for the reversal of sterilization was emphasized in an international program to determine the reversibility of female sterilization in Asia using microsurgical technique. Rock and associates reported that 111 of 219 patients (51%) conceived following tubal anastomosis; of these, 79 had a living child. The overall cumulative probability of conception at the end of the follow-up period as deter-

TABLE 19–7
Pregnancy Success Following Tubal Anastomosis
Using Microsurgical Technique

AUTHOR (YEAR)	NO. OF CASES	PERCENT OF LIVE BIRTHS	PERCENT OF ECTOPIC PREGNANCY
Silber, Cohen (1980)	25	56	4
Patterson (1980)	50	40	4
Winston (1980)	126	58	2
Gomel (1980)	118	64	1
Grunert et al (1981)	40	57	3
Seiler (1983)	73	64	2
Paterson (1985)	147	59	5
Rock et al (1987)	246	53	4
Chang, Kim (1986)	250	44	5
	1075	55%	3%

TABLE 19–8
Pregnancy Success Following Reversal of Sterilization at the
Johns Hopkins Hospital, 1976–1983

PROCEDURE	NO. OF PATIENTS	PERCENT OF PATIENTS PREGNANT	LIVE BIRTHS	ECTOPIC PREGNANCY
Unipolar cautery	96	54	35	8
Pomeroy	54	72	32	1
Irving	12	58	5	0
Partial salpingectomy	38	71	22	1
Falope ring	45	86	35	1
Clip	1	100	1	0
Total	246	67	130 (53%)	11 (4%)

mined by life table analysis was 63%. The success of this program demonstrated that sophisticated technological advances can be adopted and applied in developing countries.

Bibliography

Acland RD. Microsurgery practice manual. Louisville, Ky.: University of Louisville Microsurgery Laboratory, Price Institute of Surgical Research, 1977.

Adhesion Study Group. Reduction of postoperative pelvic adhesions with intraperitoneal 32% dextran 70: a prospective randomized clinical trial. Fertil Steril 1983;40:612.

Altemus R, Charles D, Yoder VE. Conventional hysterosalpingography used in the evaluation of sterility problems. Fertil Steril 1967; 18:713.

American Fertility Society. The AFS classification of adnexal adhesions, distal tubal occlusion, tubal occlusion secondary to tubal ligation, tubal pregnancies, müllerian anomalies and intrauterine adhesions. Fertil Steril 1988;49(6):944.

Arronet GJ, Eduljee SY, O'Brien JR. A nine-year survey of fallopian tube dysfunction in human infertility: diagnosis and therapy. Fertil Steril 1969;20:903.

Baibot S, Parent B, Dubuisson JB, Aubriot FX. A clinical study of the CO_2 laser and electrosurgery for adhesiolysis in 172 cases followed by early second-look laparoscopy. Fertil Steril 1987; 48(1):140.

Boeckx W, Gordts KB, Brosens I. Reversibility after female sterilization. Br J Obstet Gynaecol 1986;93:839.

Boer-Meisel ME, teVelde ER, Habbena JDF, Kardaun JWPF. Predicting the pregnancy outcome in patients treated for hydrosalpinx: a prospective study. Fertil Steril 1986;45(1):23.

Bonney V. The fruits of conservationism. J Obstet Gynaecol Br Commonw 1937;44:1.

Boyd IE, Holt EM. Tubal sterility: patency tests and results of operation. J Obstet Gynaecol Br Commonw 1973;80:142.

Buncke HJ, Chater NL, Zoltans S. Manual of microvascular surgery. San Francisco: R.K. Davies Medical Center, Microsurgical Unit, Davis & Geck distributor, 1975.

Cary WH. Note on determination of patency of the fallopian tubes by the use of collargol and x-ray shadow. Am J Obstet Gynecol 1914;69:426.

Chang YS, Kim JG. Microsurgical reversal of tubal sterilization. Asia-Oceania J Obstet Gynaecol 1986;12(4):457.

Confero E. Friberg J. Bleicher W. Preliminary experience with transcervical balloon tuboplasty. Am J Obstet Gynecol 1988; 159(2):370.

Crane M, Woodruff JD. Factors influencing the success of tuboplastic procedures. Fertil Steril 1968;19:810.

Cullen TS. A normal pregnancy following insertion of the outer half of a fallopian tube into the uterine cornu. Bull Johns Hopkins Hosp 1922;33:344.

Diamond E. A comparison of gross and microsurgical techniques for repair of cornual occlusion in infertility: a retrospective study, 1968–1978. Fertil Steril 1979;32:370.

Donnez J. Casanas-Roux F. Prognostic factors of fimbrial microsurgery. Fertil Steril 1986;46(2):200.

Donnez J, Casanas-Roux F, Ferin J. Macroscopic and microscopic studies of fallopian tubes after laparoscopic sterilization. Contraception 1979;20:498.

Donnez, J. Wauters M, Thomas K. Luteal function after tubal sterilization. Obstet Gynecol 1981;57:65.

Elliott GB, Brody H, Elliott KA. Implications of "lipoid salpingitis." Fertil Steril 1965;16:541.

Estes WL. A method of implanting ovarian tissue in order to maintain ovarian function. Penn Med J 1909;13:610.

Estes WL Jr, Heitmeyer PL. Pregnancy following ovarian implantation. Am J Surg 1934;24:563.

Fayez J. Comparison between tubouterine implantation and tubouterine anastomosis for repair of cornual occlusion. Microsurgery 1987;8:78.

Fjalbrant B. Tubal surgery. Acta Obstet Gynecol Scand 1975;54:463.

Garcia CR, Aller J. Surgical approach to tubal disease. Clin Obstet Gynecol 1974;17:102.

Ghosal KK. Ovarian function after Estes operation. J Obstet Gynecol India 1974;16:540.

Gomel V. Salpingostomy by laparoscopy. J Reprod Med 1977;18:265.

Gomel V. Tubal reanastomosis by microsurgery. Fertil Steril 1977;28:59.

Gomel V. Classification of operations for tubal and peritoneal factors causing infertility. Clin Obstet Gynecol 1980;23:1259.

Gomel V. Microsurgical reversal of female sterilization: a reappraisal. Fertil Steril 1980;33:587.

Gomel V. Salpingo-ovariolysis by laparoscopy in infertility. Fertil Steril 1983;40:607.

Grant A. Infertility surgery of the oviduct. Fertil Steril 1971;22:496.

Grunert GM, Drake TS, Takaki NK. Microsurgical reanastomosis of the fallopian tubes for reversal of sterilization. Obstet Gynecol 1981;58:148.

Hafez ESE, Blandau RJ. The mammalian oviduct. Chicago: University of Chicago Press, 1969.

Hafez ESE, Evans TN. Human reproduction, conception and contraception. New York: Harper & Row, 1973.

Hanton EM, Pratt JH, Banner EA. Tubal plastic surgery at the Mayo Clinic. Am J Obstet Gynecol 1964;89:934.

Hoerenz P. Magnification: loupes and the operating microscope. Clin Obstet Gynecol 1980;23:1151.

Holden FC, Sovak FW. Reconstruction of the oviducts: an improved technic with report of cases. Am J Obstet Gynecol 1932;24:684.

Horne HW Jr, Clyman M, Debrovner C, Griggs G. The prevention of postoperative pelvic adhesions following conservative operative treatment for human infertility: a final 3-year follow-up report. Int J Fertil 1973;18:190.

Hutchins CJ. Laparoscopy and hysterosalpingography in the assessment of tubal patency. Obstet Gynecol 1977;49:325.

Jansen RPS. Surgery-pregnancy time intervals after salpingolysis, unilateral salpingostomy, and bilateral salpingostomy. Fertil Steril 1980;34:222.

Jansen RPS. Tubal resection and anastomosis. Aust NZ J Obstet Gynecol 1986;26:300.

Jessen H. Forty-five operations for sterility. Obstet Gynecol Surv 1972;27:227.

Jones HW Jr, Rock JA. On the reanastomosis of fallopian tubes after surgical sterilization. Fertil Steril 1978;29:702.

Jones HW Jr, Rock JA. Reparative and constructive surgery of the female generative tract. Baltimore: Williams & Wilkins, 1983.

Keirse MJ, Vandervellen R. A comparison of hysterosalpingography and laparoscopy in the investigation of infertility. Obstet Gynecol 1973;41:685.

Kistner RW, Patton GW. Atlas of infertility surgery. Boston: Little, Brown, 1975.

Kitchin JD, Nunley WC, Bateman BG. Surgical management of distal tubal occlusion. Am J Obstet Gynecol 1986;155(3):524.

Lamb EJ, Moscovitz W. Tuboplasty for infertility. Int J Fertil 1972;17:53.

Maathuis JB, Horback JGM, Van Hall EV. A comparison of the results of hysterosalpingography and laparoscopy in the diagnosis of tube dysfunction. Fertil Steril 1972;23:428.

McComb P. The determinants of successful surgery for proximal tubal disease. Fertil Steril 1986;46:1002.

Meldrum D. Microsurgical tubal reanastomosis: the role of splints. Obstet Gynecol 1981;57:613.

Molumsky A. The prenatal diagnosis of hereditary diseases. Springfield, Ill.: Charles C Thomas, 1973.

Mulligan WJ. Results of salpingostomy. Int J Fertil 1966;11:423.

Musick JR, Behrman SJ. Surgical management of tubal obstruction at the uterotubal junction. Fertil Steril 1983;40:423.

Novy MJ, Thurmond AS, Patton P, et al. Diagnosis of cornual obstruction by transcervical fallopian tube cannulation. Fertil Steril 1988;50:434.

O'Brien JR, Arronet GH, Eduljee SY. Operative treatment of fallopian tube pathology in human fertility. Am J Obstet Gynecol 1969;103:520.

Paterson PJ. Factors influencing the success of microsurgical tuboplasty for sterilization reversal. Clin Repro Fertil 1985;3:57.

Patterson P. Reversal of sterilization. Population Reports, Population Information Program 1980;8(5).

Peel J. Utero-tubal implantation. Proc R Soc Med 1964;57:710.

Peterson EP, Musich JR, Behrman SJ. Uterotubal implantation and obstetrics outcome after previous sterilization. Am J Obstet Gynecol 1977;128:662.

Petrucco OM, Winston RML. Presented at Tenth World Congress of Fertility and Sterility, Madrid, Spain, July 7–12, 1980.

Population Reports. Reversing female sterilization, Series C, No. 8, September, 1980.

Radwanska E, Berger GS, Hammond J. Luteal deficiency among women with normal menstrual cycles requesting reversal of tubal sterilization. Obstet Gynecol 1979;54:189.

Rock, JA. Microsurgical training manual. Unpublished, 1989.

Rock, JA. Pregnancy success following salpingolysis. The Johns Hopkins Hospital (Personal Series), 1989.

Rock JA, Bergquist CA, Kimball AW Jr, et al. Comparison of the operating microscope and loupe for microsurgical tubal anastomosis: a randomized clinical trial. Fertil Steril 1984;41:229.

Rock JA, Chang YS, Limpaphayom K, et al. Microsurgical tubal anastomosis: a controlled trial in four Asian centers. Microsurgery 1984;5:95.

Rock JA, Guzick DS, Katz E, et al. Tubal anastomosis: pregnancy success following reversal of Falope ring or monopolar cautery sterilization. Fertil Steril 1987;48:13.

Rock JA, Katayama KP, Jones HW Jr. Tubal reanastomosis: a comparison of Hellman's approach without magnification and a microsurgical technique. In: Phillips JM, ed. Microsurgery in gynecology. Los Angeles: American Association of Gynecologic Laparoscopists, 1981.

Rock JA, Katayama KP, Martin EJ, et al. Factors influencing the success of salpingostomy techniques for distal fimbrial obstruction. Obstet Gynecol 1978;52:591.

Rock JA, Katayama PK, Martin EJ, et al. Pregnancy outcome following uterotubal implantation: a comparison of the reamer and sharp cornual wedge excision techniques. Fertil Steril 1979;31:634.

Rock JA, Parmley TH, King TM, et al. Endometriosis and the development of tuboperitoneal fistulas after tubal ligation. Fertil Steril 1981;35:16.

Rock JA, Siegler AM, Meisel MB, et al. The efficacy of postoperative hydrotubation: a randomized prospective multicenter clinical trial. Fertil Steril 1984;42:373.

Roe RE, Laros RK Jr, Work BA. Female sterilization: I. The vaginal approach. Am J Obstet Gynecol 1972;112:1031.

Rosch J, Thurmond AS, Uchida BT, Sovak M. Selective transcervical fallopian tube catheterization: technique update. Radiology 1988;168:1.

Rosenberg SM, Board JA. High molecular weight dextran in human infertility surgery. Am J Obstet Gynecol 1984;148:380.

Rubin IC. Roentgendiagnostik der Uterus Tumorens mit Hilfe von Intrauterine Collargol Injectionen Vorlaeufige Mitteilung. Zentralbl Gynaekol 1914;38:658.

Rubin IC. Non-operative determination of patency of fallopian tubes in sterility: intrauterine inflation with oxygen and production of a subphrenic pneumoperitoneum: Preliminary report. JAMA 1920;74:1017.

Rubin IC. Retention of lipiodol in fallopian tubes with special reference to occlusive effect in cases of permeable strictures. NY J Med 1936;36:1089.

Rubin IC. Therapeutic aspects of uterotubal insufflation in sterility. Am J Obstet Gynecol 1945;50:621.

Russell JB, DeCherney AH, Laufer N, et al. Neosalpingostomy: comparison of 24 and 72 months follow-up time shows increased pregnancy rate. Fertil Steril 1986;45:296.

Rutherford RN. The therapeutic value of repetitive lipiodol tubal insufflations. Western J Surg 1948;54:145.

Schlaff WD, Hassiokos D, Damewood MD, Rock JA. Neosalpingostomy for distal tubal obstruction. Prognostic factors and impact of surgical technique. Fertil Steril (in press).

Schroder C. Die Excision von Ovarientumoren mit Erhaltung des Ovarium. Zentralbl Gynak 1884;8:716.

Seiler JC. Factors influencing the outcome of microsurgical tubal ligation reversals. Am J Obstet Gynecol 1983;146:292.

Shapiro BS, Diamond MP, DeCherney AH. Salpingoscopy: an adjunctive technique for evaluation of the fallopian tube. Fertil Steril 1988;49:1076.

Shirodkar VN. Further experiences in tuboplasty. Aust NZ J Obstet Gynecol 1965;5:1.

Shirodkar VN. Factors influencing the results of salpingostomy. Int J Fertil 1966;2:361.

Siegler AM. Salpingoplasty: classification and report of 115 operations. Obstet Gynecol 1969;34:339.

Siegler AM, ed. Hysterosalpingography, 2nd ed. New York: Medcom Press, 1974.

Siegler AM. Tubal surgery for infertility. In: Sciarra JJ, ed. Gynecology and obstetrics. New York: Harper & Row, 1975.

Siegler AM, Perez RJ. Reconstruction of fallopian tubes in previously sterilized patients. Fertil Steril 1975;26:383.

Silber SJ, Cohen RS. Microsurgical reversal of female sterilization. Fertil Steril 1980;33:598.

Smith PC. Presented at the Microsurgery Seminar, Third International Congress of Gynecologic Endoscopy, San Francisco, 1977.

Stangel J, Settles H, Reyniak J, et al. Microsurgical anastomosis of the rabbit oviduct using 9-0 monofilament polyglycolic acid suture. Fertil Steril 1978;30:210.

Sweeney WJ III, Gepfert R. The fallopian tube. Clin Obstet Gynecol 1965;8:32.

Swolin K. Die einwirkung grossen intraperitonealen dosen glukokortikoidauf diebildungvon-postoperativen adhasionen. Acta Obstet Gynecol Scand 1967a;46:119.

Swolin K. Fertiltratsoperatronen, Teil I and II. Acta Obstet Gynecol Scand 1967b;46:204.

Swolin K. 50 Fertilitatsoperationen: Literatur und Methodik. Acta Obstet Gynecol Scand 1967c;46:234.

Tuffier T, Letulle M. Transposition de l'ovaire avec son pedicule vasculair dans canite de l'uterus apres ablation des trompes uterine pour annexites. Bull Acad Nat Med Paris 1924;3(S)91:362.

Tulandi T. Salpingo-ovariolysis: a comparison between laser surgery and electrosurgery. Fertil Steril 1986;45:489.

Tulandi T. Adhesion reformation after reproductive surgery with and without the carbon dioxide laser. Fertil Steril 1987;47:704.

Umezaki C, Katayama KP, Jones HW Jr. Pregnancy rates after reconstructive surgery on the fallopian tubes. Obstet Gynecol 1974;43:418.

Vancaillie TG, Schmidt EH. The uterotubal junction: a proposal for classifying its morphology as assessed with hysteroscopy. J Reprod Med 1988;33:624.

Vasquez G, Winston RML, Boeckx W, et al. Tubal lesions subsequent to sterilization and their relation to fertility after attempts at reversal. Am J Obstet Gynecol 1980;138:86.

VonGraff E. Operative treatment of female sterility. J Iowa Med Soc 1936;26:31.

Williams GFJ. Fallopian tube surgery for reversal of sterilization. Br Med J 1973;1:599.

Winston RML. Microsurgical reanastomosis of the rabbit oviduct in its functional and pathological sequelae. Br J Obstet Gynaecol 1975;2:513.

Winston RML. Microsurgical tubocornual anastomosis for reversal of sterilization. Lancet 1977;1:284.

Winston RML. Reversal of sterilization. Clin Obstet Gynecol 1980; 23:1261.

Winston RML. Microsurgery and the fallopian tube: from fantasy to reality. Fertil Steril 1981;34:521.

Winston RML, Magara RA. Techniques for the improvement of microsurgical tubal anastomosis. In: Microsurgery in female infertility. Second Clinical Colloquia on Reproduction. New York: Grune & Stratton, 1980.

Woodruff JD, Pauerstein CJ. The fallopian tube. Baltimore: Williams & Wilkins, 1969.

Young PE, Egan JE, Barlow JA, et al. Reconstructive surgery for infertility at the Boston Hospital for Women. Am J Obstet Gynecol 1970;108:1092.

Endometriosis

20

TIFFANY J. WILLIAMS

Sampson's description of endometriosis in 1921 has been little improved on. He described endometriosis as the

> presence of ectopic tissue which possesses the histological structure and function of the uterine mucosa. It also includes the abnormal conditions which may result not only from the invasion of organs and other structures by this tissue but also from its relation to menstruation.

Although benign, endometriosis possesses the unique ability to invade tissue and to disseminate or metastasize by hematogenous or lymphatic routes or by direct implantation. These attributes are essentially characteristic of malignancy.

Endometriosis can be divided into two distinct clinical and pathologic types that frequently appear as entirely different diseases. One is *adenomyosis,* or internal endometriosis, which is characterized by invasion of the myometrium by endometrium from within the uterine cavity. The other is *external endometriosis,* in which tissues outside the uterus are affected or the uterine serosa is involved from without rather than by direct extension from the mucosa.

ADENOMYOSIS

Adenomyosis may have two distinct forms, diffuse and local. Diffuse adenomyosis involves the walls of the uterus to various degrees (Fig. 20-1). Although usually quite diffuse, it may be relatively localized, but it is not encapsulated. The uterus itself is usually somewhat enlarged, rarely more than twice normal size, and is more or less symmetrical. Cut section of the uterine wall reveals a coarse trabecular pattern of interlacing musculature and fibrous tissue with small islands of endometrium that are often dark and hemorrhagic. In contrast, an adenomyoma is localized disease in the uterine wall; it is encapsulated much as an ordinary

intramural leiomyoma. It is located mainly within the wall of the uterus but may project into the uterine cavity, becoming a submucous adenomyoma (Fig. 20-2).

The most generally accepted theory holds that the endometrial tissue in the myometrium is of müllerian origin and is a direct downgrowth from the endometrium of the uterine cavity. Cullen, with the help of McCleary, in his treatise on adenomyoma of the uterus, showed by serial section a direct continuity between the basalis portion of the endometrium and the endometrial islands within the areas of adenomyosis. In some instances, endometrial extensions could be followed throughout the full thickness of the myometrium to the serosal surface of the uterus.

These intramural islands generally have the histologic appearance of the basalis of the endometrium and usually respond to estrogen stimulation with a proliferative pattern or, occasionally, one of cystic hyperplasia. The progestational effect on ectopic endometrium is less predictable. Secretory changes in the glands are uncommon, whereas in pregnancy a decidual reaction of the stroma is anticipated. Ectopic endometrial tissue, like that of the uterine endometrium, may be hormone sensitive. In the absence of hormonal stimulation, it will become atrophic after the menopause. Although such ectopic endometrium may be estrogen dependent and may undergo a cystic type of hyperplasia, adenomyosis rarely shows any atypical type of hyperplasia and even more uncommonly becomes malignant.

The reported incidence of adenomyosis varies widely from one institution to another, since the diagnosis is fundamentally pathologic. The frequency, which varies between 8% and 27%, depends not only on the criteria used for diagnosis but also on the thoroughness with which the removed uterus is studied. A rigid criterion has been suggested by Benson and Sneeden; namely, the area must extend into the myometrium at least 2 low-power fields (8 mm) from the basalis. The incidence reaches its peak in the fifth decade. Infertility is not common with this form of the

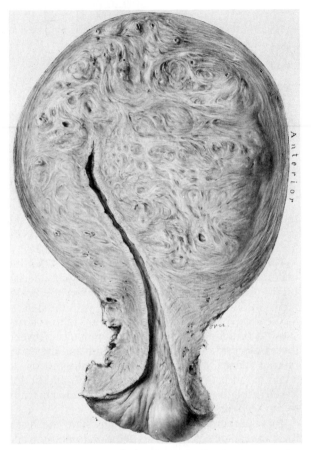

Figure 20–1. Adenomyosis of uterus (after Cullen). Typical example with complete involvement of both anterior and posterior walls. At examination, such a uterus is moderately enlarged, usually symmetrical, and very firm to palpation.

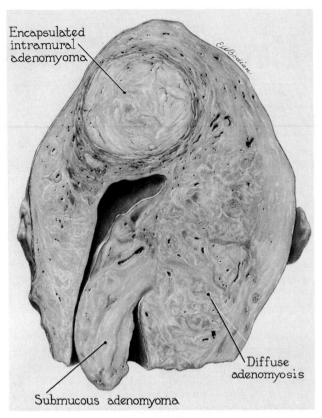

Figure 20–2. Uterus showing three types of adenomyomatous growth: encapsulated intramural adenomyoma, submucous adenomyoma, and diffuse adenomyosis of walls.

disease, and most patients are multiparous. About 12% of them have coexisting external endometriosis.

Symptoms

Adenomyosis is often an incidental pathologic finding and may be entirely asymptomatic. When involvement of the myometrium is extensive, pain and abnormal uterine bleeding, usually in the form of menorrhagia, are likely, probably because the enlarged uterine cavity has an increased surface area. Also, extensive involvement of the uterine wall may interfere with the normal uterine muscular contractility and allow excessive bleeding. Pain, when present, is usually associated with menstruation and is often severe, crampy, or knifelike. This dysmenorrheic pattern likely results from bleeding within the deep-lying islands of endo-

metrium. The pathologic basis for these symptoms is shown in Figure 20-3. The histologic features of the endometrial glands and stroma that characterize these lesions are shown in Figure 20-4. The hormonal effects of pregnancy on endometriosis are shown in Figures 20-5 and 20-6.

Pelvic Findings

The uterus may be very firm and is usually enlarged. Generally, it is not more than twice its normal size. As classically described, the uterus is likely to be more enlarged in the anterior-posterior dimension, a reflection of the more prominent involvement of the posterior uterine wall. With the diffuse type of adenomyosis, which is more common, the enlargement is likely to be symmetrical. Accordingly, the uterus is a rather globular structure. When an encapsulated adenomyoma is present, the uterus may be irregular or asymmetrical, much as it is when leiomyomata are present. At times,

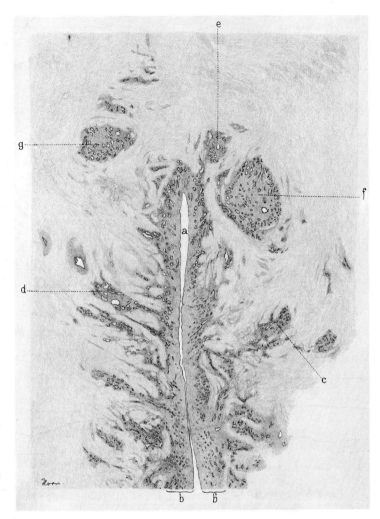

Figure 20–3. Section through central portion of uterus with adenomyosis. (*a*) Uterine cavity. (*b*) Endometrium of cavity. (*c* to *g*) Islands of displaced endometrium into which hemorrhage occurs at time of menstruation. Poor drainage of menstrual blood with increased tension explains severe menstrual pain.

particularly during menstruation, the enlarged uterus is tender to palpation.

Diagnosis

Adenomyosis should always be suspected in a woman with dysmenorrhea and menorrhagia of increasing severity in the fourth or fifth decade, particularly if the uterus is symmetrically enlarged, firm, and tender. It is difficult to be certain of the diagnosis, because functional uterine bleeding and multiple small leiomyomas may have similar findings.

Treatment

An exact preoperative diagnosis is often difficult, and it may be largely of only academic interest anyway. Only

in the rare instance when excessive myometrium is removed by the curette or a polypoid submucous adenomyoma is found can the diagnosis be confirmed without the uterus as a surgical specimen. Curettage does not aid in establishing the diagnosis and is ineffectual as treatment, even though it may be required because of abnormal bleeding. Cyclic hormonal therapy is likewise of little aid in treatment.

The need for surgery, therefore, is based on whether there is continued menorrhagia and dysmenorrhea, not on whether the uterus is thought to be normal in size or whether it contains adenomyosis or a leiomyoma. The definitive treatment is hysterectomy. The vaginal route is preferred if the size of the uterus permits and no other pelvic abnormalities are present. At times, in a younger patient who wants to retain her reproductive capability, excision of an encapsulated adenomyoma should be considered. This situation arises infrequently, because adenomyosis is generally diffuse and

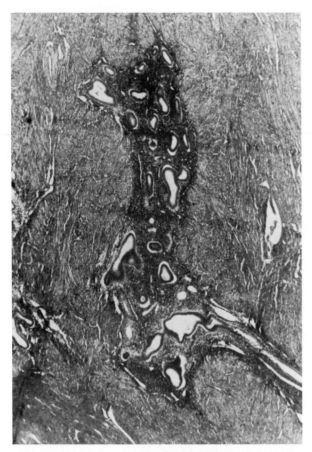

Figure 20–4. Area of adenomyosis. Compact stroma and proliferative, slightly hyperplastic glands are surrounded by hypertrophied myometrium.

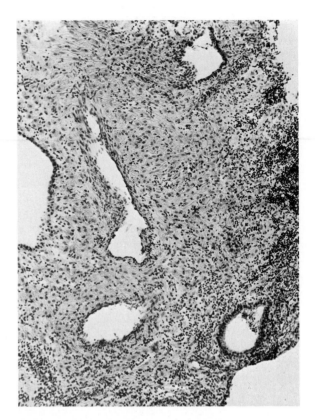

Figure 20–5. Adenomyosis in pregnancy showing decidual reaction. Note that glands still show proliferative pattern not reacting to increased progesterone stimulation.

usually occurs in multiparous women no longer interested in childbearing.

EXTERNAL ENDOMETRIOSIS

The term *endometriosis* more commonly refers to the external form, in which the ectopic endometrial tissue grows outside the uterus. The condition is more likely to be clinically symptomatic than are most cases of adenomyosis, in which there is only minimal myometrial extension and few symptoms. Infertility and symptoms of pelvic discomfort are presented to the gynecologist as diagnostic problems.

Since the first descriptions in the latter part of the 19th century, endometriosis has been recorded with increasing frequency. Increased clinical awareness, better education in gynecologic pathology, and the availability of laparoscopy have led to more frequent recognition and diagnosis. It is also probable, however,

that the disease is actually increasing in frequency. In 1977, Williams and Pratt, in reporting a prospective study involving 1000 consecutive celiotomies for benign disease, documented a 50% incidence of endometriosis. Although this figure may be biased by the type of patients referred to the Mayo Clinic, the diagnosis of endometriosis is more commonly made in high-income patients than in the indigent. The difference in observed frequency may prove to be more closely related to the patient's ability to pay for specialty medical care than to a true difference in the occurrence of the disease based on socioeconomic factors.

From a multi-institutional study reported in 1980, Simpson and associates concluded that there may be a hereditary component functioning in women with endometriosis. They postulated a polygenic and multifactorial relationship. This seemed to be particularly true among familial groups in which severe endometriosis was noted (ie, 62% as opposed to 23% of "nonfamilial" groups).

There seems to be little question that pregnancy may decrease the incidence of endometriosis and confers some protection on the parous woman. Often, 5 or

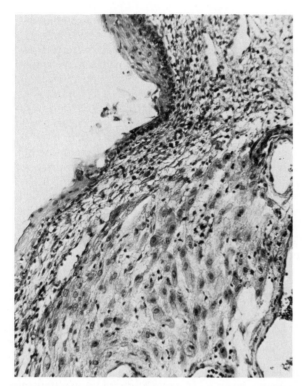

Figure 20–6. Adenomyosis in pregnancy. Decidual change in stromal cells is accompanied by glandular changes.

more years pass after a patient's last pregnancy before symptomatic endometriosis is discovered. Whether those benefits result from the hormonal changes of pregnancy or the cervical dilatation and delivery is not certain.

Although it has been widely believed that endometriosis is rare among black women, Chatman found a 22.7% incidence among black women undergoing diagnostic laparoscopy. Among poor African women, Ekwempu and Harrison reported an 8% incidence in hysterectomy specimens. Miyazawa found a 10% incidence among Oriental women and a 5% incidence for non-Oriental patients. Recent studies have also documented endometriosis in teenagers with pelvic pain, many of these instances diagnosed at a young age despite previous data suggesting that the condition occurs primarily in the middle decades of life. Many cases thought to have been infections in the past could have been endometriosis.

The ectopic endometrium, wherever it may be, depends on ovarian hormones for its maintenance and for various degrees of stimulation. In 1962, Scott and Wharton, performing studies on endometriosis in castrated rhesus monkeys, showed that estrogen was important in maintaining active endometrial implants and that when estrogen-primed implants were subjected to progesterone-induced withdrawal bleeding, implants became more active. Each implant may then respond to these hormonal stimuli as though it were a miniature uterus. Frequently, the response to progesterone is minimal, and in this respect the implants resemble the basalis portion of the uterine endometrium. But response varies greatly, depending on the distribution of estrogen and progesterone receptors. In the same patient, some areas may show a good progestational response while others show none. The implants, however, are usually capable of local withdrawal bleeding, regardless of their histologic pattern and degree of progestational response.

In pregnancy or with progestogen therapy, implants may show a marked decidual reaction of the stroma (see Figs. 20-5 and 20-6). This response, too, is not entirely predictable. Because of the decidual reaction of the implants and the absence of menstruation, the general impression had been that endometriosis improves during pregnancy. This concept was questioned by McArthur and Ulfelder, who, in a review of reported cases, found that pregnancy had nearly similar effects in regression and progression on endometriosis.

Laboratory studies involving the cytosol estrogen and progesterone receptors have shown a difference between the receptors present in endometriosis and those in the endometrium itself. Bergqvist and associates found markedly lower receptor content for estrogen in endometriotic tissue. Data on the cytoplasmic progesterone receptors for endometriosis were conflicting. The conclusion, however, was that a functional difference existed between the endometriotic tissue and the endometrium. Jänne and associates documented similar findings. These data are in accord with the often favorable but variable response noted to hormonal treatment of endometriosis and tend to explain the discrepancy.

The fact that endometriosis depends on ovarian hormones generally confines its clinical importance to the reproductive era of a woman's life. It has not been reported before menarche, and the implants become atrophic after the menopause. Endometriosis has its peak incidence in the fourth decade. Scott and associates found that 49.5% of their cases were in this age group and that 83.1% occurred before age 40. Thus, the classic patient with endometriosis is a nulliparous, high-income woman in her fourth decade of life.

Many studies have attempted to explain why some women present with endometriosis and others do not. A specific possibility is alteration in the body's immune mechanism. Dmowski and Radwanska showed that, as measured by lymphocyte response to autologous antigens, immune response among monkeys having endometriosis was decreased. Further studies reported an increase in autoantibodies, primarily IgG and IgA, to endometrium and ovary in patients with endometriosis. Other studies had different results, and in several reports, complement—mainly C3 and C4—was increased in both serum and peritoneal fluid. HLA antigens did not, however, seem to be related to endometriosis. At this time, conflicting reports do not allow a definitive answer to this intriguing relationship of immune status to endometriosis. The basic tenet is logical, and further elucidation is expected.

Also of interest relative to immune situation and endometriosis is the status of monoclonal antibodies, specifically CA125. Although an increase in CA125 appears relevant to ovarian malignancy specifically, increases were also noted in patients having endometriosis. Slight increases of CA125 were noted in stage I and stage II disease, but significant increases were seen only in stages III and IV. Serum levels have been consistently reported as being increased with greater degrees of endometriosis. Surprisingly, study of peritoneal washings evaluated for CA125 did not show differences between controls and patients having endometriosis. Treatment of endometriosis by surgery or by danazol showed lowering of CA125 levels, whereas treatment with progesterone compounds did not, despite similarity of response. The monoclonal antibody test may be of some use in evaluating the extent of endometriosis but, unfortunately, may not be of help in monitoring the response to treatment.

Studies of the cellular components of the peritoneal fluid have been made in an attempt to explain further not only the cause of endometriosis but also the apparent relation to infertility. Macrophages were significantly increased among patients with endometriosis. Prostaglandins and complement factors were also increased, the latter in serum as well. Further increases were noted in comparisons of fertile and infertile individuals. Prostaglandin levels seemed to be more increased when dysmenorrhea was significant. The increase in the macrophages with resultant prostaglandin changes might affect sperm as well as tubal motility. In laboratory animals, factors present in peritoneal fluid seemed to impair ovum capture by coating the fimbria and preventing contact with the cumulus. There are no data correlating such a factor in the human female. Tumor necrosis factor, shown to be increased in women with endometriosis, may also have an effect on fertilization as a function of the macrophage system. Cytotoxicity can affect sperm, oocytes, and embryos irrespective of the cause of the increase in macrophages. The increases in macrophage numbers seem cyclic, and release of still other factors may be related to infertility.

Studies relating prostaglandins to increased macrophages, dysmenorrhea, and endometriosis have supported such a relationship. Antiprostaglandins, however, have not been effective in pain relief, and not all studies have been able to confirm the increases in prostaglandins. One must await further information before accepting this logical progression of substance, symptoms, and disease as fact.

Plasminogen activator factors could also be implicated in endometriosis and infertility relative to adhesion formation. Conflicting reports about increased levels, however, do not allow a conclusion to be made about any significance. Serum and peritoneal prolactin hormone levels have been studied. When prolactin levels were increased, there appeared to be a reduction of the prolactin levels with treatment (danazol). There was no decrease if levels were normal, however, and increased levels could not be related to the presence of endometriosis.

Distribution and Gross Pathology

Endometrial implants and growths have been described in a variety of places, primarily within the pelvis. Ovarian disease is noted most frequently. The incidence seems to decrease as the centrifugal distance from the uterus increases. The distribution is illustrated in Figure 20-7 diagrammatically. The numerical incidence of endometriosis in the various pelvic and other abdominoperineal structures is shown in Table 20-1. In addition to these common sites, some rare locations have been reported, including the extensor carpi radialis muscle and the thigh.

Ovary

The lesions encountered on the ovary vary in size from tiny spots to masses larger than 10 cm in diameter. The small superficial lesions are more often noted on the surface of the ovary; they vary from dusky red to brownish black, depending on the state of preservation of the contained blood (Fig. 20-8). The larger cysts often have a rather thick wall and the dull white of the ovarian cortex; where the capsule is thinned, the dark chocolate-colored contents may darken the wall to brown or almost black (Fig. 20-9).

The cysts characteristically perforate when the pressure resulting from intracystic hemorrhage becomes sufficiently great. Organization of the extruded blood seals over the defect in the cyst wall, and blood then accumulates anew within the cavity until perforation again takes place. This discharge of blood and subsequent organization result in adhesions about the ovary to the parietal peritoneum, usually the posterior leaf of the broad ligament and cul-de-sac.

The peritoneum, irritated by this blood, becomes

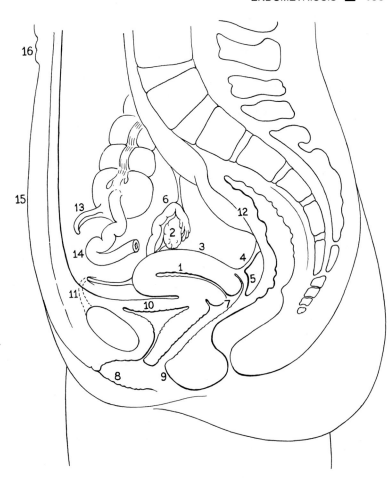

Figure 20–7. Schematic drawing of sites of endometriosis (numbered, beginning with the ovary, in approximate order of frequency): (*1*) Adenomyosis site. (*2*) Ovary. (*3*) Serous surface of uterus. (*4*) Uterosacral ligament. (*5*) Cul-de-sac. (*6*) Tube. (*7*) Cervix. (*8*) Vulva. (*9*) Perineum. (*10*) Bladder. (*11*) Extraperitoneal portion of round ligament. (*12*) Rectosigmoid. (*13*) Appendix. (*14*) Ileum. (*15*) Abdominal scar. (*16*) Umbilicus.

hyperemic and thickened. When the peritoneal cavity is opened after recent rupture, the characteristic finding is old blood or chocolate-colored material lying free within the cavity. Usually it is scanty, but in rare instances, as much as 100–200 ml may be present. When the cyst is dissected free, the point or points of previous perforations are inevitably entered, and the cyst contents spill. Generally, the material is a thick brown fluid, from which the name *chocolate cyst* has been derived, but it may be very thick, tenacious, and almost black. German authors have called these *tar cysts* and, indeed, the contents may resemble tar more than chocolate.

The presumptive diagnosis is endometrial cyst if, when an adherent ovary or ovarian cyst is dissected free, chocolate or tarry substance appears. This rule is not invariable, since hemorrhage into the corpora lutea and into other types of ovarian cysts may give a somewhat similar picture. The tissue in the wall of the cyst, however, is that of the friable corpus luteum rather than that of the more fibrotic endometrioma. In addition, the blood in a corpus luteum hematoma is much more apt to form a clot than to remain a thick fluid, as in an endometrial cyst. Hemorrhage into any cystadenoma may give a chocolate color to the contents; but the blood, becoming mixed with the contents, is not usually sufficient to alter the consistency of the original fluid content.

Rupture and leakage are assumed to occur frequently, and the secondary irritation is thought to be responsible for some of the symptoms. However, this may not be the case. Of 325 patients with endometriosis who were studied by Williams, 277 had endometriosis on the ovary and 132 had endometrioma. In eight of these patients, leakage or rupture was found at the time of surgery. Only one of these patients had pain that could have been attributed to that leakage. Abdominal pain associated with rupture of an endometrial cyst is generally thought to be caused by peritoneal reaction to hemolyzed blood.

Uterus

Second to the ovary, the uterus is involved most frequently. The serosal surface of the uterus is often the

TABLE 20–1
Location of External Endometriosis

TYPE	SITE	NUMBER	PERCENT*
Ovarian	One ovary	285	55.2
	Both ovaries	127	24.6
Superficial and small spots on serosa	Diffuse scattered pelvic	171	33.1
	Uterine surface	73	14.1
	Tubal surface	71	13.7
	Posterior cul-de-sac	24	4.7
	Uterosacral ligaments	19	3.7
	Anterior cul-de-sac	11	2.1
	Omentum	3	0.6
	Round ligaments	2	0.4
	Broad ligaments	1	0.2
	Small intestine	1	0.2
	Appendix	7	1.4
Intra-abdominal nodules	Rectovaginal septum	8	1.6
	Rectovaginal septum with rectosigmoid involvement	20	3.9
	Rectovaginal septum with vaginal extension	9	1.8
	Sigmoidal	4	0.8
	Anterior cul-de-sac	2	0.4
	Anterior cul-de-sac with bladder involvement	5	1.0
	Tube	8	1.6
	Broad ligament	4	0.8
	Round ligament	3	0.6
Extraperitoneal	Cervix	13	2.5
	Inguinal	4	0.8
	Umbilical	4	0.8
	Incisional—ventral	4	0.8
	Incisional—vulval	1	0.2

*Total is more than 100% because of multiple lesions.

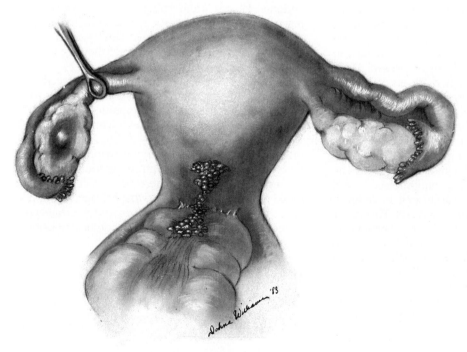

Figure 20–8. Typical picture of old pelvic endometriosis. The ovary, uterosacral ligament, posterior surface of uterus, and rectal wall are involved. An atraumatic small ring forceps (Williams's clamp), as shown on the left utero-ovarian ligament, is used for traction when necessary.

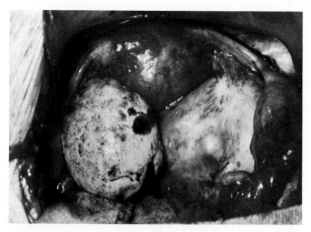

Figure 20–9. Typical bilateral endometrial cysts of ovary almost completely destroying ovarian tissue. Old blood is disseminated on pelvic peritoneum as well.

site of multiple implants. They are usually very small, but on occasion they can form dark vesicles up to 4 or 5 mm in diameter (see Fig. 20-8). Where the endometrial lesion occurs on these serosal surfaces, there is likely to be a characteristic puckering or scarring of the adjacent serosa about the small, dark lesion. Implants on the anterior surface of the uterus sometimes cause adhesions between it and the peritoneal surface of the bladder or any other adjacent structure. There may be invasion of the bladder extending through the entire thickness of the vesical wall (Fig. 20-10).

The lesions of endometriosis are more common on the posterior surface of the uterus, especially on the lower and more dependent portion. The cul-de-sac is a favorite place for endometrial implants. Accordingly, the posterior wall of the vagina and the cervix may become densely adherent to the anterior rectal wall and completely obliterate the cul-de-sac.

Uterosacral Ligaments

The uterosacral ligaments on either side of the cul-de-sac are commonly involved with the endometriosis, which forms small, puckered, shotty nodules along the course of the ligaments. Downward extension of the invasive endometrial process from the cul-de-sac and the uterosacral regions proceeds into the rectovaginal septum. Here the endometriosis can involve the anterior rectal wall and, at times, penetrate the mucosa of the posterior vaginal vault. This growth may be not only palpable but also visible as a dark nodular mass posterior to the cervix (Fig. 20-11).

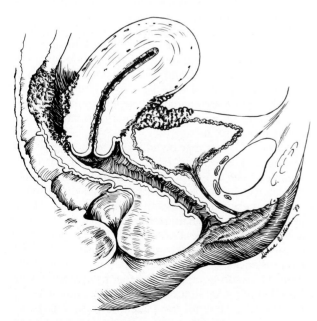

Figure 20–10. Endometriosis involving bladder wall, posterior uterus, uterosacral ligaments, and rectosigmoid colon.

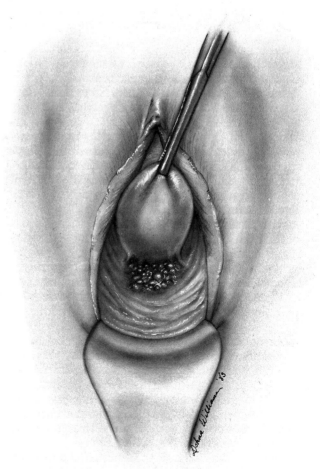

Figure 20–11. Endometriotic lesions in posterior vaginal fornix extending from cul-de-sac endometriosis.

Round Ligaments

Small endometrial implants may occur on the serosal surface of the round ligaments at any place within the peritoneal cavity. A lesion of special interest was described by Cullen in 1896. In this lesion, the extraperitoneal portion of the round ligament is involved in an endometriotic process, forming a nodule in the region of the inguinal ring. Such a nodule may vary from 1 to 3 cm in diameter and usually blends diffusely into the surrounding adipose tissue. These round ligament growths show hypertrophy of the adjacent smooth muscle along with islands of glands and stroma. The tissues may be darkened by evidence of old or recent hemorrhage. The inguinal mass is usually associated with pain, and there may also be cyclic enlargement. The pain may mimic that of musculoskeletal conditions, although there is no direct bony involvement and excision is curative.

Peritoneum

All peritoneal surfaces, both parietal and visceral, may show the same stigmata of endometriosis described for other organs. Of particular interest are the subtle or minimal lesions that have come to be appreciated by use of the laparoscope and operating microscope. Jansen and Russell confirmed not only whitish opacified lesions but also red, flamelike areas and pale translucent areas similar to endometrium itself. Yellowish brown peritoneal patches could be confirmed as endometriosis in nearly one half of cases.

Retroperitoneum

Significant involvement of the uterosacral ligaments extending toward the pelvic wall may not only mimic the findings of malignancy but also affect the retroperitoneal tissues. Sciatic pain (usually cyclic) and neurologic defect, such as foot drop, may occur. Lymph node involvement was infrequently recorded by Moore and associates, and most instances were in women 40 years old and older.

Intestine

In addition to involvement of the anterior rectal wall and invasion of the rectovaginal septum, a prominent lesion in the upper rectum or sigmoid is not uncommon. Such lesions usually result in a thickening and proliferation of the muscularis of the bowel. The degree of involvement may be great enough that encroachment on the bowel lumen produces partial or even complete obstruction.

Usually, the invasion extends through the serosa to the muscularis, but the mucosa is not directly involved by the endometriosis. This is an important diagnostic point in the differentiation of endometriosis from carcinoma of the bowel. In the latter, since the carcinoma arises from the mucosa, barium enema and proctoscopy are very helpful. Endometriosis, however, can involve the full thickness of the intestinal wall and even produce polypoid growths within the bowel lumen. Cyclic bleeding usually occurs, and the diagnosis can be made by proctoscopy or sigmoidoscopy with a biopsy of the lesion. Barium enema and proctoscopy as diagnostic procedures yielded positive results in less than 10% of women having intestinal endometriosis. If these have not been done, it may be difficult to distinguish bowel endometriosis from carcinoma at surgery. Endometriosis elsewhere in the pelvis generally gives a clue to the bowel lesion. Even if there is no actual involvement of the mucosa by the endometriosis, cyclic hematochezia may occur, and careful inspection of the mucosa reveals a defect contiguous with the adjacent endometriosis. It must be remembered that endometriosis is the third most common benign tumor of the colon.

In a study by Williams of 325 consecutive cases of endometriosis in which the female genital tract was involved, the intestinal tract was found to have endometriosis in 41% of cases. The sigmoid was involved in 84% and the ileum in only 9%. Obstructive symptoms, however, were far more frequent with ileal endometriosis (25% of cases) than with colonic (6%).

The appendix, cecum, and ileum are frequently involved in the process of endometriosis but rarely to the degree seen in the sigmoid and rectum. In the appendix, involvement is usually an incidental pathologic finding with appendectomy. However, the marked decidual reaction and changes that occur with pregnancy may result in spontaneous perforation of the appendix and the signs and symptoms of acute abdominal distress. Similar complications have been reported with endometriosis involving the colon, but these are merely curiosities that must be kept in mind. An extensive growth of endometriosis on an appendix is illustrated in Figure 20-12.

A loop of ileum may be adherent in the pelvis, producing angulation and obstruction, either partial or complete. The gross appearance of the lesion is usually typical of endometriosis. Biopsy of the lesion, however, may be necessary to establish the benignity of the implant. Bowel resection or excision of the involved area should be done if obstruction is present or if the caliber of the lumen shows compromise. Under such circumstances, castration alone is not adequate treatment, since subsequent fibrosis may further narrow the bowel lumen. The sequelae of intestinal endometriosis may not appear until the patient is postmenopausal. Although the endometriosis may have become inactive,

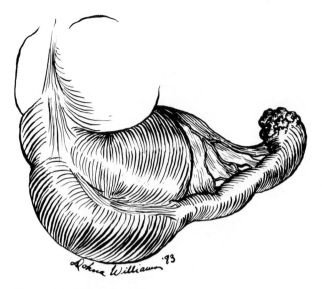

Figure 20—12. Endometriosis at tip of appendix.

the resulting cicatrization leads to a decrease in the bowel lumen and to symptoms of obstruction.

It is interesting that Krebs and Goplerud, in reviewing 368 patients with gynecologic disease and intestinal obstruction, did not mention endometriosis. When, however, extensive endometriosis involves the intestine and constricts the lumen or malignant disease cannot be excluded, resection of the diseased area and the definitive gynecologic operation of total abdominal hysterectomy and bilateral salpingo-oophorectomy are indicated to avoid the necessity of reoperation for recurrence. Taylor and associates (unpublished data) further demonstrated that definitive treatment could be accomplished at one operation with only infrequent complications.

Bladder

The urinary tract is involved less frequently than the bowel. Peritoneal implants on the bladder may infiltrate partially or completely into the bladder wall, where they cause symptoms of vesical irritability and, occasionally, hematuria. Vesical endometriosis may occur by direct implantation after vaginal hysterotomy for abortion. The frequency of this complication is so high that in Sweden, vaginal hysterotomy has been discontinued as a method of midtrimester interruption of pregnancy.

Cytologic evaluation of the urine may show endometrial cells, but the diagnosis usually requires cystoscopy and biopsy. Cystography may document a filling defect, but it, like ultrasound, is nonspecific. Segmental resection of the lesion is preferable to attempts at hormone management.

Ureter

A more serious situation arises when the ureter is compressed by an endometrial cyst or is directly invaded by endometriosis in the pelvis. Either of these leads to ureteral obstruction and subsequent loss of renal function (Fig. 20-13). Early diagnosis and treatment are required to avoid loss of the kidney. Scarring and continued obstruction require not only definitive surgery with castration but also excision of the diseased ureter with anastomosis or implantation into the bladder. Only some 100 cases are recorded in the literature, and in general surgical management is recommended. In four cases, however, successful management with progestational agents and with danazol is documented. This approach may allow a period of temporization should the obstruction occur in a young woman wanting to bear a child.

Kidney

Ten cases of renal endometriosis have been reported. This condition may result from passage of fragments of endometrium up the ureter or, more likely, by lymphatic or vascular metastasis along or in the ureteral wall. The symptom is vague flank discomfort, occasionally with hematuria. Roentgenograms indicate an expansive lesion suggesting a diagnosis of malignancy.

Incisional Scars

Scars from operations are occasionally the sites of endometriotic implantation. Perineal, vaginal, or vulvar scars—particularly episiotomies, colporrhaphies, and Bartholin's gland excisions—are likely areas for involvement by endometriosis. The hormonal effects of pregnancy on the endometrium may produce adverse conditions for implantation and growth. Otherwise, one could expect nearly all episiotomies to be potential sites of endometriosis, whereas fewer than 100 cases are recorded in the literature.

When an incisional scar becomes a site of endometriosis, there is frequently a history of delayed wound healing. The growths appear as either deep-lying or subcutaneous nodules infiltrating the fat, fascia, and muscle. Bleeding into the tissues at the time of menstruation may cause cyclic local pain, tenderness, and discoloration of the tissues; however, the nodule may lie too deep for detection of any color change through the skin. If the nodule is very superficial, cyclic bleeding or ulceration may be apparent.

In most instances, incisional endometriomas have followed surgical procedures that violated the uterine cavity and allowed the lining endometrium to be transplanted. Wespi and Kletzhändler suggested that the fre-

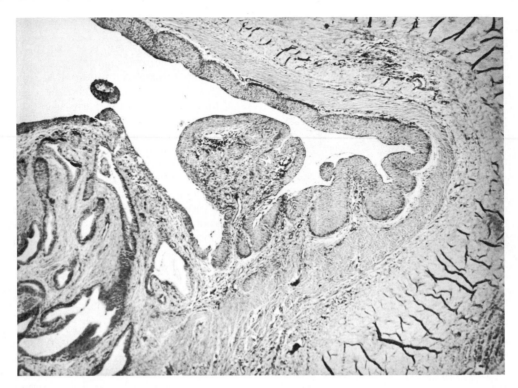

Figure 20–13. Compression and invasion of ureteral wall by endometriosis.

quency might approach 5% among patients having cesarean section or hysterectomy. Chatterjee reported an incidence of 1% of scar endometriosis among patients having hysterectomy and described associated pelvic endometriosis in 24% of 17 patients. Indeed, endometriosis has been recorded along the needle tracts after amniocentesis or saline injection for abortion.

Careful flushing and irrigation of the abdomen and of the incision during closure should minimize the chance of contamination when incision into the uterine cavity is required. Metroplasty and myomectomy as well as cesarean section and hysterotomy increase the risk of incisional endometriosis. Episiotomy scars and cervical and vaginal lacerations also serve as implantation sites after delivery. The number is significantly increased when curettage is done after delivery. Paull and Tedeschi reported 15 instances in 2208 deliveries when curettage was carried out and none in 13,800 without curettage. One might infer that the basalis component of the endometriosis is required for implantation.

Management, usually best carried out by local excision, is both diagnostic and curative. The use of various hormone regimens may be proper if it is necessary to avoid surgery. However, it must be remembered that malignancy can occur in each area of ectopic endome-triosis, and histologic confirmation of the tentative diagnosis is preferable.

Umbilicus

Endometriosis involving the umbilicus accounts for about 1% of cases. It presents the problem of differential diagnosis from metastatic cancer. Here the endometrial tissue infiltrates the surrounding tissues and, with hemorrhage, forms bluish nodules, sometimes visible through the skin (Fig. 20-14). There may be little or no associated pelvic endometriosis, and the symptoms may be cyclic, related to the periods, or completely absent save for an umbilical mass.

Thorax

In 1981, Foster and associates tabulated 65 cases of thoracic endometriosis. They described two categories of involvement, the pleura and the lung parenchyma. These areas of involvement presented different findings. In patients with pleural disease, there was pain with right-sided pneumothorax or pleural effusion in 93% of the cases. These instances were believed to be secondary to tubal regurgitation and transport through diaphragmatic defects to give implantation onto the

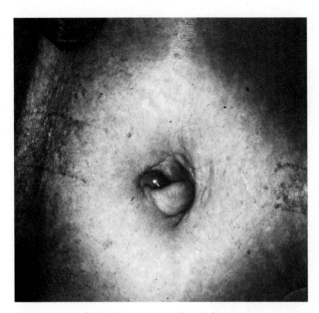

Figure 20–14. Endometriosis of umbilicus.

pleura. The authors pointed out that a preponderance of defects in the right diaphragm correlated with this local predominance of endometriosis. They found that women with pleural endometriosis were younger than those having parenchymal disease. Previous pelvic surgery was more common among women who had parenchymal endometriosis; however, pelvic endometriosis was found more often in those with pleural disease. Cases involving the pleura produced pleuritic pain or pleural effusions, whereas those involving the lung parenchyma produced hemoptysis rather than the pleuritic symptoms.

Catamenial pneumothorax or hemoptysis should alert the physician to the possibility of thoracic endometriosis. The chest roentgenogram is usually of little value in the diagnosis; however, cytology, aspiration biopsy, and pleuroscopy may be used to confirm it. Massive effusion and bleeding may occur, but they suggest even more the possibility of a malignancy.

Histology

Endometriosis in its different sites may present a variety of histologic patterns. In many instances, particularly when the location is the ovary, there are typical glands with an abundance of characteristic endometrial stroma (Fig. 20-15). In large chocolate cysts, the epithelium lining the cavity may be thinned by pressure, often to the point of being unrecognizable. Indeed, in some areas the epithelium may be entirely lacking. Stromal cells may be scanty in many of the lesions, and one may be forced to search diligently for enough stroma to identify the tissue. In many such situations, hemosiderin phagocytosis may be the most prominent feature.

When endometriosis grows in a setting of smooth muscle, such as on the round ligament or on the surface of the uterus or the bowel, it seems to stimulate the proliferation of the smooth muscle. The muscular components may grow in whorls between bits of endometrial tissue, so that histologically the growth resembles that of adenomyosis.

In many instances, the glands and the stroma go through the same cyclic changes as the endometrium in its normal site. During pregnancy, a full decidual reaction is frequently noted, and such responsive endometriosis seems common in the ovary (see Figs. 20-5 and 20-6). The typical cyclic menstrual changes are not seen universally, and the histologic pattern of the ectopic tissue may be purely proliferative with no progestational change. In some instances, the typical pattern of hyperplasia is present. This is usually cystic, and adenomatous or atypical change is infrequent.

In some cysts, the epithelial lining resembles tubal epithelium, with ciliated and nonciliated cells. Both Sampson in 1922 and Everett described this, and the former suggested the term *endosalpingosis*. Some cysts have been seen in which one part of the wall is lined by typical endometrium and another part is lined by epithelium of the tubal type.

Examination and comparison of the eutopic and ectopic endometrium by electron microscopy further support the variable patterns of hormonal response. Schweppe and associates documented this variation among ectopic implants and between them and the normal endometrium as well. Their elegant studies show a predominantly mixed pattern with differences between adjacent glands and even within the same gland. In the secretory phase of the cycle, one half of the glands were irregularly differentiated, some proliferative and some completely nonresponsive. Indeed, secretory activity was noted in endometriosis even during the proliferative phase. Their data fit with the information available on the steroid receptors found in endometriosis.

Vasquez and associates used the scanning electron microscope to help differentiate three morphologically different types of endometriotic lesions. Their description of the intraperitoneal polypoid lesions without glandular opening but with deeper endometriotic tissue; foci with surface epithelium, glands, and stroma; and retroperitoneal foci with few glands and stroma further serves to support some minimal or subtle features in endometriosis.

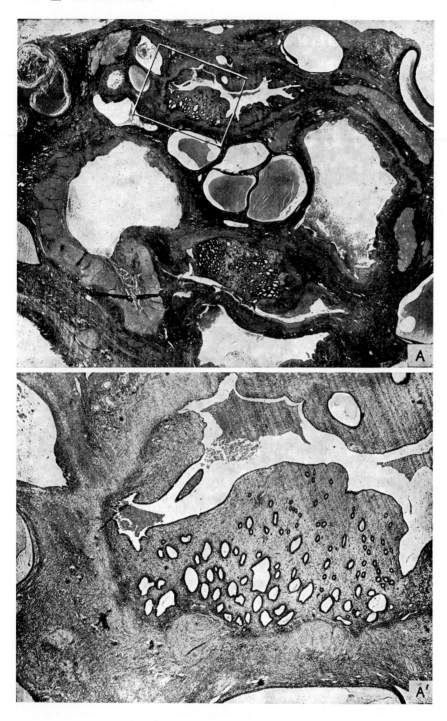

Figure 20–15. Multiple endometrial cysts of ovary. *A,* Lower-power section of most of ovary. *A',* Higher-power section of one area of cyst wall.

Histogenesis

The classic reports of Cullen in 1897 and Russell identified ectopic endometrial tissue as müllerian in origin. These lesions show all variations of response to the ovarian hormones characteristic of endometrium in its normal site. Cullen and Russell believed that the ectopic endometrial tissue was the result of misplaced embryonic müllerian rests but made no attempt to explain the mechanism by which the endometrial tissue was disseminated.

Not until 1921, with Sampson's contribution, did gynecologists begin to study seriously the histogenesis of this disease. The problem has not been solved completely by any single theory. The theory generally considered Sampson's most important contribution holds that the menstrual endometrium flows in a retrograde manner through the tubes and implants itself to proliferate and grow in the pelvic viscera.

Sampson briefly stated his implantation theory as follows:

Ovarian and other forms of peritoneal endometriosis arise from the implantation of bits of müllerian mucosa, of either uterine or tubal origin, which, having been carried with menstrual blood escaping through patent tubes into the peritoneal cavity, have lodged on the surfaces of the various pelvic structures. The ectopic mucosa in these implants, regardless of their size or situation, may become additional foci for the spread of the endometriosis by direct extension and also by the implantation of bits of müllerian tissue which escape from them during their reaction to menstruation. The latter phenomenon is most spectacular in the ovary where ectopic endometrial cavities may attain a much larger size than elsewhere, forming the well-known endometrial cysts of that organ.

Sampson originally believed that the ovary acted as an incubator or hotbed for the development of implants on the peritoneum and that it might even impart greater virulence to the müllerian epithelium growing in it. He based this belief on the finding that, in the cases he studied up to 1922, the endometriosis seemed to be more extensive and more invasive in cases associated with endometrial cysts of the ovary. However, the study of more material showed him that extensive pelvic endometriosis may occur without ovarian involvement; hence, he later considered unwarranted his earlier suggestion that the ovary imparts greater virulence to the müllerian epithelium.

Sampson deliberately operated on many patients during menstruation and frequently observed blood coming from the ends of the tubes. This observation has been substantiated by many gynecologists. Blumenkrantz and associates noted intraperitoneal bleeding immediately before and during menstruation among women undergoing dialysis. In 90% of women evaluated, Halme and associates further documented the presence of blood at laparoscopy performed during the perimenstrual period. It had been suggested that retroposition of the uterus would augment this flow. It seems more likely, however, that the retroposition so commonly noted with endometriosis is the effect of scarring pulling the uterus into the cul-de-sac. In 1927, Sampson reported and showed fixed and sectioned fallopian tubes with blood in them and demonstrated endometrial tissue; he believed this endometrial mucosa to be viable (Fig. 20-16).

Sampson's theory is undoubtedly the most widely accepted explanation of the phenomenon of pelvic endometriosis. Repeated observation at the operating table has shown that endometrial cysts of the ovary are associated with pelvic adhesions that may be the result of organization of old blood. If one couples this observation with the fact that many of these adhesions, when sectioned, show endometrial tissue, it is difficult to escape the conclusion that the peritoneal endometrial plaques are implants from the bloody contents of cysts. The question is whether the endometrium-lined cysts of the ovaries are the result of implantation of bits of cast-off menstrual endometrium that traveled through the tube.

Although experimental studies have shown beyond doubt that endometrium taken from the uterine lining and transplanted into the pelvic cavity or other areas will grow, until recently no unimpeachable experiments had been done to show whether the cast-off particles of menstrual endometrium were capable of implantation and growth. Therein lies the crux of the entire Sampson theory, for, as Sampson himself recognized, if endometrium passed into the peritoneal cavity is always dead, the implantation theory is also dead. Even the opponents of Sampson's theory admitted that if it could be shown that cast-off menstrual endometrium is viable, Sampson's hypothesis would be greatly strengthened.

Novak in his textbook summarized objections that have been raised to Sampson's theory:

(1) Retrograde menstruation, although it may occur, is a rarely observed phenomenon, in contrast to the great frequency of endometriosis; (2) it is difficult to believe that endometrium thrown off in the uterus could enter the small uterine orifice of the tube, travel outward against the current, and still be capable of implanting itself and growing on the pelvic structures; (3) endometrium thrown off at menstruation is already degenerated or dead, so

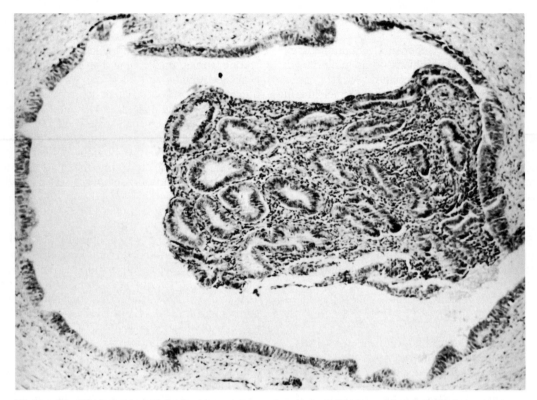

Figure 20–16. Fragment of shed endometrium within lumen of human fallopian tube.

that it is not easy to conceive of its taking root in the peritoneum; (4) such experiments as those of Jacobson, showing that endometrium can grow in the peritoneum, have dealt with the normal, healthy endometrium of animals; (5) experiments such as those of Heim in monkeys, in which a uteroabdominal fistula was created, all failed to show any development of endometrium despite the fact that the menstrual blood was emptied freely into the abdomen; and (6) Sampson's theory could not explain endometriosis in some locations, such as the umbilicus.

Most of those who have been reluctant to accept Sampson's theory as reported in 1927 have championed that of Iwanoff and of Meyer in one of its modifications. These two investigators independently presented the idea that aberrant endometrium originates from abnormal differentiation of the coelomic epithelium, from which all the genital mucous membrane arises. This theory in its various modifications suggests that the pelvic peritoneum under certain stimuli—inflammatory, hormonal, or other—may develop into endometriumlike tissue. It has not seemed logical that inflammation can be such a stimulus. Pelvic endometriosis is least likely to be found in patients who have pelvic inflammatory disease, and

the converse is also true. Intraperitoneal injection of blood during menstruation also does not seem to incite endometriosis, and although Merrill was able to produce structures similar to endometrial glands outside of Millipore filters, true endometriosis with typical endometrial glands and stroma has not been produced outside of the filters. It therefore seems quite clear that although coelomic metaplasia may occur and may explain some cases of pelvic endometriosis or endometriosis elsewhere in the body, it has yet to be demonstrated experimentally and proved. No factor, be it hormonal, inflammatory, or exogenous, has been shown as yet to incite the development of typical endometriosis.

Halban's theory of dissemination through the lymphatic system appears to be relevant in only a few cases of endometriosis. The usual pelvic lesions of endometriosis do not follow the paths of the lymphatics. Endometrium has been found occasionally in the pelvic lymph nodes at operation, as reported by Javert, but does not usually produce clinical endometriosis. Dissemination through the lymphatic system, however, appears to be the best explanation for endometriosis of the umbilicus, since in 1955 Scott and Wharton showed in rhesus monkeys that there is lymphatic involvement with endometriosis. Lymphatics of the anterior abdominal wall may drain from the pelvis to the umbilicus.

Desquamated human endometrium was grown successfully on tissue culture by Keettel and Stein. The cultured cells had the appearance of fibroblasts and epithelial cells. In short, all these studies have given strong support to Sampson's theory of retrograde menstruation and implantation and have shown that menstruating endometrium is not only viable but also capable of growing and causing endometriosis.

Scott and associates reported experimental work demonstrating that desquamated menstrual endometrium is capable of growth. The uterus of each of 10 rhesus monkeys was divided from its vaginal attachment and rotated on its ovarian axis to allow intraperitoneal menstruation to occur; the menstrual flow spilled in the cul-de-sac or up toward the diaphragm (Fig. 20-17) . In six of the 10 animals, typical areas of endometriosis developed within the peritoneal cavity. Growing endometrium was found from 75 to 963 days after the reversal operation. The other four animals did not survive. The uterus of another monkey was rotated 90°, and the cervix was brought through the anterior abdominal wall so that menstruation could occur at the site (Fig. 20-18). The uterus subsequently retracted, leaving a sinus tract in the anterior abdominal wall. Endometriosis was found in this sinus tract. In two additional animals, the rotated cervix was implanted into the rectus muscle so that menstruation could occur in an area entirely free from peritoneum or from tissue arising from the coelomic epithelium. Endometriosis was found adjacent to the reversed cervix within 12–19 months after the original operation.

It had been suggested that, by itself, blood originating from the rupture of ovarian follicles or corpora lutea or escaping from the fimbriae of fallopian tubes during menstruation might incite metaplasia of the peritoneum and produce endometriosis. To test this possibility, Scott and associates injected venous blood obtained during episodes of menstruation into the peritoneal cavities of four monkeys; in no instance did endometriosis develop.

Dizerega and associates, in further primate studies, demonstrated the need for steroid supplementation in development of endometriosis. Without steroids, viable endometriosis was not encountered, and once implanted, the endometriosis required steroids (estradiol or progesterone or both) for maintenance.

In 1958, Ridley and Edwards documented similar findings in women. For 12 hours, they collected the menstrual flow in eight women through cervical cannulas. This material was centrifuged, and the sediment was injected into the rectus muscle of the same patient, who in each case was to have an abdominal operation 90–180 days after the single injection. Six of these patients did not have endometriosis in the injection site at laparotomy, one had a definite area of endometriosis

175 days after injection, and the eighth patient had an area suggestive of endometriosis at 110 days.

Four women accidentally provided a natural clinical experiment. Three of them had a noncommunicating horn of a double uterus. In these women, the only exit of the menstrual flow from the noncommunicating horn was through the fallopian tube, and endometriosis developed in each woman in the ovary on the side of the rudimentary horn. The fourth patient was an unmarried woman of 40 in whom dysmenorrhea and eventually amenorrhea developed, but with recurring monthly pain. Examination showed the upper vagina to be obliterated completely by adhesions, and laparotomy showed endometriosis of the posterior surface of the uterus and cul-de-sac. Such situations can occur as a complication of cervical agenesis with functioning endometrium and ovarian tissue. Endometriosis can occur from the retrograde flow, although this anomaly is very rare. Cervical stenosis as a complication of dilatation and curettage may also produce such a situation (Fig. 20-19).

The preceding experiments give no support to the theory of serosal metaplasia, but they give more or less conclusive support to Sampson's theory of retrograde menstruation. However, this theory does not explain the occurrence of endometriosis at the umbilicus. Because of the lymphatic drainage from the pelvic region to the umbilicus through the route to the urachus and obliterated hypogastric vessels, it seems likely that endometrial particles are deposited in the umbilicus by way of the lymphatic channels. This hypothesis is strengthened by the results of one of Scott and associates' experiments. Extensive endometriosis of the pelvis developed in a monkey and completely obstructed one ureter. An autopsy revealed endometriosis in the nonfunctioning kidney, probably the result of deposits of endometrial particles from the pelvis by way of the periureteral lymphatics. The rare occurrence of endometriosis in the lung, forearm, and thigh is certainly not explained by natural flow; the only possible route would seem to be hematogenous. It is of historical interest that Sampson in the early days of his histologic studies believed that endometrial particles could be disseminated through the bloodstream, and indeed this is the only way in which some instances of endometriosis can be explained. If malignant cells can be shed into the bloodstream by uterine manipulation, it is surprising that more instances of distant endometriosis are not appreciated.

Symptoms

Pain

Pain is the most constant single symptom of endometriosis. Scott and associates found that pain, exclusive of

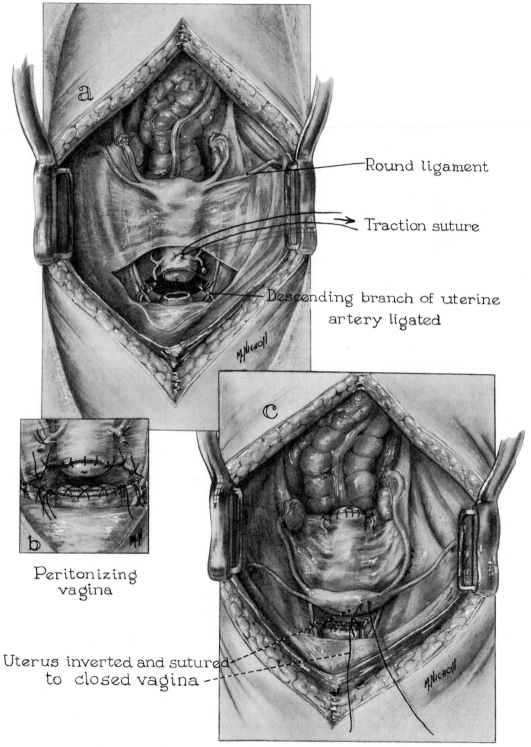

Round ligament

Traction suture

Descending branch of uterine artery ligated

Peritonizing vagina

Uterus inverted and sutured to closed vagina

Figure 20–17. Experimental surgical procedure on monkeys to allow intra-abdominal menstruation. Entire uterus is separated from vagina and rotated 180° to allow menstruation into peritoneal cavity.

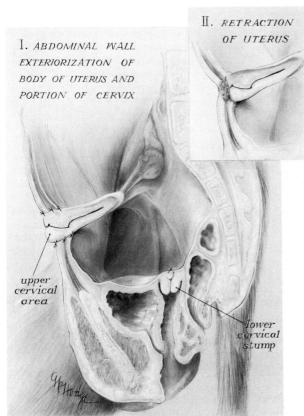

I. *ABDOMINAL WALL EXTERIORIZATION OF BODY OF UTERUS AND PORTION OF CERVIX*

II. *RETRACTION OF UTERUS*

upper cervical area

lower cervical stump

Figure 20–18. Uterus, except for distal portion of cervix, was brought out through anterior abdominal wall. *Inset* shows retraction of uterus and scarring in anterior abdominal wall.

dysmenorrhea, was present in 57.6% of 243 patients operated on primarily for endometriosis. On the other hand, in the prospective study by Williams and Pratt, pain exclusive of dysmenorrhea occurred in 6% of all patients with endometriosis and in 8% of patients without endometriosis. Dysmenorrhea, however, was present in 17% of patients with endometriosis but in only 8% of those without it.

Despite the frequency of pain in patients with endometriosis, many women with extensive endometriosis report not even the slightest discomfort. Conversely, some women with only a few small endometrial implants in the pelvis complain of very severe pain. Since the lesions vary so much in size, number, and location, it is quite natural that the pain arising from them should vary in both location and nature, but the pain is chiefly in the lower abdomen. The pain may be either unilateral or bilateral, but it is more often diffuse and tends to be aggravated premenstrually or menstrually, leaving residual postmenstrual pelvic soreness.

Endometrial cysts are inclined to rupture or leak some of their entrapped blood into the peritoneal cavity. Leakage may occur suddenly and dramatically or intermittently. In either case, the blood may produce a chemical peritonitis, with severe pain, rebound tenderness, and all other signs of peritoneal irritation. On the other hand, patients have had documented rupture of an ovarian endometrial cyst with absolutely no related signs or symptoms.

Dysmenorrhea

Dysmenorrhea is a common symptom of endometriosis. Although acquired dysmenorrhea is usually thought to be characteristic of this disease, an analysis of the cases of endometriosis does not substantiate this pattern. In their study of 243 patients with endometriosis, Scott and associates found that 51.4% had had nonprogressive dysmenorrhea and only 9.1% acquired dysmenorrhea—probably coinciding with the development of endometriosis. The prospective evaluation of Williams and Pratt documented that dysmenorrhea as a symptom was nearly twice as likely in patients with endometriosis as in those without endometriosis. Therefore, the combination of pain and dysmenorrhea should alert the gynecologist to the possibility of endometriosis.

Dyspareunia

Involvement of the cul-de-sac or the uterosacral ligaments or both may lead to dyspareunia and possibly to low backache. Dyspareunia was recorded by Williams and Pratt in about 6% of patients with endometriosis but in only 1% of those without it. Along with dysmenorrhea and the various pain symptoms, dyspareunia is significant for endometriosis.

Cyclic Pain

When endometriosis involves a scar in the abdominal wall, umbilicus, inguinal region, or perineum, there usually is a nodule that undergoes painful swelling at intervals corresponding to menstruation. If these lesions are superficial, there may be a bluish discoloration from hemorrhage into the tissues and, at times, cyclic external bleeding if there is a break in the epithelium. Hematuria, generally cyclic, as well as dysuria has been noted with bladder involvement.

When the anterior rectal wall is involved, rectal pressure and painful defecation are common. With invasion of the mucosa of the sigmoid or rectum, bleeding per rectum and diarrhea can occur at menstruation. With more extensive bowel infiltration, intestinal obstruction may result (Fig. 20-20). Even though there may be no overt mucosal involvement, careful examination of

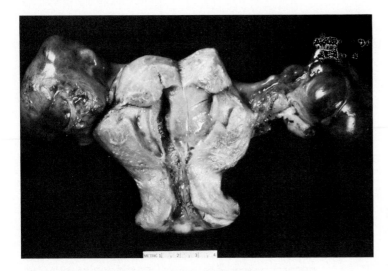

Figure 20–19. Bilateral endometrial cysts 1 year after dilatation and curettage. Scarring and stenosis can be seen at internal os. Patient had cyclic monthly pain despite amenorrhea.

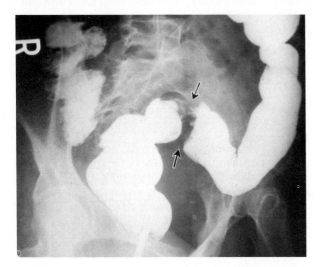

Figure 20–20. Barium enema in patient with obstructive lesion (*arrows*) due to endometriosis. Lesion was resected by surgeon who believed it to be carcinoma.

the colon will reveal a communication from the lumen to the endometrioma in patients with cyclic rectal bleeding.

The disparity between the extent of the endometriosis and the severity of the pain remains without adequate explanation. Sturgis and Call suggested that superficial implants may expand more easily with hormonal stimulation, whereas the deeper islands of ectopic endometrium tend to be encased in fibrous tissue that makes distention more difficult and more painful. This is logical and may be a valid assumption, but supporting evidence is not convincing.

Abnormal Uterine Bleeding

Abnormal uterine bleeding is often associated with endometriosis. It may be menorrhagia or metrorrhagia, or both. Scott and associates encountered abnormal bleeding in 26.6% of patients operated on primarily for endometriosis. In further study of these patients, some associated lesions were found that obviously explained the bleeding. This finding reduced the incidence of abnormal bleeding with no cause other than endometriosis to 14.4%. The menorrhagia and, in some instances, the metrorrhagia may result from ovarian dysfunction secondary to ovarian involvement. At celiotomy, one frequently finds old blood in the peritoneal cavity, and the intermenstrual spotting could be due to the escape of the chocolate contents of the ovarian cysts into the abdomen and out through the uterus by way of the tubes in an anterograde fashion. The prospective evaluation reported by Williams and Pratt found that among these consecutive patients, the frequency of menorrhagia was identical among those with and without endometriosis. Of patients treated by resection of endometriosis, 14% had menometrorrhagia; 12% of the control group had the symptoms. When hysterectomy was carried out as treatment, menorrhagia was present as a symptom in 42% of both those with and those without endometriosis. Therefore, the belief is that there is *no* increase in this symptom complex of menometrorrhagia among patients with endometriosis.

Infertility

Infertility is another common and important symptom in endometriosis. Among all couples, the infertility rate is generally estimated to be approximately 10%.

With endometriosis, it is generally conceded that this rate is much higher. At the Johns Hopkins Hospital, the absolute sterility rate was 33.3% and the relative sterility rate was 46%. Counseller reported rates of 32.1% and 48.9%, respectively. Haydon reported a 53% relative infertility rate.

The cause of infertility may or may not be apparent. Clinical investigators believe that about 30% of patients with infertility have endometriosis as the only predominant cause. Tubal occlusion may occur, but most women with pelvic endometriosis have patent tubes unless peritubal adhesions have caused angulation and obstruction. Extensive destruction of ovarian tissue or replacement by endometrial cysts may interfere with ovulation, and extensive periovarian adhesions can prevent the normal egress of the ovum. In addition, the numerous pelvic adhesions probably interfere with ovum pickup and prevent the normal migration of the ovum from the ovary to the uterus through the tube.

Although impossible to prove, it seems likely that the hemolyzed peritoneal blood entering the tubal lumen could interfere with the action of the tubal epithelial cilia in propelling the ovum. Dyspareunia is known to limit sexual exposure. These theories aside, however, there still are many instances in which minimal endometriosis appears to cause infertility without any apparent mechanical or endocrine abnormality. Conversely, endometriosis does not preclude pregnancy. Many women with endometriosis have had several pregnancies. Prostaglandins have been implicated in this relationship between endometriosis and infertility. Rock and associates, however, found no significant difference in either the amount of peritoneal fluid present or the concentration of prostaglandins with or without endometriosis. At this point, the question and its significance remain unresolved.

Kaunitz and Di Sant'Agnese considered the possibility of a relationship between unruptured luteinized follicles and endometriosis and infertility. They thought that with the unruptured follicle, progesterone levels were lower, and they suggested that higher levels would kill endometrial cells. The net result of unruptured follicles would then be low levels of progestational hormones; hence, endometriosis and the subsequent decrease in fertility would present. Thus, the endometriosis would be the consequence of the ovulation defect and its resultant infertility and not the cause of infertility.

Abortion rates have been believed to be increased among women having endometriosis. Naples and associates noted a significant increase in spontaneous abortion and in addition found a decrease in the abortion rate after conservative surgery. Theoretically, the increased prostaglandins could be related to the increased abortion rate. Pittaway and associates, however, presented data reflecting a relationship between endometriosis and increased abortions, and they thought this was also characteristic of other infertility subgroups and not of endometriosis itself.

Soules and associates related ovulation to the infertility associated with endometriosis. Marik and Hulka further described the luteinized unruptured follicle in relation to endometriosis. The concept is intriguing, but the data are not entirely convincing. The studies are generally laparoscopically controlled, and we do not know how long it takes to peritonize the stigma after ovulation. Hence, the records may be erroneous. Koninckx and associates postulated a reverse mechanism, that implantation of endometriosis is prevented by the specific steroidal hormone environment. When this environment is abnormal, as it is with the unruptured follicle, the endometriotic implantation can occur. Pittaway and associates were not able to relate luteal phase defects to endometriosis. Diagnostic methods recommended in addition to laparoscopy are ultrasound examination and determination of progesterone levels in peritoneal fluid; these levels are decreased in association with the luteinized unruptured follicle. Dhont and associates, however, concluded that these tests are of no value. Convincing data are awaited.

Diagnosis

The symptoms described should always suggest endometriosis, but any or most of them may be present with other pelvic conditions. There is *no* history sufficiently typical of endometriosis to justify the diagnosis on this basis alone, and a gynecologist operating without confirmatory pelvic findings often finds grossly normal pelvic organs.

If a cystic hemorrhagic nodule is visible at the umbilicus, in an abdominal scar, in the perineum, or in the vaginal vault, the diagnosis of endometriosis can be made with relative certainty, particularly if there is cyclicity to the signs and symptoms. In the usual case of intra-abdominal endometriosis, the diagnosis must be aided by bimanual examination. The finding of adherent adnexa during the menstrual years in a woman in whom venereal, tubercular, or other infection can be excluded with reasonable certainty should cause one to consider endometriosis. Shotty induration in the cul-de-sac, in the uterosacral ligaments, or on the posterior surface of an adherent retroposed uterus is the single most suggestive pelvic finding of endometriosis. These nodular areas are frequently tender, particularly just before menstruation. When these findings are coupled with an enlarged ovary or an adherent ovarian cyst, the diagnosis is almost a certainty, within the 85th percentile of accuracy. Carcinoma of the ovary can reproduce most of these findings, except that the nodules of metastatic carcinoma in the cul-de-sac usually are not tender, particularly if they are examined during the cyclic changes. If symptoms are cyclic, examination is best performed at the time of the symptoms rather than during asymptomatic periods, when there may be quiescent disease.

When the rectovaginal septum is involved, the pelvic and rectal findings may stimulate carcinoma of the bowel or the induration and scarring of diverticulitis. With cancer, however, the rectal examination should suggest a mucosal component that is uncommon with endometriosis. In diverticulitis, the mass usually has a popcornlike feeling, and the nodularity is less tender except during acute flare-up of the inflammation. At this time, induration is likely to be a significant finding along with a more diffuse tenderness and with evidence of peritoneal irritation. Bluish cysts in the posterior vaginal vault may be very helpful in deciding in favor of endometriosis (see Fig. 20-11). Moreover, they are in a readily accessible biopsy site for pathologic confirmation of the diagnosis. Histologic confirmation of the diagnosis is mandatory along with continued follow-up, since the rectovaginal septum is the second most common site of malignancy developing in endometriosis. If the rectal mucosa is involved, colon roentgenograms are helpful, and proctoscopy with biopsy of the lesion establishes the diagnosis.

A group of women remains who have severe pelvic pain and other symptoms suggestive of endometriosis but who lack definitive pelvic findings on examination. If the cul-de-sac is free from adhesions, culdoscopy may be a very helpful procedure, particularly in extremely obese women. Since the cul-de-sac, however, is often involved in endometriosis and since infertility is a symptom in many women with endometriosis, laparoscopy is a much more practical approach to the diagnosis of endometriosis. In the infertile patient and in the patient with severe pelvic pain and few, if any, findings on pelvic examination, ovarian endometriosis, peritubal adhesions, and endometriosis in the cul-de-sac can be seen and biopsy documentation usually obtained by the laparoscope. In some instances, small areas of endometriosis may be fulgurated or vaporized through the laparoscope. Women with minimal degrees of symptomatic endometriosis can then be differentiated from those whose symptoms are psychosomatic and in whom there is a complete absence of findings for organic disease.

Other noninvasive tests, such as computed tomography and ultrasound scans, have been recommended. Our experience has been that such tests are not helpful in making a diagnosis. They may document and record the size and position of ovarian enlargements but can-

not be definitive. Figure 20-21 shows a scan from the patient in Figure 20-9 with bilateral endometriomas. Intracystic echoes suggest shadows from old blood.

Staging

One of the difficulties in the management of endometriosis is the evaluation of various treatments. The protean nature of the condition not only in symptoms but also in extent of disease complicates the selection of appropriate therapy.

In an attempt to simplify and organize the different classifications of endometriosis, the American Fertility Society devised a staging form, which has been revised, that grades the extent of the disease into mild, moderate, and severe (Fig. 20-22). This form can be filled out easily at the time of surgery, and point scores can be applied to different areas and amounts of endometriosis. Although the areas and numerical equivalents have been arbitrarily stated, they can serve as a guide and can be further revised in the future as more information becomes available. On the basis of such accurate data, prospective information can be obtained and the true relationship of endometriosis to infertility can be better assessed.

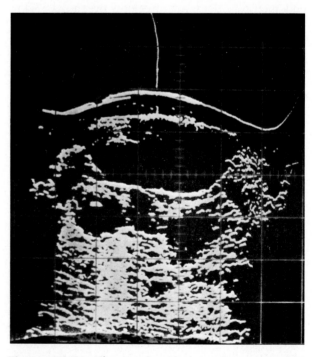

Figure 20–21. Ultrasound study in patient with pelvic masses (same patient as in Fig. 20–9). Although echoes are seen within ovarian cysts and may be from clotted blood, malignancy cannot be excluded.

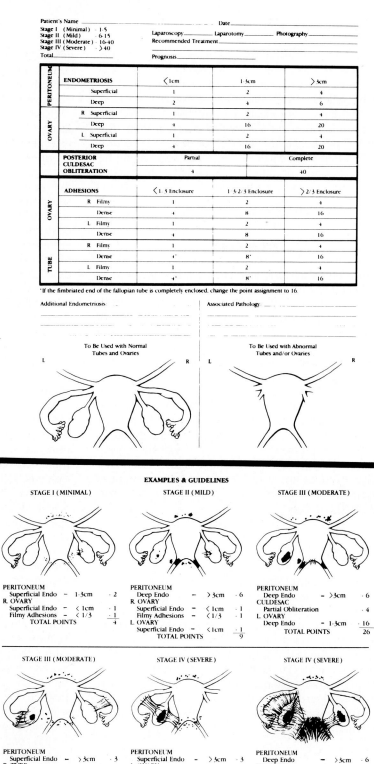

Figure 20–22. American Fertility Society classification of endometriosis. (From The American Fertility Society: Revised American Fertility Society classification of endometriosis: 1985. Fertil Steril 1985; 43:351. Reproduced with permission of the publisher, The American Fertility Society.)

The pelvic organs should be inspected in routine fashion so that all areas are evaluated in the same way each time. Point scores are assigned based on the number of lesions and bilaterality. The uterine implants are considered peritoneal. The size of lesions and the organs of involvement are weighted to determine the severity and, hence, the stage of disease. It is recommended that a standardized approach and staging be used so that data on different therapeutic approaches and successes can be compared.

Treatment

Since endometriosis is generally a benign process that becomes quiescent with the menopause, its presence is not necessarily an indication for surgery. The need for treatment depends on the severity and type of symptoms, the extent of the disease, the age and the general physical condition of the patient, the patient's desire to preserve childbearing function, the psychological evaluation of the patient, and the presence or absence of other disease in the reproductive tract. In the absence of palpable pelvic disease, particularly in the adnexal area, exploratory celiotomy on the basis of symptoms alone is rarely required. Moderately extensive but asymptomatic endometriosis may not require treatment, provided that the diagnosis is certain.

Four courses are available for the management of endometriosis: observation, hormonal therapy, surgery, and irradiation.

Observation

In the absence of any significant symptoms and in the absence of an adnexal mass that might suggest an ovarian neoplasm, observation is the treatment of choice for endometriosis. Analgesics can be used satisfactorily to control dysmenorrhea and pelvic discomfort. If infertility is an important factor, active treatment is sometimes indicated. García and David, however, recorded that even among patients with infertility and mild to moderate degrees of endometriosis, a relatively high percentage was able to conceive without operative intervention.

Hormonal Therapy

Suppression of ovulation and menstruation, either by pregnancy or by the use of exogenous hormones, has been observed to alleviate symptoms and at times to bring about clinical improvement. Estrogens, pro-gestogens, and androgens have been used. Danazol (Danocrine), an antigonadotropin and a derivative of a 17α-ethinyl testosterone, has also been shown to be effective in the treatment of endometriosis.

Hormonal therapy has been used rather extensively. Estrogens were the first endocrine preparations used. Estrogens in sufficient doses both inhibit ovulation and suppress menstruation. They do not induce a pseudopregnancy state, at least from the histologic aspect of the endometrium. If estrogens are used, diethylstilbestrol is the drug of choice. Karnaky recommended starting at 0.5 g daily for 3 days and then increasing the dose rather rapidly to suppress breakthrough bleeding. Frequently, doses of 100 mg daily are reached, ultimately to produce a period of amenorrhea for a total time of 3–6 months. General experience has shown this method of treatment to be unsatisfactory. The diethylstilbestrol causes nausea and, frequently, severe bleeding. Furthermore, it appears to effect at best only temporary symptomatic relief and is not in any sense a cure. The areas of ectopic endometrium not only do not regress but also may frequently show areas of cystic hyperplasia, as one would expect. In general, this form of therapy is rarely used and has few advocates.

Androgens, usually orally administered methyltestosterone, also may be used to treat endometriosis. When sublingual doses of 10 mg daily are used, ovulation and menstruation can be suppressed, but mild hirsutism may occur when the monthly dose reaches or exceeds 300 mg. Patients usually are not treated for more than 3–6 months because of the potential, if not actual, virilizing effects of this hormone. Another dosage schedule of 5 mg daily for up to 6 months may be efficacious. At this dosage level, there is usually menstruation and sometimes ovulation. Patients should therefore use a barrier method of contraception or stop the medication if menses are late or irregular. Androgen ingestion during pregnancy will result in masculinization of the external genitalia of a female fetus. Pelvic pain has been relieved at least temporarily, with Hammond and associates reporting 75% success but with subsequent recurrence. Pregnancies can occur after such therapy, but usually additional surgical treatment is required. Histologically, the endometriosis appears to be unaffected, and the mechanism whereby this form of treatment achieves its results is not clear. Although androgens appear to achieve short-term palliation, one cannot use them for prolonged therapy, and, hence, this form of therapy has definite limitations.

A popular form of hormonal treatment has been the use of the progestational agents. These synthetic progesteronelike steroids are frequently combined with an estrogen, such as mestranol or ethinyl estradiol. Some are given parenterally (hydroxyprogesterone caproate and medroxyprogesterone acetate), but most are taken orally, the most frequently used being norethynodrel and norethindrone.

Any of the currently used contraceptive pills combining a progesterone and an estrogen may be used to suppress ovulation and produce amenorrhea. The dose of the preparation selected should be minimal at the start, doubled at the end of 4 weeks, and increased thereafter by one pill monthly (or weekly, if necessary) for at least 12 months, to suppress not only ovulation but also breakthrough bleeding until amenorrhea and anovulation have been achieved. In fact, dosage may be continued for 2 or 3 years, if need be. In addition to amenorrhea and anovulation, a pseudopregnancy state with decidual reaction involving the uterine endometrium and the ectopic endometrium can be achieved. In 110 patients, Kistner reported an improvement rate of 83%, with remissions as long as 52 months and a 47% pregnancy rate in those trying to conceive. Despite these impressive results, endometrial implants often become active after the cessation of the pseudopregnancy. The patients to be treated by progestogens must be selected carefully, and permanent cure should not be expected. The prime indication for this mode of treatment appears to be symptomatic endometriosis recurrent after surgery.

About 15% of users of these hormones discontinue the medication because of the side-effects, which are usually those of early pregnancy. Another 15% or more of patients have an initial response level and then an apparent loss of effect. Overall, about a 50% success rate with progestational compounds seems to be a reasonable expectation in alleviation of symptoms or in allowing subsequent pregnancy. Moghissi and Boyce reported a 90% pregnancy success rate with this type of treatment when other factors were excluded.

Currently, danazol is often recommended as an "antigonadotropin" in the treatment of endometriosis. The effects are likely multifactorial, however, involving the hypothalmic-pituitary axis, binding with steroid receptors, and effects on ovarian function itself. Changes in lipoprotein cholesterol also occur and would seem to be of concern if long-term therapy is planned. Administration should begin immediately after a menstrual cycle. The medication serves as a contraceptive during the time of administration. Not all studies, however, show a benefit from danazol therapy, particularly in mild disease.

Danazol is expensive and has a high incidence of side-effects. Barbieri and associates quoted an 85% incidence; they also recorded a 46% pregnancy rate and 33% recurrence. Greenblatt and Tzingounis thought the side-effects were less significant, but the pregnancy rate was lower (30%) and the recurrence rate was identical. Currently, danazol seems to be the medication of choice when there is moderate disease and surgery is not required. Interestingly, the presence of increased estrogen and progesterone receptors in endometriosis did not show a change in receptor activity with treatment by either progesterone or danazol.

The recent use of gonadotropin-releasing hormone analogues to create a hypogonadic state has shown some advantage in the treatment of endometriosis. This appears to allow a reversible down-regulation of the pituitary-ovarian axis, with prompt return of ovarian function. The need for injection has generally been well accepted by patients; hot flashes are the main complaint. Increased calcium excretion and bone loss may be expected with prolonged administration. Relief of pain is usually prompt, and histologic study demonstrates atrophic and inactive disease.

Hormonal therapy is not indicated in women having adnexal masses, since no one can be certain that the adnexal masses are, indeed, endometriosis rather than ovarian malignancies. Further, hormonal therapy will not cause an established endometrial cyst to regress. Since all forms of hormonal therapy, with the exception of low-dose testosterone therapy, inhibit ovulation during the course of therapy, this form of treatment delays the desired result of pregnancy. Neither estrogen or progestin therapy nor administration of the newer "antiestrogens" is indicated in older women who have a limited time remaining to achieve pregnancy. Such hormonal manipulation, however, seems particularly useful in women approaching the menopause. In them, temporizations can be obtained in anticipation of spontaneous improvement with the menopause. A summary of results of hormonal therapy in the treatment of infertile patients with endometriosis is given in Table 20-2.

The lack of controlled prospective studies continues to hamper knowledge about even the need for treatment when infertility and endometriosis are related. The information that is available suggests that with mild and perhaps even moderate endometriosis, observation alone gives results as good as those with either surgery or hormonal manipulation. Seibel suggested an observation period of at least 6 months after diagnosis before any interventional therapy is begun. Similar data by Portuondo and associates reported in 1983 resulted in a recommendation of no therapy for 18 months. When pregnancy occurred, the chances of a subsequent pregnancy remained good.

Newer technology has achieved successful pregnancy as well in patients with infertility and endometriosis. With in vitro fertilization, Chillik and Rosenwaks had a 48% success rate with minimal and mild endometriosis but only a 15% rate in moderate and severe stages. They thought that the difference might be not only the smaller numbers of oocytes retrieved but also their poor quality. Success has likewise been recorded with gamete intrafallopian transfer.

TABLE 20–2
Pregnancy in Patients with Endometriosis After Hormonal Therapy

HORMONAL AGENT	REFERENCE (YEAR)	INFERTILE PATIENTS (NO.)	PATIENTS ACHIEVING PREGNANCY (NO.)	RATE OF PREGNANCY (%)
Stilbestrol	Karnaky (1948)	37	5	14
	Haskins and Woolf (1955)	15	3	20
	Total	52	8	15
Progestins	Riva et al. (1961)	83	4	5
	Kistner (1962)	38	18	47
	Kistner (1965)	22	11	50
	Williams (1967)	11	8	73
	Andrews and Larsen (1974)	31	8	26
	Total	185	49	26
Methyltestosterone	Hirst (1947)	19	2	11
	Creadick (1950)	25	5	20
	Preston and Campbell (1953)	80	48	60
	Katayama et al. (1976)	64	12	19
	Total	188	67	36
Danazol	Friedlander (1973)	22	9	41
	Greenblatt et al. (1974)	21	9	43
	Total	43	18	42

(From Katayama KP, Manuel M, Jones HW Jr, et al. Methyltestosterone treatment of infertility associated with pelvic endometriosis. Fertil Steril 1976; 27:83. Reproduced with permission of the publisher, The American Fertility Society.)

Surgery

An operation may be considered conservative when the reproductive potential is retained, semiconservative when the reproductive ability is eliminated but ovarian function is retained, and radical or definitive when ovarian function is ablated along with the uterus, which is the source of the endometriosis.

Surgery is still considered the best form of therapy in most cases of symptomatic endometriosis. Definitive treatment consisting of abdominal hysterectomy and bilateral salpingo-oophorectomy is preferred in women with extensive endometriosis involving the pelvic structures and both ovaries, particularly if the patient is over 40 years of age and past the reproductive years. When infertility surgery is planned because of endometriosis, a complete infertility evaluation is required preoperatively for both partners, and the risks, benefits, and alternatives must be thoroughly discussed. Unfortunately, there are younger women, a few in their twenties, whose ovaries have been so destroyed by endometriosis that little or no functional ovarian tissue can be salvaged.

One should not hesitate to use estrogens for menopausal symptoms in younger women after removal of both ovaries. It has been shown that delaying the start of hormone therapy for 3–4 months after operation allows estrogen replacement and minimizes chances of recurrent disease stimulated by the estrogens themselves. Medroxyprogesterone acetate (Provera) may be used during this time to help alleviate hot flashes should they be a significant problem. Theoretically, estrogens can reactivate endometriosis, but the occurrence has been less than 5% in the reported cases.

The variation in the estrogen receptors found in endometriosis could explain this discrepancy. Most of the current literature documents a decrease in both estrogen and progesterone receptors in endometriotic lesions but not in the endometrium itself. In addition, there seems to be a difference in the luteinizing hormone receptors. These, however, show variation with the menstrual cycle.

Conservative Surgery

Many women with endometriosis are quite young and want to retain their ability to reproduce or, when infertility is a problem, to enhance fertility. In the latter situation, a thorough infertility study must be done to exclude other causes before the lack of pregnancy is attributed to endometriosis alone. When this has been done, or when there are other symptoms of endometriosis sufficient to require treatment, conservative surgery is advised. This generally consists of a celiotomy with the intent of destroying by resection or fulguration all areas of endometriosis. Large endometrial implants or endometrial cysts of the ovaries are managed by resection. The smaller superficial implants may be fulgurated, and the many adhesions characteristic of endometriosis, involving the cul-de-sac, posterior surface of the uterus, and adnexa, are lysed and excised. It is particularly important in problems of infertility to release any peritubal and periovarian adhesions that might interfere with ovum transport. To prevent the uterus from becoming readherent on the cul-de-sac, uterine suspension is performed, and frequently an ovarian suspension is done as well (Fig. 20-23). Optical augmentation by loupes or the operating microscope enables one to find areas of endometriosis that might otherwise escape detection. Careful rinsing of powder from gloves, irrigation with physiologic solution, avoidance of sponging and its trauma, and nonreactive absorbable sutures are recommended. Catgut, silk, and the like have little place in conservative surgery on the pelvic organs of young women.

An important step in these conservative procedures is a presacral neurectomy. This should be done in all cases in which midline cramping dysmenorrhea is present and perhaps in all instances of infertility, for should further endometriosis develop, this procedure may prevent it from becoming symptomatic. Prevention of dyspareunia by such procedures may reduce abstinence and increase chances for pregnancy. Data on this possibility, however, are inconclusive, so that presacral neurectomy appears to be indicated only for relief of pain.

Figure 20-24 shows the anatomy of the presacral dissection. After the bowel is packed well into the upper abdomen, the rectosigmoid is drawn to the left. A midline incision is made in the posterior parietal peritoneum beginning from a point in the hollow of the sacrum opposite the third or fourth sacral vertebra to a point 1 or 2 cm above the bifurcation of the aorta. The retroperitoneal exposure is made by placing stay sutures on the edges of the peritoneum or by holding the edges apart with Allis clamps. Usually, exposure of the right ureter and the inferior mesenteric vessels on the left is accomplished easily.

Beginning above the bifurcation of the aorta, usually a single nerve trunk network can be seen as it passes over the bifurcation and divides into right and left nerve bundles. The nerve trunk should be transected completely from the lower end of the aorta and the proximal portion of the common iliac vessels. The proximal (cephalic) end of the nerve bundle should be ligated. The distal (pelvic) end of the nerve trunk should be retracted with firm tension, and the entire plexus with its left and right nerve trunks should be dissected thoroughly from the presacral region.

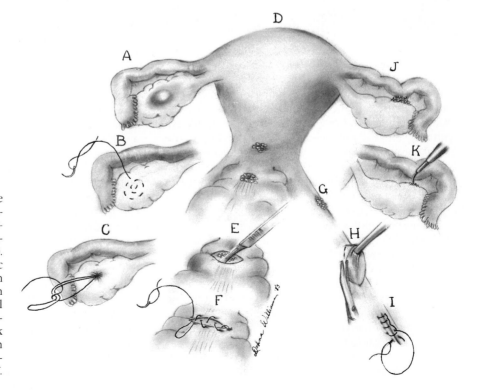

Figure 20–23. Conservative surgery for endometriosis. Endometrioma of ovary *A,* with excision and purse-string concentric closure of defect (*B* and *C*). Posterior uterus and cul-de-sac endometriosis *D,* with excision *E,* and inverting baseball stitch closure of serosa *F.* Uterosacral endometrium *G,* with sharp dissection *H,* and continuous lock suture closure *I.* Tubo-ovarian endometriosis *J,* with microcautery excision and destruction *K.*

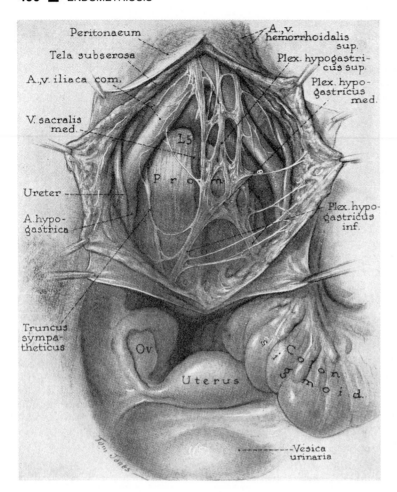

Figure 20–24. Presacral nerves in relation to peritoneal tissues. Anterior view of pelvis. Removal of the peritoneum and the retroperitoneal tissues shows the relation of the more prominent autonomic nerves to the pelvic anatomy. (From Curtis AH, Anson BJ, Ashley FL, Jones T. The anatomy of the pelvic autonomic nerves in relation to gynecology. Surg Gynecol Obstet 1942; 75:743. Reproduced by permission of the journal.)

By careful retraction of the sigmoid mesentery and the inferior mesenteric vessels by means of a narrow Deaver retractor, the entire plexus can be visualized, with the left and right pelvic ureters serving as the lateral margins of the dissection. The blunt dissection is continued along the medial aspect of the right ureter, with removal of all retroperitoneal connective tissue and nerve fibers from the presacral space to the region of the medial aspect of the left ureter.

The nerve bundles are transected at the level of the third sacral vertebra, and the distal ends are ligated. Blunt dissection is best for this and minimizes bleeding. Two distinct layers of nerve-connective tissue are usually recognized during the dissection. The upper layer must be dissected free from the peritoneum, and the deeper layer, which contains the main nerve trunks, is dissected from the vessels and the presacral anterior longitudinal ligament.

Bleeding must be meticulously controlled by fine ties or electrocautery. The operator must avoid injury to the inferior mesenteric artery and its superior hemorrhoidal branch. Protection can be accomplished best by retracting the vessels within the sigmoid mesentery away from the operating field. The middle sacral artery, which is closely attached to the bony structures, emerging onto the sacrum from beneath the left common iliac vein, usually escapes injury with careful blunt dissection. To avoid injury, the middle sacral artery and vein can be ligated initially or clipped with small vascular clips either before the presacral space is dissected or as soon as these vessels come into operative view during the procedure. If they should be injured, usually bleeding can be controlled easily by exerting firm pressure directly against the adjacent bony structures and then occluding them with small vascular clips. On rare occasions, it may be necessary to place Gelfoam or microfibrillar collagen (Avitene) in the retroperitoneal space to control oozing. This carries the risk of continued bleeding, and a pelvic hematoma may occur. After removal of the connective tissue and the nerve tissue, hemostasis is assured and the peritoneal margins are approximated with a continuous suture of nonreactive material such as polyglactin.

If low back pain is the predominant symptom, it is advisable to include a resection of the uterosacral ligaments and Frankenhauser's plexus as a part of the operative procedure. This is done by grasping, with a Babcock or an Allis clamp, each uterosacral ligament as it emerges from the posterior aspect of the lower uterine segment. Care should be taken to identify the lower portion of the pelvic ureter, which should be lateral to the uterosacral ligament but can be dangerously close to it when pelvic endometriosis has involved the cul-de-sac. The ligament should be divided completely, with resection of approximately 0.5–1 cm. The free ends are ligated with permanent suture but, to avoid regeneration of nerve fibers, are not approximated. The sacral portion of the uterosacral ligament may be sutured to the posterior surface of the cervix to avoid retrodisplacement of the uterus after surgery. However, in most instances the shortened ligaments cannot be made to reach the cervix and are left to retract beneath the pelvic peritoneum. The operative defect is then closed by approximation of the cul-de-sac peritoneum to the back of the cervix, particular care being taken to avoid damage to the adjacent pelvic ureter. The success of this procedure is related to the amount of nerve fiber that is removed in the resected uterosacral ligament; therefore, the procedure should be thorough, even if the resected ligament is not long enough to reapproximate to the posterior cervix for support of the uterus.

Patients with extensive cul-de-sac endometriosis with involvement of the rectovaginal septum may require simultaneous transvaginal and transabdominal approaches. With the patient positioned in stirrups, an assistant may push a sponge forceps up against the posterior fornix to lift the cul-de-sac into the abdominal field above to facilitate dissection. This maneuver will allow careful delineation of the lower border of the lesion. A smooth bougie may also be inserted in the rectum to delineate the position of the involved rectum.

With conservative surgery, there is always the risk of recurrence of endometriosis. The risk, however, seems to be relatively small. Gray noted a 4% rate, and Scott and Burt found a 2.7% rate, whereas McCoy and Bradford reported a 21% rate. In contrast, these authors reported pregnancy rates of 51%, 64.1%, and 63%, respectively. These figures are considerably better than those recorded with progestogen therapy. In general, an overall 40% to 50% pregnancy rate can be expected, as opposed to a 10% to 12% recurrence rate of endometriosis that is likely to require an additional operation. Studies by Buttram and others showed that the stage of the disease is correlated with the success rates of pregnancy from surgery. Surgery, since it can not

only remove the endometriosis but also correct the mechanical problems caused by it, remains the logical choice in the treatment of infertility, particularly as the patient's age increases. For a very young patient, a trial of medical management may be appropriate.

Surgical therapy for endometriosis is often cytoreductive treatment. Microscopic disease with implants of less than 200 μm has been documented by Murphy and associates. The significance of microscopic and atypical presentations of endometriosis has not been determined. Some authors have suggested that preoperative and postoperative hormonal therapy may be warranted to treat these minute implants. However, there are no randomized clinical trials to support this therapeutic regimen.

Some women with symptomatic endometriosis are in a category between those treated conservatively and those requiring a complete and definitive procedure. These women, usually in their middle to late thirties, have completed their childbearing but want to avoid premature menopause. In these women, Cashman's concept of removal of the uterus and other areas of pelvic endometriosis with preservation of some ovarian tissue has much to recommend it. Such a procedure may seem illogical, since the retention of ovarian function might permit continued activity and, therefore, symptoms from any residual endometriosis. This problem, however, arises infrequently, as shown by Scott and associates, who found that only 4.1% of such patients later required further surgery. This concept is further supported by the data of Williams and Pratt, which showed that subsequent surgery for endometriosis was required in 6%. In comparison, the figures were 16% in patients having resection only and 0% in those with complete operations. Hammond and associates, however, found need for further surgery in 60% of patients. If there is progression of disease in the retained ovary, subsequent surgery is required, and it is frequently more difficult and hazardous to the patient. The rate of recurrence of symptoms is usually a reflection of the extent of the surgical dissection and adequacy of removal of all viable and palpable endometriosis.

Definitive Surgery

Removal of the uterus eliminates not only dysmenorrhea but also any possible abnormal bleeding. In addition, it removes the main source of the ectopic endometrium. Endometrial implants themselves probably can spread to cause daughter implants, but spreading may not occur very often.

When endometriosis causes ureteral or bowel obstruction, release of the obstruction is essential, since the problem is mechanical and neither hormonal therapy nor castration relieves it. In fact, the fibrosis and scarring after castration may aggravate the obstruction. This accounts for the fact that bowel obstruction secondary to endometriosis may be encountered in the postmenopausal patient.

If the kidney has normal function, the ureter should be released from its adhesions. Scarring involving the ureteral wall usually shows evidence of proximal dilatation from obstruction. In such cases, the obstructed region must be resected, and a ureteroureteral anastomosis should be done to preserve kidney function. If the kidney has no function on the involved side and the other kidney has normal function, nephrectomy may be necessary. There is little excuse, however, for allowing endometriosis to progress to this extent. In instances of obstruction, total abdominal hysterotomy and bilateral salpingo-oophorectomy are recommended along with release or excision of the damaged ureter.

When there is extensive endometriotic involvement of the bowel wall, stenosis of the bowel lumen may occur. For this reason, obstructive lesions of the intestinal tract due to endometriosis, wherever they may occur, should be treated by resection and reestablishment of bowel continuity by an anastomosis. This treatment is appropriate when small bowel is involved and when the colon is compromised. When only the anterior wall of the rectosigmoid is extensively involved, a wedge resection of this segment of bowel with approximation of the normal bowel wall is sufficient to preserve and restore an adequate bowel lumen.

If the history or findings on physical examination suggest partial obstruction or endometriosis involving the bowel, preoperative roentgenographic and endoscopic examinations should be done. It is wise to plan early admission to the hospital for preoperative bowel preparation when findings suggest intestinal involvement with endometriosis. However, even if the surgeon is surprised at the time of operation, resection should be carried out as indicated.

Other endometrial lesions involving the bladder wall, peritoneal surfaces, or rectovaginal septum may be removed and ovarian conservation practiced if justifiable. Endometriotic lesions involving abdominal or other scars of the umbilicus, the vulva, or the inguinal regions are infiltrating and should be excised by a wide margin so that no endometrial remnants are left to cause further problems.

It should be stressed that surgery for endometriosis can be very difficult. The adhesions may be extremely dense, often much more so than the usual inflammatory or postoperative type of scar. Sharp dissection is often necessary, especially in freeing the uterus from the anterior rectal wall. Fortunately, the rectal wall is often thickened by fibrosis, so that perforation is rare. Nevertheless, in making the dissection, it is better to err

by leaving a bit of uterine tissue on the rectum than by inadvertently perforating it.

Another point to be stressed is that resection of part of an ovary is worthwhile in young women. Generally, with other ovarian tumors, a complete oophorectomy is preferable to resection if the opposite ovary is normal. This dictum does not apply in endometriosis, in which bilateral ovarian involvement occurs in about 25% of the cases.

Because of the extensive adhesions and scarring with endometriosis, fragments of ovarian tissue may remain adherent to pelvic peritoneum. Neovasculature may allow even small fragments of ovarian tissue to persist and function. This "ovarian remnant syndrome" is manifested by cyclic symptoms of pain and mass if examined at the proper time. Reoperation and removal usually are required; such ovarian remnants often are entrapped as well. Endometriosis may continue to be stimulated by the fragments. The microscope may be helpful in attempts to excise all remnants. If recurrent symptoms still persist after the reoperation, radiation may be useful in effecting the necessary castration.

As mentioned earlier, optical augmentation helps identify areas of endometriosis requiring excision. In addition, more complete excision or destruction is possible with minimal trauma to adjacent tissues. Fine, nonreactive sutures, such as those made of polyglutamic and polyglycolic acids, are recommended. Catgut sutures have little place in conservative surgery on the pelvic organs.

Gordts and associates had a success rate that was nearly identical among stages of endometriosis when microsurgical techniques were used. Laboratory study in rats with induced endometriosis also documented few adhesions when microsurgical techniques were used.

Microcautery is a helpful adjunct to sharp surgical dissection and removal of areas of endometriosis. The CO_2 laser speeds the destruction of endometriosis by vaporization. Care is still essential, however, to protect other pelvic organs. The danger to tissues is similar regardless of the source (ie, light or electricity), as demonstrated by Luciano and associates.

Although the CO_2 laser remains the workhorse for laser technology in management of endometriosis, whether by laparoscopy or celiotomy, other laser techniques are available. Keye and associates reported that the argon laser has the specific advantages of a flexible fiberoptic source and an affinity for hemosiderin, which would be logical improvements over the CO_2 techniques. The neodymium:yttrium-aluminum-garnet laser coagulates rather than vaporizes, so that it has a technical advantage in not requiring smoke and vapor evacuation. The potassium-titanyl-phosphate (KTP 532) laser also has flexible delivery and allows vaporization as well as coagulation. Costs, however, are significant factors with these techniques, and there are no data on long-range effects on patient and surgeon.

Kistner and others have used progestogen therapy before proposed exploration for endometriosis and after conservative surgery. Preoperative hormonal therapy is thought to make the dissection easier and the implants easier to find and softer from the decidual reaction. Although our policy has been not to use this combined treatment preoperatively, it may be considered unless there is an ovarian mass or evidence of urinary or intestinal obstruction. Since the possibility always exists that the ovarian mass may be carcinoma rather than an endometrial cyst, exploration should not be delayed by attempts at hormonal manipulation. Also, such preoperative treatment may mask areas of endometriosis that might otherwise be found and excised; hence, an incomplete surgical procedure may result.

Ranney gave these reasons for not using preoperative progestational treatment: (1) increased friability of tissues interferes with clear dissection, (2) increased bleeding increases blood loss and slows surgery, and (3) softening of tissues affects accurate palpation and delineation of the borders of the lesion.

Danazol given preoperatively may not have vascular and softening effects on tissues but may very well mask lesions. Batt and Naples found the conception rate to be lower and the stillbirth rate to be higher after preoperatively administered danazol. For preoperative medication as a routine, the disadvantages seem to outweigh the advantages. Grunert and Franklin demonstrated improvement in conception rates when danazol was used preoperatively in moderate disease but not in severe disease. They did believe that the operations were technically easier. Other studies showed improvement in such results with postoperatively administered danazol. Studies of danazol alone and conservative surgery alone for what seems comparable disease seem to show similar results. Patient preference and age may be the leading factors for the final decision.

Generally, we do not advocate hormonal therapy after conservative surgery, particularly in patients with infertility. Both the surgeon and the patient are usually concerned that she become pregnant as soon after surgery as reasonable, and we see no advantage in delaying this by progestogen-induced anovulation. As is true for tubal reconstructive surgery, conception is highest during the first 6 months after conservative surgery, before the reestablishment of peritubal adhesions. Indeed, the data by Andrews and Larsen and others show definitely that the pregnancy rate is less when surgery is combined with postoperatively administered hormones than when surgery alone is used. With danazol, however, as reported by Wheeler and Malinak, some improvement in the pregnancy rate does appear to take place. Among patients with severe endometriosis, the pregnancy rate was 30% when surgery alone was carried out and 79% when danazol was given postoperatively. Our policy with patients having severe endometriosis and conservative surgery has been to consider a 3-month course of danazol after the operation, particularly if there is concern about the completeness of the surgery. This approach has been recommended by Buttram.

Because of the significant concerns of infertile women with endometriosis, some patients request a second conservative operation for the condition. Schenken and Malinak found that only 12% of patients so managed were able to achieve pregnancy. Wheeler and Malinak reported that after conservative surgery, recurrence rates of endometriosis were 13.5% and 40.3% at 3 and 5 years, respectively. It is interesting that the severity of the initial disease was not productive of recurrence. They presented a success rate of 47% for pregnancy after a second conservative operation for recurrence. Of the patients, 20% required a third major procedure.

Irradiation

Castration by external irradiation treats endometriosis quite effectively. There are, however, very limited indications for this now rarely used method of treatment. One suitable circumstance is symptomatic endometriosis, recurrent after and proved by operation, in a patient who is too poor a medical risk for definitive surgical treatment. Another acceptable reason is continued symptoms despite complete surgery. In some cases, ovarian remnants may persist and be responsible for continued pain. When this situation persists even after appropriate reoperation for the residual ovary syndrome, radiation may be quite effective. This is particularly true when no pelvic masses can be found on roentgenography, ultrasound, or computed tomography scan and hormone assay supports the presence of functioning ovarian tissue.

Malignancy in Endometriosis

Ectopic endometrium may become malignant in rare instances but has no more, and perhaps less, proclivity to do so than endometrium within the uterine cavity.

In 1925, Sampson, in reporting seven cases of ovarian carcinoma of possible endometrial origin, outlined the criteria to establish such a diagnosis: (1) Benign and malignant tissues must coexist in the same ovary and have the same histologic relationship to each other as that in carcinoma of the body of the uterus. (2) The carcinoma must arise in the benign tissue and not invade it from some other source. (3) Additional supportive evidence includes the presence of tissue resembling endometrial stroma about characteristic epithelial glands and the finding of old hemorrhage rather than fresh.

Among 516 cases of endometriosis reported by Scott and associates, there were only eight cases of ovarian malignancy. Three of these were papillary serous cystadenocarcinomas, two were epidermoid carcinomas arising in dermoid cysts, and one was a granulosa cell tumor. The remaining two cases were adenocarcinomas; in neither could the transition from benign endometriosis to carcinoma be shown, but the histologic features of each tumor suggested that it might be of endometrial origin. In 1957, Thompson collected 20 reported cases of ovarian malignancy arising in ovarian endometriosis. Most of these malignant tumors were adenocarcinoma (one was a carcinosarcoma). Thompson also reported 17 cases of ovarian adenocanthoma, seven of which definitely arose from endometriosis. Other, sporadic cases have been reported since that time, and it is thought that malignancy is an uncommon complication of endometriosis.

There have been many reports, however, of ovarian carcinomas with microscopic features of uterine endometrial carcinoma. These have been designated by the name *endometrioid carcinoma,* and they may or may not be associated with or originate from endometriosis. Although the World Health Organization histologic classification includes the category of endometrioid carcinoma, this does not presuppose that the tumors arise from endometriosis but is merely descriptive of the microscopic findings.

There are also very unusual instances of extraovarian malignancy arising in endometriosis in the rectovaginal septum. Dockerty and associates described two cases in 1954, Lash and Rubenstone reported one case in 1959, and more recently Granai and associates published a report. The rectovaginal septum is the second most common site of malignancy arising from endometriosis. Even though a diagnosis of endometriosis is made, careful follow-up is required because of this association. Interestingly, the prolonged use of exogenous estrogens has been common among most of the reported cases of endometrial rectovaginal malignancy. Endometriosis in the rectovaginal septum may be a further relative contraindication to estrogen treatment. Kapp and associates recorded long-term survival for patients with malignant rectovaginal endometriosis treated by irradiation.

It seems justifiable to conclude that endometriosis is capable of malignant change, but the incidence is extremely low and is of little significance in the clinical management of patients with this condition. Of greater clinical importance is the common finding of considerable enlargement of one or both ovaries in a patient with obvious endometriosis. The much more likely possibility of a coexisting ovarian malignancy unrelated to endometriosis must be considered, and exploratory celiotomy is then indicated, even though the patient may have absolutely no symptoms.

Of more concern is the differential diagnosis of an adnexal mass. It is believed that ovarian masses should not be needled, ruptured, or "tapped" in either diagnostic or therapeutic attempts. Spread of malignant cells and peritoneal contamination compromise survival should the lesion be malignant, and infection from aspiration has been recorded, with subsequent abscess formation and the need for more complicated surgical management.

Bibliography

Addison A, Dodson WC, Fortier KJ, Livengood CH III. Disposition of the normal-appearing ovary during surgery intended to cure endometriosis externa: a case report. J Reprod Med 1984;29:281.

Allen E. Endometrial transplantation. Am J Obstet Gynecol 1932;23:343

Andrews WC, Larsen GD. Endometriosis: treatment with hormonal pseudopregnancy and/or operation. Am J Obstet Gynecol 1974;118:643.

Åstedt B, Nordenskjöld F. Plasminogen activators in endometriosis. Acta Obstet Gynecol Scand [Suppl] 1984;123:23.

Awadalla SG, Friedman CI, Haq AU, Roh SI, Chin NW, Kim MH. Local peritoneal factors: their role in infertility associated with endometriosis. Am J Obstet Gynecol 1987;157:1207.

Barbieri RL, Evans S, Kistner RW. Danazol in the treatment of endometriosis: analysis of 100 cases with a 4-year follow-up. Fertil Steril 1982;37:737.

Barbieri RL, Ryan KJ. Medical therapy for endometriosis: endocrine pharmacology. Semin Reprod Endocrinol 1985;3:339.

Bartosik D. Immunologic aspects of endometriosis. Semin Reprod Endocrinol 1985;3:329.

Batt RE, Naples JD. Conservative surgery for endometriosis in the infertile couple. Curr Probl Obstet Gynecol 1982;6:45.

Batzofin JH, Holmes SD, Gibbons WE, Buttram VC Jr. Peritoneal fluid plasminogen activator activity in endometriosis and pelvic adhesive disease. Fertil Steril 1985;44:277.

Benson RC, Sneeden VD. Adenomyosis: a reappraisal of symptomatology. Am J Obstet Gynecol 1958;76:1044.

Bergqvist A, Bergqvist D, Lindholm B, Linell F. Case report: endometriosis in the uterosacral ligament giving orthopedic symptoms through compression of the sciatic nerve and surgically treated via an extraperitoneal approach keeping the pelvic organs intact. Acta Obstet Gynecol Scand 1987;66:93.

Bergqvist A, Carlström K, Jeppsson S, Ljungberg O. Histochemical localization of specific estrogen and progesterone binding in human endometrium and endometriotic tissue: a preliminary report. Acta Obstet Gynecol Scand [Suppl] 1984;123:15.

Bergqvist A, Jeppsson S, Ljungberg O. Histochemical demonstration of estrogen and progesterone binding in endometriotic tissue and in uterine endometrium: a comparative study. J Histochem Cytochem 1985;33:155.

Bergqvist A, Rannevik G, Thorell J. Estrogen and progesterone cytosol receptor concentration in endometriotic tissue and intrauterine endometrium. Acta Obstet Gynecol Scand [Suppl] 1981;101:53.

Blumenkrantz MJ, Gallagher N, Bashore RA, Tenckhoff H. Retrograde menstruation in women undergoing chronic peritoneal dialysis. Obstet Gynecol 1981;57:667.

Brosens IA, Koninckx PR, Corveleyn PA. A study of plasma progesterone, oestradiol-17β, prolactin and LH levels, and of the luteal phase appearance of the ovaries in patients with endometriosis and infertility. Br J Obstet Gynaecol 1978;85:246.

Butler L, Wilson E, Belisle S, et al. Collaborative study of pregnancy rates following danazol therapy of stage I endometriosis. Fertil Steril 1984;41:373.

Buttram VC Jr. Conservative surgery for endometriosis in the infertile female: a study of 206 patients with implications for both medical and surgical therapy. Fertil Steril 1979;31:117.

Caffier P. Uber Endometriumexplanation: Bisherige Ergebnisse, Wachstumsmechanik und Kritik. Zentralbl Gynakol 1928;52:63.

Cashman BZ. Hysterectomy with preservation of ovarian tissue in the treatment of endometriosis. Am J Obstet Gynecol 1945;49:484.

Chatman DL. Endometriosis and the black woman. J Reprod Med 1976;16:303.

Chatman DL, Ward AB. Endometriosis in adolescents. J Reprod Med 1982;27:156.

Chatterjee SK. Scar endometriosis: a clinicopathologic study of 17 cases. Obstet Gynecol 1980;56:81.

Chillik C, Rosenwaks Z. Endometriosis and in vitro fertilization. Semin Reprod Endocrinol 1985;3:377.

Counseller VS. Surgical procedures involved in the treatment of endometriosis. Surg Gynecol Obstet 1949;89:322.

Creadick RN. Non-surgical treatment of endometriosis: preliminary report on use of methyl testosterone. N Carolina Med J 1950;11:576.

Cullen TS. Adeno-myoma of the round ligament. Johns Hopkins Hosp Bull 1896;7:112.

Cullen TS. Adeno-myoma uteri diffusum benignum. Johns Hopkins Hosp Rep 1897;6:133.

Cullen TS. Adenomyoma of the uterus. Philadelphia: WB Saunders, 1908.

Curtis AH, Anson BJ, Ashley FL, et al. The anatomy of the pelvic autonomic nerves in relation to gynecology. Surg Gynecol Obstet 1942;75:743.

Daniell JF, Miller W, Tosh R. Initial evaluation of the use of the potassium-titanyl-phosphate (KTP 532) laser in gynecologic laparoscopy. Fertil Steril 1986;46:373.

Dawood MY, Khan-Dawood FS, Wilson L Jr. Peritoneal fluid prostaglandins and prostanoids in women with endometriosis, chronic pelvic inflammatory disease, and pelvic pain. Am J Obstet Gynecol 1984;148:391.

Dhont M, Serreyn R, Duvivier P, et al. Ovulation stigma and concentration of progesterone and estradiol in peritoneal fluid: relation with fertility and endometriosis. Fertil Steril 1984;41:872.

Dizerega GS, Barber DL, Hodgen GD. Endometriosis: role of ovarian steroids in initiation, maintenance, and suppression. Fertil Steril 1980;33:649.

Dmowski WP, Cohen MR. Treatment of endometriosis with antigonadotropin, danazol: a laparoscopic and histologic evaluation. Obstet Gynecol 1975;46:147.

Dmowski WP, Radwanska E. Current concepts on pathology, histogenesis and etiology of endometriosis. Acta Obstet Gynecol Scand [Suppl] 1984;123:29.

Dockerty MB, Pratt JH, Decker DG. Primary adenocarcinoma of the rectovaginal septum probably arising from endometriosis: report of two cases. Cancer 1954;7:898.

Eisermann J, Gast MJ, Pineda J, et al. Tumor necrosis factor in peritoneal fluid of women undergoing laparoscopic surgery. Fertil Steril 1988;50:573.

Ekwempu CC, Harrison KA. Endometriosis among the Hausa/Fulani population of Nigeria. Trop Geogr Med 1979;31:201.

Everett HS. Probable tubal origin of endometriosis. Am J Obstet Gynecol 1931;22:1.

Ferrari BT, Shollenbarger DR. Abdominal wall endometriosis following hypertonic saline abortion. JAMA 1977;238:56.

Foster DC, Stern JL, Buscema J, et al. Pleural and parenchymal pulmonary endometriosis. Obstet Gynecol 1981;58:552.

Furman WR, Wang KP, Summer WR, Terry PB. Catamenial pneumothorax: evaluation by fiberoptic pleuroscopy. Am Rev Respir Dis 1980;121:137.

García C-R, David SS. Pelvic endometriosis: infertility and pelvic pain. Am J Obstet Gynecol 1977;129:740.

García C-R, Mastroianni L Jr. Microsurgery for treatment of adnexal disease. Fertil Steril 1980;34:413.

Gleicher N, Dmowski WP, Siegel I, et al. Lymphocyte subsets in endometriosis. Obstet Gynecol 1984;63:463.

Golan A, Dargenio R, Winston RML. Fulguration versus resection of experimental endometrial peritoneal implants in the rat. Aust NZ J Obstet Gynaecol 1984;24:286.

Goodall JR. A study of endometriosis, endosalpingiosis, endocervicosis, and peritoneo-ovarian sclerosis: a clinical and pathologic study. Philadelphia: JB Lippincott, 1943.

Goodman JD, Macchia RJ, Macasaet MA, Schneider M. Endometriosis of the urinary bladder: sonographic findings. AJR 1980;135:625.

Gordts S. Boeckx W, Brosens I. Microsurgery of endometriosis in infertile patients. Fertil Steril 1984;42:520.

Gould SF, Shannon JM, Cunha GR. Nuclear estrogen binding sites in human endometriosis. Fertil Steril 1983;39:520.

Granai CO, Walters MD, Safaii H, Madoc-Jones H, Moukhtar M. Malignant transformation of vaginal endometriosis. Obstet Gynecol 1984;64:592.

Granberg I, Willems JS. Endometriosis of lung and pleura diagnosed by aspiration biopsy. Acta Cytol 1977;21:295.

Gray LA. Endometriosis of the bowel: role of bowel resection, superficial excision and oophorectomy in treatment. Ann Surg 1973;177:580.

Greenblatt RB, Tzingounis V. Danazol treatment of endometriosis: long-term follow-up. Fertil Steril 1979;32:518.

Grunert GM, Franklin RR. Preoperative Danocrine therapy as an adjunct to conservative surgery for endometriosis: a preliminary report [Abstract]. Fertil Steril 1984;(suppl)41:74.

Guastella G, Comparetto G, Gullo D, et al. Gamete intra-fallopian transfer (GIFT): a new technique for the treatment of unexplained infertility. Acta Eur Fertil 1985;16:311.

Guzick DS, Rock JA. A comparison of danazol and conservative surgery for the treatment of infertility due to mild or moderate endometriosis. Fertil Steril 1983;40:580.

Halban J. Hysteroadenosis metastatica (die lymphogene Genese der sog. Adenofibromatosis heterotopica). Wien Klin Wochenschr 1924;37:1205.

Halme J, Becker S, Wing R. Accentuated cyclic activation of peritoneal macrophages in patients with endometriosis. Am J Obstet Gynecol 1984;148:85.

Halme, J, Hammond MG, Hulka JF, et al. Retrograde menstruation in healthy women and in patients with endometriosis. Obstet Gynecol 1984;64:151.

Hammond MG, Hammond CB, Parker RT. Conservative treatment of endometriosis externa: the effects of methyltestosterone therapy. Fertil Steril 1978;29:651.

Haney AF, Handwerger S, Weinberg JB. Peritoneal fluid prolactin in infertile women with endometriosis: lack of evidence of secretory activity by endometrial implants. Fertil Steril 1984;42:935.

Harbitz HF. Clinical pathogenetic and experimental investigation of endometriosis especially regarding the localisation in the abdominal wall (laparotomy scars) with a contribution to the study of experimental transplantation of endometrium. Acta Chir Scand 1934;74(suppl 30):1.

Haskins AL, Woolf RB. Stilbestrol-induced hyperhormonal amenorrhea for the treatment of pelvic endometriosis. Obstet Gynecol 1955;5:113.

Haydon GB. A study of 569 cases of endometriosis. Am J Obstet Gynecol 1942;43:704.

Heneghan MA, Teixidor HS. Pleuroperitoneal endometriosis. AJR 1979;133:727.

Hibbard J, Schreiber JR. Footdrop due to sciatic nerve endometriosis. Am J Obstet Gynecol 1984;149:800.

Hirsch EF, Jones HO. The behavior of the epithelium in explants of human endometrium. Am J Obstet Gynecol 1933;25:37.

Irani S, Atkinson L, Cabaniss C, Danovitch SH. Pleuroperitoneal endometriosis. Obstet Gynecol 1976;47(suppl 1):72.

Iwanoff NS. Drüsiges cystenhaltiges uterusfibromyom complicirt durch sarcom und carcinom (adenofibromyoma cysticum sarcomatodes carcinomatosum). Monatsschr Geburtsh Gynak 1898;7:295.

Jacobson VC. The autotransplantation of endometrial tissue in the rabbit. Arch Surg 1922;5:281.

Jacobson VC. Intraperitoneal transplantation of endometrial tissue. Arch Pathol Lab Med 1926;1:169.

Jänne O, Kauppila A, Kokko E, et al. Estrogen and progestin receptors in endometriosis lesions: comparison with endometrial tissue. Am J Obstet Gynecol 1981;141:562.

Jansen RPS, Russell P. Nonpigmented endometriosis: clinical, laparoscopic, and pathologic definition. Am J Obstet Gynecol 1986;155:1154.

Javert CT. Observations on pathology and spread of endometriosis based on theory of benign metastasis. Am J Obstet Gynecol 1951;62:477.

Kapp DS, Merino M, LiVolsi V. Adenocarcinoma of the vagina arising in endometriosis: long-term survival following radiation therapy. Gynecol Oncol 1982;14:271.

Karnaky KJ. The use of stilbestrol for endometriosis: preliminary report. South Med J 1948;41:1109.

Katayama KP, Manuel M, Jones HW Jr, et al. Methyltestosterone treatment of infertility associated with pelvic endometriosis. Fertil Steril 1976;27:83.

Kaunitz A, Di Sant'Agnese PA. Needle tract endometriosis: an unusual complication of amniocentesis. Obstet Gynecol 1979;54:753.

Keettel WC, Stein RJ. The viability of the cast-off menstrual endometrium. Am J Obstet Gynecol 1951;61:440.

Keye WR Jr, Hansen LW, Astin M, Poulson AM Jr. Argon laser therapy of endometriosis: a review of 92 consecutive patients. Fertil Steril 1987;47:208.

King WLM. Metastatic endometriosis in abdominal scars. Can J Surg 1979;22:579.

Kistner RW. The effects of new synthetic progestogens on endometriosis in the human female. Fertil Steril 1965;16:61.

Koninckx PR, Ide P, Vandenbroucke W, Brosens IA. New aspects of the pathophysiology of endometriosis and associated infertility. J Reprod Med 1980;24:257.

Krebs H-B, Goplerud DR. Mechanical intestinal obstruction in patients with gynecologic disease: a review of 368 patients. Am J Obstet Gynecol 1987;157:577.

Langmade CF. Pelvic endometriosis and ureteral obstruction. Am J Obstet Gynecol 1975;122:463.

Lash SR, Rubenstone AI. Adenocarcinoma of the rectovaginal septum probably arising from endometriosis. Am J Obstet Gynecol 1959;78:299.

Lomano JM. Nd:YAG laser ablation of early pelvic endometriosis: a report of 61 cases. Lasers Surg Med 1987;7:56.

Long ME, Taylor HC Jr. Endometrioid carcinoma of the ovary. Am J Obstet Gynecol 1964;90:936.

Luciano AA, Randolph J, Whitman G, et al. A comparison of thermal injury, healing patterns, and postoperative adhesion formation following CO_2 laser and electromicrosurgery. Fertil Steril 1987;48:1025.

Maathuis JB, Van Look PFA, Michie EA. Changes in volume, total protein and ovarian steroid concentrations of peritoneal fluid throughout the human menstrual cycle. J Endocrinol 1978;76:123.

Madsen H, Hansen P, Andersen OP. Endometrioid carcinoma in an operation scar. Acta Obstet Gynecol Scand 1980;59:475.

Malinak LR, Wheeler JM. Association of endometriosis with spontaneous abortion, prognosis for pregnancy, and risk for recurrence. Semin Reprod Endocrinol 1985;3:361.

Marik J, Hulka J. Luteinized unruptured follicle syndrome: a subtle cause of infertility. Fertil Steril 1978;29:270.

Markee JE. Menstruation in intraocular endometrial transplants in the rhesus monkey. In: Contributions of embryology, No. 177. Washington DC: Carnegie Institution of Washington, 1940 (publication no. 518):221.

Martino CR, Haaga JR, Bryan PJ. Secondary infection of an endometrioma following fine-needle aspiration. Radiology 1984;151:53.

Maslow LA, Learner A. Endometriosis of kidney. J Urol 1950;64:564.

Mathur BB, Shah BS, Bhende YM. Adenomyosis uteri: a pathologic study of 290 cases. Am J Obstet Gynecol 1962;84:1820.

McArthur JW, Ulfelder H. The effect of pregnancy upon endometriosis. Obstet Gynecol Surv 1965;20:709.

McCoy JB, Bradford WZ. Surgical treatment of endometriosis with conservation of reproductive potential. Am J Obstet Gynecol 1963;87:394.

Meek SC, Hodge DD, Musich JR. Autoimmunity in infertile patients with endometriosis. Am J Obstet Gynecol 1988;158:1365.

Meigs JV. Endometriosis: etiologic role of marriage age and parity; conservative treatment. Obstet Gynecol 1953;2:46.

Meldrum DR. Clinical management of endometriosis with luteinizing hormone-releasing hormone analogues. Semin Reprod Endocrinol 1985;3:371.

Merrill JA. Endometrial induction of endometriosis across Millipore filters. Am J Obstet Gynecol 1966;94:780.

Meyer R. Ueber eine adenomatöse Wucherung der Serosa in einer Bauchnarbe. Ztschr Geburtsh Gynakol 1903;49:32.

Meyer R. Uber entzündliche heterotope epithelwucherungen im weiblichen genitalgebiete und über eine bis in die wurzel des mesocolon ausgedehnte benigne wuocherung des darmepithels. Virchows Arch Pathol Anat 1909;195:489.

Miyazawa K. Incidence of endometriosis among Japanese women. Obstet Gynecol 1976;48:407.

Moghissi KS, Boyce CR. Management of endometriosis with oral medroxyprogesterone acetate. Obstet Gynecol 1976;47:265.

Moore JG, Binstock MA, Growdon WA. The clinical implications of retroperitoneal endometriosis. Am J Obstet Gynecol 1988;158:1291.

Moretuzzo RW, DiLauro S, Jenison E, Chen SL, Reindollar RH, McDonough PG. Serum and peritoneal lavage fluid CA-125 levels in endometriosis. Fertil Steril 1988;50:430.

Murphy AA, Green WR, Bobbie D, et al. Unsuspected endometriosis documented by scanning electron microscopy in visually normal peritoneum. Fertil Steril 1986;46:522.

Naples JD, Batt RE, Sadigh H. Spontaneous abortion rate in patients with endometriosis. Obstet Gynecol 1981;57:509.

Novak E. The significance of uterine mucosa in the fallopian tube, with a discussion of the origin of aberrant endometrium. Am J Obstet Gynecol 1926;12:484.

Novak E. Gynecological and obstetrical pathology: with clinical and endocrine relations. Philadelphia: WB Saunders, 1940.

Olive DL, Weinberg JB, Haney AF. Peritoneal macrophages and infertility: the association between cell number and pelvic pathology. Fertil Steril 1985;44:772.

Paull T, Tedeschi LG. Perineal endometriosis at the site of episiotomy scar. Obstet Gynecol 1972;40:28.

Pellegrini VD Jr, Pasternak HS, Macaulay WP. Endometrioma of the pubis: a differential in the diagnosis of hip pain; a report of two cases. J Bone Joint Surg [Am] 1981;63:1333.

Pittaway DE, Maxson W, Daniell J, et al. Luteal phase defects in infertility patients with endometriosis. Fertil Steril 1983;39:712.

Pittaway DE, Vernon C, Fayez JA. Spontaneous abortions in women with endometriosis. Fertil Steril 1988;50:711.

Portuondo JA, Agustin A, Herran C, Echanojauregui AD. The corpus luteum in infertile patients found during laparoscopy. Fertil Steril 1981;36:37.

Portuondo JA, Echanojauregui AD, Herran C, Alijarte I. Early conception in patients with untreated mild endometriosis. Fertil Steril 1983;39:22.

Punnonen R, Klemi P, Nikkanen V. Recurrent endometriosis. Gynecol Obstet Invest 1980;11:307.

Ranney B. The prevention, inhibition, palliation, and treatment of endometriosis. Am J Obstet Gynecol 1975;123:778.

Ridley JH. The validity of Sampson's theory of endometriosis. Am J Obstet Gynecol 1961;82:777.

Ridley JH. The histogenesis of endometriosis: a review of facts and fancies. Obstet Gynecol Surv 1968;23:1.

Ridley JH, Edwards IK. Experimental endometriosis in the human. Am J Obstet Gynecol 1958;76:783.

Riva HL, Wilson JH, Kawasaki DM. Effect of norethynodrel on endometriosis. Am J Obstet Gynecol 1961;82:109.

Rivlin ME, Krueger RP, Wiser WL. Danazol in the management of ureteral obstruction secondary to endometriosis. Fertil Steril 1985;44:274.

Rock JA, Dubin NH, Ghodgaonkar RB, et al. Cul-de-sac fluid in women with endometriosis: fluid volume and prostanoid concentration during the proliferative phase of the cycle—days 8 to 12. Fertil Steril 1982;37:747.

Rönnberg L, Kauppila A, Rajaniemi H. Luteinizing hormone receptor disorder in endometriosis. Fertil Steril 1984;42:64.

Rosenfeld DL, Jacob J. Subsequent pregnancies in previously infertile women with endometriosis. Obstet Gynecol 1988;72:908.

Russell WW. Aberrant portions of the Müllerian duct found in an ovary. Johns Hopkins Hosp Bull 1899;10:8.

Sampson JA. Perforating hemorrhagic (chocolate) cysts of the ovary: their importance and especially their relation to pelvic adenomas of endometrial type ("adenomyoma" of the uterus, rectovaginal septum, sigmoid, etc.). Arch Surg 1921;3:245.

Sampson JA. The life history of ovarian hematomas (hemorrhagic cysts) of endometrial (Müllerian) type. Am J Obstet Gynecol 1922;4:451.

Sampson JA. Endometrial carcinoma of the ovary, arising in endometrial tissue of that organ. Arch Surg 1925;10:1.

Sampson JA. Peritoneal endometriosis due to menstrual dissemination of endometrial tissue into peritoneal cavity. Am J Obstet Gynecol 1927;14:422.

Sampson JA. The development of the implantation theory for the origin of peritoneal endometriosis. Am J Obstet Gynecol 1940;40:549.

Schenken RS, Malinak LR. Reoperation after initial treatment of endometriosis with conservative surgery. Am J Obstet Gynecol 1978;131:416.

Schriock E, Monroe SE, Henzl M, Jaffe RB. Treatment of endometriosis with a potent agonist of gonadotropin-releasing hormone (nafarelin). Fertil Steril 1985;44:583.

Schweppe K-W, Wynn RM, Beller FK. Ultrastructural comparison of endometriotic implants and eutopic endometrium. Am J Obstet Gynecol 1984;148:1024.

Scott RB, Burt JH. Clinical experimental endometriosis: fifteen years experience at University Hospitals of Cleveland. South Med J 1962;55:129.

Scott RB, Te Linde RW, Wharton LR Jr. Further studies on experimental endometriosis. Am J Obstet Gynecol 1953;66:1082.

Scott RB, Wharton LR Jr. The effects of excessive amounts of diethylstilbestrol on experimental endometriosis in monkeys. Am J Obstet Gynecol 1955;69:573.

Scott RB, Wharton LR Jr. The effect of testosterone on experimental endometriosis in rhesus monkeys. Am J Obstet Gynecol 1959;78:1020.

Scott RB, Wharton LR Jr. Effects of progesterone and norethindrone on experimental endometriosis in monkeys. Am J Obstet Gynecol 1962;84:867.

Seibel MM. Minimal pelvic endometriosis and infertility. Semin Reprod Endocrinol 1985;3:307.

Simpson JL, Elias S, Malinak LR, Buttram VC Jr. Heritable aspects of endometriosis. I. Genetic studies. Am J Obstet Gynecol 1980;137:327.

Simpson JL, Malinak LR, Elias S, et al. HLA associations in endometriosis. Am J Obstet Gynecol 1984;148:395.

Soules MR, Malinak LR, Bury R, Poindexter A. Endometriosis and anovulation: a coexisting problem in the infertile female. Am J Obstet Gynecol 1976;125:412.

Stanley KE Jr, Utz DC, Dockerty MB. Clinically significant endometriosis of the urinary tract. Surg Gynecol Obstet 1965;120:491.

Steingold KA, Cedars M, Lu JKH, et al. Treatment of endometriosis with a long-acting gonadotropin-releasing hormone agonist. Obstet Gynecol 1987;69:403.

Strasser EJ, Davis RM. Extraperitoneal inguinal endometriosis. Am Surg 1977;43:421.

Sturgis SH, Call BJ. Endometriosis peritonei: relationship of pain to functional activity. Am J Obstet Gynecol 1954;68:1421.

Suginami H, Yano K. An ovum capture inhibitor (OCI) in endometriosis peritoneal fluid: an OCI-related membrane responsible for fimbrial failure of ovum capture. Fertil Steril 1988;50:648.

Sully L. Endometrioma of the perineum associated with episiotomy scars. Scott Med J 1977;22:307.

Tamaya T, Motoyama T, Ohono Y, et al. Steroid receptor levels and histology of endometriosis and adenomyosis. Fertil Steril 1979;31:396.

Te Linde RW, Scott RB. Experimental endometriosis. Am J Obstet Gynecol 1950;60:1147.

Thompson JD. Primary ovarian adenocanthoma: its relationship to endometriosis. Obstet Gynecol 1957;9:403.

Traut HF. Adult human endometrium in tissue culture. Surg Gynecol Obstet 1928;47:334.

Vasquez G, Cornillie F, Brosens IA. Peritoneal endometriosis: scanning electron microscopy and histology of minimal pelvic endometriotic lesions. Fertil Steril 1984;42:696.

Vernon MW, Beard JS, Graves K, Wilson EA. Classification of endometriotic implants by morphologic appearance and capacity to synthesize prostaglandin F. Fertil Steril 1986;46:801.

Vierikko P, Kauppila A, Rönnberg L, Vihko R. Steroidal regulation of endometriosis tissue: lack of induction of 17β-hydroxysteroid dehydrogenase activity by progesterone, medroxyprogesterone acetate, or danazol. Fertil Steril 1985;43:218.

Von Recklinghausen FD. Die Adenomyome und Cystadenome der Uterus-und Tubenwandung: Ihre Abkunft von Resten des Wolff'schen Körpers. Berlin: August Hirschwald, 1896.

Wallace AM, Lees DAR, Roberts ADG, et al. Danazol and prolactin status in patients with endometriosis. Acta Endocrinologica 1984;107:445.

Wespi HJ, Kletzhändler M. Uber Narbenendometriosen. Mschr Geburtsh Gynakol 1940;111:169.

Wheeler JM, Malinak LR. Postoperative danazol therapy in infertility patients with severe endometriosis. Fertil Steril 1981;36:460.

Wheeler JM, Malinak LR. Recurrent endometriosis: incidence, management, and prognosis. Am J Obstet Gynecol 1983;146:247.

Williams BFP. Conservative management of endometriosis: follow-up observations of progestin therapy. Obstet Gynecol 1967;30:76.

Williams HE, Barsky S, Storino W. Umbilical endometrioma (silent type). Arch Dermatol 1976;112:1435.

Williams TJ. The role of surgery in the management of endometriosis. Mayo Clin Proc 1975;50:198.

Williams TJ, Pratt JH. Endometriosis in 1,000 consecutive celiotomies: incidence and management. Am J Obstet Gynecol 1977;129:245.

Application of Laser in Gynecology

21

JAMES H. DORSEY

HISTORY OF THE LASER

The term laser is an acronym for the words *l*ight *a*mplification by *s*timulated *e*mission of *r*adiation. In 1917 Albert Einstein described the process of stimulated emission of radiation, but it was not until 1973 that Charles Townes and coworkers produced a device called a maser, which amplified microwaves by stimulated emission of radiation. In 1958 Schawlow and Townes published a hypothesis that described the laser in general terms, and finally, in 1960, Theodore Maimman actually constructed the first working laser, consisting of a ruby crystal that was stimulated to emit laser energy by pumping with light from a xenon flash lamp. The carbon dioxide laser was developed by Patel in 1964, and in 1965 this laser was used for the first time in experimental surgery. In 1973 the laser was first used in gynecology for vaporization of infected cervical tissue. Since that time a large number of reports concerning the use of CO_2 laser for lower reproductive tract surgery have accumulated. During the late 1970s the CO_2 laser was coupled to the laparoscope, and the first successful operative laparoscopies were performed with this new modality.

Other lasers that have proved useful in gynecologic surgery have wavelengths that are conducted by quartz fibers. In 1963 the neodymium:yttrium-aluminum-garnet (Nd:YAG) laser was developed at Bell Laboratories. The useful wavelengths of the argon laser were discovered in 1964, and in 1984 the frequency-doubled YAG wavelengths of KTP 532 became available for clinical trials. Each of these "fiberoptic" lasers currently is used successfully in gynecology, particularly in the field of operative endoscopy, where fiberoptic delivery simplifies the application of laser energy.

LASER PHYSICS

Laser light is most often described in terms of its wave characteristics or wavelength. Wavelength is the distance between two successive crests or troughs; it determines the color of light. Wavelengths usually are measured in microns or nanometers. One micron (μm) equals $1/1000$ mm, and 1 nanometer (nm) equals $1/1,000,000$ mm. Electromagnetic waves often are referred to as light, although visible light occupies only a small portion of the electromagnetic spectrum. CO_2 laser energy in the mid-infrared portion of the spectrum, although invisible to the eye, may therefore be correctly thought of as light energy (Table 21-1).

An atom is composed of a positively charged nucleus surrounded by electrons, which orbit the nucleus. Each electron orbit can be described in terms of energy levels. As orbital distance from the nucleus increases, the energy level increases. When an electron moves from a higher-energy orbit to a lower-energy orbit, the atom loses a specific amount of energy in the form of a photon, which also has a specific wavelength.

Lasers contain the active lasing medium, a collection of atoms or molecules that are housed in an optically resonant cavity. This active medium is stimulated or "pumped" by an external energy source such as electricity or light, which stimulates the active lasing medium to higher energy levels. As decay back to resting energy levels occurs, photons of energy are released into the optical cavity. Electrons that are still in excited or higher orbital energy levels also can be stimulated by bombardment with these photons, so that they undergo identical decay and emit an identical photon. This is called stimulated emission because one photon has stimulated the production of another photon. In the

TABLE 21–1
Laser Colors and Wavelengths

NAME	COLOR	WAVELENGTH (nm)
Excimers	Ultraviolet	200–400
Argon	Blue-green	488 nm/515
KTP 532	Green	532
Krypton	Green-yellow	532 nm/568
Dye Laser	Yellow-green-red	577 nm/630
Helium Neon	Red	632
Gold Vapor	Red	630
Krypton	Red	647
Ruby	Deep red	694
Nd: Yag	Infrared-infrared	1064 nm/1318
CO_2	Infrared	10,600

same way that sound waves can be made to resonate back and forth between the walls of a closed cavity, so light can resonate. The optical cavity of the laser tube is closed at both ends by a mirror. One of these mirrors is totally reflective, but the other is semitransparent. Although photon direction in the tube is random, a certain number of photons will be emitted in the axis of the optical cavity and the others are focused by the mirrors, so that the majority are resonating or bouncing back and forth along the axis of the cavity. Some of these photons emerge through the semitransparent mirror at the end of the optical cavity and are emitted as light. This laser light has three special characteristics: it is monochromatic, parallel, and coherent for both time and space. Monochromaticity results because the photons are all identical. Parallelism of laser rays is produced by limitation of energy egress from the optical cavity to those photons traveling in one direction (ie, the optical axis of the cavity). Coherence is governed by wave resonance within the optical cavity, and all of the light waves are perfectly aligned, so that each trough or peak passes the same point at exactly the same time. The laser thus creates a light that travels in a tight beam over infinite distances. Laser power is measured in terms of watts (W), and laser energy is expressed in terms of joules (J). One joule equals 1 W for 1 second.

Lasers are named after the active lasing medium within the optical cavity. In the case of the carbon dioxide laser, the optical cavity contains two other gases, nitrogen and helium, which aid in the transfer of vibrational energy to and from the CO_2 molecule.

The pumping mechanism for both CO_2 and argon lasers is electricity. In contrast, the Nd:YAG laser is optically pumped. The Nd:YAG wavelength of 1064 nm can be altered by passage through a crystal of potassium (K) titanyl (T) phosphate (P). This results in

doubling the frequency but halving the wavelength to 532 nm, an emerald green light. These four wavelengths, CO_2, argon, KTP 532, and Nd:YAG, currently are commercially available for use in gynecology.

Power Density and Transverse Electromagnetic Mode

As a result of coherence of laser radiation, much of the energy from the laser can be collected and focused into a relatively small spot size. For any given power setting, the smaller the spot size, the higher the power density. The focal spot size varies directly with the focal length of the laser lens. Power density is expressed as watts per square centimeter (W/cm^2). Because the calculation of power density is relatively complicated, most surgeons prefer to note the power setting on the laser and the effective spot size used for surgery.

For the CO_2 laser, energy is not completely uniform throughout the cross-sectional diameter of the beam. The term transverse electromagnetic mode refers to the energy distribution of the cross-sectional diameter of the beam. For most CO_2 surgical lasers, the energy distribution is greatest at the center of the beam and decreases toward the periphery. If one graphs the energy distribution of the cross-sectional beam diameter of the CO_2 laser, the resultant curve is bell-shaped. Knowledge of the ways in which the shape of this curve is influenced by power selection and focal spot size is crucial for the CO_2 laser surgeon, if satisfactory results are to be obtained (Fig. 21-1).

The other surgical lasers whose wavelengths can be conducted through a quartz fiber do not demonstrate this same pattern of energy distribution. In the case of YAG, KTP 532, and argon, energy transmission through the fiber results in a loss of coherence and parallelism. The beam diverges from the tip of the fiber at a 15-degree angle. Power density is highest at the end of the fiber but, because of beam divergence, rapidly decreases as distance from the tip increases.

LASER TISSUE INTERACTION AND BEAM MANIPULATION

The primary tissue effects of the surgical lasers used in gynecology are produced by laser heat energy. Water content of soft tissue is about 80% by volume, and if the latent heat or vaporization of water is delivered by the beam, tissue is vaporized. The shape of the crater produced by this process reflects the intensity profile of the

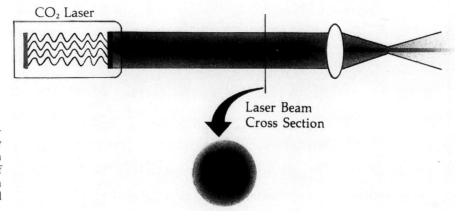

Figure 21–1. Transverse electromagnetic mode. Laser energy distribution is not uniform throughout the cross section of the beam. Energy concentration is highest at the beam center and decreases toward the periphery.

incident energy (Fig. 21-2). Some of the tissue at the periphery of the lesion that does not receive enough energy to become vaporized will be damaged. When tissue is heated to about 57° C, irreversible damage occurs and the cell dies. Thus between 57° and 100° C there will be tissue death without vaporization. Additional tissue damage also results from lateral conduction of heat away from the laser impact site. The amount of damage done by heat conduction is directly proportional to the amount of time spent in lasing. There are, therefore, three zones of laser tissue damage that may be defined: the area vaporized, the area of tissue death that results from heating tissue short of vaporization, and the area of tissue damage caused by conduction of heat away from the lased site (Fig. 21-3).

CO_2 Laser Tissue Effects

CO_2 laser energy is almost completely absorbed by a thin layer of water. Because of the high water content of cells, penetration into tissue is minimal, and most laser energy is absorbed in vaporization. Tissue may thus be vaporized accurately, since the surgeon views the process through an operative microscope and there is little fear of deep thermal damage. This margin of safety has contributed to the popularity of CO_2 laser surgery. The concept of beam geometry control has been emphasized by Reid, and is an important part of laser surgery. The sharply focused beam has a narrow spot diameter with a high-power density, and will produce an impact crater that resembles a drill hole. This is perfect for

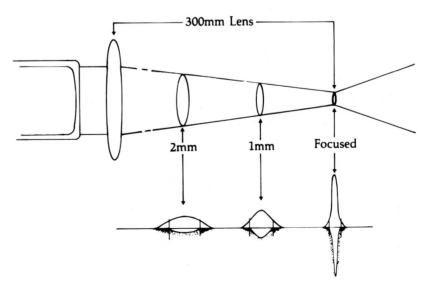

Figure 21–2. Beam profile variations. For any given power setting, beam profile (the shape of the gaussian curve) can be altered by changing spot size diameter. The small spot size results in a steep curve, which is used for cutting. Larger spot sizes produce flatter curves suitable for vaporization. Tissue damage and crater shape mirror the energy distribution.

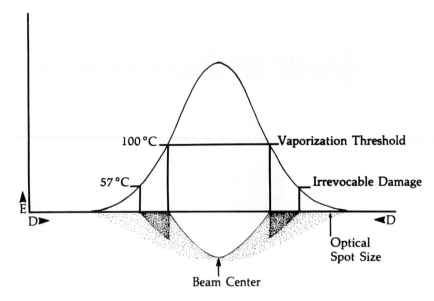

Figure 21–3. Beam profile and tissue damage. Laser wounds produce three zones of tissue damage: the vaporization crater, the area of tissue necrosis caused by heating tissue to temperatures between 57° and 100° C, and the area of damage resulting from heat conduction. Higher power settings produce more rapid vaporization of tissue and lessen the secondary thermal damage.

cutting, and lateral tissue damage is minimized. On the other hand, enlarging the spot diameter by partially defocusing the beam reduces the central amplitude of the gaussian curve, and results in a larger spot size that is more easily controlled when vaporization is desired. The surgeon selects the proper power setting and spot diameter to effect the desired result.

YAG Laser Tissue Effects

YAG laser energy is able to penetrate tissue to a much greater depth than does CO_2 laser energy, since it passes through intracellular and extracellular water. Exposure to YAG laser energy may result in tissue damage to depths up to 4 mm. The YAG often is used in a liquid medium, as exemplified by YAG laser endometrial ablation. Because it penetrates water so well, the YAG is not a good laser for vaporization. It is an effective coagulator, however, as it passes deeper into tissue before absorption occurs. YAG energy also scatters in tissue, so thermal damage is greater than with CO_2 energy.

The tissue effect of YAG laser energy can be altered by applying artificial sapphire tips to the end of the fiber. The sapphire changes the pattern of energy egress from the fiber and greatly enlarges the scope of YAG laser surgery (Fig. 21-4). Various configurations of the sapphire tip allow the surgeon to use the YAG as a scalpel, and a precise hemostatic incision can be made. Other tips enhance the coagulating or vaporizing efficiency of the YAG. In general, sapphire tips limit the penetration

of YAG energy to tissue depths of 1 mm or less. Hemostasis can be achieved, however, by coagulation of smaller vessels with the heated sapphire. The laparoscopic uses of the YAG also have been greatly expanded with the application of sapphire tips, since it is now much safer to use this laser for intra-abdominal surgery.

Argon and KTP Tissue Effects

The argon laser produces a blue-green light that has two distinct bands at 488 nm and 515 nm on the electromagnetic spectrum. Because colored laser light traverses water very well. This laser also is a photocoagulator, since its energy is absorbed preferentially by its opposite color, red or black. Argon is located somewhere between CO_2 and YAG in its ability to produce vaporization and coagulation. The laser will vaporize tissue, but this is not as rapidly achieved as with CO_2. Coagulation extends deeper into tissues than with CO_2 because of the penetrability of its beam.

The KTP 532-nm wavelength is emerald green, and its tissue effects are similar to those produced by the argon laser. The KTP 532 can be used to vaporize or to coagulate, and the end of the fiber can be used to cut tissue. Again, because of its penetration, its tissue effects often extend 1 to 2 mm into the irradiated target. This laser has been effectively used for both lower reproductive tract and endoscopic surgery. Fibers of 200 to 600 μm in diameter are available, so that with power settings of 15 to 20 W, higher power densities are available. Both argon and KTP work well when used under water.

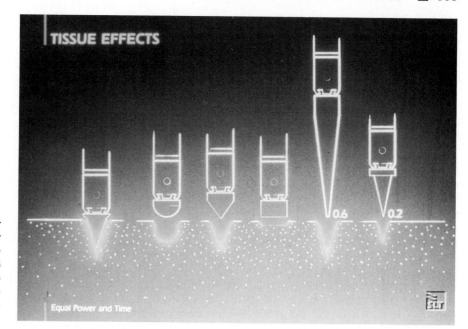

Figure 21–4. Sapphire tips for Nd:YAG laser. Sapphire tips alter the energy egress from the YAG quartz fiber. Here tissue effects are shown to vary with changes in sapphire design. Sharp tips make good scalpels. Rounded tips are used for vaporization.

LASER DELIVERY SYSTEMS

CO_2 laser energy is propagated through air to the target site. The CO_2 laser beam is delivered through a tubular arm, and the direction of the beam is changed by mirrors. The beam is focused by lenses mounted in several different useful devices: (a) the micromanipulator, in which a joystick is used to move a mirror that is located past the focusing lens and the beam, is thus directed to the target. Micromanipulators are mounted on colposcopes or operative microscopes and provide a highly accurate method of beam control; (b) a laser handpiece, which houses a short focal length lens, is capable of producing the smallest focal spot sizes, making it ideal for fine incisions; (c) the CO_2 laser operative laparoscope and laser laparoscopic probes. Irrespective of the delivery system used, the beam can be focused or defocused, depending on the surgeon's desires. When the beam is in focus, the focal point of the beam is in contact with the target tissue and the power density is highest for that particular lens and power setting. Laser incisions are, therefore, three dimensional, in that they have length, depth, and width. The width of the incision is equal to the focal spot size. Incisional depth depends on the time that the laser energy is applied to target tissue.

Micromanipulators may be fitted with a system of focusing lenses that are similar to the zoom lens of a camera, so that the spot can be varied in size without changing the optical focus for the surgeon.

Fiberoptic lasers are much easier to use in endoscopes and handpieces, since beam delivery is through fibers that are 200 to 600 μm in diameter. The beam diverges from the cable at 15 degrees, so that power density is greatest just off the tip of the fiber, and the beam can be defocused by moving the tip of the fiber further away from the target tissue.

LOWER REPRODUCTIVE TRACT LASER SURGERY

The vast majority of lower reproductive tract laser surgery has been directed at the treatment of intraepithelial neoplasia and clinically evident human papillomavirus (HPV) infection. Because it is now known that certain HPV types are more likely to produce the dysplastic epithelial changes, it has been the practice of some laser surgeons to treat all evidence of papillomavirus infection with the laser. It is now apparent that although the laser provides a highly effective and accurate method of treating intraepithelial neoplasia and clinically evident papillomavirus infection (ie, warts), the laser does not eradicate the virus from the lower reproductive tract.

Colposcopy has provided the most accurate technique for identifying lesions of intraepithelial neoplasia and HPV, and laser surgery for this spectrum of disease has most often been carried out with a CO_2 laser mounted on a colposcope. An alternative method of laser surgery includes the use of the laser handpiece while the surgeon visualizes the operative field through the colposcope. In either case a variable magnification colposcope is a *must*. It is this microsurgical approach to the lower reproductive tract that has made the laser so effective.

Laser Surgery of the Cervix

Although cervical intraepithelial neoplasia (CIN) has been described as a surface phenomenon, it is well known that it involves the endocervical crypts. In 1978 Malcolm Anderson measured the depth of crypt involvement, and found that 99% of CIN extends no further than 4 mm from the surface epithelium into the cervical crypt. A logical assumption could then be made that if an area of intraepithelial neoplasia on the cervix is either excised or vaporized to a depth greater than 4 mm, virtually all the neoplastic process would be irradiated. This concept of depth of crypt involvement is extremely important to the laser surgeon, particularly when the cervix is to be vaporized rather than a conization specimen excised. Atypical epithelial changes almost always start in the transformation zone. Additionally, intraepithelial neoplasia is almost always found in contact with the original squamous epithelium of the cervix. The neoplastic process does not arise in isolated foci of metaplasia found elsewhere in the transformation zone or in the endocervical canal. Thus multifocal CIN or skip lesions (lesions not in contact with the main focus on CIN) are rare. It follows that if the lesion of intraepithelial neoplasia is visualized in its entirety— that is, if the borders of the lesion are clearly seen on the cervix and the lesion does not extend up into the canal—then the entire lesion can be biopsied and correctly diagnosed as intraepithelial neoplasia. This assumption provides the justification for all ablative procedures used to destroy intraepithelial disease.

The reserve cells and columnar cells of the transformation zone constitute the cell population at risk for the development of atypical squamous metaplasia and CIN. In the early days of laser surgery surgeons attempted to destroy only the visible lesion and not the entire transformation zone. Unfortunately this practice has been associated with a high rate of persistence or recurrence of the CIN, a fact that rapidly became apparent to early users of the laser. Since 1978 surgeons have made it a practice to destroy the entire transformation zone, including the visible lesion, to a measured depth.

Cervical conization has been defined as an operation that removes a volume of tissue from the central longitudinal axis of the cervix; this includes the external os and a certain length of endocervical canal. The actual shape of the volume of tissue removed should be determined by the distribution of the lesion and not by some preconceived geometric shape. Conization, then, is a generic term, and does not necessarily imply that a perfect cone-shaped defect has been produced in the cervix. Cones can be asymmetric, and are short, long, thin, or cylindrical, or any other shape that accomplishes the intended goal of complete removal of the lesion and the tissue at risk. A number of techniques have been used to perform conization operations. In laser surgery the instrument may be used as a scalpel to excise. The end results of either excisional laser conization or laser vaporization for CIN are essentially the same. There is a central defect in the longitudinal axis of the cervix surrounding the cervical canal that has been created by the laser, and the cervical stroma has been coagulated for hemostasis by laser heat energy. The term vaporization conization is, therefore, often used to describe the laser vaporization procedure performed on the cervix for the treatment of CIN.

CIN that involves the endocervical canal, and for that reason cannot be entirely visualized, or a neoplasm that cannot be properly diagnosed for any reason must not be treated by an ablative procedure. Although the visible lesion may be intraepithelial, the nonvisualized lesion in the canal may be invasive. The requirements for vaporization conization are listed in Table 21-2.

Vaporization Conization

Vaporization conization may be performed in the office, the clinic, or the operating room. We have used the CO_2 laser coupled to the colposcope by micromanipulator for the vast majority of cervical conizations; however, we also have performed successful vaporization conizations using a KTP laser with the laser handpiece and colposcope. General anesthesia usually is not required for cervical vaporization, particularly if the patient has been carefully reassured about the laser surgery and the nature of her disease. Preoperative medication may include antiprostaglandins, which may reduce the cramping that accompanies the laser ablation. Local anesthesia may be directly injected into the cervix. We use a 10-ml syringe and inject lidocaine 1% into the cervix in 1-ml aliquots around the circumference and into the stroma. Some patients demand general anesthesia, and this is done on an outpatient basis.

TABLE 21–2
Vaporization Conization Requirements

The lesion must be completely visualized.
The transformation zone must be completely seen.
There is no doubt as to the intraepithelial nature of the disease.
Adenocarcinoma of the endocervical canal has been ruled out.

The patient is placed in the dorsal lithotomy position, and a bivalve speculum is inserted into the vagina. No drapes are used and no prep is necessary. The cervix is cleaned with a 4% acetic acid solution, and the lesion again identified. The margin is outlined by a series of "dots," using short bursts of laser energy (Fig. 21-5A). The entire transformation zone is included in the area to be vaporized, and a margin of at least 2 mm allowed peripheral to the lesion.

The dots are then connected so that the cone is completely outlined (Fig. 21-5B). A spot size of about 2 mm is appropriate to this vaporization operation. We prefer power settings of about 25 W; however, the laser surgeon should select a power setting that is comfortable to use. High power settings mean that the surgery must be carried out quickly, whereas lower power settings mean greater ease of vaporization and accurate observation of the depth of the defect. The defect is carried to 7 mm, and the surgeon should attempt to measure the depth accurately. The cervix and the area of the external os often are not flush, and an accurate measurement of depth of vaporization may be difficult. For this reason, it seems more accurate to divide the cervix into four quadrants and then destroy the tissue quadrant by quadrant (Fig. 21-5C). In this way part of the normal cervical anatomy is preserved throughout the operation, and even though the topography of the cervix may change, the exact depth of destruction can always be measured for each quadrant. When all four quadrants have been vaporized to 7 mm, we then vaporize an additional 2 to 3 mm up into the endocervical canal. This technique has been used to avoid a prolapse of the endocervical canal, which often is seen when the vaporization defect is totally cylindrical with a flat base (Fig. 21-6). It is desirable to place the new squamocolumnar junction just inside the external os, so that metaplastic epithelium is not constantly bathed in the same vaginal milieu that initiated the development of

CIN. Although the location of the new squamocolumnar junction is at times unpredictable, the laser surgery produces a more predictable end result than do other methods of conization.

Bleeding may be encountered during vaporization procedures, particularly in the large chronically infected cervix. If bleeding does occur, a cotton-tipped applicator is used to tamponade the vessel. The power density is lowered by defocusing the beam or by slightly reducing power, and the bleeding point is coagulated by using a rapid circular motion to surround the vessel. If bleeding is more active, or if there is a "pumper" in the cervical stroma, other forms of coagulation should be considered. If bleeding is particularly worrisome, a small figure-of-eight stitch with a fine suture material will ensure hemostasis.

Excisional Conization of the Cervix

The goals of excisional conization are to produce a conization biopsy specimen that is adequate for pathologic examination and, if possible, to excise all disease. The indications for laser excisional conization are the same as for cold-knife conization and are given in Table 21-3.

The average excisional conization penetrates the cervical stroma more deeply than vaporization conization, and the patient may experience more discomfort as well as more bleeding with this procedure. Although excisional conization may be satisfactorily performed with local anesthesia, we do not hesitate to perform this procedure on an outpatient basis under general anesthesia. Before starting an excisional conization, the surgeon must decide on the size of the cone, which, again, is tailored to fit the patient and the lesion. Some surgeons who are adept at endoscopy believe that the lesion in the canal can be evaluated by contact hysteroscopy. In any case, the endocervical canal should be

Figure 21–5. Cervical vaporization for CIN. The cervix is reexamined with the colposcope and A, the margin of the vaporization conization outlined by a series of "dots," B, the dots are connected and the cervix divided into the four quadrants, and C, the tissue is vaporized quadrant by quadrant to a depth of 7 mm.

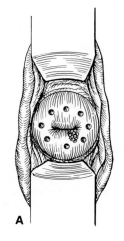
A

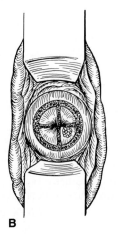
B

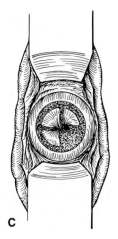
C

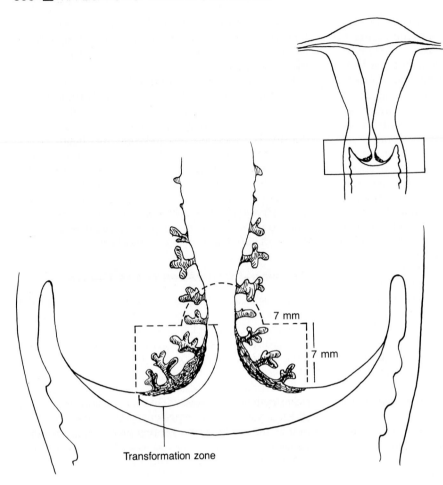

7 mm

7 mm

Transformation zone

Figure 21–6. Cervical vaporization defect. After the cervix has been vaporized to the appropriate depth, an additional 3 mm of endocervical canal is vaporized to avoid endocervical prolapse and to ensure that the new squamocolumnar junction is just inside of the external os.

TABLE 21–3
Indications for Excisional Conization

The lesion disappears into the canal.
The entire transformation zone cannot be visualized.
Abnormal cytologic smear in the absence of positive colposcopic findings cannot be explained.
The endocervical curettage is indicative of disease in the canal.
Invasive cancer has not been ruled out by biopsy.

sounded; severe dysplasia with obvious worrisome canal involvement will require a larger and deeper cone specimen.

A weighted posterior retractor is placed in the vagina and the anterior lip of the cervix grasped with a single-toothed tenaculum. The surgeon may choose to use either the CO_2 laser with micromanipulator or the YAG laser with the sapphire scalpel tip. The cervix is painted with 4% acetic acid and the patient recolposcoped. The visible borders of the lesion are again carefully noted, and the external cervical margin of the cone is outlined. In the excisional procedures, high power and small spot size are used for cutting, so that hemostatic effect is minimized. For this reason, a dilute solution of vasopressin 1.5% is injected through a 25-gauge needle at 1-ml increments around the cervix. With the CO_2 laser set for 25 to 50 W and a spot size of 0.5 to 1.0 mm, the incision is made straight into the cervical stroma and deepened to 3 to 4 mm. Superpulse for the CO_2 laser also may be effectively used to reduce lateral thermal damage. Smoke evacuation is carried out by an assistant who holds a suction wand close to the target zone. The stromal edge of the incision is grasped with a single-toothed forceps or a laser conization hook. Gentle traction is applied to facilitate laser cutting and allow the surgeon to view the depth of the incision. The cone specimen is peeled away from the cervical stroma as the laser beam slices through the tissue and works toward the canal. After removal of the cone specimen, spot size is enlarged to 2 mm and the stroma coagulated superficially to prevent delayed hemorrhage.

Laser Combination Conization Procedures

Vaporization procedures and excisional conization may be performed together for the diagnosis and treatment of certain cases of CIN. Large areas of intraepithelial neoplasia or multifocal lesions that involve much of the cervix, including the endocervical canal, and then extend into the vagina or even involve the vulva are best treated by combination laser procedures. The endocervical lesion must be removed by laser excisional conization, but the peripheral portions of the lesion that have been previously biopsied and proved benign may be vaporized. Thus the indications for both excisional and vaporization conization have been met and a conservative procedure has been carried out. Baggish and Dorsey have shown that the volume of tissue removed by a combination of vaporization and excision is far less than that removed by excision alone. Combination procedures constitute the most conservative operation possible, since the operation is microsurgical and tailored to fit each situation. The pathologist must be aware that the peripheral margin of the excisional cone may be positive for intraepithelial disease.

Postoperative Instructions

Patients who undergo cervical vaporization or excisional procedures usually require little postoperative care. We instruct our patients to avoid coitus for at least 4 weeks and to report any unusual fever or bleeding. About 15% of these patients have some vaginal bleeding; however, the amount is only significant in about 2% of the patients. The patient is asked to inform the physician if the bleeding becomes heavier than with a normal menstrual period. She is allowed to return to work within 48 hours. There are definite advantages associated with laser conization. These are listed in Table 21-4.

Results of Laser Surgery of the Cervix

In the early days of laser surgery, before 1982, a number of authors reported disappointing results with laser surgery for intraepithelial neoplasia. As techniques of laser surgery became better defined and understood, the results have improved. Baggish and Dorsey reported a series of more than 4000 cases of CIN treated by CO_2 laser with an overall success rate above 95% in those patients followed by colposcopy, cytology, and biopsy for a year or more. Vaporization and excisional conization procedures seem to produce about the same cure rate. In addition, cure rates do not

TABLE 21-4
Advantages of Laser Conization

Less bleeding occurs than with a scalpel.
Less tissue damage occurs than with the electric cautery.
The procedure can be done with much more precision, and results are better for lesions of all sizes than with cryosurgery.
Morbidity is low.
All types and extent of intraepithelial neoplasia can be treated.
The most conservative procedures can be carried out utilizing combinations of vaporization and excision.

vary when degree of CIN is taken into consideration. Other authors, such as Burke and coworkers, report success rates between 95% and 98%.

Cure is a somewhat difficult term to define. Most laser surgeons have used colposcopy and cytology to evaluate the cervix at the end of 1 year, and if no intraepithelial neoplasia can be demonstrated, "cure" is presumed. On the other hand, it has become obvious in our own large series that although intraepithelial neoplasia may not be present, evidence of HPV has not disappeared from the lower reproductive tract as a result of the lasing. It, therefore, remains to be seen how many of these patients will once again develop intraepithelial neoplasia from viral persistence or repeat exposure. It appears that by placing the transformation zone higher in the endocervical canal, the incidence of recurrence of CIN becomes small.

Laser Surgery of the Vulva

Unlike the cervix, the vulva often is the site of multifocal disease, and HPV and vulvar intraepithelial neoplasia (VIN) remain the most common target of the laser. There is no doubt that the importance of identification of disease and depth of destruction also must be applied to the therapy of VIN. Vulvar disease and vulvar laser surgery should be done with the aid of the colposcope, and we usually prefer to use the micromanipulator. It also is absolutely imperative that the surgeon who performs laser surgery on the vulva or the vagina have a working knowledge of vulvovaginal histology and of the thickness of normal and abnormal neoplastic vulvovaginal epithelium.

Vulvar skin is composed of two layers, epidermis and dermis (Fig. 21-7). The margin between epidermis and dermis is an irregular one because of the rete ridges. Between the rete ridges are projections of dermis known as dermal papillae. The dermis can be divided into two layers, the superficial papillary layer and the deeper reticular layer. There also are skin appendages, such as pilosebaceous follicles, eccrine sweat glands,

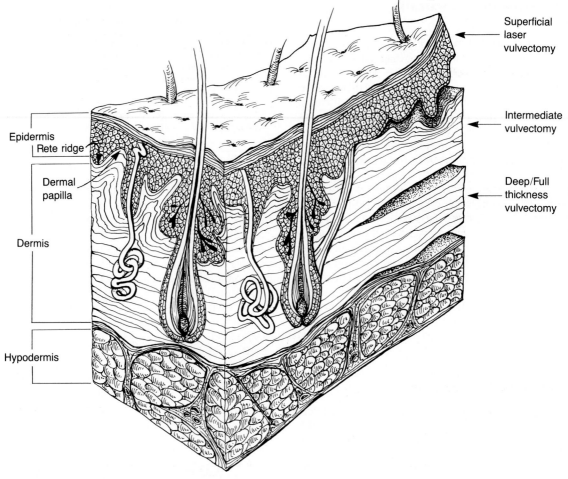

Figure 21–7. Vulvar skin. Vulvar skin is composed of epidermis and dermis plus the skin appendages. Complete removal of the epidermis and partial removal of the dermis still results in reepithelialization of the wound because of squamous recolonization from the skin appendages.

and apocrine glands, which project deep into the dermis. VIN, as well as HPV, may involve skin appendages as well as epidermis. Although the thickness of the epidermis may be a fraction of a millimeter, the dermis may measure 7 to 8 mm in thickness, and skin appendages may involve full thickness. It is the goal of the laser surgeon to remove the involved epidermis as well as a portion of the skin appendage, which also may be involved in the disease process.

In plastic surgery when a split-thickness graft is removed from a donor site, or in laser surgery when the entire epidermis is removed by a vaporization procedure, the operative site heals without replacement by a skin graft because the skin appendages located in the dermis have not been completely destroyed. Each skin appendage serves as a source of squamous epithelium, so that when reepithelialization takes place, the process proceeds from the skin appendages as well as from the periphery. On the other hand, if the entire thickness of the dermis is taken and the skin appendages are completely destroyed, the operative site must be grafted if the defect is large.

Unlike cervical vaporization, the depth of the vaporization on the vulva cannot be measured. The expert laser microsurgeon is able to recognize the depth of ablation and removes epidermis so accurately that the papillary dermis is not destroyed. The papillary dermis is identified at colposcopic magnifications. Reid has suggested that four surgical planes can be identified. The first surgical plane represents the epidermis down to the basement membrane. The second surgical plane is described as extending into the papillary layer of the dermis, so that the laser surgeon removes both the epidermis and the papillary dermis. The third surgical plane reaches well into the reticular dermis and uncovers the coarse collagen bundles that can be seen through the colposcope as grayish white fibers. The fourth surgical plane involves complete removal of the skin right down to the underlying subdermal fat.

Condylomata Acuminata

The papillomavirus involves the epidermis and also may involve the superficial portions of the skin append-ages. One of the common mistakes of the novice sur-geon is to go too deeply into the dermis in an attempt to destroy condylomas. Although only the warty lesion itself plus the surrounding epidermal margin need to be destroyed, a power density that is sufficient to ac-complish this maneuver without creating excessive car-bonization at the impact site must be used. Power densi-ties below 600 W/cm^2 cause excessive carbonization, and irradiance of carbonized surface of the vulva will raise laser impact site temperatures to more than 600° C. The power densities that we like to use are between 600 and 1500 W/cm^2, and a 2- to 3-mm focal spot size with a power setting of 15 to 30 W will accomplish this. Each condyloma should be identified and the laser beam directed to the center of this target. Laser heat energy collapses the tissues inwardly as vaporization occurs. The surrounding skin is then rapidly brushed with the beam. The char and debris are wiped away and the proper surgical level colposcopically identified. Va-porization is taken to the papillary dermis (second surgical plane). Cold saline solution is used to cool the vulvar skin, as cooling helps to reduce the heat diffu-sion and, therefore, resultant tissue injury lateral to the laser impact site.

Vulvar Intraepithelial Neoplasia

It is impossible to differentiate colposcopically be-tween some forms of HPV lesions that occur on the vulva and significant VIN. It is, therefore, extremely important to biopsy the vulva in as many areas as necessary to correctly identify the pathology before laser surgery. Local or general anesthesia may be used for vulvar laser surgery. In the case of multiple lesions or very large areas of involvement, general anesthesia is more practical. Despite extensive vulvar laser surgery, patients usually are allowed to return home on the day of the operation.

The vulva is recolposcoped with 4% acetic acid ap-plied to demonstrate areas and borders of neoplastic or viral involvement. The larger areas are outlined in the same way as described for CIN. If a lesion is very large, it may be divided into smaller areas for lasing, as this provides a more accurate approach. As soon as the laser beam is passed over the surface of the tissue, all land-marks disappear. Proper identification and marking of the limits of the disease by the laser is a highly neces-sary step in treatment. Again, a spot size of 2 to 3 mm and a power setting of 15 to 50 W may be used. Although destruction needs to be carried to the third surgical plane—that is, the reticular dermis—the first step in vulvar laser surgery always involves identifying the pap-illary dermis. When the tiny micropapules of this layer are seen, the laser surgeon again ablates through this most superficial dermis, wiping away char and identify-ing the underlying reticular dermis. Often intermittent pulses of laser energy can improve surgical control of the laser beam. Instead of reducing the power of the beam, it is possible to use the mechanical timer on the laser console to reduce exposure by delivering 1/10- to 1/20-second bursts of laser energy. This technique per-mits the surgeon time to react and maintain a satisfac-tory rate of energy delivery. This technique also re-duces char and residual thermal damage.

Postoperative Care

If the lasing has been extensive, a Foley catheter may be required to avoid the immediate discomfort caused by urinary salts on the denuded vulvar surface. Cathe-ters can be placed either through the urethra or supra-pubically. Suprapubic drainage avoids the deposit of urinary salts on the wound, which reduces pain and the risk of possible infection.

Customarily, an antibacterial cream or ointment such as sulfadine cream or bacitracin ointment is applied to the laser wound to protect the raw surface from aggluti-nation and to help prevent superficial infection. The patient must be given instructions to keep the vulvar folds separated, and the application of this medication helps in this respect. An ice pack is placed on the vulva on leaving the operating room. Sitz baths begin on the first day after laser surgery, and are continued three times a day until the patient is no longer uncomfortable and the vulvar area is well on the way to reepithelializa-tion. The patient is seen in a week to make sure there is no agglutination of vulvar folds. Because it is possible for new lesions to appear during the healing period, weekly colposcopic inspection helps to identify this problem immediately, so that adjunctive therapy may begin.

Results of Vulvar Laser Surgery

The results of laser surgery on the vulva have been quite satisfactory. It appears that there are some defi-nite advantages to using the CO_2 laser for this disease. In our own series of more than 100 patients with intra-epithelial neoplasia, 1-year cure rates have been over 90%. Other lower reproductive tract laser surgeons report similar rates. One of the greatest benefits of vulvar laser surgery is that normal vulvar anatomy is maintained. This may not be possible if conventional techniques, such as skinning vulvectomy, are used.

Vaginal Laser Surgery

Vaginal intraepithelial neoplasia (VAIN) and associated HPV infections are among the most difficult of lower reproductive tract intraepithelial neoplasias to treat for a number of reasons: (a) the vagina has a large surface area that is difficult to screen colposcopically; (b) there are many rugae and folds in the vagina; (c) the angle of the vaginal axis makes it difficult to treat by perpendicular beam impact; (d) the vaginal fornices are difficult to stabilize, as they are quite distensible and the cervix may hide portions of the fornices; (e) the colposcopic appearance of VAIN is tremendously varied and often goes unrecognized even by the expert colposcopist.

Colposcopically, VAIN does not demonstrate mosaic patterns except in areas of adenosis. One often sees coarse punctation, but the lesion may vary in color from a pale grayish white to the intense whiteness produced by hyperkeratosis and acanthosis. Most often the lesions are multifocal and the borders usually are distinct, although the lesions may be somewhat serpiginous.

The laser microsurgeon must be particularly aggressive in obtaining adequate biopsies from VAIN. If the patient has had a hysterectomy, the lateral fornix may contain a dimple that must be everted for adequate visualization and biopsy. A laser hook or a skin hook may be used to evert this area and stabilize the tissue, so that appropriate biopsy can be obtained. Once again, it must be emphasized that the surgeon should be absolutely sure of the diagnosis before vaporization is performed. If the surgeon is not sure, then the vaginal lesion must be excised.

Technique for Vaporization of VAIN

The squamous epithelium of the vaginal mucous membrane rests on a basement membrane. Below this is the lamina propria, which corresponds to the dermis of the vulvar skin. Below the lamina propria is a layer of muscle and loose connective tissue and fat. When the vaginal epithelium is destroyed, there must be a visual identification of the underlying lamina propria, since, as in the case of the vulva, it is impossible to accurately measure the depth of destruction in this irregular area. Because the vaginal squamous epithelium is only a fraction of a millimeter thick and there are no skin appendages in the vagina, ablation is a superficial operation.

Lasing the vagina is painful for the vast majority of patients, and although some small lesions in the vaginal vault can be vaporized without anesthesia, the chances of producing pain with vaginal laser surgery are high. The manipulation of the speculum also can be painful to the patient. In an effort to manipulate the target into a position that is perpendicular to the laser beam, the surgeon often cocks the speculum to one side and shoots through the open sides. The vaginal rugae also must be ironed out to ensure even laser energy application; all of this is most uncomfortable. For this reason, the majority of my patients treated for VAIN have undergone general anesthesia on an outpatient basis.

The micromanipulator is preferred, as it eliminates bulky and unnecessary instrumentation from the vagina. We prefer to use a spot size of 2 mm and power settings of 20 to 30 W. Large areas are subdivided so that more accurate ablation can be performed. The laser beam is rapidly passed over the area and the epithelium lifted away from the underlying lamina propria. A wet sponge or cotton swab is used to wipe away char and coagulated epithelium. Many surgeons find that the tops or rugae have been removed, but the troughs or valleys in between still contain viable dysplastic epithelium. By proper use of the speculum and other instruments this problem is easily overcome. Adequate margins of 5 mm or more are always planned.

Postoperative Care

Most of the discomfort encountered in postoperative vaginal laser surgery stems from laser wounds in the vaginal introitus. Because VAIN and VIN often are multifocal diseases, many of these patients will have had extensive laser surgery of the entire lower reproductive tract. In addition to sitz baths and protective vulvar creams, we also use daily vaginal applications of either estrogen or sulfa cream or some other bacteriostatic preparation. The patient also should be examined on a weekly basis to make sure that vaginal coaptation is not occurring. Vaginal healing usually takes place from the periphery of the wound because of the lack of skin appendages in the vaginal mucosa. If the laser surgeon has been thorough and the denuded area is large, healing often is delayed and granulation tissue may result. The granulation tissue may be removed and the wound then touched with a silver nitrate stick.

Results of Laser Vaporization of VAIN

We have recently analyzed a series of 60 patients treated in our clinic with CO_2 laser for VAIN. Although Townsend has reported satisfactory cure rates in the laser therapy of this disease, our recurrence rates for multifocal HPV associated VAIN are about 30% within the first year. On the other hand, unicentric VAIN has a better than 90% chance of cure with one laser surgery.

As is the case with the vulva, if patient and physician are willing to retreat and use some adjunctive therapeutic measures, the 1-year cure rates are above 95%.

Indications for Laser Surgery and HPV Infection

Although 1-year cure rates produced by laser surgery for lower reproductive tract intraepithelial neoplasia have been satisfactory, particularly in the case of the cervix, the persistence or recurrence of wart virus lesions has been discouraging to patient and physician alike. Our inability to cure HPV manifestations has led many laser surgeons to question the indications for laser surgery for this disease. Most agree that intraepithelial neoplasia should be treated; however, disagreement concerning the advisability or necessity for therapy of minor HPV infection prevails. For example, patients who have evidence of HPV infection found on a cytologic smear or who have whitish change in the vaginal introitus after application of acetic acid are debatable candidates for laser surgery. Because recurrence or persistence of subclinical HPV is so common, it seems more logical to follow these patients carefully but not subject them to surgery unless significant change occurs.

Adjunctive Therapy in Laser Surgery

Because of the disappointing recurrence rates of clinically evident wart virus infection, other methods of treating the disease often are combined with laser surgery. This is particularly true when the patient is aware of her clinical disease and wishes that every possible effort be made to rid her of its manifestations. We often use local applications of trichloroacetic acid (TCA) and 5-fluorouracil (5-FU). TCA is a caustic agent that precipitates the proteins in the epithelium at the site of application. Our patients are colposcoped on a weekly basis during the healing period, and obvious lesions are carefully touched with 90% TCA. The application is limited to a very small area, and often needs to be repeated on a weekly basis until success is achieved. The beneficial effect of the application is achieved almost instantaneously, and if the patient complains of burning, sodium bicarbonate on a cotton swab is applied to the area. This immediately neutralizes the acid.

5-FU has been used by dermatologists to treat superficially invasive neoplasms since the early 1960s. As reported by Krebs, topical 5-FU penetrates abnormal skin and inhibits both DNA and RNA synthesis as well as having an immunostimulatory action. 5-FU is available in a 5% cream in a hydrophilic base (Efudex). After vulvovaginal laser surgery in patients with extensive disease, the 5-FU cream is applied to the vulva and vagina by means of a vaginal applicator once a week for a 10-week course. Most patients tolerate this treatment well. Some patients can tolerate an application two times a week. This type of aggressive adjunctive therapy seems to eliminate clinical disease in a high percentage of patients. The use of 5-FU in the reproductive-age group has been of some concern, and patients must be strongly warned concerning the possible teratogenic effects of the compound. It is wise to have this group of patients sign an informed consent relating to this therapy.

Several clinical trials are under way to evaluate the use of interferon in the treatment of recurrent or persistent warts. A certain subset of patients seems particulary unable to develop the immune response necessary to control HPV infection. Interferon plus laser cytoreductive surgery appears to be a promising approach for such cases.

Anal Intraepithelial Neoplasia

Because of the high frequency of multifocal disease, colposcopic examination is not complete without inspection of the perianal tissue and the anal canal. Exactly the same techniques are used for the diagnosis and treatment of intraepithelial neoplasia and HPV in this region, as described previously. A pediatric speculum can be used to inspect the anal canal. The surgeon should be careful to avoid lasing into hemorrhoids, but if bleeding does occur, it usually is easily controlled by laser or by a stitch. A theoretical hazard of laser surgery in this region is the ignition or possible explosion of methane gas from the bowel. We often have used a wet gauze sponge inserted into the rectum to keep stool out of the field; this also guards against methane gas explosion. In our clinic we have never experienced this complication.

Lower Reproductive Tract Laser Surgery with the Fiberoptic Lasers

The desire to find the perfect laser suitable for all surgical operations continues to spur the usage of other laser systems for gynecologic laser surgery. The advantages of the fiberoptic lasers (ie, less bulky delivery systems and greater ability to coagulate) make them an attractive alternative for some lower reproductive tract procedures. The argon and KTP 532 lasers produce effective vaporizing wavelengths and, because of deeper penetration of laser energy, also provide an excellent mechanism for coagulation. Vaporization conization can be carried out in a manner similar to that of CO_2 laser conization. The 600-μm fiber is used with a laser handpiece and the operative procedure performed under colposcopic magnifications, using 15 to 20 W of power. The tip of the fiber should be held just off the surface of the cervical tissue. Results of conization procedures are the same as for CO_2 laser vaporization, and hemostasis and cervical healing are excellent.

We also have used the KTP 532 in the treatment of VAIN, VIN, and condylomas of the lower reproductive tract. Because of the deeper tissue penetration, one must be careful in treating these lesions. Of our first 50 patients treated for lower reproductive tract lesions with KTP laser, all patients were followed for at least 1 year. Biopsy done at the time of surgery on our first ten patients showed that there was definitely a zone of coagulation necrosis in the papillary dermis that measures about 1 mm. There seems to have been less pain in patients treated with KTP 532, perhaps because of this thin layer of coagulation. Healing is slightly slower than with CO_2 laser vulvectomy. The end result, however, is similar to that in CO_2 laser patients.

Excisional conizations done with the argon and KTP lasers are a bit more difficult, since the fiber does not cut cervical stroma particularly well. Cold-knife conization of the cervix followed immediately by laser coagulation of the cervical stroma has produced a satisfactory alternative.

YAG laser also has been used with success on lower reproductive tract lesions. Because YAG does not vaporize well, some surgeons prefer to use YAG to coagulate large condylomas and allow the necrotic debris to slough. This result does not seem to be as satisfactory as that of CO_2 vaporization. On the other hand, the advent of the sapphire tip applied to the YAG fiber has tremendously increased its usage for the lower reproductive tract. The YAG scalpel can be used to produce a satisfactory cone specimen, and the hemostatic effect of the YAG continues to be an advantage. For vaporization, the rounded sapphire tip dispenses YAG energy over its surface and produces good contact vaporization with concomitant hemostasis.

INTRA-ABDOMINAL LASER SURGERY

Intra-abdominal laser surgery in gynecology began in the late 1970s, and by the first part of the 1980s, there were a substantial number of reports from both Europe and the United States dealing with CO_2 laser usage for adhesiolysis and infertility surgery. The laser has offered an entirely new dimension to open abdominal infertility surgery, since it can be mounted on an operative microscope and the beam directed by a micromanipulator located above and out of the operative site.

Alternatively, it can be used with a handpiece in conjunction with either the microscope or surgical loops. It also can be coupled with the operative laparoscope or used with an intra-abdominal probe. This is perhaps the most exciting and promising use of lasers in the abdominal cavity.

OPEN ABDOMINAL LASER SURGERY

The great majority of laser laparotomies reported in the literature have been carried out by gynecologic surgeons using the CO_2 laser. Safety, small residual thermal damage, and great variability of focal spot size contribute to the appeal of this instrument.

In the abdominal cavity, laser surgery and conventional techniques go hand in hand. The laser surgeon uses the same microsurgical instrumentation as in conventional microsurgery but has added some special instruments for use with the laser. Although the laser has been used for many types of intra-abdominal procedures, we have found it to be most useful for (a) adhesiolysis, particularly the filmy types of adhesions that often distort the adnexa; (b) ablation of endometriosis; and (c) certain types of tubal reconstructive procedures, such as neosalpingostomy.

There are a number of possible equipment variations for CO_2 laser surgery at laparotomy. Some surgeons prefer to use the hand-held laser with magnification supplied by the operative microscope. In our clinic we prefer this method, since the laser handpiece can be used with a short focal length focusing lens, producing an impact diameter of less than 0.2 mm.

General Principles

Paper drapes should not be used by the laser surgeon. The newer, disposable laparotomy drapes are flame-resistant, and although the drape may literally melt, there is no danger of fire. Protective wet cotton packs are always used for the wound edges and the bowel and other exposed organs. Laser energy may be reflected from polished instruments, and all delicate surfaces should be protected.

The proper power density must be selected for each laser procedure. In general, power densities used in intra-abdominal laser surgery are relatively low, varying between 5 and 30 W. Superpulse often is used for cutting to further limit lateral thermal damage, but the use of continuous wave gated pulses also may give greater control for the laser surgeon when either vaporizing or cutting.

Because laser energy continues to travel and damage background tissue once it cuts through the target, the surgeon often must select an appropriate backstop. Various microsurgical dissecting rods are available to use as both dissecting tools and laser backstops. In general, glass, Pyrex, and quartz rods should be avoided, since they shatter under the intense heat of the laser. The surgeon must always keep the temperature of the dissecting rod at appropriate levels by constant irrigation and cleansing of char. Titanium or smooth blackened rods serve as excellent backstop dissectors.

Although the laser is superb for coagulating tiny bleeders, vessels larger than 0.5 mm in diameter may be difficult to coagulate with the CO_2 laser. If it is not immediately apparent that the laser is achieving hemostasis without significant damage to tissue, conventional methods of hemostasis should be used. The surgeon should not hesitate to use a bipolar electrode or precise atraumatic microsurgical suturing to minimize tissue damage. Char must always be cleared or washed away from lased tissue. Not only are carbon particles incorporated into the peritoneal scar, but scorched tissue impedes healing and decreases the ability of the surgeon to visually recognize tissue planes. Wet cotton-tipped applicators help in gentle removal of char and often serve as excellent backstops.

The laser mirror also is an instrument that may allow the surgeon to operate in inaccessible areas. For example, the ovary that is adherent to the lateral pelvic wall often may be freed by visualizing the adherent surface in the mirror and then directing the laser beam from the mirror to the adhesion. The best mirrors have polished gold reflecting surfaces. Dental mirrors cannot be used because of the possibility of shatter. Mirrors tend to be clouded rapidly by laser smoke and other debris, so that constant polishing and wiping are required.

Removal of the laser plume is extremely important, as the smoke is unpleasant to breathe and may carry some health hazards.

CO₂ Laser Adhesiolysis

Adhesiolysis with the laser has been performed mainly by reproductive surgeons to enhance fertility. There are few published studies that attempt to prove efficacy of the CO_2 laser over conventional surgery for adhesiolysis. In addition, few surgeons use a system of grading adhesions, and it is, therefore, difficult to accumulate statistically meaningful numbers of equivalent patients in study subsets. Differences in technique and abilities of surgeons also make comparisons less meaningful.

There are a number of techniques that are useful in laser adhesiolysis. The operation varies with the type of adhesion. In general, three maneuvers are used:

1. Laser incision of thick adhesions is performed using a small spot size and high-power density. Dense adhesive bands usually are cut with spot sizes of 0.2 to 1.0 mm and power settings in the 20- to 30-W range.
2. Filmy adhesions are vaporized and divided with much lower power density. The defocused beam often is used, and when the appropriate backstop is applied, the adhesion can literally be made to disappear without damage to underlying structures.
3. Thick adhesions between delicate structures, such as tube and ovary, may be lased with intermediate power density and spot size. Gentle traction and a good assistant who is knowledgeable in the use of the dissecting rods and backstops can present the adhesions to the surgeon, and by exerting gentle traction the adhesion is vaporized with minimal or no residual tissue damage.

Laser Laparotomy for Endometriosis

Endometrial implants can be effectively vaporized by CO_2 laser energy. Implants and endometriomas that are large may be more effectively excised by CO_2 laser or by conventional instrumentation. Incomplete vaporization often results in persistence of disease. We prefer to excise all endometrial ovarian cysts rather than vaporize them, since these bulky lesions have a tendency to recur. Small spot size and high-power density are used for excision. Endometrial ovarian cysts resected with a CO_2 laser may require suturing; raw surfaces of the peritoneum and other structures should be closed by conventional microsurgical techniques when possible. The results of laser surgery for patients with endometriosis seem comparable to the results produced by other careful operative procedures using conventional techniques. Pregnancy rates and recurrence rates are essentially the same. Many laser surgeons, however, believe that laser surgery speeds the operative procedure.

Laser Surgery of the Tube

There has been tremendous progress in the surgical treatment of tubal disease over the past 15 years because of the adaptation of microsurgical principles for cases of tubal infertility. Laser vaporization and excision add new dimensions to the practice of microsurgery. As with conventional microsurgery, three types of laser tubal microsurgical procedures usually are described, depending on the anatomic region of the tube involved. These are terminal tuboplasty, tubotubal anastomosis, and tubouterine anastomosis.

Terminal salpingostomy is suitable for laser surgery. The success of this procedure is related to the amount of terminal tube that has to be removed to effect satisfactory neostomy. The best result depends on identifying the original site of the tubal ostium and then opening this area with the focused laser beam and freeing what is left of the fimbria. The tube is gently distended by intrauterine injection of dilute indigo carmine solution or methylene blue, so that use of a backstop is not necessary. As laser incision of this area proceeds, the lumen is immediately identified as the dye appears. Three or four radial incisions may be made in the clubbed tube, so that satisfactory eversion of the mucosa results. The defocused laser beam also may be applied to the tubal serosa, which contracts, thereby producing mucosal eversion. We have found that it usually is more satisfactory to use 9-0 nylon sutures to effect a permanent eversion of the fimbria or ampullary mucosa.

Preparing the tubes for tubal reanastomosis also can be performed by laser tubal resection. Once again, the focused beam with small spot size of 0.2 mm and power setting of 10 W on the superpulsed beam is used to cut through the tube. Hemostasis usually results; however, if bleeding occurs in the mesosalpinx, conventional hemostasis is used. Suture with 9-0 nylon through the muscularis is used, as with conventional microsurgical techniques, to effect the anastomosis. Ampullary-to-ampullary, ampullary-to-isthmic, and isthmic-to-isthmic anastomosis are done in exactly the same way as described in earlier chapters.

We have carried out a number of tubouterine anastomoses for patients with proximal tubal obstruction. The cornual shave technique is the preferred method, and we have found no advantage of laser over microelectrode or the knife.

The results of CO_2 laser surgery often are compared with the results of tubomicrosurgery with microelectrode. Bellina has reported excellent results with CO_2 laser that are comparable to those achieved by conventional microsurgical methods. He also believes that operative time has been reduced by using the CO_2 laser. On the other hand, it appears that expert microsurgeons who champion a particular method have developed a tremendous confidence with their favorite tool. Superiority of one modality over the other remains to be established. It appears that microsurgical technique and a competent surgeon plus extent of the disease are the most important factors in tubal reconstructive surgery.

Laser Myomectomy

The CO_2 laser as well as the fiberoptic lasers have been used effectively for myomectomy. A 1.5% solution of vasopressin is injected into the surrounding myometrium and incision is made by laser. The superficial vessels on the leiomyoma can be coagulated by the defocused beam, and whether one uses the CO_2 laser or KTP, argon, or the YAG laser scalpel, hemostasis is greatly enhanced by the use of laser energy to perform the dissection.

Summary

The use of the laser in open abdominal surgery has produced encouraging results, but convincing data on laser benefit is still lacking. The laser is only one of the several tools that may be useful to the reproductive surgeon during reconstructive surgery in the open abdomen; there have been no carefully designed randomized clinical trials to demonstrate a clear advantage for laser. Perhaps an additional reason for gaining expertise in open abdominal laser surgery is that it provides appropriate background for the surgeon who wants to apply laser techniques in advanced operative laparoscopy.

LASERS IN GYNECOLOGIC ENDOSCOPY

Operative endoscopy is one of the most challenging and rapidly expanding fields in contemporary gynecologic surgery. The development of magnificent fiberoptic telescopes, safe and rapid methods for distention of both the abdominal cavity and the uterine cavity, and the design of sophisticated endoscopic accessory instruments have allowed the gynecologic surgeon to perform complicated procedures that previously required laparotomy.

Gynecologic Laser Laparoscopy

Until relatively recently, operative laparoscopy in the United States had been limited to tubal sterilization and minor types of adhesiolysis or fulguration of endometriosis. In the late 1970s Semm described techniques of laparoscopic vessel ligation and suturing, and in 1978 Bruhat used the CO_2 laser by way of the laparoscope. By the beginning of this decade laparoscopic surgeons had at their command all of the conventional ways of achieving hemostasis. This ability to reasonably assure control of hemorrhage is the key to advanced operative laparoscopic surgery (Table 21-5).

The laser alone is not adequate to ensure the type of hemostasis often needed for major laparoscopic surgery. The conventional methods of hemostasis, including suturing, ligation of vessels, and bipolar coagula-

TABLE 21–5
Methods for Achieving Laparoscopic Hemostasis

Bipolar electrocoagulation
Laser coagulation
Endoloop, endosuture, endoknot
Microsurgical sutures and ties
Endocoagulation (Semm)
Hemoclip

TABLE 21–6
CO_2 Laser Laparoscopy Disadvantages

Poor hemostasis
Cumbersome equipment
Difficult to align beam
Often difficult to identify HeNe beam
Produces much laser plume

tion, also must be mastered by the laser laparoscopist. For example, control of bleeding from the infundibulopelvic ligament during laparoscopic salpingo-oophorectomy cannot be achieved by laser. On the other hand, laser vaporization, incision, and tissue coagulation have the advantage of speed and ease when used in many of the most commonly encountered laparoscopic procedures. Most operative laparoscopies for endometriosis, adhesiolysis, ectopic pregnancy, or even ovarian cystectomy can be efficiently completed by expert use of laser alone.

CO_2 Laser Laparoscopy

The CO_2 laser can be connected to an operative laparoscope or to laparoscopic handpieces through a laser coupler that transmits the beam through a focusing lens and then down a special channel in the instrument. Laser couplers may be direct or require adjustment of the beam by means of a joystick, which is then fixed in position once the beam has been aligned with the operative channel. There usually are interchangeable lenses that provide focal lengths commensurate with the length of the laparoscope or the handpiece. Focal spot sizes produced by these systems usually are a bit less than a millimeter in diameter. The CO_2 laser is an excellent laser for laparoscopic usage, as it cuts quickly, produces little thermal damage, can be used for vaporization, coagulation, or excision, and is safe because of its absorption in water. On the other hand, there are some definite disadvantages to CO_2 laser laparoscopy, and these are listed in Table 21-6.

The mirrors in the CO_2 laser arm must be carefully aligned or the arm will lack rotational stability; when the arm is rotated, the aiming beam as well as the CO_2 beam become misaligned. The resultant reflection of the beam within the arm itself produces distortion of beam energy and significant power loss. Helium-neon (HeNe) aiming beams also are often difficult to see, particularly in a brightly lighted peritoneal cavity. Because of these difficulties, efforts to develop a fiber that will carry CO_2 laser energy have continued. Flexible, hollow waveguides, as well as stainless steel probes, currently are available. Use of these waveguide systems eliminates some of the problems with CO_2 laser en-

ergy delivery. The 2- to 3-mm diameter waveguides fit nicely through smaller operative scopes and also will pass through the smaller secondary puncture trocar sheaths.

KTP 532 and Argon Laser Laparoscopy

The fiberoptic lasers have some great advantages over CO_2, since the laser energy passes down a quartz fiber and endoscopic delivery is greatly simplified (Table 21-7). The blue or the green aiming beams of these lasers are more easily seen against the red background of the abdominal organs than is the HeNe beam. The quartz laser fibers can pass through an 18-gauge or smaller needle, so that handpieces designed for suction and irrigation also may have a central channel that accommodates the fiber. This enables the surgeon to use suction, irrigation, and laser energy through one handpiece; these handpieces fit easily through a 5-mm trocar sheath. The disadvantages of fiberoptic lasers are that they do not cut quite as well as CO_2 laser energy and they are less safe because of their penetration of both tissue and water.

YAG Laser Laparoscopy

The YAG laser has been used through the laparoscope since 1982. Most laser surgeons have considered the delivery of YAG energy by bare fiber rather dangerous for use in the abdominal cavity, since YAG energy penetrates up to 4 mm into the tissue. With the advent of effective artificial sapphire tips, the possibility for intra-abdominal YAG procedures has been greatly expanded. We have now used this type of equipment in

TABLE 21–7
Advantages of Fiberoptic Laser Laparoscopy

Equipment less cumbersome
Aiming beam easily seen
Accurate targeting
Less plume
Better hemostasis
Smaller channel needed for fibers

a number of laparoscopic situations, and the techniques seem quite promising.

Techniques of Laser Laparoscopy

Irrespective of the type of laser used, the surgeon needs to remove laser flume effectively. This makes maintenance of pneumoperitoneum difficult. The newer, rapid-fill automatic insufflators are highly desirable, since they can be set to maintain a constant intra-abdominal pressure and deliver a flow of CO_2 of up to 6 liters per minute. A high-intensity light source also is of

great importance. We attach a video camera to the laparoscope, and most operative endoscopy in our clinic is performed while watching a monitor (Fig. 21-8). The greatest advantage of video usage is that the entire operating room becomes a team. The assistant is always aware of the progress of the operation, and the surgeon is able to stand erect while inspecting all parts of the abdominal cavity. The patient is placed in a modified lithotomy position, so that the thigh is almost level with the patient's abdomen. This enables the surgeon to direct the laparoscope cephalad. This maneuver may be important not only for exploration, but also

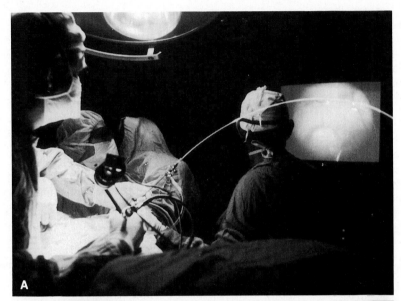

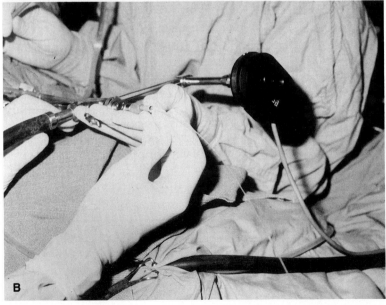

Figure 21–8. Fiberoptic laser laparoscopy. Some of the advantages of fiberoptic lasers are A, the ease with which the fiber is used in either the operative laparoscope or through a suction irrigation handpiece, and B, the uncluttered area surrounding the operative site. Here a quartz fiber of a KTP laser is passed into the laparoscope, which is equipped with an optical filter. The video camera will be attached over this filter.

for operating at the pelvic brim. If the hip is flexed and the thighs are elevated, the scope and perhaps the accessory instrumentation cannot be manipulated freely, as they will be in contact with the patient's thighs.

The vast majority of our advanced operative laser laparoscopic procedures require three incisions. The laparoscope is inserted through a transverse incision in the umbilicus and two other incisions are made in the lower abdomen on either side of the midline. The anterior abdominal wall is transilluminated by the laparoscopic light to localize the inferior epigastric vessels, so that they are not damaged by the secondary incision. If these incisions are placed too low, accessory instrumentation may not reach over the uterus into the cul-de-sac or to the lateral pelvic walls. Instruments that are used through these 5-mm trocar sheaths are the CO_2 laser waveguide, fiberoptic laser suction irrigation cannulas, and various Semm-type instruments, such as scissors, forceps, suture passers, and needle holders. We try to avoid the need for elevating the uterus with one of our abdominal instruments. A Rubin's cannula or other intrauterine manipulator is placed in the uterine cavity, and if the patient's buttocks are far enough down the table, the uterus can be elevated by an assistant from below, thus leaving the intraabdominal instrumentation free for laparoscopic surgery. Although the laser surgeon may need to make only two incisions—one for the operative scope and the other for smoke evacuation and manipulation—the majority of more complicated laparoscopic surgical procedures require a total of three and sometimes four incisions. In our clinic about 1700 laparoscopies are performed each year. More than half of these are operative laparoscopies. Common advanced laparoscopic procedures for the combination of laser plus conventional techniques are listed in Table 21-8. Percentages refer to relative frequencies of the procedures but do not add up to 100%, since two or more procedures often may be performed during the same operation.

TABLE 21–8
Frequency of Use of Laser Laparoscopy Procedures

PROCEDURE	PERCENTAGE
Fulguration or excision of endometriosis	68
Lysis of adhesions	62
Ovarian cystectomy	31
Division of uterosacral ligaments	30
Removal of adnexa	11
Removal of ectopic pregnancy	9
Myomectomy	4
Neosalpingostomy	4

Fulguration or Excision of Endometriosis

The smaller implants of mild to moderate endometriosis can be effectively vaporized, coagulated, or excised with either the CO_2 or the fiberoptic laser. Laser vaporization is rapid and usually hemostatic. Even small endometrial implants are surrounded by subclinical endometriosis, so that a margin of vaporization or coagulation is planned around the endometrial implant. Implants that are located over the ureter may be safely vaporized by various methods. The ureter is always identified by the laparoscopic surgeon. It usually is easier to visualize the ureter at the bifurcation of the common iliac artery as it passes into the pelvis. The ureter is then traced down to the cardinal ligament, where it usually is more difficult to identify. Often the ureter can be moved beneath the peritoneum, so that the endometrial implant no longer lies directly over it. In CO_2 laser surgery, injection of saline retroperitoneally into the broad ligament or the lateral pelvic sidewall provides a watery backstop that helps with dissection in addition to increasing safety. This is not protective for fiberoptic laser energy, and more care must be exerted not to damage the ureter.

The laser surgeon rapidly develops the ability to excise peritoneum; this technique should be used for the removal of endometriomas. The peritoneum may be incised by laser energy, using a focused laser beam. This puncture is enlarged with the suction irrigator, and dissection can be carried bluntly by the instrument or with the aid of the irrigating fluid itself. Forceps are then used to elevate the peritoneum, and the laser is used to complete the excision. Results of reported series of endometriosis treated laparoscopically have been compiled by Martin and Diamond. These compare favorably with results produced by conventional surgery at laparotomy (Table 21-9).

Ovarian Cystectomy

Resection of an ovarian cyst at laparoscopy is a controversial subject. Many surgeons believe that spillage of a stage I malignant neoplasm or an epithelial tumor of borderline malignancy may result in spread of the disease. Unfortunately most ovarian tumors are not discovered when they are at an early stage. Because the vast majority of young women who have cystic adnexal masses will not have ovarian tumors, it seems desirable to make an attempt at diagnosis and extirpation by the laparoscopic approach. To minimize mistakes, the cystic mass should always be evaluated by noninvasive means, such as sonography or magnetic resonance imaging. Tumor markers also are obtained, and finally a laparoscopic diagnosis is attempted.

TABLE 21–9
CO$_2$ Laser Laparoscopy for Endometriosis

AUTHOR	PATIENTS		MINIMAL/MILD		MODERATE		SEVERE/EXTENSIVE	
	Number	*Pregnant*	*Number*	*Pregnant*	*Number*	*Pregnant*	*Number*	*Pregnant*
Endometriosis in all Patients								
Kelly, 1983	10	6 (60%)	3	3 (100%)	7	3 (43%)	0	0 (0%)
Feste, 1985	140	82 (59%)	106	62 (58%)	31	18 (58%)	3	2 (67%)
Daniell, 1985	48	26 (54%)	24	16 (67%)	15	7 (47%)	9	3 (33%)
Martin, 1986	115	54 (47%)	56	23 (41%)	45	22 (49%)	14	9 (64%)
Davis, 1986	64	37 (58%)	31	20 (65%)	26	15 (58%)	7	2 (29%)
Nezhat, 1986	102	65 (64%)	24	18 (75%)	51	32 (63%)	27	15 (56%)
Adamson, 1986	156	86 (55%)	133	77 (58%)	20	7 (33%)	3	0 (0%)
Bowman, 1986	35	18 (51%)	19	12 (63%)	13	4 (31%)	3	2 (67%)
Donnez, 1987	70	40 (57%)	42	26 (62%)	21	11 (52%)	7	3 (43%)
Paulsen, 1987	431	225 (52%)	257	144 (56%)	174	81 (47%)	0	0 (0%)
Gast, 1988	122	57 (47%)	105	49 (47%)	17	8 (47%)	0	0 (0%)
Nezhat, 1989	243	168 (69%)	39	28 (72%)	86	60 (70%)	118	80 (68%)
Total	1536	864 (56%)	839	478 (57%)	506	268 (53%)	191	116 (61%)
Endometriosis as an Isolated Factor								
Feste, 1985	60	42 (70%)	44	3 (70%)	14	10 (71%)	2	1 (50%)
Martin, 1985	34	23 (67%)	13	9 (69%)	11	6 (55%)	10	8 (80%)
Nezhat, 1986	102	65 (64%)	24	18 (75%)	51	32 (63%)	27	15 (56%)
Adamson, 1986	60	39 (65%)	47	31 (66%)	11	7 (61%)	2	0 (0%)
Paulsen, 1987	228	169 (74%)	140	109 (78%)	88	60 (68%)	0	0 (0%)
Gast, 1988	27	7 (26%)		NA		NA	0	0 (0%)
Nezhat, 1989	243	168 (69%)	39	28 (72%)	86	60 (70%)	118	80 (68%)
Total	754	513 (68%)	307	226 (74%)	261	175 (67%)	159	104 (65%)

NA = not available

(Adapted from Martin DC, Diamond MP. Operative laparoscopy: comparison of lasers with other techniques. Curr Prob Obstet Gynecol Fertil 1986; 9:564. With permission from Martin DC: Laparoscopic treatment of endometriosis. In: Intraabdominal laser surgery. 2nd ed. Memphis: Resurge Press, 1989.)

Ovarian endometriomas should be excised rather than vaporized. We have experienced a high incidence of recurrence when endometriomas of more than 2 cm have been opened and vaporized rather than excised. Then, too, the universal rule of laser surgery applies to the laparoscopic as well as to the lower reproductive tract surgeon. Vaporization should never be carried out in the absence of a pathologic diagnosis. We, therefore, prefer to evacuate the endometrioma and remove it by stripping the cystic capsule away from ovarian stroma (see Chapter 16 for a more detailed description of these aspects of operative laparoscopy). We try to avoid suturing the ovary, since suture material may produce adhesions. One effective technique for reducing the size of the ovarian wound is to irradiate the bed of the excised cyst with laser energy. Superficial desiccation of the ovarian stroma may produce a contraction or shrinkage of tissue, which pulls the cortex together. It is relatively rare that the ovary needs to be closed with sutures.

Lysis of Adhesions

Adhesions between the omentum and the anterior abdominal wall usually are handled rapidly and efficiently by laser energy. In the case of the fiberoptic lasers, the fiber should be held in direct contact with the adhesion to produce rapid cutting. Blood vessels that are seen in the adhesions often can be coagulated with the defocused laser beam before cutting. Bowel adhesions are a more difficult problem. If a backstop can be manipulated between loops of bowel, or if the loop of bowel can be held gently apart, so that the laser energy is directly applied to the adhesion without fear of bowel damage, then laser adhesiolysis is feasible. On the other hand, sharp and blunt dissection with laparoscopic forceps, scissors, or microscissors often provides a safer procedure. When thick bands of adhesions are attacked with any of the lasers, the power should be turned up. We use 15 W on the fiberoptic laser and up to 30 or 40 W on the CO$_2$ laser, depending on the focal spot size. The laser surgeon rapidly becomes accustomed to the effects of various power settings. It is particularly helpful if the laparoscopic surgeon is familiar with open laser laparotomy techniques.

One of the rare complications of laser surgery has been bowel perforation. In general, small bowel should not be subjected to the laser beam. The wall of this organ is too thin, and delayed postoperative perforation may occur. The large bowel is much thicker, and the expert laser surgeon comes to appreciate how much CO_2 laser dissection and vaporization are possible on areas such as the rectosigmoid. The fiberoptic lasers should be used with extreme care even on large bowel, as these lasers produce energy that penetrates too deeply for safe application.

Uterosacral Ligament Division

Little has been written about the uterosacral ligament division for the treatment of pelvic pain. Pain stimuli originating from the uterus usually are registered through the sacral sympathetic chain and conducted through the uterosacral ligaments to the sacral sympathetic plexus by way of nerve roots S-2, S-3, and S-4. Although results remain controversial, Feste has reported relief of dysmenorrhea in more than 70% of the women who underwent CO_2 laser division of the uterosacral ligaments and who have been followed for more than a year. Lichten, in a prospective series, reported a success rate in excess of 80% of patients followed more than a year. In our series of 60 patients undergoing uterosacral ligament division for either primary dysmenorrhea or dysmenorrhea associated with endometriosis, 70% of women followed over the course of a year claimed complete or significant pain relief. The true value of the procedure remains to be elucidated by carefully designed randomized clinical trials.

Sometimes the uterosacral ligament can be confused with the ureter, so the latter structure must always be positively identified. We identify the ureter at the bifurcation of the common iliac and trace it into the pelvis to a point where it disappears in the cardinal ligament. At the same time that the uterosacral ligament is identified, the division is planned close to its insertion into the uterus. Uterosacral ligaments vary tremendously in size and structure. The division should begin at the posterior uterine wall and a section of about 1 cm of uterosacral ligament vaporized in its entire thickness. Just lateral to the uterosacral ligament lies a branch of the uterine artery as well as the ureter, so one should attempt to stay medial. Power settings of 20 W may be used on the CO_2 laser, and on the fiberoptic lasers, 10 to 15 W will suffice.

Terminal Salpingostomy

Laser laparoscopy for terminal salpingostomy is carried out in a manner similar to that described for laser laparotomy. We prefer to use CO_2 laser with a small spot size or a KTP laser fiber of 100 μm. Linear incisions are made as described after the tube has been filled with indigo carmine dye and the scar marking the previous ampullary opening has been identified. The CO_2 laser is used at 20 to 40 W, whereas the KTP setting is at 15 to

20 W. The tubes can be held gently with atraumatic forceps while the laser beam is applied through either the operative scope or one of the secondary puncture sites. In 1983 Fayez and colleagues reported a postoperative patency rate of 31% in 19 patients followed more than 1 year by hysterosalpingography. Two of the 19 patients conceived, but both had ectopic gestations. Daniell reports better results attained using the CO_2 and KTP lasers. Tubal patency at 6 weeks out of a total of 140 patients treated by either CO_2 or KTP laser was 83%; the overall percentage of intrauterine pregnancies was 28%, with a tubal pregnancy rate of 13% and an abortion rate of 12% (also discussed in Chapter 19).

Myomectomy

The indications for a laparoscopic myomectomy are the same as the indications for myomectomy in general. Significant size, rapid growth, pressure symptoms, and heavy bleeding have all been acceptable indications for surgical intervention. The role of myomectomy for the infertile patient currently is a matter of discussion. There have been conflicting reports concerning the advisability of myomectomy for this indication, and once again, no convincing data can be presented to support the superiority of endoscopic removal versus the open abdominal approach as far as subsequent fertility or adhesion formation is concerned. Pedunculated leiomyomas may be easily removed at laser laparoscopy, but intramural leiomyomas may pose a real challenge.

Our technique uses percutaneous injection of a dilute solution of vasopressin to the base of the leiomyoma and the surrounding myometrium. The uterus usually can be manipulated just under the needlestick and adequate infiltration obtained. Three lower abdominal accessory punctures are used. The capsule of the leiomyoma is incised with the laser. Two lateral forceps are used to grasp the capsule of the leiomyoma, and this is gently stripped away from the underlying myoma, much in the way an orange is peeled. The laser is used to coagulate vessels on the surface of the leiomyoma and, as the base is approached, to coagulate and cut vessels in that area. If excessive bleeding is encountered, laser coagulation is attempted, but if this fails, bipolar coagulation, the crocodile forceps with the endocoagulator of Semm, or endoscopic suturing will almost always control the bleeding. Constant traction can be placed on the leiomyoma as it is being removed through the third 5-mm accessory incision, which usually is located near the midline. A small myoma corkscrew instrument can be used through this trocar to stabilize it and exert the necessary traction. After removal of the leiomyoma the myometrium is trimmed and, if necessary, closed with sutures.

The pedunculated leiomyoma is removed in the

same way. These usually are not as difficult as intramural leiomyomas, since the pedicle often can be coagulated and cut with the laser or ligated with an endoloop.

We have removed intramural leiomyomas of up to 10 cm in diameter using these techniques and have not had to perform a laparotomy, nor have we encountered major complications. The surgery must be carefully done, and hemostasis must be complete at the end of the procedure.

It is possible to remove these leiomyomas in several ways. Morcellation may be carried out through an 11-mm trocar sheath, using the instrument designed by Semm. Smaller leiomyomas also may be removed by slightly enlarging the 11-mm umbilical incision. An alternative method is to leave the intact leiomyoma within the abdominal cavity until the uterine wound is satisfactorily closed; then the leiomyoma is removed through a colpotomy incision. The leiomyoma occasionally must be morcellated to effect vaginal delivery (also discussed in Chapter 26).

Tubal Pregnancy

Laparoscopic laser surgery for tubal pregnancy was reported by Bruhat in 1978; this was one of the first procedures done by advanced laser laparoscopy. Ampullary ectopic pregnancies usually are interstitial rather than intraluminal, and this is the perfect setting for a laser incision. Once again, a dilute solution of vasopressin can be delivered percutaneously to the tube, and the laser is used for the linear salpingostomy. Hemostasis usually is achieved by any of the lasers; however, bipolar coagulation may be necessary for very active bleeding. The pregnancy usually is extruded from the tube as the incision is made. Gentle traction with an atraumatic forceps may help. It is not necessary or desirable to curette the tube in an effort to remove the contents. It is essential to follow any conservatively treated tubal pregnancy with postoperative human chorionic gonadotropin titres to rule out persistent trophoblastic disease.

Sometimes partial salpingectomy is necessary. This may be particularly true of isthmic tubal pregnancies. Pregnancies in this region of the tube usually are intraluminal, and although they are not as frequently encountered as ampullary pregnancies, segmental rupture may occur earlier and recanalization of the tube is infrequent. For this reason, excision of the segment may be desirable; this can be carried out by coagulation on either side of the ectopic and then excision with laser or with laparoscopic scissors. Bipolar coagulation may be necessary because of the bleeding, despite the use of vasopressin. Future microsurgical reanastomosis will be required if the opposite tube is damaged and pregnancy is desired.

Salpingectomy is used when the tube is destroyed or when future pregnancy is not desired. This procedure is quickly done through the laparoscope, using the conventional laparoscopic operative technique (also discussed in Chapter 18).

HYSTEROSCOPIC LASER SURGERY

The fiberoptic lasers have been used successfully through the hysteroscope. Hysteroscopic laser surgery includes YAG endometrial ablation, metroplastic procedures such as division of a uterine septum or synechiae, and other miscellaneous procedures, such as laser excision of submucous leiomyomas (also discussed in Chapter 17).

Endometrial Ablation

YAG laser endometrial ablation was reported by Goldrath and coworkers in 1981. Because of its ability to penetrate tissue, the YAG represents an ideal laser for this purpose. Myometrium normally is about 2 to 3 cm thick except at the cornu, where it may be significantly thinner. Endometrial thickness usually can be measured in terms of a few millimeters. Because YAG laser energy penetrates about 4 mm, the YAG can be used to effectively coagulate the endometrium and the inner layers of the myometrium. The risk of damage to tissues outside the myometrium is minimal.

All patients for endometrial ablation must have a dilatation and curettage to rule out tumors or premalignant lesions. Adenomatous hyperplasia should not be ablated with the YAG. After curettage, patients are given danazol, 800 mg/day, for at least 1 month to thin out the endometrium. At the time of laser surgery the cervix is dilated, so that the distending medium, saline solution, is able to flow out of the cervix past the hysteroscope. This rapid flow of saline in and out of the uterine cavity makes visualization easy in the presence of active bleeding. We ablate the endometrial cavity by using the "touch technique"; that is, the endometrium is actually in contact with the fiber. Fifty watts of power are used, and an effort is made to destroy all the endometrium. The ablation is carried out using a system of wavy strokes that completely cover the endometrial cavity. The destruction is taken to just past the level of the internal os.

Goldrath and associates have reported excellent results in 203 of the first 218 patients undergoing YAG endometrial ablation in their clinic. In more than 100 YAG endometrial ablations performed in our clinic, satisfactory results were achieved in 80%. In the 20% of patients in the unsatisfactory result group, the vast majority had a decrease in menstrual flow but were unhappy because they wanted complete cessation of uterine bleeding.

Laser Metroplasty

Any of the fiberoptic lasers can be used for cutting of uterine septa and synechiae. Although KTP 532 and argon do not penetrate the endometrium and myometrium far enough for satisfactory ablation, contact cutting with these fibers produces good results. The YAG fiber also can be used. It should be emphasized that when septa are divided, concomitant laparoscopy should be performed to make sure that perforation does not occur.

We have used both the YAG and the KTP lasers to do successful myomectomies. Pedunculated leiomyomas usually are easily removed by division of the pedicle. Submucous leiomyomas that protrude deep into the myometrium are much more difficult to remove and are better handled by resectoscopic procedures.

LASER SAFETY

Many volumes have been written about the safe use of surgical lasers. The hazards of laser usage may be divided into two categories: those common to lasers in general and those associated with the specific wavelength and power output of the laser. By far, the most common causes of injury with lasers are careless or uninformed usage by surgeons or operating room personnel. Education is the most important step in the avoidance of laser injury. All lasers produce heat and are, therefore, capable of producing fire. Flammable liquids, paper drapes, and other flammable material may be ignited. Because electricity is used to produce laser energy in many surgical lasers, electrical hazards from the high voltages generated in the instruments are always possible.

A great deal of concern has been caused by the identification of viral DNA sequences in laser smoke. The possibility of transmission of HPV or human immunodeficiency virus by way of laser plume currently is under investigation. Although several studies show the harmful effects of laser smoke on lung tissue, actual infection by transmitted viral particles has not been proved. Careful evacuation and filtration of laser smoke should greatly reduce this health hazard. It has been conclusively shown that the effectiveness of smoke evacuation is inversely proportional to the distance of the suction device from the target tissue. An effort should be made to collect smoke no further than 2 cm from the target site.

Various types of thermal injury result from specific wavelengths. CO_2 laser energy may produce eye injury by damaging the cornea. Protective glasses, colposcopes, and the operative lenses of laparoscopes shield the laser surgeon's eyes from CO_2 laser injury. But the fiberoptic lasers that penetrate water and clear glass also penetrate the eye, so that retinal damage may occur when eye protection is not used. Each of these lasers is absorbed by a specific color, so in each case special glasses or filters are used to protect the eye. Endoscopic surgery with the fiberoptic lasers usually involves the use of an optical filter coupled to the ocular of the telescope; this filter is activated when the surgeon steps on the laser foot pedal.

Avoidance of surgical mishap with the laser is best achieved by careful education of the laser surgeon and all other operating room personnel. Because many aspects of gynecologic laser surgery are not currently taught in residency programs, a special effort to acquire proper training has been required of the gynecologic laser surgeon. Courses designed to support credentialing requests must include instruction in the proper care and safe handling of laser devices. More emphasis has recently been placed on the education of the laser safety officer and the rest of the operating room staff. To minimize liability and promote high-quality patient care, many hospitals are making an effort to educate staff and develop acceptable and rational credentialing criteria for laser surgery.

SUMMARY

Laser surgery of the lower reproductive tract has proved to be a highly efficient means of surgical treatment for intraepithelial neoplasia and related viral disease. The microsurgical delivery systems as well as the variety of tissue effects that the knowledgeable laser surgeon is able to produce afford tremendous variation in the attack on these disorders. Results are excellent from the standpoint of both apparent cure and conservative anatomic result. Controversy over the choice of instrument with which to treat lower reproductive tract intraepithelial neoplasia continues, as some surgeons still prefer the knife or the cryosurgical probe. Proper laser usage has the great advantage of applicability to almost all cases, whereas other instruments can only be used with careful case selection.

Laser endoscopy has been enthusiastically used by a relatively few pioneering gynecologic surgeons, and methodology as well as some of the results appear to significantly enlarge the scope of the operative endoscopist. Tremendous emphasis has been placed on the conservative treatment of many conditions previously assumed to require laparotomy and hysterectomy. Advanced operative laparoscopy is not a discipline that is readily learned by all surgeons. Procedures such as laparoscopic ovarian cystectomy, myomectomy, and adnexectomy require a great deal of judgment and surgical ability. Although most of these procedures have been done with more conventional instrumentation, the laser often has afforded a more rapid endoscopic technique, since incision, excision, vaporization, and coagulation can be carried out almost simultaneously. The laser should be recognized as a tool that aids the laparoscopic surgeon in the performance of some tasks, and not as an instrument to replace all others. It is abundantly clear that the endoscopist who wants to perform advanced operative laparoscopy must understand the advantages of other, more conventional instrumentation. The laser is used in conjunction with these instruments.

For many procedures the specific benefits of endoscopic laser surgery and its long-term results remain to be documented by carefully designed randomized clinical trials. These trials often are influenced by the abilities of the surgeon, the variation in the techniques used, and the extent of the disease. Certainly the concept of replacing many open abdominal operations by advanced laparoscopic procedures is appealing, since the oft-quoted advantages of reduction of the magnitude of surgery, operative time, recovery time, and cost seem obvious. Before enthusiasm leads to the replacement of tried and proven operations, however, certain criteria should be applied to make a more valid judgment (Table 21-10). One of the most compelling questions involves the need for subsequent surgery after the advanced laparoscopic procedure. Only time will establish the ultimate position of this type of surgery.

Clearly, the limits of operative endoscopy have not yet been defined. Endoscopic procedures that seemed inadvisable or impossible several years ago are now routinely used by conservative gynecologists. Technological advances have provided much of this capability to the surgeon, and laser ranks high on the list of technical achievements used to advantage by our specialty. Tunable lasers that produce a range of wavelengths and tissue effects, vastly improved delivery systems, and the increasing sophistication of endoscopic instrumentation all point to increasing laser application and an exciting future.

TABLE 21–10
Criteria for Evaluation of New Surgical Procedures

Obvious advantages
Comparable or improved results
Low risk, great benefit
Technically mastered by most surgeons

(Modified from Rock JA, Katayama KP, Martin EJ, et al. Pregnancy outcome following uterotubal implantation: a comparison of the reamer and sharp wedge excision techniques. Fertil Steril 1979;31:634.)

Bibliography

Adamson GD, Lu J, Subak LL. Laparoscopic CO_2 laser vaporization of endometriosis compared with traditional treatments. Fertil Steril 1988;50:704.

American College of Obstetricians and Gynecologists Committee Statement. Committee on Gynecologic Practice Report on Carbon Dioxide Laser. April 1984.

Anderson MC, Hartley RB. Cervical crypt involvement by intraepithelial neoplasia. Obstet Gynecol 1980;55:546.

Apfelberg DB, Mittelman H, Chadi B. Carcinogenic potential of in vitro carbon dioxide laser exposure of fibroblast. Obstet Gynecol 1988;61:493.

Baggish MS. Carbon dioxide laser treatment for condylomata acuminata venereal infections. Obstet Gynecol 1980;55:711.

Baggish MS. High power density carbon dioxide laser therapy for early cervical neoplasia. Am J Obstet Gynecol 1980;36:117.

Baggish MS. Complications associated with carbon dioxide laser surgery in gynecology. Am J Obstet Gynecol 1981;139:568.

Baggish MS. Management of cervical intraepithelial neoplasia by carbon dioxide laser. Obstet Gynecol 1982;60:379.

Baggish MS. Treating viral venereal infections with CO_2 laser. J Repro Med 1982;27:737.

Baggish MS. Laser endoscopy in obstetrics and gynecology. Clin Obstet Gynecol 1983;26:2.

Baggish MS. Status of the carbon dioxide laser for infertility surgery. Fertil Steril 1983;40:442.

Baggish MS, Baltoyannis P. Carbon dioxide laser treatment of cervical stenosis. Fertil Steril 1987;48:24.

Baggish MS, Chong AP. Carbon dioxide laser microsurgery of the uterine tube. Obstet Gynecol 1981;58:111.

Baggish MS, Chong AP. Intraabdominal surgery with the CO_2 laser. J Reprod Med 1983;28:269.

Baggish MS, Dorsey JH. CO_2 laser for the treatment of vulvar carcinoma in situ. Obstet Gynecol 1981;57:371.

Baggish MS, Dorsey JH. The laser combination cone. Am J Obstet Gynecol 1985;151:23.

Baggish MS, Sze E, Badawy S, Choe J. Carbon dioxide laser laparoscopy by means of a 3.0-mm diameter rigid wave guide. Fertil Steril 1988;50:419.

Bellina JH. Microsurgery of the fallopian tube with CO_2 laser—82 cases with follow-up. Laser Surg Medo 1982;36:129.

Bellina JH. Microsurgery of the fallopian tube with the carbon dioxide laser: analysis of 230 cases with a two-year follow-up. Laser Surg Med 1983;3:255.

Bellina JH, Hemmings R, Voros JI, Ross LF. Carbon dioxide laser and electrosurgical wound study with an animal model: a comparison of tissue damage and healing patterns in peritoneal tissue. Am J Obstet Gynecol 1984;148:327.

Bellina JH, Voros JL, Fick AC, Jackson JD. Surgical management of endometriosis with the carbon dioxide laser. Microsurgery 1984;5:4.

Bellina JH, Voros JI, Fick AC, Jackson JD. Surgical management of endometriosis with the carbon dioxide laser. Microsurgery 1984;5:197.

Boeckx W, Gordts S, Vasquez G, Brosens I: Microsurgery in gynecology. Int Surg 1981;66:47.

Brosens IA, Cornillie F, Koninckx P, V.asquez G. Evolution of the Revised American Fertility Society Classification of Endometriosis (letter). Fertil Steril 1985;44:714.

Bruhat MA. Pregnancy following salpingostomy: comparison between CO_2 laser and electrosurgery procedures. Fertil Steril 1983; 40:472.

Bruhat MA, Mage G: Use of CO_2 laser in salpingotomy. In: Kaplan I, ed.

Laser Surgery III, pt 1. Jerusalem: Jerusalem Academic Press, 1979:271.

Bruhat MA, Mage G, Manhes M. Use of the CO_2 laser via laparoscopy. Proceedings of the third annual meeting of the International Society of Laser Surgery, Tel Aviv, 1979:275.

Burke L, Covell L, Antonioli D. Laser therapy of cervical intra-epithelial neoplasia: factors determining success rate. Laser Med Surg 1980;1:113.

Buttram VC Jr. Surgical treatment of endometriosis in the infertile female: a modified approach. Fertil Steril 1979;32:635.

Buttram VC Jr. Evolution of the revised American Fertility Society classification of endometriosis. Fertil Steril 1985;43:347.

Byrne MA, Taylor-Robinson D, Wickenden C, et al. Prevalence of human papillomavirus types in the cervices of women before and after laser ablation. Br J Obstet Gynecol 1988;95:201.

Choe JK, Dawood MY, Andrews AH. Conventional versus laser reanastomosis of rabbit ligated uterine horns. Obstet Gynecol 1983;61:689.

Chong AP. Infertility amendable to laser surgery. Basic Adv Laser Surg Gynecol 1985;279:296.

Chong AP, Baggish MS. The use of carbon dioxide laser in tubal surgery. Int J Fertil 1983;28:24.

Chong AP, Baggish MS. Management of pelvic endometriosis by means of intraabdominal carbon dioxide laser. Fertil Steril 1984;41:14.

Daniell JF. The role of lasers in infertility surgery. Fertil Steril 1984;42:815.

Daniell JF, Brown DH. Carbon dioxide laser laparoscopy: initial experience in experimental animals and humans. Obstet Gynecol 1982;59:761.

Daniell JF, Diamond MP, McLaughlin DS, et al. Clinical results of terminal salpingostomy using the CO_2 laser: report of the intraabdominal laser study group. Fertil Steril 1986;45:175.

Daniell JF, Herbert CM. Laparoscopic salpingostomy utilizing the CO_2 laser. Fertil Steril 1984;41:558.

Daniell JF, Pittaway DE. Use of the CO_2 laser in laparoscopic surgery: initial experience with the second puncture technique. Infertility 1982;5:15.

David SS. Microsurgical management of distal tube disease. In: Reyniak JV, Lauersen NH, eds. Principles of microsurgical techniques in infertility. New York: Plenum, 1982:161.

Davis GD, Brooks RA. Excision of pelvic endometriosis with the carbon dioxide laser laparoscope. Obstet Gynecol 1988;72:816.

DeCherney AH. The leader of the band is tired. Fertil Steril 1985;44:299.

Department of Health, Education, and Welfare/Food and Drug Administration. Report on laser products. Fed Register 1975;40(July pt 2):148.

Diamond E. Microsurgical reconstruction of the uterine tube in sterilized patients. Fertil Steril 1977;28:1203.

Diamond MP, Daniell JF, Feste J, et al. Pelvic adhesions at early second look laparoscopy following carbon dioxide laser surgery procedures. Infertility 1984;7:39.

Diamond MP, Daniell JF, Martin DC, et al. Tubal patency in pelvic adhesions at early second look laparoscopy following intraabdominal use of the carbon dioxide laser: initial report of the intraabdominal laser study group. Fertil Steril 1984;42:717.

Dorsey JH. Excisional conization of the cervix. In: Andrews AH, Polanyi TG, eds. Microscopic and endoscopic surgery with the CO2 laser. Boston: John Wright, 1982.

Dorsey JH. Nomenclature and cervical conization. Colpos Gynecol Laser Surg 1984;1:161.

Dorsey JH. Recurrent cervical intraepithelial neoplasia (CIN) and the endocervical button. Colpos Gynecol Laser Surg 1984;1:221.

Dorsey JH. The education of the gynecologic laser surgeon and a board of laser surgery. Colpos Gynecol Laser Surg 1984;1:83.

Dorsey JH. Marsupialization techniques with the CO_2 laser: methods and case reports. Colpos Gynecol Laser Surg 1986;2:113.

Dorsey JH. The CO_2 laser as a surgical instrument: some thoughts about comparing the CO_2 laser with the cryosurgical probe. Colpos Gynecol Laser Surg 1986;2:1.

Dorsey JH. The evolution of operative colposcopy. Colpos Gynecol Laser Surg 1986;2:65.

Dorsey JH, Baggish MS. Vaginal intraepithelial neoplasia. II. Indications and technique for total vaginectomy with split thickness graft replacement. Colpos Gynecol Laser Surg 1984;1:149.

Dorsey JH, Baggish MS. Initiating a CO_2 laser program. Basic Adv Laser Surg Gynecol 1985;373:381.

Dorsey JH, Baggish MS. Laser laparoscopy with the KTP laser. Clin Pract Gynecol, Elsevier Science Publishing Co. (in press).

Dorsey JH, Baggish MS. Indications and Contraindications. Clin Pract of Gynecol, Elsevier Science Publishing Co. (in press).

Dougherty TJ, Kaufman JE, Goldfarb A, et al. Photoradiation therapy for the treatment of malignant tumors. Cancer Res 1978;38:2628.

Fayez JA, Collazo LM, Vernon C. Comparison of different modalities of treatment for minimal and mild endometriosis. Am J Obstet Gynecol 1988;159:927.

Feste JR. Laser laparoscopy: a new modality. Fertil Steril 1984;41:74S.

Fuller TA, Nadkarni VJ, et al. Carbon dioxide laser fiber optics. Bio-Laser News 1985;4:1.

Goldrath M, Fuller T, Segal S. Laser photo-vaporization of endometrium for the treatment of menorrhagia. Am J Obstet Gynecol 1981;140:14.

Gomel V. Causes of failure of reconstructive infertility microsurgery. J Reprod Med 1980;24:239.

Gomel V. Microsurgical reversal of female sterilization: a reappraisal. Fertil Steril 1980;33:587.

Gordts S, Boeckx W, Brosens I. Microsurgery of endometriosis in infertile patients. Fertil Steril 1984;42:520.

Grosspietzsch R. Microtubular reanastomosis in animal model and early human results. In: Bellina JH et al, eds. Gynecological laser surgery. New York: Plenum, 1981.

Grosspietzsch R, et al: Experiments on operative treatment of tubal sterility by CO_2 laser technique. Proceedings of the third International Congress of Laser Surgery, Tel-Aviv, 1979:256.

Grosspietzsch R, Inthraphuvasak I, Klink F, Oberheuser F. Experiments on CO_2 laser techniques for operative treatment of tubal sterility. In: Bellina JH et al, eds. Gynecologic laser surgery. New York: Plenum, 1981.

Guzick DS, Bross DS, Rock JA. Assessing the efficacy of The American Fertility Society's classification of endometriosis: application of a dose-response methodology. Fertil Steril 1982;38:171.

Hahn GA. Carbon dioxide laser surgery in treatment of condylomata. Am J Obstet Gynecol 1981;141:1000.

Haney AF, Weinberg JB. Reduction of the intraperitoneal inflammation associated with endometriosis by treatment with medroxyprogesterone acetate. Am J Obstet Gynecol 1988;159:450.

Hulka JF, Omran K, Bergen GS. Classification of adnexal adhesions: a proposal and evaluation of its prognostic value. Fertil Steril 1978;30:661.

Jordan JA. Laser treatment of cervical intraepithelial neoplasia. Obstet Gynecol 1979;34:831.

Kable WT III, Yussman MA. Fertility after conservative treatment of endometriosis. J Reprod Med 1985;30:857.

Kaplan I, Goldman J, Ger R. The treatment of erosions of the uterine cervix by means of the CO_2 laser. Obstet Gynecol 1973;41:795.

Kelly RW. Laser surgery for adhesions. Basic Adv Laser Surg Gynecol 1985;323:329.

Kelly RW, Roberts DK. CO_2 laser laparoscopy: a potential alternative to danazol in treatment of stage I and II endometriosis. J Reprod Med 1983;28:638.

Kelly RW, Roberts DK. Experience with the carbon dioxide laser in gynecologic microsurgery. Am J Obstet Gynecol 1983;146:586.

Keye WR, Dixon J. Photocoagulation of endometriosis by the argon laser through the laparoscope. Obstet Gynecol 1983;62:383.

Keye WR Jr, Hansen LW, Astin M, Poulson AM Jr. Argon laser therapy of endometriosis: a review of 92 consecutive patients. Fertil Steril 1987;47:208.

Klink F, Grosspietzsch F, Klitzing LV, et al. Animal in vivo studies and in vitro experiments with human tubes for end-to-end anastomotic operation by a CO_2 laser technique. Fertil Steril 1978;30:100.

Krebs Hans-B. The use of topical 5-fluorouracil in the treatment of genital condylomas. Obstet Gynecol Clin North Am 1987;559:567.

Larsson G, Alm P, Grundsell H. Laser conization versus cold knife conization. Surg Gynecol Obstet 1982;154:59.

Lobraico RV. Lasers in gynecology. Med Instrum 1983;17:411.

Lomano JM. Photocoagulation of early pelvic endometriosis with the Nd-YAG laser through the laparoscope. J Reprod Med 1985;30:77.

Lomano JM. Ablation of the endometrium with the neodynium: YAG laser: a multi-center study. Colpos Gynecol Laser Surg 1986;4:203.

Lorincz AT. Detection of human papillomavirus infection by nucleic acid hybridization. Obstet Gynecol Clin North Am 1987;451:468.

Luciano AA, Turksoy RN, Carleo J. Evaluation of oral medroxyprogesterone acetate in the treatment of endometriosis. Obstet Gynecol 1988;72:323.

McCoy TD, Martin DC, Poston W. Reanastomosis of rat uterine horn following laser and sharp incisions. Fertil Steril 1984;41:805.

McLaughlin DS. Evaluation of adhesion reformation by early second look laparoscopy following microlaser ovarian wedge resection. Fertil Steril 1984;42:531.

MacLean AB, Murray EL, Sharp F, More IA. Residual cervical intraepithelial neoplasia after laser ablation. Lasers Surg Med 1987;7(3):278.

Mage G, Bruhat MA. Pregnancy following salpingostomy: comparison between CO_2 laser and electrosurgery procedures. Fertil Steril 1983;40:472.

Mage G, Canis M, Pouly JL, et al. CO_2 laser laparoscopy: a ten-year experience. Eur J Obstet Gynecol Reprod Biol 1988;28(2):120.

Mage G, Chany Y, Bruhat MA. Intra-abdominal conservative surgical treatment for endometriosis by CO_2 laser. Contrib Gynecol Obstet 1987;16:297.

Mage G, Pouly JL, Bruhat MA. Laser microsurgery of the oviducts. Basic Adv Laser Surg Gynecol 1985;299:321.

Maiman TH. Stimulated optical radiation in ruby. Nature 1960;187:493.

Martin DC. Interval use of the laser laparoscope for endometriosis following danazol therapy. Fertil Steril 1984;41:74S.

Martin DC. Laser techniques for pelvic adhesions. Basic Adv Laser Surg Gynecol 1985;331:340.

Martin DC. Laparoscopic and vaginal colpotomy for the excision of infiltrating cul-de-sac endometriosis. J Reprod Med 1988;33:806.

Martin DC, Diamond MP: Operative laparoscopy: comparison of lasers with other techniques. Curr Prob Obstet Gynecol Fertil 1986;9:564.

Mylotte MJ, Allen JM, Jordan JA. Regeneration of cervical epithelium following laser destruction of intraepithelial neoplasia. Obstet Gynecol Surg 34:859.

Nezhat C, Crowgey SR, Garrison CP. Surgical treatment of endometriosis via laser laparoscopy and videolaseroscopy. Contrib Gynecol Obstet 1987;16:303.

Nezhat C, Winer WK, Nezhat F, et al. Smoke from laser surgery: is there a health hazard? Lasers Surg Med 1987;7(4):376.

Nowroozi K, Chase JS, Check JH, Wu CH. The importance of laparoscopic coagulation of mild endometriosis in infertile women. Int J Fertil 1987;32(6):442.

O'Shea RT, Jones WR. Danazol: objective assessment in the treatment of endometriosis. Clin Reprod Fertil 1985;3(3):205.

Patel CKN. High-power carbon dioxide lasers. Sci Am 1968;219:23.

Peterson EP, Musich JR, Behrman SJ. Uterotubal implantation and obstetric outcome after previous sterilization. Am J Obstet Gynecol 1977;128:662.

Pittaway DE, Maxon W, Daniell JE. A comparison of the CO_2 laser and electrocautery on postoperative intraperitoneal adhesion formation in rabbits. Fertil Steril 1983;39:402.

Pittaway DE, Maxson WS, Daniell JF. A comparison of the CO_2 laser and electrocautery on postoperative intraperitoneal adhesion formation in rabbits. Fertil Steril 1983;40:366.

Polanyi TG, Bredemeier HC, Davis TW. A CO_2 laser for surgical research. Med Biol Eng 1970;8:541.

Rettenmaier MA, Berman ML, DiSaia PJ, et al. Photoradiation therapy of gynecologic malignancies. Gynecol Oncol 1984;17:206.

Ried R. Physical and surgical principles governing expertise with the carbon dioxide laser. Obstet Gynecol Clin North Am 1987;513:533.

Rock JA, Katayama KP, Martin EJ, et al. Pregnancy outcome following uterotubal implantation: a comparison of the reamer and sharp wedge excision techniques. Fertil Steril 1979;31:634.

Schawlow AL. Advances in optical lasers. Sci Am 1963;209:36.

Schawlow AL, Townes CH. Physiol Rev 1985;112:1940.

Schellhas JF. Laser surgery in gynecology. Surg Clin North Am 1978;48:151.

Strully KJ, Yahr W. Biologic effects of laser radiation enhancements by selective stains: discussion. Fed Proc 1965;24(3):S-81.

Swolin K. Fifty fertility operations: literature and methods. Acta Obstet Gynecol Scand 1967;46:234.

Tadir Y, Kaplan I, Zuckerman Z, et al. New instrumentation and technique for laparoscopic carbon dioxide laser operations: a preliminary report. Obstet Gynecol 1984;63:582.

Tadir Y, Ovadia J, Magara R, et al. Intraperitoneal adhesiolysis by CO_2 laser microsurgery. Laser—Tokyo '81.—Tokyo:—Japanese Society for Laser Medicine, 1981:27.

Trofatter K Jr. Interferon. Obstet Gynecol Clin North Am 1987;569:578.

Wheeler JM, Malinak LR. Postoperative danazol therapy in infertility patients with severe endometriosis. Fertil Steril 1981;36:460.

Woodruff JD, Paurstein CJ. The fallopian tube. Baltimore: Williams & Wilkins, 1969:336.

Wright VC: Laser vaporization of the cervix for the management of cervical intraepithelial neoplasia. Basic Adv Laser Surg Gynecol 1985;207:215.

22

Surgery for Benign Disease of the Ovary

JOHN A. ROCK

The gynecologist frequently is confronted with the challenge of ovarian reconstruction for benign disease. The ovary and fallopian tube are sensitive to ischemia, which may result from the trauma of surgery, and secondary adhesions may develop. Furthermore, the anatomic relations among the tube, ovary, and uterus may be altered. Therefore, the gynecologist must possess a clear understanding of the anatomy and embryology of the ovary and master the principles and skills of ovarian reconstructive surgery. This chapter addresses the embryology and anatomy of the ovary. The evaluation and management of the adnexal mass is stressed. Finally, surgical methods for reconstruction of the ovary are discussed.

EMBRYOLOGY

During gestation the gonadal ridges arise as thickenings on the medial aspect of the coelomic cavity adjacent to the mesonephros. Gonadal outgrowth, composed of coelomic epithelium and underlying mesenchyme projecting into the future peritoneal cavity, usually develops at 4 to 5 weeks. The gonadal primordia are composed of epithelial and mesenchymal cells of mesodermal origin. Large spherical ovoid germ cells that originate extragonadally in the wall of the yolk sac migrate to the developing gonads. The gonads of the two sexes remain morphologically indistinguishable until 6 weeks of gestation. When the first evidence of testicular differentiation is noted, the presumptive ovaries remain undifferentiated until the onset of meiosis at the end of the first trimester. The mechanisms responsible for gonadal sex differentiation are unknown.

Some authors have theorized the presence of a testicular determining factor (H-Y cell surface antigen present on the short arm of the Y chromosome) that is elaborated by a specific gene. An in-depth discussion of the theories of mechanisms of testicular differentiation is beyond the scope of this review.

During the early prefollicular stage the ovarian cortex is characterized by germ cells and granulosa cells organized in cords and sheets without specific conformation. The first distinctive change in the fetal ovary is the onset of meiosis, which occurs at 11 to 12 weeks of gestation. This phenomenon is preceded by differentiation of primitive germ cells into actively dividing cells, the oogonia. The mitotic divisions of the oogonia are associated with complete separation at telophase, leaving the daughter cells connected by intracellular bridges. After a series of mitotic divisions, there is progressive entry into meiosis by cell groups, beginning in the innermost cortex and gradually extending to the periphery. These cells are now designated oocytes and pass through various stages of the first meiotic prophase. By late gestation all oocytes have advanced to the diplotene stage. Differentiation is then arrested and does not resume until ovulation.

A meiosis-inducing substance and a meiosis-preventing substance produced by cells derived from mesonephric structures adjacent to the gonad are involved in regulating ovarian and testicular germ cell differentiation. The balance between these two substances varies in the two sexes at different stages of development, with the meiosis-inducing substance predominating in the fetal ovary.

Ovarian hormone production is not required for the differentiation of the female reproductive tract. Ultrastructural studies have shown no specific changes in the fetal granulosa cells associated with steroid hormone secretion such as seen in the fetal Leydig cells. Thecal cells, which play an essential role in steroid synthesis in the adult ovary, do not appear until late gestation, and even then retain a relatively undifferentiated appearance.

Fetal pituitary gonadotropin production begins as early as 10 weeks, with peak levels occurring at midgestation. Although gonadotropins have a major influence on follicular development in the adult ovary, evidence for a similar function in the fetus is lacking.

Follicular formation begins at 18 to 20 weeks of gestation and continues throughout the remaining fetal development. All surviving oocytes are surrounded by adjacent granulosa cells, and oocyte and follicular growth are well established by the late fetal and early neonatal period. There is a constant degeneration and loss of oocytes before incorporation into the follicles; however, several hundred thousand follicles are present in the newborn ovary.

ANATOMY

The ovary is almond-shaped, and about half the size of the testis. The dimensions of the adult ovary vary from individual to individual but usually are about 3 to 5 cm long, 2 to 3 cm wide, and 1 to 2 cm thick, with a weight of 3 to 8 g. The surface of the ovary is pinkish-gray to white and markedly wrinkled. The ovaries normally are smooth in childhood, but their surface becomes pitted from follicular maturation and atresia.

The size, shape, and position of the ovary in the pelvis are variable. Furthermore, the consistency and follicular changes in the ovary vary with the stage of the menstrual cycle. The typical position of the ovary is on the sidewall of the pelvis, lying in the shallow peritoneal fossa of Waldeyer and the angle between the external iliac vein and the ureter. This close relation between the ovary and the ureter highlights the importance of identifying the ureter before dissecting the ovary off the pelvic sidewall.

The ovary is connected to the uterus by the ovarian ligament, to the back of the broad ligament by the mesovarium, and into the lateral pelvic sidewall by the infundibulopelvic ligament (Fig. 22-1). The mesovarium is the mesentery of the ovary. Each ovary is attached at the hilum.

The ovary, like the testis, migrates downward from high in the abdomen during embryonic life. The infundibulum of the fallopian tube extends onto the ovary and is attached at its most distal pole. The structure has been termed the fimbria ovarica. The relation of the ovary to the fimbria and to the utero-ovarian ligament are crucial, and should be maintained during ovarian reconstruction.

During embryogenesis the ovary may assume an unusual appearance and position (Fig. 22-2). The accessory ovary (Fig. 22-2A) contains ovarian tissue and must be situated very close to or connected with a normally placed ovary. The accessory ovary can be connected with the broad utero-ovarian or infundibulopelvic ligament. An accessory ovary usually is in close approximation to the normal ovary. A supernumerary ovary (Fig. 22-2B), however, must have an independent embryologic origin, and therefore develops from a separate primordium, such as arrested migrating gonadocytes. The supernumerary ovary is a structure that contains typical ovarian tissue and has no connection with a normally placed ovary. There must be no direct or ligamentous connection with a normally placed ovary. Therefore, a supernumerary ovary is a third ovary that is independent and at some distance from a normally placed ovary.

Finally, ovarian malposition (Fig. 22-2C) may occur as a result of the lack of a descent of the ovary into the pelvis to assume its normal location. The ovary normally is elongated, and may measure up to 15 cm in length. The ovary may be found adjacent to the liver or spleen, but is attached to the uterus by the utero-ovarian ligament and to the fallopian tube by the fimbria ovarica. The fallopian tube may be 20 to 26 cm long, almost twice its normal length.

The ovary itself is covered with a surface epithelium consisting of a single layer of flattened cells termed the germinal epithelium. This layer is continuous at the hilus with peritoneal epithelium of the posterior leaf of the broad ligament. Beneath the germinal epithelium is a strong layer of condensed ovarian stroma, which is the fibrous capsule of the tunica albuginea. The area where the vessels and nerves find entrance and exit is called the hilum of the ovary. Immediately around the hilum and extending into the substance of the ovary is an area known as the medulla, which is covered by the cortex. The medulla is composed of fibrous tissue unlike the specific stroma of the ovarian cortex. The medulla contains no follicles, only blood vessels and the remnants of the tubular structure that in the male develops into the testes (ie, the rete ovarii).

The ovarian artery arises on each side of the abdominal aorta just below the renal arteries. The artery descends at the site of the aorta, and crosses the ureter obliquely to enter the infundibulopelvic ligament on its course to the ovary. In the broad ligament the ovarian artery gives off branches to the tube and ovary, and finally anastomoses directly with the uterine artery to form a continuous arcade in the broad ligament. The ovarian veins are situated mainly in the mesosalpinx,

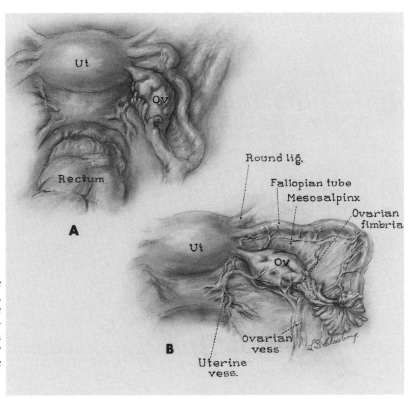

Figure 22–1. Normal anatomy of the ovary. *A,* Anatomic relations of the uterus, tube, and ovary. *B,* The infundibulum of the oviduct extends onto the ovary and is attached at its most distal pole (ovarian fimbria). The mesovarium is the mesentery of the ovary. Each ovary is attached at the hilum.

where they give rise to the pampiniform plexus. At the outer end of the broad ligament this plexus coalesces to form a single ovarian vein. The ovarian vein accompanies the ovarian artery to terminate into the inferior vena cava on the right and to the renal vein on the left.

The lymphatics of the ovary drain in three directions. The main group accompanies the ovarian vessels in the infundibulopelvic ligament, so as to eventually reach the periaortic nodes near the kidney. Additional channels communicate with those of the opposite ovary by crossing the fundus of the uterus through the ovarian ligament. Some channels drain through the ovarian and the round ligaments into the superficial inguinal nodes in the groin. The ovary is supplied by both motor and sensory parasympathetic and sympathetic nerves, which accompany the ovarian vessels from the abdomen to pass into the infundibulopelvic ligament to reach the hilum of the ovary. The segmental nerves supply the ovary from T-10 and T-11.

ADNEXAL MASS

The uterine adnexa consist of the ovaries, fallopian tubes, and uterine ligaments. Although much of adnexal pathology involves one of these structures, the contiguous tissues also may be involved. The bimanual examination is the most practical method of screening for an adnexal mass. When an adnexal mass is found, its characteristics should be carefully described initially, so that any subsequent change can be appreciated and its nature possibly ascertained. The description should include location, size (in centimeters), consistency, shape, movability, tenderness, bilaterality, and associated findings (eg, fever, ascites).

Adjunctive diagnostic techniques such as sonography, magnetic resonance imaging (MRI) and computed tomography (CT) may be helpful in delineating the nature of adnexal enlargement. Pelvic ultrasonography is an accurate means of determining the location, size, extent, and consistency of pelvic masses. Furthermore, ultrasonography may be used to detect obstructive uropathy, ascites, and metastasis (Chapter 12). Other special diagnostic procedures may be necessary for the evaluation of an adnexal mass (Table 22-1).

CT can detect and measure with precision pelvic masses 2 cm or greater in diameter. This technique has been particularly useful in gynecologic oncology because it defines the extent of paracervical and parametrial involvement and determines the resectability of malignant neoplasms. More recently MRI has allowed the measurement of adnexal masses with increased precision. It also allows a clear definition of the relations of adjacent organs.

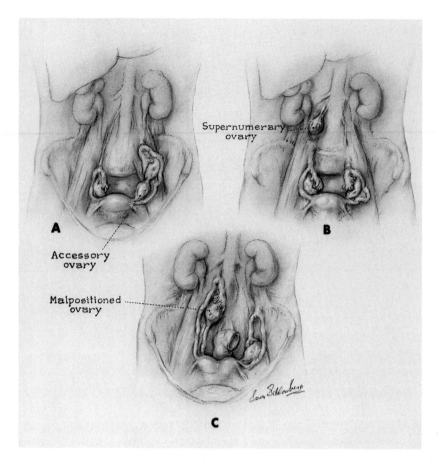

Figure 22–2. Ovarian anomalies. *A*, Accessory. *B*, Supernumerary. *C*, Malpositioned.

TABLE 22–1
Special Diagnostic Procedures for Adnexal Mass

1. Nonoperative/noninvasive
   a. Abdominal and pelvic radiography
   b. Barium enema
   c. Excretory urography
   d. GI series with small bowel follow-through
   e. Pelvic and vaginal ultrasonography
   f. CT scan
   g. Magnetic resonance imaging
   h. β-HCG
   i. CA-125
2. Nonoperative/invasive
   a. Culdocentesis
   b. Hysterosalpingography
   c. Pelvic arteriography
3. Operative/noninvasive
   a. Abdominal and pelvic examination under anesthesia
4. Operative/invasive
   a. Culdoscopy
   b. Laparoscopy
   c. Exploratory posterior colpotomy
   d. Exploratory laparotomy

An adnexal mass may be of gynecologic or nongynecologic origin (Table 22-2). It is important to establish whether the mass is of ovarian origin. A mass that causes enlargement of the ovary to greater than 6 cm in diameter should be considered potentially malignant until proved otherwise. The most common ovarian mass is the physiologic ovarian cyst. This cyst may result from failure of the follicle to rupture or regress. Failure of the corpus luteum to regress in a nonpregnant patient may result in development of a corpus luteum cyst. Physiologic cysts normally are less than 6 cm in diameter, and may be associated with menstrual irregularity. These cysts are smooth, mobile, and slightly tender to palpation, and usually contain straw-colored fluid. They usually regress by absorption of fluid or spontaneous rupture. In a premenopausal patient, an adnexal cyst less than 6 cm in diameter may be managed conservatively with monthly rectovaginal pelvic examination over two menstrual cycles. If regression fails to occur during this period of observation, or if enlargement is noted, exploratory laparotomy is indicated.

TABLE 22–2
Classification of Adnexal Masses

GYNECOLOGIC ORIGIN	NONGYNECOLOGIC ORIGIN
Nonneoplastic	Nonneoplastic
Ovarian	Appendiceal abscess
Physiologic cysts	Diverticulosis
Follicular	Adhesions of bowel and omentum
Corpus luteum	Peritoneal cyst
Theca lutein cyst	Feces in rectosigmoid
Luteoma of pregnancy	Urine in bladder
Polycystic ovaries	Pelvic kidney
Endometriosis	Urachal cyst
Inflammatory cysts	Anterior sacral meningocele
Nonovarian	Neoplastic
Ectopic pregnancy	Carcinoma
Congenital anomalies	Sigmoid
Embryologic remnants	Cecum
Tubal	Appendix
Pyosalpinx	Bladder
Hydrosalpinx	Retroperitoneal neoplasm
Neoplastic	Presacral teratoma
Ovarian (see Chapter 44)	
Nonovarian	
Leiomyoma	
Paraovarian cyst	
Endometrial carcinoma	
Tubal carcinoma	

(Adapted from Hall DJ, Hurt WG. The adnexal mass. J Fam Pract 1982; 14:135.)

Alternatively, oral contraceptives have been suggested for the treatment of patients with functional cysts. The ingestion of combination-type oral contraceptives results in negative feedback on the pituitary gland to decrease gonadotropin stimulation of the ovary, and in the regression of the cyst. Recently, however, Steinkampf and coauthors noted that the rate of disappearance of functional ovarian cysts was not affected by estrogen/progestin treatment. Nevertheless, a patient taking oral contraceptives rarely develops physiologic cysts. The presence of an ovarian cyst in a patient taking oral contraceptives should be thoroughly investigated.

The corpus luteum varies in size, depending on the amount of blood within the cyst. The corpus luteum may rupture and cause intraperitoneal hemorrhage. Amenorrhea or irregular uterine bleeding may accompany a corpus luteum cyst. A sensitive pregnancy test, laparoscopy, and ultrasonography may be used to differentiate an ectopic pregnancy from a persistent corpus luteum. There is no indication for oophorectomy based on the presence of the corpus luteum.

A thecal luteum cyst may be associated with gestational trophoblastic disease or pregnancy. This cyst results from luteinization of the ovary by human chorionic gonadotropin (HCG). Many of these cysts are bilateral and multicystic. A reduction in HCG levels usually leads to spontaneous regression of the cyst.

Polycystic ovarian disease is associated with bilaterally enlarged ovaries with a smooth surface. The ovaries contain multiple follicular cysts; many patients are obese and hirsute and have accompanying anovulation.

Endometriosis is a common cause of adnexal mass. Endometrial cysts of the ovary may turn into endometriomas and become quite large. Leakage of blood from the cyst may cause peritoneal irritation, dense adhesions, and pelvic organ fixation (Chapter 20). Tubo-ovarian inflammatory complex usually results from incompletely treated or unresolved subacute chronic pelvic inflammatory disease. The inflammatory cyst or tubo-ovarian abscess results from the walled-off area surrounded by pelvic structure (Chapter 24). The abscess occurs as a fluctuant mass, usually above the inguinal ligament or in the cul-de-sac and upper rectovaginal septum. A pyosalpinx or hydrosalpinx may be unilateral or bilateral. These findings usually are associated with the sequelae of acute and chronic pelvic inflammatory diseases. A hydrosalpinx usually is asymptomatic; however, it may be associated with chronic pelvic pain, dyspareunia, and a sense of pelvic pressure. A potentially serious nonneoplastic nonovarian mass may be the result of ectopic pregnancy.

The physician should have a high index of suspicion in any patient with irregular bleeding, pain, and an adnexal mass. Interestingly, more than 50% of women with tubal pregnancy have no palpable adnexal mass. Adnexal mass is an unusual finding when the tubal pregnancy is very early. β-HCG, laparoscopy, and ultrasonography are useful in confirming the diagnosis (Chapter 18).

Congenital anomalies of the müllerian systems and vestigial remnants of the wolffian system should be considered in the differential diagnosis of an adnexal mass. Uterine anomalies usually are associated with cyclic pain because of the development of hematometra. Alternatively, enlargement of a paraovarian cyst may be asymptomatic.

An adnexal mass may be noted in the presence of an acute abdomen. The differential diagnosis should include adnexal torsion, ruptured hemorrhagic cyst, degenerating leiomyomas, ectopic pregnancy, unruptured tubo-ovarian abscess, acute appendicitis with or without abscess formation, and diverticular disease of the sigmoid colon. A careful physical examination and history, including radiologic imaging techniques, often allows a prompt diagnosis of the origin of the adnexal mass (see Chapter 12).

Ultimately, surgery may be required to determine the nature of the adnexal mass. Laparoscopy may be useful to exclude benign ovarian neoplasms or nonovarian benign neoplasms. Indications for visualization of an adnexal mass with laparoscopy, exploratory laparotomy, or posterior colpotomy include the following:

Any ovarian mass or cyst that assumes a size greater than 6 cm in diameter
Any adnexal mass greater than 10 cm in diameter
Any adnexal mass that first develops after menopause
Failure to determine the nature of the mass (ie, myoma) with radiologic or sonographic techniques

Nonneoplastic Ovarian Masses

Ovarian neoplasms are either benign or malignant. Some clinical findings may help to differentiate a malignant from a benign neoplasm (Table 22-3). All ovarian neoplasms that are solid or greater than 6 cm in diameter require immediate investigation. The postmenopausal ovary usually is small and nonpalpable. Enlargement of the postmenopausal ovary necessitates immediate investigation. Symptoms of ovarian neoplasms usually are dependent on their size, rate of growth, and position in the pelvis or abdomen. Symptoms may be vague, and consist of lower abdominal fullness or pelvic discomfort owing to pressure. Larger masses rise out of the true pelvis, and may cause ab-

TABLE 22–3
Clinical Findings Suggestive of Benign or Malignant Adnexal Masses

BENIGN	MALIGNANT
Unilateral	Bilateral
Cystic	Solid
Mobile	Fixed
Smooth	Irregular
No ascites	Ascites
Slow growth	Rapid growth
Young patient	Older patient

dominal enlargement with varicosities and edema of the lower extremities. Most ovarian neoplasms are asymptomatic until they enlarge or involve adjacent organs and structures.

Nonneoplastic Nonovarian Masses

Uterine fibromyomata result in nodularity and, thus, irregularity of the uterus. The uterus may become enlarged, and present as an abdominal mass. Inability to distinguish a leiomyoma from an ovarian tumor on pelvic examination is indication for additional diagnostic procedures to establish the origin of the adnexal mass. Paraovarian cysts arise from wolffian remnants in the broad ligaments. Their diagnosis usually requires laparoscopy or exploratory laparotomy.

In patients with carcinoma of the rectum, appendix, or bladder, adnexal enlargement may result. These patients may present with a variety of symptoms, depending on the organs involved. A complete and thorough evaluation is necessary to delineate the cause of the neoplasm. After age 40 most women with a left adnexal mass should have a barium enema before surgery, to address the possibility of cancer of the rectosigmoid.

The evaluation of a patient with an adnexal mass requires individual management; however, some general recommendations may be suggested. Expectant management is justified only when an asymptomatic, physiologic cyst is suspected. Most cysts that are greater than 6 cm in diameter require a thorough evaluation, usually including exploratory laparotomy. Imaging techniques are invaluable for characterizing the nature of the adnexal enlargement, but these procedures do not replace a careful medical history and thorough physical and pelvic examination.

OVARIAN REMNANT SYNDROME

The ovarian remnant syndrome occurs in a patient who previously underwent bilateral oophorectomy with or without total abdominal hysterectomy. The patient may have presented with or without a palpable mass or with a palpable pelvic mass but no symptoms. Pathologic investigation confirms the presence of ovarian tissue when there should be none. The ovarian remnant syndrome differs from the residual ovarian syndrome, in which the ovary is purposely saved and a pathologic process subsequently develops in the ovary.

The ovarian remnant syndrome represents a complication of oophorectomy. Symmonds and Petit suggest that there are three major factors that complicate the initial surgery and make it difficult or impossible for the surgeon to appreciate that all ovarian tissue has not been removed: (1) increased pelvic vascularity, which renders hemostasis difficult; (2) the existence of adhesions, which distort the anatomy and make the dissection difficult; and (3) alteration of the anatomy by neoplasm. The most common preexisting disease is endometriosis, followed in frequency by pelvic inflammatory disease. Many patients with ovarian remnant syndrome present with pelvic pain and a mass. The quality of the pain varies and is often cyclic, ranging from a pressure sensation to a dull aching to a severe stabbing pain.

Excision of ovarian tissue may require a retroperitoneal dissection to define the relation of the ureter to the bowel and ovary. Care should be taken to carefully define all anatomic relations before extirpation of the remnant.

The clinical diagnosis of ovarian remnant syndrome may be difficult. A finding of premenopausal levels of follicle-stimulating hormone (FSH) may facilitate the diagnosis. Sonography (especially vaginal) may be of value in establishing the diagnosis (Fig. 22-3). CT scan or MRI may be useful in defining the relation of the ovarian remnant to surrounding structures.

The treatment of choice is adequate excision of the ovarian remnant with removal of contiguous adherent tissue such as pelvic peritoneum, bowel serosa, and underlying involved ligament, aveolar, and vascular tissues (Fig. 22-4).

RESIDUAL ADNEXA

The gynecologic surgeon may consider ovarian conservation at the time of abdominal hysterectomy for benign disease (Chapter 27). Advocates of prophylactic oophorectomy have noted the incidence of malignant neoplasm in retained ovaries. Others have noted the presence of "residual ovary syndrome" characterized by either recurrent pelvic pain or a persistent pelvic mass. Funt followed 922 patients after conservation of one or both ovaries at the time of hysterectomy. No patient developed ovarian malignancy; 1.4% of women required subsequent operation for adnexal pathology.

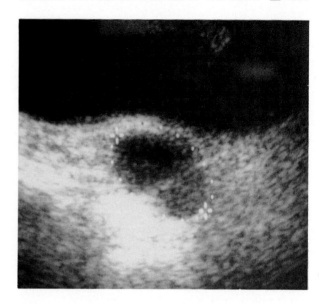

Figure 22–3. Abdominal sonogram showing a residual ovary with presumed follicular activity.

Thus it appears that the benefits of ovarian function outweigh the risks of the development of ovarian pathology requiring further surgery. The gynecologic surgeon should discuss the pros and cons of castration with the patient, to allow the patient to participate in the decision as to the fate of her ovaries at the time of surgery.

SURGERY ON THE OVARIAN SURFACE

Commonly, the gynecologist is required to remove adhesions and/or endometriosis from the ovarian surface. Adhesions may be filmy and vascular between the medial surface of the ovary and the broad ligament (Fig. 22-5A). These may be excised with fine electrocautery or vaporized with the CO_2 laser (Fig. 22-5B). More extensive adhesions may completely cover the ovarian surface. These adhesions may be thick and avascular (Fig. 22-5C and D). Care must be taken in developing the plane between the broad ligament or pelvic sidewall and the adhered ovarian surface, so as not to remove or damage peritoneum while excising the adhesion (Fig. 22-5D).

When multiple small adhesions are noted over the ovarian surface, their removal may be facilitated by applying a defocused CO_2 laser energy beam. The coagulated adhesions may be wiped off the ovary without trauma to the ovarian cortex. Alternatively, these adhesions may be coagulated with monopolar cautery and then removed.

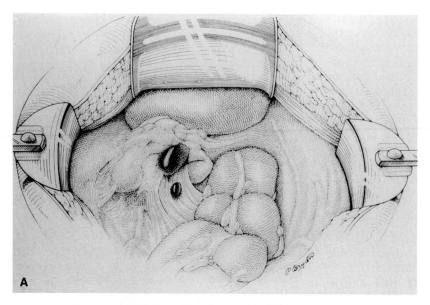

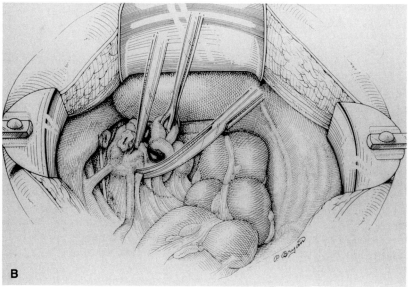

Figure 22–4. *A,* Not infrequently, the ovarian remnant may be adhered to the bowel and the pelvic sidewall peritoneum. *B,* The ureter must be visualized and its relation to the bowel and ovarian remnant established. This may require the development of the pararectal and rectovaginal spaces.

If the lateral aspect of the ovary is densely adhered to the broad ligament, it may be necessary to dissect the ovary free. In some instances a large area of the sidewall or the broad ligament may be denuded, requiring reperitonealization with fine 7-0 nonreactive suture material.

Small endometrial implants may be fulgurated or vaporized. The small ovarian defect usually does not require closure. Care should be taken to assure that the endometriosis is superficial for, in some instances, the implant is the tip of a large endometrioma within the substance of the ovary.

RECONSTRUCTION OF THE OVARY

After resection of pathologic tissue the gynecologist may be required to reconstruct the entire ovary. Before resecting ovarian tissue, mobilization of the ovary and establishment of the normal anatomic relations should be accomplished.

Ovarian surgery for the treatment of infertility usually is limited to resection of benign cysts (ie, functional or endometrial cysts) or wedge resection for the induction of ovulation in the polycystic ovary syndrome. A common indication for ovarian surgery is endometrio-

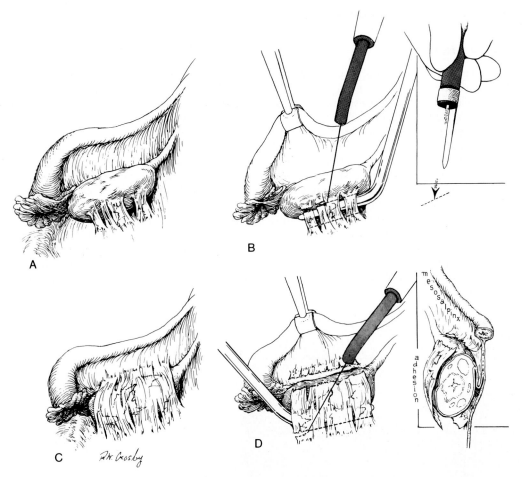

Figure 22–5. Ovarian adhesions. *A*, Filmy adhesions between the medial aspect of the ovary and the pelvic sidewall. *B*, These may be removed with the CO_2 laser or fine electrocautery, using a quartz or glass rod, respectively, as a backstop. *C*, The ovary may be enveloped by adhesions. *D*, Care should be taken to tent up the adhesions so that the peritoneum is not damaged or incised.

sis. In addition, the lysis of periovarian adhesions resulting from chronic pelvic inflammatory disease or endometriosis may be performed in an effort to enhance fertility (Chapter 20). In ovarian reconstructive surgery atraumatic technique cannot be overemphasized. Extensive periovarian and peritubular adhesions may result after reconstruction if adequate attention is not given to meticulous approximation of the cortex, hemostasis, and atraumatic technique. Pelvic lavage with 5000 units of heparin and a liter of lactate Ringer's solution before closing the abdomen is helpful in removing tiny clots while assuring that hemostasis is adequate at the suture line. In the process of removing a benign cyst or performing wedge resection, conserva-

tion of ovarian cortex and primordial follicles is important. Reconstruction of the ovary, therefore, must be performed with meticulous attention to tissue approximation while restoring a normal configuration to the adnexa.

Interceed (TC 7) recently was approved by the Food and Drug Administration for the prevention of postsurgical adhesions. This absorbable oxidized, regenerated cellulose barrier promotes a negligible tissue response while reducing postsurgical adhesions when placed between the ovary and the pelvic sidewall. This adjunctive therapy should be considered when adhesion formation is thought likely to result from ovarian reconstructive surgery.

Resection of Benign Cysts

Functional Ovarian Cysts

Physiologic enlargement of the ovary may occur as a result of failure of either follicular or corpus luteum regression. The vast majority of these cysts regress, but on occasion they may persist, varying in size from 3 to 8 cm in diameter. These physiologic nonneoplastic ovarian cysts do not require surgery; however, because of their large size and the resulting pain suffered by the patients, removal may be necessary. A cyst may adhere to the posterior broad ligament, requiring removal of the cyst, ovarian reconstruction of the peritoneal defect, and reperitonealization. If the cyst is quite large, the fallopian tube may be splayed across the ovarian cyst, with marked distortion of tubal architecture.

Surgical Technique. An elliptical incision is made through the thin ovarian cortex of a benign cyst (Fig. 22-6*B*). The end of the knife handle may then be inserted and a plane developed over the cyst wall (Fig. 22-6*C*). Alternatively, fine-needle electrocautery or the CO_2 laser may be used to develop a plane, and fine microsurgical scissors may be used to separate the cyst wall from the ovarian cortex. Surgical loupes are useful to assist the surgeon in identifying the correct plane between the cyst wall and the ovarian parenchyma. After the cyst wall has been completely separated from its adhesive attachments to the thin ovarian cortex, it may be shelled out without rupture (Fig. 22-6*C*). On occasion, however, even with the gentlest technique, because of the friable cyst wall, rupture may occur. It is of utmost importance before shelling the cyst to pack the cul-de-sac with moist, lint-free pads, so that if rupture occurs, spillage will not contaminate the cul-de-sac. After the cyst has been removed the dead space may be obliterated with a purse-string suture of 7-0 nonreactive suture (Fig. 22-6*D*). Alternatively, placing 5-0 non-

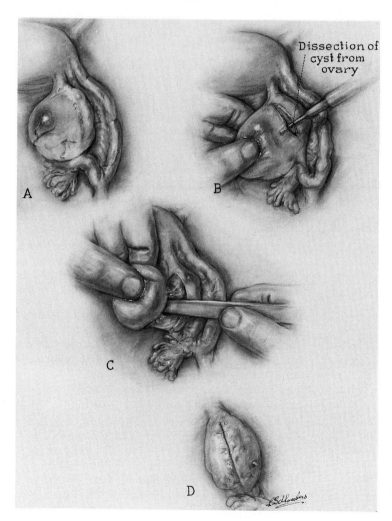

Dissection of cyst from ovary

A

B

C

D

Figure 22–6. Resection of benign cyst. *A*, Thin-walled ovarian cyst. *B*, An incision is made through the cortex. *C*, A plane is developed using blunt dissection. The inner ovarian stroma may be approximated with a purse-string of 5-0 nonreactive suture material. *D*, The ovarian cortex is approximated using 7-0 nonreactive suture material.

reactive vertical mattress sutures (Fig. 22-7A) and/or figure-of-eight sutures (Fig. 22-7B) may approximate the lateral walls of the ovary. The ovarian surface is then neatly approximated with a subcortical running suture of 7-0 nonreactive suture (Fig. 22-7C). If the cortex is quite friable, it may be necessary to place interrupted sutures of 7-0 to achieve approximation. Some authors advocate leaving the ovary open; they have noted that in their personal experience, adhesion formation did not occur after the procedure. There are no control trials at this writing that document the extent of postoperative adhesion formation when the ovary is not closed.

In some instances there is excessive redundant thin cortex, which may present a special problem in ovarian reconstruction. The amount of cortex removed depends on the position of the cyst, as well as its overall size. A careful study of the ovary before making the initial incision is necessary. An incision of the ovarian cortex should allow a symmetric reconstruction when possible. The redundant cortex, however, may be removed and the dead space obliterated with an internal closure such that suture material does not penetrate the ovarian cortex, thus avoiding ischemia and formation of adhesions. The infolding technique recommended by Kistner and Patton may result in anatomic distortion and puckering of the ovarian cortex. It is our view that the fewer suture lines used, the less likely are bleeding and adhesion formation to occur. Concern over ovarian surgery was voiced by Van der Wat. Of 36 young women operated on for ovarian cysts, 45% complained of infertility at a later date. The author made a plea for surgeons not to interfere with functional cysts in normal ovaries, as resulting adhesion formation may compromise fertility. Benign ovarian cysts should not be removed at the time of surgery for other indications unless they are sufficiently large to interfere with tubal function or cause discomfort to the patient. The vast majority of functional cysts resolve with observation and require no therapy.

Endometrial Cysts

Large endometrioma may distort the ovarian cortex. Peritubular adhesions may be present. Often the lateral side of the ovary is adhered to the pelvic sidewall or posterior broad ligament.

Surgical Technique. Initially, the normal relations between the tube, ovary, and uterus should be established. Once the ovary is mobilized, it may be placed on a rubber platform for reconstruction. Frequent irrigation is necessary to avoid drying of the serosa of the tube and ovarian cortex. An elliptical incision is made over the endometrioma along the axis between the utero-ovarian ligament and the fimbria ovarica (Fig. 22-8A). A suture may be placed in the cyst wall for traction (Fig. 22-8B). The endometrial cyst is mobilized with sharp dissection using fine scissors, fine-needle electrocautery, or the CO_2 laser (Fig. 22-8C). Once the endometrial cyst is removed, a large ovarian defect may be observed, depending on the size of the endometrioma. This space may be obliterated with a pursestring suture of nonreactive suture material (Fig. 22-8D). Redundant ovarian stroma may be approximated with a running suture and/or vertical mattress suture of 5-0 nonreactive suture material (Fig. 22-8E and F). The ovarian surface is closed by approximating the cortex with a running subcortical suture of 7-0 nonreactive suture material (Fig. 22-8G). Great care should be taken to avoid trauma to the cortex and oviduct, as these structures are most susceptible to adhesion formation. Microsurgical principles should be strictly observed.

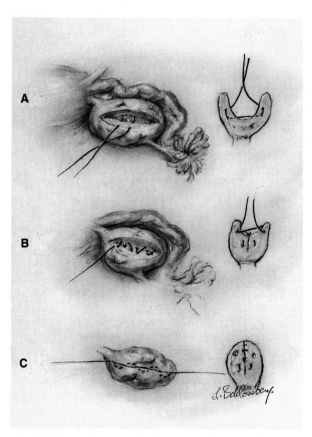

Figure 22–7. Suture placement for ovarian reconstruction. A, Vertical mattress suture. B, Figure-of-eight suture. C, The cortex is approximated with a suture of running 7-0 nonreactive suture material.

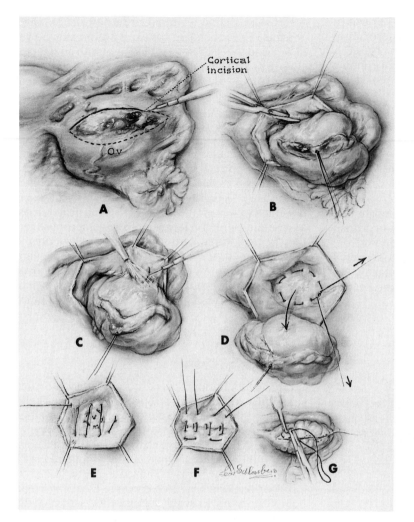

Figure 22–8. Removal of ovarian endometrioma. *A*, An elliptical incision is made over the endometrioma. *B* and *C*, The endometrial cyst is mobilized using sharp dissection and traction from a suture placed through the cyst wall. Irrigation is useful to prevent drying of tissues. *D*, Once the cyst is removed, the defect is closed. First, the base of the defect is closed with a purse-string suture of nonreactive 5-0 suture material. *E*, The rest of the defect is closed with running suture or *F*, a vertical mattress suture of 5-0 nonreactive suture material. *G*, The cortex is approximated with a running suture of 7-0 nonreactive suture material.

Wedge Resection for Polycystic Ovarian Disease

The polycystic ovary is a sign, not a diagnosis. It usually is accompanied by some degree of hirsutism, infertility, and, in most cases, ovulatory failure. The polycystic ovary may result from virilizing ovarian and adrenal tumors or congenital adrenal hyperplasia (polycystic ovary syndrome), or it may result from a suboptimal hypothalamic-pituitary function at puberty (polycystic ovarian disease). The exact mechanism for the development of ovulatory failure has been attributed to androgen overproduction and its effect on the hypothalamic-pituitary axis. The discussion of the hypothalamic-pituitary ovarian dysfunction is beyond the scope of this chapter.

The histologic findings in a polycystic ovary cover a broad spectrum. The spectrum extends from the typical Stein-Leventhal type of polycystic ovary with a large number of follicular cysts and few atretic cysts, in which there is marked stromal hyperplasia and hyperthecosis, to a smaller ovary with a few follicular cysts, atretic follicles, and stromal hyperplasia. The polycystic ovary may exhibit microscopic islands of luteinized thecal cells scattered in the stroma, but usually there is a thickened fibrosed tunica with a large number of cystic follicles beneath this thickened capsule.

There are several hypotheses as to the mechanism by which wedge resection of the polycystic ovary resolves ovulatory failure. The theory stating that the fibrous capsule acts as a mechanical barrier to the ovulatory follicle has been refuted. Evidence against this theory consists of the observation that if one ovary is removed, ovulation occurs from the other. In addition, the use of clomiphene citrate results in ovulation through an intact capsule. Some have stated that neonatal androgen may cause an abnormal hypothalamic-pituitary axis, resulting in abnormal gonadal patterns. This theory is not widely accepted. Neonatal androgen treatment in rats is associated with masculinization of the hypothalamus and ovulatory failure with polycystic ovaries. In the human with virilizing congenital adrenal hyperplasia in which there are both intrauterine and neonatal androgen excess, ovulatory cycles are established with cortisone replacement at puberty.

The more commonly held theory, by which wedge resection results in resumption of ovulatory cycles, notes that the removal of androgen-secreting stroma and theca reduces the amount of abnormal steroid production in the ovary. After wedge resection there usually is a decrease in the mean level of 17-hydroxyprogesterone, dehydroepiandrosterone, delta^4-androstenedione, and testosterone, and a transitory decrease in estradiol. This reduction in the steroidogenesis of androgens, allowing a normalization of the luteinizing hormone (LH)-FSH ratio, results in a resumption of ovulatory cycles.

There is some debate as to the amount of ovarian mass that should be removed at the time of wedge resection. Halbe and coauthors attempted to clarify this question by removing different amounts of ovarian substances from a random selection of patients with polycystic ovarian disease. Thirty-eight of 62 patients were interested in conception. The 38 patients were divided into three groups, the first of which was characterized by removal of not greater than one-fifth of the original ovarian size. The second group had one-third of the ovarian mass removed, and the third group had half to three-fourths of the original ovarian size reduced. Resumptions of ovulatory cycles were recorded as 53%, 71%, and 91%, respectively. The pregnancy rates were 50%, 53%, and 92%, respectively. The authors concluded that the best ovulatory rate and pregnancy rate resulted after removal of at least half of the ovarian medulla.

Stein and Leventhal thought that the size of the ovary was an important factor in patient selection; others, however, have found no relation between the results after surgery and the size of the ovaries. Because the size of the ovary may vary with the spectrum of the polycystic ovary syndrome, this usually has no bearing on the selection of patients for wedge resection.

Indications for Wedge Resection

The introduction of clomiphene citrate has changed the management of polycystic ovarian disease in patients who desire a pregnancy. Johnson reported ovulation in 359 of 436 patients with Stein-Leventhal syndrome with the first course of therapy. An additional 58 patients ovulated after two or more cycles. The conception rate with clomiphene (50%–60%) is, however, less than the 86% pregnancy rate reported by Stein and Leventhal for wedge resection. The incidence of post-clomiphene birth defects (3.1%) is not increased as compared with commonly quoted rates for populations at large. There are some patients, moreover, in whom ovulation seems to be achieved with clomiphene and a pregnancy does not occur. Kistner and Patton recommended wedge resection in those patients who have not conceived after seven or eight cycles of treatment with clomiphene. More often wedge resection is reserved for women who are unresponsive to clomiphene at all dose ranges and when combined with HCG.

Furthermore, some patients may not want to accept the risks of multiple birth or hyperstimulation associated with pure FSH or FSH and LH ovulation induction. Although ovulation induction with the gonadotropin-releasing hormone pump usually avoids these risks, this technique may be cost-prohibitive for some women. In any event the need for wedge resection of the polycystic ovary is much less with the development of the newer reproductive technologies. Nevertheless, this procedure may be the only option for some patients.

Babaknia and coauthors have reported an incidence of 17% of coincidental ovarian tumors in patients operated on for relief of symptoms of Stein-Leventhal syndrome. In planning therapy, consideration should be given to the possibility of an ovarian neoplasm.

Surgical Technique

About 50% of the ovarian substance should be removed with the wedge. A 2- to 3-cm incision is made through the thickened cortex (Fig. 22-9A). The incision is made over the convexity of the ovary, with particular attention to the direction of the incision so as to create a small V-shaped segment of ovarian tissue. Care is taken to avoid the hilus of the ovary, as excessive bleeding may occur. The ovary may be held with the hand or with the thumb and first finger. Through this small incision a portion of the medulla is removed, preserving as much cortex as possible (Fig. 22-9B). The ovarian defect is then closed in two layers, the first consisting of a purse-string suture of 5-0 nonreactive suture, such as polydioxanone material (Fig. 22-9C). The second layer consists of interrupted figure-of-eight 5-0 nonreactive suture, which approximates the ovarian stroma (Fig. 22-9D). A running suture of 7-0 nonreactive suture material is used to approximate the surface of the cortex (Fig. 22-9E). If the dead space is completely obliterated, the likelihood of an ovarian hematoma is small. In addition, with careful approximation and complete hemostasis, the risk of adhesion formation is minimal.

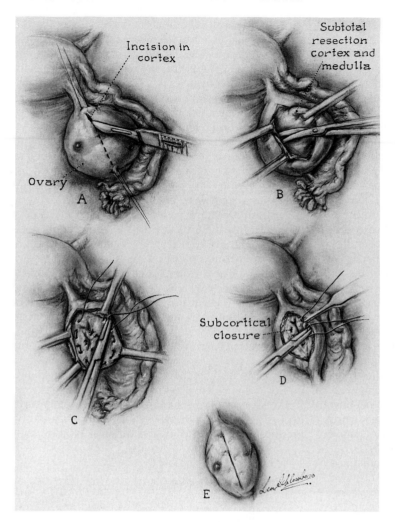

Figure 22–9. Wedge resection of the polycystic ovary. *A*, A small elliptical incision is made over the convexity of the ovary. *B*, Through this incision the medulla is incised and removed, preserving as much cortex as possible. *C*, The defect is closed with a purse-string of 5-0 nonreactive suture material. *D*, Additional vertical mattress sutures may be needed to approximate the stroma. *E*, The ovarian surface has been approximated with 7-0 nonreactive suture material.

Results

In a recent review of the literature Goldzieher reported 1079 cases of wedge resection in 187 references. Postwedge-resection resumption of regular menstrual cycles may be anticipated to follow a mean frequency of 80%, the range being 6% to 95%. The pregnancy success rate does not exceed an average of 63%, the range being 13% to 89%.

Adashi and coauthors observed a resumption of menses in 91% of patients treated by bilateral ovarian wedge resection. Furthermore, within the ovulatory group, 26 patients were characterized by oligo-ovulation and a reduced conception rate (29%), as compared with that of 56 normo-ovulatory counterparts (60%). Persistent oligo-ovulation and anovulation and the presence of concurrent tuboperitoneal adhesions were the most important determinants of the likelihood of conception.

There is concern over adhesion formation after wedge resection. Toaff and coauthors noted extensive peritubular and periovarian adhesions in seven patients who did not conceive after bilateral wedge resection. Four of these patients had reconstructive surgery and three conceived and delivered. Bilateral ovarian atrophy was noted in one patient and unilateral ovarian atrophy was noted in two patients. The authors recommend laparoscopy in cases of unsuccessful ovarian resection. Weinstein and Polishuk noted that of 57 patients treated with bilateral resection, 38 conceived, for a pregnancy rate of 67%. Eight of the 19 patients who did not conceive had extensive adhesion formation. Neither Toaff and colleagues nor Weinstein and Polishuk reported the incidence of adhesion formation in the patients who conceived.

A minimum incidence of 7.8% was documented at the Johns Hopkins Hospital for acquired post-bilateral ovarian-wedge-resection pelvic disease. It is our belief that gentle technique, the use of fine suture with minimal reactivity, and meticulous hemostasis should minimize adhesion formation after wedge resection.

PARADOXICAL OOPHORECTOMY

The value of paradoxical oophorectomy has been debated. Jeffcoate suggested that in a patient with one functional tube, her fertility should be improved by making her ovulate repeatedly from the ovary alongside the patent tube by removing the opposite ovary. Scott and coauthors reported a series of 24 patients with unilateral tubal patency confirmed by retrograde injection at laparotomy. Contralateral oophorectomy or salpingo-oophorectomy was performed, and subsequently 21 pregnancies resulted in 16 women, for a pregnancy rate of 67%. The authors suggest that the frequency at which transperitoneal migration occurs may be a factor. Hallet noted that one in five tubal ectopic pregnancies had a corpus luteum in the contralateral side. Jansen noted a pregnancy success rate of 18.7% (n = 91) after bilateral salpingostomy for hydrosalpinges, whereas the pregnancy rate was 43.8% (n = 16) with unilateral salpingostomy with bilateral division of adhesions, which was comparable to that after bilateral salpingolysis. The mean surgery-pregnancy interval was longer after unilateral salpingostomy (104 weeks) than after bilateral salpingolysis (45 weeks). The author suggests that salpingo-oophorectomy may be preferable to salpingoneostomy for unilateral hydrosalpinx. Randomized, carefully controlled clinical trials should be performed to establish the efficacy of paradoxical oophorectomy.

Increased pregnancy success after in vitro fertilization correlates with the number of cleaving embryos placed in the uterus. The number of mature eggs retrieved after superovulation usually is a reflection of the number of ovaries available for stimulation. Thus ovarian conservation is desirable. Until the efficacy of paradoxical oophorectomy is clearly established, a normal ovary should not be removed. Of course, there is always the risk of something happening to the remaining ovary, removal of which would result in premature castration.

LAPAROSCOPIC OVARIAN RECONSTRUCTION

Minor adhesive disease and endometriosis on the surface of the ovary may be treated laparoscopically. Endometriosis and/or adhesions may be fulgurated with electrocautery or vaporized using the CO_2 laser. This may avoid a major laparotomy and decrease morbidity from the procedure. Removal of a cyst, a der-

moid, or an endometrioma from the ovary, however, usually results in a large cavity within the ovary that must heal as a secondary process unless the ovarian defect is approximated using a vertical mattress suture. The exposure of suture material through the cortex predisposes to adhesion formation. Furthermore, a large open defect also may result in severe adhesive disease. Nonetheless, a small endometrioma may be easily removed (Fig. 22-10) by incision of the ovarian cortex, grasping the endometrial cyst with forceps. Twisting the forceps may separate the cyst wall from the surrounding ovarian tissue (Fig. 22-10D), facilitating cyst removal. Once the cyst wall has been twisted free (Fig. 22-10D), the cyst wall may be removed (Fig. 22-10E). At this writing there are no carefully controlled data comparing traditional microsurgical ovarian reconstruction with laparoscopic removal of ovarian cysts. With new methods of adhesion prevention and documentation of efficacy of the laparoscopic enucleation of ovarian cysts without ovarian closure, this new approach may supplement traditional microsurgical techniques.

Polycystic Ovaries Treated by Laparoscopic Surgery

Interest has been generated in laparoscopic surgery for polycystic ovarian disease with the publication of reports describing the efficacy of destruction of a small percentage of the ovarian cortex and subcortical tissue by electrocautery, laser vaporization, endocoagulation, or multiple-punch resection. Gjonnaess described a laparoscopic technique in which three to eight monopolar cauterization points 3 mm in diameter and 2 to 3 mm in depth were placed in each ovary of 35 anovulatory infertile women. He reported that 24 patients became pregnant (69%). An additional four patients conceived after the introduction of clomiphene citrate therapy postoperatively, for a cumulative pregnancy rate of 80%. In a subsequent study Aakvaag and Gjonnaess documented ovulation in 59 of 72 women within 4 weeks of laparoscopic cautery. Daniell and Miller used the argon, CO_2, and potassium-titanyl-phosphate (KPT) lasers to vaporize and drain small visible subcapsular cysts of each ovary and randomly drill "craters" in the ovarian stroma. The 2- to 4-mm vaporization sites numbered between 25 and 40 per each ovary in a group of 38 patients who failed to ovulate preoperatively with clomiphene citrate. Postoperatively, 20 women ovulated spontaneously and 17 of the remaining 18 patients ovulated when given clomiphene citrate. Twenty-five of the 38 patients (66%) conceived. Similar results were reported by Huber and coworkers using the Nd:YAG laser to create 6 to 10 incisions of 5 to 10 mm in depth in each ovary in women with polycystic ovarian disease. Finally, Sumioki and coauthors used laparoscopic mul-

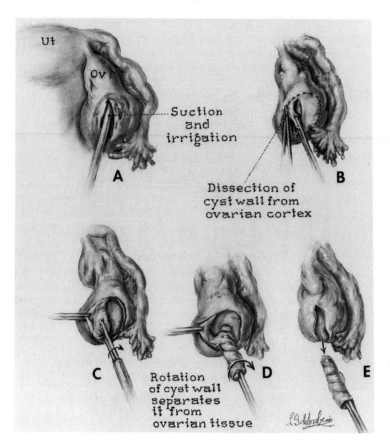

Figure 22–10. Removal of a small ovarian endometrial cyst through the laparoscope. *A,* After incision of the ovarian cortex, the contents of the endometrioma are removed with suction and irrigation. *B,* The plane between the ovary and the cyst wall is developed by using traction and twisting the forceps clockwise. *C,* The endometrial cyst wall is grasped with forceps. *D,* The cyst wall separates from the ovarian tissue using a twisting motion. The ovarian defect may be left open to heal by second intention or be closed with vertical mattress sutures. *E,* The cyst wall is removed.

tiple-punch biopsy to perform 6 to 10 superficial biopsies per woman in seven women with polycystic ovarian disease who failed to ovulate with medical treatment. Eighty-six percent resumed spontaneous ovulation and 57% of patients conceived.

Despite these promising data regarding laparoscopic treatment of polycystic ovarian disease, there is concern about the propensity toward adhesion formation. Lyles and coauthors noted ovarian adhesions of variable extent in all cases of patients treated with electrocautery or laser. Also of concern is the possibility of premature ovarian failure if a large portion of the ovarian cortex is destroyed. The efficacy of this innovative approach remains to be established in carefully designed clinical trials.

Bibliography

Aakvaag A, Gjonnaess H. Hormonal response to electrocautery of the ovary in patients with polycystic ovarian disease. Br J Obstet Gynaecol 1985;92:1258.

Adashi E, Rock JA, Wentz A, et al. Fertility after bilateral ovarian wedge resection: a critical analysis of 90 consecutive cases of polycystic ovarian disease. Fertil Steril 1981;36:320.

Adhesion Barrier Study Group. Interceed (TC-7). Prevention of post surgical adhesions by Interceed (TC-7). Fertil Steril 1989;51:933.

Babaknia A, Panayotis C, Jones HW Jr. The Stein-Leventhal syndrome and coincidental ovarian tumors. Obstet Gynecol 1976;47:223.

Burns RK Jr. The origin and differentiation of the epithelium of the urogenital sinus in the opossum, with a study of the modifications induced by oestrogens. Contrib Embryol 1942;30:63.

Burns RK Jr. Hormones versus constitutional factors in the growth of embryonic sex primordia in the opossum. Am J Anat 1956;98:35.

Christ JE, Lotze EC. The residual ovary syndrome. Obstet Gynecol 1973;46:551.

Daniell JF, Miller W. Polycystic ovaries treated by laparoscopic laser vaporization. Fertil Steril 1989;51:232.

Fayez A, Jonas HS. Assessment of the role of laparoscopic ovarian biopsy. Obstet Gynecol 1976;48:397.

Ford CE. The cytogenetics of germ cells and testes in animals. In: The human testes. New York: Plenum Press, 1970.

Funt MI. The residual adnexal—asset or liability? Am J Obstet Gynecol 1977;129:251.

Gillman J. The development of the gonads in man, with a consideration of the role of fetal endocrines and the histogenesis of ovarian tumors. Contrib Embryol 1948;32:81.

Gjonnaess H. Polycystic ovarian syndrome treated by ovarian electrocautery through the laparoscope. Fertil Steril 1984;41:20.

Goldzieher JW. Polycystic ovarian disease. In: Lehrman SJ, Kistner RW, eds. Progress in infertility. Boston: Little, Brown, 1975: 325.

Greenblatt RB. The polycystic ovary syndrome. Md State Med J 1961;10:120.

Grogan RH. Reappraisal of the residual ovary. Am J Obstet Gynecol 1967;97:124.

Halbe HW, da Fonseca AM, Silva P deP, et al. Stein-Leventhal syndrome. Am J Obstet Gynecol 1972;114:280.

Hall DJ, Hurt WG. The adnexal mass. J Fam Pract 1982;14:135.

Hallet JC. Repeat ectopic pregnancy: a study of 123 consecutive cases. Am J Obstet Gynecol 1975;122:520.

Hernandez E, Miyazawa K. The pelvic mass: patients' ages and pathologic findings. J Reprod Med 1988;33:361.

Herrmann JB, Kelly RJ, Higgins GA. Polyglycolic acid sutures: laboratory and clinical evaluation of a new absorbable suture material. Arch Surg 1970;100:486.

Huber J, Hosmann J, Spona J. Polycystic ovarian syndrome treated by laser through the laparoscope. Fertil Steril (in press).

Jansen RPS. Surgery pregnancy time intervals after salpingolysis, unilateral salpingostomy and bilateral salpingostomy. Fertil Steril 1980;34:222.

Jeffcoate TA. Principles of gynecology. London: Butterworth, 1975.

Johnson JE Jr. Outcome of pregnancies following clomiphene citrate therapy. Proceedings of the Fifth World Congress on Fertility and Sterility. Amsterdam: Excerpta Medica, 1967:101.

Judd HL, Lee RA, Anderson DC, Yen SS. The effects of ovarian wedge resection on circulating gonadotropin and ovarian steroid levels in patients with polycystic ovary syndrome. J Clin Endocrinol Metab 1976;13:347.

Katz M, Carr PJ, Cohen BM, Millar RP. Hormonal effects of wedge resection of polycystic ovaries. Obstet Gynecol 1978;51:437.

Killackey MC, Neuwirth RS. Evaluation and management of the pelvic mass: a review of 540 cases. Obstet Gynecol 1988;71(Pt 1):319.

Kistner RW, Patton GW. Surgery of the ovary. In: Atlas of infertility surgery. Boston: Little, Brown, 1975:105,177.

Lyles R, Goldzieher JW, Betts JW, et al. Early second-look laparoscopy after the treatment of polycystic ovarian disease with laparoscopic ovarian electrocautery and/or Nd:YAG laser photocoagulation. Abstract presented at the 45th Annual Meeting of the American Fertility Society, November 1989.

McKay DG, Hertig AT, Adams EC, Danziger S. Histochemical observations on the germ cells of human embryos. Anat Rec 1953;117:201.

Oelsner G, Graebe RA, Boyers SP, et al. A comparison of three techniques for ovarian reconstruction. Am J Obstet Gynecol 1986;154:569.

Scott JS, Lynch EM, Anderson JA. Surgical treatment of female infertility: value of paradoxical oophorectomy. Br Med J 1976;1:631.

Stein JF, Leventhal ML. Amenorrhea associated with bilateral polycystic ovaries. Am J Obstet Gynecol 1935;29:191.

Steinkampf MP, Hammond KR, Blackwell RE. Hormonal treatment of functional ovarian cysts: a randomized prospective study. Fertil Steril 1990;54(5):775.

Sumioki H, Utsunomyiya T, Matsuoka K, et al. The effect of laparoscopic multiple punch resection of the ovary on hypothalamo-pituitary axis in polycystic ovarian syndrome. Fertil Steril 1988;50:567.

Symmonds RE, Petit P. Ovarian remnant syndrome. Obstet Gynecol 1979;54:175.

Terz J, Barber H, Bronschwig A. Incidence of carcinoma in the retained ovary. Am J Surg 1967;113:511.

Toaff R, Toaff ME, Peyer MR. Infertility following wedge resection of the ovaries. Am J Obstet Gynecol 1976;124:2.

Turner CD, Asakawa H. Experimental reversal of germ cells in ovaries of fetal mice. Science 1964;143:1344.

Van der Wat JJ. The mutilated ovary syndrome. S Afr Med J 1970;44:687.

Verhoeven ATM, Mastboom JL, Van Leusden HAIM, van der Velder WHM. Virilization in pregnancy co-existing with an ovarian mucinous cystadenoma. A case report and review of virilizing ovarian tumors in pregnancy. Obstet Gynecol Surv 1973;28:597.

Weinstein D, Polishuk WZ. Role of wedge resection of the ovary as a cause for mechanical sterility. Surg Gynecol Obstet 1975;141:417.

Witschi E. Migration of the germ cells of human embryos from the yolk sac to the primitive gonadal folds. Contrib Embryol 1948;32:69.

Witschi E. Embryology of the ovary. In: The ovary. Baltimore: Williams & Wilkins, 1962:1.

Zdanovsky BM, Anshine MB, Semendiaev AA, et al. Treatment of polycystic ovarian syndrome by pelviscopic ovarian endocoagulation. Abstract presented at the World Congress of Gynecologic Endoscopy, September 1989.

23

Persistent or Chronic Pelvic Pain

HOWARD A. ZACUR

The intent of this chapter is to discuss the management of patients whose pelvic pain remains unresolved. Chronic pelvic pain is described as the persistence for more than 6 months of pelvic pain that remains both *unexplained* and *without evidence of active disease.* To understand this condition fully, it is necessary to review the pelvic pain pathways. This review is followed by a description of various causes of pelvic pain. Lastly, evaluation and therapy for these conditions are discussed.

PELVIC PAIN PATHWAYS

Pain sensations from the pelvis result from nociceptive (noxious) stimuli transmitted by thinly myelinated or nonmyelinated pain fibers (A delta and C fibers). These pain fibers may be activated in somatic structures (skin, muscles, bones, joints, and parietal peritoneum) or visceral structures (uterus, fallopian tubes, and ovaries). Types of stimuli that may activate these pain fibers include pressure, ischemia, chemical irritation, and injury.

Neuroanatomy for Pelvic Pain Sensations

Because the neuroanatomy for pelvic pain sensations is complex, as shown in Figure 23-1, precise localization of pain complaints may be difficult. For example, pelvic pain sensations may be transmitted from pelvic structures by way of fibers traveling with sympathetic nerves that communicate with the spinal cord dorsal horn entering at spinal cord segments T-10, T-11, T-12, L-1, and L-2. In this situation ovarian afferents would enter at T-10, and uterine afferents at T-12; bladder and vaginal afferents would enter at L-1. Pelvic organs also are innervated by pain fibers that accompany parasympathetic nerves entering the spinal cord at S-2, S-3, and S-4 with the pudendal nerve. As a result, pain sensations in the same organ may be perceived by two nociceptive systems that have different reflex arcs in the spinal cord. Complicating matters, these pelvic pain impulses intermingle with afferent neuronal input from various pelvic plexi involving the uterus, cervix, hypogastric nerve, and lumbar and lower thoracic sympathetic chain. As a result, referred pain from the site of origin frequently is experienced (eg, ovarian pain may be referred as periumbilical pain or uterine pain as lower abdominal pain).

Processing of Pain Impulses

Perception of pelvic pain is further complicated by processing of the pain impulses. As the A delta and C fibers enter the dorsal root, they synapse with other cells that affect or modulate the pain signals. For example, activation of the large myelinated fibers may inhibit pain transmission at the spinal cord level by the A delta and C fibers (Fig. 23-1). Purposeful activation of these larger myelinated pain fibers probably explains the pain-relieving "powers" of massage, acupuncture, and transcutaneous electrical nerve stimulation (TENS).

The body's ability to recognize and respond to pain is further aided by descending neural pathways, which modulate pain response by increasing or decreasing nociceptive transmission. The opioid-mediated analgesia system is one example. This system relies on endogenous opioids or endorphins within the brain to activate descending neurons, which rely in turn on

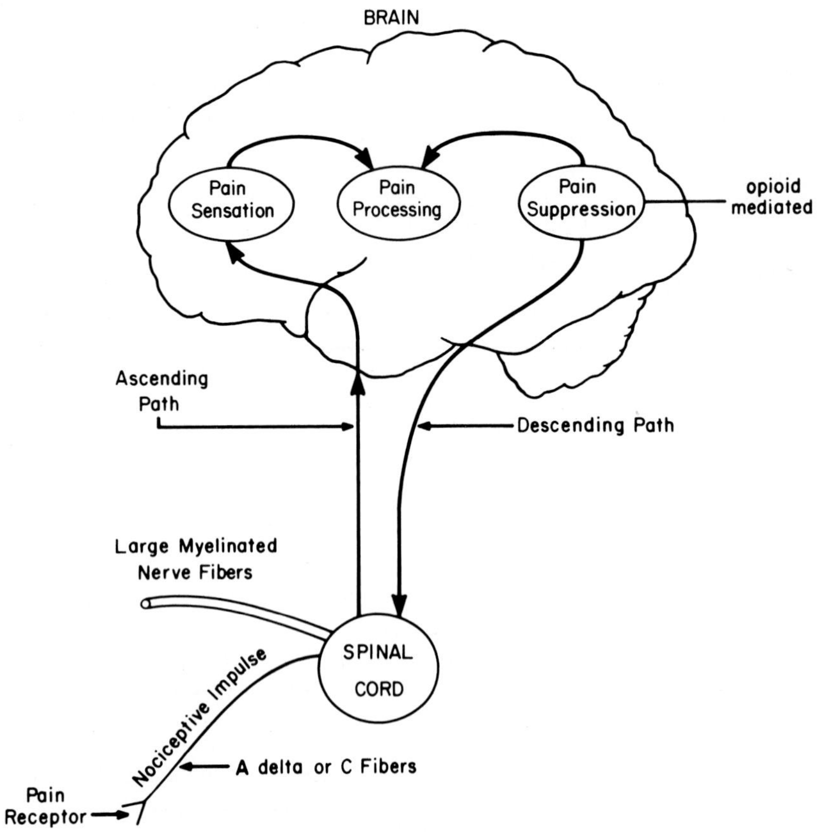

Figure 23–1. Neuronal afferents and ascending and descending neural pathways responsible for modulating pelvic pain sensation.

serotonin to cause analgesia (Fig. 23-1). Another example involves a nonopioid descending pathway using norepinephrine as the neurotransmitter that inhibits nociceptive neuronal firing. Activation of these descending analgesic pathways might vary from person to person, explaining individual differences in the ability to tolerate pain. Reduction in the activity of the pain-suppressing systems could decrease pain tolerance, which could also account for differences between individuals to tolerate the same pain stimulus.

CLINICAL FEATURES

The typical patient with chronic pelvic pain is in the reproductive age range (20–40 years) and is most likely to be married and to be parous. Menstrual cycles may be described as either regular or irregular. Similarly, dysmenorrhea, in addition to the pelvic pain complaint, may be present or absent. Pain symptoms have been reported to last from 6 months to 20 years and frequently are described as being dull with intermittent sharp exacerbations. Location of the pelvic pain may be specific, generalized, or variable, and may not

ultimately be useful as a distinguishing feature in dealing with chronic pelvic pain.

CAUSES OF CHRONIC PELVIC PAIN

An initial search for the cause of otherwise unexplained chronic pelvic pain may be organized by systematically investigating pelvic structures. In brief, this would include peritoneum, uterus, fallopian tubes, ovaries, other pelvic organs, pelvic musculature, and vasculature. Other causes of pelvic pain include neurologic and skeletal malfunction within or outside the pelvis as well as metabolic and psychologic destruction occurring outside the pelvis. Table 23-1 summarizes the various causes of pelvic pain.

Peritoneum

Irritation of parietal or visceral peritoneum may result in the transmission of pain impulses. Common peritoneal chemical irritants include blood and purulent material, which, when present, usually result in

TABLE 23–1
Causes of Pelvic Pain

Peritoneum

Irritation by blood or purulent material
Lacerations or tears
Endometriosis
Adhesions

Uterus

Leiomyomata
Adenomyosis

Fallopian Tubes

Tubal injury from infection, surgery, or endometriosis
Tubal ligation

Ovary

Cysts or neoplasms
Polycystic ovaries

Other Abdominal Organs

Spastic or irritable colon
Chronic appendicitis
Cholecystitis

Pelvic Musculature

Spasm

Neurologic and Skeletal Causes

Lumbar disk disease
Multiple sclerosis

Metabolic Disturbances

Acute intermittent porphyria
Familial Mediterranean fever
Sickle cell disease
Hematochromatosis

Vasculature

Pelvic congestion

Psychogenic

---

acute rather than chronic pelvic pain. Diagnosis may be made either by clinical evaluation alone (eg, anemia or sepsis) or by invasive techniques such as culdocentesis or laparoscopy.

An early attempt to explain chronic pelvic pain on the basis of a chronic peritoneal irritant was described by Allen and Masters. In their report they evaluated 28 patients with chronic pelvic pain who exhibited a "universal-joint" cervix on bimanual examination. In this examination the uterine fundus was in severe third-degree retroversion and the junction of the cervix to the lower uterine segment was "ill-defined." On manipulation of the cervix (up, down, lateral) there was minimal to absent responsive movement by the uterine fundus. While the examiner was manipulating the cervix in this manner, the patient frequently experienced severe pain, especially if the cervix was lifted anteriorly. On exploratory laparotomy 22 of the 28 patients studied demonstrated bilateral broad ligament "tears" or "lacerations." In the remaining six cases four had a right broad ligament laceration and two had a left broad ligament laceration. All lacerations were repaired at surgery. An example of a broad ligament laceration and its repair as presented by Allen and Masters is given in Figure 23-2. The response to surgery was beneficial for all patients studied. Confirmation of Allen and Masters' findings that more than 75% of women with chronic pelvic pain complaints have broad ligament lacerations remains to be reported (also see Chapter 27).

Although Allen and Masters reported that these lacerations resulted from childbearing, alternative explanations have been offered. Chatman has suggested that these lacerations, or "peritoneal windows," are manifestations of scarring from endometriosis. Chatman found that 25 of 635 patients undergoing laparoscopy for chronic pelvic pain had these peritoneal defects, and 17 of these 25 patients had pelvic endometriosis documented by biopsy. Batt and Smith, on the other hand, have postulated that the peritoneal defects described by Chatman and others represent a congenital anomaly owing to the rudimentary duplication of the müllerian system during organogenesis. Furthermore, Batt and Smith believe that peritoneal windows are not analogous to the traumatic lacerations identified by Allen and Masters, since not one of the 28 patients reviewed by Allen and Masters had endometriosis. An example of the peritoneal window described by Batt and Smith is found in Figure 23-3.

Ectopic endometrium or endometriosis may be found on peritoneal surfaces. It is well known that a strong correlation does not exist between the amount of endometriosis and the degree of pelvic pain. The cause of the pelvic pain observed in patients with endometriosis is only partly understood. Although the existence of adhesions or endometriomas may explain pain in some cases, these explanations cannot be invoked for the pelvic pain patient who exhibits only one or two visible implants of endometriosis. Pelvic pain in these patients may possibly be explained by the release of prostaglandins or inflammatory mediators (eg, interleukins) from ectopic endometrium.

Existence of pelvic adhesions has been reported from laparoscopic studies of women with chronic pelvic pain. The cause of adhesion formation may be related to previous pelvic infection or surgery. As with endometriosis, the exact cause of the pelvic pain remains unclear. Adhesion formation may result in the tugging or pulling of the peritoneum or involved ab-

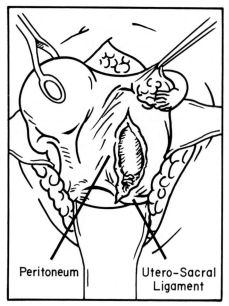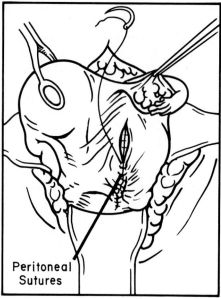

Peritoneum | Utero-Sacral Ligament

Peritoneal Sutures

Figure 23–2. Laceration of the broad ligament and its repair. (Modified from Allen WM, Masters WH. Traumatic laceration of uterine support—the clinical syndrome and the operative treatment. Am J Obstet Gynecol 1955;70:500)

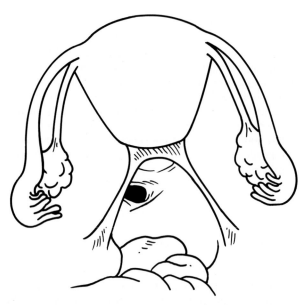

Figure 23–3. A peritoneal window. (Modified from Batt RE, Smith RA. Embryologic theory of the histogenesis of endometriosis and peritoneal pockets. Obstet Gynecol Clin 1989; 16:15)

dominal organs. Relief of pain has been mentioned after lysis of adhesions for some, but not all, patients. Alternatively, clinical studies such as that of Rapkin, in which laparoscopic results from 100 pelvic pain patients versus 88 infertility patients not complaining of pelvic pain revealed no difference in the density or location of adhesions, suggest that adhesions alone may not be responsible for producing the pelvic pain.

Uterus

Existence of pelvic pain has been reported by Buttram and Reiter in 34% of 1698 women found to have leiomyomata. Many of these patients had coexisting tubal disease, adhesions, or endometriosis. The precise cause of the pain complaint from leiomyomata may be unclear, although uterine pressure or compression of adjacent organs may be responsible. Infarction and degeneration of leiomyomata have been suggested as causes of acute pelvic pain in some patients or chronic pain in others. Yet Persaud and Arjoon failed to find a relation between frequency of pelvic pain and presence of degenerative changes in leiomyomata.

Adenomyosis is a condition of the uterus that has been termed benign invasion of the endometrium into the uterine musculature. Microscopically, this is characterized by the presence of endometrium in the myometrium 1 high-power field below the basal endometrium. Demonstration of adenomyosis has been reported in up to 50% or more of all uteri, but is believed to be much more common in uteri removed from multiparous women. Classic symptoms of adenomyosis include progressive menorrhagia and dysmenorrhea with symmetric uterine enlargement. Interestingly, hormonal treatment of these patients with cyclical estrogen and progesterone has not proved effective. In fact, use of estrogen therapy in the luteal phase (Halban's test) has been reported to worsen the degree of menorrhagia. The use of newer hormonal therapies designed to cause a medical oophorectomy (gonadotropin-releasing hormone [GnRH] analogue therapy) remains to be assessed in terms of efficacy. Total hysterectomy has been reported to be an effective form of treatment.

Simple retroversion of the uterus occurs in about 20% of women, and represents a normal anatomic variation. Despite occasional anecdotal claims to the contrary, substantiated evidence does not appear to exist to support the charge that simple uterine retroversion is a cause of chronic pelvic pain. In some patients, however, the posterior uterine fundus may become adherent to the posterior pelvic wall as a result of pelvic inflammatory disease or endometriosis conditions, which may indeed be responsible for causing chronic pelvic pain.

Adnexal Disorders

Fallopian Tube

Injury or damage to the fallopian tube resulting from infection, previous surgery, or endometriosis may cause hydrosalpinx or tubal adhesions. This may result in chronic pelvic pain. An interesting cause of chronic pelvic pain resulting from tubal injury has been proposed by those investigating late sequelae of tubal ligation. In the study by Neil and associates several women complained of chronic pelvic pain after laparoscopic tubal ligation. The cause of this late postoperative complication remains unclear, although organ torsion and ischemia have been suggested as possible factors.

Ovary

Cysts and neoplasms of the ovary may result in pain owing to compression, torsion, or hemorrhage. The identification and treatment of ovarian cysts and neoplasms are thoroughly discussed in other sections of this textbook. An interesting but unexplained cause of pelvic pain from an ovarian source is chronic anovulation (formerly known as polycystic ovarian disease). In this condition follicular development remains uncompleted, so that ovulation does not occur. As a result the ovary contains multiple follicles in early development, causing ovarian enlargement and producing a "cystic appearance."

Other conditions that involve the ovaries and are associated with chronic pelvic pain include the supernumerary and accessory ovary, retained ovary syndrome, and ovarian remnant syndrome. Each of these conditions is different and is briefly described. More complete descriptions of the retained ovary and ovarian remnant syndromes are included Chapter 22.

The supernumerary ovary is one of the rarest gynecologic conditions, with less than 15 cases reported in the English literature. This represents a situation in which a third ovary is found entirely separate from the normally placed ovaries. It apparently develops from a separate anlage. Located at various sites within the pelvis, these "ectopic" ovaries may become enlarged and compress adjacent organs, causing pain. Related to the supernumerary ovary is the accessory ovary, which, although rare, is more common than the supernumerary ovary. In this condition accessory ovarian tissue is located contiguously to the normal ovary and almost always is 1 cm or less in diameter. Abnormalities may arise within this tissue, producing pelvic pain.

The retained ovary syndrome refers to patients complaining of pelvic pain who have previously undergone total abdominal hysterectomy. The cause of the pain remains unknown, but coexistent pelvic adhesions, follicular cysts, or hemorrhagic corpora lutea involving the retained ovaries have been suggested as explanations for the pain experienced by these patients.

The ovarian remnant syndrome occurs in patients who have previously undergone bilateral oophorectomy. Chronic lower abdominal pain is reported in 75% of these cases. Retention of ovarian tissue after bilateral oophorectomy may occur because of pelvic vascularity, adhesions, or neoplasm present at the time of initial surgery. In most cases endometriosis and pelvic inflammatory disease were present at the time of the initial surgery. Because of the extensive scarring and adhesions, diagnostic laparoscopy may be of little help in the diagnosis and treatment of this condition.

Other Abdominopelvic Organs

Diagnosis of a chronic pelvic pain complaint may depend on determining that the source of pain does not reside within the reproductive tract, but in an adjacent organ. Spastic colon, ureteral stricture, and chronic appendicitis may all produce chronic pain. Bowel disorders caused by allergens or lactose intolerance also may result in chronic pelvic pain complaints, although these usually are accompanied by gastrointestinal difficulty (eg, diarrhea). In some clinical studies a diagnosis of irritable bowel syndrome could be made in 30 (60%) out of 50 patients with chronic abdominal pain with no evidence of disease on laparoscopy. Constipation also may produce pelvic pain by allowing a firm and distended rectosigmoid colon to compress adjacent organs. An unusual cause of pelvic pain may be referred pain from the upper abdomen. This may result from either chronic cholecystitis or pleural problems.

Pelvic Musculature

Muscle spasms may result in pain. Just as myalgias commonly occur in the muscle groups of the arms or legs after heavy exercise or labor, myalgias of the muscles of the pelvic floor have been reported as a cause of pelvic pain. A complex of symptoms that result in pelvic pain, including spasm of the levator ani and coccygeus muscles, has variably been called pyriformis syndrome, levator ani spasm syndrome, diaphragm pelvis spastica, and coccygodynia. The pain usually is described as an "aching" in the rectum, pelvis, and/or lower back. Symptoms of pelvic musculature myalgia as described in 94 patients by Sinaki and colleagues are listed in Table 23-2. Tenderness of the pelvic floor muscles is reported on rectal examination. Interestingly, tenderness of pelvic floor musculature does not depend on the presence of the uterus, fallopian tubes, and ovaries, since it has been reported in women who had previously undergone hysterectomy as well as in men. Therapy has included transrectal massage of the muscles as advocated by Thiele, as well as heat therapy, use of muscle relaxants, and relaxation exercises.

Neurologic and Skeletal Causes of Chronic Pelvic Pain

A detailed accounting of the various neurologic and skeletal causes of chronic pelvic pain is beyond the scope of this chapter. Lumbar disk disease and degenerative joint disease of the lower spine are but two common neurologic and skeletal causes of lower abdominopelvic pain that should not be forgotten. An additional neurologic cause of pelvic pain has been suggested by Slocumb to include trigger points within the vagina or on the surface of the abdominal wall. Pressure on these points results in pelvic pain that can be alleviated by local administration of anesthetics. Particularly in cases of otherwise unexplained chronic pelvic pain, neurologic or skeletal causes must be excluded and neurologic or orthopedic consultation may be required. An unusual cause of pelvic pain in a young woman was recently reported by Miro and colleagues. A 17-year-old girl with pelvic pain was found to have multiple sclerosis, a condition known to produce a variety of paroxysmal manifestations (eg, tonic seizures and limb pain). Use of carbamazepine for these conditions in multiple sclerosis patients has been reported to elicit positive response and was found to be of benefit in this case.

Metabolic Causes of Abdominopelvic Pain

Rarely, abdominopelvic pain complaints may result from metabolic causes and not from direct injury to a pelvic organ. Acute intermittent porphyria is one such example. In this condition, which is transmitted as an autosomal dominant disorder, a decrease in the level of uroporphyrinogen I synthetase in liver, red cells, fibroblasts, and lymphocytes is seen. As a result of this enzyme deficiency, increased porphyrin precursors are produced, including aminolevulinic acid (ALA) and porphobilinogen (PBG). During an acute attack, which may be induced spontaneously or after drug ingestion (eg, barbiturates), increased levels of ALA and PBG are detected. Also occurring at the time of an acute attack, neurologic dysfunction, resulting in abdominopelvic pain, is observed, particularly in the autonomic nervous system. The precise cause for the neurologic dysfunction remains unknown, although ALA and PBG neurotoxicity have been suggested.

Other unusual causes of abdominal pain include familial Mediterranean fever, sickle cell disease, and hematochromatosis. The cause of familial Mediterranean fever remains unknown, but the disorder is found in families with Sephardic Jewish, Armenian, or Arab heritage. Diagnosis of sickle cell disease should be considered in some patients and hemoglobin electrophoresis ordered to confirm this disorder.

Pelvic Congestion and Pelvic Pain

Pelvic congestion as a cause of chronic pelvic pain was aptly described by Taylor in 1949 in a series of three papers presented to the American Gynecologic Society. Yet this disorder had been known to gynecologists previously and was described as early as 1831 by Gooch, according to the excellent historical review of Theobald. Although the specific identifiable clinical characteristics such as age, parity, and location of pain

TABLE 23–2
Common Symptoms for Patients with Tension Myalgia of Pelvic Floor

Low back pain
Heavy feeling in pelvis
Leg pain (unilateral or bilateral)
Pain with bowel movement
Constipation
Coccyx pain
Dyspareunia

vary, a consensus does emerge as to a description of the typical patient thought to have pelvic congestion syndrome. In brief, the patient has chronic pelvic pain of no apparent cause for at least 6 months and is in the reproductive age range. Pelvic pain and/or heaviness is described that worsens premenstrually, after standing, or after intercourse. Pelvic examination reveals tender parametrial areas and severe pain on elevation of the cervix by the examining fingers. At surgery the uterus frequently is retroverted and surprisingly large amounts of straw-colored fluid are found in either anterior or posterior cul-de-sacs. The major hypothesis for this disorder is that stasis of the pelvic venous system causes congestion within the pelvic organs, producing pain either spontaneously or after manipulation.

Scientific evidence in support of pelvic varicosities as a cause of pelvic pain has been provided by Beard and colleagues, who performed venography by injecting contrast medium into the myometrium, using a transcervically passed cannula. In this study women with chronic pelvic pain were found to have a wider diameter ovarian vein than control patients and also had delayed disappearance of contrast medium from the pelvic vascular system. Conversely, dye disappearance from the pelvic circulation has been reported to be delayed in postpartum patients not complaining of pain. In nine patients with congenital arteriovenous malformation of the female pelvis reported by Beller and colleagues, chronic pelvic pain was not a common complaint. These reports would confirm the controversy surrounding the relation between pelvic vasculature disturbances and pelvic pain.

Psychogenic Causes

Descending analgesic neuronal pathways exist that suppress ascending pain inputs. One of these descending neuronal pathways appears to emanate from the periaqueductal gray region of the midbrain and is activated by opiates. Biogenic amines also act as neurotransmitters for these descending analgesic pathways, and drugs that potentiate biogenic amines (eg, tricyclic antidepressants) may in turn potentiate the activity of the analgesic pathway.

Theoretically, it would not seem inappropriate to postulate that failure to activate the descending analgesic neural pathway centrally could result in heightened pain awareness. Psychological causes for patients complaining of chronic pelvic pain have long been suggested and have even been thought to be responsible for affecting the autonomic nervous system, resulting in the pelvic congestion syndrome. Patients complaining of chronic pelvic pain have been reported to be more depressed and neurotic than normal controls. These patients also have been reported to use repression and denial as defense mechanisms. Nevertheless, caution must be exercised before assuming a cause-and-effect relation, since persistent and unremitting pelvic pain could in itself be responsible for some of the observed psychological difficulties.

Of particular interest are recent reports stating a high incidence of childhood sexual abuse in patients complaining of chronic pelvic pain. Gross and associates, in a study of 25 patients with chronic pelvic pain, reported that 9 of these patients presented with a history of incest. In this context, incest was defined as the physical contact of sexual organs between family members for purposes of sexual stimulation. Estimates of the number of adults who have been sexually abused as children have ranged from 15% to 38%. This large a range may reflect the lack of a uniform definition of sexual abuse. Higher estimates of abuse are generated if fondling, genital viewing, and urogenital contact are included in addition to coitus.

Acts of childhood sexual abuse may have acute or remote consequences in the affected children. Acutely anxious behavior, anger, nightmares, and exhibitionism may be seen in the sexually abused child. As adults, these people seem strongly predisposed toward depression and display low self-esteem. Substance abuse and sexual dysfunction also are observed quite frequently in these patients. As mentioned in a recent ACOG Technical Bulletin article on chronic pelvic pain, however, studies have not yet been reported describing the prevalence of chronic pelvic pain in women with histories of sexual abuse or sexual dysfunction.

EVALUATION OF THE PATIENT WITH CHRONIC PELVIC PAIN

The evaluation of the patient with chronic pelvic pain should begin with the taking of a thorough medical history and performance of a complete physical and pelvic examination before ordering diagnostic tests (Table 23-3). A detailed description of the patient's pain should be obtained, with attention to location, onset, relation to menstrual cycle, and factors that worsen or diminish pain. Family background and occupational description should be obtained to exclude unusual metabolic and environmental causes of abdominopelvic pain. An attempt to determine a previous history of sexual abuse should be made by asking the patient if she was sexually abused or raped as a child or adult. If sexual abuse is mentioned, the physician should attempt to learn the type of problem that occurred, when it occurred, who instigated it, and the patient's reaction.

Past methods of contraception should be queried, for example, previous intrauterine device use or tubal liga-

TABLE 23–3
Diagnostic Options for Evaluation
of Chronic Pelvic Pain

1. History, physical and pelvic examinations
   a. Inquire about past history of sexual abuse
2. Laboratory tests
   a. Hematologic evaluation
   b. Urinalysis with total porphyrin determination if appropriate
   c. Serum CA-125
3. Radiographic studies
   a. Sonography of pelvis and upper abdomen
   b. Intravenous pyelography
   c. Barium enema
4. Surgical evaluation
   a. Diagnostic laparoscopy

tion. Pelvic adhesions after subclinical infections have been alleged for some intrauterine device users, and tubal ischemia as a delayed sequela of tubal ligation also has been suggested, although controversy exists for both issues.

During the physical and pelvic examination an effort should be made to determine as precisely as possible the location of the pain. Existence of abdominal masses or organomegaly should be sought. On pelvic examination uterine size and position should be carefully noted. Elicitation of the pelvic pain may be attempted by anterior elevation of the cervix. On rectovaginal examination uterosacral nodularity and pain and/or spasm of the levator muscles should be evaluated.

Laboratory Tests and Diagnostic Procedures

After the initial history and pelvic examination additional relevant information may be obtained through various tests. An association between the menstrual cycle and the occurrence of pelvic pain may be determined by having the patient keep a basal body temperature chart and pain diary.

Appropriate initial laboratory studies include hematologic evaluation to exclude anemia and infection, blood chemistry evaluation to exclude systemic metabolic diseases, and urinalysis to exclude infection and increased excretion of porphyrins. Radiographic studies include abdominopelvic sonography to exclude pelvic mass and gallbladder, liver, and pancreatic disorders. Computed tomography scan with contrast or magnetic resonance imaging provides additional information or clarification of sonographic data. Chest radiography, upper GI series, barium enema, and intravenous pyelography may all be ordered to exclude pulmonary, gastrointestinal, and urologic disorders, respectively. Interestingly, a recent review by Johnson and

Laube concluded that unselected use of radiographic procedures was not helpful. For example, after 100 barium enemas in patients with pelvic pain, 94 were normal and 4 patients thought to have an abnormal examination were "normal" at laparoscopy. In 96 patients who had an intravenous pyelogram no abnormality was found in 92, 3 had incidental abnormalities not thought to be a cause of pain, and 1 patient had a bladder-filling defect with reflux, but her pain did not ultimately appear to be related to this urologic abnormality.

The usefulness of the diagnostic laparoscopy as an investigative procedure in the workup of the chronic pelvic pain patient is not controversial. Numerous clinical studies have testified to the fact that abnormalities such as adhesions and endometriosis may be detected by laparoscopy (Table 23–4). What remains less clear is how these conditions cause pelvic pain in some patients but not in others. Performance of the diagnostic laparoscopy early or late in the evaluation of the patient with chronic pelvic pain varies, depending on the patient. In an older woman with recent onset of severe chronic pelvic pain, diagnostic laparoscopy may be performed quite promptly, in view of the concern for pelvic cancer. In the younger patient with a normal pelvic examination in whom endometriosis is suspected, a trial of medical therapy to provide symptomatic relief (eg, oral

TABLE 23–4
Laparoscopic Findings in Patients with Chronic Pelvic Pain ($n = 1864$ Patients)

FINDING	PERCENTAGE OF PATIENTS
Peritoneal	44
Pelvic inflammation (18%)	
Lacerations (0.05%)	
Endometriosis (7%)	
Adhesions (19%)	
Uterine	4
Leiomyomata	
Ovarian	11
Cysts/masses	
Other abdominal organs	1
Appendicitis	
Pelvic congestion	2
Other	2
Normal	36

(Data tabulated from clinical studies of Bahary CM, Gorodeski IG. The diagnostic value of laparoscopy in women with chronic pelvic pain. Am Surg 1987; 53:672; Cunanan et al. Laparoscopic findings in patients with pelvic pain. Am J Obstet Gynecol 1983; 146:487; Johnson SR, Laube DW. Chronic pelvic pain: Evaluation and treatment. Iowa Med 1986; 76:572; Kresch AJ et al. Laparoscopy in 100 women with chronic pelvic pain. Obstet Gynecol 1984; 64:672; Levitan et al. The value of laparoscopy in women with chronic pelvic pain and a "normal pelvis." Int J Gynaecol 1985; 23:71; and Rapkin AJ. Adhesions and pelvic pain: A retrospective study. Obstet Gynecol 1986; 68:13.)

contraceptive pills) might be considered before resorting to surgery, particularly if the patient is apprehensive about operative intervention. Measurement of serum CA-125, a cell surface antigen, in chronic pelvic pain patients has been advocated as a screening tool, since a high degree of sensitivity, specificity, and accuracy in detecting endometriosis in women with pelvic pain has been demonstrated using this assay.

Treatment

Management of the patient with chronic pelvic pain depends on the identification of the cause of the pain. Peritoneal irritation from endometriosis may be treated medically either symptomatically or therapeutically. Combination-type oral contraceptive pills may be used to provide symptomatic pain relief. Use of progestational agents (eg, medroxyprogesterone acetate), androgen derivatives (eg, danazol), or analogues to GnRH may provide therapeutic benefit as well as symptomatic relief. Surgery to treat the patient with endometriosis and pelvic pain also may be performed. Recurrence of pelvic pain symptoms owing to endometriosis has been observed after medical or surgical therapy. Some studies, for example, have reported that by 3 years post surgery, 40% of patients had experienced a recurrence in their symptoms of endometriosis.

Uterine causes of pelvic pain may be treated medically, but surgical therapy remains the mainstay. Leiomyomata may be reduced in size with GnRH analogue therapy, but regrowth is the norm after cessation of treatment. Anecdotal reports attest to the efficacy of progestational agents or danazol in treatment of leiomyomata and adenomyosis, but a consensus does not exist to recommend these therapies on a routine basis. Myomectomy and hysterectomy remain remedies of choice for more sustained treatment of leiomyomata and adenomyosis that cause pelvic pain. Surgery also is the usual recommended therapy for adnexal disorders such as ovarian cysts or torsion.

Therapy for patients diagnosed with pelvic congestion syndrome as a cause of chronic pelvic pain remains difficult. Psychotherapy has been recommended for some women, with mixed results. Sclerotherapy to occlude pelvic varicosities has been recommended, but definitive clinical studies demonstrating the efficacy of this treatment are lacking. Hysterectomy also has been advocated as a principal form of therapy for this condition, but good prospective studies documenting the efficacy of this form of therapy are needed.

Nonextirpative operative management of chronic pelvic pain has consisted of presacral neurectomy (see Chapter 20). Central pelvic pain in the patient with endometriosis responds best to presacral neurectomy, but results of therapy become difficult to interpret when the therapy is used to treat chronic pelvic pain owing to other causes.

Lysis of pelvic adhesions is another form of nonextirpative operative therapy that may be considered in selected patients. A major difficulty in assessing the effectiveness of this form of therapy is that the cause of pelvic pain in patients with pelvic adhesions remains undetermined. Studies demonstrating the effectiveness of laparoscopy or laparotomy in lysis of pelvic adhesions to alleviate pelvic pain are lacking. Furthermore, studies do exist that document that significant pelvic adhesions may be present in patients who do not complain of pelvic pain.

Identification of psychological causes of chronic pelvic pain is especially difficult if pertinent historical questions are not asked by the examining physician (eg, past and present sexual abuse). Psychotherapy to improve self-image and self-worth and to convince the patient that she was not at fault for being sexually abused is extremely helpful. Consultation with mental health practitioners may be especially useful.

Mention should be made of the recent success obtained using tricyclic antidepressants in the treatment of chronic pelvic pain. Like chronic headache or lower back pain, chronic pelvic pain without apparent organic cause has been labeled by some as a form of masked depression. Tolerance of pain is determined in part by activation of the descending analgesic neural pathways mentioned previously. Neuronal triggering of these pathways may in part be due to serotonergic stimulation. Tricyclic antidepressants such as imipramine and amitriptyline block neuronal uptake of serotonin and have been reported to be effective in treating some patients with chronic pelvic pain. Use of tricyclic antidepressants in this manner demonstrates that as our understanding of the neurologic mechanisms responsible for producing pain sensations improves, so will our ability to devise newer and more appropriate therapies to treat these disorders.

Management of the patient with significant and persistent pelvic pain without pelvic pathology who remains unresponsive to the therapies discussed above represents a difficult clinical problem. Some have advocated performance of a hysterectomy for this condition, but this must be viewed as an empiric form of therapy, since the success of this therapeutic approach has not been documented.

Bibliography

Allen WM. Chronic pelvic congestion and pelvic pain. Am J Obstet Gynecol 1971;109:198.

Allen WM, Masters WH. Traumatic laceration of uterine support—the clinical syndrome and the operative treatment. Am J Obstet Gynecol 1955;70:500.

Anonymous. Chronic pelvic pain. ACOG Tech Bull 1989;No. 129 (June).

Anonymous. Enigmatic pelvic pain [Editorial]. Br Med J 1978;2:1041.

Aronoff GM, Witkower AB. Chronic pain: common problems and practical solutions. Resident Staff Physician 1988;34:43.

Bachmann GA, Moeller TP, Bennett J. Childhood sexual abuse and the consequence in adult women. Obstet Gynecol 1988;71:631.

Badawy SZA, Freedman L, Numann P, et al. Diagnosis and management of intestinal endometriosis: a report of five cases. J Reprod Med 1988;33:851.

Bahary CM, Gorodeski IG. The diagnostic value of laparoscopy in women with chronic pelvic pain. Am Surg 1987;53:672.

Batt RE, Smith RA. Embryologic theory of the histogenesis of endometriosis in peritoneal pockets. Obstet Gynecol Clin 1989;16:15.

Beard RW, Belsey EM, Leiberman BA, Wilkinson JCM. Pelvic pain in women. Am J Obstet Gynecol 1977;128:566.

Beard RW, Highman JH, Pearce S, Reginald PW. Diagnosis of pelvic varicosities in women with chronic pelvic pain. Lancet 1984;2:946.

Beard RW, Reginald PW, Wadsworth J. Clinical features of women with chronic lower abdominal pain and pelvic congestion. Br J Obstet Gynaecol 1988;95:153.

Beller U, Rosen RJ, Beckman EM, et al. Congenital arteriovenous malformation of the female pelvis: a gynecologic perspective. Am J Obstet Gynecol 1988;159:1153.

Beresin EV. Case report: imipramine in the treatment of chronic pelvic pain. Psychosomatics 1986;27:294.

Bonica JJ. Neurophysiologic and pathologic aspects of acute and chronic pain. Arch Surg 1977;112:750.

Buttram VC, Reiter RC. Uterine leiomyomata: etiology, symptomatology and management. Fertil Steril 1981;36:433.

Chatman DL. Pelvic peritoneal defects and endometriosis: Allen-Masters syndrome revisited. Fertil Steril 1981;36:751.

Chatman DL, Zbella EA. Pelvic peritoneal defects and endometriosis: further observations. Fertil Steril 1986;46:711.

Christ JE, Lotze EC. A residual ovary syndrome. Obstet Gynecol 1975;46:551.

Cunanan RG Jr, Courey NG, Lippes J. Laparoscopic findings in patients with pelvic pain. Am J Obstet Gynecol 1983;146:589.

Dawood MY, Khan-Daywood FS, Ramos J. Plasma and peritoneal fluid levels of CA 125 in women with endometriosis. Am J Obstet Gynecol 1988;159:1526.

Eschenback DA. Epidemiology and diagnosis of acute pelvic inflammatory disease. Obstet Gynecol 1980;55(suppl):142.

Farquhar CM, Reginald PW, Beard RW. Irritable bowel syndrome as a cause of chronic pain in women attending a gynaecology clinic. Br Med J 1987;294:1228.

Feinmann C. Pain relief by antidepressants: possible modes of action. Pain 1985;23:1.

Fields HL. Neurophysiology of pain and pain modulation. Am J Med 1984;77(3A):2.

Gidro-Frank L, Gordon T, Taylor HC Jr. Pelvic pain and female identity. Am J Obstet Gynecol 1960;79:1184.

Goldstein DP, deCholnoky C, Leventhal JM, Emans SJ. New insights into the old problem of chronic pelvic pain. J Ped Surg 1979; 14:675.

Gross RJ, Doerr H, Caldirola D, et al. Borderline syndrome and incest in chronic pelvic pain patients. Int J Psychiatry Med 1980;10:79.

Guzinski GM. Advances in the diagnosis and treatment of chronic pelvic pain. Adv Psychosom Med 1985;12:124.

Harrop-Griffiths J, Katon W, Walker E, et al. The association between chronic pelvic pain, psychiatric diagnoses and childhood sexual abuse. Obstet Gynecol 1988;71:589.

Henker FO. Diagnosis and treatment of nonorganic pelvic pain. South Med J 1979;72:1132.

Hobbs JT. The pelvic congestion syndrome. Practitioner 1976; 216:529.

Hogston P. Irritable bowel syndrome as a cause of chronic pain in women attending a gynecology clinic. Br Med J 1987;294:934.

Hopkins MP, Smith DH. Chronic pelvic pain, profile of a resident teaching clinic. Am J Gynecol Health 1989;3:17.

Jeffcoate TNA. Pelvic pain. Br Med J 1969;3:431.

Johnson SR, Laube DW. Chronic pelvic pain: evaluation and treatment. Iowa Med 1986;76:572.

Kresch AJ, Seifer DB, Sachs LB, Barrese I. Laparoscopy in 100 women with chronic pelvic pain. Obstet Gynecol 1984;64:672.

Lee RB, Stone K, Magelssen D, et al. Presacral neurectomy for chronic pelvic pain. Obstet Gynecol 1986;68:517.

Levine J. Pain and analgesia. The outlook for more rational treatment. Ann Intern Med 1984;100:269.

Levitan Z, Eibschitz I, DeVaries K, et al. The value of laparoscopy in women with chronic pelvic pain and a "normal pelvis." Int J Gynecol Obstet 1985;23:71.

Lundberg WI, Wall JE, Mathers JE. Laparoscopy in evaluation of pelvic pain. Obstet Gynecol 1973;42:872.

Magni G, Andreoli C, deLeo D, et al. Psychological profile of women with chronic pelvic pain. Arch Gynecol 1986;237:165.

Malinak LR. Operative management of pelvic pain. Clin Obstet Gynecol 1980;23:191.

Manning AP, Thompson WG, Heaton KW, Morris AF. Towards positive diagnosis of the irritable bowel. Br Med J 1978;2:653.

Miro J, Garcia-Monco C, Leno C, Berciano J. Pelvic pain: an undescribed paroxysmal manifestation of multiple sclerosis. Pain 1988;32:73.

Neil JR, Hammond GT, Noble AD, et al. Late complications of sterilisation by laparoscopy and tubal ligation—a controlled study. Lancet 1975;2:699.

Persaud V, Arjoon PD. Uterine leiomyomata: incidence of degenerative change and correlation of associated symptoms. Obstet Gynecol 1970;35:432.

Pettit PD, Lee RA. Ovarian remnant syndrome: diagnostic dilemma and surgical challenge. Obstet Gynecol 1988;71:580.

Pittaway DE, Douglas JW. Serum Ca-125 in women with endometriosis and chronic pelvic pain. Fertil Steril 1989;51:68.

Quan M. Chronic pelvic pain. J Fam Pract 1987;25:283.

Rapkin AJ. Adhesions and pelvic pain: a retrospective study. Obstet Gynecol 1986;68:13.

Rapkin AJ, Kames L. The pain management approach to chronic pelvic pain. J Reprod Med 1987;32:323.

Rapkin AJ, Kames LD. New hope for patients with chronic pelvic pain. Female Patient 1988;13:100.

Raskin DE. Diagnosis in patients with chronic pelvic pain [Letter to the Editor]. Am J Psychiatry 1984;141:824.

Reading AE. A critical analysis of psychological factors in the management and treatment of chronic pelvic pain. Int J Psychiatry Med 1982;12:129.

Renaer M. Chronic pelvic pain without obvious pathology: diagnosis, etiology and management. In: Dawood MY, McGuire JL, Demers LM, eds. Premenstrual syndrome and dysmenorrhea. Baltimore: Urban & Schwarzenberg, 1985:147.

Renaer M. Chronic pelvic pain without obvious pathology in women—personal observations and a review of the problem. Eur J Obstet Gynecol Reprod Biol 1980;10:415.

Renaer M, Guzinski GM. Pain in gynecologic practice. Pain 1978;5:305.

Renaer M, Vertommen H, Nijs P, et al. Psychological aspects of chronic pelvic pain in women. Am J Obstet Gynecol 1979;134:75.

Rosenthal RH, Ling FW, Rosenthal TL, McNeeley SG. Chronic pelvic pain: psychological features and laparoscopic findings. Psychosomatics 1984;25:833.

Sinaki M, Merritt JL, Stillwell GK. Tension myalgia of the pelvic floor. Mayo Clin Proc 1977;52:717.

Slocumb JC. Neurological factors in chronic pelvic pain: trigger points and the abdominal pelvic pain syndrome. Am J Obstet Gynecol 1984;149:536.

Symmonds RE, Pettit PDM. Ovarian remnant syndrome. Obstet Gynecol 1979;54:174.

Taylor HC Jr. Vascular congestion and hyperemia: their effect on structure and function in the female reproductive system. Pt 1. Physiologic basis and history of the concept. Am J Obstet Gynecol 1949;57:211.

Taylor HC Jr. Vascular congestion and hyperemia: their effect on structure and function in the female reproductive system. Pt 2. The clinical aspects of the congestion-fibrosis syndrome. Am J Obstet Gynecol 1949;57:637.

Taylor HC Jr. Vascular congestion and hyperemia: their effect on structure and function in the female reproductive system. Pt 3. Etiology and therapy. Am J Obstet Gynecol 1949;57:654.

Taylor HC Jr. The syndrome of pelvic pain in women. Aust NZ J Obstet Gynaecol 1961;1:5.

Theobald GW. The pelvic sympathetic syndrome. J Obstet Gynaecol Br Emp 1951;58:733.

Theobald GW. Cortical pain image or pain-sensitivity panel. Br Med J 1965;2:330.

Thiele GH. Coccygodynia and pain in the superior gluteal region and down the back of the thigh. JAMA 1937;109:1271.

Wharton LR. Two cases of supernumerary ovary and one of accessory ovary, with an analysis of previously reported cases. Am J Obstet Gynecol 1959;78:1101.

24

Pelvic Inflammatory Disease

JOHN D. THOMPSON
MICHAEL R. SPENCE

In 1910, Howard Kelly said, "The history of pelvic abscess is fraught with deepest interest, for it exhibits in miniature all the phases of the growth of gynecology at large."

Until the mid-nineteenth century, there was little knowledge of the pathology of infections within the pelvis. Between 1830 and 1840, Recamier, a French gynecologist, was the first to practice vaginal drainage of pelvic abscess. The practice was picked up by Wells and Savage of England and by Sims and Emmett in the United States. Lawson Tait performed the first abdominal removal of a tubo-ovarian abscess in 1872. After this, evidence accumulated rapidly that pelvic abscess usually resulted from a primary infection in the fallopian tube. The etiology and pathogenesis of various forms of pelvic infection evolved gradually. The organism responsible for gonococcal infection was discovered by Neisser in 1879. In 1886, Westermark demonstrated *Neisseria gonorrhoeae* organisms in exudate from the tube. In 1894, Wertheim demonstrated these organisms invading tubal tissues. In 1921, Curtis isolated *Neisseria* organisms from the endometrium and the tubes. And in 1946, Falk demonstrated that access of the organism to the fallopian tube could be prevented by resection of the interstitial portion of the tube. Since the beginning of the antibiotic era in 1942 with the discovery of penicillin, studies of pelvic infections have concentrated on microbial etiology, effective antimicrobial therapy, the indications for surgery, identification of asymptomatic carriers, and the importance of the control of pelvic infections to the public's health.

The relationship between sexual activity and the development of pelvic inflammatory disease was recognized by Howard Kelly. In 1898, he described pelvic inflammatory disease as an ascending gonorrheal infection leading to the development of pyosalpinx and hydrosalpinx, and suggested that gonorrheal infections in women resulted from gonorrheal infections in their sexual partners. In 1941, Stemmer reported that pelvic inflammatory disease was very uncommon among nuns.

It is estimated that over 1 million women are treated in the United States for acute salpingitis each year. The incidence is greatest among teenagers and young women under age 25. This condition or its complications result in over 2.5 million office visits and 150,000 surgical procedures each year. The costs for this care exceed $3 billion annually. *N. gonorrhoeae* and *Chlamydia trachomatis* are the two microorganisms most commonly associated with acute salpingitis. Less commonly, pelvic inflammatory disease is also known to be caused by *Mycoplasma hominis, Bacteroides fragilis,* and β-hemolytic streptococcus. There are approximately 3 million infections caused by gonococci and 4 million caused by chlamydia in the country each year. Two thirds of the infections occur in individuals between the ages of 16 and 24 years. Chlamydial infections are three times more common in teenagers than in women 20 years of age and older. Although these rates stabilized between 1986 and 1989, they have not decreased significantly. Thus, this young population constitutes the majority of individuals at risk for salpingitis. Hence, American gynecologists will continue to see the significant morbidity associated with the late sequelae of this disease for many years to come. Approximately 15% of women with untreated endocervical gonorrhea will develop salpingitis. Almost 250,000 women, accounting for as many as one fifth of the gynecologic admissions to some large public hospitals, are admitted with acute salpingitis, tubo-ovarian abscess, or pelvic abscess. Although mortality is low, these patients experience considerable morbidity. The major clinical significance of this acute and chronic infectious disease is that the fallopian tubes develop scar tissue, intraluminal adhesions, fibrosis of the tubal wall, partial or complete obstruction, and peritubular adhesions. After salpingitis, the risk for ectopic pregnancy may be increased tenfold. With a history of pelvic inflammatory disease, the risk of ectopic pregnancy is increased sixfold. The rate of ectopic pregnancy in the United States appears to have increased 250% since 1965. This increase roughly parallels that in pelvic inflammatory disease over this same time span. The risk of infertility is also increased. Salpingitis is responsible for 20% or more of all infertility cases. Westrom has carefully studied the influence of sexually transmitted diseases on sterility and ectopic pregnancy. In addition to gonorrhoeae and chlamydia, infectious salpingitis has been associated with other microorganisms as well as instrumentation of the genital tract. Types of pelvic infection are listed in Table 24-1.

As a public health problem of major proportions, salpingitis is difficult to control. Many factors contribute to this difficulty. For example, *C. trachomatis* organisms are difficult and expensive to culture. *N. gonorrhoeae* organisms have a short incubation period. There is a lack of natural or acquired resistance to these organisms. Many women and men have been found to be asymptomatic carriers. There is a decreasing sensitivity of gonorrhea to penicillin. According to a 1986 report by Rice and Thompson, the number of penicillinase-producing *N. gonorrhoeae* increased enormously from 1976 to 1985. Also, changing sexual mores seem to influence control of sexually transmitted diseases adversely. The Centers for Disease Control (CDC) reports that a larger percentage of teenagers were initiating sexual intercourse at younger ages in 1988 than in 1982. In the 1980s, crack cocaine became an important contributor to high-risk sexual activity, such as the exchange of sex for drugs. Recent surveys do suggest, however, that fear of sexually transmitted diseases has caused increased concern about personal sexual behavior in both men and women. Pelvic inflammatory disease is one of the most widespread and debilitating diseases affecting women today and unfortunately will probably become an even greater problem in the future.

The prevalence in the population of organisms causing sexually transmitted diseases increases the risk of pelvic inflammatory disease among the sexually active members of society. Women in unstable relationships who have multiple sexual partners, or women whose single sexual partner has multiple sexual contacts will have a higher risk of acquiring pelvic inflammatory disease. Women who are in stable single-partner relationships have a lower risk for pelvic inflammatory disease. Women with multiple sexual partners have the highest relative risk for pelvic inflammatory disease. Younger women, nulliparous women, women who use an intrauterine device, and lower-socioeconomic-class women are also at greater risk. Women who are not sexually active have a low risk of contracting pelvic inflammatory disease. Since it is difficult to be certain, the use of barrier contraception (especially condoms) should be encouraged as protection against sexually transmitted diseases.

TABLE 24–1
Types of Pelvic Infection

Sexually transmitted infections
Infections caused by the introduction of foreign material into the
   uterus. Etiologies include
   Intrauterine device use
   Hysterosalpingogram
   Tubal insufflation
   Dilatation and curettage
   Pregnancy interruption
Pelvic infections following major gynecologic surgery
Puerperal and postabortal infections
Septic pelvic thrombophlebitis
Pyometra
Infections in the pelvis due to primary pathology in the
   gastrointestinal tract
Tuberculosis
Tropical infections

CLASSIFICATION, TERMINOLOGY, AND GRADING OF PELVIC INFLAMMATORY DISEASE

Some types of pelvic infection, such as postabortal and postoperative infections, are discussed in other chapters. Those pelvic infections caused primarily by sexually transmitted agents and by tuberculosis will be discussed in this chapter. Discussions of septic pelvic thrombophlebitis and septic shock are also included in this chapter.

Many physicians use the term *pelvic inflammatory disease* (PID) to describe a variety of infections in the pelvis: acute or chronic, surgical, sexually transmitted infections, tuberculosis, and others. The term is nonspecific and is inaccurate in that an inflammation does not necessarily result from infection. Different clinical criteria to diagnose pelvic inflammatory disease are used by clinicians and by investigators, which often results in confusing and contradictory conclusions. Whenever possible, the term *pelvic inflammatory disease* should be replaced by more appropriate and descriptive terminology, such as *acute salpingo-oophoritis, pyosalpinx with pelvic peritonitis, acute tubo-ovarian abscess,* and other, more acceptable terms. However, this is not always possible. In those circumstances where accurate anatomic descriptions cannot be used, Hager and associates have developed diagnostic criteria for acute salpingitis. To fulfill these criteria, the patient should have all three of the following: (1) abdominal tenderness (direct and/or rebound; unilateral or bilateral), (2) cervical motion tenderness, and (3) adnexal tenderness. In addition, at least one and preferably two or more of the following should be present:

Oral temperature ≥ 38°C (100.4°F)
Leukocytosis ≥ 10,000 per cubic millimeter
Gram-negative, intracellular diplococci or *C. trachomatis* by rapid diagnostic test in the cervical exudate
Pus in the peritoneal cavity
Unilateral or bilateral adnexal mass(es)

It must be remembered that pelvic inflammatory disease is a diagnosis of exclusion and that the presence of a pregnancy (especially extrauterine) and other conditions must be ruled out with either a pregnancy test, a sonogram, or other appropriate diagnostic tests.

Hager and associates have suggested a system for grading salpingitis by clinical examination. A modified version of this system is used in this chapter.

GRADING OF ACUTE PELVIC INFLAMMATORY DISEASE BY CLINICAL EXAMINATION

   I. Uncomplicated salpingitis or salpingo-oophoritis, unilateral or bilateral
      A. Without pelvic peritonitis
      B. With pelvic peritonitis
  II. Complicated salpingitis, salpingo-oophoritis, pyosalpinx, or tubo-ovarian abscess, with inflammatory adnexal mass(es), unilateral or bilateral
      A. Without pelvic peritonitis
      B. With pelvic peritonitis
 III. Large (≥8 cm in diameter) tubo-ovarian or pelvic abscess(es), spread of infection to upper abdomen, or ruptured tubo-ovarian abscess

---

A schematic representation of the progressive and recurrent nature of pelvic inflammatory disease is presented in Figure 24-1.

CONTRACEPTION AND PELVIC INFLAMMATORY DISEASE

Although intrauterine devices are infrequently employed now in the United States, they were once a very popular method of contraception. They are still in widespread use in developing countries. Many studies question the advisability of their use in some populations because of the possibility of greater frequency of associated pelvic infection. Whether they deserve the notoriety they have received is highly controversial.

In 1980, Senanayake and Kramer reviewed 16 published reports of the relationship between intrauterine device use and acute pelvic infection. Ory found that intrauterine device users have three to five times more risk of pelvic infection than nonusers. More recent data from CDC suggest that the risk is only 1–2.6 times higher among IUD users. The risk is higher for young women. The risk is greatest for women with many sexual partners and in a population with a high incidence of sexually transmitted diseases.

More recent and accurate epidemiologic studies indicate that the risk of acquiring pelvic inflammatory disease with intrauterine device use is much lower than previously thought. The increased risk seems to be limited to the first 4 months after insertion. Although it was formerly thought that the risk of infection increased with duration of use, this is now known to be incorrect. For women with only one sex partner, the risk is not increased even in the first 4 months.

Formerly, it was thought that the IUD tail acted as a wick to draw bacteria into the uterine cavity. This may have been the case with the multifilament sheath-tailed Dalkon shield. Monofilament tails are less likely to act as a wick. There is apparently no difference in infection rates among women wearing tailed or tailless devices. Mishell found bacteria in the uterine cavity only immediately following intrauterine device insertion. No bacteria were found 30 days after insertion. According to Guderian and Trobough, inflammatory residues in the fallopian tubes and tubal infertility in intrauterine device users are caused not by the intrauterine device but by both overt and silent chlamydial infections. In about 5% of removed intrauterine devices, colonization with *Actinomyces israelii* can be demonstrated. We have seen Actinomyces in tubo-ovarian abscesses in patients with an intrauterine device in place, although true pelvic actinomycosis is rare. Unfortunately, we have seen many young women with serious pelvic infections associated with intrauterine device use. Because of this, our policy is to restrict the use of intrauterine contraceptive devices to older women who have completed their families and are presumed to have a stable marital relationship. All patients who have an intrauterine device are carefully instructed to report immediately any

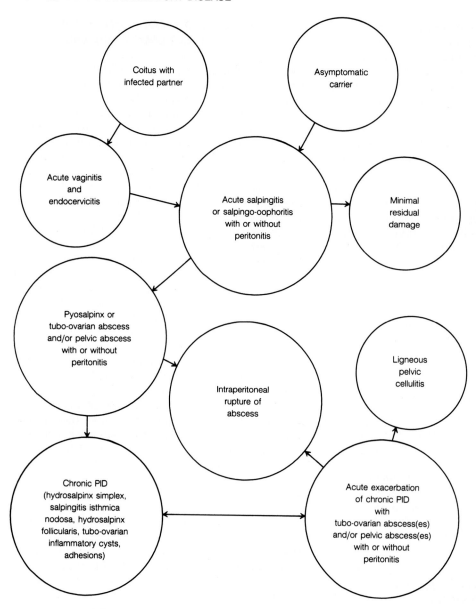

Figure 24–1. Sequential development of pelvic inflammatory disease.

abnormal vaginal discharge or lower abdominal discomfort, especially when associated with fever. Such patients should be carefully evaluated for possible pelvic infection. If the slightest suspicion is present, antibiotics should be administered, the device should be removed, and follow-up examinations should be performed to be certain the infection has cleared.

Senanayake and Kramer have analyzed reports comparing the relative risks of pelvic inflammatory disease in users and nonusers of the oral contraceptive pill. With one exception, these studies show that the risk of pelvic inflammatory disease among users is 0.3–0.9 times that for nonusers, indicating that this method of

contraception has a protective effect. This prevails in face of the analysis conducted by Washington demonstrating that pill users were more likely to be harboring *C. trachomatis* in their cervices. The mechanism of protection is not known. Eschenbach has theorized that the increased density of the cervical mucus plug caused by the oral contraceptive pill may inhibit the entry of bacteria into the uterus. Data from Toth and associates support this hypothesis by demonstrating that bacteria have difficulty in vitro penetrating cervical mucus under the influence of progestins.

In a 1980 study, Wolner-Hanssen and associates demonstrated that oral contraceptive use may modify the clinical manifestations of chlamydial pelvic inflammatory disease. Oral contraceptive use decreased both the degree of inflammation seen in acute salpingitis and the number of patients with perihepatitis. Mechanisms to explain this modifying effect of oral contraceptives on acute chlamydial infection are unknown but may be related to suppression of immune reactions.

The relationship between use of barrier contraceptive methods and pelvic inflammatory disease has been studied by Kelaghan and associates and by Stone and associates. It was found that condoms, diaphragms, and chemical barrier methods provide significant protection. The prevention of pelvic inflammatory disease and its sequelae is one of the most important noncontraceptive benefits of barrier methods of contraception. They should be prescribed for women with pelvic inflammatory disease, even those women whose infection has caused sterility from bilateral tubal occlusion, to reduce the possibility of recurrent infection and to reduce the possibility of transmission to others. Barrier methods of contraception should also be advised for all sexually active men and women to prevent sexually transmitted diseases.

ACUTE SALPINGITIS

Microbial Etiology of Acute Salpingitis

Sophisticated studies by Sweet, Monif, Chow, Cunningham, Eschenbach, Mardh, Estrom, their associates, and many others have produced important information about the bacterial etiology of acute salpingitis (grade I disease).

N. gonorrhoeae is frequently isolated from the endocervices of women with acute salpingitis. The organism is most commonly found in inner-city U.S. women, where it is isolated from up to 80% of these individuals. However, in other U.S. women, the number of positive endocervical cultures for *N. gonorrhoeae* with acute salpingitis is lower, and the organism is present in only 10% to 20% of Scandinavian women with acute salpingitis.

The presence of *N. gonorrhoeae* in an endocervical culture is not absolute proof that the organism has also caused salpingitis. Fallopian tube cultures obtained by laparoscopy and peritoneal fluid cultures obtained by culdocentesis and laparoscopy do not always show correlation with cultures obtained from the endocervix. The isolation of *N. gonorrhoeae* is dependent on the stage of infection. As demonstrated by Curtis in 1921, the organism is present when the fallopian tube is acutely inflamed, but is not found in patients who have been afebrile for 14 days. Sweet and associates found *N. gonorrhoeae* in 70% of patients presenting within 24 hours of the onset of symptoms. After 48 hours, *N. gonorrhoeae* was found in only 19% of patients. *N. gonorrhoeae* is isolated less frequently in older women with salpingitis and in women who have recurrent infections. Even among women with positive cultures for *N. gonorrhoeae,* other bacteria may also be cultured from the fallopian tubes and peritoneal fluid.

The pathogenesis of salpingitis with *N. gonorrhoeae* is not completely understood. Sexual transmission between infected partners is well documented. The organism remains localized in the cervix for a varying period. It may gain access to the uterine cavity during midcycle, when the cervical mucus is thin and penetrable by sperm and microorganisms. The organism(s) may flourish in the uterine cavity during menstruation, since menstrual blood is an excellent culture medium. Inoculation of the fallopian tubes may be facilitated by retrograde menstruation. Women who are amenorrheic rarely develop acute salpingitis. The cervical mucus mechanical barrier is more impenetrable in anovulatory women. This barrier may be temporarily lost, however, during menstruation, even in anovulatory cycles. Different types of gonococci vary in their ability to cause salpingitis, and migration of the organism to the fallopian tube during menses is facilitated by the absence of a bactericidal antibody against *N. gonorrhoeae.* The organism can also gain access to the upper genital tract by passive transport. This organism can attach to the tail of spermatozoa. Once attached, gonococci can virtually ride to the midportion of the fallopian tube on the sperm cell after either natural or artificial insemination. Once it has arrived in the tube, the organism can disembark and initiate an inflammatory response.

Presence of the gonococcus in the fallopian tube causes an intense inflammatory reaction. Work by McGee has demonstrated that the gonococcus elaborates an endotoxin that can damage cells of the endosalpinx and cause a loss of cilia. The fallopian tube becomes erythematous and swollen. A purulent exudate develops in the tubal lumen. This exudate has ready access to the peritoneal cavity and explains the common association of pelvic peritonitis. The inflammatory process spreads to adjacent surfaces of the ovary, omentum, and bowel, causing adhesions to form between these structures. Inflammatory adhesions also form between the mucosal folds of the endosalpinx within the tube and at the fimbriated end, resulting in complete or partial closure of the tubal lumen.

The findings of Cunningham, Eschenbach, Sweet, and their coworkers demonstrate clearly the polymicrobial etiology of acute pelvic inflammatory disease. Cunningham and associates studied peritoneal fluid obtained by culdocentesis in 133 women with acute pelvic inflammatory disease. *N. gonorrhoeae* was isolated from the lower genital tract in over half of these women and cultured from the peritoneal fluid in 22%. *N. gonorrhoeae* and other organisms were recovered from 32%. Nongonococcal organisms alone were recovered in 46%. These investigators believe that *N. gonorrhoeae* initiates most cases of pelvic inflammatory disease and that suprainfection with nongonococcal organisms, which occurs later, may interfere with the recovery of gonococci. Chow, Monif, and others agree with this concept, but some do not.

Eschenbach's studies confirmed this work and showed that mixed anaerobic and aerobic bacterial peritoneal infection was common in nongonococcal pelvic disease. The most common species recovered in his studies were *B. fragilis*, Peptostreptococci, and Peptococci. Eschenbach proposed that tuboperitoneal gonococcal infection probably causes pelvic inflammatory disease in most patients with cervical gonococcal infection, whereas polymicrobial tuboperitoneal infection probably causes most nongonococcal cases.

Sweet and associates found the gonococcus and anaerobic bacteria, either alone or together, in the fallopian tube in the initial episodes of salpingitis. Their findings suggest that the gonococcus may be important in initiating acute salpingitis in some patients and in establishing conditions that will facilitate subsequent invasion by other organisms present in the cervix and vagina. However, their findings also suggest an important primary role for mixed aerobic and anaerobic bacteria in the pathogenesis of acute salpingitis. A mixed anaerobic and aerobic infection causes more tubal destruction and subsequent infertility and is less likely to show a prompt and complete response to antibiotics. Indeed, the old idea that the gonococcus was always the initial invader to be followed by other bacteria invading secondarily is probably not true, as indicated by studies that demonstrate other bacteria present in cases of acute salpingitis.

C. trachomatis has received recent attention as an important agent in the microbial etiology of acute salpingitis and is now accepted as a major cause of pelvic inflammatory disease. Indeed, *C. trachomatis* is now thought by some to be the most common sexually transmitted disease in the United States and in Western industrialized society. It is estimated that over 4 million infections occur each year in the United States in men (urethritis and epididymitis), women (urethritis, mucopurulent cervicitis, and salpingitis), and children (neonatal conjunctivitis, chlamydial pneumonia). Washington and associates at the Centers for Disease Control estimated in 1987 that the economic cost of chlamydial infections in the United States was over $1.4 billion annually, with infections in women accounting for 79% of this cost. The highest rates of infection are found in sexually active teenagers in inner-city urban clinics,

including pregnant teenagers. In addition to being a major cause of acute salpingitis, chlamydial scarring of the fallopian tubes is a major cause of infertility and tubal pregnancy, often in the absence of prior clinical evidence of acute salpingitis in spite of serologic evidence of past chlamydial infection. Chlamydial salpingitis is generally associated with milder symptoms, higher costs for screening and diagnosis, and longer course of therapy for cure. For these and other reasons, it is difficult to achieve public health control. Since this is a substantial threat to the reproductive health of women, there is reason to be pessimistic about the future.

The cervix is the most common site of chlamydial infection in the female. The urethra is also a common site, and infection may occur in both sites simultaneously. Since the organism will not grow on the squamous epithelium of the ectocervix, the infection occurs in the endocervical columnar epithelium. A mucopurulent endocervicitis is evident by a yellow mucopurulent discharge through the external cervical os, although gonococcal endocervicitis may present in a similar manner. In as many as 40% of women, chlamydial and gonococcal infections may be present in the cervix simultaneously.

Mycoplasmas are the smallest known free-living organisms. They lack a cell wall. Three mycoplasmas have been implicated in acute salpingitis: *M. hominis, Ureaplasma urealyticum,* and *M. fermentans.* These organisms can be isolated from the cervix, cul-de-sac fluid, and fallopian tubes in patients with acute salpingitis. Serologic evidence also suggests that acute salpingitis can be caused by mycoplasma. The role of the genital tract mycoplasma in acute salpingitis remains unclear because of the difficulty in determining whether these organisms cause tissue damage in the fallopian tube.

Actinomyces israelii is a gram-positive, nonacidfast, anaerobic bacterium. It is classified as transitional between true bacteria and the complex fungi. Pelvic actinomycosis was formerly considered a rare disease, most often secondary to a primary infection in the intestinal tract, but foreign bodies in the genital tract have also been associated with actinomycosis infection. Recently, *A. israelii* infections have been noted in patients with an intrauterine contraceptive device. A few patients have had very serious and even fatal infections. Although an infection with this organism may be acute, more frequently it runs a subacute, indolent course. In most cases, diagnosis has been based on histologic identification of the organism in cytology smears or tissue sections.

At the Karolinska Institute in Stockholm, Brihmer and associates studied the microbiology of confirmed acute salpingitis cases. *C. trachomatis* was isolated in 12%; *Bacteroides* in 5%; *N. gonorrhoeae* in 2%; *A.*

israelii in 2%; and *U. urealyticum* in 1%. Serologic samples, drawn on admission and 2–3 weeks later, indicated chlamydial infection in 51%.

Brunham and associates in Winnipeg isolated the following organisms from 50 patients with acute pelvic inflammatory disease: *N. gonorrhoeae* in 36%; *C. trachomatis* in 10%; both organisms in 6%; and various other pathogens. In 25%, no pathogens were isolated. Women with pathogens other than *N. gonorrhoeae* or *C. trachomatis* more often had tubal abscesses.

In San Francisco, Sweet and associates studied 104 women with acute salpingitis. Forty-two percent had gonococcal infection; 27% had chlamydial infection; and 14% had both. Forty-six percent of patients had only other aerobic and anaerobic bacteria in the tubes. Bacteria were recovered from all patients.

From the three studies cited here and from others, one may conclude that the frequency with which common pathogens are involved in acute salpingitis varies from one geographic location to another.

In 1985, Lehtinen and associates reported herpes simplex virus isolation from various sites in the genital tract in four women with acute salpingitis. The significance of this finding is not clear.

Some common pathogens isolated in pelvic inflammatory disease are listed in Table 24-2.

Clinical Features and Diagnosis of Acute Salpingitis

Acute salpingitis can be seen in any sexually active reproductive-age female. It is rarely seen in premenarchal girls, postmenopausal women, and pregnant women, presumably because of absent menstruation and ovulation. It is uncommon in women who are anovulatory because of polycystic ovarian disease or because of oral contraceptive pills.

The clinical presentation of acute salpingitis may vary from nearly asymptomatic to obviously serious pelvic infection. Patients with acute salpingitis usually have an illness of moderate severity. It must be understood that the clinical diagnosis of acute salpingitis is difficult. Even with laparoscopy the diagnosis will be confirmed in only two thirds of suspected cases. Also, serious acute salpingitis may be found in some patients who have few symptoms and signs. The diagnosis of acute salpingitis can be a serious challenge to the clinical acumen of the gynecologist.

Since sexually transmitted infections of the lower genital tract almost always follow direct sexual contact, it is important to determine if the patient has had recent sexual activity. Although the risk of transmission of the disease to the female from an infected male is approx-

TABLE 24–2
Some Common Pathogens Isolated in Pelvic Inflammatory Disease

Neisseria gonorrhoeae
Chlamydia trachomatis
Aerobic bacteria
  Gardnerella vaginalis
  Gram-negative enterobacteriaceae:
    Escherichia coli
    Klebsiella species
    Proteus mirabilis
  Group B streptococci (*Streptococcus agalactiae*)
Anaerobic bacteria
  Peptostreptococcus species
  Peptococcus species
  Bacteroides species
    B. fragilis
    B. bivius
    B. disiens
    B. melaninogenicus
Mycoplasma hominis and *Mycoplasma fermentans*
Ureaplasma urealyticum
Actinomyces israelii
Mycobacterium tuberculosis

imately 80% to 90%, only 10% to 20% of the infected cases become clinically manifest as endometritis, salpingitis, and pelvic peritonitis. It is of clinical interest that the spectrum of primary infection sites of sexually transmitted disease has broadened in recent years, with gonococcal infections of the rectum and pharynx occurring with increasing frequency. The incidence of anal gonorrhea in women with positive *N. gonorrhoeae* cultures from the cervix varies between 30% and 60%. Pharyngeal infections are detected in women examined in venereal disease clinics in 3% to 11% of cases. Consequently, in a patient with the common symptom of acute pelvic pain, identification of other glandular sites of infection—namely, the vestibular glands of the vagina and urethra, the anal crypts, and the pharynx—are of as much clinical importance as the endocervix. The diagnostic accuracy of cultures for *N. gonorrhoeae* is improved significantly when two sterile swabs are cultured from the endocervical and anal canals, approaching 99% as reported by Dans. Newer developments in microbiology techniques have provided a better growth potential for and a greater accuracy in detection of the gonococcus. A Gram's stain of cervical secretions may show intracellular gram-negative diplococci resembling, but not necessarily diagnostic of, *N. gonorrhoeae.*

In obtaining a cervical culture for *N. gonorrhoeae,* it is important to clean the cervix lightly with a sponge and to leave the sterile swab in the endocervical canal for a few seconds, rotating it through 360° four or five times. A second swab should also be used to increase the rate of detection of this fastidious organism. Culture of the anal canal may be obtained by applying a sterile swab well above the anal sphincter in order to remain in contact with the rectal crypts for a few seconds and rotate the swab against the mucosa through 360° four or five times. Care should be taken to avoid gross fecal contamination. If this occurs, the swab should be discarded and the specimen retaken. The urethra may also be cultured. A specimen from the pharynx should be obtained whenever the sexual history indicates that oral-genital contact has taken place. A carrier medium is less effective than direct plating of the culture material on modified Thayer-Martin media (modified Thayer-Martin VCN media), but should this not be available, a transport medium such as Stewart's or Transgrow medium should be used with early inoculation of the material on the culture media in the laboratory. Sexually transmitted diseases rarely occur as single entities. Therefore, all individuals in whom a gonorrheal infection is suspected should have a serologic test for syphilis performed as part of their diagnostic evaluation. A Gram stain of the endocervical exudate should also be made. If examined by an experienced technician, it may show gram-negative intracellular diplococci. The average physician will identify the organism on smear in less than 50% of the cases that ultimately prove to have a positive cervical culture. Technicians are more likely to be adept in identifying this organism than physicians.

Efforts to positively diagnose and specifically treat and control chlamydial infections have been difficult because an inexpensive, simple, and reliable diagnostic test is not available. Cultures for *C. trachomatis* require sophisticated microbiologic resources that are not commonly available. Growth of the organism on tissue culture is the "gold standard" for diagnosis. Because of expense, this technique and methods of serologic testing are generally reserved for research studies. Cytologic methods of chlamydial infections lack sensitivity other than for diagnosing neonatal conjunctivitis. With Giemsa stains or stains for fluorescent antibodies, cytology of cervical smears is only about 50% sensitive in diagnosing chlamydia. In recent years, antigen detection methods have offered the best alternative to tissue-culture techniques. These techniques are simple and cost effective and can be used for screening in populations where the disease is prevalent. When compared to tissue culture, these tests have acceptable sensitivity, specificity, and positive predictive value. Although there are some false-positive reactions, the rates are relatively low.

If routine aerobic and anaerobic cultures are taken from the endocervix and vagina, a multitude of bacteria characteristically found in these locations will be reported. This information is not clinically useful.

The onset of symptoms of acute salpingitis will usually follow within 2 weeks of sexual exposure and just after the menstrual flow has ceased. Although initial location of this disease is usually confined to the endocervix with the production of increased cervical discharge, the spread of infection to the endometrium and tubes is commonly associated with the onset of menstruation. Menstruation itself may provide a method of spread of this ascending disease through the reflux of menstrual blood into the oviduct. The localized endometritis produces irregular endometrial shedding, prolongation of bleeding, and intermenstrual bleeding. These local endometrial tissue reactions produce a wide variety of menstrual irregularities as a common clinical feature of this acute event. Endosalpingitis is clinically evident by the gradual onset of lower abdominal discomfort that becomes progressively severe until pelvic peritonitis ensues and spreads to the upper abdomen.

Sweet and associates studied the temporal pattern of the onset of acute salpingitis in relation to menses. They found that the majority of patients with chlamydial and gonococcal acute salpingitis had the onset of their symptoms within 1 week of menses. Very few women with nonchlamydial, nongonococcal salpingitis reported onset of symptoms within 1 week. However, regardless of this temporal difference, all acute salpingitis cases should be assumed to be polymicrobial and managed accordingly.

Although many patients with acute salpingitis may present with symptoms of urinary frequency, urgency, and dysuria, cystitis is rare. Usually the symptoms are associated with urethritis. However, urinary tract symptoms may be the only reason the patient seeks medical treatment. A urine culture and antibiotic sensitivity studies should be done to differentiate a true bacterial cystitis from gonococcal urethritis.

Abdominal examination of the patient reveals generalized direct tenderness in both lower quadrants with occasional rebound tenderness demonstrating pelvic peritonitis. The uterus also may be quite tender on manipulation, which is an important clinical sign. The adnexa are exquisitely tender, which makes the pelvis difficult to truly evaluate for the presence or absence of an adnexal mass. Since the differential diagnosis of the patient with acute pelvic and abdominal pain must include acute salpingitis, ectopic pregnancy, acute appendicitis, and other causes of pelvic pain, an accurate assessment of the adnexa is important. Acute salpingitis patients will not always have bilateral adnexal tenderness. The infection may be less severe or even absent on one side, especially in patients with an intrauterine device in place.

Usually, the picture of bilateral pelvic peritonitis is helpful in identifying an acute salpingitis infection, which is often associated with a higher temperature and white blood cell count than is seen in a patient with an ectopic pregnancy or appendicitis. Rectal examination of the cul-de-sac produces exquisite tenderness from peritonitis, which, in the absence of palpable fluid in the pelvis, is helpful in differentiating inflammatory disease from a ruptured tubal pregnancy. Hematoperitoneum in the presence of a ruptured tubal pregnancy may cause referred shoulder pain, which is usually absent with acute salpingitis except in the case of the Fitz-Hugh-Curtis syndrome of fibrinous perihepatitis.

The laboratory data are also helpful, but not necessarily diagnostic. The white blood cell count may be elevated with a shift to the left, whereas the erythrocyte sedimentation rate may be normal or slightly elevated. A serum pregnancy test is quite accurate and may be performed to rule out the diagnosis of an ectopic pregnancy.

If pelvic findings remain unclear, a laparoscopic examination of the pelvis may be employed. In many clinics, the clinical diagnosis of salpingitis has been proved erroneous by the use of laparoscopy. During the 1960s, a series of laparoscopic studies by Falk and by Jacobson and Westrom resulted in a revision of the clinical characteristics of salpingitis and the problems of differential diagnosis of acute pelvic disease. Laparoscopy offers an excellent means of diagnosis of acute salpingitis whenever the diagnosis is uncertain, especially since a rapid and accurate diagnosis must be made if the serious late sequelae are to be prevented by the early use of effective antibiotic therapy. Ledger has discussed the risk/benefit ratio of laparoscopy when acute salpingitis is suspected. He suggested that it be used more frequently, especially in patients whose illness is severe enough to require hospitalization. Laparoscopy has a major disadvantage of requiring anesthesia and an operating room. In many large public hospitals, laparoscopy for the large number of patients seen daily with suspected acute salpingitis would be difficult. Therefore, a more convenient outpatient procedure such as microscopic examination of peritoneal fluid obtained by culdocentesis should be developed.

Fitz-Hugh-Curtis Syndrome

Perihepatitis is an inflammation of the liver capsule. An acute inflammation is followed by adhesions between the liver and the adjacent parietal peritoneum. Although it was first described in 1920 by Stajano, perihepatitis in association with acute salpingitis is called the Fitz-Hugh-Curtis syndrome after Fitz-Hugh and Curtis, who redescribed the association in 1930 and 1934. Perihepatitis can be suspected in any sexually active woman who complains of right upper abdominal quadrant and right pleuritic pain, aggravated by respiration. In over half the patients, the evidence of perihepatitis occurs at the time of lower abdominal pain caused by acute salpingitis. In some patients, the right upper quadrant pain does not appear until after the acute salpingitis has subsided. The severity of the right upper quadrant pain is variable from absent or minimal discomfort to a dramatic onset of severe pain. Either *N. gonorrhoeae* or *C. trachomatis* cultures of the cervix may be positive in approximately one half of patients. Among 274 patients with salpingitis verified by laparoscopy, Onsrud found symptomatic perihepatitis in 9% and asymptomatic perihepatitis in 5%. Although the organisms may spread from the pelvis to the liver by hematogenous or lymphatic channels, it is more likely that the organisms spread transperitoneally. The perihepatitis is most severe in the posterior subhepatic space, which, in the supine position, is the most dependent part of the peritoneal cavity above the pelvis. An inflammatory exudate from the pelvis is more likely to collect behind the liver. As pointed out by Wolner-Hanssen, oral contraceptive use provides significant protection against perihepatitis in patients with acute salpingitis.

In a patient with right upper quadrant pain, the differential diagnosis may include pneumonia, pleuritis, cholecystitis, appendicitis, and pyelonephritis. If a surgical abdomen is present, laparoscopy or laparotomy may be necessary to make the correct diagnosis. If perihepatitis of the Fitz-Hugh-Curtis syndrome is found, the antibiotics appropriate for acute salpingitis will usually be adequate.

Acute Salpingitis in Pregnancy

According to Blanchard and associates, acute salpingitis complicating pregnancy, although uncommon, probably occurs more often than previously thought. There have been very few reports in the literature. We believe it is a rare complication of intrauterine pregnancy, although some cases may not be recognized. It is conceivable that infecting organisms can be transmitted to the fallopian tube when fertilization occurs or before the pregnancy completely fills the uterine cavity after the first trimester. Presumably, when the uterine cavity is filled, organisms can gain access to the tubes by lymphatic or vascular channels. Obviously, the tubes also may be infected by septic abortion or by appendicitis.

The diagnosis of acute salpingitis is not often made in a pregnant patient. The signs and symptoms of pelvic peritonitis (lower abdominal and pelvic pain and tenderness, fever and leukocytosis, adnexal tenderness) may not be overlooked, but are usually attributed to other more likely causes, such as appendicitis. A purulent cervicitis with gram-negative intracellular diplococci will be helpful in making a correct diagnosis. But because acute salpingitis is rare in pregnant patients and the signs and symptoms are variable, the diagnosis is most often made at surgical exploration. Antibiotic therapy is generally effective against the infection, but spontaneous abortion is common.

Treatment of Acute Salpingitis

The primary treatment of acute salpingitis is medical. Unfortunately, considerable long-term morbidity and sequelae may result if the treatment is delayed, inadequate, or ineffective. According to Eschenbach, 15% of patients will develop chronic pain; 20% to 25% will have subsequent attacks of pelvic infection; infertility will result in 10% to 15% with one episode of acute salpingitis, 25% to 35% with two episodes, and 50% to 75% with three episodes; and 7% of patients will have an ectopic pregnancy with the first subsequent pregnancy. Whether or not the fallopian tubes will be occluded will depend not only on the number of episodes of salpingitis, but also on the type of organism(s) causing the infection and the effectiveness of the treatment prescribed. Polymicrobial infections are more likely to cause tubal occlusion. Abnormal findings on hysterosalpingogram are much more likely if the patient has developed an adnexal mass. Inadequate treatment may result in progression of the disease to more serious stages. Because outpatient treatment regimens have a failure rate of up to 20%, and to avoid late sequelae, the majority of patients with pelvic inflammatory disease should be hospitalized for intravenous antibiotic therapy. If that is not possible, those who receive outpatient treatment must be followed very closely. If there is no response to ambulatory therapy within 48 hours or if the disease is judged to be more severe before that time, prompt admission to the hospital should be arranged in an effort to prevent the serious sequelae of acute salpingitis with parenteral antibiotics. Hospitalization is also advisable if an intrauterine device is present; if an adnexal mass suggestive of a pyosalpinx or tubo-ovarian abscess is suspected; if a complicating medical disease such as diabetes is present; if pregnancy is diagnosed; if peritonitis is present; or if the patient's cooperation in taking medication and returning for follow-up is difficult to obtain. This may be a special problem for drug-addicted patients and adolescents with acute salpingitis. All adolescents with salpingitis should be hospitalized. When the diagnosis of acute salpingitis is questionable, hospitalization for laparoscopy may also be desirable.

The Centers for Disease Control (CDC) guidelines for the antibiotic treatment of patients with acute salpingitis were published in 1989 (Table 24-3). It is recommended that all patients receive minimally one dose of a beta-lactamase-resistant cephalosporin in a full therapeutic dose (ie, ceftriaxone 250 mg IM). Therapy for *C. trachomatis* (ie, doxycycline 100 mg b.i.d. for 7–10 days) should also be provided. Other agents in the regimen should be broad spectrum and provide adequate coverage for gram-negative organisms as well as the anaerobes (Table 24-4).

The treatment of acute salpingitis may include the employment of two or three antibiotics as maintenance therapy after the initial β-lactamase-resistant cephalosporin has been administered. The drugs are administered by the parenteral route in full therapeutic doses. Broad-spectrum regimens, as described for patients with pelvic abscesses (see later discussion), should be employed. Since both aerobic and anaerobic bacteria have been recovered from the pelves of patients with acute salpingitis and an average of five different species are recovered from each patient, broad-spectrum agents effective against these bacteria must be employed. A combination of penicillin or ampicillin plus clindamycin and an aminoglycoside such as gentamicin have been popularized at Grady Memorial Hospital. The efficacy of this regimen against *C. trachomatis* has not been documented, but good clinical responses have been achieved. Regimens that have been popular and effective in Baltimore and Philadelphia have included high doses of ampicillin (12 g/d) in combination with metronidazole or doxycycline after the initial administration of ceftriaxone 250 mg IM. The combination of cefoxitin and metronidazole has also been efficacious. Recent attention has turned to some of the long-half-life cephalosporins, extended-spectrum penicillins, and imipenems. These have also been shown to be effective in a wide variety of study settings. We are now fortunate in that our antibiotic arsenal is comprised of a diverse group of very effective agents. The newer drugs are so effective that our considerations in choosing therapy should now also be directed toward drug toxicities and cost.

It should be emphasized that the most important point in the successful management of acute pelvic inflammatory disease is the administration of adequate appropriate antibiotic therapy in the early stages of the disease before a pelvic mass (abscess) develops. This means that a larger number of patients with acute salpingitis should be admitted to the hospital for treatment with effective intravenous antibiotics. Some patients are notoriously difficult to treat or follow for response to treatment in an outpatient setting. These include adolescent patients, patients with drug addiction, and many others seen in inner-city hospitals and clinics.

TABLE 24–3
Some Current (1989) CDC Recommendations for Antibiotic Treatment

I. Uncomplicated urethral, endocervical, or rectal infections with *N. gonorrhoeae* in nonpregnant adult females:
Ceftriaxone 250 mg IM once
    plus
Doxycycline 100 mg orally b.i.d. × 7 days

II. Uncomplicated urethral, endocervical, or rectal infections with *C. trachomatis* in nonpregnant adult females:
Doxycycline 100 mg orally b.i.d. × 7 days
    or
Tetracycline 500 mg orally q.i.d. × 7 days

III. Pelvic inflammatory disease
A. Ambulatory management
Cefoxitin 2 g IM
    plus
Probenecid 1 g orally
    plus
Doxycycline 100 mg orally b.i.d. × 10–14 days
    or
Tetracycline 500 mg orally q.i.d. × 10–14 days
(Patients who do not respond to therapy within 72 hours should be hospitalized for parenteral therapy.)
B. In-patient management
1. Recommend Regimen A
Cefoxitin 2 g IV q 6 hr
    or
Cefotetan IV 2 g q 12 hr
    plus
Doxycycline 100 mg q 12 hr orally or IV
(The preceding regimen is given for at least 48 hours after the patient clinically improves.)
After discharge, continue doxycycline 100 mg orally b.i.d. × 10–14 days
2. Recommend Regimen B
Clindamycin IV 900 mg q 8 hr
    plus
Gentamicin loading dose IV or IM
(2 mg/kg) followed by a maintenance dose (1.5 mg/kg) q 8 hr
(The preceding regimen is given for at least 48 hours after the patient clinically improves.)
After discharge, continue doxycycline 100 mg daily b.i.d. × 10–14 days

(Centers for Disease Control, MMWR, 1989. Sexually Transmitted Disease Treatment Guidelines. 38:21, 1989)

ACUTE PELVIC ABSCESS

Clinical Features

Patients whose acute salpingitis has progressed or recurred may be found to have an acute pelvic abscess (grade II disease); a bilateral or unilateral tubo-ovarian abscess; or an extratubal collection of pus in the pelvis, usually located in the cul-de-sac. Such patients are usually in the third or fourth decade of life, although we have seen large pelvic abscesses in girls as young as 13. A pelvic abscess in a postmenopausal woman is usually associated with disease of the intestinal tract such as a ruptured appendix or a ruptured sigmoid diverticulum. One third of the patients are nulliparous but many will have been pregnant within the previous 2 years. One third will have a history of pelvic inflammatory disease, and some will have a history of previous hospitalization for pelvic abscess. Many will have received antibiotics recently for acute salpingitis. Of 100 patients with pelvic inflammatory disease studied by Goldenberg and Benigno, 42% had been treated on an outpatient basis within 2 weeks of hospitalization. Bilateral lower abdominal pain and tenderness, anorexia, and fever were present for several days.

On examination, the patient with acute pelvic abscess appears ill. She may walk slowly with a hand placed over her lower abdomen and her abdomen flexed. Abdominal distention and direct and rebound tenderness in the lower abdominal quadrants are present. The pelvic examination must be done carefully because of

(text continues on page 568)

TABLE 24–4

Bacterial Susceptibilities to Antibiotic Agents Used in Gynecology

	ANAEROBES		AEROBES					
DRUG	Peptococci Peptostreptococci Bacteroides species	Bacteroides fragilis	Enterococci	Enterobacteriaceae E. coli Klebsiella Proteus Enterobacter	Nonenterococcal Streptococci	Staphylococcus aureus (Methicillin-sensitive)*	Neisseria gonorrhoeae	Chlamydia trachomatis
Penicillin	++++	—	++ (in combination with aminoglycoside)	—	++++	+ (rare susceptible strain)	++++ (An increased number of strains are highly resistant due to β-lactamase production.)	—
Ampicillin	++++	—	+++ (better in combination with aminoglycoside)	++	++++	+ (rare susceptible strain)	++++ (Some strains minimally resistant due to chromosomal resistance.)	—
Carbenicillin Ticarcillin	++++	++	+	+++	++++	+ (rare susceptible strain)	++++	—
Piperacillin	++++	++ to +++	++ (better in combination with aminoglycoside)	+++ to ++++	++++	+ (rare susceptible strain)	++++	—

Imipenem	++++	++++	++ (better in combination with aminoglycoside)	++++	++++	++++	+++	
Cephalothin	+++	—	—	++	++++	++++	++	—
Cefazolin	+++	—	—		++++	++++	++	—
Cephamandole	++++	+++ to ++++	—	+++	++++	++++	++	—
Cefoxitin	++++	+++ to ++++	—	+++	++++	+++	++++	—
Cefotetan	++++		—	+++	++++	++	++++	—
Cefotaxime	++++	+	—	++++	+++ to +++++	+++	++++	—
Ceftriaxone	++++	+	—	++++	++++	+++ to ++++	++++	—
Clindamycin	++++	++++	—	—	—	+++ to ++++	—	—
Chloramphenicol	++++	++++	—	+++	++++	+++	++++	+/—
Metronidazole	+	++++	—	—	—	—	+/—	
Doxycycline	+++	++ to +++	+	++	+++	++	++++ (some resistance)	++++ (Erythromycin is an acceptable alternative in patients who do not tolerate doxycycline.)
Aminoglycosides	—	—	(only in combination with Penicillin G, Ampicillin, or Piperacillin)	++++	—	++ to +++	+/—	+/—

— Not effective.
+/— Variable.
+ to ++++ (Estimate of susceptibilities of strains in most hospitals (++++ being most susceptible; + being least susceptible).
*Methicillin-resistant strains should be treated with Vancomycin.
(Courtesy of Jonas A. Shulman, MD, Division of Infectious Diseases, Department of Medicine, Emory University School of Medicine.)

acute pelvic tenderness. Even the slightest motion of the cervix may cause extreme pain. Tissues in the cul-de-sac and on each side of the uterus may feel firm and indurated. An irregular, tender, fixed, inflammatory mass may be felt on one or both sides of the pelvis. The outline and dimensions of the mass are sometimes indistinct. The mass is usually composed centrally of an infection in and around the fallopian tube and ovary, with components of intestine, mesentery, and omentum surrounding it. The mass may be relatively small or may extend out of the pelvis into the lower abdomen. It may extend into the cul-de-sac and appear to dissect the rectovaginal septum on rectovaginal examination. The temperature, pulse, white blood cell count, and erythrocyte sedimentation rate are usually elevated. Even in the face of dehydration, anemia is frequently found. Anemia is more common in patients who have had a chronic abscess for many weeks. The anemia of chronic abscess does not respond well to the replacement of nutrients and is associated with low levels of erythropoietin. Although the commercially available erythropoietin has been employed to treat anemia of chronic disease, this is costly and not without hazard. The best results will be obtained by removing the underlying process. An abdominal x-ray is helpful to assess the degree of intestinal distention and to serve as a baseline should intestinal obstruction develop. Pelvic ultrasonography examinations during the course of medical management also will allow a more objective evaluation of the response to treatment if an abscess or inflammatory mass is seen. Taylor and colleagues reported excellent results with gray-scale ultrasonography in the detection and localization of abdominal and pelvic abscesses. Studies by Koehler and Moss, Halber and associates, and others have demonstrated the value of computerized tomography in diagnosing intra-abdominal and pelvic abscesses.

Paavonen and associates reported that 32% of patients with acute pelvic inflammatory disease had elevated tumor antigen CA 125. Compared with patients with normal CA 125 levels, patients with elevated CA 125 were older, were more often users of intrauterine contraceptive devices, had longer duration of symptoms, had higher erythrocyte sedimentation rates, and more often had an adnexal mass on pelvic examination. In most patients, the serum levels of CA 125 decreased during treatment.

General Management of Acute Pelvic Abscess

Patients with an acute pelvic abscess, usually an acute exacerbation of chronic pelvic inflammatory disease with bilateral tubo-ovarian abscesses, should be admitted to the hospital for management. They should be placed at bedrest with the head elevated in a semi-Fowler's position. Intravenous fluids should be administered and electrolytes should be replaced. Blood transfusions are seldom necessary but may be needed if severe anemia is present. Because of the potential contamination of the blood supply with the human immunodeficiency virus (HIV), the risks of blood and blood product transfusion must be carefully weighed against the potential benefits or the risks of not transfusing except as a lifesaving measure. Once the underlying disease process is corrected, the anemia will be self-correcting, thus alleviating the need for blood replacement. In the presence of a pelvic abscess, anemia usually will not respond to oral iron replacement, although it should usually be given. Suction through a nasogastric tube or a long intestinal tube should be used as indicated, depending on the degree of abdominal distention. Other complicating medical problems should be considered. For example, response to treatment will be inadequate if the patient has diabetes that is not well controlled. The rate of intrauterine device use in our patients with acute pelvic abscess is twice the rate among women seeking contraception in the Family Planning Program of our hospital. This may be an indication that patients with salpingitis who have an intrauterine device in place may not respond as well to antibiotics. If an intrauterine device is present in a patient with an acute pelvic abscess, it should be removed, but, to avoid septicemia, one should probably wait for several hours after intravenous antibiotics are started.

Appropriate intravenous antibiotics must be administered to patients with an acute pelvic abscess. Usually when antibiotics are used to treat an infection, the microorganisms causing the infection are identified from a smear or culture, their sensitivity to a variety of antibiotics is tested, and the correct antibiotics are chosen based upon these laboratory data. However, in the case of an acute pelvic abscess, a culture of the cervix will not be helpful. There is little correlation between microorganisms found in the cervix and microorganisms found in the pelvic abscess. A culture of fluid obtained from the cul-de-sac also will not be helpful, since, as shown by Sweet, contamination by microorganisms of the vagina is common. Needle aspiration of the cul-de-sac in a patient with an acute pelvic abscess could also rupture the abscess wall, resulting in spillage of the infected exudate into the general peritoneal cavity. Even if culture material could be obtained, sophisticated microbiologic laboratory facilities and several days are required to identify all the organisms causing the infection and to test their sensitivity to antibiotics. One cannot afford to wait this long before initiating therapy. The polymicrobial etiology of acute pelvic abscess is well known (see Table 24-2). Etiologic agents include *N. gonorrhoeae, C. trachomatis,* anaerobic bacteria (which include bacteroides and gram-positive cocci), facultative gram-negative rods (such as *E. coli*), *A. israelii, M. hominis,* and *U. urealyticum* and others. In the individual patient, it is impossible to differentiate among these agents at the time a treatment regimen is chosen. No single antibiotic is active against the entire spectrum of pathogens. Therefore, antibiotic treatment regimens should be chosen that are active against the broadest possible range of pathogens. Several antimicrobial combinations do provide a broad spectrum of activity against the major pathogens in vitro and have also been found to be fairly effective in clinical use. Landers and Sweet report a greater success when the drug regimen includes clindamycin. At Grady Memorial Hospital, we have used a three-drug regimen consisting of intravenous ampicillin, clindamycin, and gentamicin with good results. If response is inadequate, chloramphenicol has been substituted with success. The CDC has listed several other combination regimes with broad activity against the major pathogens in this disease (see Table 24-3). They include the following: doxycycline plus cefoxitin, clindamycin plus gentamicin or tobramycin, and doxycycline plus metronidazole. We have had a satisfactory experience with doxycycline plus metronidazole, which has the additional advantage of being less expensive.

Patients must be followed carefully for evidence of response. Abdominal and pelvic examinations should be done each day. A scoring sheet (Fig. 24-2) is used as an index of disease severity, progression, or response. Its use will assist the physician in determining whether patients are responding to treatment, require a change in antibiotics, or require surgical intervention. Careful observations must be made for signs indicating possible rupture of the pelvic abscess, which would require immediate operation.

Although antibiotics alone are effective in treating an acute pelvic abscess, antibiotics combined with surgical drainage are even more effective. Drainage of a pelvic abscess through a posterior colpotomy incision or through a gridiron incision in one or both lower abdominal quadrants will bring about a rapid improvement in the patient's condition. Occasionally, an abscess too high in the cul-de-sac to drain through a posterior colpotomy incision will drain spontaneously through the rectum and the patient's condition will improve dramatically. One should not attempt a posterior colpotomy when the abscess has drained spontaneously into the rectum, because of the possibility of creating a rectovaginal fistula. A pelvic abscess never drains through the vagina spontaneously unless the patient has had a previous posterior colpotomy for a pelvic abscess. Under these circumstances, the recurrent abscess may dissect along the tract of the previous posterior colpotomy and eventually drain spontaneously through the vagina.

Sometimes abscesses will not present for extraperitoneal surgical drainage. Experience with percutaneous drainage of intra-abdominal and pelvic abscesses under ultrasonographic or computed tomography guidance has been reported by Olak and associates, by Rosen and Roven, and by others. Worthen and Gunning used percutaneous catheter drainage of eleven abscesses in nine patients with 77% cure. Two patients required surgical intervention subsequently. In 19 patients, simple percutaneous aspiration of 23 abscesses was successful with 94% cure. The attempt at aspiration failed in seven patients (Fig. 24-3). Our experience, reported by Tyrrel and associates, is similar. Computed tomographic guided percutaneous drainage in eight patients with tubo-ovarian abscess resulted in recovery without surgery in seven. One patient had marked clinical improvement but still required a posterior colpotomy. No complications occurred. Loy and associates

	1	2	3	4	5	6	7	8
Hospital day								
Temperature (°C.)								
Physical findings								
Abdominal tenderness								
Rebound tenderness								
Bowel sounds (3 = absent, 2 = minimal, 1 = moderate, 0 = normal)								
Pain on cervical motion								
Adnexal tenderness—R								
Adnexal tenderness—L								
Adnexal enlargement—R								
Adnexal enlargement—L								
Total severity score								
Percentage change in severity score								

Figure 24–2. Scoring system for evaluating the severity of pelvic inflammatory disease and for progression or response to treatment. (For each finding, 0 = absent, 1 = minimal, 2 = moderate, 3 = marked.)

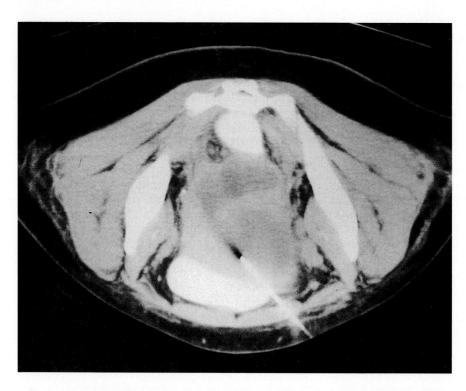

Figure 24–3. Transabdominal needle aspiration of a pelvic abscess under guidance of computed tomography. Drainage tube is also placed.

have reported that simultaneous use of real-time pelvic ultrasonography can facilitate transvaginal drainage of a pelvic abscess. If patients do not respond to intravenous antibiotics and percutaneous drainage or aspiration, surgical intervention will be required.

If the diagnosis of acute pelvic abscess is uncertain, laparoscopy or laparotomy may be required. Although laparoscopy may be a satisfactory procedure for diagnosis in patients with acute salpingitis, more severe forms of pelvic infection may make laparoscopy more difficult, more hazardous, and less satisfactory as a diagnostic procedure. There may be adhesions that make insertion of the trocar or laparoscope difficult or impossible and cause similar problems with visualization of the pelvic organs. In cases in which the diagnosis of acute unruptured pelvic abscess is questionable, a diagnostic laparotomy may be the better procedure.

Henry-Suchet and associates reported the successful use of laparoscopy to diagnose and drain tubo-ovarian abscesses in 50 women. Adhesions were lysed and the abscesses were drained through the laparoscope. All patients received intravenous antibiotics. Forty-five (90%) of the 50 patients were cured. Reich and McGlynn had a similar experience in 25 women with pelvic abscess treated laparoscopically. Four of seven women desiring pregnancy conceived, and two women had unplanned pregnancies.

Conservative management with intravenous broad-spectrum antibiotics and drainage of the abscess, when possible, has resulted in a satisfactory resolution of acute pelvic abscesses in the majority of patients at Grady Memorial Hospital, as reported by Franklin and associates. Our experience confirms that conservative management is the treatment of choice except in cases of questionable diagnosis, suspected rupture, or failure of the abscess to respond to initial conservative management. Use of the severity score sheet will allow a more objective evaluation of the patient's response. If the patient has not shown an improvement of greater than 30% in the severity score by the third or fourth day of treatment, a change of antibiotics or surgical intervention is usually necessary. Serial pelvic ultrasonography will also allow an objective evaluation of the response of the abscess to antibiotic therapy. When medical management is successful, ovarian function is conserved, even though tubal function may be destroyed by the infection and most patients will remain infertile. We were surprised to find that of 97 patients treated conservatively, 10 subsequently became pregnant with no reported ectopic pregnancies. One patient had two successful pregnancies after colpotomy drainage of 500 ml of purulent material. Rivlin reported that five of 40 potentially fertile patients (12.5%) had successful pregnancies at a later date following vaginal drainage of a pelvic abscess.

When there has been an adequate response to therapy, oral antibiotics may be continued as an outpatient procedure. Doxycycline is given by mouth for a total of

2 weeks. Patients are seen frequently for evaluation of continued response. It has been suggested that the use of oral contraceptive pills to prevent ovulation and to cause the formation of a thick cervical mucous plug may help prevent recurrent infections. To our knowledge their effectiveness for this purpose has not been evaluated clinically. Patients must still be instructed to use barrier methods of contraception assiduously in order to reduce the risk of reinfection.

Also important in reducing the risk of recurrence of the pelvic infection is the examination of all sexual partners of the patient for evidence of sexually transmitted disease agents. Those affected should be treated promptly with a regimen effective against uncomplicated gonococcal and chlamydial infection. Unfortunately, attention to this important aspect of clinical care is often inadequate.

If a patient has required hospitalization on several occasions for acute exacerbation of pelvic inflammatory disease with bilateral tubo-ovarian abscesses to the point where she is more often sick than well, definitive surgical intervention may be indicated. The operation should be done when the infection is quiescent. The surgery may still be difficult, but complications will be less frequent than when patients are operated on in the acute phase of the infection. The timing of the operative intervention is important. There should be complete absorption of the inflammatory exudate surrounding the focus of the infection. Bimanual pelvic examination should be possible without producing a marked or persistent febrile response. We suggest that definitive surgery should be delayed for 2–3 months following the recent exacerbation for more complete resolution of the infection. Ideally, the patient should have a normal erythrocyte sedimentation rate, white blood cell count, and hematocrit, and a relatively nontender pelvis.

Conservative medical management of acute unruptured pelvic abscess is not uniformly accepted. Kaplan and associates recommended a more aggressive management in patients who exhibit either no clinical response or only partial response after 24 to 72 hours of medical management. This more aggressive surgical approach, which included a total abdominal hysterectomy and bilateral salpingo-oophorectomy, was thought to reduce the protracted period of intensive medical therapy in a group of patients who may eventually require surgery. They noted that conservative management of their cases usually resulted in protracted periods of intensive care and repeated hospital admissions, and rarely in subsequent pregnancies. However, Kaplan's early surgical intervention was associated with six incidences of injury to the bowel and additional postoperative complications. Unfortunately, patients with acute pelvic abscess are frequently young, and

future childbearing is often desired, even though it may be impossible for most patients. Conservation of ovarian function for these young women is an important benefit of medical management. Some differences in the percentage of patients responding to conservative management in different studies and different geographic locations might be explained by differences in the predominant microorganisms causing the infection and their sensitivity to the antibiotics used.

Older studies of the management of patients with pelvic abscess, which emphasized the early use of surgery, are no longer pertinent, since modern antibiotic drugs were not then available. Collins and Jansen in 1959 had an early failure rate for conservative medical therapy of 10%. However, 113 of their 174 patients required later surgery, a late failure rate of 65%. In 1980, Ginsburg and associates reviewed 160 patients treated for tubo-ovarian abscess during the years 1969–1979. The early failure rate with broad-spectrum antibiotics was 31%, whereas the late failure rate was 21%. In an averaged follow-up period of 25.5 months, 48% required no surgery later. Subsequent reports by Hager and by Landers support conservative management. Our recent experience is similar.

In 1986, Dodson and associates, from Houston, reported on the use of a new monocyclic beta-lactam antibiotic, aztreonam, in combination with clindamycin to treat 42 patients with acute pelvic inflammatory disease. Fifty-one percent of patients had ultrasound findings consistent with a pelvic abscess. One patient with a tubo-ovarian abscess palpable to the umbilicus became afebrile and improved on treatment but ultimately was treated surgically. All other patients responded rapidly to the aztreonam-clindamycin regime, giving a 97.7% cure rate. Poindexter and associates found a satisfactory response to cefotetan treatment in 51 of 52 patients with pelvic inflammatory disease. Cefotetan was well tolerated. The twice-daily dosage schedule was a decided cost benefit.

Johnson reported on long-term follow-up of patients with tubo-ovarian abscesses who were successfully treated with conservative medical therapy. Of 37 patients followed for 5–10 years, only two patients required surgery for recurrent pelvic abscess. Twenty-three pregnancies and 17 term deliveries occurred in nine patients. These results indicate the value of such therapy.

When complicating medical disease such as diabetes are present, when the abscess is large (8 cm or more in diameter), and when the patient is perimenopausal with a history of repeated acute exacerbations of infection, response to medical therapy may not be satisfactory. However, it should be emphasized again that most patients will respond to medical therapy. Some authorities believe that patients who respond and are "cured" do not have true abscesses. Instead, what may seem to be an abscess is probably a complex mass of edematous tube, other pelvic tissues, intestine, and omentum that become adherent during the acute inflammatory reaction. Current experience with antibiotic therapy for patients who began with obvious pelvic abscesses on ultrasonography and/or computed tomography exams and are cured would seem to refute this notion.

When an acute pelvic abscess does not respond to intensive medical therapy, posterior colpotomy, or extraperitoneal abdominal drainage, laparotomy with or without definitive surgery may be necessary. In most patients who have extensive bilateral adnexal disease where tubo-ovarian conservation is not feasible, or in older patients past the reproductive age, we feel the operation of choice is total abdominal hysterectomy and bilateral salpingo-oophorectomy. In younger patients with extensive adnexal disease requiring bilateral salpingo-oophorectomy, the uterus may be left in place for the possible future use of new reproductive technologies to accomplish pregnancy. Occasionally, an uninvolved ovary or tube and ovary on one side may be conserved.

Surgical Management of Acute Pelvic Abscess

Posterior Colpotomy

In a classic article, Wharton described various techniques of vaginal drainage of pelvic abscess. Today, posterior colpotomy is done to evacuate pus and to establish drainage from a pelvic abscess that presents in the cul-de-sac.

There are three requirements for colpotomy drainage of a pelvic abscess: the abscess must be midline or nearly so; it should be adherent to the cul-de-sac peritoneum and dissecting the rectovaginal septum to assure the surgeon that the drainage will be extraperitoneal and that pus will not be disseminated transperitoneally; and it should be cystic or fluctuant to assure adequate drainage. Occasionally, a cul-de-sac abscess may be successfully drained without dissecting the septum. However, the serosal surface of the abscess should be adherent to the cul-de-sac peritoneum. Ultrasonography may be helpful in locating the pockets of pus.

After adequate anesthesia, the patient is placed in the lithotomy position. It is essential that a thorough examination of the pelvis be made under anesthesia so that the operator will have in mind the size and position of the mass that is to be drained.

After preparation and draping in the dorsal lithotomy position, the posterior lip of the cervix is grasped with a tenaculum and drawn down and forward. The vaginal

mucosa of the posterior vaginal fornix is incised just below the reflection of the vaginal mucosa onto the cervix, and the transverse incision is widened with a pair of long scissors (Fig. 24-4A). The incision must be large enough to allow adequate exploration and drainage of the abscess cavity with the index finger. The cul-de-sac peritoneum and abscess wall are punctured with a long Kelly clamp (Fig. 24-4B). As the abscess wall is perforated, there is a definite sensation of puncturing a cystic cavity. If blood or pus is present, this is soon seen in the upper vagina. The jaws of the clamp are spread, and the flow of liquid from the cul-de-sac is increased. A

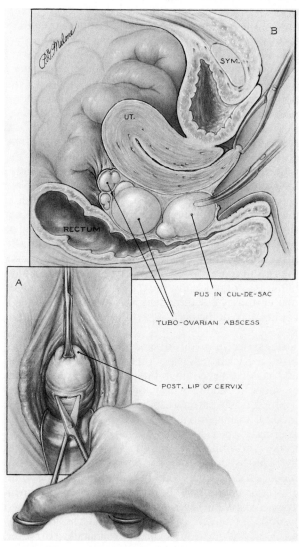

Figure 24–4. Posterior colpotomy. *A*, A transverse incision is made through the vaginal mucosa at the junction of the posterior vaginal fornix with the cervix. *B*, A Kelly clamp is thrust through the abscess wall.

sample of the purulent exudate is sent to the microbiology laboratory for appropriate culture and sensitivity. Collection of the specimen anaerobically employing a capped syringe with rapid transport to the laboratory will allow the more fastidious flora to be defined. A direct smear for Gram's stain is also made from the pus and examined for predominating organisms.

There may be more than one compartment in an abscess cavity (Fig. 24-5). It is desirable to insert an index finger in the cavity and explore. Fibrous adhesions within the cavity can be gently broken. If another abscess wall is felt, it can often be cautiously and safely punctured under the guidance of a finger. Exploration and manipulation should be done carefully to avoid intraperitoneal rupture of the abscess or perforation of the bowel. To allow adequate drainage, the vaginal incision should be at least 2 cm wide. If pus has been obtained, one or two drains are inserted into the abscess cavity and anchored with fine absorbable suture to permit easy removal. Penrose or closed suction drainage systems can be used. These are left for several days or longer. If a mushroom (Malecot) catheter is employed for drainage, it should be removed in 48–72 hours to prevent significant fibrosis that could hinder removal. Wharton emphasizes the importance of prolonged drainage. A suture or two may be required to control bleeding from the vaginal mucosa.

Extraperitoneal Abdominal Drainage

An unruptured pelvic abscess that fails to present in the cul-de-sac may occasionally require abdominal drainage for control of a septic clinical course. A puerperal infection may progress into a parametritis and tubo-ovarian abscess that remains localized in the region of the broad ligament. A gridiron or stab wound incision in the lower quadrant of the abdomen provides an excellent retroperitoneal approach to pelvic abscess. Care must be taken in directing a long Kelly clamp beneath the peritoneum into the pelvis to avoid trauma to the iliac vessels and the ureter, which cross the pelvic brim in this region. The closed suction drain is placed deep into the abscess cavity and sutured to the skin to avoid displacement by movement of the patient (Fig. 24-6).

Exploratory Laparotomy

The patient may be positioned in the Allen Universal stirrups for laparotomy. A lower abdominal transverse Maylard incision is ideal, since it affords good exposure to the lateral adnexal pelvic organs and pelvic sidewalls. Pelvic adhesions should be released and the bowel should be packed off before the pelvic dissection commences. During the dissection, free pus will often be

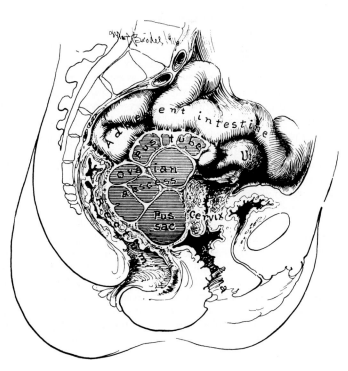

Figure 24–5. Pus may be contained within the tubo-ovarian abscess and within other pockets in the pelvic cavity.

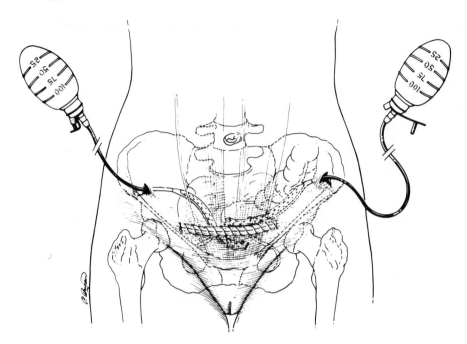

Figure 24–6. Bilateral transabdominal drainage through stab wounds. A closed suction drainage system is preferred.

spilled and the upper abdomen should be isolated from this, if possible. When a ruptured abscess is encountered, the exudate is collected and sent immediately to the laboratory for anaerobic and aerobic cultures and antimicrobial sensitivity studies. The easiest way to collect the material for anaerobic culture is simply to collect it in an airtight syringe and to submit a small piece of the abscess wall in an airtight container. The easiest place to begin the dissection is the round ligament, which is the most consistently available and identifiable landmark. Following the round ligament medially will always lead to the uterine corpus. Variations in the usual technique for the operation may be required because of extensive disease, dense adhesions, indurated and edematous tissue, and distorted anatomy. For example, it is sometimes convenient to perform the central dissection first; that is, a subtotal hysterectomy. This will allow more space and adequate exposure to do the required adnexal surgery. Tuboovarian inflammatory masses may be found densely adherent in the cul-de-sac, behind the uterus, to the posterior surface of the broad ligament, and to the lateral pelvic sidewall. There is risk of injury to the ureters, sigmoid, rectum, and small intestines. The method of dissection used will depend on the nature of the adhesions. Soft, fresh adhesions can be broken gently and easily with finger dissection. Dense fibrotic adhesions must be carefully dissected and cut with scissors. The dissection may be especially difficult and risky if pelvic tissues are intensely indurated, as in ligneous pelvic

cellulitis. If the infundibulopelvic ligament can be clamped, cut, and securely ligated, one may gain access to the lateral retroperitoneal space and identify the ureter. This will facilitate a safe dissection of the abscess wall away from the ureter. In cases with extensive disease involving one or both adnexa, the use of preoperative ureteral catheterization may be helpful in identifying the location of the pelvic ureters. With tubo-ovarian abscess, the anatomical limits of the ovary may be difficult to define. If the ovary is to be removed, it should be removed completely to prevent subsequent development of the ovarian remnant syndrome.

When both adnexa must be removed, a hysterectomy should usually be performed. In some cases, only a subtotal hysterectomy is feasible. Usually, the cervix may be excised following removal of the adnexa and the uterine corpus. The vaginal vault is left open for drainage. A Penrose drain may be inserted and then removed several days later. Suspension of the vaginal vault and reperitonization of the pelvis are accomplished in the usual manner, if possible. A routine closure of the abdominal incision is performed. Jackson Pratt suction drains are often placed above the fascia and brought out through a separate incision.

Since the patient has been placed in the Allen Universal stirrups for laparotomy, ureteral integrity can be confirmed as discussed in Chapters 27 and 29. Five cc of indigo carmine is given intravenously and a cystoscope is placed in the bladder. Blue dye can then be seen to flow from each ureteral orifice.

Formerly, it was standard practice to do a bilateral salpingo-oophorectomy in almost all patients who had a laparotomy for acute pelvic abscess. This practice was based on the belief that the disease is almost always severe in both adnexa. Recently, studies have suggested that as many as 25% to 50% of patients will have a relatively normal tube and ovary on one side. This may be true especially of patients whose infection is associated with intrauterine device use. Golde and associates reported that 37 of 85 patients (44%) with tubo-ovarian abscesses confirmed at operation had unilateral abscesses; 20 were using an intrauterine contraceptive device. The studies of Landers and Sweet, Hager and Majmudar, and Ginsburg and coworkers also found a higher percentage than previously reported of unilateral adnexal disease. As a consequence of these findings, conservative adnexal surgery should be performed if possible. We have no hesitation in leaving in a relatively normal tube and ovary at the time of hysterectomy with removal of the opposite adnexa for acute pelvic abscess, including leaving adnexa with a small hydrosalpinx and periovarian adhesions. Since the uterus is also removed and the continuity between the conserved tube and the lower genital tract is interrupted, there is no risk of a new infection. If a strictly unilateral pelvic abscess is found at laparotomy in a young woman, removal of the affected tube and ovary only, leaving in the uterus and the opposite adnexa, is acceptable in a patient who wishes to preserve fertility, even if in vitro fertilization techniques are required to accomplish pregnancy. However, it should be recognized that such a patient does have a risk of recurrent tubo-ovarian abscess. It is especially important that her sexual partner(s) be examined and receive treatment when indicated.

In recent years, there have been advances in reproductive technology that allow infertile patients to conceive and carry pregnancies to term under most extraordinary circumstances. It has been possible, for example, to accomplish a successful pregnancy in a woman who has a uterus and no ovaries by instillation of a donated fertilized ovum into a suitably prepared uterus. Such a sophisticated procedure is not available to a large audience of patients. However, mostly for medicolegal reasons, the option of leaving in the uterus when bilateral salpingo-oophorectomy is to be performed should be discussed with the patient, especially if she is young and nulliparous.

In summary, patients with acute pelvic abscess should be hospitalized for treatment with parenteral broad-spectrum antibiotics. Surgery is indicated if the abscess presents for extraperitoneal drainage; if the diagnosis is uncertain; if intraperitoneal rupture is diagnosed or suspected; or if the patient fails to respond to medical management.

RUPTURED TUBO-OVARIAN OR PELVIC ABSCESS

A tubo-ovarian or pelvic abscess may rupture spontaneously into the rectum or sigmoid colon, into the bladder, or into the free peritoneal cavity. A pelvic abscess never ruptures spontaneously into the vagina unless the patient has a previous posterior colpotomy for drainage of an abscess. Under these circumstances, a recurrent pelvic abscess may dissect along the tract of the previous posterior colpotomy incision and drain spontaneously through the vagina.

Spontaneous drainage through the rectum or sigmoid colon usually occurs in a patient whose abscess is too high to drain with a posterior colpotomy. In other words, although the abscess is fluctuant and midline, it is not yet dissecting the rectovaginal septum. While waiting for the abscess to come down, a sudden unexpected improvement in the patient's condition will be noted, and she will confirm that pus has begun to drain through the anus. Further improvement in her condition will usually occur. A posterior colpotomy will not be needed and, indeed, is contraindicated, since doing so could cause a rectovaginal fistula to form.

Spontaneous drainage through the bladder is rare. It occurs more commonly in elderly women with chronic abscesses developing from ruptured sigmoid diverticula. Only rarely will a chronic tubo-ovarian or pelvic abscess rupture and drain through the bladder. Obviously, the bladder will be secondarily infected. When the abscess is removed with laparotomy, a defect in the bladder wall will be noted. The indurated tissue around the defect should be removed and the defect closed with No. 3-0 delayed-absorbable suture in two layers. A Foley catheter may be left in place for 10–14 days while healing of the bladder wall takes place.

Of all the complications that can result from pelvic inflammatory disease, intra-abdominal rupture of a tubo-ovarian abscess (grade 3 disease) is the most life-threatening. The mortality from this complication is due to septic shock and from the complications of generalized peritonitis and should not exceed 10% in patients with warm shock.

Abscesses may rupture spontaneously or as the result of bimanual examination or accidental trauma. Bacteriologic study of the contents of the abscess has historically been unrewarding; a specific organism has been isolated in less than 50% of the cases. The gonococcus is rarely identified in a pelvic abscess. Careful aerobic and anaerobic cultures demonstrate the frequent presence of a mixed infection that includes anaerobic organisms. As reviewed by McNamara and Mead, the results of three separate studies demonstrated 31 positive isolates of anaerobes in 30 patients with a pelvic abscess. Landers and Sweet have confirmed this in their series.

Diagnosis of Ruptured Tubo-ovarian Abscess

The major clinical symptom of ruptured tubo-ovarian abscess is acute, progressive pelvic pain, which is usually so severe that the patient can accurately identify the time and place of its occurrence. In the series from the Johns Hopkins Hospital reported by Vermeeren and Te Linde, the average age of patients with a ruptured tubo-ovarian abscess was 33 years, which is at least 10 years older than the average age of patients with acute pelvic inflammatory disease. Approximately 2% of these patients are postmenopausal. To our knowledge, only two cases of ruptured tubo-ovarian abscess in a pregnant patient have been reported. Often, there is a history of recurrent attacks of pelvic inflammatory disease, with a sudden increase in the severity and extent of abdominal pain during a recent exacerbation of infection. On examination, the patient will appear seriously ill and dehydrated, with rapid, shallow respirations. The abdomen will be distended and quiet, with diminished or absent bowel sounds. Signs of generalized peritonitis, direct and rebound tenderness, muscle rigidity, and shifting dullness may be noted. A pelvic mass is palpable in over 50% of cases. Tachycardia is common. Shock may be present or may develop while the patient is under observation. It is due to accumulation of fluids in peripheral tissues and later failure of compensatory vasoconstrictor mechanisms. The temperature is usually over 101°F but can also be normal and even subnormal late in the course. The leukocyte count is likely to be over 15,000 but also may be normal. Severe leukopenia is an ominous sign. A culdocentesis is a valuable diagnostic aid and was positive for purulent material in 70% of cases in the Mickal and Sellmann series. An abdominal x-ray usually shows a paralytic ileus and sometimes evidence of free fluid in the peritoneal cavity and atelectasis in the lung bases.

Treatment of Ruptured Tubo-ovarian Abscess

The longer the delay in the operative treatment of ruptured tubo-ovarian abscess, the higher is the primary mortality. In the Vermeeren and Te Linde series from the Johns Hopkins Hospital, death occurred less than 90 hours after the time of rupture in 88% of fatal cases, both operative and nonoperative.

As time passes after rupture of a tubo-ovarian abscess, septic peritonitis becomes more severe and generalized. The passage of time allows development of septic shock from greater absorption of bacteria and bacterial endotoxins, and secretion of great quantities of fluid into the peritoneal cavity across inflamed peritoneal surfaces. Fluid shifts from the intravascular compartment to interstitial spaces as a result of increased vascular permeability of inflammation of the peritoneal membrane. This leads to hypovolemia, decreased cardiac output, decreased central venous pressure, hypotension, vasoconstriction, increased peripheral resistance, decreased tissue perfusion, metabolic acidosis, adult respiratory distress syndrome, decreased renal glomerular perfusion and filtration with decreased urine flow, severe hypoxemia, multiple organ system failure, and death. The prompt diagnosis and treatment of intraperitoneal rupture of a tubo-ovarian abscess is essential to minimize the mortality of generalized peritonitis.

The treatment of patients with ruptured tubo-ovarian abscess may be divided into three phases: the preoperative, the operative, and the postoperative.

Preoperative Phase

Operation should be undertaken after rapid but adequate preoperative preparation. The patients should be typed and cross-matched with two to four units of packed red blood cells. Monitoring of central venous pressure is essential for proper evaluation of the hemodynamics of this condition because many patients will be dehydrated, in shock, and anemic. Swan-Ganz catheter placement may be preferable, since it will also allow pulmonary capillary wedge pressure and pulmonary artery pressure determinations that will be helpful in assessing the adequacy of fluid replacement and in detecting fluid overload. Variable amounts of fluid, sometimes tremendous, will have been lost into the peritoneal cavity and intestinal tract because of peritonitis. Emergency blood chemistry determinations (eg, serum electrolytes, creatine, glucose, bilirubin, and alkaline phosphatase) are obtained and intravenous fluids are started immediately, preferably Ringer's lactate. Crystalloid solutions for fluid volume resuscitation are preferred for most patients with septic peritonitis. It may be advantageous to use partial colloid resuscitation in some patients with evidence of cardiopulmonary dysfunction, since a smaller total volume is required. An excess of intravenous crystalloid solution may result in fluid overload.

Vigorous broad-spectrum intravenous antibiotic therapy should be instituted. An indwelling urethral catheter is used to monitor fluid intake with hourly urine output. Generally, it is advantageous to insert a Cantor or Miller-Abbott intestinal tube before operation to decompress distended bowel. Combating shock is a primary concern throughout treatment. Clinical assessment of respiratory function should be made. A distended tender abdomen may cause rapid shallow respirations and use of accessory muscles for ventilation. Arterial blood gases may indicate mild hypoxemia, in which case oxygen should be administered and ventilator support provided. Blood transfusion should be started before surgery. When the patient has been properly prepared, immediate surgery should be undertaken. The results of treatment will be better if major metabolic and hemodynamic problems are corrected prior to operation, but one cannot waste time in a critically ill patient with septic peritonitis.

Operative Phase

The anesthetic of choice depends on the preference and experience of the anesthesiologist and the medical condition of the patient.

The operation should be performed as rapidly as possible. Since speed as well as access to the upper abdomen may be required, a lower midline incision should be used. It can be quickly extended above the umbilicus if necessary. The patient should not be put in the Trendelenburg position until the abdomen is packed off, and no more of a dependent position should be used than is needed to prevent further dissemination of pus into the upper abdomen. When the abdomen is opened, one should note any odor present. An unpleasant putrid odor is indicative of infection with anaerobic organisms. Pus from the abdomen should be collected correctly for both aerobic and anaerobic cultures and for Gram's stain, and promptly transported to the laboratory. Organisms grown should be tested for sensitivity to various antibiotics.

The operation of choice is removal of the free pus, together with the abscess, the uterus, the tubes, and usually the ovaries. Only occasionally is it possible to leave an ovary in a patient with a ruptured pelvic abscess. If rupture has occurred from a strictly unilateral tubo-ovarian abscess, with a relatively normal tube and ovary on the opposite side, a unilateral salpingo-oophorectomy may be done, especially if the patient is young. However, the risk of a recurrent abscess in the opposite tube and ovary will be high if the uterus is also left in place. When the uterus is removed along with the tubo-ovarian abscess, the risk of recurrent abscess in the opposite adnexa is reduced. When hysterectomy is performed, usually a total hysterectomy can be done. However, even in the best surgical hands, a subtotal hysterectomy is faster than a total one and is sometimes justified. It is probable that the mortality rate would be increased if one always insisted on doing a total hysterectomy. Although we believe firmly in total hysterectomy, we do not believe in persisting in it when the danger of total hysterectomy exceeds the danger from a retained cervix. Except in the young female, it is better to remove the corpus than to perform a unilateral adnexectomy alone. Furthermore, the opposite adnexa will be significantly involved in the majority of patients, and subsequent operation may be necessary if conservation of one side is practiced, as was required in 35% of Pedowitz and Bloomfield's cases.

The technical performance of the procedure may be difficult. Anatomy is distorted; dependable landmarks are obscured; tissues are thick, edematous, friable, and inflamed. Loops of densely adherent intestine must be separated carefully to avoid injury. Injury to the serosa of distended bowel occurs commonly and sometimes requires repair. An entry into the lumen of the bowel must be recognized and repaired. The most dependable anatomic landmark is the round ligament. Followed medially, it will always lead to the uterine corpus. Retroperitoneal planes of dissection may be employed to advantage in identifying the ureters and removing inflammatory adnexal masses. Otherwise, it is likely that fragments of ovary will be left behind and may subsequently cause signs and symptoms of the ovarian remnant syndrome. As much as possible of the remaining abscess wall should be removed without causing unnecessary additional bleeding. Pieces of the abscess wall may be left adherent to the pelvic sidewall and cul-de-sac. Oozing of blood from all dissected tissue has been likened to "cinder bed bleeding" and is difficult to control.

In 1977, Rivlin and Hunt used conservative pelvic surgery combined with intra- and postoperative peritoneal lavage with antibiotics in 113 women with generalized peritonitis caused by ruptured tubo-ovarian abscess. The uterus, ovaries, and tubes were retained whenever possible. Either one or both of the adnexa were retained in whole or in part, and hysterectomy was performed in only four cases. All loculations of pus were opened and aggressive lavage of the peritoneal cavity with gentamicin was carried out for several days postoperatively. The mortality rate was 7.1% and further surgery was required in only 17.5%. We have had no experience with this method of management of ruptured tubo-ovarian abscess.

Before the incision is closed, the abdominal cavity should be irrigated with copious quantities of sterile saline to remove remaining bacteria and debris. When generalized septic peritonitis is also present, large volumes of warm saline should also be used to irrigate the upper abdomen. There is always some fear of dissemination of the infection by copious irrigation. However, this disadvantage is far outweighed by diluting and removing bacteria and necrotic debris. "The solution to pollution is dilution." We do not add antiseptics or antibiotics to the irrigating solution. If hemostasis is poor or if considerable necrotic material is left behind, there may be some benefit from peritoneal drainage with closed suction catheters. Closed suction drains may be placed through a separate stab wound in the abdominal wall, through the cul-de-sac, or through the vaginal vault when a total hysterectomy has been done, but the drainage of free peritoneal exudate in the upper abdomen is of no therapeutic value.

The upper abdomen should be carefully explored for collections of pus in the subdiaphragmatic and sub-hepatic regions. If an upper abdominal abscess is found, it may be necessary to place a closed suction drain into the abscess cavity through the upper abdominal wall.

The abdominal incision may be closed with a Smead-Jones technique or with a continuous suture taking large bites of tissue. A monofilament suture of polypropylene or nylon should be used. Retention sutures may be placed but are not usually necessary. The incision should be irrigated with warm saline. When there has been gross contamination of the incision, the subcutaneous fat and skin should be left open and packed lightly with gauze soaked in an antibiotic solution. The wound is repacked daily and inspected. In 4–5 days, if the tissues are healthy, the incision may be closed secondarily with sutures. Alternatively, the edges may be drawn together with sterile adhesive strips.

Postoperative Phase

Postoperative care should consider shock, infection, ileus, and fluid imbalances. Complications of the late postoperative period include pelvic and abdominal abscesses, intestinal obstruction, intestinal fistulas, incisional breakdown with or without evisceration, pulmonary embolus, continued sepsis, and disseminated intravascular coagulation. Serious medical diseases such as uncontrolled diabetes or renal or pulmonary failure (ARDS) further complicate recovery from this potentially lethal disease.

Septic shock should be combated with blood, when indicated due to a hemoglobin less than 7.0 g, Ringer's lactate, respiratory support, and if necessary, vasoactive substances (see Septic Shock in this chapter). Infection is controlled by the continued, aggressive use of broad-spectrum intravenous antibiotics until the patient can take antibiotics orally. When the results of the antibiotic sensitivity studies on the operative specimen are available, one should consider changing to more effective agents, but only if the patient shows evidence of continued sepsis. Antibiotics should not necessarily be changed on the basis of sensitivity studies if the patient is improving clinically. Sometimes the patient's condition will improve initially only to show signs of recurring intra-abdominal infection in the second week after operation. Under these circumstances it is appropriate to change antibiotics. Antibiotics should be continued until the patient is afebrile with only a mild leukocytosis and able to eat a regular diet. A long period of treatment with antibiotics may result in complications such as pseudomembranous enterocolitis.

The semi-Fowler's position may help prevent subphrenic and subdiaphragmatic abscess formation. Patients with signs of continued intra-abdominal sepsis should have CT scans to identify collections of pus. If found, CT-directed drainage may be possible.

Constant intestinal suction by means of a long intestinal tube is a very important feature of postoperative care. Adynamic ileus persists postoperatively for a variable period and is best treated with the long intestinal tube until there is evidence of peristalsis and the patient is passing flatus.

Close attention to fluid balance and blood chemistry determinations is mandatory. Frequently, patients with ruptured tubo-ovarian abscess have poor kidney function. The fluid output and serum creatinine should be followed closely.

The results of the preceding therapeutic measures have been gratifying. At Grady Memorial Hospital, the current mortality rate for this formerly lethal disease is 3.5%.

PRIMARY OVARIAN ABSCESS

A primary ovarian abscess is a distinctly different entity from tubo-ovarian abscess. A tubo-ovarian abscess is one in which the abscess wall is composed of fallopian tube and ovarian parenchyma. A primary ovarian abscess, on the other hand, is one in which the infection occurs in the parenchyma of the ovary. Unlike tubo-ovarian abscess, it is an unusual condition. Interest in primary ovarian abscess was stimulated by the 1964 report of Willson and Black. According to a review by Wetchler and Dunn, 120 cases had been reported by 1985.

Although bacteria may gain access to the ovarian parenchyma by hematogenous or lymphatic spread, it is probable that the majority of primary ovarian abscesses occur because bacteria present around the ovary gain access to the parenchyma through a break in the ovarian capsule. The capsule may be broken naturally by ovulation, or it may be broken by a surgical procedure. Bacteria may come from the fallopian tube, from the vagina during or after hysterectomy, from intrauterine infection associated with intrauterine device, or from appendicitis, diverticulitis, or any other condition that is associated with peritonitis. A primary ovarian abscess is usually unilateral. However, its occurrence simultaneously in both ovaries and during pregnancy seems to support the occasional occurrence of hematogenous and/or lymphatic spread. Primary ovarian abscess has been reported secondary to infections at distant sites (tonsillitis, typhoid, parotitis, and tuberculosis). A mixed flora of anaerobic and aerobic bacteria is usually present. *A. israelii* with sulfur granules has also been identified in a few cases.

Diagnosis of an unruptured primary ovarian abscess can be difficult because of the variable clinical presentation. Lower abdominal pain and fever are usually present. Lower abdominal and pelvic tenderness and an adnexal mass may be present, but the pelvic exam is sometimes not helpful. Although an event predisposing to primary ovarian abscess (eg, surgery, IUD use, appendicitis, and systemic infection) may be uncovered in the history, the event is sometimes remote. Ultrasonography and computed tomography can be helpful in identifying an abscess cavity. When the ovarian abscess ruptures, the clinical picture is much the same as in ruptured tubo-ovarian abscess with abdominal distention, direct and rebound tenderness, ileus, and sometimes shock. The patient appears gravely ill, and the need for immediate surgery is usually obvious.

The management of patients with primary ovarian abscess is similar to the management of patients with acute tubo-ovarian abscess. If the abscess is not ruptured, medical management with antibiotics for both anaerobic and aerobic organisms (ampicillin, gentamicin, and clindamycin) plus supportive care is indicated. A failure to respond or deterioration in the patient's condition will suggest alteration in antibiotic coverage and/or possible exploratory surgery to remove the abscess. Ruptured ovarian abscess requires immediate laparotomy after a brief but intense effort to stabilize the patient and start antibiotic therapy. At operation, only the affected ovary need be removed. The tubes may be conserved as well as the uterus. If both ovaries are involved, they should both be removed. In a patient who is not interested in conception in the future, the uterus and both tubes may also be removed. If the patient is interested in pregnancy, one may elect to leave the uterus and fallopian tubes in place for possible implantation of a donated egg in future years.

SURGERY FOR CHRONIC PELVIC INFLAMMATORY DISEASE

Although the gonococcus may be responsible for initiating acute salpingitis, which is short-lived, the residual chronic salpingitis is usually due to secondary invaders, both aerobic and anaerobic, or perhaps to an initial infection with *C. trachomatis*. As a result of the initial infection or from subsequent secondary exacerbations, the fimbria may become occluded and the tubes bound to the ovaries with adhesions. In addition, the bowel may become adherent to the broad ligament and the adnexal structures, and the fascia and loose connective tissue of the broad ligament may be converted into an indurated, brawny structure typical of ligneous induration. This may extend to include tissues beneath the peritoneum on the lateral pelvic sidewall, where ligneous pelvic cellulitis may cause ureteral obstruction. If the chronic infection persists, serious effusion from the inflammatory process within the endosalpinx will produce a hydrosalpinx that may ignite periodically with secondary subacute pelvic infection or may progress to produce a pyosalpinx and tubo-ovarian abscess. If the subacute infection is left untreated or is treated inadequately, spontaneous intra-abdominal rupture or leakage of an old tubo-ovarian abscess may occur. In a review of this subject, Heaton and Ledger have identified this problem principally in premenopausal women, with only 1.7% of patients with a tubo-ovarian abscess being postmenopausal.

The signs and symptoms of chronic pelvic inflammatory disease that most frequently require surgical treatment include severe, persistent, and progressive pelvic pain, usually bilateral, although occasionally localized in one of the lower abdominal quadrants; repeated exacerbations of pelvic inflammatory disease requiring multiple hospitalizations and recurrent medical treatment; progressive enlargement of a tubo-ovarian inflammatory mass, especially if it cannot be distinguished from a neoplastic tumor of the ovary; severe dyspareunia related to the chronic pelvic infection; and bilateral ureteral obstruction from ligneous cellulitis. It was formerly accepted that a history of previous colpotomy for drainage of pelvic abscess was sufficient reason in itself to justify definitive abdominal surgery later for removal of the uterus and adnexa. We have seen several patients who have become pregnant following posterior colpotomy for drainage of a cul-de-sac abscess and who have remained relatively free of symptoms for long periods. Today, previous posterior colpotomy for pelvic abscess drainage is not a sufficient indication by itself for definitive abdominal surgery.

Selection of Operation

The final decision on the proper operation for the surgical management of chronic pelvic inflammatory disease is usually made with the abdomen open. Consideration must be given not only to the pathologic lesions found at operation but also to the patient's age, parity, desire for children, previous history of pelvic disease, and other associated pelvic disease and symptoms. Because a knowledge of all these is essential to the best surgical judgment, the operator should be thoroughly familiar with the patient, her history, and her desires.

In the surgical management of chronic pelvic inflammatory disease, the question of the removal or retention of the ovary at the time of hysterectomy and

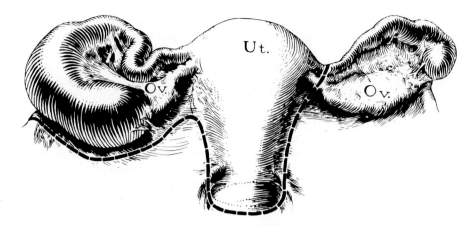

Figure 24–7. Total abdominal hysterectomy and unilateral salpingo-oophorectomy from extensive chronic salpingo-oophoritis. A small hydrosalpinx on the opposite side may be left in to preserve blood supply to the ovary.

salpingectomy has been left open to conjecture and individual surgical opinion in most instances. This question was the subject of a study by Weiner and Wallach of the ovarian histology in ovaries removed from patients with pelvic inflammatory disease. They found that in 40 consecutive women who underwent oophorectomy during surgical treatment of pelvic inflammatory disease, nearly 50% of the removed ovaries were free of inflammatory disease and demonstrated normal follicular activity. The study concluded that ovarian histology was more often normal among patients who gave no history of dysfunctional uterine bleeding. Therefore, the menstrual history of such patients should be helpful in the decision regarding ovarian conservation or ablation. Kirtley and Benigno have reviewed our experience with ovarian conservation at the time of surgery for pelvic inflammatory disease. In this series, 98 (82%) patients who required surgery had a total abdominal hysterectomy and bilateral salpingo-oophorectomy. In 22 patients (18%), either part or all of an ovary was retained. Of the 22 patients, 15 were available for follow-up hormonal assays. The mean follow-up time was 58 months. Cyclic ovarian function could be confirmed in all but two patients. In the two patients with ovarian failure, other significant disease processes were also present. No patient suffered a complication as a result of adnexal conservation. We believe that normal ovarian tissue should be conserved at the time of definitive surgery for pelvic inflammatory disease. A small hydrosalpinx on the same side as the normal ovary may also be left in place so that ovarian blood supply will not be disturbed in any attempt to remove the tube.

The release of peritubal adhesions for mild chronic pelvic inflammatory disease is indicated occasionally in women in whom future childbearing is desired, provided the tubes can be shown to be patent, usually by transfundal chromotubation after the lower uterine isthmus is occluded by a Ziegler clamp. This type of procedure, more fully discussed in Chapter 19, pro-

vides the most rewarding pregnancy rate of all types of tubal reconstructive surgery. More frequently, one tube is hopelessly closed and the opposite tube is patent after release of adhesions. In such a case, unilateral salpingectomy may be required if reconstructive surgery is not possible. Many other procedures are available in the treatment of this disease, including salpingo-oophorectomy with or without hysterectomy (Figs. 24-7 and 24-8).

In a majority of instances of surgery for chronic pelvic inflammatory disease, total abdominal hysterectomy and bilateral salpingo-oophorectomy is necessary to remove the primary tubal pathology because of inflammatory damage of both tubes and ovaries. The total abdominal hysterectomy and bilateral salpingo-oophorectomy illustrated in Figure 24-9 was done for severe actinomycosis infection.

Should the uterus be removed and an ovary preserved, it may be preferable to leave the entire adnexa in place in the absence of active tubal infection rather than to compromise the venous drainage or the arterial blood supply to the ovary with subsequent cystic changes that may require an additional operative procedure later. Once the continuity of the tubal lumen from the uterine cavity is broken, the chronically in-

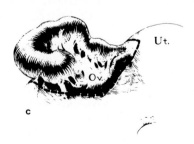

Figure 24–8. When significant chronic pelvic inflammatory disease involves only one adnexa and preservation of uterine function is indicated, a unilateral salpingo-oophorectomy only may be done.

flamed tube does not usually produce subsequent symptoms, as shown by Falk in his series of cases with interstitial tubal resection. When it is considered advisable to remove both adnexa owing to the extent of the tubo-ovarian disease, a total hysterectomy is also advisable unless the uterus is hopelessly encased in pelvic scar tissue and densely adherent to the pelvic viscera. Usually the uterus can be removed without difficulty, thus providing an easier opportunity to peritonize the operative site and avoid additional postoperative adhesions. However, there is a place for mature surgical judgment in this instance, and discretion will dictate whether a subtotal hysterectomy rather than a total hysterectomy is surgically advisable.

In the optimum case, especially in a young woman who wishes to establish or maintain the possibility of future fertility, conservative surgery may be desirable, with the hope that pregnancy can be accomplished through in vitro fertilization techniques. In this situation, the uterus and one adnexa should be conserved, and the ovary should be positioned in the pelvis so an ovum can be harvested later through the laparoscope or through the vagina. As mentioned earlier, if the patient wishes, the uterus may be left in place even though both tubes and ovaries have been removed.

Salpingectomy for Chronic Salpingitis

At the time of surgery for the treatment of chronic pelvic inflammatory disease, every effort should be made to retain uninvolved organs. Unilateral salpingectomy should be considered when the oviduct is hopelessly destroyed by the disease process and is a large hydrosalpinx.

The abdomen is entered through a transverse Maylard incision. The adhesions binding the tube are cut and the tube is freed. It is held by a Kelly clamp placed on the mesosalpinx just beneath the fimbriated end. The mesosalpinx is then clamped and cut, taking a succession of small bites as close to the tube as possible (Fig. 24-10A).

Keeping the operative trauma as far as possible from the ovary that is to be retained lessens the danger of imperiling its blood supply. Experience has shown that the ovary whose tube has been removed is more apt to become cystic than the ovary whose tube has been left undisturbed. Therefore, it would seem logical to interfere as little as possible with the blood supply of the ovary by hugging the tube closely when excising it.

The tube is excised at the uterine cornu in a wedge-shaped manner, as indicated by the dotted line in Figure 24-10A. A wide, figure-of-eight No. 2-0 delayed-absorbable suture is placed in the cornu before the wedge is excised and is tightened as the interstitial portion of the tube is removed. If there is palpable extension of the inflammation at the uterine cornu (salpingitis isthmica nodosa, so-called), the wedge may be large.

The wound in the uterus is closed with one or more No. 2-0 delayed-absorbable figure-of-eight sutures (Fig. 24-10B). The vessels in the mesosalpinx are ligated with transfixion No. 3-0 delayed-absorbable sutures. The transfixion suture has the advantage that it will not slip off the tissue when tied as the clamp is withdrawn (Fig. 24-10C).

A mattress of No. 3-0 delayed-absorbable suture is taken to bring the broad and round ligaments over the cornual wound (Fig. 24-10D). This suture passes just beneath the round ligament, so that the ligament will not be strangulated when the suture is drawn tight. When this suture is tied, the cornual wound is covered with the broad ligament, and to some extent the uterus is suspended in a manner similar to that used in the Coffey suspension.

Usually a second mattress or interrupted suture is necessary to cover over the mesosalpinx completely, as shown in Figure 24-10E.

Salpingo-oophorectomy for Chronic Salpingitis

As in the case of salpingectomy, the abdomen is entered through a transverse Maylard incision. The chronic tubo-ovarian inflammatory mass is first dis-

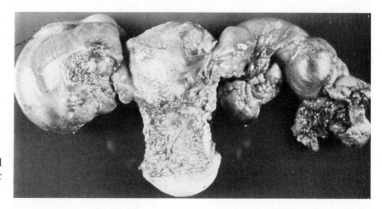

Figure 24–9. Total abdominal hysterectomy and bilateral salpingo-oophorectomy for severe pelvic actinomycosis.

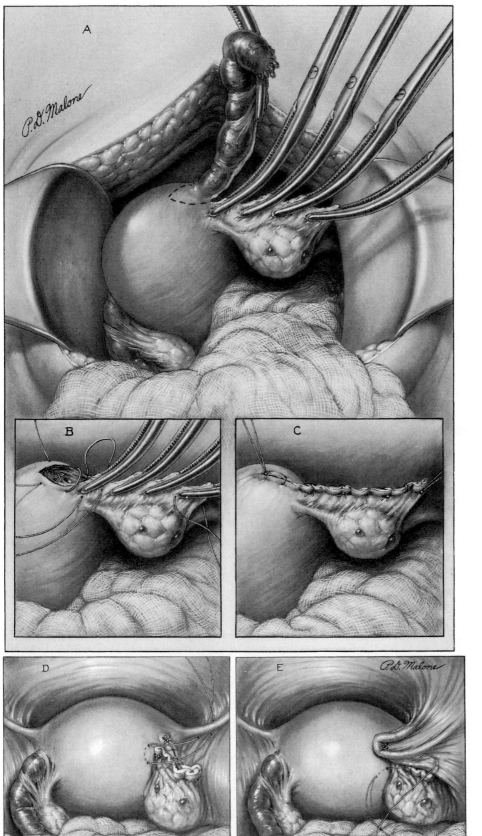

Figure 24–10. Salpingectomy. *A*, Mesosalpinx is clamped with multiple Kelly clamps and cut. Dotted lines indicate cornual excision, which is elective. *B*, Cornual wound is closed with No. 2-0 delayed absorbable suture. *C*, Mesosalpinx vessels are transfixed. *D*, Mattress suture is placed to cover operative area. *E*, Round ligament and broad ligaments cover operative area.

sected free and the infundibulopelvic ligament is identified. It is doubly clamped with Ochsner clamps and a third clamp is applied to control back-bleeding (Fig. 24-11A). The ureter must be identified before the infundibulopelvic ligament is clamped, cut, and ligated.

After the infundibulopelvic ligament is cut and ligated, the remainder of the broad ligament attachment of the tube and the ovary is clamped, cut, and ligated. The uterine end of the tube and the ovarian ligament are excised from the uterus in a wedge-shaped manner. The ascending uterine vessels are ligated just below the cornual wound, and the cornual incision is closed with a No. 2-0 delayed-absorbable figure-of-eight suture (Fig. 24-11B).

The infundibulopelvic ligament is doubly ligated with No. 2-0 delayed-absorbable suture, and the vessels in the broad ligament are ligated with No. 3-0 delayed-absorbable suture. The cornual wound is peritonized, and the uterus is suspended to some degree by bringing the round and the broad ligaments over the uterine cornu with a mattress suture of No. 2-0 delayed-absorbable suture, as shown in Figure 24-11C. An attempt should be made to remove the tubo-ovarian inflammatory complex completely. If a fragment of ovary is left attached to the lateral pelvic peritoneum or the broad ligament, the ovarian remnant syndrome may develop later. To prevent this, a retroperitoneal approach may be required.

Identification of the Ureter

Identification of the course of the ureter in a pelvis where the anatomy has become obliterated as a result

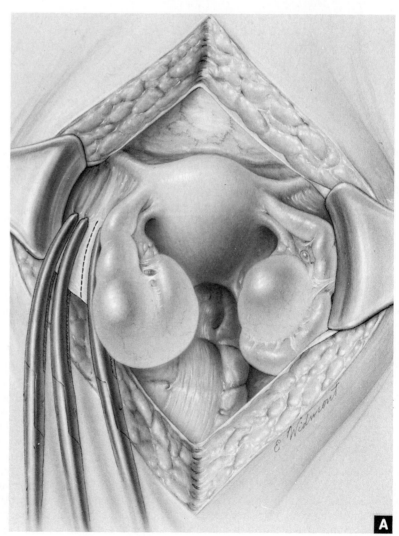

Figure 24–11. Salpingo-oophorectomy. *A*, The infundibulopelvic ligament is doubly clamped. Another clamp is placed to control back-bleeding. Dotted line indicates incision. (*continued on next page*)

A

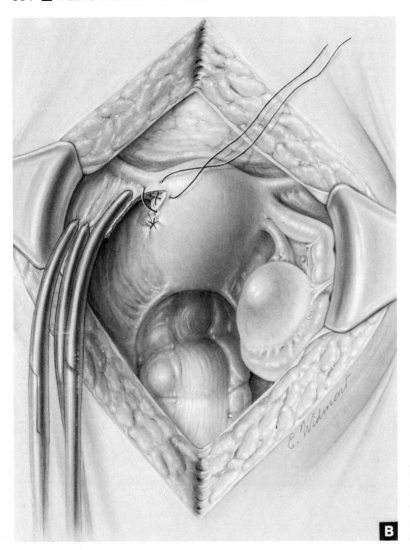

Figure 24–11. (continued) *B*, A suture has been placed so as to ligate the ascending uterine vessels just below cornual incision. The cornual incision is being closed with a figure-of-eight of No. 2-0 delayed-absorbable suture.

of pelvic inflammatory disease is one of the most important responsibilities of the gynecologist. In the surgical treatment of this disease, one may find a tuboovarian inflammatory mass that is located between the leaves of the broad ligament and extends to the lateral pelvic wall. It is not uncommon for the ligneous induration of the thickened parietal peritoneum to obscure completely the location and course of the pelvic ureter so that dissection of the diseased adnexa produces a surgical risk to the urinary tract, requiring great technical skill to avoid ureteral injury. Knowledge of the normal anatomic location of the pelvic ureters, as discussed in Chapters 4 and 29, is essential so that these vital structures can be identified before attempting to remove the adnexal masses. Dividing the round ligament allows access to the lateral pelvic wall beneath the peritoneum. After the round ligament is divided, the

peritoneum is incised inferiorly toward the internal cervical os and superiorly just lateral to the infundibulopelvic ligament. The peritoneum can be easily reflected medially away from the pelvic sidewall with finger dissection and the ureter identified. It remains attached to the peritoneum. If there is difficulty, the ureter can usually be identified as it crosses over the common iliac artery just above its bifurcation, and traced downward.

Such patients may have a preoperative ureteral catheterization when there is clinical evidence of large, adherent adnexal masses. However, if such an anatomic problem is encountered at the time of laparotomy, an incision may be made in the dome of the bladder that will allow the passage of ureteral catheters. If the patient has been positioned in the Allen Universal stirrups for operation, intraoperative cystoscopy with passage of

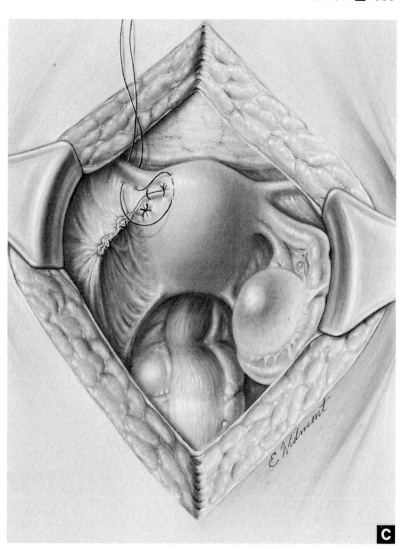

Figure 24–11. (continued) *C*, The infundibulopelvic ligament and the rest of the broad ligament vessels have been ligated. Cornual wound is being covered with the round and the broad ligament by use of a mattress suture of No. 2-0 delayed-absorbable suture.

C

ureteral stents may be easily accomplished. At the end of the operation, 5 cc of indigo carmine is given intravenously. With a cystoscope in the bladder, the dye can be seen to effuse from both ureteral orifices confirming that the ureters have not been injured or compromised.

Drainage at Laparotomy for Pelvic Abscess

Views on drainage at laparotomy for pelvic inflammatory disease have changed during the past several years. Whereas drainage was an everyday occurrence in gynecologic operating rooms in the 1950s, it is used only occasionally today. Several factors are responsible for this change. Operations for acute and subacute pelvic inflammatory disease are avoided by aggressive medical management; hence, pus is encountered less frequently. Even where small pockets of pus are encountered, experience has shown that the pus may be suctioned away, the peritoneum irrigated thoroughly with saline, and the abdomen closed with impunity without drainage. Antibiotic therapy has also reduced the indications for drainage. The operator is justified in depending on postoperative antibiotics to combat the infection.

When an abscess is densely adherent to the bowel wall or the region of the ureter, a thorough removal of all the abscess wall might result in damage to a viscus and bleeding. In such cases small portions of necrotic abscess wall may be left in situ and a closed suction drain placed against the area. The ideal exit for a drain is through the cul-de-sac, as shown in Figure 24-12. Sometimes the cul-de-sac is completely obliterated by adhe-

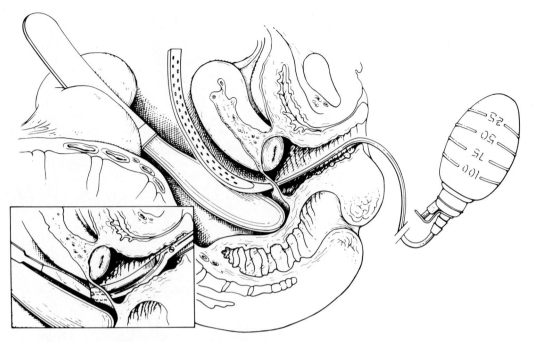

Figure 24–12. Drainage of pelvis through cul-de-sac. A long Kelly clamp is inserted into the vagina and opened slightly as the posterior vaginal fornix is pushed upward. The scalpel incises between the jaws of the clamp. The drain is clamped and withdrawn through the vagina.

sions between the anterior rectal wall and the cervix. In such instances the use of the posterior vaginal fornix for drainage may not be feasible. When drainage is indicated under such circumstances, it should be done through a small stab wound in whichever lower quadrant is most directly above the point to be drained (see Fig. 24-6). We dislike drainage through the primary incision because of the danger of hernia formation and incisional infection. When the large bowel has been entered accidentally and a perfectly satisfactory closure effected, the abdomen is closed without drainage and the patient is placed on antibiotic therapy. If the condition of the large bowel wall is such that satisfactory closure cannot be done, temporary colostomy above the injury may be preferable to the risk of an abscess and intestinal fistula.

When pus is spilled and gross contamination of the operative field is present, a closed suction drainage system can also be installed in the incision above the fascia with exit through a separate stab wound. This is especially important in diabetic and obese patients. Alternatively, the incision above the fascial closure can be packed open for a few days and closed secondarily to avoid incisional breakdown from infection.

SEPTIC PELVIC THROMBOPHLEBITIS

In three classic reports in 1951, Collins and associates at Tulane University and Charity Hospital in New Orleans described the pathology and clinical features of suppurative pelvic thrombophlebitis and reported their experience with its surgical management by vena caval and bilateral ovarian vein ligation. Experience at Grady Memorial Hospital and Emory University Hospital with septic pelvic thrombophlebitis and its medical management with antibiotics and heparin was reported by Josey and Cook and by Josey and Staggers.

Septic pelvic thrombophlebitis is much more common among obstetric patients than it is among gynecologic patients. It is more likely to be seen after septic abortion, after abdominal or vaginal delivery with postpartum endomyometritis, or with infected retained placental fragments. In gynecologic patients, septic pelvic thrombophlebitis is seen rarely with pelvic inflammatory disease, ovarian abscess, ligneous pelvic cellulitis, postoperative pelvic infections, and radium insertion.

Septic (or suppurative) pelvic thrombophlebitis is a serious but fortunately uncommon complication of pelvic infection. With equal frequency, both hypogastric and ovarian veins are involved. Initially, the septic process in the uterus or adnexa extends to the veins of the myometrium and broad ligament. A thrombus forms at the site of damage to the intima of the vein. Subsequently, bacteria invade the thrombus. Septic thrombi develop at multiple sites in the pelvis and may extend along the hypogastric veins into the common iliac veins and may progress into the inferior vena cava. By retrograde extension, the femoral vein may also be thrombosed. Massive infected thrombi may form in the ovarian veins and extend to the level of the renal veins. These pelvic veins are thick, enlarged, firm, and filled with infected clots. Fragments of thrombi containing bacteria may break away to form septic emboli to the lungs and other organs. The septic thrombi and emboli are the source of a bacteremia. If uncontrolled or unresponsive to treatment, the process may be fatal.

The clinical features of septic pelvic thrombophlebitis have been fully described, although it must be understood that only in cases where surgical exploration of the pelvis has been carried out can the diagnosis be absolutely confirmed. Typically, an already septic patient will develop chills with a characteristic and erratic, high-spiking fever, an elevated-plateau pulse, and a protracted course. The patient will appear amazingly well in spite of serious manifestations of infection. She will not complain of pain, and abdominal and pelvic examination will elicit minimal tenderness. On careful pelvic examination, one may be able to feel thrombi in pelvic veins. This, however, is quite uncommon. Blood cultures may be positive for a variety of bacteria. Reliable evidence of septic pelvic thrombophlebitis is the occurrence of a septic embolism, usually to the lung, in a patient who has a pelvic infection. These septic emboli may be multiple but are not often fatal initially. Usually one has time to make the diagnosis and institute effective therapy. One of the most reliable signs of septic pelvic thrombophlebitis is the failure of a patient with pelvic sepsis to respond to antibiotics that are usually effective.

Computed tomography and ultrasonography can be helpful in diagnosing septic pelvic thrombophlebitis, especially if contrast medium (iothalamate meglumine) is given intravenously to assist in visualizing the veins. One may see enlargement of the thrombosed vessel, a low-density mass distending the vessel lumen, and enhancement of the vessel wall with the use of intravenous contrast medium. Thrombi in the lower-extremity veins, pelvic veins, ovarian veins, and inferior vena cava can be demonstrated using the technique described by Bauer and Flynn.

When the diagnosis of septic pelvic thrombophlebitis is made or suspected, heparin therapy should be instituted. The response and improvement will often be prompt and dramatic. The temperature and pulse will quickly return to normal. The dramatic response to heparin therapy is so consistent that its absence may indicate that the patient does not have septic pelvic thrombophlebitis.

Collins and his colleagues advised immediate vena caval and bilateral ovarian vein ligation when a diagnosis of septic pelvic thrombophlebitis was made. Currently, conservative medical therapy is recommended for patients with a clinical diagnosis of septic pelvic thrombophlebitis. This should include anticoagulation with heparin. Intravenous antibiotics, preferably a combination effective against anaerobic and aerobic organisms, should be used. If used early, anticoagulation should prevent septic embolization and hasten recovery from this debilitating pyosepticemia. Surgery should be reserved for those few patients who do not respond to medical management or who continue to show evidence of septic emboli. Under these circumstances, surgery may be lifesaving and should be done without hesitation. The operation should include vena caval ligation or clipping plus bilateral ovarian vein ligation. The level of vessel ligation will depend on how far the thrombus has extended. Hysterectomy and removal of adnexal organs will depend on the nature and extent of the pelvic infection. Antibiotics should be continued, and adjunctive anticoagulation is recommended to inhibit further thrombus formation and propagation. When in the course of this disease a pelvic abscess is found that is amenable to drainage, it should be drained. Drainage of a pelvic abscess adds greatly to the successful resolution of pelvic infection.

Instead of vena caval ligation, one may elect to insert a Mobin-Udlin umbrella into the vena cava through the internal jugular vein. This device is made of stainless steel Silastic-coated alloy and becomes fixed in the wall of the vena cava. The vena cava usually remains partially patent. A stainless steel Greenfield vena cava filter may be inserted through the femoral vein or the internal jugular vein. It will entrap emboli greater than 3 mm in diameter and will maintain a greater degree of patency. Obviously, placement of these devices in the inferior vena cava will not prevent pulmonary emboli that originate from thrombosed veins in the infundibulopelvic ligament. These devices have not been extensively used and evaluated in patients with septic pelvic thrombophlebitis.

According to Hammond and associates, the most common cause of suppurative thrombophlebitis is related to intravenous catheter use. Suppurative thrombophlebitis occurs in 0.2% of patients receiving IV therapy; such patients may have local signs of infection at the IV site but commonly show signs of serious systemic infection. The diagnosis can be confirmed by aspirating pus from the infected vein. The blood cultures are usually positive. Definitive treatment includes antibiotics and surgical excision of the infected vein in advanced cases. The incidence of IV-related suppurative thrombophlebitis and associated morbidity and mortality can be reduced by careful attention to a septic technique when inserting an intravenous line; rotation of intravenous sites every 3 days or earlier if there are signs of irritation or infection; avoidance of injection of highly irritating substances (antibiotics, potassium, or other drugs) through the IV site; and avoidance of the lower extremity as a site of continuous intravenous therapy.

SEPTIC SHOCK

In 1951, Waisbren pointed out the specific shocklike picture in patients with gram-negative bacteremia. The effect of the endotoxin produced from the degenerating bacterial cell wall was first proposed by Borden and Hall in 1951 and later confirmed by Braude and associates in 1953.

The report of the European Conference on Septic Shock by Ledingham and associates provided useful definitions of terminology. *Bacteremia* indicates the presence of potentially pathogenic bacteria in the blood without signs of infection. *Endotoxinemia* describes the presence of measurable amounts of endotoxin (lipopolysaccharide) in the systemic circulation. *Sepsis* denotes infection due to a variety of microorganisms or their toxins, associated with fever and toxic reactions. *Septicemia* is a clinical syndrome commonly caused by gram-negative or gram-positive bacteria, comprising several of the following features: fever, hyperdynamic or hypodynamic circulatory shock, oliguria, thrombocytopenia, lactic acidosis, pulmonary edema, and intravascular coagulation. Finally, *septic shock* is the end result of an infective process originating in one or multiple foci that, apparently by means of endotoxin entering the systemic circulation, affects all organ systems of the body. By following the definition of these terms, one can understand the progressively more serious stages of infection.

Shock develops in 25% to 50% of patients with gram-negative bacteremia. The mortality ranges from 40% to 60%. Between 2% and 6% of patients with septic abortion will develop septic shock. In addition, septic shock is a recognized complication of advanced pelvic neoplastic disease, ruptured tubo-ovarian abscess, chronic chorioamnionitis, and acute pyelonephritis. This complication is usually associated with some precipitating event such as pelvic surgery, instrumentation of the urinary tract, immunosuppression, or—in the case of septic abortion—secondary intrauterine infection following instrumentation. Elderly patients and patients with urinary tract infection, diabetes, or hepatic disease are also more susceptible to septic shock. Although a less severe form can be caused by gram-positive organisms, the condition is usually caused by an endotoxin liberated by lysis of gram-negative bacteria, such as *E. coli, B. fragilis, Aerobacter aerogenes, Proteus mirabilis,* or *Pseudomonas aeruginosa.* A more lethal and less common exotoxin is synthesized and excreted by *Clostridium perfringens. S. Aureus* also produces an exotoxin and profound septic shock. Although *E. coli* accounts for more than 50% of the cases of septic shock, almost any microorganism can cause this disease. Many causative organisms are a part of the host's normal flora, including skin, colon, and vagina. Therefore, the finding of *C. perfringens* on a Gram's stain or culture from exudate in the vagina or cervical canal does not provide absolute evidence of a gas gangrene infection in the uterus. Since isolated intrauterine cultures are difficult to obtain without contamination, serial blood cultures, both aerobic and anaerobic, are required at 4- and 6-hour intervals and at the peak of a temperature rise for bacteriologic diagnosis. Although a single gram-negative organism will usually be found, more than one organism will be isolated in a few cases.

Endotoxins are circulating lipopolysaccharides. They are derived from the membrane of gram-negative bacteria and are the most important biologic factor in septic shock. Their effect is primarily on the microvasculature. Reacting with the endothelium, endotoxins cause damage and desquamation of endothelial cells and interaction with blood components to form platelet and leukocyte aggregates and increased capillary permeability, preferentially in the postcapillary venules.

Pathophysiology of Septic Shock

Septic shock occurs in two phases. Vasodilatation occurs initially (the hyperdynamic phase) with high cardiac output and low peripheral resistance. Later, capillary leakage from the peripheral vascular bed and peripheral vascular pooling leads to hypovolemia. Advanced shock results, which is often irreversible.

The important targets of septic shock are the cardiac output and the microcirculation of the peripheral capillary bed. Myocardial dysfunction is common and may be responsible for a transition between the hyperdynamic and hypodynamic phase of septic shock and for a failure of response to some aspect of therapy. Prior to the development of clinical shock, the endotoxemia produces an increase in cardiac output and a decline in peripheral vascular resistance, which are associated with hyperventilation and mental confusion, yet warm extremities. The duration of the warm phase varies from 30 minutes to 16 hours, and response to treatment is good. As the shocklike picture progresses, the peripheral resistance invariably increases and intense vasoconstriction results, with peripheral vascular pooling, hemoconcentration, decreased venous return, and ultimately, diminished cardiac output and lactic acidosis. Decrease in systemic tissue perfusion is related to deficits in oxygen utilization and lactic acidosis early in the course of septic shock. Peripheral vascular failure is associated with severe peripheral vasodilatation and increasing blood lactate levels, indicative of prolonged tissue hypoxia. Progression to the hypodynamic phase of shock is associated with decreased cardiac output and peripheral vasoconstriction. The lower the cardiac output, the more likely it is that lactic acidosis will be fatal. Weil and Nishijama have shown that the cardiac output is a valuable prognostic indicator of the severity of the disease and the ultimate outcome of treatment. It is important to understand that the hemodynamic state of the patient prior to treatment as well as the treatment itself significantly influences the recovery and the mortality rates from this septic complication.

Disseminated intravascular coagulation (DIC) is a common sequela of septic shock. The effects of endotoxin on the clotting, fibrinolytic, and kinin systems are interrelated and involve the factors in the intrinsic clotting pathway. Factor XII is activated by the endotoxin, following which the extrinsic pathway may also be activated, particularly factor VII. Plasmin (fibrinolysin) and other proteolytic enzymes are released by activated factor XII through the kinin system. When plasmin circulates in high concentration, as in septic shock, it has an effect on several physiologic systems. Fibrin degradation products that result from excessive fibrinolysin activity play a role in the occlusion of the microcirculation and may be involved in lysis of platelets and red blood cells. Both accelerated intravascular coagulation with depletion of the circulating fibrinogen and an acceleration of the degradation of the fibrin clot lead to excessive bleeding. Since both the clotting and fibrinolytic systems may be activated by endotoxin, either thrombosis or hemorrhage may occur, depending on which system is dominant. Further, the sludging blood flow in the microcirculation caused by hypotension and peripheral pooling may activate the extrinsic coagulation pathway and accelerate the effect of various stimuli on the intrinsic pathway. As a result of these coagulation changes, multiple laboratory tests are required to document this clotting abnormality. Although the clotting time may be normal, clot retraction is poor and fibrinogen is usually decreased. Prothrombin time, which measures the extrinsic coagulation pathway, is usually prolonged, as is the partial thromboplastin time (PTT), which measures the intrinsic pathway. Platelets are usually decreased, and platelet adhesiveness is frequently increased. In the advanced stages of disseminated intravascular coagulation, fibrin-split products are frequently found in the blood. Euglobulin lysis time, which measures fibrinolytic activation, is useful in determining the presence of active fibrinolysis. A shortened euglobulin lysis time reflects excessive fibrinolytic activity.

Aggregates of platelets and leukocytes produce microembolism with loss of autoregulation of capillary flow and shunting. The endotoxin produces profound effects on the microcirculation and endothelial wall that result in capillary leaks. With the increased capillary permeability in the lung, fluid collects in the interstitium and alveoli and destroys the surfactant. Respiratory distress may result from progressive pulmonary edema, atelectasis, perfusion/ventilation disturbances, and finally severe hypoxemia from the development of Adult Respiratory Distress Syndrome (ARDS). As many as 25% to 50% of patients in profound septic shock will develop ARDS, and among these, the mortality rate may exceed 50%.

As the shocklike state progresses, vasoconstriction increases, producing impairment of blood flow to vital organs, acidosis, peripheral vascular pooling, hemoconcentration, and decreased venous return to the heart, with a diminished cardiac output. As the clinical picture worsens, the increased peripheral resistance results in a paralysis and relaxation of the afferent arterioles while the smooth muscle of the venous capillary sphincters continues to constrict. Extensive pooling of the capillary bed may progress to impairment of perfusion of the coronary and cerebral vessels, at which time irreversible circulatory failure develops. The end stage of irreversible septic shock is manifested by unresponsive hypotension, progressive coma, renal failure, cardiac failure, and eventually death.

According to Vadas and associates, the circulating lipolytic enzyme phospholipase A_z is a mediator of circulatory collapse in experimental endotoxic shock and may also play a role in the pathogenesis of the hemodynamic and pulmonary derangements in gram-negative septic shock. Serum levels of phospholipase A_z are consistently elevated in septic shock, with a progressive fall during convalescence.

Clinical Features of Septic Shock

Variability in the clinical features of septic shock is common and depends on the patient's condition at the onset. The volume status of the patient (normovolemic vs hypovolemic) is one variable that affects the clinical presentation. If hypovolemia is present at the onset, more advanced features of septic shock will be manifest earlier.

The earliest symptoms of septic shock are rarely

recognized by either the clinician or the patient. They include mild anxiety, mental confusion, and later, disorientation. The earliest clinical signs are of respiratory distress with hyperventilation due to increased levels of norepinephrine, which may be clinically misinterpreted as atelectasis, pneumonia, possible pulmonary embolism, or even myocardial infarction. Patients may also have a transient subnormal temperature, which may coincide with a low white blood cell count. A favorable outcome to treatment can be expected if the disease is detected at this early stage. The early clinical signs include endotoxin-induced hyperventilation associated with respiratory alkalosis, a normal or high central venous pressure, low peripheral resistance, hypotension, oliguria, and warm, dry extremities. These changes result from an increased cardiac output at the onset of this disease and a striking decline in calculated peripheral resistance, as initially documented by Blain and associates. This hyperdynamic and alkalotic state is manifested by warm extremities and is frequently called warm shock. However, progression of the shock state is typically followed by more usual signs of hypotension, shaking chills, spiking fever frequently above 104°F, and cool, cyanotic extremities. Acidemia results as vascular perfusion fails and lactic acidosis supervenes. This late stage of endotoxic shock is described, physiologically, as stagnant shock and is due to pro-

longed tissue anoxia and acidosis as a result of increased venous (efferent) constriction of the capillary bed while the afferent arteriolar sphincter loses its tonicity with progressive acidosis (Fig. 24-13). These hemodynamic changes allow blood to enter the peripheral circulation, which is then trapped in the microcirculation, producing massive peripheral pooling and reduced venous return to the heart. The trapped blood ultimately causes the plasma to be forced into the extravascular space and interstitial tissues by the increased hydrostatic pressure. The circulating blood volume is thereby decreased and hemoconcentration occurs. Nausea, vomiting, and diarrhea, occasionally bloody, are clinical manifestations of vasospasm involving the intestinal tract. Oliguria and subsequent anuria present clinical signs of advanced vasoconstriction and renal ischemia.

When septic shock results from the exotoxin secreted by *C. perfringens,* the histotoxic effect of the gram-positive, encapsulated bacillus produces not only profound vasomotor collapse but also massive intravascular hemolysis with secondary anemia. The exotoxin also has a specific nephrotoxic effect, resulting in acute tubular necrosis and prolonged anuria that frequently requires renal dialysis. The tissue effect of gas gangrene is that of anaerobic myositis, including both skeletal and myocardial muscle. The very high mortality

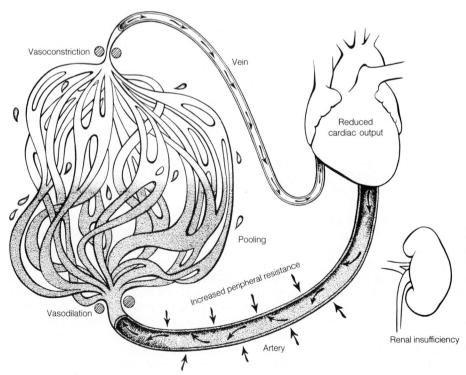

Figure 24–13. Late (stagnant) septic shock with vasodilatation of afferent arteriole, peripheral pooling in micro circulation due to vasoconstriction of efferent capillary, tissue acidosis and reduced venous return to heart. These hemodynamic changes impair circulation to the kidney, lung, heart, brain, intestines, and other vital organs.

of advanced septic shock caused by a clostridial infection is often due to cardiac arrhythmia and, finally, cardiac arrest.

Treatment of Septic Shock

Early recognition and prompt therapy are the keys for successful outcome in the treatment of septic shock. The basic treatment protocol should have two separate objectives—initially, to control the infectious process primarily with antibiotics, and second, to return the altered hemodynamic state to normal. Such therapy includes provision of adequate intravascular volume, support of vascular tone, and maintenance of cardiopulmonary function.

The treatment of hemorrhagic shock is discussed in Chapter 8. However, there are special considerations that must be given to septic shock that differ from hemorrhagic shock. These include the use of aggressive antibiotic therapy. Further, the ventilation-infusion-pump (VP) concept of septic shock treatment should be implemented. This implies the correction of early changes of arteriovenous shunting by proper ventilation and oxygenation, adequate fluid replacement before the use of vasopressor or vasodilator agents, and clinical monitoring of cardiopulmonary status. The initial therapeutic goal should concentrate on improving cardiac output and oxygen delivery in order to reverse tissue perfusion failure and lactic acidosis as rapidly as possible. The objective is to increase cardiac output while maintaining adequate arterial blood pressure.

Intravascular fluid volume expansion can be carried out rapidly in an attempt to improve venous return to the heart. Infusions of isotonic saline or Ringer's lactate at rates of 1000 ml/hr can be given to patients who do not have congestive heart failure as defined by central venous pressures equal to or less than 10 cm water or pulmonary wedge pressure less than 12 mm Hg. Patients with elevated CVP levels should receive a more gradual intravascular infusion of fluid at no more than 150 ml/30 min and should be carefully monitored. Close supervision is required for the early detection of heart failure. It is our position that a Swan-Ganz catheter should always be used in patients with septic shock so that fluid replacement, pulmonary artery pressure, arterial blood gases, and cardiac output can be carefully evaluated. A standard technique of fluid challenge is recommended. Fluid is infused at rates ranging from 5 ml/min to 20 ml/min for a period of 10 minutes. If the pulmonary artery wedge or diastolic pressure increases by more than 7 mm Hg, the infusion is discontinued. If the pressure does not increase by more than 3 mm Hg after 10 minutes of fluid infusion, or if it decreases to less than the initial value over a subsequent

10-minute rest, a second challenge is administered over a 10-minute period. This "7-3 rule" has been found to be very helpful in giving rapid volume replacement to patients in septic shock. Plasma volume expansion may be accelerated with the use of 5% human serum albumin, plasmanate (plasma protein fraction) or dextran 40, not to exceed 10 ml/kg/hr. For patients with anemia, one should use package red blood cells to provide the oxygen-carrying capability.

Modig compared dextran-70 with Ringer's acetate on pulmonary function, hemodynamics, and survival in experimental septic shock. The survival rate was significantly higher in the dextran-treated group, presumably because of better tissue perfusion leading to better tissue oxygenation. Dextran may reduce fibrin and granulocyte entrapment in the lungs and protect against endotoxin-induced pulmonary and cardiovascular failure characteristic of adult respiratory distress syndrome.

Antibiotic treatment in most clinics includes high-dose penicillin, an aminoglycoside, and an anaerobic antibacterial agent. Penicillin-G, sodium, 10 million units, intravenously every 4 hours, combined with gentamicin 2.0 mg/kg initially and then 1.5 mg/kg every 8 hours thereafter will usually control the growth of *E. coli, Proteus mirabilis,* and *Pseudomonas* microorganisms. The gentamicin dosage should be adjusted according to the creatinine level. Clindamycin, 600 mg intravenously every 6–8 hours is effective against anaerobes such as *Bacteroides* and *Clostridium* organisms. However, if the patient has liver disease, clindamycin is not the drug of choice; for those cases, anaerobic bacterial coverage can be achieved with metronidazole, 500 mg intravenously every 8 hours. In critical cases in which clindamycin or metronidazole have not been effective, chloramphenicol, 1 g intravenously every 6 hours may be substituted. In many clinics, only penicillin and an aminoglycoside in high dosage are given initially until the presence of anaerobic bacteria is established. Since *Bacteroides* occurs in no more than 10% of the cases of septic shock, this approach seems quite reasonable.

Vasoactive Drugs

Decreased perfusion of vital organs and muscles is a pathophysiologic feature of septic shock. The use of vasopressors, although tempting, is unphysiologic and may increase the hypoxemia and acidosis of the tissues rather than improve the condition. The increased peripheral resistance in advanced or late septic shock is caused by a high degree of sympathetic neuron stimulation of the vasculature, especially the precapillary arterioles. Agents with α-adrenergic activity (metaraminol, levarterenol) cause excessive vasoconstriction and have not proven particularly useful in the treatment of bacteremic shock. Although metaraminol is known to have a beneficial inotropic effect of improving coronary perfusion and cardiac output, these agents are used only if peripheral perfusion cannot be maintained by any other method.

Antiadrenergic drugs, including α-adrenergic blocking agents and β-adrenergic stimulants, are more beneficial than potent vasoconstrictors. Chlorpromazine has had wide clinical use and is an effective beta blocker that produces splanchnic vasodilatation and improvement in urinary output. We use this drug frequently for improvement in peripheral circulation.

Dopamine (3,4-dihydroxyphenethylamine) has distinct β-adrenergic stimulatory action that increases heart contractility more than heart rate. In low doses (up to 3 μg/kg/min) dopamine can stimulate specific vascular "dopaminergic" receptors and cause dilatation of the splanchnic, mesenteric, and renal vasculature. This vascular response is beneficial in improving renal perfusion and the perfusion of other vital organs. In moderate doses (3–15 μg/kg/min) the dopaminergic action lessens and the primary effect is of a β_1-adrenergic agonist, affecting heart contractility more than heart rate. Large doses of dopamine (greater than 15–20 μg/kg/min) release more epinephrine from storage sites in the adrenergic nervous system and the drug acts as a vasoconstrictor. When used, dopamine should be initiated as a constant infusion at a rate of 3 μg/kg/min, and that infusion rate should be increased every 5–10 minutes until the desired effect is achieved.

Meadows and associates recently studied the use of norepinephrine therapy in 10 patients with intractable septic shock. They found that norepinephrine can reverse hypotension in severe septic shock when used even as a last resort after dopamine and dobutamine have failed. No patient died of refractory hypotension; four of the 10 patients recovered. The major hemodynamic effect was an increase in systemic vascular resistance. Lee and associates prefer to use phenylephrine before using norepinephrine.

Corticosteroids

Although controversial, some authors believe that megadoses of corticosteroids may be lifesaving in the treatment of septic shock. The improvement in cardiac output produced by the positive inotropic effect on the heart, the promotion of gluconeogenesis with enhancement of the availability of glucose to the central nervous system, and the inhibition of the intense inflammatory reaction mediated by the complement cascade and leukocyte aggregation all produce favorable effects on the patient in septic shock. Methylprednisolone, 125 mg as an initial intravenous loading dose followed by 30 mg/kg/24 hr in continuous infusion, is recommended. Cavanagh recommends the use of a high-dose dexamethasone (6 mg/kg/24 hr) and reports only one maternal death in 31 patients with septic shock during the decade of 1965–1976. Glucosteroids decrease capillary leaks, particularly in the pulmonary-capillary bed. This is particularly beneficial in preventing interstitial edema, which may result in ARDS.

Recently, there is strong clinical evidence that high-dose corticosteroids provide no benefit in the treatment of septic shock. In 1987, a controlled clinical trial of high-dose methylprednisolone in the treatment of septic shock was reported by Bone and associates for the Methylprednisolone Severe Sepsis Study Group. In a large series of patients with severe sepsis, septic shock developed as often in the methylprednisolone-treated group as in the placebo-treated group. Also, there were no treatment differences between the two groups in the reversal of septic shock. The mortality rate tended to be increased at 14 days among the methylprednisolone-treated patients, and especially for those patients with elevated creatine concentrations. According to this report, this prospective, randomized, placebo-controlled, double-blind multicenter trial in patients with severe sepsis and septic shock showed no benefits from the use of high doses of corticosteroids. The authors state, "When coupled with a lack of documented efficacy, the potential for an increased incidence of death due to secondary infections strongly argues against the prophylactic use of corticosteroids in sepsis."

Removal of Focus of Infection

To eliminate the adverse effect of endotoxin on the microvascular circulation, it is important to control the release of endotoxin from the site of infection, wherever it may be. When the supportive measures outlined earlier have been instituted, the intrauterine nidus of infection should be eliminated by a suction curettage, followed by sharp curettage at the earliest time that the patient's condition will permit. Many clinicians would attempt to evacuate the septic uterus immediately; however, we recommend that a more conservative approach should be taken, with instrumentation of the uterus being avoided until a therapeutic tissue level of antibiotics has been achieved. In general, we defer evacuation of the uterus for a period of at least 4–6 hours, but not more than 12 hours, following the initiation of antibiotic therapy, during which time metabolic fluid imbalance is treated. In the event that the clinical picture worsens and the hypotension becomes more progressive and refractory to treatment, evacuation of the uterus may become more immediately necessary.

In our experience, aggressive medical therapy has been effective in more than 85% of the cases. However, if the patient does not respond to any supportive measure, including curettage, or if *C. perfringens* is found in the endometrial cavity or in a blood culture, a hysterectomy may become necessary. When a rising arterial blood lactate level, progressive acidosis, deepening shock, and cardiopulmonary decompensation follow all clinical measures of management, a hysterectomy may become essential as a lifesaving procedure. When suppuration has extended to the broad ligament, bilateral salpingo-oophorectomy should also be performed. In the presence of septic thrombophlebitis, both ovarian veins should be ligated prior to extirpation of the uterus and adnexa. Previously, it was our position that when any of four life-threatening conditions was associated with septic shock, an immediate hysterectomy and adnexectomy were essential. These included uterine perforation, *C. perfringens* infection, advanced endometritis-myometritis from long-standing infection, and use of a corrosive toxic douche. Fortunately, these are no longer associated with bacteremic shock with great frequency. As a consequence, a more conservative treatment with high-dose multiagent antibiotic therapy is attempted before surgery is undertaken. Patients with advanced clostridial infection who fail to respond rapidly to aggressive medical therapy must not have undue delay in removing the source of exotoxin by hysterectomy; however, one or perhaps both adnexa may be saved. The use of lye as an abortifacient is rare, but when a patient is seen with a chemical toxin and shock, aggressive surgical treatment is needed.

Septic shock is a perplexing and difficult condition to treat. However, there have been major advances recently in the successful treatment of this disease. As a result, the mortality rate has been reduced to 1% to 2% in bacteremic patients without shock and to less than 10% in patients with warm shock. It remains more than 50% in patients with cold, irreversible shock. Fortunately, most cases of septic shock are diagnosed and treated before the onset of the late phase.

PELVIC TUBERCULOSIS

Pelvic tuberculosis in the female is confined principally to the reproductive tract, particularly the endometrium and fallopian tubes. This disease has become much less frequent during recent decades and today probably accounts for less than 1% of all pelvic infections except in those cities with a large number of immigrants.

The incidence and number of cases of systemic tuberculosis in the United States has declined dramatically since 1900. Between 1966 and 1985, the incidence declined an average of approximately 5% per year. In 1986, 22,768 cases were reported to the Centers for Disease Control (9.4/100,000). An increased incidence of tuberculosis has been noted with advancing age, male gender, and nonwhite race. An increased incidence has also been noted among certain U.S. subpopulations, including Hispanics, American Indians, Alaskan Natives, Asians, Pacific Islanders, homeless populations, blacks, and persons infected with the human immunodeficiency virus (HIV-1) or persons having the acquired immunodeficiency syndrome (AIDS). Although the incidence of tuberculosis is declining in the United States and many other developed countries in the world, it remains a major public health problem in developing countries. The large number of immigrants who come to the United States from developing countries will require continued vigilance in detecting and treating this disease.

Because of the decrease in systemic disease, there has been a decline in the incidence of genital tuberculosis. Pelvic tuberculosis is found in approximately 1% of infertility patients in the United States, and there is an international incidence of genital tuberculosis of 5% to 10% in infertility patients. An average of about 8% of women who die of pulmonary tuberculosis are found to have pelvic tuberculosis.

Pathogenesis of Pelvic Tuberculosis

Tuberculosis is caused by infectious agents in the mycobacteria class. The mycobacteria are obligate aerobes distinctive for their acid-fast staining characteristic. Tuberculosis is usually caused by *Mycobacterium tuberculosis*. In developing countries without effective tuberculosis control programs for cattle and facilities to pasteurize milk, *M. bovis* may also cause tuberculosis.

With rare exceptions, tuberculosis of the female pelvis is secondary to a tuberculous infection elsewhere, usually the lungs. From a primary pulmonary infection, mycobacteria spread by the lymphatic system from the Ghon focus to the regional lymph nodes at the hilum of the lung and then to more distant sites. The more dramatic spread is hematogenous from the primary pulmonary complex. This produces acute miliary disease. Miliary spread of tuberculosis is more common within the first year of primary pulmonary infection. No location in the body is immune to the development of metastatic foci of infection. Patients may develop tuberculosis of the bone, meninges, kidney, epididymis, and fallopian tubes as well as other sites. At some sites of miliary spread, the lesions may remain

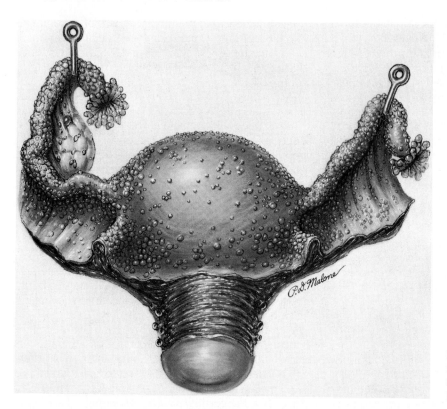

Figure 24–14. Typical specimen of tuberculosis of reproductive organs as part of generalized tuberculous peritonitis.

quiescent for long periods before reactivation and further spread of the disease. Direct extension from one organ or system to an adjacent organ or system may also occur. Organs of the female reproductive tract are usually infected from a hematogenous miliary spread from a primary pulmonary lesion, from hematogenous spread from a secondary miliary site, from lymphatic spread from a primary pulmonary site to intestinal lymph nodes and then to the pelvis, or by direct extension from adjacent abdominal organs (small intestines, appendix, rectum, bladder) that are the site of tuberculous infection. Fistulas between the intestinal tract and the fallopian tubes have been reported with pelvic tuberculosis.

A venereal transmission of the disease has been reported, with primary genital infection in the woman following coitus with a sexual partner who has tuberculosis of the genitourinary tract. According to Sutherland and MacFarlane, it is not possible to prove conclusively that genitourinary tuberculosis in the male can be transmitted to the female through sexual intercourse. Since it has been shown that *M. tuberculosis* is present in the sperm of men with urogenital tuberculosis, the possibility of transmission through intercourse to the pelvic organs of the female must be accepted, and Sutherland presents five cases in which sexual transmission of genitourinary tuberculosis from

male to female presumably occurred. However, of 128 husbands of women with genital tuberculosis, only five (3.9%) were found to have active genitourinary tuberculosis. When tuberculosis of the vulva, vagina, and cervix is present without evidence of tuberculosis elsewhere in the body, venereal transmission should be suspected.

Pathology of Pelvic Tuberculosis

Both fallopian tubes are involved in almost all patients with pelvic tuberculosis. About one half of patients with tuberculous salpingitis will have tuberculous endometritis. Tuberculosis of the cervix is present in 5% of cases. The vagina and vulva are rarely involved. At operation, one may find evidence of generalized tuberculous peritonitis with small grayish-white tubercles covering all peritoneal surfaces of the abdominal and pelvic organs. The mucosa of the fallopian tubes may not be involved in generalized serosal tuberculous infection. At a later state of infection, tuberculous salpingitis may grossly resemble other forms of pelvic inflammatory disease involving the adnexa. Unless tubercles are seen, the diagnosis may not be apparent until microscopic sections are examined by the pathologist. A large pyosalpinx may contain the caseous

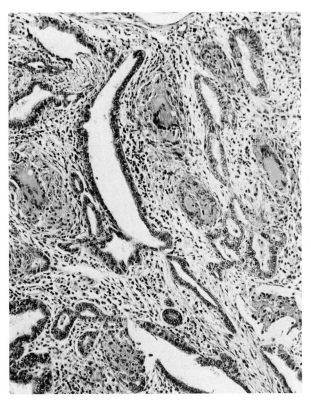

Figure 24–15. Tuberculosis of the Fallopian tube. Note the multinucleated giant cells.

material of a tuberculous infection but may also contain the purulent exudate of a secondary infection with other common organisms. Tubercles form in the lining of the tube. Some have caseation at the center, with giant cells and epithelioid cells. A proliferation of the mucosal lining of the fallopian tube may resemble a primary tubal carcinoma microscopically and may be confusing to the pathologist.

Tuberculous peritonitis is commonly associated with tuberculosis of the pelvis. Clinically, tuberculous peritonitis can be divided into two groups. In "wet" peritonitis, there is an outpouring of straw-colored fluid into the peritoneal cavity, producing ascites. The peritoneum of the parietal wall and viscera is covered with innumerable small tubercles (Fig. 24-14). The tubes, in addition to being covered with miliary tubercles on the serosal surface, are usually slightly enlarged and distended. In contrast to other forms of salpingitis, the fimbriae may be patent. Within the tubal wall and tubal mucosa, the histology is typical of tuberculosis, with tubercle formation, multinucleated giant cells, and epithelioid reaction (Fig. 24-15). In advanced cases, frank caseation is present. This pattern is more classically associated with hematogenous spread of the tu-

berculous organism to the peritoneal surfaces and the pelvic organs.

Another type of tuberculous peritonitis encountered in the female is the "dry" or adhesive type. Bowel adheres to bowel by innumerable dense adhesions that blend with the musculature. The muscle of the bowel is often invaded to some degree by the tuberculous process. Separation of these adhesions is extremely difficult surgically, and accidental injury to the bowel is common. The pelvic organs show evidence of tuberculous salpingitis with enlargement of the tubes, and occasionally pyosalpinges, and even tubo-ovarian abscess formation. This dry variety may represent the healed fibrotic end result of the wet ascitic pattern.

Tuberculous involvement of the myometrium is rare. Tuberculous endometritis, however, is common, occurring in 60% to 70% of women with pelvic tuberculosis. Microscopically, tubercles may be seen scattered throughout the endometrium, but they may be scanty. Tubercles are often seen in the endometrium removed by curettage in the premenstrual phase and are more commonly located in the endometrium adjacent to the tubal ostia. Apparently, the uterine cavity is protected from advanced tuberculous infection by the cyclic shedding of endometrial tissue in the reproductive years. Even in advanced pelvic tuberculous infections, evidence of caseation and fibrosis and calcification is rarely seen in the uterine cavity. Occasionally, the endometrial cavity is obliterated by extensive adhesions. Total destruction of the endometrium may result in amenorrhea. Especially in postmenopausal women with an occluded internal cervical os, tuberculous pyometra may develop.

Tuberculous lesions of the cervix are rare. They may be either ulcerative or exophytic and may resemble a primary cervical malignancy or granuloma inguinale of the cervix. When there is a tuberculous lesion of the cervix, the cervical biopsy frequently reveals tubercles.

A tuberculous infection of the ovary usually involves only the surface of the ovary and represents simply an extension of infection from the peritoneal cavity and the adjacent fallopian tubes. The infection is usually limited to a perioophoritis. Extension of the tuberculous infection to the ovarian parenchyma may be prevented by the tunica albuginea. Tuberculous caseation may be found within the ovarian parenchyma, although this is uncommon. Presumably, it occurs as a result of hematogenous spread to the ovarian parenchyma rather than by direct extension through the ovarian capsule. However, a break in the tunica by ovulation may also allow the tubercular bacilli to gain access to the ovarian parenchyma. The ovaries are involved in approximately 25% of cases of pelvic tuberculosis.

It is uncommon for tuberculosis to involve the vulva and vagina. It is seen in only 2% of patients with pelvic tuberculosis. The gross appearance may be ulcerative with multiple sinuses, hypertrophic with elephantiasis, or similar to carcinoma.

Throughout the pelvic organs, the microscopic picture is similar, with tubercles of granulomatous inflammation, Langhans' giant cells, epithelioid cells, and central caseation associated with chronic inflammation. With special stains, acid-fast bacilli can be demonstrated on careful microscopic examination of the tubercles.

Clinical Features of Pelvic Tuberculosis

Pelvic tuberculosis occurs most frequently in patients between the ages of 20 and 40. The age incidence of gynecologic tuberculosis has changed in recent years; the proportion of patients over 40 years of age is now much higher than in the past. Falk and associates found that the incidence of pelvic tuberculosis in postmenopausal Swedish women is increasing. This was also the opinion of Sutherland, who reported an investigation from Glasgow in which 26 of 701 patients (3.7%) with proved gynecologic tuberculosis were postmenopausal.

The most common clinical symptoms of pelvic tuberculosis include pelvic pain, general malaise, menstrual irregularity, and infertility. Brown and associates found that menstrual irregularity occurred in nearly 50% of patients, whereas amenorrhea or oligomenorrhea was present in 27%. A low-grade fever that on occasion may produce a fulminating septic course is noted in most cases of active or subacute disease. The failure of fever to subside with high doses of broad-spectrum antibiotics is a classic feature of pelvic tuberculosis. A clinical course that is refractory to antibiotic therapy for the usual pelvic inflammatory disease should always alert the clinician to the possibility of tuberculosis.

Among patients with pulmonary tuberculosis, the incidence of pelvic tuberculosis generally varies between 10% and 20%. Falk and associates noted that 38% of women with genital tuberculosis had previously had tuberculosis in other organs, usually the lungs. Many times, the patient's clinical course is that of a chronic indolent illness.

Diagnosis of Pelvic Tuberculosis

The clinical symptoms and signs of pelvic tuberculosis should direct the clinician to the diagnosis. Today the disease is so infrequent that it is seldom encountered in the usual gynecologist's practice and, quite naturally, the clinical index of suspicion is generally low. In many cases, the clinical presentation is obscure and the diagnosis is delayed. Howard Kelly once said that when competent gynecologists disagree about the diagnosis of an obscure pelvic condition, it usually is diagnosed as either an old ectopic pregnancy or pelvic tuberculosis.

More than two thirds of the cases are diagnosed at the time of laparotomy performed for some other indication, or at the time of investigation for infertility or abnormal uterine bleeding. The most common symptom is infertility and the second most common symptom is lower abdominal and pelvic pain. Some patients are completely asymptomatic and are found to have pelvic tuberculosis in connection with investigation for other disorders such as infertility. A dilatation and curettage or endometrial biopsy will be diagnostic in some cases, especially if performed in the late premenstrual phase of the menstrual cycle. In addition to standard microscopic sections, the specimen may be examined by fluorescent antibody technique. Acid-fast staining of tissue or culture of menstrual blood is effective in detecting the organism in approximately 10% of cases, according to Overbeck. Guinea pig inoculation with menstrual blood may be even more effective. The menstrual blood may be collected in a cervical cap. The culture or inoculation may be repeated many times before a positive result is obtained. Acid-fast stains of tissue suspected of tuberculous infection are important to confirm the diagnosis. Since some acid-fast bacilli are not tuberculous bacilli, it is important to obtain a positive culture whenever possible. A negative evaluation of the endometrium does not rule out pelvic tuberculosis, since the disease may be present in the fallopian tubes without tuberculous endometritis in 30% to 40% of cases.

On pelvic examination, bilateral adnexal tenderness is the rule. The tenderness is usually less marked than with acute gonococcal or streptococcal infections. Occasionally, a large tuberculous tubo-ovarian abscess may be palpated on pelvic examination and even felt through the abdominal wall. The classic doughy feel of the broad ligament suggests a tuberculous inflammatory disease that is produced by a combination of thickening of the broad ligament, adherent bowel, and some ascitic fluid. On occasion, cul-de-sac nodules representing tubercles on the serosal surfaces of pelvic organs can be felt. The clinical detection of ascites is the strongest evidence obtainable in favor of pelvic tuberculosis. It was present in one fifth of the cases reported by Brown and associates. However, other causes of ascites must be considered, including ovarian carcinoma and cirrhosis of the liver. In differentiating tuberculous salpingitis from neisserial infections, the finding of a virginal outlet in the presence of obvious tubal inflammation should lend strength to the diagnosis of pelvic tuberculosis.

The diagnosis of tuberculosis cannot be made with certainty from a hysterosalpingogram, but it may be helpful. The radiographic criteria for a suspicion of pelvic tuberculosis by hysterosalpingogram have been described by Klein and associates as follows: calcified lymph nodes or smaller, irregular calcifications in the adnexal areas; obstruction of the fallopian tube in the zone of transition between the isthmus and the ampulla; multiple constrictions along the course of the fallopian tube; endometrial adhesions or deformity or obliteration of the endometrial cavity in the absence of a history of curettage or abortion; and vascular or lymphatic extravasation of contrast material. Although a conclusive diagnosis of pelvic tuberculosis can be made only from a positive culture, these authors conclude that hysterosalpingography is a useful aid, especially in patients who are asymptomatic except for infertility.

When the diagnosis of pelvic tuberculosis cannot be made in other ways, laparoscopy has been used. Because of the possibility that numerous adhesions may be present to make the introduction of the trocar hazardous, we believe laparoscopy should be used with particular care. If it can be done, biopsies of tubal fimbriae or other suspicious areas may be examined histologically or cultured to confirm the diagnosis. In addition to numerous adhesions, laparoscopy may reveal widespread miliary tubercles involving the omentum and peritoneal surfaces. Matted adnexal masses may be seen. Microscopic examination of peritoneal fluid will show a predominance of lymphocytes.

Vaginal cytology is of limited value in diagnosing tuberculosis. The cytologist must be familiar with the morphology of epithelioid cells in the vaginal smear. Only in cases of tuberculosis of the cervix may cytology be helpful. Patients with pelvic tuberculosis should also have an examination and special diagnostic procedures to rule out tuberculous infections in the sites. Chest x-ray; tuberculin skin test; pelvic ultrasonography; intravenous pyelogram; and urine, gastric, and sputum cultures for *M. tuberculosis* should be done. In some patients, exploratory laparotomy will be needed to make the diagnosis.

Treatment of Pelvic Tuberculosis

Before the advent of antituberculous drug therapy, surgery was often used in the treatment of pelvic tuberculosis. Primary surgical treatment was technically difficult, sometimes ineffective, and associated with a high risk of fistula formation and persistent draining sinuses. With the advent of effective drug therapy, the surgical treatment for genital tuberculosis has been restricted to specific indications. Beginning first with streptomycin over 30 years ago, and later isoniazid and para-am-

inosalicylic acid, it became evident that many cases of pelvic tuberculosis could be cured or controlled with antituberculous drug therapy. There have been major advances in the antibiotic treatment of this disease, which include, principally, the use of isoniazid with rifampin, with or without ethambutol, given sometimes for a period of 2 years or longer. In 1977 and again in 1981, Sutherland analyzed the results obtained with various drug schedules.

The drugs that have been used to treat tuberculosis are isoniazid, rifampin, streptomycin, ethambutol, and pyrazinamide. Isoniazid and rifampin are the most effective currently available with the lowest toxicity and should be the foundation of most drug regimens. The addition of ethambutol may not be of benefit, at least not in pulmonary tuberculosis. Severe and sometimes fatal hepatitis, which may develop even after months of treatment, has been associated with isoniazid therapy. The risk of developing hepatitis increases with age and with daily consumption of alcohol. Liver function studies should be done before treatment is started, and patients should be carefully monitored with liver function studies throughout the course of therapy and later. The current recommendations of the American Thoracic Society and the Centers for Disease Control for the treatment of tuberculosis are given in Table 24-5.

The therapeutic success of modern antituberculous drug treatment regimes is difficult to assess in view of the limited number of cases available in the literature.

TABLE 24–5

Current Recommendations of the American Thoracic Society and the Centers for Disease Control for the Treatment of Tuberculosis

---

1. A 6-month regimen consisting of isoniazid, rifampin, and pyrazinamide given for 2 months followed by isoniazid and rifampin for 4 months is effective treatment in patients with fully susceptible organisms who comply with the treatment regimen. It may be advisable to include ethambutol in the initial phase when isoniazid resistance is suspected.
2. A 9-month regimen consisting of isoniazid and rifampin is also highly successful. The need for an additional drug in the initial phase is not certain unless isoniazid resistance is suspected, in which case ethambutol should be included until susceptibility tests have been reported.
3. In the presence of documented resistance to isoniazid, rifampin and ethambutol, perhaps supplemented initially by pyrazinamide, should be given for a minimum of 12 months.
4. Extrapulmonary tuberculosis should be managed according to the principles and with the drug regimens outlined for pulmonary tuberculosis.
5. The major determinant of the outcome of treatment is patient compliance. Careful attention should be paid to measures designed to foster compliance and to ensure that patients take the drugs as prescribed.

(American Review of Respiratory Disease. 134(2):355.)

The cure rate varies in the literature from 65% to 95%. Kardos removed the fallopian tubes from 168 patients after medical treatment for 10 months and found active tuberculosis in 35% of the surgical specimens. The experience of Sutherland suggests, however, that the results of treatment may be improved with newer drugs. The patients under treatment must be followed closely for evidence of regression or remission of the pelvic tuberculosis. Only approximately 50% of patients with genital tuberculosis have the disease in the endometrial cavity, and therefore, repeat endometrial biopsies and culture of menstrual egress will provide only limited diagnostic information. The progress of the disease can be monitored closely with the evaluation of the size of adnexal masses by pelvic examinations and ultrasonography, as well as the erythrocyte sedimentation rate, white blood cell count, and temperature response. Prolonged follow-up is probably indicated in all cases, since recurrence of the tuberculous pelvic lesion 5 and even more years after the end of drug treatment has occasionally been found.

Surgery in the management of patients with pelvic tuberculosis should be reserved for specific indications, as outlined by Schaefer and by Sutherland. In general, surgery is reserved for those patients who have failed to respond to an adequate trial of medical therapy. Our indications for the surgical treatment of pelvic tuberculosis include:

1. Persistence or enlargement of an adnexal mass after 4–6 months of antituberculous antibiotic therapy. The rare possibility of an ovarian tumor must always be considered, even though pelvic tuberculosis is also present. In a 1980 report by Sutherland, the persistence or development of substantial pelvic masses was the indication for surgery in 36 of 91 women with proved tuberculosis of the genital tract treated by surgery. Pelvic ultrasonography should be useful in following the response of adnexal masses to treatment.

2. Persistence of pelvic pain or recurrence of pelvic pain while on medical therapy. In Sutherland's report, 40 of 91 patients were operated on because of pain.

3. Primary unresponsiveness of the tuberculous infection to antibiotic therapy, as evidenced by persistent spiking temperature, leukocytosis, elevated sedimentation rate, and evidence on biopsy of continued endometrial infection. Of the 91 women in Sutherland's report, 10 were operated upon because of persistence of endometrial tuberculosis.

4. Difficulty in obtaining patient cooperation for continued long-term therapy. In these cases, we are accustomed to giving a brief course of strep-

tomycin, 0.5 g/12 hr intramuscularly for 1 week prior to surgery, to perform definitive surgery, and then give 0.5 g/24 hr in the postoperative period for 2 weeks. A persistent effort should be made to obtain the patient's cooperation for continued antituberculous therapy postoperatively. It is advisable to continue treatment for a year or longer. Isoniazid and rifampin should be used if possible. A common reason for failure of treatment is a tendency to discontinue drugs after only a few months because the patient appears well.

The preferred surgical treatment includes total abdominal hysterectomy and bilateral salpingo-oophorectomy. The very nature of this inflammatory disease may make this operative procedure technically difficult, with an increased risk of injury to bowel and bladder. Consequently, in the event of a frozen pelvis from pelvic tuberculosis, it is occasionally necessary to perform only a subtotal abdominal hysterectomy and adnexectomy. Adhesions, which are invariably present and usually widespread, may make the dissection more difficult and injury more likely. However, it is usually possible to do this operation without a high incidence of bowel fistulas and other significant complications. In 1980, Sutherland reported the results of surgery in 77 patients operated on while antituberculous therapy was being administered. There were no deaths, no fistulas, and few late complications.

For young patients who are anxious to attempt future childbearing, conservative adnexectomy should be carried out only if it is possible to do so after carefully evaluating the extent of the adnexal disease and finding it minimal. It is unwise for the surgeon to be committed to a specific operative procedure prior to the time of surgery, since conservative pelvic surgery for tuberculosis may constitute poor surgical judgment once the operative findings are known. The patient should be forewarned that conservative surgery will be performed only if the disease is minimal and such surgery is considered medically advisable.

Conservation of ovaries at the time of operation for pelvic tuberculosis is occasionally possible if the ovary is involved only on the surface. On the other hand, if one finds gross evidence of ovarian enlargement or other gross evidence of infection deep in the ovarian parenchyma, the ovary should be removed. Bisection of ovaries to assess the presence of disease deep in the ovarian parenchyma is not advisable.

Reactivation of silent pelvic tuberculosis following tubal reconstructive surgery has been reported by Ballon and associates and others. We believe reconstructive tubal surgery has no place in the management of patients who are infertile because of bilateral tubal obstruction from tuberculous salpingitis.

Pregnancy Following Pelvic Tuberculosis

It is evident from the literature, including the studies of both Schaefer and Sutherland, that only approximately 5% of patients with genital tuberculosis are capable of becoming pregnant, and only 2% will carry a pregnancy to term. It is also evident that in the presence of tuberculous tubo-ovarian abscesses, pregnancy is extremely rare and conservative surgery for the purpose of preserving fertility is unwarranted. Only when there is minimal pelvic disease without adnexal masses should conservative surgery be considered.

Bibliography

Angrish K, Verma K. Cytologic detection of tuberculosis of the uterine cervix. Acta Cytol 1981;25:160.

Ballon SC, Clewell WH, Lamb EJ. Reactivation of silent pelvic tuberculosis by reconstructive tubal surgery. Am J Obstet Gynecol 1975;122:991.

Bauer AR, Flynn RR. Computed tomography diagnosis of venous thrombosis of the lower extremities and pelvis with contrast material. Surg Gynecol Obstet. 1988;167:12.

Bazaz-Malik G, Maheshwari B, Lal N. Tuberculous endometritis: a clinico-pathological study of 1000 cases. Br J Obstet Gynaecol 1983;90:84.

Berger GS, Keith L, Moss W. Prevalence of gonorrhea among women using various methods of contraception. Br J Vener Dis 1975; 51:307.

Bhambhanis S, Das DK, Singh V, Luthra UK. Cervical tuberculosis with carcinoma in situ: a cytodiagnosis. Acta Cytol 1985;29:87.

Bircher E. Die chronische Bauchfelltuberkulose, ihre Behandlung mit Roetgenstrahlen. Zentralbl Gynakol 1908;32:31.

Blain CM, Anderson TO, Pietras RJ, et al. Hyperimmediate hemodynamic effects of gram-negative versus gram-positive bacteremia in man. Int Med 1970;126:260.

Blanchard AC, Pastorek JG, Weeks T. Pelvic inflammatory disease in pregnancy. South Med J 1987;80:1363.

Bone RC, Fisher CJ, Clemmer TP, et al. A controlled clinical trial of high-dose methylprednisolone in the treatment of severe sepsis and septic shock. N Engl J Med 1987;317:653.

Borden GW, Hall WH. Fatal transfusion reactions from massive bacterial contamination of blood. N Eng J Med 1951;245:760.

Braude AI, Siemienski J, Williams D, Sanford J. Overwhelming bacteremic shock produced by gram-negative bacilli. A report of four cases with one recovery. Univ Mich Med Bull 1953;19:23.

Braude AI, Williams D, Siemienski J, et al. Shock-like state due to transfusion of blood contaminated with gram-negative bacilli. Arch Intern Med 1953;92:75.

Brenner RW, Gehring SW. Pelvic actinomycosis in the presence of an endocervical contraceptive device. Obstet Gynecol 1967;29:71.

Brihmer C, Kallings I, Nord C-E, Bruundin J. Salpingitis; aspects of diagnosis and etiology: a 4-year study from a Swedish capital hospital. Eur J Obstet Gynecol Reprod Biol 1987;24:211.

Brill NE, Libman E. Pyocyaneus bacillianemia. Am J Med Sci 1899;228:153.

Brown AB, Gilbert RA, Te Linde RW. Pelvic tuberculosis. Obstet Gynecol 1953;2:476.

Brunham RC, Binns B, Guijon F, et al. Etiology and outcome of acute pelvic inflammatory disease. J Infect Dis 1988;158:510.

Burkman RT. Intrauterine device use and the risk of pelvic inflammatory disease. Am J Obstet Gynecol 1980;138:861.

Burkman RT, Schlesselman S, McCaffrey L, et al. The relationship of genital tract actinomyces and the development of pelvic inflammatory disease. Am J Obstet Gynecol 1982;143:585.

Cavanagh D. Septic shock in pregnant or recently pregnant women. Postgrad Med 1977;62:62.

Cavanagh D, McLeod GW. Septic shock in obstetrics and gynecology: evaluation of metaraminol therapy. Am J Obstet Gynecol 1966; 96:913.

Cavanagh D, Rao PS, Comas MR. Septic shock in obstetrics and gynecology. Philadelphia: WB Saunders, 1977.

Chipperfield EJ, Evans BA. Effect of local infection and oral contraception on immunoglobulin levels in cervical mucus. Infect Immun 1975;11:215.

Chow AW, Carlson C, Sorrell TC. Host defenses in acute pelvic inflammatory disease. Am J Obstet Gynecol 1980;138:1003.

Chow AW, Malkasian KL, Marshall JR, et al. The bacteriology of acute pelvic inflammatory disease. Am J Obstet Gynecol 1975;122:876.

Chow AW, Pattern V, Marshall JR. Bacteriology of acute pelvic inflammatory disease. Am J Gynecol Obstet 1979;133:362.

Christy JH. Treatment of gram-negative shock. Am J Med 1971;50:77.

Collins CG. Suppurative pelvic thrombophlebitis. A study of 202 cases in which the disease was treated by ligation of the vena cava and ovarian vein. Am J Obstet Gynecol 1970;108:681.

Collins CG, Ayers WB. Suppurative pelvic thrombophlebitis. III. Surgical technique. Surgery 1951;30:319.

Collins CG, Jansen FW. Management of tubo-ovarian abscess. Clin Obstet Gynecol 1959;2:512.

Collins CG, MacCallum EA, Nelson EW, et al. Suppurative pelvic thrombophlebitis. I. Incidence, pathology, and etiology. Surgery 1951;30:298.

Collins CG, Nelson EW, Collin JH, et al. Suppurative pelvic thrombophlebitis. II. Symptomatology and diagnosis. Surgery 1951; 30:311.

Cunningham FG, Hauth JC, Gilstrap LC, et al. The bacterial pathogenesis of acute pelvic inflammatory disease. Obstet Gynecol 1978;52:161.

Cunningham FG, Hauth JC, Strong JD, et al. Evaluation of tetracycline or penicillin and ampicillin for treatment of acute pelvic inflammatory disease. N Engl J Med 1977;296:1380.

Curran JW. Economic consequences of pelvic inflammatory disease in the United States. Am J Obstet Gynecol 1980;138:848.

Curtis AH. A cause of adhesions in the right upper quadrant. JAMA 1930;94:1221.

Curtis AH. Bacteriology and pathology of fallopian tubes removed at operation. Surg Gynecol Obstet 1921;33:621.

Curtis AH. Chronic pelvic infections. Surg Gynecol Obstet 1926;42:6.

Dans PE. Gynecological anorectal infections. Clinic Obstet Gynecol 1975;18:103.

Deane RM, Russell KP. Enterobacillary septicemia and bacterial shock in septic abortion. Am J Obstet Gynecol 1960;79:528.

Dodson MG, Faro S, Gentry LO. Treatment of acute pelvic inflammatory disease with aztreonam, a new monocyclic B-lactam antibiotic, and clindamycin. Obstet Gynecol 1986;67:657.

Douglas GW, Beckman EM. Clinical management of septic abortion complicated by hypotension. Am J Obstet Gynecol 1966;96:633.

Duff P. Pathophysiology and management of septic shock. J Reprod Med 1980;24:109.

Durfee RB. Infections of the female genital tract. In: Hoeprich PD, ed. Infectious diseases. New York: Harper & Row, 1972.

Edelman DA, Berger GS. Contraceptive practice and tubo-ovarian abscess. Am J Obstet Gynecol 1980;138:541.

Eschenbach DA. New concepts of obstetric and gynecologic infection. Arch Intern Med 1982;142:2039.

Eschenbach DA, Buchanan TM, Pollock HM, et al. Polymicrobial etiology of acute pelvic inflammatory disease. N Engl J Med 1975; 293:166.

Eschenbach DA, Harnisch JP, Holmes KK. Pathogenesis of acute pelvic inflammatory disease: role of contraception and other risk factors. Am J Obstet Gynecol 1977;128:838.

Falk HC. Cornual resection for the treatment of recurrent salpingitis. Am J Surg 1951;81:595.

Falk V. Interpretation of the pathogenesis of pelvic infection as determined by cornual resection. Am J Obstet Gynecol 1946;52:66.

Falk V. Treatment of acute non-tuberculous salpingitis with antibiotics alone and in combination with glucocorticoids. Acta Obstet Gynecol Scand 1965;44(suppl)6:1.

Falk V, Ludviksson K, Agren G. Genital tuberculosis in women. Am J Obstet Gynecol 1980;138:974.

Fine J. Intestinal circulation in shock. Gastroenterology 1967;52:454.

Fitz-Hugh T Jr. Acute gonococcic peritonitis of the right upper quadrant in women. JAMA 1934;102:2094.

Franklin EW, Hevron JE, Thompson JD. Management of the pelvic abscess. Clin Obstet Gynecol 1973;16:66.

Ginsburg DS, Stern JL, Hamod KA, et al. Tubo-ovarian abscess: a retrospective review. Am J Obstet Gynecol 1980;138:1055.

Gjonnaess H, Dalaker K, Anestad G, et al. Pelvic inflammatory disease: etiologic studies with emphasis on chlamydial infection. Obstet Gynecol 1982;59:550.

Golde SH, Israel R, Ledger WJ. Unilateral tubo-ovarian abscess: a distinct entity. Am J Obstet Gynecol 1977;127:807.

Goldenberg H, Benigno B. Inpatient management of acute pelvic inflammatory disease at Grady Memorial Hospital. Resident Research Day, Emory University School of Medicine, unpublished material, 1976.

Greenfield LJ, Zocco J, Wilk J, et al. Clinical experience with the Kim-Ray Greenfield vena cava filter. Ann Surg 1977;185:692.

Grimes DA. Intrauterine devices and pelvic inflammatory disease: recent developments. Contraception 1987;36:97.

Grimes DA. Nongonococcal pelvic inflammatory disease. Clin Obstet Gynecol 1981;24:1227.

Grimes DA, Blount JH, Patrick J, Washington AE. Antibiotic treatment of pelvic inflammatory disease: trends among private physicians in the United States, 1966 through 1983. JAMA 1986;256:3223.

Guderian AM, Trobough GE. Residues of pelvic inflammatory disease in intrauterine device users: a result of the intrauterine device or *Chlamydia trachomatis* infection? Am J Obstet Gynecol 1986;154:497.

Hager WD, Eschenbach DA, Spence MR, et al. Criteria for diagnosis and grading of salpingitis. Obstet Gynecol 1983;61:113.

Hager WD, Majmudar B. Pelvic actinomycosis in women using intrauterine contraceptive devices. Am J Obstet Gynecol 1979;133:60.

Halber MD, Daffner RH, Morgan CL, et al. Intraabdominal abscess: current concepts in radiologic evaluation. Am J Radiol 1979;133:9.

Halbrecht I. Latent female genital tuberculosis. Int J Fertil 1965;10:157.

Hammond JS, Varas R, Ward CG. Suppurative thrombophlebitis: a new look at a continuing problem. South Med J 1988;81:969.

Hardaway RM. Syndromes of disseminated intravascular coagulation: with special reference to shock and hemorrhage. Springfield, Ill.: Charles C Thomas, 1966.

Heaton FC, Ledger WJ. Postmenopausal tubal ovarian abscess. Obstet Gynecol 1976;47:90.

Hemsell DL, Cunningham FG. Combination antimicrobial therapy for serious gynecological and obstetrical infections—obsolete? Clin Ther 1981;(suppl A)4:81.

Henderson DN, Harkins JL, Stitt JF. Pelvic tuberculosis. Am J Obstet Gynecol 1966;94:630.

Henderson SR. Pelvic actinomycosis associated with an intrauterine device. Obstet Gynecol 1973;41:726.

Henry-Suchet J, Catalan F, Loffredo V, et al. Microbiology of specimens obtained by laparoscopy from controls and from patients with pelvic inflammatory disease or infertility with tubal ob-

struction. *Chlamydia trachomatis* and *Ureaplasma urealyticum*. Am J Obstet Gynecol 1980;138:1022.

Holmes KK, Eschenbach DA, Knapp JS. Salpingitis: overview of etiology and epidemiology. Am J Obstet Gynecol 1980;138:1022.

Hunt JB, Rivlin ME, Clarebout HJ. Antibiotic peritoneal lavage in severe peritonitis. S Afr Med J 1975;49:233.

Hutchins CJ. Tuberculosis of the female genital tract—a changing picture. Br J Obstet Gynaecol 1977;84:534.

Innes JA. Non-respiratory tuberculosis. J R Coll Physicians Lond 1981;15:227.

Jacob HS, Craddock PR, Hammerschmidt DE, et al. Complement-induced granulocyte aggregation: an unsuspected mechanism of disease. N Engl J Med 1980;302:789.

Jacobson L. Differential diagnosis of acute pelvic inflammatory disease. Am J Obstet Gynecol 1980;138:1006.

Jacobson L, Westrom L. Objective diagnosis of acute pelvic inflammatory disease. Am J Obstet Gynecol 1969;105:1088.

Johnson CG. Discussion of Kaplan AL, Jacobs WM, Ehresman JB: aggressive management of pelvic abscess. Am J Obstet Gynecol 1967;98:486.

Johnston RF, Wildrich KH. "State of the ART" review: the impact of chemotherapy on the care of patients with tuberculosis. Am Rev Resp Dis 1974;109:636.

Jones NC, Savage EW, Salem F, et al. Tuberculosis presenting as a pelvic mass. J Natl Med Assoc 1981;73:758.

Josey WE, Cook CC. Septic pelvic thrombophlebitis: report of 17 patients treated with heparin. Obstet Gynecol 1970;35:891.

Josey WE, Staggers SR. Heparin therapy in septic pelvic thrombophlebitis: a study of 46 cases. Am J Obstet Gynecol 1974;120:228.

Kaplan AL, Jacobs WM, Ehresman JR. Aggressive management of pelvic abscess. Am J Obstet Gynecol 1967;98:982.

Kaplan RL, Sahn SA, Petty TL. Incidence and outcome of the respiratory distress syndrome in gram-negative sepsis. Arch Intern Med 1979;1939:867.

Kardon F. Late results in women with genital tuberculosis. Obstet Gynecol 1967;29:247.

Kelaghan J, Rubin GL, Ory HW, et al. Barrier-method contraceptives and pelvic inflammatory disease. JAMA 1982;248:184.

Kelly H. Operative gynecology. Vol II. New York: Appleton, 1898:199, 212, 374, 412, 432, 433.

Kimball MW, Knee S. Gonococcal perihepatitis in a male. The Fitz-Hugh-Curtis syndrome. N Engl J Med 1970;284:1082.

Kirtly L, Benigno BB. The residual adnexa following surgery for pelvic inflammatory disease. Resident Research Day. Emory University School of Medicine, Gynecology and Obstetrics Department. 1979, unpublished data.

Klein TA, Richmond JA, Mishell DR Jr. Pelvic tuberculosis. Obstet Gynecol 1976;48:99.

Koehler PR, Moss AA. Diagnosis of intra-abdominal and pelvic abscesses by computerized tomography. JAMA 1980;244:49.

Kraus GW, Yen SSC. Gonorrhea during pregnancy. Obstet Gynecol 1968;31:258.

Landers DV, Sweet RL. Tubo-ovarian abscess: contemporary approach to management. Rev Infect Dis 1983;5:876.

Ledger WJ. Laparoscopy in the diagnosis and management of patients with suspected salpingo-oophoritis. Am J Obstet Gynecol 1980;138:1012.

Ledingham I, Messmer K, Thijs L. Report on the European conference on septic shock of the European Society of Intensive Care Medicine and the European Shock Society, Brussels, Belgium, March 1–2, 1987. Intensive Care Med 1988;14:181.

Lee J, Warner L, Khaleghian R. Sonographic features of tuberculous endometritis. J Clin Urol 1983;11:331.

Lee NC, Rubin GL, Ory HW, et al. Type of intrauterine device and the risk of pelvic inflammatory disease. Obstet Gynecol 1983;62:1.

Lee W, Clark SL, Cotton DB, Gonik B, Phelan J. Septic shock during pregnancy. Am J Obstet Gynecol 1988;159:410.

Leff A, Lester TW, Addington WW. Tuberculosis: a chemotherapeutic triumph but a persistent socioeconomic problem. Arch Intern Med 1979;139:1375.

Lehtinen M, Rantala I, Teisala K, et al. Detection of herpes simplex virus in women with acute pelvic inflammatory disease. J Infect Dis 1985;152:78.

Loy RA, Gallup DG, Hill JA, Holzman GM, Geist D. Pelvic abscess: examination and transvaginal drainage guided by real-time ultrasonography South Med J 1989;82:788.

MacIntosh OC, Saxon RD. Endometritis due to mycobacterium tuberculosis. Can Med Assoc J 1985;133:667.

MacLean LD, Mulligan WG, McLean APH, et al. Patterns of septic shock in man: a detailed study of 56 patients. Ann Surg 1967;166:543.

Mardh P. An overview of infectious agents of salpingitis, their biology, and recent advances in methods of detection. Am J Obstet Gynecol 1980;138:933.

Mardh P, Ripa T, Svensson L, et al. Chlamydia trachomatis infection in patients with acute salpingitis. N Engl J Med 1977;296:1377.

McGee JA, Johnson AP, Taylor-Robinson D. Human fallopian tubes in organ culture: preparation, maintenance, and quantitation of damage by pathogenic micro-organisms. Infect: Immunol 1976;13:608.

McGowan L. Use of posterior colpotomy in the diagnosis and treatment of pelvic disease. Obstet Gynecol 1963;21:108.

McKay DG. Disseminated intravascular coagulation: an intermediary mechanism of disease. New York: Paul B Hoeber, 1965.

McNamara MT, Mead PB. Diagnosis and management of the pelvic abscess. J Reprod Med 1976;17:299.

Meadows D, Edwards JD, Wilkins RG, Nightingale P. Reversal of intractable septic shock with norepinephrine therapy. Crit Care Med 1988;16:663.

Mickal A, Sellmann AH. Management of tubo-ovarian abscess. Clin Obstet Gynecol 1969;12:252.

Mickal A, Sellmann AH, Beebe JL. Ruptured tubo-ovarian abscesses. Am J Obstet Gynecol 1968;100:432.

Mishell DR, Bell JH, Good RG, Moyer DL. The intrauterine device: a bacteriologic study of the endometrial cavity. Am J Obstet Gynecol 1966;96:119.

Modig J. Comparison of effects of dextran-70 and Ringer's acetate on pulmonary function, hemodynamics, and survival in experimental septic shock. Crit Care Med 1988;16:266.

Monif GRG. Clinical staging of acute bacterial salpingitis and its therapeutic ramifications. Am J Obstet Gynecol 1982;143:489.

Monif GRG. Significance of polymicrobial bacterial superinfection in the therapy of gonococcal endometritis-salpingitis-peritonitis. Obstet Gynecol 1980;55:154S.

Monif GRG, Welkos SL, Baer H, et al. Cul-de-sac isolates from patients with endometritis-salpingitis-peritonitis and gonococcal endocervicitis. Am J Obstet Gynecol 1976;126:158.

Morris CA, Boxall FN, Cayton HR. Genital tract tuberculosis in subfertile women. J Med Microbiol 1970;3:85.

Nobles ER. Bacteroides infections. Ann Surg 1973;177:601.

Olak J, Christon NV, Stein LA, Casola G, Meakins JL. Operative vs. percutaneous drainage of intra-abdominal abscesses. Arch Surg 1986;121:141.

Onsrud M. Perihepatitis in pelvic inflammatory disease associated with intrauterine contraception. Acta Obstet Gynecol Scand 1980;59:69.

Ory HW. A review of the association between intrauterine devices and acute pelvic inflammatory disease. J Reprod Med 1978;20:200.

Osborne NG. The significance of mycoplasma in pelvic infection. J Reprod Med 1977;19:39.

Overbeck L. Is tuberculosis of the female urogenital tract an entity? J Obstet Gynaecol Br Commonw 1966;73:624.

Paavonen J, Miettinen A, Heinonen PK, et al. Serum Ca125 in acute pelvic inflammatory disease. Br J Obstet Gynaecol 1989;96:574.

Pedowitz P, Bloomfield R. Ruptured adnexal abscess (tubo-ovarian) with generalized peritonitis. Am J Obstet Gynecol 1964;88:721.

Poindexter AN, Sweet R, Ritter M. Cefotetan in the treatment of obstetric and gynecologic infections. Am J Obstet Gynecol 1986;154:946.

Rackow EC, Astiz ME, Weill MH. Cellular oxygen metabolism during sepsis and shock: the relationship of oxygen consumption to oxygen delivery. JAMA 1988;259:1989.

Reef E. Gonococcal bartholinitis. Br J Vener Dis 1967;43:150.

Reich H, McGlynn F. Laparoscopic treatment of tuboovarian and pelvic abscess. J Repro Med 1987;32:747.

Rice RJ, Arol SO, Blount JH, Zaidi AA. Gonorrhea in the United States 1975-1984: Is the giant only sleeping? Sex Transm Dis 1987;14:83.

Rice RJ, Thompson SE. Treatment of uncomplicated infections due to Neisseria gonorrhoeae. A review of clinical efficacy and in vitro susceptibility studies from 1982 through 1985. JAMA 1986;255:1739.

Rivlin ME. Clinical outcome following vaginal drainage of pelvic abscess. Obstet Gynecol 1983;61:169.

Rivlin ME, Hunt JA. Ruptured tubo-ovarian abscess: Is hysterectomy necessary? Obstet Gynecol 1977;50:518.

Rosen RJ, Roven SJ. Pecutaneous drainage of abscesses and fluid collections. Urology (Special Issue) 1984;23:54.

Rozin S. Genital tuberculosis. In: Berman SJ, Kistner RW, eds. Progress in infertility. 2nd ed. Boston: Little, Brown, 1975.

Rubin GL, Ory HW, Layde PM. Oral contraceptives and pelvic inflammatory disease. Am J Obstet Gynecol 1982;144:630.

Santos GH, Lansman S. Prevention of pulmonary embolism with use of Mobin-Uddin filter. NY State J Med P 1982;82:185.

Schaefer G. Female genital tuberculosis. Clin Obstet Gynecol 1976;19:223.

Schumer W. Steroids in the treatment of clinical septic shock. Ann Surg 1976;183:333.

Senanayake P, Kramer DG. Contraception and the etiology of pelvic inflammatory disease: new perspectives. Am J Obstet Gynecol 1980;138:852.

Shafer M, Irwin CE, Sweet RL. Acute salpingitis in the adolescent female. J Pediatr 1982;100:339.

Sheagren JN. Septic shock and corticosteroids. N Engl J Med 1981;305:456.

Shubin H, Weil MH, Carlson RW. Bacterial shock. Am Heart J 1977;94:112.

Sibbald J, Anderson RR, Reid B, et al. Alveolocapillary permeability in human septic ARDS: effect of high-dose corticosteroid therapy. Chest 1981;79:133.

Simpson FF. Choice of time for operation for pelvic inflammation of tubal origin. Trans Gynecol Soc 1909;34:161.

Spence MR. The role of the gonococcus in salpingitis. J Reprod Med 1977;19:31.

Spink WW. The pathogenesis and management of shock due to infection. Arch Intern Med 1960;106:433.

Stajano C. La maccion frencia en ginecologia. Sem Med B Air 1920;27:243.

Stemmer VW. Uber die Ursacgen von Einleiterentzundungen. Zentralbl Gynak 1941;22:1061.

Stone KM, Grimes DA, Magder LS. Personal protection against sexually transmitted diseases. Am J Obstet Gynecol 1986;155:180.

Struthers BJ. Pelvic inflammatory disease, intrauterine contraception, and the conduct of epidemiologic studies. Adv Contracept 1985;1:63.

Sutherland AM. Laparoscopy in diagnosis of pelvic tuberculosis. Lancet 1979;2:95.

Sutherland AM. Postmenopausal tuberculosis of the female genital tract. Obstet Gynecol 1982;59:54S.

Sutherland AM. Surgical treatment of tuberculosis of the female genital tract. Br J Obstet Gynaecol 1980;87:610.

Sutherland AM. The management of genital tuberculosis in women. Gazzet San 1970;19:180.

Sutherland AM. The treatment of tuberculosis of the female genital tract with rifampicin, ethambutol, and isoniazid. Arch Gynecol 1981;230:315.

Sutherland AM. Twenty-five years experience of the drug treatment of tuberculosis of the female genital tract. Br J Obstet Gynaecol 1977;84:881.

Sutherland AM, MacFarlane JR. Transmission of genitourinary tuberculosis. Health Bull (Edinb) 1982;40(2):87.

Svensson L, Westrom L, Ripa KT, et al. Differences in some clinical and laboratory parameters in acute salpingitis related to culture and serologic findings. Am J Obstet Gynecol 1980;138:1017.

Sweet RL, Blankfort-Doyle M, Robbie MO, Schacter J. The occurrence of chlamydial and gonococcal salpingitis during the menstrual cycle. JAMA 1986;255:2062.

Sweet RL, Draper DL, Hadley WK. Etiology of acute salpingitis: influence of episode number and duration of symptoms. Obstet Gynecol 1981;58:62.

Sweet RL, Draper DL, Schachter J, et al. Microbiology and pathogenesis of acute salpingitis as determined by laparoscopy: What is the appropriate site to sample? Am J Obstet Gynecol 1980;138:985.

Sweet RL, Mills J, Hadley K, et al. Use of laparoscopy to determine the microbiologic etiology of acute salpingitis. Am J Obstet Gynecol 1979;134:68.

Swenson RM, Michaelson TC, Daly JJ, et al. Anaerobic bacterial infections of the female genital tract. Obstet Gynecol 1973;42:538.

Taylor ES, McMillan JH, Greer BE, et al. The intrauterine device and tubo-ovarian abscesses. Am J Obstet Gynecol 1975;123:338.

Thompson SE, Hager WD. Acute pelvic inflammatory disease. Sex Transm Dis 1977;4:105.

Thompson SE, Hager WD, Wong K, et al. The microbiology and therapy of acute pelvic inflammatory disease in hospitalized patients. Am J Obstet Gynecol 1980;36:179.

Toth A, O'Leary WM, Ledger W. Evidence for microbial transfer by spermatozoa. Obstet Gynecol 1982;59:556.

Tyrrel RT, Murphy FB, Bernardino ME. Tubo-ovarian abscesses: CT-guided percutaneous drainage. Radiology 1990;175:87.

U.S. Department of Health and Human Services. Sexually transmitted diseases treatment guidelines 1982. MMWR 1982;31(suppl 2S).

Vadas P, Pruzanski W, Stefanski E, et al. Pathogenesis of hypotension in septic shock: correlation of circulating phospholipase A2 levels with circulatory collapse. Crit Care Med 1988;16:1.

Vermeeren J, Te Linde RW. Intraabdominal rupture of pelvic abscesses. Am J Obstet Gynecol 1954;68:402.

Waisbren BA. Bacteremia due to gram-negative bacilli other than salmonella: a clinical and therapeutic study. Arch Int Med 1951;88:467.

Walzer A, Koenigsberg M. Ultrasonographic demonstration of pelvic tuberculosis. J Ultrasound Med 1983;2:139.

Wang S, Eschenbach D, Holmes K, et al. Chlamydia trachomatis infection in Fitz-Hugh-Curtis syndrome. Am J Obstet Gynecol 1980;138:1034.

Washington AE, Johnson RE, Sanders LL. Chlamydia trachomatis infections in the United States: What are they costing us? JAMA 1987;257:2070.

Weil MH, Nishijima H. Cardiac output in bacterial shock. Am J Med 1978;64:920.

Weil MH, Shubin H, Biddle M. Shock caused by gram-negative microorganisms: analysis of 169 cases. Ann Intern Med 1964;60:384.

Weiner S, Wallach EE. Ovarian histology in pelvic inflammatory disease. Obstet Gynecol 1974;43:431.

Westrom L. Clinical manifestations and diagnosis of pelvic inflammatory disease. J Reprod Med 1983;28:703.

Westrom L. Incidence, prevalence, and trends of acute pelvic inflammatory disease and its consequences in industrialized countries. Am J Obstet Gynecol 1980;138:880.

Westrom L. Influence of sexually transmitted diseases on sterility and ectopic pregnancy. Acta Eur Fertil 1985;16:21.

Wetchler SJ, Dunn LJ. Ovarian abscess: report of a case and a review of the literature. Obstet Gynecol Survey 1985;40:476.

Wharton LR. Pelvic abscess: a study based on a series of 716 cases. Arch Surg 1921;2:246.

Whittington WL, Knapp JS. Trends in resistance of *Neisseria gonorrhoeae* to antimicrobial agents in the United States. Sex Transm Dis 1988;15:202.

Willson JR, Black JR. Ovarian abscess. Am J Obstet Gynecol 1964;90:34.

Wolner-Hanssen P, Marcd P, Svensson L, et al. Laparoscopy in women with chlamydial infection and pelvic pain: a comparison of patients with and without salpingitis. Obstet Gynecol 1983;61:299.

Wolner-Hanssen PW, Westrom L, Mardh PA. Perihepatitis and chlamydial salpingitis. Lancet 1980;1:901.

World Health Organization. Mechanism of action, safety, and efficacy of intrauterine devices. Technical Report Series 753. Geneva: World Health Organization, 1987:70.

Worthen NJ, Gunning JE. Percutaneous drainage of pelvic abscesses: management of the tubo-ovarian abscess. J Ultrasound Med 1986;5:551.

Wright NH, Laemmle P. Acute pelvic inflammatory disease in an indigent population. Am J Obstet Gynecol 1968;101:979.

25

Surgery for Anomalies of the Müllerian Ducts

JOHN A. ROCK

Maldevelopment of the müllerian ducts occurs in a variety of forms and, although each anomaly is distinctive, some generalizations may be made. Although classification of vaginal anomalies based on certain anatomical findings may be useful in organizing the type of malformation, there are usually exceptions to each rule. Thus, after a preliminary diagnostic evaluation is performed, what would appear to be an apparently isolated vaginal malformation may be found to have an associated uterine or renal anomaly. Although a comprehensive preoperative evaluation of patients with suspected malformations of the müllerian ducts is essential, a clear understanding of the anomaly may not finally be established until the time of surgical correction. It is therefore important that the reproductive surgeon be skilled in both uterine and vaginal reconstruction.

The patient with a uterovaginal anomaly often relies on her physician to clarify the reproductive consequences associated with her diagnosis. The physician will allay anxiety by prompt evaluation and accurate description of the reproductive implications or the obstetric consequences of a particular uterovaginal anomaly.

CLASSIFICATION OF UTEROVAGINAL ANOMALIES

Past classifications for uterovaginal anomalies were organized on a clinical basis. More recently, with improved understanding of embryologic development, most uterovaginal anomalies are now explainable on this basis. Alternatively, the recent American Fertility Society classification of müllerian anomalies (Table 25-1) is based on the degree of failure of normal development, and thus separates the anomalies into groups with similar clinical manifestations, treatment, and prognosis for fetal salvage. The classification system is weighted primarily toward disorders of lateral fusion. The classification does not include associated vaginal anomalies. The scheme allows the user to describe anomalies involving the vagina, tubes, and urinary tract as associated malformations.

A classification of müllerian maldevelopment, however, can scarcely pivot on the uterus. Many times the vagina, and sometimes the tubes, are also involved. The following is a suggested classification of uterovaginal anomalies based on embryologic considerations that comprises four groups, as outlined in Table 25-2.

Class I. Dysgenesis of the Müllerian Ducts

Dysgenesis of the müllerian ducts or agenesis of the uterus and vagina (Mayer-Rokitansky-Küster-Hauser syndrome) is an impairment of the reproductive system and is characterized by no reproductive potential other than that achieved by in vitro fertilization to a host uterus.

Class II. Disorders of Vertical Fusion of the Müllerian Ducts

Disorders of vertical fusion may be considered to represent faults in the junction between the down-

TABLE 25–1
American Fertility Society Classification of Müllerian Anomalies*

CLASSIFICATION	ANOMALY
Class I.	Segmental Müllerian Agenesis/Hypoplasia
	A. Vaginal
	B. Cervical
	C. Fundal
	D. Tubal
	E. Combined anomalies
Class II.	Unicornuate
	A. Communicating
	B. Noncommunicating
	C. No cavity
	D. No horn
Class III.	Didelphus
Class IV.	Bicornuate
	A. Complete (division down to internal os)
	B. Partial
Class V.	Septate
	A. Complete (septum to internal os)
	B. Partial
Class VI.	Arcuate
Class VII.	DES drug-related

*This classification allows the user to indicate the malformation type as well as additional findings to describe associated variations involving the vagina, cervix, tubes (right, left), and kidneys (right, left)

(Adapted from the American Fertility Society Classification of Müllerian Anomalies, Fertil Steril 1988; 49(6):944, with permission.)

growing müllerian ducts (müllerian tubercle) and the up-growing derivative of the urogenital sinus. Typically, these disorders are characterized by patients with an atretic portion of the vagina. This segment of vagina may be quite thick, extending through more than half the distance of the vagina or a small obstructing membrane. Regardless of the length of the septum, these disorders should be regarded as a transverse vaginal septum and are classified as either obstructed or nonobstructed. The so-called partial vaginal agenesis with uterus and cervix present is probably a misnomer but represents a large segment of atretic vagina. Also included in this group are patients with cervical agenesis or dysgenesis.

Class III. Disorders of Lateral Fusion of the Müllerian Ducts

Disorders of lateral fusion of the two müllerian ducts may be symmetric-unobstructed, as with the double vagina, or asymmetric-obstructed, as with patients with unilateral vaginal obstruction. Obstructed lesions associated with disorders of lateral fusion are particularly noteworthy in that they are observed clinically only

TABLE 25–2
Classification of Uterovaginal Anomalies

Class I. Dysgenesis of the Müllerian Ducts
Class II. Disorders of Vertical Fusion of the Müllerian Ducts
    A. Transverse vaginal septum
      1. Obstructed
      2. Unobstructed
    B. Cervical agenesis or dysgenesis
Class III. Disorders of Lateral Fusion of the Müllerian Ducts
    A. Asymmetric-obstructed disorder of uterus or vagina usually associated with ipsilateral renal agenesis
      1. Unicornuate uterus with a noncommunicating rudimentary anlagen or horn
      2. Unilateral obstruction of a cavity of a double uterus
      3. Unilateral vaginal obstruction associated with double uterus
    B. Symmetric-unobstructed
      1. Didelphic uterus
        a. Complete longitudinal vaginal septum
        b. Partial longitudinal vaginal septum
        c. No longitudinal vaginal septum
      2. Septate uterus
        a. Complete
          (1) Complete longitudinal vaginal septum
          (2) Partial longitudinal vaginal septum
          (3) No longitudinal vaginal septum
        b. Partial
          (1) Complete longitudinal vaginal septum
          (2) Partial longitudinal vaginal septum
          (3) No longitudinal vaginal septum
      3. Bicornuate uterus
        a. Complete
          (1) Complete longitudinal vaginal septum
          (2) Partial longitudinal vaginal septum
          (3) No longitudinal vaginal septum
        b. Partial
          (1) Complete longitudinal vaginal septum
          (2) Partial longitudinal vaginal septum
          (3) No longitudinal vaginal septum
      4. *T*-shaped uterine cavity (DES drug-related)
      5. Unicornuate uterus
        a. With a rudimentary horn
          (1) With endometrial cavity
             (a) Communicating
             (b) Noncommunicating
          (2) Without endometrial cavity
        b. Without rudimentary horn
Class IV. Unusual Configurations of Vertical/Lateral Fusion Defects

(Modified from the American Fertility Society Classification of Müllerian Anomalies, Fertil Steril 1988; 49(6), with permission.)

when obstruction is unilateral. Unilateral obstruction is almost invariably associated with absence of the ipsilateral kidney. It is thought that bilateral obstruction is associated with bilateral kidney agenesis with subsequent nonviability of the developing embryo.

The three varieties of asymmetric obstruction with ipsilateral renal agenesis are (1) a unicornous uterus with a noncommunicating horn, which contains menstruating endometrium; (2) unilateral obstruction of a cavity of a double uterus; and (3) unilateral vaginal obstruction. Symmetric-unobstructed disorders of lateral fusion include five groups of disorders. The didelphic (first group), bicornuate (second group), and septate uterus (third group) are each a type of double uterus. The differentiation between a septate and a bicornuate uterus requires visualization of the fundus. The T-shaped uterine cavity (fourth group), which may be hypoplastic and irregular, is associated with diethylstilbestrol (DES) exposure in utero. The fifth group is the unicornous uterus, which may be associated with or without a rudimentary horn.

The septum within the septate uterus may be complete or partial. When the septum is complete, there are inevitably two cervices with a longitudinal vaginal septum that may extend to the introitus or partially down the vagina. The bicornuate uterus also may have a partial or almost complete separation of the uterine cavities. An *arcuate uterus* is primarily a radiologic term referring to a slight septum in the uterine fundus. There must be a clear separation of the uterine cavities. This type of uterus is usually included under the category "partial septate uterus."

The unicornous uterus may have an attached horn with a cavity that communicates with the unicornous uterus. Alternatively, there may be no uterine horn, or a uterine horn with no cavity. Some debate has focused on whether the unicornous uterus with a communicating horn may represent a hypoplastic side of a bicornuate uterus.

Class IV. Unusual Configurations of Vertical/Lateral Fusion Defects

The final category includes combinations of uterovaginal anomalies and other disorders. Unusual uterovaginal configurations have been described that do not fit a particular category or example; that is, vertical and lateral fusion disorders may coexist.

Obstructive lesions require immediate attention to relieve the retrograde flow of trapped mucus and menstrual blood, and the increasing pressure on surrounding organs and structures. When no obstruction is present, attention may not be required immediately but will be required eventually to establish or improve reproductive or coital function.

EMBRYOLOGY

The reproductive organs in the female (indeed, also in the male) consist of external genitalia, gonads, and an internal duct system between the two. These three components originate embryologically from different primordia and in close association with the urinary system and hindgut. Thus, the developmental history is complex. Even in the 4–5 mm embryo, it is possible to recognize bilateral thickenings of the coelomic epithelium medial to the mesonephros (primitive kidney) in the dorsum of the coelomic cavity. These thickenings are the gonadal ridges (Fig. 25-1). At about the sixth week, in the 17–20 mm embryo, the gonad can be distinguished as either a testis or an ovary.

In the female, the labia minora and majora develop from the labioscrotal folds, which are ectodermal in origin. The phallic portion of the urogenital sinus gives rise to the urethra. The müllerian (paramesonephric) duct system is stimulated to develop preferentially over the wolffian (mesonephric) duct system, which regresses in early female fetal life. The cranial parts of the wolffian ducts may persist as the epoophoron of the ovarian hilum; the caudal parts may persist as Gartner's ducts. The müllerian ducts persist and attain complete development to form the fallopian tubes, the uterine corpus and cervix, and a portion of the vagina.

Origin of the Müllerian Ducts

About 37 days after fertilization, the müllerian ducts first appear lateral to each wolffian duct as invaginations of the dorsal coelomic epithelium. The site of origin of the invaginations remains open and ultimately forms the fimbriated end of the fallopian tubes. At their point of origin, the müllerian ducts each form a solid bud. Each bud penetrates the mesenchyme lateral and parallel to each wolffian duct. As the solid buds elongate, a lumen appears in the cranial part, beginning at each coelomic opening. The lumina extend gradually to the caudal growing tips of the ducts.

Eventually, the caudal end of each müllerian duct crosses the ventral aspect of the wolffian duct. The paired müllerian ducts continue to grow in a medial and caudal direction until they eventually meet in the midline and become fused together in the urogenital septum. A septum between the two müllerian ducts gradually disappears, leaving a single uterovaginal canal lined with cuboidal epithelium. Failure of reabsorption of this septum can result in a septate uterus. The most cranial parts of the müllerian ducts remain separate and form the fallopian tubes. The caudal segments of the müllerian ducts fuse to form the uterus and part of the vagina. The cranial point of fusion is the site of the future fundus of the uterus. Variations in this site of fusion can result in an arcuate or bicornuate uterus. Complete failure of fusion can result in a didelphic uterus.

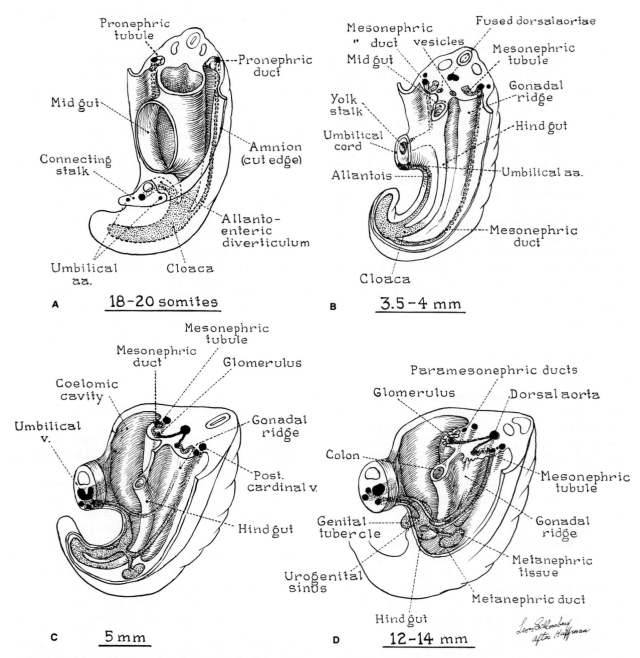

Figure 25–1. Diagrammatic representation of the development of the female reproductive organs and structures in early embryogenesis. *A,* At the 18–20 somite stage (fourth week) the gonadal ridges have not yet begun to form. *B,* In the 3.5–4 mm embryo (fifth week) the gonadal ridges can be recognized as thickenings of the coelomic cavity just medial to the mesonephric tubules. Gonadal differentiation into either testis or ovary does not occur until the sixth week of development. The allantoenteric diverticulum is joined caudally to the dilated cloaca. *C* and *D,* The genital tubercle and labial folds form in the region just anterior to the cloaca. The cloaca later divides into the ventral urogenital sinus and the dorsal rectum.

The development of the urinary system closely parallels that of the reproductive system. The nonfunctioning pronephric tubules shown in *A,* develop to form the mesonephric ducts shown in *B* and *C.* The permanent kidneys eventually develop from the metanephric tissue, and the urinary collecting system develops from the metanephric ducts. The paramesonephric (müllerian) ducts are apparent by the 12–14 mm stage (*D*). Their subsequent development is illustrated in Figure 20–2.

Development of the Vagina

The vagina is formed from the lower end of the uterovaginal canal, developed from the müllerian ducts and the urogenital sinus (Fig. 25-2). The point of contact between the two is the müllerian tubercle. A solid vaginal cord results from proliferation of the cells at the caudal tip of the fused müllerian ducts. The cord gradually elongates to meet the bilateral endodermal evaginations (sinovaginal bulbs) from the posterior aspect of the urogenital sinus below. These sinovaginal bulbs extend cranially to fuse with the caudal end of the vaginal cord, forming the vaginal plate. Subsequently, canalization of the vaginal cord occurs, followed by epithelialization with cells derived mostly from endoderm of the urogenital sinus. Recent proposals hold that only the upper one third of the vagina is formed from the müllerian ducts, with the lower vagina developing from the vaginal plate of the urogenital sinus. Recent studies also suggest that the vaginal canal is actually open and connected to a patent uterus and tubes, even in early embryonic life, and that the vagina does not form and later become canalized from an epithelial cord of squamous cells growing upward from the urogenital sinus. Most investigators now suggest that the vagina develops under the influence of the müllerian ducts and estrogenic stimulation. There is general agreement that the vagina originates as a composite formed partly from the müllerian ducts and partly from the urogenital sinus.

At about the 20th week, the cervix takes form as a result of a condensation of stromal cells at a specific site around the fused müllerian ducts. The mesenchyme surrounding the müllerian ducts becomes condensed early in embryonic development and eventually forms the musculature of the female genital tract. The hymen is the embryologic septum between the sinovaginal bulbs above and the urogenital sinus proper below. It is lined by an internal layer of vaginal epithelium and an external layer of epithelium derived from the urogenital sinus (both of endodermal origin) with mesoderm between the two. It is not derived from the müllerian ducts.

Anomalies in Organogenesis of the Vagina

Anomalies in the organogenesis of the vagina are easily understood. Should there be a failure in the development of the müllerian ducts at any time between their origin from the coelomic epithelium at 5 weeks of embryonic age and their fusion with the urogenital sinus at 8 weeks, the sinovaginal bulbs will fail to proliferate from the urogenital sinus and the uterus and vagina will fail to develop. The Mayer-Rokitansky-Küster-Hauser syndrome is the most common clinical example of this anomaly. The uterus is absent with congenital absence of the vagina.

Transverse Vaginal Septum. A transverse vaginal septum can develop in any location in the vagina, but is more common in the upper vagina at the point of junction between the vaginal plate and the caudal end of the fused müllerian ducts. This defect is caused, presumably, by a failure of absorption of the tissue that separates the two or a failure of complete fusion of the two embryologic components of the vagina. A large segment of vagina may be atretic. In past reviews, this has been termed "partial vaginal agenesis with a uterus present." It may be more difficult to elucidate the origin of the high transverse vaginal septum. A local abnormality of the vaginal mesoderm or failure of canalization of the epithelial vaginal plate may provide the answer. Why the abnormality occurs at this particular site is not evident. The proportion of the vagina originating from the urogenital sinus may at times be considerably more than one fifth, and thus a high transverse vaginal septum may represent the junction of an abnormally long urogenital sinus contribution and a short müllerian portion. Alternatively, the high transverse septum could be the sequela of a local infection of the septum at the end of the vagina. Septa in other areas of the vagina are left unexplained by this theory, which has not gained widespread acceptance.

Disorders of Sexual Differentiation with Ineffective Suppression of Müllerian Ducts. In cases of abnormal gonadal development in which the müllerian ducts have been ineffectively suppressed, the development of ambiguous external genitalia frequently will be accompanied by a small rudimentary uterus or a partially developed vagina. Additionally, when there is a genetic loss of cytoplasmic receptor proteins within androgenic target cells, such as occurs in the androgen insensitivity syndrome (formerly called testicular feminization syndrome), it is understandable that the vagina will not be completely developed, because in this XY female the existing male gonads have suppressed the development of the müllerian ducts. Because these genetic male patients are seen clinically as phenotypic females without a completely formed vagina, it is important that a vagina be surgically constructed so that these patients may function satisfactorily sexually in their female gender role.

Congenital rectovaginal fistula, imperforate (covered) anus, hypospadias, and a variety of anatomical variants of cloacal dysgenesis also may occur. These anomalies may be associated with maldevelopment of the müllerian and mesonephric duct derivatives.

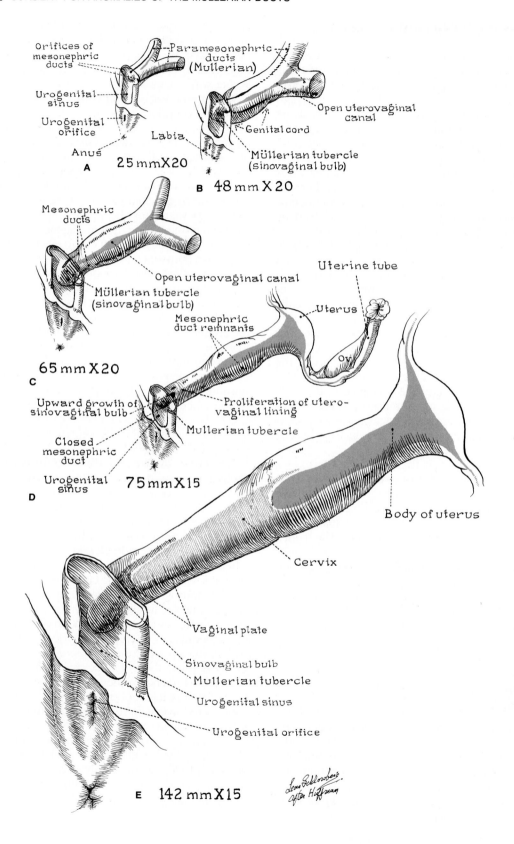

Orifices of mesonephric ducts
Paramesonephric ducts (Mullerian)
Urogenital sinus
Open uterovaginal canal
Urogenital orifice
Genital cord
Anus
Labia
Müllerian tubercle (sinovaginal bulb)

A 25 mm X 20

B 48 mm X 20

Mesonephric ducts
Open uterovaginal canal
Müllerian tubercle (sinovaginal bulb)
Uterine tube
Uterus
Mesonephric duct remnants
Ov

65 mm X 20

C

Upward growth of sinovaginal bulb
Proliferation of utero-vaginal lining
Closed mesonephric duct
Mullerian tubercle
Urogenital sinus

75 mm X 15

D

Body of uterus
Cervix
Vaginal plate
Sinovaginal bulb
Mullerian tubercle
Urogenital sinus
Urogenital orifice

E 142 mm X 15

Lore Schlossberg.
after Huffman

Müllerian Duct Abnormalities

Abnormalities in the formation or fusion of the müllerian ducts can result in a variety of anomalies of the uterus and vagina—single, multiple, combined, or separate. The entirely separate origin of the ovaries from the gonadal ridges explains the infrequent association of uterovaginal anomalies with ovarian anomalies (see Ch. 22). The close developmental relationship of the müllerian ducts and the wolffian ducts can explain the frequency with which anomalies of the female genital system and urinary tract are associated. Failure of development of a müllerian duct is likewise associated with failure of development of a ureteric bud from the caudal end of the wolffian duct. Thus, the entire kidney may be absent on the same side as agenesis of a müllerian duct.

Depending on the time when the teratogenic influence may be operative, renal units may be absent, fused, or in unusual locations in the pelvis. Ureters may be duplicated or may open in unusual places such as the vagina or uterus. Jones and Rock have pointed out that failure of lateral fusion of the müllerian ducts with unilateral obstruction is associated consistently with absence of the kidney on the side with obstruction. Bilateral obstruction has not been observed clinically, presumably because it would be associated with bilateral renal agenesis, a condition that would not allow the embryo to develop. According to Thompson and Lynn, 40% of female patients with congenital absence of the kidney will be found to have associated genital anomalies.

CONGENITAL ABSENCE OF THE MÜLLERIAN DUCTS

The disorders of müllerian agenesis include congenital absence of the vagina and uterus. Although often referred to in the literature as congenital absence of the vagina or vaginal agenesis, this condition can be more accurately labeled aplasia, or dysplasia, of the müllerian ducts because patients with this condition generally have a normal lower vagina but the middle and upper two thirds are missing. Despite the absence of the uterus, rudimentary uterine primordia are found that are comparable in size and appearance. Tubes and ovaries in patients with congenital absence of the müllerian ducts are usually normal. This syndrome usually is referred to as the Mayer-Rokitansky-Küster-Hauser syndrome (Table 25-3). This syndrome may be associated with the heterogeneous group of disorders with a variety of genetic, endocrine, and metabolic manifestations and associated anomalies of other body systems.

For purposes of classification, patients with partial agenesis of the vagina with the uterus present, or a transverse vaginal septum, fall in the category of disorders of vertical fusion. These patients have a low incidence of urinary tract anomalies, another circumstance that sets them apart from patients with Mayer-Rokitansky-Küster-Hauser syndrome.

Realdus Columbus first described congenital absence of the vagina in 1559. In 1829, Mayer described congenital absence of the vagina as one of the abnormalities found in stillborn infants with multiple birth defects. Rokitansky in 1838 and Küster in 1910 de-

TABLE 25–3
Characteristics of Women with Müllerian Agenesis

Congenital absence of the uterus and vagina (small rudimentary uterine bulbs are usually present with rudimentary fallopian tubes)
Normal ovarian function, including ovulation
Sex of rearing—female
Phenotypic sex female (normal development of breasts, body proportions, hair distribution, and external genitalia)
Genetic sex female (46XX karyotype)
Frequent association of other congenital anomalies (skeletal, urologic, and especially renal)

◄ **Figure 25–2.** Further development of the paramesonephric (müllerian) ducts and the urogenital sinus. *A*, Early development of the paramesonephric ducts. The cranial ends of the paramesonephric ducts develop first. These ends remain open to form the fimbriated end of the fallopian tubes. The paramesonephric ducts grow caudally, cross the mesonephric ducts ventrally, and *B*, Eventually fuse together to form the uterovaginal canal. *C*, Further development caudally brings this structure into contact with the wall of the urogenital sinus, producing the müllerian tubercle. The caudal ends of the fused paramesonephric ducts form the uterine corpus and cervix. Together with the urogenital sinus, they also form the vagina. The cranial point of fusion of the paramesonephric ducts marks the location of the future uterine fundus. The fallopian tubes form from the unfused cranial parts of the paramesonephric (müllerian) ducts. The proliferation of the lining of the uterovaginal canal above and the upward growth of the sinovaginal bulb from below (*D*) form the vaginal plate (*E*) which later becomes canalized to leave an open vaginal canal. Thus, the vagina is of composite origin. The mesonephric ducts in the female degenerate but may persist into adult life as Gartner's ducts.

scribed an entity in which the vagina was absent, a small bipartite uterus was present, the ovaries were normal, and anomalies of other organ systems (renal and skeletal) were frequently observed. Hauser and associates emphasized the spectrum of associated anomalies. Pinsky suggested that congenital absence of the vagina is part of a symptom complex and not a true syndrome. Over the years, the disorder has come to be known as the Mayer-Rokitansky-Küster-Hauser syndrome or the Rokitansky-Küster-Hauser syndrome or simply as the Rokitansky syndrome (Fig. 25–3).

Counseller found that the condition occurred once in 4000 female admissions to the Mayo Clinic. Evans estimated that vaginal agenesis occurred once in 10,588 female births in Michigan from 1953 to 1957.

Individuals with an absent vagina and the classic Mayer-Rokitansky-Küster-Hauser syndrome usually are brought to the gynecologist at age 14 to 15 years when the absence of menses gives the parents concern. Such young women have a normal complement of chromosomes (46XX) and usually have normal ovaries and secondary sex characteristics, including external genitalia. Menstruation does not appear at the usual age because the uterus is absent, but ovulation occurs regularly. Some exceptions to the rule of normal ovaries have been noted. For example, polycystic ovaries and gonadal dysgenesis have been reported in patients with congenital absence of the vagina.

Etiologic Factors

An exclusive genetic etiology cannot be ascribed to vaginal agenesis, because almost all patients have a

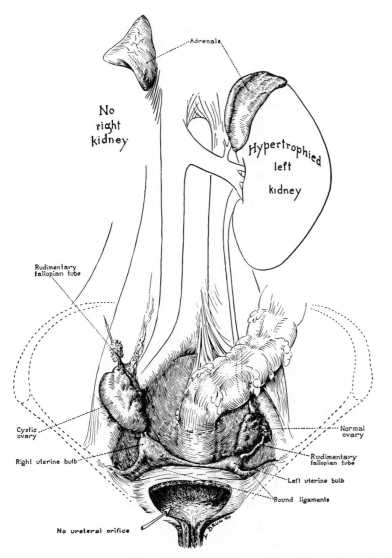

Figure 25–3. Typical findings in a patient with Mayer-Rokitansky-Küster-Hauser syndrome. Note absence of the right kidney and right ureteral orifice. The uterus is represented by bilateral rudimentary uterine bulbs joined by a band behind the bladder. The ovaries appear normal. There is malposition of the right ovary.

normal karyotype (46XX). Also, the discordance of vaginal agenesis in three sets of monozygotic twins has been reported. The occurrence of complete vaginal agenesis in sisters with a 46XX karyotype suggests an autosomal mode of inheritance for these patients. Shokeir investigated the families of 13 unrelated females with aplasia of müllerian duct derivatives. Similarly affected females were found in 10 families. Usually there was an affected female paternal relative, suggesting female-limited autosomal dominant inheritance of a mutant gene transmitted by male relatives.

Other investigators point to the variety of associated anomalies as support for the etiologic concept of variable expression of a genetic defect possibly precipitated by teratogenic exposure operative between the 37th and the 41st gestational day, the period during which the vagina is formed. Knab has suggested that five possible etiologic factors of the Mayer-Rokitansky-Küster-Hauser syndrome are (1) inappropriate production of müllerian regressive factor in the female embryonic gonad, (2) regional absence or deficiency of estrogen receptors limited to the lower müllerian duct, (3) arrest of müllerian duct development by a teratogenic agent, (4) mesenchymal inductive defect, and (5) sporadic gene mutation. Knab believes that the teratogenic and the mutant gene etiologies are the most probable.

Anomalies Associated with Müllerian Agenesis

A significant number of patients with müllerian agenesis will have associated anomalies of the upper müllerian duct system as well as associated anomalies of other organ systems. By gentle rectal examination, the physician can feel an absence of the midline müllerian structure that should represent the uterus. Instead, the physician feels a smooth band (possibly a remnant of the uterosacral ligaments) that extends from one side of the pelvis to the other. In Mayer-Rokitansky-Küster-Hauser syndrome, the uterus is represented by bilateral rudimentary uterine bulbs that may vary in size, are not usually palpable, are connected to small fallopian tubes, and are located on the lateral pelvic side wall adjacent to normal ovaries. Depending on their size, these rudimentary uterine bulbs may or may not contain a cavity lined by endometrial tissue (Fig. 25-4). If present, the endometrial tissue may appear immature or, rarely, may show evidence of cyclic response to ovarian hormones. The endometrial cavity does not communicate often with the peritoneal cavity because the tube may not be patent at the point of junction between the tube and the rudimentary uterine bulb. However, in rare instances, active endometrium may exist within the uterine anlagen and the endometrial cavity, enabling communication with the peritoneal cavity through patent fallopian tubes. Reports have described several patients with functioning endometrial tissue in one or both rudimentary uterine bulbs (Fig. 25–4*B*). The patient may develop a large hematometra due to cyclic accumulation of trapped blood. Cyclic abdominal pain is relieved with the excision of the active uterine anlagen. A patient with Mayer-Rokitansky-Küster-Hauser syndrome has been reported who had a 4-cm endometrioma removed from the left ovary by laparotomy at the time of operation to

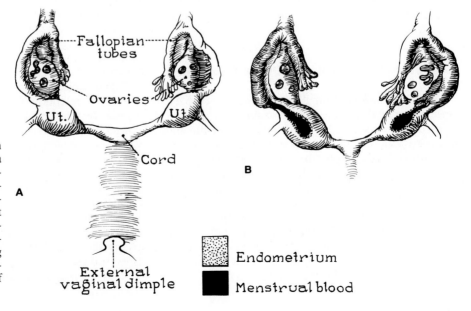

Figure 25–4. Patients with congenital absence of the vagina may show variations in the development of the upper müllerian ducts. *A*, Bilateral rudimentary uterine bulbs without endometrium. *B*, Bilateral rudimentary uterine bulbs containing a cavity lined by functioning endometrial tissue. Cross-section view shows presence of menstrual blood.

create a vagina. Myomas have been known to form in the muscular wall and mild dysmenorrhea has been attributed to their presence. A small myoma has been found, in addition to the tube and ovary, in the inguinal canal or in an inguinal hernia sac.

The potential for function from the rudimentary bulbs has been clearly demonstrated by Chakravarty, Gun and Sarkar and by Singh and Devi. These authors have attempted to use these rudimentary uterine bulbs to reconstruct a midline uterus. The reconstructed uterus is then connected to the newly constructed vagina. A surprising number of patients who have undergone this procedure have experienced cyclic menstruation, although recurrent stenosis and obstruction of the rudimentary horns is the most common outcome of such efforts. The editors of this book have had no experience with this technique and question its usefulness. However, these rudimentary uterine bulbs usually are insignificant structures that cause no problems.

Associated Urologic and Renal Anomalies

Fore and associates reported that 47% of patients in whom evaluation of the urinary tract was performed had associated urologic anomalies. In other studies, approximately one third of patients with complete vaginal agenesis were found to have significant urinary anomalies, such as unilateral renal agenesis, unilateral or bilateral pelvic kidney, horseshoe kidney, hydronephrosis, hydroureter, and a variety of patterns of ureteral duplication. A significant number of patients with partial vaginal agenesis also will have associated urinary tract anomalies.

Associated Skeletal and Other Anomalies

Associated skeletal anomalies have been recognized since congenital absence of the vagina was first described. In a review of 574 reported cases, Griffin and associates found a 12% incidence of skeletal abnormalities. Most of these involve the spine (wedge vertebrae, fusions, rudimentary vertebral bodies, and supernumerary vertebrae), but the limbs and ribs also can be involved. Other anomalies include syndactyly, absence of a digit, congenital heart disease, and inguinal hernias, although inguinal hernias are apparently more often present in patients with androgen insensitivity syndrome than in patients with the Mayer-Rokitansky-Küster-Hauser syndrome (see Table 25-3).

Treatment for Disorders of Müllerian Agenesis

Preoperative Considerations

If functioning endometrial tissue is present with the anlagen, then symptoms from cryptomenorrhea will begin shortly after female secondary sex characteristics develop. Prompt removal of the active uterine bulbs affords complete relief of symptoms.

Occasionally, older patients with the classic Mayer-Rokitansky-Küster-Hauser syndrome consult a gynecologist, either before or after marriage, because of difficult or painful intercourse. The indication for operation in these patients is also obvious. Of all patients, they are the most satisfied with the operative results.

Most commonly, patients aged 14 to 16 years are seen by a gynecologist because of primary amenorrhea. An examination may not have been done by a previous physician because the patient was "too young," but various hormonal medications may have been given with hope that menstruation would begin. An inaccurate examination may have led to a mistaken diagnosis of imperforate hymen. Futile attempts to incise the hymen may have resulted in scarring of the apex of the vaginal dimple before a correct diagnosis of congenital absence of the vagina was finally made.

Formerly, it was customary to advise a delay in operating to create a vagina for these young patients until just before their marriage. This custom led to difficulties at times, particularly when complications developed that required delay in the marriage until the vagina healed completely. More recently, the procedure has been performed when the patient is aged 17 to 20 years, at which time it is clearly evident that she is emotionally mature and intellectually reliable enough to manage the vaginal form without difficulty. In addition, at this age, a delay in healing of the newly constructed vagina most likely would not create any unnecessary emotional trauma for the patient or her family.

Psychologic Preparation of the Patient. Probably insufficient attention has been given to the psychologic aspects of this problem. Obviously, the patient with congenital absence of the vagina cannot be made into a whole person simply by creating a perineal pouch for intercourse. Establishment of sexual function is only one concern and may be the easiest problem to correct. Evans reported that 15% of his patients have real psychiatric difficulty. He and David and associates suggest that psychiatric help should be initiated before the operation. Learning about this anomaly, especially at a young age, is a shock and is accompanied by diminished self-esteem. Such patients may be encouraged by their gynecologist with the offer of appropriate surgery to establish coital function. The gynecologist may point out that, functionally, the patient will be like thousands of young women who have had a hysterectomy because of serious pelvic disease and who also have satisfied their desire to be a parent through adoption.

Patient Cooperation. Regardless of which operative technique is chosen, the patient must cooperate if the operation is to be successful. When a McIndoe operation is performed, patients must understand the need to wear a form continuously for several months and intermittently for several years until the vagina is no longer subject to constriction and regular intercourse is taking place. The operation should not be done until it is certain in preoperative interviews that the patient understands her essential role in its success. This is especially important when the patient is a young teenager. The single most important factor in determining the success of vaginoplasty is the psychosocial adjustment of the patient to her congenital vaginal anomaly.

Laboratory and Diagnostic Testing

A buccal smear should be done to determine the presence or absence of the chromatin body. If the chromatin body is absent, or there is a suspicion of ovarian dysgenesis, androgen insensitivity syndrome, or some aberration of the classic Mayer-Rokitansky-Küster-Hauser syndrome, then a complete chromosomal analysis should be done. Obviously, an intravenous pyelogram should be done preoperatively. This also will provide an adequate survey for anomalies of the spine. If a pelvic mass is present, then additional special studies, including ultrasonography, should be performed to differentiate between hematometra, hematocolpos, endometrial and other ovarian cysts, and pelvic kidney.

Evaluation of Cyclic Pain

Some patients without a pelvic mass will complain of cyclic pain. This pain may be ovulatory or possibly a result of dysmenorrhea originating in well-developed rudimentary uterine bulbs. The physician can differentiate between the two by asking the patient to keep a basal body temperature chart and marking the days when pelvic pain is present. Occasionally, there may be a question about whether a patient has congenital absence of the vagina or an imperforate hymen with cryptomenorrhea. The diagnosis may be clarified simply by placing a metal catheter or similar instrument in the urethra and a finger in the rectum. If the metal instrument in the urethra can be easily felt through the anterior rectal wall, then the vagina is probably absent. On the other hand, if there is an intervening mass

between the rectal finger and the instrument in the urethra, this may represent a hematocolpos behind an imperforate hymen. The hymen will bulge from the force of accumulated blood in the vagina, especially when the hematocolpos is palpable suprapubically.

METHODS OF CREATING A VAGINA

Even today there is no unanimity of opinion regarding the correct approach to the problem of vaginal agenesis. A review of the methods devised for the formation of a vagina follows.

Nonsurgical Methods

In 1938, Robert Frank described a method of formation of an artificial vagina without operation. In 1940, he reported remarkably satisfactory results in eight cases treated by this method. His follow-up study showed that a vagina formed in this manner remained permanent in depth and caliber, even in patients who neglected dilatation for more than 1 year. It has been emphasized that the pelvic floor itself may be embryologically deficient in some patients. Indeed, the ease with which some patients are able to create a vagina with intercourse alone or with other intermittent pressure techniques may be explained on this basis. Five patients have even been reported to have developed enteroceles, one following coitus alone, three following a Williams vulvovaginoplasty, and three following a McIndoe operation. This complication may develop when the vaginal mucosa is brought in close proximity to the pelvic peritoneum, but it also may be contributed to by a relative embryologic weakness or absence of endopelvic fascia.

Rock and associates at the Johns Hopkins Hospital reported that an initial trial of vaginal dilatation was successful in 9 out of 21 patients. Prompted by the rewarding results of Broadbent and Woolf, Ingram has described a passive dilatation technique of creating a new vagina. Using dilators especially designed for use with a bicycle seat stool, Ingram was able to produce satisfactory vaginal depth and coital function in 10 out of 12 patients with vaginal agenesis and 10 out of 14 patients with various types of stenosis.

The Frank dilatation technique requires active manipulation by the patient to dilate the neovaginal space. In a teenager, such manipulation is difficult even with careful instruction. Since the introduction of Ingram's passive dilatation technique at the Johns Hopkins Hospital, 8 out of 10 women with congenital absence of the vagina have obtained a neovagina of sufficient length and width for comfortable sexual relations. With congenital absence of the vagina with a vaginal pouch or dimple, it is appropriate to encourage passive vaginal dilatation. Often, a major surgical procedure may be avoided. In case of failure, a surgical procedure can be done at a later time.

Surgical Methods

During the past three decades, experience has crystallized physicians' ideas so that they tend to believe that one method of dealing with complete absence of a vagina is superior to others in the majority of cases: the Abbe-Wharton-McIndoe operation, more popularly called the McIndoe operation. In special circumstances, the vulvovaginal pouch of Williams or the sigmoid transplant of Pratt may be indicated.

Historical Development of Surgical Procedures

In 1907, Baldwin used a double loop of ileum to line a space dissected between the rectum and bladder, leaving the mesentery connected to the bowel. The continuity of the intestinal tract was reestablished by an end-to-end anastomosis. He reported that the new vagina was absolutely normal in every way. In 1910, Popoff constructed a vagina using a portion of the rectum that was moved anteriorly. This operation was modified by Schubert in 1911. The rectum was severed above the anal sphincter and moved anteriorly to serve as the vagina. The sigmoid was sutured to the anus and the continuity of the intestinal tract was thus reestablished. The high mortality and morbidity of both operations were a sobering influence and their popularity declined. Today, segments of sigmoid are used more often to create a vaginal pouch or extend vaginal length in patients who have lost vaginal function because of extensive surgery or irradiation for pelvic malignancy.

Less formidable procedures, consisting of dissection of a space between the bladder and rectum and lining this space with flaps of skin from the labia or inner thighs, also were tried. Marked scarring resulted and hair usually grew in the vagina. Extensive plastic procedures to construct a vagina are no longer necessary or desirable and have been discarded in favor of safer procedures, unless the physician is faced with the problem of maintaining a vaginal canal in a patient who is having an extensive exenterative operation for pelvic malignancy. In this case, the physician may wish to consider using the gracilis myocutaneous flap technique described by McCraw and associates in 1976.

The Abbe-Wharton-McIndoe Operation

Genesis of the Procedure. The operation that is most popular today for creating a new vagina began with simple surgical attempts to create space between the bladder and the rectum. The earlier attempts were often in patients with cryptomenorrhea. However, such a space usually would constrict because of a failure to recognize the importance of prolonged continuous dilatation until the constrictive phase of healing was complete. Wharton in 1938, at the Johns Hopkins Hospital, combined an adequate dissection of the vaginal space with continuous dilatation by a balsa form covered with a thin rubber sheath and left in the space. Rather than using a split-thickness skin graft, Wharton based his operation on the principle that the vaginal epithelium has remarkable powers of proliferation and in a relatively short time will cover the raw surface. Recalling that a similar process occurs in the fetus when the epithelium of the sinovaginal bulbs and urogenital sinus form the vaginal canal, Wharton merely applied this same principle in the adult. This simple procedure is entirely satisfactory as long as the space is kept dilated long enough to allow the epithelium to grow in. But occasionally, even after several years, the vault of the vagina remains without epithelial covering. Coital bleeding and leukorrhea result from the persistent granulation tissue and there is a tendency for vaginas constructed by this method to be constricted from scarring in the upper portion. In Counseller's 1948 report from the Mayo Clinic of 100 operations to construct a new vagina, 14 were done by Wharton's method, with excellent results in all 14 patients. It was stated that the disadvantages of persistent granulation tissue with bleeding and leukorrhea were of no consequence. This has not been the experience of the editors of this book.

When inlay skin grafts were first used to construct a new vagina, the results were poor because the necessity for dilatation of the new vagina was not recognized. Severe contraction, uncontrolled by continuous or intermittent dilatation, almost invariably spoiled the results. Although Heppner, Abbe, and others had preceded him by many years in using a skin-covered prosthesis in neovaginal construction, it was Sir Archibald McIndoe at the Queen Victoria Hospital in England who popularized the method and gave it substantial clinical trial. He emphasized the three important principles used today in the operation for vaginal agenesis: (1) dissection of an adequate space between the rectum and the bladder, (2) inlay split-thickness skin grafting, and (3) the cardinal principle of continuous and prolonged dilatation during the contractile phase of healing.

Other tissues such as amnion and peritoneum have

been used to line the new vaginal space, but usually without substantial success. However, Tancer, Katz, and Veridiano reported good results with human amnion. Karjalainen and associates stated that a more physiologic result was achieved with an amnion graft than with a skin graft. Nevertheless, concerns about the transmission of human immunodeficiency virus with human amnion will limit this option.

Technique of the Abbe-Wharton-McIndoe Operation

TAKING THE GRAFT. After a careful pelvic examination is done under anesthesia to verify previous findings, the patient is then positioned for taking a skin graft from the buttocks. For cosmetic reasons, the graft should not be taken from the thigh or hip unless for some reason it cannot be obtained from the buttocks. Patients may be asked to sunbathe in a brief bathing suit before coming to the hospital so that its outline can be seen; an attempt should be made to take the graft from both buttocks within these borders. The quality of the graft will determine to a great extent the success of the operation. We have found the Padgett's electrodermatome to be the most satisfactory instrument for taking the graft. With relatively little experience and practice, the gynecologic surgeon can cut a graft successfully. A graft of controlled width and thickness can be cut (Fig. 25-5). The instrument is set and checked for taking a graft approximately 0.018 inch thick and 8–9 cm wide. The total graft length should be 16–20 cm. If the graft cannot be taken from one buttock, then a graft 8–10 cm long will be needed from each buttock.

The skin of the donor site is prepared with an antiseptic solution (povidone iodine), which should be thoroughly washed away. It is then lubricated with mineral oil. Assistants steady and stretch the skin tight.

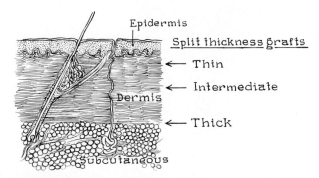

Figure 25–5. The skin graft should be uniform in thickness. Padgett's electrodermatome is set to take a graft approximately 0.018 inch thick. A graft that is a little too thick is better than a thin graft.

Considerable pressure is made uniformly across the dermatome blade. The thickness of the graft must have minimal variation. A graft that is a little too thick is better than one a little too thin. There should be no breaks in the continuity of the graft. The graft is placed between two layers of moist gauze and the donor sites are dressed. The donor site is soaked with a dilute solution of epinephrine for hemostasis and a sterile dressing is applied. A pressure dressing is then placed over the site and may be removed on the seventh postoperative day. The sterile dressing will dry in place over the donor site and ultimately will fall off of its own accord. Moistened areas on the dressing may be dried with cool air. If there is separation and evidence of some superficial infection, then mebromin may be applied to these areas.

CREATING THE NEOVAGINAL SPACE. The patient is placed in the lithotomy position and a transverse incision is made through the mucosa of the vaginal vestibule as shown in Figure 25-6A. The space between the urethra and bladder anteriorly and the rectum posteriorly is dissected until the undersurface of the peritoneum is reached. This step may be made safer by placing a catheter in the urethra and sometimes a finger in the rectum to guide the dissection in the proper plane. After incising the mucosa of the vaginal vestibule transversely, the physician often is able to create a channel on each side of a median raphe (Fig. 25-6B), starting with blunt dissection and then dilating each channel with Hegar's dilators or with finger dissection. In some instances, it may be necessary to develop the neovaginal space by dissecting laterally and then bringing the fingers toward the midline. The median raphe is divided (Fig. 25-6B), thus joining the two channels. This maneuver is helpful in dissecting an adequate space without injury to surrounding structures.

To avoid subsequent narrowing of the vagina at the level of the urogenital diaphragm, it may be helpful to incise the margin of the puborectalis muscles bilaterally along the midportion of the medial margin (Fig. 25-7). Although useful in all patients, incising the puborectalis muscle is particularly important in the patient with the androgen insensitivity syndrome, who has an android pelvis where the levator muscles are more taut against the pelvic diaphragm, rather than in the patient who has a gynecoid pelvis. The patient experiences no difficulty with fecal incontinence with this procedure and it has significantly improved the ease with which the vaginal form can be inserted into the canal in the postoperative period. Use of this procedure also has eliminated the problem of contracture of the upper vagina because of a poorly applied form. The dissection should be carried as high as possible without entering the peritoneal cavity and without cleaning away all tissue beneath the peritoneum. A split-thickness skin graft will not take

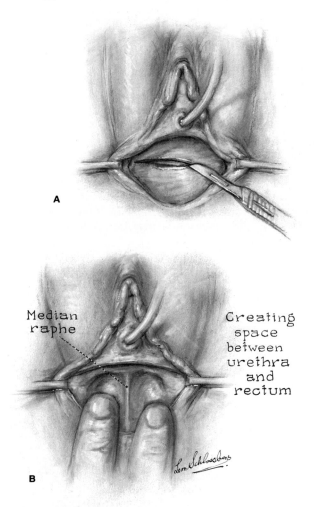

A

B

Median raphe

Creating space between urethra and rectum

Figure 25–6. The McIndoe procedure. *A*, A transverse incision is made in the apex of the vaginal dimple. *B*, A channel can usually be dissected on each side of a median raphe. The median raphe is then divided. Careful dissection will prevent injury to the bladder and rectum.

well when applied against a base of thin peritoneum. Care must be taken to ligate all bleeders. They are clamped and tied with very fine sutures. It is essential to have the vaginal cavity dry to prevent bleeding beneath the graft. Bleeding will cause the graft to separate from its bed, resulting in the inevitable failure of the graft to implant in that area and in local graft necrosis.

PREPARING THE VAGINAL FORM. Formerly, the skin graft was placed over a balsa form. Balsa has many advantages. It is an inexpensive, easily available, and light wood, and it can be sterilized without difficulty. It also can be whittled easily in the operating room to a proper shape to fit the new vaginal space. However, in some instances, pressure from the form will cause the skin graft to slough in places. Furthermore, if there are

pressure spots there is an increased risk of fistula formation. In place of a rigid form, the physician can use the Counseller-Flor (1957) modification of the McIndoe technique (Fig. 25-8), which uses a foam rubber mold covered with a condom. A form for the vaginal cavity is shaped from a foam rubber block (Fig. 25-8*A*). The material is gas sterilized in blocks measuring approximately $10 \times 10 \times 20$ cm. The block is shaped with scissors to approximately twice the desired size and compressed by covering it with a condom (Fig. 25-8*B*). The compressed form is placed into the neovagina (Fig. 25-8*C*). The form is left in place for 20–30 seconds with a condom open to allow the foam rubber to expand and conform to the neovaginal space (Fig. 25-8*D*). The condom is then closed and the form is withdrawn. The external end is tied with No. 2-0 silk and an additional condom is placed over the form (Fig. 25-8*E*) and tied securely (Fig. 25-8*F*).

SEWING THE GRAFT OVER THE VAGINAL FORM. The skin graft may then be placed over the form and its undersurface exteriorized and sewn over the form with interrupted vertical mattress No. 5-0 nonreactive sutures (Fig. 25-8*G*). Where the graft is approximated, the undersurfaces of the sutured edges are also exteriorized.

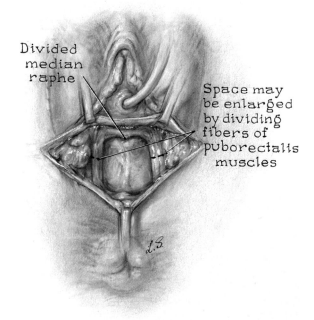

Divided median raphe

Space may be enlarged by dividing fibers of puborectalis muscles

Figure 25–7. The McIndoe procedure. A space between the urethra and bladder anteriorly and the rectum posteriorly is dissected until the undersurface of the peritoneum is reached. Incision of the medial margin of the puborectalis muscles will enlarge the vagina laterally.

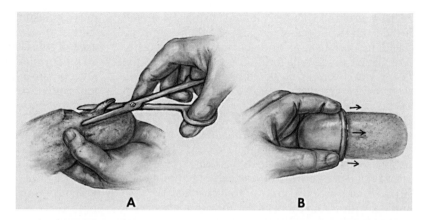

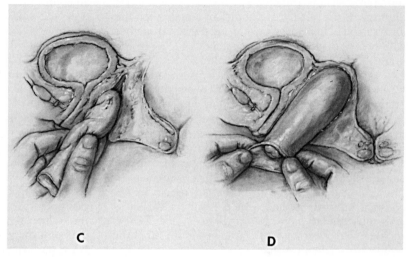

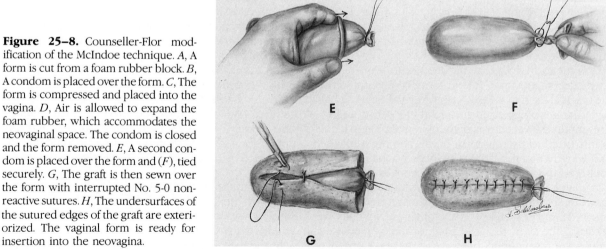

Figure 25–8. Counseller-Flor modification of the McIndoe technique. *A,* A form is cut from a foam rubber block. *B,* A condom is placed over the form. *C,* The form is compressed and placed into the vagina. *D,* Air is allowed to expand the foam rubber, which accommodates the neovaginal space. The condom is closed and the form removed. *E,* A second condom is placed over the form and (*F*), tied securely. *G,* The graft is then sewn over the form with interrupted No. 5-0 nonreactive sutures. *H,* The undersurfaces of the sutured edges of the graft are exteriorized. The vaginal form is ready for insertion into the neovagina.

The graft should not be "meshed" to make it stretch farther, and the edges of the graft should be approximated meticulously around the form without gaps. Granulation tissue will form at any place where the form is not covered with skin. Contraction usually will occur where granulation tissue forms. Once the form has been placed in the neovaginal space, the edges of the graft are sutured to the skin edge with No. 5-0 nonreactive absorbable suture, allowing sufficient space between sutures for drainage to occur. The physician must be careful not to have the form so large as to cause undue pressure on the urethra or rectum. A balsa form should have a groove to accommodate the urethra. With a foam rubber form, this is unnecessary. A suprapubic silicone catheter is placed in the bladder for drainage. If the labia are of sufficient length, then the form can be held in place by suturing the labia together with two or three nonreactive sutures.

REPLACING WITH A NEW FORM. After 7–10 days, the form is removed and the vaginal cavity is irrigated with warm saline solution and inspected. Usually this can be done with the use of mild sedation and without an anesthetic. The cavity should be inspected carefully to determine if the graft has taken satisfactorily in all areas of the new vagina. Any undue pressure by the form should be noted and corrected. It is especially important that the form not make too much pressure superiorly against the peritoneum of the cul-de-sac. Such a constant upward pressure could result in weakness with subsequent enterocele formation. A new form is molded with a sterile sheath cover (condom) to fit the size of the vaginal canal.

The patient is given instructions on its daily removal and reinsertion and taught how to administer a low-pressure douche of clear warm water. She is advised to remove the form at the time of urination and defecation, but otherwise to wear it continuously for 6 weeks. A neopreme form, which is much easier to remove and keep clean than a foam rubber form, is substituted for the original form in 6 weeks. However, the new vaginal cavity must be inspected frequently to detect and to prevent pressure necrosis of the skin graft. The patient is instructed to use the form during the night for the following 12 months. If there has been no change in the caliber of the vagina by that time, then it is unlikely to occur later and the insertion of the form at night may be done intermittently until coitus is a frequent occurrence. However, if there is the slightest difficulty in inserting the form, then the patient should be advised to use the form continuously again. Most patients are able to maintain the form in place by simply wearing a panty girdle and perineal pad. Douches are advisable while there is residual vaginal healing and discharge.

Results and Complications. The serious complications formerly associated with the McIndoe operation have been significantly reduced in recent years by improvements in technique and greater experience. Results also have improved. Recently reported percentages of satisfactory results have ranged from 80% to 100%. Serious complications still occur, including a 4% postoperative fistula rate (urethrovaginal, vesicovaginal, and rectovaginal). Postoperative infection, intraoperative and postoperative hemorrhage, and failure of graft take are still reported as occasional complications. Failure of graft take often will lead to the development of granulation tissue, with the possible requirement for reoperation, curettement of the granulation tissue down to a healthy base, and even regrafting. Minor granulation may be treated with silver nitrate application. The functional result is more important than the anatomical result in evaluating the success of this operation. Although a vagina of only 4 cm may be adequate for some couples, in most instances, a vagina of < 4 cm causes major problems.

Because of the excellent results obtained following a modified McIndoe vaginoplasty, this operation is recommended as the procedure of choice in women who are unable or unwilling to obtain a neovagina using dilatation methods. Women with a flat perineum with no dimple or pouch have no alternative other than the McIndoe vaginoplasty to obtain a neovagina for comfortable sexual relations.

Between 1950 and 1989, the McIndoe operation was done on 94 patients at the Johns Hopkins Hospital. The postoperative results have improved significantly since the balsa vaginal form has been replaced by a foam rubber form. In the 39 years in which this operation has been performed at this institution, 83% of the 94 patients had a 100% take of the graft; in only three cases was there a significant area where the graft failed.

Urethrovaginal fistula has become even more infrequent since the introduction of the suprapubic catheter and the foam rubber form. The catheter is removed when the patient is voiding well and has no residual urine. In general, the patient is able to void without difficulty within the first few days following the procedure. Use of prophylactic broad-spectrum antibiotics, started within 12 hours before surgery and continued for 7 days, is of definite value in reducing the incidence of graft failures from infection in the operative site.

It is important that a McIndoe operation be done correctly the first time. If the vagina becomes constricted because of granulation tissue formation, injury to adjacent structures, or failure to use the form properly, then subsequent attempts to create a satisfactory vagina will be more difficult. The first operation has the best chance of success.

DEVELOPMENT OF MALIGNANCIES. At least 10 case reports exist of malignant disease developing in a vagina created by various techniques; these reports were reviewed by Gallup, Castle, and Stock. The authors reported a patient who was initially treated for intra-epithelial malignancy by total vaginectomy combined with a split-thickness skin graft vaginoplasty to reconstruct a functional vagina. The authors noted a lesion in her vaginal apex 7 years later. These findings suggest that epithelium transplanted to the vagina also may assume the oncogenic potential of the lower tract. It is therefore important that patients have long-term follow-up examinations following split-thickness skin graft vaginoplasty.

The Williams Vulvovaginoplasty

Although construction of a "perineal bridge" to help contain the vaginal mold was a routine part of the operation described by McIndoe, it was not adopted subsequently by others. However, Williams described a similar vulvovaginoplasty procedure in 1964 and advised that it could be used to create a vaginal canal. In 1976, he reported that the procedure was unsuccessful in only 1 out of 52 patients. Feroze, Dewhurst, and Welply reported that the anatomical results were good in 22 out of 26 patients. According to these authors, the advantages of the Williams operation are its technical simplicity, the absence of serious local complications even when the operation is done as a repeat procedure, the ease of postoperative care, the absence of postoperative pain and the speed of recovery, the absence of a need of dilators and the consequent applicability of the operation to patients who do not intend to have regular intercourse in the near future, and the higher success rate of primary and repeat procedures. The technique is not applicable to patients who have poorly developed labia. It does result in an unusual angle of the vaginal canal, which is reported to straighten out to a more normal direction with intercourse. If a very high perineum is created, urine may momentarily collect in the pouch following urination, giving the impression of postvoid incontinence. Failure of the suture line to heal by primary intention will result in a large area of granulation tissue and most likely an unsatisfactory result.

Williams believes that if the urethral meatus is patulous, a vulvovaginoplasty should not be done because of the possibility that the urethra will be stretched farther by coitus. He suggests that deficiencies in muscular and fascial tissue may be the reason that some patients with uterovaginal agenesis are able to develop a satisfactory vaginal canal with simple intermittent pressure with coitus and some are prone to develop enteroceles.

The technique of vulvovaginoplasty, as described by Williams, is as follows. A horseshoe-shaped incision is made in the vulva. It extends across the perineum and up the medial side of the labia to the level of the external urethral meatus. The success of the operation depends on the appropriation of sufficient skin to line the new vagina. For this reason, the initial mucosal incisions are made as close to the hairline as possible and approximately 4 cm from the midline. After complete mobilization, the inner skin margins are sutured together with knots tied inside the vaginal lumen (Fig. 25-9A). A second layer of sutures approximates subcutaneous fat and perineal muscles for support (Fig. 25-9B). Finally, the external skin margins are approximated with interrupted sutures (Fig. 25-9C). If the procedure is properly done, it should be possible to insert two fingers into the pouch for a depth of 3 cm. An indwelling bladder catheter is used. The patient is confined to bed for 1 week in an effort to avoid tension on the suture line. Examinations are avoided for 6 weeks, at which time the patient is instructed to use dilators.

Capraro and Gallego have advised a modification of this technique. They make the U-shaped incision in the skin of the labia majora at the level of the urethra or even lower. It is claimed that this modification will result in a vulva that is more normal to sight and to touch, that trapping of stagnant urine in the vaginal pouch will be avoided, and that the vagina will still be satisfactory for intercourse. Other modifications have been made by Feroze and associates.

The Williams vulvovaginoplasty is a useful operation and should certainly be considered as the operation of choice in patients who may need a supplement to an unsatisfactory McIndoe operation or a supplement to a small vagina resulting from extensive surgery or radiation therapy, Rarely will a patient with a solitary kidney low in the pelvis not have room for dissection of an adequate vaginal space.

Acquired Vaginal Inadequacy

Although unusual types of infection and atrophy may result in closure of part of the vagina, although rarely, acquired vaginal inadequacy most often results from the treatment of various gynecologic malignancies with surgery or radiation or a combination of both. The maintenance or restoration of vaginal function is now considered an important part of the treatment plan for such malignancies, especially when the patient is young and otherwise healthy. The techniques of vaginal reconstruction in gynecologic oncology have been reviewed by Magrina and Masterson, by Pratt, and by McCraw and associates.

DISORDERS OF VERTICAL FUSION

The problems associated with vertical fusion include transverse vaginal septum with or without obstruction. Although imperforate hymen is a vertical fusion problem, the hymen is not a derivative of the müllerian

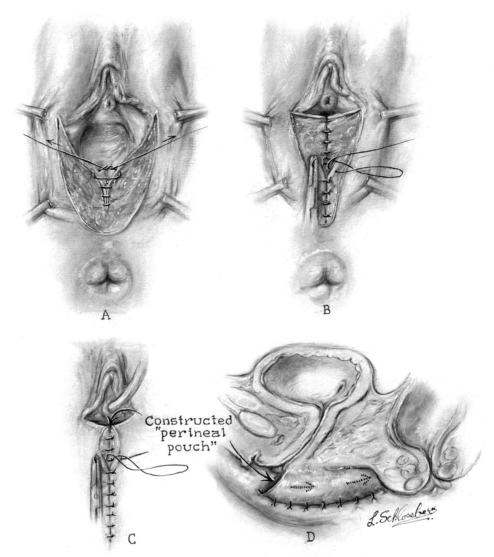

Figure 25–9. The Williams vulvovaginoplasty. *A–C,* No. 3-0 polyglycolic acid sutures may be used throughout to close both inner and outer skin margins and the tissue between. *D,* The entrance to the pouch should not cover the external urethral meatus.

ducts; therefore, this condition is discussed elsewhere (see Ch. 40).

Transverse Vaginal Septum

No reliable epidemiologic data exist regarding the incidence of transverse vaginal septum. Reported incidences vary from 1 in 2100 to 1 in 72,000. It is probably less common than congenital absence of the vagina and uterus. It has been diagnosed in newborns, infants, and older adolescent girls. Its etiology is unknown, al-

though McKusick has suggested that in some and perhaps most cases it results from a female sex-limited autosomal recessive transmission. Obviously, there is a developmental defect in vaginal embryogenesis that leads to an incomplete fusion between the müllerian duct component and the urogenital sinus component of the vagina. The incomplete vertical fusion results in a transverse vaginal septum (AFS Class IA). The septum varies in thickness. It can be located at almost any level in the vagina (Fig. 25-10). Lodi has reported that 46% occur in the upper vagina, 40% in the midvagina, and 14% in the lower vagina. Rock and Associates have

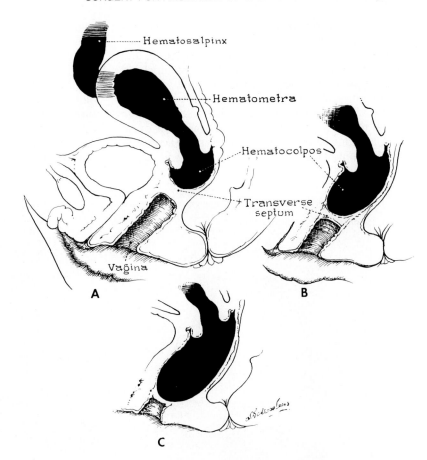

Figure 25–10. Positions of a septum responsible for complete vaginal obstruction. *A*, High, *B*, mid, and *C*, low transverse vaginal septum. Note the position of the hematocolpos. Lower vaginal septa allow more blood to accumulate in the upper vagina. The vaginal mass shown in *C* may be more readily appreciated on rectovaginal exam.

noted septa in the upper, middle, and lower thirds of the vagina in 46%, 35%, and 19% of patients, respectively. In general, the thicker septum is noted to be more common closer to the uterine cervix. In contrast to congenital absence of the müllerian ducts, the transverse vaginal septum is associated with few urologic or other anomalies. Imperforate anus and bicornuate uterus may be found, as reported by Mandell, Stevens, and Lucey. The lower surface of the transverse septum is always covered by squamous epithelium. The upper surface may be covered by glandular epithelium, which is likely to be transformed into squamous epithelium by a metaplastic process after correction of the obstruction.

In neonates and young infants, imperforate transverse vaginal septum with obstruction may lead to serious and life-threatening problems caused by the compression of surrounding organs by fluid that has collected above the septum. The fluid undoubtedly comes from endocervical glands and müllerian glandular epithelium in the upper vagina that have been stimulated by the placental transfer of maternal estrogen. Continued fluid collection in infants even after the first year also has been reported; thus the physician should consider the possibility of a fistula between the upper vagina and the urinary tract. The distended upper vagina creates a large pelvic and lower abdominal mass that may displace the bladder anteriorly; displace the ureters laterally with hydroureters and hydronephrosis; compress the rectum with associated obstipation and even intestinal obstruction; and limit diaphragmatic excursion, compress the vena cava, and produce cardiorespiratory failure. Fatalities have been reported. The hydrocolpos develops along the axis of the upper vagina and, therefore, may not cause the outlet or perineum to bulge when there is compression of the mass from above. After careful preoperative radiologic and endoscopic investigations of the infant, the septum should be removed through a perineal approach. Bilateral Schuchardt's incisions may be required to ensure that the septum has been removed. Because of a subsequent tendency for vaginal stenosis and reaccumulation of the fluid in the upper vagina, follow-up studies to assess the recurrence of urinary obstruction are important. Vaginal reconstruction may be required in later years to allow satisfactory menstruation and coitus.

A hematocolpos may not develop until puberty. Patients with this problem will present with cyclic lower abdominal pain, no visible menstrual discharge, and gradual development of a central lower abdominal and pelvic mass. Sometimes a small tract will open in the septum, some menstrual blood will escape periodically, and symptoms will be variable. A septum large enough to allow pregnancy to occur may still cause dystocia during labor. Cyclic hematuria may be present if a communication between the bladder and upper vagina exists. The pelvic organs of a woman who had a transverse vaginal septum are shown diagrammatically in Figure 25-11. The woman had difficulty at the time of onset of menstruation with the development of severe cyclic pain, but no external bleeding. Finally, menstrual blood began to flow externally through the small sinus shown in Figure 25-11A. Pelvic examination per rectum revealed a cervix and a normal-sized corpus. The ovaries were palpable, but adherent, probably because of organized blood from hematosalpinx and hema-

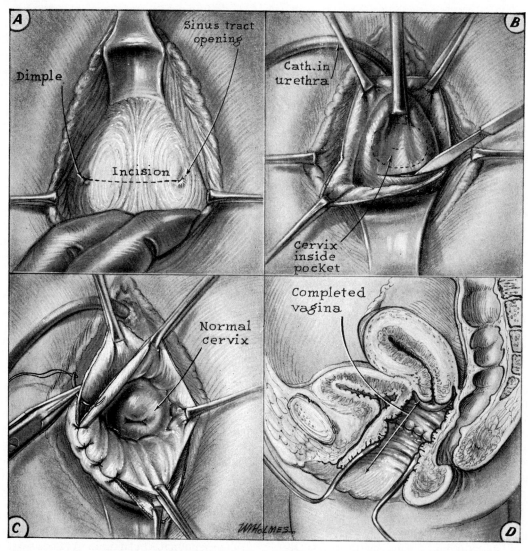

Figure 25–11. Surgical correction of transverse vaginal septum. *A*, The upper end of a short vagina. The small sinus tract opening, through which the patient menstruated, is shown. The line of incision is drawn through the mucous membrane between the vaginal dimple and the sinus. *B*, Areolar tissue is dissected through to the pocket of mucosa which covered the cervix. The mucosa is incised. *C*, An anastomosis is made between the lower vagina and the upper vagina. *D*, Completed vagina. It is slightly shorter than normal but of normal caliber.

toperitoneum. Remarkably, the woman had little dysmenorrhea after beginning to menstruate externally. Coitus was fairly satisfactory before surgical correction, but the shortness of the vagina was something of a handicap. The obstructing membrane was excised and an anastomosis of the upper and lower vagina performed (Fig. 25-11*B–D*).

Reported experiences at the Johns Hopkins Hospital among 26 patients with complete transverse vaginal septum have indicated findings of associated congenital anomalies of the urinary tract, coarctation of the aorta, atrial septal defect, and malformations of the lumbar spine. Vaginal patency and coital function were successfully established in all patients, and 7 out of 19 patients attempting pregnancy eventually had children. The incidence of endometriosis and spontaneous abortion was high. A lower pregnancy rate and more extensive endometriosis were present when the transverse septum was located high in the vagina, suggesting that retrograde flow through the uterus and fallopian tubes occurs earlier in these patients. More extensive dissection between the bladder and rectum is required to identify the upper vagina when the septum is thick and high. In five patients, an exploratory laparotomy was necessary to guide a probe through the uterine fundus and cervix and to assist in locating a high hematocolpos.

Surgical Technique for a Transverse Vaginal Septum

A transverse incision is made through the vault of the short vagina (Fig. 25-11*A*). A probe can be introduced through the septum after a portion of the barrier has been separated by sharp and blunt dissection. The physician usually finds some areolar tissue in dissecting the space between the vagina and the rectum. Palpation of a urethral catheter anteriorly and insertion of a double-gloved finger along the anterior wall of the rectum posteriorly will provide the proper surgical guidelines so that the bladder and rectum can be avoided during this blind procedure. After the dissection is continued for a short distance, the cervix can usually be palpated, and continuity can be established with the upper segment of the vagina (Fig. 25-11*B* and *C*). The lateral margins of the excised septum are extended widely by sharp knife dissection to avoid postoperative stricture formation. The edges of the upper and the lower vaginal mucosa are undermined and mobilized enough to permit anastomosis, using interrupted delayed-absorbable sutures (Fig. 25-11*C*). Figure 25-11*D* shows the completed anastomosis with a vagina that is of normal caliber but slightly shorter than the average length. A soft foam rubber vaginal form covered with a sterile latex sheath may be placed in the vagina and removed in 10 days for evaluation of the healing process. The form may be worn for 4–6 weeks until complete healing has occurred. After this, coitus is permitted. If the patient is not sexually active, then vaginal dilatation may be necessary to maintain established patency. Alternatively, a silicone elastomer (Silastic) vaginal form may be inserted at night until the constrictive phase of healing is complete.

High Transverse Vaginal Septum. If the length of the obstructing transverse vaginal septum is such that reanastomosis of the upper and lower vagina is impossible, as is the case with a high transverse vaginal septum where a significant portion of vagina is atretic, then a space is created between the rectum and bladder to permit identification of the obstructed vagina. The mass that has resulted from accumulated menstrual blood must be distinguished from the bladder anteriorly and the rectum posteriorly, a process that may be facilitated by the mass itself (Figs. 25-12 and 25-13). When differentiation is impossible, however, exploratory laparotomy may be performed. During this procedure, a probe is passed through the fundus of the uterus to tent out the vaginal septum (Fig. 25-13*B*), enabling the surgeon to incise it from below and resect it safely. In most surgical procedures to remove the high transverse vaginal septum, the obstructing membrane may be readily identified, after which the operator may probe the mass with an aspirating needle to identify old menstrual blood (Fig. 25-12*C*). The upper vagina is then opened and the septum excised.

Because the distance between the septum and the upper vagina is too great to permit an anastomosis, an indwelling acrylic resin (Lucite) form (Fig. 25-13*C*), consisting of a bulbous end and a channel through which menstrual blood may drain, is placed into the vagina and anchored with a retaining harness. The bulbous end of the form will in most instances be retained in the upper vagina and should be left in place for 4–6 months while epithelialization is accomplished. Following removal of the acrylic resin (Lucite) form, vaginal dilatation should be practiced on a daily basis for 2–4 months to prevent contracture of the space. Alternatively, the physician may consider the use of a split-thickness graft to bridge the gap. The graft is usually sutured in situ in the vagina rather than suturing it to a form. It is essential to the success of the operation that the new space not become constricted; to avoid constriction, the form must be worn for many months during the constrictive phase of healing. Alternatively, a rather ingenious but complicated *Z*-plasty method of bridging the gap has been described by Garcia and by Musset. A simpler flap method was described by Brenner, Sedlis, and Cooperman.

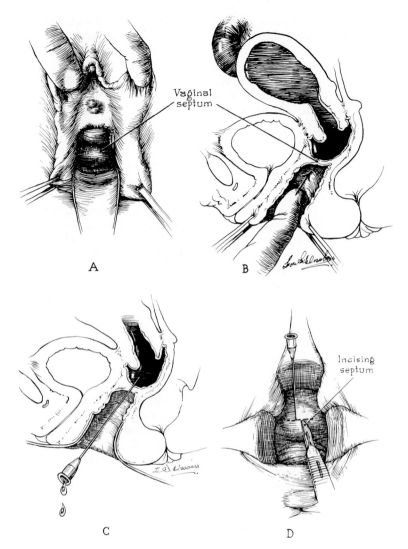

Figure 25–12. A high transverse vaginal septum. *A*, The neovaginal space is dissected, revealing a high obstructing vaginal membrane. *B*, This may be palpated with the middle finger. *C*, A needle is then placed into the mass, over which the incision is made with a sharp knife (*D*).

Congenital Absence or Dysgenesis of the Cervix

Agenesis or atresia of the cervix (AFS Class IB) is a relatively infrequent müllerian anomaly. When this anomaly does occur, it is often in association with absence of a portion or all of the vagina. In many cases of cervical agenesis or atresia, retention of menstrual blood initiates symptoms of cyclic lower abdominal pain without menstrual flow, resulting in the patient seeking gynecologic evaluation and care. The diagnosis of cervical agenesis or atresia is usually difficult before operation. In the past, diagnosis was suspected on the basis of a history and physical findings but was not proven until the time of surgery. The possibility of making a correct diagnosis before surgery offers signif-

icant advantages in patient care, the most important of which is effective presurgical planning and preparation.

Diagnosis of Cervical Dysgenesis

Patients with congenital absence of the cervix present a diagnostic challenge. Patients with cervical aplasia with a functioning midline uterine corpus have aplasia of the lower two thirds of the vagina with an upper vaginal pouch. Similarly, some patients will have a considerable atretic segment of vagina and an upper vaginal pouch with a properly developed uterine cervix and corpus above. Differentiation of these two müllerian anomalies is essential. Ultrasonography may be helpful. Valdes, Malini, and Malinak have reported use of preoperative ultrasonography in the evaluation of

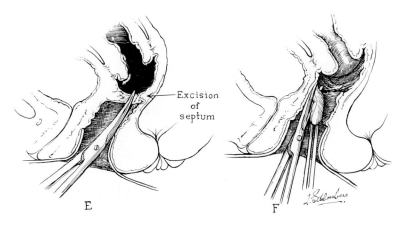

Figure 25–12. (continued) *E* and *F*, The high transverse vaginal septum is usually thick and considerable bleeding may occur when excised with Mayo scissors. *G*, After the septum is removed, the wall of the septum is oversewn with interrupted sutures of No. 2-0 chromic catgut. Because the distance between the septum and the upper vagina is too great to allow anastomosis, an acrylic resin (Lucite) form is placed in the vagina such that epithelialization may occur over the form while vaginal patency is maintained. *H*, The form is in place and fitted with a plastic retainer. Rubber strips may be placed through the retainer and attached to a waist belt to allow constant upper pressure so that the form is retained in the upper vagina. Modification of this method includes a small adapter to allow drainage through the acrylic resin (Lucite) form, preventing the accumulation of old blood and mucus in the upper vagina. (Rock J: Anomalous development of the vagina. Seminars in Reproduction. Endocrinology 1986;4:24.)

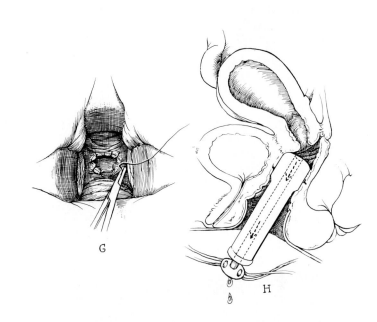

two patients with atresia of the vagina and the cervix. Magnetic resonance imaging (MRI) has been found to be helpful in confirming this diagnosis, as reported by Markham and associates. The lower uterine segment and cervical tissue may be carefully examined as demonstrated in Figure 25-14. With cervical dysgenesis, there is no vaginal dilatation with the accumulation of blood as seen with a high transverse vaginal septum. Both ultrasonography and MRI are most helpful when they are correlated with the findings of a careful pelvic examination under anesthesia.

Anatomical Variations of Congenital Cervical Anomalies

Cervical anomalies have been observed in three basic configurations (Fig. 25-15). In the first type, there is

total absence (aplasia) of the uterine cervix. There is a narrowing of the lower uterine segment terminating in a peritoneal sleeve at a point well above the normal communication with the vaginal apex (Fig. 25-15A). A second variety has been identified where there are small inclusions of endocervical-type tissue within a bed of fibrous tissue (Fig. 25-15B). Finally, in rare instances, there is total atresia of the endocervical canal with cervical stroma being present but without canalization of the internal and external os (Fig. 25-15C). There is a unique histologic finding of muscle bundles extending as an uninterrupted bridge around the closed end of the cervical canal. Microscopic sections through the cervix reveal endocervical glands within the normal lamina propria. However, the muscle bundles deeper in the cervix are more linearly arranged than is normally found and then extended as a complete

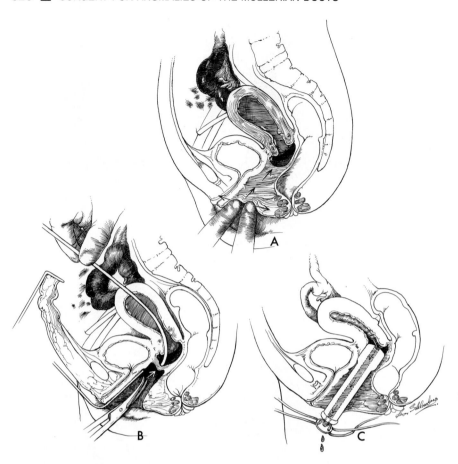

Figure 25–13. Correction of an atretic vagina. *A*, A large portion of atretic vagina is palpated with two fingers. Once the vaginal space is developed, it may be necessary to open the abdomen and pass a probe through to the uterine fundus (*B*) to tent out the septum, which may then be safely excised. *C*, The acrylic resin (Lucite) form is then placed into the upper vagina and secured with rubber straps.

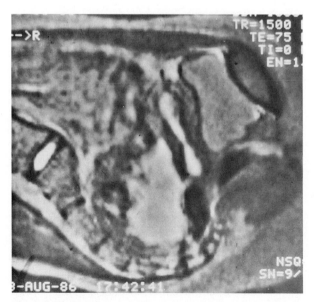

Figure 25–14. MRI T1 image showing atretic segment of distal cervix. The tip of an atretic cervix (*arrow*) is shown. There is no vagina noted.

uninterrupted bridge around the closed end of the cervical canal. This observation may explain the difficulty in reestablishing the endocervical canal in cases of distal cervical atresia.

Treatment

When the vagina and cervix are both absent and a functioning uterine corpus is present, it is difficult to obtain a satisfactory fistulous tract through which menstruation may occur. Many methods have been tried, most involving the creation of a passage through the dense fibrous tissue between the uterine cavity and the vagina with placement of a stent to keep the tract open. Occasionally, success in maintaining an open passageway has been reported and patients have experienced a normal cyclic menstruation. However, endocervical glands do not develop and there is no way to compensate for the absence of the cervical mucus, which plays an important role in sperm transport. Even though cyclic ovulatory periods can be achieved with a few patients, pregnancy will be unlikely. Eventually, the

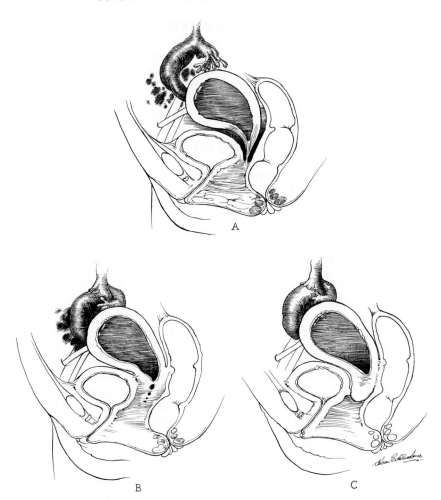

Figure 25–15. Congenital absence of dysgenesis of the cervix. *A,* Cervical agenesis. *B,* Malformed cervix with islands of endocervical glands present. *C,* A bulbous cervical stroma without an endocervical canal.

uterovaginal tract closes from constriction by fibrous tissue. Endometriosis may develop along the tract. Endometriosis also may develop in ovaries and other pelvic sites because of retrograde menstruation. Recurrent and severe pelvic infection is a common problem and may require total hysterectomy and removal of both ovaries. With the advent of in vitro fertilization and the prospect of having a host uterus possibly carry a pregnancy to term, procedures to establish a fistulous tract largely have been abandoned. Nevertheless, Cukier and associates reported treating a patient with congenital absence of the cervix by construction of a splint that extends into the neocervical canal such that a split-thickness skin graft could actually be placed within the endocervical canal. This patient has continued to menstruate without difficulty, although pregnancy has not been accomplished.

Many authors have recommended that a patient with a functioning uterine corpus who has congenital absence of a cervix and a vagina should have a hysterectomy as an initial procedure. A hysterectomy will eliminate much needless suffering from cryptomenorrhea, sepsis, and endometriosis, as well as multiple operations. If a hysterectomy can be done soon enough, then it may be possible to conserve the ovaries and their useful functions for years to come. Despite recommendations to the contrary in articles by Farber and Marchant and Farber and Mitchell, most authors agree with Geary and Weed, Maciulla, Heine, and Christian, Dillon, Mudaliar, and Wingate, Niver, Barrette, and Jewelewicz, and Jones and Rock that a recommendation for a hysterectomy as an initial primary therapy in these cases seems realistic with few exceptions. The reconstructive surgeon should be prepared to perform a vaginoplasty using a split-thickness graft if hysterectomy is performed. This is particularly true if there has been a vaginal dissection. If the neovaginal space is allowed to close and scar, then future operations to develop an adequate neovagina are associated with increased risks of graft failure and fistula formation.

DISORDERS OF LATERAL FUSION

The final group in the classification of vaginal anomalies results from failure of lateral fusion of the two müllerian ducts, which may be obstructed or unobstructed.

Unobstructed Lateral Fusion Disorders

Double Uterus (Bicornuate, Septate, or Didelphic Uterus)

Complete failure of medial fusion of the two müllerian ducts may result in a complete duplication of the vagina, cervix, and uterus. A partial failure of fusion may result in a single vagina with a single or duplicate cervix and complete or partial duplication of the uterine corpus. A failure of absorption of the uterine septum between the two fused müllerian ducts may result in the septum persisting inside the uterus to a variable extent while the external appearance is that of a single uterus. The septum may be so complete that it divides both the uterine cavity and endocervical canal into two equal or unequal components. More commonly, incomplete disappearance of the septum may leave only the upper uterine cavities divided. Each of these and a variety of other forms of "double uteri" have their own special clinical significance. When no obstruction is present, surgical reconstruction has been done primarily for difficulties with reproduction.

Some aspects of this subject remain controversial because information is still inaccurate or incomplete. Many reports are based on small samples of selected patients, patients have been diagnosed to have one anomaly or another based on incomplete data, and some patients have received unification operations without preliminary studies to rule out other causes of reproductive difficulty. A comparison of results from one series to the next may be difficult because authors have used different classifications based on a variety of embryologic, anatomical, physiologic, functional, or radiologic considerations. An unknown number of uterine anomalies escape detection, especially if the patient has an acceptable reproductive performance and no gynecologic difficulties.

Historical Development of Surgical Procedures. Ruge, in 1882, first reported excision of a uterine septum in a woman who had undergone two abortions. The woman subsequently carried a pregnancy to term. Paul Strassmann of Berlin and later Erwin Strassmann, his son, were strong advocates of uterine unification operations. The studies of Jones and Jones have greatly improved the understanding and management of patients with uterine anomalies. Their studies began with a report in 1953 of a series that was started in 1936. Updates have been published from time to time. Wheeless, Rock, Andrews, and others have joined in these reports.

Diagnosis of Uterine Anomalies. If a uterine anomaly is associated with obstruction of menstrual flow, then it will cause symptoms that will come to the attention of the gynecologist shortly after menarche. Unobstructed uterine anomalies will be diagnosed later in a variety of circumstances. Young girls may notice difficulty in using tampons or later in coitus if a longitudinal vaginal septum is present. This can lead to the diagnosis of an associated uterine anomaly. A patient with an anomalous upper urinary tract on intravenous pyelogram may be found to have a uterine anomaly when referred for gynecologic evaluation. A uterine anomaly may occasionally be found when a patient complains of dysmenorrhea or menorrhagia or when a dilation and curettage (D & C) is done for abortion or some other indication. A palpable mass may be found to be a uterine anomaly when confirmed by ultrasonography, by hysterography, or by laparoscopy. As Semmens has pointed out, the diagnosis of uterine anomaly may result from the astute observation of an abnormal uterine contour during pregnancy, either in the antepartum period or at the time of abdominal or vaginal delivery. The abnormal contour is caused by a combination of fetal malpresentation and an anomalous uterus. An anomalous uterus may be diagnosed when a patient becomes pregnant despite the presence of an intrauterine contraceptive device. Persistent postmenopausal bleeding despite recent D & C may lead to a diagnosis of an anomalous uterus. Sometimes the diagnosis is made as an incidental finding at laparotomy. However, most uterine anomalies are diagnosed as a result of hysterosalpingography to evaluate patients with infertility or reproductive loss, usually repeated spontaneous abortion.

Uterine Anomalies and Reproductive History. Although some uterine anomalies may cause infertility, the vast majority of patients with uterine anomalies are able to conceive without difficulty. There is no question that uterine anomalies may be associated with a perfectly normal reproductive performance. Overall, however, the incidence of spontaneous abortion, premature birth, fetal loss, malpresentation, and cesarean section is clearly increased when a uterine anomaly is present. Unfortunately, it is impossible to predict which patients with uterine anomalies will have these problems.

ETIOLOGY OF REPRODUCTIVE FAILURE. The etiology of reproductive failure in patients with uterine anomalies remains unclear. Mahgoub considers that the presence of a uterine septum may lead to abortion because of diminished intrauterine space for fetal growth or because of implantation of the placenta on a poorly vascularized septum. Mizuno and associates have attached importance to the inadequacy of vascularization of the uterine septum. Associated cervical incompetence, luteal phase insufficiency, and distortion of the uterine milieu have all been implicated in the etiology of increased reproductive loss. However, it is as yet unexplained why some patients with a uterine anomaly have normal reproductive function whereas others abort early in pregnancy. Interestingly, it has been reported that the chance for a liveborn child increases with each pregnancy loss. It is unknown whether this conditioning of the uterus is due to better vascularization, better myometrial stretching and accommodation, or some other factor.

A patient with a history of three or more spontaneous abortions or premature labor should undergo hysterosalpingography to determine if structural abnormalities of the uterus are present. An abnormality will be found in about 10% of such patients. Among chronic early second-trimester aborters, the incidence may be higher. The etiology of spontaneous abortion is complex, and a complete work-up should be done even when an anomalous uterus has been found. A careful history should include a detailed discussion of each previous pregnancy loss; inquiry about DES exposure; drug and chemical toxicity; specific medical illnesses; and exposure to contagious diseases. A family history should emphasize reproductive failures among family members of the patient and the husband. Specific medical diseases such as thyroid disease, diabetes mellitus, renal disease, and systemic lupus erythematosus should be ruled out. The possibility of infection, including such agents as *Neisseria gonorrhoeae*, Chlamydia, Mycoplasma, Toxoplasma, and Listeria, should be considered. Chromosome analysis should be done with the expectation of finding abnormalities in up to one fourth of couples with a history of habitual abortion and with the understanding that in >50% of spontaneous abortions, chromosomal abnormalities are found in the aborted tissue. Identifying such couples makes it possible to offer genetic counseling for subsequent pregnancies. Uterine leiomyomas, especially lower uterine segment and submucous leiomyomas, may cause spontaneous abortion. Basal body temperature charts, serum progesterone determinations, and endometrial biopsies timed in the luteal phase will help determine the presence of luteal phase deficiency. The cervix should be studied for incompetence. Couples with multiple etiologies for reproductive loss should have all other problems corrected before metroplasty is considered.

Correcting other factors first may, indeed, correct the problem of reproductive loss without a metroplasty. Rock and Jones reported seven patients with anomalous uterine development who also were found to have ex-

trauterine factors in the etiology of their reproductive loss. These patients had had 16 pregnancies of which five (31%) resulted in a liveborn child. After therapy to correct the extrauterine factor, the success rate increased to 71%. Stoot and Mastboom reported an impressive improvement in reproductive performance among uterine anomaly patients simply by improving abnormal carbohydrate metabolism.

HYSTEROGRAPHIC STUDIES. The technique of performing hysterosalpingography to diagnose uterine anomalies is important. The hysterogram must be taken at right angles to the axis of the uterus so that a true assessment of the deformity can be made. The study is best done under fluoroscopy. The distinction between a septate uterus and a bicornuate uterus cannot be made with hysterogram alone (Fig. 25-16). The external uterine configuration also cannot usually be determined by pelvic examination alone, but some idea of the configuration may be obtained by ultrasonography. McDonough and Tho have suggested the use of double-contour pelvic pneumoperitoneum-hysterographic studies for precise identification of müllerian malformations. Of course, laparoscopy is even more certain. The physician must be prepared to correct either anomaly depending on the findings at laparotomy, if the uterine corpus has not been previously visualized.

ADDITIONAL TESTING. A complete investigation should also include the assessment of tubal patency, and an intravenous pyelogram. A variety of upper urinary tract anomalies are seen, including absence of one kidney, horseshoe kidney, pelvic kidney, duplication of the collecting system, and ectopically located ureteral orifices. The lower urinary tract (bladder and urethra) is much less often anomalous.

Effect of Double Uterus on Obstetric Outcome. The percentage of full-term pregnancies in an unselected series of women with various types of double uterus who have not been operated on is unknown. For all types combined, it is probably approximately 25%. In patients selected for operation, it probably increases from approximately 5% to 10% to approximately 80% to 90%. Because patients with uterine anomalies who have relatively normal obstetric histories cannot be identified, there is confusion in the literature about which anomalies are more often associated with obstetric difficulties and which are relatively benign in their effect. Special diagnostic procedures to detect uterine anomalies are not usually done before reproductive performance is tested. The didelphic uterus is an exception. This anomaly can be diagnosed easily by identifying two complete cervices and perhaps a longitudinal vaginal septum as well on routine pelvic exam. A study by Heinonen in Finland of 182 women with uterine anomalies indicated that pregnancies in the septate uterus had a better fetal survival rate

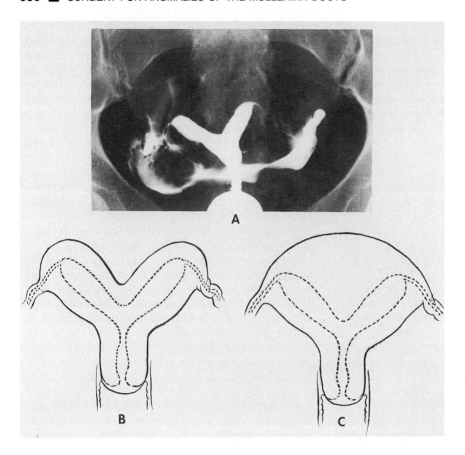

Figure 25–16. *A,* A hysterogram of a double uterus. A bicornuate (*B*) and a septate (*C*) uterus are types of double uteri. Visualization of the fundus is required to determine the type of uterus.

(86%) than in the complete bicornuate uterus (50%) or the unicornuate uterus (40%). These findings differ from the prevalent opinion that the septate uterus is associated with the highest reproductive loss, as proposed by Jones and Jones.

In 1968, Capraro, Chuang, and Randall reported seeing 85 patients with uterine anomalies between 1962 and 1966. One uterine anomaly was seen for every 645 admissions (0.145%). In only 14 (16%) of these 85 patients was metroplasty considered necessary. According to Jones and Jones, only one third of patients with a double uterus have important reproductive problems. In most instances, the presence of a double uterus is not in itself an indication for metroplasty.

In 1980, Jewelewicz, Husami, and Wallach estimated the spontaneous abortion rate to be 33.8% in women with a bicornuate uterus, 22.2% in those with a septate uterus, and 34.6% in those with a unicornuate uterus. More recently, Ludmir and associates' reported that high-risk obstetric intervention did not significantly increase the fetal survival rate for uncorrected uterine anomalies. Capraro and associates found a preoperative fetal salvage rate of 33.3% for the septate uterus, 10% for the bicornuate uterus, and 0% for the didelphic

uterus. Postoperatively, the fetal salvage rate was 100% for the bicornuate uterus, 80% for the septate uterus, and 66% for the didelphic uterus. The report gives the improved salvage figures after abdominal metroplasty from several previous studies.

THE DIDELPHIC UTERUS. A didelphic uterus with two hemicorpora is easily diagnosed because all patients will be found to have two hemicervices visible on speculum examination, and most, if not all, will have a longitudinal sagittal vaginal septum. In the series reported by Heinonen, Saarikoski, and Pystynen, all 21 patients with a didelphic uterus had a vaginal septum. Conversely, a patient with a longitudinal vaginal septum will usually, but not always, be found to have a didelphic uterus. The indication for uterine unification is related to the role of this anomaly as an etiologic factor in reproductive loss. Of all the uterine anomalies (except an arcuate uterus), the didelphic uterus is associated with the best possibility of a successful pregnancy. However, there is still some increase in perinatal mortality, premature birth, breech presentation, and cesarean section for delivery. Heinonen and associates reported a fetal survival of 64% without metroplasty. Musich and Behrman stated that the didelphic uterus was found to give the best chance for a successful pregnancy (57%) and was not considered an appropriate indication for metroplasty. However, W.S. Jones considered the didelphic uterus to give the worst obstetric outcome. In the opinion of the editors of this book, a unification operation for a didelphic uterus is not indicated often and the results may be disappointing, especially when an attempt is made to unify the cervix. Not only is this procedure technically difficult in a complete didelphic anomaly, but it also may result in cervical incompetence or cervical stenosis.

THE SEPTATE UTERUS. Most patients who are evaluated for repeated abortion and are found to have a uterine anomaly will have a septate uterus. A few will have other anomalies, mostly bicornuate uterus. In the experience of this author, fetal survival rates are higher after the repair of a septate uterus than after repair of other types of anomalies. Rock and Jones reported that, at the Johns Hopkins Hospital, of 43 patients with septate uteri selected for Jones metroplasty, 95% became pregnant postoperatively, 73% of pregnancies were carried to term, and 77% of patients had a liveborn child. Similar results have been reported following hysteroscopic or resectoscopic incision of the uterine septum.

Uterine Anomalies and Menstrual Difficulties. Dysmenorrhea and abnormal and heavy menstrual bleeding have been reported to occur more frequently in patients with any form of double uterus and to be relieved after unification operations. Capraro and associates reported several cases in which dysmenorrhea was cured by metroplasty. Erwin Strassmann also believed that all cases of dysmenorrhea and menorrhagia in conjunction with uterine anomalies were relieved by unification of the two uterine cavities. Generally, however, dysmenorrhea and menorrhagia are inappropriate indications for uterine unification and the physician should hesitate to do the operation solely for these reasons.

Uterine Anomalies and Infertility. Opinions differ considerably in terms of whether infertility is a proper indication for metroplasty. Erwin Strassmann stated that primary infertility could be cured in 60% of patients with uterine anomaly provided all other causes of infertility were excluded. Strassmann reported doing eight metroplasties for "primary sterility." These operations yielded nine pregnancies and seven liveborn children, although the number of patients who conceived was not given. Similar reports of small numbers of patients can be found throughout the literature. Heinonen and Pystynen indicated that uterine anomalies are rarely the reason for infertility. Nonuterine causes of infertility must be ruled out before, as a last resort, metroplasty is considered.

Certainly, a full infertility investigation must be done first to rule out other causes of infertility before the anomalous uterus is blamed. Even then, if no other cause for infertility is found and the uterus is septate or bicornuate, then the physician may not have a proper indication for metroplasty. This question simply has not yet been answered, and the decision is therefore difficult. The physician has an even more difficult decision to make if an infertility patient with a septate or bicornuate uterus requires laparotomy for some other reason, such as endometriosis or tubal occlusion.

Surgical Technique for Uterine Unification

Traditionally, the septate uterus has been unified with either the Jones or the Tompkins procedure. Clinical reports by Chervenak and Neuwirth, Daly and coauthors, DeCherney and associates, and Israel and March have compared favorably hysteroscopic or resectoscopic incision of the septum of a septate uterus with the traditional transabdominal approach. Term pregnancy rates following this procedure have approached 80%–85%. In patients with a wide septum, several attempts may be necessary to incise the septum, although in most instances the septum may be incised completely at the first operation.

Transcervical Lysis of the Uterine Septum. Abdominal metroplasty for transfundal incision or excision of the septum associated with the septate uterus generally has been abandoned. Although the hysteroscope and scissors have been used for cutting the septum, recently use of the resectoscope has been found to be comparable. The optics are excellent and the septum may be electrosurgically incised with little difficulty. Alternatively, with the hysteroscopic scissors, the procedure may be tedious, especially with a large, broad septum.

Before transcervical lysis of a uterine septum, the patient is placed on danazol or a GnRh agonist for 2 months. This drug reduces the amount of endometrium that may obscure the surgeon's view during the procedure. Transcervical lysis is usually performed in conjunction with laparoscopy under general endotracheal anesthesia. The uterine cavity is distended with Hyskon (dextran 70, Pharmacia, Piscataway, NJ) by way of the resectoscope (R. Wolf Co., Rosemont, IL), which is inserted into the cervix. The septum is then electrosurgically incised by advancing the cutting loupe using the trigger mechanism of the resectoscope. The uterine septum is incised until the tubal ostia may be visualized and there is no appreciation of the septum by the surgeon. The procedure is performed under simultaneous laparoscopy to limit the risks of uterine perforation. The laparoscopic light may be turned off so that the light from the hysteroscope may be clearly visualized through the fundus. Most patients may be discharged within 4 hours of the procedure. Patients are placed on antibiotics before the procedure and the medication is continued for 5 days following surgery to limit the risks of infection. No intrauterine devices are used. If excessive bleeding occurs after the procedure, a Foley catheter should be placed into the uterine cavity for tamponade and removed in 4–6 hours.

Transcervical lysis also may be performed to repair a complete septate uterus, that is, a single fundus with two cavities with two cervices. In this instance, a No. 8 Foley catheter may be inserted into one cervix and indigo carmine injected into the cavity. The left cavity may be distended with Hyskon by way of the resectoscope. The septum may be electrosurgically incised at a point above the internal cervical os until the Foley bulb catheter is visualized. The septum may then be incised in a superior direction until the tubal ostium may be visualized and there is no appreciation of the septum (Fig. 25-17).

Following a transcervical lysis of a uterine septum, a 2-month delay before attempting pregnancy is suggested to allow complete resorption of the septum. These patients may deliver vaginally. The Jones procedure may be used for the repair of a septate uterus where a particularly broad septum may not be easily incised with the resectoscope. The Strassmann procedure is used for unification of a bicornuate uterus.

The Modified Jones Metroplasty. The modified Jones unification operation is demonstrated in Figure 25-18. The abdomen is generally opened through a transverse incision. If a unification operation only is planned, then a Pfannenstiel's incision is permissible. The pelvic viscera are inspected. The septate uterus may demonstrate a median raphe across the fundus, but it is surprising how often the corpus looks normal. To facilitate manipulation, a traction suture of heavy silk is placed through the top of the septum. The site of this suture will be removed when the septum is excised.

No attempt is made to stain the uterine cavity with methylene blue. The normal unstained endometrial tissue can be easily differentiated from the myometrium. There are essentially two methods to control bleeding during this procedure. For hemostasis, a tourniquet may be applied at the junction of the lower uterine segment and cervix by inserting a 0.5-Penrose drain through an avascular space in the broad ligaments just lateral to the uterine vessels on each side. The tourniquet is placed around the lower uterine segment and is tied anterior to the uterus. Because the uterine corpus receives a significant blood supply through the ovarian arteries, tourniquets should also

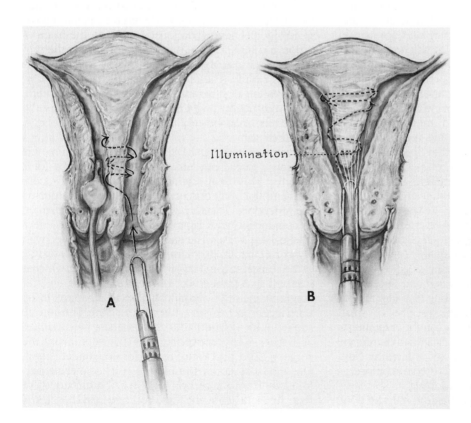

Figure 25–17. Resectoscopic metroplasty. *A*, A Foley catheter is placed in one cavity of a complete septate uterus (AFS Class VA uterus). The resectoscope is inserted in the opposite cavity and the septum incised until the Foley is visualized. The septum is then incised. The septum may be easily incised with the resectoscope until both internal oses are visible. *B*, A septate uterus with a single cervix. The septum may be incised with the straight loupe of the resectoscope.

be tied around the infundibulopelvic ligaments on each side, using the same hole in the broad ligament. All tourniquets must be tied tightly enough to occlude both the arterial supply to and the venous drainage from the uterus. If only the venous drainage is occluded, then the corpus will become engorged and congested and bleeding will be increased. If the arterial supply is occluded, then the uterus will blanch and the bleeding will be minimal. A sterile Doptone can be used to establish disappearance of uterine artery pulsations. The use of hypotensive anesthetic techniques in conjunction with the tourniquets will allow a uterine unification operation to be accomplished with negligible blood loss. Alternatively, up to 20 units of vasopressin diluted in 20 ml of saline may be injected into the anterior and posterior walls of the uterus before making the incision.

The uterine septum should be surgically excised as a wedge (Fig. 25-18D). The incisions begin at the fundus of the uterus. In approaching the endometrial cavity, care must be taken that the cavity is not transected (Fig. 25-18E). The original incisions at the top of the fundus are usually within 1 cm, and sometimes even less, of the insertion of the fallopian tubes. If the incision is directed toward the apex of the wedge, however, there seems to be little danger of transecting the tube across its interstitial transit in the myometrium.

After the wedge has been removed, the uterus may be closed in three layers with interrupted stitches; No. 2-0 nonreactive suture on an atraumatic tapered needle is convenient. Two sizes of needles are used: (1) a half-inch needle for the inner and intermediate layers and (2) a large needle, three fourths half-round, for the outer muscular layer. The inner layer of stitches must include about one third of the thickness of the myometrium, because the endometrium itself is too delicate to hold a suture and it will cut through. The suture is placed through the endometrium/myometrium in such a way that the knot is tied within the endometrial cavity (Figs. 25-18G and H). While the suture is being tied, an assistant presses together the two lateral halves of the uterus both manually and with the guy sutures to relieve tension on the suture line and reduce the possibility of cutting through. The stitches are placed alternatively anteriorly and posteriorly. After the first few stitches are placed and before the first layer is completed, the second layer can be started to reduce tension.

As the operation proceeds, the third layer can be inserted in the serosa both anteriorly and posteriorly (Figs. 25-18I–K). Finer, nonreactive suture may be used to approximate the serosal edges of the uterus more precisely and to prevent adhesion formation to the suture line (Figs. 25-18K and L). At the conclusion, the uterus appears near normal in its configuration. The striking feature is usually the proximity of the insertions of the fallopian tubes. Special care must be exercised not to obstruct the interstitial portions of the fallopian tubes while placing the fundal myometrial and serosal sutures.

The final size of the uterine cavity seems to be unimportant. Many times the constructed cavity is quite small compared with the normal uterus. Of more importance seems to be the symmetry. Whether the surgeon removes the septum with the Jones procedure or lyses the septum transcervically, often postoperative hysterogram films will show small dogears that are leftover tags from the original bifid condition of the uterus. Such dogears do not seem to interfere with function, although postoperative roentgenogram after such an operation cannot be considered normal in the sense that it appears as a normal endometrial cavity. If a double cervix is present, then the physician should not attempt to unify the cervix because an incompetent cervical os will result. To allow the uterine incision the best possible opportunity to heal, a delay of 4–6 months in attempting pregnancy is advised after abdominal metroplasty.

THE JONES METROPLASTY COMPARED WITH THE TOMPKINS PROCEDURE. The technique of modified Jones metroplasty is a compromise between the classic Jones metroplasty and the Tompkins metroplasty. In the Jones operation, the entire septum is removed. In the Tompkins operation, a single median incision divides the uterine corpus and septum in half. The incision is carried inferiorly until the endometrial cavity is reached. Each lateral septal half is then incised up to within 1 cm of the tubes. No septal tissue is removed. The myometrium is reapproximated, taking care not to place sutures too close to the interstitial portion of the tubes. Proponents of this technique suggest that it is simpler. It conserves all myometrial tissue and leaves the uterotubal junction in a more normal and lateral position. Good results with this technique have been reported by McShane, Reilly, and Schiff.

THE WEDGE METROPLASTY COMPARED WITH TRANSCERVICAL LYSIS. There are obvious advantages to a transcervical incision of a uterine septum for patients with a septate uterus. There is a decreased morbidity following the procedure and patients may deliver vaginally at term. Term pregnancy rates are comparable with those following abdominal metroplasty for repeated pregnancy wastage. Nevertheless, certain patients with a broad uterine septum may benefit from the wedge metroplasty. Reconstructive surgeons should continue to be knowledgeable in the performance of a wedge metroplasty to remove a large septum. The majority of the septa associated with a septate uterus may be cut through the cervix by way of the hysteroscope or the resectoscope.

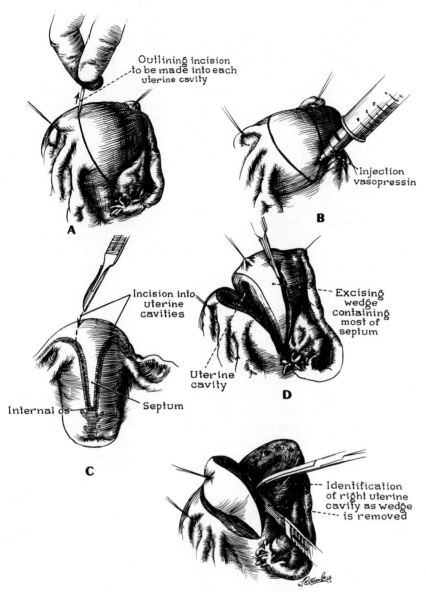

Outlining incision to be made into each uterine cavity

A

Injection vasopressin

B

Incision into uterine cavities

Internal os Septum

C

Excising wedge containing most of septum

Uterine cavity

D

Identification of right uterine cavity as wedge is removed

E

Figure 25–18. The modified Jones metroplasty. See the text for a full description of the various steps in the operative repair of a septate uterus by excision of a wedge.

The Strassmann Metroplasty. The Strassmann procedure is not easily adapted to the septate uterus, but it is the procedure of choice for unification of the two endometrial cavities of an externally divided uterus—bicornuate or didelphic (Fig. 25-19). A bicornuate uterus cannot be repaired through transcervical lysis, because perforation will result. When there has been failure of fusion of the two müllerian ducts, inspection of the pelvic cavity often will reveal a broad peritoneal band that lies in the middle between the two lateral hemicorpora (see Fig. 25-19). This rectovesical

ligament is attached anteriorly to the bladder, folds over and is attached between the uterine cornua, continues posteriorly in the cul-de-sac, and ends with its attachment to the anterior wall of the sigmoid and rectum. It is not invariably present, but when it is, the physician cannot help but wonder about its possible significance in the etiology of this anomaly, possibly by preventing the two müllerian ducts from joining. It must be removed before a unification procedure can be done.

Then, for hemostasis, tourniquets are used in a manner similar to that described for the modified Jones

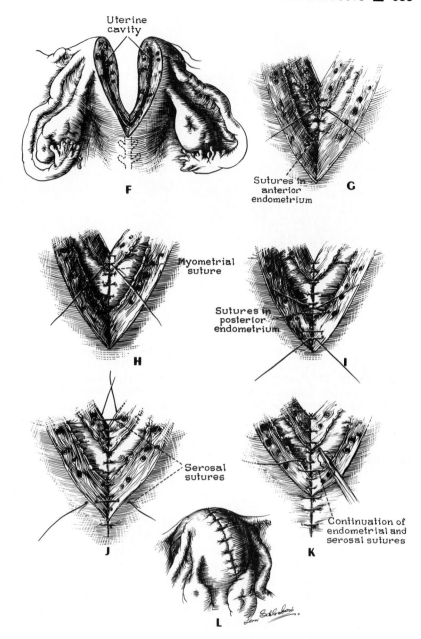

Figure 25–18. (continued)

procedure. The two uterine cornua are incised on their median sides in their longitudinal axes, deeply enough to expose the uterine cavities (Fig. 25-19B). Superiorly, the incision must not be too close to the interstitial portion of the fallopian tubes. Inferiorly, the incision is carried far enough to join the two sides into a single endocervical canal. If it appears that a deeper incision will compromise the competence of the cervix, then a double cervical canal may be left. If the cervix is already duplex, then it should not be joined. As the incision in the myometrium releases the internal stresses in the walls of the hemicorpora, each one everts and is perfectly positioned for apposition, almost as if the original intention in embryologic development was finally to be realized. The suture technique for joining the two sides (Fig. 25-19C–E) is exactly the same as for the modified Jones procedure. The suture line in the uterine corpus should be observed for several minutes to determine the adequacy of hemostasis. Occasionally, it will be necessary to place one or two extra sutures to control bleeding.

A uterine suspension may be performed as necessary.

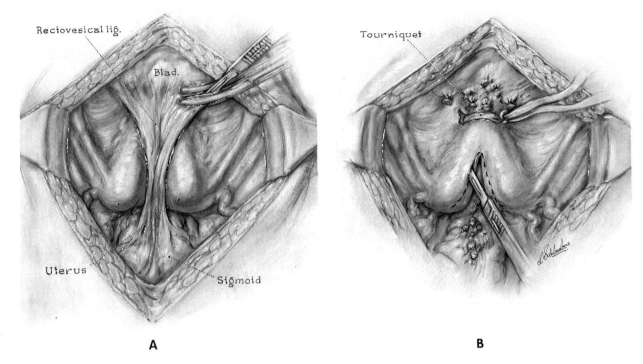

A **B**

Figure 25–19. The Strassmann metroplasty with modifications. *A*, If a rectovesical ligament is found, it should be removed. *B*, An incision is made on the medial side of each hemicorpus and carried deep enough to enter the uterine cavity. The edges of the myometrium will evert to face the opposite side. *C* and *D*, The myometrium is approximated using interrupted vertical figure-of-eight No. 3-0 polyglycolic acid sutures. Avoid placing sutures too close to the interstitial portion of the fallopian tubes. *E*, A continuous No. 5-0 polyglycolic acid subserosal suture is used as a final layer. Tourniquets are removed and defects in the broad ligament are closed.

However, in the event of pregnancy, the shortened round ligaments may produce symptoms from an enlarging uterus. Presacral neurectomy in association with uterine unification should be considered only in patients with severe midline dysmenorrhea.

The cervix should be dilated to ensure proper drainage from the uterine cavity. This can be accomplished transvaginally after the abdominal procedure or from above by inserting a dilator through the cervical canal into the vagina, to be removed later.

The operative technique used should be consistent with the goal of maintaining or enhancing fertility and the possibility of a successful pregnancy. Tissue surfaces should be kept moist throughout the procedure; instruments should be selected and used in such a way that tissue damage is minimized; abdominal packs should be placed in plastic bags to avoid adhesions or no-lint laparotomy pads (Johnson & Johnson) may be used. Talc should be carefully washed from gloves; meticulous aseptic technique should be used; and the appendix should not be removed. A solution of Ringer's

lactate containing heparin and corticosteroid may be used for peritoneal lavage throughout the procedure.

Cervical Incompetence Associated with a Double Uterus

When a patient with an anomalous uterus, with or without unification, becomes pregnant, she must be watched closely for evidence of cervical incompetence, especially if a history of previous reproductive loss suggests cervical incompetence. Heinonen and associates were able to improve fetal survival from 57% to 92% by cerclage. Cervical cerclage was used mostly in patients with a partial bicornuate uterus, in whom fetal salvage was improved from 53% before cerclage to 100% afterward. Prematurity also was decreased, from 53% to 3%. The authors stress that cervical incompetence, not the uterine anomaly, is the indication for cerclage in these patients. However, the frequency with which these problems are found together suggests the importance of doing a careful evaluation for both prob-

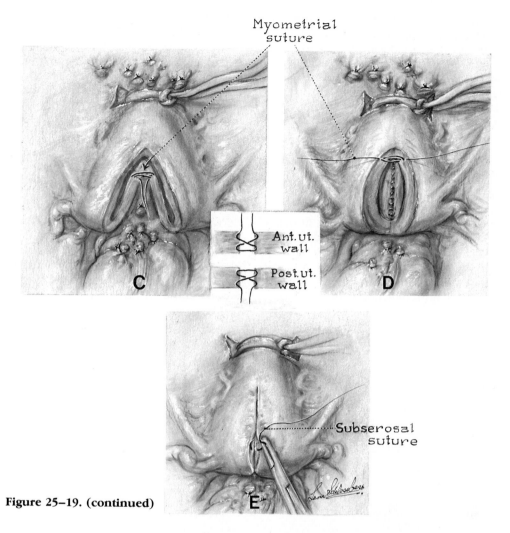

Figure 25–19. (continued)

lems. Obviously, some reproductive losses in patients with a uterine anomaly, before and after metroplasty, can be prevented by cerclage of an incompetent cervix. However, routine cerclage at the time of metroplasty is not recommended.

In addition, it is not recommended that the physician attempt to unify a double cervix or a septate cervix because of the possibility of causing cervical incompetence. However, a double or septate cervix may adversely affect the outcome of delivery if vaginal delivery is attempted. Delivery should be by cesarean section if it appears the cervix will cause dystocia.

Mode of Delivery of a Pregnancy Following Metroplasty

The scar in the myometrium following unification is as strong as, if not stronger than, that following cesarean section. The biologic conditions in which healing

occurs are entirely different in these two situations. Endomyometritis is a common complication following cesarean section but is not a complication of uterine unification. Of 71 known pregnancies in Strassmann's collected series reported in 1952, 61 were delivered per vagina. There were no cases of uterine rupture during pregnancy or delivery. Despite evidence that the uterine scar heals securely after unification operations, our policy is to recommend delivery by elective cesarean section in all patients who have undergone abdominal metroplasty. Patients may deliver vaginally following metroplasty by way of the hysteroscope or resectoscope.

Diethylstilbestrol Drug-Related Uterine Anomalies

Exposure of the female fetus to DES may result in significant anomalous development of the uterus, as reported by Kaufman and associates and by Haney and associates. The *T*-shaped uterus is the variant most commonly seen. It is associated with an increased rate of spontaneous abortion, preterm deliveries, and ectopic pregnancies. No operative procedure is indicated, but such patients must be monitored closely for evidence of dilatation and effacement of the cervix early in pregnancy. Cervical cerclage may be indicated in some patients.

Unicornuate Uterus

A unicornuate uterus may be present alone or with a rudimentary horn or bulb on the opposite side. In a series reported by Heinonen and associates, 11 out of 13 patients with a unicornous uterus had a rudimentary horn and two did not. The rudimentary anlage (uterine muscle bundle or bulb) may communicate with the unicornous uterus. In some instances, there is no cavity within the anlage or no rudimentary horn.

Most rudimentary horns are noncommunicating (90% according to O'Leary and O'Leary). The two sides may be connected by a fibromuscular band or there may be no connection and no communication between the two uterine cavities. Recently, Fedele and associates have found sonography useful in determining the presence of not only a rudimentary horn but also a cavity within.

Associated Anomalies. Urinary tract anomalies are often associated with unicornous uterus. On the side opposite the unicornous uterus may be a horseshoe or a pelvic kidney, or the kidney may be hypoplastic or absent. This is especially true if there is associated müllerian duct obstruction. When all müllerian duct derivatives and the kidney are absent on one side, the ovary may be malpositioned, because this implies failure of development of the entire urogenital ridge, including the genital ridge where the ovary forms (Fig. 25-20). Rock and associates reported a unilateral ovary located above the pelvic brim in four women with

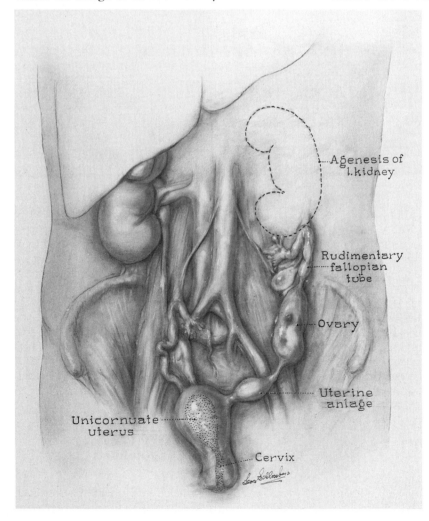

Agenesis of l. kidney

Rudimentary fallopian tube

Ovary

Uterine anlage

Unicornuate uterus

Cervix

Figure 25–20. A unicornuate uterus associated with ovarian malposition on the left. Notice the ovary and the tube are slightly above the pelvic brim. In this instance, the ovary measured 6 inches in length.

uterine anomalies. The orifice of the müllerian duct develops at about the level of the fourth thoracic vertebra (T4) in the embryo. The tip subsequently migrates along the course of the müllerian duct into the pelvis. The orifice of the duct or the fimbriated end of the tube comes to lie in the pelvis as a result of differential growth of the fetus. The subsequent differential growth is retarded so that the portion of the urogenital ridge that gives rise to both the gonad and tube does not displace into the pelvis. Thus, malposition of the ovary and tube results.

Effect on Reproductive Performance. According to Heinonen and associates, the unicornous uterus has the poorest fetal survival (40%) of all uterine anomalies. W. S. Jones reported similar findings. It has been suggested that the abnormal shape and insufficient muscular mass of the uterus, and a reduced uterine volume with inability to expand, may explain the poor obstetric outcome.

Because most patients with a unicornous uterus will have a noncommunicating rudimentary uterine horn on the opposite side, there is danger of pregnancy developing in the rudimentary horn from transperitoneal migration of the sperm or ovum from the opposite side. O'Leary and O'Leary found the corpus luteum to be on the side contralateral to the rudimentary horn containing a pregnancy in 8% of cases. Signs and symptoms of an ectopic pregnancy will develop with eventual rupture of the horn if the pregnancy is not detected early. Rupture through the wall of the vascular rudimentary horn is associated with sudden and severe intraperitoneal hemorrhage and shock. Death may occur in a few minutes. It is surprising that the current mortality has decreased to 5%. According to Holden and Hart, some 350 cases of pregnancy in a rudimentary horn have been reported since the original case report by Mauriceau in 1669.

Very little, if anything, can be done to improve the reproductive performance of patients with a unicornous uterus. The physician should observe closely for cervical incompetence and do cerclage as indicated. Andrews and Jones have suggested that removal of the rudimentary uterine horn may improve the chances of a successful pregnancy, but the experience is too small to support a definite recommendation. Asymmetric development as with unicornous uterus and an opposing rudimentary uterine horn is not amenable to unification.

Longitudinal Vaginal Septum

Failure of fusion of the lower müllerian ducts that form the vagina may result in a vagina with a longitudinal septum. The septum may be partial or complete. Young patients will have difficulty using tampons. There may be difficulty with intercourse. In patients with didelphic uterus and a longitudinal vaginal septum, one uterine hemicorpus is usually better developed than the other. If intercourse consistently occurs on the vaginal side connected to the uterine hemicorpus that is less well developed, then infertility or repeated abortion could result. For these reasons, the septum should be removed in the nonpregnant state unless there is a contraindication. It can usually be done easily with reasonable precaution against injury to the urethra, bladder, and rectum.

Asymmetric Obstruction of the Uterus or Vagina

Unicornous Uterus with a Noncommunicating Uterine Anlage that Contains Functional Endometrium

One müllerian duct may develop normally while the opposite müllerian duct may fail to develop or may develop incompletely. On one side, a relatively normal unicornous uterus is found. On the opposite side, the cervix, musculature, uterine cavity, endometrium, fallopian tube, blood supply, and ligamentous attachments may be absent or hypoplastic to a varying degree. Obstruction to menstruation may occur at any level on the side. For example, if a rudimentary uterine horn does not communicate externally but does have an endometrium lined uterine cavity, symptoms of obstructed menstruation may begin soon after menarche (Fig. 25-21). Severe dysmenorrhea will be present. Unfortunately, cryptomenorrhea may not be considered, because the patient will also experience cyclic menstruation from the opposite side. If the lumen of the tube communicates with the endometrial cavity of the rudimentary uterus, then retrograde menstruation and pelvic endometriosis will develop. It is, therefore, important to make the diagnosis as soon as possible so that reproductive potential will not be destroyed.

The findings at an operation to remove obstructed rudimentary uterine horn are illustrated in Figure 25-21. Fortunately, in this case, the fallopian tube was obstructed and retrograde menstruation was impossible. The fallopian tube connected to the rudimentary uterine horn may not be patent because of incomplete development.

Unilateral Obstruction of a Cavity of a Double Uterus

Another example of a rare obstructed lateral fusion problem is illustrated in Figure 25-22A. A complete septum was present between two uterine cavities. One cavity communicated with a cervix and the other did

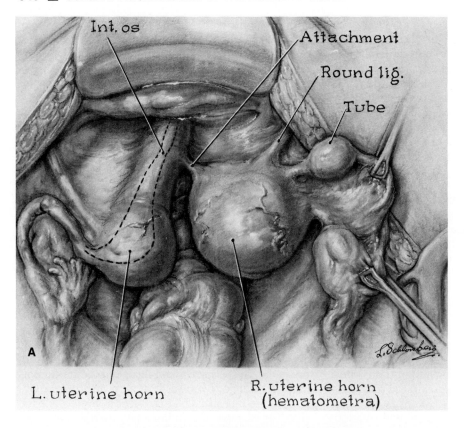

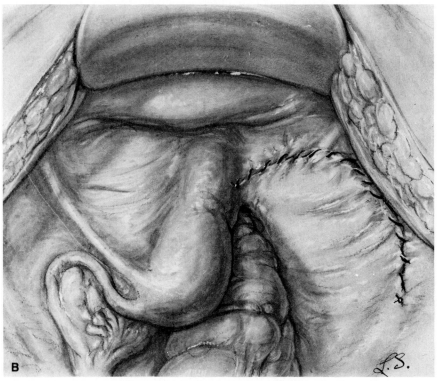

Figure 25–21. *A,* A noncommunicating rudimentary horn with functional endometrium and containing menstrual blood under pressure. Note the congenital abnormality of the fallopian tube, which prevented retrograde menstruation. *B,* The same patient following excision of the rudimentary horn.

not. This could represent an example of unilateral failure of cervical development. The patient complained of incapacitating dysmenorrhea that appeared shortly after the menarche and lasted 5 days. A tense cystic mass was palpable in the right half of the pelvis. The operation, described originally by Jones in the second edition of this book, consisted of making an incision through the anterior wall of the cystic right portion of the uterus. It was found to contain old menstrual blood. The entire septum was excised and the uterus was reconstructed by anastomosis of the two cavities. A continuous lockstitch was reinforced by interrupted myometrial sutures (Fig 25-22*B*). The plastic reconstruction of the uterus was completed by a third layer of interrupted sutures uniting myometrium and serosa (Fig. 25-22*C*).

Double Uterus Associated with an Obstructed Hemivagina and Ipsilateral Renal Agenesis

This unique clinical syndrome, consisting of the double uterus, obstruction of the vagina (unilateral, partial, or complete), and ipsilateral renal aplasia, is rare. Renal agenesis (mesonephric involution) on the side of the obstructed vagina associated with a double uterus and cervix is suggestive of an embryologic arrest occurring during 8 weeks of pregnancy that simultaneously affected the müllerian and metanephric ducts. The exact cause is unknown.

Diagnostic Groups. Depending on the uterovaginal relationships in individual patients, the clinical presentation of their symptoms varies, making diagnosis difficult. The physician can divide these patients into three groups:

1. Group 1 patients have complete unilateral vaginal obstruction without uterine communication, resulting in a paravaginal mass and the symptoms of severe dysmenorrhea and lower abdominal pain. Menses are regular.
2. Group 2 patients have an incomplete unilateral vaginal obstruction without uterine communication. Their presenting symptoms are lower abdominal pain, severe dysmenorrhea, excessive foul mucopurulent discharge, and, in some instances, intermenstrual bleeding.
3. Group 3 patients have complete vaginal obstruction with a laterally communicating double uterus. They have a paravaginal mass, lower abdominal pain, and dysmenorrhea. Menses are regular.

Because menses in patients with this syndrome are rarely regular, the physician can easily overlook the possibility of this diagnosis. To determine the correct diagnosis, a careful pelvic examination must be made. With MRI, the physician can identify the obstructed vagina, double uterus, and absence of a kidney on the side of the obstruction (Fig. 25-23). This may be impossible if there is incomplete vaginal obstruction or a uterine communication.

Complete unilateral obstruction (group 1) may go unrecognized for a number of years following the onset of menses. A large amount of blood may accumulate in the obstructed side, because the vagina is distensible and can therefore accommodate the increments of blood resulting from each menstrual cycle. There is sufficient absorption of menstrual blood between periods so that subsequent flow may add to the accumulated blood without pain. Nevertheless, once retrograde menstruation occurs, endometriosis invariably is the result.

Surgical Treatment. Careful excision of the vaginal septum is the treatment of choice for a unilateral vaginal obstruction. Prophylactic antibiotics should be administered before surgery. After opening the vaginal pouch, the surgeon should use suction and lavage to remove the pooled blood and mucus.

Because the obstructing septum is usually thick, removal may be difficult. Clamps should be used to isolate a generous vaginal pedicle while the suture is being tied in place to prevent slippage of tissue. Such pedicles generally retract during healing and formation of a vaginal stenosis is avoided. In most instances, surgery is restricted to excision of the septum and abdominal exploration is unnecessary. For patients with the previously described lateral communication of the uterine horns, uterine reconstruction is not indicated.

Reproductive Performance. Reproductive performance for patients with this disorder is usually consistent with that of patients with a double uterus, unless delay in diagnosis and resection of the obstructing septum has resulted in tubal function being destroyed or the development of endometriosis.

UNUSUAL CONFIGURATIONS OF VERTICAL/LATERAL FUSION DEFECTS

Müllerian duct anomalies may occur in association with a variety of other problems. For example, Stanton has reported that in a series of 70 patients with bladder extrophy, 30 patients (43%) had reproductive tract abnormalities. He suggested that the number may actually be higher. Müllerian abnormalities included absence of the vagina; septate vagina; unicornous, bicornuate, and didelphic uterus; and absent uterus. Fewer müllerian anomalies were seen with epispadias. Jones called attention to anomalies of the external genitalia and vagina

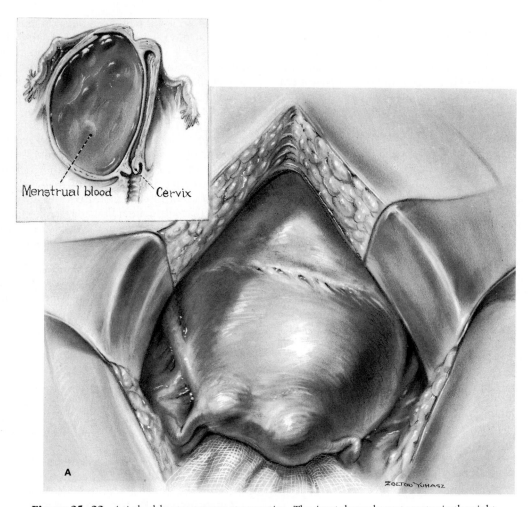

Figure 25–22. *A*, A double uterus seen at operation. The *inset* shows hematometra in the right uterine cavity, which does not communicate with the other cavity or the cervical canal. *B*, The septum of the double uterus has been excised and anastomosis is being made uniting the two cavities.

among 30 patients with bladder exstrophy seen at the Johns Hopkins Hospital, and suggested operative techniques for correction. Operative techniques for correction of these anomalies as well as for the management of other gynecologic and obstetric problems (especially uterine prolapse) also have been discussed by Weed and McKee and by Blakeley and Mills. A number of other congenital malformations of the vagina and perineum also may be associated with uterine anomalies. These rare combinations and their surgical correction, espe-cially in children, are reported by Hendren and Dona-hoe and by others.

Müllerian duct anomalies are seen in patients with the McKusick-Kaufman syndrome, an autosomal recessive disorder. Other clinical findings reported in this syn-drome include hydrometrocolpos, postaxial polydactyly, syndactyly, congenital heart disease, intravaginal displace-ment of the urethral meatus, and anorectal anomalies. Jabs, Leonard, and Phillips added an additional case to the previous cases reported in the literature.

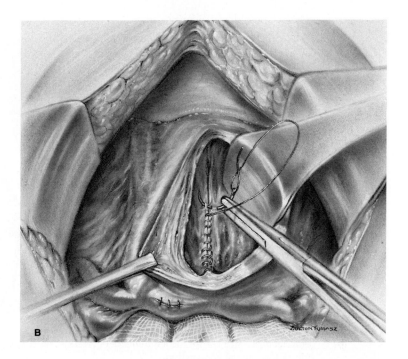

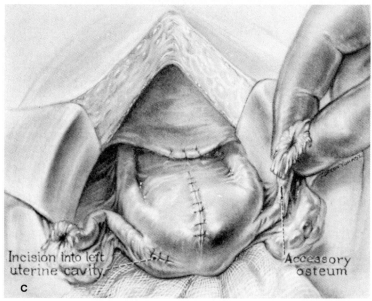

Figure 25–22. (continued) *C*, Anastomosis is completed. The small incision in the left uterine cavity was made before the septum was removed for the purpose of orientation.

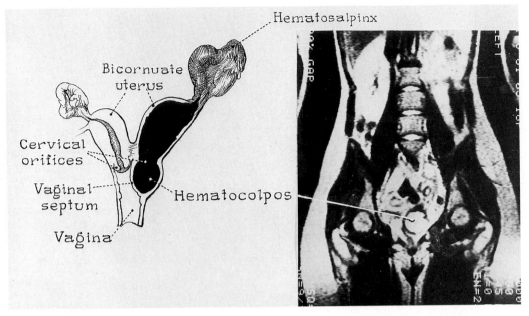

Figure 25–23. A double uterus with unilateral complete vaginal obstruction and ipsilateral renal agenesis. MRI reveals the left hematocolpos, both uteri, and absence of the left kidney on the side of the vaginal obstruction.

Bibliography

Abbe R. New method of creating a vagina in a case of congenital absence. Medical Record 1898;54:836.

American Fertility Society classification of müllerian anomalies. Fertil Steril 1988;49(6):952.

Andrews MC, Jones HW. Impaired reproductive performance of the unicornuate uterus: intrauterine growth retardation, infertility, and recurrent abortion in five cases. Am J Obstet Gynecol 1982;144:173.

Blakeley CR, Mills WG. The obstetric and gynaecological complications of bladder exstrophy and epispadias. Br J Obstet Gynaecol 1981;88:167.

Brenner P, Sedlis A, Cooperman H. Complete imperforate transverse vaginal septum. Obstet Gynecol 1965;25:135.

Broadbent TR, Woolf RM. Congenital absence of the vagina: reconstruction without operation. Br J Plast Surg 1977;30:118.

Buttram VC Jr. Müllerian anomalies and their management. Fertil Steril 1983;40:159.

Buttram VC Jr, Gibbons WE. Müllerian anomalies: a proposed classification (an analysis of 144 cases). Fertil Steril 1979;32(1):40.

Capraro VJ, Chuang JT, Randall CL. Improved fetal salvage after metroplasty. Obstet Gynecol 1968;31:97.

Capraro VJ, Gallego MB. Vaginal agenesis. Am J Obstet Gynecol 1976;124:98.

Chakravarty BN. Congenital absence of the vagina and uterus—simultaneous vaginoplasty and hysteroplasty. J Obstet Gynecol (India) 1977;27:627.

Chakravarty BN, Gun KM, Sarkar K. Congenital absence of vagina: anatomico-physiological consideration. J Obstet Gynecol (India) 1977;27:621.

Chervenak FA, Neuwirth RS. Hysteroscopic resection of the uterine septum. Am J Obstet Gynecol 1981;141:351.

Counseller VS. Congenital absence of the vagina. JAMA 1948;136:861.

Counseller VS, Davis CE. Artresia of the vagina. Obstet Gynecol 1968;32:528.

Counseller VS, Flor FS. Congenital absence of the vagina. Surg Clin North Am 1957;37:1107.

Cukier J, Batzofin JH, Conners JS, et al. Genital tract reconstruction in a patient with congenital absence of a vagina and hypoplasia of the cervix. Obstet Gynecol 1986;68:325.

Daly DC, Tohan N, Walters C, et al. Hysteroscopic resection of the uterine septum in the presence of a septate cervix. Fertil Steril 1983;39:560.

Daly DC, Walters CA, Soto-Albors CE, et al. Hysteroscopic metroplasty: surgical technique and obstetrical outcome. Fertil Steril 1983;39:623.

David A, Carvil D, Bar-David E, et al. Congenital absence of the vagina: clinical and psychological aspects. Obstet Gynecol 1975;46:407.

Davydov SN. Colpopoiesis from the peritoneum of the uterorectal space. In Proceedings of the Ninth World Congress of Obstetrics and Gynecology, Tokyo, 1979. Amsterdam Excerpta Medica 1980:793.

DeCherney A, Polan ML. Hysteroscopic management of intrauterine lesions and intractable uterine bleeding. Obstet Gynecol 1983;61:392.

DeCherney AH, Russell JB, Graebe RA, et al. Resectoscopic management of müllerian fusion defects. Fertil Steril 1986;45(5):726.

Dillon WP, Mudaliar NA, Wingate NB. Congenital atresia of the cervix. Obstet Gynecol 1979;54:126.

Evans TN. The artificial vagina. Am J Obstet Gynecol 1967;:944.

Evans TN, Poland ML, Boving RL. Vaginal malformations. Am J Obstet Gynecol 1981;141:910.

Farber M, Marchant DJ. Reconstructive surgery for congenital atresia of the uterine cervix. Fertil Steril 1976;27:1277.

Farber M, Mitchell GW. Bicornuate uterus and partial atresia of the fallopian tube. Am J Obstet Gynecol 1979;134:881.

Farber M, Mitchell GW. Surgery for congenital absence of the vagina. Obstet Gynecol 1978;51:364.

Farber M, Mitchell GW. Surgery for congenital anomalies of müllerian ducts. Contemp Obstet Gynecol 1977;9:63.

Fayez JA. Comparison between abdominal and hysteroscopic metroplasty. Obstet Gynecol 1986;68(3):399.

Fedelle L, Doeta M, Vercellini P, et al. Ultrasound in the diagnosis of subclasses of unicornuate uterus. Obstet Gynecol 1988; 71(2):274.

Feroze RM, Dewhurst CJ, Welply G. Vaginoplasty at the Chelsea Hospital for women: a comparison of two techniques. Br J Obstet Gynaecol 1975;82:536.

Fore SR, Hammond CB, Parker RT, et al. Urologic and genital anomalies in patients with congenital absence of the vagina. Obstet Gynecol 1975;46:410.

Frank RT. The formation of an artificial vagina without operation. Am J Obstet Gynecol 1938;35:1053.

Frank RT. The formation of an artificial vagina without operation. NY State J Med 1940;40:1669.

Frank RT, Geist SH. The formation of an artificial vagina by a new plastic technic. Am J Obstet Gynecol 1927;14:712.

Gallup DG, Castle CA, Stock RJ. Recurrent carcinoma in situ of the vagina following split thickness skin graft vaginoplasty. Gynecol Oncol 1987;26:98.

Garcia J, Jones HW. The split thickness graft technic for vaginal agenesis. Obstet Gynecol 1977;49:328.

Garcia RF. Z-plasty for correction of congenital transverse vaginal septum. Am J Obstet Gynecol 1967;:1164.

Geary WL, Weed JC. Congenital atresia of the uterine cervix. Obstet Gynecol 1973;42:213.

Genest D, Farber M, Mitchell GW, et al. Partial vaginal agenesis with a urinary-vaginal fistula. Obstet Gynecol 1981;58:130–134.

Graves WP. Method of constructing an artificial vagina. Surg Clin North Am 1921;1:611.

Griffin JE, Edwards C, Madden JD, et al: Congenital absence of the vagina. Ann Intern Med 1976;85:224.

Haney AF, Hammond CB, Soules MR, et al. Diethylstilbestrol-induced upper genital tract abnormalities. Fertil Steril 1979;31:142.

Hauser GA, Keller M, Koller T. Das Rokitansky-Küster Syndrom. Uterus bipartitus solidus rudimentarius cum vagina solida. Gynecologia 1961;151:111.

Hauser GA, Schreiner WE. Das Mayer-Rokitansky-Küster Syndrom. Schweiz Med Wochenschr 1961;91:381.

Heinonen PK. Longitudinal vaginal septum. Eur J Obstet Gynecol Reprod Biol 1982;13:253.

Heinonen PK, Pystynen PP. Primary infertility and uterine anomalies. Fertil Steril 1983;40:311.

Heinonen PK, Saarikoski S, Pystynen P. Reproductive performance of women with uterine anomalies. Acta Obstet Gynecol Scand 1982;61:157.

Hendren WH, Donahue PK. Correction of congenital abnormalities of the vagina and perineum. J Ped Surg 1980;15:751.

Holden R, Hart P. First-trimester rudimentary horn pregnancy: prerupture ultrasound diagnosis. Obstet Gynecol 1983; (suppl)61:56.

Ingram JM. The bicycle seat stool in the treatment of vaginal agenesis and stenosis: a preliminary report. Am J Obstet Gynecol 1981;140:867.

Israel R, March CM. Hysteroscopic incision of the septate uterus. Am J Obstet Gynecol 1984;149(1):66.

Jabs EW, Leonard CO, Phillips JA. New features of the McKusick-Kaufman syndrome. Birth Defects 1982;18:161.

Jeffcoate TNA. Advancement of the upper vagina in the treatment of haematocolpos and haematometra caused by vaginal aplasia. Pregnancy following the construction of an artificial vagina. J Obstet Gynecol Br Comm 1969;76:961.

Jewelewicz R, Husami N, Wallach EE. When uterine factors cause infertility. Contemp Obstet Gynecol 1980;16:95.

Jones HW. An anomaly of the external genitalia in female patients with exstrophy of the bladder. Am J Obstet Gynecol 1973;117:748.

Jones HW. Reproductive impairment and the malformed uterus. Fertil Steril 1981;36:137.

Jones HW, Delfs E, Jones GE. Reproductive difficulties in double uterus: the place of plastic reconstruction. Am J Obstet Gynecol 1956;72:865.

Jones HW, Jones GE. Double uterus as an etiological factor in repeated abortion: indications for surgical repair. Am J Obstet Gynecol 1953;65:325.

Jones HW, Mermut S. Familial occurrence of congenital absence of the vagina. Am J Obstet Gynecol 1972;114:1100.

Jones, HW, Rock, JA. Reparative and constructive surgery of the female generative tract. Baltimore: Williams & Wilkins, 1983.

Jones HW, Wheeless CR. Salvage of the reproductive potential of women with anomalous development of the müllerian ducts: 1868–1968–2068. Am J Obstet Gynecol 1969;104:348.

Jones TB, Fleischer AC, Daniell JF, et al. Sonographic characteristics of congenital uterine abnormalities and associated pregnancy. J Clin Ultrasound 1980;8:435.

Jones WS. Obstetric significance of female genital anomalies. Obstet Gynecol 1957;10:113.

Karjalainen O, Myllynenl, Kajanoja P, et al. Management of vaginal agenesis. Ann Chir Gynaecol 1980;69:37.

Kaufman RH, Binder GL, Gray PM, et al. Upper genital tract changes associated with exposure in utero to diethylstilbestrol. Am J Obstet Gynecol 1977;128:51.

Knab DR. Müllerian agenesis: A review. Bethesda, Maryland: Department of Gynecology/Obstetrics, Uniformed Services University School of Medicine, & Naval Hospital, 1983.

Kusuda M. Infertility and metroplasty. Acta Obstet Gynecol Scand 1982;61:407.

Lees DH, Singer A. Vaginal surgery for congenital abnormalities and acquired constrictions. Clin Obstet Gynecol 1982;25:883.

Lodi A. Contributo clinico statistico sulle malformazion della vagina osservate nella clinica Obstetrica e Ginecologica di Milano dal 1906 al 1950. Ann Ostet Ginecol Med Perinat 1951;73:1246.

Ludmir J, Samuels P, Brooks S, Mennuti M. Pregnancy outcome of patients with uncorrected uterine anomalies managed in a high risk obstetric setting. Obstet Gynecol 75(6):907, 1990.

Maciulla GJ, Heine MW, Christian CD. Functional endometrial tissue with vaginal agenesis. J Reprod Med 1978;21:373.

Magrina JF, Masterson BJ. Vaginal reconstruction in gynecological oncology: a review of techniques. Obstet Gynecol Surv 1981; 36:1.

Mahgoub SE. Unification of a septate uterus: Mahgoub's operation. Int J Gynecol Obstet 1978;15:400.

Mandell J, Stevens PS, Lucey DT. Diagnosis and management of hydrometrocolpos in infancy. J Urol 1978;120:262.

Markham SM, Parmley TH, Murphy AA, et al. Cervical agenesis combined with vaginal agenesis diagnosed by magnetic resonance imaging. Fertil Steril 1987;48(1):143.

McCraw JB, Massey FM, Shanklin KD, et al. Vaginal reconstruction with gracilis myocutaneous flaps. Plast Reconstr Surg 1976;58:176.

McDonough PG, Tho PT. Use of pelvic pneumoperitoneum a critical assessment of 12 years experience. South Med J 1974;67:517.

McIndoe A. The treatment of congenital absence and obliterative conditions of the vagina. Br J Plast Surg 1950;2:254.

McIndoe AH, Banister JB. An operation for the cure of congenital absence of the vagina. J Obstet Gynaecol Br Emp 1938;45:490.

McKusick VA. Transverse vaginal septum (hydrometrocolpos). Birth Defects 1971;7:326.

McKusick VA, Bauer RL, Koop CE, et al. Hydrometrocolpos as a simply inherited malformation. JAMA 1964;189:119.

McKusick VA, Weilbaccher RG, Gragg GW. Recessive inheritance of a congenital malformation syndrome. JAMA 1968;204:111.

McShane PM, Reilly RJ, Schiff I. Pregnancy outcomes following Tompkins metroplasty. Fertil Steril 1983;40:190.

Mizuno K, Koike K, Ando K, et al. Significance of Jones-Jones operation on double uterus: vascularity and dating of endometrium in uterine septum. Jap J Fertil Steril 1978;23:9.

Murphy AA, Krall A, Rock JA. Bilateral functioning uterine anlagen with the Rokitansky-Mayer-Küster-Hauser syndrome. Int J Fertil 1987;32(4):316.

Musich JR, Behrman SJ. Obstetric outcome before and after metroplasty in women with uterine anomalies. Obstet Gynecol 1978;52:63.

Musset R. Traitement chirurgical des cloisans transversales due vagin d'origine congenitale par la plastie en "Z" a l'Hopital Lariboisiere. Gynec et Obstet 1956;55:382.

Niver DH, Barrette G, Jewelewicz R. Congenital atresia of the uterine cervix and vagina—three cases. Fertil Steril 1980;33:25.

Nunley WC, Kitchin JD. Congenital atresia of the uterine cervix with pelvic endometriosis. Arch Surg 1980;115:757.

O'Leary JL, O'Leary JA. Rudimentary horn pregnancy. Obstet Gynecol 1963;22:371.

Pinsky L. A community of human malformation syndromes involving the müllerian ducts, distal extremities, urinary tract, and ears. Teratology 1974;9:65.

Pratt JH. Vaginal atresia corrected by use of small and large bowel. Clin Obstet Gynecol 1972;15:639.

Rock JA, Baramki TA, Parmley TH, et al. A unilateral functioning uterine anlage with müllerian duct agenesis. Int J Gynecol Obstet 1980;18:99.

Rock JA, Jones HW. The clinical management of the double uterus. Fertil Steril 1977;28:798.

Rock JA, Jones HW. The double uterus associated with an obstructed hemivagina and ipsilateral renal agenesis. Am J Obstet Gynecol 1980;138:339.

Rock JA, Jones HW Jr. Vaginal forms for dilatation and/or to maintain vaginal patency. Fertil Steril 1984;42(2):187.

Rock JA, Parmley T, Murphy AA, et al. Malposition of the ovary associated with uterine anomalies. Fertil Steril 1986;45(4):561.

Rock JA, Reeves LA, Retto H, et al. Success following vaginal creation for müllerian agenesis. Fertil Steril 1983;39:809.

Rock JA, Schlaff WD. The obstetrical consequences of uterovaginal anomalies. Fertil Steril 1985;43(5):681.

Rock JA, Schlaff WD, Zacur HA, et al. The clinical management of congenital absence of the uterine cervix. Int J Gynecol Obstet 1984;22:231.

Rock JA, Zacur HA. The clinical management of repeated early pregnancy wastage. Fertil Steril 1983;39:123.

Rock JA, Zacur HA, Dlugi AM, et al. Pregnancy success following surgical correction of imperforate hymen and complete transverse vaginal septum. Obstet Gynecol 1982;59:448.

Rotmensch J, Rosensheim N, Dillon M, et al. Carcinoma arising in the neovagina: case report and review of the literature. Obstet Gynecol 1983;61:534.

Semmens JP. Abdominal contour in the third trimester: an aid to diagnosis of uterine anomalies. Obstet Gynecol 1965;25:779.

Shokeir MHK. Aplasia of the müllerian system: evidence for probably sex-limited autosomal dominant inheritance. Birth Defects 1978;14:147.

Singh KJ, Devi L. Hysteroplasty and vaginoplasty for reconstruction of the uterus. Int J Gynecol Obstet 1980;17:457.

Stanton SL. Gynecologic complications of epispadias and bladder extrophy. Am J Obstet Gynecol 1974;119:749.

Stoot JE, Mastboom JL. Restriction on the indications for metroplasty. Acta Eur Fertil 1977;8:79.

Strassmann EO. Operations for double uterus and endometrial atresia. Clin Obstet Gynecol 1961;4:240.

Strassmann EO. Plastic unification of double uterus. Am J Obstet Gynecol 1952;64:25.

Strassmann P. Die operative vereinigung eines doppelten uterus. Zentralbl Gynakol 1907;31:1322.

Tancer ML, Katz M, Veridiano NP. Vaginal epithelialization with human amnion. Obstet Gynecol 1979;54:345.

Thompson DP, Lynn HB. Genital anomalies associated with solitary kidney. Mayo Clin Proc 1966;41:538.

Thompson JD, Wharton LR, Te Linde RW. Congenital absence of the vagina. Am J Obstet Gynecol 1957;74:397.

Tompkins P. Comments on the bicornuate uterus and twinning. Surg Clin North Am 1962;42:1049.

Ulfelder H, Robboy SJ. The embryologic development of the human vagina. Am J Obstet Gynecol 1976;126(7):769.

Valdes C, Malini S, Malinak L. Sonography in the surgical management of vaginal and cervical atresia. Fertil Steril 1983;40:263.

Weed JC, McKee DM. Vulvoplasty in cases of extrophy of the bladder. Obstet Gynecol 1974;43:512.

Wharton LR. A simple method of constructing a vagina. Ann Surg 1938;107:842.

Wharton LR. Congenital malformations associated with development defects of the female reproductive organs. Am J Obstet Gynecol 1947;53:37.

Wharton LR. Further experiences in construction of the vagina. Ann Surg 1940;111:1010.

Williams EA. Congenital absence of the vagina, a simple operation for its relief. J Obstet Gynecol Br Comm 1964;71:511.

Williams EA. Uterovaginal agenesis: Ann R Coll Surg Engl 1976;58:266.

Williams EA. Vulvo-vaginoplasty. Proc R Soc Med 1970;63:40.

Myomectomy

26

EDWARD E. WALLACH

Uterine leiomyomas are the most common pelvic tumors in women. Traditionally described as present in 20% of women over age 35, their appearance at 50% of postmortem examinations performed on women suggests a much higher frequency. These neoplasms are variously referred to as leiomyoma, fibromyoma, myoma, leiomyofibroma, fibroleiomyoma, and fibroid. The most acceptable term is leiomyoma, which most accurately describes its origin and predominant cellular composition. The term myoma, however, is widely used to describe these tumors, and is used in this chapter, whereas "fibroid" is an inaccurate descriptor. The high prevalence rate of myomas suggests that they usually have a minor influence on ability to conceive but may exhibit a profound effect on pregnancy maintenance. A genetic basis for the presence and growth of uterine myomas appears likely. For example, the incidence of myomas among black women is significantly greater than among white women. Nonetheless, the increased prevalence of myomas with age, when viewed from the perspective of the current demographic trend toward postponing childbearing, justifies concern over the effects of these tumors on reproductive performance in future years.

Uterine myomas usually are accepted as originating from smooth-muscle cells of the uterus, although in certain instances an origin from the smooth muscle of uterine blood vessels is likely. Myomas range in size from seedlings only millimeters in diameter to large uterine tumors that may not only fill the pelvis, but can reach the costal margin. These tumors may be solitary or multiple. Excessive menstrual bleeding often is the only symptom produced by myomas. Vascular alterations in the endometrium associated with myomas have been correlated with hypermenorrhea. The obstructive effect on uterine vasculature produced by intramural tumors has been associated with the development of endometrial venule ectasia. As a consequence of this phenomenon, myomas give rise to proximal congestion in the myometrium and endometrium. The engorged vessels in the thin atrophic endometrium that overlies submucous tumors contribute to excessive bleeding during cyclic sloughing of the endometrium. The increased size of the uterine cavity and the surface area of the endometrium also are contributing factors in increasing the quantity of menstrual flow. Hypermenorrhea associated with uterine myomas may be aggravated by the presence of endometritis, which frequently is observed histologically in the endometrium overlying submucous tumors.

The growth of uterine myomas is clearly related to their exposure to circulating estrogen. These tumors are most prominent and demonstrate their maximum growth during a woman's reproductive life, when ovarian estrogen secretion is maximal. They appear to exhibit a growth spurt during the fifth decade just before menopause, a phenomenon that may relate to the frequency of anovulatory cycles and unopposed estrogen action that prevail during the immediate premenopausal years. With the actual onset of menopause, myomas characteristically regress in volume. This regression often is counterbalanced by estrogen replacement therapy. Growth of myomas in the absence of hormonal treatment after menopause suggests an extraovarian source of estrogen or its elaboration from an enzymatically active ovarian stroma. Whenever myomas undergo growth after menopause, the potential for cancer must be seriously considered. Myoma growth is common during pregnancy, and occurs less frequently during the cyclic use of estrogen-progestogen preparations, such as oral contraceptive pills. The increased size of myomas during pregnancy also reflects their dependence on estrogen.

In contrast to the influence of estrogens on myomas, progesterone and progestational compounds exert an antiestrogenic effect; therefore, in view of this balance between estrogenic and progestational effects, gestational growth of myomas also must represent enhancement of uterine blood supply that accompanies pregnancy. The success of progesterone and synthetic progestogens in decreasing the size of uterine myomas supports this concept. A higher concentration of estrogen receptors has been identified in uterine myomas than in the adjacent myometrium itself and in normal uterine tissue. In addition, it has been reported that uterine myomas bind approximately 20% more estradiol per milligram of cytoplasmic protein than does normal myometrium from the same uterus. Cramer and coworkers demonstrated heterogeneity in growth potential of uterine leiomyomas when cells were cultured in the presence of hormones. During pregnancy the rapid myoma growth rate may exceed its blood supply and thereby lead to necrosis. The reduced circulation to these tumors also can result in thrombosis and extravasation of blood. The compromised tumors become dark and hemorrhagic, a characteristic finding in the red or carneous degeneration often associated with pregnancy.

PATHOLOGY

Malignant transformation of benign leiomyomas is extremely rare. The often cited statistic that 0.5% of leiomyomas are malignant tumors overstates the likelihood of malignant change. In view of the high frequency of myomas, the large number of myomas often found in a single uterus, and the rarity of metastases appearing after the removal of uteri containing multiple myomas, the frequency of sarcomatous change is undoubtedly far less than 0.5%. In a review of 13,000 myomas by Montague and colleagues from Woodruff's group at Johns Hopkins, 38 cases (0.29%) demonstrated malignant change. Even this figure appears unduly elevated in light of the high prevalence of these benign tumors and the relative rarity of leiomyosarcoma. Corscaden and Singh reported that malignant change developed in less than 0.13% of uterine myomas, with the true figure probably on the order of 0.04%.

Only a small percentage of uteri containing myomas are ever surgically removed, thus yielding a much higher denominator than that based solely on surgical procedures performed in which uterine myomas are found. Furthermore, not all of the myomas contained in the uterus removed at hysterectomy are sectioned and examined histologically. Also, unless the pathologists use strict criteria for the determination of malignancy, cellular myomas may be erroneously classified as leiomyosarcomas. Sarcomatous areas, typically in the center of the tumor, have a characteristic soft and homogeneous appearance on gross examination of the sectioned surface. In addition, leiomyosarcomas lack the characteristic whorl-like appearance of benign myomas, giving a "raw pork"-type appearance instead, as described by T. S. Cullen. Significant necrosis results in a brainlike appearance with broken-down areas, marked friability, and hemorrhage. The microscopic

diagnosis relies on the level of mitotic activity and degree of cellular atypism. The latter feature is based on the presence of nuclear hyperchromatism and pleomorphism.

Tumors with less than 5 mitotic figures per 10 high-power fields (HPF) and little, if any, cytologic atypia are classified as cellular leiomyomas; those with more than 10 mitotic figures per 10 HPF are considered malignant; those tumors with 5 to 10 mitotic figures per 10 HPF and no cellular atypia are referred to as "smooth-muscle tumors of uncertain malignant potential," whereas those with this level of mitotic activity and cellular atypia are classified as leiomyosarcoma. From a prognostic standpoint, a poor outlook can be predicted when tumors display a high mitotic count and cytologic atypia.

In contrast to leiomyosarcomas, leiomyomas are characterized microscopically by interlacing bundles of smooth-muscle cells arranged in a whorl-like pattern. Nuclei are rod-shaped and usually fairly uniform in both size and shape. The spindle shape of the cell is apparent when sectioned longitudinally, while in transverse sections the cell appears rounded or polyhedral. Smooth-muscle cells are admixed with connective tissue elements to a varying degree. An unusual atypical uterine smooth-muscle tumor has been classified as an epithelioid leiomyoma by Kurman and Norris. Its characteristic histologic feature is the mixture of rounded polygonal cells and multinucleated giant cells present in epithelioid clear cell and plexiform patterns. For the most part, these tumors behave clinically like benign lesions, but occasionally epithelioid leiomyomas with mitotic counts of less than 5 mitoses per 10 HPF may metastasize, usually after a tumor-free interval of about 5 years. These patients should, therefore, be carefully followed. Kurman and Norris suggest that epithelioid tumors with more than 5 mitotic figures per 10 HPF be considered epithelioid leiomyosarcomas. Intravenous leiomyomatosis is characterized by extension of worm-like cords of smooth muscle into venous channels in the broad ligament and parametrium. They seldom extend in a retrograde manner into the vena cava and heart. These are benign tumors that have a low mitotic index.

Leiomyomatosis peritonealis disseminata (LPD) is an unusual entity that should be distinguished from intravenous leiomyomatosis. LPD is characterized by multiple small nodules composed of either benign smooth-muscle cells or an admixture of smooth-muscle cells, fibroblasts, myofibroblasts, and decidual cells, implanted on the peritoneal surface of abdominal organs, omentum, and mesentery. This entity is a benign, self-limited process. LPD appears to be derived from subcoelomic mesenchyme through a metaplastic process. A high concentration of both estrogen and progesterone receptors has been reported in the smooth-muscle cells in LPD. An unusual predilection or selective sensitivity of the subperitoneal mesenchymal cells to estrogen and progestogen may account for development of this entity, since LPD has almost always been associated with conditions characterized by high levels of circulating estrogen, such as pregnancy, as well as in women with granulosa cell tumors and in those using oral contraceptives. After removal of hormonal stimulation, LPD spontaneously resolves.

The evolution of ultrasound as a routine diagnostic procedure during pregnancy over the past 10 to 15 years has increased our understanding of the behavior of myomas in pregnancy. Before the use of sonography, only large myomas were detectable in pregnancy and primarily by clinical examination. Aharoni and associates followed 32 myomas in 29 patients serially, using ultrasonography, and found that an increase in size was apparent in only 7, whereas 6 myomas decreased in volume and 19 changed in size by less than 10% of their initial volumes. Thus, in aggregate, 78% of the uterine leiomyomas followed sonographically failed to grow. Although these data are reassuring, the rates of certain disturbances in reproductive performance, including infertility, spontaneous abortion, and preterm delivery, are increased when uterine myomas are present. Degeneration of myomas during pregnancy, alluded to earlier, is not uncommon. Other complications associated with myomas in pregnancy include preterm premature rupture of the membranes, malpresentation, dysfunctional labor, increased abdominal delivery rate, retained placentas, postpartum hemorrhage, and puerperal uterine infections. In the series of Katz and co-workers 2% of pregnant women had uterine leiomyomas and 10% had complications related to myomas per se. Acute red degeneration often is accompanied by development of a heterogeneous pattern and anechoic or cystic spaces on ultrasonography.

The two changes in uterine myomas discussed above—malignant change and degeneration—are the most significant. Other secondary changes within myomas include hyaline degeneration, cyst formation, calcification, fatty change, infection, and necrosis unassociated with pregnancy. As myomas exhibit growth, they also risk diminution of blood supply, giving rise to a continuum of degenerative changes. The spectrum of manifestations of calcium deposition in myomas includes a thin rim of calcium on the periphery, a diffuse honeycomb pattern, a series of concentric rings, and a solid calcific mass. All of these patterns can be appreciated radiographically. Infection or suppurative change most commonly occurs when a submucous myoma protrudes through the cervix and into the vagina, as it ulcerates and becomes edematous. Infection of a submucous myoma may accompany puerperal endometritis and advance to endomyometritis with or without abscess formation. Necrosis and cystic change also are manifestations of compromised blood supply secondary to growth or to infarction accompanying torsion of a pedunculated myoma. Fatty degeneration of a myoma is relatively rare, but may accompany hyalinization of the tumor. More commonly, the yellow appearance observed macroscopically, which suggests deposition of fat, simply represents another stage of necrosis.

SIGNS AND SYMPTOMS OF UTERINE MYOMAS

Most patients with uterine leiomyomas are symptom-free. When symptoms are produced, they often relate to the location of the myomas, their size, or concomitant degenerative changes. Pain is most often experienced in patients with a pedunculated myoma as its pedicle undergoes torsion. Pain also may be attributed to cervical dilatation by a submucous myoma protruding through the lower uterine segment, or to carneous degeneration associated with pregnancy. In each of these three conditions, pain is acute and requires immediate attention. Other pathologic conditions, including ectopic pregnancy, accident in an ovarian cyst, or acute pelvic inflammatory disease, must be considered in any patient who experiences acute abdominal pain and has identifiable myomas.

More commonly encountered than pain, pressure and increased abdominal girth develop insidiously, often are less apparent, and usually are vaguely described by the patient. As myomas grow, pressure frequently is exerted on adjacent viscera. Pressure on the urinary bladder usually provokes urinary frequency, especially when the myoma is located in the subvesical region or when a large myomatous uterus fills the entire pelvis. When the myoma is located adjacent to the urethra and bladder neck, acute urinary retention with overflow incontinence is apt to occur. An enlarging myoma anatomically located just over the cervix also may cause protrusion of the base of the bladder and distention of the anterior vaginal wall, suggesting pelvic relaxation. Stress urinary incontinence also may reflect myomas situated in the vicinity of the bladder neck. Ureteral obstruction is one of the most serious consequences of chronic pressure on the urinary collecting system. Usually silent, this complication results from pressure of the myomatous uterus on the pelvic brim in the vicinity of the ureter. Unless the kidney has suffered parenchymal damage, this anatomic change is reversible once the pressure is alleviated. Chronic obstruction at the level of the bladder neck also can lead to hydroureter and hydronephrosis. Rectal pressure is rare unless the myomatous uterus is incarcerated in the cul-de-sac or contains a solitary large posterior wall myoma. Constipation or tenesmus also may be associated with a posterior myoma, representing pressure of the tumor on the rectosigmoid.

Because the incidence of malignancy in these tumors is relatively low, careful consideration must be paid to specific indications for surgery. A history of rapid growth, especially postmenopausal growth, should prompt removal, even in the absence of associated symptoms. The most common reason for rapid growth of myomas is pregnancy. Therefore, in the younger patient in whom pregnancy has been ruled out and in older patients beyond menopause, rapid growth must raise the possibility of leiomyosarcoma. Small asymptomatic myomas require only serial follow-up, initially at 1- to 2-month intervals, to establish a growth curve pattern; if the myomas are stationary in size, pelvic examinations can be repeated at 3- to 4-month intervals. Myomas often remain constant in size for many years. Because uterine size tends to vary with the phase of the menstrual cycle and response to hormonal stimulation, selection of a uniform time in the cycle for each follow-up examination is appropriate. With larger asymptomatic tumors, expectant management also may be justified, provided the examiner has reason for confidence that the pelvic mass is a myomatous uterus and does not either represent an ovarian neoplasm or obscure the detection of such a tumor. If an adnexal neoplasm is suspected, further diagnostic studies are mandatory. Exploratory laparotomy should be performed if diagnostic studies are not explicit in ruling out ovarian neoplasia.

In any event, pelvic examination may be supplemented by ultrasonography, which can provide objective information regarding the size of individual myomas. Because a mass considered on pelvic examination to be a myoma may in fact prove to be an ovarian tumor, a sonographic study demonstrating normal-appearing ovaries clearly distinct from the uterus is an invaluable piece of information. Sonography also assists in documenting growth of myomas with a finer level of discrimination than by means of serial pelvic examination. The presence of hydronephrosis also can be determined through this noninvasive technique by visualizing kidney size and shape. Conventional radiographs also may supplement pelvic examination. Characteristic radiographic findings of calcification, described previously, are reassuring. Intravenous pyelography is more precise than sonography in defining renal and ureteral characteristics. In specific cases computed tomography (CT) can supplement ultrasonography and simple pelvic x-ray studies, although Tada and colleagues have reported that 5% of patients diagnosed as having myomas by tomography were subsequently found to have an ovarian tumor at the time of surgery. Magnetic resonance imaging (MRI) provides better definition of the source of a pelvic mass. Regardless of imaging procedures, in the event of diagnostic uncertainty, laparoscopy or laparotomy should be performed.

No standard size of an asymptomatic myomatous uterus has been invoked as an absolute indication for treatment. The presence of a large myomatous uterus in an asymptomatic patient in whom dimensions have not increased and cancer is unlikely, and the patient's age, fertility status, and desire to retain the uterus or to avoid surgery must be factored into any treatment decision. A size equivalent to that of a 12-week gestation has customarily been the dividing point between surgery and a conservative approach in the asymptomatic patient. In women approaching menopause relatively large myomas often can be observed serially by pelvic examination and sonography with the confidence that they will diminish in size once ovarian function ceases. Estrogen replacement therapy during menopause, however, may offset the reduced growth that customarily accompanies cessation of ovarian function. Likewise, a conservative approach should be followed in the younger patient who wants to preserve childbearing capacity or who wants to establish a pregnancy. After menopause asymptomatic small leiomyomas usually may be left undisturbed, provided an ovarian neoplasm has been ruled out.

Careful observation is suitable management for most myomas. The majority produce no symptoms, are confined to the pelvis, should not be confused with other pathologic conditions, and are seldom malignant, especially in the absence of rapid growth rate. The major indications for aggressive management of uterine myomas are as follows:

Abnormal uterine bleeding
Rapid growth
Growth after menopause
Infertility
Recurrent pregnancy loss
Pain or pressure symptoms
Urinary tract symptoms or obstruction
Possibility of ovarian neoplasia
Iron deficiency anemia secondary to chronic blood
  loss

THERAPEUTIC APPROACHES AND INDICATIONS

The therapeutic alternatives for treatment of uterine myomas include myomectomy, hysterectomy, conservative follow-up with serial examinations, and hormonal therapy.

Myomectomy

Myomectomy should be considered whenever preservation of the uterus is desired for its childbearing function and it is specifically requested. It also is the procedure of choice for a solitary pedunculated myoma. Indications for myomectomy include interference with fertility or predisposition to repeated pregnancy loss owing to the nature or location of the myoma, single or multiple. Infertility is seldom a consequence of uterine myomas, but when a causal relation is suspected, the location of myomas usually is the significant element that interferes with establishment or maintenance of pregnancy.

Locations associated with difficulties in pregnancy include the following:

1. Directly under the endometrium, where myomas may interfere with implantation and result in infertility or impair embryonic-fetal nutrition, giving rise to early pregnancy loss. In addition, chronic endometritis is common in the tissue overlying a submucous myoma and may adversely affect implantation.
2. Impingement on the uterotubal junction, which may cause intramural obstruction of the fallopian tube
3. A broad ligament site, where a myoma can distort the anatomic relation between the tubal ostium and the ovary
4. Supracervical, where myomas can alter the position of the cervix within the vagina, thereby interfering with the opportunity for the cervical os to be bathed in the ejaculate after coitus, and thus prevent normal insemination

Indications for myomectomy are listed in Table 26-1. The desire for uterine retention in our culture cannot be underestimated. Current technology enables the uterus of a woman who lacks ovaries to serve as a

TABLE 26–1
Indications for Myomectomy

Pedunculated subserous myoma
Submucous myoma with hypermenorrhea
Rapidly enlarging myoma
Infertility secondary to myomas
Desire to retain fecundity
Desire to retain uterus

gestational vehicle through in vitro fertilization, endometrial preparation with exogenous hormonal therapy, and embryo donation. Furthermore, the Hysterectomy Educational Resource Service (HERS), an active educational resource, perhaps sensitized to public concern over unnecessary hysterectomy, has significantly influenced women's decisions regarding uterine retention in the presence of benign pathology. Wide dissemination of such attitudes may render myomectomy an even more prevalent procedure in the near future than it is today.

Hysterectomy

With few exceptions, removal of the uterus is the procedure of choice whenever surgery is indicated for myomas and when childbearing has been completed. Hysterectomy also is the favored procedure whenever there is a reasonable likelihood of malignancy within a myoma (eg, rapid enlargement). If myomectomy is not technically feasible, hysterectomy should be carried out (eg, in the presence of diffuse leiomyomatosis of the uterus). Although it is unusual for myomectomy to be technically implausible, the procedure may be difficult, time-consuming, and associated with a substantial complication rate. Therefore, to balance the risks of performing a difficult and potentially complicated myomectomy, sufficient indication for uterine preservation should be evident. Hysterectomy usually is a simpler procedure than multiple myomectomy, as well as the procedure to which most gynecologists are more accustomed.

Conservative Follow-up with Serial Examinations

If surgery is not performed for myomas, serial follow-up should be carried out with precise and objective documentation of uterine size and configuration. Examination and sonography performed initially at 1- to 2-month intervals can provide the physician with a reasonable appreciation of whether the myomas are enlarging and, if so, at what rate. If the size appears stationary, serial examinations at 3- to 4-month intervals are reasonable. Temporizing also is appropriate if the patient is in the immediate premenopausal age range. Nevertheless, prediction of age at menopause in individual patients often is unreliable.

Hormonal Therapy

Despite the fact that the endocrine alterations associated with pregnancy may favor the growth of uterine myomas and be associated with profound alterations (enlargement, edema, and degeneration), progestational agents alone seem to have a salutary influence on myoma growth. Progestational therapy has been successful, using norethindrone, medrogestone, and medroxyprogesterone acetate to achieve diminution in aggregate size of the myomatous uterus. These compounds produce a hypoestrogenic effect by inhibiting gonadotropin secretion and suppressing ovarian function. Progestational compounds also may exert a direct antiestrogenic effect at the cellular level.

Gonadotropin-releasing hormone agonists (GnRHa) have been successfully used to achieve hypoestrogenism in various estrogen-dependent conditions (eg, endometriosis, precocious puberty, and uterine leiomyomas). Patients with uterine myomas who have been treated with this approach have experienced significant reduction in tumor size. This approach offers great promise as a primary means of conservative therapy or as an adjunct to surgical myomectomy. The effects of either progestational therapy or GnRHa treatment are transient, and within several cycles after therapy is discontinued, myomas tend to return to their pretherapy size. Adjunctive therapy with a 3- to 4-month course of GnRHa should reduce myoma size and render surgery easier, accompanied by less blood loss. This approach has special advantages in facilitating a hysteroscopic resection of a submucous myoma, since the time consumed in the hysteroscopic resection itself is largely a function of tissue volume.

An original concern that the tissue plane separating the myoma from surrounding myometrium is more fibrotic and less precise after GnRHa therapy has not been borne out by our own experience. After the patient receives a course of GnRHa, the myomectomy is performed through a hypovascular myometrium, theoretically reducing blood loss. Long-term treatment of young patients is neither practical nor desirable because of the possibility of bone loss as a consequence of hypoestrogenism during prolonged therapy with GnRHa. Pretreatment with GnRHa, however, not only facilitates the myomectomy itself, but also provides an amenorrheic interval before surgery during which hemoglobin levels can be restored in the hypermenorrheic anemic patient, enabling presurgical blood donation for subsequent autotransfusion. Because short-term use is desirable, GnRHa also may be applied to perimenopausal women in whom reduction in myoma volume may stabilize when menopause occurs shortly thereafter. In the study of Andreyko and associates a daily dose of 800 mg of nafarelin for 6 months caused a mean decrease in uterine volume of 57% in 10 patients followed by serial MRI. Maheux and coworkers reported a mean decrease of 71% in myoma size after treatment with intranasal buserelin in nine patients.

Schlaff and colleagues used leuprolide in a double-blind placebo-controlled study and demonstrated a 42.7% and 30.4% decline in nonmyoma and myoma volume, respectively, through serial MRI studies. Results in clinical studies of GnRHa therapy for myomas are variable, and accurate prediction of responders to GnRHa appears to be impossible.

ABDOMINAL MYOMECTOMY

Preoperative Evaluation

Once a decision has been made to perform myomectomy, the surgeon must carry out a careful preoperative appraisal. As with any gynecologic surgical procedure, evaluation of the cervix by Papanicolaou smear is mandatory. Use of imaging to evaluate the size and location of myomas may be helpful but is not essential. Sonography alone may suffice to delineate the topography of the myomatous uterus. If adnexal neoplasia is a possibility, CT or MRI is helpful to confirm whether adnexal pathology or normal ovarian tissue is present. In cases of hypermenorrhea and other forms of abnormal bleeding, evaluation of the endometrium is necessary before performing definitive surgery. In the younger patient, who is without significant risk of endometrial cancer, office biopsy, aspiration, or curettage should suffice. In the patient over 35 years of age thorough curettage is warranted. In either event a patient with myomas and abnormal bleeding for whom myomectomy is contemplated should have a hysteroscopic examination to determine size, shape, and location of submucous myomas, as well as feasibility of hysteroscopic resection. At the time of hysteroscopy a thorough endometrial sampling can be performed. Definitive surgery should be deferred until 4 to 6 weeks after hysteroscopy and curettage, to minimize the chance of disseminated infection through contamination of the endometrium.

Hysterography is especially helpful before myomectomy because it provides a permanent record of the size and outline of the endometrial cavity. This procedure also enables the surgeon to evaluate tubal patency and the proximity of submucous myomas to the interstitial portion of the tubes or tubal ostia. Laparoscopic examination is indicated whenever the nature of the pelvic mass is unclear or adnexal neoplasia is a strong possibility. If the mass is larger than the equivalent of a 10-week gestation, laparoscopy may be technically difficult and usually is unnecessary. If sizable myomas or broad ligament extension is present, exploratory urography provides information regarding location of the ureters and presence of obstruction to the renal outflow tract.

Hematologic status, especially when heavy or prolonged bleeding is present, should be appraised well in advance of surgery. A patient with a normal hemoglobin level should have 2 units of her own blood obtained 2 weeks before surgery and stored, while she undergoes treatment with supplemental iron. If the patient is anemic, pretreatment with GnRHa or progestational agents can produce an amenorrheic state during which iron stores can be replenished. The hemoglobin level should return to normal at the end of a hormonally induced 4- to 6-month interval of amenorrhea, and preparations for phlebotomy and storage of blood for autotransfusion may be made.

Because many patients use analgesics for pelvic pain, cramping, or pressure associated with myomas, a determination of history of drug use is important. If salicylates have been taken, they should be discontinued for a minimum of 2 weeks before elective surgery. Aspirin has an irreversible influence on platelet aggregation. Two weeks is ample time to reduce the likelihood of unnecessary blood loss related to medication, since a new population of unexposed platelets normally is generated within 9 days.

Even with stored autologous blood, typing and crossmatching additional units of blood provide protection against the hazards of significant blood loss during surgery.

Principles and Technique

Preoperative hysterography and hysteroscopy can be used to delineate the location and size of myomas in preparation for their surgical removal. These parameters influence the site for the abdominal incision. The finding of a uterus with an aggregate size larger than the equivalent of a 12-week gestation or one containing prominent broad ligament myomas usually necessitates a vertical abdominal incision to facilitate exposure. A transverse lower abdominal incision should be contemplated only in the presence of a uterus less than the equivalent of a 12-week gestation. No discussion of myomectomy is complete without paying homage to William Alexander, who described the first multiple myomectomy; to Victor Bonney, who felt that myomectomy is a preferable procedure to hysterectomy; and to I. C. Rubin, who championed the procedure of multiple myomectomy. The general principles for myomectomy involve adequate exposure, hemostasis, and adhesion prevention. More specific principles are summarized in Table 26-2.

Once the abdomen has been opened, the intra-abdominal viscera should be explored, as during any abdominal operation. To optimize exposure, selection of an expedient abdominal incision, use of appropriate

TABLE 26–2
Principles of Surgical Technique

Single incision
Anterior incision
Incision into myoma to establish plane
Removal of as many myomas as possible
Hemostasis
Uterine suspension
Adjuvant therapy

retractors, and elevation of the uterus in the pelvis and abdomen by preoperative insertion of a vaginal pack are helpful adjuncts.

To minimize blood loss and preserve the strength of the uterine musculature postoperatively, the site for the uterine incision should be carefully selected so as to facilitate removal of the maximum number of myomas and to minimize the need for multiple uterine incisions. The incision into the uterus should be made as close to the midline as possible (Fig. 26-1A). Use of a vertical incision in the midline, although not always possible, can eliminate the need to incise vascular areas of the uterus and help to reduce blood loss. Injury to the interstitial portion of the fallopian tube also may be avoided with a vertical midline incision. An anterior uterine incision has the advantage of minimizing the possibility of incorporating the adnexal structures in adhesions which may form postoperatively and usually adjacent to a posterior uterine incision.

After selecting an anterior myoma located close to the midline and in proximity to other myomas, the surgeon makes an incision in the serosa overlying the tumor and extends it into the substance of the myoma itself (Fig. 26-1B). By incising progressively deeper into the myoma, the surgeon usually can identify the plane between the tumor and the myometrium by dissecting bluntly or with a knife (Fig. 26-1C and D). Allis clamps or towel clips are then placed on each half of the bisected myoma. While applying traction with the clamps, the surgeon can identify the base of the myoma. Hemostasis is achieved once the myoma is removed and when all other adjacent myomas have been excised through the same uterine incision.

Many techniques have been used to lessen blood loss during myomectomy. An assistant may apply pressure to the edges of the uterine incision to limit blood loss. A clamp designed by Bonney may be used to encompass and compress both uterine arteries at the base of the broad ligament. Alternatively, rubber-shod right-angle clamps can be used. Application of a hemostatic rubber tourniquet inserted through the broad ligament and encircling the uterine vessels also has been described. In this case the tourniquet is twisted and drawn taut posterior to the uterus, grasped with a clamp, and then

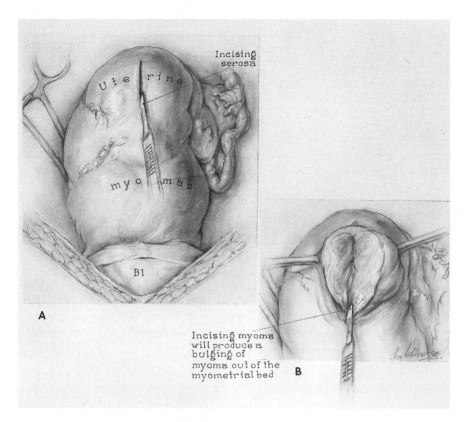

Incising
serosa

Uterine

myomas

B1

A

Incising myoma
will produce a
bulging of
myoma out of the
myometrial bed   B

Figure 26–1. Technique of multiple myomectomy. *A*, A vertical incision is made over a myoma on the anterior surface of the fundus as close to the midline as possible. Many myomas can be removed through this single incision. *B*, The incision is extended into the substance of the myoma.

loosened periodically to prevent uterine ischemia. Lock suggested using ring forceps placed bilaterally across the infundibulopelvic ligament and lower portion of the broad ligament for hemostasis. These approaches may help to reduce blood loss from the myomectomy site yet preserve integrity of the blood supply to the remainder of the uterus. Operating with a Bonney clamp or tourniquet to grasp the uterine vessels usually is unnecessary, and these previously described maneuvers tend to be traumatic, especially in a procedure invoked for its conservatism. Rapid, but careful, surgery usually accomplishes the same objective without additional traumatic injury to the uterus. Hemostatic agents such as adrenalin and vasopressin can be injected locally. Vasopressin (1 ampule in 20 mL of lactated Ringer's solution or normal saline solution) may be injected into the myometrium to limit blood loss. Many surgeons have found this method satisfactory; however, I have natural concerns over the possibility of delayed bleeding and a false sense of security with these agents. If this method is used, the surgeon should pay careful attention to oozing from the sutured uterine surface before abdominal wall closure, which may signify hematoma formation in the myometrium.

After the removal of as many myomas as possible through a single uterine incision, the myoma bed is closed in layers of nonreactive interrupted absorbable suture material (Fig. 26–1*E* and *F*). It is virtually impossible to identify discrete vessels throughout the myometrium, and a series of figure-of-eight or mattress sutures placed in the remaining defect usually is effective in controlling bleeding and obliterating dead space. A purse-string suture also may be used to obliterate a deep cavity in the myometrium. When the dead space is obliterated and the serosal region is reached, a continuous suture is placed in the subserosal tissue, using a "baseball"-type stitch (Fig. 26-1*G* and *H*). This continuous suture traverses the inner aspect of the serosa and is then carried through the superficial surface on each side throughout serosal closure. Alternatively, a subserosal suture of No. 5-0 or 6-0 nonreactive absorbable material may be used to approximate the serosal edges. If the uterus begins to engorge after serosal approximation, the surgeon should suspect continued bleeding into the myoma bed secondary to inadequate hemostasis. In this case the sutures should be removed and the uterine defect reexamined and resutured to achieve hemostasis.

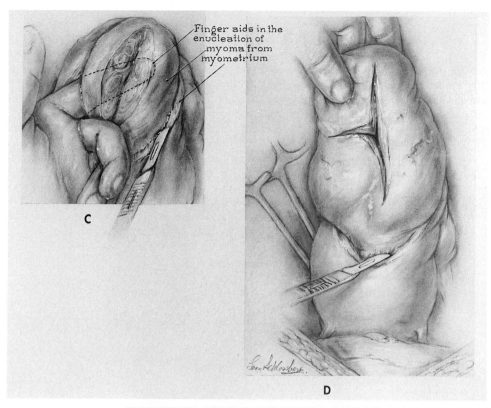

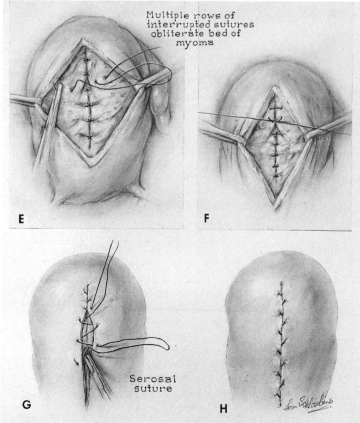

Figure 26–1. (continued) *C,* By incising progressively deeper into the myoma, the surgeon can identify and bluntly dissect the plane between myoma capsule and myometrium. *D,* Sharp dissection may be necessary to separate the myoma from its capsule at its base. *E,* After the removal of as many myomas as possible, the remaining cavity is obliterated and hemostasis secured. *F,* Multiple rows of nonreactive interrupted absorbable suture material are used to close the cavity. *G,* When the "dead space" has been obliterated, the serosa is closed with a continuous "baseball"-type suture of No. 5-0 or 6-0 nonreactive absorbable material. *H,* This type of closure approximates the serosal edges.

Prevention of Adhesions

Adhesion prevention may be accomplished by careful packing of viscera, using laparotomy pads contained in plastic bags. This step reduces dissemination of lint throughout the abdomen. During the procedure irrigation is carried out using heparinized Ringer's lactate (5000 IU heparin/1000 mL of Ringer's lactate). The irrigant can be delivered by syringe or through a hand-held apparatus attached to an intravenous bottle and tubing.

As mentioned, use of the anterior uterine incision is helpful in reducing the formation of adhesions, including those that involve adnexal structures. This principle was described in 1898 by Alexander of Liverpool, who stressed the concept of a single anterior uterine incision and removal of all tumors wherever they may be located. A posterior incision is more likely to lead to postoperative adhesions that incorporate the fallopian tubes and ovaries. An anterior hood-type incision, as described by Bonney, may be useful in avoiding the need for a posterior fundal uterine incision when approaching posterior fundal myomas (Fig. 26-2A and B). This procedure can be accomplished by extending the myometrial incision overlying the myoma to the fundal or posterior fundal region (Fig. 26-2C and D), creating a posterior flap that is subsequently folded over the anterior uterine wall (Fig. 26-2E–G). A posterior cervical

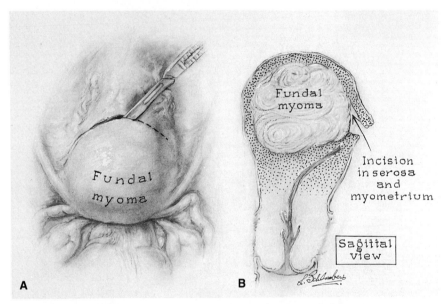

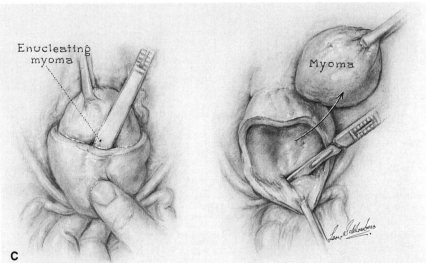

Figure 26–2. Technique of myomectomy using an anterior hood-type of incision as described by Bonny. *A*, A transverse incision is made in the anterior fundal wall over the myoma. *B*, Sagittal view of the location of the incision. *C*, Using blunt and sharp dissection, the surgeon enucleates the myoma from its bed.

myoma usually cannot be reached through Bonney's hood approach. If the anterior incision is made low enough on the uterine corpus, the peritoneum of the bladder flap may be used to cover it. The uterus can be suspended by plication of the round ligaments, by attachment of the round ligaments to the anterior rectus sheath (Olshausen technique), or by a Gilliam technique with absorbable suture material such as chromic catgut, polyglycolic acid (Dexon), or polyglactin 910 (Vicryl).

Adjuvant antiadhesion medications should be considered as with reconstructive tubal surgery. I favor a combination of dexamethasone (20 mg) and promethazine (25 mg) administered intravenously just before surgery and then at 4-hour intervals postoperatively for nine additional doses. The same doses of the two agents, diluted in 75 to 100 mL of Ringer's lactate solution, also are placed intraperitoneally just before the last peritoneal suture. This antiadhesion regimen was originally described by Replogle and coworkers. Others favor the use of intraperitoneal low molecular weight dextran.

A material has recently been described that can be placed on traumatized tissues to separate raw edges and act as a barrier to the formation of adhesions in reconstructive surgery on the reproductive tract. INTERCEED (TC7), for example, a fabric composed of oxidized, regenerated cellulose, can be placed on the deperitonealized area of the pelvic sidewall before closure, to reduce the extent of adhesion formation. Omental grafts should be avoided because of their adhesion-provoking tendency.

No regimen to prevent adhesion formation after reconstructive surgery on the reproductive tract has been validated. Because of the heightened risk of infection developing in potential blood-filled spaces in the myometrium, preoperative antibiotics should be administered prophylactically and continued for at least 1 to 2 days after surgery.

VAGINAL MYOMECTOMY

Submucous myomas also can be surgically managed with a vaginal approach in certain instances. Some pedunculated submucous tumors present themselves

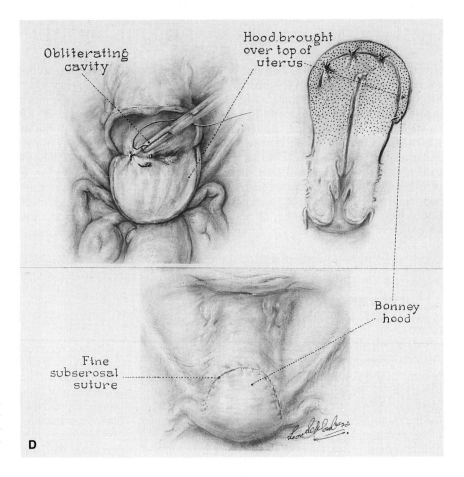

Figure 26–2. (continued) *D*, Excess hypertrophied myometrium may be trimmed and removed before closure of myometrium and serosa.

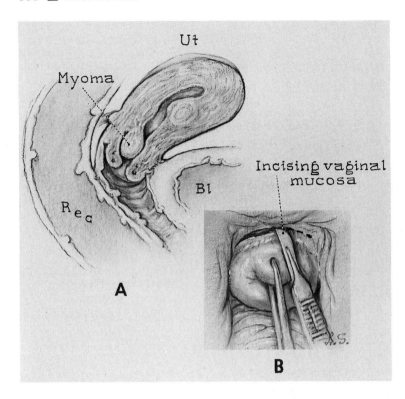

Figure 26–3. Transvaginal removal of a pedunculated submucous myoma that presents itself at the external cervical os. *A,* Sagittal view of uterus, demonstrating the location of the myoma originating on the posterior wall of the fundus just above the cervix. *B,* A transverse incision is made anteriorly through the vaginal mucosa at the cervicovaginal junction.

at or through the cervix (Fig. 26-3*A*). This type of tumor can be removed transvaginally through an already dilated cervix by advancing the bladder and making an anterior midline cervical incision (Fig. 26-3*B* and *C*), or by vaginal hysterotomy. The pedicle of the myoma is identified as high as possible, clamped close to its base, and transfixed (Fig. 26-3*D*). If the cervix was vertically incised, it is reapproximated with interrupted sutures of No. 0-0 absorbable, nonreactive material and the overlying vaginal epithelium is reapproximated with interrupted No. 3-0 sutures (Fig. 26-3*E* and *F*). Preoperative and perioperative antibiotic therapy is essential in this approach because of the hazards of disseminating infection from the prolapsed, inflamed myoma.

HYSTEROSCOPIC RESECTION OF UTERINE MYOMAS

Use of hysteroscopic resection of certain submucous myomas prevents the need for an abdominal incision, eliminates the necessity for hysterotomy, and reduces the length of hospital stay. Technologic advances in fiberoptic light sources offer the opportunity to visualize the endometrial cavity directly, evaluate the extent of the myomas, and identify bleeding sites. The development of instruments to resect tissue and electrosurgi-

cal means to secure hemostasis also have made hysteroscopic excision of submucous myomas possible. A resectoscope and a cutting loop are adaptations of instruments used for transurethral prostatectomy. Delicate scissors also can be used to shave off portions of the myoma. The medium for distending the uterus, 32% dextran 70, helps the surgeon to visualize the tumor despite bleeding and washes away blood before cauterization. In most instances laparoscopy should be done simultaneously to reduce the hazards of uterine perforation. Although it is a useful technique, hysteroscopic resection of myomas should not be undertaken by any surgeon who is not skilled in operative hysteroscopy and use of the specialized equipment needed to accomplish the procedure.

Technique

Once the resectoscope or hysteroscope is introduced into the uterus, the submucous myoma may be shaved and portions of the myoma removed (Fig. 26-4*A*). The loop of the resectoscope is placed at the most distant reachable portion of the myoma and drawn toward the surgeon. In the process the operator exerts similar pressure as with a curette in performing a curettage. With repeated strokes of the loop the excised

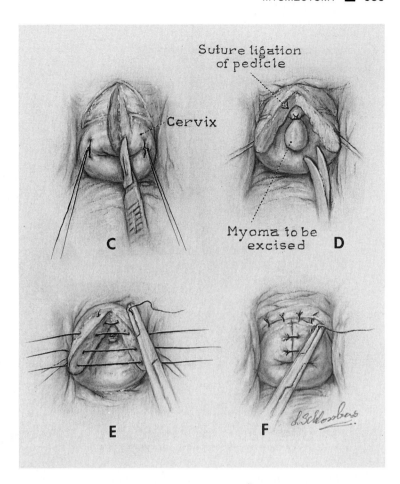

Suture ligation
of pedicle

Cervix

Myoma to be
excised

Figure 26–3. (continued) *C*, After the bladder is advanced bluntly, the cervix is incised anteriorly in the midline. *D*, The myoma and its pedicle are exposed, and the pedicle is suture ligated for hemostasis. *E*, After the myoma is excised, the cervix is reapproximated with interrupted suture of No. 0-0 absorbable, nonreactive material. *F*, The overlying vaginal mucosa is sutured with interrupted No. 3-0 absorbable sutures.

slices of tissue float in the medium (32% dextran 70) and flow out from the uterine cavity as the resectoscope is periodically removed. A grasping forceps also can be used to reduce the number of fragments of myoma in the cavity. A forceps may be used to twist off the residual myoma from its pedicle (Fig. 26-4*B*). Reinsertion of the telescope enables the surgeon to evaluate the extent of the resection. Seldom is it necessary to remove the entire myoma. The remaining portion usually is passed through the cervix 2 to 3 weeks after the procedure. Most small pedunculated myomas may be easily removed through the cervix.

Indications for Hysteroscopic Resection

The hysteroscopic approach is not applicable to all myomas, and should be reserved for submucous tumors that are simple or multiple yet not extensive, as well as for pedunculated myomas. Selection of patients should be focused on women who desire to retain childbearing capacity, women with a history of hypermenorrhea secondary to submucous myomas, and those for whom laparotomy might be hazardous (eg, the obese). The patient and the operating team should be prepared in each case for the possibility of laparotomy.

Adjunctive Measures

Pretreatment with GnRH analogs can facilitate hysteroscopic resection of myomas by diminishing their size, thereby reducing operating time. Bleeding also may be lessened after a preliminary 2- to 3-month course of GnRH analogs. Postoperatively, hemostasis can be achieved by insertion of a balloon catheter into the endometrial cavity. Inflation of the balloon tamponades the bleeding sites. The balloon can be deflated several hours after surgery and removed if bleeding has ceased.

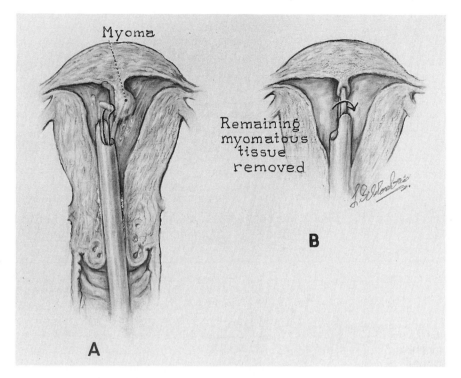

Figure 26–4. Hysteroscopic removal of a submucous myoma. *A*, After insertion of the resectoscope, the submucous myoma is removed by progressive shaving. The loop of the resectoscope is placed at the most distant portion of the myoma and the current applied as the resectoscope is drawn toward the surgeon. Pressure is exerted by the loop against the myoma with each stroke. *B*, A grasping forceps is used to twist off the remaining tissue once the size has been appreciably reduced.

MYOMECTOMY BY LASER VAPORIZATION

The carbon dioxide laser has been used as a surgical adjunct for myomectomy. During laparotomy small myomas have been directly vaporized with the laser, and both medium and large myomas were excised in McLaughlin's series. This series cited improved hemostasis; greater precision, which enables removal of only abnormal tissue; and the ability to remove myomas from previously inaccessible areas as definite advantages of this technique, but acceptance of this technique must await long-term results through extended follow-up in a larger series of patients, as the author indicates.

Baggish and associates have described treatment of submucous myomas with the neodymium:yttrium-aluminum-garnet (Nd:YAG) laser. One approach involves multiple passes with the clear fiber into the substance of the myoma. This maneuver devascularizes the myoma, thereby destroying its blood supply. Alternatively, the base may be transected with the laser and the myoma removed or left in the cavity to be expelled. Slicing the lesion plane by plane reduces the size of the myoma. Elements of the myoma can be removed with a sponge forceps or left to be passed spontaneously. As with the operating hysteroscope, concomitant laparoscopy is advisable.

COMPLICATIONS OF MYOMECTOMY

Multiple myomectomy usually is a more difficult and time-consuming procedure than hysterectomy. It frequently is accompanied by significant blood loss, a greater need for blood replacement, a higher frequency of postoperative anemia, paralytic ileus, and pain, and necessitates a longer hospital stay (Table 26-3). Long-term complications also must be considered. The need for future uterine surgery to manage recurrence of myomas is high. Roughly 20% to 25% of patients who have undergone myomectomy will ultimately require another surgical procedure, usually hysterectomy, for recurrences. The recurrence rate for

TABLE 26–3
Immediate Morbidity Associated with Myomectomy as Compared with Hysterectomy

1. ↑ Blood loss
2. ↑ Operating time
3. ↑ Postoperative morbidity
   a. Fever
   b. Ileus
   c. Anemia
4. ↑ Hospital stay
5. ↑ Pain

patients with solitary myomas is lower than that in women with multiple myomas (26.8% versus 58.8%).

With deep or multiple intramural myomectomy, delivery by cesarean section is advisable after establishment of pregnancy. Abdominal delivery is the procedure of choice whenever extensive dissection of the myometrium has been necessary. This rule of thumb should supersede the classic adage that cesarean section is indicated whenever the endometrial cavity has been entered. The incidence of late intestinal obstruction is higher after myomectomy than it is after hysterectomy, and pelvic adhesions are not uncommon, occasionally serving as a newly acquired factor in infertility. Anatomic impairment of the interstitial portion of the oviduct as a result of dissection in this location may represent an additional cause of postoperative infertility (Table 26-4). The patient contemplating myomectomy should be aware of the hazards of this "conservative" surgery as compared with those associated with hysterectomy for myomas. She also should be advised of the possibility that hysterectomy may be required rather than the proposed myomectomy. The reason for this note of caution is that myomectomy may not always be feasible. Unfortunately the surgeon cannot infallibly predict the feasibility of uterine conservation because unforeseen technical factors may accompany the excision of myomas. Despite these drawbacks, most patients who want to retain their childbearing function select myomectomy over hysterectomy when given the option. For those who want to conceive, a delay of 4 to 6 months until attempting pregnancy is advisable after the surgical procedure, since the myometrium is significantly disrupted during myomectomy.

RESULTS OF MYOMECTOMY

Evaluation of the outcome after myomectomy must be based on the specific indication for the surgery. Subsequent fertility, diminution of hypermenorrhea, achievement of a term pregnancy, alleviation of pain or pressure symptoms, and recurrence rate of myomas can each individually serve as a useful index of success-

TABLE 26–4
Long-term Complications Associated with Myomectomy

Intestinal obstruction
Recurrence of myomata
↑ Need for subsequent surgery
Infertility secondary to procedure
Disruption of uterine scar in pregnancy
↑ Need for cesarean section

ful outcome when keyed to the reason or reasons for surgery. The removal of submucous myomas should result in diminished menstrual blood loss in virtually all cases in which the bleeding has been related to their presence. Regression in size of the uterus usually is apparent immediately, but because of postoperative edema and absorption of blood from intercellular spaces, uterine size does not completely regress until about 12 weeks after surgery. The gynecologist may want to reevaluate the uterine cavity by hysterography after myomectomy, but the procedure should be deferred until 4 to 6 months have elapsed from the time of surgery, when the shape of the endometrial cavity can be truly appreciated. Distortion of the cavity related to the surgical procedure itself persists for a long time and can be misleadingly troublesome when hysterography is performed within 1 to 2 months of myomectomy.

In the series of 139 patients reported on by Ingersoll and Malone not all were married and desirous of childbearing when surgery was originally performed. Most patients under age 30 conceived, and 45% of those between ages 31 and 35 established a pregnancy. None of those older than 39 years of age at the time of surgery subsequently became pregnant. Of those conceiving, 70% did so within 2 years. In the series of Ranney and Frederick 28 of 34 married patients of reproductive age (82.4%) gave birth to a total of 48 babies after myomectomy. Berkeley and colleagues reported that 25 of 50 patients in their series conceived a total of 36 pregnancies, resulting in 24 term and 3 premature viable infants. A striking finding, however, was that only 16% of women with a myomatous uterus who underwent myomectomy for infertility eventually conceived. These data are in contrast to those of Babaknia and associates, who reported a term pregnancy rate of 38% among 34 patients with primary infertility who underwent myomectomy and of 50% in 12 patients with secondary infertility. None of the six women over age 35 conceived. The myomectomy-to-conception interval was short, with 73% conceiving within 1 year. The figures of Babaknia and coworkers are in line with those of Lock, who, after presenting his own experience and reviewing the literature, concluded that when multiple myomectomy is performed for primary infertility in the absence of other causal factors, between 40% and 50% of patients will subsequently become pregnant.

Buttram and Reiter reviewed 18 studies encompassing 1193 women in whom myomectomy was performed for infertility; 480 (40%) of these women conceived postoperatively. The same authors reviewed 1941 cases of myomectomy and compared preoperative and postoperative abortion rates. The reduction in abortion rate after myomectomy from 41% to 19% suggests improvement in reproductive salvage through the use of this procedure.

Bibliography

Aharoni A, Reiter A, Golan D, et al. Patterns of growth of uterine leiomyomas during pregnancy. A prospective longitudinal study. Br J Obstet Gynaecol 1988;95:510.

Alexander W. Enucleation of uterine fibroids. Br Gynaecol J 1898; 14:47.

Andreyko J, Blumenfeld Z, Marshall L, et al. Use of an agonistic analog of gonadotrophin-releasing hormone (nafarelin) to treat leiomyomas: Assessment by magnetic resonance imaging. Am J Obstet Gynecol 1988;158:903.

Babaknia A, Rock JA, Jones HW Jr. Pregnancy success following abdominal myomectomy for infertility. Fertil Steril 1978;30:644.

Baggish MS, Sze EHM, Morgan G. Hysteroscopic treatment of symptomatic submucous myomata uteri with the Nd:YAG laser. J Gynecol Surg 1989;5:27.

Berkeley A, DeCherney A, Polan M. Abdominal myomectomy and subsequent fertility. Surg Gynecol Obstet 1983;156:319.

Bonney V. The technique and results of myomectomy. Lancet 1931;1:171.

Briggs DW. Abdominal myomectomy in the treatment of uterine myomas. Am J Obstet Gynecol 1966;93:769.

Brown AB, Chamberlain R, Te Linde RW. Myomectomy. Am J Obstet Gynecol 1956;71:759.

Buttram VC Jr, Reiter RC. Uterine leiomyomata: Etiology, symptomatology, and management. Fertil Steril 1981;36:43.

Coddington CC, Collins RL, Shawker TH, et al. Long-acting gonadotropin hormone-releasing hormone analog used to treat uteri. Fertil Steril 1986;45:624.

Corscaden JF, Singh BP. Leiomyosarcoma of the uterus. Am J Obstet Gynecol 1958;75:149.

Coutinho EM, Goncalves MT. Long-term treatment of leiomyomas with gestrinone. Fertil Steril 1989;51:939.

Cramer S, Robertson A, Ziats N, Pearson O. Growth potential of human uterine leiomyomas: Some in vitro observations and their implications. Obstet Gynecol 1985;66:36.

Davids AM. Myomectomy. Surgical treatment and results in a series of 1,150 cases. Am J Obstet Gynecol 1952;63:592.

Dearnley G. The place of myomectomy in the treatment of primary infertility. Proc R Soc Med 1956;49:252.

Donnez J, Schrurs B, Gillerot S, et al. Treatment of uterine fibroids with implants or gonadotropin-releasing hormone agonist: Assessment by hysterography. Fertil Steril 1989;51:947.

Farber M, Conrad S, Heinrichs WI, et al. Estradiol binding by fibroid tumors and normal myometrium. Obstet Gynecol 1972;40:479.

Farrer-Brown G, Beilby W, Tarbit M. Venous changes in the endometrium of myomatous uteri. Obstet Gynecol 1971;38:743.

Fujii S. Leiomyomatosis peritonealis disseminata. In: Williams CJ et al, eds. Textbook of Uncommon Cancer. 1988 New York: John Wiley & Sons, 1988: 133.

Goldzieher J, Maqueo M, Ricaud L, et al. Induction of degenerative changes in uterine myomas by high-dosage progestin therapy. Am J Obstet Gynecol 1966;96:1078.

Healy D, Fraser H, Lawson S. Shrinkage of a uterine fibroid after subcutaneous infusion of a LHRH agonist. Br Med J 1984; 289:1267.

Ingersoll F, Malone L. Fertility following myomectomy. Fertil Steril 1963;14:596.

Ingersoll F, Malone L. Myomectomy: An alternative to hysterectomy. Arch Surg 1970;100:557.

INTERCEED (TC7) Adhesion Barrier Study Group. Prevention of postsurgical adhesions by INTERCEED (TC7), an absorbable adhesion barrier: A prospective, randomized multicenter clinical study. Fertil Steril 1989;51:933.

Katz VL, Dotters DJ, Droegemueller W. Complications of uterine leiomyomas in pregnancy. Obstet Gynecol 1989;73:593.

Kelly HA, Cullen TS. Myomata of the Uterus. Philadelphia: WB Saunders, 1907.

Kurman RJ, Norris HJ. Mesenchymal tumors of the uterus. VI. Epithelioid smooth muscle tumors including leiomyoblastoma and clear cell leiomyoma. Cancer 1976;37:1853.

Letterie GS, Coddington CC, Winkel CA, et al. Efficacy of a gonadotropin-releasing hormone agonist in the treatment of uterine leiomyomata: Long-term follow-up. Fertil Steril 1989;51:951.

Lev-Toaff AS, Coleman BG, Arger PH, et al. Leiomyomas in pregnancy: Sonographic study. Radiology 1987;164:375.

Lock F. Multiple myomectomy. Am J Obstet Gynecol 1969;104:642.

McLaughlin D. Micro-laser myomectomy technique to enhance reproductive potential: A preliminary report. Lasers Surg Med 1982;2:107.

Maheux R, Lemay A, Merat P. Use of intranasal luteinizing hormone-releasing hormone agonist in uterine leiomyomas. Fertil Steril 1987;47:229.

Montague A, Swartz A, Woodruff J. Sarcoma arising in a leiomyoma of the uterus. Am J Obstet Gynecol 1965;92:421.

Neuwirth RS. Hysteroscopic management of symptomatic submucous fibroids. Obstet Gynecol 1983;62:509.

Pfeffer WH. Adjuvants in tubal surgery. Fertil Steril 1980;33:245.

Ranney B, Frederick I. The occasional need for myomectomy. Obstet Gynecol 1979;53:437.

Replogle RL, Johnson R, Gross RE. Prevention of postoperative intestinal adhesions with combined promethazine and dexamethasone therapy. Ann Surg 1966;163:580.

Rubin I. Progress in myomectomy. Am J Obstet Gynecol 1942;44:196.

Schlaff WD, Zerhouni EA, Huth JAM, et al. A placebo controlled trial of a depot GnRH analog (leuprolide) in the treatment of uterine leiomyomata. Obstet Gynecol (in press).

Sutherland JA, Wilson EA, Edger DE, Powell D. Ultrastructure and steroid binding studies in leiomyomatosis peritonealis disseminata. Am J Obstet Gynecol 1980;136:1992.

Tada S, Tsukioka M, Ishii C, et al. Computed tomographic features of uterine myoma. J Comput Assist Tomogr 1981;5:866.

Wallach EE. Evaluation and management of uterine causes of infertility. Clin Obstet Gynecol 1979;22:43.

Hysterectomy

27

JOHN D. THOMPSON

James Johnson, editor of the *London Medico-Chirurgical Review,* said in 1825,

> We consider extirpation of the uterus, not previously protruded or inverted, one of the most cruel and unfeasible operations that ever was projected or executed by the head or hand of man. We are very far from discouraging bold or untried operations, but there is a limit beyond which it may not be prudent to go.

Only 150 years later, hysterectomy was the most common operation performed in the United States, accounting for approximately 750,000 operations in 1975. A thoughtful and critical review of hysterectomy was written recently by Bachman.

The history of hysterectomy has been reviewed by several authors including Leonardo, Mathieu, Henrotin, Noble, and Cianfrani. Although significant advances in the technique of hysterectomy did not occur until the 19th century, earlier attempts are recorded. Vaginal hysterectomy was performed many centuries before abdominal hysterectomy was attempted. Some reference to hysterectomy was made in B.C. 5th century, in the time of Hippocrates. Soranus of Ephesus is said to have amputated a gangrenous uterus vaginally in A.D. 2nd century. An Italian, Jacopo Berengario de Capri, performed a vaginal hysterectomy in A.D. 1517 and again later, using the technique developed by his father. In 1560, Andrea della Croce of Spain, performed a vaginal hysterectomy. In 1600, Schenck of Grabenberg, collected and reported 26 cases of vaginal hysterectomy. Midwives also performed some operations. These earliest hysterectomies were vaginal and usually were done for uterine prolapse or uterine inversion. According to Mathieu, "These people saw an inverted or prolapsed uterus protruding from the vagina, and not recognizing its nature, foolhardily cut it off. It is miraculous that any of the heroic patients survived this formidable ordeal." Some women with uterine prolapse even performed the operation on themselves.

Vaginal hysterectomies were done sporadically through the 17th and 18th centuries. Between 1800 and 1816, Baudelocque of France performed 23 vaginal hysterectomies. Eight vaginal hysterectomies were performed by Osiender of Gottingen. In 1810, Wrisberg presented a paper to the Vienna Royal Academy of Medicine recommending vaginal hysterectomy for uterine cancer. Langenbeck, a German surgeon, did a successful vaginal hysterectomy for uterine cancer in 1813. Sauter was the first to use ligatures on the broad ligaments in 1822. In 1829, Recamier in France performed a vaginal hysterectomy with good results. Also in 1829 in the United States, the first vaginal hysterectomy was performed by John Collins Warren of Harvard University, but the patient died on the fourth postoperative day. A successful vaginal hysterectomy for uterine cancer was performed in 1832 in Pittsburgh by Herman and Werneberg. In the late 19th century, the technique of vaginal hysterectomy was systematically studied and developed by Czerny, Billroth, Mikulicz, Schroeder, Kocher, Teuffel, and Spencer Wells.

The earliest attempts to perform abdominal hysterectomy usually involved cases in which uterine leiomyomas were misdiagnosed as large ovarian cysts. In the early 19th century, laparotomy for ovarian cysts was still considered a dangerous operation despite the initial success of McDowell in America in 1809 and Emiliami in Europe in 1815. Abdominal removal of the uterus for leiomyomas or any other reason was considered impossible to accomplish successfully. Of course, removal of pedunculated leiomyomas was more easily accomplished. Many of the earliest myomectomies consisted of removal pedunculated tumors. The first vaginal myomectomy was done by Amussat in France in 1840. In 1843, Esselman of Nashville successfully removed an inverted myomatous uterus vaginally. Washington L. Atlee of Lancaster, Pennsylvania did the first successful abdominal myomectomy on August 28, 1844. He became known for his boldness and success in removing uterine tumors. However, among his first 125 "abdominal sections" was not a single attempt to remove the whole uterus.

In 1825, Langenbeck made the first attempt to remove the uterus through an abdominal incision. The operation was done for advanced cervical cancer in 7 minutes and the patient died several hours later. An abdominal hysterectomy was performed by Charles Clay in Manchester, England, in August 1843. In November 1843 in Manchester, A.M. Heath also performed an abdominal hysterectomy. Both patients were thought to have ovarian tumors, but were found at operation to have leiomyomas. Both patients died of postoperative hemorrhage. Heath was the first to ligate both uterine arteries, a novel idea at the time that was forgotten for almost 50 years as hemorrhage continued to be a common and often lethal operative and postoperative problem. In January 1844, Clay performed another operation on a patient who had a large leiomyomatous uterus and bilateral ovarian cysts. The uterus and both ovaries were removed. The patient was recovering until dropped by the nurse on the 13th day. She died on the 15th day.

The first deliberately planned abdominal hysterectomy for uterine leiomyomas was performed in 1846 by John Bellinger of Charleston, South Carolina. The patient died on the fifth postoperative day. In 1848 in Boston, Massachusetts, Samuel Parkman's patient died of hemorrhage 12 hours after abdominal hysterectomy. Walter Burham of Lowell, Massachusetts, however, is credited with performing the first successful, although unplanned, hysterectomy for uterine leiomyomas on June 26, 1853. The preoperative diagnosis was ovarian tumor. After the abdominal incision was made, the patient vomited and extruded the leiomyomatous uterus through the incision. It could not be replaced and therefore was removed. The patient survived.

On September 1, 1853, G. Kimball of Lowell, Massachusetts, was the first person to deliberately and successfully perform an abdominal hysterectomy for a correct preoperative diagnosis of uterine leiomyomas. In a formal paper, he advocated the operation, although he had only one success in his first four operations. According to Storer, only 6 of the first 24 patients who had abdominal hysterectomy lived. Of the 18 patients who died, 11 died of hemorrhage and shock.

As time passed, needed improvements were made in the technique of abdominal hysterectomy. Hemorrhage was almost impossible to control until 1864 when Koeberle of France published a landmark paper on hysterectomy and introduced his method of securing the large vascular pedicle of the lower uterus with his serreneud. This *ligature en masse* around the lower uterus with the corpus amputated above was the usual technique of controlling bleeding with hysterectomy in the earliest years. The stump thus formed was such a large mass of tissue that it could not always be safely returned to the peritoneal cavity because of the danger of intraperitoneal bleeding, and often was fixed extraperitoneally in the incision so that it was available for hemostatic clamping should the need arise. In 1889, Stimson described a technique for secure individual ligation of uterine and ovarian arteries that was responsible for reducing the incidence of postoperative hemorrhage. Kelly published a similar technique with illustrations in 1891. Of course, abdominal hysterectomy was more common by this time. The first successful total abdominal hysterectomy in the United States was done by Mary Amanda Dixon Jones in 1888, although it seems that the uterine corpus was removed abdominally and the cervix was removed vaginally.

According to Cullen, 969 abdominal hysterectomies for uterine leiomyomas were done at The Johns Hopkins Hospital between 1889 and 1906 with a mortality of 5.9%, a remarkable achievement considering that many patients were in poor health. Between 1906 and 1909, the mortality was reduced to < 1%. In 1909, Cullen wrote,

> It was my good fortune to come to Baltimore in 1891, shortly after the hospital opened. At that time many cases of myoma were considered inoperable, and even when hysterectomy was undertaken it was only in the cases in which a stout rubber ligature could be temporarily tied around the cervix; and when, as happened in some cases, this ligature slipped, alarming hemorrhage followed. Then came the systematic controlling of each cardinal vessel; later the bisection, and finally the transverse severance of the cervix as a preliminary feature of the operation in exceptionally difficult cases, until at present a myomatous uterus that cannot be removed is almost unheard of. I have watched the gradual simplifications of the surgical procedures with the greatest interest. Many American surgeons have had much to do with the wonderful advance in this direction, but I know of no other man, either here or abroad who has done as much toward this advancement as Howard A. Kelly.

In the early decades of the 20th century, hysterectomy began to be used more often in the treatment of gynecologic disease and symptoms. During this period, gynecology as a specialty was developing from its infancy. The surgical treatment of gynecologic disease received major emphasis for understandable reasons. Little else was available to gynecologists to help their patients. For example, estrogen and progesterone were not discovered until the late 1920s and early 1930s. Major discoveries and concepts of reproductive organ physiology and pathology were just beginning. As surgery became safer, skillful gynecologists concentrated on developing newer surgical procedures to help their patients. Noteworthy contributions were made to the techniques of gynecologic surgery by Sims, Wertheim, Schauta, Kelly, Bonney, Clarke, Mayo, Meigs, and many others. In retrospect, it is probably true that some operations were done in that era for incorrect indications. Although some may say that these unnecessary operations were done because of the gynecologist's preoccupation with the personal development of surgical skills and operative techniques, it is also likely that it was related to the unavailability of proper information about the physiology and pathology of the reproductive organs and the clinical manifestations of pelvic disease.

Through the remainder of the century, as gynecology matured as a specialty in medicine, knowledge of reproductive organ function and disease became more complete; special and more accurate diagnostic techniques were developed (the intravenous pyelogram, for example, was developed in 1923); and effective nonsurgical methods of therapy were discovered. Currently, in the modern practice of gynecology, appropriate use of this knowledge and advanced modern diagnostic technologies allow a more correct choice of treatment and the use of surgical therapy only when indicated.

With better recognition and treatment of complicating medical diseases, with proper use of blood transfusions and antibiotics, and with improvements in anesthetic techniques, a hysterectomy can be done fairly safely by the skillful gynecologic surgeon of today. Mortality from hysterectomy in most medical centers is 1 to 2 per 1000. It is possible to report no mortalities in a series of several thousand hysterectomies. However, morbidity continues to be a problem. Complications of some sort may occur in as many as 25% of patients undergoing vaginal hysterectomy and 50% of those undergoing abdominal hysterectomy. Some complications may be serious (eg, infection, hemorrhage, urinary tract and intestinal tract injury, and pulmonary embolus). In the hands of the occasional operator, mortality and the incidence of significant complications are likely to be higher. However, the rate of complications should always be as low as possible. It should be emphasized that the ability to perform several hundred hysterectomies with a low mortality and morbidity rate, although extremely desirable, is not ipso facto evidence that gynecologic surgery is being practiced correctly. In addition to a low morbidity and mortality rate, the physician also must be certain that only patients with proper indications are chosen for surgical treatment.

The knowledge that is needed to formulate proper "indications for hysterectomy" includes primarily a thorough understanding of the physiology and pathology of the female reproductive organs, the clinical manifestations of pelvic disease, and normal and abnormal psychosocial-sexual development. This basic and thorough knowledge and understanding is the absolute foundation upon which the "pyramid of successful practice of gynecologic surgery" is built (Fig. 27-1). It is from this knowledge (and sometimes wisdom) that the physician must draw in deciding that a patient should be offered surgical therapy, remembering that it is only the occasional gynecologic patient who requires surgery for relief. Then, after the right patient has been selected for operation, the right operation must be selected for the patient. For example, it is a mistake to do an abdominal hysterectomy when better results can be obtained by performing a vaginal hysterectomy. The pyramid of successful practice of gynecologic surgery is complete with proper preparation of the patient for operation, proper performance of the operation, and proper postoperative care. In the practice of gynecologic surgery, most mistakes are made by those physicians who may know "how" but may not understand "when" and "why." In referring to this point, the late Dr. Richard W. TeLinde, Professor of Gynecology at The Johns Hopkins University and originator of this book, said,

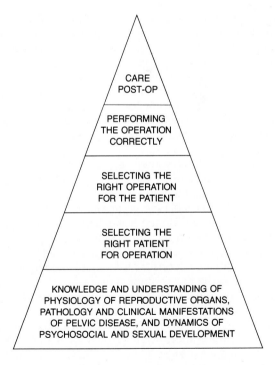

Figure 27–1. Pyramid of successful practice of gynecologic surgery.

The ease with which the average hysterectomy may be done has proven both a blessing and a curse to womankind. There is no doubt that a hysterectomy done with proper indications may restore a woman to health and even save her life. However, in the practice of gynecology, one has ample opportunity to observe countless women who have been advised to have hysterectomies without proper indications. . . . I am inclined to believe that the greatest single factor in promoting unnecessary hysterectomies is a lack of understanding of gynecologic pathology. The greatest need today among those who are performing pelvic surgery is a better knowledge of gynecologic pathology.

Certainly, many women have benefited enormously from a hysterectomy properly indicated and properly performed. However, considerable concern has been expressed that this same operation is overused and not always done for proper indications. The medical profession has a strong tradition of accountability for the quality of care given to patients, evident in daily rounds and conferences, chart reviews, audits, hospital tissue and credential committees, specialty and subspecialty board certification and recertification, specialty society activities, rules and regulations of the Joint Commission on Accreditation of Hospitals, licensure, continuing medical education requirements, and so forth. Nevertheless, accusations of unnecessary operations, including unnecessary hysterectomies, still come from unions, insurance companies, consumer groups, the media, state and federal agencies, the U.S. Congress, and also from members of the medical professions.

From a National Center for Health Statistics report, Pokras and Hufnagel cited some interesting statistics for a study period between 1965 and 1984:

Of the 97 million women aged 15 years or older in the United States in 1985, approximately 18.5 million have had a hysterectomy.

Between 1965 and 1984, approximately 12.5 million women in the United States had a hysterectomy.

Hysterectomy was the most common major surgery each year after 1965 until 1981, when an increase in cesarean section for births supplanted hysterectomy as the most common major surgery. Hysterectomy remained the second most common major surgery from 1981 through 1985.

The largest number of hysterectomies occurred in 1975, when there were 725,000, or 8.6 per 1000 women aged 15 years and older. Since 1975, the annual number and rate have declined slightly and leveled off to approximately 650,000 hysterectomies, or 7 per 1000 women, in the 1980s.

The average age of patients undergoing hysterectomy during the 20-year period studied was 42.7 years, median 40.9 years.

From 1970 through 1984, the most common indications for hysterectomy were leiomyomas (26.8%), prolapse (20.8%), endometriosis (14.7%), cancer (10.7%), and endometrial hyperplasia (6.2%). The remaining 20.7% included disorders of menstruation and abnormal bleeding; diseases of the parametrium or pelvic peritoneum; infectious and other diseases of the cervix, ovaries, or fallopian tubes; obstetrical catastrophe; and benign neoplasms other than leiomyomas.

From 1965–67 to 1982–84, the rate of hysterectomies for endometriosis increased 2.2-fold.

By 1985, approximately 65% of women aged 60–64 years had intact uteri.

Assuming constant age-specific hysterectomy rates, the number of hysterectomies will increase over the next 20 years as the population of women in the age group 30–49 years increases. The number of hysterectomies will rise, from approximately 670,000 in 1985 to an estimated 810,000 in 1995 and 854,000 in the 2005.

The age-specific rate for hysterectomy is low (1 per 1000) in women under age 25 years, but rises (16 per 1000) for women over age 35 years. After age 35 years, women usually have completed childbearing and also have a higher incidence of significant gynecologic disease.

The mortality risk of hysterectomy in the United States has been studied by several authors. At the Hutzel Hospital in Detroit, 6435 hysterectomies were performed between 1965 and 1974. Seventeen deaths occurred for a rate of 26.4 per 10,000 women having a hysterectomy, according to Amirika and Evans. Ledger and Child studied 12,026 hysterectomies done in 1970. There were 20 deaths for a rate of 16.6 per 10,000 women. The most comprehensive recent study was reported in 1985 by Wingo and associates from the Centers for Disease Control (CDC). During 1979 and 1980, they found 477 deaths among 317,389 women having abdominal hysterectomies and 46 deaths among 119,972 women having vaginal hysterectomies. The mortality rates for hysterectomy were higher for procedures associated with pregnancy or cancer than for procedures not associated with these conditions (29.2, 37.8, and 6.0 per 10,000 hysterectomies, respectively). In general, mortality rates for hysterectomies performed by the abdominal approach were higher than rates for hysterectomies performed by the vaginal approach. Excluding pregnancy and cancer-related cases, the mortality rate for abdominal hysterectomy was 8.6 and for vaginal hysterectomy was 2.7 per 10,000 women having hysterectomies. Overall, mortality rates increased with age, particularly after age 57 years. Because of significant rates of mortality and morbidity in all age groups, hysterectomy cannot be thought of as a low-risk operation that can be done to treat relatively minor gynecologic symptoms or disease.

UNNECESSARY HYSTERECTOMIES, SECOND OPINIONS, AND AUDITS

In 1946, Miller reviewed patients who had undergone hysterectomy and reported that "in 33.1% of the cases, there was either no disease, or else disease contraindicating hysterectomy, such as unsuspected pregnancy, infected retained secundines, etc." He further stated, "If what we have observed in this look behind the scenes is confirmed by further studies, then we may be sure when the curtain rises we shall witness a tragedy painful and far-reaching in its implications."

Indeed, further studies did seem to confirm Miller's findings and prophecy. Doyle reported in 1953 that 39% of hysterectomies were unnecessary. Trussell, Morehead, and Ehrlich reported in 1962 that > 30% of hysterectomies were unnecessary. Fine and Morehead reported in 1971 that "case records were reviewed by board certified specialists who felt that 43% of hysterectomies were unjustified." These and other data led to a study of voluntary and mandatory second opinions by McCarthy and Kamons. Patients who were advised to have a hysterectomy agreed voluntarily to obtain a second opinion. In 43.9% of the voluntary second opinions obtained, the physician rendering the second opinion did not agree that a hysterectomy was needed. When the second opinion was mandatory, 20.2% of the opinions were unconfirmed. Although the study was criticized, many unions and insurance companies, in an attempt to control costs, subsequently insisted that patients obtain second opinions before hysterectomy and other selected surgical procedures. The investigation and report of the U.S. House of Representatives Interstate Commerce Committee Subcommittee on Oversight and Investigation on Unnecessary Surgery brought on a storm of protests about the validity of the statistics and conclusions drawn in the report. Nevertheless, because of the report, the federal Medicare and Medicaid programs began to require recipients to obtain second opinions before hysterectomy and other selected operations.

The validity of the studies that showed a high rate of unnecessary hysterectomies was challenged. The Hysterectomy Subcommittee of the Quality Care Committee of the New York Medical Society reported that only "3.1% of hysterectomies were judged unacceptable based on close scrutiny of medical records." In 1977, Emerson and Creedon reported that

when 1,901 hysterectomies were evaluated and the documented indications measured against present criteria, including pathologic confirmation, two operations were not justified and nine were questionable. On review, the nine cases were found acceptable by the hospital review committees. Even if these operations were unjustified, the total number of cases considered unjustified was less than 1 percent.

A proper Tissue Committee audit and retrospective review of records must use clear-cut preestablished criteria as indications for the operation. These criteria must be agreed to and used consistently by all members of the committee. In addition, a sufficient number of reviewers within the specialty of the procedure under review must be included in the committee. Richardson reported that, for gynecologic cases, 28 reviewers would be required to produce a composite judgment of the quality of care of a single patient with a 95% confidence level. Clearly, such completeness and accuracy in reviews is impractical and is rarely achieved in hospital audit committees. Studies also are hampered by the term "unnecessary hysterectomy" itself. As stated by Rutkow and Zuidema, "The term 'unnecessary surgery' has no value without an adequate definition and, at present, a suitable one has not been found." Nevertheless, in Whitelaw's medico-legal perspective of hysterectomy, a total of 17% of legal suits were based on an allegation of unnecessary hysterectomy.

To determine the percentage of preoperative diagnoses that were confirmed by pathologic examination, Lee and associates analyzed data from the Collaborative Review of Sterilization (CREST study), a multicenter prospective study conducted by the Division of Reproductive Health of the CDC, to examine the health effects of hysterectomies and tubal sterilizations in women aged 15 to 44 years. Of the 1851 women included in the study from 1978 to 1981, 1283 (69%) had abdominal hysterectomies and 568 (31%) had vaginal hysterectomies. Overall, 52% of the hysterectomies were performed for a preoperative diagnosis that could potentially be confirmed by pathologic examination. Pathologic examination actually confirmed the preoperative diagnosis of endometrial hyperplasia in 95% of the cases, cervical intraepithelial neoplasia in 89%, leiomyomas in 84%, pelvic inflammatory disease in 75%, adenomyosis in 48%, and endometriosis in 47%. Among all the potentially confirmable diagnoses, 80% were confirmed. The remaining 48% of the women who had hysterectomies had preoperative diagnoses that were not amenable to confirmation by pathology. Most of these hysterectomies were for one of three diagnoses: (1) menstrual bleeding disorders, (2) pelvic pain, or (3) pelvic relaxation. In 47% of these cases, pathologic examination showed leiomyoma or adenomyosis; no abnormalities were found in 38% of these cases.

In 1946, Miller found the clinical diagnosis was confirmed by pathologic examination in 246 hysterectomies. In 31%, the hysterectomy specimen showed no abnormality. Other series by Ojeda, by Doyle, and by D'Esopo found that 9%–15% of specimens were normal. Studies of vaginal hysterectomy for sterilization purposes by Atkinson and Chappell, by Hubbard, and by Van Nagell and Roddick found that 81%–94% of the uteri were normal. Foster found that 82 (16.9%) of 485 uteri removed were considered anatomically normal.

It should be obvious to members of hospital tissue committees, audit committees, and quality assurance committees that a variety of circumstances and conditions in gynecology require removal of a uterus that may show no evidence of gross or microscopic pathology when examined later by the pathologist. Depending on a variety of circumstances, removal of a normal uterus may sometimes be indicated and permitted in the surgical treatment of ovarian tumors (benign or malignant); fallopian tube cancer; vaginal cancer; pelvic inflammatory disease; endometriosis; pelvic relaxation and genital prolapse; dysfunctional uterine bleeding; ectopic pregnancy; pelvic pain; pelvic tuberculosis; postpartum hemorrhage; and sterilization.

Since 1970, the Division of Reproductive Health of the CDC has provided valuable epidemiologic surveillance information of hysterectomies performed on women in the United States. Most of their studies are limited to women in the 15–44 year age group. According to the CDC, in the period from 1970 to 1982, an estimated 5,170,000 women aged 15–44 years underwent hysterectomy in non-Federal, short-stay U.S. hospitals. The number of hysterectomies increased from a low of 306,000 in 1970 to a high of 442,000 in 1977 and then declined to 421,000 in 1981 and 407,000 in 1982. The hysterectomy rate in 1981 was 7.9 per 1000 women aged 15–44 years; in 1982, the rate was 7.5 per 1000 women, the lowest rate since 1970. Women in the Northeast had the lowest hysterectomy rates; women in the South had the highest hysterectomy rates (2.5 times that of women in the Northeast).

In addition, the CDC reported that the average age at the time of hysterectomy was similar in all geographic areas, ranging from 34.2 years in the South to 36.6 years in the Northeast. In 1981 and 1982, 27% and 24%, respectively, of all hysterectomies were performed vaginally. There were substantial regional differences in the percentage of hysterectomies done vaginally (14% in the Northeast compared with 33% in the West). The authors of the report believe patient-related factors may

include regional differences in the incidence of gynecologic conditions and in general attitudes toward surgery or sterilization during the reproductive years. For example, a population that comprises a higher percentage of black women can expect a larger number of patients requiring hysterectomy for symptomatic and large leiomyomas. A population that includes a larger number of indigent women can expect to have a larger number of operations for salpingo-oophoritis and cervical neoplasia. Regionally, hysterectomy rates in the United States dropped from 6.4 to 3.8 per 1000 women aged 15–44 between 1972 and 1984 in the Northeast. During the same period in the South, hysterectomy rates decreased from 11.7 to 10 per 1000 women aged 15–44.

In Canton Ticino, Switzerland, a public information campaign focused on a 57% increase in hysterectomy rates between 1977 and 1982. The subject received wide publicity in six local newspapers and in the broadcast media during 9 months in 1984. By the end of 1985, the annual rate for hysterectomy had fallen by 25.8%. In the reference area (Canton Bern), where no information was given to the public, hysterectomy rates increased by 1%. This campaign showed the sensitivity of the health-care market to an informational campaign on common surgical procedures and an increased awareness among physicians of the difficulties associated with defining and using appropriate indications for surgery. According to Dyck and coworkers, following a program of surveillance in the Canadian province of Saskatchewan, the number of hysterectomies there decreased dramatically. Marked variations in hysterectomy rates exist both within and between countries with similar populations having no major differences in health status. For example, the hysterectomy rate per 10^5 women was 979 in Canada in 1971, 651 in the United States in 1973, 126 in Sweden in 1977, 456 in New South Wales (Australia) in 1979, 391 in the Netherlands in 1981, and 260 in England and Wales in 1983, according to Dickinson and Hill. Such wide differences in rates are difficult to explain and understand. As pointed out by Domenighetti (1988),

> international and regional variations in the frequency of hysterectomy and of the most common surgical procedures seem to be best explained by factors such as medical and surgical bed density, insurance and payment systems, professional uncertainty, surgeon's sex, control and review of surgical indications, medical auditing, and second opinion programs, than by differences in morbidity, mortality, and other sociodemographic characteristics of the population studied.

It is appropriate for the medical profession to regulate its own affairs if outside intervention, which may be detrimental to the welfare of patients, is to be avoided. Peer review medical audits should be carried out at the local hospital level and members of such hospital committees should have legal protection to be effective.

An excellent example of an attempt to validate the indications of hysterectomy and to establish a workable quality assurance process was described by Gambone and associates in 1989. Pointing out that more indications are listed for hysterectomy than for any other major operation and that the problem is confounded by the common but questionable practice of combining several indications (any one of which would be insufficient justification if listed alone), these authors required the surgeon to select preoperatively only one designated indication for each hysterectomy performed. The process of using only a single designated indication and reviewing only two documents in the record (the pathology report and the surgeon's preoperative note) greatly simplified the quality assurance process. The authors recommend that hospital quality assurance committees use their method to easily monitor the appropriateness of indications for hysterectomy.

On the other hand, Ranney points out that seldom does a gynecologic patient who needs a hysterectomy have a single diagnosis. Among 2892 patients who needed a hysterectomy, only 127 had a single diagnosis. The remainder had 2 to 10 separate diagnoses. Therefore, as Ranney suggests, chart reviews, coding systems, or computer systems that are limited to a few diagnoses will be incomplete, inaccurate, and misleading.

A competent gynecologist who has followed a patient for several years, has kept careful records of findings and treatment, and has the patient's full confidence is probably able to make the most accurate judgment about the necessity for hysterectomy. In some circumstances, however, a second opinion should still be sought, especially if there is the slightest doubt or question about the necessity for operation. Significant complications and morbidity still occur with hysterectomy. Anesthetic accidents, postoperative pulmonary emboli, hemorrhage, wound complications, injuries to the ureters and bladder, and especially infection are definite surgical risks. If a patient has a serious complication, then it is important to have the previously recorded opinion of another physician that the operation was necessary. Certainly, any time the patient requests consultation with another physician, the request should be honored. The consulting physician should be a qualified physician of the same specialty who provides similar services under approximately similar conditions. If more second opinions are obtained voluntarily, it should be less likely that second opinions will be mandated for all hysterectomies. It is to be hoped that the greatest benefit of a second opinion will be to the patient, by providing improved care and performing surgery only for appropriate indications. In a study of second opinions for elective surgery, Gertman and associates concluded that many unconfirmed second opinions were due to honest differences of opinions about indications for surgery. These authors estimated that second opinion programs would produce only modest direct savings to third-party payers, but probably would offer important improvements in the quality of health care.

The appropriateness of indications for hysterectomy is of great concern to third parties that pay for health care and must keep costs within reasonable limits. Utilization reviewers for third-party payers determine the appropriateness of hospital admissions and place limits on the length of hospital stay. Their decisions are based on the initial opinion of the patient's physician and also on second and sometimes third opinions regarding appropriateness of planned treatment. They are also based on advisory guidelines set by the medical profession usually through various medical specialty organizations. This sometimes results in reviewers haggling with the patient's physician over the need for operation. Private and government health insurers, faced with the prospect of continued increases in the cost of health care (including women's health care) are dissatisfied with the results of current methods of review. In the future, physician's treatment decisions (including the decision to perform a hysterectomy) will be more closely scrutinized. Increasingly, patients will be forced to pay for the cost of health care judged by third-party payers to be inappropriate.

A new era in utilization review and clinical practice standards is approaching. Very likely, a computerized product called "decision review protocols" that comprise detailed sets of clinical indications will be used to more aggressively prejudge and monitor the appropriateness of treatment, including hysterectomy. The standards (parameters) that are used may provide adequate clarity to allow a general understanding, provide a comprehensive list of indications, and provide a willingness to identify overuse. But patients present in highly individual and sometimes ambiguous ways; can objective appropriateness criteria be subjective and inclusive enough to replace clinical judgment by the individual physician? Also, a system of appropriateness review that does not consider underuse as well as overuse, that does not identify patients who need procedures but do not get them, that does not consider the clinical outcome of the case when the operation is approved and especially when the operation is not approved, may not result in an improved quality of patient care. In other words, when considering ways to control the economic costs of hysterectomies in the United States, there must be concomitant concern for improving the quality of care that each patient receives.

The frequent performance of hysterectomy has come under closer scrutiny in the past 20 years and continues today. The indications for the operation have been questioned; the motives of the surgeons have been questioned. Such doubts have been supported by the points discussed so far. Also, whether the health benefit is worth the economic cost has been questioned. The cost of hysterectomies in 1985 in the United States was $3 billion, for hospital costs only. It is now universally agreed that resources available to meet all demands for health care are unavailable. Hard decisions regarding the rationing and allocation of limited health resources will be made. Resource-allocation decisions made by private industry, union, and governmental health planners, administrators, and providers will be guided by considerations of cost compared with expected benefits. In this environment of cost-cutting and benefit-analysis, it will be incumbent upon gynecologic surgeons to prove to what degree their procedures are cost effective and are necessary to save or enhance the quality of life of the patients they serve. Certainly, the first of all considerations is performing hysterectomies only when they are indicated and clearly justified.

As stated by Bunker,

When it is agreed to make "necessary" medical care available to every citizen as a right, decisions will have to be made regarding what is necessary and what is not. There can, of course, be little question of the necessity of hysterectomy in the treatment of cancer of the endometrium; large, painful, or bleeding fibroids; or uterine prolapse. At issue will be the allocation of public funds for a procedure when it appears neither necessary nor clearly beneficial to health, but more in the nature of a convenience or personal preference, and when this allocation competes with growing demands for funds to pay for other medical uses, many of which may present stronger claims.

TERMINOLOGY

The only suitable terms to modify the word "hysterectomy" are "total" or "subtotal" and "vaginal" or "abdominal." Terms that are confusing or inappropriate include "panhysterectomy," "complete hysterectomy," "incomplete hysterectomy," "supravaginal hysterectomy," and "supracervical hysterectomy."

The term "hysterectomy" is a noun that cannot be converted into a verb (eg, "hysterectomize"). Removal of the adnexal organs should be specified separately as "bilateral" or "unilateral" and as "salpingectomy," "oophorectomy," or "salpingo-oophorectomy."

APPROPRIATE INDICATIONS FOR HYSTERECTOMY

Without question, a properly indicated and properly performed hysterectomy can be of enormous benefit to properly informed patients with significant gynecologic symptoms or disease. It must never be done, however, without proper indications. In the final analysis, as once explained by J.M.T. Finney of The Johns Hopkins University, the indications for surgical procedures fall into the following broad categories:

To save life
To relieve suffering
To correct deformity

The following discussion represents the author's opinion regarding appropriate indications for hysterectomy. Admittedly, there is room for other opinions.

Benign Disease or Symptoms of Uterine Origin

Dysfunctional Uterine Bleeding

Dysfunctional uterine bleeding is defined as heavy, prolonged, or frequent bleeding (ie, menorrhagia, metrorrhagia, or polymenorrhea) of uterine origin in the absence of infection, tumors, pregnancy, or associated medical conditions. It is usually present with anovulation and irregular shedding or maturation of the endometrium. Some patients will be found to have endometrial hyperplasia in one or another of its several forms. Dysfunctional uterine bleeding is more completely discussed in Chapter 13.

Although formerly it was not an uncommon indication for hysterectomy, in the modern practice of gynecology, it is almost always possible to treat dysfunctional uterine bleeding successfully with hormonal therapy. Endometrial curettage is sometimes necessary and is indicated especially in older women in the decade before menopause to rule out the diagnosis of endometrial cancer. Curettage to remove retained secundines or a placental polyp also may be indicated when abnormal uterine bleeding follows a recent pregnancy. Hysteroscopy and hysterography may be helpful in locating unusual pathology in the uterine cavity such as endometrial polyps or submucous leiomyomas. Endometrial ablation or resection through the hysteroscope has been found to be effective in treatment, thus avoiding the need for hysterectomy in some patients (see Ch. 17). Hysterectomy is not indicated unless the bleeding is recurrent, severe, and unresponsive to hormonal therapy and endometrial curettage on several occasions. When hysterectomy is necessary, it usually can be done vaginally unless otherwise contraindicated. Recalcitrant dysfunctional uterine bleeding is not an indication for bilateral oophorectomy at the time of hysterectomy. In young women, hysterectomy should almost never be done to treat dysfunctional uterine bleeding.

Adenomyosis

Dysmenorrhea, uterine tenderness, menorrhagia, and uterine enlargement usually symmetrical and most prominent in the anteroposterior dimension may indicate adenomyosis. Depending on the severity of symptoms, hysterectomy may be indicated after failure of response to more conservative measures, such as hormonal therapy or uterine curettage. Either vaginal or abdominal hysterectomy may be done if necessary.

It should be emphasized that adenomyosis is not a common indication for hysterectomy. Deep myometrial involvement with endometrium and associated myometrial hypertrophy is uncommon. A preoperative diagnosis of adenomyosis may not be confirmed pathologically, and minimal adenomyosis found by careful pathologic study is probably of no significance clinically. In a study of validation of hysterectomy indications by Gambone and associates, adenomyosis represented the least verified indication with only 38% of pathology reports providing confirmation. These authors stated that adenomyosis should no longer be considered a reliable indication for hysterectomy and recommended that patients suspected of having adenomyosis should be considered under other categories (ie, chronic pelvic pain or recurrent uterine bleeding). I do not agree that adenomyosis should no longer be mentioned as an appropriate indication for hysterectomy, but do agree that it should be an uncommon indication. Adenomyosis is discussed in Chapter 20.

Physicians should be cautioned that the symptom of menorrhagia is difficult to evaluate. Some women who give a history of heavy menstrual flow will be found to have a normal amount of menstrual blood loss on careful evaluation. On the contrary, other women who give a history of normal menstruation may be found to have an excessive flow. The physician should not expect to always get accurate information about the amount of menstrual flow by simply asking, "Is your menstrual flow normal?" More detailed questions must be asked. There is a great need in the clinical practice of gynecology for a simple, practical, convenient, and accurate method to estimate menstrual blood loss. Such a method would greatly assist the gynecologist in deciding when to recommend hysterectomy for recurrent or persistent menorrhagia.

Symptomatic Vaginal Relaxation, Uterine Descensus, and Prolapse

Symptomatic descent or prolapse of the uterus, usually associated with symptomatic vaginal wall relaxation (ie, cystourethrocele, enterocele, and rectocele) with or without stress urinary incontinence, is a common indication for vaginal hysterectomy with restoration of normal anatomy and proper support to the vaginal outlet, vaginal walls, and vaginal vault. It should be emphasized that this operation is indicated only if symptoms are severe enough to justify the risk involved; if conservative measures, such as Kegel exercises or vaginal estrogen, have failed to give sufficient comfort; and, most of all, *if the patient is asking for relief.* An operation to correct asymptomatic and mild-to-moderate anatomic relaxation of the vaginal walls and uterine descensus is rarely indicated. Too many operations are done for this indication in patients who are asymptomatic. Unfortunately, some asymptomatic patients may be caused to have symptoms by an ill-advised operation.

Hysterectomy is not a necessary part of surgical procedures to correct stress urinary incontinence. For example, if a suprapubic colpourethropexy is indicated to correct stress urinary incontinence, then hysterectomy is not indicated unless other conditions are present. Vaginal repair of a large symptomatic cystocele and enterocele is usually done better if vaginal hysterectomy is also done at the same time.

Uterine Leiomyomas

Uterine leiomyomas are common benign tumors of the myometrium that usually do not cause symptoms or require removal. The patient with small, asymptomatic uterine leiomyomas may be followed with periodic pelvic exams. If symptoms do not appear before menopause, then it is unlikely that a hysterectomy will be needed after menopause. No new myomas appear after menopause, and myomas already present cease to grow and usually become smaller.

Uterine leiomyomas are the most common reason for hysterectomy. Abdominal or vaginal hysterectomy may be indicated if there is associated discomfort, urinary frequency or obstruction, menorrhagia, or metrorrhagia. If the uterus is not too large, then a conservative approach with uterine curettage rather than hysterectomy should be tried first. If a submucous myoma is found by hysterography, hysteroscopy, or uterine curettage, it is unlikely that conservative measures will relieve the patient's bleeding. Depending on the circumstances, a submucous myoma may be removed with the hysteroscope, with myomectomy, or with hysterectomy.

Rapid enlargement of a leiomyomatous uterus may indicate sarcomatous change. In young women, it is more commonly an indication of associated pregnancy. In this situation, a pregnancy test is indicated before hysterectomy is recommended.

It is possible for a leiomyomatous uterus to be rather large and still cause no symptoms. When it reaches the size of a 12- to 14-week pregnant uterus, a recommendation for removal may be made based on size alone. If a decision is made not to operate but to follow such a patient, then the physician must be extremely careful that all components of the pelvic mass are indeed benign uterine leiomyomas. There is always the possibility that one or more of the components of the mass is an ovarian tumor—the removal of which should not be delayed. Some idea of the various components of the mass may be obtained from computerized tomography (CT) or ultrasonography scans of the pelvis. False positive and false negative findings are possible with these studies, as indicated in Chapter 12. Although an abdominal approach is preferred when hysterectomy is indicated for large leiomyomas, vaginal hysterectomy may be preferred when symptomatic leiomyomas are small. Extensive morcellation may be required to remove a leiomyomatous uterus vaginally.

A submucous pedunculated leiomyoma protruding through the cervical os is always infected and should be removed by vaginal myomectomy to prevent unavoidable bacterial contamination of the peritoneal cavity with abdominal removal. Several weeks later, if there is still significant enlargement of the uterus or persistent symptoms, an abdominal or vaginal hysterectomy may be recommended at a later date after the risk of peritonitis has passed. A more complete discussion of uterine leiomyomas can be found in Chapter 26.

Obstetric Problems

Hysterectomy in obstetric practice was reviewed by Hill and Beischer. Uncontrollable postpartum hemorrhage, uterine rupture, uterine inversion, and interstitial, abdominal, or cervical pregnancy are obstetrical catastrophes that may require abdominal hysterectomy to prevent death from hemorrhage.

Septic abortion is usually treated successfully with antibiotics and evacuation of retained infected placental and fetal parts. Few patients are unresponsive to medical therapy and curettage. However, occasionally, the physician also may need to do an abdominal hysterectomy when there is severe infectious septic shock, peritonitis, and impairment of renal function perhaps associated with infection with clostridia microorganisms.

Nonneoplastic Diseases of the Tubes and Ovaries in Which the Uterus Is Not Primarily Involved

In the circumstances discussed in the sections that follow, the uterus may be removed as part of an operation to remove the diseased adnexa even though there is no pathology in the uterus itself. If, during an operation for pathology primarily in the tubes or ovaries, or both, it appears that the patient will be unable to conceive, it is also appropriate to remove the uterus. Exceptions to this recommendation can be made in young women who would like to attempt pregnancy through the application of one of the many newer reproductive technologies. Young women should be advised of this option of uterine conservation before the operation is done. Specific permission for removal of the uterus should be obtained in such young women in case it becomes absolutely necessary to perform hysterectomy.

Pelvic Inflammatory Disease

As discussed in Chapter 24, an acute exacerbation of chronic pelvic inflammatory disease with bilateral tubo-ovarian abscesses can usually be treated successfully with conservative medical management including antibiotics for polymicrobial infection and drainage of pus when this is possible by either posterior colpotomy or CT-guided needle aspiration. In our experience, 80% of patients will respond to this management. For the 20% of patients who do not respond, for patients with a ruptured tubo-ovarian abscess, or for patients with significant symptoms of chronic pelvic inflammatory disease, operation may be recommended. Usually, a bilateral salpingo-oophorectomy will be necessary because extensive adnexal disease will be found bilaterally. Occasionally, it is possible to conserve the function of one ovary. Hysterectomy also is usually recommended in women who are not interested in taking advantage of the new reproductive technologies for achieving pregnancy. For those who are, the uterus may be left in place even though both tubes and ovaries have been removed.

Pelvic Endometriosis

Extensive pelvic endometriosis not responsive to hormonal therapy may require surgery for relief. Young women who have not completed childbearing should have conservational surgery, including removal of all visible and palpable endometriosis, possible presacral neurectomy, and possible uterine suspension and cervical dilatation. For older women who have no desire for future pregnancies or for patients whose symptoms and pelvic findings of endometriosis have recurred following a previous conservationistic operation (or operations), a more definitive operation may be needed. Under these circumstances, abdominal hysterectomy with bilateral salpingo-oophorectomy is the procedure of choice unless the patient insists on the uterus remaining for the purpose of utilizing new reproductive technologies to achieve conception. The surgical management of pelvic endometriosis is discussed in Chapter 20.

Ectopic Pregnancy

Certain ectopic pregnancies may require hysterectomy. A hysterectomy may be required for cervical pregnancies, interstitial pregnancies, or abdominal pregnancies when the placenta cannot be removed without removing the uterus. It also may be permissible to perform a hysterectomy in a patient who has had repeated tubal pregnancies that have completely destroyed both fallopian tubes to the point that their function cannot be restored and whose condition during surgery is completely stable. Again, it is necessary for the patient to give specific permission for hysterectomy after being fully informed of all options for future reproduction. The surgical management of ectopic pregnancies is discussed in Chapter 18.

Neoplastic Diseases

Cervical Intraepithelial Neoplasia

Under well-controlled circumstances, cervical intraepithelial neoplasia may be adequately treated in most patients with cervical cauterization, cryosurgery, laser surgery, or cervical conization (see Ch. 41). Hysterectomy is sometimes recommended for patients who do not desire or are incapable of having (more) children, and for patients whose severe cervical dysplasia or carcinoma in situ is too extensive to be removed with cervical conization or other local treatment modalities. Vaginal hysterectomy is preferred unless contraindicated by adnexal disease, uterine enlargement, or other circumstances. A vaginal cuff should be removed with the uterus when the carcinoma in situ extends close to or on to the adjacent vaginal fornix.

Early Invasive Cervical Cancer

Under special circumstances, a simple, total hysterectomy and partial vaginectomy may be an adequate operation for very early invasive disease if an adequate cervical conization has been thoroughly examined and shows minimal, superficial, microscopic stromal invasion limited to a depth of invasion not > 3 mm below the surface. There must be no confluence of tumor in the stroma and no evidence of invasion of vessels. Abdominal hysterectomy is usually done.

Most patients with Stage IB and IIA carcinoma of the cervix should be treated with extensive abdominal hysterectomy, bilateral pelvic lymphadenectomy, and partial vaginectomy, as discussed in Chapter 42. Treatment with primary surgery rather than irradiation is especially indicated in premenopausal women because of the opportunity to conserve the function of normal ovaries.

Endometrial Adenomatous Hyperplasia, Adenocarcinoma, and Sarcoma of the Uterus

Adenomatous hyperplasia of the endometrium with atypical changes is considered by most authorities to be a precursor to endometrial adenocarcinoma and, therefore, an appropriate indication for hysterectomy. Less severe forms of hyperplasia usually are reversible and do not require hysterectomy.

Endometrial adenocarcinoma and sarcomas of the endometrium and myometrium must be treated with total abdominal hysterectomy and bilateral salpingo-oophorectomy. Even though various combinations of adjuvant irradiation and chemotherapy also may be used, the most important part of the treatment is the hysterectomy. Para-aortic and pelvic lymph nodes may be sampled in selected cases and enlarged nodes should be examined, but complete pelvic lymphadenectomy is not required. Peritoneal washings should be sent for cytologic examination. A complete discussion can be found in Chapter 43.

Ovarian and Fallopian Tube Neoplasms

Malignant neoplasms of the ovaries and fallopian tubes are treated surgically with or without adjuvant chemotherapy and occasionally irradiation. In addition to bilateral salpingo-oophorectomy, a total abdominal hysterectomy is almost always done. A subtotal rather than total hysterectomy may be done when extensive disease is spread throughout the abdomen, the cervix is encased in tumor, and removal of the cervix does not help with efforts to decrease the bulk of the tumor. In special circumstances of limited disease, conservation of the function of the uterus and the opposite ovary may be indicated in a young nulliparous woman. The surgical treatment of ovarian malignancies is discussed in Chapter 44.

Trophoblastic Disease

Trophoblastic disease of the uterus is usually treated successfully with chemotherapeutic agents. Hysterectomy is rarely necessary. It may be done in patients with a persistently elevated human chorionic gonadotropin titer after chemotherapy when there is suspicion that the only disease still left remaining is in the uterus, perhaps deep in the myometrium. Also, a total abdominal hysterectomy may be the quickest and safest treatment for a high parity patient with a hydatidiform mole distending the uterus, especially if uterine bleeding becomes difficult to control.

Malignant Disease of Other Adjacent Pelvic Organs

When malignant disease of other adjacent organs is treated surgically, a hysterectomy may be done for the operation to be technically adequate. This is frequently true of carcinoma of the rectum, but may also be true of carcinomas of the cecum, sigmoid, or bladder that may be adherent to the uterus. Hysterectomy may be required in operations for retroperitoneal tumors.

Miscellaneous and Unusual Indications

Cervical Problems

Usually in postmenopausal patients, cervical stenosis with recurring pyometra following unsuccessful attempts to keep the cervix open may require abdominal hysterectomy for final solution. Not infrequently, malignancy will be found in the uterine cavity or endocervical canal.

Rarely, an anomalous development of the müllerian duct system may leave the patient with a uterine corpus and uterine cavity lined with functioning endometrium, but with congenital absence of the cervix and vagina. It is almost impossible to create a suitable endocervical canal and functional vagina at menarche to allow a permanently patent external exit for the menstrual flow. Hysterectomy will be necessary to prevent recurrent hematometra and possibly endometriosis from retrograde menstrual flow.

Chronic Pelvic Pain

In the absence of specific pelvic pathology, chronic pelvic pain should not be treated with hysterectomy except under very unusual circumstances. In caring for patients with chronic pelvic pain, there are a number of important points to emphasize (see Ch. 23). Take time to evaluate patients carefully. Psychiatric problems are common. Do not hesitate to use the laparoscope to look for evidence of pelvic pathology. Hysterectomy for relief of chronic pelvic pain in the absence of organic pelvic pathology should not be done unless the symptoms are severe and not relieved by more conservative measures including psychiatric therapy.

Numerous studies have described the difficulty of providing relief of pelvic pain with hysterectomy, especially in the absence of uterine pathology. Waldemar and Boysen concluded that many patients who complain of pelvic pain in the absence of uterine pathology were probably suffering from "somatization disorder" characterized by multiple recurrent somatic symptoms for which medical attention is sought but for which no physical disorder is found. This is but one example of the difficulty faced by the gynecologic surgeon in trying to decide which patients with pelvic pain will benefit from surgery.

The Pelvic Congestion Syndrome and the Allen-Masters "Universal Joint" Syndrome

In 1949, in a series of three papers, Taylor described a syndrome of vascular congestion and hyperemia of the pelvis. In 1955, Allen and Masters described their "universal joint" syndrome most frequently occurring in postpartum women who had evidence of lacerations of the fascial tissue layers in the broad and cardinal ligaments sometimes extending into the uterosacral ligaments.

There is some overlap of symptoms in these two syndromes. Patients complain of dyspareunia, dysmenorrhea, excessive tiredness, heavy menstrual flow, backache, pelvic aching, and chronic headaches. With the Allen-Masters syndrome, they may have a history of difficult or precipitate obstetric delivery. Also, the uterus is found in severe third-degree retroversion and the cervix can be moved independently in all directions in the pelvis as a "universal joint," associated with severe pain.

These syndromes have been controversial since they were first described. The diagnosis is difficult to make. They are rarely appropriate indications for hysterectomy.

Surgical Sterilization

When requested and indicated, surgical sterilization usually should be accomplished by tubal ligation instead of hysterectomy. Hysterectomy for sterilization is inappropriate except in carefully selected patients in whom there is clear indication that significant disease or symptoms are present that, in all likelihood, will require hysterectomy in the near future. For example, a 30-year-old patient with a 10-week–sized myomatous uterus and menorrhagia who requests sterilization may be advised to have a total hysterectomy rather than tubal ligation and myomectomy. A 40-year-old patient with severe cervical dysplasia who requests surgical sterilization may be advised to have a hysterectomy rather than tubal ligation and cervical conization. A 35-year-old patient with symptomatic uterine descensus and vaginal relaxation who requests surgical sterilization may be advised to have a vaginal hysterectomy and repair rather than a tubal ligation.

The risk of complications following hysterectomy is greater than the risk of complications following tubal ligation; therefore, hysterectomy should not be chosen as the most acceptable method of surgical sterilization unless significant gynecologic disease or symptoms are present. This recommendation also should apply to patients who request surgical sterilization at the time of cesarean section or elective termination of pregnancy. All patients requesting surgical sterilization should be evaluated carefully before a final recommendation is made regarding which operation to perform. The subject of tubal ligation versus hysterectomy for sterilization is also discussed in the section The Concept of Elective Hysterectomy in this chapter.

INAPPROPRIATE INDICATIONS FOR HYSTERECTOMY

Hysterectomies are sometimes done for inappropriate indications as described in the following sections.

Management of the Menopause

Hysterectomy should not be done so that menopausal patients can be given estrogen without risk of developing endometrial hyperplasia or cancer, or having annoying episodes of postmenopausal bleeding.

Leukorrhea and Chronic Cervicitis

Depending on the results of diagnostic studies, specific therapy for leukorrhea should be prescribed. Cervical cauterization or cryosurgery is the most appropriate treatment for chronic cervicitis. Certainly these problems can be managed without hysterectomy.

Primary Dysmenorrhea

Although primary dysmenorrhea can be severe and debilitating in some patients, hysterectomy is not indicated. This symptom usually may be relieved with conservative medical therapy and cervical dilatation.

Premenstrual Syndrome

Patients may be extremely uncomfortable with premenstrual syndrome (PMS) symptoms. However, most of these symptoms are related to the ovarian cycle and cannot be relieved by hysterectomy. Backstrom, Boyle, and Baird found only a small improvement in symptoms of PMS in most women following hysterectomy and concluded that "neither the presence of the uterus nor the occurrence of menstruation are necessary for the manifestation of the premenstrual tension syndrome and support the view that it has a hormonal basis."

Mild Urinary Incontinence

As many as 50% of women will admit to occasional involuntary loss of urine. Such mild incontinence should be managed without surgery that might include a hysterectomy.

Postmenopausal Bleeding

A single episode of postmenopausal bleeding is not an indication for hysterectomy. It is an indication for careful pelvic examination and curettage. Some patients with postmenopausal bleeding will be found to have atrophic vaginitis, cervical polyp, or urethral caruncle for which local treatment is sufficient. Some patients will be found to have endometrial polyps for which uterine curettage, not hysterectomy, is needed. Approximately 10%–20% of patients with postmenopausal bleeding will be found on pelvic examination or uterine curettage to have a cervical or endometrial malignancy. If the diagnosis of malignant disease is made preoperatively, an extensive hysterectomy may be indicated..

Abnormal Vaginal/Cervical Cytology

A hysterectomy should never be done just because the pap smear report is abnormal. Additional studies such as colposcopy, cervical biopsy, endocervical scrape, and endometrial biopsy or curettage are indicated to determine the reason for the abnormality.

Cervical Dysplasia

For patients with mild and moderate cervical dysplasia, hysterectomy is not indicated. Cervical cauterization, cryosurgery, laser surgery, or cervical conization with follow-up examinations usually is sufficient.

Multiple Minor Problems

Not infrequently, a physician may see a multiparous patient with a small asymptomatic myoma in the uterine fundus, chronic cervicitis with leukorrhea, inflammatory atypia on vaginal cytology, significant symptoms of PMS with dysmenorrhea, and mild stress urinary incontinence with minimal anterior vaginal wall relaxation. None of these problems by itself, even though bothersome, is an appropriate indication for hysterectomy, and combining the problems also does not constitute an appropriate indication for hysterectomy even when they are all present in the same patient. Specific nonsurgical therapy can be prescribed for each problem listed, and chances are good that the small myoma will never cause the patient a significant problem. It also does not help to add the "useless uterus syndrome" in an attempt to justify hysterectomy in a patient with mild gynecologic symptoms and minimal findings who has already had a tubal ligation. The indications for hysterectomy that are appropriate are the same for all patients regardless of whether a tubal ligation has been performed previously. Mention of the "useless uterus syndrome" as an indication for hysterectomy should be avoided and completely eliminated.

When surgery (including bilateral salpingo-oophorectomy) is required for benign gynecologic disease, hysterectomy may not be indicated in a young premenopausal patient who has not completed childbearing. Even when surgery is required for certain limited malignant gynecologic disease, the uterus may be left in place in a young premenopausal patient who has not completed childbearing. Use of new reproductive technologies now may allow in vitro fertilization of a donor ovum with subsequent transfer of the embryo to the endocrinologically prepared uterus. According to Asch and associates and others, new reproductive technologies (ie, in vitro fertilization using donated oocytes and intrauterine or intrafallopian tube gamete transfer in a patient whose uterus is hormonally prepared) can establish fertility in agonadal patients.

THE CONCEPT OF ELECTIVE HYSTERECTOMY

Perhaps more than any other, the concept of elective hysterectomy, usually done in women between ages 35 and 45 years who request surgical sterilization or relief from pelvic discomfort and gynecologic symptoms associated with menstruation, has resulted in wide disagreement among gynecologists. This concept also has resulted in criticism of gynecologists from other quarters who claim that elective hysterectomy is unnecessary surgery. On the other hand, some women believe that hysterectomy should be available "on request."

That this is not an inconsiderable problem is indicated by Travis who, based on an analysis of data from a variety of sources, estimated that 25% of hysterectomies (approximately 159,500 per year) performed in the United States are elective. Using a mortality rate of 20 per 10,000 hysterectomies, an average patient age of 40 years, and a life expectancy of 78 years, she estimated that 319 deaths occur annually in the United States among women undergoing elective hysterectomy—an annual loss of 12,122 woman years. Of course, with lower or higher mortality figures, the outcome could be better or worse. The mortality rate of performing elective hysterectomies probably is much lower (approximately 3 per 10,000 procedures), given that almost all patients would have insignificant pathology and could have the operation performed vaginally. The economic costs of performing 159,500 elective hysterectomies are considerable today, amounting to approximately $2 billion for hospital costs and surgeon's fees alone, excluding the other economic costs of lost wages, complications, and other costs.

Travis defines *elective hysterectomy* as one performed for "conditions or symptoms that are neither life threatening nor indicative of tissue pathology where alternative management is a viable option. Elective procedures are performed primarily for symptom relief rather than organic disease." Often, the operation is done as much to accomplish permanent sterilization as to provide relief of symptoms. In his report, Richards stated that 260 of 340 (76.5%) hysterectomies were "elective," according to his definition as "patient-indicated hysterectomy for disability and quality of life considerations" or "prophylactic hysterectomy."

Various arguments to support the concept of elective hysterectomy have been proposed. One is the idea of surgical prophylaxis against cancer, which began in earnest in gynecology when total hysterectomy rather than subtotal hysterectomy was proposed and became the procedure of choice nearly 50 years ago. As a result, cancer of the cervical stump was almost eliminated and the value of prophylactic removal of a normal but "useless and potentially cancer-bearing organ" was clearly demonstrated. There has been little controversy about or objection to this idea of total rather than subtotal hysterectomy.

Gradually, the concept of surgical prophylaxis against cancer was extended to include hysterectomy when bilateral salpingo-oophorectomy was necessary for bilateral tubo-ovarian abscess, endometriosis, or ovarian cysts; hysterectomy in women who required operation for significantly symptomatic vaginal relaxation problems; and in other circumstances. Quite naturally, the idea also has been extended to include those women who requested surgical sterilization. The ultimate extension of this philosophy was expressed seriously in the gynecologic literature by the suggestion that every woman should have an elective hysterectomy and even bilateral salpingo-oophorectomy a few months after the last pregnancy and delivery. Wright in 1969 said, "The uterus has but one function: reproduction. After the last planned pregnancy, the uterus becomes a useless, bleeding, symptom-producing, potentially cancer-bearing organ and therefore should be removed." Although he apparently was willing to conserve the ovaries, his statement nonetheless was criticized vigorously. Critics pointed out that the uterus to many women is important to gender identity, sexuality, relationships, and self-concept, much more than simply reproductive function and much more than a potentially problem-producing foreign body after reproduction is finished. Earlier, in 1953, Thomas also was criticized for his statement that "panhysterectomy is to be preferred to tubectomy for prevenception insurance because there are no failures and more importantly, there is no chance for subsequent development of serious uterine disease." Critics stated that this was like removing a perfectly normal breast because a cancer might later develop in it.

Although tubal ligation is a simpler and safer operation, some gynecologists also recommend elective hysterectomy for surgical sterilization because of the frequent occurrence of the so-called post-tubal ligation syndrome. As defined, the *post-tubal ligation syndrome* consists of functional menstrual disturbances or pelvic pain, discomfort, or dysmenorrhea of progressively increasing severity in the absence of obvious pelvic pathology or other significant history, except for previous tubal ligation. The incidence is not known. The pelvic discomfort and pain, although undoubtedly present, is difficult to explain. Possible explanations include foci of endosalpingiosis, adhesions to the site of tubal ligation, congestion of pelvic veins, torsion of the adnexa lateral to the point of ligation, hydrosalpinx involving the distal segment of the tube, or coincidental Allen-Masters syndrome or pelvic congestion. Endometriosis and salpingitis are rarely found as a cause of chronic pelvic pain following tubal ligation. To explain functional menstrual disturbances, a post-tubal ligation luteal phase deficiency presumably related to interference with utero-ovarian blood supply has been postulated, but evidence for this explanation is conflicting. Donnez, Wauters, and Thomas reported decreased midluteal

phase levels of serum progesterone following tubal sterilization by coagulation techniques but normal values with Hulka clip application to occlude the tubes. Corson and associates were unable to confirm a post-tubal ligation decreased secretion of progesterone in the luteal phase.

Conflicting opinions also surround changes in menstrual patterns following tubal ligation. Some studies have reported an increase in menstrual disturbances and the amount of menstrual flow (Sachs and LaCroix, and Neil and associates). Other studies have reported no increase (Bhiwandiwala, Mumford, and Feldblum, Kasonde and Bonnar, Stock, and Rubinstein and associates). An interesting study by Neil and associates matched patients who had undergone tubal ligations with control subjects whose husbands had had vasectomies. A significant increase in the incidence of menorrhagia and pelvic pain was found in the tubal sterilization group compared with the controls. Three percent required hysterectomy within the succeeding 28 months. Muldoon confirmed the findings of previous investigators (Weed; Pletsch and Sandberg; and Montague) that women who have a tubal ligation at the time of cesarean section are even more likely to have a major gynecologic problem subsequently that may require hysterectomy. It has even been suggested that elective hysterectomy rather than tubal ligation be done to accomplish voluntary sterilization at the time of the last delivery by cesarean section. We believe the higher incidence of complications with cesarean/hysterectomy precludes its use as an appropriate operation for this purpose, and to date it has not been widely adopted in the United States.

Our controlled study at Emory University indicates no increase in the incidence of menstrual disturbances or pelvic pain following tubal ligation. The incidence of pelvic pain may be slightly increased after tubal ligation, but frankly, we believe the post-tubal ligation syndrome is an as yet unproven entity, although certainly continued study is needed.

Haynes and Wolfe reviewed 489 patients who had undergone tubal sterilization operations at least 3.5 years earlier. Subsequently, surgical procedures were necessary in 37.2%, including hysterectomy in 13% and vaginal repair in 14%. Muldoon followed 374 patients for at least 10 years after tubal ligation. A subsequent gynecologic operation was required in 37.2%: 18.7% were hysterectomies and 5.9% were vaginal repairs. In a well designed epidemiologic study, Cohen analyzed the long-term risks of hysterectomy after tubal sterilization among a large group of women in the province of Manitoba, Canada. For women aged 30 years and older, tubal ligation was not a risk factor for subsequent hysterectomy in either the short or long term. However, for women aged 25–29 years, there was a 1.6% increase in risk of having a hysterectomy following tubal ligation. A recent study by Stergachis and associates confirmed that younger women age 20 to 29 years were 3.4 times more likely to have a subsequent hysterectomy compared to a population-based cohort of nonsterilized women. These authors also found that married women who are sterilized at age 30 years and older are not an increased risk of subsequent hysterectomy.

Unfortunately, it seems that in patients with dysfunctional uterine bleeding and pelvic discomfort who have had a previous tubal ligation, physicians may resort more quickly to hysterectomy without first trying more conservative measures. Hysterectomy for functional menstrual disturbances and pelvic pain following tubal ligation should be recommended only when symptoms are persistent and severe and conservative measures have failed. The same indications that are appropriate for hysterectomy for all patients are also appropriate for patients who have had a previous tubal ligation. In the CDC CREST study of women aged 15–44 years who had undergone a hysterectomy, 41% had undergone a tubal ligation before the hysterectomy. This finding is alarming and difficult to explain. Templeton and Cole also believe that hysterectomy is recommended more often in patients who have had a previous tubal ligation.

Possible reasons why hysterectomy is done more frequently following tubal ligation include

Tubal ligation failure (2–10 per 1000 cases)
Development of new gynecologic disease after tubal ligation
Concurrent gynecologic disease overlooked at the time of tubal ligation
"Post-tubal ligation syndrome"
More liberal indications for hysterectomy following tubal ligation

According to Thorsteinsson and Pratt, tubal ligation for surgical sterilization was first suggested by Von Blundell in 1834. Hysterectomy was first suggested for surgical sterilization by Rein in 1876. That tubal ligation (ie, interval, postpartum, with cesarean section, vaginal, abdominal, and laparoscopic, all by a variety of techniques) has gained acceptance for voluntary permanent sterilization is evident in the 640,000 tubal sterilizations that were performed in the United States in 1987, according to a study by the Association for Voluntary Surgical Contraception and the CDC. There are no reliable estimates of the number of hysterectomies for sterilization performed annually because, in some cases, the real purpose of the operation, that is, sterilization, may not be mentioned in the record as an indication. However, the gynecologic literature over the past 30–40 years gives clear indication that hysterectomy has received greater attention because associated

morbidity and mortality of the operation has been reduced somewhat. In 1975, Little, in his review of 4270 female sterilization procedures, indicated a progressive increase in the percentage of elective hysterectomies for sterilization from 7% in 1967 to 27% in 1973. Hibbard reported a sevenfold increase in elective hysterectomy for sterilization in 1972 compared with a 1968 review of 2060 sterilization procedures. Ballard reported using vaginal hysterectomy for simultaneous indications of abortion and sterilization. Stumpf, Ballard, and Lowensohn reported 500 consecutive abdominal hysterectomies for abortion and sterilization in a predominantly indigent population at the Los Angeles County–University of Southern California Medical Center. This procedure was done in selected patients as an alternative to suction curettage and tubal ligation. Thirty-two percent of patients had a significant febrile episode, 6.8% had transfusions, four had accidental cystotomy, two had pulmonary emboli, and one sustained a ureteral injury.

In 1972, 115 vaginal hysterectomies done for sterilization by nine vaginal surgeons working in a regional military hospital were analyzed by Atkinson and Chappell. Vaginal hysterectomy was offered to patients as one option to accomplish sterilization because it "not only offers complete protection against childbearing but prevention from future benign and malignant uterine disease." Significant complications occurred in 11.3% of patients, and one patient died of cerebral edema, brain stem infarction, and pulmonary emboli. The authors concluded that these data reinforced "the concept that vaginal hysterectomy is the preferred method of sterilization in the young female who has completed her family and wants to be protected against future benign and malignant uterine disease and be spared the drudgery of menses for a 15–20 year period."

Tubal ligation is a safer operation than hysterectomy, including vaginal hysterectomy. The mortality and morbidity rates are lower for tubal ligation. The postoperative course of 846 women who were sterilized by various surgical techniques was described by Poulsen in 1973. The morbidity rate was 4.2% for interval abdominal tubal ligations, 2.6% for vaginal tubal ligations, and 2.4% for postpartum tubal ligations. The highest morbidity rate (10.5%) was found among women sterilized by vaginal hysterectomy. One of the vaginal hysterectomy patients died of postoperative sepsis and hepatic complications.

Laros and Work studied 111 cases of vaginal hysterectomy performed for sterilization at the University of Michigan. Immediate morbidity (ie, urinary tract infections, pelvic cellulitis, abscess requiring antibiotics, postoperative hemorrhage, and additional surgical procedures) occurred in 89 (90%) of patients. These authors found that these data compared most unfavorably with the morbidity of interval tubal ligation.

Advocates of hysterectomy argue that a significant number of patients will develop gynecologic disease, sometimes even life-threatening disease, after tubal ligation, which could be avoided by removing the uterus. It is mentioned that the benefits accrued are even greater when the patient is young. Even though the failure rate of tubal ligation is low, the failure rate of hysterectomy is even lower. On the other hand, proponents of tubal ligation point to safety, lower cost, and less emotional trauma.

In a complicated analysis of cost effectiveness, Deane and Ulene concluded that, at a market rate of interest between 5% and 15% (the range most likely to contain the real rate of interest as determined by market forces), a tubal ligation is to be preferred to a hysterectomy regardless of the age at the time of the procedure. These authors believe that this conclusion holds both from the point of view of society and from the point of view of an individual, and "the downstream savings due to avoidance of selected gynecologic disease often attributed to a hysterectomy is not large enough to offset the higher initial cost and risk of death associated with this procedure, even when considering the less than 100% success expected of sterilization by tubal ligation." Deane and Ulene admit that there are "instances when care should be exercised in applying the conclusions of the analysis to each individual in the population being considered."

The direct mortality rate for tubal ligation is approximately 4 per 100,000 women. The rate for a similar group of women undergoing vaginal hysterectomy would be approximately 30 per 100,000 women undergoing the procedure. Even though tubal ligation is a safer operation for surgical sterilization than hysterectomy, there are definite disadvantages. For example, it is well known that long periods of infertility imposed by tubal ligation may predispose a patient to development of uterine leiomyomas, especially among black women. Also, it is most regrettable when advanced cancer of the cervix is diagnosed in a patient with a history of tubal ligation. Haynes and Wolfe, Muldoon, and Stock have reported this unfortunate occurrence, and it has been seen too often, especially by gynecologists who work with indigent clinic patients. Women sometimes stop having annual gynecologic examinations with cervical cytology after having a tubal ligation. Stock reported that 22% of private practice patients undergoing tubal sterilization failed to continue their previously routine periodic pelvic examination and pap smear. Of course, the cervix should be evaluated carefully at the time of tubal ligation, and the patient should be instructed about the need for periodic examinations.

In a review of 108 cases of consecutively selected women undergoing hysterectomy for nonmalignant disease, O'Herlihy and Chandler found that more than one third of the patients or their husbands had previously been sterilized. They found, in many instances, the gynecologic problem necessitating hysterectomy antedated the sterilization procedure. These authors suggested that a careful gynecologic evaluation should be done before surgical sterilization of either partner. Vas ligation is a much safer operation than tubal ligation, and certainly much safer than elective hysterectomy, and should be used as often as possible to provide permanent sterilization in a stable marriage.

Despite these problems, we believe *tubal ligation is the correct operation to accomplish surgical sterilization in most gynecologically asymptomatic patients who have a normal examination, even in a high-risk indigent population.*

Paterson published a thoughtful review of the advantages and disadvantages and risks and benefits of tubal ligation or hysterectomy to accomplish sterilization. He reviewed morbidity, mortality, hospital stay, subsequent pregnancy rate, unexpected uterine pathology, and psychologic sequelae of the two procedures. He concluded that "sterilization by tubal methods should be recommended to the majority of patients because of its lower morbidity, mortality, and psychologic sequelae. Nevertheless, an attempt should be made to identify those patients most at risk of subsequently requiring major gynecological surgery."

Paterson, Laros and Work, and many others, agree that tubal ligation is the most appropriate operation to accomplish surgical sterilization in the majority of women. It has lower morbidity and mortality rates and a lower incidence of psychologic sequelae. It is somewhat disturbing that such a large number of patients require major gynecologic operations subsequent to tubal ligation, sometimes even shortly after the procedure. In this regard, all patients requesting surgical sterilization should have a careful gynecologic evaluation to rule out abnormalities of the menstrual flow, uterine leiomyomas, significant symptomatic anatomic relaxations, serious cervical dysplasia, pelvic discomfort, urinary incontinence, adnexal disease, and other problems. If a patient has a gynecologic problem that is likely to require an operation for relief, she should be offered hysterectomy as the most appropriate method to accomplish sterilization. But it should be understood that the operation is being done primarily for elective sterilization, and it is not being done "under the guise of mild symptomatic pelvic disease," as stated by Atkinson and Chappell. For example, a patient with an approximately 10-week–sized asymptomatic leiomyomatous uterus who requests surgical sterilization should be offered a hysterectomy rather than tubal ligation. Of course, the risks and benefits and advantages and disadvantages of tubal ligation versus hysterectomy (usually vaginal) should be presented carefully to each patient. Even if there seems to be a reasonable indication for hysterectomy, the final decision rightfully will be the patient's decision.

According to Braun and Druckman, if all women in the United States had a hysterectomy at age 35 years, the life expectancy of the total group would be increased by 2 months. This is about the length of time it takes for a complete recovery from the operation. The increased life expectancy does not accrue to the total group but only to those who might have died in future years of cancer of the uterine corpus or cervix. Considering the enormous cost, economic and otherwise, it hardly seems worth it.

In the matter of the decision for or against elective hysterectomy, there are also ethical issues that involve the patient's right to have what she wants and feels is proper for her. In modern societies, it is possible for a woman to request voluntary termination of an early pregnancy and have it done. She can request breast augmentation, abdominoplasty, and other procedures to improve her self-image. She can request voluntary sterilization and it can be done, usually by tubal ligation. What if she requests that the surgical sterilization be done with vaginal hysterectomy because she has decided not to have (more) children, she would like to be relieved of the inconvenience and discomfort of monthly menses, she would like to eliminate the risk of benign and malignant uterine disease in future years, and she wants to be able to take estrogen after menopause without having to take progesterone and worry about having endometrial biopsies periodically, and she is willing to pay for the procedure herself when told that her health insurance will not? Gynecologists cannot be judgmental in such matters. Modern women are different from women of previous decades. They have different desires and beliefs and aspirations. They feel differently about reproduction, abortion, contraception, career, relationships, and marriage. They have different ideas about their sexuality and different ways to express their femininity. In short, modern women have different ways to satisfy their human need to be creative and a greater variety of options from which to choose.

The physician must listen to the patient who requests elective hysterectomy. The advantages and disadvantages and risks and benefits of such an operation should be explained carefully. Hopefully, her gynecologist will be familiar with the psychology of the decision-making process, will point out the difference between "the odds" and "the risks," and will be willing to carefully examine his or her own position in this ethical dilemma before deciding whether or not to accede to her request.

PREPARATION FOR HYSTERECTOMY

A gynecologist should talk with his or her patient while trying to decide whether a hysterectomy is indicated. Fortunately for the patient and the gynecologist, in almost every instance, time for talking is available. Not very often is hysterectomy an emergency. Unfortunately, the time may not be used or used properly.

Based on their survey of women who had undergone hysterectomy, Neefus and Taylor concluded that "there is an urgent need for patient education on the physical, psychological, and sexual aspects of hysterectomy." Ninety-four percent of women wanted information before entering the hospital, especially information about the physical and sexual effects of surgery. According to Neefus and Taylor, "The systematic provision of such information to these patients appears uncommon and sporadic."

Often, the need for hysterectomy is obvious. There is a complete prolapse, or a large and symptomatic leiomyomatous uterus, or an endometrial cancer. Under these and other obvious circumstances, the patient may be told early that a hysterectomy is recommended and why. The indication for surgery must be explained clearly and in language that the patient can understand. The risks, benefits, and side effects must be reviewed, but in such a way that the patient will not be unduly alarmed. Then the patient and the physician must spend the time necessary to discuss all the ancillary points that patients will bring up and need to discuss, including details about the operation and how long it will take, the period of recuperation required in the hospital and at home, whether or not function of normal ovaries should be conserved, whether hormones will be needed after surgery, what will fill the vacant space after the uterus is removed, what will happen to all the ova released from the ovaries when there is no place for them to go, what will be the effect of the operation on sexual function and femininity, and whether there will be a tendency to gain weight. These are but a few of the issues that patients must be allowed and encouraged to discuss before the operation is performed. The gynecologist must have the time and patience to acknowledge and explore the patient's questions and discuss her feelings with her in a nonjudgmental and nonpaternalistic manner.

In circumstances in which the indication for hysterectomy is not as clear or as urgent, it is more important that the decision to do or not to do a hysterectomy be made only after the patient has made several visits and had several examinations. This is especially true when pelvic pain is an important component of the complaint. It is amazing how often the patient's symptoms will change and even the physical findings will vary from visit to visit. Not only does it take time for the physician to evaluate the patient, but it also takes time for the patient to evaluate the physician. It takes time for her to decide if she can talk honestly and confidentially to a physician she may have never seen before. After a relationship of mutual respect and confidence has been achieved, information exchanged is more accurate and better decisions can be made. The patient can be encouraged as much as possible to participate in the decision making process and to make a correct choice between alternative forms of treatment. She becomes more informed about the nature of the problem, the solution, and what her role will be in helping to ensure a successful outcome. She must never feel that she has no control over what will happen to her. She must be told that nothing will be done to her without her understanding and agreement. She must feel free to make suggestions, to make decisions, and to express her feelings. It is easier for patients to make proper adjustments if they are given correct information before the operation. Gynecologists owe it to their patients to help them do this. Special help will be needed for young women and for those who have not had children.

Data from extensive literature indicate that hysterectomy may lead to an emotional crisis (though rarely serious enough to require psychiatric care in a mental hospital) in at least a small percentage of women. According to Raphael, it was stated as early as 1890 by Krafft-Ebing that psychoses were more frequently caused by hysterectomy than by other procedures. Lindemann concluded that 40% of pelvic operations may be followed by depressive reaction that could lead to impairment of mental health, social maladjustment, and the need for institutional care in some patients. Thirty-three percent of patients experienced depression within 3 years following hysterectomy, according to Richards's report. These studies and others too numerous to cite are included in excellent reviews by Raphael, by Richards, by Roeske, by Polivy and by others. The gynecologic surgeon is encouraged to become thoroughly familiar with this information. Raphael concludes

that a hysterectomy may produce for a woman a crisis situation: a situation in which she will experience a variety of helpful and unhelpful interactions and possibly some unmet needs. She will appreciate an opportunity to ventilate her anxieties and fears, her positive and negative feelings about the operation, and relationships which offer her support and encouragement to do this. Practical help and reassurance are important to her, as are empathy and the opportunity for identification with others sharing this experience. She has particular concern about the effect of the operation on her marital relationships and her concepts of herself as a feminine person. She considers the discussion of such concerns as of positive value to her. She expects from her surgeon, apart from his technical skill, an adequate and appropriate explanation beforehand and empathetic support and understanding subsequently. The woman experiencing many unhelpful interactions and many unmet needs is at high risk of malresolution.

Bernal, in her bioethical investigation of hysterectomy, emphasizes the ethical imperative of promoting the patient's *autonomy,* defined as "an individual's exercise of the capacity to form, revise, and pursue personal plans for life." This, according to the President's Commission, is a central goal in health care. According to Bernal, "Physician attitudes toward hysterectomy and the hysterectomy patient can have a major influence on patient self-determination." The physician can assist in the promotion of self-determination by providing, within the context of a decision for hysterectomy, informed consent that includes "balanced information and supportive exploration of the woman's values, goals, and life plan."

The knowledgeable and empathetic gynecologic surgeon will be aware of his or her patient's concerns. The surgeon will find time in preoperative conversations to identify cultural, religious, and personal beliefs and other risk factors that may cause depression or other difficulty in posthysterectomy adjustment, especially in younger women and those who have not completed their families. Misconceptions and fears will be dispelled, if possible, preferably before the patient is admitted to the hospital, even though it may take so much time that admission may have to be postponed in a nonemergency situation. The gynecologic surgeon will not adopt a "cut and run" attitude, but instead will find time to assist the patient through difficult times, asking for advice and consultation from colleagues when the need arises. A consideration of the emotional needs of patients is necessary to the correct practice of gynecologic surgery, perhaps more so than to other surgical specialties. A thorough discussion of this subject is found in Chapter 2.

Unfortunately, a woman who has had an emergency hysterectomy will not have had the time to participate in preoperative counseling or extended decision making. She will require special attention in the postoperative period to assure appropriate adjustment to her sudden change. According to Lalinec-Michaud and Engelsmann, "The shorter the interval from the decision to operate until the operation, the greater the incidence of depression." It may even be advisable to allow an appropriate interval for some nonemergency patients to allow better accommodation to the idea of hysterectomy.

A simple total hysterectomy must always be preceded by a study of the cervix to rule out invasive cancer. Even though the cervix is normal to inspection and palpation, it may contain an invasive carcinoma. Except for the most minimal and superficial stromal invasion, a simple total hysterectomy is inadequate treatment for invasive carcinoma of the cervix. Proper radiation therapy is difficult to give after a total hysterectomy has been done. Therefore, if the presence of an invasive cervical cancer is detected, then the patient must be treated in some other way. Preoperative cervical cytology examination usually will suffice, but only if the cytology is of good quality. Otherwise, cervical biopsy with endocervical scrape must be done.

When patients have a menstrual flow that is heavy (menorrhagia), prolonged (metrorrhagia), or frequent (polymenorrhea), a chronic blood loss iron deficiency may exist with or without anemia. If bleeding is severe, curettage and cyclic hormonal therapy may be indicated to control the bleeding, rule out malignancy, and provide time before hysterectomy to correct the anemia with oral ferrous sulfate therapy. Preoperative transfusions with packed red blood cells are seldom necessary and should be reserved for those patients whose severe anemia is associated with symptoms of hypovolemia or patients who have an aregenerative form of anemia, as discussed in Chapter 8. Most patients with severe iron deficiency anemia can be managed conservatively with oral iron therapy and without transfusion. Anemia often can be corrected in a few weeks and hysterectomy performed without transfusion. Even menorrhagia patients without iron deficiency anemia should be given ferrous sulfate preoperatively so that the preoperative hematocrit can be as high as possible before the operation. Attention to this detail may help avoid intraoperative transfusion or post-operative anemia. The advantages of preoperative deposit for possible autologous blood transfusion intraoperatively are discussed in Chapter 8. In order to avoid interference with platelet production, patients should be asked to avoid aspirin and aspirin-like medications before operation.

A general medical history and physical examination will determine the necessity for preoperative evaluation by other medical specialists, and the necessity for special preoperative studies. Pulmonary function studies, CT of the abdomen and pelvis, cardiology consultation, mammography, coagulation profile, colonoscopy, cystoscopy, excretory urography, and other studies may be needed in selected patients. In 1988, Simel, Matchar, and Piscitelli studied the cost-effectiveness of routine intravenous pyelograms before hysterectomy for benign disease to reduce the incidence of ureteral injury. At a baseline ureteral incidence injury rate of 0.5%, these investigators found that the marginal cost-effectiveness ratio indicated that 833 pyelograms would be needed to prevent a single ureteral injury, $166,000 would be spent to avoid a single ureteral injury, and $3,330,000 would be spent to avoid a single death assuming that approximately 5% of ureteral injuries end in death. Women with normal gynecologic examinations are much less likely to have ureteral abnormalities discovered by excretory urography. Therefore, these investigators recommend selectively limiting preoperative excretory urography to patients with either a large leiomyomatous uterus or an adnexal mass. Of course, preoperative excretory urography has never been conclusively proven to prevent ureteral injury. However, preoperative excretory urography should be performed when there is extensive or strategically located pelvic disease that may compromise the ureters, when an extensive pelvic dissection is anticipated, when anomalous development of the müllerian duct system may be associated with an anomalous development of the upper urinary collecting system, or when there is a history of previous pelvic surgery that may have injured or involved the ureters without being recognized.

Patients are asked to avoid eating solid foods and start a liquid diet 24 hours before the operation is scheduled. Nothing should be taken by mouth after midnight before surgery the next day. Enemas are given the evening before surgery. More than one will be needed to ensure that the lower colon is empty of fecal material. Enemas should be evacuated completely before the patient arrives in the operating room. Nothing is more disconcerting than defecated stool contaminating the operative field. A complete mechanical bowel cleansing with electrolyte solution and antibiotics is unnecessary for the usual abdominal or vaginal hysterectomy unless involvement of the bowel by pelvic pathology is likely. For example, it may be considered advisable in a patient whose operation is done for extensive endometriosis or suspected ovarian malignancy.

Infection is the most frequent complication of hysterectomy, either abdominal or vaginal. The incidence of postoperative infectious morbidity from all causes may exceed 50%. The principal microorganisms responsible are commonly found in normal vaginal flora and include aerobic streptococci, mainly groups B and D; anaerobic streptococci; aerobic gram-negative bacilli, most notably *Escherichia coli*; and *Bacteroides* species. Other organisms may be found in immunocompromised patients.

In addition to measures to improve the patient's general health and nutrition, a variety of methods to reduce postoperative infectious morbidity following hysterectomy have been tried. These include perioperative antibiotics, *T*-tube suction drainage through the vaginal cuff, and even topical irrigation of the operative field with an antibiotic aerosol spray. Vaginal suppositories with antibiotics are not ordinarily prescribed before surgery unless there is evidence of bacterial vaginosis. A vaginal douche and thorough bath with phisohex or povidone-iodine (betadine) is prescribed the evening before surgery. Zakut, Lotan, and Bracha used preoperative vaginal and perineal scrubbing with 10% povidone-iodine solution 12 hours before operation and a tampon soaked in 15 cc of 10% solution left in the vagina until 10 minutes before operation. This local preparation of the vagina was more effective than perioperative ampicillin in reducing the incidence of postoperative infectious morbidity in their patients.

According to Eschenbach, patients with bacterial vaginosis who undergo hysterectomy are at a considerably increased risk of postoperative infection. Patients who are about to undergo hysterectomy should be examined for bacterial vaginosis and, if it is present, should be treated preoperatively. The diagnosis usually can be made clinically by detecting a thin, watery vaginal discharge coating the vaginal wall; a vaginal $pH >$ 4.5; a fishy, amine odor with the addition of KOH; and the presence of clue cells on microscopic examination of a saline wet mount. Patients are treated with oral metronidazole. Condoms are advised for the patient's sexual partner.

The risks of postoperative infectious morbidity (eg, cuff cellulitis, pelvic abscess, wound infection, or urinary tract infection) depends on many variables. These include the patient's age, duration of the operation, the pathology found, the injection of vasoconstrictors into tissues dissected, the duration of hospitalization before surgery, the indication for the operation, the type of operation performed, the administration of perioperative prophylactic antibiotics, and other factors. The use of perioperative prophylactic antibiotics to reduce the incidence and severity of postoperative infections is based on the signal works of Miles and later Burke, who demonstrated that the preoperative administration of antibiotics will improve the host defense against bacteria inoculated into the wound. The important principle is to have the antibiotic present in the tissue before the bacteria are introduced, although Bates and associates have shown that antibiotics administered intraoperatively are also effective. Prophylactic perioperative antibiotics are most effective when used in premenopausal patients undergoing vaginal hysterectomy. It has been more difficult to show a favorable effect in postmenopausal patients undergoing vaginal hysterectomy or in premenopausal or postmenopausal patients undergoing abdominal hysterectomy. Senior and Steigrad reviewed 18 different reports on prophylactic antibiotics in abdominal hysterectomy patients. Twelve studies showed a beneficial effect and six did not. It appears that perioperative prophylactic antibiotics have

not consistently reduced the incidence of pelvic cellulitis after total abdominal hysterectomy and, therefore, should not be used routinely unless the patient population served has an inherently high risk of postoperative sepsis. Of course, perioperative antibiotics should be used on an individual basis when there is evidence of interference with natural host defenses in any patient. In 1983, Hemsell and associates also suggested that individual determination is required with elective abdominal hysterectomy.

Cefotetan, a semisynthetic derivative of oganomycin G produced by *Streptomyces organonesis,* is stable to β-lactamases of gram-negative bacteria and is particularly active against *E. coli, Hemophilus influenzae, Klebsiella* sp., *Proteus mirabilis,* and indole-positive *Proteus.* It is not active against *Streptococcus faecalis* or *Pseudomonas.* It is a new, broad spectrum, long-acting cephalosporin. It can be given intravenously (IV) as a single 2 g dose 30–60 minutes before operation. It has been shown by Orr and associates to be effective in reducing postoperative infectious morbidity in total abdominal hysterectomy patients.

Usual practice is to use prophylactic perioperative antibiotics in all patients before vaginal hysterectomy, although it is difficult to find incontrovertible evidence of their usefulness in postmenopausal patients. Perioperative antibiotics should always be used in premenopausal patients undergoing vaginal hysterectomy. Our practice is to give the first dose of cefazolin 0.5 g on call to the operating room and two additional doses 6 and 12 hours after the first dose, as described by Holman, McGowan, and Thompson. Several studies indicate that a single preoperative dose is equally effective in reducing postoperative infectious morbidity in patients having vaginal hysterectomy. Hemsell and associates reported the use of a single 1 gm cefazolin IV or IM administration preoperatively for prophylaxis at hysterectomy. The overall incidence of major operative site infection requiring parental antimicrobial therapy in evaluable women was 7.2%:7.6% for 539 women undergoing abdominal hysterectomy and 6.3% for 207 women undergoing vaginal hysterectomy.

The lower abdominal, pubic, and vulva hair should not be shaved the night before surgery or even in the operating room. If the pubic hair is profuse and thick, the patient may be given a scissors and asked to cut short the pubic hair, being careful not to injure the skin. Shaving the pubic hair the night before operation increases the incidence of wound infection. In addition, the patient will experience more discomfort when the pubic hair grows back.

Again with the idea of reducing the incidence of postoperative infectious morbidity, it has been suggested that hysterectomies in premenopausal patients should be done in the preovulatory phase of the menstrual cycle. In a premenopausal patient undergoing hysterectomy, a fresh corpus luteum may allow access of organisms into the ovarian parenchyma with subsequent development of ovarian abscess. If the gynecologic surgeon can conveniently do so, he or she should schedule the operation in the preovulatory phase of the cycle. However, the surgeon should not hesitate to also consider other factors, such as patient convenience, operating schedules, the patient's condition, and diagnosis, in choosing the date for operation.

ABDOMINAL HYSTERECTOMY VERSUS VAGINAL HYSTERECTOMY

In the early history of operative gynecology, valiant attempts were made to remove the uterus vaginally because of the unacceptably high mortality and morbidity associated with abdominal operations. As abdominal surgery became safer, interest in vaginal hysterectomy waned. Originally an enthusiastic supporter of the vaginal approach, Howard Kelly was more in favor of the abdominal approach in later years. In the mid-20th century, vaginal hysterectomy regained its popularity and became the operation of choice again for a variety of conditions. During the past decade, however, the percentage of hysterectomies done vaginally has declined again to the consternation of vaginal hysterectomy advocates. Today, approximately 25%–30% of hysterectomies are done vaginally. The vaginal hysterectomy and the abdominal hysterectomy are entirely different operations and are not done on comparable patients. Certainly, it is clear that postoperative morbidity is lower with vaginal hysterectomy, but patients with more serious disease are operated on abdominally.

Ranney has documented a reduction in the number of patients with symptomatic vaginal relaxation problems and uterine prolapse requiring vaginal hysterectomy and repair. He believes that steady improvements in obstetric delivery techniques and increasing rates of delivery by cesarean section in the past 40 years are responsible for this reduction.

Once a proper indication for hysterectomy exists, the gynecologic surgeon must decide whether to remove the uterus abdominally or vaginally. In most situations, the decision is not difficult. In others, a proper choice can require experience, mature judgment, and a careful evaluation of the patient and the surgeon's technical skills. There are distinct advantages to the patient when the hysterectomy can be done vaginally without compromising safety.

Experienced gynecologic surgeons can point to the following seven reasons why vaginal hysterectomy is superior to abdominal hysterectomy:

1. Vaginal hysterectomy is an almost entirely extraperitoneal operation. The peritoneum is opened to only a minimal extent and little packing of the intestines away from the operative field is necessary. Because there is less manipulation of the intestines, postoperative ileus is much less common than with abdominal hysterectomy.
2. With vaginal hysterectomy, the morbidity associated with making an abdominal incision (eg, infection, dehiscence, evisceration, discomfort, or hernia) is avoided. Patients are pleased not to have a scar on the abdomen. Avoidance of an abdominal incision also reduces the depth and length of anesthesia.
3. Extreme obesity increases the technical difficulties of both abdominal and vaginal hysterectomy, but the technical difficulties are less with vaginal hysterectomy.
4. Postoperatively, patients are able to ambulate earlier and better and to care for themselves. The need for nursing care is reduced. Bowel function returns sooner, patients can be fed sooner, and parenteral fluid therapy is minimized. There is less interference with pulmonary function. The incidence of postoperative infectious morbidity is less than half that of abdominal hysterectomy, and the need for postoperative antibiotics is reduced. The need for postoperative pain medication is reduced. Vaginal hysterectomy patients are generally discharged from the hospital earlier.
5. Vaginal hysterectomy is better tolerated by elderly patients and those with complicating medical diseases.
6. Needed repair of vaginal wall relaxations is easier with vaginal hysterectomy.
7. Fewer postoperative adhesions develop after vaginal hysterectomy.

Bezdek, Grigarova, and Kleisl reported their experience with 6106 women who had a hysterectomy between 1964 and 1982. Of those hysterectomies, 82.4% were done vaginally and 17.6% abdominally. In addition to the usual indications, these authors did not hesitate to operate on patients with endometriosis, pelvic inflammatory disease, large myomas, and corpus cancer vaginally. Only 0.14% of hysterectomies begun vaginally were completed abdominally; 0.14% of vaginal hysterectomy patients died and 0.56% of abdominal hysterectomy patients died. In addition, 0.09% of patients developed ureterovaginal fistulas and 0.56% developed vesicovaginal fistulas after total abdominal hysterectomy; 0.14% developed ureterovaginal fistulas and 0.04% developed vesicovaginal fistulas following vaginal hysterectomy. Febrile morbidity was less after vaginal hysterectomy. These authors use vaginal hysterectomy more liberally than most gynecologists.

Vaginal hysterectomy is done most often for benign disease including recurrent and severe dysfunctional uterine bleeding unresponsive to hormonal therapy and uterine curettage; serious symptoms of uterine prolapse, usually associated with relaxation of the vaginal walls (cystocele, urethrocele, enterocele, rectocele, or a combination of any of these); small, symptomatic uterine leiomyomas causing excessive uterine bleeding; and cervical intraepithelial neoplasia, particularly carcinoma in situ. These are the main indications for vaginal hysterectomy, although other indications may be justified occasionally. In each instance, the patient must have completed her childbearing career because alternative therapies that allow conservation of uterine function (eg, endometrial ablation, myomectomy, or cervical conization) are available. When hysterectomy is indicated in these situations, vaginal hysterectomy is preferred over an abdominal procedure because of a lower rate of postoperative complications.

Contraindications to the vaginal approach exist and should be respected. If there is suspected pathology in the adnexal organs (eg, benign or malignant ovarian neoplasms, tubo-ovarian inflammatory cysts, or endometriosis of the ovaries or uterosacral ligaments), then exploratory laparotomy should be done. If pelvic pain of unknown etiology is a significant component of the patient's symptomatology, then the vaginal approach usually will not allow sufficient exposure for an adequate exploration of the pelvis to determine its cause. Surgery for invasive cervical cancer and endometrial cancer is done abdominally except in the most unusual circumstances. Extensive pelvic endometriosis, ectopic pregnancy, severe acute or chronic pelvic inflammatory disease, and suspected intra-abdominal disease of the bowel, appendix, or other organs that may require exploration or surgery are all contraindications to the vaginal approach. Except in the first trimester for legitimate reasons, vaginal hysterectomy is contraindicated in pregnant patients. A history of previous abdominal or pelvic surgery is not a contraindication to vaginal hysterectomy except for previous uterine suspension, especially previous ventral fixation to the anterior abdominal wall.

However, nulliparity or absence of uterine descensus are not in themselves contraindications to vaginal hysterectomy. On those few occasions when hysterectomy has been indicated in a nulliparous patient without descensus, it has been accomplished vaginally without difficulty. A history of previous cesarean section is not a contraindication to the vaginal approach. Indeed, the difficulty encountered in dissecting the bladder from the lower uterine segment, sometimes experienced in abdominal hysterectomy in a patient who has had a previous cesarean section, may be easier to accomplish with a vaginal approach.

Although some expert vaginal surgeons may remove a large (ie, up to 500 g) leiomyomatous uterus vaginally, it may be safer for other surgeons to do an abdominal hysterectomy to remove a uterus this large. The decision regarding the correct approach will depend on the technical skill and experience of the surgeon, the size of the uterus, and a careful assessment of other patient characteristics. For example, the subpubic arch must not be too narrow. Palpation of the subpubic arch and estimation of the distance between the ischial tuberosities will give an impression of how much room is available for operating. Obviously, removal of a large uterus will be more difficult if the patient has had no vaginal deliveries; if there is no descensus; if adhesions from previous pelvic surgery, pelvic inflammatory disease, or endometriosis are present; or if the patient is obese. The obesity that makes abdominal hysterectomy more difficult also makes vaginal hysterectomy more difficult.

TOTAL VERSUS SUBTOTAL ABDOMINAL HYSTERECTOMY FOR BENIGN CONDITIONS OF THE UTERUS

Total hysterectomy has always been the procedure of choice for malignant disease of the uterus. As abdominal hysterectomy has become a relatively safe operation in the hands of competent gynecologists, there has been a uniform shift toward total rather than subtotal hysterectomy for benign disease in recent decades. Until 50 years ago, total abdominal hysterectomy was considered a much more serious operation reserved by technically skilled gynecologic surgeons mostly for the surgical management of malignant disease of the uterus. In the first 50 years of the 20th century in the United States, many subtotal hysterectomies were performed. Many women had retained cervices, some without their knowledge. As a result of thoughtful debates regarding the advantages and disadvantages of removal of the cervix, the issue was settled in favor of total hysterectomy based mostly on a desire to eliminate the most unfortunate occurrence of death from carcinoma of the cervical stump. In 1946, Miller reported 69% subtotal and 31% total hysterectomies. At the Mayo Clinic, 666 total abdominal hysterectomies and 115 subtotal hysterectomies were done in 1944. According to Pratt and Jefferies, these numbers had changed to 472 total abdominal and 16 subtotal abdominal hysterectomies by 1953. Johnson, Moll, and Post reported 1246 abdominal hysterectomies done on the Tulane Service at Charity Hospital between 1952 and 1954. None was a subtotal hysterectomy. Indeed, Dr. Conrad Collins, Chief of the Tulane Service at Charity Hospital, was a leader in the crusade to gain acceptance for total rather than subtotal hysterectomy as the preferred method of removal of the uterus.

Currently, in most clinics in the United States, > 99% of all abdominal hysterectomies are total. In a recent series of 4341 abdominal hysterectomies at Grady Memorial Hospital, only 40 (0.9%) were subtotal. At the Milwaukee County Medical Complex, the cervix is retained in < 0.5% of all cases undergoing an abdominal hysterectomy. This standard of almost routine removal of the cervix is justified, although it should not be absolutely mandatory in every case. In comparing the two procedures, the gynecologic surgeon should balance the advantages of removal of the cervix against the possibilities of an increased morbidity and mortality for the total operation. To some extent, this comparison is difficult to make because subtotal hysterectomy is currently performed infrequently and usually only in patients with serious pelvic disease. Therefore, one might expect postoperative mortality and morbidity rates from subtotal abdominal hysterectomy that are higher than for total abdominal hysterectomy, but for reasons that have nothing to do with whether the cervix was removed. The advantages of removal of the cervix are principally that its removal eliminates it as a possible source of troublesome discharge or bleeding and especially as a site where carcinoma may develop. Indeed, in the United States, the number of patients with carcinoma of the cervical stump has been reduced significantly by the almost routine practice of total rather than subtotal hysterectomy. The incidence of the development of carcinoma is no greater in the retained cervical stump than in the cervix of an intact uterus. However, carcinoma diagnosed in a cervical stump presents challenging treatment problems. The anatomy is distorted, the relationship of the bladder to the top of the cervical stump is abnormal, and there may be dense adhesions between the cervix and the intestines. Treatment by surgery or irradiation may not be as successful and may be associated with more complications.

The incidence of carcinoma in a cervix that has had repeated negative cytologic evaluation is extremely low, and even lower if the endocervical canal and exocervix has been cauterized at the time of subtotal hysterectomy or soon thereafter. In 1982, Kilkku and associates reported on subtotal hysterectomies in 2712 Scandinavian patients and found the incidence of carcinoma of the cervical stump was only 0.11% compared with the usual incidence of 0.4–1.9% as reported by Tervila. The low incidence reported by Kilkku and associates may have been due to their routine cauterization of the retained cervix. Although there is a recognized false-negative rate of vaginal cytology of approximately 10%–15%, repeated cytologic study and clinical evaluation of the cervix reduces the risk of advanced cervical cancer. There is still a requirement for continued clinical and cytologic follow-up after subtotal abdominal hysterectomy especially in high-risk populations. This is a major disadvantage of subtotal hysterectomy because many patients do not understand this requirement following subtotal hysterectomy. If the cervix is left in at the time of abdominal hysterectomy, then the patient must be told and the need for subsequent cytologic follow-up emphasized.

The rationale for the removal of the cervix at the time of abdominal hysterectomy for benign disease must be based on the disease process that necessitates the hysterectomy and on the risk of complications that may result from attempting to remove the cervix from its anatomical location between the bladder above, the rectum below, and the ureters on each side. As pointed out in Chapters 29 and 30, injury to the urinary tract in gynecologic surgery occurs most often during removal of the cervix with abdominal hysterectomy, although such injury is an uncommon occurrence.

When the gynecologic surgeon encounters intraoperative technical difficulty or is informed by the anesthesiologist that the patient's condition is critical, a subtotal amputation of the uterine corpus may be performed quickly. This is in the best interest of the patient. Subtotal hysterectomy also may be performed in patients with severe pelvic inflammatory disease, advanced pelvic endometriosis, widespread tumor involvement in the cul-de-sac from ovarian cancer, and other conditions in which anatomical relationships around the cervix are not clearly defined and removal of the cervix is not essential to the solution of the patient's primary problem. Even in these circumstances, however, an experienced gynecologic surgeon can usually remove the cervix without danger of injury to surrounding structures. This subject is thoughtfully discussed by Baker.

Total abdominal hysterectomy is thought to have some disadvantages with respect to sexual responsiveness, but it has been difficult to sort out the most important influences and components as evidenced by studies by Zussman and associates, Dennerstein, Wood, and Burrows, by Utian, and by Sloan. Previous psychosexual dynamics, the nature of pelvic pathology, the operative technique used, the removal or conservation of functioning ovarian tissue, estrogen replacement therapy, age, the attitude of the sexual partner, and other conditions of social circumstances and health all are factors that may influence sexual responsiveness following hysterectomy. Kilkku and associates have made a determined effort to analyze the long-term morbidity other than carcinoma of total versus subtotal hysterectomy. They reported that the subtotal operation gave greater relief from pollakiuria, nocturia, sensation of residual urine, and incontinence. There was no difference in libido between the total and subtotal operations. Removing of the cervix did decrease the frequency of orgasm. Although there is disagreement, some believe that cervical secretory functions and mobility during coitus with a partner, or with masturbation, do play a role in determining some degree of sexual pleasure. Dyspareunia may be less common after subtotal hysterectomy because leaving the cervix in place may help keep the ovaries away from the vaginal vault so that deep penile thrusting will not cause pain. With total hysterectomy the ovaries should not be left in the cul-de-sac or just above the vaginal vault.

Langer and associates studied the effect of total abdominal hysterectomy on bladder function in women who were urologically asymptomatic preoperatively. No clinical symptoms of frequency, nocturia, urgency, or urge or stress incontinence were found postoperatively, and there were no significant differences from preoperative values for cystometry, uroflometry, and urethral pressure profiles. The authors concluded that urinary dysfunction should not be a consequence of an uncomplicated total abdominal hysterectomy for benign conditions in women who were previously free of urinary symptoms.

Regarding the effect of hysterectomy on bladder function, Sand and associates found that previous total hysterectomy increased the risk of subsequent failure of surgery for urinary incontinence. Citing the work of Snooks et al., these investigators suggested that extensive dissection of the bladder pillars during extrafascial total hysterectomy causes partial denervation of the bladder. Whether such an effect of total hysterectomy could be prevented by an intrafascial technique of removing the cervix or by performing subtotal hysterectomy instead is unknown.

The decision to perform subtotal rather than total hysterectomy is also based on the surgical risk involved in removing the cervix, because the current standard of care in performing hysterectomy is for a total hysterectomy. This decision may be delayed until the uterine vessels have been ligated. At that moment, the gynecologic surgeon should weigh the advantages and disadvantages in each individual patient, and decide whether to remove the cervix. The surgical risk of removing the cervix should be significant before a decision is made to retain it. Although the number of patients with carcinoma developing in a cervical stump has been remarkably reduced in recent years, it is unfortunate that there are still women who die of this disease when it could have been avoided by spending a few extra minutes to do a total rather than subtotal hysterectomy. Although there is some risk of vesicovaginal and rectovaginal fistula and ureteral injury with removal of the cervix, these complications should rarely occur, especially in the absence of significant pelvic disease, if proper surgical technique is used. This potential risk should not be a deterrent to removing the cervix at the time of the usual abdominal hysterectomy. Only when the danger of removing the cervix exceeds the danger of leaving it in should the subtotal operation be done. Because these circumstances are uncommon, the cervix is usually removed when an abdominal hysterectomy is performed.

There is one unusual circumstance in which the danger of removing the cervix is definitely greater than the danger of leaving it in. A patient who has cirrhosis of the liver with ascites who also must have a hysterectomy should have a subtotal operation if possible. If the cervix is removed and the vaginal apex does not heal securely, then the ascitic fluid will drain through the vagina and drain despite attempts to close the drainage site. The patient may die eventually of malnutrition. Therefore, cirrhosis of the liver with ascites is an almost absolute indication for the subtotal operation when hysterectomy must be done.

Pratt and Jefferies reported on the Mayo Clinic experience with the retained cervical stump. Between 1949 and 1973, 262 were removed—208 vaginally and 54 abdominally. Many were removed incidentally during an operation for pelvic mass or pelvic relaxation, but there were 46 cases of cervical malignancy. In the absence of a clear indication for removal, a normal cervical stump may be allowed to remain in place but regular examinations and cervical cytology should be performed.

If the surgeon decides to leave the cervix in place at the time of hysterectomy, the upper endocervical canal may be removed as described in the technique of subtotal hysterectomy. Later, the exocervix may be cauterized or treated with cryosurgery. Such treatment, if adopted routinely, will reduce the risk of malignancy in a retained cervix.

THE TECHNIQUE OF TOTAL ABDOMINAL HYSTERECTOMY FOR BENIGN DISEASE

Assuming there are proper indications for surgery and the patient has been properly prepared, from a purely technical standpoint, the objectives to be accomplished in performing abdominal hysterectomy are as follows:

To remove the uterus through an abdominal incision
To avoid excessive or unnecessary blood loss
To avoid bacterial contamination of the operative site by maintaining strict aseptic technique
To avoid unnecessary injury to tissues and adjacent structures
To restore normal anatomy to the degree possible

To conserve or improve useful function and avoid postoperative dysfunction

To detect and possibly correct other diseases and abnormalities

A variety of carefully considered techniques of abdominal hysterectomy allow the accomplishment of these objectives. The Mayo Clinic technique described by Lee is a notable example, although there are some important differences when compared with the technique of abdominal hysterectomy presented in this chapter—a technique that was described originally in 1929 by Dr. Edward H. Richardson, to whom this book was originally dedicated by Dr. Richard Te Linde. The Richardson technique is regarded as classic and some of his original illustrations by Brodel are included to emphasize some of the important and time-honored features of the procedure.

In expressing dissatisfaction with the techniques in vogue at that time and as justification for publishing the description of his new technique so methodically and meticulously developed over many years, Dr. Richardson stated,

> The vast majority of total hysterectomies can be comfortably and satisfactorily executed by one of several established methods. But we are less interested today in the large percentage of successes than can be legitimately credited to the end-results of an operative procedure than we are in the smaller number of technical difficulties, complications, and failures that persistently crop up to mar our records. Such deficiencies in no inconsiderable number are to be found recorded in every tabulated statistical study of the end-results of abdominal hysterectomy that I have reviewed. It is highly improbable, therefore, that any experienced pelvic surgeon will deny that, by any technique now in vogue, occasionally he finds this operation difficult of execution; that hemorrhage is frequently troublesome, and occasionally embarrassing, even to the extent of jeopardizing one or both ureters in the urgent necessity of its immediate control; that measures to combat or prevent postoperative shock are now and again required; that actual damage to the ureters still occur; and that, in rare instances, a fulminating streptococcus peritonitis brings a rapid exodus to his patient and profound mortification to himself.

Thus, Dr. Richardson emphasized an obsessive attention to detail in every case, and a carefully planned and technically correct anatomical dissection to reduce to an absolute minimum even the most unusual complication of abdominal hysterectomy. His basic and standard technique has been used by thousands of gynecologic surgeons throughout the world with excellent success. Its steps and principles can be illustrated and taught and learned with relative ease and easily modified when special circumstances prevent the carrying out of the uniform standard procedure. The gynecologic surgeon, however, should have some standard plan to begin with and be thoroughly familiar with the plan to facilitate modifications when needed.

A. Cullen Richardson, Lyon, and Graham of Atlanta have presented evidence that meticulous dissection, careful handling of tissues, and other measures can result in a low rate of morbidity and complications and reduced hospital stay and costs when abdominal hysterectomy is performed. Abdominal hysterectomy for benign disease is done most often for leiomyomas. The great variation in size and shape of the uterus with leiomyomas makes it necessary to occasionally deviate from any standard surgical technique and frequently to improvise as the surgeon proceeds. Also, the complication of adnexal disease may prevent the carrying out of a uniform procedure. Although this procedure is presented as it might be done in the surgical treatment of leiomyomatous uteri, this method is also used for the surgical treatment of other benign pelvic disease including pelvic endometriosis, pelvic inflammatory disease, adnexal tumors, and other benign pathology.

After the patient has been correctly identified and placed on the operating table, a satisfactory level of anesthesia is obtained. The patient's legs are then placed in Allen universal stirrups with the thighs flexed approximately 15° in relation to the abdomen and the knees separated 30° (Fig. 27-2A). The bladder is emptied with a catheter, and a pelvic examination, including a bimanual recto–vaginal–abdominal examination, is always done before the patient is prepared and draped. A pelvic examination under anesthesia became a routine procedure before each gynecologic operation at The Johns Hopkins Hospital after an 1890 study by Hunter Robb demonstrating its value in 240 cases. Without question, pelvic examination under anesthesia is the best time to evaluate pelvic pathology and it should be done routinely. The bladder has just been emptied with a catheter, the bowel has been emptied with an enema, and presumably the anterior abdominal wall is relaxed with anesthesia. Useful information is obtained about the size, location, and mobility of pelvic tumors and their proximity to organs and structures in the pelvis such as bladder, ureters, and rectum. The choice of incision can be made from findings on pelvic examination under anesthesia. Previously unknown new pathology may be discovered. Comparing the findings under anesthesia with the operative findings is an excellent way to learn the proper interpretation of abnormal findings on pelvic examination.

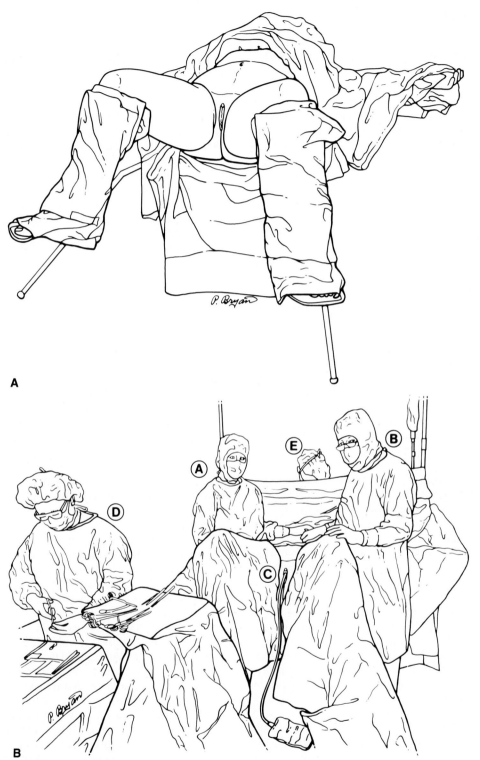

Figure 27–2. *A*, Patient is positioned on the operating table for pelvic laparotomy. The legs are placed in Allen universal stirrups and the patient is draped to allow access to the vaginal introitus and external urethral meatus. *B*, Members of the operating team are positioned as follows: *A*, the operator stands on the patient's right side. *B*, the first assistant stands on the patient's left side. *C*, the second assistant, if available, stands between the patient's legs. *D*, the instrument nurse. *E*, the anesthesiologist.

Positioning patients in the Allen universal stirrups for pelvic laparotomy has a number of advantages, including the following four:

1. With the legs flexed approximately 15°–20° on the abdomen, there is less strain on the patient's lumbar spine than there is from lying flat on the operating table for 1, 2, or 3 hours at a time, or longer.

2. In this position in stirrups, the vaginal introitus is available for instrumentation should there be a need intraoperatively. An empty sponge forceps placed through the introitus to the top of the vagina can aid in the identification of its anatomical limits. When there is endometriosis in the cul-de-sac, an instrument can push up on the posterior vaginal fornix and elevate the cul-de-sac into the operative field for easier removal of the endometriosis. Should there be a need to drain the pelvis through the posterior vaginal fornix, the drainage incision can be more accurately placed by cutting down on an instrument that has been placed in the vagina from below to elevate the posterior vaginal fornix. When a suprapubic colpourethropexy is done, fingers of the operators's hand placed in the vagina can elevate the anterior vaginal wall on each side of the urethra into the space of Retzius above, allowing more accurate placement of sutures for suprapubic colpourethropexy.

3. The availability of the urethral meatus in the operative field allows the placement of instruments into the bladder to determine its anatomical limits or to detect an area of weakness or injury. Should the need arise, intraoperative cystoscopy with placement of ureteral catheters is possible without the need for repositioning the patient or the need for a cystotomy incision. Most important, as the abdominal incision is closed, 5 cc of indigo carmine dye can be injected IV, 200 cc of sterile saline can be instilled in the bladder through the urethra, and in 3–5 minutes, the dye can be observed to efflux from both ureteral orifices, thus proving ureteral integrity. This routine for proving ureteral integrity after each operation is possible when patients are positioned in stirrups for pelvic laparotomy.

4. If one is fortunate enough to have a second assistant for the operation, that person can stand between the patient's legs and from this vantage point can see the operative field better and provide better assistance than if standing by the patient's side but distant from the operative field (Fig. 27-2B).

After the patient is positioned in stirrups and the pelvic examination under anesthesia is completed, special attention is given to cleaning the depths of the umbilicus with cotton applicators. Providone-iodine (betadine) is used for skin preparation, first with a 5-minute wash and then with four sponges on long sponge forceps. The area prepared includes the entire skin from the rib cage to the level of the mid-thigh, anterior, medial, and lateral. Special emphasis is given to the mons, labia, clitoris, buttocks, and vagina and perineum, including the anus last. The deepest portions of the vaginal fornices are cleaned with several soaked sponges on long sponge forceps. Although it is impossible to sterilize all the rugae of vagina, it is important to render this area surgically clean before the procedure. Dry sponges should be used to remove excess preparation solution from the vagina. Towels are placed around the operative field, which includes the lower abdomen, mons, and vulva. At least two thicknesses of drapes cover the abdomen and legs. A double-gloved assistant then places the indwelling Foley catheter in the bladder. It drains straight down to a bag on the floor.

To facilitate the operative procedure and to avoid injury to vital structures, adequate exposure through an incision in the lower abdomen is mandatory. The lower abdominal transverse Maylard incision is preferred for reasons stated in Chapter 11. Occasionally, a lower midline incision may be necessary. The exposure afforded by a Pfannenstiel's or Kustner's incision is usually inadequate for performance of abdominal hysterectomy. Although a modest Trendelenburg position may be helpful to facilitate exposure, an exaggerated or steep Trendelenburg position can and should be avoided.

After the incision is made, the upper abdomen is explored. Standing on the patient's right side, the operator inserts the right hand into the upper abdomen. The right kidney, liver, gallbladder, pancreas, stomach, left kidney, and para-aortic lymph nodes are palpated in sequence, and abnormalities are noted. Some type of self-retaining retractor is inserted to expose the pelvic contents. The O'Connor-O'Sullivan or Balfour self-retaining retractors may be used with a longitudinal incision. However, it is preferable to use the Bookwalter self-retaining retractor with a transverse Maylard incision. Regardless of the incision or the type of retractor used, the lateral blades must not be allowed to press against the femoral nerves. When a Bookwalter retractor is used with a Maylard incision, lateral blades are not needed. Adhesions must be released before the intestines can be placed in the upper abdomen and held there with tagged laparotomy packs. Restoration of pelvic anatomy by release of adhesions also will facilitate the operative procedure.

At this point in the procedure, the surgeon should pause and assess the nature and extent of pelvic pathology; of the anatomical relationships, with particular reference to the ureters, bladder, and rectum; and of the operative procedure to be performed. "Totalabdominalhysterectomybilateralsalpingo-oophorectomy" is not one word. A separate decision must be made about each part and whether it is to be removed or retained. Many different circumstances must be considered to fit the operation to the individual patient, her pathology, her symptomatology, and her future.

The Ochsner's clamp (also called Kocher's clamp), both straight and curved, is commonly used throughout in performing abdominal hysterectomy. The Masterson clamp is specially designed for hysterectomy and is quite satisfactory.

The operation usually begins with the round ligaments. Even in patients with every extensive pathology and distorted anatomy, the round ligaments can be identified laterally. Following the round ligaments medially will always lead to the uterine corpus. One of the round ligaments is grasped with a curved Ochsner's clamp near the uterine cornu, cut with the scalpel or scissors, and ligated a short distance lateral to the clamp with No. 0 or No. 2-0 delayed-absorbable suture (Fig. 27-3). Thus, the anterior leaf of the broad ligament is opened. The anterior leaf of the broad ligament is incised to the point of reflection of the bladder peritoneum on the uterus (Fig. 27-4). Beneath the utero-

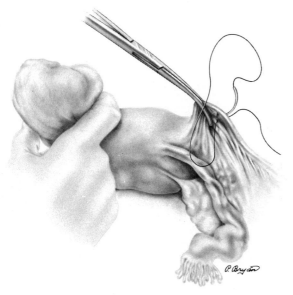

Figure 27–3. The technique of abdominal hysterectomy begins with the round ligament. The ligament is clamped, ligated with a transfixion suture, and cut. The broad ligament is opened.

ovarian ligament, the posterior leaf of the broad ligament is pushed forward with the surgeon's fingers (Fig. 27-5). This portion of the broad ligament is quite avascular. It is incised with the scissors, thus making a window in the broad ligament.

If the tubes and ovaries are to be conserved, the tube and the utero-ovarian ligament are triply clamped (Fig. 27-6). The clamps should be placed as close to the uterine corpus as possible so that blood vessels in the mesosalpinx and mesovarium will not be interfered with. The clamp closest the uterus is to control back bleeding and to provide traction on the uterus; therefore, the incision with the scalpel is made between it and the middle clamp. Thus, the vessels are doubly clamped as they extend from the uterine artery and vein to the tube and ovary. Double clamping of these vessels is the usual routine and it is an excellent precaution in that it prevents slipping and retraction of the cut vessels with the formation of a broad ligament hematoma. Further, the ligation must be in the nature of a mass tie, and the crushing of the tissues by means of the most lateral clamp affords a groove in which to tie the first ligature. This lateral clamp on the cut pedicle is removed as a free ligature is tied around it, and the proximal clamp is kept in place. A free-tie ligature of No. 0 or No. 2-0 delayed-absorbable suture is used initially to avoid trauma to the vessels in the vascular pedicle. These vessels must be occluded by ligation first so that the pedicle may be safety secured again distal to the tie with a transfixion suture. A No. 0 or No. 2-0 delayed-absorbable suture is placed medial to the first ligature in the center of the pedicle beneath the remaining clamp, passing the free ends of the suture around the tip and heel of the clamp before tying. The clamp is then removed (Fig. 27-7). There are instances in which the double clamp technique cannot be used, but when it is feasible, it is a worthwhile precaution.

If the tube and the ovary are to be removed with the uterus, the infundibulopelvic ligament portion of the broad ligament is clamped with three curved Ochsner's clamps (Fig. 27-8). The surgeon should locate the ureter before placing clamps on the infundibulopelvic ligament. The tip of each clamp is placed through the open window in the broad ligament. The clamp that is the most lateral is placed first with conscious attention to the position of the ureter. The ureter should be visualized. The other two clamps are placed above the first. The ligament is divided between the middle and medial clamp, and double ligation of the ovarian vessels by No. 0 or No. 2-0 delayed-absorbable ligature is carried out. The initial ligature around the lateral clamp on the cut pedicle is a free tie, and the second tie is a transfixion suture placed distal to the first tie through the center of the pedicle behind the remaining middle clamp. Clam-

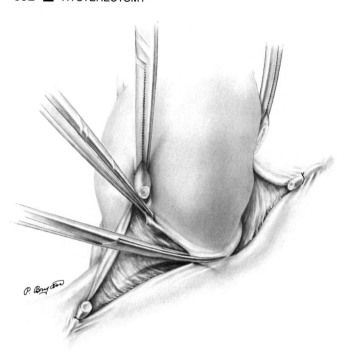

Figure 27–4. Abdominal hysterectomy. The anterior leaf of the broad ligament is incised to the point where the bladder peritoneum is reflected onto the anterior lower uterine isthmus in the midline. To avoid unnecessary blood loss, the bladder is not dissected away from the uterus at this point.

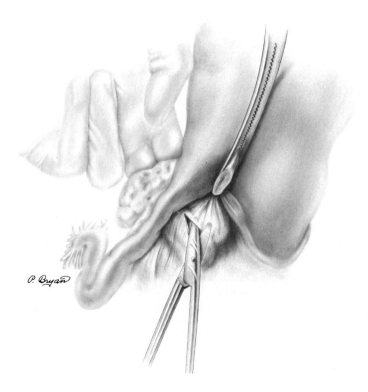

Figure 27–5. Abdominal hysterectomy. Two fingers push the posterior leaf of the broad ligament forward. An incision is made to develop a window in the broad ligament.

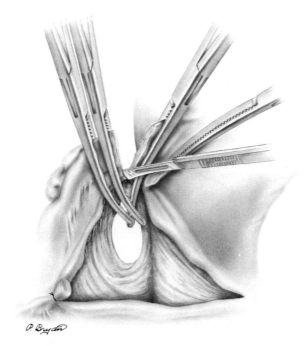

Figure 27–6. Abdominal hysterectomy. If the tube and ovary are to be conserved, three Ochsner's clamps are placed across the tube and utero-ovarian ligament as close to the uterus as possible. An incision is made between the middle and the medial clamp.

ping, cutting, and ligating of the round ligament, the uterine end of the tube, and ovarian ligament or of the infundibulopelvic ligament are carried out in the same manner on the opposite side as indicated. In general, it is good policy to ligate the clamped ovarian vessels as they are cut rather than to leave all the clamps on the pedicles until after the uterus is removed. Likewise, sutures used to ligated pedicles are cut and are not held. Clamps and long pedicle ligatures should not be allowed to clutter the operating field and interfere with exposure.

The midline reflection of the bladder peritoneum onto the uterus is now freed by extending the incision in the anterior leaf of the broad ligament medially across the anterior lower uterine isthmus. It is technically easier to incise and free the bladder peritoneum from the lower portion of the uterus by continuing the dissection of the anterior leaf of the broad ligament medially from the point where each round ligament is cut rather than by initiating the dissection in the midline. The incision in the anterior peritoneal leaf of the broad ligament is simply extended medially and inferiorly toward the midportion of the lower uterine segment where the incisions meet in the midline. A subperitoneal tissue plane is easily obtained by sliding the Metzenbaum scissors, with the curvature facing up-

ward, beneath the peritoneum before incising the peritoneum. If the dissection is made just through the peritoneum, a good line of cleavage is entered; if the dissection goes too deeply, bleeding will be encountered (see Fig. 27-4). At this point, the bladder should be separated from the lower uterine segment and upper cervix by careful sharp dissection of the fascial fibers beneath the bladder wall (Fig. 27-9). Complete mobilization of the bladder away from the cervix and upper anterior vaginal wall will be needed eventually. However, to avoid unnecessary blood loss, a complete dissection and mobilization of the bladder may be done later. Using a sponge on a sponge forceps to push the bladder down may cause unnecessary trauma to the bladder musculature, especially if the bladder is unusually adherent to the cervix. Usually, the bladder can be dissected away and displaced into the lower pelvis quite easily, but if it is adherent, it should be surgically released with Metzenbaum scissors and not bluntly forced.

The posterior leaf of the broad ligament is incised on either side parallel with the lateral side of the uterus down to the point of origin of the uterosacral ligaments behind the cervix (Fig. 27-10). Incising the anterior and posterior broad ligament peritoneum will allow the uterine vessels to be exposed and skeletonized before they are clamped.

Before clamping and cutting the uterine vessels, it is always advisable to palpate the lower portion of the pelvic ureters as they course beneath the uterine artery, lateral to the internal cervical os, and pass medially and anteriorly through the base of the broad ligament to enter the trigone of the bladder. With wide mobilization and displacement of the bladder base from the cervix, and with upward traction on the uterine corpus, the ureters are usually 1.5–2.0 cm lateral and inferior to the point of clamping of the uterine vessels. However, they may be displaced by pelvic disease and induration of paracervical tissue, particularly in the presence of endometriosis and pelvic inflammatory disease, and should be identified before the uterine artery clamps are placed in this vulnerable area.

The uterine vessels are completely skeletonized and exposed and are then triply clamped bilaterally with curved Ochsner's clamps (Fig. 27-11). It is desirable to have these clamps slide off the edge of the cervix. It is important to remember three rules in clamping uterine vessels: (1) the lowest clamp is placed initially, (2) this clamp is placed at the level of the internal cervical os, and (3) it is placed at right angles to the lower uterine segment. If the surgeon places clamps on uterine vessels in this way, injury to the ureter should be avoided.

The upper clamp is intended to prevent back bleeding from the uterus, and the two lower clamps doubly occlude the uterine vessels. The vessels are cut with the

(*text continues on page 696*)

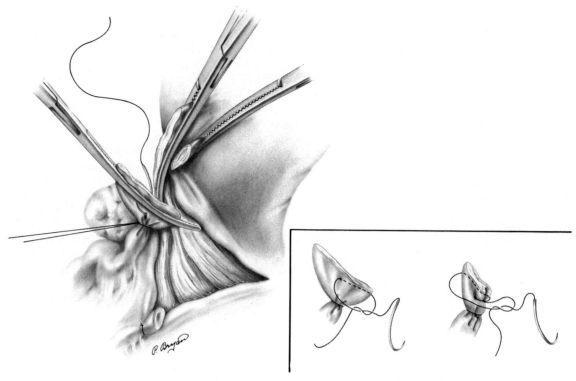

Figure 27–7. Abdominal hysterectomy. The lateral clamp is replaced with a free tie that completely surrounds the pedicle and occlues the vessels. The middle clamp is replaced by a transfixion suture ligature that is tied securely around both sides of the pedicle.

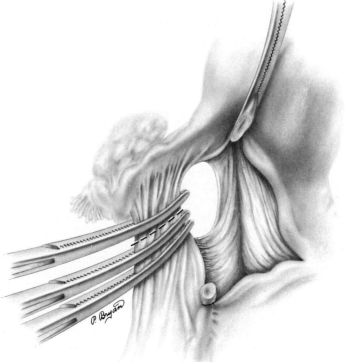

Figure 27–8. Abdominal hysterectomy. If the tube and ovary are to be removed, three Ochsner's clamps are placed across the infundibulopelvic ligament, using the window in the broad ligament. After the ureter is located, the lateral-most clamp is placed first. The ligament is incised at the dotted line, and the pedicle is doubly ligated with No. 0 delayed-absorbable suture as illustrated in Figure 27–7.

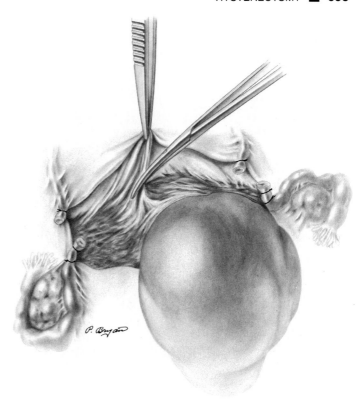

Figure 27–9. Abdominal hysterectomy. The bladder must be mobilized inferiorly by sharp dissection away from the cervix. To avoid unnecessary bleeding, this step may be done in stages as necessary.

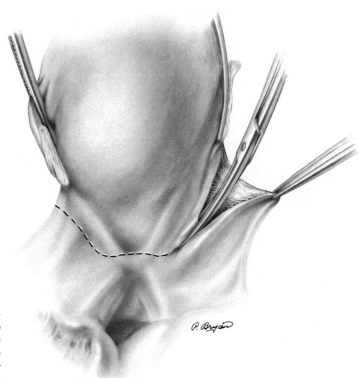

Figure 27–10. Abdominal hysterectomy. The posterior leaf of the broad ligament is incised down to the point where the uterosacral ligaments join the cervix (*dotted lines*). Dissection across the back of the cervix can be delayed until later to avoid unnecessary bleeding.

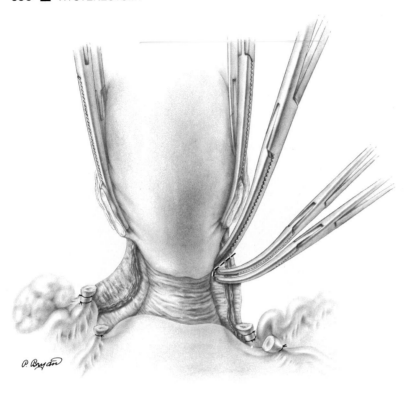

P. Bryan

Figure 27–11. Abdominal hysterectomy. After the uterine vessels are skeletonized, they are triply clamped and cut along the dotted lines. To avoid clamping the ureter, the lowest clamp is placed first, at the level of the internal cervical os and at right angles to the lower uterine isthmus. The lowest two clamps are replaced by No. 0 delayed-absorbable suture ligatures.

scalpel between the upper and middle clamps and freed from the uterus by extending the incision around the tip of the middle clamp. This separates the vessels from the uterus and permits direct ligation of the vascular pedicles. This step also provides access to the upper portion of the cardinal ligament. Care should be taken to avoid incising the tissue beyond the tip of the lowest clamp, because doing so could permit bleeding from collateral vessels that are not included in the clamp. The sutures must be placed precisely in the angle of the incision and the tip of the clamp to be certain that all of the vessels in the clamp are secured by the ligature.

The uterine vessels are doubly ligated with No. 0 delayed-absorbable suture with ligation of the tissue within the lowest clamp initially. As the first suture is tied, the clamp is removed; if the bite of tissue is large, it may be well to loosen the middle clamp slightly and then again close the ratchet to permit the tissue to be compressed tightly by the ligature. As the second ligature is placed and tied, the middle clamp is removed. Double clamping is of great value here, because if only one clamp is used and the tissue slips out of the ligature and retracts, the uterine vessels must be caught again to control the bleeding. Attempts at clamping retracted uterine vessels in the base of the broad ligament may result in injury to the ureter.

Following ligation of the uterine vessels, a straight Ochsner's clamp may be placed between the uterine

vessels and the side of the uterus (Fig. 27-12). The tissue clamped is the uppermost part of the cardinal ligament. The incision is made in such a way that a fringe of tissue remains distal to the clamp. This will enhance the security of its ligation and will allow the uterine vessel pedicle to drop further laterally.

The uterus is pulled forward and upward to expose and stretch the uterosacral ligaments posteriorly. The incisions in the posterior peritoneum of the broad ligaments are carried transversely through the uterine reflection of the cul-de-sac peritoneum between the attachments of the two uterosacral ligaments. The peritoneal flap is mobilized initially from its attachment to the cervix and posterior vaginal fornix with the Metzenbaum scissors (Fig. 27-13). Each uterosacral ligament is clamped with a curved Ochsner's clamp, with particular care being taken to avoid the pelvic portion of the ureter as it courses along the base of the broad ligament. The anterior rectal wall also must be avoided. The uterosacral ligaments are then clamped, incised, and ligated with No. 0 or No. 2-0 delayed-absorbable suture (Fig. 27-14). Continued sharp and blunt dissection posteriorly and inferiorly in the midline between the ligated uterosacral ligaments will develop a plane between the cervix and vagina anteriorly and the anterior rectal wall posteriorly. This is the entrance to the rectovaginal space (Fig. 27-15). Usually there is no bleeding if a proper loose areolar plane is entered and care is

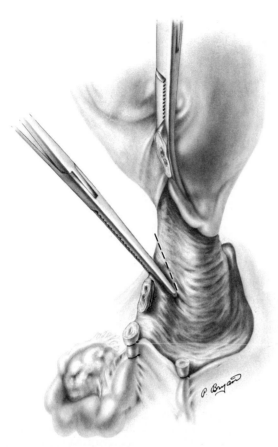

Figure 27–12. Total abdominal hysterectomy. If a total hysterectomy is to be done, the uterine vessels are dropped away by placing an Ochsner's clamp across the upper cardinal ligament between the uterine vessels and the lower uterine isthmus. The tissue is cut along the dotted line and ligated.

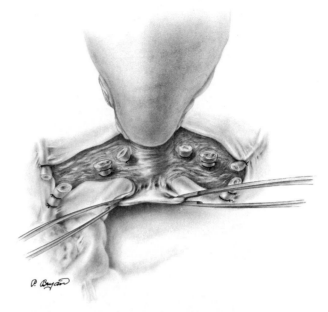

Figure 27–13. Total abdominal hysterectomy. A flap of peritoneum is dissected from the cervix posteriorly. This will allow the uterosacral ligaments to be isolated and the rectovaginal space to be entered behind the cervix.

taken to avoid extensive lateral dissection where the hemorrhoidal vessels insert into the rectum (Fig. 27-16).

At this point, dissection of the bladder base away from the anterior vaginal wall must be completed (Fig. 27-17). Inadequate dissection and mobilization of the bladder inferiorly and laterally is one of the most frequent causes of inadvertent injury to the bladder wall. Bladder injury may result in a vesicovaginal fistula if the injury is not recognized and repaired at the time of surgery. With the uterus under firm traction, the two index fingers or the thumb and index finger from the same hand may be readily opposed below the cervix, and further dissection and mobilization of the base of the bladder anteriorly and the rectum posteriorly can be accomplished if needed (Fig. 27-18).

It is important to call particular attention to the pubovesicocervical fascia, which was described by Richardson in 1929 and reviewed by Jaszczak and Evans. This fascia contains many small arteries and venous plexus that provide collateral circulation to the base of the bladder, cervix, and upper vagina. It is part of the endopelvic fascia that surrounds the cervix and blends with the cardinal ligaments, the uterosacral ligaments, and the broad ligaments and extends to the lateral pelvic wall. To avoid these vessels and to provide protection to the base of the bladder and the adjacent ureter, a *T*-shaped or *V*-shaped incision is made in the pubovesicocervical fascia anterior to the cervix just below the level of the internal cervical os and the ligated uterine vessels (Fig. 27-19). As the edges of the incised fascia retract laterally, a pale avascular area of the anterior surface of the cervix can be seen. Care should be taken to avoid incising too deeply into the cervix because this will produce additional bleeding, the loose fascial plane will be missed, and the dissection will be difficult and bloody. The blunt end of the scalpel is useful in dissecting the loosened fibers of the pubovesicocervical fascia away from the cervix. The dissection can be continued until the fascia has been reflected laterally off the anterior surface of the cervix and upper vagina.

As this dissection progresses, the whitish fascial plane of the vagina comes into view and gives clear evidence to the operator that the plane of dissection is correct. Dissection of the remaining portion of the

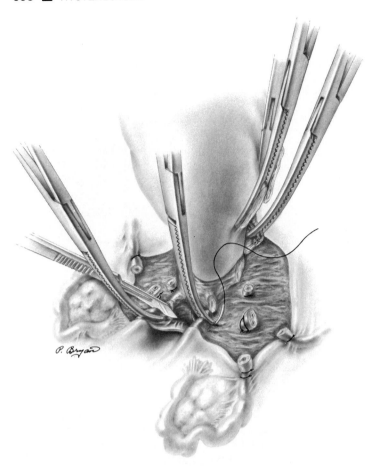

Figure 27–14. Total abdominal hysterectomy. The uterosacral ligaments are clamped, cut, and ligated adjacent to the cervix. Each clamp is replaced by a No. 0 delayed-absorbable suture.

cardinal ligament is carried out by placing straight Ochsner's clamps inside the rectovaginal space posteriorly and inside the cut edges of the pubovesicocervical fascia anteriorly (see Fig. 27-19). Usually two or three bites are required on either side of the cervix until the pale white tissue of the vaginal wall representing the lateral vaginal fornix is identified. Each clamp is replaced by a No. 0 or No. 2-0 delayed-absorbable suture ligature. Occasionally, the lateral fornix is entered when the lower portion of the cardinal ligament is incised, clearly defining the vaginal apex.

This technique of removing the cervix by placing clamps on the cardinal ligament beneath the pubovesicocervical fascia is called the *intrafascial technique of total abdominal hysterectomy*. It can be used in almost every case when hysterectomy is done for benign disease. It is the safest technique of removing the cervix. As pointed out previously, most injuries to the bladder and ureters occur with removal of the cervix. If the bladder is properly mobilized laterally and inferiorly, and if the pubovesicocervical fascia is properly developed and clamps are placed beneath the fascia,

the risk of urinary tract injury is reduced. The bladder and ureters have never been found beneath the pubovesicocervical fascia.

The intrafascial technique of total hysterectomy is appropriate only for benign disease of the uterus. Otherwise, we use an extrafascial technique to remove the cervix. Few comparisons have been made of extrafascial versus intrafascial abdominal hysterectomy. Hinojosa, Arechiga, and Aguilera reported a 38% morbidity for extrafascial abdominal hysterectomy and a 32% morbidity for intrafascial abdominal hysterectomy.

The anterior and posterior walls of the vagina may be clamped together at each lateral vaginal angle as shown in Figure 27-20 using an Ochsner's clamp, or the uterus may be removed by a circumferential incision in the vagina close to the cervix, being certain that the entire cervix is removed with the uterine corpus (Fig. 27-21). As the anterior, posterior, and lateral angles of the vagina are opened, straight Ochsner's clamps are used to secure the vaginal margins. If Ochsner's clamps are placed on the lateral vaginal angles, they are replaced with transfixion sutures (Fig. 27-22).

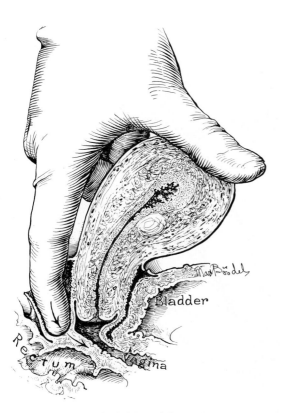

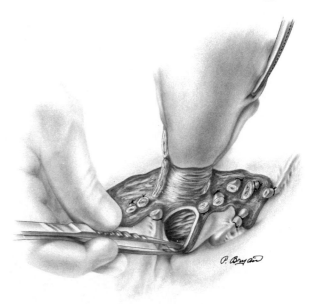

Figure 27–16. Total abdominal hysterectomy. Dissection between the ligated uterosacral ligaments behind the cervix will enter the rectovaginal space. This step is also illustrated in Figure 27–15.

Figure 27–15. Total abdominal hysterectomy. A sagittal view showing the bladder dissection completed and indicating depth and direction of the posterior dissection into the rectovaginal space. (Reprinted from Richardson EH. A simplified technic for abdominal panhysterectomy. Surg Gynecol Obstet 1929; 48:248, with permission.)

The original Richardson technique used routine vaginal drainage, which was considered a major contribution to this procedure. Although surgeons formerly practiced tight closure of the vaginal vault for most cases, the open cuff technique also advised by Gray and others has recently regained popularity as a method of allowing better extraperitoneal drainage. When the vaginal vault is left open, the incidence of cuff cellulitis, abscess, and hematoma is reduced. The open cuff does remain patent for a sufficient time to serve as a useful conduit for serum or blood that may accumulate gradually above the vaginal vault. However, if better drainage is required for a longer time, then the addition of a small closed suction drain may be used but is rarely needed.

After the vaginal angle clamps have been replaced with transfixion sutures, the free margin of the vagina is reefed with a continuous locking suture of No. 2-0 delayed-absorbable suture (see Fig. 27-22). The vaginal vault should not be sutured closed, although doing so

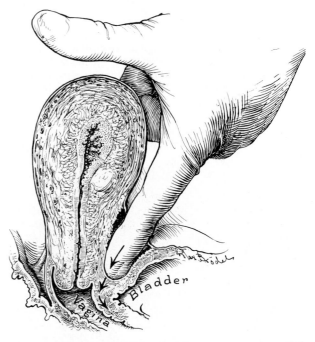

Figure 27–17. Total abdominal hysterectomy. A sagittal view showing depth and direction of the vesicocervicovaginal dissection. This step serves to displace the bladder and the ureters still further away from the danger zone. (Reprinted from Richardson EH. A simplified technic for abdominal panhysterectomy. Surg Gynecol Obstet 1929; 48:248, with permission.)

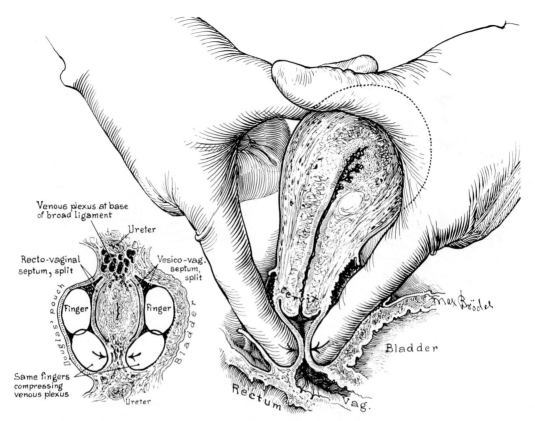

Figure 27–18. Total abdominal hysterectomy. Testing the depth of the anterior and posterior dissections. The *inset* shows the method of segregating the vascular plexus on each side into a narrow zone adjacent to the basal segment of the broad ligament. (Reprinted from Richardson EH. A simplified technic for abdominal panhysterectomy. Surg Gynecol Obstet 1929; 48:248, with permission.)

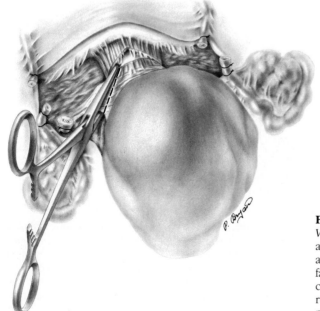

Figure 27–19. Total abdominal hysterectomy. A *T*-shaped or *V*-shaped incision is made in the pubovesicocervical fascia anterior to the cervix. Straight Ochsner's clamps are placed across the cardinal ligaments lateral to the cervix and inside the fascia in such a way that the fascia is actually peeled off the cervix. An incision is made at the dotted line and the clamp is replaced with a No. 0 delayed-absorbable suture. Several bites may be needed in each cardinal ligament.

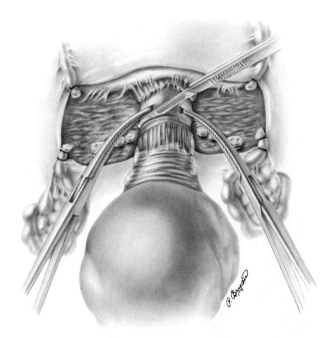

Figure 27–20. Total abdominal hysterectomy. After the surgeon determines with certainty that the bladder and rectum have been completely dissected away from the vagina, curved Ochsner's clamps are placed across the vaginal angles and the uterus is removed by incising the vagina below the cervix.

usually will not cause harm. It is simply unnecessary. There is a good reason to leave the cuff open—for drainage. There is no good reason to close it.

In 1975, Gray reported his series of total abdominal hysterectomy in 2421 patients. The vaginal cuff was left open in all patients. There were no postoperative vaginal cuff abscesses and febrile morbidity was recorded in 20.8%. Large quantities of serosanguinous fluid can be suctioned from the space above a closed vaginal cuff in the immediate postoperative period, as shown by the studies of Swartz and Tanaree. Such a closed space is an ideal location for the growth of anaerobic bacteria. Leaving the cuff open will facilitate drainage of this fluid and allow the space to close gradually. However, it should not lead to a false sense of security since collections of fluid and pus may still occur laterally.

Because of the possibility of vaginal vault prolapse or enterocele in subsequent years after total abdominal hysterectomy, careful attention must be paid to the support of the vaginal vault. A new step may be added to the standard Richardson technique at this point. It is the performance of a posterior culdoplasty as illustrated in Figure 27-23. A No. 0 polydioxanone suture is passed first through the uterosacral ligament on one side. The suture then passes in and out of the posterior vaginal fornix and through the uterosacral ligament on the

opposite side. When tied, this suture approximates the uterosacral ligaments behind the upper posterior vagina and pulls the posterior vaginal fornix in a posterior direction (Fig. 27-24). More than one suture may be used if the posterior fornix appears unduly relaxed. Care must be taken to avoid the ureters when placing the sutures in the uterosacral ligaments. If additional support of the posterior vagina is needed, the surgeon might consider obliteration of a deep cul-de-sac by the Moschcowitz or Halban technique at this point in the procedure. Obliteration of the cul-de-sac will tend to isolate and protect a weakened and relaxed upper posterior vaginal wall from the constant pressure of intraabdominal contents with occasional intermittent spikes of greater pressure associated with coughing, sneezing, and straining. Also, ovaries cannot prolapse behind the vagina if the cul-de-sac has been obliterated.

Additional suspension of the vaginal vault is combined with a peritonization suture. This technique places the free margins of the vascular pedicles beneath the peritoneum so that any postoperative bleeding will be contained retroperitoneally in the base of the pelvis and avoid dangerous occult intraperitoneal bleeding. The technique uses a continuous No. 0 or No. 2-0 delayed-absorbable suture that first pierces the anterior vaginal wall laterally and passes through the free margin of the cardinal ligament, avoiding the uterine vessel pedicle. The suture then passes through the anterior bladder peritoneum near the round ligament; continues through the round ligament and the remaining edge of the anterior leaf of the broad ligament; continues posteriorly along the cut edge of the posterior leaf of the broad ligament, incorporating the uterosacral ligament; and finally, pierces the posterior edge of the vaginal wall laterally (Fig. 27-25). A similar suture is placed on the opposite side of the pelvis, and both ligatures are tied firmly. These sutures accomplish vaginal vault suspension and peritonization on each side. If the ovaries have been preserved, the tip of the pedicle is closed separately with a purse-string suture of No. 3-0 delayed-absorbable suture and the free margin of the pedicle is buried beneath the peritoneum. By this technique, the ovaries are retained against the pelvic wall and are not anchored to the vaginal vault. This technique is advised to avoid subsequent dyspareunia and overstretching of the ovarian vessels with possible thrombosis, ischemia, and cystic change of the ovary. If the ovaries have been removed, the infundibulopelvic ligament pedicle is likewise buried beneath the peritoneum with a No. 3-0 delayed-absorbable purse-string suture.

Reperitonization is completed by suturing the bladder peritoneum to the cul-de-sac peritoneum with No. 3-0 delayed-absorbable suture. This suture is initiated near the point where the round ligament joins the angle

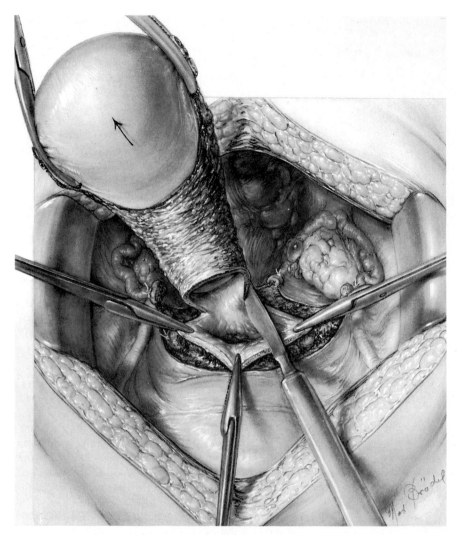

Figure 27–21. Total abdominal hysterectomy. The dissection completed, the amputation across the vaginal vault is shown here. This should be done as closely as possible to the cervix to avoid shortening the vagina. The four quadrants of the vaginal vault are held with straight Ochsner's clamps for subsequent placement of sutures. (Reprinted from Richardson EH. A simplified technic for abdominal panhysterectomy. Surg Gynecol Obstet 1929; 48:248, with permission.)

of the vagina. The anterior peritoneal edge is sutured to the posterior peritoneal flap (Fig. 27-26). The suture is tied, which ensures that the vascular pedicles remain beneath the peritoneum, and is then continued to the opposite angle of the vagina as a continuous suture, approximating the bladder and cul-de-sac peritoneum. If preferred, interrupted No. 3-0 delayed-absorbable sutures may be used. If there has been repair of a bladder injury, or if there is any question in the operator's mind about the integrity of the bladder wall, the edge of the peritoneum behind the bladder should be sutured to the anterior vaginal cuff to prevent superimposition of the weakened bladder wall against the vaginal apex (see Ch. 30).

If elective appendectomy is indicated, it is carried out at this point in the procedure (see Ch. 36). Upon completion of the appendectomy, the operator returns to

make a final inspection of the pelvis to be certain that hemostasis is secure. The pelvis should be irrigated with warm sterile saline. In 1984, Nelson and associates reported on the use of intraoperative intraperitoneal irrigation with a solution of 500 ml of normal saline containing 2 mg of ampicillin and 2 g of streptomycin in 171 patients undergoing abdominal hysterectomy. The percentage of patients with a diagnosis of postoperative cuff cellulitis was reduced from 27.0 to 4.7. This routine might be worthy of adoption especially because perioperative antibiotics are of questionable value in abdominal hysterectomy.

The sigmoid colon should be placed in the pelvis ahead of loops of small intestine, and the omentum should be placed over the colon. The ovaries are placed over the omentum. If there is a tendency for the ovaries to fall into the cul-de-sac, then the surgeon may elect to

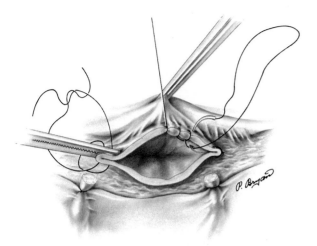

Figure 27–22. Total abdominal hysterectomy. The clamps on the lateral vaginal angles are replaced by No. 0 delayed-absorbable transfixion sutures. A No. 2-0 delayed-absorbable continuous locking suture is placed around the vaginal margin. Again, the bladder must be completely mobilized and retracted inferiorly.

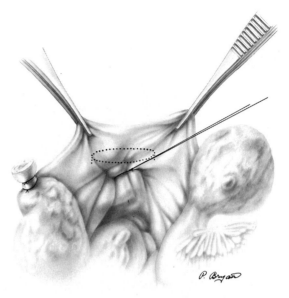

Figure 27–24. Total abdominal hysterectomy. When the posterior culdeplasty suture is tied, the posterior vaginal fornix is pulled in a more natural direction toward the sacrum.

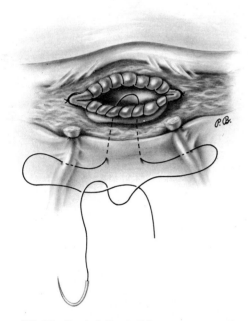

Figure 27–23. Total abdominal hysterectomy. Taking care to avoid the ureters, No. 0 polydioxanone suture is passed through both uterosacral ligaments and the posterior vaginal fornix.

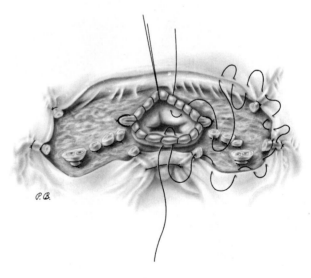

Figure 27–25. Total abdominal hysterectomy. Further suspension and reperitonization of the pelvis is accomplished by a continuous No. 0 delayed-absorbable suture that includes the anterior vagina, the cardinal ligament, the anterior edge of broad ligament peritoneum, the round ligament, the utero-ovarian or infundibulopelvic ligament, the posterior edge of broad ligament peritoneum, the uterosacral ligament, and the posterior vagina. A similar suture is placed on the opposite side. To avoid leaving the ovaries above the vaginal vault, the utero-ovarian ligaments should be extraperitonized as separate structures.

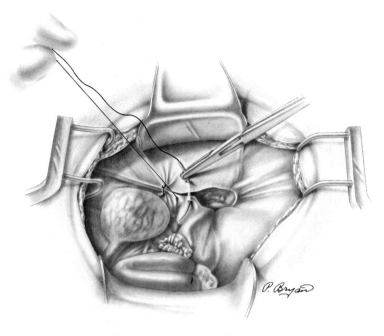

Figure 27–26. Total abdominal hysterectomy. Reperitonization is completed with a continuous No. 3-0 delayed-absorbable suture that approximates the edge of the bladder peritoneum to the edge of the cul-de-sac peritoneum. The ovaries should be left laterally.

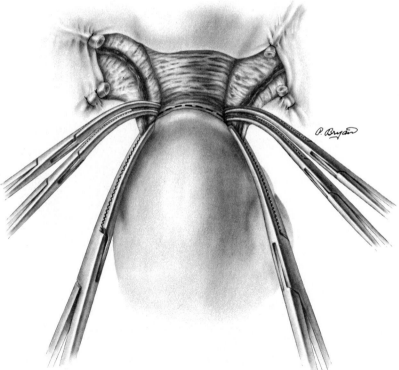

Figure 27–27. Subtotal abdominal hysterectomy. If a subtotal hysterectomy is to be done, the uterine corpus can be amputated by cutting across the cervix at the level of the internal os (*dotted line*).

close the cul-de-sac with a Moschcowitz procedure or to suspend the ovaries to the round ligament. All laparotomy pads are removed before closing the incision.

In our hands, this technique of total abdominal hysterectomy has proven to be superior to any thus far described. It is logically planned to ensure complete

hemostasis, to keep the pelvis free of interfering clamps at all times, and to use all ligamentous supports for the vagina. Basically, it is quite similar to the original Richardson procedure and has been modified only minimally from its original description.

Again, for the purpose of allowing a determination of

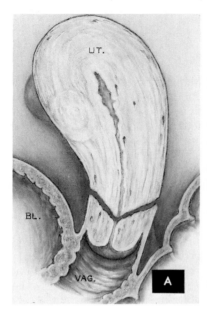

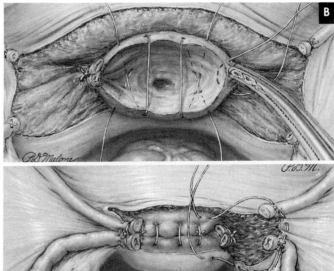

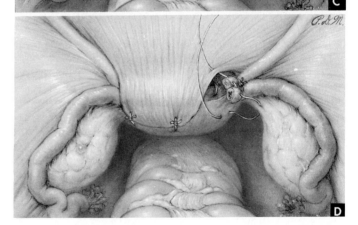

Figure 27–28. Subtotal abdominal hysterectomy. *A,* Method of coning out cervix to facilitate closing. *B,* Method of ligating the uterine vessels and suturing the cervix. *C,* Method of suspending the cervix and partial peritonization. *D,* Peritonization is completed by suturing the bladder peritoneum to the posterior surface of the cervix.

ureteral integrity before the incision is closed, 5 cc of indigo carmine is injected IV. Approximately 200 cc of clear sterile saline is instilled into the bladder through the Foley catheter, and the catheter is removed. A cystoscope is placed in the bladder. Within 3–5 minutes, the blue dye will be seen spurting from each ureteral orifice. The procedure is easy and takes little time, especially if the patient has been positioned in the Allen universal stirrups for operation. It provides reassurance that both ureters are functioning normally. The urethral catheter is replaced but is removed early in the morning of the first postoperative day.

THE TECHNIQUE OF SUBTOTAL ABDOMINAL HYSTERECTOMY

The technique of a subtotal abdominal hysterectomy is identical to that for a total abdominal hysterectomy until ligation of the uterine arteries has been performed. In the usual subtotal hysterectomy, the bladder need not be freed extensively from the cervix. Bleeding is prevented by avoiding unnecessary dissection of the bladder from the cervix; however, when a low amputation of the cervix is desired, freeing of the bladder must be carried out as low as necessary to perform the amputation. Following ligation of the uterine arteries, the corpus is amputated as indicated by the dotted line in Figure 27-27. The level of this amputation should always be below the internal cervical os to avoid bothersome cyclic menstrual bleeding from remnants of endometrium. It is well to make a V-shaped cut in the cervical stroma and endocervix (Fig. 27-28A) to facilitate the closure of the stump and ensure that the endometrium has been removed as well as much of the endocervical canal. The part of the lower endocervical canal left remaining should be cauterized with the electrosurgical (Bovie) unit. The cervical stump is then closed, using figure-of-eight sutures of No. 0 or No. 2-0 delayed-absorbable suture, as illustrated in Figure 27-28B. A cutting needle may facilitate placement of this suture, although it is usually unnecessary.

The cervical stump is suspended by suturing the various ligaments to it as described for a total hysterectomy. Figure 27-28C shows this step when the adnexa on both sides have been saved. The suture is first placed through the anterior surface of the cervix. It then picks up the anterior peritoneum and the round ligament. A bite or two is taken in the peritoneum between the round ligament and the tube. The tube to which the ovarian ligament has been tied is included next. One or two bites are taken in the posterior leaf of the broad ligament. In picking up the broad ligament, the surgeon should be careful to include only the peritoneal edge under vision because of the risk of kinking or ligating the ureter with the suture if wide bites are taken. Finally, a bite is taken in the posterior surface of the cervix. An assistant grasps the ends of the round ligament and the tube and the suspension suture is tied over them. This suture not only suspends the cervix, but also partially peritonizes the pelvis.

If the adnexa have been removed, the suspension and the peritonization are done somewhat differently. The infundibulopelvic ligament may be sufficiently mobile to be brought down to the cervix without tension, but often it is not. In such cases, the cut edges of the broad ligament may be closed separately with a continuous No. 2-0 delayed-absorbable suture as previously described and the stump of the infundibulopelvic ligament buried beneath the peritoneum by a purse-string suture.

The peritonization of the cervical stump is carried out by suturing the edge of the bladder peritoneum to the cul-de-sac peritoneum using either interrupted or continuous No. 3-0 delayed-absorbable sutures. To ensure that the cut ends of the ligaments and the tubes are covered, it is often desirable to pick up the structures at the angles of the vagina with the suture as indicated in Figure 27–28D, to cause them to invert beneath the peritoneum.

THE TECHNIQUE OF TOTAL VAGINAL HYSTERECTOMY FOR BENIGN DISEASE

Assuming there are proper indications for surgery and the patient has been properly prepared, from a purely technical standpoint, the objectives to be accomplished in performing vaginal hysterectomy are as follows:

To remove the uterus through the vagina
To avoid bacterial contamination of the operative site by maintaining strict aseptic technique
To avoid unnecessary injury to tissues and adjacent structures
To restore, conserve, or improve useful function and avoid postoperative dysfunction
To restore normal anatomy to the degree possible
To detect and possibly correct other diseases and abnormalities

As with abdominal hysterectomy, a variety of carefully considered techniques of vaginal hysterectomy allow accomplishment of these objectives. In the United States, Price, Mayo, Heaney, Falk, Gray, Pratt, Te Linde, and many others have published techniques of vaginal hysterectomy, all of which have variations. The technique described by Nichols and Randall is a another notable example, although there are important differences when compared with the technique described in this chapter. The technique in this chapter, described previously by Smith and Thompson, has evolved as a result of experience of the author for > 30 years and has been taught to many others in training. It is based on careful anatomic dissection, meticulous attention to detail, steps done in logical sequence, and concern for prevention of immediate and late complications. It is a standard plan that can be modified as long as essential steps and principles are not omitted or compromised. After the uterus is removed, restoration of normal anatomy and support must be a major concern. Support for the vaginal vault and upper posterior vaginal wall especially must be provided in such a way that the vagina will remain in its normal position for the remainder of the patient's life.

After satisfactory anesthesia is obtained, the patient is placed in the dorsal lithotomy position in stirrups with her hips at the edge of the operating table and her thighs well flexed on the abdomen. The knee and hip joints should be well flexed, but the hip joints must be in only minimal external rotation. Placing a patient improperly in the dorsal lithotomy position in stirrups has been implicated in injury to the sciatic, peroneal, and femoral nerves. It is essential to use a position in stirrups that does not stretch the sciatic nerves. Assistants should be warned not to lean on the patient's inner thighs or press the legs against the stirrups. Sciatic, peroneal, and femoral nerves injury as a complication of vaginal surgery has been reviewed by Burkhart and Daly, by McQuarrie and associates, and by Batres and Barclay. Fortunately, prognosis for recovery is favorable.

The external urethral meatus is prepared with povidone-iodine (Betadine) and the bladder is emptied with a straight catheter. A careful and complete pelvic examination, including a rectovaginal abdominal examination, is always performed next. This step should not be omitted because it may give valuable information about previously unrecognized pelvic pathology, about the best operative approach, and about the degree of difficulty to be expected. The lower abdomen, mons, vulva, vagina, cervix, upper medial thighs, perineum, and perianal skin are thoroughly scrubbed and prepared with povidone-iodine, and the operative field is covered with sterile drapes except for the vaginal introitus. A silk suture on a cutting needle is used to anchor the drape to the perineal skin just above the anus to help protect the operative field from contamination by discharge from the anus.

A narrow subpubic arch or a tight vaginal introitus occasionally may limit exposure sufficient to require a median episiotomy or Schuchardt's incision (see Ch. 11). Although not often needed, either incision should be made without hesitation if, by so doing, the technical performance of the operation will be facilitated. After hemostasis is satisfactory, the incision is simply left open until it is closed at the end of the operation.

A weighted speculum of proper size is placed in the vagina. It may be connected to suction or attached to a glove. Its bill should not be so long that it prevents the cervix from being pulled toward the introitus. Lateral vaginal retractors will facilitate exposure of the operative field. The cervix is grasped with a Jacob's tenaculum and pulled strongly into view. These retractors and the cervical tenaculum may be moved around during the operation to provide optimum exposure. The proper use of these instruments for traction and countertraction is essential for the correct performance of the operation. A variety of retractors are available, but Breisky-Navratil retractors of different sizes are preferred. The instruments should preferably have curved shanks and should be long enough to keep the handles away from the vaginal introitus. Exposure of the operative field in the top of the vagina thus will be enhanced.

Approximately 100–200 mm of sterile saline is injected beneath the vaginal mucosa around the cervix (Fig. 27-29). This facilitates dissection in the proper

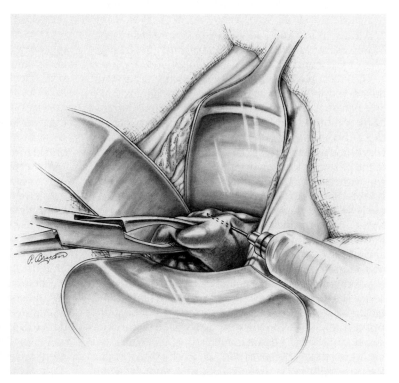

Figure 27–29. The anterior cervix is grasped with a tenaculum and sterile saline is injected beneath the vaginal mucosa around the cervix.

plane and also acts as an internal tourniquet, decreasing blood loss. Several investigators have reported decreased blood loss if the saline solution also includes vasoconstrictors. However, in a randomized well-controlled study, England, Randall, and Graves of the Department of Gynecology and Obstetrics, Emory University School of Medicine, found that injecting saline with vasoconstrictors did not decrease blood loss more than injecting saline without vasoconstrictors. They did find an important and significant increase in the incidence of postoperative infectious morbidity and vaginal cuff cellulitis among patients who were injected with a sterile saline solution containing vasoconstrictors. It has been clearly shown that host tissue defense mechanisms against infection are inhibited by injecting vasoconstricting agents. Host tissue defense mechanisms affected by vasoconstrictors include

Induction of tissue hypoxia
Decreased tissue opsonization potential
Decreased leucocytic chemotaxis
Inhibition of intracellular peroxidide production in the leucocyte, thereby reducing its intracellular killing potential
Inhibition of distribution of antibiotic into ischemic area
Inhibition of antibiotic effectiveness and increased antibiotic degradation as a result of acidosis, which is produced by vasoconstrictor-induced ischemia

Because there is no additional benefit of decreased blood loss and there is a definite harmful effect, injection of vasoconstricting agents is unjustified.

The incision is first made posterior to the cervix. With the cervix pulled forward, the posterior vaginal fornix is exposed. A semilunar incision in the vaginal mucosa of the posterior fornix is made at the point of attachment to the cervix. Making the incision behind the cervix first assures better visibility because blood pools in the posterior fornix when the dissection begins anterior to the cervix. Because the posterior fornix is usually relaxed in multiparous patients, sometimes conspicuously so, the excess vaginal mucosa may be excised by making a U-shaped incision, the apex of which extends into the posterior vaginal fornix (Fig. 27-30). This was also advised by Torpin as a part of his technique of providing better support to the posterior vaginal fornix.

Although this dissection may be done with scissors or scalpel, we prefer to use the cutting current of the electrocautery (Bovie) unit. The blade tip is bent approximately 45°. The dissection is made with brief strokes through the tissue in much the same manner as an artist strokes a canvas with a brush. With proper traction on the cervical tenaculum and countertraction with a retractor, the tissue will fall away when only

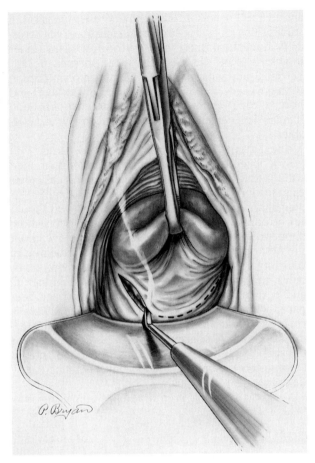

Figure 27–30. With the blade tip on the electrocautery Bovie unit, a *U*-shaped incision is made in the posterior vaginal fornix.

lightly touched with the Bovie blade. This technique of dissection minimizes bleeding. Small bleeders may be quickly cauterized as they are encountered.

Dissection in the proper plane will lead directly to the cul-de-sac peritoneum, which should be incised with scissors (Fig. 27-31). The dissection must be done carefully to avoid injury to the rectum. If the rectum is injured, it should be repaired as suggested in Chapter 34. The cul-de-sac peritoneum is grasped with forceps and incised with scissors rather than the Bovie blade. Once the cul-de-sac is identified, the peritoneal incision is extended laterally up to the attachment of the uterosacral ligaments on each side. The posterior cul-de-sac is explored with the operator's index finger for evidence of adhesions or other pathology. The information gained will allow the operator to make another judgment regarding the feasibility of continuing the vaginal approach. Not every hysterectomy begun vaginally must be completed vaginally. On rare occasions, the

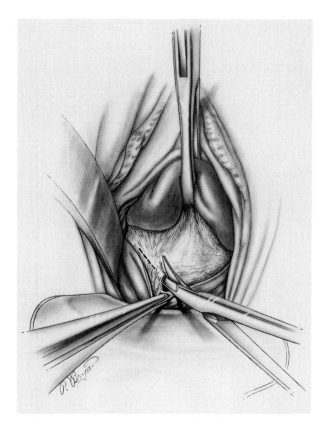

Figure 27–31. Dissection in the proper plane will lead to the peritoneum, which should be incised with scissors. The peritoneal incision is extended laterally as far as the attachments of the uterosacral ligaments. Bleeding must be controlled.

surgeon may decide that it would be safer for the patient to complete the hysterectomy abdominally. Under these circumstances, the operating room team must have the capability to immediately convert from a vaginal to abdominal approach. In a lifetime of gynecologic surgery, even the most experienced gynecologic surgeons will do this, but only a few times.

The unexpected finding of obliteration of the cul-de-sac from endometriosis, pelvic inflammatory disease, or adhesions is not always necessarily an indication to abandon the vaginal approach. The hysterectomy can still be done vaginally using a mostly extraperitoneal approach beneath the posterior serosal surface of the uterus until free peritoneal space is encountered.

Bleeding from the posterior vaginal cuff must be controlled before proceeding anterior to the cervix. If the cuff is allowed to bleed throughout the remainder of the operation, considerable blood will be lost unnecessarily.

The incision in the vaginal mucosa is extended around anterior to the cervix. The level of the incision is

critical to finding the correct plane of dissection between the bladder and the lower uterine segment. The point of attachment of the vaginal mucosa to the cervix can be demonstrated by moving the cervix up and down several times. The incision should be made 2–3 mm above the border between the smooth cervical mucosa and the vaginal rugae. Then, with strong traction on the cervical tenaculum downward and counter traction with a retractor lifting up on the anterior vaginal wall, the proper plane of dissection between the bladder and cervix is found using the blade tip of the Bovie unit (Fig. 27-32). Scissors dissection also may be used if the handles are elevated and the points directed downward against the uterus (Figs. 27-33 and 27-34). Pushing upward with a gauze covered index finger may cause too much tissue trauma, but gentle finger dissection without gauze may be helpful (Fig. 27-35).

Dissection in the wrong plane will cause more than the usual amount of bleeding. If the incision in the vaginal mucosa is too high, the wall of the bladder might be injured. The dissection may be difficult if the patient has had previous lower uterine segment cesarean sections causing abnormal adherence between the bladder and uterus. In this circumstance, an instrument placed through the external urethral meatus will help locate the bladder in relation to the plane of dissection. Instilling a few milliliters of methylene blue in the bladder will stain the bladder mucosa. The blue color will assist in identifying a more correct plane of dissection and may prevent an entry into the bladder. An injury to the bladder wall or an entry into the bladder should be recognized and repaired (see Ch. 30). If the incision in the vaginal mucosa is too low, the plane of dissection may go too deep in the cervix causing unnecessary bleeding and difficulty finding the right plane between the bladder and cervix.

After the fascial attachment between the bladder and the cervix has been incised, the peritoneal reflection of the anterior cul-de-sac can be seen. The surgeon should avoid pushing the peritoneum away with the gloved finger. A small incision is made in the peritoneum (Fig. 27-36). The surgeon should identify loops of small intestine or omentum to confirm that the peritoneal cavity rather than the bladder has been entered. Then the incision in the peritoneum can be extended laterally on each side (Fig. 27-37). A retractor can then be placed into the anterior cul-de-sac to retract the bladder superiorly and place the lateral uterine attachment on tension. If entering the anterior cul-de-sac is difficult, it may be delayed until later, until just before the uterine vessels are clamped and ligated. After releasing the cardinal, uterosacral, and vesicouterine ligaments in sequence from the lower uterine segment bilaterally, the anterior peritoneal reflection will be easier to iden-

(*text continues on page 713*)

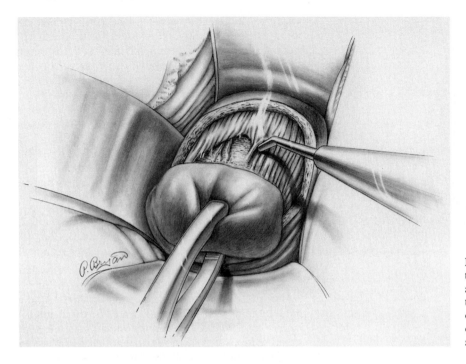

Figure 27–32. The incision in the vaginal mucosa is extended anterior to the cervix. The blade tip of the Bovie unit is used to dissect the bladder away from the cervix and lower anterior uterine segment.

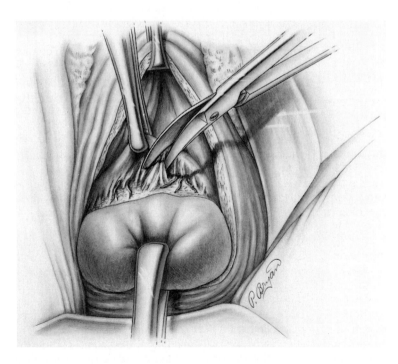

Figure 27–33. Scissors dissection also may be used to find the proper plane.

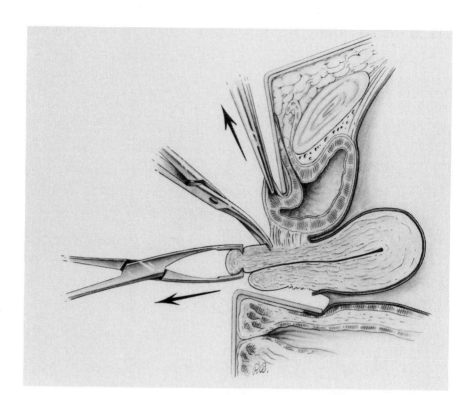

Figure 27–34. The handle of the scissors should be elevated and the points directed downward against the uterus. Strong traction and countertraction will facilitate the dissection.

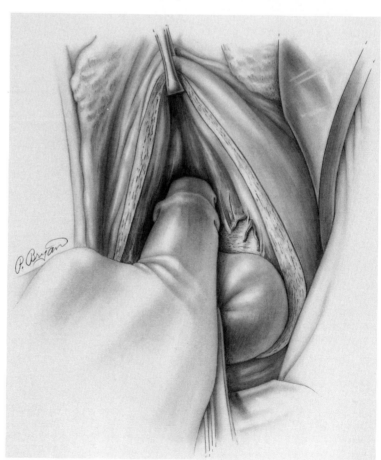

Figure 27–35. Gentle finger dissection can be helpful in identifying the proper plane.

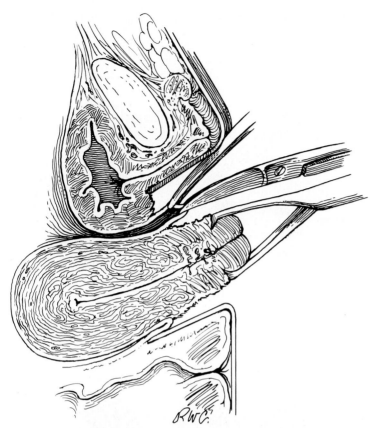

Figure 27–36. A small incision is made in the peritoneal reflection between the bladder and the uterus.

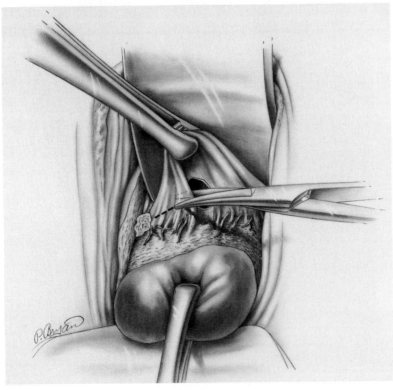

Figure 27–37. If the surgeon is certain that the peritoneal cavity has been entered, then the incision in the peritoneum can be extended laterally. If entering the peritoneal cavity anteriorly is difficult, then it can be delayed until later but should be done before the uterine vessels are clamped and ligated.

tify and incise. The index and middle fingers can sometimes be inserted through the posterior cul-de-sac and brought over the top of the broad ligament to push downward against the anterior peritoneal reflection, thus permitting an incision of the peritoneum under direct vision (Fig. 27-38).

The operation proceeds by successively clamping, cutting, and ligating the cardinal, uterosacral, and uterovesical ligaments. Each pedicle is clamped with a single Heaney clamp. Heaney clamps are heavier than most clamps and are designed to be used as single clamps on pedicles. If more than one clamp is to be used on a single pedicle, then one that is narrower than a Heaney clamp should be selected. Two Heaney clamps are too broad when placed side by side on a single pedicle. The most lateral clamp comes too close to the ureter. The bottom jaw of the clamp is placed behind the cervix into the posterior cul-de-sac first. The tip of the anterior jaw slides off the anterior lower uterine

segment as the clamp is closed. Only small bites of tissue should be taken. The tissue is cut to the point of the clamp and close to the uterus so that a fringe is left for more secure ligation. No. 0 or No. 2-0 delayed-absorbable suture attached to a control release needle is used to ligate each pedicle. The Heaney transfixion stitch is used. The knots are tied tight as the tissue is released from the clamp (Fig. 27-39). At least two ligatures on each side are held long for use later in suspending the vaginal vault: one is from the uterosacral ligament pedicle and one is from the cardinal ligament pedicle. Later, the utero-ovarian ligament pedicle ligatures also will be held for use in suspending the vault.

Firm downward traction on the cervix exaggerates the curvature (the so-called "knee") of the ureters as they course beneath the uterine vessels and through the cardinal ligaments. The ureters lie close to the lower uterine isthmus. For this reason, the clamps must be placed as close to the uterus as possible. For greater

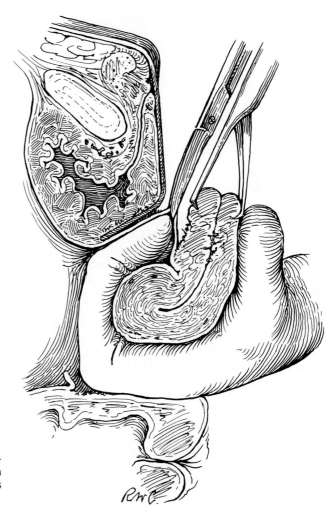

Figure 27–38. Lateral view of posterior cul-de-sac approach for identification and incision of bladder peritoneum between index and middle fingers. In difficult cases, this approach is sometimes helpful.

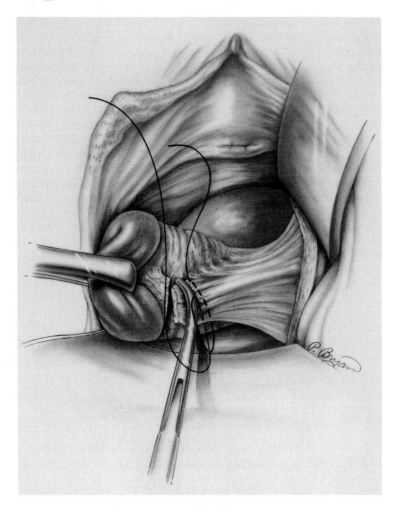

Figure 27–39. Staying as close to the uterus as possible, the paracervical uterosacral and cardinal ligament tissue is successively clamped, cut, and ligated with a Heaney clamp and a Heaney transfixion stitch. This ligature is held long for later use in suspending the vaginal vault.

exposure, the Jacob's tenaculum on the cervix should be moved to the side where the tissue is being clamped. Also, the vesicouterine ligaments should be clamped as separate structures after palpating the ureters (Figs. 27-40 and 27-41). after the vesicouterine ligaments are divided, the ureters can be retracted further laterally from the uterus. Routine dissection of the ureters with vaginal hysterectomy has been recommended by Cruikshank, but not by us. An intrafascial technique of removing the cervix with vaginal hysterectomy has been described by Jaszczak and Evans, but has not found practical application.

After ligating the cardinal, uterosacral, and vesicouterine ligaments, the uterine vessels are ligated. If the anterior peritoneum has not been opened, it must be before the uterine vessels are ligated (Fig. 27-42). The uterine vessel pedicle, which contains the uterine artery and vein and the broad ligament peritoneum anterior and posterior to these vessels, is clamped with a single Heaney clamp and ligated with a single liga-

ture. A transfixion suture ("Heaney stitch") should not be used on this vascular pedicle because of the possibility of injuring a vessel and causing a broad ligament hematoma.

After ligating the uterine vessels bilaterally, the operator may again consider if the operation can be completed vaginally. If the cervix is large and interferes with exposure, it may simply be removed by cutting across the lower uterine isthmus below the point of uterine vessel ligation. This is done with reluctance when, on rare occasions, the vaginal hysterectomy is done for malignant disease of the cervix or corpus. Alternatively, the cervical tenaculum on the cervix may be used for traction while the volume of a large uterine corpus is reduced by intramyometrial coring (Fig. 27-43). This technique was introduced by Lash and subsequently described by Nichols and Randall and by Kovac. A uterine sound is used to find the direction and depth of the uterine cavity. Using a scalpel, a cylindrical core of the uterus is progressively removed as firm traction is

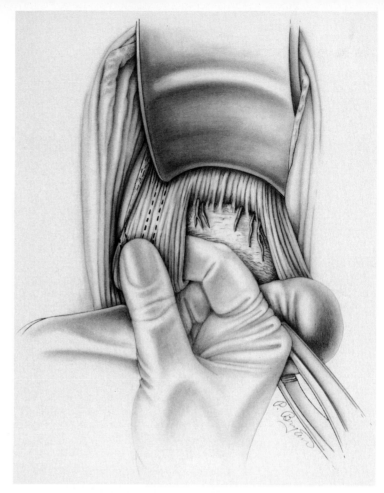

Figure 27–40. The ureters (*dotted lines*) may be palpated in the vesicouterine ligament.

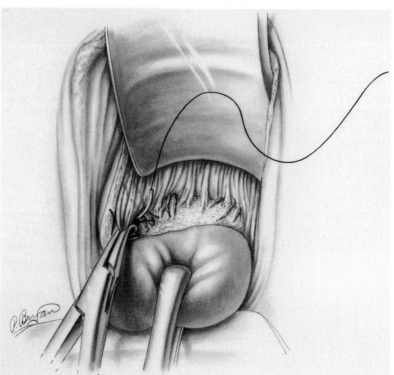

Figure 27–41. To allow retraction of the ureters away from the operative field, the vesicouterine ligaments may be clamped, cut, and ligated as close to the uterus as possible.

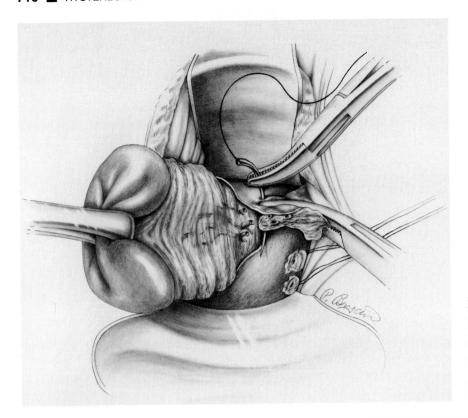

Figure 27–42. The uterine vessels are clamped with a single Heaney clamp, which also includes the anterior and posterior peritoneum. A transfixion "Heaney stitch" should not be used to ligate this vascular pedicle.

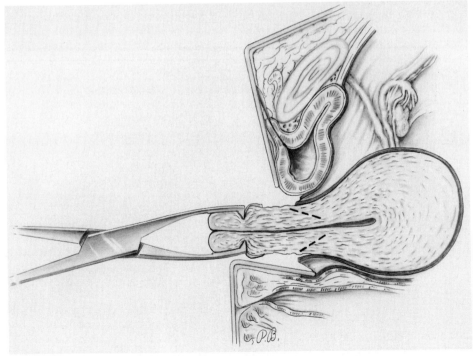

Figure 27–43. Intramyometrial coring is a suitable technique to reduce the size of a large volume uterus. The incision is made initially below the level of the ligated uterine vessels.

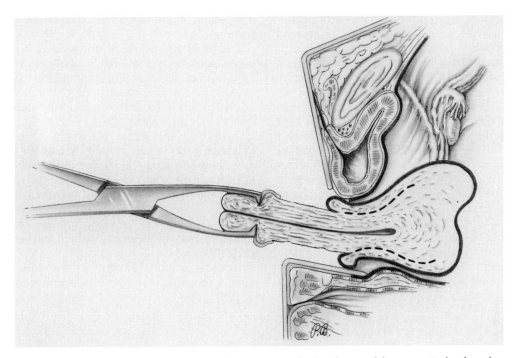

Figure 27–44. With strong traction on the cervix, a cylindrical core of the uterus is developed within the serosal surface of the uterus.

made on the cervix. With experience, this core can be removed without entering the endometrial cavity, staying safely within the serosal surface of the uterus (Fig. 27-44). Always, the dissection must be done with adequate visualization. Because the uterine vessels have been previously ligated, the amount of bleeding is minimal and limited only to the blood supply to the uterine corpus through the ovarian arteries.

If the uterus is larger than expected, removing small pieces by morcellation also may be appropriate. A simple method is to amputate the cervix with a wedged-shaped incision into the uterine corpus and then to bisect the remaining corpus if necessary. This allows better access to the upper broad ligament attachments for secure ligation. A major danger in reducing the size of the uterine corpus by morcellation, wedging, intra-myometrial coring, or bisection is an accidental injury to a loop of intestine that may be near or adherent to the serosal surface of the uterus. A careful watch for adherent intestine is mandatory. If injury does occur, hopefully it will be recognized and repaired properly through the vagina. Otherwise, immediate laparotomy will be required.

Another danger of removing the uterus in pieces involves the patient who has an undiagnosed and unexpected malignancy of the uterine cervix or corpus.

Preoperative diagnosis is unfortunately not possible in every case. We have recently seen a patient with a massive and widespread intra-abdominal sarcoma recurrent following vaginal hysterectomy with morcellation. Leiomyosarcoma arising in the myometrium was found on routine section of several morsels. Leibsohn and associates studied 1429 women who had hysterectomies for presumed uterine leiomyomata. Histologic diagnosis of leiomyosarcoma was made in 7 patients (0.49%).

After the uterine vessels are ligated on each side, the remaining portions of the broad ligament attachments are clamped, cut, and ligated, including the anterior and posterior peritoneum of the broad ligaments and the round ligaments on each side. Again, the clamps should be placed close to the side of the uterus. Usually, several bites are required before the top of the broad ligament is reached. As much as possible should be done from below before attempting to turn the uterus for delivery anteriorly or posteriorly, whichever seems easiest. Leahey thyroid clamps may be used for this purpose. Any adherence of intestine or omentum to the uterine fundus should be released carefully.

The remaining portion of the broad ligament attachment to the uterus contains the fallopian tubes and utero-ovarian ligaments. Because this pedicle contains large vessels, it should be doubly clamped with Heaney clamps. This can be done without danger of ureteral injury, but the surgeon must be certain that omentum or intestine has not been included in the clamp. This is the only time during the technique of vaginal hysterectomy that the surgeon secures pedicles—vascular or otherwise—with two clamps rather than one. To avoid interfering with ovarian blood supply, the Heaney clamps should be placed as close to the uterine fundus as possible. This pedicle is doubly ligated by replacing the lateral clamp (the one closest to the ovary) with a free ligature (Fig. 27-45). This tie occludes all vessels in the pedicle. The remaining clamp (the one closest to the uterus) is replaced with a transfixion suture ligature placed on the uterine side of the previously placed free tie. The transfixion suture ligature is held long for later use in vaginal vault suspension.

After removal, the uterus is opened and carefully examined in the operating room. Suspicious findings may require consultation with a pathologist and frozen section.

The tubes and ovaries are inspected. This may require adjustment of the lights, gentle traction on the tubo-ovarian pedicles, and some packing away of the intestine for adequate visualization. Our policy is to leave normal ovaries in place in premenopausal patients and to remove them in postmenopausal patients if it can be done safely through the vagina. If removal of the adnexa is indicated, it can usually be done with gentle traction on the tubo-ovarian pedicle so that the infundibulopelvic ligament can be doubly clamped and doubly ligated (Fig. 27-46A and B). When the ovaries are removed vaginally, it is difficult to extraperitonize the infundibulopelvic ligament—this is a distinct disadvantage. The surgeon, therefore, must be absolutely certain that hemostasis is perfect before the last tie is cut.

By using careful technique and two experienced vaginal surgeons as assistants, Smale and associates were

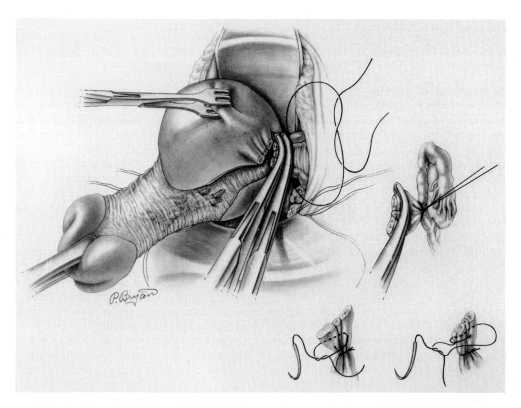

Figure 27–45. Two Heaney clamps may be used on the upper broad ligament pedicle that includes the fallopian tube and utero-ovarian ligament. The pedicle is doubly ligated by replacing the lateral clamp with a free-tie ligature and the medial clamp with a transfixion suture. This tie is held long for later use in suspending the vaginal vault.

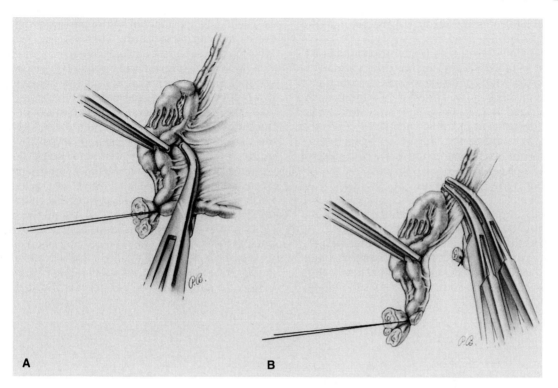

A   **B**

Figure 27–46. *A,* If the ovaries are to be removed, then clamps are placed across the meso-salpinx and then across the infundibulopelvic ligament, *B*. These pedicles must be securely ligated.

able to report 355 vaginal hysterectomies with adnexal removal with only a single instance of hemorrhage from ovarian vessels requiring laparotomy. Obviously, the surgeon must use judgment in deciding whether the ovaries can and should be removed vaginally. In a patient of high parity, several previous vaginal deliveries, and uterine descensus, removal of both tubes and ovaries with vaginal hysterectomy may be accomplished easily. In a nulliparous obese patient with no uterine descensus and extensive adnexal adhesions, it may be impossible to remove adnexa safely through the vagina. Releasing adnexal adhesions vaginally must be done cautiously and gently to avoid injury to surrounding structures and bleeding.

In reconstructing and supporting the vaginal vault, it is important to consider the following six points:

1. The surgeon must attempt insofar as possible to restore vaginal anatomy to normal.
2. The upper vagina is the roomiest part of the vagina. It should not be unnecessarily constricted.

3. When considering the roominess of the upper vagina, the surgeon must consider the adequacy of the vaginal fornices and the vaginal depth.
4. The cervix actually comes through the anterior vaginal wall. The highest and deepest point of the vagina is the posterior vaginal fornix and this is the point where the vagina should be suspended to achieve the greatest depth.
5. The upper vagina points mostly posteriorly in the direction of the sacrum at about S-3 or S-4.
6. The most frequent reason for unsatisfactory support following vaginal hysterectomy is the failure to detect and to correct a beginning enterocele in the cul-del-sac.

The following technique described is based on these important principles. The patient is placed in a slight Trendelenburg position. A pack is placed deep in the pelvis and elevated away from the cul-de-sac by a large broad right angle retractor. On each side, three ligatures have been held long for use later to support the vaginal vault (Fig. 27-47). These ligatures contain the uterosacral ligaments, the cardinal ligaments, and the top of the broad ligaments.

The next step is to reconstruct and suspend the vaginal vault at its highest point (the posterior vaginal fornix) and to close the cul-de-sac to prevent subsequent enterocele formation. The posterior culdoplasty technique described by McCall suspends the posterior vaginal fornix to the uterosacral ligaments and closes the cul-de-sac by bringing the uterosacral ligaments together in the midline. In our modification of the McCall culdoplasty, one to three No. 2-0 polydiaxinone sutures are used depending on the degree of relaxation of the posterior fornix.

The first suture is placed through the apex of the posterior vaginal fornix at a point that will become the deepest point of the vagina. The suture goes into the cul-de-sac through the peritoneum, avoiding the anterior rectal wall. The same suture then passes through one uterosacral ligament, continues across the cul-de-sac reefing the peritoneum before passing through the uterosacral ligaments on the opposite side. Carefully avoid placing sutures too deeply into the anterior rectal wall when crossing the cul-de-sac. The suture then continues back through and out the posterior vaginal fornix approximately 1 cm from its point of entry (Fig. 27-47). This suture is held long to be tied later. When the suture is passed through the uterosacral ligament, the ureter is in danger of ligation or kinking if the suture passes too high on the lateral pelvic sidewall.

After placement of the culdoplasty sutures, the next step is to close the peritoneum. Many techniques advise peritoneal closure with a 360° purse-string suture. This tends to constrict the upper vagina, brings the ovaries closer to the midline, and should not be used. A 360° purse-string suture to close the peritoneum is also not used in the technique of total abdominal hysterectomy and for the same reasons. Our technique of peritoneal closure requires two No. 2-0 delayed-absorbable su-

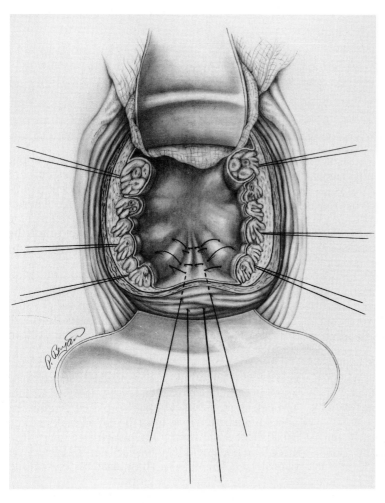

Figure 27–47. Support of the vaginal vault begins by placing posterior culdeplasty sutures to approximate the uterosacral ligaments, obliterate the cul-de-sac, and suspend the posterior vaginal fornix as high as possible. One, two, or three sutures may be used, and tied later.

tures to effect an *H*-shaped closure of the peritoneum (Fig. 27-48). The suture picks up the peritoneum over and between each pedicle on each side. After the pack is removed, each suture is tied. Closure is completed by a transverse suture approximating the edge of peritoneum behind the bladder to the peritoneum of the cul-de-sac (Fig. 27-49). Make certain that the fallopian tubes are left in an intraperitoneal location and not allowed to prolapse through the peritoneal closure.

It is extremely important to fix the pedicle stumps in an extraperitoneal position. This step avoids occult, insidious, and dangerous intraperitoneal bleeding in the immediate postoperative period. If there is postoperative bleeding from a pedicle, then it will be transvaginal and visible rather than intra-abdominal and hidden.

Although this method of peritoneal closure may require several more minutes to complete than a purse-string suture closure, it does have the distinct advantage of allowing the vaginal apex to retain its normal config-

uration. It also avoids bringing the ovaries toward the midline. A purse-string closure, which tends to constrict the vaginal apex and draw the ovaries toward the midline, may increase the possibility of postoperative dyspareunia.

To support the lateral vaginal fornices and to securely fix the pedicles laterally and extraperitoneally on each side, the ligatures that were held long on each side are threaded beneath the vaginal mucosa for several centimeters down the vagina. They are then tied. These suture ligatures are passed underneath the vaginal mucosa in a posterior direction below an imaginary line drawn horizontally across the open vaginal apex from the 3 o'clock to the 9 o'clock positions (see Fig. 27-49). Directing the sutures posteriorly will avoid the possibility of ureteral injury. This method of support also leaves the ovaries in the most lateral position possible in relation to the vaginal vault. It is preferred not to crisscross ligatures and pedicles from one side to the other. As described in other techniques, this tends to

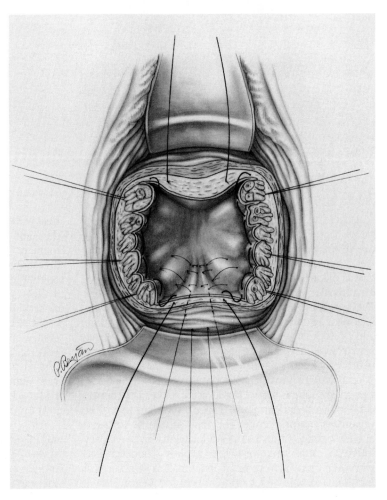

Figure 27–48. An *H*-shaped closure of the peritoneum is accomplished by suturing the peritoneum over and between each pedicle on each side.

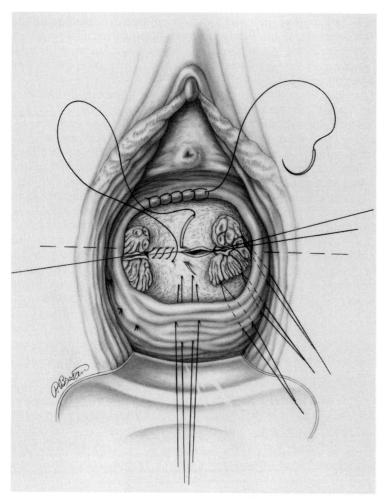

Figure 27–49. After each lateral peritoneal suture is tied, anterior and posterior peritoneal edges are sutured together. The ends of the pedicles are thereby extraperitoneal in location. The pedicle ligatures are threaded in a posterior direction beneath the vaginal mucosa.

constrict the upper vagina and also draws the ovaries closer to the midline, increasing the risk of postoperative dyspareunia.

A continuous locking No. 3-0 delayed-absorbable suture is placed in the edge of the vaginal mucosa around the vaginal apex to establish hemostasis (see Fig. 27–49). This leaves the apex open for drainage and reduces the incidence of cuff hematoma, cellulitis, abscess formation, and postoperative infectious morbidity. There is no reason to close the vaginal vault; there is an important reason to leave it open. Closure of the vaginal vault creates a potential space in which blood, necrotic tissue, and foreign body suture material will accumulate. It is always contaminated and an ideal space in which anaerobic organisms can proliferate. The vault should be irrigated and left open to drain and to gradually heal by secondary intention. This same principle applies whenever and wherever there is potential contamination of a surgical incision; it should be left open to heal secondarily. It will

heal with a strong transverse scar that may add support to the vault. According to a 1970 study by Kral in our department, postoperative infectious morbidity was 69.9% with the vaginal cuff closed and 44.1% with the vaginal cuff left open. Kuhn and deCrespigny reported febrile morbidity in 70% of patients undergoing vaginal hysterectomy with closed cuffs.

Finally, the posterior culdoplasty sutures are tied (Fig. 27-50). Tying these sutures approximates the uterosacral ligament in the midline, closes the cul-de-sac, and suspends the vagina at its highest point—the posterior vaginal fornix. In our experience, this has greatly reduced the risk of subsequent vaginal vault prolapse and enterocele formation.

This technique for supporting the vaginal vault is sufficient for most patients unless uterine descensus is severe. When there is significant descensus or complete uterine prolapse, additional support and suspension of the vaginal vault may be obtained by

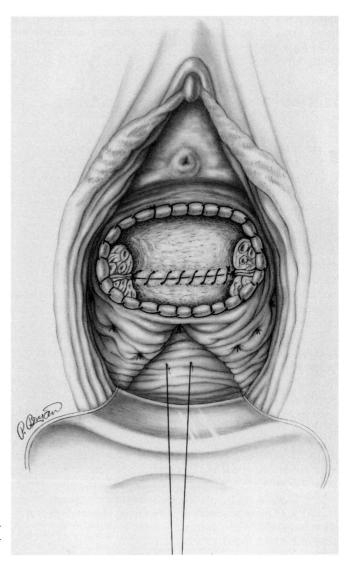

Figure 27–50. The vaginal vault is left open. A continuous lock stitch provides hemostasis. Finally, the posterior culdeplasty sutures are tied.

Excision of the cul-de-sac peritoneum with closure as high as possible

Reduction in the caliber of the upper vagina by excision of excess vaginal mucosa

Use of perirectal fascia for support of the vaginal vault

Sacrospinous ligament fixation of the upper vagina (see Ch. 32)

Before the operation is completed, ureteral integrity should be proved. This can be done quickly and satisfactorily by injecting IV 5 ml of indigo carmine dye and 200 cc of sterile saline in the bladder. With a cystoscope, blue dye can be observed to efflux from each ureteral orifice in 3–5 minutes. This should be done routinely in each case. A transurethral Foley catheter is inserted and removed when the patient is alert and awake.

Although not described here, an anterior and posterior colporrhaphy may be indicated in some patients, depending on the coincidental presence of a symptomatic or anatomically significant cystocele, rectocele, or relaxed vaginal introitus. Our philosophy is to regard each as a separate operation requiring separate justification.

The details of the operative procedure described here are all important in its correct performance and in consistently achieving good results in maintaining normal anatomy. The technique will prevent subsequent enterocele and vault prolapse if essential steps are not omitted or oversimplified. Careful attention to details and correct technical performance are essential to achieving a low rate of postoperative complications and good long-term support.

MANAGEMENT OF NORMAL OVARIES AT HYSTERECTOMY

The history of oophorectomy has been reviewed by Longo. The first successful procedure for oophorectomy was performed by Ephraim MacDowell in 1809. The operation was done for an enormous ovarian cystoma and was definitely indicated. In the 19th century, the removal of normal ovaries was practiced widely for various inappropriate indications, including insanity and convulsive disorders. Although the original procedure was known as the Battey operation, Battey himself performed fewer oophorectomies than others and cautioned that the operation was being performed too frequently and for indications that were too general. Tait frequently performed the operation in England. Enthusiasm for the operation waned as reports of a 25% mortality rate and only 25% success rate in relieving symptoms began to appear in the medical literature. By the turn of the century, many textbooks of gynecology did not mention Battey's operation.

In the early 20th century, as ovarian physiology began to be understood, an era of ovarian conservation began. At the same time, however, the concept of prophylactic surgery (ie, prophylactic removal of the appendix, uterus, and cervix) was gaining acceptance. Gynecologic surgeons, frustrated mostly by the difficulty of diagnosing and curing ovarian cancer, debated the merits of prophylactic removal of normal ovaries in premenopausal and postmenopausal women at the time of hysterectomy.

There are still no uniformly acceptable and established criteria for removal or retention of normal ovaries at the time of abdominal hysterectomy. Although a surprisingly large number of gynecologists leave in normal ovaries in postmenopausal women according to Randall, most advocate routine prophylactic oophorectomy at the time of abdominal hysterectomy in the menopausal or postmenopausal patient. Most gynecologists also advocate ovarian conservation in premenopausal women younger than age 40 years at the time of abdominal hysterectomy. However, according to the study by Dicker and associates of the National Center for Health Statistics Data for 1970 through 1978, nearly 50% of women aged 40–44 years undergoing abdominal hysterectomy had a concurrent bilateral oophorectomy. According to Pokras and Hufnagel, in 1965, 25% of women with a hysterectomy also had both ovaries removed; this increased to 41% in 1984. Performing this combined procedure for women aged 45–64 years increased from 35% in 1965 to 66% in 1984. It is unknown how many of these oophorectomies were done for primary or associated ovarian pathology and how many were prophylactic to prevent ovarian cancer. In 1952, Doyle reported that 704 normal ovaries were removed from 546 patients at the time of hysterectomy. In none of the patients were there associated lesions to justify oophorectomy.

In consideration of the age at which oophorectomy should be recommended at the time of hysterectomy, there are several questions that must be asked and answered.

Do Ovaries Continue to Function Normally After Hysterectomy?

When normal ovaries are conserved at the time of abdominal hysterectomy in premenopausal women, normal hormonal function will continue unaltered in a cyclic fashion in almost all until the natural age of menopause, at which time they will cease to produce 17-β estradiol and progesterone. Burford and Diddle and Te Linde and Wharton showed that in the *Mecaca* rhesus and irus monkeys, normal ovarian function continues after hysterectomy with no evidence of altered arrangement of the follicular or corpus luteum development, maturation, or regression and no evidence of detectable changes in the ovarian stroma. Bancroft-Livingston, in 1954, and Randall and associates, in 1977, using vaginal cytology, concluded that normal ovaries, if conserved at hysterectomy, may continue to function for > 15 years. Because the ovary may not be the only source of estrogen affecting vaginal cytology, it has been necessary to confirm these findings with endocrine assays. Beavis, Brown, and Smith studied 69 patients who had partial or total ovarian conservation at the time of hysterectomy at age 25–48 years. Ovarian function was monitored by weekly urinary estrogen and pregnanediol determinations for periods of 4–6 weeks at intervals for up to 2.5 years. In the group with total conservation of the ovaries, ovarian function continued normally until the expected time of menopause. In a study of premenopausal patients who had had extensive surgery for invasive cervical carcinoma, in whom the normal ovaries were conserved, Thompson and coworkers found normal estrogen values in all patients and also evidence of continued ovulation in these young women. Cyclic ovarian function continued until the expected menopausal age, and patients were spared the physical and psychologic discomfort of a premature and acute surgical menopause.

Souza and associates studied ovarian biopsies before and 12 months after total abdominal hysterectomy in 25 patients with symptomatic uterine myomas. After hysterectomy, the ovarian biopsies showed stromal cell hyperplasia, thickening of the tunica albuginea, and a significant decrease in follicular reserve, follicular cysts, and corpora albicantia. There was no significant difference in the number of atretic follicles and corpora lutea. The serum levels of all hormones studied were unchanged. According to Riedel, Leihmann-Willenbrock, and Semm, levels of progesterone and estrogen concentrations were lower in women who had had hysterectomy with ovarian conservation compared with controls, even though biphasic cycles were present in most patients.

Siddle, Sarrel, and Whithead found that the mean age of the natural menopause in 226 women was 49.5 ± 4.04 years, compared with 45.4 ± 4.0 years among 90 women who had had a hysterectomy. Although their statistical methods were questioned by Machin and Williams, they suggest that hysterectomy may advance the time of ovarian failure in some women, usually a minority.

Some have suggested that one normal ovary should be removed and one preserved. Beavis and associates demonstrated that the frequency of anovulatory cycles is increased significantly when only one ovary is preserved. Also, one residual normal ovary assumes sole function less effectively in older than in younger women. Contrary to popular belief, a gynecologic surgeon cannot reduce the potential for subsequent development of ovarian cancer by 50% by removing one ovary. The remaining ovary will still have the same potential as both ovaries had.

Stone, Dickey, and Mickal and Janson and Jansson have studied the acute effect of hysterectomy on ovarian blood flow and ovarian function. A transient reduction in ovarian blood flow and steroidogenesis was found and could possibly explain the transient appearance of vasomotor hot flushes in approximately 40% of women following hysterectomy with ovarian conservation. From their studies, Menon and associates believe that menopause does not increase in frequency following simple hysterectomy with ovarian conservation. However, they believe that a "subtle diminution in estrogenization" occurs frequently and may explain the hot flushes experienced by some patients after hysterectomy. These and other studies suggest that concentrations of estradiol and gonadotropins, and perhaps basal body temperature records, should be obtained in patients following hysterectomy with ovarian conservation. Any evidence of hypoestrogenicity might deserve supplemental estrogen therapy.

Obviously, if normal ovaries did not function normally following hysterectomy, then a recommendation for their removal would be appropriate. The weight of evidence suggests, however, that they usually do continue to function normally, or occasionally at a slightly reduced level.

At What Age Does the Human Ovary Cease to Function?

Most of the controversy involves the establishment of an arbitrary age during the fifth decade when prophylactic oophorectomy will be practiced. It is amazing how often women beyond age 40 years are considered by their gynecologist to be menopausal with only a few years of ovarian function left. Such a view is incorrect for a great majority of women. According to Coulam, Adamson, and Annegers, only 0.88% of women will go through a natural menopause between ages 40 and 44 years. Of 737 patients who were premenopausal at age 40, only 28 (3.8%) were postmenopausal by age 45; 711 (96.2%) were still premenopausal.

According to Willett and associates in 1983, the median age of menopause for registered nurses in the United States who never smoked was 52.4 years. The mean age of menopause in 6000 Dutch women with no known diseases was 51.4 years, according to a 1979 report by Bjoro. According to Novak, 23% of women show histologic evidence of ovulation after age 50 years. As the general health of American women has improved, apparently menopause has occurred at a later age. Women who have bilateral oophorectomy between ages 40 and 45 years may lose 10 or more years of normal ovarian function.

Are There Significant Health Hazards When Normal Ovaries Are Removed from Premenopausal Women?

After hysterectomy, of course, the role of the ovaries in the process of reproduction is irrelevant unless ova are to be harvested for donation. However, the ovaries of premenopausal women play an active role in many basic metabolic processes throughout the body through secretion of estrogen, progesterone, and androgens. Bilateral oophorectomy in premenopausal women causes a sudden decline of estrogen and progesterone levels. The biochemical, physiologic, and psychologic effects of this loss have been studied thoroughly. What has not been acknowledged and appreciated is the significant decrease in plasma testosterone that also occurs when both ovaries are removed. Although the role of androgen production in women is not as well understood, Sherwin and Gelfand presented data suggesting that reduced levels of circulating testosterone subsequent to bilateral oophorectomy may play an important role in the development of physical and psychologic symptoms that are frequent sequelae of this surgical procedure. Their findings suggest that premenopausal women who need to undergo bilateral salpingo-oophorectomy may be excellent candidates for a combined estrogen–testosterone hormone therapy regimen "in an attempt to mitigate symptoms that may be a consequence of their sudden and drastically altered endocrine status postoperatively." Currently, not many premenopausal women who have been castrated are receiving such combined therapy that includes androgens.

Ovarian hormones influence protein, calcium, bone, potassium, and carbohydrate metabolism, among others, and lipoproteins and triglycerides. Montgomery and associates reported that plasma triglycerides increased by 60% within 6 weeks of bilateral oophorectomy, but plasma total and lipoprotein cholesterol levels as well as apolipoprotein markers for low-density lipoprotein and high-density lipoprotein (HDL) were unaffected. The absence of ovarian function over a period of years has been implicated in the pathogenesis of osteoporosis, coronary artery disease, and cerebrovascular accidents. Of course, there are many other interrelated factors that influence the development of these diseases. The extent to which long-term estrogen replacement therapy with or without progesterone and testosterone may avert these problems in the premenopausal woman who has had bilateral oophorectomy is not completely determined.

Can the General Metabolic Effects of Ovarian Function Be Replaced After Bilateral Oophorectomy?

To attempt replacement of normal ovarian steroidogenesis, exogenous hormone replacement therapy would have to be given for a long time. Several dozen naturally occurring estrogens, progesterone, and androgens in correct balance at normal levels would be needed on a daily basis. The usual conjugated estrogen treatment after surgical menopause in itself does not represent physiologic hormone replacement therapy, if defined as the dosage required to maintain premenopausal circulating concentrations of reproductive hormones, according to Utian and associates. Ovarian function plays a role in regulating nitrogen, phosphorus, calcium, cholesterol, lipid, triglyceride, and carbohydrate metabolism. Ovarian function plays a role in regulating function of other endocrine organs (eg, adrenal cortex, pituitary, thyroid, and pancreas). Ovarian function provides protection against diabetes, atherosclerosis, and osteoporosis. Belief that long-term exogenous estrogen replacement therapy (with or without progesterone and androgens) is a safe and effective way to completely replace normal ovarian

function in a woman who has had hysterectomy and bilateral oophorectomy would favor "prophylactic" removal of both normal ovaries. Otherwise, a recommendation for ovarian conservation would be more appropriate.

For patients who undergo bilateral oophorectomy, the role of compliance in taking estrogen postoperatively must be considered. According to Speroff and associates, such compliance is not perfect. From a review of 10 published studies, they report that for groups of women with bilateral oophorectomy, commencement of estrogen ranges from a low of 31% to a high of 89%, with 13% to 71% maintaining estrogen replacement for 5 years. This must be taken into account when deciding whether or not to remove normally functioning premenopausal ovaries.

Are There Significant Health Hazards Associated with Long-term Replacement Therapy with Estrogen with or without Progesterone or Androgens?

Even though it is considered desirable to give cyclic estrogen replacement therapy with or without progesterone to women who have been castrated, such therapy is not always well tolerated or without adverse side effects. Some premenopausal women tolerate an artificial menopause with few symptoms. Indeed, de-Neef and Hollenbeck reported that only 50% of premenopausal women subjected to bilateral oophorectomy experienced menopausal symptoms. However, in our experience many premenopausal women undergo great discomfort, both physical and emotional, as a result of acute surgical castration. Low-dose cyclic replacement therapy appears to be safe and well tolerated by most premenopausal castrated women and is indicated in most women to delay the appearance of osteoporosis and atrophy of the mucosa of the vagina and lower urinary tract regardless of the presence or absence of vasomotor symptoms.

However, there are definite risks involved. The risk for development of breast cancer is still controversial, but probably insignificant. Hypertension may develop in some patients, although the risk ratio is low and the hypertension should subside if estrogen treatment is discontinued. In the Boston Collaborative Drug Surveillance Program, a 2- to 3-fold increase in the risk of surgically confirmed gall bladder disease in women receiving post-menopausal estrogeus was reported. The annual incidence of gallbladder disease for estrogen users was 218 per 100,000. For nonusers it was 87 per 100,000. In the premenopausal woman who has had a hysterectomy and bilateral salpingo-oophorectomy, low-dose cyclic estrogen may be given so long as the patient understands and accepts her increased risk for gallbladder disease, the blood pressure is checked periodically, the breast examination is performed frequently, and estrogen treatment is discontinued if hypertension or breast tumors appear. The extent to which the adverse effect of long-term estrogen replacement treatment can be eliminated by the simultaneous use of progesterone has yet to be determined. Although some have objected to the validity of his data, Gambrell reports that the incidence of breast cancer is lower in estrogen-progestogen users (67.3 per 100,000) than in untreated women (342.3 per 100,000). The question of ovarian hormonal replacement for the surgically castrated premenopausal woman is a complicated one. When it is necessary to remove both ovaries, such replacement should be given, but is not always well tolerated and certainly cannot and should not be depended on to replace the useful function of normal ovaries to such an extent that premenopausal patients can be routinely castrated when abdominal hysterectomy is done.

In addition, Bush and associates in 1983 reported the results of a study of the association of exogenous estrogen use and hysterectomy status with all-cause mortality in 2269 white women aged 40–69 years. The relative risk of death in estrogen users compared with nonusers was 0.54 in gynecologically intact women, 0.34 in women with a history of previous hysterectomy, and 0.12 in women who had had both ovaries removed. Bush et al. believe some of the lower risk of mortality in estrogen users can be accounted for by increased levels of HDL cholesterol. For whatever reason, it is certainly important for women who have been castrated prematurely to be placed on long-term, estrogen replacement therapy unless there are contraindications.

How Much Can Routine Prophylactic Castration at the Time of Hysterectomy Reduce the Number of Deaths from Ovarian Cancer?

The major risk of ovarian conservation at the time of hysterectomy is the risk that ovarian cancer, an admittedly devastating disease, will develop subsequently. Ovarian cancer remains one of the most lethal tumors of the female reproductive tract. Currently in the United States, approximately 11,000 women die annually from this disease. The ovary is hidden in the pelvis and is difficult to assess critically on pelvic examination. Few early warning signals accompany ovarian cancer, and in > 60% of cases, the cancer has spread beyond the boundaries of the ovarian capsule and beyond a reasonably curable stage at the time of its detection. Although there is no evidence to suggest that retained ovaries have a greater risk of neoplasia than do ovaries attached to an intact uterus, the gynecologist may decide to accept the responsibility of assuring the patient that continued hormonal function of the ovary has greater importance to the patient than the small risk of subsequent ovarian neoplasm.

Counseller, Hunt, and Haigler at the Mayo Clinic studied 1500 patients with ovarian cancer and found that 4.5% had previously undergone hysterectomy for benign disease. Terz, Barber, and Brunschwig found an incidence of 5.1% and Fagan and coworkers reported an incidence of 7.5%. Among 200 patients with ovarian carcinoma in a study at The Johns Hopkins Hospital, 15 (nearly 8%) had previously experienced a pelvic laparotomy. None of these patients would have developed ovarian cancer had the ovaries been removed at laparotomy. However, it should be noted that in many of the patients studied, the hysterectomy was performed vaginally. For reasons of technical difficulty, the routine removal of normal ovaries is done less frequently with a vaginal than with an abdominal hysterectomy. In many cases, the hysterectomy was performed when the patient was younger than age 40 years, an age when gynecologists would agree that normal ovaries should be retained. As shown in Table 27-1, ovarian cancer among hysterectomy patients with retained ovaries is uncommon, occurring in approximately 0.1% of such cases.

McGowan studied 291 women with epithelial ovarian cancer. Forty-one (14%) had a prior hysterectomy. The interval between hysterectomy and discovery of ovarian cancer was 10 years in the vaginal hysterectomy group and 18 years in the abdominal hysterectomy group. Women who had their ovaries retained at hysterectomy and later developed invasive ovarian cancer had approximately an 80% mortality. Similar results were reported by Finazzo and associates. Fifteen percent of the patients in their study theoretically would not have had ovarian cancer if prophylactic oophorectomy had been carried out at the time of pelvic surgery at age 36 years or older.

Randall and Gerhardt, basing their assessment on the statistics of the health departments of the states of Connecticut and New York (excluding New York City), have calculated that the probability of a 40-year-old woman developing cancer of the ovary is 0.9%. That probability remains at 0.9% until the woman reaches her 45th year, after which it begins to decline (0.82% at age 50 years; 0.7% after age 60; and 0.3% after age 70). Data from Randall and Gerhardt's study would indicate that of the women over age 50 years, 15 out of 1000 (1.5%) will develop an ovarian neoplasm. Of these, nine (60%) will be malignant and six (40%) will be benign. Randall and Gerhardt have further stated that if, in the 15 per 1000 women who had a pelvic laparotomy, both normal ovaries were removed, the incidence of ovarian cancer might be reduced from nine cases to seven cases per 1000 women. Hollenbeck concluded that prophylactic

TABLE 27–1
Ovarian Cancer in Retained Ovaries

STUDY (YR)	NO. OF HYSTERECTOMIES	CANCER IN RETAINED OVARIES	%
Randall (1963)	915	2	0.2
Gevaerts (1962)	300	0	0.0
Reycraft (1955)	4500	9	0.2
Funck-Brentano (1958)	580	1	0.2
Whitelaw (1959)	1215	0	0.0
Ranney and Abu-Ghazaleh (1977)	2136	4	0.2
Funt (1977)	992	0	0.0
Total	10,638	16	0.1

oophorectomy might conceivably save three patients from ovarian cancer if it were done routinely in 10,000 women who have a hysterectomy, although this question may require a complex equation for statistical validity. The conclusion is that, because the incidence of ovarian cancer after hysterectomy is 0.1% of all females, even universally practiced prophylactic oophorectomy would not reduce the incidence significantly. Even Grogan and Duncan, who were early advocates of oophorectomy, expressed the belief that prophylactic oophorectomy cannot be justified on the basis of its effect in reducing the incidence of ovarian malignancy.

Some surgeons are of the opinion that the problem of ovarian conservation and ovarian cancer subsequent to hysterectomy can be solved by conservation of only one ovary instead of two, apparently feeling that the incidence of subsequent ovarian cancer will be reduced by 50% and that the function of one ovary is as good as two. There is no statistical data to support this view. Realistically, to retain one ovary is to retain 100% of the malignant potential of both ovaries. Also, it has been shown that the incidence of anovulatory cycles increases and that menopause occurs at an earlier age if only one ovary is conserved. When it comes to the question of conservation of normal ovarian function, two normal ovaries are better than one. By conserving two normal ovaries at the time of hysterectomy, the incidence of subsequent ovarian cancer is not known to be increased.

Four case-control studies that found a lower risk of ovarian cancer among women who had a history of previous hysterectomy have been analyzed by Weiss and Harlow. They believe the difference is explained by "screening" for visible ovarian malignancy, which generally occurs at the time of hysterectomy by those gynecologic surgeons who do not routinely remove both ovaries if they are normal. Those women whose ovaries have been examined and found not to contain malignancy will have a reduced risk of ovarian cancer subsequently when compared with women whose ovaries have not been subjected to the same screening procedure. This lower risk will only last a few years, however.

What is the Incidence of Nonneoplastic Problems in Preserved Ovaries?

Interest in the residual ovary (or more properly called residual adnexal syndrome) began in 1955 with a report by Grogan and Duncan that 19 (5.1%) of 391 patients who had abdominal hysterectomy with ovarian conservation subsequently required removal of the ovaries because of an adnexal mass, severe pain, dyspareunia, or generalized pelvic discomfort. Another 20 patients developed similar problems of a less severe degree that did not require surgery. Grogan and Duncan stated that the interest of the patient was best served by prophylactic castration, mostly because of the frequency with which such conserved ovaries would subsequently show problems. In 1975, Christ and Lotze reported 202 (3.3%) cases of the residual ovary syndrome among 6188 patients with hysterectomy and ovarian conservation.

Ranney and Abu-Ghazaleh conserved ovaries in 1557 (72%) of 2153 patients who had a hysterectomy. Only 14 (0.9%) patients required a second operation to remove the conserved ovaries. Bukovsky and associates reported six (1.8%) patients with the residual adnexal syndrome among 329 patients who underwent hysterectomy with preservation of one or both ovaries. Of 922 patients who had one or both ovaries conserved at the time of abdominal hysterectomy at Grady Memorial Hospital, Funt, Benigno, and Thompson reported that 13 (1.4%) patients required subsequent operation for pathology of the conserved adnexal tissue. These and other data suggest that 1%–2% of patients who have one or both ovaries conserved at the time of hysterectomy will subsequently require operation for a problem with an ovary or tube. The pathology in the few residual adnexa requiring removal will usually show nothing more than a physiologic cyst, a small hydrosalpinx, or adhesions. The management of patients with physiologic cysts of the ovary should remain the same whether the patient has had a previous hysterectomy or not. Unfortunately, it seems that a patient who develops a small functional cyst in an ovary retained after hysterectomy is operated on more often and sometimes unnecessarily. Few patients with the residual adnexal syndrome will be found to have a malignancy of the ovary.

The etiology of the residual adnexal syndrome is unknown. It seems to be more common following abdominal hysterectomy than vaginal hysterectomy. A permanent disturbance of blood flow to the ovary at the time of hysterectomy may explain its occurrence. Symptoms also may be related to an abnormal position of the ovary just above the vaginal vault. A dysfunctional cyst in a normally placed ovary may not be as symptomatic as a dysfunctional cyst in an ovary adherent to the apex of the vagina.

Can Improvements in the Operative Technique Reduce the Magnitude and Effect of Operative Trauma and Damage to the Ovary?

If the ovary is to be conserved when hysterectomy is done, every attempt should be made to preserve its blood supply. The infundibulopelvic ligament containing the ovarian vessels must not be twisted or stretched. Clamps that are used to separate the ovary from the uterus should be placed as close to the uterine corpus as possible so that the arcade of vessels in the meso-salpinx that supply the ovary will not be interfered with (Fig. 27–51). Normal tubes should be left with the ovary. Attempts to remove the tube could interfere with ovarian blood supply. The surgeon might even elect to leave in a small hydrosalpinx, because its removal might jeopardize the blood supply to its companion ovary.

The blood supply to the ovary has been the subject of too few investigations. The general opinion is that the uterine artery supplies the medial half of the ovary and the medial two thirds of the fallopian tube, the rest of the blood supply coming from the ovarian artery. The distribution of these arteries, however, shows great variation according to the studies of Borell and Fernstrom, ranging from cases in which the ovarian artery supplies the entire tube and ovary to cases in which the blood supply of these organs is solely derived from the uterine artery. If a significant portion of the blood supply to the ovary is derived from the uterine artery, continued normal ovarian function might be impossible after a hysterectomy because of ligation of both uterine arteries.

When plastic surgeons have concern about the adequacy of the blood supply to a myocutaneous flap, fluorescent dye is injected IV and its presence in the flap determined with a Wood's light. General surgeons also use the same method to determine the adequacy of blood supply to the intestine. We have used this fluorescene dye/Wood's light technique to access the adequacy of blood supply to ovaries conserved at the time of hysterectomy. The sterile Doptone can be used to find ovarian artery blood flow in the infundibulopelvic ligament. These measures may allow intraoperative

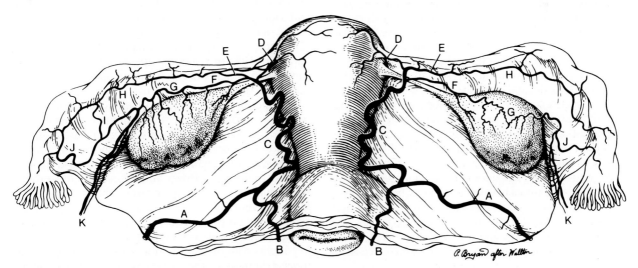

Figure 27–51. Normal uterus and adnexa with schematic representation of the usual ovarian and uterine artery branches. Many variations exist. *A,* uterine artery in parametrium. *B,* cervico-vaginal branch. *C,* uterine artery along lateral margin of the uterus. *D,* fundal branch. *E,* medial tubal branch. *F,* medial ovarian branch. *G,* ovarian arcade. *H,* tubal arcade. *I,* lateral tubal branch. *J,* infundibular branch. *K,* ovarian artery.

recognition and removal of ischemic ovaries, hopefully to prevent the subsequent development of the residual adnexal syndrome.

In addition to preservation of blood supply to the ovary, the residual adnexal syndrome may be prevented by suspending the ovaries away from the vaginal vault when hysterectomy is done. If the ovaries are allowed to become fixed over the vaginal vault, pain may be produced from penile thrusting during intercourse. The utero-ovarian ligaments should be extraperitonized separately.

Should Prophylactic Oophorectomy Be Practiced at Any Age?

Although we cannot subscribe to routine castration of premenopausal women undergoing abdominal hysterectomy, we cannot conceive of a good reason to conserve the ovaries of a woman who is menopausal or postmenopausal. A much lower level of estrogen production and the absence of ovulation after menopause does not justify preservation of the normal postmenopausal ovaries. Even though many menopausal and postmenopausal women have cytologic evidence of estrogen effect in the vaginal mucosa, it is clear that the ovary is not the source of the estrogen. Estradiol production rates are not significantly altered by removal of postmenopausal ovaries, according to Barlow, Emerson, and Saxena. Similarly, estrone production rates in postmenopausal women with intact ovaries and in those whose ovaries have been removed were found to be comparable by Siiteri and MacDonald. On the basis of differences in ovarian vein and peripheral vein concentrations, Judd and associates concluded that the postmenopausal ovary continues to secrete a large amount of testosterone and a moderate amount of androstenedione, but only minimal ovarian estrogen secretion was found. According to studies by Mikhail, by Greenblatt, Colle, and Mahesh, and by Vermeulen, the adrenal cortex is almost the exclusive source of plasma estradiol, estrone, and progesterone and is the most important source of plasma dehydroepiandrosterone in postmenopausal women. On the basis of these and other confirmatory investigations, it is concluded that there is no logical reason for conservation of ovaries at the time of abdominal hysterectomy in menopausal and postmenopausal women. Bilateral oophorectomy does eliminate the small chance of ovarian neoplasia developing subsequently, and it does not seem to cause the same psychologic and physiologic disturbance as in younger women.

Garcia and Cutler, on the other hand, pointed to the increased quantity of stroma of postmenopausal ovaries as steroidogenic with increased capacity to synthe-size androstenedione, the hormone that, in the menopausal woman, is converted to estrone in the fat depots of the body. He points out that this pathway can be significant in preventing osteoporosis and believes the practice of routine prophylactic oophorectomy at the time of hysterectomy in postmenopausal women be reexamined as the evidence for postmenopausal ovarian function accumulates.

The decision to recommend removal or conservation of normal ovaries of a premenopausal women who is undergoing hysterectomy in the fifth decade of her life presents a difficult choice for the thoughtful gynecologic surgeon. It is difficult to believe that gynecologic surgeons help a premenopausal woman in any way, either physically or psychologically, by removing her normal ovaries. *An evaluation of the available evidence suggests that the grossly normal ovaries of premenopausal women should be conserved when hysterectomy is done. The decision to remove them should not be based on some arbitrary age in the fifth decade. Rather, a decision to leave in or remove the ovaries should be based on an assessment of their functional status. Although the patient's wishes must always be considered, prophylactic oophorectomy is not advised at the time of abdominal hysterectomy in premenopausal women until they are within 1 or 2 years of the mean age of menopause (age 51 years). Normal ovaries usually should be removed when abdominal hysterectomy is done on the postmenopausal woman. The same recommendations are made for women undergoing vaginal hysterectomy provided the ovaries can be removed safely and without technical difficulty.*

In this matter of removing or retaining ovaries, there are exceptions to any general rules. For example, Allen and Hertig found a family history of malignancy in 12.5% of their patients with cancer of the ovary. Counseller and associates found a family history of malignancy in 19% of patients with cancer of the ovary. Families in which women have an especially high genetic risk of ovarian cancer have been described by Lynch and associates, Fraumeni and associates, Lurain and Piver, and others. In such families, one often encounters women with early onset ovarian carcinoma as well as one or more of the cardinal tumors of the family cancer syndrome, namely, endometrial, breast, and colonic carcinoma. O'Brien and associates and others have concluded that primary carcinoma of the ovary is five times more frequent among women with previous carcinoma of the colon and rectum. A similar increase in the frequency of ovarian malignancy has been found in patients with breast carcinoma. Ovarian neoplasia is more common in the presence of the Peutz-Jeghers syndrome. *Therefore, bilateral prophylactic oophorectomy should be done when hysterectomy is indicated in premenopausal patients with the Peutz-Jeghers syn-*

drome; with a personal history of breast, colon, or rectal cancer; or with a strong family history of ovarian cancer.

Unfortunately, prophylactic oophorectomy in women who have a high genetic risk for ovarian malignancy will not always accomplish the protection desired. Tobacman, Tucker, and Kase have reported performing prophylactic oophorectomy in 28 female members of 16 families at high risk for ovarian carcinoma. Three of these women subsequently developed disseminated intraabdominal malignancy indistinguishable histopathologically from ovarian carcinoma. These authors suggest that in cancer-prone families, the susceptible tissue is not limited to the ovary but also includes other derivatives of the coelomic epithelium, from which primary peritoneal neoplasms may arise following prophylactic oophorectomy. Woodruff has hypothesized that ovarian cancer with intra-abdominal spread may actually represent multicentric neoplasia derived from the embryonic mesothelium or celomic epithelium. The peritoneum and the germinal epithelium of the ovary have a common embryologic origin.

Caucasian women, women who have difficulty conceiving, and women who have not born children have a greater risk of ovarian cancer. Women who have a relatively lower risk for ovarian cancer include those who are black, multiparous, and long-time users of oral contraceptives.

Hysterectomy with bilateral oophorectomy does decrease the risk of breast cancer in women younger than age 55 years, according to a study by Irwin and associates. However, the risk was lowest in women who had their surgery before age 40 years or 15 or more years in the past, at an age when prophylactic oophorectomy would be contraindicated for a number of other reasons.

With few exceptions, both ovaries should be removed in postmenopausal and premenopausal patients with endometrial and ovarian malignancy. Young women who have extensive abdominal hysterectomy and bilateral lymphadenectomy for early invasive cervical cancer may have both normal ovaries conserved (see Ch. 42). When an ovary is severely involved by a tumor, cyst, infection, adhesions, or endometriosis, or when its blood supply is compromised, it should be removed. If an ovarian cystectomy is done, the ovary should be meticulously repaired with fine suture material to eliminate interstitial dead space and minimize adhesions. If more than two thirds of the ovarian parenchyma has been removed, the entire ovary should be removed. During vaginal hysterectomy, the ovaries are examined. They may or may not be removed vaginally depending on an assessment of the technical difficulties. If the ovaries are accessible, the same guidelines for prophylactic oophorectomy should apply to the menopausal and postmenopausal patient at the time of vaginal hysterectomy. If it is important to remove the ovaries because of gross pathology or to resect an ovarian lesion, it should usually be done through an abdominal incision.

If a bilateral oophorectomy is done, whether for prophylactic reasons or because of pathology of the ovaries or uterus, the ovaries should be removed completely. If a remnant of ovarian parenchyma is left remaining in a premenopausal woman, especially if it is left in an extraperitoneal location, it may eventually cause symptoms such as pelvic pain or dyspareunia. A tender mass may be palpable on the pelvic sidewall. Ureteral obstruction may be found on excretory urography, as discussed by Phillips and McGahan. Plasma follicle-stimulating hormone, luteinizing hormone, and estrogen levels will confirm the presence of functioning ovarian tissue. Symmonds and Pettit reviewed their experience with 20 cases of ovarian remnants at the Mayo Clinic and described the difficult technical problems encountered in operative removal. The ovarian remnant syndrome is more likely to follow a difficult abdominal hysterectomy and bilateral salpingo-oophorectomy for extensive pelvic endometriosis or pelvic inflammatory disease.

Despite these exceptions, the golden rule of pelvic surgery is the conservation of useful organ function. The conservation of both normal ovaries in premenopausal women at the time of abdominal hysterectomy does represent conservation of useful function, in our opinion. Of course, it is important to establish a frank and open dialogue with each patient. The advantages and disadvantages of ovarian conservation should be honestly and fairly presented. The patient must be allowed to have her questions answered and must be given time to express her feelings before a final recommendation is made. If the ovaries are conserved, the patient should be informed of the necessity for subsequent periodic follow-up examinations.

A survey of the practice of prophylactic oophorectomy by 1142 fellows and members of the Royal College of Obstetricians and Gynaecologists was carried out by Jacobs and Oram. The percentage of respondents who said they would usually remove apparently normal ovaries at the time of abdominal hysterectomy from premenopausal women in age groups 35–39, 40–44, 45–49, and over 49 years was 0.4%, 2%, 20%, and 51%, respectively, and from postmenopausal women, 85%.

OTHER CONSIDERATIONS

Routine postoperative care is discussed in Chapter 6. A variety of specific postoperative complications are covered in other chapters (postoperative infections in

Chapter 9; postoperative hemorrhage in Chapter 8; surgical injury of the bladder in Chapter 30; surgical injury of the ureters in Chapter 29; thromboembolic disease in Chapter 6; incisional complications in Chapters 10 and 11; postoperative vaginal vault prolapse in Chapter 32; and intestinal complications in Chapter 37). These problems are not discussed again here. Other problems, however, are mentioned below.

When patients return for routine examination 4–6 weeks after surgery, the vaginal vault may or may not be completely healed. A small line of granulation tissue may be present. It may be touched with silver nitrate and the patient instructed to douche with warm water to encourage the final stages of healing to be complete.

Granulation tissue in the vaginal apex may be mistaken for prolapse of the fallopian tube. According to Dao and Cartwright, only approximately 70 cases of fallopian tube prolapse have been reported up to 1985, most of which followed vaginal hysterectomy. The majority of cases are the result of faulty surgical technique in that the peritoneum was not closed securely or did not heal securely because of infection or hematoma. Patients will complain of persistent and profuse vaginal discharge, sometimes blood-tinged. Lower abdominal discomfort is common. Dyspareunia is seen occasionally. After the red bud of tissue that appears to be granulation tissue persists for several weeks, an attempt is usually made to remove it in the office or clinic. At that moment, the diagnosis will become obvious. If the red bud of tissue is granulation tissue, it can be removed with biopsy forceps painlessly. On the other hand, any attempt to remove a piece of prolapsed fallopian tube with biopsy forceps without anesthesia will cause extreme pain. Anesthesia will be required before the prolapsed tube can be removed. This can usually be accomplished vaginally, sometimes also with the aid of laparoscopy. Laparotomy will be necessary in a few cases. Pathologic examination will confirm that the tissue is fallopian tube.

Spontaneous and traumatic rupture of the vaginal vault following vaginal or abdominal hysterectomy with or without evisceration may occur but is rare. A severe and sudden increase in intra-abdominal pressure may cause disruption of an incompletely healed fresh vaginal vault incision. Traumatic vault rupture following coitus also has been reported by Hacker, Charles, and Scnage, by Powell, by Hall et al., and by others. Bleeding may or may not be profuse. Repair may usually be accomplished vaginally but laparotomy with hypogastric artery ligation to control profuse bleeding may be required. All posthysterectomy patients should be given careful instructions before leaving the hospital, including instructions to avoid coitus until postoperative pelvic examination shows a properly healed vaginal vault incision.

The sensitive gynecologist will spend sufficient time with patients in the postoperative recovery period to be certain that no serious adverse psychologic reaction to hysterectomy has occurred. If significant depression is recognized early, psychiatric consultation and counseling may be more effective. Likewise, postoperative sexual dysfunction should be recognized and treated before serious consequences develop.

Finally, recent epidemiologic studies have suggested that women who have had hysterectomy before age 45 years may have an increased relative risk of coronary heart disease, hypertension, and cardiac arrhythmia, regardless of whether the ovaries were removed at the same time. Such findings of Punnonen, Ikalainen, and Seppala and of Centerwall suggest that the uterus may have a hormonal or other secretory function (ie, prostaglandins) that may influence ovarian function or prevent cardiovascular disease in premenopausal women by some other mechanism. If future studies confirm this association, special recommendations for care will be needed for premenopausal women who require hysterectomy.

Bibliography

Ackner B. Emotional aspects of hysterectomy. Adv Psychosom Med 1960;1:248.

Adams TW. Female sterilization. Am J Obstet Gynecol 1964;89:395.

Alderson M, Donnan S. Hysterectomy rates and their influence upon mortality from carcinoma of the cervix. J Epidemiol and Community Health 1978;32:175.

Allan MS, Hertig AT. Carcinoma of the ovary. Am J Obstet Gynecol 1949;58:640.

Allen JL, Rampone JF, Wheeless CR. Use of prophylactic antibiotics in elective major gynecologic operations. Obstet Gynecol 1972;39:218.

Allen WM, Masters WH. Traumatic laceration of uterine support: The clinical syndrome and the operative treatment. Am J Obstet Gynecol 1955;70:500.

Amirikia H, Evans TN. Ten-year review of hysterectomies: trends, indications, and risks. Am J Obstet Gynecol 1979;134:431.

Annegers JF, Strom H, Decker DG, et al. Ovarian cancer, incidence and case-control study. Cancer 1979;43:723.

Aravantinos DJ. Keeping or removing the ovaries at the time of hysterectomy. Eur J Obstet Gynecol Reprod Biol 1988;28:146.

Asch RH, Balmaceda JP, Ord T, et al. Oocyte donation and gamete intrafallopian transfer in premature ovarian failure. Fertil Steril 1988;49:263.

Atkinson SM, Chappell SM. Vaginal hysterectomy for sterilization. Obstet Gynecol 1972;39:759.

Atlee WL. Case of successful extirpation of a fibrous tumor of the peritoneal surface of the uterus by the peritoneal section. Am J Med Sci 1845;9:26.

Bachmann GA. Hysterectomy: a critical review. J Reprod Med 1990; 35:839.

Backstrom CT, Boyle H, Baird DT. Persistence of symptoms of premenstrual tension in hysterectomized women. Br J Obstet Gynaecol 1981;88:530.

Baker HW. Selective indications for subtotal abdominal hysterectomy. J Kentucky Med Assoc 1985; 83:355.

Ballard CA. Therapeutic abortion and sterilization by vaginal hysterectomy. Am J Obstet Gynecol 1974;118:891.

Bancroft-Livingston G. Ovarian survival following hysterectomy. J Obstet Gynaecol Br Commonw 1954;61:628.

Bang J, Dragsted V, Halse C. Hysterectomy: a prospective psychiatric and gynecologic investigation. Ugeskr Laeger 1981;143:3035.

Barclay DL, Hawks BL, Frueh DM, et al. Elective cesarean hysterectomy: a 5-year comparison with cesarean section. Am J Obstet Gynecol 1976;124:900.

Barker MG. Psychiatric illness after hysterectomy. Br Med J 1968;2:91.

Barlow JJ, Emerson K, Saxena BB. Estradiol production after ovariectomy for carcinoma of the breast. N Eng J Med 1969;280:633.

Bates T, Siller G, Crathesu BC, Bradley SP, Zlotnik RD, Couch C, James RDG, Kay CM. Timing of prophylactic antibiotics in abdominal surgery: Trial of pre-operative versus an intra-operative first dose. Br J Surg 1989;76:52.

Batres F, Barclay DL. Sciatic nerve injury during gynecologic procedures using the lithotomy position. Obstet Gynecol 1983;62(suppl):92S.

Batty LH, Williams SB, Krantz KE. Laparoscopic repair of the prolapsed fallopian tube. J Reprod Med 1980;24:244.

Beavis ELG, Brown JB, Smith M. Ovarian function after hysterectomy with conservation of the ovaries in premenopausal women. J Obstet Gynaecol Br Commonw 1969;76:969.

Bernal EW. Hysterectomy and autonomy. Theor Med 1988;9:73.

Bezdek J, Grigarova H, Kleisl R. Vaginal hysterectomy—technique and results in the last 19 years. Sb Ved Pr Lek Fak Univ Karlovy 1985;28:31.

Bhiwandiwala PP, Mumford SD, Feldblum PJ. Menstrual pattern changes following laparoscopic sterilization. J Reprod Med 1982;27:249.

Bjoro K. Klimakteriet. In: Bjoro K, Kolstad P, eds. Gynaekologi. Oslo, Norway: Universitetsforlaget, 1979:.

Borell V, Fernstrom I. The adnexal branches of the uterine artery: an artriographic study in human subjects. Acta Radiol 1953;40:561.

Boston Collaborative Drug Surveillance Program. N Engl J Med 1974;290:15.

Braun P, Druckman E. Public health rounds at The Harvard School of Public Health. N Engl J Med 1976;295:264.

Bukovsky I, Liftshitz Y, Langer R, et al. Ovarian residual syndrome. Surg Gynecol Obstet 1988;167:132.

Bunker JP. Elective hysterectomy: pro and con. N Engl J Med 1976;295:264.

Bunker JP. Surgical manpower: a comparison of operations and surgeons in the USA and in England and Wales. N Engl J Med 1970;282:135.

Burchell RC. Decision regarding hysterectomy. Am J Obstet Gynecol 1977;127:113.

Burford TH, Diddle AW. Effect of total hysterectomy upon the ovary of the Macacus Rhesus. Surg Gynecol Obstet 1936;62:701.

Burke JF. The effective period of preventive antibiotic action in experimental incisions and dermal lesions. Surgery 1961;50:161.

Burke JF. Preventive antibiotic management in surgery. Am Rev Med 1973;24:289.

Burke JF, Miles AA. The sequence of vascular events in early infective inflammation. J Pathol Bacteriol 1958;76:1.

Burkhart FL, Daly JW. Sciatic and peroneal nerve injury: a complication of vaginal operations. Obstet Gynecol 1966;28:99.

Burnham W. Extirpation of the uterus and ovaries for sarcomatous disease. Lancet 1854;8:147.

Bush T, Cowan LD, Barett-Connor E, et al. Estrogen use and all-cause mortality. JAMA 1983;249:903.

Carenza L. Keeping or removing the ovaries at the time of hysterectomy. Eur J Obstet Gynaecol Reprod Biol 1988;28:155.

Centers for Disease Control. Cancer and steroid hormone study: Oral contraceptive use and the risk of ovarian cancer. JAMA 1983;249:1596.

Centerwall BS. Premenopausal hysterectomy and cardiovascular disease. Am J Obstet Gynecol 1981;139:58.

Christ JE, Lotze EC. The residual ovary syndrome. Obstet Gynecol 1975;46:551.

Christian DD. Ovarian tumors: an extension of the Peutz-Jegher's syndrome. Am J Obstet Gynecol 1971;111:529.

Ciannhfrani TA. Short history of obstetrics and gynecology. Springfield, Illinois: Charles C. Thomas, 1960.

Cohen MM. Longterm risk of hysterectomy after tubal sterilization. Am J Epidemiol 1987;125:410.

Cole P, Berlin J. Elective hysterectomy. Obstet Gynecol 1977;129:117.

Copenhaver EH. Vaginal hysterectomy: an analysis of indications and complications among 1000 operations. Am J Obstet Gynecol 1962;84:123.

Copenhaver EH. Vaginal hysterectomy, past, present and future. Surg Clin North Am 1980;60:437.

Coppen A, Bishop M, Beard RJ, et al. Hysterectomy, hormones, and behavior. Lancet 1981;1:126.

Corson SL, Levinson CJ, Batzer FR, et al. Hormonal levels following sterilization and hysterectomy. J Reprod Med 1981;26:363.

Coulam CB, Adamson SC, Annegers JF. Incidence of premature ovarian failure. Obstet Gynecol 1986;67:604.

Counseller VS, Hunt W, Haigler FH. Carcinoma of the ovary following hysterectomy. Am J Obstet Gynecol 1955;69:538.

Cruikshank SH. Avoiding ureteral injury during total vaginal hysterectomy. South Med J 1985;78:1447.

Dao AH, Cartwright PS. Fallopian tube prolapse following abdominal hysterectomy. J Tenn Med Assoc 1987;80:141.

Deane RT, Ulene A. Hysterectomy or tubal ligation for sterilization: a cost-effective analysis. Inquiry 1977;14:73.

Defore WW, et al. Necrotizing fascitis: a persistent surgical problem. J Am Coll Emerg Phys 1977;6:2.

deNeef JC, Hollenbeck ZJR. The fate of ovaries preserved at the time of hysterectomy. Am J Obstet Gynecol 1966;96:1088.

Dennerstein L, Wood C, Burrows GD. Sexual response following hysterectomy and oophorectomy. Obstet Gynecol 1977;49:92.

D'Esopo DA. Hysterectomy when the uterus is grossly normal. Am J Obstet Gynecol 1962;83:113.

DeStefano F, Greenspan JR, Dicker RC, et al. Complications of interval laparoscopic tubal sterilization. Obstet Gynecol 1983;61:153.

DeStefano F, Huezo CM, Peterson HB, et al. Longterm risk of menstrual disturbances after tubal sterilization. Am J Obstet Gynecol 1985;152:835.

Dexeus S, Munos A, Tusquets JM. Preservation of the ovaries: a controversial subject. Eur J Obstet Gynaecol Reprod Biol 1988;28:146.

Dicker RC, Greenspan JR, Strauss LT, et al. Complications of abdominal and vaginal hysterectomy among women of reproductive age in the United States. Am J Obstet Gynecol 1982;144:841.

Dicker RC, Scally MJ, Greenspan JR, et al. Hysterectomy among women of reproductive age: trends in the United States, 1970–1978. JAMA 1982;248:323.

Dickinson JA, Hill AM. The incidence of hysterectomy and its effect on the probability of developing uterine cancers. Community Health Studies 1988;12:176.

Domenighetti G, Luraschi P, Gutzwiller F, et al. Effect of information compaign by mass media on hysterectomy rates. Lancet 1988;2:1470.

Domengihetti G, Luraschi P, Marazzi A. Hysterectomy and the sex of the gynecologist. N Engl J Med 1985;313:1482.

Donnez J, Wauters M, Thomas K. Luteal function after tubal sterilization. Obstet Gynecol 1981;57:65.

Doyle JC. Indications for and contraindications to ovariectomy. Ann West Med Surg 1952;6:411.

Doyle JC. Unnecessary hysterectomies: a study of 6,248 operations in 35 hospitals during 1948. JAMA 1953;151:360.

Doyle JC. Unnecessary ovariectomies: study based on removal of 704 normal ovaries from 546 patients. JAMA 1952;148:1105.

Duff P. Antibiotic prophylaxis for abdominal hysterectomy. Obstet Gynecol 1982;60:25.

Dyck FJ, Murphy FA, Murphy JK, et al. Effect of surveillance on the number of hysterectomies in the Province of Saskatchewan. N Engl J Med 1977;296:1326.

El-Minawi MF, Mashhaor N, Reda MS. Pelvic venous changes after tubal sterilization. J Reprod Med 1983;28:641.

Emerson RS, Creedon JJ. Unjustified surgery dilemma. NY State J Med 1977;77:784.

England GT, Randall GW, Graves WL. Impairment of soft tissue defenses by vasoconstrictors in vaginal hysterectomy. Obstet Gynecol 1983;61:271.

Eschenbach DA, Davick PR, Williams BL, et al. Prevalence of hydrogen peroxide-producing *Lactobacillus* species in normal women and women with bacterial vaginosis. J Clin Microbiol 1989;27:251.

Eschenback DA, Hillier S, Critchlow C, et al. Diagnosis and clinical manifestations of bacterial vaginosis. Am J Obstet Gynecol 1988;158:819.

Escobedo LG, Peterson HB, Gruff GS, et al. Case-fatality rates for tubal sterilization in U.S. hospitals, 1979 to 1980. Am J Obstet Gynecol 1989;160:147.

Fagan GE, Allen ED, Klawans AH. Ovarian neoplasms and repeat pelvis surgery. Obstet Gynecol 1957;7:418.

Falk HC, Soichet S. The technique of vaginal hysterectomy. Clin Obstet Gynecol 1972;15:703.

Faro S. Prevention of infections after obstetric and gynecologic surgery. J Reprod Med 1988;33:154.

Feichtinger W, Kemeter P. Pregnancy after total ovariectomy achieved by ovum donation. Lancet 1985;2:722.

Fernstrom I. The normal anatomy of the uterine artery. Acta Radiol 1955;122(suppl):21.

Fifer WR, Rovinsky JJ, Easterling WE Jr. In an audit of hysterectomy for leiomyoma, whither went the issues? Am Coll Obstetricians and Gynecologists Qual Rev Bull 1977;March:12.

Finazzo MS, Hoffman MS, Roberts WS, et al. Previous pelvic surgery in patients with ovarian cancer. South Med J 1988;81:1518.

Fine J, Morehead MA. Study of peer review of inhospital patient care. NY State J Med 1971;71:804.

Fortney JA, Cole LP, Kennedy KI. A new approach to measuring menstrual pattern change after sterilization. Am J Obstet Gynecol 1983;147:830.

Foster HW. Removal of the normal uterus. South Med J 1976;69:13.

Fraumeni JF Jr, Grundy GW, Creagan ET, et al. Six families prone to ovarian cancer. Cancer 1975;36:364.

Funk-Brentano P. The remaining ovary after hysterectomy. Rev Fr Gynecol Obstet 1958;53:217.

Funt MI, Benigno BB, Thompson JD. The residual adnexa—asset or liability? Am J Obstet Gynecol 1977;129:251.

Gambone JC, Lench JB, Slesinski MJ, et al. Validation of hysterectomy indications and the quality assurance process. Obstet Gynecol 1989;75:1045.

Gambrell RD, Maier RC, Ganders BI. Decreased incidence of breast cancer in postmenopausal estrogen-progesterone users. Obstet Gynecol 1983;62:435.

Garcia C, Cutler WB. Preservation of the ovary: a reevaluation. Fertil Steril 1984;42:510.

Gerhard G. Sur les variations d'origine et de nombre des arteres genitales, spermatiques ou ovariennes de l'homme. Comp Rend Soc Biol 1913;74:778.

Gertman PM, Stackpole DA, Levenson DK, et al. Second opinions for elective surgery: The mandatory Medicaid program in Massachusetts. N Engl J Med 1980;302:1169.

Gevaerts PO. Abdominale totale uterus extirpatie of supravaginalis uterus amputatie [Dissertation]. Holland: 1963, Faculteit der Geneeskunde Rijksuniversiteit te Leiden.

Goldman JA, Feldberg D, Dicker D, et al. Femoral neuropathy subsequent to abdominal hysterectomy: a comparative study. Eur J Obstet Gynaecol Reprod Biol 1985;20:385.

Grammatikati J. Experimentelle Untersuchungen uber das weitere Schickal der Ovarien and Tuben nach der Totalexstirpation des Uterus bei Kaninchen. Centralblatt fur Gynakologie 1889;7:195.

Graves WP. Transplantation and retention of ovarian tissue after hysterectomy. Surg Gynecol Obstet 1917;25:315.

Gray LA. Indications, techniques, and complications in vaginal hysterectomy. Obstet Gynecol 1966;28:714.

Gray LA. Open cuff method of abdominal hysterectomy. Obstet Gynecol 1975;46:42.

Gray LA. Vaginal hysterectomy. Springfield, Illinois: Charles C Thomas, 1963.

Greenblatt RB, Colle ML, Mahesh VB. Ovarian and adrenal steroid production in the postmenopausal woman. Obstet Gynecol 1976;47:383.

Greenhalf JO. Vaginal vault granulation tissue following total abdominal hysterectomy. Br J Clin Pract 1967;6:247.

Grodin JM, Siiteri PI, MacDonald PC. Source of estrogen production in postmenopausal women. J Endocrinol Metabol 1973;36:207.

Grogan RH. Reappraisal of residual ovaries. Am J Obstet Gynecol 1967;97:124.

Grogan RH, Duncan CJ. Ovarian salvage in routine abdominal hystrectomy. Am J Obstet Gynecol 1955;70:1277.

Hacker NF, Charles EH, Scnage EW. Postcoital posthysterectomy vaginal vault disruption with hemorrhagic shock. Aust N Z J Obstet Gynaecol 1980;20:182.

Hall BD, Phelan JP, Pruyn SC, et al. Vaginal evisceration during coitus: a case review. Am J Obstet Gynecol 1978;131:155.

Haynes DM, Martin BR Jr. Cesarean-hysterectomy: a 25-year review. Am J Obstet Gynecol 1979;134:393.

Haynes DM, Wolfe WM. Tubal sterilization in an indigent population. Am J Obstet Gynecol 1970;106:1044.

Heaney NS. A report of 565 vaginal hysterectomies performed for benign pelvic disease. Am J Obstet Gynecol 1934;28:751.

Hemsell DL, Heard MC, Nobles BJ, et al. Single-dose prophylaxis for vaginal and abdominal hysterectomy. Am J Obstet Gynecol 1987;157:498.

Hemsell DL, Reisch J, Nobles B, et al. Prevention of major infection after elective abdominal hysterectomy: individual determination required. Am J Obstet Gynecol 1983;147:520.

Hemsell DL, Johnson ER, Hemsell PG, Nobles BJ, Heard MC. Cefazolin for hysterectomy prophylaxis. Obstet Gynecol 1990;76:603.

Henrotin F. Vaginal hysterectomy. In: Kelly HA, Noble CP, eds. Gynecology and abdominal surgery. Philadelphia: WB Saunders, 1910:759.

Hibbard LT. Sexual sterilization by elective hysterectomy. Am J Obstet Gynecol 1972;112:1076.

Hill DJ, Beischer NA. Hysterectomy in obstetric practice. Aust N Z J Obstet Gynecol 1980;20:151.

Hinojosa RR, Arechiga MAE, Aguilera CH. Histerectomia abdominal extrafascial vs subfascial: estudio comparativo. Ginecol Obstet Mex 1986;54:236.

Hollenbeck ZJR. Ovarian cancer: prophylactic oophorectomy. Am J Obstet Gynecol 1955;21:442.

Holman JF, McGowan JE, Thompson JD. Perioperative antibiotics in major elective gynecologic surgery. South Med J 1978;71:417.

Howkins J, Williams DK. Vault granulations after total abdominal hysterectomy. J Obstet Gynaecol Br Commonw 1968;75:84.

Irwin KL, Lee NC, Peterson HB, et al. Hysterectomy, tubal sterilization, and the risk of breast cancer. Am J Epidemiol 1988;127:1192.

Irwin KL, Peterson HB, Hughes JM, et al. Hysterectomy among women of reproductive age, United States, update for 1981–1982. CDC Morbidity and Mortality Weekly Report 1986;35:1SS.

Isaacs JH. Vaginal hysterectomy and vaginal repair. In: Breen JL, Osofsky HJ, eds. Current concepts in gynecologic surgery. Baltimore: Williams & Wilkins, 1987:81.

Jackson MN, LoFerto JP, Diehr P, et al. Elective hysterectomy: a cost-benefit analysis. Inquiry 1978;15:275.

Jacobs I, Oram D. Prevention of ovarian cancer: a survey of the practive of prophylactic oophorectomy by fellows and members of the Royal College of Obstetricians and Gynaecologists. Br J Obstet Gynaecol 1989;96:510.

Janson PO, Jansson I. The acute effect of hysterectomy on ovarian blood flow. Am J Obstet Gynecol 1977;127:349.

Jaszczak SE, Evans TN. Intrafascial abdominal and vaginal hysterectomy: a reappraisal. Obstet Gynecol 1982;59:435.

Jenkins VR II. Unnecessary-elective-indicated? Audit criteria of the American College of Obstetricians and Gynecologists to assess abdominal hysterectomy for uterine leiomyoma. Am Coll Obstetricians and Gynecologists Qual Rev Bull 1977;May:7.

Johansson BW, et al. On some late effects of bilateral oophorectomy in the age range 15–30 years. Acta Obstet Gynecol Scand 1975;54:449.

Johnson CG, Moll CF, Post L. An analysis of 6,891 hysterectomies for benign pelvic disease. Am J Obstet Gynecol 1956;71:515.

Judd HL, Judd GE, Lucas WE, et al. Endocrine function of the postmenopausal ovary: concentration of androgens and estrogens in ovarian and peripheral vein blood. J Clin Endocrinol Metab 1974;39:1020.

Kaltreider NB, Wallace A, Horowitz MJ. A field study of the stress response syndrome: young women after hysterectomy. JAMA 1979;242:393.

Kannitz AM, Thompson RJ, Kannitz KK. Mental retardation: a controversial indication for hysterectomy. Obstet Gynecol 1986;68:436.

Kasonde JM, Bonnar J. Effect of sterilization on menstrual blood loss. Br J Obstet Gynaecol 1976;83:572.

Kasper AS. Hysterectomy as a social process. Women Health 1985;10:109.

Keith C. Discussion group for posthysterectomy patients. Health Soc Work. 1980;:59.

Kelly HA. Conservatism in ovariotomy. JAMA 1896;26:249.

Kelly HA. Ligature of the trunks of the uterine and ovarian arteries as a means of checking hemorrhage from the uterus and broad ligaments in abdominal operations. The Johns Hopkins Hospital Reports 1891;2:220.

Kelly HA. Operative gynecology. New York: Appleton, 1896.

Kelly HA. Operative gynecology. Vol 2. New York: Appleton and Company, 1901:.

Kelly HA, Cullen TS. Myomata of the uterus. Philadelphia: WB Saunders, 1909.

Kelly HA, Noble CP. Gynecology and abdominal surgery. Vol 1. Philadelphia: WB Saunders, 1907.

Kilkku P. Supravaginal uterine amputation vs hysterectomy: effects on coital frequency and dyspareunia. Acta Obstet Gynecol Scand 1983;62:141.

Kilkku P. Supravaginal uterine amputation vs hysterectomy with reference to subjective bladder symptoms and incontinence. Acta Obstet Gynecol Scand 1985;64:375.

Kilkku P, Gronroos M. Preoperative electrocoagulation of the endocervical mucosa and later carcinoma of the cervical stump. Acta Obstet Gynecol Scand 1982;61:265.

Kilkku P, Grourros M, Hirvonen T, et al. Supravaginal uterine amputation vs hysterectomy: effects on libido and orgasm. Acta Obstet Gynecol Scand 1983;62:147.

Kilkku P, Gronroos M, Rauramo L. Supravaginal uterine amputation with preoperative electrocoagulation of endocervical mucosa. Acta Obstet Gynecol Scand 1985;64:175.

Kilkku P, Hirvonen T, Gronroos M. Supra vaginal uterine amputation vs abdominal hysterectomy: the effects on urinary symptons with special reference to pollakiuria, nocturia and dysuria. Maturitas 1981;3:197.

Korenbrot C, Flood AB, Higgins M, et al. Case study #15. Elective hysterectomy: Costs, risks, and benefits. Washington, DC: US Government Printing Office, 1981; Case Studies of Medical Technologies.

Kovac SR. Intramyometrial coring as an adjunct to vaginal hysterectomy. Obstet Gynecol 1986;67:131.

Krailo MD, Pike MC. Estimation of the distribution of age at natural menopause from prevalence data. Am J Epidemiol 1983;117:356.

Kral R. Post-operative morbidity incident to vaginal hysterectomy. Unpublished 1970.

Kuhn RJP, deCrespiguy LC. Vault hematoma after vaginal hysterectomy: An invariable sequel? Austral and NZ J Obstet Gynecol 1985;25:59.

Kvist-Poulsen H, Borel J. Iatrogenic femoral neuropathy subsequent to abdominal hysterectomy: incidence and prevention. Obstet Gynecol 1982;60:516.

Lalinec-Michaud M, Englesmann F. Depression and hysterectomy: a prospective study. Psychosomatics 1984;25:550.

Lalinec-Michaud M, Engelsmann F, Marino J. Depression after hysterectomy: a comparative study. Psychosomatics 1988;29:307.

Langer R, Neuman M, Rouel R, et al. The effect of total abdominal hysterectomy on bladder function in asymptomatic women. Obstet Gynecol 1989;74:205.

Laros RK, Work BA. Female sterilization III. Vaginal hysterectomy. Am J Obstet Gynecol 1975;122:693.

Lash AF. A method for reducing the size of the uterus in vaginal hysterectomy. Am J Obstet Gynecol 1941;42:452.

Lash AF. Vaginal hysterectomy: a technique for removal of abnormally large uteri without entering the cavities. Clin Obstet Gynecol 1961;4:210.

Lash AF, Stepto RC. Chicago technique for vaginal hysterectomy at the Cook County Hospital. Clin Obstet Gynecol 1972;15:755.

Lazarus ML, Levanthol ML. Total abdominal and vaginal hysterectomy, a comparison. Am J Obstet Gynecol 1985;61:2.

Ledger WJ, Child MA. The hospital care of patients undergoing hysterectomy: an analysis of 12,026 patients from the Professional Activities Study. Am J Obstet Gynecol 1973;117:423.

Ledger WJ, Gee C, Lewis WP. Guidelines for antibiotic prophylaxis in gynecology. Am J Obstet Gynecol 1975;121:1038.

Ledger WJ, Sweet RI, Headington JT. Prophylactic cephaloridine in the prevention of postoperative pelvic inspections in premenopausal women undergoing vaginal hysterectomy. Am J Obstet Gynecol 1973;115:766.

Lee NC, Dicker, RC, Rubin GL, et al. Confirmation of the preoperative diagnoses for hysterectomy. Am J Obstet Gynecol 1984;150:283.

Lee RA. Abdominal hysterectomy (simple). In: Breen JL, Osofsky HJ, eds. Current concepts in gynecologic surgery. Baltimore: Williams & Wilkins, 1987:151.

Leibsohn S, d'Ablaing G, Mishell DR Jr, Schlaerth JB. Leiomyosarcoma in a series of hysterectomies performed for presumed uterine leiomyomas. Am J Obstet Gynecol 162:968, 1990.

Leonardo RA. History of gynecology. New York: Froben Press, 1944.

Lindemann E. Observations on psychiatric sequelae of surgical operations in women. Am J Psychiatry 1941;98:132.

Little WA. The selection and application of various surgical methods of sterilization. Am J Obstet Gynecol 1975;123:12.

Longo LD. The rise and fall of Battery's operation: a fashion in surgery. Bull Hist Med 1979;53(2):244.

Lurain JR, Piver MS. Familial ovarian cancer. Gynecol Oncol 1979;8:185.

Lutjen P, Trounson A, Leeton J, et al. The establishment and maintenance of pregnancy using in vitro fertilization and embryo donation in a patient with primary ovarian failure. Nature 1984;307:174.

Lynch HT, Albano WA, Lynch JF, et al. Surveillance and management of patients at high genetic risk for ovarian carcinoma. Obstet Gynecol 1982;59:589.

Lynch HT, Harris RE, Guirgis HA, et al. Familial association of breast/ovarian carcinoma. Cancer 1978;41:1543.

Lynch HT, Lynch PM. Tumor variation in the cancer family syndrome: ovarian cancer. Am J Surg 1979;138:439.

Lyon JL, Gardner JW. The rising frequency of hysterectomy: its effect on uterine cancer rates. Am J Epidemiol 1977;105:439.

Machin D, Williams JD. The effect of hysterectomy on the age at ovarian failure. Fertil Steril 1988;49:378.

MacMahon B, Worcester J. Age at menopause, United States 1960–1962. Washington, DC: National Center for Health Statistics, 1966; DHEW publication no (HSM) 66-1000. (Vital and health statistics; Series 11, data from the National Health Survey; No. 19).

Mathieu A. History of hysterectomy. West J Surg Obstet Gynecol 1934;42:2.

Mattingly RF, Huang HY. Steroidogenesis in the menopausal and postmenopausal ovary. Am J Obstet Gynecol 1969;103:679.

McCall ML. Posterior culdoplasty. Obstet Gynecol 1957;10:595.

McCall ML, Keatty EC, Thompson JD. Conservation of ovarian tissue in the treatment of carcinoma of the cervix with radical surgery. Am J Obstet Gynecol 1958;75:590.

McCarthy EG, Kamons AS. Voluntary and mandatory presurgical screening programs: an analysis of their implications. Presented at American Federation for Clinical Research, Clinical Epidemiology, Health Care Research, Atlantic City, New Jersey, May 2, 1972.

McGowan L. Ovarian cancer after hysterectomy. Obstet Gynecol 1987;69:386.

McPherson K, Wennberg JE, Howard OB, et al. Small-area variations in the use of common surgical procedures: an international comparison of New England, England, and Norway. N Engl J Med 1982;307:1310.

McQuarrie HG, Harris JW, Ellsworth HS, et al. Sciatic neuropathy complicating vaginal hysterectomy. Am J Obstet Gynecol 1972;113:223.

Mead PB, Eschenbach DA, Ledger WJ, et al. Reconsidering bacterial vaginosis. Contemp Obstet Gynecol 1989;34:76.

Meikle S. The psychological effects of hysterectomy. Can Psychol Rev 1977;18:128.

Menon RK, Okonofua FE, Agnew JE, et al. Endocrine and metabolic effects of simple hysterectomy. Int J Gynecol Obstet 1987;25:459.

Mikhail G. Hormone secretion by the human ovaries. Gynecol Invest 1970;1:5.

Miles AA, Niven JSF. The enhancement of infection during shock produced by bacterial toxins and other agents. Br J Exper Pathol 1950;31:73.

Miles AA, Miles EM, Burke J. The value and duration of defence reactions of the skin to the primary lodgement of bacteria. Br J Exper Pathol 1957;38:79.

Miller NF. Hysterectomy: therapeutic necessity or surgical racket? Am J Obstet Gynecol 1946;51:804.

Mocquot P, Rouvillois C. La vascularisation arterielle de l'ovarie etudie en vue de la chirurgie conservatrice. J Chir 1938;51:161.

Montague CF. Cesarean hysterectomy: its value as a sterilization procedure. Obstet Gynecol 1959;14:28.

Montgomery JC, Crook D, Godsland IF, et al. Plasma lipid risk factors in oophorectomized women. Br J Obstet Gynaecol 1989;96:1236.

Moschowitz AV. The pathogenesis, anatomy, and cure of prolapse of the rectum. Surg Gynecol Obstet 1912;15:7.

Muldoon MJ. Gynaecological illness after sterilization. Br Med J 1972;1:84.

Muntz HG, Falkenberry S, Fuller AF. Fallopian tube prolapse after hysterectomy: a report of two cases. J Reprod Med 1988;33:467.

Neefus M, Taylor M. Educational needs of hysterectomy patients. Patient Counseling Health Ed 1981;3:150.

Nehra PC, Loginsky SJ. Pregnancy after vaginal hysterectomy. Obstet Gynecol 1984;64:735.

Neil JR, Noble AD, Hammond GT, et al. Late complications of sterilization by laparoscopy and tubal ligation. Lancet 1975;2:699.

Nelson KJ, Gallup DG, Gibbs R, et al. Intraoperative antibiotic irrigation as prophylaxis in abdominal hysterectomy: a preliminary report. South Med J 1984;77:700.

Nichols DH, Randall CL. Vaginal surgery. 3rd ed. Baltimore: Williams & Wilkins, 1989.

Nichols DH, Willey PS, Randall CL. Significance of restoration of normal vaginal depth and axis. Obstet Gynecol 1970;36:251.

Noble CP. Abdominal hysteromyomectomy and myomectomy. In: Kelly HA, Noble CP, eds. Gynecology and abdominal surgery. Philadelphia: WB Saunders, 1910:660.

Notelovitz M, Gudat JC, Ware MD, et al. Lipids and lipoproteins in women after oophorectomy and the response to estrogen therapy. Br J Obstet Gynaecol 1983;90:171.

Novak ER. Ovulation after fifty. Obstet Gynecol 1970;36:903.

Novak ER, Williams TJ. Autopsy comparison of cardiovascular changes in castrated and normal women. Am J Obstet Gynecol 1960;80:863.

O'Brien PH, Newton BB, Metcalf JS, et al. Oophorectomy in women with carcinoma of the colon and rectum. Surg Gynecol Obstet 1981;153:827.

O'Herlihy C, Chandler C. Hysterectomy following sterilization. Int J Gynecol Obstet 1979;17:263.

Ohm MJ, Galask RP. The effect of antibiotic prophylaxis on patients undergoing total abdominal hysterectomy. I. Effect on morbidity. Am J Obstet Gynecol 1976;125:442.

Ojeda VJ. The pathology of hysterectomy specimens. N Z Med J 1979;89:169.

Orr JW, Varner RE, Kilgore LC, et al. Cefotetan versus cefoxitin as prophylaxis in hysterectomy. Am J Obstet Gynecol 1986;154:960.

Paloucek FP, Randall CL, Graham JB, et al. Cancer and its relation to abnormal vaginal bleeding and radiation. Obstet Gynecol 1963;21:530.

Paterson PJ. Sterilization—tubal approach or hysterectomy? Aust N Z J Obstet Gynecol 1975;15:36.

Patterson R, Craig JB. Misconceptions concerning psychological effects of hysterectomy. Am J Obstet Gynecol 1963;85:104.

Phillips HE, McGahan JP. Ovarian remnant syndrome. Radiology 1982;142:487.

Pitkin RM. Vaginal hysterectomy in obese women. Obstet Gynecol 1977;49:567.

Pletsch TD, Sandberg EC. Cesarean hysterectomy for sterilization. Am J Obstet Gynecol 1963;85:254.

Pokras R, Hufnagel VG. Hysterectomy in the United States, 1965–84. AJPH 1988;78:852.

Pokras R, Hufnagel VG. National Center for Health Statistics, 1965–84. Washington, DC: US Government Printing Office, December 1987; DHHS publication no. (PHS) 87-1753. (Vital and health statistics; series 13; No. 92).

Polivy J. Psychological reactions to hysterectomy: a critical review. Am J Obstet Gynecol 1974;118:417.

Poma PA. Tubal sterilization and later hospitalizations. J Reprod Med 1980;25:272.

Porges RF. Changing indications for vaginal hysterectomy. Am J Obstet Gynecol 1980;136:153.

Poulson AM Jr. Analysis of female sterilization technics. Obstet Gynecol 1973;42:131.

Powell JL. Vaginal evisceration following vaginal hysterectomy. Am J Obstet Gynecol 1973;115:276.

Pratt JH, Galloway JR. Vaginal hysterectomy in patients less than 36 and more than 60 years of age. Am J Obstet Gynecol 1965;93:812.

Pratt JH, Jefferies JA. The retained cervical stump: a 25-year experience. Obstet Gynecol 1976;48:711.

Pratt JH. Common complications of vaginal hysterectomy: thoughts regarding their prevention and management. Clin Obstet Gynecol 1976;19:645.

Pratt JH. Vaginal hysterectomy by morcellation. Mayo Clin Proc 1978;43:374.

Punnonen R, Ikalainen M, Seppala E. Premenopausal hysterectomy and the risk of cardiovascular disease. Lancet 1987;1:1139.

Radwanska E, Headley SK, Dwowski P. Evaluation of ovarian function after tubal sterilization. J Reprod Med 1982;27:376.

Randall CL, Birtch PK, Harkins JL. Ovarian function after the menopause. Am J Obstet Gynecol 1957;74:719.

Randall CL, Gerhardt PR. The probability of occurrence of the more common types of gynecologic malignancies. Am J Obstet Gynecol 1954;68:1378.

Randall CL, Hall DW, Armenia CS. Pathology in the preserved ovary after unilateral oophorectomy. Am J Obstet Gynecol 1962;84:1233.

Randall CL, Paloucek FP. The frequency of oophorectomy at the time of hysterectomy. Am J Obstet Gynecol 1968;100:716.

Ranney B. Multiple diagnoses and procedures during hysterectomy. Int J Gynecol Obstet 1990;33:325.

Ranney B. Decreasing numbers of patients for vaginal hysterectomy and plasty. So Dakota Jo Med 1990;43:7.

Ranney B, Abu-Ghazaleh S. The future function and fortune of ovarian tissue which is retained in vivo during hysterectomy. Am J Obstet Gynecol 1977;128:626.

Ranney B, Leonardson G. Volume reduction of the uterus during and soon after hysterectomy. Am J Obstet Gynecol 1986;155:354.

Raphael B. The crisis of hysterectomy. Aust N Z J Psychiatry 1972;6:106.

Rapp RP, Connors JE, Hager WD, et al. Comparison of single-dose moxalactam and a three-dose regimen of cefoxitin for prophylaxis in vaginal hysterectomy. Clin Pharm 1986;5:988.

Reiter RC, Lench JB, Gambone JC. Consumer advocacy, elective surgery, and the "golden era of medicine." Obstet Gynecol 1989;74:815.

Report by the Subcommittee on Oversight and Investigations of the Committee on Interstate and Foreign Commerce. Cost and quality of health care: unnecessary surgery. House of Representatives, Ninety-fourth U.S. Congress, Second Session, January, 1976.

Report of the Hysterectomy Subcommittee of the Quality Care Committee. NY Med J 1972;28:17.

Richards BC. Hysterectomy: from women to women. Am J Obstet Gynecol 1978;131:446.

Richards DH. A post-hysterectomy syndrome. Lancet 1974;2:983.

Richards DH. Depression after hysterectomy. Lancet 1974;2:430.

Richardson AC, Lyon JB, Graham EE. Abdominal hysterectomy: relationship between morbidity and surgical technique. Am J Obstet Gynecol 1973;115:514.

Richardson, EH. The effect of hysterectomy upon ovarian function. Trans Am Gynecol Soc 1918;43:114.

Richardson EH. A simplified technique for abdominal panhysterectomy. Surg Obstet Gynecol 1929;48:248.

Richardson FM. Peer review medical care. Med Care 1972;10:29.

Riedel H-H, Leihmann-Willenbrock E, Semm K. Ovarian failure phenomena after hysterectomy. J Reprod Med 1986;31:597.

Ringrose CAD. Posttubal ligation menorrhagia and pelvic pain. Int J Fertil 1974;19:168.

Roeske NCA. Hysterectomy and other gynecological surgeries: a psychological view. In: Notman MT, Nadelson CC, eds. The woman patient: medical and psychological interfaces. New York: Plenum Press, 1978:217.

Roy S, Wilkins J, Hemsell DL, et al. Efficacy and safety of single-dose ceftizoxime vs multiple-dose cefoxitin in preventing infection after vaginal hysterectomy. J Reprod Med 1988;33:149.

Rubin GL, Org HW, Layde PM. The mortality risk of voluntary surgical contraception. Biomed Bull Assoc Voluntary Steril 1982;3:1.

Rubinstein LM, Lebherz TB, Kleinkopf V. Laparoscopic tubal sterilization: Long-term postoperative follow up. Contraception 1976;13:631.

Russell KP. Current trends in indications for female sterilization. Am J Obstet Gynecol 1968;101:348.

Rutkow IW, Zuidema GD. Unnecessary surgery: an update. Surgery 1978;84:671.

Sacks S, LaCroix G. Gynecologic sequelae of postpartum tubal ligation. Obstet Gynecol 1962;19:22.

Sand PK, Bowen LW, Ostergard DR, et al. Hysterectomy and prior incontinence surgery as risk factors for failed retropubic cystourethropexy. J Reprod Med 1988;33:171.

Sattin RW, Rubin GL, Hughes JM. Hysterectomy among women of reproductive age, United States Update for 1979–1980. CDC Morbidity and Mortality Weekly Report 1983;32:15S.

Schwartz DB, Wingo PA, Antars LL, et al. Female sterilization in the United States, 1987. Fam Plann Perspect 1989;21:209.

Senior CC, Steigrad SJ. Are preoperative antibiotics helpful in abdominal hysterectomy? Am J Obstet Gynecol 1986;154:1004.

Sherwin BB, Gelfand MM, Brender W. Androgen enhances sexual motivation in females: a prospective, crossover study of sex steroid administration in the surgical menopause. Psychosom Med 1985;47:339.

Sherwin BB, Gelfand MM. Differential symptom response to parenteral estrogen and/or androgen administration in the surgical menopause. Am J Obstet Gynecol 1985;151:153.

Sherwin BB, Gelfand MM. Sex steroids and effect in the surgical menopause: a double-blind, cross-over study. Psychneuroendocrinology 1985;10:325.

Shoemaker ES, Forney JP, MacDonald PC. Estrogen treatment of postmenopausal women: benefits and risks. JAMA 1977;238:1524.

Siddle N, Sarrel P, Whithead M. The effect of hysterectomy on the age at ovarian failure: identification of a subgroup of women with premature loss of ovarian function and literature review. Fertil Steril 1987;47:94.

Simel D, Matchar DB, Piscitelli JT. Routine intravenous pyelograms before hysterectomy in cases of benign disease: possibly effective, definitely expensive. Am J Obstet Gynecol 1988;159:1049.

Siiteri PK, MacDonald PC. Role of extraglandular estrone in human endocrinology. In: Greep RO, ed. Handbook of physiology: the female reproductive system. Vol 2. Bethesda: American Physiology Society, 1973:.

Sloan D. The emotional and sexual aspects of hysterectomy. Am J Obstet Gynecol 1978;131:598.

Smale LE, Smale ML, Wilkening RL, et al. Salpingo-oophorectomy at the time of vaginal hysterectomy. Am J Obstet Gynecol 1978;131:122.

Smith GR Jr, Monson RA, Ray DC. Psychiatric consultation in somatization disorder. A randomized controlled study. N Engl J Med 1986;314:1407.

Smith HO, Thompson JD. Indications and technique for vaginal hysterectomy. Contempt Ob-Gyn 1986:28:125.

Snooks SJ, Badenoch DF, Tiptaft RC, et al. Perineal nerve damage in genuine stress urinary incontinence. Br J Urol 1985;57:422.

Soderstrom RM. Sterilization failures and their causes. Am J Obstet Gynecol 1984;152:395.

Souza AZ, Fonseca AM, Izzo VM, et al. Ovarian histology and function after total abdominal hysterectomy. Obstet Gynecol 1986;68:847.

Speroff T, Dawson NV, Speroff L, Haber RJ. A risk-benefit analysis of elective bilateral oophorectomy: effect of changes in compliance with estrogen therapy on outcome. Am J Obstet Gynecol 1991;164:165.

Steiner M, Aleksandrowicz DR. Psychiatric sequelae to gynaecological operations. Isr Ann Psychiatry 1970;8:186.

Stergachis A, Kirkwood KS, Grothaus LC, et al. Tubal sterilization and the long-term risk of hysterectomy. JAMA 1990;264:2893.

Stimson LA. On some modifications in the technique of abdominal surgery, limiting the use of the ligature en masse. Trans Am Surg Assoc 1889;7:65.

Stock RJ. Evaluation of sequelae of tubal ligation. Fert Steril 1978;29:169.

Stock RJ. Sequelae of tubal ligation: an analysis of 75 consecutive hysterectomies. South Med J 1984;77:1255.

Stone SC, Dickey RP, Mickal A. The acute effect of hysterectomy on ovarian function. Am J Obstet Gynecol 1975;121:193.

Storer HR. Successful removal of uterus and ovaries. Am J Med Sci 1986;51:110.

Studd J. Prophylactic oophorectomy. Br J Obstet Gynaecol 1989;96:506.

Stumpf PG, Ballard CA, Lowensohn R. Abdominal hysterectomy for abortion—sterilization: a report of 500 consecutive cases. Am J Obstet Gynecol 1980;136:714.

Swartz WH, Tanaree P. Suction drainage as an alternative to prophylactic antibiotics for hysterectomy. Obstet Gynecol 1975;45:305.

Swartz WH, Tanaree P. T-tube suction drainage and/or prophylactic antibiotics. Obstet Gynecol 1976;47:665.

Symmonds RE, Pettit PDM. Ovarian remnant syndrome. Obstet Gynecol 1979;54:174.

Taylor HC. Discussion of paper by D'Esopo. Am J Obstet Gynecol 1962;83:113.

Taylor HC Jr. Vascular congestion and hyperemia. Part II. The clinical aspects of the congestion fibrosis syndrome. Am J Obstet Gynecol 1949;57:637.

Taylor HC Jr. Vascular congestion and hyperemia. Part III. Etiology and therapy. Am J Obstet Gynecol 1949;57:654.

Te Linde RW. Hysterectomy, present day indications. J Mich State Med 1949;48:829.

Te Linde RW, Wharton LR Jr. Ovarian function following pelvic operation: an experiment on monkeys. Am J Obstet Gynecol 1960;80:844.

Templeton AA, Cole S. Hysterectomy following sterilization. Br J Obstet Gynaecol 1982;89:845.

Tervila L. Carcinoma of the cervical stump. Acta Obstet Gynecol Scand 1963;42:200.

Terz JJ, Barber HRK, Brunschwig A. The incidence of carcinoma in the retained ovary. Am J Surg 1967;113:511.

Thomas WL. Prevenception insurance: panhysterectomy versus tubectomy. South Med J 1953;46:787.

Thompson JD. Fallopian tube prolapse after abdominal hysterectomy. Aust N Z J Obstet Gynecol 1980;20:187.

Thompson JD, Birch HW. Indications for hysterectomy. Clin Obstet Gynecol 1981;24:1245.

Thompson JD, Caputo TA, Franklin EW, et al. The surgical management of invasive cancer of the cervix in pregnancy. Am J Obstet Gynecol 1975;121:853.

Thorsteinsson VT, Pratt JH. Gynecologic operations for sterilization. Minn Med 1972;55:204.

Tobacman JK, Tucker MA, Kase R. Intra-abdominal carcinomatosis after prophylactic oophorectomy in ovarian cancer-prone families. Lancet 1982;2:795.

Torpin R. Excision of the cul-de-sac of Douglas for the surgical care of hernias through the female caudal wall, including prolapse of the uterus. J Int Coll Surg 1955;24:322.

Travis CB. Medical decision making and elective surgery: the case of hysterectomy. Risk Anal 1985;5:241.

Trussel RE, Morehead MA, Ehrlich J. The quantity, quality, and costs of medical and hospital care secured by a sample of teamster families in the New York area. New York: Columbia University School of Medicine of Public Health and Administrative Medicine, 1962.

Utian WH. Effect of hysterectomy, oophorectomy and estrogen therapy In libido. Int J Gynecol Obstet 1975;13:97.

Utian WH, Goldfarb JM, Kiwi R, et al. Preliminary experience with in vitro fertilization—surrogate gestational pregnancy. Fertil Steril 1989;52:633.

Van Nagell JR Jr, Roddick JW Jr. Vaginal hysterectomy as a sterilization procedure. Am J Obstet Gynecol 1971;111:703.

Vermeulen A. The hormonal activity of the postmenopausal ovary. J Clin Endocrinol Metabol 1976;42:247.

Waldemar G, Werdelin L, Boysen G. Neurologic symptoms and hysterectomy: a retrospective survey of the prevalence of hysterectomy in nuerologic patients. Obstet Gynecol 1987;70:559.

Weed JC. The fate of the postcesarean uterus. Obstet Gynecol 1959;14:780.

Weiss NS, Harlow BL. Why does hysterectomy without bilateral oophorectomy influence the subsequent incidence of ovarian cancer? Am J Epidemiol 1986;124:856.

Wetchler SJ, Hurt WG. A technique for surgical correction of fallopian tube prolapse. Obstet Gynecol 1986;67:747.

Wheelock JB, Schneider V, Goplerud DR. Prolapsed fallopian tube masquerading as adenocarcinoma of the vagina in a postmenopausal woman. Gynecol Oncol 1985;21:369.

White SC, Wartel LJ, Wade ME. Comparison of abdominal and vaginal Histerectomies: A review of 600 operations. Obstet Gynecol 1971;37:530.

Whitelaw JM. Hysterectomy: A medical-legal perspective, 1975 to 1985. Am J Obstet Gynecol 1990;162:1451.

Whitelaw RG. Ovarian activity following hysterectomy. J Obstet Gynaecol Br Emp 1958;65:917.

Whitelaw RG. Pathology and the conserved ovary. J Obstet Gynaecol Br Emp 1959;66:413.

Willett W, Stampfer MJ, Bain C, et al. Cigarette smoking, relative weight, and menopause. Am J Epidemiol 1983;117:651.

Wingo PA, Huezo CM, Rubin GL, et al. The mortality risk associated with hysterectomy. Am J Obstet Gynecol 1985;152:803.

Woodruff JD. The pathogenesis of ovarian neoplasia. Johns Hopkins Med J 1979;144:177.

Wright RC. Hysterectomy: past, present, and future. Obstet Gynecol 1969;33:560.

Wynder EL, Dodo H, Barber HRK. Epidemiology of cancer of the ovary. Cancer 1969;23:352.

Zakut H, Lotan M, Bracha Y. Vaginal preparation with povidone-iodine before abdominal hysterectomy: a comparison with antibiotic prophylaxis. Clin Exp Obstet Gynecol 1987;14:1.

Zussman L, Zussman S, Sunley R, et al. Sexual response after hysterectomy-oophorectomy: recent studies and reconsideration of psychogenesis. Am J Obstet Gynecol 1981;140:725.

Evolving Aspects of Reparative Surgery

HOWARD W. JONES, JR.

By the 1970s it had been established that the application of then standard operative techniques by open laparotomy had a certain usefulness in treating infertility caused by obstructed fallopian tubes, congenital anomalies of the müllerian ducts, endometriosis, polycystic disease of the ovaries, pelvic adhesive disease, and other conditions. Microsurgical technology with a compound microscope or surgical loupes was developed during the 1970s and widely practiced in the early 1980s. Assisted reproduction, that is, in vitro fertilization (IVF) and its associated techniques, began to play a role in the early 1980s and heavily influenced reparative surgery in the late 1980s. Also in the 1980s, surgical manipulation through the laparoscope became popular as an approach to pelvic diseases and as a substitute for open operation. Grafted onto this in the late 1980s was the use of laser technology, particularly through the laparoscope and, to a lesser extent, by an open operation, as an approach to conditions in the pelvis amenable to surgery. This chapter traces the influence of these techniques on the indications for various surgical procedures.

IN VITRO FERTILIZATION AND ALLIED TECHNOLOGIES

To accomplish the purpose of this chapter and this volume, it is not necessary to dwell on the minute details of the technology of IVF or the allied procedures of gamete intrafallopian transfer (GIFT), zygote intrafallopian transfer (ZIFT), or others. Rather, it seems more useful to emphasize those factors that allow one to estimate for a particular patient the probabilities of a pregnancy and term delivery by IVF or an allied procedure. Only in this way can a judgment be made whether the best interests of the patient can be served by a surgical procedure or by assisted reproduction.

Procedures

Essentially all programs of assisted reproduction imply ovarian stimulation with the aim of harvesting multiple eggs because increasing pregnancy rates are directly related to the transfer of increasing numbers of fertilized eggs. It should be noted that as the number of transferred eggs goes up, so does the multiple pregnancy rate. To prevent high-order multiple births, many programs limit the number of transferred pre-embryos to three or, at most, four.

Ovarian stimulation usually is accomplished by the use of clomiphene citrate, human menopausal gonadotropins in a $1:1$ mixture of follicle-stimulating hormone (FSH) and luteinizing hormone (LH), or sometimes FSH alone. There has recently been increasing concomitant use of a gonadotropin releasing hormone agonist (GnRHa) such as leuprolide acetate. The GnRHa improves the control of ovarian stimulation by suppressing pituitary gonadotropin output. This allows for improved synchrony of nuclear oocyte maturation while blocking any premature and, therefore, detrimental LH surge.

The patient's response to stimulation is monitored by serum estradiol (E_2) values and ultrasound examination with a vaginal transducer. After suitable follicular growth and proper elevation of the serum E_2, final maturation of the oocytes can be induced by administration of exogenous human chorionic gonadotropin (hCG) as a surrogate for the LH surge, which is suppressed by the GnRHa and exogenous gonadotropins. Mature oocytes are collected about 34 to 36 hours after hCG administration.

Almost all programs now use ultrasound-directed transvaginal needle aspiration of the follicles as the method of oocyte collection. If GIFT of ZIFT is selected, a laparoscopy is necessary.

Oocytes in meiosis II can be inseminated as soon as convenient after harvest. Oocytes in meiosis I or prophase need to be allowed to mature to meiosis II before insemination (Fig. 28-1). Centrifugation and a "swim-up" technique are used to prepare the sperm if the semen examination is normal. The insemination culture medium is supplemented with protein support such as fetal cord serum or patient serum. With a normal semen examination 50,000 motile sperm per milliliter of culture medium seems adequate, but with compromised sperm examination a larger number of sperm seems to be helpful. Transfer by the transcervical route occurs about 48 hours after insemination, when the pre-embryos are in the four- to six-cell stage. ZIFT requires a laparoscopy to transfer the fertilizing egg at the pronuclear stage, about 24 hours after insemination.

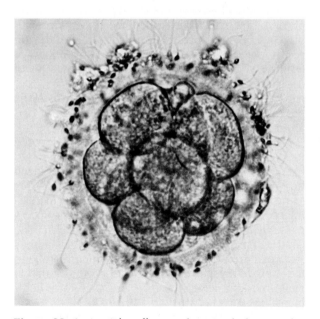

Figure 28–1. An eight-cell pre-embryo just before transfer. Note the large number of sperm adherent to the outer surface of the zona pellucida.

Prognostic Factors for Pregnancy

The Male

For both surgery and assisted reproduction, an adequate semen specimen is essential. It is no longer appropriate to eliminate from the evaluation of surgical results those patients with a complicating "male factor." Such patients can and should be suspected preoperatively, and appropriate alternate therapy should be used. If treatment of the male is unsuccessful—as it mostly is—IVF is helpful in patients with oligospermia, provided the total motile sperm population is not less than 1.5 million. Efforts to achieve pregnancy with an extremely low count, by micromanipulation of the oocyte or by injection of sperm into the oocyte, must be considered experimental.

Age

It has been observed by a number of investigators that the IVF pregnancy rates decrease and abortion rates increase in patients over age 40 (Table 28-1). This is probably true of surgical results as well, although reported surgical results are seldom stratified by age.

Patient Response

It was observed early in the IVF experience that patients responded differently to the same gonadotropin stimulation. This led to the classification of patients into low, intermediate, or high responders. Further study revealed that standardized basal FSH values correlated quite well with response—the higher the basal FSH value, the lower the response. With the use of GnRHa, started in the latter part of the luteal phase of the cycle preceding the stimulated cycle, larger numbers of better synchronized oocytes are harvested in the intermediate- and high-responder groups. This has led to substantially enhanced pregnancy and take-home baby rates in these groups. Luteal administration of GnRHa in the low-responder groups is of only marginal assistance, however, although follicular

TABLE 28–1
Pregnancy and Term Delivery Rate, Norfolk, 1989—Luprolide Before Gonadotropin Stimulation

AGE (YR)	NUMBER	% PREG/TR	% DEL/TR
<26	7	28.6	28.6
26–30	82	41.8	34.2
31–35	241	36.5	22.2
36–39	187	32.9	25.0
≥40	34	29.6	11.0

GnRHa, administered according to the "flare-up" technique, seems to be an improvement over stimulation without GnRHa. This enhanced result is probably accounted for, at least in part, by the suppression of the undesirable spontaneous LH surges. Such surges are particularly characteristic of low responders, and compromise the biologic potential of the oocytes.

Pregnancy Rates

There is no such thing as an IVF pregnancy rate against which surgical results can be compared. If the male is compromised to the point where pregnancy is unlikely to occur if all else is normal, IVF should be recommended, regardless of the surgical problem. Among husbands with normal sperm, however, there are categories of patients with well-determined prognostic characteristics that enable the observer to estimate with considerable accuracy the expectancy of pregnancy in a good IVF program. This anticipated take-home baby rate may vary from around 11% in patients over 40 years of age to well over 50% per cycle among high responders who use cryopreservation (Tables 28-1 and 28-2). It is against this individualized prognosis that the choice of surgery or assisted reproduction must be made.

SALPINGECTOMY

For many years it was taught and practiced that salpingectomy, as for ectopic pregnancy or pyosalpinx, was done by excising a generous portion of the intramural portion of the tube and closing the myometrium with interrupted stitches. The purpose of this technique was to prevent an interstitial abscess postoperatively when operating for a pyosalpinx or to prevent an interstitial pregnancy postoperatively. Both of these are well-recognized conditions in the older literature. With the widespread use of perioperative antibiotics, postoperative interstitial abscesses have disappeared, and interstitial pregnancies are so rare that a reevaluation of interstitial excision was the subject of a review. The difficulty is that after deep cornual resection, there is a measurable incidence of uterine rupture at that point, with a subsequent intrauterine pregnancy. This problem may be aggravated by the widespread use of assisted reproduction when intrauterine pregnancies occur after bilateral salpingectomy. Therefore, it seems appropriate that the technique of salpingectomy be modified for whatever indication and to recommend, for the reasons mentioned above, that if salpingectomy is carried out, a traditional cornual resection is inappropriate. A superficial resection at the

TABLE 28–2
Effect of the Use of Cryopreservation in an IVF Program, Norfolk, 1989— Luprolide Before Gonadotropin Stimulation

	NO. OF PREOVULATORY OOCYTES		
	1–5	6–10	>10
Peak E_2 (mean; pg/mL)	789	1,113	2,108
Preovs retrieved (mean)	3.7	7.7	15.8
Fertilization (%)	90.1‡	87.9†	84.3*
No. preovulatory oocytes frozen/cryopreservation cycle	1.0	2.8	7.6
Fresh Cycles			
Implantation (sacs/embryo; %)	13.4	11.2	12.4
Pregnancy rate/retrieval (%)	32.6	36.4	33.6
Ongoing pregnancy rate/retrieval (%)	23.4	22.2	22.7
Fresh + Cryopreservation Cycles (to date)			
Pregnancy rate/stimulation cycle (%)	32.6*	43.2	49.1†
Ongoing pregnancy rate/stimulation cycle (%)	23.4*	24.4*	35.5†
Projected Cumulative Performance (fresh + all cryopreservation cycles)			
Pregnancy rate (pregnancy/cycle; %)	32.6*	50.4†	75.7‡
Ongoing pregnancy rate/cycle (%)	23.4*	29.5*	54.1†

*<
†<
‡p < 0.05 (chi-square).

uterine attachment, removing none of the myometrium, is all that currently is required, with closure of the peritoneal defect by two or three interrupted stitches of very fine caliber.

TUBAL SURGERY

End Results

Because the evaluation of end results from tubal surgery is subject to a large number of variables, it is exceedingly difficult to be confident that any end result is a consequence of the procedures being tested. There are at least four major concerns: diagnosis, clinical material, operative technique, and presentation of end results.

Diagnosis. How is the diagnosis of tubal obstruction made? Neither hysterosalpingography nor laparoscopy with hydrotubation is free from technical problems and misinterpretations. As a general rule, one should be hesitant to offer or carry out an operative procedure based on a single diagnostic technique at a single examination. This caution about diagnostic dependability applies particularly to obstruction at the proximal end of the tube, especially when the tube appears otherwise normal at laparoscopic examination. A false-positive result may come from thickened endometrium in the premenstrual period, technical details with the apparatus, transient debris in the uterus or isthmic portions of the tube, or other conditions that can be quite different at a second examination with completely different findings.

Clinical Material. It is difficult to be confident in a test and control series that the clinical material is similar. Pelvic disease is so variable in its manifestations that no two cases are exactly alike. Furthermore, certain populations are more prone to reinfection, which surely influences end results.

Operative Technique. Many times an operative technique is the variable being tested in one of the two arms of a study population. It is not unusual, however, for the procedure itself to evolve during the course of a test, so that the results often do not express the technique. In this connection, ancillary matters often creep in, such as the routine use of prophylactic antibiotics, change in size of the suture material, and so forth, any of which can influence the end result.

Presentation of End Results. Of all the variables, the method of the presentation of end results is the most troublesome. It can be stated without question that the only meaningful methods for the evaluation of end results are by a cumulative pregnancy rate per month or year of exposure (a modified life table technique) or the calculation of a fecundity rate (ie, pregnancy per menstrual cycle of exposure). Despite this, even contemporary clinical trials often present results as a percentage of patients who are pregnant after a follow-up of some arbitrary minimum interval, usually 1 year. This has only limited value. The bibliography at the end of this chapter gives preference to those articles in which the end results are presented in a meaningful manner. It is not always possible to do this, simply because the data are not available.

Tubal Disease

Cornual Obstruction

As mentioned above, the diagnosis of cornual obstruction is tricky, and a single hysterogram or a single laparoscopic examination with apparent cornual obstruction cannot be relied on. When cornual obstruction is identified, if the distal tube appears normal by laparoscopy, and operative relief is considered, the diagnosis is almost always salpingitis isthmica nodosa. Because of poor results, the time has now passed when surgical relief for a tube with both distal and cornual obstructions should be undertaken. Results from assisted reproduction are far superior to the results obtained by surgery when the obstruction is at more than one site in the fallopian tube. An understanding of the causes of cornual obstruction can be obtained by a review of the histopathologic findings after excision of obstruction. Several of these studies have found either no demonstrable lesion obstructing the lumen or endosalpingosis or a related condition. The cases with no demonstrable obstruction or other pathologic lesion attest to the fickleness of the diagnostic accuracy of cornual obstruction.

For many years the reamer technique with excision of the obstructed portion of the proximal portion of the tube was carried out. The results from this type of macrosurgery were reasonably acceptable, even by contemporary standards, with a cumulative pregnancy rate of about 40% after 4 years and an even higher percentage if the isthmic portion of the tube was sacrificed and the ampullary portion of the tube was introduced through the reamer defect. Despite these good results, uterine rupture after tubal reimplantation was a troubling complication. For this reason, this procedure must be considered of historical interest only. An alternate surgical technique wherein a tubocornual anastomosis is carried out seems to avoid the complication of uterine rupture. One of the preoperative variables in this condition is the question of visualization of the intramural tube by hysterosalpingography before surgery. In an informative study Donnez and Casanas-Roux pointed out that the best results could be obtained if the intramural portion was visualized before surgery. Unfortunately these results are not presented by the life table technique, but the gross pregnancy rate was 44%. The practical point is that Donnez and Casanas-Roux advocated a surgical attempt even if the intramural portion could not be visualized preoperatively, pointing out that most often after amputation of the tube, patency of the intramural portion proved to be satisfactory despite preoperative information to the contrary.

Transuterine catheterization of the tube has been advocated as a method of overcoming proximal tubal obstruction. This currently must be considered an experimental approach. A study of the histopathologic material from cornual obstruction would lead to the suspicion that transuterine tubal catheterization would be likely to succeed when there was no intrinsic pathologic lesion. It would be difficult to imagine that permanent relief of obstruction owing to endosalpingosis or infection could be overcome by catheterization even if it were accompanied by dilatation. Practical results are not yet available in sufficient numbers to properly evaluate this approach to the problem. All of these techniques must be evaluated against the prospects of pregnancy by IVF.

Reanastomosis

Of all the therapeutic options available for various types of tubal disease, open surgical reanastomosis after surgical tubal interruption is perhaps the least controversial. It is the shining example of the best there is of microsurgical technique. Tubal anastomosis is not a single operative procedure. The technique used depends on the type of anastomosis required, for example isthmic-isthmic, ampullary-isthmic, or ampullary-ampullary.

Isthmic-Isthmic Anastomosis

The isthmic-isthmic anastomosis is one of the most satisfactory of the tubal procedures. With this situation there is no tubal or muscular disparity, and the operative procedure seldom takes more than 30 or 40 minutes for each tube. After excision of the stump of the tubes and the identification of the adequacy of the two lumina, the mesosalpinx can be brought together with a few interrupted stitches of No. 000000 or higher braided dacron or similar material. The tubal ends can be approximated by three or four muscle-to-muscle stitches, care being taken not to enter the lumen of the tube, as this seems to result in an undesirable endosalpingial reaction with postoperative obstruction. After approximation of the muscularis, the serosa can be brought together with three or four interrupted fine stitches. The operative procedure can be carried out either with or without a stent introduced through the lumen of the tube. Most surgeons prefer to remove the stent at the end of the procedure, but I have, for a number of years, left a coiled stent within the endometrial lumen, removing it a few weeks after the primary operation.

Isthmic-Ampullary Anastomosis

Isthmic-ampullary anastomosis requires the approximation of lumina with different diameters. There are various techniques to accomplish this. One commonly used method is to open the isthmic end longitudinally for a short distance, thus artificially increasing the lumen of the proximal stump. After this has been accomplished, the anastomosis is carried out with a technique essentially identical to that used in the isthmic-isthmic anastomosis. An alternate technique uses an Intracath with a needle perforating the proximal end of the distal portion of the tube to give a lumen essentially the same as that of the proximal stump. With this technique it usually is necessary for the suture to penetrate the lumen of the distal stump because of the thinness of the muscularis at this point. Despite this theoretical disadvantage, this technique has given excellent results, although the sudden change in luminal size would seem to predispose to ectopic pregnancy. This concern is not borne out in fact.

Ampullary-Ampullary Anastomosis

As has been mentioned, it is undesirable to enter the tubal lumen with the fine suture. The fact is that the muscularis in the ampullary portion of the tube often is so thin that a good bit of tearing will occur unless the endosalpinx or serosa is involved in the suture. Because results are satisfactory, one should not hesitate to do this in indicated situations. Indeed, through-and-through sutures in the ampullary portion of the tube often are required because of the delicacy of the tissues. In this technique a minimum bite should be taken on both sides of the anastomosis to prevent a diaphragmlike effect at the site. Seven or eight interrupted stitches are required around the circumference of the lumen for a satisfactory anastomosis. The results of this surgery are reasonably good, but the number of cases in which this is required is minimal, as this is an undesirable place to interrupt the tube and most often is used after interruption by the occasional operator or under special circumstances.

Contraindications to Tubal Reanastomosis

Tubal reanastomosis after surgical interruption is an extremely satisfactory operation. With the availability of assisted reproduction, however, there are certain situations in which it should not be recommended. The principal situation has to do with the residual length of the ampullary portion of the tube. A number of studies have indicated that if the residual ampulla is less than 4 cm, the expectancy of pregnancy is greatly diminished. The conclusion is obvious: Unless one can have at least 4 cm of ampulla after anastomosis, the patient should seek to solve her problem with IVF.

There has been some evidence to suggest that reanastomosis after interruption for a period more than 5 years had a decreased chance of success. Personal experience casts doubt on this conclusion. Thus prolonged surgical interruption may not be an absolute contraindication to surgical reanastomosis, provided there is adequate tubal length.

There is some evidence to suggest that the technique by which the tube is interrupted is reflected in ultimate pregnancy rates. Thus interruption by cautery seems to carry an ultimate pregnancy rate inferior to that of interruption by clips or bands. Although these data state the facts, it may well be that interruption by cautery results in a shortened ampullary length on reanastomosis, and that the inferior results are related to the length of the residual tube rather than to the technique of interruption. Nevertheless, if interruption has been by cautery, special attention needs to be paid to the residual length of the tube. If one has doubts in surveying the patient before recommending a technique for overcoming the tubal obstruction, IVF may represent a more reliable alternative to surgical reanastomosis.

Use of the Microscope

Microsurgical techniques are said to involve more than the use of magnification. These include meticulous handling of tissue, use of special light instruments, and use of very fine sutures—No. 000000 and smaller. In a randomized trial of end results comparing a compound microscope with an optic visor and loupe, no difference in success rates could be shown in terms of subsequent pregnancies. In this connection it is of interest that in an early series using fine suture material, a high pregnancy rate was obtained without the use of either loupe or microscope.

Distal Tubal Obstruction

Distal tubal obstruction represents the major portion of tubal obstructive disease. There are various alternate applicable techniques: macrosurgery, microsurgery, laparoscopic surgery with or without laser, and assisted reproduction. Data are not yet available to show a clear superiority of any one method of surgical treatment, but certain general facts have emerged.

Macrosurgery. Macrosurgery necessarily forms the base against which subsequent techniques must be compared. A number of series of salpingostomy using macrosurgical techniques have resulted in rather uniform pregnancy rates around 30% after 4 to 5 years.

Microsurgery. Microsurgical techniques have likewise resulted in pregnancy rates of around 30%. It was furthermore shown by Tulandi and colleagues that with open microsurgery, carbon dioxide laser salpingostomy had essentially the same pregnancy rate as microdiathermy. Other groups have shown the same results.

Operative Laparoscopy. It is remarkably difficult to find references to good studies of terminal salpingostomy by operative laparoscopic techniques. There are some reports in non–peer review journals; the results indicate that the expectancy of pregnancy is not too different from that reported from macrosurgical and microsurgical techniques. It is to be noted, however, that with open surgical procedures, there is little case selection, whereas laparoscopic operative techniques are selectively applied. It follows that laparoscopic operative procedures are being carried out on the most favorable cases, and the results must be viewed with this in mind.

Pregnancy Outcome in Relation to Extent of Disease. A number of studies with open operative techniques have related the pregnancy rates to the extent of tubal disease. They are in agreement, although it is difficult to compare one study with another because of varying techniques in classifying the extent of disease. In a study of 87 cases Rock and Jones showed that with mild disease a pregnancy rate of 87% was found, with moderate disease 30%, and with severe disease only 5%. About half of the patients (45/87) were in the category of mild and moderate degree of disease. Mage and coworkers showed essentially the same results. Although these workers divided the grades of disease into four categories, 42/76 (55%) cases were in the lesser grades with a pregnancy rate of 18/42 (43%), whereas in the severer categories among 34 patients there were but two pregnancies (6%).

Recommendations in Regard to Distal Salpingostomy. Current evidence fails to indicate any superiority of any one surgical technique on an end result basis. Laparoscopic approaches may have some advantage in length of hospital stay, hospital costs, quick return to work, and so on. Because of the difficulties of evaluating the data, it is premature to conclude that laparoscopic salpingostomy offers the patient the best possible chance to get pregnant. This, after all, should be the main goal of reparative surgery of the tubes. It seems clear from the data that success, as measured by pregnancy outcome from operative treatment of tubal disease, is related more to extent of disease than to operative technique. Furthermore, in severe tubal disease surgical treatment yields results that are inferior to those obtainable by IVF. For these reasons it is not difficult to recommend that in distal tubal obstruction, considerable care be exercised in the selection of patients for operative treatment. Patients with severe tubal disease should be offered IVF as primary therapy. This recommendation seems to apply to about half of all patients with distal obstruction.

Fimbrioplasty and Salpingolysis

By definition, the tubes in this group of patients are open when examined by hysterosalpingography or by hydrotubation at laparoscopy. There are pelvic adhesions of various degrees, however, and many times phymosis impeding the free motion of the fimbria. Thus these conditions are considered together, as seldom does one occur without at least some degree of the other. In these patients there is truly a choice between open operation, laparoscopic surgery with or without the laser, and assisted reproduction.

It is not easy by a review of the literature to determine past and current experience. In the older literature, with open operative procedure in which results are not expressed by the life table method, a postsalpingolysis pregnancy rate of 50% to 60% or somewhat higher is quite common. Lavy and associates found that in five series using macrosurgery, reporting a total of 465 patients, there was a pregnancy rate of 42%. When microsurgery was used among 271 patients, there were 142 pregnancies, or 52%. With laparoscopic techniques in about 100 patients, the pregnancy rate was 61%. There were no statistically significant differences among any of these series. Furthermore, Tulandi and colleagues were unable to show any difference in the subsequent intrauterine pregnancy rate between the use of microdiathermy and the carbon dioxide laser.

With results in the 50% to 60% range, an operative procedure with one of the techniques discussed above would seem preferable to the use of assisted reproduction in this particular clinical situation.

Reiterative Surgery for Tubal Disease

Second operations in patients who have failed to conceive after a primary tuboplasty have yielded very poor results. For this reason, with few exceptions, failed tuboplasty is a strong indication for the use of assisted reproduction.

OVARIAN PLACEMENT AT PELVIC LAPAROTOMY

Operations because of pain caused by extensive pelvic disease often involve not only the release of pelvic adhesions, but also removal of one or both fallopian tubes. At the end of the operative procedure the surgeon has certain options in the placement of the ovary. Clearly, if both tubes have been removed or if one is removed and the other is nonfunctional, assisted reproduction offers the patient an opportunity to achieve her family goals. In the interval when laparoscopic egg harvest was routinely being done, there were persuasive reasons to locate the remaining ovary as high in the pelvis as possible. In fact, a location in the region of the cornu of the uterus was far better than having the ovary in its normal position against the lateral pelvic wall.

The now widespread use of transvaginal ultrasonic-guided oocyte retrieval makes the high placement of the ovary a disadvantage. It is far better to locate the ovary low in the pelvis, in the cul-de-sac region, attached with one or two sutures to the posterior surface of the uterus in the neighborhood of the uterosacral ligaments, so that it will be immediately adjacent to the cul-de-sac for oocyte retrieval (Fig. 28-2).

TREATMENT OF ENDOMETRIOSIS

There is as much uncertainty now as ever concerning the optimum treatment for endometriosis. It has been difficult to show that treatment of stage I and II endometriosis is beneficial. Sometimes it has been concluded from such data that minimal endometriosis is not associated with infertility. An alternate and more likely conclusion is that the treatment of minimal endometriosis is not efficacious. This conclusion is supported by the fact that patients with mild endometriosis, treated or untreated, have a low fecundity level, which is probably explained on the basis of the endometriosis.

For more advanced disease, treatment apparently needs to be modulated according to whether or not there are endometriomas, as it usually is agreed that endometriomas larger than 1 or 2 cm are not favorably influenced by standard hormonal treatment for endometriosis. Therefore, with ovarian involvement, some type of surgical approach is useful. This has traditionally been by open operation, but in more recent years operative laparoscopy has been considered an alternative (see Ch. 16, 20, and 21).

Nevertheless, surgical therapy of whatever kind or medical treatment is not always successful. In that circumstance assisted reproduction, especially IVF, offers the possibility of therapy (Table 28-3). An additional point is that although fertility lessens with age, particularly past age 35, the expectancy of pregnancy with IVF does not diminish much until age 40 (see Table 28-1). In view of the delay that is necessarily involved in the medical management of endometriosis and, to a lesser extent, in the surgical management, consideration

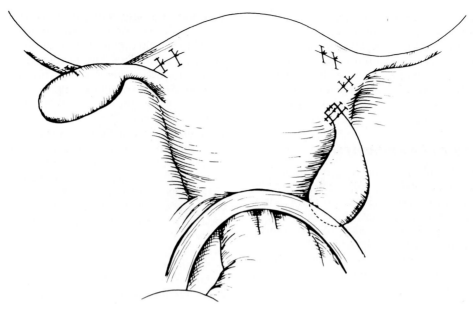

Figure 28–2. Pelvis after a bilateral salpingectomy. On the left, the utero-ovarian ligament is undisturbed, but the ovary is suspended to the round ligament to provide maximum access for laparoscopic approach. With anticipated transvaginal ultrasound-guided oocyte aspiration, this is no longer a desirable operative procedure. On the right, the utero-ovarian ligament has been divided and the ovary placed low in the pelvis for easy access from the vagina. It is not always necessary to sever the utero-ovarian ligament.

TABLE 28–3
Pregnancy Rate by Patient, Cycle, and Transfer of Preovulatory Oocytes According to the Stage of Endometriosis*

GROUP	NO. CYCLES	NO. TRANSFERS (%)	NO. PREGNANCIES	PREGNANCY RATE (%) PER		
				Patient	*Cycle*	*Transfer of Preovulatory Oocytes*
1†	54	50 (92.6)	9	39.1	16.7	20.0
2‡	191	168 (87.9)	46	50.5	24.1	28.4
3§	35	31 (88.6)	7	31.8	20.0	23.3

*No significant differences between the groups.
† Previous history of endometriosis but normal pelvis at laparoscopic oocyte retrieval.
‡ Stages I–II endometriosis (revised American Fertility Society classification).
§ Stages III–IV endometriosis.
Oehninger SO et al. In vitro fertilization and embryo transfer (IVF/ET): An established and successful therapy for endometriosis. J In Vitro Fert Embryo Trans 1988; 5:252.

needs to be given to the use of assisted reproduction as the primary method of therapy in patients over age 35.

CHANGING INDICATIONS FOR HYSTERECTOMY

For many years it was considered good practice to do a prophylactic hysterectomy when removing both fallopian tubes or when it otherwise appeared that future reproduction was impossible. The reason for this was to prevent the subsequent development of uterine cancer. The use of IVF has shown that fallopian tubes are not required for normal intrauterine pregnancies. Therefore, in deciding whether or not a hysterectomy should be done prophylactically in association with operations for benign pelvic disease, the future reproductive potential of the patient and her partner must be considered. In our litigious society malpractice suits have been brought against surgeons who have done a hysterectomy under these circumstances, wherein the plaintiff has taken the position that the surgeon should have realized that IVF would have made it possible for her to achieve a pregnancy. This thought can be extended even to patients in whom oophorectomy is necessary for whatever reason. With donor eggs, and exogenous hormonal stimulation, reproduction is possible if the uterus is in place. Therefore, hysterectomy must be carefully evaluated in all patients and a clear understanding arrived at before surgery as to whether or not the uterus will be retained. It is desirable that these considerations be clearly set forth in the operative permit, so that there will be little opportunity for misunderstanding after the operative procedure.

Bibliography

Daniell JF, Diamond MP, McLaughlin DS, et al. Clinical results of terminal salpingostomy with the use of the CO$_2$ laser: Report of the intraabdominal laser study group. Fertil Steril 1986;45:175.

Donnez J, Casanas-Roux F. Prognostic factors in fimbrial microsurgery. Fertil Steril 1986;46:200.

Donnez J, Casanas-Roux F: Prognostic factors influencing the pregnancy rate after microsurgical cornual anastomosis. Fertil Steril 1986;46:1089.

Ferraretti AP, Garcia JE, Acosta AA, Jones GS. Serum luteinizing hormone during ovulation induction with human menopausal gonadotropin for in vitro fertilization in normally menstruating women. Fertil Steril 1983;40:742.

Garcia JE, Jones HW Jr, Acosta AA, Andrews MC. Reconstructive pelvic operations for in vitro fertilization. Am J Obstet Gynecol 1985;153:172.

Jacobs LA, Thie J, Patton PE, Williams TJ. Primary microsurgery for postinflammatory tubal infertility. Fertil Steril 1988;50:855.

Jones HW Jr, Rock JA: On the reanastomosis of the fallopian tubes after surgical sterilization. Fertil Steril 1978;29:702.

Jones HW Jr, Rock JA: Reparative and Constructive Surgery of the Female Generative Tract. Baltimore: Williams & Wilkins, 1983:96, Table 7.8.

Lavy G, Diamond MP, DeCherney AH. Ectopic pregnancy: Its relationship to tubal reconstructive surgery. Fertil Steril 1987;47:543.

Mage G, Pouly JL, Boulet de Joliniere J, et al. Preoperative classification to predict intrauterine and ectopic pregnancy rates after distal tubal microsurgery. Fertil Steril 1986;46:807.

Mohlen K, Shortle B. Cornual resection as prophylaxis against interstitial pregnancy: Is it necessary or dangerous? A review of the literature. Eur J Obstet Gynecol Reprod Biol 1984;17:155.

Muasher SJ, Oehninger S, Simonetti S, et al. The value of basal and/or stimulated serum gonadotropin levels in prediction of stimulation response and in vitro fertilization outcome. Fertil Steril 1988;50:298.

Rock JA, Bergquist CA, Kimball AW Jr, et al. Comparison of the operating microscope and loupe for microsurgical tubal anastomosis: A randomized clinical trial. Fertil Steril 1984;41:229.

Rock JA, Katayama KP, Martin EJ, et al. Factors influencing the success of salpingostomy techniques for distal fimbrial obstruction. Obstet Gynecol 1978;52:591.

Rock JA, Katayama KP, Martin EJ, et al. Pregnancy outcome following uterotubal implantation: A comparison of the reamer and sharp cornual wedge excision techniques. Fertil Steril 1979;31:634.

Rock JA, Parmley TH, King TM, et al. Endometriosis and the development of tuboperitoneal fistulas after tubal ligation. Fertil Steril 1981;35:16.

Shortle B, Jewelewicz R. Uterine rupture following tubal reimplantation: Review of the literature and report of three additional cases. Obstet Gynecol Surv 1984;39:407.

Sulak PJ, Letterie GS, Coddington CC, et al. Histology of proximal tubal occlusion. Fertil Steril 1987;48:437.

Thurmond AS, Rosch J, Patton PE, et al. Fluoroscopic transcervical fallopian tube catheterization for diagnosis and treatment of female infertility caused by tubal obstruction. Radio Graphics 1988;8:621.

Tulandi T, Farag R, McInnes RA, et al. Reconstructive surgery of hydrosalpinx with and without the CO$_2$ laser. Fertil Steril 1984;42:839.

van Uem JF, Acosta AA, Swanson RJ, et al. Male factor evaluation in in vitro fertilization: Norfolk experience. Fertil Steril 1985;44:375.

Vasquez G, Winston RML, Boeckx W, Brosens I. Tubal lesions subsequent to sterilization and their relation to fertility after attempts at reversal. Am J Obstet Gynecol 1980;138:86.

29

Operative Injuries to the Ureter: Prevention, Recognition, and Management

JOHN D. THOMPSON

The subject of ureteral injury and repair has stimulated the concern and inventive genius of pelvic surgeons for a century or more. During these past 100 years, contributions too numerous to recount have added to our knowledge of the etiology, prevention, diagnosis, and treatment of ureteral injuries. The interest of gynecologists has coincided, understandably, with the development of operative management of gynecologic disease. For example, it was not until the technique of vaginal hysterectomy was developed and used that Tuffier and Levi were able to report in 1895 a series of 20 cases of ureterovaginal fistula following vaginal hysterectomy. Since the earliest recorded ureteral injury repairs of Berard (1841) and Simon (1869), early studies were made by Tuffier, Kelly, Sampson, Wertheim, Schauta, Stoeckel, Mackenrodt, and many others to the present.

From a historical viewpoint, the importance of the ureters in the surgical management of gynecologic disease has always been recognized. However, the first systematic studies of the ureter were done by John Sampson in the early twentieth century while he was still a young faculty member at Johns Hopkins. These studies are classics and are still very pertinent. They are recommended reading, especially for those beginning their careers in pelvic surgery. Intravenous pyelography, introduced in the 1920s, was not commonly used until the 1930s. As a noninvasive procedure, it became a most useful diagnostic tool in gynecologic surgery.

Injury to the ureter is one of the most serious complications of gynecologic surgery. It is a constant threat—a sword of Damocles hanging over every major operative procedure in the pelvis.* Fortunately, such injury is uncommon, occurring on the average between 0.1% and 1.5% of all cases of pelvic surgery. The ureter lies very near the female reproductive organs throughout its course from the pelvic brim to the bladder. Gynecologic disease can involve the ureters directly or can cause the course of the ureters to deviate. Various gynecologic operations come very close to the ureters. Even their normal anatomic relationships in the pelvis may vary. In spite of these close associations, the fact that injury to the ureter occurs infrequently is noteworthy and is a credit to the skill and attention given the ureter by gynecologic surgeons. Even so, injuries to the urinary tract during gynecologic operations represent the most common reason for medicolegal action against gynecologic surgeons. However, ureteral injury may be almost unavoidable in some situations, even in the

---

*Damocles was a courtier of the Greek tyrant Dionysius of Syracuse. Damocles talked so much about the happiness of kings that Dionysius decided to teach him a lesson. He invited Damocles to sit at the king's place at a banquet. Damocles was horrified to find a sword suspended by a single hair above his head. Dionysius thus showed the uncertainty of his life even when he seemed to be secure. "The sword of Damocles" came to be used for a dreaded tragedy that may happen at any moment.

hands of the most skilled and experienced gynecologic surgeon.

Ureteral injuries are far more serious and troublesome than injury to either the bladder or the rectum, the other two important sites of potential surgical trauma during pelvic surgery. Unrecognized ureteral injury is often associated with high morbidity, ureterovaginal fistulas, and the potential loss of kidney function. The risk of impairment or loss of kidney function is greatly increased when ureteral injury is not recognized until the postoperative period, when ureteral obstruction and/or urinary leakage are diagnosed.

This chapter emphasizes the prevention and early recognition of ureteral injury. Management of simple intraoperative injuries required of gynecologic surgeons is discussed. More complicated injuries that require especially skilled and experienced pelvic surgeons for proper management are also discussed.

EMBRYOLOGY AND ANATOMY OF THE URETERS

Because of the close relationship of the genital and urinary tracts, a clear understanding of the embryology and anatomy of ureters is essential. The urethra, bladder, and pelvic portion of the ureters represent the lower urinary tract portion of the urogenital system.

Embryology

Beginning at the fourth week of embryonic development, the cloaca is divided by the urorectal septum, which completely separates the rectum posteriorly from the urogenital sinus anteriorly by the eighth week. The urogenital sinus later develops into the urethra, bladder, and lower portion of the vagina in the female fetus. At the fifth week of development, when the mesonephric ducts from above join the cloaca below, the ureteric buds arise from the posterolateral wall of each mesonephric duct. Each ureteric bud elongates and develops into a ureter that eventually fuses with the developing metanephros (kidney) on the same side (Fig. 29-1).

By virtue of the close development and proximity of these urogenital organ systems, alterations in anatomy and physiologic function may occur in one system in the presence of pathology or disease in the other system. It is well known clinically that diseases of the reproductive organs may present with urinary tract signs or symptoms; the opposite may also occur. An abnormality or disease process of one system—such as congeni-

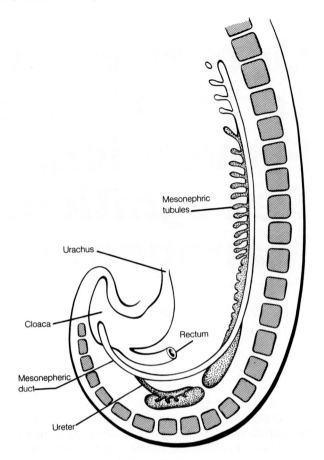

Figure 29–1. Embryologic development of the urinary and genital systems (32 days). (From Mattingly and Borkowf, 1974.)

tal malformations, anatomic variants, infection, neoplasm, or injury—may affect the function of the other system. For example, 35% to 40% of patients with congenital absence of one kidney will have anomalous development of the mullerian ducts. Moreover, when significant parts of one or both mullerian ducts are missing (as in congenital absence of the vagina and uterus) or obstructed (as in uterine didelphys with unilateral hematocolpos), major anomalies of the upper urinary collecting system will be found in 35% to 40% of patients.

In avoiding and managing ureteral injuries, the gynecologic surgeon must be aware of the possibility of anomalous development of the upper urinary collecting system and must be familiar with the following terminology:

Duplex kidney—a kidney with two pyelocaliceal systems.

Bifid system—two renal pelves joining at the uretero-pelvic junction (bifid pelvis) or two ureters joining above the bladder (bifid ureter).

Double ureters—complete duplication with two ureters on the same side draining the same kidney. The ureter draining the upper pole of a duplex kidney is the *upper-pole ureter,* and its orifice in the bladder is the *upper-pole orifice.* Similarly, the lower-pole pelvis is drained by the *lower-pole ureter,* and its orifice is the *lower-pole orifice.* In *double ureters,* the orifice of the upper-pole ureter has the more caudal and medial position in the bladder. The orifice of the lower-pole ureter has the more cranial and lateral position in the bladder. Exceptions to this relationship are so rare that it has been called the *Weigert-Meyer law.*

Approximately 1% of women have duplications of the ureter(s). Unilateral duplication is much more common than bilateral. In most instances, ureteral duplication is an incidental finding causing no symptoms. However, it is extremely helpful, especially in performing difficult gynecologic surgery, to know if ureteral duplication is present. If a ureteral catheter is placed preoperatively in only one ureter of a duplicated system, the ureter without the catheter is more likely to be injured. The gynecologic surgeon should keep in mind the possibility of ureteral duplication on one or both sides of the pelvis. If one ureter is identified, it cannot be assumed that it is the only one present on the same side.

An ectopic ureteral orifice, whether associated with a duplex or single drainage system, may be located caudal to the bladder trigone in the bladder neck or the urethra. In its embryologic development, failure of the ureter to separate from the mesonephric duct results in drainage through the genital tract structures derived from the paramesonephric (mullerian) ducts (ie, uterus, cervix, or vagina). In addition, extraurinary tract drainage of urine may rarely be established by way of a connection between an ectopic ureter and Gartner's duct, a vestigial remnant of the degenerated mesonephric duct in the female. The commonly accepted explanation for duplication and the other anomalies of the ureters is a variation in the origin of the ureteral bud(s) from the mesonephric ducts.

If a congenital anomaly is responsible for the kidney being located in the pelvis in a patient who is having a gynecologic operation, the course of the ureter can be unpredictable. To avoid injury, it may be necessary to dissect the ureter carefully and completely. Preoperative placement of a ureteral catheter may also be helpful. It is especially important to be careful with the ureter of a solitary pelvic kidney.

Anatomy

Three anatomic layers can be identified in the ureter: the transitional epithelium lining the lumen; the smooth muscle of the ureteral wall composed of longitudinal, circular, and spiral fibers to provide regular and efficient peristaltic waves several times each minute; and an adventitial sheath surrounding the ureter and containing and protecting its blood vessels.

In its course from the renal pelvis to the bladder, the ureter is divided anatomically into two major components: abdominal and pelvic. The ureter measures approximately 25–30 cm in length, depending on the height of the patient. In most people, the abdominal and pelvic components are approximately equal in length, 12–15 cm each. The abdominal ureter passes along the anterior surface of the psoas muscle to the pelvic inlet. The right ureter is located close to the lower portion of the vena cava, where this vessel rests on the medial border of the psoas muscle. The ureters enter the pelvis by coursing over the iliac vessels at the point of division of the common iliac artery into the external iliac and hypogastric vessels. The pelvic ureter passes along the posterolateral pelvic wall, adjacent to the anterior border of the greater sciatic notch and slightly anterior to the hypogastric artery until it reaches deep in the pelvis at the level of the ischial spine. In this area, the ureter lies medial to the branches of the anterior division of the hypogastric artery and lateral to the peritoneum of the cul-de-sac of Douglas (Fig. 29-2).

The ureter can usually be conveniently identified in its retroperitoneal location as it crosses the common iliac artery at the pelvic brim to enter the upper pelvis. Here the ureter tends to elevate the thin and transparent peritoneum and is both visible and palpable unless the peritoneum is thickened or involved in a disease process. On the left side, the position of the ureter in relation to the common iliac artery may be obscured by the sigmoid colon. When the anatomy is normal, the ureter can usually be followed visually from the pelvic brim throughout its course beneath the peritoneum along the lateral wall of the true pelvis until it disappears beneath the uterine vessels and into the "tunnel" through the cardinal ligament before entering the bladder. On the pelvic sidewall beneath the peritoneum, peristalsis can be seen in the ureter, and this is helpful in its identification. Ureteral peristalsis can be stimulated by simply stroking it longitudinally along its course; it is not necessary to pinch the ureter to stimulate peristalsis (Fig. 29-3).

When the peritoneum is opened above the ureter, the ureter's course can be easily traced along the lateral pelvic wall. Deep in the pelvis the ureter courses along the lateral side of the uterosacral ligament to enter the

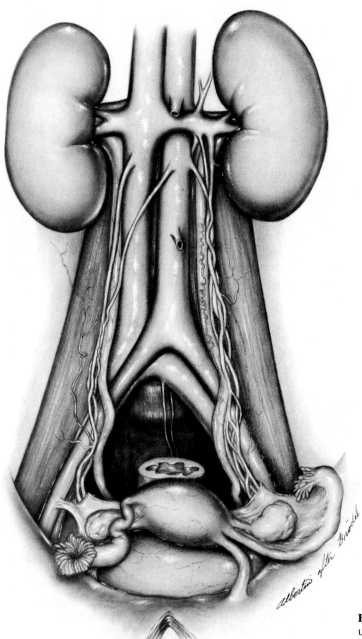

Figure 29–2. Abdominal and pelvic portions of the ureter showing relationship to aorta, psoas muscle, vena cava, and common iliac artery and vein.

base of the broad ligament (the cardinal ligament). The ureter passes beneath the uterine artery approximately 1.5 cm lateral to the cervix at the level of the internal cervical os (Figure 29-3). As the distal portion of the ureter approaches the bladder, it passes medially over the anterior vaginal fornix before entering the wall of the bladder, just above the trigone (Figs. 29-4 *A–B* and 29-5). This angulation in the lower part of the ureter as it passes beneath the uterine vessels and turns to join

the bladder is sometimes referred to as the knee of the ureter. The lowest 1–2 cm of the ureter can sometimes be felt by examination through the vagina.

Freund and Joseph (1869) provided one of the earliest anatomic descriptions of the ureters and their normal relation to the various structures in the pelvis. These anatomists emphasized that the course of the two ureters was not always symmetrical and demonstrated that the left ureter was frequently closer to the cervix than

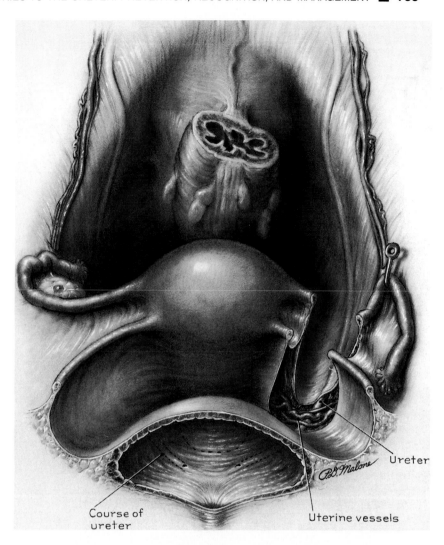

Figure 29–3. Dissection showing relation of ureters to pelvic viscera.

Course of ureter

Ureter

Uterine vessels

the right. As shown by the classic study of Sampson (1904), the proximity of the ureter to either side of the cervix may vary considerably with the position of the uterus in the pelvis, even in the absence of pathology (Fig. 29-6). With displacement of the uterus to one side or the other by parametrial scarring or disease, the ureter may be drawn closer to or displaced farther from the lateral wall of the cervix.

Cinefluoroscopic studies of the topography of the pelvic ureters by Hofmeister confirmed this asymmetry of the terminal ureters and demonstrated that the average distance of the ureter from the cervix of a normal-sized uterus at the level of the uterine artery was approximately 2.1 cm. The important clinical consideration for the pelvic surgeon to understand is the close approximation of the terminal ureter to the cervix and to the vaginal fornices as it passes medially to enter the bladder (see Figs. 29-4, 29-5, and 29-6). This close

relationship was reemphasized by Hofmeister, who found by cinefluoroscopy during an anterior colporrhaphy that the ureter was only 0.9 cm from the surgeon's needle at the closest point in the upper one third of the vagina.

Blood Supply

The ureter has the advantage of a blood supply from multiple sources, which gives it preferential healing capabilities should injury occur. A freely anastomosing arterial network supplies the superior segment of the ureter with branches from renal and ovarian arteries. The middle segment derives its blood supply directly from aortic branches and from a vessel from the common iliac artery. The pelvic ureter is nourished by multiple anastomosing vessels, including branches from the uterine,

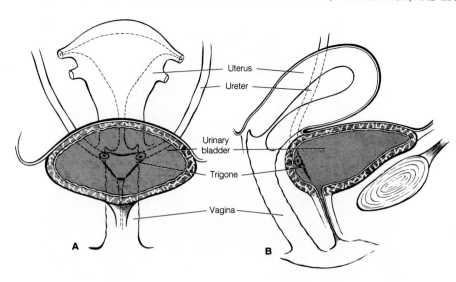

Figure 29–4. *A*, Anterior view of the normal anatomy of ureter and bladder. The terminal end of the ureter passes medially from the lateral pelvic wall and crosses over the anterior fornix, where it enters the trigone of the bladder, which rests on the upper one third of the anterior vaginal wall. *B*, Sagittal view of anatomic relationship of ureter and bladder base. Note that the ureter enters the trigone in the area of the upper one third of the vagina.

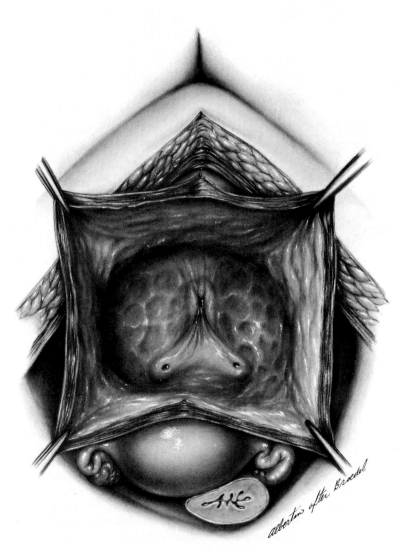

Figure 29–5. Opened view of bladder showing relationship of trigone and bladder base to adjacent uterus and vagina.

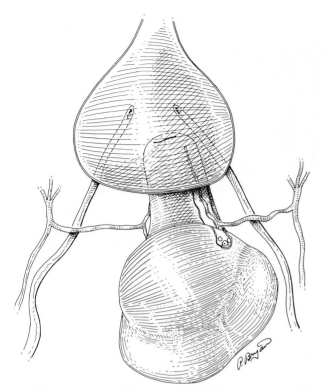

Figure 29–6. The distance between the uterine isthmus and the ureter is not always the same on each side. As illustrated here, the right ureter is closer to the uterus than the left.

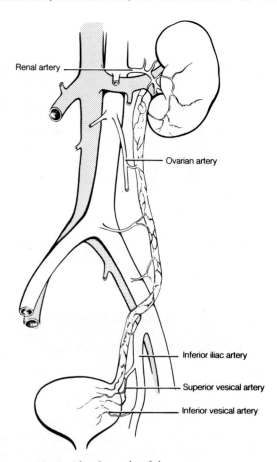

Figure 29–7. Blood supply of the ureter.

vaginal, middle hemorrhoidal, and vesical arteries. A rather constant branch arises from the hypogastric artery near its origin. This vessel is frequently seen in the course of dissections to remove pelvic lymph nodes. Ureteral veins follow a similar intercommunicating network. Both arteries and veins can be easily demonstrated by the prominent longitudinal vessels that course within the adventitia of the ureter (Fig. 29-7). Because the blood supply to the upper and middle portions of the ureter is from its medial side, ureteral exploration or an incision into the ureter is made preferably along the *lateral* margin, taking care not to injure the longitudinal arteries and veins. Since the pelvic ureter derives its blood supply principally from the lateral side, it would be logical to dissect along the medial side in an effort to produce the least vascular damage. Because of the proximity of branches of the hypogastric artery and vein, the pelvic ureter must be dissected carefully to avoid bleeding. The rich collateral blood supply permits extensive mobilization of the ureter from its retroperitoneal course so long as the longitudinal blood supply within the periureteral adventitia is not traumatized.

As shown in Figure 29-8 *A–B*, the ureteral vessels anastomose freely with each other in the surrounding adventitia. Waldeyer (1892) described this loose connective tissue adjacent to the muscular wall of the ureter, noting the longitudinal course of the small arteries and veins that intercommunicate along the entire ureter. Sampson (1904) emphasized the efficiency of this periureteral arterial plexus and the importance of its preservation, especially in the more extensive operations for gynecologic malignancies. Interference with these vessels by trauma or skeletonization of the ureter by removal of this pseudo-periureteral sheath may produce local ischemia of a segment of the ureter and subsequent necrosis with rupture of the ureteral wall, or fibrosis with periureteral scarring, stenosis of the lumen, and hydroureter.

According to Sampson (1904), the ureter, through its peristalsis, forms a pseudo-sheath from the tissues about it. The sheath varies with the tissue along its course and cannot be considered a distinct structure belonging to the ureter. It should not be mistaken for Waldeyer's sheath, which extends only a short distance

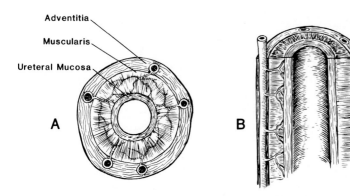

Adventitia
Muscularis
Ureteral Mucosa

A   B

Figure 29–8. Cross section (*A*) and sagittal (*B*) views of the longitudinal arteries and veins in the adventitia provide the important collateral circulation along the course of the ureter.

above the bladder and consists mostly of bundles of smooth muscle. The pseudoperiureteral sheath blends with the sheath of Waldeyer and encloses its lower end just above the bladder.

GYNECOLOGIC DISEASES AND OTHER CONDITIONS THAT MAY OBSTRUCT THE URETER

In their course through the pelvis the ureters are susceptible to involvement and compression by a variety of normal physiologic and pathologic conditions that affect the other structures and organs in the pelvis. These include pregnancy, both normal and abnormal; benign and malignant tumors; vascular anomalies; retroperitoneal collections of lymph, blood, or pus; organ displacement; and a miscellaneous variety of other conditions. The experienced gynecologic surgeon will understand when the symptoms or pelvic findings suggest ureteral involvement and the appropriateness of additional preoperative studies or preparation. Frequently, ureteral compression with dilatation above results from a large intraperitoneal tumor resting against the ureter at the pelvic brim. Simply lifting the tumor up and off the ureter will relieve the obstruction. This is common with a large leiomyomatous uterus. At other times, a disease process may cause ureteral obstruction by actually involving periureteral tissues and the ureteral wall. This requires greater technical skill and precise dissection to free the ureter from the disease that surrounds it.

A normal intrauterine *pregnancy* may be associated with ureteral obstruction, more commonly present on the right than on the left. An enlarging gravid uterus and the distended ovarian vessels in the right infundibulopelvic ligament may compress the right ureter at the pelvic brim while the left ureter is protected from compression by the sigmoid colon. High levels of progesterone in pregnancy have also been implicated in causing ureteral ectasia. Such normal physiologic dila-

tation is rarely the cause of clinically significant signs or symptoms in the absence of other urinary tract disease. The ectasia promptly disappears after delivery. An abdominal pregnancy or chronic tubal pregnancy that ruptures between the leaves of the broad ligament can be associated with ureteral obstruction.

Large pelvic tumors, most commonly uterine leiomyomas and large benign or malignant, solid or cystic ovarian tumors are commonly associated with ureteral obstruction by extrinsic compression. Especially notable are leiomyomas that arise in the cervix or lower uterus and cause direct compression of the bladder trigone and lower ureters. Over a period of months such tumors can cause uremia.

Of all *gynecologic malignancies* that can be associated with ureteral obstruction, invasive cervical cancer is the most notorious. Indeed, bilateral ureteral obstruction with uremia is a frequent cause of death with cervical cancer. Dilatation of the ureters in patients with cervical cancer is an ominous sign ordinarily associated with advanced disease. Endometrial adenocarcinoma and uterine sarcoma may involve the ureters, but not as commonly. The ureters may be compressed and deviated anteriorly and medially in their course by a variety of retroperitoneal tumors and by tumor metastatic to retroperitoneal lymph nodes. Excretory urography can be a most rewarding diagnostic procedure in determining that a pelvic mass is retroperitoneal, but to demonstrate the ureteral displacement commonly associated with such tumors, lateral and oblique films must be included in the study.

Most patients with *endometriosis* show no involvement of the ureters. In the presence of extensive endometriosis, the ureters may be encased in tissue hardened by invasive endometriotic implants and intense fibrosis to the point of causing even complete obstruction. Since most of these patients will have had few symptoms referable to the urinary tract, the diagnosis must be based on a high index of suspicion. The finding on pelvic examination of an enlarged, adherent, irregular and tender ovarian mass or of tender nodularity in the cul-de-sac or along the uterosacral ligaments or in the wall of the rectosigmoid colon should lead one to suspect ureteral involvement as well. The routine use of excretory urography in such cases will warn the gynecologic surgeon of the difficult dissection that will be encountered. The ovary, sigmoid colon, uterosacral ligament, and uterine artery and vein will all be found gathered together with the ureter in a firm, irregular mass of endometriosis in which planes of dissection are obscure and exposure is difficult. To avoid ureteral damage in the attempt to remove all the endometriosis, the ureter, it is hoped, can be identified in more normal tissue above and then carefully traced downward and freed. A ureteral catheter and/or magnification with loupes may facilitate dissection. Occasionally, the ureter is obstructed by infiltration of its wall and sheath by endometriosis. In this case, ureterolysis will not be sufficient. Transection of the ureter above the point of obstruction with ureteroneocystostomy will be required.

Hydroureteronephrosis may be found in association with active *tubo-ovarian abscess(es)*. The obstruction may be unilateral, but it is commonly bilateral. If the infection has extended to involve retroperitoneal spaces, ligneous peritonitis with ureteral obstruction may result. The obstruction is often relieved when the infection is successfully treated with antibiotics and/or surgery. At operation, dissection of the ureter is not done to relieve obstruction as much as to ensure that the ureters will not be injured. If present, the ureteral obstruction will usually disappear after the tubo-ovarian abscess is removed and the induration of periureteral tissues resolves. To avoid injury, however, dissection may be needed for ureteral identification. Sometimes the best way to remove the abscess is an extraperitoneal approach that would allow ureteral identification at the same time.

Marked dilatation of both ureters is uniformly present when complete *uterine procidentia* has been chronic over many months or years. Lesser degrees of descensus may be associated with lesser degrees of dilatation. Urography and anatomic studies have suggested that the obstruction lies at the point where the ureters course beneath the uterine vessels and through the lateral cervical attachments. As the uterus and bladder descend through the vaginal introitus and beyond, the knee of the ureter is greatly exaggerated, to the point that the ureters may actually be dragged outside the body. Symptoms related to the hydroureter are usually absent unless impairment of renal function occurs in longstanding cases. Because hydroureteronephrosis is such a standard and consistent finding in patients with procidentia, urologic investigations are not commonly done or needed. The obstruction is easily relieved by colporrhaphy and surgical correction of the prociden-

tia. When surgical correction is not appropriate, a pessary may be used to replace the uterus and relieve the ureteral obstruction.

It has been suggested that the right ureter can be obstructed by the ovarian veins where they cross the ureter on a course to join the inferior vena cava and that this may be associated with right-sided flank pain and recurrent urinary tract infections. We doubt the existence of this so-called *ovarian vein syndrome* and believe that surgery for this condition is rarely, if ever, justified. On the other hand, when a postpartum patient develops suppurative pelvic thrombophlebitis and ovarian vein thrombophlebitis, definite ureteral obstruction occurs from extension of the inflammatory process to periureteral tissues.

Other rare gynecologic diseases may also involve the ureters. An *ovarian remnant* may cause hydroureter. Indeed, the first case of *ovarian remnant syndrome* was reported by Kaufman, a urologist who made the discovery of ovarian remnants during the investigation of two patients with ureteral obstruction. Major and others have reported ureteral obstruction in patients with ovarian remnants. Pettit and Lee have emphasized how tedious the ureteral dissection in these patients is. Three of nine patients had dilatation of ureters on preoperative excretory urography, and two additional patients had ureteral distortion on CT scan.

A *pelvic hematoma* that develops after delivery or after a surgical procedure may cause deviation and obstruction of the ureter. These same changes can be seen in a patient who develops a lymphocyst following an extensive operation for pelvic malignancy.

TYPES AND ANATOMIC LOCATIONS OF URETERAL INJURY

There are six types of operative trauma to the ureter: crushing from misapplication of a clamp(s); ligation with suture; transection (either partial or complete); angulation with secondary obstruction (either partial or complete); ischemia that results from stripping the ureteral wall of its blood supply for a short distance; and resection of a segment of ureter, usually intentional in the course of an extensive operation for malignant disease. Of course, combinations of these may also occur. An injury may result from difficult or careless surgery. It may occur unexpectedly during a routine procedure. The significance of the injury can be compounded if it occurs in a pelvis with active infection, previous irradiation, or other disease, such as endometriosis, that may have already caused periureteral fibrosis or ischemia. Injuries may be bilateral or unilateral, the former being much less frequent but much more serious than the latter. Obviously, unilateral ureteral injury in a patient with absent or poor function of the contralateral kidney is also more serious.

Ureteral injury with gynecologic operations usually occurs in one of four locations (see Fig. 29-3): (1) in the base of the broad ligament, where the ureter passes beneath the uterine vessels; (2) beyond the uterine vessels as the ureter passes through its tunnel in the cardinal ligament and turns anteriorly and medially to enter the bladder; (3) at or below the infundibulopelvic ligament; and (4) along the course of the ureter on the lateral pelvic sidewall just above the uterosacral ligament. In our experience the majority of ureteral injuries involve the lowest 3 cm, between the uterine vessels and the bladder. This site of injury is more common, but injury to the ureter along the lateral pelvic sidewall or beneath the infundibulopelvic ligament can also occur. Actually, the ureter may be injured at any point along its course.

OPERATIVE PROCEDURES INVOLVED IN URETERAL INJURY

Although ureteral injuries may occur with colorectal surgery for cancer and inflammatory bowel disease, with appendectomy, with iliac endarterectomy, and with procedures done by urologic surgeons, about 75% of injuries result from gynecologic operations. Of these, about three fourths of ureteral injuries occur during an abdominal gynecologic procedure. About one fourth occur during a vaginal procedure. Almost any gynecologic operation can result in ureteral injury. The incidence is highest (1.0%–2.0%) with extensive abdominal operations for invasive cancer of the cervix. The incidence is higher for abdominal hysterectomy (0.5%–1.0%) than for vaginal hysterectomy (0.1%). This difference in frequency of injury between abdominal and vaginal hysterectomy is due primarily to the fact that an abdominal hysterectomy is often done in patients with extensive disease adjacent to the ureters, which places them at greater risk. In general, a vaginal hysterectomy is more commonly performed in patients with symptomatic vaginal relaxation and uterine prolapse. These patients do not have pelvic disease that would distort the location of the lower ureter unless complete uterine procidentia is present. The incidence of ureteral injury with adnexal surgery or with suprapubic urethropexy operations is below 0.1%. The ureter may be at greater risk of injury when an operation is done to remove a tubo-ovarian abscess, extensive pelvic endometriosis, an intraligamentary leiomyoma, an adherent residual adnexa, an ovarian remnant, or presacral nerves. In our experience, the risk of ureteral injury is especially high when a partial vaginectomy is done with either abdominal or vaginal hysterectomy or

when an extrafascial technique of removing the cervix is more appropriate (as in patients with endometrial malignancies) than the customary intrafascial technique for performing total abdominal hysterectomy for benign disease. Sutures placed in the uterosacral ligaments to support the vaginal apex after the uterus is removed either abdominally or vaginally can kink or obstruct the ureters. If not done carefully, the Moschcowitz technique of closing the cul-de-sac can cause the same problem. Laparoscopy with use of electrocoagulation or laser for fulguration of endometriosis, lysis of adhesions, transection of uterosacral ligaments, and even tubal sterilization must be done carefully to avoid damage to the ureter. Above the pelvis, more ureteral injuries can be expected as para-aortic node samplings are done more frequently in patients with gynecologic malignancies.

The ureter is rarely injured during obstetric operations. However, when total abdominal hysterectomy is done at the time of cesarean section or in the immediate postpartum period, ureteral injury may occur, because the cervix is larger and closer to the lower ureters, especially if dilatation and effacement of the cervix have begun. In a series of 1000 consecutive cesarean hysterectomies at Charity Hospital in New Orleans, Barclay reported two ureteral injuries among 200 emergency operations and only two ureteral injuries among 800 elective operations. Plauche reported a literature review of the surgical complications of cesarean hysterectomies between 1951 and 1984. Among 5220 operations there were 23 (0.44%) ureteral injuries and 5 (0.1%) ureterovaginal fistulas. Deep lacerations through the cervix and lateral vaginal fornix from difficult forceps deliveries can also involve the ureter, as reported by Feiner.

General reports of the incidence of ureteral injury will vary according to the experience of the surgeons, the number of patients in the series with advanced pelvic disease, and the number of extensive operations

TABLE 29–1
Gynecologic Procedures Associated with Ureteral Injury*

OPERATIVE PROCEDURE	INCIDENCE OF URETERAL INJURY (PERCENT)
Abdominal hysterectomy	0.5–1.0
Vaginal hysterectomy	0.1
Extensive Wertheim hysterectomy	1.0–2.0
Adnexectomy	0.1
Marshall-Marchetti-Krantz procedure	<0.1

*Data derived from current literature.

for malignant disease included in the series (Table 29-1). Some reports have suggested that the incidence of ureteral injury has increased during the past four to five decades since removal of the uterine cervix has become a standard procedure with abdominal hysterectomy. In our series of ureteral injuries, none occurred among patients who had subtotal abdominal hysterectomy. It is obviously the removal of the cervix that is the most risky part of the total abdominal hysterectomy procedure, since most injuries occur in the lowest 3 cm of ureter just above the bladder. Current data, however, do not support the view of an increasing incidence. Sampson's original review in 1902 reported ureteral injury in 0.78% of patients in a series of 4086 major gynecologic operations at the Johns Hopkins Hospital. In 1939, Newell reported 0.4% ureteral injuries among 3144 hysterectomies. This percentage was similar to that found by Benson and Hinmann, who noted in 1955 a percentage of 0.58 in 6211 major gynecologic operations. In 1956, Everett and Mattingly observed ureteral injury in 0.26% of 15,000 major pelvic operations at the Johns Hopkins Hospital. Their data showed that 60% of these injuries occurred following abdominal procedures and 40% followed vaginal operations, including 500 vaginal hysterectomies. In our series of 9171 major gynecologic operations done at Grady Memorial Hospital between 1959 and 1977, 43 ureteral injuries occurred in 39 patients, a percentage of 0.43. Thirty-five were unilateral and four were bilateral. Abdominal surgery accounted for 77% of the injuries and vaginal surgery was associated with 23%. When extensive operations for gynecologic malignancies were not included, ureteral injury occurred in 0.37% of abdominal operations and in 0.22% of vaginal operations. The most current series was reported by Mann and others from the State University of New York at Stony Brook. Between 1980 and 1987, 17 ureteral injuries occurred during 3185 major gynecologic operations. Fourteen (0.4%) were "accidental." Indeed, the general incidence of ureteral injury with major gynecologic surgery has not changed in the past 50 years.

Extensive hysterectomy with pelvic lymphadenectomy for invasive cervical carcinoma has contributed more to ureteral injury than any other pelvic operation. The dissection of the pelvic ureters as originally done in this operation resulted in a high incidence of injury, even when the operation was performed by an experienced pelvic surgeon. Wertheim himself reported in his experience with 500 cases that 10% developed ureteral fistulas. Meigs revived interest in primary surgery for invasive cervical cancer in 1945 and reported ureteral fistulas in 7.2% in a series of 85 operations. In a 1955 report by Liu and Meigs of 473 "radical" hysterectomies, fistulas remained essentially unchanged at 7.4%. With more recent improvements in technique of extensive hysterectomy, operative injury to the ureters should be only slightly more frequent than that for hysterectomy for benign disease and should be seen in no more than 1% to 2% of such cases. This is confirmed by recent reports by Hatch and associates from the University of Alabama, by Larson and associates from the M.D. Anderson Hospital and Tumor Institute, and by our own experience at Emory University. It should be emphasized that the type of ureteral injury that occurs with an extensive hysterectomy is associated with a complete dissection of the lowest 4–6 cm of each ureter with the possibility of stripping the ureter of its blood supply sufficient to cause ischemia, necrosis, and rupture of the ureteral wall with subsequent formation of a urinoma that eventually dissects its way to the vaginal cuff for drainage and fistula formation. Even without fistula formation, a stenosis of the lumen of the lower ureter may lead to hydroureter, hydronephrosis, and gradual impairment of kidney function. Obviously, this may portend more serious consequences for continued normal renal function, especially if both lower ureters become stenotic.

SEQUELAE OF URETERAL INJURY

Depending on a variety of circumstances, the following sequelae of ureteral injury can be described:

1. *Spontaneous resolution and healing.* When injury to the ureter has been minor, only temporary and minimal interference with function may result. A suture placed too close to the ureter may cause a minor degree of kinking and obstruction that may disappear in time. Careful dissection of the lower ureter from its bed may be associated with transient periureteral edema and scarring, resulting in some dilatation of the ureter that usually disappears in a few weeks. Spontaneous healing of a ureterovaginal fistula without residual impairment of ureteral function is possible but highly unlikely and should not be expected.

2. *Posthydronephrotic renal atrophy with or without sepsis.* With complete ligation of a ureter, unrecognized at operation or in the postoperative period, it is inevitable that the kidney function will gradually and silently disappear, sometimes without clinical signs and symptoms. No one can be certain how often this occurs. Newell in 1939 reported six cases of ligated ureters found at autopsy. In none of the cases was injury to the ureters suspected prior to autopsy. Although such undoubted cases as these and others have been reported, it must be a rare occurrence. We reviewed several thousand autopsy findings in female patients who died of general causes at

Grady Hospital over a 25-year period and were unable to find a single case of silent atrophy of the kidney following gynecologic surgery. Excretory urograms taken routinely in large numbers of asymptomatic patients following gynecologic operations show very little evidence of unrecognized ureteral obstruction. A silent atrophy is possible only if there is no infection. When infection is present, the problem is immediately evident and quickly diagnosed. We do not agree with Hofmeister and others that the majority of ureteral injuries today are asymptomatic, unrecognized, and therefore unreported.

A frequently asked question is, "For how long can a kidney be completely obstructed and subsequently return to normal function after relief of obstruction?" Animal experiments suggest that there is rarely any return of renal function with complete ureteral obstruction of more than 40 days. However, there is clinical evidence of recovery of renal function in the human after longer periods of ureteral obstruction. Three cases reported by Shapiro and Bennett showed recovery of renal function following apparent occlusion for periods ranging from 28 to 158 days. The major problem in defining the absence of renal function in these and other cases is the imprecision of most diagnostic techniques. Although excretory urograms and renograms are helpful clinical tests, they may not document a complete absence of renal function or a complete return of function after obstruction is relieved. There have been reports of cases of apparent renal obstruction lasting more than 100 days in which relatively normal kidney function returned after relief of the ureteral obstruction (eg, those reported by Everett and Williams). Based on this information, if any evidence of renal function is present within 3 months following apparent complete ureteral obstruction, it is reasonable to attempt to salvage the kidney by relieving the obstruction if other circumstances of the patient's clinical condition are appropriate to such an attempt.

3. *Ureteral necrosis with urinary extravasation.* A ureter that has been ligated does not usually stay ligated. The ureteral wall eventually necroses and urine escapes. In fact, it is somewhat difficult to ligate a ureter intentionally and have it stay permanently ligated. Numerous inventive techniques of intentional ligation have been tried, usually to no avail. After ligation, the ureteral lumen dilates to an extreme degree. Intraluminal pressure pushes the thinned-out ureteral wall against the suture ligature and rupture of an ischemic area eventu-

ally occurs with subsequent urinary extravasation into periureteral tissues. If the ureter is injured at an operation that does not include a fresh incision into the peritoneal cavity or into the vagina (as in extraperitoneal pelvic lymphadenectomy), then the extravasated urine may form a urinoma. If the urinoma becomes infected, a retroperitoneal abscess is likely to form. If the ureter is injured at an operation that includes a fresh incision in the peritoneum but not in the vagina (as in removal of an adherent residual adnexa), the urine will extravasate into the peritoneal cavity with urinary ascites and possible peritonitis. If the ureter is injured at an operation that includes a fresh incision into the vagina (as in total abdominal hysterectomy), the extravasated urine will eventually find its way to the vaginal vault for drainage, creating a ureterovaginal fistula.

Of course, ureteral necrosis with rupture and extravasation of urine can occur when the ureter is stripped of its blood supply, as in performing a dissection of the lower ureter in extensive hysterectomy for invasive cancer of the cervix. The sequence of events in this situation is illustrated by Sampson's work (Fig. 29-9).

4. *Secondary stenosis of the ureteral lumen at the site of injury and/or stenosis of the fistula tract with silent atrophy of the kidney or pyoureteronephrosis.* The stenosis that develops at the site of injury is one of the most important events in the pathogenesis of subsequent insidious loss of kidney function. The stenosis is associated with gradually increasing hydroureter and hydronephrosis. When the stenosis of a ureterovaginal fistula tract is complete, urine leakage through the fistula ceases. The kidney function is in imminent danger of being lost if the obstruction is not relieved.

5. *Uremia.* Uremia results from bilateral ureteral injury with obstruction. Although rare, suppression of contralateral kidney function can result from unilateral ureteral injury. Of course, ligation of the ureter of a solitary kidney also results in uremia.

With bilateral ureteral ligation, the patient is anuric immediately following surgery. For the first 24–48 hours, anuria is usually the only symptom, but soon thereafter the blood urea nitrogen and creatine levels begin to rise and the patient shows increasing signs of uremia. Intervention is necessary to reestablish urinary drainage. Sometimes drainage is established spontaneously by the development of a ureterovaginal fistula on one or both sides, but normal renal function is still in jeopardy.

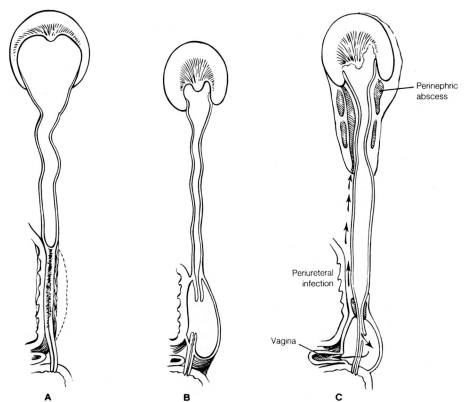

Figure 29–9. Sampson's canine experiments showing the pathogenesis of ureteral stenosis and fistula from injury and ischemia. *A,* Ureteral necrosis and occlusion 3 weeks following stripping of periureteral arterial-venous plexus for 1 cm. *B,* Similar experiment in dog in which ureteral necrosis results in loss of ureteral wall with urinoma formation. *C,* Similar experiment with necrosis of ureteral wall due to localized ischemia with secondary periureteral ascending infection and perinephric abscess formation. Ureterovaginal fistula has also formed.

The pathophysiology of urinary obstruction was recently reviewed by Gillenwater. The normal mean pressure in the lumen of the ureter and renal pelvis is approximately 6.5 mm Hg. With complete ureteral obstruction, pressure may rise to 50–75 mm Hg within an hour. Patients experience flank pain at the higher pressures. The pressure tends to decrease with time. Histologically demonstrable atrophy in the distal renal nephron begins in the first week and extends to the cortical region by the second week. Glomeruli are not damaged until later. If a renal biopsy is done, however, protein casts deposited in Bowman's space of the glomeruli can be seen and are pathognomonic of ureteral obstruction if ureterovesical reflux can be ruled out. Pyelocanalicular and pyelosinus backflow of urine occurs initially with acute obstruction. When pressure in the renal pelvis increases further, urine escapes through both the lymphatic and venous systems. There is vasoconstriction of the afferent arterioles. Total renal blood flow and glomerular filtration rates are reduced. If ureteral obstruction is incomplete, renal function may be destroyed slowly, but even incomplete obstruction can destroy all renal function given sufficient time.

Gillenwater explains that recovery of renal function is possible after the release of either unilateral or bilateral ureteral obstruction. The recovery potential depends on many factors, including the length of time the kidney has been obstructed, the completeness of the obstruction, the severity of the renal injury, the presence or absence of infection, presence of an intrarenal or extrarenal pelvis in the kidney, or the degree of pyelolymphatic or pyelovenous backflow. Interestingly, greater recovery of function in an obstructed kidney is stimulated if function of the opposite kidney is impaired. However, most postobstructed kidneys demonstrate a residual impairment of function, including a reduction in glomerular filtration rates, renal blood flow, concentrating ability, hydrogen ion clearance, and phosphate excretion. Sodium reabsorption is mildly impaired, whereas urinary dilution remains normal.

From this discussion it is clear that impairment of renal function begins very soon after ureteral obstruction and may not return to completely normal if relief of the obstruction is delayed. Certainly, the longer the obstruction is allowed to exist, the more likely the kidney function is to be severely and permanently impaired.

PREVENTION OF URETERAL INJURIES

The most important aspect of the subject of ureteral injury is *primary prevention*–prevention of the injury before it occurs. Assuming the gynecologic surgeon understands the anatomy and physiology of the ureter and how it is involved in gynecologic disease and gynecologic surgery, prevention of ureteral injuries should not be a difficult task in almost every operation.

Primary prevention of ureteral injury begins preoperatively with a careful evaluating of the patient's gynecologic disease and recognition of the risk to the ureter of the surgical procedure planned. In our judgment, preoperative excretory urography is useful, but it is not done routinely in every patient before a major gynecologic operation. It is possible to be selective and avoid unnecessary, expensive, time-consuming, and potentially hazardous preoperative studies by using sound clinical judgment based on one's own experience or advice from experienced consultants. However, a preoperative excretory urogram may be helpful in evaluating kidney location and function, dilatation or displacement of ureters, encroachments on the bladder, and anomalies of the upper collecting system. Especially in doing an extensive hysterectomy and pelvic lymphadenectomy, it is important to know preoperatively if a double urinary collecting system is present on one or both sides and to know if the ureters are dilated. Preoperative excretory urography should be obtained in any patient who is to have an extensive operation for either benign or malignant disease. If disease in the pelvis is extensive or strategically located in an area that is likely to involve the ureter (experienced pelvic examiners can usually determine this), preoperative excretory urograms may be helpful. They may also be done in a patient with anomalous development of the mullerian ducts, since anomalies of the upper urinary tracts are often associated. For medicolegal as well as for other reasons, an excretory urogram might be considered in a patient who has had previous pelvic surgery in order to detect previously unrecognized urinary tract injury, the presence of which should be documented before another operation is performed. Other procedures, such as cystoscopy with retrograde pyelography, computerized tomography, and magnetic resonance imaging scans of the abdomen and pelvis, can also be helpful in special circumstances and may be done in addition to or instead of an excretory urography.

In a study at the Duke Medical Center, Piscitelli and her associates asked, "Who should have an intravenous pyelogram before hysterectomy for benign disease?" A preoperative excretory urogram was performed on 299 (60.6%) of 493 selected cases of abdominal and vaginal hysterectomy. Abnormalities in the preoperative excretory urogram were noted in 77 patients (26%). There was a 6% prevalence of congenital anomalies, 10.6% ureteral dilatation, and 4.7% ureteral deviation, findings compatible with previous studies. Uterine size of 12 weeks or larger and adnexal masses 4 cm or larger were most often associated with an increased incidence of abnormal excretory urogram findings. Patients with normal pelvic examinations were found unlikely to have excretory urogram findings of practical significance to the pelvic surgeon. The authors concluded that there is no proof yet that a preoperative excretory urogram reduces the risk of ureteral injury. However, many surgeons feel that preoperative knowledge of the lower urinary tract anatomy does help to avoid such injuries. When proper clinical judgment is used, only those patients who are more likely to have significant abnormalities will have a preoperative excretory urogram, thereby reducing the number of unnecessary studies, decreasing cost, and avoiding some adverse reactions.

There is controversy among gynecologic surgeons regarding the value of preoperative ureteral catheterization. Most experienced gynecologic surgeons prefer not to use ureteral catheters because of the possibility that manipulation of a ureter with a hard catheter in its lumen will cause more damage to the wall of the ureter. In our experience, ureteral catheters have been helpful in only a very small number of cases and usually only those with very unusual and difficult and complicated problems. We use preoperative ureteral catheterization in less than 5% of major gynecologic operations performed. They are never used with extensive abdominal hysterectomy for invasive cervical cancer. Unless a large cervical or intraligamentous component is present, they are not usually necessary in a patient with a large leiomyomatous uterus, even when ureteral compression and dilatation are present. They may be helpful when operating for the ovarian remnant syndrome, when the ureter is involved in retroperitoneal fibrosis from radiation or endometriosis or infection (so-called ligneous pelvic cellulitis), when dissecting around a retroperitoneal tumor, or when debulking an extensive ovarian malignancy. If a ureteral catheter is needed and has not been placed preoperatively, it can be easily threaded up the ureter through a cystotomy incision. Alternatively, if the patient is positioned in stirrups for laparotomy, the external urethral meatus is available to pass a ureteral catheter through a cystoscope, thus avoiding a cystotomy incision. In our experience, lighted ureteral catheters are unnecessarily cumbersome and time-consuming. To see the illumination of the catheter, the operating room lights must be turned away. Then it is not possible to see to operate. A lighted ureteral catheter offers little or no advantage.

When ureteral catheter placement in the immediate preoperative or intraoperative period is deemed appropriate, the catheters should be No. 6 French in size. Smaller catheters are difficult to palpate; larger catheters may cause trauma to the ureteral mucosa. The "right" and "left" catheters should be marked in some suitable way to allow their individual identification, should this be required during the operation or later. Both ureteral catheters should be tied securely to an indwelling Foley catheter as closely as possible to the external urethral meatus to avoid inadvertent removal.

Primary prevention includes first and foremost the maintenance of an appropriate level of consciousness of the risk of injury to the ureters throughout the entire pelvic dissection, especially at certain key points in each operation. The ureters must not be hidden in the operator's unconscious mind. If a ureter is hidden from view on the lateral pelvic sidewall or not easily palpable in paracervical cardinal ligament tissue, the operation usually should not proceed until it can be clearly seen or definitely palpated. Failure to observe this rule has resulted in many ureteral injuries. Taking a chance that the ureter is in its usual location has caused others.

It is an important axiom in all surgical procedures that an adequate incision must be made so that proper exposure can be accomplished. Proper exposure is needed to perform the operation safely and to avoid injury to surrounding structures and organs, including the ureters. In our opinion, the usual Pfannenstiel incision does not provide the exposure necessary to do major pelvic surgery. A Pfannenstiel incision provides limited exposure, usually adequate to do limited pelvic operations. Depending on the circumstances, the exposure needed for major gynecologic surgery can be provided by either the transverse Maylard incision or an adequate lower midline incision. After an adequate incision is fashioned, exposure is enhanced by the placement of a self-retaining retractor such as a Balfour or Bookwalter retractor. Providing adequate exposure through an adequate incision is the first step in preventing ureteral injuries. Exposure of important structures in the pelvis must never be limited by a limited incision.

It is another axiom in surgery that important structures in the operative field that are at risk of injury should always be dissected sufficiently to allow their identification and retraction out of harm's way throughout the operation. This axiom certainly applies to the ureter in pelvic operations. In most gynecologic operations done abdominally, the ureters can be visualized easily through the intact peritoneum along the lateral pelvic sidewall. If visualization is difficult because of extensive pathology, the broad ligament can be opened by transecting the round ligament and extending the incision superiorly along the lateral border of the infundibulopelvic ligament. By reflecting the peritoneum medially away from the lateral pelvic sidewall, the ureter can be visualized attached to the undersurface of the peritoneum. If identification is still difficult, the ureter can be located at the pelvic brim as it comes into the pelvis just at the point of bifurcation of the common iliac artery into its external and internal branches. Having identified the ureter, it can be traced inferiorly to the point where it passes beneath the uterine artery and vein. Dissection of the ureter beyond this point may also be done, but it is usually more difficult and may itself result in injury and bleeding if not done carefully. Fortunately, in most cases the ureter can be felt in the paracervical cardinal ligament. Palpation of the ureter in this location is advisable in every case. Symmonds and others have emphasized routine dissection and palpation of the ureter in every abdominal gynecologic operation as the most effective way to prevent ureteral injury. We support this opinion.

Several key points in gynecologic operations done abdominally are especially important. The distance between the infundibulopelvic ligament clamps and the ureter may be only 1 cm or less (see Fig. 29-3). The ureter can be seen easily in this location in most cases. However, a short infundibulopelvic ligament may result from distortion of the normal anatomy by a variety of disease processes, such as a large ovarian tumor, a paraovarian cyst, pelvic endometriosis, or a tubo-ovarian abscess. The clamp placed on the ovarian vessels in such cases may include the underlying ureter unless it is carefully identified. Before clamping the infundibulopelvic ligament, the surgeon must identify the location of the ureter as it enters the pelvis and make certain that the pedicle clamp does not encroach upon the underlying ureter. The location of this segment of the ureter should be verified by opening the peritoneum lateral to the bifurcation of the common iliac artery and reflecting the peritoneum medially until the ureter comes into full view. With this anatomic security, a distorted ovarian pedicle can be developed, safely clamped, and doubly ligated with minimal risk of injury to the adjacent ureter. If an ovary is to be removed and the infundibulopelvic ligament containing the ovarian vessels is to be ligated, the first clamp placed across the infundibulopelvic ligament should be the lowest clamp, and it should be placed after a conscious thought regarding the location of the ureter. After the lowest clamp has been placed correctly, the other clamp(s) can be placed above it without danger of ureteral injury (see Fig. 27-8). The ureter is in even greater danger of injury when the uterine vessels are clamped and ligated. After these vessels have been skeletonized, three rules about the placement of clamps should be followed:

1. Place the lowest clamp on first.
2. Place it on at a right angle to the uterus.

3. Place it on at the level of the *internal* cervical os, usually identified as the narrowest width in the lower uterine segment.

After the ureter has been palpated in the cardinal ligament and this first clamp has been placed correctly, the remaining clamp(s) can be placed above it without danger of ureteral injury. The ligatures should contain only the uterine vessels. After ligating the uterine vessels, the distance between the ureters and the cervix may be increased if the upper part of the cardinal ligament is clamped, cut, and ligated at this point (see Fig. 27-12).

As stated previously, the most common site of injury is in the distal, terminal 3–4 cm of ureter between the uterine artery and the bladder. In a difficult pelvic dissection where the bladder base and adjacent ureters have not been displaced adequately from the upper vagina and base of the cardinal ligament, the paracervical and paravaginal clamps or sutures may crush or ligate the ureter as it passes medially to enter the bladder. The safe placement of these clamps and sutures as close as possible to the cervix is always facilitated if one can feel the ureter and even attempt to push it laterally. In a total abdominal hysterectomy for benign uterine disease, ureteral injury between the uterine artery and the bladder base can be avoided by adherence to the Richardson intrafascial technique of removing the cervix. If the pubovesicocervical fascia is developed sufficiently to allow placement of the clamps and sutures within and beneath the fascia, injury to the ureter is much less likely (see Fig. 27-19). Regardless of the particular technique used in total abdominal hysterectomy, care should be taken to dissect the bladder well away from the upper vaginal wall, both inferiorly and laterally (see Figs. 27-9, 27-17, 27-18, and 27-20), before excising the cervix from the vaginal fornices. The surgeon should note carefully what is included in each stitch as the vagina is sutured and suspended, always with the location of the ureter consciously in mind. Palpation of the ureters in paracervical tissues should always be done before placement of clamps and sutures. Locating the ureter by palpation may be difficult if paracervical tissue is indurated from previous surgery, recent infection, or recent cervical conization. When there is induration and fibrosis of paracervical tissue, the ureters may be drawn abnormally close to the cervix and will not fall away from the cervix and vagina as the dissection proceeds. The intrafascial technique can be helpful in such cases. Location of the ureter with dissection may be needed. Remember also the variation in the anatomic relationship between the ureter and the cervix demonstrated by Sampson (see Fig. 29-6).

The normal course of the ureter comes close to the uterosacral ligaments. In suspending the vaginal apex after removal of the uterus, the uterosacral ligaments are often used. The sutures to accomplish this suspension must incorporate only the uterosacral ligaments. If they are placed higher and more laterally on the pelvic sidewalls, the ureters may be kinked or ligated. One must be careful also in placing sutures to reperitonize the pelvis. The ureter is very close to the edge of the posterior leaf of the broad ligament. It may also be compressed against the pelvic brim by a peritoneal closure that is too tight or under tension.

With large pelvic tumors, especially those that have developed between the leaves of the broad ligament, freeing the tumor from the sidewall of the pelvis may endanger a ureter if it is adherent. Although the broad ligament is the least common site of ureteral injury, identification and exposure of the pelvic ureter will be necessary in such cases. It is important to locate the ureter at the pelvic brim, open the peritoneum on the lateral side of the ureter, and leave the pelvic peritoneum and periureteral tissue attached to the ureter, for in this tissue lie the important blood vessels that supply the ureter. Every gynecologic surgeon should be able to trace the course of the pelvic ureter skillfully without separating it widely from its peritoneal attachment or jeopardizing its blood supply.

Ureters are sometimes injured when trying to control intraoperative bleeding by placing clamps blindly on bleeding vessels deep in the pelvis in a pool of blood. Hemorrhage can usually be avoided by careful dissection, but it is inevitable in an occasional case with extensive pathology. Using the pressure of a pack or stick sponge or finger to control the bleeding temporarily will allow the surgeon time to get the situation under control, to arrange for proper exposure and suction, to organize an approach that is most likely to be successful, to replace blood if necessary, to request the proper instruments and sutures, and to ligate the vessel as exactly and securely as possible without injuring adjacent structures.

Differently, trauma to the distal ureter that occurs during an extensive hysterectomy for cervical cancer usually results from stripping the blood vessels too close to the ureteral wall for several centimeters where the ureter is covered by Waldeyer's sheath just before entering the bladder. The important longitudinal veins and arteries provide an excellent collateral blood supply to the dissected ureter. However, should these vessels be traumatized, thrombosed, or ligated in dissecting the ureter from its tunnel through the cardinal ligament (the web), a segment of ureter may become avascular. Depending on the extent of the injury, fibrosis and stenosis and hydroureter and hydronephrosis may develop. In more severe injuries, necrosis and fistula formation may be followed by fibrosis and stenosis and hydroureter and hydronephrosis. In a previously irradiated pelvis, the biologic effect of radiation causes obliterative endarteritis of the nutrient vessels of the ureter and reduces its blood supply. Any additional surgical dissection often robs the ureter of the remainder. Dissection of the lower ureter from an irradiated bed must be done with great care and even then almost inevitably results in stenosis of the ureteral lumen.

Although most ureteral injuries occur during abdominal gynecologic operations, the gynecologic surgeon must also be aware of the possibility of ureteral injury during the performance of vaginal surgery. The gynecologist must be "ureter conscious" when operating vaginally as well as abdominally. As stated previously, in approximately one fourth of ureteral injuries, the injury will occur during a vaginal procedure.

The primary prevention of ureteral injury with vaginal surgery should also begin preoperatively with a careful assessment of the extent of pelvic disease, preoperative cystoscopy and excretory urography when indicated, and preoperative ureteral catheterization in selected patients. However, preoperative excretory urograms and preoperative ureteral catheterization are not as often necessary before vaginal operations. In the performance of vaginal hysterectomy, the vesicouterine space must be developed adequately to allow displacement of the ureters away from clamps and sutures by downward traction on the cervix and countertraction upward beneath the bladder. The ureters are caught beneath the uterine vessels on each side of the uterus. Traction on the cervix exaggerates the "knee" of the ureter and brings it more into the field of operation. Complete development of the vesicouterine space and countertraction beneath the bladder facilitates the displacement of the ureters away from clamps and sutures. Ureters are protected better if only small bites of paracervical and parametrial tissue are clamped, cut, and ligated adjacent to the uterus. The "bladder pillars" between the bladder and the uterus on each side of the vesicouterine space should be clamped as separate structures as close to the uterus as possible (see Fig. 27-41). These steps allow the ureters to be further retracted out of harm's way. Locating the ureter by palpation within the "bladder pillar" can be helpful in proper placement of the clamp (see Fig. 27-40). Double clamping of cardinal ligaments and uterine vessels should be avoided, since the most lateral of the two clamps usually come too close to the ureter. If a unilateral or bilateral salpingo-oophorectomy is done vaginally, it should be remembered that Hofmeister measured the distance between the ureter and the clamp on the infundibulopelvic ligament as only 1 cm when operating vaginally. He found that only 0.9 cm separated the ureters and sutures in performing an anterior colporrhaphy. It is especially important to be careful when placing the sutures in the uterosacral ligaments for a posterior culdoplasty. The ureters are located along the lateral pelvic sidewalls just above the uterosacral ligaments. Sutures placed too high in tissue above the uterosacral ligaments can incorporate the ureters. In our experience, when a partial vaginectomy is done with vaginal hysterectomy, the risk of ureteral injury is significantly increased. To avoid this, it is important to release paravaginal tissue laterally first before clamping the cardinal ligaments.

Cruikshank has described a surgical dissection method of identifying the ureters during total vaginal hysterectomy and has recommended that it be done routinely to avoid ureteral injuries. However, Cruikshank's method does not expose the ureter in its most vulnerable part between the ureterovesicle junction and the uterine artery. Exposure of the ureter in this location can best be accomplished according to the classic technique of ureteral dissection in the Schauta-Amreich extensive vaginal hysterectomy, but it is not recommended as a routine procedure in vaginal hysterectomy for benign disease.

Secondary prevention of ureteral injury involves the recognition of the injury at the operation of injury so that immediate repair can be done. This is extremely important to prevent serious postoperative morbidity and to reduce the possibility of loss of kidney function. In our series of ureteral injuries, when the injury was recognized and repaired at the operation of injury, no kidneys were lost and only one reoperation was required. In 22 ureteral injuries discovered in the postoperative period, six kidneys were lost. When ureteral injury is not diagnosed and repaired at the operation of injury and a ureterovaginal fistula develops subsequently, nephrectomy is frequently necessary. Lee and Symmonds, in a review of 68 ureterovaginal fistulas, reported that nephrectomy was necessary in 34 (50%). Clearly, the best chance of avoiding serious postoperative morbidity and loss of kidney function when the ureter is injured is to diagnose and repair the injury at the operation of injury. It is important to keep in mind the timeless statement that has benefitted so many pelvic surgeons: "The venial sin is injury to the ureter; the mortal sin is failure of recognition." Although ureteral injury most commonly occurs concurrently with extensive and strategically located pelvic disease, of near equal frequency is the inadvertent trauma to the ureter in the absence of significant pelvic disease or bleeding complications. Symmonds, who studied 600 patients with genitourinary fistula referred to the Mayo Clinic from throughout the Western Hemisphere, concluded that "the easy hysterectomy (or other straightforward gynecologic operation), not the hazardous and difficult dissection, is responsible for most of the genitourinary tract injuries (and fistulas) in this country." Unfortunately, in these cases, ureteral damage may not be recognized until several days or weeks following surgery.

Ureteral injury is now among the most common and serious of all the complications of pelvic surgery. It is one of the most frequent reasons for medicolegal action by the patient. So important is this complication that it is critical for a gynecologic surgeon to become "ureter conscious" and to develop a routine method of ensuring the integrity of both ureters before concluding a major operative procedure in which there is a risk of ureteral injury. Whether by direct palpation, mobilization and inspection, ureteral catheterization, or some other means of ureteral identification, the surgeon should develop some fail-safe method of evaluating integrity of the pelvic ureter before the operative procedure is terminated. An intravenous chromogen test has proven to be an effective and convenient method of providing this assurance. Before closing the incision when operating abdominally, the surgeon may quickly ascertain bilateral ureteral integrity by inspecting the ureteral orifices in the bladder trigone with a cystoscope or some other suitable endoscope after an intravenous bolus of 5 cc of indigo carmine or methylene blue has been injected. The dye will usually spurt from each ureteral orifice within about 3–5 minutes. If it takes longer, the intravenous fluids may be given more rapidly or a rapidly acting diuretic may be given, although often neither procedure is necessary. This simple procedure is facilitated by instilling 200 cc of clear sterile saline into the bladder and by having the patient in stirrups for the laparotomy. The external urethral meatus is readily available for passage of the cystoscope if the patient is in stirrups. Of course, vaginal operations are no problem, since the external urethral meatus is always a part of the operative field and available for passage of a cystoscope at any time during the procedure.

Should a ureteral orifice fail to spurt dye after the patient has been adequately hydrated, the ureter should be explored along its course. If the operation was done abdominally, the exploration should be done through the abdominal incision. If the operation was done vaginally, exploration through the vaginal vault should be carried out. In either case, if it is difficult to find the point of obstruction, a ureteral catheter should be passed as far as possible up the ureter through the cystoscope or through a cystotomy incision in the anterior extraperitoneal bladder wall. Survey of the damage should be followed by appropriate repair.

Of course, if the ureter has been transected partially or completely without ligation, urine may escape into the operative field. Or the surgeon may notice gradually increasing ureteral dilatation above a site of obstruction. It will then be necessary to determine the site of injury by dissecting the ureter, possibly aided by passage of a ureteral catheter through a cystoscope or through a cystotomy incision. In our experience, intraoperative excretory urography is cumbersome, time-consuming, and not often helpful.

TREATMENT OF OPERATIVE INJURY OF THE URETER

The treatment of ureteral injuries should be considered in the two groups into which they naturally fall: those recognized at the operating table and those discovered postoperatively.

Injuries Recognized at Operation

It is a regrettable fact that no more than 30% of ureteral injuries are recognized at the time of occurrence during surgery, although intraoperative recognition may be improving, as suggested by the report of Mann and associates. When a clamp or a ligature is discovered on a ureter during an operation, it should be removed immediately and the ureter should be inspected carefully. In many instances, damage will not have been severe enough to prevent normal function of the ureter. If the damage is slight but the operator feels uneasy about the condition of the ureter, a stab wound may be made and a drain placed extraperitoneally, adjacent to the injury site, as a safety valve. The peritoneum should be closed over this site, so that if there is leakage, it will be extraperitoneal. If the operator feels uneasy about simple pelvic drainage, the prudent approach is to intubate the ureter for 7–10 days while revascularization takes place. This can be done by means of water cystoscopy and retrograde catheterization of the ureter. This should be done at the time of surgery to make certain that the area of trauma can be bypassed by the ureteral catheter. Intraoperative cystoscopy can be easily accomplished if patients are positioned in stirrups for pelvic laparotomy (see Fig. 27-2). If there is difficulty with insertion of the catheter by cystoscopy, the bladder dome should be opened and a soft, pliable Silastic catheter should be inserted through the ureteral orifice to a position in the renal pelvis well beyond the damage site of the ureter. Recent developments in indwelling ureteral stents have made temporary indwelling ureteral intubation more practical. A J-shaped stent that passes up the ureter and anchors firmly in the renal pelvis is a satisfactory method of ureteral intubation.

A ureter that has been partially or completely ligated may appear normal immediately after the suture is removed. However, over time, the ureteral wall may separate at the point of ligation. Simple disligation of the ureter is therefore usually insufficient by itself. The additional procedures described earlier should also be done.

Obviously, there is room for judgment on the seriousness of the damage. If the ureter is discovered to be cut, or if extensive damage following clamping or ligation makes spontaneous healing unlikely, the operator has two choices. The severed or damaged lower ureter may be implanted into the bladder. A ureteroureteral anastomosis of the upper ureter may be done. The ideal repair should preserve normal kidney function and restore continuity of the ureter. Implantation of the lower ureter into the bladder offers a closer approach to this ideal than ureteroureteral anastomosis. Therefore, if the injury to the ureter is within 4–5 cm from the ureterovesical junction, implantation into the bladder is the preferred procedure. If the injury is in the region of the pelvic brim and too high for implantation, ureteroureteral anastomosis is the preferred treatment. The psoas muscle hitch procedure, in which the bladder wall is mobilized widely and the bladder dome is sutured to the psoas muscle near the pelvic brim, affords the opportunity for direct ureterovesical anastomosis of a ureter that has been damaged extensively within the lower half of the broad ligament.

Injuries to the ureter near the pelvic brim may also be anastomosed to the bladder dome by means of a bladder flap (Boari) procedure. Many clinicians have found this technique to be useful in performing a ureteroneocystostomy when the ureter is short, since a lengthy segment of a distended bladder wall can be fashioned in a tubular manner and the ureter can be brought into the end of the bladder flap in a submucosal fashion. If a submucosal implant is used with the bladder flap procedure, vesicoureteral reflux can be avoided. Others have found that the limited blood supply in a lengthy bladder flap leads to a higher risk of impairment of healing, which may result in ureteral stenosis, obstruction, or leakage. For these reasons, we prefer a ureteroureteral anastomosis in cases where the proximal and distal segments of the ureter are normal. Injuries to large segments of the ureter at the pelvic brim that leave only the upper half of the ureter intact rarely fall into the domain of the gynecologic surgeon. In such cases, a transperitoneal anastomosis to the opposite ureter has proven to be a satisfactory method of providing continuity and drainage to a very short ureter.

Anastomosis of the ureter to the intact sigmoid colon even as a temporary expedient is not appropriate.

Only rarely is intentional ligation of the injured ureter justifiable, namely, in cases of advanced pelvic cancer where the life expectancy of the patient would not be enhanced by an extensive effort to reestablish ureterovesical or ureteroureteral continuity. In most cases of ureteral injury, a skin ureterostomy as a last resort is preferable to permanent ligation. Before deliberate ligation is done, one should have information concerning the function of the opposite kidney, preferably by a preoperative excretory urogram. In the absence of such information, the damaged ureter should be anastomosed to the bladder or to the remaining segment of the pelvic ureter. If neither procedure seems reasonable, because of the patient's condition, a skin ureterostomy is an acceptable alternative. Experience has shown that ureteral ligation when the urine is uninfected usually results in an asymptomatic death of the kidney. On the other hand, if infection supervenes, the patient may experience a dramatic and serious septic course possibly requiring nephrectomy as a life-saving measure. If intentional ligation of the ureter is chosen as the most appropriate procedure, it should be done with several strong, nonabsorbable sutures after the ureter has been doubled back on itself.

Bilateral damage to the ureters is rare. Still more uncommon is the discovery of this situation at the operating table. When one is confronted with such a serious accident during an operation, ureteroureteral anastomosis or ureterovesical implantation must be done. In case the patient's condition does not permit repair of both ureters, one ureter may be repaired and the opposite ureter brought out as a skin ureterostomy, to permit adequate function of that kidney until it can be repaired later. In such a serious case, diverting temporary percutaneous nephrostomies also may be appropriate.

Injuries Unrecognized at Operation

Unilateral ureteral injury may become apparent during the postoperative period by symptoms of pyelitis and flank pain, by evidence of ureterovaginal fistula, or by appearance of a tender abdominal mass in the kidney region resulting from hydronephrosis. In general, a postoperative excretory urogram should be obtained if any unusual clinical conditions, symptoms, or signs become evident postoperatively. Indications for postoperative excretory urography include the following:

Loin or costovertebral angle tenderness
Unexplained or persistent fever, with or without chills
Persistent abdominal distention
Unexplained hematuria
Escape of watery fluid through the vagina
Appearance of lower abdominal or pelvic mass after operation

Oliguria or elevated serum creatinine levels

Any operation with extensive pelvic disease that distorts the ureters

Any question of ureteral integrity

Complete and permanent occlusion of one ureter in the absence of infection may, on rare occasions, lead to renal atrophy without symptoms. In most instances, however, ureteral injury is accompanied by acute symptoms. The appearance of fever and costovertebral angle tenderness may indicate an acute pyelitis, but when these symptoms and signs occur following pelvic surgery, the possibility of ureteral injury should be considered and excretory urography should be obtained. If the pyelogram shows unilateral impairment of kidney function, or hydronephrosis, ureteral catheterization by cystoscopy will confirm whether the ureter has been damaged. If one is fortunate enough to catheterize the ureter and bypass the obstruction, the catheter should be left in place for 14 days or longer to permit drainage of the kidney and healing of the injured ureter. Kaplan and associates have reported dilation of a ligated ureter through a percutaneous nephrostomy. If the ureteral catheter will not pass the area of obstruction, either immediate ureteral repair or a percutaneous nephrostomy should be done to preserve the kidney function. When temporary, percutaneous nephrostomy is done, surgery should be deferred for 6–8 weeks. At that time, reexploration may be undertaken and a ureteroplastic procedure performed when the patient's local and general condition can better ensure the success of the necessary repair.

There is still controversy regarding the management of a ureteral injury when it is noted in the immediate postoperative period, 1 week, or even 2–3 weeks postoperatively. Early disligation has been championed by many gynecologists and urologists; others have taken a more conservative approach to this difficult complication. At present, there is some support for early disligation or reimplantation if the ureteral injury is diagnosed within the first 48–72 hours following surgery. However, if the diagnosis is made 2–3 weeks postoperatively, percutaneous nephrostomy is the treatment of choice, with definitive repair delayed until 6–8 weeks later. Frank contraindications to immediate ureteral repair include those cases in which extensive devascularization and injury are likely to have occurred, namely, following extensive hysterectomy for invasive cervical cancer. In these cases, skeletonization of the distal ureter usually has occurred and extensive retroperitoneal fibrosis, cellulitis, and induration may be expected as a result of the extensive pelvic dissection. In other cases of delayed recognition, where retroperitoneal cellulitis or abscess formation has occurred prior to diagnosis of the ureteral injury, temporary percutaneous nephrostomy and delayed ureteral repair are preferable to an attempt at immediate anastomosis. Ureteral repair should also be deferred in debilitated patients with a chronic disease process, since such patients may have poor healing of tissues until their general medical and nutritional status is improved.

Our conservative position on the timing of the repair of operative injuries of the ureter has been modified somewhat in recent years. The experience in Flynn and associates, Winters and associates, and Beland has suggested that prompt repair should be carried out whenever feasible. In a young, healthy patient with an otherwise normal urinary tract without pelvic induration and cellulitis, immediate repair of a distal ureteral injury that requires only ureteroneocystostomy might be considered and performed with relative safety within the first 10–14 days following the original surgery. The use of wide mobilization of the bladder base combined with a psoas muscle hitch procedure and a submucosal tunnel ureteral anastomosis has made the repair of the damaged pelvic ureter a relatively uncomplicated operation. If necessary, with early ureteral repair, up to 3–4 cm of distal ureter can be sacrificed with excellent healing and anatomic results. In this select group of healthy women in whom injury to the terminal ureter occurred following total hysterectomy, immediate ureteral reimplantation is preferable to a 6–8-week delay. If there is a lengthy delay, drainage of urine from the vagina or the nephrostomy tube may prove to be a serious hardship to some patients. However, surgery should be delayed in the presence of significant pelvic infection, cellulitis, or postoperative abscess formation or in any patient with a chronic, debilitating disease in whom primary healing of the reimplanted ureter may be impaired. Broad-spectrum antibiotics that inhibit both aerobic and anaerobic bacteria have improved the resolution of pelvic cellulitis and have aided in the prompt healing of ureterovesical anastomosis. In cases in which ureteral injury has occurred near the pelvic brim and ureteroureteral anastomosis is required, every effort should be made to delay surgery and maintain kidney drainage by percutaneous nephrostomy for 6–8 weeks or longer if the pelvic cellulitis has not resolved. Ureteral stenosis and obstruction are serious complications of a ureteroureteral anastomosis that can be avoided by delaying surgery until an adequate blood supply is assured and all clinical evidence of infection has resolved.

Ureterovaginal Fistula

The appearance of urine in the vagina may give the first intimation of ureteral injury. If the ureter has been cut without ligation, the urine may appear almost immediately postoperatively. However, this is rare, as transection of the ureter is usually the result of clamping the ureter within a tissue pedicle. In most instances, when a ureter has been cut or incorporated in a ligature, 10–14 days pass before necrosis of the wall occurs or the suture loosens from shrinkage and retraction of the pedicle. When the ureteral damage is the result of stripping the ureter of its blood supply, as in extensive hysterectomy for cervical cancer, a longer period may elapse before ischemia has progressed to the point of necrosis of the ureteral wall and fistula formation.

The classic canine experiments of Sampson (1909) provide the most descriptive information of the pathologic changes in the ureter that precede fistula formation. As described by Sampson, the most important factor is the extent of damage to the periureteral arterial plexus (see Figs. 29-7 and 29-8). As a result of localized ischemia, a hemorrhagic infarct occurs in the ureteral wall, beginning first in the submucosa. The size of the infarct and the extent of the process depend on the severity of the ureteral trauma and circulatory impairment. These changes in the submucosa provide an anatomic explanation for the early obstruction of the ureteral lumen that makes retrograde catheterization either extremely difficult or impossible when the injury is diagnosed in the postoperative period. Although necrosis and fistula formation usually result from the process of hemorrhagic infarction, a fistula will not occur if the necrosis is not extensive or if the ureteral wall becomes adherent to adjacent pelvic organs and develops a collateral blood supply. If a fistula does not occur, scarring and stricture are equally damaging and, if uncorrected, may produce progressive hydroureteronephrosis with impairment of renal function. Should secondary infection occur in the operative site or from within the urinary tract, bacteria may be seeded into the periureteral lymphatics and produce pyelonephritis or a perinephric abscess that will further endanger the kidney (see Fig. 29-9).

After a total hysterectomy, urine from a ureteral defect enters the vagina through a small fistula tract above the vault. In most cases, the appearance of the fistula is preceded by an attack of pyelitis, including a spiking temperature and unilateral costovertebral angle tenderness. The onset of vaginal drainage afforded by the fistula may result in subsidence of pain and temperature. The evidence of pyelitis may reappear after the fistula has occurred, for there is a tendency for a fistulous opening to contract and to produce ureteral obstruction. Depending on the location and extent of ureteral injury and the health of periureteral tissues, the fistula may close spontaneously with reestablishment of the ureteral lumen, but this is unlikely. A reasonable period of expectant treatment is permissible before kidney drainage is established by nephrostomy. This conservative approach to management of a ure-

teral injury may be rewarded, rarely, by spontaneous healing if there is evidence of ureteral continuity by retrograde pyelography or excretory urography studies. If the policy of watchful waiting is pursued for several weeks, particularly if delayed repair of the ureter is planned, excretory urography studies should be done repeatedly at 2–3-week intervals to make certain that there is adequate kidney drainage and that there is no increase in the initial degree of hydronephrosis (Fig. 29-10). If the hydronephrosis becomes progressive, as it usually does, nephrostomy or surgical repair of the ureter should be done without delay. Which of these two procedures is chosen depends on the local condition of the tissues and the general condition of the patient. The spontaneous cessation of vaginal drainage of urine may indicate complete obstruction of the ureter from scar formation and is usually an ominous sign. Occasionally, the urine will be diverted elsewhere, such as into the retroperitoneal space (urinoma) or, rarely, into the peritoneal cavity, as has been reported by Hunner and Everett. Only when excretory urography demonstrates normal kidney function with an intact ureter can the cessation of urinary drainage into the vagina be considered beneficial.

Excretory urography is one of the first studies indicated after the appearance of urine in the vagina. The objective is to show whether the fistulous tract communicates with the bladder or the ureter. The most common pyelogram abnormality that results from a ureteral injury is the impairment of kidney function and the finding of hydroureteronephrosis. A convenient way to determine whether there is also a bladder injury is to place a gauze sponge or tampon into the vagina and fill the bladder with a weak solution of methylene blue. If the vaginal sponge or tampon remains free of methylene blue after ambulation, the evidence points to a ureteral fistula.

The location of the fistula can be identified more accurately by water cystoscopy with inspection of the ureteral orifices and by passage of a ureteral catheter on the suspect side. As a rule, the ureteral orifice will not spurt urine on the affected side, and it is impossible to force the catheter past the point of injury. The impasse is usually due to the submucosal infarction, edema, stricture formation, and angulation of the ureter. If, by good fortune, the catheter is made to pass the injured area of the ureter, it should be left in the ureter for 14 days or longer, during which time the ureteral wall will usually heal. A retrograde pyelogram should be done to demonstrate an intact ureter with healing of the fistula before the catheter is removed. Before the operation for repair or implantation of the ureter that is associated with secondary kidney damage is undertaken, an excretory urogram and differential kidney function studies should be done to determine beyond

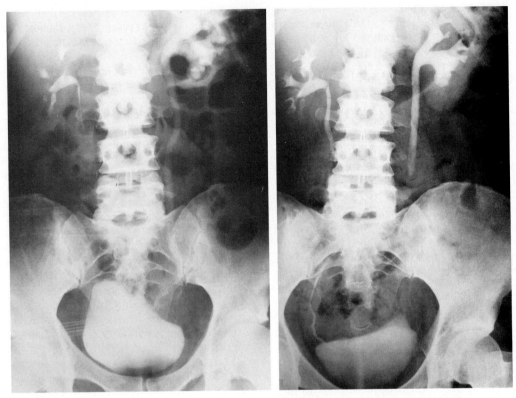

Figure 29–10. (Left) Urogram taken 2 weeks after operative injury to left ureter. Hydronephrosis is stationary, but the patient is still draining urine from the vagina. Ureter was reimplanted 6 weeks after injury. (Right) Urogram taken 5 weeks after implantation of injured left ureter into bladder, showing ultimate result. Note the delicate caliber of the pelvic ureter.

question the function of the kidney on the uninjured side. Knowledge of the function of the opposite kidney is invaluable to the surgeon in making a decision on how to treat the injured ureter.

Only when the operation is finally undertaken, and after investigating the local conditions from within the pelvis, can one decide on the exact procedure that must be done. If the injury is at the level of the uterine vessels or within 4–5 cm from the ureterovesical junction, ureterovesical implantation is preferable to ureteroureteral anastomosis. In some instances when the shortened ureter near the pelvic brim does not quite reach the bladder, the bladder may be elongated by rolling up a flap (Boari technique). If the blood supply of the unirradiated bladder is abundant, this generally may be accomplished without fear of sloughing. However, it is not necessary to use the Boari method often because the usual site of injury to the terminal ureter makes direct ureterovesical anastomosis a preferable procedure. In our experience, ischemia of an elongated flap and secondary stenosis of the anastomosis have produced more complications with the bladder flap procedure than with alternative techniques.

Bilateral Ureteral Ligation

Bilateral ureteral ligation is an extremely rare operative complication that is soon apparent when the patient is discovered to be anuric immediately following surgery. For the first 24–48 hours, anuria is usually the only symptom, but soon thereafter the blood urea nitrogen and creatinine levels begin to rise and the patient shows increasing signs of uremia. Back pain and bilateral costovertebral angle tenderness are usually present but are frequently obscured by the administration of postoperative analgesics. If the obstructions are unrelieved, progressive uremia and renal failure will result. If there was no evidence of kidney disease in the preoperative studies and the operative procedure was not associated with excessive blood loss, hypovolemia, or prolonged hypotension, one can be reasonably certain that anuria for 24–48 hours postoperatively signifies bilateral ureteral obstruction. Ureteral obstruction is easily demonstrated by excretory urography, which will show evidence of either a bilateral faintly visible nephrogram or a hydroureter and hydronephrosis in delayed films. An excretory urogram should always be obtained when the surgeon is concerned about the possibility of ureteral ligation. As Sampson succinctly put it, one of the greatest aids in the diagnosis of ureteral ligation is "the conscience of the operator." Before resorting to emergency surgery, it is our custom to attempt to insert ureteral catheters to confirm the presence of ureteral obstruction and, as is occasionally possible, to pass the catheter beyond the areas of obstruction. When one is certain that the condition exists, the earlier that treatment is instituted, the better. If discovered within 48–72 hours following surgery and before the patient is profoundly ill from uremia, immediate disligation is the treatment of choice to reestablish ureteral patency. However, bilateral percutaneous nephrostomies are preferable to at-

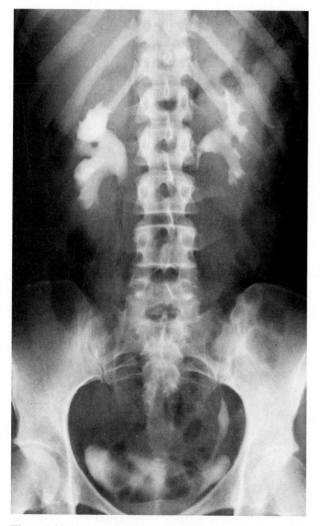

Figure 29–11. Excretory urogram taken several months after bilateral ureterovesical anastomosis, following bilateral ligation.

tempting disligation or anastomosis in a seriously ill patient who is not an appropriate candidate for surgery. This percutaneous procedure can be done easily with the aid of fluoroscopy and ultrasound or computerized tomography, using a needle trocar (2.8 mm) and a small radiopaque catheter (1.8 mm). Nephrostomy can also be accomplished surgically through bilateral flank incisions. After nephrostomy drainage is established, ureteral repair may be deferred for 6–8 weeks or, if a longer period of renal recovery is required, until the patient is a good surgical candidate. With bilateral nephrostomies, the patient soon begins to pour forth large quantities of urine, and the blood urea nitrogen and creatinine levels fall rapidly. Occasionally, the ureteral continuity may become spontaneously reestablished after nephrostomy or pyelostomy. If not, an additional attempt should be made to pass a ureteral catheter beyond the areas of obstruction, although such attempts usually fail. This attempt may be made through the nephrostomy tube or through a cystoscope. If catheterization is unsuccessful, a laparotomy should be performed 6 weeks or later after the nephrostomy, and a ureteroplastic procedure should be done. The condition of the patient and her tissues will be good enough, it is hoped, to permit the painstaking surgical work that is necessary to restore normal ureteral drainage and kidney function. In cases where disligation has been successful by means of immediate reoperation, it is advisable to place a catheter in each ureter by means of water cystoscopy or direct catheterization by cystotomy at the time of surgical repair. The ureters should remain intubated for 10 days to 2 weeks while the surgical trauma and ureteral edema gradually resolve. Renal function and regression of the ureteral obstruction should be followed carefully with frequent excretory urography studies (Fig. 29-11). If one or both ureters have been cut or irreparably damaged close to the bladder, bilateral ureterovesical anastomosis may be required.

Principles of Ureteral Surgery

The principles of ureteral surgery have been discussed by Koontz, Klein, and Smith and are summarized below. A number of factors affect the healing of the ureter after injury and repair. The ureter should always be handled gently, preferably with noncrushing clamps and forceps. Dissection of the ureter free from its bed should be limited to that required for the operation. Unnecessary dissection should be avoided but should always be sufficient to accomplish repair without tension on the suture line. The ureter is capable of closing its own defect by regenerating all its own components.

Several factors will encourage uroepithelial growth. If careful mucosa-to-mucosa approximation is done, if urinary leakage is minimal, and if there is no tension on the suture line, the defect can be bridged by new growth of transitional epithelium in less than 2 weeks. The growth of new smooth muscle across the gap will complete the repair. If the periureteral tissue is rigid and fibrotic, healing of the repair site may be better if the ureter can be wrapped in omental fat. Resumption of electric and peristaltic activity across the repair site usually is seen in approximately 1 month.

Although controversy exists regarding the use of stents in repairing ureteral injuries, most gynecologic and urologic surgeons believe that stents will stabilize and immobilize the ureter during healing, will allow orderly regeneration of uroepithelium and smooth muscle, will help prevent urinary extravasation through the suture line, will help maintain a normal lumen within the ureter and prevent stenosis, and will minimize any tendency of the ureter to become angulated. The stent must be a correct size, one that fits comfortably in the lumen without distending the ureteral wall. According to other surgeons, stents are associated with inflammation and stricture at the repair site plus accumulation of deposits. Silastic tubing is a suitable material for ureteral stents. However, at body temperature, silastic tubing becomes soft and pliable and may be expelled if not tied to holding catheters such as a transurethral Foley catheter. The single- or double-ended pigtail or J-catheters are also popular, since they are less likely to migrate up or down the ureter. A plastic infant feeding tube has also been used as a ureteral stent.

The surgeon must decide if diversion of the urinary stream above the repair is necessary. If the injury is a simple one and the repair is technically satisfactory, only brief and minimal periureteral urinary extravasation will occur. Diversion of the urinary stream with percutaneous nephrostomy is not usually necessary unless the defect is large, the ureter has been completely transected, or the ureter lies in a bed of inflammation. If extravasated urine leaks through the repair site for many days, healing may not be satisfactory. Drainage of this extravasated urine will prevent its accumulation in the retroperitoneal tissues. A Jackson-Pratt drain placed retroperitoneally at the repair site is preferred.

Nonabsorbable, permanent suture material should never be used to repair ureteral injuries; No. 4-0 delayed-absorbable sutures are preferred. Careful approximation (not strangulation) without tension should be the objective. We agree with Ponig that magnification is helpful in repairing ureteral injuries. The magnification provided by surgical loupes is usually sufficient and the operating microscope is not necessary.

Ureteroureteral Anastomosis

Ureteroureteral anastomosis may be done at the time of injury or at the time of subsequent delayed repair. The procedure is usually performed for ureteral injuries that occur near or above the pelvic brim. Ureteroureteral anastomosis in the lowest 3–4 cm is technically difficult, and the results are not satisfactory.

If diagnosed and repaired at the time of injury, the intraoperative trauma is usually due to transection of the middle or upper segment of the ureter. A ureteral catheter, possibly a silicone (Silastic) tube with multiple drainage holes in its wall (internal diameter 0.078 in), is threaded into the upper and the lower segments of the ureter and then into the bladder, where it is permitted to curl up as shown in Figure 29-12. The

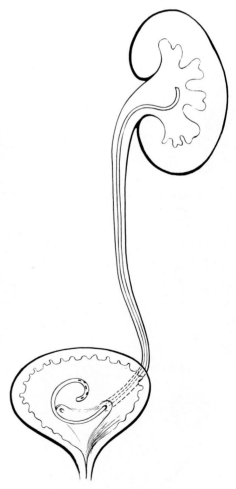

Figure 29–12. Splinting ureteral tube (silicone, internal diameter, 0.078 in), which is threaded into renal pelvis and coiled in bladder. This is used for ureterovesical or ureteroureteral anastomosis.

Silastic tube is inert, soft, and pliable. It can be left in the ureter for long periods without obstructing or creating a foreign-body reaction in the operative site. Reinforcement of the wall of the soft Silastic stent with finely coiled stainless steel wire has improved the efficiency of the indwelling catheter in draining the ureter. Alternatively, a double-J stent can be used and may be retained better than a Silastic catheter.

If the ureteral anastomosis is done at some time subsequent to the original injury, a No. 7 French whistle-tip catheter is passed into the ureter by cystoscopy until it meets the site of obstruction. By retaining the stent in the lower ureter the operator can identify the lower segment of the ureter easily at the time of operative repair. Edema and infection in the surrounding tissues may make ureteral identification difficult without the aid of the catheter. When ureteral injuries are repaired abdominally, we prefer to use the transperi-

toneal approach rather than the retroperitoneal approach because the transperitoneal approach provides much greater exposure of the operative field. The peritoneum is incised and reflected along the lateral side of the injured ureter. The ureter is opened at the site of injury and the area of the traumatized tissue is excised (Fig. 29-13A). If there is a question regarding the adequacy of the blood supply to the ends of the ureter, fluorescein dye and a Wood's lamp may be used for confirmation. The ureter above and below the site of injury must have good blood supply and must be mobilized sufficiently to allow an anastomosis without tension. A Silastic tube is passed into the kidney pelvis. The other end of the tube is threaded through the lower ureter and into the bladder. It can be left indwelling for 2–3 weeks and then removed with cystoscopy later. A suture placed in the bladder end of the Silastic stent will assist in identifying the free end at cystoscopy should

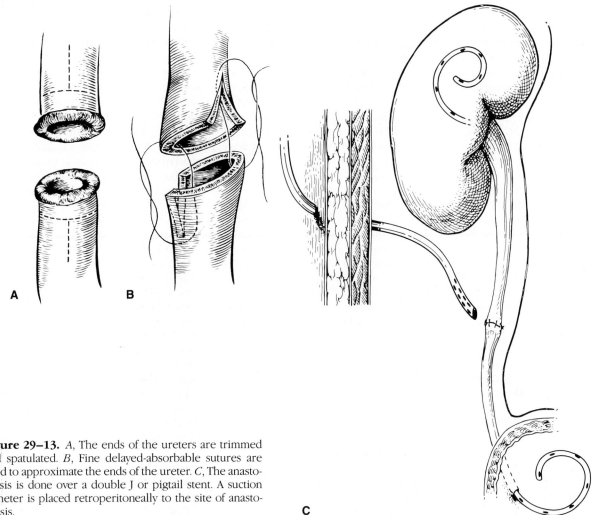

Figure 29–13. *A*, The ends of the ureters are trimmed and spatulated. *B*, Fine delayed-absorbable sutures are used to approximate the ends of the ureter. *C*, The anastomosis is done over a double J or pigtail stent. A suction catheter is placed retroperitoneally to the site of anastomosis.

the catheter need to be exteriorized for irrigation. After the ureteral ends are excised to the level of viable tissue, the free ends are spatulated for 5 mm and cut obliquely to ensure a wide anastomosis site. With the ureter splinted by the Silastic tubing, the two ends are drawn together and united by four to six interrupted sutures of No. 4-0 delayed-absorbable sutures placed through the seromuscular wall of the ureter. The ureteral closure should be reasonably watertight, although too many sutures can produce a ureteral stricture. The sutures are tied gently and without undue tension (Fig. 29-13B). We have found the use of No. 4-0 delayed-absorbable suture will enhance the integrity of the ureteral suture line without undue scarring or stricture formation. If the ureteral wall is thin and attenuated, sutures are placed through full thickness of the ureteral wall to ensure adequate approximation. Before the abdomen is closed, drainage is established extraperitoneally by placement of a Jackson-Pratt drain through a small stab wound (Fig. 29-13C). The drain is easily placed under direct vision to a point near the site of anastomosis. Then the peritoneum is closed over the ureter. If, during the postoperative course, there is any reason to believe that the Silastic tubing in the ureter is not draining adequately, the end of the tubing can be grasped through a cystoscope and brought out through the urethra and irrigated.

This technique is suitable in the usual case, but there is a special precaution that should be taken when, owing to the condition of the ureter, it is feared that the anastomosis is not as satisfactory as one might desire. In such a case, when urinary leakage at the anastomosis seems likely, it may be desirable to leave the indwelling ureteral tubing in place for more than the usual 14 days. To assist further in decompressing the suture line, a pyelostomy tube can be placed at the time of the ureteral procedure and exteriorized through the flank to provide a safety valve for urinary drainage should the ureteral tube become obstructed. If the anastomosis is satisfactory, we prefer to use only the indwelling Silastic stent. Some gynecologists and urologists remove the stent at the completion of the procedure, although we prefer to leave it in.

Submucosal Tunnel Ureteroneocystostomy

The submucosal tunnel technique of ureteroneocystostomy has been found to be most useful in restoring the intramural anatomy of the ureter and in avoiding vesicoureteral reflux, one of the complications of ureterovesical anastomosis (Fig. 29-14). Although it is questionable whether minimal ureteral reflux will produce long-term renal complications, recurrent pyelone-

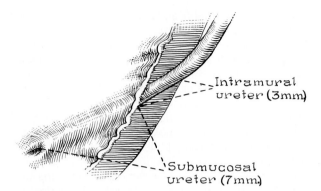

Figure 29–14. Normal anatomy of the intramural ureter.

phritis in conjunction with ureteral reflux can prove to be a difficult clinical problem in the presence of a previously damaged kidney. Consequently, it is important to consider the use of a submucosal tunnel procedure to avoid this complication. A transabdominal approach has been used for the repair of most ureteral injuries. The distal ureter is carefully dissected from the site of trauma in order to preserve as much of the distal ureter as possible for anastomosis, excising all areas of devitalized tissue. The anastomosis must be done without tension. Both sides of the bladder base and adjacent peritoneum are mobilized widely. If necessary, the mobilized bladder dome should be sutured to the psoas muscle near the pelvic brim to accommodate implantation of a shortened ureter (psoas muscle hitch) (see Fig. 29-18 later in the chapter). The submucosal tunnel to be created in the bladder for placement of the ureter should be at least 1–1.5 cm long in order to prevent reflux with voiding. After the dome of the bladder is opened transversely, the most dependent portion of the bladder wall that will reach the ureter without undue tension is selected for the site of the submucosal tunnel (Fig. 29-15A). The tunnel is then initiated from inside the bladder by making two small, 5-mm parallel mucosal incisions, one approximately 1.5 cm above the other, that outline the upper and lower margins of the tunnel (Fig. 29-15 B–C). The upper incision is extended through the bladder wall with a small scalpel blade and the free end of the ureter is drawn into the bladder by a traction suture. The submucosal tunnel is developed between the two mucosal incisions, following which the ureter is guided through the submucosal tunnel and sutured to the margins of the lower incision, thereby establishing the submucosal implantation (Fig. 29-15D).

This mucosa-to-mucosa anastomosis of ureter to bladder is performed using interrupted No. 4-0 delayed-absorbable sutures over an indwelling Silastic tube (Fig. 29-15E). The Silastic tube is either left coiled

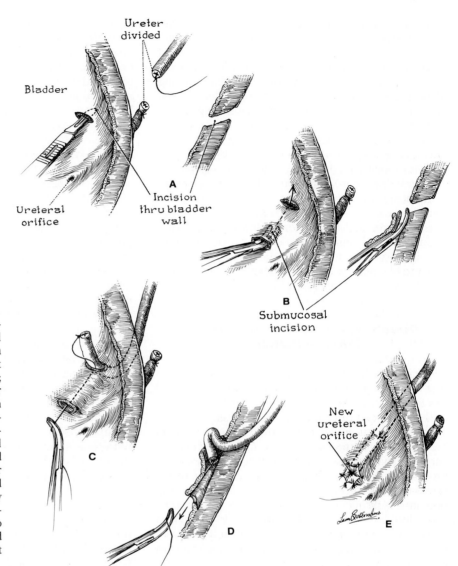

Figure 29–15. Submucosal tunnel technique of ureterovesical implantation. *A*, Bladder mucosa is incised above trigone at planned site of implantation; oblique incision through bladder wall made from exterior. *B*, Adson clamp is inserted through new orifice and tunneled beneath mucosa for 1.5 cm to upper mucosal incision. *C*, Ureter is guided through bladder wall and upper mucosal orifice and gently guided through submucosal tunnel *D* by traction suture. *E*, Mucosa-to-mucosa anastomosis of ureter to bladder; upper incision is closed with fine suture. A Silastic stent should be left indwelling.

in the bladder or passed through the urethra and tied to an indwelling urethral catheter. The upper mucosal incision of the tunnel is closed with two or three interrupted sutures. The anastomosis is supported with No. 4-0 delayed-absorbable sutures placed in the muscularis of the bladder and the seromuscular layer of the ureter. The bladder wall should be anchored firmly to the musculature of the adjacent pelvic wall or psoas muscle (psoas muscle hitch) with No. 3-0 delayed-absorbable sutures to make certain that there is no tension on the suture line. The transverse incision in the dome of the bladder is closed longitudinally in a double layer with No. 3-0 delayed-absorbable suture, using a continuous through-and-through, mucosa–inner muscularis suture for the first layer and interrupted

seromuscular sutures for the second layer. If the transverse cystotomy incision is closed longitudinally, the bladder can be drawn upward and sutured to the psoas muscle with less tension on the suture line. The operative site is then reperitonized by approximating the cul-de-sac and bladder peritoneum and closing the peritoneum over the ureter. The Silastic catheter is left in the ureter for at least 2 weeks. The anastomosis site should always be drained retroperitoneally, with the Jackson-Pratt drain exteriorized through a stab wound that is separate from the abdominal incision.

An alternate method may be used to produce a submucosal tunnel for ureteral implantation from the external surface of the bladder wall. After the location of the ureterovesical anastomosis is established and the dome of the bladder is opened transversely, a small, 1-cm transverse muscular incision is made in the posterior wall of the bladder (Fig. 29-16A) and extended obliquely to the submucosa. After an Allis clamp is placed on either side of the incision for traction, a long Adson clamp is inserted beneath the bladder mucosa for a distance of 1.5 cm, thereby establishing a submucosal tunnel (Fig. 29-16B). The mucosa is tented slightly by elevating the tip of the clamp and a 5-mm mucosal opening is made under direct vision with scalpel. With a small straight rubber catheter as a guide, the catheter is drawn through the tunnel and muscular wall by retracting the Adson clamp (Fig. 29-16C). At this point, the catheter is sutured to the free end of the excised ureter and the ureter is drawn through the bladder wall and tunnel by traction on the rubber catheter (Fig. 29-16D). A mucosa-to-mucosa anastomosis of ureter to bladder is accomplished with No 4-0 delayed-absorbable suture (Fig. 29-16E).

Direct Implantation of the Ureter into the Bladder

Because of the associated risk of vesicoureteral reflux, direct ureter implantation into the bladder is used less frequently today, although it has served as a time-honored procedure for many gynecologic surgeons and is still an effective method. We have found that, in the absence of previous urinary tract infections or chronic renal disease, urinary reflux has not usually produced subsequent clinical problems such as recurrent ascending infection or loss of renal function. The operation is frequently referred to as the "fish-mouth" procedure because the ends of the ureter are incised and splayed on each side for approximately 5 mm to produce ureteral flaps that are sutured to the inside of the bladder wall.

The ureter is dissected free from the site of injury and mobilized from its bed for a sufficient distance to permit its implantation into the bladder without tension. Usually the bladder can be brought up to the shortened ureter if the ureter cannot be brought down to the bladder in its usual position. There is no advantage in performing the implantation retroperitoneally. The implantation should be done as close to the base of the bladder as possible (Fig. 29-17A).

After each side of the lower end of the ureter is split for about 5 mm, a substantial bite is taken into each ureteral flap with No. 4-0 delayed-absorbable sutures. A Silastic tube is threaded into the ureter and is used as a guide for the suture placement. A small opening is made directly through the full thickness of the bladder wall at the point selected for the implantation, preferably as close to the base of the bladder as can be done

without tension. The bladder base should be freed, mobilized, and advanced to facilitate this anastomosis. The edges of the bladder opening are held with Allis clamps, and the end of the catheter is introduced into the bladder. The anastomosis is performed by using the two traction sutures that were previously placed in the lower end of each ureteral flap. Each suture is introduced through the small opening into the lumen of the bladder and passed through the full thickness of the bladder wall, from serosa to mucosa, as shown in Figure 29-17B. The sutures are placed on opposite sides of the bladder incision so as to hold apart the slit ends of the ureter. A grooved director placed through the cystotomy incision will facilitate their correct placement. These sutures are tied, thus drawing the ureter into the bladder and against the mucosal surface. Anchoring sutures are placed in the seromuscular layer of the bladder and the adventitia of the ureter to fix the ureter to the bladder wall. These stitches pass through the edges of the incision in the bladder wall and pick up the sheath of the ureter (Fig. 29-17C). Any residual opening in the bladder wall is closed with interrupted No. 3-0 delayed-absorbable sutures. The bladder wall should be anchored to the pelvic wall as close as possible to the anastomosis, to relieve the tension on the ureterovesical suture line. Ordinarily, the cul-de-sac or bladder peritoneum is advanced over the operative site to maintain the suture line beneath the peritoneum. A retroperitoneal Jackson-Pratt drain is placed in the area of the anastomosis and brought through a stab wound incision in the lower abdomen.

The Silastic tubing used for splinting the anastomosis may be notched several times for improved drainage, coiled in the bladder, and left in place for about 2 weeks or longer, or it may be brought out through the urethra and tied to the urethral catheter. During the time that the ureteral stent is in place, it is irrigated only if it fails to drain freely, and then only 5 ml of 1% neomycin solution is used. The urethral catheter may be left in the bladder for a few additional days after removal of the ureteral splint while ureteral drainage becomes well established.

Ureterovesical Anastomosis of the Short Ureter

For the ureter that is badly traumatized within the broad ligament with an injury more than 5 cm above the ureterovesical junction, the technique of the psoas muscle hitch, as popularized by Harrow and others, permits ureterovesical anastomosis of a shortened ureter. This procedure also avoids the necessity of a ureteroureteral anastomosis. After assessing the extent of devitalization of the pelvic ureter, it is important to

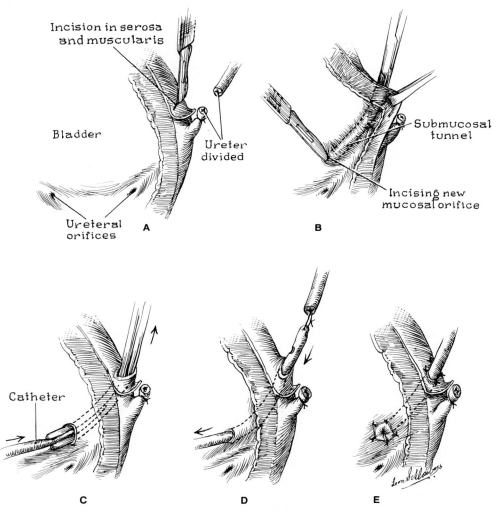

Figure 29–16. Submucosal tunnel procedure for ureterovesical anastomosis, external technique. *A*, Oblique incision through bladder wall initiated on external surface. *B*, Adson clamp passed through muscular wall and beneath mucosa for 1.5 cm (tunnel formation); bladder mucosa incised over tip of clamp at site of new ureteral orifice. *C*, Small, straight rubber catheter drawn through tunnel and bladder wall. *D*, Catheter sutured to excised ureter; ureter guided through bladder wall and tunnel by traction on catheter. *E*, Mucosa-to-mucosa anastomosis of ureter to bladder.

determine if a ureterovesical anastomosis can be performed without undue tension on the anastomosis. If the ureter does not reach the bladder wall, the lateral bladder peritoneum can be incised from each side of the inferior ramus of the pubis and the bladder base sharply dissected and mobilized from its fascial attachments to the upper vagina. To facilitate mobility of the bladder, the bladder wall should be freed from its peritoneal attachment on both sides. A horizontal incision is made in the anterior bladder wall. With a finger placed inside the bladder, the cornu can be elevated

and anchored to the psoas muscle near the pelvic brim with No. 3-0 delayed-absorbable suture to assure firm fixation (Fig. 29-18*A*). The horizontal incision is subsequently closed vertically. Care must be taken to avoid damage to the adjacent iliac vessels and genitofemoral nerves during this procedure.

Following the mobilization, funneling, and anchoring of the bladder wall to the psoas muscle, a ureteral anastomosis may be performed by one of the methods described earlier, including a direct mucosa-to-mucosa anastomosis, a fish-mouth procedure, or, preferably,

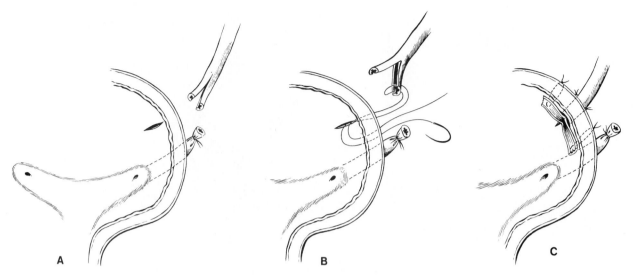

Figure 29–17. Ureterovesical implantation, fish-mouth technique. *A*, Excised free end of ureter is spatulated for 1–2 cm. New ureteral orifice has been made by scalpel above the trigone in position to reach excised ureter. *B*, Each end of ureteral flap is anchored with a mattress suture of No. 4-0 delayed-absorbable suture and passed through new ureteral orifice and full thickness of bladder wall. *C*, Bladder flaps are tied on external surface of the bladder and reinforced with seromuscular sutures in bladder wall and ureter at site of implantation.

the submucosal tunnel procedure. A fine suture of No. 4-0 delayed-absorbable suture is used to suture the ureteral and bladder mucosa, and an indwelling Silastic tube with multiple fenestrations is inserted to the renal pelvis and coiled in the bladder for postoperative drainage. The angles of the bladder incision are closed with interrupted seromuscular sutures. The implant is supported by three or four anchoring sutures of fine, delayed-absorbable suture in the serosa-muscularis layer of the bladder and ureter (Fig. 29-18*B*). This technique is superior to the Boari bladder flap procedure, as the latter is frequently associated with reflux and is subject to ischemia with secondary stenosis or necrosis of the flap if it is lengthy or if the pelvis has received radiation.

Vaginal Repair of Ureteral Injuries

Credit is given to Mackenrodt for the original method of vaginal repair of ureterovaginal fistulas by a technique of "entropionizing." Kelly was an advocate of the vaginal approach. In 1901, he wrote that one must not open the abdomen to repair a ureterovaginal fistula if a simple anastomosis can be affected per vaginum. This advice has certainly not been followed since.

Current reports of ureteral injury repair seldom mention the possibility that such repairs may be done vaginally at the time of operation of injury or even later

if the injury is not discovered immediately. However, our experience, first reported in 1971 and extended since then, suggests that simple injuries to the terminal (lowest 3 cm) ureter can be repaired vaginally and sometimes more easily than with an abdominal approach. The initial report of vaginal repair of eight ureteral injuries in seven patients was successful with satisfactory results in all but one case. These transvaginal operations included simple disligation (two), disligation with ureteroureterostomy (two), and ureteroneocystostomy (four). The interval between the operation of injury and the operation of repair varied between 0 and 46 days.

In some cases, the injured ureter is found without difficulty. In others, some search is necessary. If more adequate exposure can be achieved with a Schuchardt incision (Figs. 11-21*A* and 11-21*B*), it should be made without hesitation. Knowing the anatomy of the ureter as seen through the vagina is helpful. Developing the paravesicle space will facilitate the dissection and make it possible to locate the dilated ureter above the site of injury. A timid dissection limited to a small area around an indurated fistulous tract will make ureteral identification and repair more difficult. On the other hand, a careless and random dissection in indurated tissue and distorted anatomy increases the possibility that the bladder and/or rectum will be injured. Injecting certain tissues with normal saline may help the dissection. Identification of the ureter is facilitated if by cystoscopy

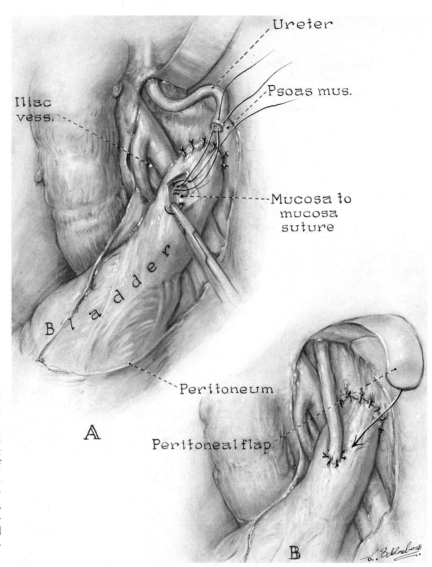

Figure 29–18. Ureterovesical anastomosis of the short ureter–psoas muscle hitch procedure. *A,* Bladder peritoneum is incised from lateral pelvic wall, and bladder is mobilized and anchored to psoas muscle at pelvic brim (psoas muscle hitch) near site of planned ureterovesical anastomosis. Mucosa-to-mucosa anastomosis of ureter to bladder is performed. *B,* Ureterovesical anastomosis is reinforced with fine serosal sutures and peritoneum is advanced over anastomotic site.

a catheter can be passed up the injured ureter to the point of obstruction, even if it is for only a centimeter or less. Once a structure is dissected and identified as the ureter, this can be confirmed by doing a retrograde pyelogram on the operating table or by injecting indigo carmine intravenously.

After the ureteral injury has been examined, a decision regarding the proper operative procedure for repair is made. Depending on the extent and location of the injury, decision will usually be a choice between simple disligation, disligation with repair of a defect in the ureteral wall, disligation with ureteroureterostomy, or disligation with ureteroneocystostomy. If the ureter has been partially or completely ligated, very often a defect will be obvious in the ureteral wall upon

removal of the suture. A ureteroureterostomy may be done, provided the distal ureter does not seem damaged or stenosed. A catheter splint is left indwelling. This operation has the advantage of preserving the normal ureterovesical junction. If the ureter has only recently been partially obstructed and angulated by the pull of an adjacent suture, it will generally not yet have become stenotic from fibrous tissue formation. In such a case, simply releasing the ureter from the suture and inserting an indwelling ureteral catheter for several days will suffice.

If a ureteroneocystostomy is to be performed, the end of the ureter is freshened, split on each side for 0.5 cm, and then drawn into the bladder through a small incision in the bladder base. The bladder base is the most optimal anatomic location for reimplanting a ureter. When operating vaginally, the bladder base is the only location available for reimplantation (Fig. 29-19). Usually, two 3-0 delayed-absorbable sutures are used to anchor the ureter inside the bladder, and the anastomosis is reinforced with a few additional sutures approximating periureteral and perivesical tissues, carefully placed so as not to kink or obstruct the ureter. An indwelling ureteral catheter is used and left in place for 2–3 weeks. A double-ended pigtail catheter has the advantage of better retention. However, since the lowest end is coiled within the bladder, it is not available for irrigation should this be necessary to reestablish drainage. A soft silastic tube that fits snugly but without distending the lumen of the ureter may be brought out through the urethra and tied to an indwelling Foley catheter. It may be irrigated at any time the drainage seems slow. A ureteral catheter with a pigtail in the renal pelvis and a lower end brought out through the urethra has the advantage of better retention and the possibility of irrigation when needed.

On occasion it may be deemed appropriate for the site of repair to be reinforced by developing a bulbocavernosus fat flap from the labia and transposing it to the bladder base. Lapides and Caffery have suggested that the healing of a ureteral injury might be facilitated if the site of repair could be surrounded by fat. This fat flap will also serve as a protective shield between the ureteral repair site and the vaginal vault (see Fig. 30-10). The vault should, of course, be left open for drainage.

Varying circumstances will dictate how long a ureteral splinting catheter should be left indwelling. In general, it should be left in for several weeks, until, it is hoped, the ureter has healed without stenosis. Urinary antibiotics and an adequate urine output will help prevent serious urinary tract infection. Excretory urography is done shortly after the ureteral catheter is removed, periodically for several years, and at any time there is a suggestion of inadequate drainage through the repaired ureter.

Almost all ureteral injuries sustained at the time of vaginal surgery will be located in the very lowest part of the ureter, and depending on circumstances, should be accessible for repair through a vaginal approach. If the injury results from abdominal hysterectomy, it may be more difficult to repair transvaginally unless it can be demonstrated with certainty that the injury is in the very lowest part of the ureter and circumstances are otherwise optimal. The skill and experience of the operator will have a great impact on whether to use the transvaginal or the transabdominal approach.

If the integrity of the ureters is determined at the end of each vaginal surgery that places the ureters at risk of injury, then the proper repair of an injury can be done immediately through the vagina with ease and with better results to be anticipated. This prompt identification of ureteral injury can be achieved by simply injecting 5 cc of indigo carmine intravenously and watching the dye spurt from each ureteral orifice with a cystoscope. This can be routinely done at the end of each

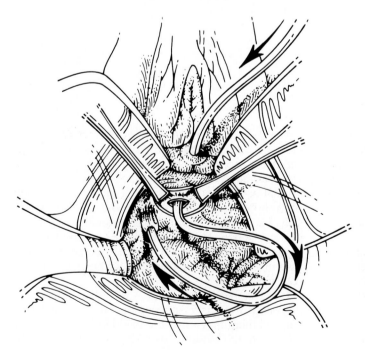

Figure 29–19. After the ureter is identified, debrided, mobilized, spatulated, and catheterized, the catheter is brought into the bladder and out through the ureter through a cystostomy incision. A ureteroneocystostomy is then performed.

vaginal operation. Of course, it can also be done at the end of each abdominal operation, provided the patient has been positioned in Allen stirrups for the procedure.

Other Procedures

Other more complicated procedures usually beyond the scope of most gynecologic surgeons have been used in the management of ureteral injuries.

Transureteroureterostomy (ie, anastomosis of the upper ureter on one side to the intact ureter on the opposite side) may be done through a tunnel beneath the peritoneum if the ureter above the injured site is long enough to reach across but for some reason cannot or should not be implanted into the bladder. The decision to use this technique should be made with great care, since there is the potential for compromising the normal function of the contralateral urinary tract. The technique has been used successfully in carefully selected cases, however.

Renal autotransplantation into the pelvis offers the potential for excellent results in the hands of an experienced renal transplant surgeon. It is a method to be considered in a patient who has no possibility of repair of the injured ureter and poor function of the contralateral kidney. It is an advantage that the risk is limited to the kidney on the affected side.

Ingenious techniques have been devised for substituting a segment of ileum for a ureter that has been damaged too extensively to be repaired or implanted into the bladder (Fig. 29-20). In 1970, Krupp and associates reported their experience with this operation in 19 gynecologic patients. Indeed, the ileum may be used to replace the entire ureter from the kidney to the bladder. Of course, both ureters may be anastomosed to an ileal conduit that may then be anastomosed to an intact and properly functioning bladder or to the skin, as in the Bricker pouch, if the bladder is not present or is unsuitable. In exenteration procedures a sigmoid conduit may be used (see Fig. 45-7).

As proposed by Turner-Warwick, repair of difficult ureteral injuries may be more successful if the site of repair can be wrapped with a vascularized omental pedicle. He points out that healing of the ureter is fundamentally dependent on the condition of the tissues surrounding the ureter. In the presence of inflammation and fibrosis of the periureteral tissues, healing may be impaired. The support of an omental wrap is infinitely better, according to Turner-Warwick.

Percutaneous nephrostomy done under the guidance of computerized tomography has become the procedure of choice in almost all cases of urinary tract obstruction requiring temporary nephrostomy drainage, as pointed out by Hedegaard and Wallace. The percutaneous nephrostomy can provide temporary de-

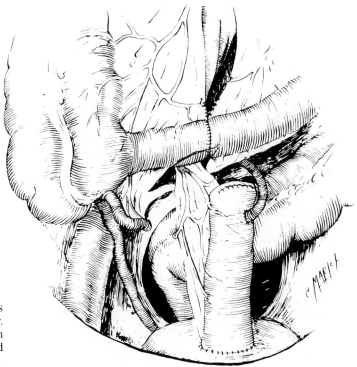

Figure 29–20. A segment of terminal ileum has been used to substitute for the lower ureter. (Krupp P, Hoffman M, Roeling W. Terminal ileum as ureteral muscle: relationship to intubated ureterotomy. J Urol 1955;73:47.)

compression of the kidney to preserve function while other therapy is planned. The procedure is done under local anesthesia, a major advantage in a seriously ill patient. The percutaneous nephrostomy tract also allows the passage of stents and catheters down the ureter and sometimes beyond the point of ureteral obstruction and into the bladder.

Results of Ureteral Plastic Surgery

The long-term results of any type of ureterovesical anastomosis are good if the proper procedure has been chosen and performed with meticulous surgical skill. Healing will fail only when there has been an error in surgical judgment or when ischemia or irreversible ureteral damage has occurred at the site of anastomosis. Vesicoureteral reflux may be associated with the fish-mouth anastomosis. Although recently there has been concern about the detrimental effect of reflux on the upper urinary tract, our past experience with the fish-mouth procedure has been favorable without evidence of progressive infection or deterioration of kidney function. However, there is no question that the submucosal tunnel technique of implantation is more physiologic, and in the presence of chronic urinary tract infection it is obviously preferable.

The success rate with ureteroureteral anastomosis has been improved in recent years by the careful selection of cases for this procedure and improvements in the operative technique used. In general, the indwelling Silastic catheter has helped to ensure a dry anastomotic site. The stent can be left in place for long periods until ureteral healing has been complete without creating a foreign-body effect on the anastomotic site. Only when the blood supply of the ureter has been seriously compromised or more than 1.5 cm of ureter has been resected has there been an increased risk of failure of healing with secondary fistula formation or ureteral stricture. Such cases require drainage of the kidney for an extended time and should probably have a protective pyelostomy to enhance healing of the suture line. Alternatively, a J-tube inserted in the ureter at the time of anastomosis will be better retained in the renal pelvis and can be left to drain into the bladder for long periods.

Excretory urography will be indicated for several months or longer to be assured of satisfactory long-term results.

Even though challenged by a variety of pathologic conditions and surgical procedures, the integrity of the urinary tract can usually be maintained or reconstructed without loss of function if the gynecologic surgeon will:

Learn the anatomy and physiology of the ureter.
Avoid ureteral injury by careful pelvic dissection.

Make every effort to recognize ureteral injury at the operation of injury so that appropriate repair can be performed immediately.
Recognize signs of ureteral injury as early as possible in the postoperative period so that measures can be taken to minimize impairment of renal function with ultimate restoration of ureteral integrity.

Bibliography

Barclay DL. Cesarean hysterectomy at Charity Hospital in New Orleans—1000 consecutive operations. Clin Obstet Gynecol 1969; 12:635.

Beland G. Early treatment of ureteral injuries found after gynecological surgery. J Urol 1977;118:25.

Benson RC, Hinmann F, Jr. Urinary tract injuries in obstetrics and gynecology. Am J Obstet Gynecol 1955;70:467.

Bergman H, ed. The ureter. New York: Springer-Verlag, 1981.

Blandy JP. Operative urology. Oxford: Blackwell, 1978.

Boari A. Chirugia dell'uretere, con prefazione del Dott: I. Albarran, 1900, Contributo sperimentale alla plastica delle uretere. Atte Dell'a Acad Delle Science Med e Naturali di Ferrara 1894; Seduta 27, May, 14:444.

Boyce WH. Use of the internal ureteral stent in surgery of the kidney and ureter. In: Boyarksy S, Gottschalk EA, Tanagho EA, et al, eds. Urodynamics: hydrodynamics of the ureter and renal pelvis. New York: Academic Press, 1971.

Bright TC, Peters PC. Ureteral injuries secondary to operative procedures. J Urol 1977;9:22.

Brudenell M. The pelvic ureter. Proc R Soc Med 1977;70:188.

Cruikshank SH. Surgical method of identifying the ureters during total vaginal hysterectomy. Obstet Gynecol 1986;67:277.

Ehrlich RM, Melman A, Skinner DG. The use of vesicopsoas hitch in urologic surgery. J Urol 1978;119:322.

Everett HS, Mattingly RF. Urinary tract injuries resulting from pelvic surgery. Am J Obstet Gynecol 1956;71:502.

Everett HS, Williams TJ. Urology in the female. In: Campbell MF, Harrison JB, eds. Urology. 3rd ed. Philadelphia: WB Saunders, 1970.

Feiner D. Operative injuries of the ureter. SGO 1938;66:790.

Flynn JT, Tiptaft RC, Woodhourse CR, et al. The early and aggressive repair of iatrogenic ureteric injuries. Brit J Urol 1979;51:454.

Freund WA, Joseph L. Ueber die Harnleiter—Gebarmutter—Fistel nebst neuen Unntersnchungen uber das normale Verhalten der Harnleiter im Weiblichen Becken. Berlin Klin Wochenschrift 1869;6:504.

Fry DE, Milholen L, Harbrecht PJ. Iatrogenic ureteral injury: options in management. Arch Surg 1983;118:454.

Gillenwater JY. The pathology of urinary obstruction. In: Walsh, Gittes, Perlmutter, and Stomey, eds. Urology. 5th ed. Philadelphia: WB Saunders, 1986.

Glenn JF, ed. Urologic surgery. 3rd ed. Philadelphia: JB Lippincott, 1983.

Harrow BR. A neglected maneuver for ureterovesical implantation following injury at gynecologic operation. J Urol 1968;100:280.

Hatch KD, Parham G, Shingleton HM, et al. Ureteral strictures and fistulae following radical hysterectomy. Gynecol Oncol 1984; 19:17.

Hedgegaard CK, Wallace D. Percutaneous nephrostomy: current indications and potential uses in obstetrics and gynecology. Literature review and report of a case. Obstet Gynecol Surv 1987; 42:671.

Hofmeister FJ. Pelvic anatomy of the ureter in relation to surgery performed through the vagina. Clin Obstet Gynecol 1982;25:821.

Hunner GL, Everett HS. Ureteroperitoneal fistula with urinary ascites and chronic peritonitis. JAMA 1930;95:327.

Kaplan JO, Winslow OP, Sneider SE, et al. Dilatation of a surgically ligated ureter through percutaneous nephrostomy. Am J Roentgenol 1982;39:188.

Kaufman JJ. Unusual cause of extensive ureteral obstruction. J Urol 1962;87:319.

Kaye KW, Goldberg ME. Applied anatomy of the kidney and ureter. Urol Clin North Am 1982;9(1):3.

Kelly HA. Operative gynecology. Vol. 1. New York: Appleton-Century-Crofts, 1901.

Koontz WW, Klein FA, Smith MJ. Surgery of the ureter. In: Walsh, Gittes, Perlmutter, Stamey, eds. Urology. 5th ed. Philadelphia: WB Saunders, 1986.

Krupp P, Hoffman M, Roeling W. Terminal ileum as ureteral substitute. Obstet Gynecol 1970;35:416.

Lapides Jr, Caffery EL. Observations on healing of ureteral muscle: relationship to intubated ureterotomy. J Urol 1955;73:47.

Larson DM, Malone JM, Jr, Copeland LJ, et al. Ureteral assessment after radical hysterectomy. Obstet Gynecol 1987;69:612.

Lee RA, Symmonds RE. Ureterovaginal fistula. Am J Obstet Gynecol 1971;109:1032.

Lewis HY, Pierce JM. Return of function after complete ureteral obstruction of 69 days duration. J Urol 1962;88:377.

Liu W, Meigs JV. Radical hysterectomy and pelvic lymphadenectomy. Am J Obstet Gynecol 1955;69:1.

Major FJ. Retained ovarian remnant causing ureteral obstruction. Obstet Gynecol 1968;32:748.

Mann WJ, Arato M, Patsner B, et al. Ureteral injuries in an obstetrics and gynecology training program: etiology and management. Obstet Gynecol 1988;72:82.

Marmar JL. The management of ureteral obstruction with silicone rubber splint catheters. J Urol 1970;104:386.

Mattingly RF, Borkowf HI. Lower urinary tract injuries in pregnancy. In: Barber HK, Graber EA, eds. Surgical disease in pregnancy. Philadelphia: WB Saunders, 1974.

Meigs JV. The Wertheim operation of carcinoma of the cervix. Am J Obstet Gynecol 1945;49:542.

Newell QU. Injury to ureters during pelvic operation. Ann Surg 1939;109:48.

Notley RG. Ureteral morphology: anatomic and clinical considerations. Urology 1978;12:9.

Notley RG. Anatomy and physiology of the ureter. In: Blandy JP, ed. Urology. London: Blackwell, 1976.

Pettit PD, Lee RA. Ovarian remnant syndrome: diagnostic dilemma and surgical challenge. Obstet Gynecol 1988;71:580.

Piscitelli JT, Simel DL, Addison WA. Who should have intravenous pyelograms before hysterectomy for benign disease? Obstet Gynecol 1987;69:541.

Plauche WC. Cesarean hysterectomy: indications, technique, and complications. Clin Obstet Gynecol 1986;29(2):318.

Ponig BF, Jr. Microsurgical ureteroureterostomy in ureteral injuries. J Urol 1982;128:594.

Prout GR, Jr, Koontz WW, Jr. Partial vesical immobilization: an important adjunct to ureteroneocystostomy. J Urol 1970;103:147.

Sampson JA. Ligation and clamping of the ureter as complications of surgical operations. Am Med 1902;4:693.

Sampson JA. The relation between carcinoma cervicis uteri and the ureters and its significance in the more radical operations for that disease. Johns Hopkins Med Bull 1904;156:72.

Sampson JA. Ureteral fistulae as sequelae of pelvic operations. Surg Gynecol Obstet 1909;8:479.

Shapiro SR, Bennett AH. Recovery of renal function after prolonged unilateral ureteral obstruction. J Urol 1976;115:136.

Shoenwald MB, Orkin LA. Bilateral intravesical ureteral ligation. Complication of Cooper's ligament suspension. J Urol 1974;3:787.

Symmonds RE. Ureteral injuries associated with gynecologic surgery: prevention and management. Clin Obstet Gynecol 1976;19:623.

Thompson IM. Bladder flap repair of ureteral injuries. Urol Clin North Am 1977;4(1):51.

Thompson IM, Ross G, Jr. Long-term results of bladder flap repair of ureteral injuries. J Urol 1974;111:483.

Thompson JD, Benigno BB. Vaginal repair of ureteral injuries. Am J Obstet Gynecol 1971;3:601.

Thompson RH. Ureteral injuries in pelvic surgery. Bull Dept Gynecol OB Emory U 1980;11(2):93.

Tuffier T, Levi C. Etude sur les fistules ureterovaginales (etiologie et traitement). Ann Gynecol Obstet 1895;43:382.

Turner-Warwick R. The use of pedicle grafts in the repair of urinary tract fistulae. Br J Urol 1972;44:644.

Turner-Warwick R, Worth PH. The psoas bladder hitch procedure for the replacement of the lower third of the ureter. Br J Urol 1969;41:701.

Van Nagell JR, Jr, Roddick JW, Jr. Vaginal hysterectomy, the ureter and excretory urography. Obstet Gynecol 1972;39:784.

Waldeyer W. Uber die sogenannte Ureterscheide (Verhandlugen der Anatomischen Gesellschaft). Anatomischer Anzeiger 1892;9:259.

Wertheim E. Zur Frag der Radikaloperation beim Uteruskrebs. Arch Gynak 1900;61:627.

Wesolowski S. Bilateral ureteral injuries in gynaecology. Br J Urol 1969;41:666.

Witters S, Cornelissen J, Vereecken R. Iatrogenic ureteral injury: aggressive or conservative treatment. Am J Obstet Gynecol 1986;155:582.

30

Vesicovaginal Fistulas

JOHN D. THOMPSON

Before the 17th century, vesicovaginal fistula was considered a hopeless condition. The more practical-minded of those times devoted their efforts to making receptacles to catch urine, thus making the life of the victim more endurable.

The first real attempt to repair a vesicovaginal fistula surgically was made by a Dutchman, H. van Roonhuyse, whose contribution was far in advance of his time. In 1676, van Roonhuyse recommended placement of the patient in a lithotomy position, satisfactory exposure of the fistula by a retracting speculum, thorough denudation of the margins of the fistula, approximation of the denuded edges by means of quills thrust through the edges of the wound and held in place by silk threads, dressing of the wound with balsam and absorbent vaginal dressings, and quiet bedrest until the parts had healed.

In 1839, George Hayward, of Boston, described the important technical point of separating the vagina from the bladder. In 1840, John Mettauer, of Virginia, first used twisted metal (lead) sutures. In 1845, Jobert de Lamballe described his incision for relieving tension on the suture line. In 1852, Wutzer, of Bonn, reported curing 11 of 35 patients. He was the first to use suprapubic drainage.

McGregor has written an interesting account of female disorders and 19th-century medicine with special emphasis on obstetric care, vesicovaginal fistula, and the work of J. Marion Sims (generally considered the father of surgery for vesicovaginal fistula in America) and Thomas A. Emmet at the Woman's Hospital in New York City. Sims's first paper on vesicovaginal fistula appeared in 1852. There is no doubt that he attained greater success than anyone up to his time, although his results were certainly not perfect. It is interesting that his operation was not new. Each step had been used and described before by other surgeons. The only innovation that Sims contributed was the use of silver wire suture, which was, in truth, a great step forward in fistula repair. Sims should be given credit for enunciating clearly many principles of vesicovaginal fistula repair that are still appropriate today.

The transvesical approach was described by Trendelenburg in 1890. In 1893, von Dittel described the transperitoneal approach, dissecting the bladder from the uterus and the vagina and closing the opening in the bladder from above. Maisonneuve, and later Mackenrodt, made a contribution to the technique that was of great importance. He incised the vagina in the midline across the fistula and then, with the knife and forceps, split the margins of the fistula so as to separate completely the bladder from the vaginal wall. He then closed the bladder and vaginal incisions separately. This procedure, also described by Mackenrodt, approximated broad raw surfaces for healing and more nearly approached our modern methods than any technique previously described.

In 1896, Kelly described a method of closing a large bladder defect by freeing the bladder from the cervix all the way up to the peritoneum. In the same communication, Kelly mentioned using preoperative ureteral catheterization to avoid injury of the ureters, although Pawlik first recommended ureteral catheterization in vesicovaginal fistula repair in 1882. In 1906, Kelly described a suprapubic route of operating for vesical fistulas and reported 12 different surgical approaches for closure of vesicovaginal fistulas.

Most of this early experience with vesicovaginal fistula repair was derived from operating on patients whose fistula resulted from an obstetrical etiology. In 1914, Latzko described a technique suited to cases of vesicovaginal fistula resulting from total hysterectomy. Modified from the original description by Simon, it consisted of obliteration of the vaginal vault with approximation of broad areas of denuded tissue. In 1942, he reported on 31 cases of vesicovaginal fistula treated by this method, with cure in 29 cases, improvement in one case, and failure in another. Latzko's contribution has been a truly great one, and in recent years its value has been magnified because of the increase in the number of fistulas that followed the introduction of the total hysterectomy. Many others, including Garlock, Ingelman-Sundberg, Martius, Bastiaanse, and O'Connor, have contributed special techniques of vesicovaginal fistula repair. Robert Zacharin has written an interesting review of the history of obstetric vesicovaginal fistula.

ETIOLOGY

Vesicovaginal fistulas, as seen today, result chiefly from obstetric injury; operative accidents, mostly those during total abdominal or vaginal hysterectomy; extension of carcinoma of the cervix or the radiation therapy for treating this disease; and miscellaneous causes. Formerly, those following obstetric injury formed the largest group, but the improvement in obstetric methods has greatly reduced their number in many countries in the world. However, vesicovaginal fistulas from obstetric causes are still common in developing countries, especially in Africa and Asia. The tragic social and medical circumstances of these young women have been studied by Murphy. Tahzib studied the epidemiologic determinants of vesicovaginal fistulas in northern Nigeria between 1969 and 1980. There were 1443 patients in the series, the largest series of vesicovaginal fistula patients ever reported. Eighty-three percent resulted from prolonged obstructed labor. Thirteen percent resulted from gishiri cut, a traditional tribal practice of cutting the anterior vagina with a razor blade to treat a variety of conditions, including obstructed labor, infertility, dyspareunia, backache, goiter, and a number of other complaints. Only 1% of fistulas in this study resulted from surgical trauma. Vesicovaginal fistulas are still a major cause for concern in many developing countries. Measures for prevention must include universal education, an improved status of women, and improved and accessible medical services, including contraceptive services. The considerable efforts of Lawson in Ibadan (Nigeria), of the Hamlins in Addis Ababa (Ethiopia), and of many others toward the alleviation of this problem are indeed laudable.

The uniform use of total rather than subtotal hysterectomy has resulted in an increase in postoperative fistulas. There is very little risk of injury to the bladder when a subtotal hysterectomy is performed. It is the removal of the cervix that increases the risk of injury to the bladder during the performance of total hysterectomy.

Everett and Mattingly reviewed 149 cases of bladder fistulas operated on at the Johns Hopkins Hospital between 1933 and 1953. Of these, 44% followed gynecologic surgery, 20% resulted from obstetrical injury, 32% were related to carcinoma of the cervix and its radiation treatment, and 4% were from miscellaneous causes. Since that report, there has been a further reduction both in the number of vesicovaginal fistulas caused by gynecologic cancer and its treatment with radiation or surgery and in the number caused by obstetric trauma. In the last 30 years at Grady Memorial Hospital in Atlanta, no vesicovaginal fistulas have occurred during 180,000 obstetric deliveries in a predominantly black and indigent population. In the United States, about three fourths of the vesicovaginal fistulas seen are small fistulas in the vaginal vault that appear after total abdominal and vaginal hysterectomy for benign disease. Lee and associates reported the etiology of vesicovaginal fistulas seen in 156 patients at the Mayo Clinic between 1970 and 1985. One hundred thirty-two followed abdominal hysterectomy, 20 followed vaginal hysterectomy, 4 followed radical hysterectomy, 3 followed vaginal repair, 5 followed cesarean section, 6 followed cesarean section/hysterectomy, 8 followed forceps delivery, 6 followed trauma/fulguration, and 6 followed radiation.

ANATOMIC CONSIDERATIONS

Fistulas may be located at any point along the anterior vaginal wall and may include any part or all of the bladder base and urethra (Fig. 30-1). They may be single or multiple. Although there may be a single orifice on one side and multiple orifices on the other, this is unusual.

High fistulas with the uterus in situ may be obstetric in etiology and may include the anterior cervical lip. High fistulas that result from radiation may also include the cervix. When a fistula follows total hysterectomy, it is high in the vaginal vault. Its posterior margin coincides with the transverse scar in the vault that results from removal of the cervix. The high fistulas are always supratrigonal in location, that is, above the interureteric ridge, although the ureteral orifices may be located near the lower edge of a high fistula. This is an important anatomic point to remember in avoiding ureteral obstruction during repair of a high vesicovaginal fistula.

Midvaginal fistulas may be located below the interureteric ridge and usually are caused by a misplaced radium applicator or anterior colporrhaphy. Difficult forceps operations may also cause midvaginal lacerations and fistulas.

Obstetric fistulas are most commonly located in the *bladder neck and upper urethra*. Fistulas in this location damage the tissue responsible for maintaining normal urinary continence. During prolonged obstructed labor, pressure necrosis of the bladder wall caught

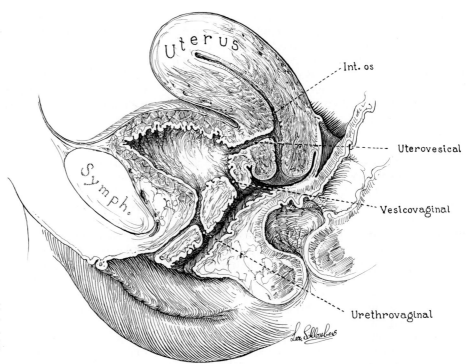

Int. os

Uterovesical

Vesicovaginal

Urethrovaginal

Figure 30–1. Diagrammatic sagittal section showing locations of vesicocervical, vesicovaginal, and urethrovaginal fistula.

between the fetal head and the pubic symphysis may result in vesicovaginal fistulas. Difficult forceps operations, anterior colporrhaphies, and irradiation may cause fistulas in this location.

Massive fistulas involve loss of most or all of the vaginal wall. The anterior cervical lip, the bladder base including the trigone, and the upper urethra may be lost in extreme cases. The ureteral orifices are easily identified, spurting urine at the margins of the fistula. The dome of the bladder may prolapse through the fistula. Moir has described a circumferential vesicovaginal fistula owing to extreme cases of prolonged obstructed labor. Both the anterior bladder wall behind the symphysis and the posterior bladder wall undergo pressure necrosis and slough, leaving a large area of exposed pubic bone. This obviously creates special technical problems in repair.

PREVENTION

The first and essential step in limiting the morbidity of vesicovaginal fistulas is prevention. In the United States, major contributors to prevention have been improved obstetric management and techniques of delivery, especially the more liberal use of cesarean section for delivery, with a concomitant decrease in the number of difficult forceps maneuvers, and the im-

provements in labor management. Because of this, few American gynecologists have experience in the repair of vesicovaginal fistulas of obstetric etiology unless the experience was gained abroad, as reported by Elkins and associates.

Today the most important measures in further reducing the incidence and morbidity of vesicovaginal fistulas must be directed toward proper techniques of gynecologic operations, especially total vaginal and abdominal hysterectomy, and toward immediate recognition and repair of bladder injury at the operation of injury so that a fistula will not develop. Mattingly and Borkowf have written a complete review of this subject. Gynecologic surgery is the most common etiology of vesicovaginal fistulas in the United States and in many other developed countries in the world, and the bladder is the most common site of urinary tract injury during gynecologic surgery. The bladder is rarely injured during subtotal abdominal hysterectomy. Among 75 posthysterectomy vesicovaginal fistulas reported by Miller and George, none followed subtotal hysterectomy, 54 followed total abdominal hysterectomy, 18 followed vaginal hysterectomy, and 3 followed radical abdominal hysterectomy. Since the advent of the total abdominal hysterectomy, the incidence of injury to the bladder base has increased; it occurs in approximately 0.5% to 1% of patients undergoing a total abdominal hysterectomy. To reduce the risk of vesicovaginal fistulas, Baker has suggested that the surgeon consider leaving the cervix in place by doing a subtotal hysterectomy when the cervix is benign, when removing the uterine corpus will remove the patient's pathology, and when there are conditions such as endometriosis or tuboovarian abscess that may increase the risk of bladder injury when the cervix is removed. We subscribe to this principle of using good surgical judgment but believe it should be possible for an experienced gynecologic surgeon to remove the cervix in almost all patients and without injury to the bladder. However, if in the judgment of the gynecologic surgeon, the danger of removing the cervix is greater than the danger of leaving it in, then a subtotal hysterectomy should be done.

The bladder is very closely related developmentally to the uterus, cervix, and vagina and is especially vulnerable to injury when a total hysterectomy is done. The base of the bladder rests on the anterior lower uterine isthmus and the cervix. The trigone of the bladder, however, is found at a level below the cervix. It is attached to the upper one third of the anterior vaginal wall, beginning at about the anterior vaginal fornix and below, and therefore is less susceptible to injury. If the bladder is injured during its dissection away from the cervix and upper vagina, the injury will be located above the interureteric ridge in almost all cases. This anatomic relationship is extremely important to keep in mind (see Chapters 4 and 29).

Injury to the base of the bladder is three times more common with total abdominal hysterectomy than with vaginal hysterectomy. The usual cause of such injury is inadequate mobilization of the bladder inferiorly and laterally or vigorous and blunt dissection in an improper plane between the bladder base and the protective pubovesicocervical fascia covering the cervix. Dissection in the proper plane to separate the bladder from the cervix and upper vagina should be done sharply and carefully with fine scissors. The use of blunt dissection, especially pushing down against the vesicocervical attachment with a sponge stick, should be discouraged, since this technique can weaken the integrity of the bladder wall. An intrafascial technique of removing the cervix, utilizing an inverted T or V incision in the pubovesicocervical fascia covering the cervix anteriorly, should be used whenever possible to prevent injury to the bladder and the ureters (see Chapter 27). Before clamps can be safely placed on the cardinal ligaments and before an incision is made through the anterior vaginal wall, the bladder must be thoroughly mobilized *inferiorly* and *laterally* and the vesicocervicovaginal space must be completely developed (see Chapter 27). Constant traction of the uterus superiorly and retraction of the bladder inferiorly with accurate placement of clamps and sutures will help prevent bladder injury. Some vesicovaginal fistulas are caused

by placement of suture(s) through the bladder base when the vaginal cuff is sutured. This is usually the result of inadequate mobilization of the bladder inferiorly and laterally away from the upper vagina or of inadequate exposure and retraction. In this instance, usually unrecognized, gradual necrosis of the bladder wall will lead to the development of a vesicovaginal fistula most commonly within the first week after surgery, when the patient will notice incontinence of urine through the vagina.

During the past three to four decades, the more frequent use of vaginal hysterectomy for the correction of anatomic pelvic relaxation and treatment of benign gynecologic disease has resulted in an increase in the number of injuries to the base of the bladder from vaginal hysterectomy. The location of the injury is identical to that which occurs with a total abdominal hysterectomy. The vast majority of such injuries are in the supratrigonal portion of the bladder base, although in rare instances when a cystocele repair has also been done, the injury may occur lower in the trigone. The correct anatomic plane between the bladder and the cervix and uterine isthmus in the midline is ordinarily easy to find and is relatively avascular. Sharp dissection in this plane with traction on the cervix inferiorly and retraction of the bladder superiorly will locate the vesicouterine fold of peritoneum promptly (see Chapter 27). After a small incision is made in the peritoneum, loops of small intestine or omentum should be identified to confirm that the peritoneal cavity rather than the bladder has been entered. Only then should the peritoneal incision be enlarged. A retractor kept beneath the bladder will protect it from harm. However, when development of the vesicocervical space is difficult or misdirected, troublesome bleeding obscures the operative field. The dissection may be too anterior and superficial and the bladder wall may be weakened or the bladder actually entered. Hopefully, the operator will not extend the incision into the bladder before recognizing the error. Although most entries into the bladder are easily recognized, on occasion the operator may be misled into believing that entry into the peritoneal cavity has been made. The presence or absence of omentum or intestine seen through the entry site will distinguish between the two. Placing an instrument (Kelly clamp or uterine sound) transurethrally into the bladder helps identify a bladder entry and can be used to identify a proper plane of dissection between the bladder and cervix before an accidental entry is made. Transurethral instillation of 5 cc of methylene blue will stain the bladder mucosa and allow its identification before final entry into the bladder. This simple measure is recommended whenever it is anticipated that the proper plane of dissection will be difficult to find. Leaving some urine in the bladder during vaginal surgery may also facilitate recognition of bladder injury, since a spurt of urine will be seen if the bladder is entered. Vesicovaginal fistulas resulting from total vaginal hysterectomy are best prevented by finding the proper plane of dissection between the bladder base and the anterior lower uterine segment, opening the anterior peritoneum carefully, adequately mobilizing the bladder laterally, placing a retractor beneath the bladder, and properly placing clamps and ligatures on paracervical and parametrial tissue as close to the uterus as possible. Jaszczak and Evans have proposed an intrafascial technique for vaginal hysterectomy designed to avoid bladder injury, among other things. Although this idea may be sound, it has not been evaluated extensively by others.

Because of the frequent use of low cervical cesarean section as a method of abdominal delivery, it can be estimated that approximately one out of every five or six women in the United States who need a hysterectomy will have previously had a cesarean section. This can cause difficulty in dissection of the vesicocervical space because of unusually dense adherence of the bladder to the uterine isthmus. This difficulty can be experienced with either abdominal or vaginal hysterectomy. In our experience, the dissection is less difficult with vaginal hysterectomy because the operator can use transurethral passage of an instrument to help identify a proper plane of dissection. Certainly, a history of previous cesarean section should be a warning that the dissection must be carefully performed and the bladder tested for integrity before the operation is complete. A history of prior radiation causes similar difficulties and requires similar precautions.

Vesicovaginal fistula may be very rare when gynecologic surgery is done properly. Between 1970 and 1985, 24,883 patients underwent major gynecologic operations at the Mayo Clinic. Only one patient developed a vesicovaginal fistula (after a primary radical hysterectomy).

BLADDER INJURY

If an injury to the bladder can be recognized at the operation of injury and can be repaired properly, a vesicovaginal fistula is not likely to occur. However, since the bladder base is the most dependent portion, injuries in this location are especially likely to result in fistula formation if they are not recognized and repaired correctly. Whether the bladder wall has been weakened or the bladder has actually been entered, the extent of the injury and its proximity to the ureteral orifices should be assessed. Ordinarily, the ureteral orifices are not involved. However, if they cannot be located easily, 5 ml of indigo carmine given intravenously will cause blue urine to spurt from the orifices in only a few minutes, facilitating their identification through the cystoscope. Ureteral catheters can be passed to avoid damage to or incorporation of the ureters in the repair of the bladder defect. However, this is not often necessary, since the injury is almost always supratrigonal. After careful assessment of the extent of the injury, a continuous No. 3-0 delayed-absorbable suture may be used to invert and close the bladder mucosa, making certain that the entire defect is securely closed (Fig. 30-2). Formerly, a major concern was the inadvertent placement of sutures through the bladder mucosa during the repair of a bladder laceration. Today this is no longer a matter for concern. Healing will occur, provided there is accurate approximation of tissue layers. The first layer of closure should be reinforced by a second layer of continuous or interrupted No. 3-0 delayed-absorbable suture(s) placed in the musculofascial tissues imbricating and supporting the initial layer. A third layer may be used if necessary. The security of the closure should be tested by filling the bladder with at least 200 ml dilute methylene blue or sterile milk after the first layer of closure is completed. Any point of leakage can be identified and reinforced. The anterior peritoneal edge behind the bladder should be sutured to the anterior vaginal cuff or to the bladder wall below the defect to interpose another layer between the site of bladder repair and the vaginal vault and to relieve tension on the suture line (see Fig. 30-2). This is a very useful maneuver and should be used to reinforce any suspected area of trauma to bladder muscle even if the bladder has not actually been entered. In any case of suspected weakness of the bladder wall, the bladder muscle must not be left approximated over the vaginal apex. After injecting indigo carmine intravenously, cystoscopy should be performed to be certain the dye spurts from both ureteral orifices. If the patient has been positioned in stirrups for laparotomy (see Chapter 27), intraoperative cystoscopy can be done easily without contaminating the operative field. If the bladder injury and repair occur during vaginal hysterectomy, cystoscopy is very easily accomplished without contamination of the operative field. The bladder should be kept as empty as possible for 10 days following surgery. A suprapubic catheter may be used for drainage, especially if the defect is low and involves the vesical neck. Alternatively, a transurethral Foley catheter may be used, but one should try to avoid placing any indwelling catheter near the suture line inside the bladder.

The principles and technique of repairing an injury to the bladder are the same regardless of whether the injury has occurred with abdominal or vaginal hysterectomy. The defect is carefully and securely closed; then the edge of the bladder peritoneum is pulled over

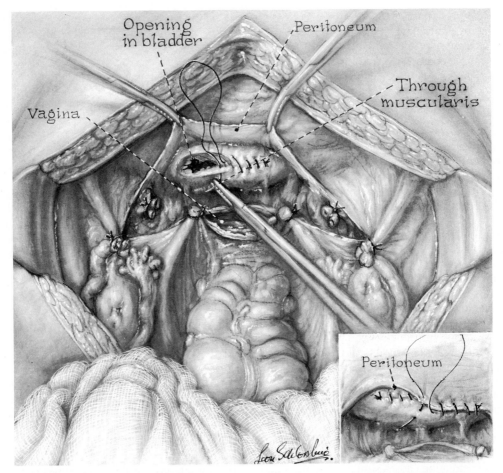

Figure 30–2. Closure of accidental opening of bladder during total abdominal hysterectomy. The bladder is closed with a continuous No. 3-0 delayed-absorbable suture, inverting mucosa into the bladder. A second muscular layer of interrupted sutures should support the initial layer. The suture line is then reinforced by bringing the peritoneum over the operative defect and suturing it in place. Advancement of the bladder peritoneum over the suture line will protect it from postoperative pelvic cellulitis and make certain that no leakage occurs into the vagina. The edge of the bladder peritoneum may also be sutured to the arterior vaginal cuff.

the defect and sutured, usually to the anterior vaginal cuff. This maneuver will interpose another layer of tissue between the site of bladder repair and the vaginal vault and help the bladder heal primarily without vesicovaginal fistula formation (see Fig. 30-2).

It is our position that the gynecologic surgeon should be technically capable of closing a bladder defect once he has created it. In this litigious era, it is important for the gynecologist to understand that the primary responsibility for the bladder injury falls on the shoulders of the surgeon who caused it and cannot be transferred to another specialist summoned to perform the repair. Injury to the urinary tract during gynecologic operations is now the leading cause of malpractice suits against gynecologists.

Other Factors Associated with Bladder Injury and Fistula Formation

When operating abdominally, the incision in the abdominal wall must be large enough to allow adequate exposure of the pelvis. Performing gynecologic operations, especially for extensive pelvic disease, through small incisions places the bladder and ureters and other adjacent structures at a greater risk of injury.

One of the most frequent sites of injury occurs in the bladder dome on opening the abdominal cavity. One must be especially careful when making an abdominal incision in a patient who has had a previous incision. Adhesions and scarring may cause difficulty. Advancing pregnancy produces alterations in the normal relationships of the bladder to the uterus and cervix and to the abdominal wall. With growth of the uterus during pregnancy, the bladder becomes an abdominal rather than a pelvic organ. These anatomic changes account for the increased susceptibility to and frequency of injury during cesarean section, especially repeat cesarean section. In this circumstance, the bladder is more susceptible to injury not only during its dissection away from the lower uterine segment, but also when the abdominal incision is fashioned. If the bladder neck has been chronically obstructed by a pelvic tumor, usually a leiomyomatous uterus, the bladder muscle may hypertrophy and the bladder may enlarge to the point of occupying the entire distance from the symphysis to the umbilicus. Under these circumstances, to avoid injury to the bladder, it may be necessary to enter the peritoneal cavity *above* the umbilicus. Failure to empty the bladder completely before surgery is one of the main errors of omission that may result in accidental bladder laceration on entering the abdomen. Insertion of an indwelling Foley catheter during the preparation of the patient for surgery is an important requirement for continued decompression of the bladder throughout the surgical procedure to avoid bladder injury. If a Foley catheter has not been inserted and intraoperative bladder distention interferes with exposure, the bladder may be easily decompressed by aspiration of the urine with a syringe and 20-gauge needle inserted through the dome of the bladder.

When the bladder dome is injured, the wall of the bladder may be easily repaired in a double-layered closure, including an initial continuous No. 3-0 delayed-absorbable suture in the bladder mucosa reinforced by another layer of continuous or interrupted sutures in the bladder muscle. An indwelling transurethral catheter should be left in place for 7–10 days postoperatively, depending on the extent of the injury, the security of the closure, and the location of the injury in the bladder dome (extraperitoneal or transperitoneal).

It should be understood that primary healing after intraoperative bladder injury is not dependent on placement of a large number of sutures in the bladder. Rather, tissue healing is enhanced by the accurate placement of the correct number of sutures that will approximate the bladder wall correctly and not interfere with its blood supply. It is comforting to know that the bladder has a rich collateral blood supply and will heal rapidly when closed correctly. Injury to the bladder need not be considered a dreaded and serious complication of gynecologic surgery. Indeed, the gynecologic surgeon can be encouraged to enter the bladder intentionally when it is necessary to do so to define the anatomic limits of pathology or operative procedures. In an analysis of 77 cases of recognized bladder entry, Everett and Mattingly found no case that failed to heal when repaired at the time of initial injury.

Although injuries to the bladder most commonly occur during total abdominal or vaginal hysterectomy, other gynecologic operations also place the bladder at risk of injury. In a subtotal abdominal hysterectomy, the bladder is usually drawn over the apex of the cervical stump to reperitonize the pelvis. The resultant alteration in the location of the bladder will render it more vulnerable to injury in any subsequent attempt to remove the cervix, whether done abdominally or vaginally. The exact boundary of the bladder wall is obscured by dense adhesions to the apex of the cervix.

In patients with congenital absence of the vagina, construction of a neovagina may result in bladder injury during the dissection of a space between the urethra and bladder anteriorly and the rectum posteriorly. Definition of the correct plane of dissection can be facilitated by placing a finger in the rectum and an instrument in the bladder. After a bladder injury has been properly repaired, it is essential to use a soft foam rubber form to carry the split-thickness skin graft into the new space and hold it there.

Total abdominal hysterectomy performed immediately after cesarean section increases the risk of bladder injury and vesicovaginal fistula formation. The tissues are soft and vascular. The anatomic limits of the bladder, cervix, and vagina may be difficult to see or feel. If the proper plane of dissection cannot be found, the bladder may be injured. If injury to the bladder is suspected, the bladder should be distended with sterile saline instilled through the Foley catheter and the bladder should be carefully inspected for defects or areas of weakness and repaired if necessary.

Endometriosis or ovarian cancer may involve the peritoneal reflection between the anterior lower uterine segment and the bladder and may make dissection of the bladder away from the uterus difficult. Various abnormal relationships of a myomatous uterus and the bladder are illustrated in Figure 30-3. These are especially dangerous situations if not recognized before the dissection begins.

A variety of operations used to correct stress urinary incontinence may result in bladder injury. Bladder injury during primary anterior colporrhaphy is infrequent but is more likely to occur when an anterior colporrhaphy is done a second time. It can be avoided altogether by a careful layered dissection of the vaginal mucosa from the underlying pubovesicocervical fascia. This can be facilitated by injecting saline beneath the vaginal mucosa. Patients with previous bladder neck surgery are at special risk of bladder injury when a repeat abdominal retropubic procedure is done to correct recurrent stress incontinence. This type of bladder injury occurs most frequently during mobilization of the adherent

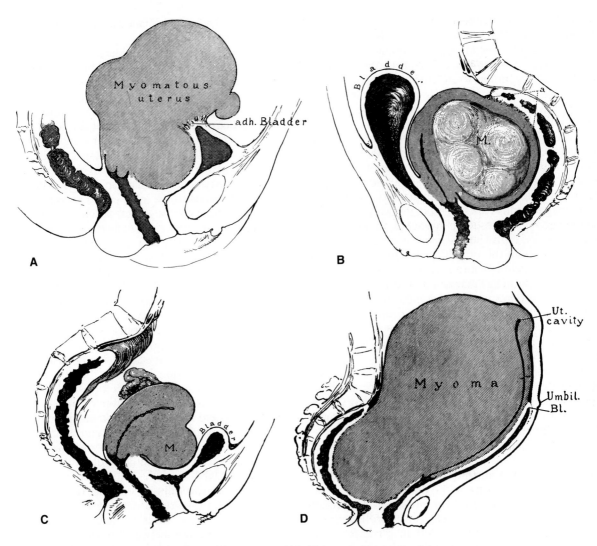

Figure 30–3. Abnormal relationships of the uterus and bladder caused by uterine leiomyomas. *A,* The bladder is abnormally adherent to the uterus. *B,* A large posterior myoma pushes the bladder against the symphysis. *C,* An anterior myoma pushes the bladder against the symphysis. *D,* A large myoma causes obstruction of the vesical neck with bladder hypertrophy extending to the umbilicus. (From Kelly HA, Cullen TS. Myomata of the uterus. Philadelphia: WB Saunders, 1909.)

bladder neck and urethra when dissecting in the retropubic space of Retzius. These injuries are particularly troublesome because their anatomic location, which limits exposure, makes them difficult to close. As a result of previous surgery, the vesical wall is frequently attenuated and friable with compromised blood supply. The surgeon should approach the scarred bladder neck with caution. Sharp, controlled dissection in the retropubic space is less hazardous in this situation than forceful, blunt separation of the dense adhesions. An inflated catheter bulb will identify the urethrovesical

junction and the location of the bladder neck. The bladder neck and the urethral margins can also be more accurately defined if the surgeon inserts the fingers into the vagina to elevate the paraurethral tissues and bladder neck into the operative field while performing the dissection and placing the sutures. When the anatomic margins of the bladder are distorted and cannot be delineated, it is preferable to open the bladder through the anterior wall and then to perform the dissection and place the sutures with greater accuracy under direct vision. Injuries to the bladder may occur during various operations to suspend the bladder neck by the retropubic placement of a fascial strap, such as in the Goebell-Frangenheim-Stoeckel operation. If cystoscopy can be routinely performed as the last step in all these procedures, an assessment of the presence or absence and extent of bladder injury can be made and appropriate repair carried out when necessary.

In every series of vesicovaginal fistulas, there are still many patients whose fistulas are the result of treatment of gynecologic malignancies with radiation therapy or extensive pelvic surgery. One to three percent of patients will develop vesicovaginal fistulas after extensive hysterectomy as primary therapy for cervical cancer. If the extensive hysterectomy is done in the presence of previous pelvic irradiation, the incidence of postoperative vesicovaginal fistula will be much higher. Radiation has an acute effect on tissues that lasts for several months. During this acute phase, fistula formation results from destruction and sloughing of neoplastic tissue in the vesicovaginal septum or from the acute effects of radiation on sensitive tissues. Even though most irradiated tissue may seem to recover from this acute phase, fistulas may yet appear many years later because of progressive obliterative endarteritis with resultant tissue ischemia and slough. Early evidence of this ischemia can be seen cystoscopically in patients who were irradiated for cervical cancer many years before. The bladder mucosa just above the interureteric ridge will appear pale and avascular at the point of maximum intensity of radiation in the bladder. Because of this progressive ischemia over a prolonged period, vesicovaginal fistulas may appear many years after radiation. Although the dose and distribution of radiation are important, Van Nagell and associates found that the absolute dosage did not always correlate with fistula formation, nor did the patient's weight and age, suggesting that bladder tissue sensitivity to radiation varies from patient to patient and that some patients are more susceptible to fistula formation than others. They found that patients with vascular disease, as manifested by hypertension and diabetes, were more susceptible to fistula formation than others. The importance of blood supply to the area is evidenced by a fourfold increase in fistula formation when simple hysterectomy is performed on patients who had previously had radiation therapy, as noted by Boronow and Rutledge. Hysterectomy further compromises the central pelvic blood supply already compromised by radiation. When extensive pelvic surgery is done after complete pelvic irradiation has been given, fistulas are especially likely to result. Although some postirradiation vesicovaginal fistulas are unavoidable, others could be prevented by proper irradiation dosage or distribution of rads and by use of the proper technique of extensive pelvic surgery for

gynecologic malignancies. Since these fistulas are the most difficult to close, every precaution should be taken to prevent their formation.

Petty and associates reported five patients who developed new cervical or uterine neoplasms 1–27 years after initial radiation therapy for cervical cancer. All underwent abdominal hysterectomy without postoperative vesicovaginal fistula formation. Success was attributed to cautious surgical technique and to the use of an omental pedicle graft to bring new vascularity to the vaginal apex and bladder base. Such prophylactic use of an omental pedicle graft to avoid vesicovaginal fistula in this high-risk situation makes good sense.

Various other etiologies of vesicovaginal fistulas are reported. Regrettably, a few still result from the outmoded transurethral resection of the "female prostate," erroneously thought to be the cause of bladder neck obstruction. Transurethral resections in the female should be restricted to a careful and limited resection of congenital urethral valves or folds usually found in young girls with obstruction of urinary outflow.

SYMPTOMS AND DIAGNOSIS OF VESICOVAGINAL FISTULA

When a patient develops a vesicovaginal fistula following hysterectomy, a review of the operative report and postoperative recovery record may show no apparent complication(s) that might lead one to suspect a fistula will ultimately develop. Often, however, one will find that the operation was difficult and associated with unusual bleeding and transfusion. The dissection may have been difficult because of adhesions, endometriosis, pelvic infection, malignancy, previous radiation, obesity, or poor exposure. The postoperative recovery may have been complicated by persistent fever, unusual discomfort, hematuria, or prolonged ileus. Instillation of sterile saline stained with methylene blue into the bladder through a catheter is a simple way to test for a vesicovaginal fistula in these high-risk circumstances.

The successful treatment of vesicovaginal fistula depends on an exact diagnosis. With a small fistula, the urinary leakage will be slight and, in some instances, dependent on the position of the patient. Women with such a small fistula may void a good quantity of urine, whereas in those with larger fistulas, sufficient urine does not collect in the bladder to permit voiding. Most often, patients are totally or almost totally incontinent of urine, require rubber sheets to protect the mattress, and need diapers or rubber pants to protect their clothing. With marked incontinence, the vulva usually becomes reddened, tender, and excoriated over time. The odor of urea may be so offensive as to be disgusting and embarrassing to the patient and repulsive to others.

Such patients often become reclusive and depressed. Frank psychotic depression may result from prolonged incontinence if repair is delayed too long.

Most vesicovaginal fistulas are painless. But fistulas resulting from irradiation can cause severe pain. Graham has reported 10 such cases with progressive pain, aggravated by movement or sitting. The tissues around these fistulas are very tender, and often anesthesia is required for a satisfactory examination. Bacteria in the vagina split urea and produce an alkaline medium in which crystals form. The vagina and labia have greenish-gray deposits, and in many cases there are encrustations and necrotic tissue along the margins of the fistula. Since these patients have received radiation for a gynecologic malignancy, the fistula margins must be biopsied to rule out recurrent or persistent cancer. However, not all postirradiation fistulas fall into this painful pattern.

If a fistula opening cannot be readily demonstrated by careful speculum examination, often it may be found by filling the bladder with a dilute solution of methylene blue and then inspecting the anterior vaginal wall and vaginal vault. When the fistula is small and the point of leakage is still not discovered with the patient in the dorsal lithotomy or knee-chest positions, the three-tampon test of Moir should be used. In this test, three cotton tampons are placed in the vagina in tandem. Methylene blue is instilled in the bladder. After having the patient walk about for 10–15 minutes, the tampons are removed and examined. If the lowest tampon is wet and stained blue, the patient may be presumed to have transurethral urinary incontinence and no fistula. If the upper tampon is wet and blue, a vesicovaginal fistula is indicated. If the upper tampon is wet but not blue, a ureteral fistula is the likely diagnosis. Careful inspection of the tampons with regard to their position in the vagina will give some information about the location of the vaginal orifice of the fistula.

The air method of Kelly or the carbon dioxide technique of Robertson are admirably adaptive for cystoscopic examination of these patients. Although this examination is more commonly made with a water cystoscope, difficulty is experienced in filling the bladder when the vesicovaginal opening is large unless the examination is done with the patient in the knee-chest position. It should be remembered that air cystoscopy can be performed very satisfactorily using an ordinary cystoscope with the patient in the knee-chest position, as described by Ridley. However, with either water or air cystoscopy, small fistulas are often seen only with great difficulty from within the bladder. Small fistulas can be seen more easily with the cystoscope if a probe can be passed through the fistula from the vagina into the bladder. In spite of these difficulties, the cystoscopic examination should be done to ascertain the size and the position of the fistula and, particularly, its relation to the ureteral orifices and the vesical sphincter. It must be remembered that more than one vesicovaginal fistula may be present. If a single fistula is identified, one cannot assume that it is the only one present.

When a urinary fistula develops postoperatively, the diagnostic possibilities are a vesicovaginal fistula, a unilateral ureterovaginal fistula, bilateral ureterovaginal fistulas, or various combinations. An exact determination must be made before appropriate treatment can be instituted. Recalling the details of the recent operative procedure of injury, the surgeon may be able to suspect which kind of fistula is more likely to be present. However, this suspicion should always be confirmed with appropriate studies. If the bladder is distended with methylene blue solution and the urine in the vagina is *unstained,* the communication is with the ureter(s). If the bladder is distended with methylene blue solution and the urine in the vagina is *stained,* the communication is with the bladder, but the patient might still have a ureterovaginal fistula as well. If urine in the vagina is unstained when the bladder is filled with a methylene blue solution but becomes blue when indigo carmine is injected intravenously, the communication is with the ureter, but which ureter is still unknown. The findings must be confirmed by cystoscopy, which will show a failure of the ureteral orifice on the affected side to spurt urine. Attempts to pass a catheter usually meet obstruction when the tip reaches the point of ureteral injury. Installation of radiopaque dye through the ureteral catheter may outline the tract of a ureterovaginal fistula. A ureterovaginal fistula is very commonly associated with hydronephrosis and hydroureter above because of stenosis of the ureter at the site of injury. Therefore, excretory urography should be a routine part of the investigation. A hydronephrosis and hydroureter suggest but are not diagnostic of a ureterovaginal fistula on the same side, since these changes can also result from scarring of the edges of a vesicovaginal fistula in the region of the ureteral orifice with concomitant ureteral stenosis and dilatation above. Further discussion of the differential diagnosis of urinary fistulas can be found in Chapter 29.

When vesicovaginal fistula results from gynecologic surgery, urinary leakage will be noted most commonly in the first 10 days after operation. Some patients will demonstrate incontinence between the 10th and 20th days. Rarely, the incontinence will first appear later.

MANAGEMENT PRINCIPLES OF SIMPLE VESICOVAGINAL FISTULAS

There is no standard vesicovaginal fistula. There is considerable variation among vesicovaginal fistulas in etiology, size, location, and associated features. However, most vesicovaginal fistulas seen in the United States are relatively small, simple fistulas in the vaginal vault that result from unrecognized bladder injury during total hysterectomy, abdominal or vaginal, for benign gynecologic and obstetric disease. A few fistulas result from extensive surgery or pelvic irradiation for gynecologic malignancies. The major emphasis in this discussion will be given to simple small vesicovaginal fistulas following unrecognized bladder injury during pelvic surgery. Complicated fistulas and their repairs are discussed later.

Preoperative Investigation

As described earlier, the patient must undergo a careful evaluation of the bladder, ureters, kidney function, urethra, vagina, and other pelvic organs; tissues; and disease so that the nature and extent of the fistula and associated problems can be properly assessed. This evaluation will certainly include a careful pelvic examination, cystoscopy, urethroscopy, excretory urography, biopsy of fistula margins when indicated, and other studies. Some studies done initially to make the diagnosis may need to be repeated later as circumstances change. Repair should not be attempted in the absence of current information.

Operative Considerations

Time of Repair

Formerly, most experienced gynecologists advised that, regardless of a vesicovaginal fistula's etiology or size, at least 6 months should elapse before attempting repair, so that tissues could be completely healed. With delayed repair, cure rates have varied in many series between 85% and 98%, with an average of around 90%. In the past 25 years, the 6-month rule has been challenged: Many experts now recommend waiting only 3–4 months. Some experts have advised repair even earlier. Fearl and Keizur found 2 or 3 months to be an adequate resolution time if the wound was a clean surgical one. Collins and Prent, in 1960, reported on their experience with early repair of vesicovaginal fistulas after preoperative administration of cortisone to bring about "resolution of inflammatory reaction" around the fistula. In 15 cases, all operated on within 8 weeks and most within 4 weeks of discovery of the fistula, 13 repairs were successful on the first attempt. These acute fistulas resulted from operations for benign disease. Less favorable results were obtained when early repair was attempted in patients whose fistulas resulted from radiation or extensive surgery for gynecologic malignancy. All the repairs were done

transvaginally. Continuing to use preoperative steroids and a transvaginal approach, Collins and associates reported a 72.4% success rate in 1971 on the first attempt at even earlier repair in 29 patients without malignancy. The reparative procedures were done in the first 2 weeks after fistula discovery.

In 1984, O'Quinn and associates presented an update of the Tulane University experience with early repair of vesicovaginal fistulas. Fifty-four patients with acute fistulas were operated on within 8 weeks of the discovery of the fistula. Forty-three of the 54 patients were operated on within 4 weeks. Preliminary corticosteroid treatment was used in all patients. Forty-eight of the 54 patients had successful first-attempt closure. Four patients were reoperated on 12 days later, with successful closure on the second attempt. The remaining two patients had a successful second attempt at closure 5 and 6 weeks later. All patients had a simple transvaginal operation for repair of the fistula.

In 1979, Persky and associates reported their experience with early repair (1–10 weeks after the initial surgery) in seven cases. All the repairs (except one vaginal) were done by the suprapubic transvesical approach with interposition of a flap of peritoneum or omentum between the bladder and vagina at the area of closure, and all were successful. Cruikshank has reported his experience with early repair of posthysterectomy vesicovaginal fistulas. A simple transvaginal repair was used in nine patients who had a small, simple, noncomplicated fistula. The repairs were all done between 13 and 19 days following the diagnosis, which was made from 6 to 15 days following hysterectomy. The repair was successful in all nine patients. Early repair using a combined approach (transvaginal/transvesical) in two patients with complicated fistulas was not successful initially. At Emory University, attempts to repair simple posthysterectomy vesicovaginal fistulas by a Latzko operation have been successful in 14 patients when the repair was done from 2 to 12 weeks following discovery of the fistula. Early in the series, five patients received preoperative steroids. Since success has been regularly achieved in more recent years without steroids, we are unable to confirm that they are essential in achieving success in early repair, and we no longer recommend their use. Based on our experience, we have no hesitation in repairing simple posthysterectomy vesicovaginal fistulas as soon as the diagnosis is made. A simple transvaginal Latzko partial colpocleisis will be successful in over 80% of cases.

Those who prefer to wait 3–4 months to repair a vesicovaginal fistula are especially concerned that the tissues be completely normal, and without edema and infection, so that a proper dissection, proper suturing, and proper healing will result in a successful closure.

Meanwhile, the patient is terribly uncomfortable. Collection devices and indwelling catheters usually do not keep her dry and may cause more perineal irritation. She is embarrassed, depressed, and restricted in her social and marital activities. She is not easily convinced that she should remain in this unpleasant state for months before anything is done. During this long period of watchful waiting, she is likely to become impatient and seek other advice. If patients with simple, uncomplicated posthysterectomy vesicovaginal fistulas can be offered an earlier repair with reasonable chance of success, much unpleasantness can be avoided.

Two hypothetical scenarios may be described. In the first, 100 patients with simple posthysterectomy vesicovaginal fistulas have immediate repair (within 1 month) with 80% success. The remaining 20 patients have a successful repair 3 months later. The calculated total of patient wet days in this group is 4800. In the second scenario, 100 patients with simple posthysterectomy vesicovaginal fistulas have their repair delayed a standard 3 months with 95% success. The remaining five patients have a successful repair 3 months later. The calculated total of wet days in this group is 9450. In other words, in this hypothetical comparison between early and delayed repair, the number of wet days experienced by the two groups of patients is reduced by about 50% by early repair. Although it should always be important to think in terms of doing a successful repair, it is also important to consider reducing the total number of patient wet days as much as possible. If given a choice, most patients would opt for early repair.

When a patient develops a vesicovaginal fistula, usually in the first or second week following total hysterectomy, and evaluation shows no complicating features, one may still be uncomfortable with the idea of immediate repair and prefer to wait until the tissues around the fistula are no longer indurated and infected. A large indwelling Foley catheter should be inserted for continuous bladder drainage to facilitate spontaneous healing or eventual complete epithelialization of the fistula tract. Spontaneous healing has been reported in 15% to 20% of patients. In our experience, spontaneous healing is unusual except for the very smallest fistulas only a few millimeters in diameter. Among 38 postoperative vesicovaginal fistulas, Latzko reported that 9 healed spontaneously. Greatest success was achieved when a large-caliber catheter was used and the fistula was only a few millimeters in diameter. The time required for healing varied from 17 days to 3 months. The catheter must eliminate all urine loss through the vagina if the fistulous tract is to have a chance to close spontaneously. Sometimes the spontaneous healing of a fistula is not very secure and the fistula spontaneously opens again in a few weeks. Rather than prolonged catheter drainage with the hope that a few fistulas will close spontaneously, early repair with a simple Latzko partial colpocleisis may be more acceptable.

Very few patients can tolerate a catheter connected to a leg bag for several weeks and remain relatively dry and comfortable. For those who cannot tolerate a catheter, a vaginal collecting device such as that described by Wolff and Gilliland can be constructed by gluing a Pezzer catheter to a fitted contraceptive diaphragm with rubber cement. The catheter is fitted to a leg bag and may be worn for the weeks or months before bladder repair is carried out. Patients who are postmenopausal or younger patients who have had both ovaries removed should be placed on oral estrogen. An ointment or cream containing lanolin will provide some protection for the vulva. Hot sitz baths and douches or creams containing antibacterials may help to improve tissue vascularity and reduce infection before surgery. Urinary antibiotics are generally not used unless there is clinical evidence of a urinary tract infection above the bladder. Acute cystitis is uncommon in conjunction with a vesicovaginal fistula.

After about a month of continuous catheter drainage, the catheter is removed. If the fistula persists, surgery can be planned. Generally, all uncomplicated posthysterectomy vesicovaginal fistulas will be ready for repair by the 12th postsurgical week, and most will be ready earlier. When edema, cellulitis, and evidence of tissue necrosis have resolved from the fistula margins, the patient's physical and mental well-being are better served by a simple surgical procedure to close the fistula rather than by wearing the catheter prophylactically for a longer time. It should be emphasized that complicated fistulas cannot usually be closed this soon. For example, it may take from 6 months to 2 years for the tissues around a postirradiation fistula to be ready for surgical repair.

Very rarely, a minute (<3 mm) vesicovaginal fistula may be closed by superficial bladder fulgeration. Falk and Orkin have reported success with this procedure, as have both Hyman and O'Connor. They emphasize that the tract should be free from infection and that the vesicovaginal septum should not be too thin. If this rule is not observed, fulgeration may increase, rather than decrease, the caliber of the opening. Most experts do not recommend fulgeration. Van Oyen and associates concluded that electrocoagulation and prolonged bladder drainage were only occasionally successful, even in selected cases with small-diameter fistulas. We never use it.

Choice of Operation

The choice of operative approach is all-important. We have come more and more to the conclusion that almost all vesicovaginal fistulas should be closed per vaginum. Simple posthysterectomy vesicovaginal fistulas in the vaginal vault certainly should be closed with a Latzko partial colpocleisis. The operation is rapid and recovery is prompt. Extensive transperitoneal-transvesical operations are not needed to repair these simple fistulas. Even most complicated fistulas can be approached vaginally unless there are unusual circumstances. A transperitoneal or transvesical approach may be needed when the fistula margins are near the ureteral orifices, requiring a transvesical approach to catheterize the ureters, mobilize the bladder mucosa, and close it securely without compromise of the ureters; when ureteroneocystostomy is also needed; when an omental fat flap is to be used; or when a very large fistula or contracted bladder may require bladder patching or augmentation with sigmoid colon, cecum, or ileum. We recognize that some excellent surgeons—principally urologists (eg, Pfaneuf, O'Connor, Marshall, Glenn, and Stevens)—recommend and routinely use the transvesical approach to fistula repair and are successful by that method. However, we believe that it is not the preferred method of approach for the usual gynecologic vesicovaginal fistula, and most gynecologic surgeons agree.

Patient Positioning

When the vaginal approach is used, exposure can be accomplished best by placing the patient in the dorsal lithotomy position. The Sims lateral position and the knee-chest position are rarely used. The great majority of our fistulas are repaired in the lithotomy position. Dropping the head of the table and elevating the buttocks often facilitates exposure. On those infrequent occasions when it is necessary to approach the fistula through an abdominal incision, the patient's legs should be placed in stirrups with the thighs flexed 15°. In this position, the operator or the assistant, by placing the index and middle fingers in the vagina, will be able to elevate the fistula into the abdominal operative field for better visualization. Also, in this position the external urethral meatus will be available for cystoscopic examination of the bladder and ureteral orifices when the repair is completed.

Special Instruments

It is helpful to have a cystoscope available, so that the margins of the fistula and the bladder mucosa can be examined and the location of the ureteral orifices in relation to the fistula can be determined. If necessary, ureteral catheters can be inserted. The examination is best done by a surgeon who is skilled in cystoscopy, preferably by the one who is to perform the operation. Most fistulas can be repaired correctly with a basic instrument set. It may be necessary to supplement this basic set with a few instruments that are long and thin with fine points, such as long, fine-pointed dissecting scissors; long, fine-pointed tissue forceps; long, delicate needle holders; an assortment of long scalpel handles and blades; the extender for the needle point Bovie; and an assortment of vaginal retractors. Technical difficulties encountered in the repair may be solved by obtaining better instruments and by innovations in their use, but they are more likely to be solved by improved exposure and accessibility of the fistula itself.

Fistula Exposure

Ordinary retraction of the vaginal walls is usually sufficient for adequate exposure. However, when there is a tight vaginal outlet, scarring of the vagina, a narrow subpubic arch, or a deep and fixed vaginal vault, an episiotomy or a Schuchardt incision (see Fig. 11-21) may be needed. Such an incision should be made without hesitation if exposure and accessibility will be improved. Traction on stay sutures placed in the bladder wall on each side of the fistula can be helpful. Exposure and dissection around a small fistula can be facilitated by traction on a small urethral catheter placed through the fistula and into the bladder with the catheter bulb distended inside the bladder. The Young prostatic retractor may be used in a similar fashion.

Excision of the Fistula Tract

If the fistula is fresh and the tissue is still indurated, the entire tract from the vaginal orifice to the bladder orifice should be excised during the dissection. This need not necessarily be done first, but it should be accomplished at some time during the dissection. The tract is surrounded by indurated tissue, and this should be removed so that normal tissue can be carefully approximated with sutures for better healing. Completely excising the fistula tract will inevitably result in a larger hole in the bladder, and that is as it should be. However, some surgeons are reluctant to do this, failing to understand that to be properly closed, the fistula must first be made larger by excising the indurated edges of the tract completely. On the other hand, if the fistula is mature and the tract is a fibrotic scar, one may elect not to excise the tract. It may instead be entropionized into the bladder. For example, the margins of a mature obstetric fistula do not need to be excised.

Wide Mobilization of the Vaginal Mucosa Around the Fistula

So that the repair can be done in several layers, the vaginal mucosa should be mobilized widely in all directions around the fistula. Wide mobilization will allow approximation of *broad surface to broad surface without tension,* an important principle in all fistula repairs. The bladder muscularis should not be disturbed. At the same time, the vaginal mucosal flap should not be too thin. Any indurated tissue or scar tissue surrounding the fistula should be excised and completely debrided to leave healthy tissue. This dissection can be facilitated by injecting sterile normal saline just beneath the vaginal mucosa to help identify the proper tissue planes. We prefer not to add a vasopressor to the solution because of the theoretical risk that healing might be inhibited by interference with local tissue resistance to infection. Wide dissection and mobilization of the bladder base are especially important in the closure of postirradiation fistulas because the blood supply to the scar tissue surrounding the fistula is poor and healing is therefore at a great disadvantage. The farther away from the fistula opening one dissects, the better the blood supply becomes and the more secure will be the layered closure of the bladder wall over the fistula.

Choice of Sutures

The use of silver wire sutures for closure of a vesicovaginal fistula has been almost completely abandoned in favor of more modern suture materials. Over the years, catgut for the first two or three layers followed by a nonabsorbable synthetic suture material (eg, nylon, Prolene, or Dacron) in the vaginal mucosa has been a favorite choice. Of course, the nonabsorbable synthetic suture in the vaginal mucosa must eventually be removed. Today our suture preference for vesicovaginal fistula repair is for synthetic, delayed-absorbable polyglactin or polyglycolic acid sutures. These sutures retain their tensile strength longer than catgut, and the tissue reaction is less than that with catgut. A stronger cicatrix will have formed at the repair site by the time these sutures begin to lose their tensile strength. This is the greatest advantage when compared to catgut and may be responsible for better results with early repair. Our preference is for No. 3-0 delayed-absorbable suture swaged onto a fine, small-caliber, semimalleable, round needle. It is the most nearly ideal suture we have found for fistula repair. It can be used for all layers and does not need to be removed.

Closure of Bladder Mucosa

Closure of the fistula should begin by approximating the bladder mucosa with interrupted No. 3-0 delayed-absorbable sutures. Ideally, the first row should not penetrate the bladder mucosa but should be taken parallel to the edge of the fistula tract so as to invert the edge within the bladder. From a practical viewpoint, this may prove to be difficult, and direct suture approx-

imation of the bladder mucosa has not proved to be especially deleterious. The first row of sutures is the most important. Good bites should be taken in healthy tissue and the defect must be closed securely. The security of this first layer of closure should then be tested by instillation of 200 ml dilute methylene blue or sterile milk into the bladder. If any point of leakage is detected, it must be reinforced before proceeding. A vesicovaginal fistula repair will not be successful unless the urinary side of the fistula is securely closed.

Closure of Broad Surface to Broad Surface Without Tension

Once the bladder mucosa is securely closed, it is reinforced by two or three covering layers of interrupted No. 3-0 delayed-absorbable mattress sutures placed in the bladder muscularis. That closure of broad surface to broad surface must be without tension is an important axiom in all types of fistula repair. If the layers do not come together without tension, a wider dissection of the bladder base is required. The excess vaginal mucosa may be trimmed away, but generous flaps should be left for approximation without tension.

All layers should be approximated in a direction that is transverse to the longitudinal axis of the vagina. There is much less tension on the suture line when layers are approximated in this direction, and there is no advantage to alternating the direction of the layers of closure with the initial layer. Unusual circumstances may dictate an exception to this rule.

Ureteral Integrity

At the end of the repair, 5 ml indigo carmine should be injected intravenously with rapid infusion of parenteral fluids. The bladder should be instilled with 200 ml normal saline or distilled water, and with a cystoscope, the dye should be observed spurting from both ureteral orifices to be certain that the ureters are not obstructed by the fistula repair.

Bladder Drainage

It is impossible to keep the bladder completely empty and dry during the postoperative period. However, the bladder should be maintained as empty as possible and must not be allowed to become distended. Although we have always subscribed to the use of a urethral catheter for 10 days following fistula repair in order to place the operative site at rest, Falk and others have avoided the use of the postoperative catheter out of a concern over adding trauma to the bladder base. In recent years we have sometimes resolved both concerns by using suprapubic drainage. This not only avoids trauma to the operative site, but provides bladder drainage without the need for catheterization during the time the patient initiates voiding. In using this technique, care must be taken to make certain that the suprapubic catheter does not become obstructed, for many good surgical repairs of a fistula have been ruined by overdistention of the bladder. The management of the bladder after vesicovaginal fistula repair must be an individual matter. Sometimes bladder drainage will be required for 10–14 days. On the other hand, if the fistula is small and the closure is undoubtedly secure, bladder drainage may be discontinued after 1 or 2 days. For this short time, a transurethral catheter may be used. It is no longer considered advisable to make a vaginal cystotomy incision for drainage.

When the fistula is large and closure is difficult, the patient should remain in bed initially for 5–7 days. Patients with small fistulas without much scar tissue and a secure closure may be up within 24–48 hours without endangering the success of the closure. Only on very rare occasions for the most complicated fistulas do we advise that the patient remain in a prone position with a catheter coming directly through a split mattress to a drainage bottle on the floor, that the Bradford frame be used, or that the catheter be attached to suction. If adequate drainage is established so that the bladder does not become distended, the position the patient lies in postoperatively makes little difference. Bladder irrigations are not used except to clear a blocked catheter. Urinary antibiotics are unnecessary unless acute upper urinary tract infection develops. In keeping with modern theory, some surgeons have used intraoperative antibiotics to enhance tissue healing, but there have been no controlled studies to support this approach for simple transvaginal vesicovaginal fistula repair. An adequate intake of fluids is required so that an adequate urine output can be maintained. The best way to keep the catheter open and avoid urinary tract infection is to ensure a high output of dilute urine, preferably as much as 100 ml/hr.

The Modified Latzko Operation for Supratrigonal Vesicovaginal Fistula Repair

In 1913, Latzko recommended a technique of high colpocleisis, first described by Simon, as "the simplest and surest procedure for vesicovaginal fistulas following hysterectomy." In 1926, Latzko offered a modification of Simon's procedure in order to eliminate the formation of bladder diverticula. This technique is now called the Latzko operation. The principles of the operation were described in detail in 1942. Latzko reported 29 cures among 31 cases using this technique. These results are

impressive, since in the majority of his patients the fistula resulted from a radical abdominal hysterectomy for cervical cancer. Many others have reported satisfactory results since then.

The operation is basically a partial colpocleisis, an obliteration of the upper vagina for 2–3 cm around the fistula. The anterior and posterior vaginal walls with vaginal mucosa removed are easily approximated without tension, since they naturally fall together. The upper or posterior edge of the fistula always coincides with the transverse firm scar in the vault of the vagina. A fistula that follows total abdominal or vaginal hysterectomy is usually small and supratrigonal. Therefore, the ureters are generally not in danger.

The Latzko operation is the procedure of choice when a vesicovaginal fistula develops after total hysterectomy. It cannot be done if the cervix has not been removed. Since a fistula resulting from total hysterectomy is almost always small and high in the vagina, the shortening of the vagina caused by approximation of the anterior and posterior vaginal walls is slight. In our experience, no patients have complained after operation that the vagina was too short for satisfactory coitus.

If exposure is difficult, the fistula may be brought into operating range by traction sutures placed in the lateral quadrants of the vaginal vault. If difficulty is still encountered, greater exposure may be obtained by a mediolateral episiotomy or a true Schuchardt incision (see Fig. 11-21). At times the incision may be conveniently drawn down with a Young prostatic retractor or with a small (No. 8 Foley) urethral catheter placed through the fistula and inflated in the bladder.

Infiltration of sterile saline beneath the vaginal mucosa around the fistula will facilitate dissection. The incision should be approximately 1 cm from the fistula edge in all directions (Fig. 30-4A). The vaginal mucosa is mobilized as shown in Figure 30-4B. When the vaginal mucosa is being removed posteriorly, an effort should be made to avoid entry into the peritoneal cavity through the peritoneum of the cul-de-sac, although Lawson prefers to open the cul-de-sac directly. If an inadvertent peritoneal entry is made, it should be closed and the dissection carried out in another plane.

Latzko apparently did not feel it necessary to excise the fistulous tract. He operated on mature fistulas. However, we advise adding this step if the fistula is fresh, since the margins of a fresh, indurated, and necrotic fistula may not heal well when approximated with sutures, but the margins will heal if the tract is removed first. If an older scarred and epithelialized fistula tract is not excised, it should be carefully entropionized rather than suturing the edges together. If the edges of the tract are still indurated, it is important that the tract be excised back to healthy tissue. This should be done even if a larger hole results. This step is illustrated in

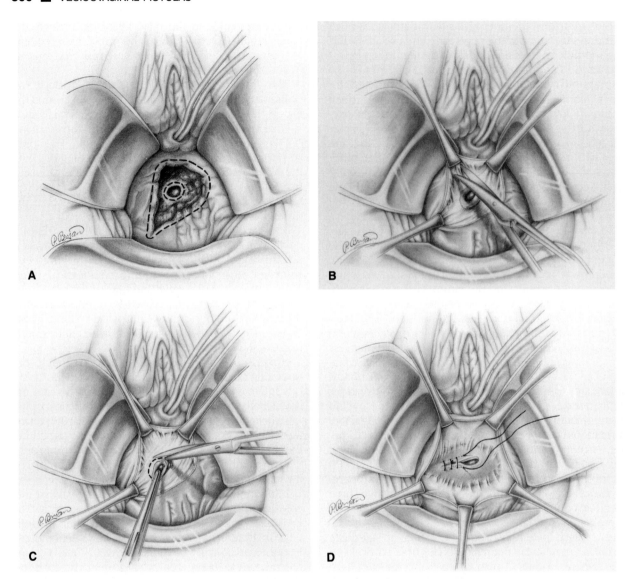

Figure 30–4. Operation for a closure of a simple posthysterectomy vesicovaginal fistula by the Latzko technique. *A,* Ureters have been catheterized to prevent encirclement of a ureter by a suture. Incisions about the fistula opening and about the indurated vaginal mucosa margin are marked by the dotted lines. *B,* The vaginal mucosa is dissected back from the fistula opening for a sufficient distance to mobilize the bladder wall about the fistula. *C,* The fistula tract is sharply and completely excised. *D,* No. 3-0 delayed-absorbable interrupted mattress sutures taken parallel to the edge of the fistula tract are used as the initial suture line, inverting tissue into the bladder. The security of the closure should be tested by instillation of 100–200 ml dilute methylene blue or sterile milk into the bladder.

Figure 30-4*C.* After excising the fistula tract, the bladder mucosal edges are approximated transversely with interrupted No. 3-0 delayed-absorbable sutures swaged onto a fine round needle (Fig. 30-4*D*). Care must be taken that the lateral margin of the bladder mucosa is closed securely by including tissue beyond the fistula margin. After placing this first line of sutures, the bladder is filled with 100–200 ml sterile evaporated milk or dilute methylene blue and tested for leakage. Points of weakness are noted and reinforced with additional sutures. This first suture line is then covered over by a second and third layer of No. 3-0 delayed-absorbable

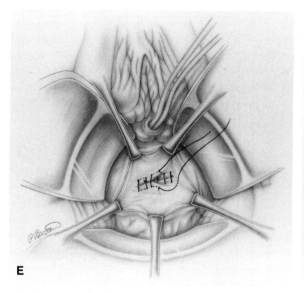

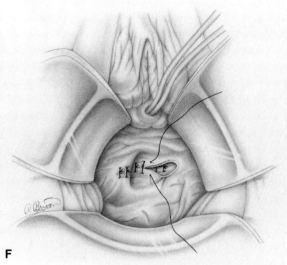

E

F

Figure 30–4. (continued) *E*, Two or three additional suture layers should approximate the bladder muscularis broad surface to broad surface without tension. No. 3-0 delayed-absorbable interrupted mattress sutures should be used. *F*, The vaginal mucosa is closed transversely with interrupted No. 3-0 delayed-absorbable sutures.

sutures, each inverting the previous line of sutures and approximating the anterior and posterior vaginal walls in the process (Fig. 30-4*E*). Further denudation of the vaginal mucosa or dissection beneath the vaginal mucosa may ultimately be required. In fact, it is often advisable not to denude at the beginning of the operation as wide an area as may ultimately be necessary. Avoiding early complete denudation prevents blood loss that may be annoying to the operator and depleting to the patient. After the last suture is placed, the vaginal mucosa is closed with interrupted No. 3-0 delayed-absorbable sutures (Fig. 30-4*F*). Monofilament nylon can also be used. It is nonreactive. Nylon sutures cause less tissue maceration than silver wire, are easier to place, and permit better patient ambulation. However, both nylon and silver wire sutures must be removed later. Delayed-absorbable sutures in the vaginal mucosa are equally satisfactory in this technique, since the success or failure of the repair has already been determined by the suture layers placed in the bladder mucosa and bladder wall before the vaginal mucosa is closed.

An indwelling catheter is left in the bladder for 1–14 days postoperatively, depending on the operator's assessment of several factors, including the size of the fistula, the health of the tissues, the security of the closure, and a history of previous unsuccessful attempts at repair.

Following an operation for fistula closure, we may use a suprapubic silicone tube for bladder drainage,

because the operative site can be traumatized by an indwelling transurethral catheter and voiding can be accomplished without catheterization. On the other hand, if it is anticipated that bladder drainage will be needed for only a few days, a transurethral catheter may be entirely satisfactory.

As mentioned earlier, the Latzko technique can give satisfactory results when a posthysterectomy vesicovaginal fistula is small, even though the tissue is still indurated. In this situation, the upper vagina must be extensively debrided of necrotic and indurated tissue. If debridement is timid and incomplete, the repair may be unsuccessful.

Standard Operation for Closure of Trigonal Vesicovaginal Fistula

The simple technique illustrated here in Figure 30-5 *A–D* may be used in closing an easily exposed fistula in which there is no excess scar tissue. It represents a more or less typical closure, if there is such a thing as a typical closure in a condition in which there is such great variation. The fistula for which this operation is done is shown in Figure 30-5*A*.

Since the fistula is close to the trigone, the ureters may be first catheterized. An incision is made about the fistulous opening, and the vaginal mucosa is dissected free from the bladder for a sufficient distance in all directions to mobilize enough bladder wall for at least a

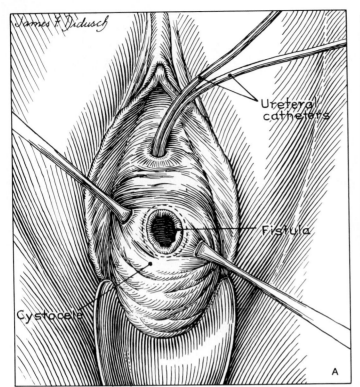
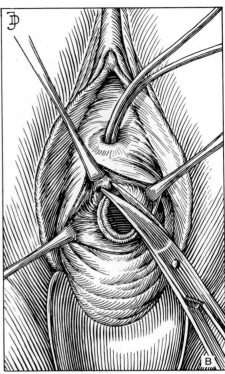

Figure 30–5. Standard operation for closure of a simple vesicovaginal fistula. *A*, Ureters have been catheterized to prevent encirclement of a ureter with a suture. An incision about the fistulous opening is marked by the dotted line. The scarred fistula tract should be excised. *B*, The vaginal mucosa is dissected back from the fistulous opening for a sufficient distance to mobilize the bladder wall about the fistula.

double line of closure without tension. Usually a zone of about 1–2 cm is sufficient (Fig. 30-5*B*). The mature fistula tract is entropionized into the bladder. Closure begins beyond the end of the fistula opening with interrupted mattress or continuous sutures (No. 3-0 delayed-absorbable) (Fig. 30-5*C*). These stitches are taken either parallel to the edges of the opening, well into the bladder wall, or alternatively, through the bladder mucosa. They should begin and end well beyond the edge of the fistula. When each suture is tied, the edges are inverted into the bladder.

At this stage of the operation, the closure is tested by introducing into the bladder about 200 ml sterilized evaporated milk (easily obtained from the hospital nursery) through a urethral catheter. The advantage of milk over methylene blue is that it does not stain the tissues if leakage occurs. A dilute solution of methylene blue also works nicely. If the suture line is not watertight, the weak point is reinforced with additional interrupted sutures, mobilizing more bladder if necessary. A second layer of No. 3-0 delayed-absorbable continuous or interrupted mattress sutures is placed in the bladder musculature, inverting the first layer (Fig. 30-5*D*). A third layer of sutures may be required. Plication of the

urethra and the vesicourethral angle may be carried out if deemed necessary. Also, a bulbocavernosus fat pad developed from the labium majus may be interposed at this point (see Fig. 30-10 *A–D*).

The vaginal mucosa is trimmed and approximated with No. 3-0 interrupted sutures. This closure should be made in the direction that gives the least amount of tension, which may be either transverse or longitudinal to the axis of the vagina. Illustrations of a longitudinal closure in the midline of the anterior vaginal wall are shown in Figure 30-6. This closure tends to provide better support to the urethrovesical angle. If ureteral catheters were previously inserted, they are now removed. A suprapubic catheter is used for bladder drainage for 14 days.

COMPLICATED VESICOVAGINAL FISTULAS

Complicated fistulas are those that are large; those that have had previous unsuccessful attempts at repair; those that involve the urethra, vesical neck, or ureters; those that are associated with intestinal fistulas; and

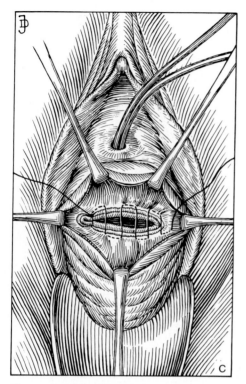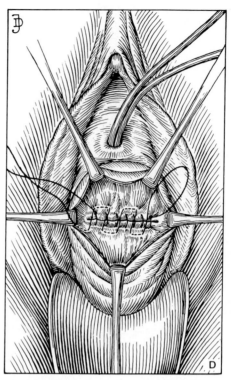

Figure 30–5. (continued) *C,* The first suture line is placed with a continuous or interrupted No. 3-0 delayed-absorbable suture, inverting tissue into the bladder. *D,* A second suture line is placed, inverting the first. Excess vaginal mucosa is trimmed and approximated with interrupted No. 3-0 delayed-absorbable sutures.

those that result from radiation for gynecologic malignancy. Although the standard principles for fistula repair still apply, and perhaps should be applied more strictly, other special techniques may be necessary to achieve continence. As mentioned earlier, a longer interval of time may be required before the tissue around the fistula is mature or healed and ready for closure. Techniques of bringing in new tissue for support and neovascularization should be considered. These include mobilization of the bulbocavernosus muscle and fat pad from the labia, the gracilis muscle from the inner thigh, or an omental fat pad. A combined transvaginal-transvesical-transperitoneal approach may be needed. The operation may need to be done in stages. For example, if a radiation-induced vesicovaginal fistula is associated with a rectovaginal fistula and bilateral ureteral stenosis, a three-stage operation may be required. The first stage may be a ureteroileocutaneous anastomosis and colostomy. The second stage would be a closure of the fistulas. If the fistulas heal, the third stage would be a closure of the colostomy and anastomosis of the ileal conduit to the bladder.

Only when the closure of a vesicovaginal fistula is considered to be technically impossible should one consider supravesical diversion of the urinary stream.

The painful postirradiation fistulas fall into this group. In former years we transplanted the ureters into the sigmoid, but experience has taught us that transplantation into the functioning bowel may shorten the patient's life. Hydronephrosis and pyelonephritis can develop, with the attendant metabolic and electrolyte disturbance of hyperchloremic acidosis. Over time, malignancy of the colonic mucosa at the site of ureteral anastomosis can develop. We now rarely perform ureterosigmoid implantations. Even in patients with postirradiation fistulas where chances for cure are not good or in whom longevity is limited by the presence of malignancy, it is preferable to anastomose the ureters to an isolated segment of ileum. When a fistula is the result of benign disease or injury but impossible to close, we believe that the implantation of the ureters into an isolated ileal loop is also the procedure of choice.

TRANSABDOMINAL CLOSURE OF VESICOVAGINAL FISTULA

In most instances, a high, small vesicovaginal fistula can be closed by the Latzko method. However, multiple previous unsuccessful attempts at closure may produce

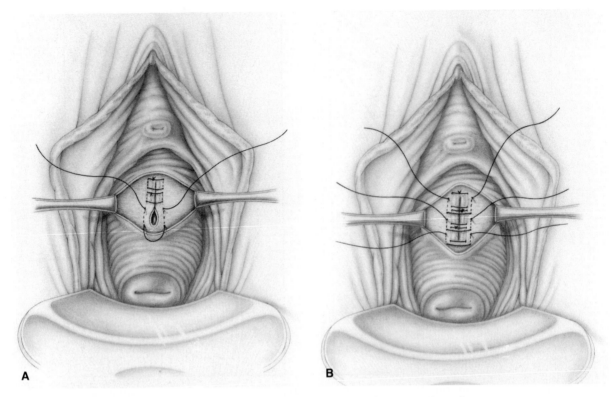

A **B**

Figure 30–6. *A,* Interrupted mattress sutures (No. 3-0 delayed absorbable) are used as a first layer to close the fistula and invert the margins. *B,* The first layer of closure is supported by two additional rows of interrupted mattress sutures before the vaginal mucosa is closed.

excessive scarring and fix the vagina so that exposure from below is extremely difficult. Under these circumstances, transabdominal closure may be necessary. This approach may also be appropriate when the margins of the fistula are close to or involve the ureteral orifice(s), or when the fistula results from irradiation.

With the patient in Trendelenburg position, the pelvis is inspected through a low transverse Maylard incision. The intestines are packed back into the abdomen. The bladder is found adherent to the apex of the vagina at the site of the fistula. The peritoneum is cut at its attachment to the vagina and dissected free. It is left attached to the bladder.

When making this dissection, it should be borne in mind that a flap of peritoneum is to be brought down later between the bladder and the vagina. After freeing the peritoneal flap, a longitudinal (vertical) incision is made in the bladder dome and is extended along the posterior wall in the midline until it reaches the bladder base and the site of the fistulous tract (Fig. 30-7*A*). Here the incision encircles the fistulous tract, including the bladder and vaginal orifices (Fig. 30-7*B*). Then the vagina is closed with interrupted No. 3-0 delayed-absorbable sutures (Fig. 30-7*C*). The bladder, which has been

sufficiently mobilized, is closed with two layers of sutures as shown in Figure 30-7*D*. If possible, the initial layer of interrupted sutures should invert the mucosal edges into the bladder cavity. The integrity of the suture line is tested by filling the bladder with sterile water through a suprapubic catheter placed in the bladder dome (Fig. 30-7*E*). The catheter is in a retroperitoneal position and exteriorized through the abdominal wall in a separate stab wound incision. It is left connected to straight drainage for 12–14 days. The second layer, which includes the muscularis, may be closed with No. 3-0 continuous or interrupted sutures (Fig. 30-7*F*). After the bladder and the vagina are closed, the peritoneal flap is brought down from the bladder reflection and sutured to the anterior vaginal wall or bladder wall so that the suture line in the bladder wall is covered. An omental pedicle graft may be obtained from the transverse colon and sutured between the bladder closure and the vagina (Fig. 30-7*G*). A retroperitoneal drain is brought out through a separate stab wound incision.

O'Connor described an abdominal operation for vesicovaginal fistula repair in 1951. Later, in a series of reports, O'Connor, Jr., has achieved excellent results with this operation. According to O'Connor, Jr.,

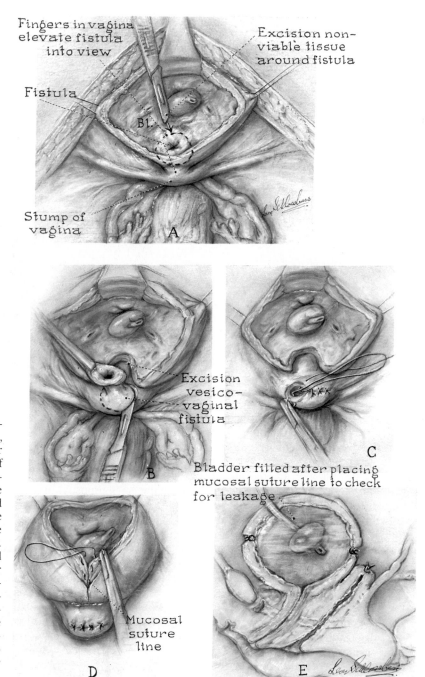

Figure 30–7. Transabdominal, transvesical closure of vesicovaginal fistula. *A,* A longitudinal incision in the bladder dome illustrates the vesical opening of the fistula and its relationship to the vagina and the ureteral orifices. *B,* The incision in the bladder wall is extended around the orifice of the fistula. The fistulous tract and its vaginal orifice are completely excised. *C,* Interrupted No. 3-0 delayed-absorbable sutures are used to close the vaginal opening in one or two layers. *D,* A continuous No. 3-0 delayed-absorbable suture closes the bladder mucosa longitudinally. *E,* A suprapubic catheter is placed through the bladder dome in an extraperitoneal location. The bladder is distended to check for security of closure. (*Figure continued on next page.*)

The key to the operative procedure is bisection of the bladder with wide mobilization of the bladder and vagina, allowing for closure of the vagina and bladder in separate planes. As much dissection as possible is done to free the posterior wall of the bladder and the bladder is then opened at the dome. From this initial incision the exposure is improved by incising vertically down to the area of the fistula. Stay sutures are placed every few centimeters on either side to allow elevation of the bladder wall and the exposure is excellent as these are lifted. The fistulous tract is excised in racquet fashion, making the lateral margin wide enough to leave viable tissue for subsequent closure. Then

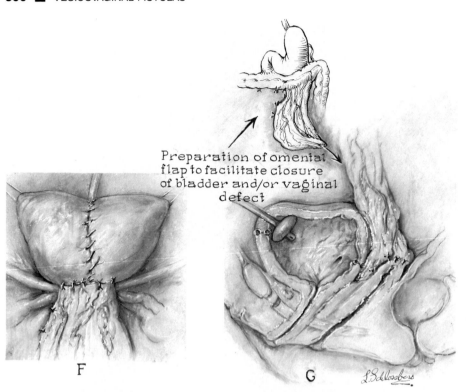

Preparation of omental flap to facilitate closure of bladder and/or vaginal defect

F

G

L. Schlossberg.

Figure 30–7 (continued) *F*, The bladder muscularis is closed with No. 3-0 delayed-absorbable continuous or interrupted sutures. *G*, In complicated fistulas, an omental flap may be developed and sutured between the bladder closure and the vaginal closure.

the exposure may be helped by inserting either a balloon catheter or a Young prostatic tractor through the fistula to elevate the bladder and vagina. After generous excision of the tract, the walls of the bladder are mobilized widely away from the vagina. If there is concern regarding the ureters, catheters can be placed to visualize these structures during this part of the dissection. All nonviable or necrotic tissue is excised and the vaginal closure is done with fresh, viable tissue in 2 layers. . . . This may be further reinforced by placing fat, peritoneum, fibrous tissue or pedicled omentum over this closure. The bladder closure is then begun carefully at the apex of the incision, using a continuous suture, starting with the original knot on the outer surface of the bladder, including all muscle layers. . . . If the defect is extensive, variations of the bladder flaps that are placed to cover the defect can be used but these are usually unnecessary if wide mobilization of the back wall of the bladder can be effected.

Glenn and Stevens, Wein and associates, Marshall, and others have reported good results with a similar operation. A transabdominal operation can be combined with the transvaginal approach, since it may be difficult to mobilize and close the vaginal side of the fistula satisfactorily through an abdominal incision. We have used the combined transabdominal and transvesical approach to advantage in several complicated cases. This technique has been described by Taylor and associates, by Weyrauch and Rous, and by Clarke and Holland. It should be reemphasized, however, that only in unusual and special circumstances is it necessary to repair a vesicovaginal fistula abdominally.

Autograft as an Aid to Fistula Closure

The tissue surrounding complicated vesicovaginal fistulas may be relatively avascular, rigid, and fibrosed. This is especially true of postirradiation fistulas where hyalinization of blood vessels and sclerotic tissue may extend for a considerable distance beyond the fistula margins. When local tissue healing is seriously impaired by irradiation, infection, diabetes, or other factors, it is usually necessary to bring fresh, normal, non-irradiated, pliable, and well-vascularized tissue into the operative field to support the repair and facilitate healing. Neovascularization from such pedicle grafts has been proved experimentally. Small arterioles migrate from the normal into the ischemic tissues of the repair site.

Various techniques of autografting have been described and reviewed by Zacharin. Kiricuta and Goldstein described a procedure for using pedicled omentum in the repair of difficult fistulas. According to these authors, the repair of the fistula does not even require the closure of the bladder defect. If it is technically impossible to close the bladder or vagina because of inaccessibility deep in the pelvis, the vaginal wound will eventually heal over the omental flap. Bastiaanse was also an advocate of pedicled omental grafts. Turner-Warwick has used them in a variety of ingenious ways to reconstruct the upper and lower urinary tract. A free graft of omentum cannot be used for this purpose, since the vascular supply and lymphatic drainage must be intact. Fleischman and Picha have described an abdominal approach for gracilis muscle interposition and repair of recurrent vesicovaginal fistulas. It may be used when an omental pedicle graft is not available.

An abdominal incision must be made if an omental pedicle graft is to be used. Other grafting techniques are available in vaginal operations. Garlock described the vaginal application of the gracilis muscle graft in 1928, and this has been modified by Ingelman-Sundberg and, more recently, by Hamlin and Nicholson. A convenient method of pedicle grafting to provide support and neovascularization for the fistula repair was described by Martius. This graft is obtained from the labium majus on one or both sides and is composed of bulbocavernosus muscle and fat (see Fig. 30-10). It is desirable to close the vaginal mucosa over a pedicle graft if possible. However, if it is not possible, the defect will become reepithelialized in time. Good results with its use have been reported by Zacharin, by Patil and associates, and by Smith and Johnson. We have also found this technique extremely useful, but do not consider it necessary in routine simple fistula repairs. The Martius graft is also very useful in urethral reconstruction, as discussed later.

VESICOUTERINE AND VESICOCERVICAL FISTULAS

Vesicouterine and vesicocervical fistulas (see Fig. 30-1) are alike in etiology, symptoms, and management. Therefore, they will be considered together. Good discussions of these fistulas have been published by Tancer and by Hache and associates.

Improved obstetric practice is responsible for a reduction in the incidence of these fistulas today as compared to a much more frequent occurrence in the nineteenth century. Although some result from instrumentation and malignancy, today almost all vesicouterine and vesicocervical fistulas are associated with injury to or necrosis of the bladder wall directly over dehiscence of a lower uterine segment cesarean section incision. When there has been inadequate mobilization of the bladder inferiorly and laterally, the bladder may

be injured with delivery of a large fetal head, or the bladder wall may be accidentally included in the sutures used to close the uterine incision. When the sutures are absorbed and a fistula forms, the patient may experience some involuntary loss of urine through the vagina or she may remain continent. She may complain of cyclic hematuria and amenorrhea. This symptom was called menouria by Youssef. In most cases, variable degrees of intermittent urinary incontinence will be present and only microscopic hematuria will be present during regular menstrual flow. Of course, vaginal examination will fail to reveal a fistula, although occasionally urine will be seen trickling through the cervical os. Cystoscopy, cystogram, and hysterogram are helpful diagnostic procedures. The vesical orifice of the fistula will always be supratrigonal in location when viewed through the cystoscope.

Although a few fistulas have been reported to close spontaneously, most often surgery is required. The operation is fairly simple to perform and almost routinely successful. Either a transvaginal or a transabdominal approach may be used. When the fistula is high and there is no uterine descensus when traction is made on a cervical tenaculum, the repair should be performed through an abdominal incision. A dissection is carried out to separate the bladder from the cervix and lower uterine segment. Following identification of the fistula tract, the uterine and bladder defects are closed separately in layers. A layer of vesical peritoneum should be interposed between the two sides. Transurethral bladder drainage should be carried out for 7–10 days postoperatively. A hysterectomy is not required for fistula repair. If hysterectomy is done, it should be indicated for some other reason, including the presence of a large defect in the uterine wall. If the uterus is left, pregnancies can and will occur unless a tubal ligation is performed or contraception is used assiduously.

COMPLICATIONS OF FISTULA REPAIR

As soon as the last repair suture is placed, 5 ml indigo carmine should be injected intravenously, the bladder should be filled with 200 ml clear sterile saline, and a cystoscope should be gently placed into the bladder. Careful examination of the repair site for evidence of bleeding should then be carried out. The dye should be seen spurting from each ureteral orifice. By this technique, two of the most common complications of vesicovaginal fistula repair—intravesical hemorrhage and ureteral obstruction—can be diagnosed at the earliest possible moment and corrected.

When intravesical bleeding still occurs in the postoperative period and threatens the integrity of the repair by obstruction of the catheter and overdistention of the bladder, gentle attempts to evacuate the clots can be made by transurethral bladder irrigations. If these are not successful, it may be necessary to perform an immediate suprapubic cystotomy to remove the clots and suture the bleeding points in the bladder mucosa. Infection is common after such events and should be combated with antibiotics. Transfusions will be needed if significant amounts of blood are lost.

If the patient exhibits signs of ureteral obstruction (persistent fever, abdominal distention, pain, and tenderness), an excretory urogram should be done immediately. Occasionally, ureteral obstruction will be temporary from tissue edema caused by the fistula repair. If a complete ureteral obstruction is diagnosed, several options are available. One might consider breaking down the repair to remove the offending suture(s). This procedure may be less hazardous in a poor-risk or elderly patient than an operation to relieve the obstruction. However, it carries with it the great disappointment of failure to establish continence, since the fistula repair will need to be redone later after a prolonged interval of waiting and may be more difficult. One also has the option of performing an abdominal operation to relieve the obstruction. After the ureter has been identified on the pelvic side wall, the choice lies between placing a T-tube in the ureter for drainage, hoping the obstruction below will be relieved spontaneously when the sutures are absorbed, or performing a ureteroneocystostomy. A percutaneous nephrostomy may be a satisfactory temporary solution attempting to preserve kidney function until a definitive repair of the ureter can be done. Sometimes a ureteral catheter can be passed down through the nephrostomy, past the point of ureteral obstruction, and into the bladder.

The most important and dreaded complication, of course, is breakdown of the repair. This usually occurs about 7–10 days after operation. If the repair breaks down, large-caliber catheter drainage should be reinstituted and continued for several weeks to provide an adequate opportunity for the fistula to heal spontaneously. Spontaneous healing, however, rarely occurs, and only under optimal conditions. A significant reduction in the size of the fistula may result so that the next attempt at repair will be easier and will be more likely to be successful.

Recurrence of the fistula months or even years after initial successful repair may occur, but this is very rare. More commonly, patients may continue to experience urinary incontinence, which will be found on careful examination to come through the intact urethra. Such incontinence may be associated with a small bladder capacity from prolonged bladder drainage through the fistula. The bladder detrusor muscle may be dysenergic after repair. Scarring at the vesical neck caused by the repair may interfere with the maintenance of normal intralumenal pressures in the upper urethra or change the normal anatomic relationship between the bladder neck and the upper urethra. Any and all of these factors can result in patients experiencing transurethral urinary incontinence after vesicovaginal fistula repair.

URETHRAL DAMAGE

Serious damage to the urethra that results in a fistula is uncommon. Formerly, obstetric injury from prolonged labor or difficult forceps delivery was the major cause of this condition. In developing countries, this is still a significant cause of urethral injury. More commonly, inadvertent urethral damage results from an unsuccessful attempt to remove an infected suburethral diverticulum. Gray reports a 25% incidence of urethrovaginal fistula in such cases, which is much higher than our own experience of 5%. Additionally, direct trauma may occur during an anterior colporrhaphy. If this is unrecognized at the time of surgery, a fistula will follow. Irradiation damage to the floor of the urethra may occur with the use of intravaginal irradiation of tumors in the lower genital tract; in most of these cases there has been extension of the tumor into the urethrovaginal septum, which subsequently breaks down with the regression of the neoplasm. We have observed ischemia of the distal half of the urethra following repeated attempts at urethral plication for urinary incontinence that have led to a severely compromised blood supply to the urethra. The urethra may also be damaged if the bulb of a Foley catheter is accidentally inflated in the urethral lumen.

The destructive effects of lymphogranuloma venereum may cause urethral loss. Finally, some patients with congenital absence of the vagina will have loss of urethral function as a result of overzealous attempts to create a vaginal cavity by the Frank method, from frequent intercourse through the urethra, or from sloughing of the distal urethra as a complication of the Abbe-Wharton-McIndoe operation.

Loss of the distal one third of the urethra is usually not associated with urinary incontinence, although it is often associated with loss of a well-defined urinary stream. Urine may spray from the urethra and down the insides of the thigh in an annoying fashion. The distal urethra can be sacrificed in extensive operations for the vagina and vulva without loss of continence.

Many of the principles outlined for vesicovaginal fistula repair are also applicable to repair of urethrovaginal fistulas. However, since urethrovaginal fistulas may be more difficult to repair successfully, the tissues must be as nearly normal as possible before repair is attempted. For this reason, after the diagnosis is made, a delay of several months may be necessary to allow the tissues to heal completely. Wide meticulous dissection and mobilization is essential, so that tissues can be approximated exactly and without tension. Pedicle grafting is frequently necessary. Suprapubic rather than transurethral catheter drainage is always preferred. The repair must be individualized to fit the special circumstances presented by each patient.

Urethral reconstruction and restoration of continence is difficult to accomplish at the same time with a single operation. Success is generally achieved in about 50% of cases. Symmonds and Hill have pointed out that successful anatomic restoration is not synonymous with restoration of physiologic function. Little is accomplished if urethral length is restored but the patient remains incontinent. Emphasis is placed on fashioning a new urethra of small caliber using as much muscular tissue as possible, plicating the vesical neck whenever appropriate, and supporting the new repair with a pedicled bulbocavernosus muscle and fat pad if necessary. It cannot be predicted if restorative operations on the urethra will establish continence. Patients in whom continence is not established should have a retropubic cystourethropexy done after waiting at least 6 months after urethral reconstruction. A Goebell-Frangenheim-Stoeckel operation (see Chapter 33) has also been used in these patients but runs the risk of interfering with the urethral blood supply and causing damage again to the urethral floor.

Operations for Restoration of Urethra

The following operations are designed for certain cases of urinary incontinence resulting from destruction of the urethra and part of the sphincter from childbirth injury, surgery, or a diverticulum.

In the standard operation for urethral reconstruction and sphincter repair, a U-shaped flap or vaginal mucosa is dissected free and held forward, thus exposing the undersurface of the trigone and sphincter region of the bladder (Fig. 30-8A). Rather deep interrupted stitches of No. 3-0 delayed-absorbable suture are taken in the sphincter region. These, when tied, tighten the internal orifice (Fig. 30-8 B–C).

The flap of mucosa is drawn downward and an area about 6 or 7 mm wide is denuded forward for a distance equal to the length of the flap (Fig. 30-8D).

The edge of the flap is held forward with a smooth dissecting forceps and is curled under, so that the raw surface of the flap may be sutured to the anterior denuded area (Fig. 30-8E). Interrupted No. 3-0 delayed-absorbable sutures are used. This is repeated on the other side, thus forming an epithelial-lined tube to serve as a urethra. This new urethral floor is supported by a layer of paraurethral fascia that is plicated beneath the urethra with No. 3-0 delayed-absorbable sutures.

The wound is closed by approximating the mucosal edges with interrupted No. 3-0 delayed-absorbable sutures. This buries the newly constructed urethra and completely closes the wound (Fig. 30-8 F–G).

To permit healing of the newly constructed urethra, a suprapubic silicone catheter is used for bladder drainage. A transurethral indwelling catheter should not be used.

We have found this procedure to be successful when used as the initial attempt to restore the floor of an extensively traumatized urethra. It has been less successful in cases where previous attempts to repair the urethra have failed owing to the compromise of the blood supply to the long mucosal pedicle. In such cases, we prefer the following technique, which reestablishes the walls of the urethra along the urethral floor, as illustrated in Figure 30-9 A and G, in cases where the walls have retracted into the roof of the urethral tube. Symmonds has had excellent success in establishing urinary continence with this method. Falk and Tancer described a similar procedure and have encouraged its use. This operation emphasizes preservation of the limited blood supply to the urethral margins. By incising the vaginal mucosa at the very lateral margin of each side of the urethral remnants along the roof of the exposed urethra, leaving no more than 2 mm of vaginal mucosa attached to the urethral walls, the edges of the retracted side walls can be freed with careful sharp dissection without encroaching too far laterally on the paraurethral blood supply (Fig. 30-9B). The dissection should mobilize enough of the urethral walls to permit snug approximation of the edges in the posterior midline with interrupted No. 3-0 delayed-absorbable sutures over a small No. 12 French catheter (Fig. 30-9C). Although a very small urethral lumen is created by this conservative dissection, this has a distinct advantage in establishing urethral continence. The adjacent urethral fascia is then freed with sharp dissection along the side of the newly created urethral tube, avoiding deep lateral dissection and interruption of the blood supply.

Interrupted No. 3-0 delayed-absorbable sutures are placed through the fascia and musculature of the urethral tube along each side of the urethra, with each suture being held until placement has been made on both sides (see Fig. 30-9C). The lower strand of each suture is then joined with the lower strand of the corresponding suture on the opposite side of the urethra and tied across the urethral floor. The upper strand of each suture is then tied in the midline. As described by Symmonds, this produces a pulley effect that approximates broad surface of fascia and urethral muscle to broad surface (Fig. 30-9D). Alternatively, vertical mat-

(text continues on page 814)

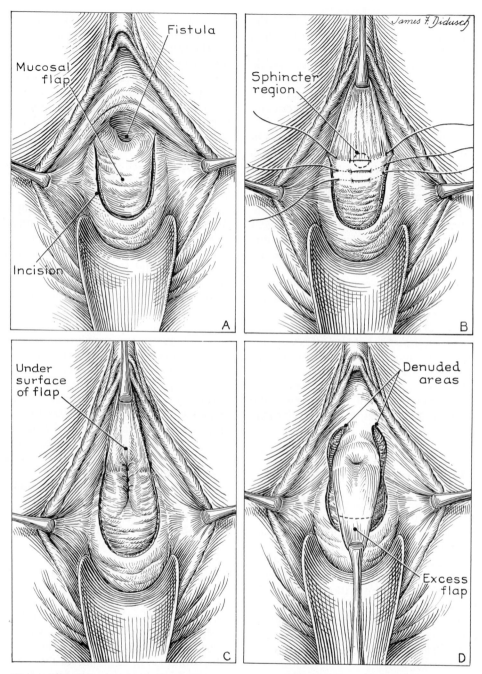

Figure 30–8. Reconstruction of urethra and repair of sphincter. *A,* A U-shaped incision is made through the vaginal mucosa. *B,* The mucosal flap has been freed and pulled forward. Three interrupted sutures of No. 3-0 delayed-absorbable suture are placed to tighten the sphincter region. *C,* The sphincter sutures have been tied, inverting the tissue. *D,* The mucosal flap has been pulled downward, and areas have been denuded anteriorly on both sides.

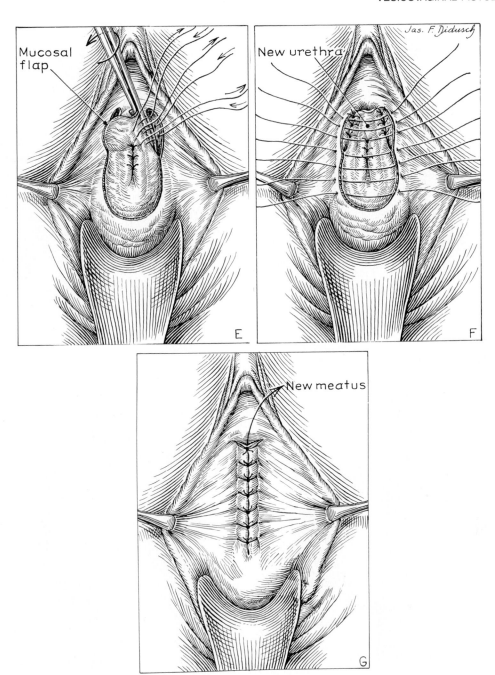

Figure 30–8 (continued) *E*, The flap is sutured anteriorly with No. 3-0 delayed-absorbable suture, rolling the flap inward so as to approximate raw surfaces. *F*, Mucosal edges are approximated over the newly formed urethra with interrupted sutures of No. 3-0 delayed-absorbable after a supporting layer of paraurethral fascia is plicated beneath the urethral floor. *G*, Completion of reconstruction of the urethra, showing interrupted suture closure of suburethral mucosa. Urethral catheter is removed after insertion of suprapubic catheter.

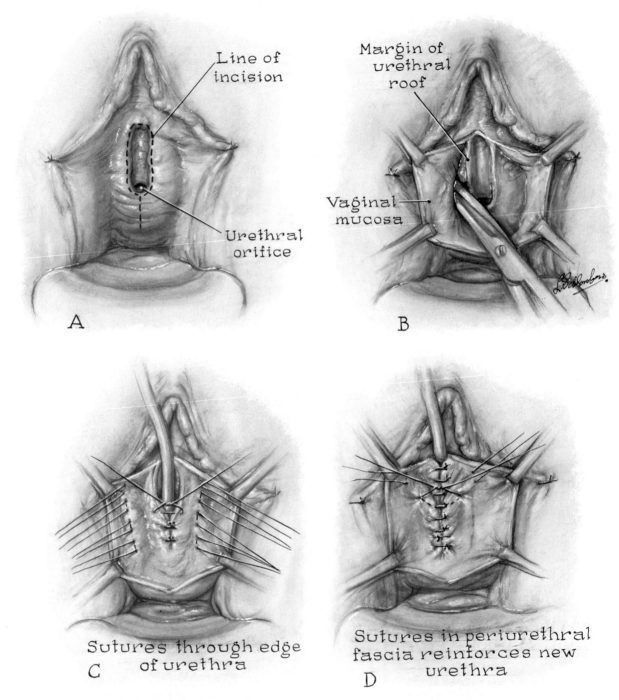

Figure 30–9. Reconstruction of total or partial loss of urethral floor. *A*, Line of incision along lateral margin of roof of urethra and beneath bladder base. *B*, Enough of the urethral margins and fascia are freed from the vagina to permit approximation of the urethral mucosa in the midline. *C*, Urethral edges are approximated in the midline over a No. 12 French catheter with interrupted No. 3-0 delayed-absorbable sutures. Mobilized urethral fascia is sutured on each side of the total length of the urethra. The lower strand of each suture is tied beneath the urethral floor *D*, and the upper strands of the two sutures are used to pull the fascia beneath the urethra, where they are tied.

Figure 30–9 (continued) *E*, The vaginal mucosa is closed without tension. The bladder is filled with sterile water before the catheter is removed and a suprapubic tube is inserted. *F*, Alternatively for additional reinforcement, a labial fat pad is developed by a U-shaped incision along the lateral and medial aspects of the labia, leaving a broad pedicle superiorly. The lateral vaginal mucosa is resected between the urethral operative site and the labial graft *G*. The skin margins of the labial graft are sutured to the vaginal margins with No. 3-0 delayed-absorbable suture. The labial skin margins are closed so as to produce a flat vulvar surface.

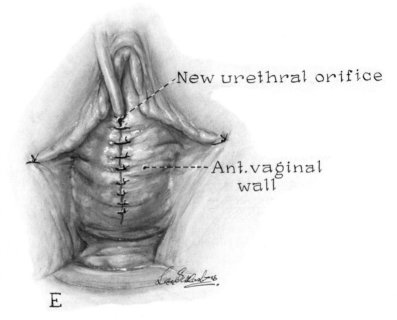

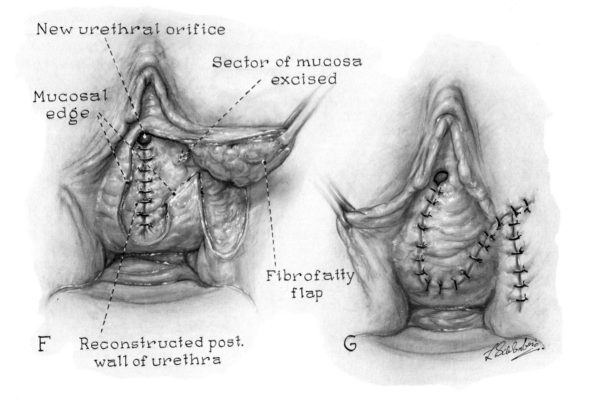

tress sutures in the fascia and adjacent urethral musculature will produce equal support to the urethral wall. The edges of the vaginal mucosa are then undermined and freed sufficiently to permit approximation in the midline without undue tension, using No. 3-0 delayed-absorbable sutures (Fig. 30-9E). It is important to remove the small urethral catheter at the completion of the procedure to avoid pressure necrosis to the suture line. It is our policy to fill the bladder with 300 ml sterile water and to insert a suprapubic silicone tube before removing the catheter because it is frequently difficult and hazardous to catheterize the newly constructed urethra. Should the suprapubic catheter become plugged, only the surgeon who understands the landmarks of the newly constructed urethral tube should attempt to catheterize this patient postoperatively. The bladder and urethra are left at rest for 12–14 days before the suprapubic catheter is clamped intermittently to initiate voiding through the reconstructed urethra.

Alternatively, before closing the vaginal mucosa, it is frequently useful to reinforce the surgical reconstruction of the urethra with a labial fat pad as shown in Figure 30-9 F–G. This modified Martius technique adds a vascularized labial graft that will provide a new blood supply to the operative site and avoid necrosis and breakdown of the ischemic urethra. By making a U-shaped incision along the lateral and medial margins of the labium majus and minus, the fat pad overlying the bulbocavernosus muscle is dissected free, leaving a wide base of the graft at the superior aspect of the labia. The vaginal mucosa is excised along the side of the urethra adjacent to the pedicle graft to accommodate the width of the pedicle and to provide a graft site for the vulvar flap (see Fig. 30-9F). The skin margins of the fat pad are then sutured to the margins of the vaginal mucosa using No. 3-0 delayed-absorbable sutures, obliterating the mucosal defect in the operative site. The vulvar skin is closed with interrupted sutures to give a flat contour to the excised labia (see Fig. 30-9G). If bleeding is excessive, the labial donor site may be drained temporarily through a small lateral incision.

POSTIRRADIATION FISTULAS

The most intractable of all fistulas are those created by the effect of ionizing irradiation on sensitive tissues. The entire urethrovaginal or vesicovaginal septum may tolerate combined radiation doses as high as 8000 rads before necrosis and fistula occur, but occasionally it is necessary to exceed the normal tissue tolerance knowingly in the treatment of certain malignancies of the lower genital tract. Fortunately, this is uncommon. A fistula may appear a few months to several years after

the radiation treatment is completed. As pointed out by Boronow in his review of radiation-induced vaginal fistula (vesicovaginal and rectovaginal) among 2756 cervical cancer patients treated with radiation at the Radiumhemmett (Stockholm), 9 vaginal fistulas occurred; among 3158 cervical cancer patients treated with radiation at the Roswell Park Memorial Institute, 13 vaginal fistulas occurred. The combined incidence is one vaginal fistula per 269 patients irradiated. The incidence of fistula is much higher if hysterectomy is done in a pelvis that has received radiation previously.

Vesicovaginal fistulas induced by radiation therapy are usually complicated and difficult to close for several reasons. The fistula is usually large and located in the apex of the vagina. If it has not been previously removed, the cervix will be a part of the fistula margin. The tissue surrounding the fistula will be fixed, relatively avascular, and fibrotic. Encrustations may cover the margins of older fistulas. Because the radiation-induced obliterative endarteritis is progressive over a period of many months, the fistula may gradually enlarge with continued ischemia and necrosis of more tissue. Many months may pass before the obliterative endarteritis and ischemia stabilize and the ultimate size of the fistula is attained. Certainly one must wait until the acute radiation injury has subsided completely.

When a radiation-induced urethrovaginal or vesicovaginal fistula does occur, the margins should be biopsied to rule out persistent or recurrent cancer. The status of the upper urinary tracts must be assessed and the proximity of the ureteral orifices to the fistula margin determined. Every effort should be made to obtain as viable a margin of tissue around the fistula as possible before attempting a surgical closure. Therefore, it is our policy to delay repair of a radiation-induced fistula for a minimum of 6 months after its occurrence and preferably for 12 months, if possible. The key to successful closure of these fistulas is the establishment of a new blood supply to the devitalized vaginal tissues.

MARTIUS BULBOCAVERNOSUS FAT PAD

We have found the Martius method to be very effective and to reduce greatly the previously high failure rate in attempted closure of these complicated fistulas. For irradiation fistulas that are located high in the vagina, we use the original Martius procedure and dissect the fat pad separately from the overlaying vulvar skin, leaving one end attached to its blood supply (Fig. 30-10A). In such cases, the mobilized fatty tissue can be tunneled beneath the labia minora and vaginal mucosa to the operative site (Fig. 30-10B). The tunnel should be large enough to allow adequate blood to flow from the

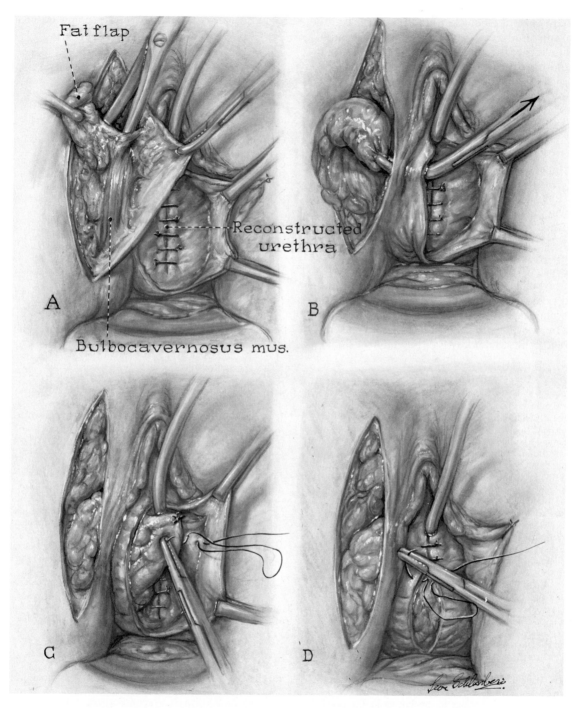

Figure 30–10. Martius bulbocavernosus fat pad graft for urethrovaginal or vesicovaginal fistula repair. *A*, The lateral margin of the labia majora is opened by a vertical incision and the fat pad adjacent to the bulbocavernosus muscle is mobilized, leaving a broad pedicle attached at the inferior pole. *B, C,* The fat pad is drawn through a tunnel beneath the labia minora and vaginal mucosa and sutured with No. 3-0 delayed-absorbable sutures to the fascia of the urethra and bladder. *D*, The vaginal mucosa is mobilized widely to permit closure in the midline. The vulvar incision is closed with interrupted No. 3-0 delayed-absorbable sutures and drained if necessary.

base to the tip of the pedicle without constriction. The pedicle should not be constricted on its base and the base should have broad attachment laterally. The pedicle is sutured to the margins of the fistulous repair (Fig. 30-10C). If the fistula is large and complicated and additional tissue is needed, the underlying bulbocavernosus muscle may be mobilized along with the fat pad. Alternatively, a bulbocavernosus fat pad may also be mobilized from each side if additional tissue is needed. The vaginal mucosa is dissected widely and approximated over the graft of fatty tissue as the final layer of closure (Fig. 30-10D). If the vaginal mucosa is insufficient or cannot be mobilized widely enough to close without tension, one may substitute labial skin attached to the labial fat pad as described by Symmonds and by Podratz and associates. A drain may be left beneath the labial incision. Prolonged suprapubic bladder drainage will usually be necessary.

Good results utilizing the Martius bulbocavernosus fat pad pedicle graft to repair radiation-induced and other complicated vesicovaginal fistulas have been reported by Boronow, by Steg and Chiche, by Betson, by Smith and Johnson, and by Patil and associates.

Bibliography

Baker HW. Selective indications for subtotal hysterectomy. J Ky Med Assoc 1985;83:355.

Bastiaanse MA, Van Bouwdyk. The treatment of vesicovaginal fistulas, including so-called radium fistulas. Proc R Soc Med 1954;47:610.

Betson JR. Bulbocavernosus fat pad transplant. Obstet Gynecol 1980;9:303.

Boronow RC. Repair of radiation-induced vaginal fistula utilizing the Martius technique. World J Surg 1986;10:237.

Boronow RC, Rutledge F. Vesicovaginal fistula, radiation, and gynecologic cancer. Am J Obstet Gynecol 1971;111:85.

Clarke DH, Holland JB. Repair of vesicovaginal fistulas: simultaneous transvaginal-transvesical approach. South Med J 1975;68:1410.

Collins CG, Prent D. Results of early repair of vesicovaginal fistula with preliminary cortisone treatment. Am J Obstet Gynecol 1960; 80:1005.

Collins CG, Collins JH, Harrison BR, et al. Early repair of vesicovaginal fistula. Am J Obstet Gynecol 1971;111:524.

Cruikshank SH. Early closure of post-hysterectomy vesicovaginal fistulas. So Med J 1988;81:1525.

Davis RS, Linke CA, Kraemer GK. Use of labial tissue in repair of urethrovaginal fistula and injury. Arch Surg 1980;115:628.

Elkins TE, Drescher C, Martey JO, Fort D. Vesicovaginal fistula revisited. Obstet Gynecol 1988;72:307.

Everett HS, Mattingly RF. Urinary tract injuries resulting from pelvic surgery. Am J Obstet Gynecol 1956;71:502.

Everett HS, Williams TJ. Urology in the female. In: Campbell MF, Harrison JB, eds. Urology. 3rd ed. Philadelphia: WB Saunders, 1970.

Falk HC, Orkin LA. Nonsurgical closure of vesicovaginal fistulas. Obstet Gynecol 1957;9:538.

Falk HC, Tancer ML. Loss of urethra: report of three cases. Obstet Gynecol 1957;9:458.

Falk HC, Tancer ML. Urethrovesicovaginal fistula. Obstet Gynecol 1969;33:422.

Fearl CL, Keizur LW. Optimum time interval from occurrence to repair of vesicovaginal fistula. Am J Obstet Gynecol 1968; 104:205.

Fleischmann J, Picha G. Abdominal approach for gracilis muscle interposition and repair of recurrent vesicovaginal fistulas. J Urol 1988;140:552.

Garlock JH. The cure of an intractable vesicovaginal fistula by the use of a pedicled muscle flap. Surg Gynecol Obstet 1928;47:225.

Glenn JF, Stevens PS. Simplified vesicovaginal fistulectomy. J Urol 1973;110:521.

Graham JB. Painful syndrome of postradiation urinary vaginal fistula. Surg Gynecol Obstet 1964;124:1260.

Gray LA. Urethrovaginal fistulas. Am J Obstet Gynecol 1968;101:28.

Hache L, Pratt JH, Cook En. Vesicouterine fistula. Mayo Clin Proc 1966;41:150.

Hamlin RHJ, Nicholson EC. Reconstruction of the urethra totally destroyed by labour. Br Med J 1969;2:147.

Harrison KA. Obstetric fistula: one social calamity too many. Br J Obstet Gynecol 1983;90:385.

Hayward G. Case of vesicovaginal fistula, successfully treated by an operation. Am J Med Sci 1839;24:283.

Hyman RM. Coagulation therapy for small vesicovaginal fistulas. Clin Obstet Gynecol 1968;8:465.

Iloabachie GC, Njoku O. Vesicouterine fistula. Br J Urol 1985;57:438.

Ingelman-Sundberg AGI. Pathogenesis and operative treatment of urinary fistulae in irradiated tissue. In: Youssef AF, ed. Gynecological urology. Springfield, Ill.: Charles C Thomas, 1960.

Jaszczak SE, Evans TN. Intrafascial abdominal and vaginal hysterectomy: a reappraisal. Obstet Gynecol 1982;59:435.

Kelly HA. The treatment of large vesicovaginal fistulae. Bull Johns Hopkins Hosp 1896;7:29.

Kelly HA. The suprapubic route in operating for vesical fistulae. Trans Am Gynecol Soc 1906;31:225.

Kelly HA. The history of vesicovaginal fistula. Trans Am Gynecol Soc 1912;37:3.

Kiricuta I, Goldstein AMB. The repair of extensive vesicovaginal fistulas with pedicled omentum: a review of 27 cases. J Urol 1972;108:724.

Kursh EC, Morse RM, Resnick MI, Persky L. Prevention of the development of a vesicovaginal fistula. Surg Gynecol Obstet 1988; 166:490.

Latzko W. Behandlung Hochsitzender Blasen-und Mastdarmscheidenfisteln nach Uterusextipation mit hohem Schedienverschluss. Zentralbl Gynak 1914;38:906.

Latzko W. Postoperative vesicovaginal fistulas. Am J Surg 1942;58:211.

Lawson JB. Management of genitourinary fistulae. Clin Obstet Gynecol 1975;5:209.

Lee RA, Symmonds RE, Williams TJ. Current status of genitourinary fistula. Obstet Gynecol 1988;72:313.

Mackenrodt A. Die operative Heilung der Harnleiterfisteln. Ein geheilter Fall von Harnleiter-Gabarmutterfistel. 261 Gynak 1894; 18:1026.

Maisonneuve JG. Clinique chirurgicale. Paris: 1863:660..

Marshall VF. Vesicovaginal fistulas on one urological service. J Urol 1979;121:25.

Martius H. Vesicovaginal therapy especially by plastic transplantation of flaps. Z Geburtsh Gynak 1932;103:22.

Mattingly RF, Borkowf HI. Lower urinary tract injuries in pregnancy. In: Barber HR, Graber EA, eds. Surgical diseases in pregnancy. Philadelphia: WB Saunders, 1974.

McCall ML, Bolten KA, ed and trans. Martius gynecological operations with emphasis on topographic anatomy. Boston: Little, Brown, 1956.

McGregor DK. Female disorders and nineteenth century medicine: the case of vesicovaginal fistula. Caduceus 1987;3:1.

Mettauer JP. Vesicovaginal fistula. Boston Med Surg J 1840;22:154.

Miller NF, George H. Lower urinary tract fistulas in women. A study based on 292 cases. Am J Obstet Gynecol 1954;68:436.

Moir JC. Vesicovaginal fistula. Proc R Soc Med 1966;59:1019.

Murphy M. Social consequences of vesicovaginal fistula in northern Nigeria. J Biosoc Sci 1981;13:139.

O'Connor VJ. Suprapubic closure of vesicovaginal fistula. Springfield, Ill.: Charles C Thomas, 1957.

O'Connor VJ, Jr. Repair of vesicovaginal fistula with associated urethral loss. Surg Gynecol Obstet 1978;146:251.

O'Connor VJ, Jr. Review of experience with vesicovaginal fistula repair. Trans Am Assoc Genito-Urinary Surgeons 1979;71:120.

O'Quinn AG, Degefu S, Batson HK, et al. Early repair of vesicovaginal fistula following preliminary corticosteroid treatment. Presented at the Society of Pelvic Surgeons, New Orleans, November, 1984.

Patil V, Waterhouse K, Laungani G. Management of 18 difficult vesicovaginal and urethrovaginal fistulas with modified Ingelman-Sundberg and Martius operations. J Urol 1980;123:653.

Pawar HN. Management of vesicouterine fistula following cesarean section. Urology 1985;25:66.

Pawlik C. Ueberdie Operation der Blasenscheidenfisteln. Ztschr F. Geburtsh U. Gynak, 1882;8:22.

Persky L, Herman G, Geurrier K. Non-delay in vesicovaginal fistula repair. Urology 1979;13:273.

Petty WM, Lowy RO, Oyama AA. Total abdominal hysterectomy after radiation therapy for cervical cancer: use of omental graft for fistula prevention. Am J Obstet Gynecol 1986;154:1222.

Pfaneuf LE. Vesicovaginal fistula management—end results. Am J Obstet Gynecol 1936;31:316.

Podratz K, Symmonds RE, Hagen JV. Vesicovaginal fistulae. Bailliere's Clin Obstet Gynecol 1987;1:4124.

Ridley JH. Indirect air cystoscopy. So Med J 1951;44:114.

Ridley JH. Surgery for vaginal fistulae. In: Ridley JH, ed. Gynecologic surgery: errors, safeguards, and salvage. 2nd ed. Baltimore: Williams & Wilkins, 1981.

Robertson JR. Vesicovaginal fistula: the gynecologist's responsibility. Obstet Gynecol 1973;42:611.

Schuchardt K. Uber die paravaginale Methode der Extirpation uteri and ihre Enderfolge beim Uteruskrebs. Monatsschr Geburtsch Gynak 1901;13:744.

Simon G. Falle von Operation bei Urinfisteln am Weibe. Beobachtung einer Harnleiter Scheidenfistel. Deutsch Klin 1856;p. 311.

Sims JM. On the treatment of vesicovaginal fistula. Am J Med Sci 1852;23:59.

Smith WG, Johnson GH. Vesicovaginal fistula repair—revisited. Gyn Oncol 1980;9:303.

Steg A, Chiche R. The challenging vesicovaginal fistula. Eur Urol 1983;9:157.

Symmonds RE. Incontinence: vesical and urethral fistulas. Clin Obstet Gynecol 1984;27:499.

Symmonds RE, Hill M. Loss of the urethra: a report on 50 patients. Am J Obstet Gynecol 1978;130:130.

Tahzib F. Epidemiological determinants of vesicovaginal fistulas. Br J Obstet Gynecol 1983;90:387.

Tancer ML. The post-cesarean fistula. Clin Obstet Gynecol 1965;8:472.

Tancer ML. The post total hysterectomy (vault) vesicovaginal fistula. J Urol 123:839, 1980.

Taylor JS, Hewson AD, Rachow P. Synchronous combined transvaginal transvesical repair of vesicovaginal fistulas. Aust NZ J Surg 50:23, 1980.

Thanos A, Pavlakis AJ, Poulias I, Davillas N. Vesicouterine fistuli. Urology 28:426, 1986.

Trendelenburg F. Operations for vesicovaginal fistula and the elevated pelvic position for operations within the abdominal cavity. Samml Vortr No. 355:3373, 1890.

Turner-Warwick R. The use of the omental pedicle graft in urinary tract reconstruction. J Urol 116:341.

Van Nagell JR, Jr, Parker JC, Jr, Maruyama Y, et al. Bladder or rectal injury following radiation therapy for cervical cancer. Am J Obstet Gynecol 1974;119:727.

Van Oyen P, Denys H, and Vergison R. Simple vesicovaginal fistula following gynaecological procedures for benign conditions. Acta Urologica Belgica 1986;54:440.

van Roonhuyse H. Medico-chirurgical observations. Englished out of Dutch by a careful hand. London: M Pitt, 1676.

Von Dittel L. Abdominale Blasenscheidenfistel-Operation. Wein Klin Wchr 1893;J26:449.

Wein AJ, Malloy TR, Carpinello VL, et al. Repair of vesicovaginal fistula by a suprapubic transvesical approach. Surg Gynecol Obstet 1980;150:57.

Weyrauch HM, Rous SN. Transvaginal-transvesical approach for surgical repair of vesicovaginal fistula. Surg Gynecol Obstet 1966; 123:121.

Wolff HD, Jr. Gililland NA. Vaginal diaphragm catheters. J Urol 1957;78:681.

Youssef AF. "Menouria" following lower segment cesarean section: a syndrome. Am J Obstet Gynecol 1957;73:759.

Zacharin RF. Grafting as a principle in the surgical management of vesicovaginal and rectovaginal fistulae. Aust NZ J Obstet Gynaecol 1980;20:10.

Zacharin RF. Obstetric fistula. New York: Springer-Verlag, 1988.

Malpositions of the Uterus

31

JOHN D. THOMPSON

RETRODISPLACEMENT OF THE UTERUS

The recognition and surgical correction of retrodisplacement of the uterus form an interesting chapter in the development of gynecology. In 1955, Frederic Fluhmann wrote a review of the subject, and in this brief historical sketch we have drawn heavily from his work. He who fails to heed the mistakes of the past is apt to repeat them. With this in mind we have considered it worthwhile to sketch briefly this history.

During the early part of the 18th century, retrodisplacement of the uterus became identified as an obstetric complication, occurring during the fourth and fifth months of pregnancy. Sometimes retrodisplacement resulted from incarceration, abortion, and secondary infection and caused death. Death also resulted from fatal injuries during forceful attempts at displacement. In 1782, Denman considered overdistention of the bladder the chief cause of the condition and recommended repeated catheterization as the essential treatment.

In Howard Kelly's review of the subject, he calls the early part of the 19th century the "pessary period." It was then that retrodisplacement became recognized in the nonpregnant state and many ingenious instruments and techniques were devised for bringing the uterus forward and holding it there. Churchill, in 1875, described the symptoms as greater menstrual flow, pelvic engorgement, greater tendency to abortion, a sensation of depression and falling of the womb, pain, difficult and frequent urination, dull backache, a sense of pressure in the rectum, pain down the thighs, leukorrhea, and interference with general health. Even then Nauche stated that the condition could exist without symptoms, but unfortunately no one heeded him. Although J. Marion Sims was a strong advocate of the use of pessaries, he cited several instances of vaginal ulceration and vesicovaginal and rectovaginal fistula resulting from their uses. He believed that no one who did not possess mechanical ingenuity should attempt to insert a pessary. He himself shaped each pessary individually to the vagina using "block tin or gutta-percha softened with a little lead."

In the latter part of the 19th century there began what Fluhmann calls the "dark ages of operative furor." Alexander and Adams are credited with doing the first abdominal uterine suspensions. Alexander performed his first one in 1881, and Adams did his first in 1882, but Adams recorded the operation first in the literature. The operation soon attained great popularity, and numerous modifications were described. In 1914, Kelly collected over 50 types of suspension; and in 1928, Hadden collected 120. Alexander became so enthusiastic about uterine suspension that on one occasion he was asked to demonstrate the operation for some visiting surgeons. He sent four assistants north, south, east, and west throughout Liverpool to find a suitable case. They returned empty-handed, saying that in all Liverpool they could find no woman who had not had the Alexander operation performed on her. Howard Kelly stated that he personally had done over 1000 suspensions, and Barton Cook Hirst reported "hundreds." By that time, and even before, skeptics were raising some questions. Scanzoni wrote in 1850, "My decided conviction is that the mechanical treatment of this affliction of retrodisplacement ... is either useless or positively mischievous." Although J. Montgomery Baldy devised a method of uterine suspension, he wrote, "Like the poor, the subject seems to be always with us.... We should not discuss the treatment of retrodisplacement but treatment of conditions with which retrodisplacements of the uterus occur as an incident."

Ventrofixation, hysterorrhaphy, and *hysteropexy* were terms applied to the earliest operations in which an attempt was made to suspend the retroplaced uterus to the abdominal wall. Howard Kelly was one of the first to attempt the operation, although the interest in the operation is now only historical.

In 1914, there was a symposium on the subject in Philadelphia. At that time Baldy said, "In my opinion nine-tenths of the operations performed on women for retrodisplacement are uncalled for.... I am sorry to say it but it looks to me as though the possible number of retrodisplacement operations performed in this country is limited only by the number of females in existence."

Despite these freely expressed criticisms, Aldridge in 1940 stated, "Retroversion of the uterus will probably always be one of the more common gynecological conditions requiring treatment and surgical intervention for the cure of symptoms in some cases."

Within the past three or four decades there has been a gradual reduction in the number of operations done. In our clinic it is a rarity to open an abdomen primarily for a uterine suspension. What factors have brought this about? In the first place, on the face of it, it seems unlikely that a condition that occurs in 20% to 30% of the population would require correction. Another factor that contributed to the rejection of the suspension operations was the failure of many operative procedures to hold the uterus in position. But more important still was the failure of relief of symptoms even when the uterus was held in perfect position. There were also a few serious postoperative complications. A better understanding of the orthopedic causes of low back pain has also kept many women from unnecessary surgery.

Fluhmann concluded his review with an expression of his own views on the subject of uterine suspension: "It is not necessary for adequate gynecologic practice. At most it occasionally may play a secondary role to other procedures such as peritonization of the pelvis, of endometriosis, correction of certain vascular disorders and plastic reconstruction of the fallopian tubes."

With this historical background, we shall attempt to express our personal views in the present chapter.

Anatomic Considerations

An explanation of the anatomic support structures of the uterus and the mechanism by which it is maintained in its normal position of anteflexion and anteversion is important for a proper discussion and understanding of uterine displacements and appropriate surgical correction. The support system includes not only the structures attached to the uterus, but support structures of the vagina and the pelvic floor and how well they resist the pressure of intra-abdominal contents.

Typically, the portio vaginalis of the cervix points posteroinferiorly, and the uterine corpus is flexed with a wide obtuse angle on the cervix, so that when the woman is standing erect, the corpus lies anteriorly and almost horizontally, resting in an anteverted position behind and on top of the bladder. Minor variations in the directions of the axis of both the cervix and the corpus should be considered within normal limits. Physiologic displacements also occur during pregnancy. In the third trimester the uterus becomes a practically vertical organ.

The fibroelastic tissue within the lower portion of the broad ligament, extending from each side of the cervix and upper vagina to the sides of the pelvis, forms the ligamenta transversalis colli (Mackenrodt's ligament), also called the cardinal ligament. Attached to the endopelvic fascia of the pelvic diaphragm, the two cardinal ligaments hold the cervix and upper vagina at that level. The lateral vaginal fornices below the cervix are also fixed to the arcus tendinei of the levator ani muscles by the fibers of Luschka.

Beneath the peritoneal folds, on either side of the cul-de-sac of Douglas, are the two fascial structures known as the uterosacral ligaments. These usually well-developed ligaments are attached to the posterolateral surface of the cervix and proceed backward on either side of the rectum, where they are inserted into the periosteum of the sacrum, thus holding back the cervix. In the normal position, with the cervix held back, the somewhat rigid corpus lies forward, so that the intra-abdominal pressure falls on the posterior surface of the corpus, maintaining and accentuating it in anteverted position. If the uterosacral ligaments are congenitally inadequate or have become so through childbirth or aging, the cervix moves forward. Under such conditions, the uterine corpus, swinging on a more or less fixed transverse axis at about the level of the internal cervical os, falls backward, and the intra-abdominal pressure falls on the anterior surface of the corpus, thus aggravating and maintaining the uterine retrodisplacement. Once retroflexion and retroversion of the uterus have begun, they can be completed easily by intra-abdominal pressure on the anterior uterine surface (Fig. 31-1). Most cases of retrodisplacement include both retroversion and retroflexion, although either may exist independently.

The round ligaments provide little or no support against uterine descent, but they do provide some support in holding the uterus in anteposition. Surgical procedures to correct uterine retroversion usually take advantage of the round ligaments. Although the round ligaments do not hold the uterus forward tautly, they assist in maintaining the forward position of the corpus while the traction of the uterosacral ligaments holds the cervix back.

The ligamentous support system of the uterus is subject to stretching from childbearing, physical work,

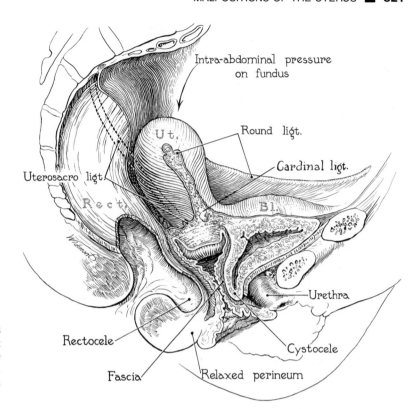

Figure 31–1. Failure of normal supports and widening of the levator hiatus permit descent of the uterus, as well as cystocele and rectocele formation. Intra-abdominal pressure directed to the anterior fundus holds to the uterus in a retroverted position.

aging, increased intra-abdominal pressure, and lack of estrogen support. The softening effect of the pregnancy hormones, the weight of the uterus in pregnancy, the stretching and tearing of the support structures during delivery, and the increased intra-abdominal pressure of straining, coughing chronically, chronic constipation, and hard work all tend to stretch the cardinal and uterosacral ligaments, permitting the cervix to become more mobile and the uterus to drop permanently to a lower level. Descent of the uterus causes the corpus to fall back from its normal anteverted position. When the ligaments that normally hold the cervix in place fail to do so, retrodisplacement often occurs.

Symptomatology in Relation to Treatment

It is generally estimated that one out of five women has a retrodisplaced uterus, either congenital or acquired. Although retroversion occurs frequently, it generally is asymptomatic. If symptoms do occur, they are usually slight or are due to associated coincidental pathology and do not justify operative intervention. Retrodisplacement of the uterus is commonly found in women who are completely free of symptoms. These women do not require surgery simply to suspend the uterus in an anterior position.

An uncomplicated, retroverted uterus is less apt to cause symptoms than one complicated by other intrapelvic disease. Among the conditions commonly associated with retrodisplacement are chronic salpingitis with pelvic adhesions, endometriosis, ovarian tumors, uterine leiomyomas, pelvic congestion syndrome, and Allen-Masters syndrome. Some of these conditions are responsible for symptoms that, in themselves, may necessitate surgery. But even in the presence of significant pelvic disease, a retrodisplaced uterus is usually asymptomatic. For example, during surgery for some other condition, one may encounter an entirely asymptomatic adherent retroverted uterus with residue of chronic salpingitis.

A word of caution about the pelvic examination findings may be appropriate. In some patients it may be difficult to be certain that the mass in the cul-de-sac is the uterine corpus. Sometimes a retroflexed uterus may be confused with even more significant pathology in the cul-de-sac, such as an ovarian tumor or a posterior leiomyoma. Determining the direction of the uterine cavity by gentle sounding through the cervix may be helpful. Vaginal ultrasonography may also be helpful.

Pelvic Discomfort. Backache and a bearing-down type of lower abdominal discomfort are frequent complaints of the erect female human biped. These symptoms, which also may be associated with uterine retrodisplacement, are noticed by women in whom the pelvic diaphragm is weakened and enlarged through repeated childbearing. Although these symptoms, which may be more severe premenstrually, tend to be aggravated by a retroverted uterus, they can occur with the uterus in a normal anteverted position. When there is no anatomic alteration in the reproductive tract to account for these symptoms, orthopedic consultation is advisable. Frequently, the etiology of low back pain will be found to be positional, occupational, or related to displacements of vertebrae with associated muscle spasm. Surgery for uterine retroversion and vaginal wall relaxation provides little relief of the symptoms in such cases.

Disturbances of Menstruation. Few menstrual symptoms can be accurately attributed to the position of the uterus. Historically, all kinds of menstrual dysfunction were commonly attributed to a retropositioned uterus. Passive venous congestion was a common explanation for increased menstrual bleeding from the uterus lying in the cul-de-sac. More current understanding of the endocrine control and cellular physiology of menstruation dispels any misconceptions about the effect of position of the uterus on menstrual flow. Menorrhagia in a patient with uterine retroversion is not an appropriate indication for uterine suspension.

Dysmenorrhea. Primary dysmenorrhea is not related to uterine position. It occurs in the anteverted as well as in the retroverted uterus. Replacement of the uterus may play some physiologic role in the symptoms of secondary dysmenorrhea, judging from the relief obtained, historically, by replacement or suspension of a retroverted uterus. It is argued that *acute retroflexion* of the uterus, which might interfere with venous drainage from the myometrium and broad ligaments, is more apt to be a factor in dysmenorrhea than *retroversion* alone without retroflexion. With retroflexion there might also be an element of relative stenosis at the internal cervical os that increases dysmenorrhea. The menstrual discomfort may take the form of cramps or sacral backache. Since it is frequently difficult to evaluate the relation of uterine retroversion to menstrual pain, a therapeutic test with a vaginal pessary is helpful.

Infertility. The finding of a uterus in retroposition in a woman complaining of infertility is not an indication that the position of the uterus has a direct relation to the problem. In such cases, a thorough investigation of all factors related to infertility must be made in both the man and the woman, without regard for the retroposition. Although infertility may be more common among women with retrodisplacement of the uterus, the relationship is difficult to prove except in cases with such other associated pathology as pelvic endometriosis or chronic salpingitis. With a retrodisplaced uterus, the cervix is positioned away from the posterior vaginal pool where semen is deposited. Some investigators consider this anatomic factor to be a serious impediment to fertility, but there is only limited scientific evidence to support this contention. Uterine suspension for the relief of infertility alone is seldom, if ever, justified. Artificial insemination can always be done if it is thought that the cervix is not positioned properly in relation to the posterior vaginal pool of semen.

Abortion. It is doubtful that uterine retroposition is ever the cause of abortion, unless incarceration of the uterus and compromise of the blood supply have occurred. Although chromosomal abnormality occurs in more than 50% of first-trimester pregnancy losses, many early abortions have an unexplained etiology. They appear to occur no more frequently in women with retropositioned uteri than in other women. When uterine incarceration occurs during early pregnancy, with the uterus wedged in the pelvis, the patient should be placed in the knee–chest position and an attempt should be made by digital pressure on the uterus through the rectum to displace the uterus from the cul-de-sac and put it in an anterior position. The uterus can usually be held out of the cul-de-sac by a pessary until the first trimester of pregnancy is past, at which stage the corpus will emerge from the pelvis and rest on the brim of the pelvis. In the rare case in which the uterus remains incarcerated in the pelvis as pregnancy advances, careful and frequent observation of the patient is essential to prevent fixation and sacculation of the pregnant uterus. Rarely, a pelvic examination under anesthesia or laparotomy may be required to release the incarcerated uterus from the cul-de-sac and avoid the complications of abortion, premature delivery, fetal death in utero, fetal malformation, or uterine rupture. Uterine suspension should not be performed on the pregnant uterus.

Pelvic Congestion Syndrome. Uterine retroversion has often been associated with the pelvic congestion syndrome, although in Taylor's original description of the syndrome in 1949 only 35% of patients were found to have uterine retroversion. According to Taylor, patients with this syndrome were typically multiparous and in the reproductive years. Symptoms included diffuse suprapubic pain, dysmenorrhea, menorrhagia, premenstrual lower back pain, and dyspareunia. In addition to retroversion, the uterus was often found to be enlarged, soft, and congested. Painful "cystic" ovaries were found frequently.

Taylor believed that vascular congestion of the pelvic organs could be responsible for these complaints because of the lability of the pelvic circulation. He explained that pelvic veins can easily become dilated because they lack valves, because the surrounding adventitial tissue in the broad ligaments is weak, because they are affected by gravity and the increased intra-abdominal pressure of straining due to their location on the pelvic floor, and because they are required to dilate during pregnancy to accommodate an enormous increase in circulation to the uterus. He also believed that the veins could be damaged by infection (phlebitis), and he postulated a role for estrogen and the autonomic nervous system control of circulation to the reproductive organs.

Taylor did not recommend hysterectomy or uterine suspension for these patients. He recognized the frequency with which his patients also had psychosomatic and psychiatric complaints. He relied on psychiatric consultation and nonsurgical symptomatic treatment. It is not known how many patients with vascular congestion of pelvic organs are asymptomatic. We have great difficulty making a correct diagnosis and agree with Taylor that uterine suspension or hysterectomy is rarely indicated for pelvic congestion. The pelvic congestion syndrome has also been studied by Hobbs and by Beard and associates.

Allen-Masters Syndrome. The Allen-Masters syndrome was first described in 1955 in 28 patients, all of whom had uterine retroversion. In addition, the other hallmarks of this syndrome included broad ligament lacerations (apparently the result of traumatic delivery), a hypermobility of the cervix in all directions in the pelvis (the "universal joint"), and enlargement and engorgement of the uterus. Symptoms included chronic throbbing pelvic pain, dyspareunia, dysmenorrhea, menometrorrhagia, chronic backache, a heavy feeling that "everything is falling out," and chronic fatigue.

Allen and Masters treated their patients with an operation that included a repair of the broad ligament defects ("windows") and uterine suspension, with good relief of symptoms. Lawry treated 19 patients with the Allen-Masters syndrome with hysterectomy. Many others doubt the existence of the syndrome. In our clinic, no patient has been operated upon for a preoperative diagnosis of the Allen-Masters syndrome. On the other hand, we have seen asymptomatic patients with defects ("windows") in the broad ligament at the time of laparoscopy for tubal sterilization. We believe the Allen-Masters syndrome requires careful restudy to determine its true validity.

Indications for Uterine Suspension

Fluhmann stated that primary suspension of the retroverted uterus is not necessary for adequate gynecologic practice. Uterine suspension is most often indicated in connection with such conservative operations as those done for endometriosis or tubal pregnancy, or in microsurgical tubal reconstruction procedures for relief of infertility. To leave the uterus of an infertile patient in the cul-de-sac, where tubal adhesions may recur, while performing other conservationistic procedures would be to do incomplete surgery that may not completely relieve the primary problem.

Certainly, the mere presence of uterine retrodisplacement alone in an asymptomatic patient is not an indication for prophylactic uterine suspension. However, there are a few young women in whom the symptoms of uterine retroversion are clear-cut and severe. In such a patient, a test with a Smith-Hodge pessary should be tried. The uterus is first brought to an anterior position by manual manipulation. A pessary of proper size is then inserted to hold it in position, allowing the pressure of intra-abdominal organs to become reoriented to the posterior surface of the uterine corpus. After several months, if the symptoms are relieved and the uterus stays in an anterior position after the pessary is removed, no further action is required. If the uterus returns to a retroverted position and the symptoms return, one may have a reason to do a primary uterine suspension. In practice, there are very few occasions when this is necessary. Primary uterine suspension has almost completely disappeared from the operative schedule in most hospitals.

Uterine retroversion may be present in a patient with severely symptomatic anatomic vaginal wall relaxation and uterine descensus. In almost all such cases, when childbearing is complete and symptoms are severe, vaginal hysterectomy and repair are appropriate. However, for women with prolapse who want more children, there is still a place, infrequent though it may be, for intra-abdominal uterine suspension. It must be recognized that this will be a temporary solution to the problem. The prolapse is likely to recur after the next delivery and will eventually require a more definitive operation for final solution.

Choice of Operation

Choice of operative techniques depends to a great extent on the desirability of future pregnancies. The modified Gilliam suspension is a very good technique for suspending the uterus and preserving childbearing potential. When no future pregnancies are desired, other procedures may be more appropriate.

The modified Gilliam suspension procedure draws each round ligament through an aperture in the peritoneum near the internal inguinal ring and brings each ligament beneath the anterior rectus sheath. There the round ligament is sutured under tension so as to hold the uterus forward. Although some patients experience transient round ligament pain with vigorous physical activity or uterine enlargement, there is no evidence that the suspension is detrimental to a subsequent pregnancy.

Many surgeons have reported satisfactory results with other types of suspensions. Some techniques have been abandoned; newer procedures give better anatomic positioning with fewer complications. In Olshausen's operation, for example, the uterus is fixed to the anterior abdominal wall. This procedure precludes the possibility of a future intrauterine pregnancy because the anchored uterus will produce severe abdominal pain as the uterus enlarges with advancing pregnancy. It also broadens the exposure of the cul-de-sac to the small intestines, which creates a serious risk of enterocele formation. The operation should never be done. In the Baldy-Webster procedure, the round ligaments are passed through the anterior and posterior leaves of the broad ligament and are sutured to the posterior surface of the uterus, leaving the support of the uterus to the hammock effect of the suspending ligaments. If the round ligaments are sutured too low on the posterior surface of the uterus, the cervix will be brought forward, thus aggravating the retroversion. If the round ligaments are sutured too high on the posterior surface of the uterus, the function of the fallopian tubes may be interfered with. The extraperitoneal technique of shortening each round ligament in the inguinal canal described by Alexander and by Adams is no longer used in this country, although it is still in use in some European clinics. The operation is blind, since the uterus is not visualized unless a laparotomy is performed. The extraperitoneal approach is its only advantage. Simply shortening the round ligaments by reefing will not hold the uterus adequately in anteposition.

One of the more effective supplemental procedures for providing additional support is shortening the uterosacral ligaments. This is especially valuable when some descensus is present or when the cervix has been displaced anteriorly. Shortening the uterosacral ligaments by plication helps maintain the forward position of the uterine corpus when combined with another procedure, such as the modified Gilliam procedure. Caution should be taken to avoid excessive plication of the uterosacral ligaments, since this can result in dyspareunia and in angulation of the pelvic ureter. One or two permanent sutures that unite the uterosacral ligaments in the midline are sufficient when used in combination with another suspension procedure.

Forty to 50 years ago, vaginal repair and abdominal uterine suspension were usually recommended for a patient with symptomatic pelvic relaxation and uterine retroversion. Today, if future pregnancy is definitely not desired and a vaginal plastic operation is needed, the best operation may be vaginal hysterectomy and vaginal repair. Under these conditions, especially if dysmenorrhea and/or menorrhagia is a chronic problem

that is unresponsive to conservative therapy, there is little reason for saving the uterus. Removal of the uterus will relieve the symptoms of retroposition and insure against future trouble due to dysfunctional bleeding or uterine neoplasm. It is important that the anatomic vaginal relaxations and associated symptoms be sufficient in order to justify an operation for relief.

Technique of Modified Gilliam Suspension of the Uterus

The procedure of primary uterine suspension begins with a Pfannenstiel or Kustner incision, although a small midline incision could be used. The uterus is held forward. The middle of the round ligament is grasped with a Babcock clamp and a traction suture is placed around it. The suture should be placed to provide good uterine positioning when the ligaments are attached to the underside of the rectus sheath. The average distance is about 3–4 cm from the uterus, although exact positioning can only be determined by testing the uterine position with traction on the round ligament (Fig. 31-2A).

An Ochsner clamp is placed on the edge of the anterior rectus fascia. A Kelly clamp is placed on the peritoneal edge at the same level. Then, using blunt and sharp dissection, the rectus muscle is separated from its fascial sheath (Fig. 31-2B). At the point of separation, a long Kelly clamp is inserted along the lateral margin of the rectus muscle and beneath the peritoneum as it passes along the lateral pelvic wall to the level of the internal inguinal ring. Here the peritoneum is elevated with the tip of the clamp and the jaws of the clamp are separated slightly, so that an assistant can incise the peritoneum (Fig. 31-2C).

With the point of the Kelly clamp, the peritoneal cavity is entered and the traction suture is grasped and drawn back out of the peritoneal cavity. By bringing the round ligament through the opening in the parietal peritoneum at the point of the internal inguinal ring, a loop is brought between the rectus muscle and its anterior sheath (Fig. 31-2D). The loop of round ligament is sutured to the undersurface of the fascia, using interrupted No. 2-0 permanent suture. Suture with substantial bites into the full thickness of the ligament on both sides and at the end of the loop, taking care not to encircle and strangulate the ligament (Fig. 31-2E). The procedure is repeated on the opposite round ligament. When completed, the inside of the abdomen is inspected to be certain that no loop of bowel has been or can be caught between the ligament and the abdominal wall. Also, one should be sure that the fallopian tube was not drawn into the internal inguinal ring by excessive traction on the round ligament (Fig. 31-2F).

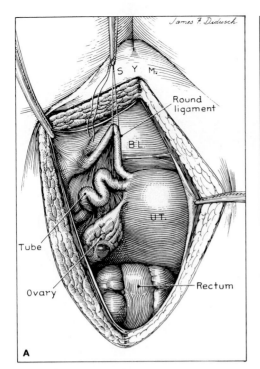

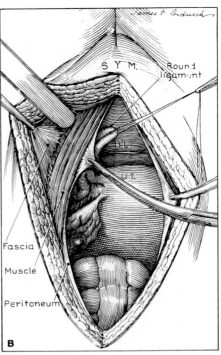

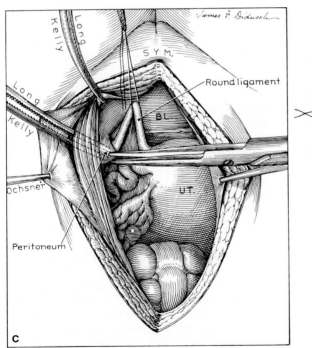

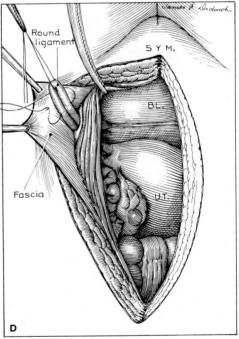

Figure 31–2. Modified Gilliam suspension of uterus. *A*, A traction suture of No. 0 delayed-absorbable material is placed about the round ligament at an appropriate point. *B*, The anterior rectus sheath is dissected from the body of the muscle. *C*, A long Kelly clamp is passed around the rectus muscle, through the internal inguinal ring. The peritoneum is cut over the tip of the clamp so that it may enter the peritoneal cavity. *D*, The traction suture is grasped by the Kelly clamp and withdrawn through the internal ring. The round ligament is sutured to the inside of the rectus sheath with medium silk sutures. *(Figure continued on next page.)*

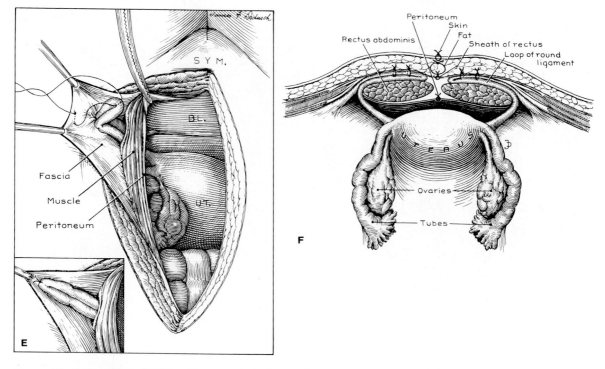

Figure 31–2. (continued) *E,* Another suture is anchoring the round ligament to the fascia. The inset shows the round ligament sutured to the fascia. All sutures transfix the round ligament. *F,* Transverse section showing final result.

Technique of Shortening the Uterosacral Ligaments

Shortening or plication of the uterosacral ligaments is easily accomplished if exposure is adequate. An assistant can hold the uterus forward by hand or with a retractor. The intestines are held back from the pelvis with a laparotomy pack.

Each uterosacral ligament is grasped with an Allis or Babcock clamp at a point just below its attachment to the uterus and the two ligaments are brought together. Using No. 2-0 permanent suture on a round needle, the ligaments are sutured together, including a bite in the posterior surface of the cervix at the midline. Usually two or three sutures plicate the ligaments together adequately (Fig. 31-3 *A–B*).

The surgeon must avoid kinking or ligating the ureter, which lies in close proximity to the lateral aspect of the uterosacral ligament. Although shortening of the ligaments is necessary to hold the cervix back and to position the fundus forward, excessive tucking or folding may result in displacement or injuries to the ureter(s).

Following abdominal hysterectomy, plication of the uterosacral ligaments may be done to support the vaginal vault and to protect against enterocele formation. The technique of using the McCall posterior culdeplasty to support the vaginal vault with abdominal hysterectomy is described in Chapter 27 (see Fig. 27-23). It may also be appropriate to close the cul-de-sac with a Moschcowitz culdeplasty at the same time (see Fig. 33-10).

PROLAPSE OF THE UTERUS

Uterine prolapse and its allied conditions and their treatment constitute a major subject in gynecology. Especially in its advanced state, uterine prolapse is a cause of serious disability and a difficult challenge to the skill of any gynecologic surgeon who attempts to correct it. It has been a controversial subject among gynecologists for the past century, especially regarding the best operation to perform and the important anatomic defects and surgical principles to emphasize. No condition has stimulated the inventive genius of gynecologic surgeons more than the management of uterine prolapse. No condition has been used to judge the skill of the gyne-

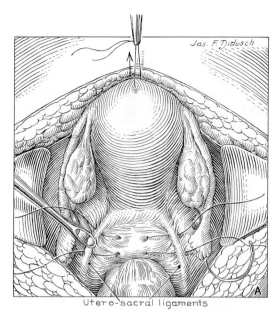

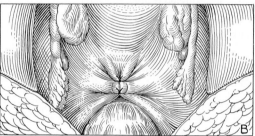

Figure 31–3. Shortening of uterosacral ligaments. *A,* Interrupted permanent sutures are passed through the uterosacral ligaments and the posterior surface of the cervix. *B,* Sutures have been tied, thus shortening the ligaments.

cologic surgeon more than the ability to provide permanent relief of this classic malady, with maintenance or restoration of normal function, it is hoped.

Important highlights in the history of treatment of uterine prolapse were described by Phaneuf, by Te Linde, by Ricci, and by others. Mentioned in the writings of Hippocrates and Galen, the condition received little attention for many centuries. Unfortunately, this is still true today in some developing countries in the world. Long before the advent of modern surgery, various supports and pessaries and other ways of maintaining the uterus in its normal position were devised. Vaginal packings, tampons, massages, and exercises were used with some degree of success. Some patients were suspended from their feet for 24 hours in an attempt to achieve cure. Rodericus A. Castro advised that prolapse should be attacked with a red hot iron as if to burn it, "when fright would cause it to recede into the vagina."

Various caustics were applied to the vagina: silver nitrate, by Meding; nitric acid, by Phillips; acid nitrate of mercury, by Lougier; red hot iron, by Velpeau, Kennedy, Dieffenbach, and Degranges; and sulfuric acid, by Selnow, Richter, Hedrich, and Rokitanski.

The fitting of pessaries became an art form and undoubtedly brought relief to many women. They were especially popular in the mid-19th century. Some were held in place by a waistband or T-bandage. In some cases, pessaries were deliberately left in until vaginal erosions developed. Their subsequent healing would be expected to decrease the caliber and increase the support of the vagina. Unfortunately, they occasionally were neglected, eroded too deep, became embedded, and were even recovered from the peritoneal cavity.

The earliest surgical attempts to relieve prolapse were relatively simple ones and included suturing the labia together or removing pieces of vaginal mucosa and suturing the edges together to reduce vaginal caliber. Heming operated on the anterior vaginal wall in 1831, but surgery for uterovaginal prolapse was not commonly done until the advent of anesthesia and antisepsis in the mid-19th century. Rizzoli published his description of an elongated and hypertrophied prolapsed cervix in 1850. In 1859, Huquer was the first to amputate the cervix, emphasizing that hypertrophy and elongation of the cervix were important factors in prolapse. The first vaginal hysterectomy for prolapse was performed by Samuel Choppin of New Orleans in 1861, although vaginal hysterectomy was not commonly performed for prolapse until much later. Martin, in Germany, described the first vaginal hysterectomy with a complete colpectomy in 1898. In America, Edebohls performed the first "panhysterocolpectomy" for procidentia in 1901.

Colporrhaphy operations were more commonly performed by Sims, Emmet, Aveling, Thomas, Simon, Hegar, and Martin. Cervical amputation was soon added. The first of the operations known today as the Manchester operation were done by Donald in 1888 and later modified by Fothergill. In addition to colporrhaphy, amputation of the prolapsed cervix allowed plication of ligaments across the uterine isthmus for better support.

In 1877, LeFort described his partial colpocleisis for prolapse. Techniques of ventral fixation of the uterine fundus to the abdominal wall were described by Harris, by Murphy, and by Kocher, and these procedures were commonly done at the end of the 19th century and into the 20th century by Pozzi, Terrier, Leopold, Kelly, and others. During this same period, another commonly performed operation was a combined vaginal and abdominal procedure consisting of dilatation and curettage, trachelorrhaphy, anterior and posterior colporrhaphy and perineorrhaphy, done vaginally; and plication of uterosacral ligaments and uterine suspension, done abdominally.

Watkins performed his first interposition operation in 1898. Wertheim described a similar operation in 1899. Designed for postmenopausal patients with a moderate prolapse and large cystocele, using the uterine corpus as an obturator for the defective pelvic diaphragm, it offered a rapid method of supporting the bladder while maintaining coital function. Although it was popular during the first three decades of the 20th century, it had serious disadvantages.

In the United States, vaginal hysterectomy plus colporrhaphy became the most popular operation for uterovaginal prolapse because of the work of Goffe, C. H. Mayo, Heaney, Kennedy, Allen, Aldridge, Edwards, Gray, Pratt, Ward, Te Linde, Symmonds, Nichols, and many others. When vaginal hysterectomy and colporrhaphy were used for advanced degrees of uterovaginal prolapse, enterocele and vaginal vault prolapse sometimes developed postoperatively. Efforts to prevent this complication by providing better support to the vault with vaginal hysterectomy were made by many, including E. H. Richardson, with the Spalding-Richardson composite operation; McCall, with the posterior culdeplasty; Thornton, with the use of pararectal fascia; and Richter and Nichols, with the sacrospinous colpopexy. Abdominal sacral colpopexy, described by Parsons and Ulfelder and by Birnbaum and Lane, has also been combined with abdominal hysterectomy and vaginal colporrhaphy with good results.

Thus, the modern surgical management of uterovaginal prolapse has evolved through interesting phases with improved results that will, it is hoped, continue to improve in the future. Today, thankfully, there continues to be discussion regarding the best operation to perform. Some operations, especially ventral fixation of the uterus, have completely lost favor, because they were found to be ineffective. In many clinics, vaginal hysterectomy with colporrhaphy is considered to be the answer to all degrees and types of prolapse and is done by a variety of techniques, each of which has its staunch advocates. In some clinics in Great Britain and continental Europe, the Manchester operation, as described by Shaw, with modifications, is thought to be preferable to vaginal hysterectomy. The Watkins-Wertheim interposition operation is no longer used in North America. The Spalding-Richardson composite operation, beautiful in concept, has lost favor because of technical difficulty in performance and other problems. The LeFort partial colpocleisis continues to be acceptable for a few patients who do not need coital function and cannot tolerate a more extensive procedure. In recent years, support of the vaginal vault by vaginal sacrospinous ligament fixation or by abdominal sacral colpopexy has gained favor. With proper assessment of each patient and the defects in her support, the gynecologic surgeon can fortunately choose from a variety of operative techniques described in this chapter and in other chapters. All problems of uterovaginal prolapse cannot be properly corrected by a single operative technique. Fitting the operation to the individual needs of the patient will provide the best results.

Anatomic Considerations

The normal position and support of the uterus, vagina, bladder, and rectum are maintained by several anatomic structures and systems that are interrelated and provide varying contributions to the support mechanisms of the uterus and other pelvic organs. The anatomic support structures responsible for maintaining the uterine corpus in its normal position of anteflexion and anteversion have been previously discussed. When these support structures hold the uterine corpus forward, intra-abdominal pressure is less likely to push the uterus through the genital hiatus. In a position of uterine retroversion, the cervix points more in the axis of the vagina, and descent through the genital hiatus can occur more easily.

The muscular, ligamentous, and fascial support structures of the pelvic organs attach to the pelvic bones. These include the sacrum posteriorly, the pubic rami and symphysis pubis anteriorly, and the ischial bones on each side of the pelvis. Pelvic bone structure and architecture can influence genital organ support. If the anterior compartment of the pelvic outlet is narrowed by a tight subpubic arch, the presenting part of a term fetus is likely to cause more stretching and tearing and damage to the posterior vaginal and rectal support mechanisms when vaginal delivery occurs, while the support of the anterior vaginal wall, the bladder floor, and the proximal urethra will be protected. On the other hand, if the sacrum and coccyx are angulated forward and the posterior compartment of the outlet is inadequate, the presenting part of the fetus will be pushed forward beneath the subpubic arch, causing more damage to the anterior vaginal wall, bladder floor, and proximal urethra. Traumatic injury and fractures of the pelvic bones can also affect genital organ support. In patients with exstrophy of the bladder, the pubic symphysis and rami are absent, causing serious deficiencies in the anterior support mechanisms of the uterus and anterior vaginal wall. A careful evaluation of the pelvic bone structure and architecture can be helpful in assessment of specific deficiencies in various genital organ support mechanisms in patients with uterine prolapse and vaginal relaxation.

The muscular floor of the pelvis (the pelvic diaphragm), which is discussed in detail in Chapter 4, is attached to the pelvic bone structure and forms the major support upon which the uterus and upper and lower vagina rests (Fig. 31-4). The middle and lower vagina is densely adherent to the puborectalis and pubococcygeus muscles, commonly called the levator crura. The anterior fibers of the pubococcygeus muscles are attached to the vagina on each side, to the perineal body, and to the anal canal. Posterior fibers of the pubococcygeus muscles are attached to the median raphe between the anus and the coccyx, the so-called levator plate formed by the midline junction of these muscles and the iliococcygeus muscles. The fibers of the puborectalis muscles are deeper and form a sling behind the rectum, holding it in a forward position toward the symphysis pubis. The most posterior component of the pelvic musculature is composed of the iliococcygeus and the coccygeus muscles. Additional support is provided by the muscles of the urogenital diaphragm and the superficial and deep perineal muscles.

The muscle components of the pelvic floor should not be thought of as a single morphologic and functional unit (often referred to as the levator muscle or levator sling), as pointed out by Critchey and associates. The component parts of the levator ani have different functions, indicated simply by their different anatomic locations. Together, they do provide resistance to the continuous downward force of intra-abdominal pressure and, acting together with muscles of the abdominal wall, deflect the direction of that pressure away from the genital hiatus through which pelvic organs otherwise might descend.

Tearing and separation of these muscles at the time of vaginal delivery will weaken the pelvic floor and widen

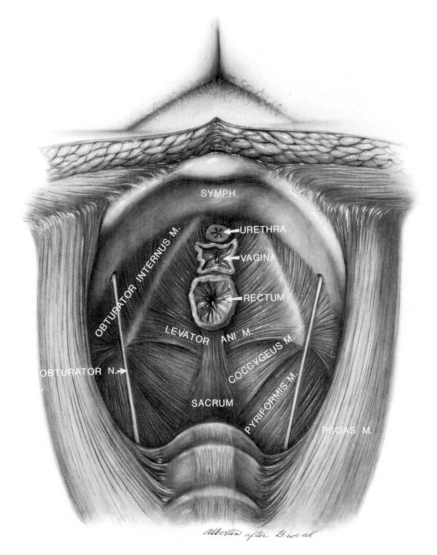

Figure 31–4. Muscular structures forming the pelvic floor in the female.

the genital hiatus. The medial fibers of the pubococcygeus and puborectalis muscles are especially likely to be torn and stretched. Contraction of these muscles, along with the bulbocavernosus muscles, constricts the vaginal lumen and elevates the anterior vaginal wall. These muscles are voluntarily contracted with the so-called perineal muscle or Kegel's exercises. These exercises should be advised following vaginal delivery so that the tone of these important muscles may be regained as much as possible. The muscle tone may also be improved by the use of vaginal cones of increasing weight, as advised by Plevnik, by Stanton, and by Olah and associates.

In addition to weakness of the muscles of the pelvic floor resulting from stretching and tearing during parturition, aging, and other factors, recent evidence suggests that nerve damage or degeneration may result in pelvic floor muscle weakness. With histochemical studies of pelvic floor muscle biopsies and pelvic floor single-fiber electromyography, Gilpin and associates and Smith and associates have demonstrated evidence of muscle fiber damage in the pelvic floor muscles of women with genital prolapse and stress incontinence of urine. Smith and associates demonstrated clear evidence of denervation damage to pelvic floor muscles in women with genital prolapse by measuring the conduction time to the pubococcygeus muscle, external urethral sphincter, and external anal sphincter after electrical stimulation of the terminal branches of the pudendal nerves.

The median raphe between the anus and coccyx is called the levator plate. It is formed by the midline fusion of the iliococcygeal muscle fibers and the posterior fibers of the pubococcygeus muscles from each side. In the standing position, the levator plate is horizontal and supports the vagina and rectum above it. Weakness of the pubococcygeus and iliococcygeal muscles may cause the levator plate to sag and descend permanently, allowing the genital hiatus to open as it does to an even greater extent with straining. This increased opening of the genital hiatus changes the normal horizontal axis of the vagina to a more nearly vertical axis. These changes are more conducive to uterovaginal prolapse (Fig. 31-5).

The superior lateral borders of the levator ani muscle components are attached to the pelvis along the arcus tendineus, which runs from the back of the pubic bones to the ischial spines on each side. The anterior sulcus of the vaginal walls is attached to the arcus tendineus. As pointed out by White, these attachments can be torn with vaginal delivery, and a cystocele can result. The paravaginal connective tissue of the lower vagina is attached laterally to the fascial sheath covering the pubococcygeus muscles by the fibers of Luschka. The upper vaginal walls are not attached to the pelvic diaphragm but normally rest over the rectum, which rests on the levator plate. The upper vagina depends on its attachment to the cervix for its support. The cervix and upper vagina are quite mobile except for limits prescribed by attachments to the uterosacral and cardinal ligaments. There is very little anatomic support for the upper posterior vaginal wall and many pelvic relaxation problems are related to this deficiency. The most common site for enterocele formation is through the upper posterior vaginal wall.

In 1953, using myography, Berglas and Rubin described the importance of the vaginal axis relative to the levator plate. In the normal erect patient, the rectum and the vagina lie horizontally upon this plate, pointing into the hollow of the sacrum. When intra-abdominal pressure increases, the vagina is pushed further back against the levator plate and away from the genital hiatus.

Radiographic colpography studies in living patients by Richter, by Nichols and associates, and by Funt and associates demonstrate the normal anatomy of the vagina better than cadaver dissection. The vagina is not a straight tube that points to the sacral promontory. The vagina is a curved organ with a lower convex perineal portion and a distinct upper portion that lies in an almost horizontal plane with the patient standing. According to Funt, the central line of the vagina measures 8.4 cm from the introitus to the most distal point in the posterior fornix, the deepest point in the vagina. The angle between the upper and lower vaginal axis measures 129.8°. The mean vector of the axis of the upper vagina points posteriorly just above the center of the fourth sacral vertebra. The most distal point of the posterior fornix extends approximately 3 cm beyond the ischial spines (Fig. 31-6). As described by Zacharin, the upper portion of the vagina is normally supported posteriorly in the presacral area by endopelvic fascia and the levator ani complex. These anatomic points are important to keep in mind when explaining the horizontal position of the upper vagina over the levator plate and in choosing an operative technique that will restore normal vaginal anatomy and axis in a patient with uterovaginal prolapse.

Over the years, there has been much debate between two main schools of thought regarding the predominant mechanism of support for the uterus. One school has emphasized that the uterus is maintained in position by support from below provided by the pelvic diaphragm and levator plate described earlier. An opposing school has maintained that primary support of the uterus is provided by the cardinal and uterosacral ligament attachments to the cervix and upper vagina. These "ligaments" consist of blood vessels, nerves, lymphatic channels, smooth muscle fibers, and connective tissue. The cardinal ligaments (also called the liga-

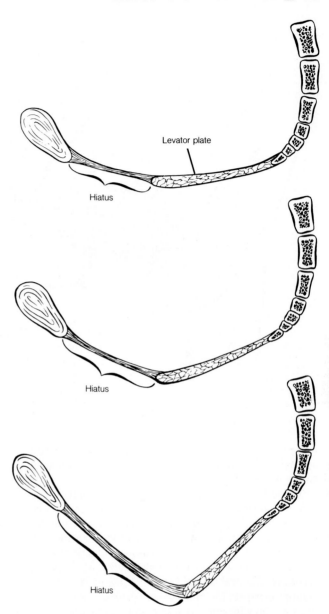

Levator plate

Hiatus

Hiatus

Hiatus

Figure 31–5. Sagittal view of pelvic floor, showing posterior rotation of the levator plate and consequent enlargement of the levator hiatus. This encourages descent of the uterus and vagina. (After Nichols DH, Randall CL. Vaginal surgery. 3rd ed. Baltimore: Williams & Wilkins, 1989.)

menta transversalis colli or Mackenrodt's ligament) are attached to the lateral margins of the cervix and upper vagina and to the endopelvic fascia of the pelvic diaphragm. They represent a condensation of the lowermost portion of the broad ligaments. Laterally, these cardinal ligaments are continuous with connective tissue that surrounds the hypogastric vessels and their branches as they course through the cardinal ligaments between the uterus and vagina and the lateral pelvic sidewall. Medially, the connective tissue of the cardinal ligaments is continuous with the connective tissue that surrounds the cervix and upper vagina, the so-called

pubovesicocervical fascia. The uterosacral ligaments, studied by Campbell, are attached to the cervix and the upper vaginal fornices posterolaterally. Posteriorly, they attach broadly to the presacral fascia in front of the sacroiliac joint. The connective tissue component of the uterosacral ligaments is continuous with that of the cardinal ligaments around the cervix. The cardinal and uterosacral ligaments hold the uterus and upper vagina in their proper place over the levator plate. They also provide a suspensory function as well and resistance to descent of these organs. Mengert proved the importance of the suspensory function when he showed in

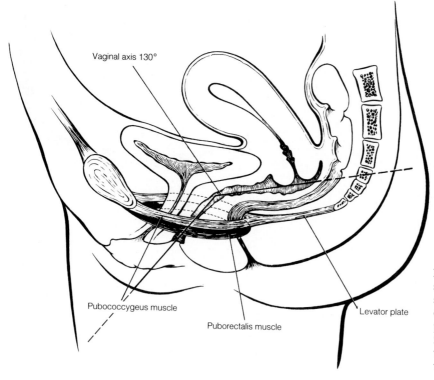

Figure 31–6. Normal axis of lower and upper vagina, which meet in a 130° angle. Upper one third of vagina rests on the levator plate in a horizontal plane that passes through the third or fourth sacral vertebra. The posterior vaginal fornix is the deepest part of the vagina.

cadavers that uterine and vaginal prolapse occurred only when the upper two thirds of the parametrial tissues were cut.

On the basis of their careful gross and microscopic studies, Range and Woodburne concluded that there was no "ligament" as such between the cervix and the lateral pelvic sidewall. According to these authors, "It would appear that the entire mass of retroperitoneal areolar connective tissue functions to support the pelvic viscera. While one isolated strand is incapable of preventing prolapse, the intact mass by means of its multitudinous attachments to the fascia lining the pelvis forms an effective and elastic support for the uterus." Ideas regarding the anatomy and function of the cardinal (transverse cervical) ligament have changed since the original description was published by Mackenrodt in 1895.

The cardinal ligaments and the various components of the pelvic fascia contribute major support to maintaining the normal nulliparous vagina in position. The cardinal ligaments are firmly attached to the upper segment of vagina and form a strong fascial sheath that inserts on the muscular pelvic wall.

Anteriorly, the pubovesicocervical fascia extends between the bladder and vagina and stretches from its origin at the symphysis pubis beneath the bladder to blend with fascia that surrounds the cervix. The most lateral part of this fascia is strengthened on each side of the proximal urethra to form the important pubourethral ligaments that support the bladder neck. The upper part of this fascia is easily seen when the bladder is dissected from the cervix and anterior vaginal fornix in a total abdominal hysterectomy.

Posteriorly, similar fascia, known as pararectal fascia, separates the vagina from the muscular wall of the rectum. The pararectal fascia supports the anterior rectal wall from bulging into the vagina. According to Milley and Nichols, the rectovaginal septum is a fusion of the walls of the fetal peritoneal pouch (an extension of the pouch of Douglas) to form the fascia of Denonvillier, which is attached caudally to the perineal body and fused posterolaterally to the endopelvic fascia. This rectovaginal septum is also fused with the fibromuscular posterior vaginal wall and gives support to it.

As the muscles of the levator crura are stretched and weakened by childbirth and aging and the genital hiatus is widened, these fascial structures and attachments become weaker and the vaginal walls lose support. As a result, rectocele, cystocele, and enterocele may develop. The pressure of intra-abdominal organs, straining, and the weight of the uterus (especially if it is retroverted) may overwhelm the fascial support of the sagging vagina and cause the vagina to become partially or entirely everted when uterine prolapse becomes complete.

The modern concept supports the view that the upper vagina and uterus are maintained in their normal position both by support from below and by suspension from above. In addition to the support mechanisms described earlier, various authors may emphasize the importance of the round ligaments, the broad ligaments, the perirectal fascia, a deep cul-de-sac of Douglas, or other mechanisms of support. Different types of genital prolapse may occur, depending on the site or sites of damage to the support mechanisms. As stated by Te Linde:

> The purpose in reviewing these points in anatomy is to emphasize that defects may occur in any or all of these supporting structures and that plastic reconstruction of the part affected is necessary to the success of the repair. This means that there is great variation in the defects and that each case should be examined carefully preoperatively to determine the exact site of the defect and its extent. Considering this, it becomes self-evident that there should be considerable variation in the surgical approach to the correction of various defects.

Etiology and Prevention

There are definite racial differences in the incidence of uterovaginal prolapse. These may be explained on the basis of inherited racial differences in pelvic architecture, the quality of supporting pelvic muscles and connective tissue, and the tendency in some races for thicker fibrous tissue to develop following injury. They also may be explained by environmental and social differences among races and cultures as well (reproductive function and care, participation in hard physical labor, pelvic infection, etc.). For example, it is a practice among the women of certain nomadic desert tribes to put salt in the vagina following delivery to cause contraction of the vaginal walls. Because of either racial or environmental factors or both, uterovaginal prolapse is said to occur more frequently among white women. It occurs less frequently among Asians and blacks.

Since there are many forms of uterovaginal prolapse, there must be multiple etiologies. It is unusual to see a patient with only a single etiologic factor. Multiple factors are usually involved in each patient, and each may be more or less evident. The most prominent of these is pregnancy, labor, and vaginal delivery, which may result in various degrees of damage to pelvic support structures, including the ligaments, fascia, and muscles and their nerve supply. More damage is caused when

the labor is prolonged, when the fetal head and/or shoulders are large, and when difficult forceps operations are required for delivery. There is tremendous individual variation in the strength and recovery of pelvic tissues, however, as indicated by the absence of prolapse in some women who have had many vaginal deliveries. The changing practices of modern obstetrics (higher rates of cesarean section for prolonged labor, fetal-pelvic disproportion, and abnormal presentation) and family planning (fewer high-parity patients) should in the future reduce further the ravages of parturition on the structures that support pelvic organs. However, previous pregnancy is not a required precondition for prolapse, since it can occur in nulliparous women when the cervix is congenitally elongated.

Any tendency to prolapse is more likely to manifest itself after the menopause, when ovarian steroidogenesis ceases and genital support tissues are no longer affected by estrogen. Such a tendency is increased by greater intra-abdominal pressure, which, in the erect female, is directed with greater force to the most dependent part of the abdominal cavity, the pelvic diaphragm. Such increases in the intra-abdominal pressure may result from chronic cough, obesity, pelvic tumors, ascites, hard physical exertion, heavy lifting, tight-fitting corsets, and straining. The constant presence of intra-abdominal pressure rises suddenly with coughing and straining. The thrust of abdominal viscera from above is directed downward against the lower anterior abdominal wall and then deflected downward and backward into the posterior cul-de-sac.

We consider chronic constipation, for whatever reason, a prime etiologic factor in uterine prolapse and allied defects of pelvic organ support. We are amazed that so many women with prolapse are found to have an unrecognized anal stenosis, producing chronic constipation and straining. Parks and associates have shown that chronic straining may be associated with an acquired neuropathy affecting the strength and function of the pelvic floor muscles. With rectocele, enterocele, and uterine retroversion, the patient may experience rectal tenesmus and chronic constipation and straining, thus further aggravating a tendency to uterine prolapse.

Most etiologies of uterine prolapse are acquired and are, therefore, subject to preventive measures. Whenever possible, patients and their physicians should direct their attention to avoiding or correcting chronic cough from chronic lung disease, nicotine abuse, or chronic bronchitis; neglected dystocia and traumatic vaginal delivery; excess weight gain; tight corsets; anal stenosis and chronic constipation; and hard physical exertion and lifting. Every effort should be made to restore the tone of pelvic floor muscles after each delivery or whenever they appear weak. Unless contraindicated, estrogen should be provided after the menopause. Obviously, any pelvic tumors should be removed. Some patients who present with fairly sudden and recent uterine prolapse will be found to have an ovarian malignancy with or without ascites. Apparently, the increased intra-abdominal pressure of the tumor and/or ascites can overcome previously satisfactory uterine support and cause prolapse in some patients.

Repeated acute exacerbations of chronic pelvic inflammatory disease and severe postabortal and puerperal sepsis can cause induration (sometimes ligneous) of paracervical and parametrial tissues. Dense intrapelvic adhesions may form. Such patients are at minimal risk of developing uterine prolapse in later years because of tissue fibrosis and low parity.

Clinical Evaluation

The correct management of patients with uterine prolapse and associated vaginal relaxations will depend on a careful evaluation of each patient, her age, desire for preservation of reproductive function, desire for preservation of coital function, general medical status, previous attempts at surgical correction, symptomatology, and physical examination. Decisions regarding management will depend as much or more on the evaluation of symptomatology as on the physical findings, but a correlation of symptoms with physical findings is not always easy. Some women who have grown accustomed to marked pelvic relaxation problems may feel very little inconvenience. Others may complain of symptoms characteristic of prolapse and be found on examination to have only minor degrees of uterine descensus and vaginal relaxation. Slowly progressing uterine prolapse is likely to cause fewer symptoms than rapidly progressing uterine prolapse. According to Nichols:

> The rate of progression may help to distinguish types of prolapse, which in reality differ both in etiology and in prognosis, i.e., slowly progressive uterovaginal prolapse is usually due to damage to the lateral supports of the cervix and upper vagina, whereas rapidly progressing prolapse is due in all probability to primary atrophic failure of all the supporting tissues, including the pelvic floor.

The most frequent symptom of uterine prolapse is an annoying protrusion at the vaginal introitus. There may also be a bearing-down sensation, a feeling that "everything is falling out." Discomfort and aching in the lower back are common. These symptoms may be aggravated by standing and may be relieved when lying down. Intercourse may be more difficult because "something

is in the way." The patient's sexual partner may also complain that the vagina is too large.

Of course, the complaint of an annoying protrusion from the vaginal introitus may also be caused by a rectocele, a cystocele, and sometimes an enterocele. It may be impossible to differentiate between these problems by taking a history, and pelvic examination will be necessary. Except for the protrusion, all three may be asymptomatic. In some cases of rectocele it is necessary to use a low enema to defecate or to evacuate stool completely from the rectum. With enterocele, a bearing-down sensation and backache are common. Rectal tenesmus and constipation may be present with both rectocele and enterocele, but are not necessary components of either. Rectocele is not a cause of constipation but may be aggravated by it.

With cystocele, in addition to an annoying protrusion, the patient may have voiding difficulties. Although the cystocele is very large and protruding, genuine stress urinary incontinence is unusual. The mechanism of urinary continence in women with severe uterovaginal prolapse was studied by Bump and associates. These investigators essentially confirmed the previous work of Richardson and associates that women with severe prolapse have an enhanced bladder-to-urethra pressure transmission ratio during dynamic urethral pressure profilometry when the prolapse is allowed to protrude. When the prolapse is reduced, the pressure transmission ratio falls significantly. These findings support the hypothesis that the urinary continence mechanism in women with severe degrees of uterovaginal prolapse results from transient obstruction of the urethra with sudden increases in intra-abdominal pressure.

Bump and associates also reported that many of their subjects had intermittent and low-flow-rate uroflowmetry, suggesting some degree of mechanical urethral obstruction. Many patients with a large protruding cystocele have learned to push it up into the pelvis to relieve the obstruction, initiate voiding, and empty the bladder completely. A persistently large residual urine volume in some patients who cannot empty completely can lead to chronic urinary tract infections.

After the history is taken in detail, a general physical examination is done. The gynecologic surgeon must make an assessment of the patient's general health before decisions can be made regarding management. Sometimes referral for medical consultation is prudent.

The patient is placed in lithotomy position for pelvic examination. The labia are spread and the protrusion is identified. The patient is asked to strain as though attempting defecation. She may also be asked to cough. The examiner is then able to determine what actually appears first at the introitus—the cervix, a cystocele, a rectocele, or an enterocele. What appears first at the introitus on straining may suggest the location of the most major defect in pelvic support mechanisms and have implications for the technique of surgical correction.

The bony structure of the pelvis, especially the outlet, should be examined. Assessment of the subpubic arch, the intertuberous diameter, and the angulation of the sacrum and coccyx is especially important in determining the most likely location of support deficiencies and the likely degree of difficulty with a vaginal procedure. The dimensions of the vaginal introitus should be estimated with the examining fingers. In virginal patients with congenital elongation of the cervix, the introitus may accept only one finger. In most patients, with relaxed vaginal outlet, it is usually possible to insert three or four fingers easily. The occasional patient will have a large, gapping vaginal introitus through which an entire hand up to the wrist can be inserted without discomfort to the patient.

Along with examination of the vaginal introitus, the examiner may wish to estimate the tone of the pubococcygeus muscles on each side of the lower vaginal walls. This can be done simply by asking the patient to contract these muscles around two fingers in the vagina as if she was attempting to stop the flow of urine during the act of voiding. Most patients with advanced degrees of uterovaginal prolapse demonstrate complete loss of function of these muscles.

The anterior and posterior vaginal walls are carefully examined and an estimation of the degree of their relaxation is made. In examining the posterior vaginal wall, a low rectocele can be easily identified with an examining finger in the rectum. The rectovaginal septum may be unusually thin. A high rectocele can also be identified, but it may be difficult to differentiate from an enterocele (Fig. 31-7). The index finger of the left hand is placed in the rectum with the tip directed forward. Two fingers of the right hand are placed in the vagina. The patient is asked to strain down. If an enterocele is present, it will bulge into the space between the rectum and upper posterior vaginal wall and can be felt between the examining fingers. Intravaginal ultrasonography can also identify loops of small intestine in an enterocele sac. Examination in the standing position may be done when unusual difficulty is encountered. We do not recommend this awkward examination as a routine but use it only occasionally and when thought necessary to demonstrate a suspected enterocele not demonstrable by usual examination methods. An enterocele that is not large enough to be found by examination in the lithotomy position is probably not clinically significant.

The degree of prolapse of the uterus should be determined with the patient in the lithotomy position, relaxed and straining. Only occasionally will it be neces-

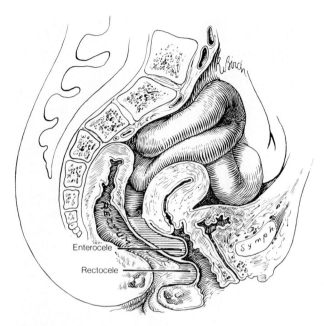

Enterocele

Rectocele

Figure 31–7. Sagittal section of pelvis, showing relative position of rectocele and enterocele.

sary to place a tenaculum on the cervix for traction to demonstrate the degree of prolapse. Even in asymptomatic patients, traction on the cervix of varying amounts can cause the cervix to descend even when support is normal. Bartscht and DeLancey studied 73 asymptomatic patients under anesthesia and found that the cervix would descend from 3.5 to 0.81 cm above the hymenal ring when traction of 4 lb was applied. In these patients, relaxation of muscular support with anesthesia may be partly responsible for the descent. Examination of the unanesthetized patient while straining in the lithotomy or standing position should give an accurate clinical assessment of the degree of prolapse. Pulling on the cervix with a tenaculum is unnecessary.

There is much confusion in the gynecologic literature regarding definitions and classifications of degrees of uterine prolapse. It would seem more sensible simply to describe the level to which the cervix descends on straining, such as, "descends to slightly below normal level," "descends to 1 inch above the introitus," "descends to the introitus," "descends to 2 inches below the introitus." The term *procidentia* should be reserved for those patients who have a total uterine prolapse with eversion of the entire vagina (Fig. 31-8). A grading or staging system seems to concentrate too much on the degree of uterine prolapse without giving sufficient attention to other aspects of the patient's vaginal relaxation problem of equal or even greater importance. Those who prefer an exact grading system may wish to refer to the one suggested by Beecham.

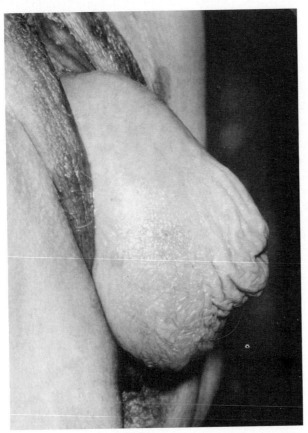

Figure 31–8. Total uterine prolapse and vaginal eversion (uterine procidentia).

An attempt should be made to evaluate the length of the cervix. In some patients, most of the prolapse is an elongated and hypertrophied cervix. In addition to bimanual palpation, sounding the uterus will be helpful in determining the length of the cervical canal. One must also be certain that the uterus is free and not fixed in the prolapsed position by intrapelvic adhesions.

The vaginal and cervical mucosa should be examined carefully for atrophy, hypertrophy, and lesions. Vaginal and cervical cytology and biopsies may be necessary, especially if lesions are present. Carcinoma of the vagina and cervix definitely can occur with procidentia, contrary to the opinion of some. With chronic neglected procidentia, the cervical and vaginal mucosa may show shallow ulcerative lesions with distinct borders. They should be biopsied. These ulcers are similar to chronic stasis ulcers of the lower extremities of patients with vascular insufficiency and are very difficult to manage.

A bimanual recto-vaginal-abdominal examination is done to detect uterine and adnexal tumors and to be sure the pelvic organs are free and not restricted by adhesions or other pathology. As stated earlier, pelvic tumors with or without ascites may cause uterovaginal prolapse. The detection of this pathology is important to make proper management decisions.

In addition to disturbances in bladder and bowel function already described, the lower ureters may be obstructed by advanced degrees of uterovaginal prolapse, especially procidentia. Reports of the prevalence of this complication vary widely, from 2% in the series by Guillemin and Cavailher to 92% in the report by Franche. The lower incidence is found in patients with milder degrees of uterovaginal prolapse, whereas the higher incidence is found among patients with procidentia. When there is procidentia, the entire bladder trigone and lower ureters are dragged outside the pelvis because of downward traction of the uterine arteries against the lower ureters as the uterus descends. The caudal displacement of the bladder trigone causes compression of the ureters between the uterus and the genital hiatus. The ureters are at high risk of being obstructed by this insidious process of uterine prolapse. Usually, the hydroureter and hydronephrosis are asymptomatic. Sometimes repeated upper urinary tract infections draw attention to the problem. Impairment of renal function may develop in some neglected cases. Renal failure caused by uterovaginal prolapse was first described by Froriep in 1824. More recent cases of progressive deterioration of urinary tract function have been reported by Hadar and Meiraz, by Mueller-Heuback, and by Riddle and associates. If obstruction has not progressed to end-stage renal parenchymal destruction, it can usually be reversed and function can be restored by surgery to correct the prolapse or even by pessary. One should be reluctant to manage a patient with uterovaginal prolapse expectantly without evidence by excretory urogram that the ureters are not obstructed. Patients with advanced degrees of uterovaginal prolapse should not be managed expectantly, because of the likely presence of impaired urinary tract function.

Finally, if a postmenopausal patient with uterovaginal prolapse complains of bleeding, an investigation should be done to determine the cause. The investigation should include cytology, biopsy of vaginal and cervical lesions, and especially dilatation and curettage, and should be done before an operation to cure the prolapse.

Choice of Treatment

Decisions regarding proper management of patients with uterovaginal prolapse should be made with the following statements in mind:

The judgement as to surgical correction should depend upon a correlation of the history and physical findings. Even marked prolapse in the absence of complaint should rarely be corrected. The patient should ask the gynecologist for relief; the gynecologist should not urge the patient to have the corrective surgery if she does not feel sufficiently uncomfortable to request it [Te Linde, 1966].

Vaginal reconstructive surgery is concerned with the return of abnormal organ relationships to a usual or normal state. There is no one site or degree of damage that must be repaired or restored; there are many and they occur in various combinations at various times of life, from different etiologic factors, in varying degrees, and with varying degrees of symptomatology and disability [Nichols and Randall, 1989].

Patients with varying degrees of uterovaginal prolapse of different etiologies and varying degrees of symptoms may be managed according to the following choices and options:

1. Expectant management
2. Surgical management
   a. Vaginal hysterectomy, posterior culdeplasty, colporrhaphy (with or without sacrospinous ligament fixation)
   b. Vaginal hysterectomy, closure of enterocele sac, total colpectomy, colporrhaphy, and colpocleisis
   c. Combined vaginal colporrhaphy with abdominal hysterectomy, Moschcowitz culdeplasty, sacral colpopexy, suprapubic urethrocolpopexy
   d. Manchester operation
   e. LeFort colpocleisis and colporrhaphy
   f. Vaginal repair and uterine suspension (with or without sacral cervicopexy)
3. Pessaries

It is difficult to present the advantages and disadvantages of all choices and options to each patient. However, the patient deserves to understand her condition as clearly as her doctor can describe it. To give an informed consent she also must know as well as possible the advantages and disadvantages of various treatment options.

Expectant Management

The largest number of patients will have mild degrees of uterovaginal prolapse perhaps discovered during a routine gynecologic examination. Such patients may have no symptoms or symptoms that are relatively mild. Under these circumstances, surgical repair is not indicated. The patient should be informed of her condition and of associated problems that could make her relaxation worse over time (eg, chronic cough, obesity, chronic constipation). Measures to prevent or correct these associated problems should be instituted. Postmenopausal women should be advised to accept estrogen replacement therapy unless contraindicated. Patients should be taught the technique of perineal muscle exercises and encouraged to do them assiduously. In addition, vaginal cones of increasing weight may be prescribed, as advised by Plevnik, Stanton, and others. Periodic examinations should be done to determine the status of uterovaginal support and symptomatology and to reinforce the patient's motivation to continue preventive measures. It is to be hoped that such an approach will prevent the need for future surgery.

Because of interference with function of the urinary tract primarily, patients with advanced degrees of uterovaginal prolapse cannot be managed expectantly.

Surgical Management

Only those patients with uterovaginal prolapse who have significant symptoms and who request relief should be considered for surgery. Even among these patients, some with mild degrees of prolapse with symptoms may be given a trial of conservative expectant management, described earlier, before acceding to a request for surgery. Indeed, surgical correction of mild degrees of uterine prolapse in the absence of other associated gynecologic problems is rarely, if ever, necessary. In some patients whose main request is for surgical sterilization, vaginal hysterectomy and repair may be selected as the appropriate method of accomplishing sterilization if symptomatic uterovaginal prolapse is also present.

Choice of Operations. Fortunately, there are a variety of operations from which to choose to correct uterovaginal prolapse. A proper choice among the various procedures will depend on a careful evaluation of the following factors:

Patient's general health status. The patient's age is not important except insofar as it may reflect a greater likelihood of associated medical diseases. A careful medical evaluation may indicate that an operation would carry a great risk and should not be done. In other patients, only local anesthesia or a brief general or conduction anesthetic should be given. Of course, in the majority of patients the general health will be good enough to allow any operation to be done that the patient needs. Most patients can tolerate an expertly administered anesthetic. Just a few patients with marked uterovaginal prolapse should have only a LeFort colpocleisis under local, brief general, or conduction anesthesia.

Degree and type of uterovaginal prolapse. Some operations are satisfactory for mild to moderate degrees of uterovaginal prolapse but will not give satisfactory results in patients with complete procidentia. For example, vaginal hysterectomy with posterior culdeplasty and colporrhaphy is likely to give satisfactory results in patients with mild and moderate degrees of prolapse but is not an effective operation in giving permanently satisfactory results if a complete procidentia is present. We never use the Manchester operation for complete procidentia. Suturing the cardinal ligaments in front of the cervix along with anterior and posterior colporrhaphy does not provide sufficient support to correct complete procidentia. With advanced degrees of prolapse, additional procedures, such as sacrospinous ligament fixation, sacral colpopexy, or colpectomy with colpocleisis will be required to give adequate support to the vaginal vault and, it is hoped, a permanently satisfactory result.

In some patients, the prolapse may be an elongated cervix. Even though the elongated cervix protrudes beyond the introitus, the uterine corpus may still be in a relatively normal position in the pelvis. We have seen a prolapsed cervix as long as 10 cm. A Manchester operation with cervical amputation, anterior plication of the cardinal ligaments, with appropriate colporrhaphies can provide proper support for such a patient. If an enterocele is present, it will be difficult to repair without removing the uterus. To repair the enterocele properly, we prefer to remove it in most patients. However, in older women without complete procidentia who are symptomatic and simply have an elongated cervix, a Manchester operation is easier to perform than other operations and is likely to give satisfactory results. Of course, a dilatation and curettage should be done first to rule out endometrial pathology. If the gross findings of the curettings are the least bit suspicious of malignancy, the operation should be delayed until the final pathology report is available.

Need for preservation of coital function. The expectations of the patient and her sexual partner for intravaginal intercourse must be discussed before an operation can be chosen and recommended. The subject must be discussed even with an elderly patient with serious medical problems and complete procidentia, for whom the standard LeFort colpocleisis might seem the most appropriate procedure. If she and her partner cannot adjust to the idea of a relationship without intravaginal intercourse, perhaps the Goodall-Powers modification of the LeFort colpocleisis can be done to leave a vagina long enough for intercourse, but obviously much shorter than normal. Frank discussions regarding sexual function are important before every operation to correct uterovaginal prolapse, since a change in vaginal caliber and direction can be expected to result from any operation. To protect against subsequent recurrent prolapse, the vagina may need to be closed so snugly that sexual intercourse is difficult and unsatisfactory. This may occur even with an expert surgeon. Symmonds preserved the vagina in 34 patients operated upon for vaginal prolapse. In 13 patients the vagina was not satisfactory for intercourse after operation.

Concomitant intrapelvic disease. All patients should be carefully evaluated for concomitant vaginal, uterine, or adnexal pathology. Large uterine leiomyomas or ovarian tumors suggest an abdominal approach for removal plus abdominal culdeplasty, suprapubic colpourethropexy, and sacral colpopexy if an advanced degree of uterovaginal prolapse is also present. Colporrhaphies that are needed should usually be done first from below before the abdominal phase of the operation is done.

Desire for preservation of menstrual and/or reproductive function. A few patients will develop symptomatic uterovaginal prolapse before childbearing is complete. Unless the problem is severe, these patients should be advised to complete their childbearing so that a definitive operation giving permanently satisfactory results can be done. Sometimes a pessary can be used to give temporary relief. However, when this advice is unacceptable and relief is needed, an abdominal round ligament (Gilliam) uterine suspension with uterosacral ligament plication and culdeplasty may be combined with suprapubic colpourethropexy and/or appropriate colporrhaphies, if needed, done first from below. A fascial strap may also be interposed between the cervix and the sacrum. The patient should be told that the results may not be permanently satisfactory and that another operation may be required later after she has had as many children as she wishes.

Some younger women with uterovaginal prolapse prefer an operation that will allow continued menstrual function even when additional pregnancies are not an issue. A Manchester operation with cervical amputation and appropriate colporrhaphies can be done, but it should be combined with vaginal or abdominal tubal ligation. When pregnancy follows a Manchester operation with cervical amputation, the frequency of cervical dystocia, cervical lacerations, cervical incompetence, and premature birth is increased. Cervical stenosis and infertility may also occur. There is an objection to cervical amputation if future childbearing is desired or even possible, as indicated by the report of Fisher and of others. For this reason, there is less objection to the Manchester operation with cervical amputation when the patient is postmenopausal, and it should include tubal ligation when done in premenopausal patients. Another approach to the preservation of uterine and reproductive function in young women with prolapse is the use of transvaginal sacrospinous uterine fixation as reported by Richardson and associates.

Other considerations. Operations that provide the strongest support should be favored when conditions that predispose to recurrent prolapse are likely to continue. The obese patient may lose weight, but the weight loss may not be permanent. A chronic cough related to nicotine abuse may continue even though every effort is made to convince the patient to stop smoking. And the straining of chronic constipation may not be completely eliminated by measures to relieve it. Those patients who must return to employment that includes straining and heavy lifting should also have an operation that provides the strongest support.

Surgical Principles. In considering surgery for the correction of uterovaginal prolapse, the gynecologic surgeon is well advised to think in terms of surgical principles rather than think only about a particular operative technique. For example:

Remember that the uterus is not the cause of uterovaginal prolapse. Uterine prolapse is the result but not the cause. Doing only a hysterectomy will not solve the problem of prolapse. Indeed, it may not be absolutely necessary to remove the uterus in all cases. Removal of the uterus will facilitate repair of an enterocele. Leaving the uterus in place can facilitate repair of a cystocele. Support for the vaginal walls, vaginal vault, and vaginal outlet is the most important part of the operation, not hysterectomy, although it is generally desirable to remove the uterus for other reasons.

Repair all relaxations, even though they are minor. Minor relaxations (defects in support) will likely become major problems in the future if not repaired.

Whenever possible, attempt to re-create normal anatomy. Maintain normal vaginal length. A shortened vagina is more likely to prolapse again. Suspend the vagina in its normal posterior direction over

the levator plate. Avoid suspending the vaginal vault anteriorly to the abdominal wall. Ventral fixation of the vaginal apex is an unanatomic position that exposes the upper posterior vaginal wall to intra-abdominal pressure and increases the risk of subsequent enterocele formation.

Narrow the caliber of a large vagina, but not so much that intercourse will be difficult, painful, or even impossible. Results of the operation will be better, however, if a large-caliber vagina is narrowed.

Evaluate the strength of various support structures. If they are weak, do not depend on them to provide dependable support in reconstruction. For example. if the uterosacral ligaments are weak, use them but do not depend on them to provide support needed. Use other techniques for support as well.

Close the cul-de-sac and repair an enterocele in all cases, if possible. This should be done even when doing a total colpectomy and colpocleisis, and especially when a Burch suprapubic colpourethropexy is done.

Do a posterior colpoperineorrhaphy in all cases, if possible. Repair of the lower posterior vaginal wall provides some support to the anterior vaginal wall and lengthens the vagina. It must be done carefully to avoid unnecessary constriction of the introitus and vagina.

Support the urethrovesical angle separately to correct or prevent genuine stress urinary incontinence. It is especially important to do a Burch suprapubic colpourethropexy when a sacral colpopexy is performed. It is also important to do an anterior colporrhaphy when the vagina is suspended to the sacrospinous ligament.

Make an independent decision about each part of the operation. Each operation should be individualized according to the symptoms and physical findings in each case. But the most important requirement for satisfactory support and a good result is a vagina that is normal in caliber and length with its apex secured at an appropriate position posteriorly over the levator plate and into the hollow of the sacrum.

Regarding this philosophy of applying surgical principles, Bonney made the following colorful statement:

A surgeon who proclaims that the operation he employs for prolapse is Jones's or Smith's or Robinson's also proclaims himself as belonging to that considerable section of mankind who prefer to get someone else to think for them. Fancy a tailor who advertised that he corrected the bad fit of a pair of trousers by Jones's method! Gentlemen, in the matter in hand we are all tailors, and our aim should be not to carry out any particular preconceived set operation, but, in the words of Gilbert's immortal Lord High Executioner, "to make the punishment fit the crime" by employing just those dissections, excisions, readjustments, and suturings that will, if possible, leave the parts concerned "as good as new."

Surgical Techniques. As we express our opinion on the various operations, we realize fully that there is room for honest difference of opinion on this subject. Without doubt, in many cases, equally satisfactory results may be obtained by more than one method. If this were not true, there would not be such strong advocates of the different types of procedures. It is assumed that each surgeon who strongly defends a particular operation does so believing that the procedure is giving satisfactory results in his hands. There is no doubt that the skill of the individual operator, in a particular operation, is a great factor in the results. But no matter how skillful a surgeon may become in a favorite procedure, he or she should not permit enthusiasm for it to overcome judgment as to its indication.

VAGINAL HYSTERECTOMY, POSTERIOR CULDEPLASTY, AND COLPORRHAPHY (WITH OR WITHOUT SACROSPINOUS LIGAMENT FIXATION). Since the mid-20th century, we have observed the increasing use of the vaginal hysterectomy as the major method of surgical treatment of symptomatic uterine prolapse in conjunction with the presence of a cystocele, rectocele, and/or enterocele. Originally, we held a very conservative view toward the benefits of this procedure, as we were concerned that it may have been performed more frequently than the indications warranted. Today, with a wider experience with this operation, we are in agreement that it has achieved a position of primacy in the treatment of mild and moderate degrees of prolapse of the uterus. When performed properly, with meticulous attention to the anatomic details associated with the pelvic relaxation, it has become a valuable tool in the management of this condition. The major complication that led to failure with this procedure in earlier years was the inadvertent oversight of a coexisting enterocele. Failure to correct this anatomic defect when present produced a high incidence of prolapse of the vaginal vault. Time and experience have improved this risk and have relegated this operation to its proper place in gynecologic surgery. Despite our previous skepticism for the operation as a cure-all for uterine prolapse, we are most enthusiastic about its use in properly selected cases.

Most premenopausal patients with significant symptoms and physical findings of uterovaginal prolapse select an operation that includes removal of the uterus in order to be relieved of tiresome heavy menstruation and dysmenorrhea and the need for contraception. Most postmenopausal patients also opt for hysterectomy so that estrogen replacement can be taken without progesterone, without monthly periods, and without the need for periodic endometrial biopsies. In addition, there is the benefit of removing an organ that can be the future site of malignancy. Important incidental uterine and adnexal pathology may be found in some patients (as many as 50%, according to Falk and associates). Krige found unsuspected and symptomless gross pathology in 36 of 200 postmenopausal patients who underwent repair of genital prolapse combined with vaginal hysterectomy. Most of the patients would have needed treatment later if the uterus had not been removed. Of course, operations for uterovaginal prolapse should be preceded by a curettage. If the gross findings of the curettings are ever suspicious of malignancy, the operation should be stopped until the final answer concerning the pathology of the endometrium is reported. Accurate frozen section diagnosis of endometrial pathology is difficult even in the most experienced hands.

The technique of vaginal hysterectomy and posterior culdeplasty is described in detail in Chapter 27, since the operation is commonly used for a variety of conditions other than uterovaginal prolapse. Some additional comments regarding its use specifically in the surgical correction of uterovaginal prolapse may be appropriate here.

Removal of the uterus in patients with procidentia is usually accomplished without difficulty. However, two specific and unique problems may be encountered. In chronic complete uterovaginal prolapse, the vagina and uterus are in a chronically dependent position. Obstruction at the genital hiatus causes venous congestion. Constant bleeding from large dilated veins can be a problem during dissection. The amount of blood loss can be controlled by injecting normal saline submucosally, by dissecting in proper planes, and by quickly ligating or coagulating persistent bleeders. The most important way to control the amount of blood loss may be to complete the operation without delay. The amount of blood lost should be carefully monitored and replaced when necessary, preferably with predeposited autologous blood.

The second problem is the frequent finding of an elongated cervix. Successive and multiple clamping and ligating of tissues on each side of the cervix may be required before opening the cul-de-sac and before the uterine vessels and upper broad-ligament structures can be clamped and ligated.

Since most operations for advanced prolapse are done in postmenopausal women, it is perfectly acceptable and usually possible to remove both tubes and ovaries vaginally at the same time (see Fig. 27-46), thus eliminating the possibility of ovarian cancer developing later.

When vaginal hysterectomy is done for other indications in the absence of uterine prolapse and vaginal relaxation problems, the normal vaginal caliber should not be constricted, especially in the vault. This is discussed in Chapter 27. Constriction of the vault could result in dyspareunia. With uterovaginal prolapse, plication of ligaments across the midline, from one side to the other, and 360° closure of the peritoneum can still predispose to dyspareunia by bringing the ovaries into a position over the vaginal apex and should be avoided when possible in premenopausal women. In postmenopausal patients with uterovaginal prolapse in whom the ovaries are atrophic and/or removed, a technique of closing the vaginal apex that results in some constriction may be chosen to give better vault support. This is especially appropriate when the uterovaginal prolapse is advanced and the upper vaginal space needs to be reduced to a normal caliber while preserving length.

As stated previously, we do not believe a standard technique of vaginal hysterectomy and colporrhaphy alone will provide sufficient long-lasting support when done for advanced uterovaginal prolapse. With mild and moderate degrees of prolapse, a posterior culdeplasty should also always be done to close the cul-de-sac, plicate the uterosacral ligaments in the midline, and suspend the posterior vaginal fornix (the deepest part of the vagina) to these ligaments. Up to three culdeplasty sutures may be needed to close the cul-de-sac and support the vault. The technique of posterior culdeplasty is described in Chapter 27. Hirsch reports that the McCall posterior culdeplasty is the primary procedure used in his clinic in Tubingen to support the vaginal vault and as prophylaxis against posthysterectomy enterocele with vaginal and abdominal hysterectomy. In 186 procedures, the only complication was kinking of the ureter in one case. Given described the use of McCall's posterior culdeplasty in patients with enterocele and complete procidentia. Torpin's culdeplasty may also be used.

With advanced degrees of uterovaginal prolapse, the vaginal vault should still be supported with a posterior culdeplasty, but the vault also should be suspended to the sacrospinous ligament according to the technique described by Nichols in Chapter 32. The combination of posterior culdeplasty and sacrospinous ligament fixation will give the best chance of a successful result. We do not agree, however, that sacrospinous ligament suspension should be done in all patients who have vaginal hysterectomy for prolapse of a mild or moderate degree. Posterior culdeplasty usually provides sufficient support in these patients. Among 135 patients undergoing vaginal hysterectomy, Cruikshank and Cox performed sacrospinous ligament fixation in 48 patients who demonstrated moderate or severe uterovaginal prolapse. These authors believe that this procedure should be used as a prophylaxis against posthysterectomy vault prolapse if there is loss of pelvic support structures (uterosacral-cardinal ligament complex).

Thornton and Peters utilize perirectal fascia to support the vaginal vault at the time of hysterectomy in patients with prolapse of the uterus in whom high approximation of the cardinal and uterosacral ligaments after vaginal hysterectomy does not adequately support the vault. According to these authors, the distal perirectal fascia is sutured to the uterosacral ligaments in the vault and closed across the midline to the level of the levator ani muscles, using interrupted 2-0 silk sutures. This maintains the horizontal axis of the vagina and obliterates potential space for subsequent development of an enterocele or vault prolapse. The perirectal fascia continues cephalad as the endopelvic fascia, as illustrated by Uhlenhuth and associates.

Appropriate anterior and posterior colporrhaphies must also be done. These are described in Chapters 33 and 34, respectively.

VAGINAL HYSTERECTOMY, EXCISION AND HIGH LIGATION OF THE CUL-DE-SAC PERITONEUM, TOTAL COLPECTOMY, ANTERIOR AND POSTERIOR COLPORRHAPHY, AND COLPOCLEISIS. This operation may be the procedure of choice in older women when an advanced degree of uterovaginal prolapse (procidentia) is present, when maintenance of coital function is unnecessary, when the operator feels that proper support cannot be achieved by the previously described techniques, and when the patient's medical condition will tolerate the additional procedure. Colpectomy may be required in the presence of an advanced, chronic, and neglected uterovaginal prolapse with extensive chronic ulceration of the vaginal mucosa that will not heal. Following removal of the uterus vaginally (and possibly the tubes and ovaries), the peritoneum of an enterocele or deep cul-de-sac should be dissected free and excised. The peritoneum should be closed with a 360° purse-string suture of No. 2-0 polydioxanone as high as possible. Excess peritoneum below this closure may be excised and/or used again for another reinforcing 360° purse-string suture. The anterior colporrhaphy is done next. The anterior vaginal mucosal flaps are completely excised. Dissection of the posterior vaginal wall begins just inside the vaginal introitus. Generous injection of sterile saline beneath the mucosa will facilitate removal of the posterior and lateral vaginal walls completely to the apex of the vagina. Significant bleeding should be quickly controlled and the dissection completed without delay. Posterior colporrhaphy begins at the vaginal apex by plicating perirectal fascia in the midline in front of the rectum down to the level of the puborectalis and pubococcygeus muscles. The uppermost plicating sutures may be used for additional support of the bladder base by including the uterosacral ligaments and the bladder base. The vaginal space is obliterated by closing the pubococcygeus muscles, the remaining lower vaginal mucosa, and finally the perineal muscles and skin in the midline. If hemostasis is satisfactory, a pack or drain will not be needed. A transurethral Foley catheter or suprapubic catheter is used for bladder drainage. A technique of vaginal hysterectomy with colpectomy and colpocleisis is illustrated in Figures 31-9 *A–D,* and may vary, depending on circumstances.

According to Percy and Perl, priority for complete removal of the uterus and vagina for the correction of uterovaginal prolapse belongs to Martin, who, in 1894, performed vaginal hysterectomy and colpectomy for prolapse. In 1901, Edebohls published the first well-documented case reports of complete vaginal obliteration after "panhysterocolpopectomy." Total colpectomy was sometimes done without removing the uterine corpus, something that would be considered unacceptable today. Moreover, appropriate emphasis was not always given to obliteration of an enterocele or repair of other vaginal wall relaxations. Subsequent troublesome herniations can develop postoperatively if the enterocele, cystocele, and rectocele are not attended to. Simultaneous repair of the cystocele with "panhysterocolpopectomy" was first reported by Masson and Kuepper in 1938 in 38 operations for procidentia. Other refinements were offered by Williams, by Ricci and Thom, by Thompson and associates, and by others. A more modern series of surgical repair of complete procidentia was published by Barclay in 1989. Vaginal hysterectomy with vaginectomy was done successfully in 41 patients.

An operation for prolapse that does not maintain or restore continued coital function is considered by some to be a destructive operation and an admission of defeat. Certainly, such an operation would be inappropriate when continued coital function is desirable. However, under the strictly defined circumstances outlined earlier, we believe vaginal hysterectomy, excision and high ligation of enterocele sac, total colpectomy, colporrhaphy, and colpocleisis can give excellent and permanently satisfactory results.

COMBINED VAGINAL COLPORRHAPHY WITH ABDOMINAL HYSTERECTOMY, CULDEPLASTY, SACRAL COLPOPEXY, AND SUPRAPUBIC COLPOURETHROPEXY. A combined abdominal and vaginal operation may be chosen to correct advanced uterovaginal prolapse in some patients. The operation consists of several parts and is essentially the same procedure as that described by Hendee in

Chapter 32 for vaginal vault prolapse. Beginning vaginally, appropriate colporrhaphies are done first, but vaginal constriction should be avoided. After packing the vagina to hold the uterus and cervix in place, an abdominal incision, usually a transverse Maylard, is fashioned, removing a fascial strip from the aponeurosis of the anterior rectus sheath on the way in. The strip of fascia should be about 10 cm long and 2 cm wide. A total abdominal hysterectomy (with bilateral salpingo-oophorectomy in postmenopausal patients) is followed by excision of redundant anterior and posterior vaginal walls. The vault may be closed longitudinally to preserve vaginal length. The deep cul-de-sac is obliterated by a bilateral hemi-Moschcowitz technique using 2-0 polydioxanone suture (see Fig. 33-10). A sacral colpopexy (see Chapter 32) is followed by closure of the pelvic peritoneum. Suprapubic colpourethropexy is also usually done (see Chapter 33).

This abdominal procedure is longer than the previously described vaginal operations and is usually not the operation of choice in older women in poor health. In healthy patients it gives excellent results. It is the procedure of choice when pelvic tumors must also be removed or when suprapubic urethrocolpopexy must be done. If previous colporrhaphies have been done and the vagina cannot tolerate additional constriction, the abdominal approach allows preservation of vaginal function with greater certainty.

MANCHESTER OPERATION AND COLPORRHAPHY. In 1888, Donald, of Manchester, began treating prolapse of the uterus by the combination of anterior and posterior colporrhaphy and amputation of the cervix. This operation continues to be performed in Manchester and other areas of England by a number of gynecologists. Before Fothergill modified the operation, the procedure included amputation of the cervix by the Schroder method, followed by an anterior colporrhaphy. Fothergill made the incision for the anterior repair triangular in shape with the base at the cervix and then carried the incision around the cervix to perform the amputation. This exposed the bases of the broad ligaments to better advantage than the method previously employed and facilitated the approximation of these supporting structures in front of the cervix. This operation, with slight variation, has been done by different members of the Manchester staff since 1888. Descriptions of its technique, which have appeared in the literature, vary as to detail. The operation as done in our clinic is described here. The fundamental principles underlying the procedure are exactly as in the operation described by Shaw from the Manchester Clinic in 1933, but certain details differ slightly, especially if the posterior cul-de-sac is opened for enterocele repair.

Despite the favorable Manchester experience in previous years, we are not convinced that the operation is

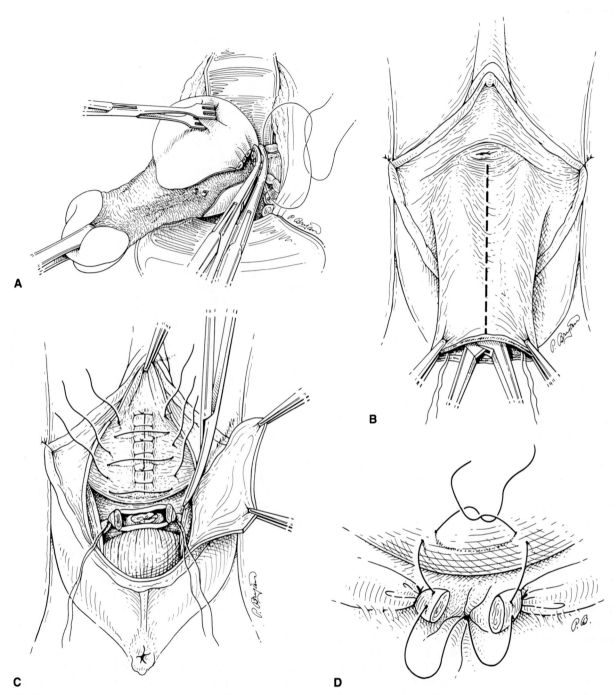

Figure 31–9. Technique of vaginal hysterectomy with colpectomy and colpocleisis for uterovaginal prolapse. *A*, The prolapsed uterus is removed vaginally. The enterocele sac is ligated as high as possible and the excess sac is dissected free and removed (see Fig. 33-11*A*). *B*, The anterior vaginal wall is dissected away from the bladder in preparation for an anterior colporrhaphy. *C*, Two or three rows of 2-0 delayed-absorbable mattress sutures elevate the cystocele. The posterior vaginal wall is dissected free from the perineum to the vaginal apex. The vaginal mucosa is removed. *D*, Additional support for the vaginal apex may be obtained by suturing the bladder base, paracervical ligaments, and enterocele sac closure together. Following a rectocele repair (see Fig. 34-4), the anterior and posterior vaginal walls are closed together as in a LeFort colpocleisis (see Fig. 31-12).

the one of choice in "all patients with prolapsed uteri, irrespective of age, social position or parity." It is our opinion that the Manchester operation has a limited place in modern gynecology when (1) there is a cystocele associated with a prolapse of first or second degree, (2) childbearing no longer needs to be considered, and (3) the uterus is not in marked retroposition or when the retrodisplaced uterus is a small atrophic structure and not contributory to the patient's symptoms. The operation is particularly satisfactory under the preceding conditions when much of the apparent prolapse is due to cervical elongation. Although the indications are quite different in Britain, its use in the United States is infrequent and it is usually done for expediency's sake where the patient is a surgical risk for prolonged surgery.

We believe that there is a definite objection to the operation when future pregnancy is likely, because of the amputation of the cervix. Leonard found that, following cervical amputation, the incidence of sterility was abnormally high, premature delivery between the sixth and eighth months increased, and cervical dystocia was common. Shaw's own results would seem to condemn the operation during the childbearing period, as few of his patients subsequently had children.

The patient is placed on the table in lithotomy position and cleaned up for operation with the usual technique. Dilatation and curettage are done for two reasons: (1) a dilatation of the cervical canal is desirable at a later stage of the operation when the posterior flap of mucosa is drawn into the cervical canal; and (2) since the body of the uterus is to be saved, it is well to make certain that no malignancy exists. If the endometrium obtained looks at all abnormal grossly, it is best to proceed no further with the operation until microscopic examination of the curettings has been made.

Traction is made on the cervix by a Jacobs clamp, and a transverse incision is made through the anterior vaginal mucosa. A midline incision is made from cervix to urethral meatus, dissecting beneath the mucosa with the curved scissors or scalpel as illustrated in the operation for cystocele (see Chapter 33). Injection of normal saline facilitates dissection in the proper plane.

The flaps of vaginal mucosa are dissected laterally, and the bladder is dissected up from its attachment to the cervix. In the beginning the separation of the bladder from the cervix must be done by sharp dissection. However, usually after a few "snips" with the scissors the bladder may be freed from the uterus by dissection with the scissors up to the vesicouterine reflexion of the peritoneum. The bladder is held up anteriorly with a thin-bladed retractor, as illustrated in Figure 31-10A. The anterior cul-de-sac is not entered.

The transverse cervical incision through the mucosa is then carried posteriorly, completely circumcising the cervix. The posterior flap of mucosa is dissected free from the cervix until a flap has been mobilized sufficiently to cover easily the posterior lip of the shortened cervix. With the mucosa about the cervix freed, the attenuated cardinal ligament is seen. Contained in it is the cervical branch of the uterine vessels. The lateral cardinal ligament is clamped en masse, with an Ochsner clamp parallel with and close to the cervix, cut and tied (see Figs. 31-10 A–B). When the cervix is markedly elongated so that a great length must be amputated, two tandem bites of the ligament may be necessary. This is repeated on the opposite side. To control the cervical blood supply further, a suture ligature of No. 1 delayed-absorbable suture is placed through the side of the cervix bilaterally, just above the point of intended amputation.

The cervix is amputated as indicated by the dotted line in Figure 31-10A, and the shortened posterior lip is covered with the posterior flap of mucosa, using a Sturmdorf suture of No. 1 delayed-absorbable suture. The ligated cardinal ligaments are then drawn together and sutured in front of the shortened cervix. It is well to bite into the anterior cervical wall with this suture in order to fix the ligaments in this position (Fig. 31-10C).

Following completion of the Manchester procedure, the anterior vaginal wall is repaired by a routine anterior colporrhaphy (as described in Chapter 33). After excising the excess vaginal mucosa, a midline closure is accomplished with interrupted suture of No. 2-0 delayed-absorbable suture (Fig. 31-10 D–E). It is usually advantageous to suture the cervical end of the mucosal incision first. In doing this, a bite is taken into the anterior lip of the shortened cervix. One or two lateral sutures are necessary to cover the cervix completely.

A posterior colporrhaphy is done with appropriate technique to cure the rectocele and relaxed vaginal outlet (see Chapter 34).

One of the serious disadvantages of the classical Manchester operation is the lack of attention given to an enterocele or deep cul-de-sac that may be present. For this reason we do not recommend this operation to patients with advanced degrees of uterovaginal prolapse who are also likely to have a large enterocele. Recognizing this deficiency, Solomons designed a technique to prevent recurrence of enteroceles after the Manchester operation. The cul-de-sac is opened, the peritoneum is excised, and the uterosacral ligaments are approximated. O'Leary and O'Leary have also "extended" the Manchester operation to include opening the posterior cul-de-sac, excising the enterocele sac and closing the cul-de-sac at a high level with a purse-string suture that included the uterosacral ligaments and the uterine serosa. This technique of culdeplasty was employed in 150 of 289 Manchester procedures. Only one patient developed recurrent prolapse. A technique of

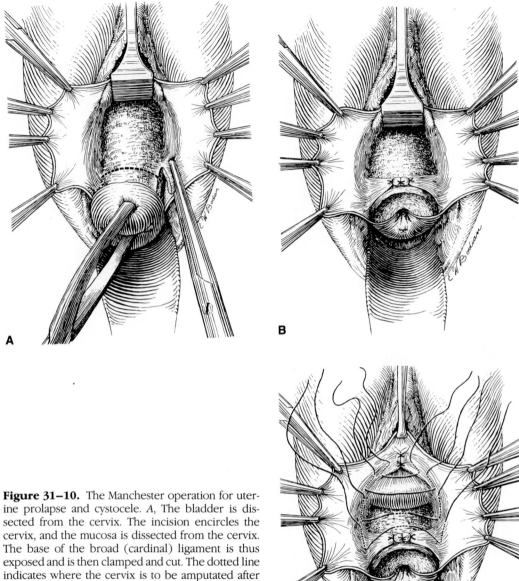

Figure 31–10. The Manchester operation for uterine prolapse and cystocele. *A,* The bladder is dissected from the cervix. The incision encircles the cervix, and the mucosa is dissected from the cervix. The base of the broad (cardinal) ligament is thus exposed and is then clamped and cut. The dotted line indicates where the cervix is to be amputated after the cervical branch of each uterine artery is ligated. *B,* The cervix is amputated, and the posterior lip is covered with a flap of mucosa. The bases of the broad ligaments are sutured to the anterior surface of the cervix. *C,* Pubovesicocervical fascia is approximated in the midline beneath the urethra and the base of the bladder. Note that the lower sutures bite into the anterior wall of the cervix. *(Figure continued on next page.)*

closing an enterocele and repairing a rectocele with the Manchester operation is illustrated in Figure 31-11 *A–B.*

Tipton and Atkin presented a long-term follow-up (6–12 years) of 82 patients treated for prolapse with the Manchester operation between the ages 29 and 52 years. After the operation, 34 patients (41%) had uterine disease or unwanted pregnancy. Two patients developed uterine carcinoma and one of these patients died. Seventeen patients (21%) required uterine operations,

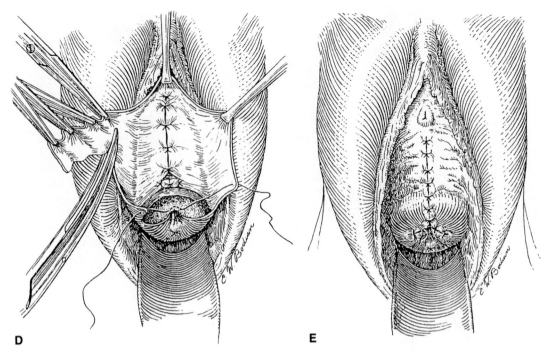

D   **E**

Figure 31–10. (continued) *D*, The fascia approximation has been completed. Excess vaginal mucosa is being excised. The first suture has been placed through flaps of the mucosa, biting into the cut surface of the shortened cervical lip to cover it with mucosa. *E*, The operation on the anterior wall has been completed. It is to be followed by a posterior colporrhaphy (see Fig. 34-4).

including eight hysterectomies. Contraception and fear of pregnancy were problems in many cases. Many patients said that they would have welcomed a hysterectomy at the time the Manchester operation was done. This study and others like it suggest that operations for uterovaginal prolapse should usually include hysterectomy, because future uterine disease is prevented.

LEFORT COLPOCLEISIS AND COLPORRHAPHY. The original operation, as described by Neugebauer and later by LeFort, was used for the treatment of total uterine procidentia and consisted of denuding a long, narrow triangle on the anterior and posterior walls of the vagina. The base of each triangle was just below the cervix, the apex was at the outlet, and vaginal closure was brought about by approximating these denuded areas. A slightly different procedure is now used. Rectangular strips of mucosa are excised from the upper portion of the anterior and posterior vaginal walls, and the exposed submucosa and vaginal musculature are then closed.

This operation does not correct the anatomic defect associated with a complete prolapse of the uterus or vagina that is due to a large traction or pulsion enterocele. The LeFort procedure should be used only when there is a very good reason not to carry out one of the usual operations for prolapse. The operation is an admission on the part of the surgeon that there is no way to cure the prolapse by a procedure that would leave a functioning vagina. Nevertheless, it is useful in rare cases. Its virtue lies in its being perhaps the quickest of any procedure used for the cure of prolapse and in its safety. (It can be done under local anesthesia if necessary.) The procedure is generally restricted to an elderly widow who might otherwise be condemned to the indefinite use of a pessary. Regardless of the age of the patient, the closure of the vagina should never be done without a complete understanding on the part of the patient and her spouse, if living, that the procedure will terminate intravaginal intercourse.

Both stress and urge urinary incontinence may occur with the LeFort procedure, because of traction of the suture line on the trigone and bladder neck. Ridley reports an incidence of urinary incontinence of 24% following the LeFort procedure. This disadvantage can be avoided by closing only the upper one third to one half of the anterior vaginal wall, stopping short of the area that underlies the bladder neck and the urethra. Nonetheless, part of the bladder base and the entire trigone rest on the upper one third of the vagina, so it is

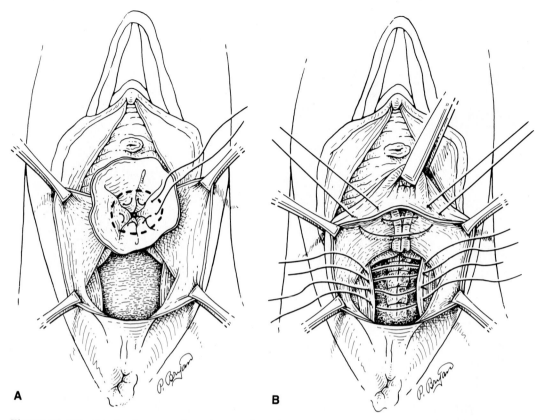

Figure 31–11. Repair of enterocele and rectocele with Manchester operation. *A*, The posterior vaginal wall has been dissected to the vaginal apex. The enterocele sac is ligated as high as possible, including bites into the posterior uterine wall. Excess enterocele sac is removed. *B*, Pararectal fascia, puborectalis muscles, and uterosacral ligaments are sutured together to support the posterior vaginal fornix and posterior vaginal wall. The posterior vaginal mucosa is closed.

difficult to close the upper vagina without placing some traction on the bladder trigone.

To avoid the risk of postoperative urinary stress incontinence, the urethra should be dissected free and a thorough plication of the vesical neck should be performed. If the patient is not sexually active, the levators are approximated very tightly, leaving only enough opening for urination. If the patient desires to retain some coital function of the vagina, the latter step is omitted, although the residual depth of the outer vagina may still preclude satisfactory coitus.

Obviously, this procedure is useful only for the postmenopausal female with total uterine prolapse where menses are absent. It is essential that the cervix and endometrial cavity be assessed fully by a cytologic smear and a dilatation and curettage to make certain that there is no evidence of occult uterine malignancy prior to closure of the vagina.

With the patient in the lithotomy position, the cervix is drawn out as far as possible. With total uterine procidentia, drawing out the cervix almost completely everts the vagina.

The area to be denuded anteriorly is marked out with the scalpel as indicated by the dotted line in Figure 31-12A. Sufficient mucosa should be left laterally to form a canal for drainage of cervical secretions. The area to be denuded extends to within 2 cm of the tip of the cervix and to within 5 cm of the urethral meatus, remaining away from the location of the vesical neck. To avoid incorporating the bladder neck and posterior urethra in the operative site, a balloon-filled urethral catheter should be used to delineate the location of the urethrovesical junction.

The mucosa is denuded from the anterior vaginal wall by sharp dissection (Fig. 31-12B). An area of mucosa of equal size and shape is denuded from the posterior vaginal wall (Fig. 31-12C). Injection of sterile saline beneath the mucosa will facilitate dissection in

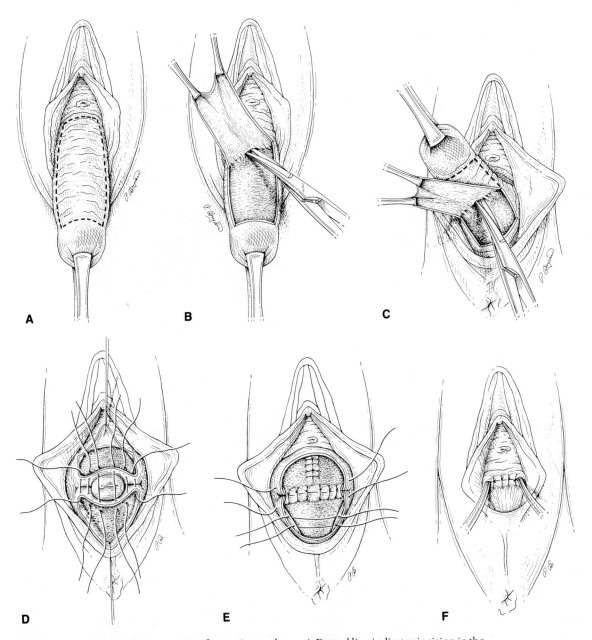

Figure 31–12. The LeFort operation for uterine prolapse. *A*, Dotted line indicates incision in the anterior vaginal mucosa. *B*, The vaginal mucosal flap is removed, leaving the fascia attached to the bladder. *C*, A similar flap is excised from the posterior vaginal wall. *D*, The vaginal mucosal edge is approximated in front of the cervix at the upper margin of the excised mucosa. *E*, The denuded areas of anterior and posterior vaginal walls are approximated with horizontal layers of interrupted 2-0 delayed-absorbable sutures. Plication mattress sutures are placed beneath the bladder neck and across the lower anterior rectal wall. *F*, The outer mucosal edges are closed. Note the tunnels that remain on either side of the vagina, demonstrated by Kelly clamps.

the proper plane. As illustrated in Figure 31-12*E,* plication sutures should be placed beneath the bladder neck and in the anterior rectal wall.

The mucosal edges are approximated transversely below the cervix with interrupted sutures of No. 2-0 delayed-absorbable suture (Fig. 31-12*D*). Beginning at the top, the denuded areas are approximated with No. 2-0 interrupted sutures (Fig. 31-12*E*). Mucosa-lined tunnels left on both sides are demonstrated by the Kelly clamps (Fig. 31-12*F*).

VAGINAL COLPORRHAPHY AND UTERINE SUSPENSION (WITH OR WITHOUT SACRAL CERVICOPEXY). Formerly, vaginal colporrhaphy with uterine suspension was fairly common, but this operation has now fallen into almost complete disfavor because the results are not permanently satisfactory. A definitive reoperation will likely be needed for early recurrence of the prolapse. We would not recommend this operation to a patient expecting permanently satisfactory results.

Occasionally, however, a young woman will suffer through one or two pregnancies with the cervix protruding through the introitus. A donut pessary may have been used to hold the cervix in the vagina during the first half of pregnancy or until the uterus was large enough to rest on the brim of the pelvis. Following delivery, the prolapse and discomfort may have recurred. Such a patient may not tolerate further use of the pessary and may not allow a definitive operation that includes hysterectomy, because she would like to have more children. For this reason also a Manchester operation should not be done. Under these well-defined circumstances, one might recommend a modified Gilliam round ligament suspension, plication of uterosacral ligaments, and colporrhaphy only if definitely needed.

We have seen a few young patients with congenital anomalies (eg, sacrum, bladder exstrophy) who had associated uterine prolapse with the cervix protruding beyond the vaginal introitus. In these patients, a modified Gilliam suspension was combined with a sacral cervicopexy with satisfactory long-term results. A strip of fascia is harvested from the anterior rectus sheath. One end is sutured behind the cervix and the other end is sutured to the presacral fascia. The strap should be just tight enough to hold the cervix in the middle to upper vagina. A similar technique of constructing a sacrocervical "ligament" using fascia from the external oblique aponeurosis was described by Stoesser in 1955. Another technique was described in 1980 by Dewhurst and associates. These authors used polyvinyl sponge (Ivalon) rather than fascia.

The surgical management of symptomatic uterovaginal prolapse in young women is a special problem, especially when the patient wishes to maintain uterine function, childbearing potential, and of course a functional vagina. Richardson and associates recently have reported using transvaginal sacrospinous uterine fixation with good results in five young women. In addition to suturing the uterosacral ligaments to the right sacrospinous ligament, enterocele repair, urethropexy, and colporrhaphy were done when appropriate. Since the procedure is performed transvaginally, trauma to the fallopian tubes and the potential for intra-abdominal and pelvic adhesion formation is avoided, as is the morbidity of major abdominal surgery. Also attempting surgical correction of uterine prolapse in young women, Williams used a modified Manchester operation with plication of the uterosacral ligaments posterior to the cervix and plication of the cardinal ligaments anterior to the cervix. The cervix was not amputated. In 19 patients with follow-up, there were three failures and six patients were delivered of full-term pregnancies.

HISTORICAL OPERATIONS FOR UTERINE PROLAPSE. In 1937, Edward Richardson devised a composite operation that used and improved on the principles and techniques of various procedures already in use. Richardson's procedure included amputation of the cervix; removal of the corpus at any level desired; utilization of the isthmic portion of the uterus with its broad and uterosacral ligament attachments for vault support; and, finally, approximation in the midline of the pubocervical fascia beneath the urethra, the base of the bladder, and the retained portion of the isthmus of the uterus.

Richardson's plan had the following objectives: (1) to remove the hypertrophied vaginal portion of the cervix; (2) to extirpate the corpus uteri, together with the tubes and the ovaries if indicated; (3) to destroy or excise any remaining cervical canal epithelium; (4) to minimize trauma and devitalization of structures, so they could later be used for reconstruction purposes; (5) to preserve a blood supply to the uterine isthmus; (6) to ablate totally any associated enterocele through high obliteration of the cul-de-sac of Douglas; (7) to use rationally all supporting structures, namely, the pubocervical fascia, the cardinal ligaments, with their extraordinarily strong cervical attachments, the uterosacral and the round ligaments, the fascia of the rectovaginal septum, as well as the muscles and the fascial layers of the pelvic floor and the perineum; (8) to reestablish a vagina of normal depth and caliber; and (9) to restore normal anatomic relationships.

Richardson made no claim of originality for any of the procedures used in his operation. Many of the operative steps were already in use, independently, for various conditions in gynecologic surgery. On reading the 1937 article, Ludwig Emge communicated with Richardson, calling his attention to the description of a similar operation reported by Spalding in 1919. Spalding and Richardson each described practically identical operations. Both men were motivated by the shortcomings of the other operations for uterine prolapse in vogue at the time, and both men emphasized the same points in claiming superiority for their operations. Since the operation was described independently by the two authors, it has been called by their joint names (the *Spalding-Richardson procedure*). It is not surprising to surgeons familiar with the operation that Richardson reinvented the procedure in 1937. The remarkable fact is that an operation that had such merit had escaped the general attention of gynecologists since Spalding's original article in 1919.

Although the Spalding-Richardson procedure is rarely used today in gynecologic clinics, it is recognized as one of the major surgical contributions of its time for uterine prolapse. The details of this operation are shown in Figure 31-13 and the technique is described in the original publications and in previous editions of this text.

The *Watkins transposition operation*, an operation for cystocele and uterine prolapse, was first performed by Thomas J. Watkins in 1898, and he reported it the following year. The procedure was used extensively for uterine prolapse with a very large cystocele. In most instances the results were very satisfactory. The procedure is generally known throughout this country as the interposition operation, but Watkins preferred the term *transposition,* since the uterus was transposed beneath the bladder. Basically, the operation consisted

of amputating the elongated cervix and suturing the fundus of the uterus beneath the large cystocele. The fundus was therefore used as an obturator to fill the defect in the anterior segment of the pelvic diaphragm.

Improved techniques of vaginal hysterectomy and repair of the vagina gradually led to the abandonment of the Watkins operation, and it is unlikely that recently trained gynecologists have ever seen this procedure performed. The completed procedure is shown in Figure 31-14, and the reader interested in this operation can refer to previous editions of this text for further operative details.

Pessaries

Before the availability of surgical procedures to correct uterovaginal prolapse, all sorts of primitive mechanical devices were used by patients and by physicians to hold the uterus in place. The use of pessaries was an art that has, fortunately or unfortunately, been largely lost, since surgical procedures are so satisfactory. Nevertheless, there is even today a rare occasion when a pessary should be used. Patients who refuse surgery and those whose general health is too poor to permit surgery may be given some relief with a pessary. Those who require treatment before surgery can be done may be given some temporary relief with a pessary.

As mentioned earlier, a Smith-Hodge pessary is used in patients with uterine retroversion. Once the uterus is brought to an anterior position, it can be held there with a properly fitting Smith-Hodge pessary. If the patient has sacral backache and bearing-down discomfort in the pelvis because of uterine retroversion, these symptoms may be relieved if the uterus is held forward with a Smith-Hodge pessary. The pessary must not obstruct the urethra and interfere with voiding. An occasional douche may be required if vaginal discharge is a problem. The pessary must be removed to allow vaginal examination every few weeks. If vaginal ulcerations appear, a different type of pessary should be chosen or its use should be discontinued until the ulcerations heal.

Although a variety of pessaries are available for uterovaginal prolapse, the simple soft rubber donut pessary is the easiest and most satisfactory. As with other pessaries, it rests on the perineum and depends on support of the vaginal outlet. Otherwise, it cannot be retained within the vagina. Sometimes a simple posterior colporrhaphy done under local anesthesia to constrict the vaginal outlet will be required for the pessary to be retained. The donut pessary must also be removed and the vagina inspected occasionally. Under ordinary circumstances, it can be removed and left out overnight about every week or two. The patient may do this

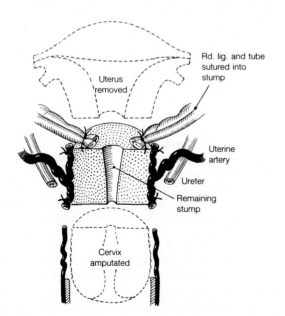

Figure 31–13. Diagram of Spalding–Richardson composite operation indicating the portion of uterus that remains. Note that the blood supply is intact.

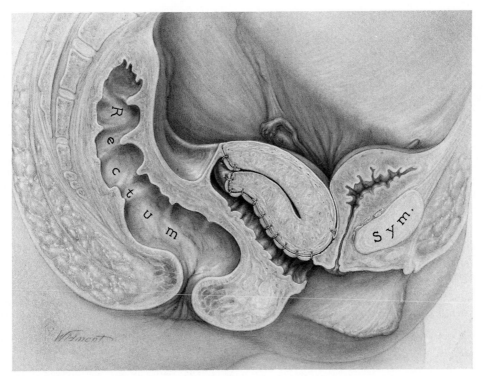

Figure 31–14. The Watkins transposition operation. The procedure is completed with the transposed uterus fixed in its new position beneath the bladder and urethra.

herself. A douche is taken and the pessary is cleaned before reinsertion. If done properly, this can be a satisfactory method of management for several years.

Bibliography

Adams JA. Cited by WP Graves. In: Graves WP. Gynecology. Philadelphia: WB Saunders, 1916.

Alexander W. Quoted by Curtis. In: Curtis AH, ed. Obstetrics and gynecology. Philadelphia: WB Saunders, 1937.

Allen WM, Masters WH. Traumatic lacerations of uterine supports: the clinical syndrome and operative treatment. Am J Obstet Gynecol 1955;70:500.

Anderson RS. A neurogenic element to urinary genuine stress incontinence. Br J Obstet Gynaecol 1984;91:412.

Averett L. Vaginal hysterectomy: indications and advantages. J Int Coll Surg 1945;8:53.

Baldy JM. Treatment of uterine retrodisplacements. Surg Gynecol Obstet 1909;8:421.

Baldy JM. Prolapse of the uterus. Trans Am Gynecol Soc 1912;27:25.

Barclay DL. Surgical correction of total procidentia and vaginal vault prolapse. J Arkansas Med Soc 1989;85:487.

Bartscht KD, DeLancey JOL. A technique to study the passive supports of the uterus. Obstet Gynecol 1988;72:940.

Beard RW, Pearce S, Highamn JH, Reginald PW. Diagnoses of pelvic varicosities in women with chronic pelvic pain. Lancet 1984; 2:946.

Beecham CT. Classification of vaginal relaxation. Am J Obstet Gynecol 1980;136:957.

Berglas B, Rubin IC. Study of the supportive structures of the uterus by levator myography. Surg Gynecol Obstet 1953;97:677.

Birnbaum SJ. Rational therapy for the prolapsed vagina. Am J Obstet Gynecol 1973;115:411.

Bonney V. The sustentacular apparatus of the female genital canal, the displacements from the yielding of its several components and their appropriate treatment. J Obstet Gynaecol Br Emp 1914; 45:328.

Bonney V. An address on genital displacements. Br Med J 1928;(March 17):432.

Bonney V. The principles that should underlie all operations for prolapse. J Obstet Gynaecol Br Emp 1934;41:669.

Bump RC, Fantl JA, Hurt WG. The mechanism of urinary continence in women with severe uterovaginal prolapse: results of barrier studies. Obstet Gynecol 1988;72:291.

Campbell RM. The anatomy and histology of the sacrouterine ligaments. Am J Obstet Gynecol 1950;59:1.

Copenhaver EH. Vaginal hysterectomy: an analysis of indications and complications among 1000 operations. Am J Obstet Gynecol 1962;84:123.

Copenhaver EH. Vaginal hysterectomy: past, present and future. Surg Clin North Am 1980;60:437.

Critchley HOD, Dixon JS, Gosling JA. Comparative study of the periurethral and perianal parts of the human levator ani muscle. Urol Int 1980;35:226.

Cruikshank SH, Cox DW. Sacrospinous ligament fixation at the time of transvaginal hysterectomy. Am J Obstet Gynecol 1990;162:1611.

Dewhurst J, Toplis PJ, Shepherd JH. Ivalon sponge hysterosacropexy for genital prolapse in patients with bladder extrophy. Br J Obstet Gynaecol 1980;87:67.

Dickinson RL. Genital prolapse: its operative correction based on a new study of cleavage lines and sliding segments. Am J Obstet Dis Wom 1910;17:17.

Donald A. A short history of the operation of colporrhaphy with remarks on the technique. J Obstet Gynaecol Br Emp 1921; 28:256.

Emge LA, Durfee RB. Pelvic organ prolapse: four thousand years of treatment. Clin Obstet Gynecol 1966;9:997.

England GT, Randall HW, Graves WL. Impairment of tissue defenses by vasoconstrictors in vaginal hysterectomies. Obstet Gynecol 1983;61:271.

Everett HS. End-result with the Watkins interposition operation. Surg Gynecol Obstet 1935;61:403.

Falk HC, Polishuk W, Solomon C. Vaginal hysterectomy for uterine prolapse. Am J Obstet Gynecol 1955;69:333.

Fisher JJ. The effect of amputation of the cervix uteri upon subsequent parturition. Am J Obstet Gynecol 1951;62:644.

Fluhmann CF. The rise and fall of suspension operations for uterine displacement. Bull Johns Hopkins Hosp 1955;96:59.

Fothergill WE. On the pathology and the operative treatment of displacements of the pelvic viscera. J Obstet Gynaecol Br Emp 1907;13:410.

Fothergill WE. Anterior colporrhaphy and amputations of the cervix combined as a single operation for use in the treatment of genital prolapse. Am J Surg 1915;29:161.

Franche O, Pak-Miong-Piv, Boga-Colman C, et al. L'état des voies urinaires dans le prolapsus genital total de la femme. Urol Int 1959;9:28.

Freund HW. Uber Moderne Prolapsoperationen. Zbl Gynak 1901; 25:441.

Funt MI, Thompson JD, Birch H. Normal vaginal axis. South Med J 1978;71:1534.

Gilliam DT. Round-ligament ventrosuspension of the uterus: a new method. Am J Obstet 1900;41:299.

Gilpin SA, Gosling JA, Smith ARB, Warrell DW. The pathogenesis of genitourinary prolapse and stress incontinence of urine. A histological and histochemical study. Br J Obstet Gynaecol 1989;96:15.

Given FT. "Posterior culdeplasty:" revisted. Am J Obstet Gynecol 1985;153:135.

Goodall JR, Power RMH. A modification of the LeFort operation for increasing its scope. Am J Obstet Gynecol 1937;34:968.

Gosling JA. The structure of the female lower urinary tract and pelvic floor. Urol Clin North Am 1985;12:207.

Graves WP. Olshauser operation for suspension of the uterus. Surg Gynecol Obstet 1931;52:1028.

Gray LA. Vaginal hysterectomy. 3rd ed. Springfield, Ill.: Charles C Thomas, 1983.

Guillemin G, Cavailher H. Les deformations vesicales et ureterales dans le prolapsus genitaux. Rev Fr Gynecol Obstet 1948;43:93.

Hadar H, Meiraz D. Total uterine prolapse causing hydronephrosis. Surg Gynecol Obstet 1980;150:711.

Hayden RC, Levinson JM. Total vaginectomy, vaginal hysterectomy, and colpocleisis for advanced procidentia. Obstet Gynecol 1960;16:564.

Heaney NS. Report of 565 vaginal hysterectomies performed for benign pelvic disease. Am J Obstet Gynecol 1934;28:751.

Heaney NS. Vaginal hysterectomy: its indications and technic. Am J Surg 1940;48:284.

Heaney NS. Techniques of vaginal hysterectomy. Surg Clin North Am 1942;22:73.

Hirsch HA. Uterosacral ligament suspension of vaginal vault (McCall's culdeplasty). Eur J Obstet Gynecol Reprod Biol 1989;32:13.

Hirst BC. A modification of the Alexander operation. Surg Gynecol Obstet 1915;20:599.

Hobbs JT. The pelvic congestion syndrome. Practitioner 1976;216:529.

Kegel AH. Progressive resistance exercise in the functional restoration of the perineal muscles. Am J Obstet Gynecol 1948;56:238.

Kegel AH. Physiologic therapy for urinary stress incontinence. JAMA 1952;10:915.

Kelly HA. Hysterorrhaphy. Am J Obstet 1887;20:33.

Kelly HA. History of retrodisplacement of the uterus. Surg Gynecol Obstet 1915;20:598.

Kelly HA. Vaginal hysterectomy. In: Kelly HA, ed. Gynecology. New York: Appleton, 1928.

Kennedy JW, Campbell AD. Vaginal hysterectomy. Philadelphia: FA Davis, 1942.

Klempner E. Gynecological lesions and ureterohydronephrosis. Am J Obstet Gynecol 1952;64:1232.

Krige CF. The repair of genital prolapse combined with vaginal hysterectomy. J Obstet Gynaecol Br Comm 1962;69:570.

Lane FE. Repair of posthysterectomy vaginal-vault prolapse. Obstet Gynecol 1962;20:72.

Langenbeck JCM. Quoted by Senn N. The early history of vaginal hysterectomy. JAMA 1950;25:476.

Lawry EV. Traumatic lacerations of uterine supports. Am J Obstet Gynecol 1968;101:315.

Lee RA, Symmonds RE. Surgical repair of post hysterectomy vault prolapse. Am J Obstet Gynecol 1972;112:953.

LeFort L. Nouveau procede pour la guerison du prolapsus uterin. Bull Gen Ther 1877;92:237.

Leonard VN. The postoperative results of trachelorrhaphy in comparison with those of amputation of cervix. Surg Gynecol Obstet 1914;18:35.

Martin A. Ueber Exstirpatio Vaginae. Berl Klin Wschr 1898;35:910.

Mattingly RF. Surgery in the aging female. Clin Obstet Gynecol 1964;7:573.

McCall ML. Posterior culdeplasty: surgical correction of enterocele during vaginal hysterectomy. A preliminary report. Obstet Gynecol 1957;10:595.

Mengert WF. Mechanics of uterine support and position. Am J Obstet Gynecol 1936;31:775.

Milley PS, Nichols DH. A correlative investigation of the human rectovaginal septum. Anat Rec 1969;163:443.

Mueller-Heuback R. Prolapsus uteri causing hydronephrosis. J Am Geriat Soc 1969;17:1055.

Nichols DH, Milley PS, Randall CL. Significance of restoration of normal vaginal depth and axis. Obstet Gynecol 1970;36:251.

Nichols DH, Randall CL. Vaginal surgery. 3rd ed. Baltimore: Williams and Wilkins, 1989.

Olah KS, Bridges N, Denning J, Farrar DJ. The conservative management of patients with symptoms of stress incontinence: a randomized, prospective study comparing weighted vaginal cones and interferential therapy. Am J Obstet Gynecol 1990;162:87.

O'Leary JA, O'Leary JL. The extended Manchester operation: a review of 289 cases. Am J Obstet Gynecol 1970;107:546.

Olshausen R. Uber Ventrale Operation bei Prolapsus and Retroversio Uteri. Zbl Gynak 1886;10:698.

Paramore RH. The supports-in-chief of the female pelvic viscera. J Obstet Gynecol Br Emp 1908;14:173.

Parks AG, Swash M, Urich M. Sphincter denervation in anorectal incontinence. Gut 1977;18:656.

Parsons L, Ulfelder H. An atlas of pelvic operations. 2nd ed. Philadelphia: WB Saunders, 1968:280.

Percy NM, Perl JI. Total colpectomy. Surg Gynecol Obstet 1961; 113;175.

Phaneuf LE. The place of colpectomy in the treatment of uterine and vaginal prolapse. Trans Am Gynecol Soc 1935;60:142.

Plevnik S. New methods for testing and strengthening the pelvic floor muscles. In: Proceedings of the 15th Annual Meeting of the International Continence Society. London, 1985, p. 267.

Porges RF. Changing indications for vaginal hysterectomy. Am J Obstet Gynecol 1980;136:153.

Randall CL, Nichols DH. Surgical treatment of vaginal inversion. Obstet Gynecol 1971;38:327.

Range RL, Woodburne RT. The gross and microscopic anatomy of the transverse cervical ligament. Am J Obstet Gynecol 1964;90:460.

Ricci JV. Uterovaginal extirpation for procidentia. Am J Surg 1952;82:92.

Ricci JV, Thom CH. Uterovaginal extirpation for procidentia. Am J Surg 1953;83:192.

Richardson DA, Bent AE, Ostergard DR. The effects of uterovaginal prolapse on urethrovesical pressure dynamics. Am J Obstet Gynecol 1983;146:901.

Richardson DA, Scotti RJ, Ostergard DR. Surgical management of uterine prolapse in young women. J Reprod Med 1989;34:388.

Richardson EH. An efficient composite operation for uterine prolapse and associated pathology. Am J Obstet Gynecol 1937;34:814.

Richter K. Lebendige anatomie der vagina. Geburts u Frauenh 1966;26:1213.

Richter K, Frick H. Die anatomie der fascia pelvis visceralis aus didakticher sicht. Geburtshilfe Frauenheilkd 1985;45:282.

Riddle PR, Shawdon HH, Clay B. Procidentia and ureteric obstruction. Br J Urol 1975;47:387.

Ridley JH. Evaluation of the colpocleisis operation: a report of 58 cases. Am J Obstet Gynecol 1972;113:1114.

Schauta F. Uber Prolapsoperationen. Gynak Rundschau 1909;3:729.

Senn N. The early history of vaginal hysterectomy. JAMA 1895;25:476.

Shaw WF. The treatment of prolapsus uteri, with special reference to the Manchester operation of colporrhaphy. Am J Obstet Gynecol 1933;26:667.

Smith ARB, Hosker GL, Warrell DW. The role of partial denervation of the pelvic floor in the aetiology of genitourinary prolapse and stress incontinence of urine. A neurophysiological study. Br J Obstet Gynaecol 1989;96:24.

Smith ARB, Hosker GL, Warrell DW. The role of pudendal nerve damage in the aetiology of genuine stress incontinence in women. Br J Obstet Gynaecol 1989;96:29.

Solomons E. The cure of uterine prolapse with special reference to the Manchester operation. Am J Obstet Gynecol 1955;70:514.

Spalding AB. A study of frozen sections of the pelvis with description of an operation for pelvic prolapse. Surg Gynecol Obstet 1919;29:529.

Stanton S, Plevnik S, Peattie A. Cones: a conservative method of treating genuine stress incontinence. In: Proceedings of the 16th Annual Meeting of the International Continence Society. Boston, 1986, p. 227.

Stoesser FG. Construction of a sacrocervical ligament for uterine suspension. Surg Gynecol Obstet 1955;101:638.

Symmonds RE, Pratt JH. Vaginal prolapse following hysterectomy. Am J Obstet Gynecol 1960;79:899.

Taylor HC, Jr. Vascular congestion and hyperemia: their effect on structure and function in the female reproductive system. Am J Obstet Gynecol 1949;57:211.

Taylor HC, Jr. Vascular congestion and hyperemia. II. The clinical aspects of the congestion fibrosis syndrome. Am J Obstet Gynecol 1949;57:637.

Taylor HC, Jr. Vascular congestion and hyperemia. Their effect on function and structure in the female reproductive organs. III. Etiology and therapy. Am J Obstet Gynecol 1949;57:654.

Te Linde RW. Prolapse of the uterus and allied conditions. Am J Obstet Gynecol 1966;94:444.

Te Linde RW, Richardson EH, Jr. End results of the Richardson composite operation for uterine prolapse. Am J Obstet Gynecol 1943;45:29.

Thompson HG, Murphy CJ, Jr., Picot H. Hysterocolpectomy for the treatment of uterine procidentia. Am J Obstet Gynecol 1961; 82:748.

Thornton WN, Peters WA, III. Repair of vaginal prolapse after hysterectomy. Am J Obstet Gynecol 1983;147:140.

Tipton RH, Atkin PF. Uterine disease after the Manchester repair operation. J Obstet Gynaecol Br Comm 1970;77:852.

Tobin CE, Benjamin JA. Anatomical and surgical restudy of Denonvilliers' fascia. Surg Gynecol Obstet 1945;80:373.

Torpin R. Excision of the cul-de-sac of Douglas for the surgical care of hernias through the female caudal wall, including prolapse of the uterus. J Int Coll Surg 1955;24:322.

Uhlenhuth E, Day EC, Smith RD, Middleton EB. The visceral endopelvic fascia and the hypogastric sheath. Surg Gynecol Obstet 1948;86:9.

Uhlenhuth E, Wolfe WM, Smith EM, Middleton EB. The rectovaginal septum. Surg Gynecol Obstet 1948;86:148.

Watkins TJ. The treatment of cystocele and uterine prolapse after the menopause. Am J Obstet Gynecol 1899;15:420.

Watkins TJ. Transposition of the uterus and bladder in the treatment of extensive cystocele and uterine prolapse. Am J Obstet Gynecol 1912;65:225.

Webster JC. A satisfactory operation for certain cases of retroversion of the uterus. JAMA 1901;37:913.

Wertheim E. Zur plastischen Verwendung des Uterus bei Prolapsen. Zbl Gynak 1899;23:369.

White GR. Cystocele—a radical cure by suturing lateral sulci of vagina to the white line of pelvic fascia. JAMA 1907;53:1707.

Williams BFP. Surgical treatment for uterine prolapse in young women. Am J Obstet Gynecol 1966;95:967.

Zacharin RF. Pulsion enterocele: review of functional anatomy of the pelvic floor. Obstet Gynecol 1980;55:135.

32

Enterocele and Massive Eversion of the Vagina

DAVID H. NICHOLS

As a greater number of women live to an older age, massive eversion of the vagina is seen more frequently by gynecologists. Although the problem does not shorten or threaten life, it subtracts significantly from the quality of life of the afflicted, because more women are interested in maintaining sexual activity beyond menopause.

Massive eversion of the vagina is a complex disorder. Prolapse of the vaginal vault may or may not coexist with cystocele, rectocele, and enterocele, and the distinction is surgically important. The disorder can be remedied by carefully selected surgery, restoring the quality of life.

That a dropped uterus is the result of a genital prolapse and not the cause has not been appreciated by surgeons who would subject a patient with uterine prolapse to a "routine" hysterectomy without special attention to supporting the vaginal vault. The vaginal prolapse persists, of course, and sometime after their primary surgery these women are seen in consultation for reoperation. It is becoming more and more difficult to justify this unnecessary double expense, risk, inconvenience, and pain in our present system of practice.

Enterocele is a peritoneum-lined sac containing small bowel or omentum. The common posterior type is located between the vagina and rectum, in contrast to the uncommon ones located at other sites, such as anterior (anterior enterocele) or lateral (pudendal enterocele) to the vagina. Enterocele may occur with or without coincident prolapse or eversion of the vaginal vault. Eversion of the vaginal vault may be seen with or without coincident enterocele (the two occur together about three quarters of the time). Being of separate etiology, each must be recognized and separately repaired during surgical reconstruction, lest the unrepaired element become obvious postoperatively and require reoperation. To repair an enterocele and neglect an obvious vault eversion is as inadequate as repairing a vault eversion while ignoring an enterocele.

A deep cul-de-sac is a potential enterocele. Enterocele occurs when the sac is filled with omentum and loops of small bowel. For the latter to happen, a pathologically long intestinal mesentery is required. Still unanswered is the question of whether this long mesentery is the cause of the enterocele or the result of the presence of the deep cul-de-sac.

The content of the sac differentiates enterocele from an unusually deep, but empty, cul-de-sac of Douglas. In fetal life, the peritoneal cavity extends to a point of continuity with the cranial part of the perineal body, but this sac generally becomes obliterated early in life. Its fused tissues probably constitute a layer of the fascia of Denonvilliers adherent to the undersurface of the posterior vaginal wall, to which it adds a measure of supportive and surgically useful strength. This fascia forms the anterior margin of the avascular rectovaginal space, which permits the rectum and the vagina to function independently of each other. When fusion of the embryologic peritoneal sac fails to occur, the upper posterior vaginal wall lacks a complete layer of the fascia, the rectovaginal septum. Under some circumstances this area of weakness may give rise to a high rectocele and account for the frequent coexistence of high rectocele with enterocele. This coexistence is so likely that when one is found, a search must be made for the other, so that it too can be repaired in any surgery that is to be done.

A number of different surgical procedures are available to the patient and surgeon who have decided on surgical relief for vaginal prolapse. A skilled surgeon will be able to choose an operation or combination of operations that best fit the patient and will not be limited to a single operation. Although a surgeon tends to concentrate on operations he or she performs best, the various combinations of damage suggest that he or she should be familiar with a spectrum of alternate techniques.

Relief of the patient's symptoms constitutes the first goal of reconstructive surgery. The symptoms should be sufficiently severe that the patient requests relief. The various options open to her should be outlined. When it appears that a surgical remedy would be the best, the operative alternatives should be described along with the surgeon's reasons for a particular recommendation.

When symptoms to be treated surgically are the consequence of damage to one organ or organ system, obvious (though asymptomatic) damage to other pelvic organs should be noted. The additional damage, if likely to progress and become symptomatic, can be repaired at the time of the primary surgical procedure.

Since another goal of reconstructive surgery is restoration of anatomy to a normal state, a clear conception of what is "normal" is essential. The vagina with a vertical axis, as depicted in many anatomy textbooks, may be usual for an aged cadaver whose pelvic muscles are not only atrophic but fixed by embalming, but the position is not the normal one for a living, mature individual whose musculature is functional and without atrophy. If a colpogram is taken of the nulliparous vagina, which has been lightly coated with a barium paste, it is seen that the upper half of the vagina has an almost horizontal axis (Fig. 32-1) that is accentuated when the patient strains, as by a Valsalva maneuver. The upper vaginal axis is horizontal because the vagina lies on an intact and more or less horizontal levator plate formed by the fused posterior portion of the pubococcygei and extending from the posterior surface of the rectum to the sacrum (Fig. 32-2). When this levator plate tips, there is a tendency for anything resting on it to be pulled by gravity and to descend; moreover, the greater the tipping, the larger is the hiatus or opening through which the organ can herniate (Fig. 32-3).

At least seven distinctive anatomic systems are responsible for pelvic support: the bony pelvis, the peritoneum and subperitoneal retinaculum, the round and broad ligament complex, the cardinal–uterosacral ligament complex, the pelvic diaphragm (the levatores ani and their investing fascia), the urogenital diaphragm, and the perineum and perineal body. Probably no single cause or defect in any one anatomic system is responsible in all persons for the varieties of prolapse that may occur. Any of these structures may be defective or damaged in almost any possible combination, and the gynecologist must skillfully and clearly identify each site of damage and its probable cause.

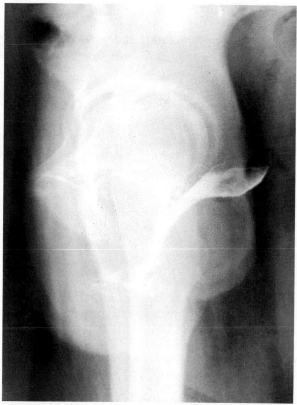

Figure 32–1. A normal vaginal depth and axis. Colpogram of a healthy, 25-year-old nulligravida standing at rest. The inferior margin of the pubis is seen in the half-circle to the left. The perineal curve of the lower vagina is shown along the more horizontal axis of the upper vagina. (From Nichols DH, Milley PS, Randall CL. Significance of restoration of normal vaginal depth and axis. Obstet Gynecol 1970; 35:251. With permission of the American College of Obstetricians and Gynecologists.)

CAUSES AND TYPES OF DAMAGE TO PELVIC SUPPORTS

The combination of etiologic factors includes congenital weakness, parity, aging, and life-style. A genetic contribution may be suggested by the presence of a family history of the condition.

Support factors in the pelvis are not always within our control, as congenital defects of tissue strength and muscular innervation may be more common than previously thought. An otherwise strong levator ani with a congenital or acquired unsatisfactory innervation may not function well. Chronically increased intra-abdominal pressure plays a role in genital prolapse, as in the person who wears a girdle or corset that is too tight, someone who does heavy manual labor, or a person

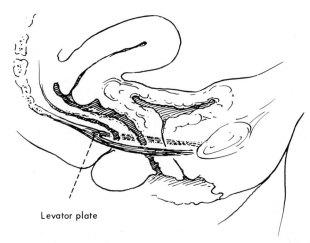

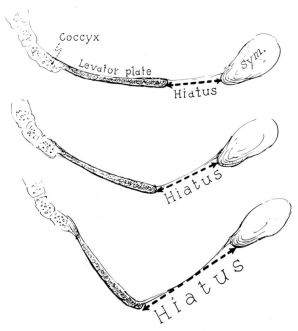

Figure 32–2. Drawing of normal vaginal axis, showing almost horizontal upper vagina and rectum lying upon and parallel to the levator plate. (From Nichols DH, Milley PS, Randall CL. Significance of restoration of normal vaginal depth and axis. Obstet Gynecol 1970; 36:251. With permission of the American College of Obstetricians and Gynecologists.)

Figure 32–3. As the levator plate tips, the genital hiatus becomes larger, as shown. In addition, the pull of gravity and the forces of intra-abdominal pressure accentuate the strain on the pelvic suspensory system. (From Nichols DH, Randall CL. Vaginal surgery. 3rd ed. Baltimore: Williams & Wilkins, 1989:336. With permission.)

who is responsible for the daily care of an infirm patient who must be lifted to and from bed, bathtub, and commode. Nursing professionals are at risk, as they are often responsible for moving and lifting heavy patients without adequate help. Chronic coughing or obstructive pulmonary disease increases intra-abdominal pressure.

Obstetric damage is sometimes predictable. Bearing down prior to full dilatation of the cervix pushes the cervix ahead of the baby, at times stretching beyond capacity those pelvic connective tissues concerned with support of the cervix and the upper vagina.

The degenerative features of aging and menopause are evident. Aging may be a factor in at least two ways: the loss of estrogenic support of tissue consequent to the menopause and the inability of the tissue to repair effectively or replicate essential structural components consequent to natural biologic exhaustion of these qualities within an individual. That there is a loss of pelvic tissue elasticity with menopausal aging is clear. Probably this process can be effectively slowed or at times reversed by adequate long-term estrogen supplementation. Although no one can stop aging, some of the atrophic effects within the vaginal skin may be minimized by appropriate estrogen replacement therapy.

Massive eversion of the vagina can occur in both young and old persons, whether the uterus is present or not. It is more common in the white person than the black for reasons not totally understood. In many instances, unrepaired genital descent will progress to procidentia, the displacement of the entire uterus outside of the pelvic cavity.

Because various etiologic factors are at work, restoration requires different surgical procedures.

Figure 32-4 depicts descent of the uterus and an obvious enterocele. This is the most common type of uterine prolapse. The cervix is outside the pelvis, and there is a cystocele and enterocele but no rectocele. The relationship between the cervix and the anterior wall of the rectum is changed, because the cul-de-sac and its peritoneum have dissected between the rectum and vagina. The latter actually slides along the anterior wall of the rectum, the vaginal opposite of rectal prolapse.

Figure 32-5 shows an obvious protrusion of the cervix beyond the vulva. Notice the rectocele and cystocele without an enterocele. This condition represents the less common *general* prolapse, which is usually postmenopausal, and includes weakness of all the pelvic supporting tissues, with consequent descent of the cul-de-sac. All the genitalia have dropped, but the relationship between the anterior rectal wall and the back of the uterus is unchanged, being the same as when the genitalia were higher within the pelvis. There is displacement of the cul-de-sac, but it does not dissect between the rectum and vagina, as would be true of an enterocele. One must make this distinction, because both

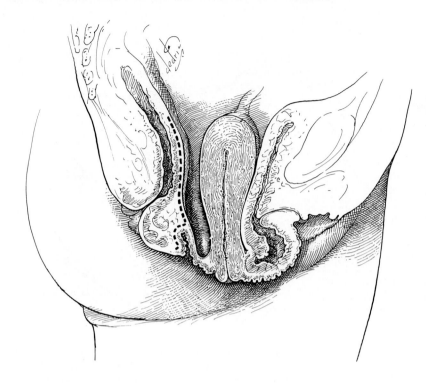

Figure 32–4. Uterovaginal or sliding prolapse is depicted. Enterocele is present, but no rectocele. The rectovaginal septum and position of the anterior rectal wall are indicated by the dotted lines. (After Halban and Tandler, from Nichols DH, Randall CL. Vaginal surgery. 3rd ed. Baltimore: Williams & Wilkins, 1989:79. With permission.)

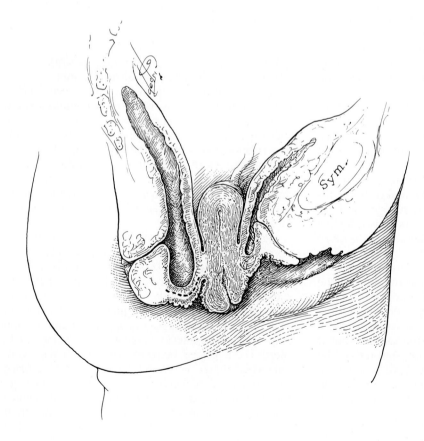

Figure 32–5. This illustration depicts a general postmenopausal prolapse resulting from atrophy and weakening of all the endopelvic supporting tissues. A rectocele is present but no enterocele. The rectovaginal septum in the anterior rectal wall is indicated by the dotted line. (From Nichols DH, Randall CL. Vaginal surgery. 3rd ed. Baltimore: Williams & Wilkins, 1989:80. With permission.)

etiology and surgical therapy of the condition shown in Figure 32-4 are entirely different from the usual uterovaginal or "sliding" prolapse.

TYPES OF ENTEROCELE

One must consider the different types of enterocele that may result from either a single or combined source of damage to understand why the treatment of each type must be different. The location correlates with the cause and determines the treatment of enterocele (Table 32-1). In these three examples, massive eversion of the vagina is developing. For the sake of simplicity, the uterus in Figure 32-6 has been removed. Congenital enterocele results from failure of fusion or reopening of the previous fusion of the peritoneum so that the bowel-filled cul-de-sac may extend by dissection all the way to the perineal body. The surgical treatment is that of exposing and mobilizing the sac, ligating the neck, and excising the sac.

With a pulsion type of enterocele the vault of the vagina is probably being pushed and everted by chronic increases in intra-abdominal pressure as with heavy lifting. Among other causes, the patient may have asthma, emphysema, hay fever, vasomotor rhinitis, or any number of respiratory difficulties. She may be a smoker whose chronic coughing has pushed the vaginal vault down. As it descends, the vault will ultimately bring along with it the structures to which the vagina is attached. If one were to treat this patient by the same operation as that used to correct congenital enterocele,

one would likely resect the loose or unsupported portion of the upper vagina, leaving, to the chagrin of both surgeon and patient, a very short vagina. This patient requires suspension or fixation of the vaginal vault as a means of restoring vaginal depth.

When cystocele and rectocele coexist with enterocele and eversion of the vault, this type might be characterized as a traction descent of the vault wherein it may have been pulled down consequent to a general soft tissue weakness associated with this cystocele and rectocele. This circumstance requires colporrhaphy as well as colpopexy to reestablish both vaginal depth and axis.

The fourth type of enterocele is iatrogenic, usually following a surgically produced change in vaginal axis (such as a vesicourethral "pin-up" operation like those of Burch or Marshall-Marchetti-Kranz or a ventral suspension), which leaves the cul-de-sac unprotected. It is important to distinguish pseudoenterocele from enterocele.

Figure 32-7 illustrates pseudoenterocele in a patient whose midvaginal rectocele was not treated, although a simple perineorrhaphy had been performed. A precept in rectocele repair is that the repair should begin at a point cranial to the site of damage.

There are partial degrees of eversion that, if undiagnosed or ignored at hysterectomy or left otherwise unattended, will generally progress (Fig. 32-8). Without cystocele or rectocele a poorly supported vault may be pushed down. In the presence of progressive cystocele and rectocele an unsupported vault may be pulled down.

TABLE 32–1
Correlation Between Etiology, Location, and Treatment of Enterocele

CAUSE	LOCATION	TREATMENT
Congenital	Sac between posterior vaginal wall and anterior rectal wall	Excision of the sac with high ligation of its neck; approximation of uterosacral ligaments
Pulsion (pushed)	With eversion of vaginal vault	Restore vault depth by shortening cardinal-uterosacral ligaments or cul-de-plasty if ligaments are strong
		If ligaments are of poor quality, do sacrospinous fixation or sacrocolpopexy; coincident hysterectomy often desirable
Traction (pulled)	Lower eversion (cystocele and rectocele) pulling vault into eversion	Use same procedure as above plus anterior and posterior colporrhaphy
Iatrogenic	Anterior to vagina or posterior from change in vaginal axis	Excise or obliterate sac and restore normal vaginal axis if it is defective

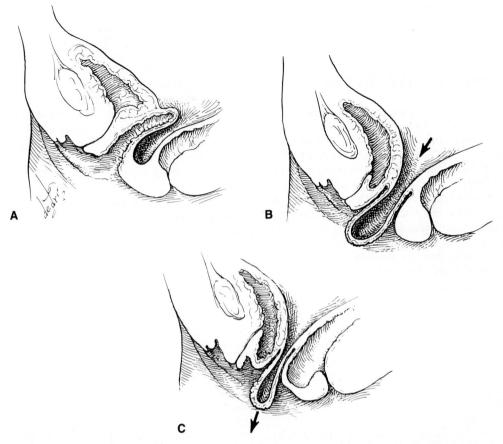

Figure 32–6. *A,* Posterior enterocele, probably congenital, without eversion of the vagina. *B,* The *arrow* indicates increased intra-abdominal pressure. The vagina is everted and the pulsion enterocele sac follows the everted vault. Cystocele and rectocele are minimal. *C,* There is eversion of the vagina with traction enterocele, cystocele, and rectocele. The *arrow* indicates traction to the vault of the vagina. (From Nichols DH. Types of enterocele and principles underlying the choice of operation for repair. Obstet Gynecol 1972; 40:257. With permission of the American College of Obstetricians and Gynecologists.)

SYMPTOMS

It is unlikely that one can improve by surgery the comfort of an asymptomatic patient, but if symptoms are present, one must decide if they are sufficiently disabling to require surgery and match the symptoms of the disorder to the surgery. Enterocele and vault prolapse are often associated with a feeling of pelvic heaviness and pressure. The bearing-down sensation, often exacerbated with prolonged standing, results from the pull of gravity stretching the mesentery of the sac contents. If the cardinal and uterosacral ligaments are involved in the prolapse, downward traction on the uterosacral ligaments often gives rise to backache, which may worsen as the day goes on and is relieved somewhat by lying down. There may be vaginal discomfort from the presence of a protruding vulvar mass. Coincident dyspareunia is common, accentuated by dryness of the exteriorized vagina. If the vaginal skin is ulcerated, there may be troublesome discharge and bleeding. When rectocele coexists, the patient may experience difficulty emptying the bowel, incomplete movements, and postevacuation aching.

Urinary complaints are uncommon unless displacement cystocele coexists and there is inability to empty the bladder, resulting in stagnation of urine with overflow incontinence. Urinary stress incontinence is uncommon but may result from a coincident hypermobile urethra. Thoughtful and appropriate primary reconstructive genital surgery should provide relief from the discomfort and distress of all these symptoms.

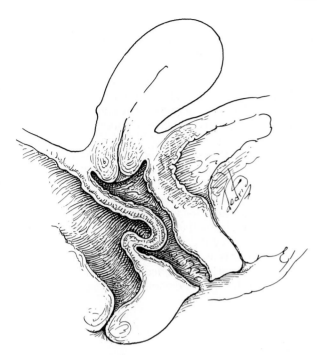

Figure 32–7. A perineorrhaphy may hide an unrepaired midvaginal rectocele. Effective repair must always begin proximal to the point of weakness. (From Nichols DH, Randall CL. Vaginal surgery. 3rd ed. Baltimore: Williams & Wilkins, 1989:276. With permission.)

DIAGNOSIS AND TREATMENT

Physical Examination

A careful overall assessment of the patient's general physical health should be made, including a measurement of her blood pressure, weight, and height without shoes (noting at each annual examination any possible changes indicative of vertebral compression), auscultation of the lungs and heart, and inspection and palpation of the breasts. One should note the patient's posture, and the presence and width of abdominal wall striae, which indicate the elasticity of the patient's connective tissue. The genitalia should be inspected and any degree of vulvar atrophy or genital prolapse should be noted.

Bonney described two general systems maintaining pelvic integrity: the upper suspensory system and lower supportive system. After the prolapsed organs have been gently replaced even in a person with total eversion of the vagina, the patient is asked to bear down, as in a Valsalva maneuver. The site of primary damage will appear first at the vulva, followed by the sites of secondary damage. When damage to the upper suspensory system is primary, the cervix or vaginal vault will appear first followed by any cystocele and rectocele. With primary damage to the lower supportive system, a cystocele and rectocele will appear first, followed by the cervix or vaginal vault. For those patients to whom surgery will be recommended, the gynecologist should take special note of the site of primary damage. In planning the patient's operation, the surgeon should remember Bonney's rule: the primary site of damage should be identified and overrepaired to lessen the chance of recurrence. Beyond this generic classification of upper and lower factors with pelvic support, one can define the seven separate anatomic systems described earlier that may be damaged either singly or in any combination. An effort should be made to determine the specific site of primary damage as well as the nature and extent of any secondary damage to any of these systems. The patient is initially examined when she is in the lithotomy position. A careful bimanual examination is performed. On

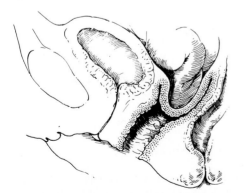
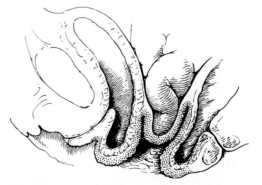

Figure 32–8. (*Left*) A partial eversion of the vagina without cystocele and rectocele is noted after hysterectomy. (*Right*) A partial eversion of the vaginal vault after hysterectomy coexists with obvious cystocele and rectocele. (From Nichols DH. Repair of enterocele and prolapse of the vaginal vault. In: Goldsmith HS. Practice of surgery. Woodbury, Conn.: Ciné-Med, 1981.)

asking the patient to contract her pubococcygei, thus squeezing the vagina, the examiner should note the strength and symmetry of contraction. A rectal examination should be performed to note any palpable pathology, the presence of any blood on the examining finger, the strength and effectiveness of the external anal sphincter, the presence of rectocele, and the presence of perineal defect. The general architecture of the patient's bony pelvis should be assessed.

Descent of the cul-de-sac without enterocele is primarily related to a major defect of the pelvic diaphragm. It is usually, although not always, seen in a postmenopausal person in whom the pelvic diaphragm sags and the levator plate tips, causing the loss of the normally horizontal axis of the upper vagina. Descent of the cul-de-sac differs from enterocele, which is an actual herniation of bowel between rectum and vagina. The proper time to make this distinction is prior to examination in the operating room, when the patient is recumbent.

Damage that is obvious when the patient is awake and straining is now less evident. One must be mindful of the findings observed previously in the examining room.

An effective way of distinguishing between enterocele, prolapse of the vaginal vault, rectocele, and combinations of these weaknesses is by supplemental examination of the unanesthetized patient in a standing position.

The patient should be asked to stand and the vaginal examination should be repeated, first with the patient at rest, then "holding," and finally straining. The presence of any vault eversion should be noted and the posterior and anterior vaginal wall and their supports should be reassessed (Fig. 32-9). One should observe how much the cystocele sags beneath the inferior margin of the pubis. If the patient complains of coincident urinary or rectal incontinence, this too should be evaluated carefully. Then the vault of the vagina should be

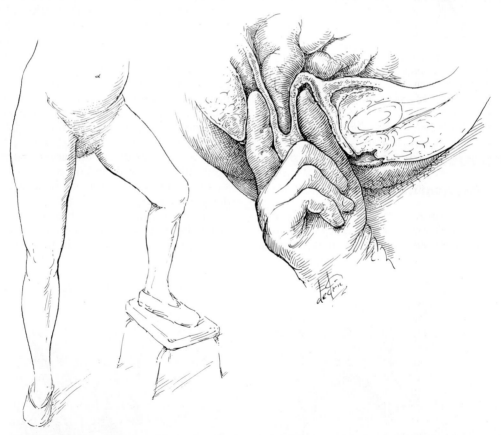

Figure 32–9. Examination of the patient in a standing position permits the thumb in the vagina to note and replace any descent of the vaginal vault, whereas the index finger introduced into the rectum permits evaluation of any possible rectocele. When the patient strains, any enterocele present is evident by palpation of a bowel-filled sac dissecting the rectovaginal septum. (From Nichols DH. Repair of enterocele and prolapse of the vaginal vault. In: Goldsmith HS. Practice of surgery. Woodbury, Conn.: Ciné-Med, 1981.)

replaced to its highest level within the pelvis, and the results should be noted when the patient is asked to bear down by a Valsalva maneuver. If in this situation a peritoneal sac containing omentum or a palpable loop of bowel comes down between the thumb and index finger, the patient has an enterocele.

Nonoperative Treatment of Genital Prolapse

Nonoperative treatment can sometimes be recommended. This may include a change in the patient's lifestyle, so that heavy lifting is eliminated. At times estrogen replacement will be recommended, and the patient may be instructed in initiating a long-term course of Kegel or perineal resistive exercises.

When symptoms of pelvic fullness, pressure, and bearing down are present but not severe enough to warrant consideration for surgery, or when for various medical or social reasons surgery is impossible, these nonoperative means can provide effective help. Improved tissue elasticity, restoration of vaginal thickness, and improved blood supply will sometimes follow long-term estrogen supplementation when given by the systemic route. The additional sustained regular use of intravaginal estrogen cream more effectively supplies a measured dose to the target tissue. For the severely atrophic birth canal one might recommend installation of 2 g of estrogen cream at bedtime, three times per week for 2–4 weeks, with gradual tapering of the dose to a maintenance level of one application at bedtime once per week. This may lessen the speed of prolapse progression and will relieve many patients of the symptoms of urinary urgency and precipitancy.

Effectively treating coincident medical problems will improve the patient's overall and gynecologic sense of well-being. The control and treatment of cardiovascular disease will be helpful, and adequate attention should be given to any symptom of chronic constipation. Chronic respiratory disease, errors in carbohydrate metabolism, arthritis, and obesity are especially responsive to careful attention and followup.

A sustained program of voluntary exercises of the muscle of the pelvic diaphragm and pelvic sphincter system by effective isometric contractions of these pelvic muscles will be helpful in strengthening tissue relationships and improving function, especially if any urinary stress incontinence is present. Improvement should be seen, especially in the patient in whom, with straining, the cystocele drops to less than 4 cm beneath the lower border of the pubic symphysis, measured when the patient strains while she is standing. An effective program of voluntary exercise of these pelvic muscles consists of 15 strong voluntary contractions, each of 3

seconds duration, six times per day (ie, on arising and at midmorning, lunchtime, midafternoon, suppertime, and bedtime). The patient should be told that these can be done even in public places and that it is unimportant whether she is standing, sitting, or lying down. Because the muscles are deep within the pelvic cavity, their exercise is not visible externally. For the sedentary person, a general improvement in muscle tone will follow a program of brisk daily exercise (eg, walking) and restoration and maintenance of good body posture.

For those patients requiring mechanical support of the prolapse, a well-fitting intravaginal pessary may be helpful. Choices range from a plastic ring, a plastic Gellhorn pessary, a rubber doughnut, or an inflatable pessary in an effective size. Some strength of the pelvic diaphragm measured at the levator "sling" or hiatus where the levator ani crosses the sides of the vagina is necessary for the patient to be able to retain a pessary comfortably. The patient should not be able to feel a properly fitted pessary. If the patient cannot remove it nightly for cleaning, this must be done, at first monthly, then quarterly by someone else who will note and treat any effect of pessary pressure upon the vagina. Since a pessary stretches the vagina in various directions and dimensions, the required size may become larger as time goes by, so that the fit must be evaluated by the examiner from time to time and the size or style changed as necessary.

Operative Approach

With increased operator skill and greater safety in anesthesia during hospitalization, an operative approach to solving a mechanical problem will often be optimal even for elderly patients. The comfort of surgical reconstruction can be extended to increased numbers of women, with the decision based not upon their age but upon their general medical health and life expectancy. To be cost effective, the right operation must be chosen on an individual basis and must be done correctly the first time. The choice may range from a perineorrhaphy done to enable the patient to retain a pessary (which can be accomplished under local anesthesia if necessary) to a hysterectomy with colporrhaphy and colpopexy for the patient with prolapse who wishes to preserve coital interest. Colpocleisis or colpectomy may be considered for the patient for whom vaginal function is not a consideration.

Vaginal hysterectomy with shortening of the cardinal–uterosacral complex support of the vaginal cuff plus colporrhaphy is the surgical treatment that responds effectively to the goals of reconstructive surgery in the majority of patients (see Chapters 27 and 31).

When uterosacral ligaments are long and strong, the addition of a McCall or New Orleans type of culdoplasty will help to reestablish vaginal length. Careful attention must be given to the presence and correlation of any enterocele, lest a posthysterectomy vaginal eversion be initiated that would complicate a number of these patients in their postoperative years. When at surgery there is insufficient cardinal–uterosacral ligament strength to which the vaginal wall can be attached with the confidence that it will remain there, the vault may be anchored to a strong nongynecologic pelvic support, such as the sacrospinous ligament. In this setting sacrospinous colpopexy as part of the primary procedure is a useful addition. When the cervix is elongated and strong cardinal uterosacral ligament support is evident, the Manchester operation consisting of cervical amputation with mobilization and attachment of the cardinal ligaments anterior to the cervix, followed by appropriate colporrhaphy, will support the vagina. One must be mindful, however, that a dropped uterus is the *result* of a genital prolapse and not the cause. Because uterine bleeding sometimes follows estrogen supplementation, this approach is not as popular in the United States as is vaginal hysterectomy.

Le Fort colpocleisis is an effective, quick, and relatively simple method of vaginal obliteration, but it has several notable disadvantages:

1. The operation removes the coital potential, disturbing the patient's concept of her femininity.
2. The operation retains the uterus, which may bleed in the future. The diagnosis of the cause of such bleeding is difficult, because access to the uterine cavity is hindered by the partial vaginal obliteration.
3. By fixing the base of the bladder and vesicourethral junction to the anterior rectal wall the surgeon may create a flattening of the posterior urethrovesical angle, permitting urinary stress incontinence, which when socially disabling will be most difficult to treat.
4. Because the Le Fort operation is extraperitoneal, any enterocele will remain untreated and will often progress, with subsequent discomfort to both the patient and her surgeon.

For the posthysterectomy patient a colpectomy removes the prolapsed vagina, and although any problems with future uterine bleeding cannot occur, the other objections to colpocleisis noted earlier still obtain. An ideal treatment to achieve the goals of reconstructive surgery for the posthysterectomy patient with vault eversion consists of effective colpopexy with appropriate colporrhaphy. An experienced vaginal surgeon can accomplish this operation through a single vaginal exposure via sacrospinous colpopexy with excision of any enterocele, and with colporrhaphy.

For the experienced abdominal operator, or in a patient with an undiagnosed adnexal mass or any other indication for abdominal exploration, transabdominal sacral colpopexy is indicated, with appropriate transvaginal colporrhaphy, though this obviously requires deeper and longer anesthesia.

No single operation for the restoration of normal anatomy will correct all the pathology that might be present in the various types of prolapse. Often a combination of procedures designed for the individual case is required. Pessaries are occasionally of temporary help in some women who are not candidates for surgery or whose personal schedule will not permit surgery because of responsibilities such as small children at home, pressing career demands, or an aging relative who requires constant care. If a pessary can be retained, it will often be the ring type, occasionally a rubber doughnut or sometimes a Gellhorn. Isometric pubococcygeal contraction exercises are helpful in restoring muscle tone but usually are not curative.

At the time of initial vaginal hysterectomy and repair, one can do much to prevent postoperative enterocele. Enterocele may be present, but not obvious, in the patient who is sound asleep in the Trendelenburg position with the pull of gravity toward the head of the table. After the uterus has been removed and before the peritoneum has been closed, one should hook a finger in the cul-de-sac to see if there is extra cul-de-sac peritoneum that should be excised. If strong uterosacral ligaments are found, they should be shortened and used to help support the vaginal vault. A culdoplasty in which sutures penetrate and attach the now shortened, but surgically useful and strong, uterosacral ligaments to the vaginal cuff will, when sutures are tied, bring the vault of the vagina back into the hollow of the sacrum, actually cranial and posterior to the point at which the peritoneum has been closed. The same stitches may be effectively used for supporting the vagina during abdominal hysterectomy. If the vagina is widened excessively, a wedge may be excised from the posterior vaginal vault followed by side-to-side approximation of the cut lateral edges of the triangle. Following vaginal hysterectomy, a high purse-string or H-closure of the peritoneal cavity is helpful in most instances. The suture used in the peritoneal closure should penetrate both uterosacral and round ligaments. The surgeon should, however, be mindful of the course of the ureters to avoid kinking them when the suture is tied. Such sutures, by incorporating the subperitoneal retinaculum to which the peritoneum is attached, bring the strength of connective tissue to a closure that would otherwise involve only a single cell layer. If a large enterocele has been resected, one might wish to use two of these purse-string sutures, one caudad to the other.

Amreich indicated the importance of preserving vaginal depth following hysterectomy. If, after removal of the uterus, the vagina is otherwise well supported and sits upon an intact levator plate, intra-abdominal pressure applied to the vagina will be countered by pressure from the pelvic diaphragm. The vagina will be compressed by these two opposing pressures and remain in place. If, however, the vagina is shortened following hysterectomy, it may in time become even shorter. Lacking the length that would place the upper vagina over the levator plate and therefore in a horizontal direction, a short vagina will have an axis that tends to be vertically directed and to end anterior to the levator plate. Increased intra-abdominal pressure will thus cause it to telescope in upon itself. An exception is the patient who has had a Wertheim or Schauta radical cancer operation in which the scarring around the vagina is so great that very little will disturb it. Preserving vaginal depth is an important prophylactic feature of all genital surgery.

Transabdominal Surgery

The difficult problem of genital prolapse may be approached by a number of abdominal procedures that result in varying degrees of success. Ventral fixation of the prolapsing uterus or vaginal vault to the anterior abdominal wall was once popular. Although the patient may be reasonably comfortable for a while, the cause of the prolapse has not been relieved, and given enough time, progression of the prolapse will continue.

By changing the axis of the vagina, ventral fixation leaves a vulnerable cul-de-sac exposed to increase in intra-abdominal pressure (Fig. 32-10). Although the uterine fundus may remain fixed, the uterus and cervix elongate until ultimately the vagina and those organs to which it is attached come down again. The patient, meanwhile, often has forgotten the nature of her surgery done so many years ago. The records have been lost, the surgeon may no longer be in practice, and one may start what appears to be a routine vaginal hysterectomy only to find on opening the peritoneal cavity that the fundus of the uterus goes all the way to the anterior abdominal wall. A confirmatory tug on the cervix at that point will produce visible dimpling in the anterior abdominal wall. The surgeon now knows the true nature of what had been done before.

When Burch presented his excellent results in treating urinary incontinence by fixation of the vagina to Cooper's ligament, it was pointed out that the incidence of subsequent enterocele was between 11% and 15%. The probable explanation was that the change in vaginal axis caused the now unprotected cul-de-sac to become directly vulnerable to increased intra-abdominal

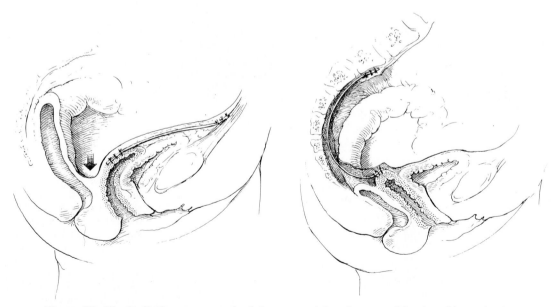

Figure 32–10. (*Left*) The unprotected cul-de-sac remaining after ventral fixation of the vagina is noted by the arrow. (*Right*) The vagina has been fixed to the promontory of the sacrum by a retroperitoneal bridge using Mersilene mesh, Gore-Tex, or of fascia. The cul-de-sac is no longer vulnerable. (From Nichols DH. Repair of enterocele and prolapse of the vaginal vault. In: Goldsmith HS. Practice of surgery. Woodbury, Conn.: Ciné-Med, 1981.)

pressure to which it may not have been previously subject. The cul-de-sac should be clearly obliterated as a separate step with any abdominal surgery that changes the normal horizontal axis of the upper vagina. After Moschcowitz introduced circumferential purse-string ligation of the cul-de-sac for treatment of rectal prolapse, some gynecologic surgeons appropriated the procedure for the treatment of genital prolapse. A number of problems emerged with the adaptation, however. Tying the top stitch at the pelvic brim is difficult, and if any central opening remains, the hole can provide access to a loop of small bowel and may cause intestinal obstruction. It unsuccessfully supports a prolapsed vagina, the failure secondary to the mobility of the rectum. Additionally, although the stitch may not be placed in the ureter itself, it may be close enough to pull or displace the tissue to which the ureter is attached. Thus, one or both ureters may be sufficiently kinked to cause obstruction. Halban suggested an alternate method of treating the cul-de-sac: five or six stitches are passed through the peritoneum of the pelvic floor in parallel sagittal planes and held untied (Fig. 32-11). When all the sutures have been placed, they are then tied very effec-

tively obliterating the cul-de-sac without compromising the position of the ureter.

The transabdominal method of retroperitoneal sacral colpopexy is a satisfactory though complex procedure. It is attractive particularly when the abdomen must be opened for an unrelated reason such as removal of an ovarian tumor. The major problem with this concept is that if cystocele and rectocele are present, they would not be effectively treated by this operation. Arthure and Savage attached the fundus of the uterus to the periosteum of the sacrum, as did Falk. Alternatively, and better, one can remove the uterus and attach the vagina to the sacrum by a retroperitoneal bridge of Mersilene mesh Gore-Tex, or a fascial graft. This procedure reestablishes a more or less horizontal vaginal axis.

Transvaginal Surgery

A frequent problem is that of an aging but sexually active patient who has vaginal eversion, cystocele, and rectocele but who is unable to retain a vaginal pessary.

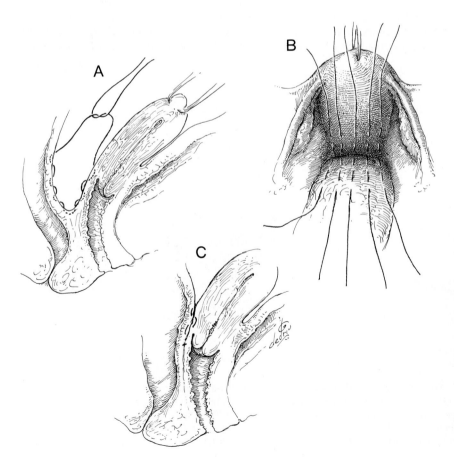

Figure 32–11. The cul-de-sac is being obliterated by a series of interrupted stitches placed from front to back. The placement of the stitches is shown in sagittal section *A,* as viewed from the abdomen, *B.* After all have been placed, they are tied, as shown in *C.* If the uterus is no longer present, stitches are placed in the posterior wall of the vagina and the anterior rectal wall. (From Nichols DH. Repair of enterocele and prolapse of the vaginal vault. In: Goldsmith HS. Practice of surgery. Woodbury, Conn.: Ciné-Med, 1981.)

Particularly in the postmenopausal patient progression of the genital prolapse may have been gradual. The prolapsed uterus can be removed, and if there are strong cardinal and uterosacral ligaments these should be shortened and used to support the vaginal vault.

Occasionally, however, it becomes evident that there is nothing of strength to which to attach the vagina with confidence that it will stay in place. Such a person demonstrates a *general* prolapse with descent of the vault, a quarter of the time without a true enterocele. This situation usually represents a major problem with the integrity of all endopelvic soft tissues and particularly of the pelvic diaphragm. When the vagina is completely everted, its lateral attachments to the arcus tendineus may have been severely compromised or avulsed. Support of the vault by colpopexy and colporrhaphy may restore vaginal support. The transvaginal paravaginal fixation suggested by White in 1909 sews the stretched fornices directly to the arcus tendineus. A very effective transvaginal operation that reestablishes a horizontal vaginal axis and returns the vagina to the hollow of the sacrum is that of sewing the vagina to the sacrospinous ligament, an operation first described in 1892 by Zweifel. The transvaginal approach permits simultaneous treatment of any cystocele and rectocele by colporrhaphy. The procedure may be effective for posthysterectomy vaginal vault eversion or in conjunction with vaginal hysterectomy in the patient whose cardinal–uterosacral ligament complex is too attenuated to be used for adequate vault support. The sacrospinous ligament is contained within the coccygeus muscle (Fig. 32-12). Having the same origin and insertion as the muscle, the ligament can be easily palpated as it runs from the ischial spine to the sacrum. To find it safely, one must understand the nature and boundaries of the connective tissue spaces and septa. A fiberoptic headlight is useful in illuminating the depths of the wound. Special retractors are helpful (Figs. 32-13, 32-14), as are long-handled ligature carriers and suture hooks, such as those shown in Figure 32-15. If the surgeon is using curved Deaver retractors, he or she must place them with special care and caution the assistant to avoid sweeping them across the anterior surface of the sacrum, risking damage to the penetrating sacral veins.

Surgical Technique of Transvaginal Sacrospinous Colpopexy

Transvaginal sacrospinous colpopexy (Fig. 32-16) immediately following vaginal hysterectomy in patients with uterine prolapse and without strong uterosacral–cardinal ligament support is surprisingly easy, because there is no scarring from previous surgery. The operation can be accomplished with an additional 15

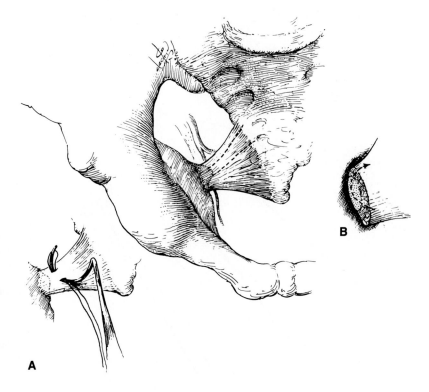

Figure 32–12. Location of the sacrospinous ligament deep within the substance of the coccygeus muscle is shown by the dotted line. The sciatic nerve and pudendal artery are shown behind the ischial spine. To avoid them, penetration of the coccygeus muscle and sacrospinous ligament is made 2–3 cm medial to the ischial spine, as indicated in *A*. Note that the ligature carrier has been placed through the muscle and ligament and not around them. The path of a ligature is shown by the dotted line in *B*; a cross section of the sacrospinous ligament is represented by the stippled area within the coccygeus muscle. (From Nichols DH. Effects of pelvic relaxation on gynecologic and urologic problems. Clin Obstet Gynecol 1978;21:770.)

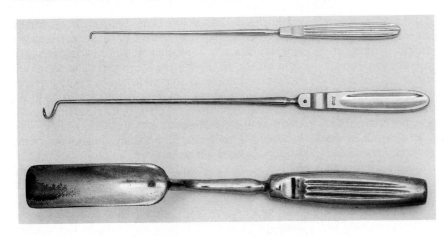

Figure 32–13. A Breisky-Navratil retractor is shown (*bottom*) along with a long Deschamps ligature carrier (*center*) for the right hand, and a small hook. (From Nichols DH, Randall CL. Vaginal surgery. 3rd ed. Baltimore: Williams & Wilkins, 1989:340. With permission.)

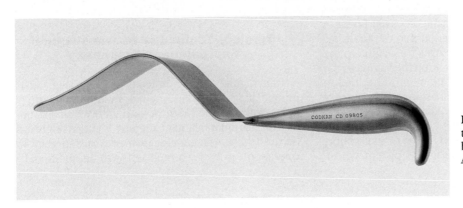

Figure 32–14. Long, straight retractor, available in various widths by special order from Codman or American V. Mueller.

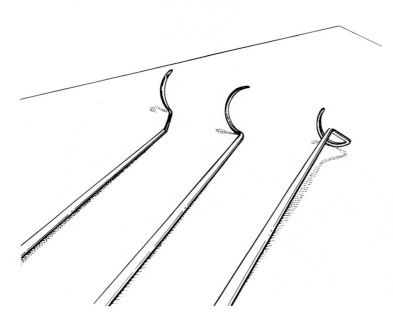

Figure 32–15. Modifications of the tips of the long-handled Deschamps ligature carrier (*center*) are shown in which repositioning the handle to the center of the arc, rather than at its periphery, causes the size of the circular excursion of the tip to be halved, as noted at the right. This is useful when operating in an unusually confined space. An angled Deschamps ligature carrier modeled after one modified by Rosenshein, noted at the left, is useful when the sacrospinous ligament is unusually deep, but there is plenty of room in which to operate. The handle must be swung through a wide arc. These instruments are available on special order from Codman or American V. Mueller.

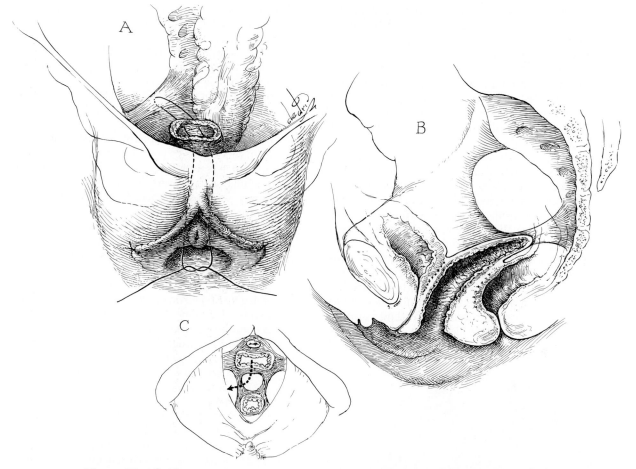

Figure 32–16. The everted vagina has been sewn to the right sacrospinous ligament, 2–3 cm medial to the ischial spine, as shown in frontal view in *A* and in sagittal view in *B*. Notice the restoration of normal vaginal depth and axis. *Dotted line* and *arrow C* trace the path of the incision from the vagina into the rectovaginal space, then through the right rectal pillar to the right pararectal space, thence to the ischial spine and sacrospinous ligament. (From Randall CL, Nichols DH. Surgical treatment of vaginal inversion. Obstet Gynecol 1971; 38:327. With permission from the ACOG.)

minutes of operating time. The sequence of events in this instance is as follows:

1. Vaginal hysterectomy.
2. Excision of any enterocele with high ligation of the sac and closure of the peritoneal cavity.
3. Anterior colporrhaphy.
4. Incision of the perineal skin and posterior vaginal mucosa to open the rectovaginal space. Penetration of the right rectal pillar overlying the right ischial spine, to enter the right pararectal space. (The ischial spine and the sacrospinous ligament–coccygeus muscle complex form a portion of the lateral wall of the pararectal space.)
5. Sacrospinous colpopexy stitches placed.

6. Repair upper part of posterior colporrhaphy.
7. Tie sacrospinous colpopexy stitches.
8. Completion of posterior colpoperineorrhaphy.

If the uterus has been removed previously and there is posthysterectomy eversion of the vaginal vault, the sequence and techniques, described for the right-handed operator, are as follows:

1. The initial surgical incision is made through the perineum and posterior vaginal wall to enter the rectovaginal space.
2. Any enterocele is identified and opened. The neck of the enterocele sac is carefully palpated for any usable uterosacral ligament strength,

which in massive eversion is usually found lacking. After the neck of the sac is closed, the sac is excised and the operator proceeds with the sacrospinous colpopexy.

3. When the rectum has been carefully displaced by an appropriate retractor to the patient's left, the right ischial spine is carefully palpated. For proper suture placement, the surgeon needs to form a window through the descending rectal septum over the ischial spine. This window can be established by blunt penetration with the operator's finger, by the closed tips of curved Mayo scissors, or by a sharp-pointed hemostat as the resistance of the tissue demands. The coccygeus muscle–sacrospinous ligament complex is palpated and usually can be visualized as it courses from the ischial spine to the sacrum.

4. Once established, the "window" is gently enlarged in the axis of the vagina (Fig. 32-17). This maneuver is usually accomplished by spreading the index and middle finger in the window to stretch the tissues, thereby providing palpable access and usually a clear view of the upper surface of the pelvic diaphragm, the ischial

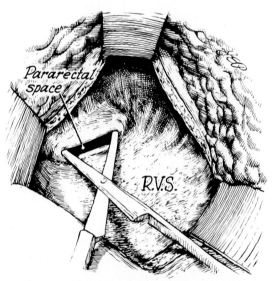

Figure 32–17. The right cardinal ligament and ureter have been displaced anteriorly by a Breisky–Navratil retractor in the 12 o'clock position, and the rectum has been displaced to the patient's left by a retractor in the 4 o'clock position. An opening is made either bluntly or by using a sharp, pointed hemostat through the descending rectal septum into the right pararectal space, at the site of the ischial spine. This opening is enlarged by spreading the point of the hemostat or of the Mayo scissors to permit access to the coccygeus muscle, which lies in the lateral wall of the pararectal space and contains within it the sacrospinous ligament. RVS = rectovaginal space. (From Nichols DH. Transvaginal sacrospinous fixation. Pelvic Surgeon 1981; 1:10. With permission.)

spine, and coccygeus muscle. One retractor is placed in the 12 o'clock position to hold the cardinal ligament containing the ureter out of harm's way. Another retractor holds the patient's rectum to the left side, and if needed, a shorter retractor may compress the distal portion of the pelvic diaphragm along the lateral wall of the pelvis. Because the surgeon is working in a confined area, essentially in the hollow of the sacrum, a fiberoptic headlight is useful. Bleeding from blood vessels is uncommon. If bleeding is present, it is usually venous can be controlled by coagulation, by suture ligation, or—most commonly—with medium-sized hemoclips.

5. At a point 2–3 cm medial to the ischial spine (Fig. 32-18), the coccygeus muscle–sacrospinous ligament complex is penetrated by the blunt tip of a long-handled Deschamps ligature carrier (Fig. 32-19) holding a full length of a synthetic suture, such as polyglycolic acid or polyglactin (Dexon or Vicryl, size 1 or 2). If visual exposure is difficult and penetration cannot be accomplished under direct vision, it can also be accomplished safely by palpation. If the penetration is made through the right sacrospinous ligament–coccygeus muscle complex, the index and middle fingers of the surgeon's left hand are inserted through the "window" in the rectal pillar into the right pararectal space (Fig. 32-20). The tip of the middle index finger is placed on the medial surface of the right ischial spine (Fig. 32-21). A long-handled Deschamps ligature carrier, holding a proper suture, is grasped in the right hand. The curved tip of the carrier is gently slid down the undersurface of the left index finger to the posteroinferior border of the sacrospinous ligament–coccygeal muscle complex (Fig. 32-22) to a point 2–3 cm medial to the ischial spine, which is still being palpated by the middle finger of the left hand (Fig. 32-23). As the tip of the ligature carrier is rotated in a clockwise direction, a significant resistance should be encountered. The resistance indicates that the carrier has been placed through the ligament, neither superficial nor deep to it (Fig. 32-24). This latter error could endanger the sciatic nerve and pudendal vessels and nerves. At the same time, the handle of the ligature carrier is moved through a larger clockwise arc beneath the palm of the left hand to permit vertical penetration of the ligament (Fig. 32-25). A gentle tug to the ligature carrier or to the suture, which has been grasped by a hook (Fig. 32-26), if it actually moves the patient a small degree on the table, indicates proper placement of the suture through the substance of the sacrospinous liga-

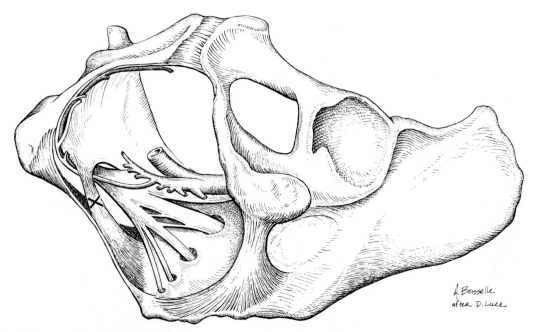

Figure 32–18. The surgical anatomy of the coccygeus muscle–sacrospinous ligament complex is identified. The pudendal artery and nerve pass beneath the ischial spine. At a distance of 3–5 cm medial to the ischial spine, at a point marked by the X, the complex should be penetrated by the tip of the Deschamps ligature carrier, safely avoiding the pudendal nerve and vessels by a wide margin. (Redrawn after Morley and Luce.)

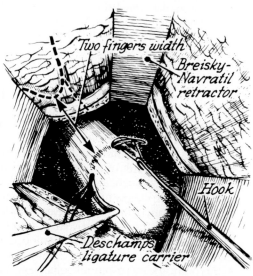

Figure 32–19. The coccygeus muscle and sacrospinous ligament have been penetrated by the blunt end of a long Deschamps ligature carrier at a point 2–3 cm medial to the ischial spine, safely away from the pudendal nerve and vessels and the sciatic nerve. The ligature carrier was previously threaded with a full uncut length of 54-in No. 2 synthetic delayed-absorbable suture, or a nonabsorbable synthetic suture, or both. Traction to the hook exteriorizes the suture, and the Deschamps ligature carrier is removed. (From Nichols DH. Transvaginal sacrospinous fixation. Pelvic Surgeon 1981; 1:10. With permission.)

ment. Direct palpation of the suture and of the ischial spine confirms the required distance of 2–3 cm between the two. If the suture seems too close to the ischial spine, traction is made upon it to identify its exact location, and a new suture is placed medial to the offending suture, which is then removed. If desired, an additional suture, usually synthetic and nonabsorbable, or two can be inserted through the muscle–ligament complex medial to the first suture.

6. Although sacrospinous colpopexy may be accomplished on both sides if the vaginal vault is very wide, such bilateral fixation is rarely done, as equally satisfactory results are obtained if unilateral colpopexy is performed. With unilateral colpopexy, however, a redundantly wide vault should be surgically narrowed. The vagina is thus converted to a cylinder of uniform diameter, as it now serves as an instrument of coitus and not of parturition.

7. With a free needle, each suture is sewn to the undersurface of the midportion of the vaginal vault (Fig. 32-27). Although polyglycolic or polyglactin acid is generally used, their long latent periods before absorption (4–6 weeks) permit development of a strong scar between the vagina and the sacrospinous ligament. Nonabsorbable size 0 monofilament synthetic sutures such as

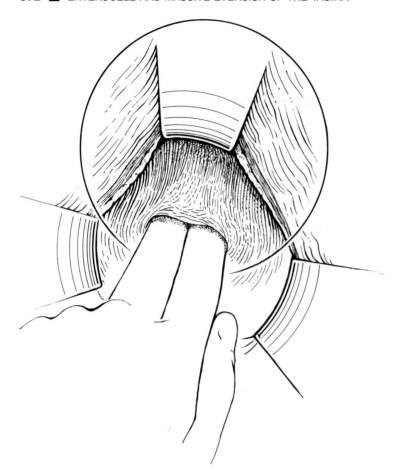

Figure 32–20. Placing the colpopexy stitches by palpation through a "window" in the descending rectal septum. When visual exposure is difficult and penetration cannot be accomplished under direct vision, it can be done safely by palpation using the following maneuver: a window has been created in the descending rectal septum between the rectovaginal space and the perirectal space. The window is of a diameter to permit two or three fingerbreadths (2–3 cm) as noted. It overlies the ischial spine, which is in the lateral wall of the perirectal space.

Prolene, Surgilene, or size CV-O Gore-Tex may be substituted in a patient with chronic respiratory disease or with rerecurrent prolapse. These permanent stitches, however, should be placed subepithelially in the vagina, so that they are buried in the fibromuscular wall. The colpopexy stitches are then held long in hemostats to be tied later in the operation.

8. Any necessary anterior colporrhaphy is now accomplished. Full-length anterior colporrhaphy with special attention to the supports of the vesicourethral junction is performed almost without exception. Plication of the pubourethral "ligament" portion of the urogenital diaphragm beneath the urethra (Fig. 32-28) with a long-acting, absorbable suture such as size 2-0 polydioxanone or polyglyconate (PDS or Maxon) will, in most instances, support the vesicourethral junction at its correct anatomic location and thus effectively treat or prevent urinary stress incontinence postoperatively. If a history of former urinary stress incontinence is obtained or

the condition is a primary symptom, a nonabsorbable synthetic suture such as Ethabond or Gore-Tex may be placed as shown in the insert of Figure 32-28.

9. The upper portion of the posterior colporrhaphy is begun at the vault of the vagina by a side-to-side, running, subcutaneous–subcuticular suture that incorporates fully the fascia and fibromuscular sheath of the posterior vaginal wall but carefully avoids the anterior wall of the rectum. This suture is continued until the midportion of the posterior vaginal wall has been reached.

10. At this point, the sacrospinous colpopexy stitches are tied to attach the vagina firmly to the surface of the coccygeus muscle–sacrospinous ligament complex with no intervening bridge of suture material.

11. The posterior colporrhaphy is completed.

12. Any necessary perineorrhaphy is accomplished.

13. Rectal examination confirms the integrity of the rectum, and if desired, a vaginal packing may be inserted for 24 hours.

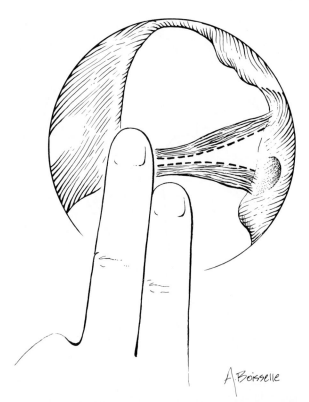

A. Boisselle

Figure 32–21. The index finger of the surgeon's left hand is inserted through the window into the perirectal space, and the tip of the middle finger is made to touch the medial surface of the right ischial spine.

When the patient has a history of previous surgery in this area, the anatomic relationships will frequently have been distorted by fibrosis and adhesions. This scarring complicates the ease with which the surgeon can find the lateral wall of the pararectal space. Nevertheless, when one follows the preceding steps, identification and entry into the pararectal space is anatomically and surgically precise.

Preoperative and Postoperative Care

Preoperative and postoperative care are the same as that for most vaginal reconstructive procedures. Estrogen replacement therapy—systemic, intravaginal, or both—is used in the postmenopausal patient. The patient begins walking the day following surgery, and normal bowel activity is stimulated then if necessary. Continuous bladder drainage is required only if anterior colporrhaphy has been performed. The average duration of hospitalization is the same as that following vaginal hysterectomy and repair.

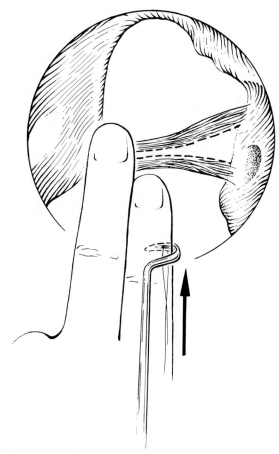

Figure 32–22. The long-handled Deschamps ligature carrier holding a full length of synthetic suture is grasped in the right hand. The curved tip of the carrier is gently slid down the undersurface of the left index finger to the postero-inferior border of the sacrospinous ligament–coccygeus muscle complex.

RECURRENT GENITAL PROLAPSE

A recurrent genital prolapse is a gynecologic tragedy. The patient deserves empathy and understanding and above all a very sophisticated reevaluation by the best and most experienced operator available. One should be mindful that each trip to surgery tends to prejudice unfavorably any subsequent operation. A special effort should be expended to identify clearly the primary weaknesses that gave rise to the prolapse, and a reevaluation of the whole patient, including her life-style and daily habits, should be accomplished. Positive ideas and findings should be most carefully noted, and a plan for reoperation should be thoughtfully developed to allow for an appropriate time and environment for adequate postoperative convalescence. The most expe-

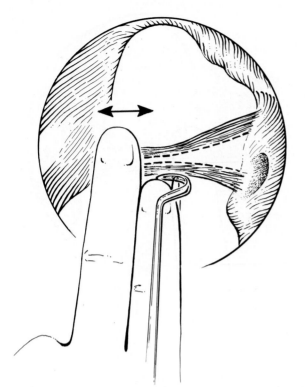

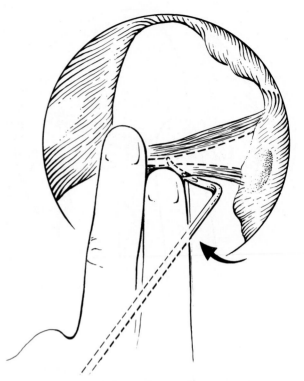

Figure 32–23. At a spot 2–3 cm medial to the ischial spine, the ligature carrier is advanced. The ischial spine is still being palpated as shown.

Figure 32–24. The middle finger palpates the ischial spine, and the index finger touches the sacrospinous ligament as shown. The handle is rotated in a clockwise direction, as shown by the curved arrow.

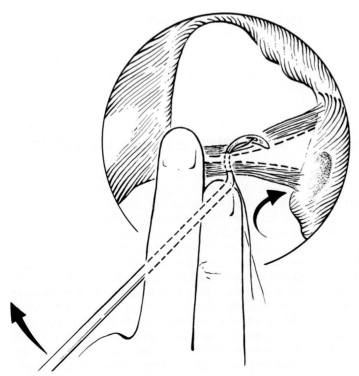

Figure 32–25. At the same time, the handle of the ligature carrier is moved in an independent clockwise direction beneath the palm of the operator's slightly raised left hand, permitting vertical penetration of the ligament as shown. As the tip of the ligature carrier also is rotated in a clockwise direction, a significant resistance should be encountered, indicating that the carrier has been placed *through* the ligament and is neither superficial to it nor beneath it.

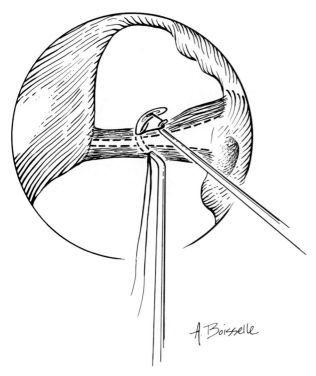

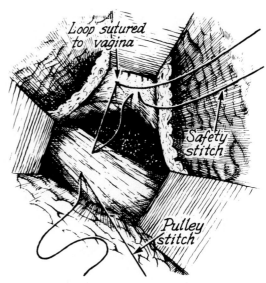

Figure 32—26. The suture is grasped and held with the hook as shown, and the ligature carrier is removed by rotating it in a counterclockwise direction.

rienced and best operative assistance should be recruited. Most important, the surgeon should be properly equipped with a resourceful armamentarium of operative techniques from which to choose so that the surgery may be tailored precisely to correct all recurrent defects. Postoperatively, adjuvant perineal resistive exercises are helpful in restoring the tone to the pelvic vasculature.

RECTAL AND PERINEAL PROLAPSE

In addition to genital prolapse, significant defect in the integrity or effectiveness of the pelvic diaphragm may have a pronounced negative effect on the rectum, particularly when the levator plate sags and allows the anus to become the most dependent portion of the patient's intergluteal area. Though initially asymptomatic, progressive excessive funneling of the levator may significantly decrease the diameter of the stool and increase the difficulties of evacuation. This result may be obstipation and impaction, requiring daily digital manipulation to empty the bowel. Untreated, this situation is often associated with progressive denervation of the levator ani and external anal sphincter followed by rectal incontinence. Evacuating through a 3-inch hole

Figure 32—27. A gentle tug to the ligature carrier or by the suture that has been grasped by the hook should actually move the patient a small degree on the table, indicating proper placement of the suture through the substance of the sacrospinous ligament. The ligature carrier is removed. Direct palpation of the suture and of the ischial spine confirms the required distance between the two. If the suture seems too close to the ischial spine, traction is made upon it and a new suture is placed medial to the offending suture, which is then removed. If desired, an additional suture or two can be inserted through the muscle—ligament complex medial to the first suture. In the patient with chronic respiratory disease, a suture or two of nonabsorbable synthetic 0 Prolene, Surgilene, or Gore-Tex may be added or substituted for the absorbable sutures. The end of one suture is threaded on a free needle, which is then sewn to the undersurface of the vaginal wall through the full thickness of the fibromuscular layer and fixed in this position by a single half-hitch. The end of the second piece of suture is stitched to the undersurface of the vagina 1 cm medial to the first. These sutures are held on hemostats until the upper posterior vaginal wall is closed for 3—5 cm. After the posterior colporrhaphy has been completed and the margins of the posterior vaginal mucosa have been approximated, the sacrospinous fixation stitches are tied, fixing the vaginal vault to the surface of the sacrospinous ligament—coccygeus muscle complex. (From Nichols DH. Transvaginal sacrospinous fixation. Pelvic Surgeon 1981; 1:10. With permission.)

in a board placed across a toilet seat may make effective counterpressure around the anus when this condition first becomes symptomatic, but the inconvenience of such measures when away from home may lead to laxative abuse to the point of discomfort or diarrhea. Straining at stool is to be avoided lest it further stretch an already attenuated pelvic diaphragm and the nerves supplying it. A long-term course of isometric perineal

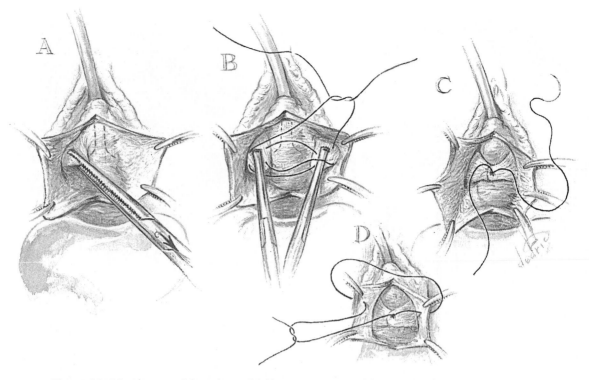

Figure 32–28. Plication of the pubourethral ligament portion of the urogenital diaphragm. The base of the bladder has been exposed through a midline incision and the paraurethral tissue of the urogenital diaphragm grasped in a forceps (*A*). Traction to the forceps will actually move the patient on the table. A long-lasting synthetic suture is passed through each end of the ligament (*B*). After the ligaments have been plicated (*C*), the same suture takes a bite of the vaginal wall, reestablishing fusion (*D*). (From Nichols DH, Randall CL. Vaginal surgery. 2nd ed. Baltimore: Williams & Wilkins, 1976:150. With permission.)

muscle exercises is often helpful as an adjunct to treatment. One procedure embracing a surgical treatment for this condition is retrorectal levatorplasty (Fig. 32-29). After any necessary transvaginal colporrhaphy, the patient is placed in a jackknife position and an incision is made between the anus and the coccyx. The damaged levator plate is bisected, and dissection proceeds directly into the retrorectal space. The posterior surface of the rectum is attached by successive plication stitches to the periosteum in the hollow of the sacrum. A series of interrupted stitches bringing the pubococcygei together behind the rectum reconstitutes the length of the levator plate. Any pathologic elongation of the levator ani may be shortened by appropriate Z stitches.

Rectal Prolapse

A defect in the supports in the rectum and sigmoid colon coincident with their elongation may lead to an obvious rectal and sigmoid intussusception, that, with straining, may project a portion of intestinal mucosa and wall up to 15 cm through the now attenuated external anal sphincter. This defect may be the product of chronic straining consequent to poor bowel habits and may first be noted in the patient's history as a decrease in sensations of rectal fullness and stool passage along with some partial incontinence and difficulty with cleansing after a bowel movement. Early in its development one may see on external inspection during physical examination the red anterior rectal wall visible through the partially dilated anal sphincter. Abnormal bowel habits should be corrected as soon as possible, but for the patient in whom intussusception and prolapse have already occurred, surgical correction is desirable. The most effective surgery is that of transabdominal proctopexy—the attaching of the rectosigmoid to the hollow of the sacrum, often by one of the perirectal sling operations. For the bedridden or the infirm, the insertion of a Thiersch wire to reinforce a

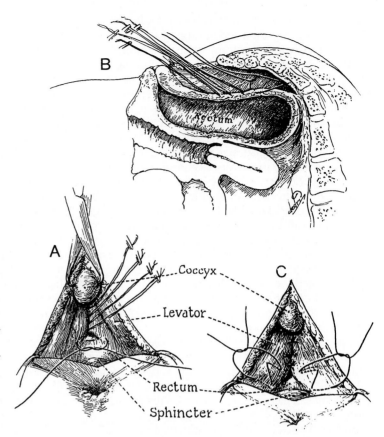

Figure 32-29. Retrorectal levatorplasty. An incision has been made between the coccyx and the anus, and the retrorectal space has been entered. Plication stitches have been placed 1 cm apart on the posterior wall of the rectum and tied as shown in *A*. These are then sewn individually to the anterior periosteum on the sacrum, as shown in *B*. The levator plate is restored and lengthened by bringing the pubococcygei of each side together in the midline between the coccyx and rectum, as shown in *C*. The bellies of the pubococcygei may be shortened by a Z stitch placed as shown in *C*. (From Nichols DH. Retrorectal levatorplasty for anal and perineal prolapse. Surg Gynecol Obstet 1982; 154:251–254. Reproduced with permission.)

weakened external anal sphincter will be helpful, though it imposes a permanent partial obstruction at the anal outlet. With a distinctive and separate etiology, rectal prolapse is quite independent of a genital prolapse, though the two may coexist. For this reason its treatment is independent of that for the genital prolapse, though it may be offered coincidentally.

SUMMARY

Genital prolapses and their symptoms may detract significantly from the quality of life experienced by women of any age, but especially among those over 50, in whom these disabilities are more common. Treatment may be nonsurgical or surgical, but for maximal effectiveness requires precision in diagnosis of damage and understanding of the probable etiology. When surgery is required, selecting the optimal procedure requires that the gynecologic surgeon be comfortable with a spectrum of operations so that, in the words of Charles Mayo, one may "make the operation fit the patient, not the patient fit the operation."

SACRAL COLPOPEXY FOR ENTEROCELE AND VAGINAL VAULT PROLAPSE

ARMAND E. HENDEE

Increasing numbers of elderly women today enjoy full and active lives. Many are sexually active into their seventh and eighth decades. At least one third of American women have had a hysterectomy by age 65. Aging and inadequate support to the vaginal vault following hysterectomy are two important factors that have led to an increased frequency of vaginal vault prolapse and enterocele, and the need for reconstructive pelvic surgery to correct this delayed complication of either abdominal or vaginal hysterectomy. The gynecologic surgeon who attempts to correct vaginal vault prolapse must understand three purposes of the operation: (1) symptoms must be relieved; (2) normal anatomy must be restored; and (3) normal function must be restored.

In 1962, Lane first described the technique of abdominal sacral colpopexy for posthysterectomy vaginal vault prolapse. In 1968 Parsons and Ulfelder, and in 1973 Birnbaum, reported and illustrated an abdominal operation for posthysterectomy vaginal vault prolapse with the "concept of posterior fixation of the vagina—holding it loosely toward the hollow of the sacrum" using a Marlex mesh graft. Addison has reported the Duke University Medical Center experience, Lansman used dura mater for support, and Maloney has reported the use of an autologous fascial graft.

Vaginal vault prolapse and vaginal enterocele are used synonymously in this discussion, although a variety of enteroceles have been described. A concomitant cystocele and rectocele will usually, but not always, be present. A massive vaginal prolapse with complete vaginal eversion will result in a distorted and greatly increased vaginal caliber. The vaginal outlet is often widely dilated. Previous surgical attempts to correct vaginal relaxation may have shortened the vaginal depth, changed the vaginal axis, narrowed the vaginal caliber, and distorted the vaginal introitus. To relieve symptoms, restore anatomy, and restore coital function, such defects must be corrected.

Some patients will have no difficulty voiding. Others will maintain a high residual urine volume with chronic cystitis. Some will learn to replace the anterior vaginal wall digitally to initiate voiding. Others will depend on intermittent self-catheterization to keep the bladder as empty as possible. A few will complain of urinary incontinence. Meticulous attention must be paid to restoring normal bladder function, recognizing that preoperative bladder dysfunction may range from bladder neck obstruction and urinary retention to proximal urethral descent with associated pressure equalization stress urinary incontinence.

Several surgical procedures are available to correct vaginal vault prolapse. In most patients we have used the abdominal sacral colpopexy with an autologous fascial graft, usually combined with transvaginal colporrhaphy to repair relaxations of the lower anterior and posterior vaginal walls and vaginal introitus and suprapubic colpopexy to correct or avoid postoperative stress urinary incontinence. A satisfactory outcome with good restoration of anatomy and function and good long-term results has been achieved in most patients.

A brief review of the anatomy of the normal vagina is necessary to understand better the rationale for this operation for the correction of vaginal vault prolapse and to compare it to other operations. Funt and associates and Nichols, Milley, and Randall have described the normal axis of the vagina and its anatomic relationships. The upper one third of the vagina is directed posteriorly toward the third and fourth sacral vertebrae. It occupies an almost horizontal position in the upright patient. The upper vagina thus lies upon the rectum and both are supported by the similarly horizontal levator plate formed posterior to the rectum by the fusion of the levator muscles in the midline. The vagina is held in the midline in this horizontal position by the lateral paravaginal attachments to the fascial sheaths of the pubococcygei and puborectalis muscles along the arcus tendineus and somewhat by the cardinal and uterosacral ligaments. A valsalva maneuver or sudden increases in intra-abdominal pressure with coughing or sneezing merely flatten the upper vagina against the strong levator plate rather than evert it through the levator hiatus. The basic defects seen in vaginal vault prolapse involve loss of support of these ligaments, which hold the vagina in this favorable position, and the laceration, stretching, and loss of tone of the levator muscles. A predisposition to vaginal vault prolapse may also result from previous surgery in which the vagina has been shortened or the axis of the upper vagina has been misdirected anteriorly, leaving the comparatively thin and unsupported upper posterior vaginal wall exposed to the pressure of intra-abdominal contents.

The abdominal sacral colpopexy with the ancillary procedures described synthesizes the advantages of several operations. A proper anatomic positioning of the upper vagina is achieved by directing the vaginal apex toward S3–4 vertebrae. The Moschcowitz and/or Halban culdoplasty obliterates the cul-de-sac, approximates the posterior vaginal wall to the anterior rectal wall and isolates it from intra-abdominal pressure, and provides a peritoneal shelf that deflects pressure away from this most dependent portion of the female pelvis. These features virtually eliminate the potential problem associated with anterior abdominal wall vaginal vault suspension, that of rendering the upper posterior vaginal wall vulnerable to enterocele formation and of elevating the base of the bladder enough to flatten the posterior urethrovesical angle significantly, thus predisposing the patient to urinary stress incontinence. An autologous fascial graft from the aponeurosis of the anterior abdominal wall is used. It is strong and easily available. Its use also eliminates the low but persistent incidence of chronic infection and sinus tract drainage associated with the use of synthetic materials. Some older women have sigmoid diverticulosis with bouts of diverticulitis. A graft of synthetic material in the pelvis could pose a potential problem when diverticulitis is present.

The posterior colporrhaphy and perineorrhaphy provide support of the middle and lower vagina and vaginal introitus by reducing the levator hiatus and strengthening the connective tissue support of the posterior vaginal wall. Thus, all components of the defect are corrected.

Technique of Abdominal Sacral Colpopexy

Preoperative preparation may include intravaginal estrogen cream if atrophy of the vaginal mucosa is present. Emphasis on weight control and cessation of smoking should begin preoperatively if appropriate. The operation will be facilitated if the intestinal tract is empty. Patients are asked to take only liquids by mouth beginning 24 hours prior to operation. Enemas until clear are given the evening before operation.

When a significant anterior vaginal wall relaxation has been prediagnosed while the patient was awake and able to do the Valsalva maneuver, repair of the cystocele and rectocele should be done initially from below. If sacral colpopexy is done first, vaginal colporrhaphy will be more difficult later and therefore should be done first. If cystocele is not a problem or will be corrected by vaginal vault suspension, then the abdominal surgery may commence initially.

The patient is placed in the lithotomy position in Allen Universal stirrups. The bladder is emptied, a pelvic examination under anesthesia is done. The vaginal

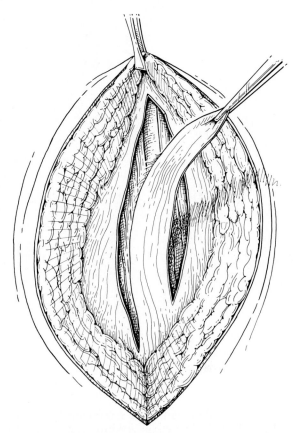

Figure 32–31. A 10 × 2.5-cm strip of fascia is then removed and saved for use later. The peritoneal cavity is entered.

vault is demonstrated, and once again defects in the vaginal support, perineal support, and vaginal and introital caliber are noted. The skin preparation extends from the lower rib cage to include the entire abdomen, mons, anterior thighs, perineum, vagina, and perianal area. The patient is then draped to allow easy access to the vagina and the lower abdomen, and a Foley catheter is inserted.

A midline lower abdominal incision is made to the fascia (Figs. 32-30 and 32-31). The fascia is cleaned widely on each side of the midline. A 2.5 × 10-cm strip of fascia is excised longitudinally and placed between saline moistened sponges. If preferred, a transverse Maylard incision may be used. An adequate fascial strip can be excised transversely. Lateral to the lateral border of the rectus abdominus muscles, the fascia is split into two layers. This does not ordinarily present a problem, however.

The peritoneal cavity is entered, the upper abdomen is explored, adhesions are lysed, the bowel is packed

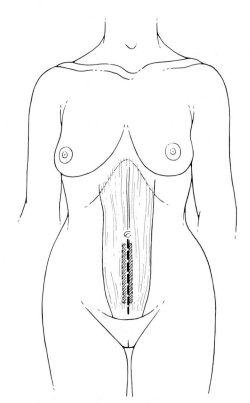

Figure 32–30. The fascia is cleaned of fat through a lower midline incision or transverse Maylard incision.

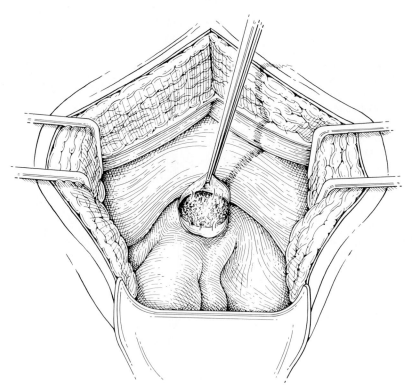

Figure 32–32. A 3×4-cm area of vaginal apex is exposed.

into the upper abdomen, and a self-retaining retractor is inserted. In postmenopausal women, atrophic ovaries are usually removed. The vagina is usually recognized easily. If there is any uncertainty, a sponge forceps inserted through the introitus can be used to elevate and manipulate the vaginal apex in the pelvis. The vaginal apex is grasped with two Allis forceps—one at each lateral angle of the vagina. The vesical peritoneum overlying the vaginal apex is incised. The bladder is freed from the anterior vaginal wall and the rectum is freed from the posterior vaginal wall so that at least a 3×4-cm area of vaginal wall at the apex is exposed (Fig. 32-32). If needed, a wedge of vaginal wall may be removed from the anterior and posterior vaginal walls to reduce the excess caliber and relaxation of the upper vaginal walls (Fig. 32-33). However, the vaginal length should not be shortened. The edges of the vaginal mucosa are approximated from side to side with No. 2-0 delayed-absorbable sutures.

A true enterocele may exist in the upper posterior vaginal wall. If so, the peritoneum lining this defect can be excised along with the excess posterior vaginal wall. The defect is further obliterated by the Moschcowitz culdoplasty.

At this point, it is helpful for the surgeon to place his or her hand in the vagina to assess the thickness of the vaginal wall. Four to five No. 2-0 figure-of-eight Tevdek sutures are placed in the thickness of the vaginal wall at

the apex in a single row from one lateral fornix to the other (Fig. 32-34). If the suture is placed into the vaginal lumen, attempting to obtain a strong purchase of the full thickness of vagina, no harm will result. Epithelialization occurs in time over these sutures in the vagina and no suture will remain exposed for very long. These sutures are held long and untied. Both free ends of each suture are then brought through one end of the fascial graft. The graft is slid down the sutures to the vaginal apex. The sutures are then tied and cut (Fig. 32-35). A second row of No. 2-0 Vicryl sutures are then placed through the graft and into the posterior vaginal wall near the apex.

Culdoplasty is an important part of this operation and can usually be accomplished best by the Moschcowitz technique, although the Halban technique also may be used. With the Moschcowitz technique, a purse-string suture of No. 2-0 Tevdek is used, beginning at the very bottom of the cul-de-sac and exercising care to include any remnant of uterosacral ligaments, the posterior vagina, only peritoneum laterally, and only shallow bites of serosa over the sigmoid colon (Fig. 32-36). When the pelvis has been encircled with this purse-string suture and traction is applied, a peritoneal shelf will obliterate the cul-de-sac. Closure of the cul-de-sac should not leave behind any defect that could result in bowel entrapment, and it should not constrict the sigmoid colon. Constriction of the sigmoid can be avoided

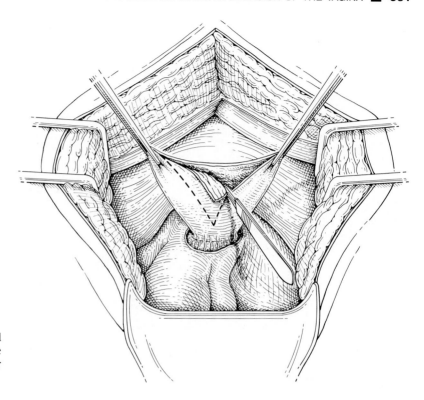

Figure 32–33. Partial colpectomy and repair may be done if needed to reduce the excess caliber of the upper anterior and posterior vaginal walls.

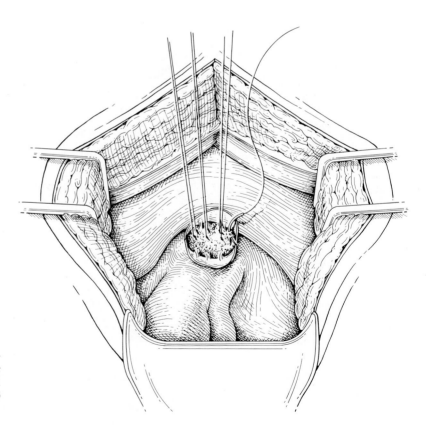

Figure 32–34. Four to five No. 2-0 figure-of-eight permanent sutures are placed in the full thickness of the vaginal wall at the apex from one lateral fornix to the other.

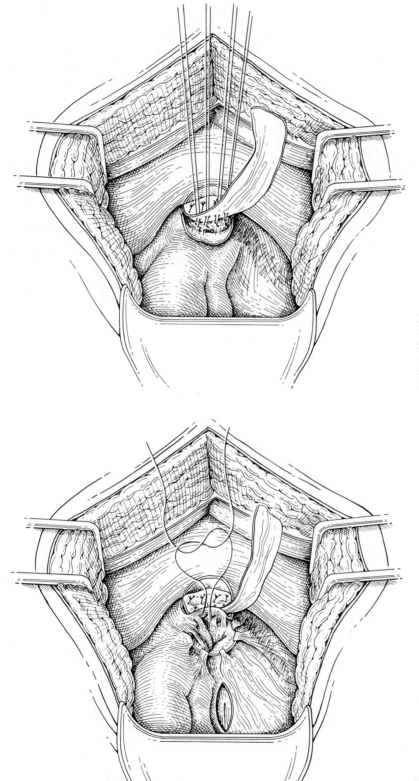

Figure 32–35. Both free ends of each suture are brought through one end of the fascial graft. The sutures are tied and cut. A second row of No. 2-0 delayed-absorbable sutures is placed to reinforce the first layer.

Figure 32–36. A continuous No. 2-0 permanent suture is used to close the cul-de-sac with a Moschcowitz technique.

by doing a hemi-Moschcowitz bilaterally on each side of the sigmoid (see Figs. 27-23 and 27-24).

With the sigmoid colon retracted to the left, the posterior parietal peritoneum overlaying the anterior sacrum is opened longitudinally in the midline from the sacral promontory caudally to a point below S-3. The anterior sacral fascia is exposed by blunt and sharp dissection, exercising care to avoid injury to the presacral vessels. Three permanent sutures (No. 2-0 Tevdek) are placed into the periosteum of the sacrum spaced about 1 cm apart in the midline overlying S-3 and S-4 vertebrae. These sutures are held long without tying. The fascial graft that was attached to the vaginal apex is now measured and trimmed to reach the exposed anterior sacrum without tension. The sutures in the sacrum are then placed securely in the sacral end of the fascial graft and tied (Fig. 32-37). The vaginal apex should not be pulled tightly toward the sacrum. The graft should not be taut but should be only tight enough to hold the vaginal apex in a normal position. The culdoplasty peritoneum will be beneath the fascial strip. The sigmoid colon should pass beneath it without undue compression.

The peritoneum is then sutured over the graft from the sacrum toward the vagina. Usually only a small segment of the graft cannot be covered and the margins of this segment should be sutured to underlying sigmoid serosa or culdoplasty peritoneum to avoid any bridging between the graft and the underlying tissues (Fig. 32-38).

After closure of the anterior peritoneum of the incision, the space of Retzius is entered and a suprapubic colpopexy is done according to a modified Burch technique, described in Chapter 33. This is considered to be a necessary part of the operation to prevent or correct stress urinary incontinence. Because of the defect in the anterior rectus aponeurosis where the fascial graft was obtained, a permanent interrupted suture or continuous prolene suture is used to approximate the fascia when closing the incision.

Following the abdominal skin closure, if the Allen Universal stirrups are used, the surgeon can proceed with vaginal surgery without repositioning and redraping the patient. A high posterior colporrhaphy and perineorrhaphy is performed in almost all cases. This reduces the enlarged levator hiatus and supports the middle and lower posterior vaginal wall while restoring a normal caliber to the vagina and vaginal introitus.

Complications and Results

One hundred and forty patients with posthysterectomy vaginal vault prolapse were treated by abdominal

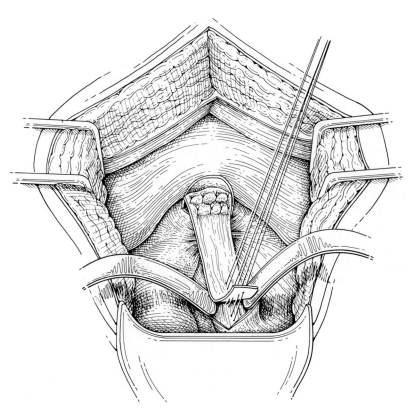

Figure 32–37. The anterior sacral fascia is exposed. Three permanent sutures are used to anchor the fascial graft to the presacral fascia at the level of S-3 or S-4.

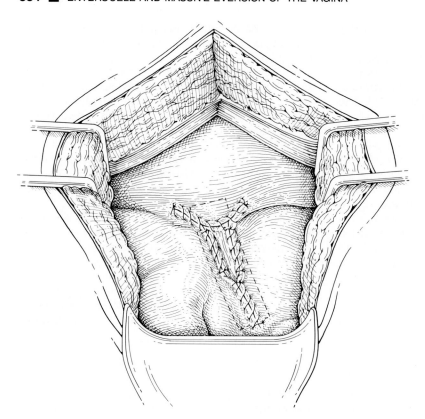

Figure 32–38. The peritoneum is closed over the graft.

sacral colpopexy at Emory University Hospital. All had been followed for over 1 year, and 60% had been followed from 3 to 11 years. Ninety-six percent had good vaginal vault suspension. The failures occurred in the earlier cases when only absorbable sutures were used to approximate the graft to a smaller area of the vaginal wall apex. This apical vaginal wall is often thin. Currently, to avoid this problem, a single row of permanent figure-of-eight sutures is placed in the full thickness of the vaginal wall at the apex from one lateral fornix to the other. A second row of delayed absorbable sutures is placed below the apical sutures and attaches the grafts to a larger area of vaginal wall. Twenty-four percent of the patients have mild to moderate cystocele, rectocele, or stress urinary incontinence postoperatively. This number can be greatly reduced by better preoperative appraisal and repair of all defects found. Any patient with more than a first-degree prolapse of the vaginal vault (upper third) should usually have a posterior colporrhaphy and perineorrhaphy.

Intraoperative complications may result from the lysis of sometimes extensive adhesions before the bowel can be packed into the upper abdomen. This increases the danger of bowel injury and bleeding. It also increases the risk of the postoperative complications of adynamic ileus and mechanical bowel obstruc-

tion. Dissection to expose the presacral fascia or periosteum must be carefully done to avoid injury to the presacral vessels. Hemorrhage from these vessels can be difficult to control. Addison reported two such cases of severe hemorrhage from injury to the presacral vessels requiring intensive effort to control bleeding and multiple units of blood replacement.

Postoperative complications may result because many of these patients are old and some have medical complications. Obesity is a frequent complication. Sixty-three percent of these patients reviewed from Emory Hospital were significantly overweight to morbidly obese.

Although this is a good operation with a high rate of success and durability, it is a long operation. Postoperative morbidity that is often associated with atelectasis, circulatory problems (including deep venous thrombosis), adynamic ileus, wound disruption, or infection may be anticipated and prevented through proper prophylactic measures.

Prevention

Prevention of posthysterectomy vaginal vault prolapse should be a consideration whenever a hysterectomy is performed. With vaginal hysterectomy the uterosacral ligaments may be sutured to the posterior upper vagina and plicated. This supports the upper vagina and closes the space where enterocele may develop. In addition, any degree of enterocele encountered with vaginal hysterectomy should be repaired with this culdoplasty. It is a modification of the McCall culdoplasty described in Chapter 27.

A posterior colporrhaphy and perineorrhaphy will reinforce the support of the middle and distal third of the posterior vaginal wall and reduce the often enlarged levator hiatus. Often vaginal vault prolapse occurs when an abdominal hysterectomy is done without correcting the anatomic changes associated with the loss of pelvic support. Whenever these findings are present, they can be corrected and vaginal prolapse often prevented by plicating the uterosacral ligaments and suturing them to the posterior upper vagina as described earlier or by the technique of culdoplasty, as described by either Moschcowitz or Halban, thus obliterating the cul-de-sac, supporting the posterior vagina, and deflecting pressure from this dependent portion of the female pelvis.

Bibliography

Addison WA, Livengood CH, Sutton GP, Parker RT. Abdominal-sacral colpopexy with Mersilene mesh in the retroperitoneal position in the management of post hysterectomy vaginal vault prolapse and enterocele. Am J Obstet Gynecol 1985;153:140.

Amreich J. Aëtiologie und Operation des Scheidenstumpf prolapses. Klin Wochenschr 1951;63:74.

Arthure HGE, Savage D. Uterine prolapse and prolapse of the vaginal vault treated by sacral hysteropexy. J Obstet Gynecol Br Emp 1957;64:355.

Baden WF, Walker TA. Physical diagnosis in the evaluation of vaginal relaxation. Clin Obstet Gynecol 1972;15:1060.

Birnbaum SJ. Rational therapy for the prolapsed vagina. Am J Obstet Gynecol 1973;115:411.

Bonney V. The sustentacular apparatus of the female genital canal, the displacements that result from the yielding of its several components, and their appropriate treatment. J Obstet Gynaecol Br Emp 1914;45:328.

Burch JC. Urethrovaginal fixation to Cooper's ligament for correction of stress incontinence, cystocele, and prolapse. Am J Obstet Gynecol 1961;81:281.

Falk HC. Uterine prolapse and prolapse of the vaginal vault treated by sacropexy. Obstet Gynecol 1961;18:113.

Funt MI, Thompson JD, Birch HW. Normal vaginal axis. South Med J 1978;71:1534.

Halban J. Gynäkologische Operationslehre. Berlin and Vienna: Urban and Schwarzenbert, 1932.

Hendee AE, Berry CM. Abdominal sacropexy for vaginal vault prolapse. Clin Obstet Gynecol 1981;24(4):1217.

Henry MM, Swash M, eds. Colpoproctology and the pelvic floor. London: Butterworths, 1985.

Kegel AH. Progressive resistance exercises in the functional restoration of the perineal muscles. Am J Obstet Gynecol 1948;56:238.

Lane FE. Repair of posthysterectomy vaginal-vault prolapse. Obstet Gynecol 1962;20(1):72.

Lansman HH. Post hysterectomy vault prolapse: sacral colpopexy with dura mater graft. Obstet Gynecol 1984;63:577.

Maloney JC, Dunton CJ, Smith K. Repair of vaginal vault prolapse with abdominal sacropexy. J Reprod Med 1990;35(1).

Marshall VF, Marchetti AA, Krantz KE. The correction of stress incontinence by simple vesicourethral suspension. Surg Gynecol Obstet 1949;88:509.

Moschcowitz AV. The pathogenesis anatomy and cure of prolapse of the rectum. Surg Gynecol Obstet 1912;15:7.

Nichols DH, Milley PS, Randall CL. Significance of restoration of normal vaginal depth and axis. Obstet Gynecol 1970;36:251.

Nichols DH. Sacrospinous fixation for massive eversion of the vagina. Am J Obstet Gynecol 1982;142:901.

Nichols DH, Julian PJ. The vaginal pessary. In: Nichols DH, Evrard JR, eds. Ambulatory gynecology. Philadelphia: Harper & Row, 1985.

Parsons L, Ulfelder H. An atlas of pelvic operations. 2nd ed. Philadelphia: WB Saunders, 1968:280.

Randall CL, Nichols DH. Surgical treatment of vaginal inversion. Obstet Gynecol 1971;38:327.

Richter K. Die operative Behandlung des prolabierten scheidengrundes nach Uterusextirpation Beitrag zur Vaginaefixatio Sacrotuberalis nach Amreich. Geburtshilfe Frauenheilkd 1967;27:941.

Sutton GP, Addison WA, Livengood CH, Hammond CB. Life-threatening hemorrhage complicating sacral colpopexy. Am J Obstet Gynecol 1981;24:1217.

White GR. Cystocele. A radical cure by suturing lateral sulci of vagina to white line of pelvic fascia. JAMA 1909;53:1707.

Zweifel P. Vorlesungen über klinische gynakologie. Berlin: Hirschwald, 1892:407.

Urinary Stress Incontinence

33

JOHN D. THOMPSON, L. LEWIS WALL, WILLIAM A. GROWDON, JOHN H. RIDLEY

CLINICAL EVALUATION OF THE INCONTINENT PATIENT

L. LEWIS WALL

Urinary incontinence has been defined by the International Continence Society as a condition in which involuntary loss of urine is a social or hygienic problem and is objectively demonstrable. Urinary incontinence is a particular medical problem for women. While involuntary urine loss is *not* a normal part of aging, it often becomes a clinical problem for the aging woman as the trauma of childbirth, the development of other acute and chronic illnesses, and the loss of estrogenic stimulation at menopause weaken pelvic support and diminish the amount of normal homeostatic reserve available to cope with the demands of bladder function. At its consensus development conference on adult urinary incontinence in October, 1988, the National Institutes of Health conservatively estimated the monetary costs of managing adult incontinence at $10.3 billion per year. As our population continues to age, and particularly as the women born in the baby boom that followed World War II reach menopause, gynecologists can expect to see the problem of urinary incontinence occupying an increasingly larger place in their practices. They must be ready to meet the medical and surgical challenges that this will present.

For conceptual purposes urinary incontinence may be divided into two broad categories based on the route of urine loss (Table 33-1). Extraurethral incontinence refers to urine loss through an abnormal opening between the urinary tract and the outside, such as from a congenital defect or a fistula. More commonly, however, urine loss occurs through the urethra for one or more reasons.

The most common form of female urinary incontinence is stress incontinence. In this condition urine loss occurs during periods of increased intra-abdominal pressure, such as sneezing, coughing, or exercise, and results from an incompetent closure mechanism at the urethra and bladder neck. A community survey of 1060 randomly selected women over the age of 18 in South Wales, for example, found that 22% of women had this complaint. The continence mechanism in women is particularly susceptible to this kind of urine loss, particularly during exercise that involves repetitive bouncing motions.

However, urine loss in women also may occur for many other reasons. Among the most common of these causes are uninhibited contractions of the bladder muscle (detrusor instability). If these contractions are caused by a neurologic lesion such as multiple sclerosis or a cerebrovascular accident, they are called *detrusor hyperreflexia*. The term *reflex incontinence* is used to refer to the hyperreflexic condition that occurs in spinal cord injury patients where involuntary urine loss occurring without urgency or a conscious need to urinate is precipitated by abnormal reflex activity in the spinal cord. When no obvious neurologic reason for detrusor instability can be found it is called *idiopathic* instability.

Other causes of transurethral urine loss include uninhibited urethral relaxation or urethral instability, which is a somewhat rare cause of incontinence and is usually associated with a neuropathic lesion. Patients who have acontractile or poorly functioning bladders may become incontinent when the bladder is overdistended. When intravesical pressure exceeds maximum urethral pressure, overflow incontinence results, without any precipitating detrusor or urethral activity. Urethral diverticula may cause incontinence by trapping urine during normal micturition and releasing it unexpectedly during other activities. Congenital abnormalities of the urethra such as epispadias also may

887

TABLE 33–1
Etiology of Urinary Incontinence

I. Extraurethral incontinence
  A. Congenital
    1. Ectopic ureter
    2. Bladder exstrophy
  B. Acquired (fistulae)
    1. Ureteral
    2. Vesical
    3. Urethral
    4. Multiple combinations
II. Transurethral incontinence
  A. Urethral sphincter incompetence
    ("Genuine stress incontinence")
  B. Detrusor instability
    1. Idiopathic instability
    2. Neuropathic instability
      a. Detrusor hyperreflexia
      b. Reflex incontinence
  C. Urethral instability
  D. Urinary retention with overflow incontinence
  E. Urethral diverticulum
  F. Congenital urethral abnormalities (*eg,* epispadias)
  G. Functional incontinence (*eg,* impaired mobility)
  H. Miscellaneous and transient incontinence

result in incontinence. Functional urinary incontinence may occur in patients with decreased mobility or debilitating diseases such as arthritis if, for example, they are unable to walk quickly enough to a toilet and undo their clothing when the need to urinate arises. Changes in the living conditions and social environment of such patients may restore continence without significant medical or surgical intervention. Other miscellaneous conditions such as untreated urinary tract infections, drugs, or the acute confusion associated with delirium may cause transient urinary incontinence that may be cured by appropriate medical treatment. This is particularly important in the elderly, where decreased physiologic reserve puts them at greater risk from such insults. In sum, urinary incontinence is a *symptom,* not a diagnosis, and the incontinent patient deserves appropriate investigation prior to the start of treatment.

Fundamental Investigations

The initial evaluation of the incontinent patient has five basic components: (1) a complete urinalysis and urine culture, (2) a thorough history, (3) a frequency/volume bladder chart, (4) a careful physical examination, and (5) urodynamic testing.

While urinalysis serves as a screening test for many relevant metabolic and urinary tract disorders, a urine culture is essential to rule out infection in any patient with urinary tract symptoms. Failure to culture the urine, even in the absence of a suspicious urinalysis,

may lead the clinician down the wrong track. Not to perform a urine culture on an incontinent patient before embarking on a series of sophisticated urodynamic investigations is akin to starting a work-up for amenorrhea without checking to see if the patient is pregnant! Where possible, infection should be eliminated prior to proceeding further with the evaluation of incontinence. The presence of unusual organisms, infections that persist after appropriate treatment, "sterile" pyuria, or other microscopic abnormalities provide reasons to pursue a more extensive investigation of the upper urinary tract.

A careful review of the patient's history of incontinence allows the physician to determine the nature of the patient's complaint and its severity and helps guide further investigations in certain directions. By itself, however, it does not allow an accurate diagnosis to be made. An adequate history should include the chief complaint (eg, urine loss with coughing), its duration (eg, "since the birth of my last child five years ago"), any special circumstances or precipitating causes (eg, associated change in medication, association with an acute illness such as bronchitis or stroke), and its progression (eg, worsening rapidly over the last 3 months). Previous attempts at therapy, either medical or surgical, should be elicited, and some idea of the severity of the complaint should be obtained. The emotional distress reported by patients does not correlate well with the amount of urine loss that can be demonstrated. Some women will be distraught at a tiny amount of urine leakage occurring during vigorous exercise, such as playing tennis; others will tolerate wearing two or three incontinence pads per day with only minor complaints. Many patients are extremely embarrassed by their urine loss and suffer needlessly for years as a result. A solicitous inquiry into this area during routine care may allow the woman to bring this problem up for discussion and avoid needless delay.

While the physiology of bladder function is still incompletely understood, in practical terms the bladder has only two functions: to store urine and then to empty it completely at a socially acceptable time and place. Doing this involves a complex interplay of afferent sensory messages and efferent motor discharges modulated and directed by an intact nervous system. Because the bladder is an involuntary organ under voluntary control, it is a unique entity, and the complex interplay between the cerebral cortex and the bladder makes symptomatology difficult to evaluate. This is not only because symptoms may have multiple causes, but also because the patient frequently presents an interpretation of her symptoms in the guise of the symptoms themselves. However, patient's symptoms are generally referable to one of four major problems: incontinence or problems with urine storage; voiding difficulty or problems emptying the bladder; problems with bladder sensation, such as pain or lack of bladder sensation; or disorders of bladder contents, such as stones, hematuria, and so on (Table 33-2).

Failure to store urine leads to incontinence. Urinary frequency is the number of times per day that the patient voids. By convention, more than seven voids per day suggests a problem with frequency, but this is highly dependent upon habit and fluid intake. Patients are notoriously inaccurate in estimating urinary frequency and should be encouraged to keep a frequency–volume bladder chart or "urinary diary" for several days as part of their initial evaluation. The volume of each void should be measured and recorded, along with the time. The time and amount of all fluid intake also can be noted if desired. It is especially useful to have the patient record any episodes of incontinence and the circumstances under which these occurred (eg, with sneezing, with urgency, while washing dishes, etc). Patients are often surprised at the patterns revealed by their bladder charts once they have kept them, and the process of doing this plays a useful role in bladder retraining later. Frequency and urgency accompanied by high urine output, for example, may represent compulsive water drinking, not a basic fault with bladder physiology. Nocturia is defined as awakening from sleep with the need to urinate. If this occurs more than once per night, it may represent an abnormality, although nocturia is highly dependent on patient age and normally increases with advancing age. Urge incontinence refers to urine loss accompanied by a powerful desire to urinate (urgency). Urgency may be due to unstable detrusor activity (motor urgency), but it also may be associated with inflammatory bladder disorders and other causes of sensory urgency. The symptom of stress incontinence refers to urine loss under conditions of increased intra-abdominal pressure. This may be due to urethral and bladder neck incompetence, but urine loss during physical exertion also may be produced by unstable detrusor contractions triggered by movement or changes of position without an accompanying sense of urgency.

Voiding difficulty in women has many causes, but only rarely is it caused by true outflow obstruction. Trouble starting the stream of urine (hesitancy), straining to void, and poor or intermittent flow can all reflect either urethral or detrusor dysfunction. Postmicturition dribbling may be a clue to the presence of a urethral diverticulum. Acute urinary retention is manifested as an inability to void that requires catheterization and results in the drainage of a large volume of urine. While this may be psychological in origin, it also may represent serious underlying pathology.

Symptoms of disordered bladder sensation are the most difficult to evaluate, since they are entirely subjective. Urgency, dysuria, and bladder pain may all be accompaniments of acute urinary tract infection; inflammatory bladder disorders, such as interstitial cystitis; psychosomatic reactions to stress; or neoplasia. Feeling of "pressure" in the lower pelvis may represent the effects of a large cystocele or other gynecologic pathology, such as a large ovarian tumor or fibroid uterus. Often such symptoms have no obvious explanation. A lack of bladder sensation or unconscious and unnoticed urine loss is worrisome, as they may represent underlying neurologic disease.

Complaints of "unusual urine" are common and are often difficult to interpret. The patient may notice an unexpected change in the color or smell of her urine, for example. Such changes may be the result of recent dietary indiscretion or the normal mechanism of urine concentration at work in the kidneys, but they also may represent underlying metabolic disease, infection, or something more sinister. Hematuria in particular requires careful evaluation by urinary cytology, culture, cystoscopy, and urography, particularly if it is not related to an acute infection that clears promptly with appropriate antibiotic therapy. Gross hematuria is related to urinary tract malignancy in 22% of patients, and persistent microscopic hematuria is also associated with a neoplasm or other significant urologic lesion in

---

TABLE 33–2
Classification of Bladder Symptoms

I. Symptoms of storage disorders
  A. Frequency
  B. Nocturia
  C. Urge incontinence
  D. Nocturnal enuresis
  E. Stress incontinence
II. Symptoms of emptying disorders
  A. Hesitancy
  B. Straining to void
  C. Poor flow
  E. Intermittent stream
  D. Postmicturition dribble
  F. Incomplete emptying
  G. Acute urinary retention
III. Symptoms of disordered sensation
  A. Urgency
  B. Dysuria
  C. Bladder pain
  D. Feelings of pressure or prolapse
  E. Decreased sensation
  F. Unconscious urine loss
IV. Symptoms of disordered contents
  A. Hematuria
  B. Abnormal color
  C. Abnormal smell
  D. Stones
  E. Foreign bodies
  F. Miscellaneous chemical and other abnormalities

over 20% of cases. Urinary tract stones and foreign bodies that have been introduced into the bladder also may present in a myriad of ways.

It is therefore clear that while symptoms provide clues to the diagnostic possibilities and help point further investigations in certain directions, they are an unreliable guide to the final diagnosis. The clinician who relies upon the history alone in making a diagnosis when dealing with the female lower urinary tract will be wrong an alarming proportion of the time. An example of this is given in Table 33-3, which compares the symptoms elicited in 100 women with genuine stress incontinence due to urethral sphincter incompetence and 100 women with urinary incontinence due to urodynamically demonstrated unstable detrusor activity. It is obvious that the overlap in symptomatology is enormous and that the history by itself does not form a reliable basis for the final diagnosis.

The question arises of whether a woman whose sole complaint is stress incontinence needs further evaluation prior to surgery. To a large degree this depends on the quality of the history taken. Careful investigation reveals that isolated symptomatology occurs only rarely. Haylen and coworkers evaluated 494 women who had complaints of stress incontinence to see how useful this symptom was in making the proper diagnosis. Careful standardized history taking revealed that only 12 (2%) of these women had monosymptomatic stress incontinence, and 482 (98%) of these patients had additional urinary complaints. Urgency and/or urge incontinence was also present in 84% of these women (417); 34% (166) also had dysuria or pain associated with micturition; and 53% (261) had combinations of symptoms that included two or more of the following besides the symptom of stress incontinence: hesitancy, poor stream, sense of incomplete emptying, or need to revoid immediately after micturition. Urine loss during the physical examination was demonstrated in only 168 of these 494 women (34%), and of the 12 women with monosymptomatic stress incontinence, urinary leakage during examination was elicited in only six. All 12 patients with the sole symptom of stress incontinence proved to have genuine stress incontinence after a full evaluation, but out of 494 women, only 290 (59%) had genuine stress incontinence as their sole urodynamic diagnosis at the completion of their testing. The authors concluded that all women should have a urodynamic investigation prior to surgery, since it was so uncommon to make the correct diagnosis on purely clinical grounds alone. Nearly 30 years ago Hodgkinson and colleagues estimated that one third to one half of all "failures" in surgery for stress incontinence were due to preoperative misdiagnosis. Surgical "failure" due to an inadequate preoperative evaluation should not be tolerated.

An appropriate history also must include previous attempts at therapy, including surgical procedures and their results and any medications used in treating bladder disorders. Many medical conditions may affect bladder function, and a neurologic history is especially important in this regard. Diabetes and diseases requiring long-term corticosteroid use will impair wound healing if surgery is undertaken, for example. Current medications taken for other, apparently unrelated con-

TABLE 33–3
The Incidence of Symptoms Associated with Genuine Stress Incontinence and Detrusor Instability in 200 Patients

SYMPTOM	GENUINE STRESS INCONTINENCE (n = 100)	DETRUSOR INSTABILITY (n = 100)
Stress incontinence	89%	49%
Diurnal and nocturnal frequency with stress and urge incontinence	19	26
Urge incontinence	55	38
Current nocturnal enuresis	14	13
Past history of nocturnal enuresis	13	24
Urinary leakage on standing up	45	31
Diurnal urinary frequency	57	79
Nocturnal urinary frequency	38	69
Diurnal and nocturnal urinary frequency	28	56
Difficulty voiding	6	9
Sensation of prolapse	42	18

(After Cardozo L, Stanton SL. Genuine stress incontinence and detrusor instability: a review of 200 patients. Br J Obstet Gynaecol 1980;87:184.)

ditions may have a significant impact on bladder function. Tricyclic antidepressants, for example, have anticholinergic side-effects that may precipitate voiding difficulty, and alpha blockers such as prazosin, used in treating hypertension, may cause drug-induced stress incontinence due to their relaxant properties on the urethra and bladder neck.

Physical examination of the incontinent patient encompasses three areas: a general physical examination, a neurologic screening examination with special emphasis on the lower extremities and perineal area, and the urogynecologic examination. The general physical condition of the patient should be evaluated, with special regard to her mobility, mental status, general level of activity, and potential fitness to undergo an operative procedure. The healthy 40-year-old female with an active life-style and mild stress incontinence requires a different management strategy from the 85-year-old, demented, bedridden nursing home patient with continuous urinary leakage. Transient urinary incontinence is a particular problem among the elderly, for example, and correlates with increasing age and frailty. Because the elderly have a diminished physiologic reserve due to the aging process, are more likely to undergo a pathologic or pharmacologic insult to their systems, and so are more prone to disorientation, sound medical management alone may cure their incontinence without resort to more drastic measures. Resnick has elegantly summarized these factors under the mnemonic *DIAPPERS* (Table 33-4).

The neurologic examination is of particular importance, as significant neurologic conditions may present initially as an isolated disorder of bladder function. While it is true that patients without an obvious neurologic deficit rarely have an occult neurologic problem, the incidence of neuropathology is higher among patients with bladder disorders than among the general population. While our understanding of the neurophysiology of lower-urinary-tract function is far from

TABLE 33–4
Causes of Transient Urinary Incontinence Among the Elderly

Delirium
Infection
Atrophic urethritis/vaginitis
Pharmacologic causes
Psychological causes
Endocrine causes
Restricted mobility
Stool impaction

(After Resnick NM. Voiding dysfunction in the elderly. In: Yalla SV, McGuire EJ, Elbadawi A, et al, eds. Neurourology and urodynamics: principles and practice. New York: Macmillan, 1988.)

complete, it is clinically obvious that normal urinary control requires an intact neurourologic axis, extending from the cerebral cortex down through the pons and midbrain, then through the spinal cord to the peripheral nerves innervating the bladder. Table 33-5 summarizes the neuropathology that may impact on bladder function. Although many authors have devoted extensive space to the description of multiple neurophysiologic "loops" and inhibitory and facilitative micturition reflexes, these remain areas of controversy even among neuroscientists. Until the neurophysiology of bladder function is more clearly understood, detailed descriptions of the processes involved belong in specialty texts that can devote appropriate space to the controversies in this area.

The neurologic examination for the incontinent patient does not have to be extensive. A general screening examination can be done in only a few minutes. If evidence of a previously unsuspected neurologic deficit is uncovered, the patient may be referred for a more extensive neurologic evaluation. Because of the importance of the "micturition center" in the sacral spinal cord, particular importance should be given to the examination of the lower extremities and the lumbosacral spine. Lower-extremity reflexes and movement of the hip, knee, ankle, and foot should be evaluated. In addition, several sacral reflexes may easily be elicited on physical examination. These include the anal wink reflex, the bulbocavernosus reflex, and the cough reflex. Lightly stroking the buttocks lateral to the anal sphincter should elicit a rapid reflex contraction, or "wink," of the external anal sphincter. Gently tapping or stroking the clitoris will elicit a similar response (bulbocavernosus reflex). A reflex contraction of the pelvic floor and perineum will normally be elicited by a cough. The presence of these reflexes provides reassurance that the sacral spinal cord is intact; failure to elicit them, however, does not confirm the presence of a neuropathy, and they should be evaluated within the context of the overall picture presented by the patient. The skin overlying the perineum, buttocks, and medial thighs is innervated by the sacral spinal cord (dermatomes S_2–S_4). Testing the sensitivity of this area to pinprick and light touch provides another means of evaluating the integrity of the sacral spinal cord.

Gynecologic examination of the incontinent patient differs only in degree from that of the continent female. Urinary leakage should be demonstrated, if possible. The condition of the external genitalia should be noted for signs of excoriation and atrophy. The condition, capacity, and mobility of the vagina should be noted, as these may have significant implications for the choice of operation if surgical management is indicated. The presence and degree of any genitourinary prolapse should be noted, which might require simultaneous

TABLE 33–5
Neurological Diseases Affecting Bladder Function

I. Diseases of the brain
  A. Dementia
    1. Neurologic causes (including Huntington's disease, Alzheimer's disease, hydrocephalus, trauma, etc)
    2. Medical causes (such as hypothyroidism, Wernicke-Korsakoff syndrome, syphilis, etc)
  B. Parkinson's disease
  C. Cerebrovascular disease
    1. Ischemic
    2. Occlusive
  D. Multiple sclerosis
  E. Brain tumors
    1. Primary
    2. Metastatic
  F. Trauma
  G. Encephalopathy
  H. Other
II. Diseases of the spinal cord
  A. Trauma
  B. Myelopathy
    1. Vitamin B_{12} deficiency and other nutritional causes
    2. Friedrich's ataxia
    3. Syphilis
    4. Cervical spondylosis
    5. Multiple sclerosis and devic's disease
    6. Amyotrophic lateral sclerosis
    7. Shy-Drager syndrome
    8. Other
  C. Spinovascular disease
  D. Ateriovenous malformations of the spinal cord
  E. Spinal arachnoiditis
  F. Myelitis

  G. Developmental abnormalities (including neural tube defects, tethered cord syndrome, etc)
  H. Spinal cord tumors
    1. Primary
    2. Metastatic
  I. Syringomelia
  J. Other
III. Diseases of the peripheral innervation of the bladder
  A. Trauma
    1. Following radical pelvic surgery
      a. Radical hysterectomy
      b. Abdominoperineal resection
      c. Other
    2. Prolapsed lumbar intravertebral disc
    3. Other
  B. Neuropathy
    1. Metabolic, including diabetes mellitus, hypothyroidism, uremia, hepatic disease
    2. Inflammatory neuropathy (*eg*, Guillain-Barré syndrome)
    3. Collagen-vascular disease
    4. Malignancy
    5. Alcoholism
    6. Infectious neuropathy (including syphilis and herpes zoster)
    7. Exogenous poisoning (*eg*, lead, arsenic, etc)
    8. Other
  C. Tumors
    1. Primary
    2. Metastatic
  D. Tethered cord syndrome
  E. Lumbar spinal stenosis
  F. Sacral agenesis
  G. Other

(After Hald T, Bradley WE. The urinary bladder: neurology and dynamics. Baltimore: Williams & Wilkins, 1982.)

correction at the time of surgery. Of particular importance is the evaluation of bladder neck and urethral hypermobility, for descent of the bladder neck below the pelvic floor appears to be one of the major factors involved in the development of genuine stress incontinence. However, hypermobility of the bladder neck may be present in otherwise normal, continent women or in incontinent women whose leakage is due to an unstable detrusor. The diagnosis of genuine stress incontinence remains a *urodynamic* diagnosis.

Urodynamic Studies

In the broadest sense, anything that provides objective information on lower-urinary-tract function may be considered a urodynamic study. A full discussion of the many complex and often controversial techniques that have been developed to look at bladder and urethral function lies beyond the scope of this chapter and may be found in a number of specialist monographs. The

most important and most useful of these techniques—the real workhorse of lower-urinary-tract investigation—remains the subtracted cystometrogram. Cystometry is the technique by which the pressure/volume relationship of the bladder is measured, and it is used to assess bladder sensation, bladder capacity, bladder compliance (change in pressure with change in volume), and detrusor activity. It is a way of attempting to reproduce the bladder cycle of filling and emptying in a clinical laboratory.

Because the bladder is a distensible organ that fills and empties regularly, much of its function may be understood by purely mechanical principles. Figure 33-1 represents the cycle of bladder filling and emptying as a simple pressure/volume loop. Initially, the bladder accommodates a gradual increase in volume without a significant rise in detrusor pressure (point 1). At a volume of approximately 150 ml (point 2) the first sensation of fullness or first desire to void normally occurs, but this is followed by a period of voluntary cortical suppression of the micturition reflex (point 3) until a socially acceptable time and place arises (point

Figure 33–1. The bladder cycle represented as a pressure/volume loop. (1) Accommodation—a gradual increase in bladder volume without a significant rise in detrusor pressure. (2) First sensation of fullness. (3) Cortical suppression of the micturition reflex. (4) Voluntary initiation of voiding. (5) Isometric pressure rise as detrusor contraction begins before the bladder neck is fully open and the pelvic floor is fully relaxed. (6) Sustained detrusor contraction resulting in complete bladder emptying. (7) Detrusor relaxation. (After Torrens MJ. Neurophysiology. In: Stanton SL, ed. Clinical gynecologic urology. St. Louis: CV Mosby, 1984.)

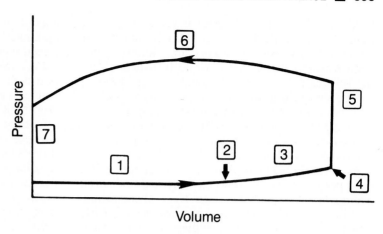

4). At this time the normal individual can generate a detrusor contraction and produce a concomitant rise in bladder pressure while relaxing the pelvic floor. This may appear as an isometric pressure rise if the detrusor contraction begins before the bladder neck is fully open (point 5). Normal voiding is then accomplished by a continuous detrusor contraction (point 6) that is sustained until the bladder is empty, at which time the bladder relaxes and the pelvic floor resumes its normal tone (point 7).

The cystometrogram is an attempt to reproduce these physiologic changes within the unphysiologic confines of a urodynamics laboratory. Pressure catheters, consisting of either fluid-filled lines or electronic microtip pressure-transducer catheters, are placed in the bladder to measure bladder pressure (Fig. 33-2).

However, since the bladder is an intra-abdominal organ, measurement of bladder pressure alone will be confounded by concurrent changes in abdominal pressure that may be mistaken for unstable detrusor activity on a simple cystometrogram. To correct for this problem, subtracted cystometry is used. Another catheter is placed in the vagina or rectum and the pressure measured there is used as an approximation of intra-abdominal pressure. The abdominal pressure (P_{abd}) is then subtracted from the intravesical pressure (P_{ves}) to arrive at the intrinsic bladder pressure or subtracted detrusor pressure (P_{det}), which represents the pressure in the bladder due to the tone or contraction of the detrusor muscle ($P_{det} = P_{ves} - P_{abd}$). The bladder is then filled at a standard rate (usually 50–100 ml/min) and the patient's sensations are recorded and corre-

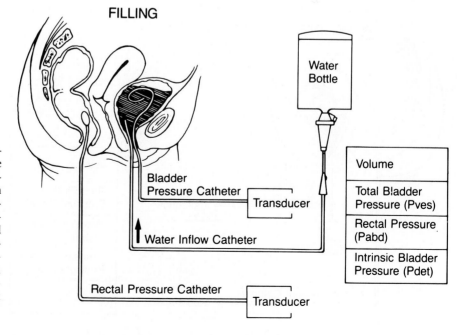

Figure 33–2. Filling cystometry. Pressure catheters are in place in the bladder and rectum. An additional filling catheter has been placed in the bladder. Volume infused, total bladder pressure, rectal (abdominal) pressure, and subtracted detrusor pressure (intrinsic bladder pressure) are recorded. (After Wall LL, Addison WA. Basic cystometry in gynecologic practice. Postgrad Obstet Gynecol 1988;8(26):1.)

lated with the subtracted detrusor pressure. During filling the subtracted detrusor pressure should remain stable, without phasic contractions, and should not normally rise more than $15 \, cmH_2$. While the patient's bladder is being filled she should cough, change position, and be subjected to various physical activities such as heel bouncing, bending over, or standing up, in an attempt to provoke unstable detrusor activity. The use of these provocative maneuvers will uncover far more pathology than supine filling alone, which may miss many unstable bladders. With the bladder full, in the erect position, the patient should cough and strain in an attempt to reproduce her leakage. The goal of cystometry is to reproduce the patient's symptoms in the urodynamics laboratory so that they can be evaluated fully in the light of bladder function. For this reason, urodynamic studies are best done by a person, preferably the treating physician, who is thoroughly familiar with her history and physical examination. Without this information urodynamic studies are difficult to interpret accurately.

When the filling lines have been removed, the patient can be placed over a urine flowmeter and a study of the emptying phase of the bladder cycle begun (Fig. 33-3). Urine flow rate is measured and correlated with changes in bladder, abdominal, and subtracted detrusor pressures. The addition of pelvic floor or urethral sphincter electromyography and fluoroscopic visualization of a contrast-filled bladder may be necessary in some cases for a complete evaluation of bladder function. Patients with low flow rates and those who void primarily by abdominal straining or urethral relaxation, for example, appear to be at higher risk for voiding dysfunction after certain kinds of anti-incontinence operations. The approximate range of normal cystometric values in women is given in Table 33-6.

Controversy exists over whether filling cystometry is best done with a gas (CO_2) or liquid (water or radiocontrast) medium. The advantages of carbon dioxide are that it is fast, relatively clean, cheap, and easy to infuse at a constant rate through small filling catheters. Because carbon dioxide is readily soluble in blood, there is little chance of causing a gas embolism. Carbon dioxide cystometry also appears to be a good provocative test for uncovering unstable detrusor activity. However, gas infusion is extremely unphysiologic, and because carbon dioxide forms carbonic acid when dissolved, it can be painful in hypersensitive bladders. Similarly, because gas is readily compressible, there is no appreciable increase in bladder mass with filling, and it becomes more difficult to evaluate bladder accommodation. Since only one catheter is commonly used in gas cystometry, it is impossible to evaluate intra-abdominal pressure, making the technique subject to artifactual error. Most important, the emptying phase of the bladder cycle cannot be evaluated using carbon dioxide, since pressure-flow voiding studies are not possible with a gas medium.

Although a constant filling rate is more difficult to achieve using a liquid medium such as normal saline, sterile water, or radiographic contrast, and although liquid cystometry is more expensive and less tidy than gas cystometry, the former technique has many advantages. Since the urothelium of the bladder normally interacts with a liquid, water cystometry is more physiologic. Bladder irritation is minimal and evaluation of

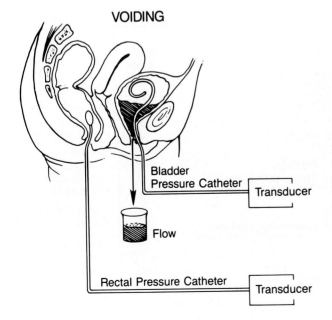

VOIDING

Bladder Pressure Catheter — Transducer

Flow

Rectal Pressure Catheter — Transducer

Volume
Total Bladder Pressure (Pves)
Rectal Pressure (Pabd)
Intrinsic Bladder Pressure (Pdet)
Flow

Figure 33–3. Pressure-flow voiding study. The filling catheter has been removed. Volume voided, urine flow rate, total bladder pressure, rectal (abdominal) pressure, and subtracted detrusor pressure (intrinsic bladder pressure) are recorded. (After Wall LL, Addison WA. Basic cystometry in gynecologic practice. Postgrad Obstet Gynecol 1988;8(26):1.)

TABLE 33–6
Approximate Normal Cystometric Values in Women

Residual urine	Less than 50 ml
First sensation	150–250 ml
Cystometric capacity	400–600 ml
Maximum detrusor pressure during filling	Less than 15 cm H_2O
Maximum detrusor pressure during voiding	Less than 70 cm H_2O
Peak urine flow rate	Greater than 15 ml/sec

temperature sensation is possible. Simultaneous measurement of bladder and rectal pressures is possible, allowing calculation of subtracted detrusor pressure. Voiding studies are also possible using a liquid medium, and if radiocontrast is used, simultaneous fluoroscopic videocystourethrography is possible to evaluate the configuration, integrity, and position of the bladder neck.

Figure 33-4 represents a stable cystometrogram in a patient with genuine stress incontinence. As the bladder is gradually filled with water (*A*) there is a slight rise in intravesical pressure. Abdominal pressure remains constant and the subtracted detrusor pressure is stable. At point *B* the patient, who has been supine, rises to a standing position. The change in position causes a rise in both intravesical and rectal pressure as the abdominal contents shift, but the subtracted detrusor pressure remains stable. Sharp pressure spikes (*C, arrows*) are generated by the patient coughing in the erect position with a full bladder. The demonstration of urinary leakage under these conditions allows the urodynamic diagnosis of genuine stress incontinence to be given.

Figure 33-5 is an example of an abnormal, unstable cystometrogram. Here during the filling phase, rectal pressure (abdominal pressure) remains low while there are phasic pressure changes in both the intravesical and detrusor pressure tracings (*A*). This demonstrates unstable detrusor activity. At point *B,* multiple

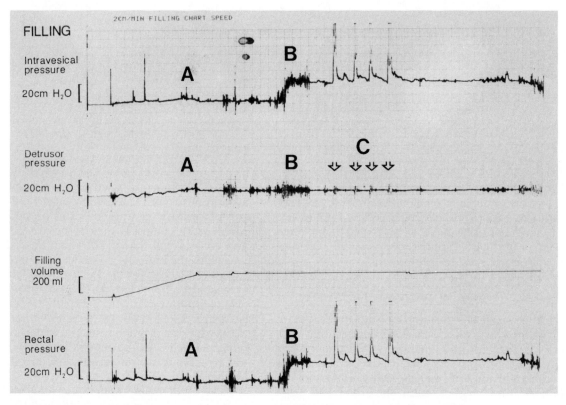

Figure 33–4. Stable filling cystometrogram showing genuine stress incontinence. During supine filling (*A*), there is no rise in detrusor pressure. When the patient stands up *B*, there is a rise in intravesical and rectal pressure as the intra-abdominal contents shift; however, the subtracted detrusor pressure remains stable. When the patient coughs in the erect position (*C, arrows*), the detrusor remains stable. Coughs appear as sharp pressure spikes on the intravesical and rectal pressure tracings. Demonstration of urine leakage under these conditions gives the urodynamic diagnosis of genuine stress incontinence.

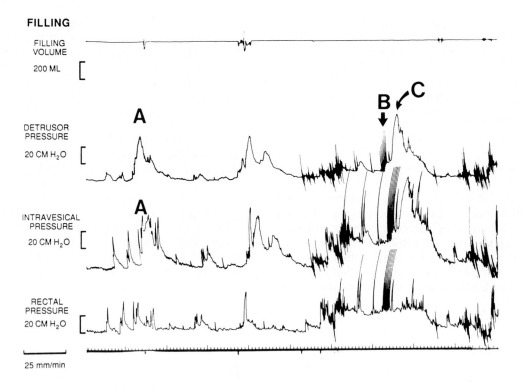

FILLING

FILLING
VOLUME

200 ML

DETRUSOR
PRESSURE

20 CM H₂O

INTRAVESICAL
PRESSURE

20 CM H₂O

RECTAL
PRESSURE

20 CM H₂O

25 mm/min

Figure 33–5. Unstable filling cystometrogram demonstrating detrusor instability. During filling, pronounced phasic detrusor contractions are demonstrated (*A*) with urine loss, making the diagnosis of detrusor instability. Sharp pressure spikes *B* represent coughs, which in this case are followed immediately by an unstable detrusor contraction *C*. Such patients may be misdiagnosed as having simple stress incontinence if urodynamic studies are not carried out.

sharp pressure spikes represent the patient coughing. In this case, coughing precipitates unstable detrusor activity (*C*). Such a patient could be mistaken for one with simple stress incontinence and could be subjected to an ineffectual and unnecessary operation if urodynamic studies are not performed.

Management of Detrusor Instability

The patient whose urinary incontinence is due to uninhibited detrusor activity needs different treatment from the patient with simple stress incontinence. The therapeutic mainstays for such patients are behavioral modification and drug therapy. Other, more complex therapies involving electrical stimulation or major urologic reconstructive surgery such as augmentation cystoplasty are available for complicated and refractory cases. These modalities are beyond the scope of this chapter, and the interested reader is referred to two recent comprehensive reviews for further information (Freeman and Malvern, 1989; Wall, 1990).

Behavioral modification, or bladder retraining for

detrusor instability, is based on the premise that the basic problem with bladder function in these patients is that the bladder has escaped from previously established cortical control. During normal development the child goes through a period of automatic bladder emptying when the urge arises. Gradually, suppression and control of bladder function is learned as the child is socialized to cultural norms. This results in the ability to postpone micturition until a socially acceptable time and place. The incontinent patient with an unstable bladder has lost this ability and must regain it. Behavioral modification for the unstable bladder is, therefore, nothing more than a refresher course in toilet training for adults.

Bladder drill regimens attempt to reestablish cortical control over bladder function, gradually lengthening the time that micturition may be postponed. Many studies have been done using both inpatient and outpatient training protocols, with excellent results. These regimens work well for patients with motor or sensory urgency, frequency, and urge incontinence, many of whom suffer from half-hourly or hourly urinary frequency and incontinence. The object of therapy is to break this vicious cycle and return them to a normal voiding pattern.

To do this the patient's baseline voiding pattern must first be established with a frequency/volume chart or urinary diary. Once this is done the patient can be instructed to start a schedule that she can manage, for example, to void every 45 minutes during the day. The patient must then void by the clock, whether she needs to or not, on a rigid schedule throughout the day. At night, she voids only as the need arises and does not maintain a fixed schedule. Thus, when the patient gets up in the morning, she voids at 6:15 AM, 7:00 AM, 7:45 AM, and so on. However, if it is 6:50 AM and she has a terrible urge to urinate, she must postpone it, even if this results in leakage. Similarly, if it is 7:45 AM and she does not feel the need to urinate, she must do so anyway. The object is to reestablish cortical control over bladder function and to put her back in charge of her bladder, rather than the other way around. When she can complete this schedule successfully for 1 week, the interval is gradually increased by 15 minutes. Week by week the voiding interval is increased by small amounts until the patient can control her bladder for 2–3 hours. These regimens are successful, but patient compliance is the absolute prerequisite for success. This can be enhanced by the unrelenting enthusiasm and support of the physician. The patient also must not try to do too much too soon. Gradual increases in the voiding interval are extremely important. As useful as this therapy is, however, some patients are unsuited to such an approach.

Drug therapy for detrusor instability is a reasonable and useful alternative to behavioral modification. All drug treatment for the unstable bladder is an attempt to interrupt the uncontrolled activity of the neuromuscular unit at some level, and since the main neurotransmitter in the bladder is acetylcholine, all drugs currently available for treating detrusor instability have anticholinergic properties and side-effects to some extent. Typical anticholinergic side-effects from these drugs include a dry mouth, from suppression of salivary and oropharyngeal secretions; constipation, resulting from decreased gastrointestinal motility; an increase in heart rate due to vagal blockade; feelings of drowsiness; and transient blurring of the vision from blockade of the sphincter of the iris and the ciliary muscle of the lens of the eye. In general, these drugs are safe and dosage is usually limited by intolerance to side-effects rather than other forms of toxicity. However, they should be used cautiously in patients with significant cardiac arrhythmias or narrow-angle glaucoma, in whom they may cause a precipitous rise in intraocular pressure.

The drugs useful in treating the unstable detrusor may be classified into four main categories (Table 33-7):

TABLE 33–7
Drug Treatment of Detrusor Instability

DRUG	DOSE*
Anticholinergic Drugs	
Methantheline bromide	50 mg po QID
Propantheline bromide	15–30 mg po QID
Antispasmodic/Spasmolytic Drugs	
Oxybutynin chloride	5–10 mg po TID/QID
Dicyclomine hydrochloride	10–20 mg po TID/QID
Flavoxate hydrochloride	200 mg po QID
Tricyclic Antidepressants	
Imipramine hydrochloride	10 mg po TID; 50 mg po BID
Doxepin	50–75 mg po QHS
Calcium Channel Blockers	
Terodiline hydrochloride	12.5–25 mg po BID

*po = by mouth, BID = twice daily, TID = three times daily, QID = four times daily, QHS = at bedtime.

anticholinergic drugs, such as methantheline or propantheline; antispasmodic or spasmolytic drugs, such as oxybutynin, dicyclomine, or flavoxate, which have a direct relaxant effect on smooth muscle in addition to anticholinergic effects; tricyclic antidepressants, such as imipramine or doxepin, which have effects on the central nervous system and alpha-adrenergic effects on the urethra and bladder neck as well as anticholinergic effects; and newer drugs, such as terodiline, a calcium channel blocker with anticholinergic properties. Some women appear to have perimenstrual exacerbation of their detrusor instability resulting from uterine prostaglandin synthesis and release. The addition of a prostaglandin synthetase inhibitor, such as mefenamic acid, around the time of menstruation may be of great benefit in selected cases. Older women with atrophic urethritis/vaginitis and detrusor instability also may benefit from appropriate hormone replacement therapy.

Factors Contributing to Genuine Stress Incontinence

As has been noted earlier, stress incontinence is the most common form of urinary incontinence in women, but the term is used to refer to three distinct entities: a symptom, a sign, and a condition. The *symptom* of stress incontinence refers only to the patient's complaint that she leaks urine when intra-abdominal pressure is increased. The *physical sign* of stress incontinence refers to demonstration of urine loss during physical examination of the patient when intra-abdominal pressure is raised, as with coughing. Both the symptom and the physical sign of stress incontinence, however, can be produced by pathologic processes other than anatomic defects of bladder neck support or failure of the sphincteric mechanism of the urethra and bladder neck. The *condition* or *diagnosis* of genuine stress incontinence is made when urine loss is demonstrated to occur when intravesical pressure exceeds the maximum urethral pressure, but in the absence of a detrusor contraction. This implies stable detrusor activity at the time of urine loss, which can only be demonstrated urodynamically. The use of the term *genuine stress incontinence* therefore implies that the patient has had a urodynamic investigation demonstrating these findings. The term *pressure-equalization incontinence* is also sometimes used for this condition because urine loss occurs when the bladder outlet and urethra cannot withstand the increased intravesical pressure generated by exercise, coughing, sneezing, straining, and so on. The sudden rise in bladder pressure generated by these activities is not transmitted adequately to the proximal urethra and bladder neck so that a positive pressure gradient is not maintained, and as bladder pressure suddenly rises higher than outlet resistance, the patient leaks a spurt of urine.

Clearly, this condition is common among women. Hodgkinson stressed that the relatively short and unprotected female urethra made all women relatively susceptible to urinary incontinence and that nearly all women experienced stress incontinence from time to time. Indeed, several surveys of otherwise young, healthy, nulliparous women have shown that 50% have experienced this symptom, and a significant number have experienced it frequently. According to the International Continence Society's definition referred to earlier, incontinence exists when urine loss becomes a social or hygienic problem. What factors push the mild, relatively common occurrence of female stress incontinence into the realm of a clinical problem?

To the best of our current knowledge, three factors are important in the development of this condition: (1) abnormal descent of the bladder neck and urethra below the zone of effective pressure transmission of the pelvic floor; (2) weakness of or damage to the intrinsic sphincter mechanism of the urethra and bladder neck itself; and (3) neurologic damage to the pelvic floor.

Hypermobility of the bladder neck and urethra is an anatomic defect that is associated with genuine stress incontinence in many cases. Laxity of support of the bladder neck and proximal urethra allows these structures to fall out of the zone of effective pressure transmission during physically stressful activities and prevents the maintenance of an effective closure pressure. Incontinence then results. Correction of the hypermobility is associated with clinical cure in the majority of cases.

Hypermobility of these structures can be evaluated by several means. The easiest is by physical examination, paying close attention to the position and mobility of the bladder neck while the patient strains during a pelvic examination with the posterior vagina retracted with a Sims speculum. A lubricated cotton-tipped applicator placed in the urethra to the level of the bladder neck (the Q-tip test) accentuates this movement and allows for better visualization of mobility. As the patient strains down, her hypermobile bladder neck will rotate downward and backward, making the Q-tip rise upward. The normally supported urethra and bladder neck will not do this. Fluoroscopic examination of the bladder filled with radiographic contrast medium also shows this mobility, and allows further observation of bladder neck opening during this process. Similar, but more limited, information can be obtained during a urethroscopic examination of the bladder neck, watching it move downward and backward under stress.

It must be carefully pointed out, however, that bladder neck hypermobility may be demonstrated in normal, continent women and that the demonstration of bladder neck hypermobility is not the same as genuine stress incontinence. Patients with a hypermobile bladder neck may be incontinent due to unstable detrusor activity or other causes and should still undergo cystometry prior to surgery.

Urinary continence is normally maintained at the level of the proximal urethra and bladder neck, and for this to occur, outlet resistance must be higher than the bladder pressure. Many factors contribute to the intraurethral pressure, which is an important part of this outlet resistance (Table 33-8). Experimental evidence suggests that one third of the total intraurethral pressure is due to the striated muscle of the urethra and pelvic floor, the rest being contributed by other factors. Although urethral pressure profilometry is now generally considered to have little role in diagnosing genuine stress incontinence, urethral pressure measurements in women with genuine stress incontinence do suggest that intrinsic urethral pressure decreases as the severity of incontinence increases and that urethral pressure

TABLE 33–8
Factors Contributing to Intraurethral Pressure

1. Striated muscle of the urethral wall
2. Smooth muscle of the urethral wall and blood vessels
3. Vascular congestion of the submucosal venous plexus
4. Elasticity of the urethral wall
5. Transmission of intra-abdominal pressure
6. Mucosal coaptation of the urothelium
7. Hormonal status
8. Autonomic (sympathetic) innervation and tone (alpha-adrenergic receptors)

decreases as the number of prior attempts at surgical cure increases. This suggests that damage to the intrinsic sphincteric unit plays a role in some cases of stress incontinence, most notably in those unfortunate women who have failed previous attempts at cure and through progressive scarring have developed a low-pressure, "drainpipe" urethra that is little more than a functionless conduit for the uncontrolled drip of urine to the outside world. Merely supporting or repositioning such a urethra and bladder neck is unlikely to result in a cure of incontinence in these patients. Fluoroscopic examination generally reveals a wide-open bladder neck with copious "gravitational" incontinence under minimal stress. Urethroscopic examination often reveals similar findings.

Evidence is increasing that suggests that denervation injury to the pelvic floor is an important component in the development of genuine stress incontinence. Studies using single-fiber electromyography, a sensitive test of denervation injury and subsequent reinnervation, have consistently shown a higher fiber density in the musculature of the pelvic floor in stress-incontinent women compared to normal controls. The normal fiber density of a motor unit is low, but increases following denervation injury due to collateral sprouting of injured nerves as they attempt to reinnervate the muscle. The higher single-fiber densities demonstrated in stress-incontinent women are direct evidence of associated pelvic neuromuscular damage. Additional evidence of this phenomenon comes from studies using the motor nerve latency of the pudendal nerve, which innervates both the external anal sphincter and the striated urethral sphincter. Using a transrectal electrode, it is possible to stimulate the pudendal nerve as it passes the ischial spine and measure the conduction latency to either the anal or urethral sphincter. Several studies have now shown prolonged latency in stress-incontinent women compared to normal controls, and these measurements have been correlated with decreased maximum urethral pressure in the incontinent patients. The available evidence suggests that this denervation is a result of pelvic trauma sustained during delivery and probably made worse in patients who have chronic tenesmus. Denervation injury of this type is also associated with idiopathic anorectal incontinence in women.

The clinical implications of these neurologic findings remain unclear. In the patient with an intact sphincteric unit, the maintenance of continence depends upon adequate transmission of pressure across the urethra and bladder neck during stress, so that outlet pressure remains higher than bladder pressure. If, as seems reasonable, the pelvic floor acts as a "trampoline" to bounce these pressure waves across this area, then neuromuscular injury probably contributes to the development of incontinence by preventing the pelvic floor from maintaining an adequate tone and decreasing the resiliency of this pressure transmission process. Obstetric injury that damages the connective tissue and fascial supports of the bladder neck and urethra further disrupts normal pressure transmission. Pudendal nerve damage leading to diminished maximum urethral pressure would similarly weaken the continence mechanism and predispose to the development of urinary incontinence. The summation of these many factors on the status of the urethra and bladder neck could ultimately diminish the patient's "margin for continence" and push her below the threshold for urinary leakage.

Nonsurgical Management of Genuine Stress Incontinence

Pelvic surgeons tend to regard the solution to the problem of genuine stress incontinence as surgical; however, surgery for urinary incontinence is almost always an elective procedure, never an emergency. It is a mistake of major proportions to pressure a patient into having surgery for her incontinence before she is ready. An operation should be carried out only when the problem has become severe enough for the patient to want to have it done. Some women may not be bothered enough by the degree of their leakage to wish to undergo the expense and convalescence of surgery. Others may not have finished childbearing and, while bothered by their leakage, may be reluctant to undergo an operation that may be damaged or undone by subsequent pregnancy, labor, and delivery. Still other incontinent women are frail and elderly and are reluctant to undergo an operation because of their general health. If nonsurgical approaches to restoring bladder neck support and urethral tone could be developed, such women could benefit greatly.

It remains unclear precisely how urethral tone, bladder neck and urethral mobility, and the state of pelvic floor innervation all interact to produce urinary continence or incontinence. Recent work on the anatomy of this region suggests that the continence mechanism is more sophisticated and elaborate than heretofore recognized; clearly, however, much of the support of this region comes from the pelvic musculature. The musculature of the levator ani complex provides substantial support for the urethra, vagina, and rectum as they descend through the pelvic floor, by its connection with the endopelvic fascia.

The periurethral levator ani muscles contain both type I (slow twitch) and type II (fast twitch) muscle fibers, which allows them to maintain tone over a long period and to increase tone suddenly to compensate for the increased abdominal pressure that occurs with coughing, sneezing, and straining. Rehabilitation of these muscle groups through exercise and physical therapy might serve to improve the continence mechanism in two ways. First, strengthening the striated urogenital sphincter could enhance its ability to constrict the urethral lumen. This might yield a higher resting pressure in the urethra and/or increase the amount of pressure generated in the urethra during a cough or other stressful situations. Second, because the levator ani muscles are important to pelvic and urethral support, an exercise program could improve the support of the proximal urethra. Since these muscles may be activated during a cough, continence might be improved without a noticeable rise in resting urethral pressure measurements.

Arnold Kegel was the first person to investigate pelvic floor muscle strengthening in a systematic fashion. His method consisted of developing the patient's awareness of the pubococcygeus muscle and then instructing her in exercises to strengthen this muscle with a crude pneumatic biofeedback device called a perineometer. Kegel originally stressed the importance of supervised instruction and encouragement in the performance of these exercises and reported good success rates in relieving symptomatic stress incontinence by his program. While nearly all gynecologists are familiar with these exercises, they rarely are taught and used as Kegel did originally, and this form of therapy has often degenerated into a few brief words of oral instruction in which the patient is told to stop and start her urine stream a few times each day while voiding. Not surprisingly, programs of this nature often have disappointing results.

For muscular rehabilitation of the pelvic floor to work, it must be supervised, done regularly, and aided by some form of feedback so that the patient can judge her progress. Bo and coworkers have clearly shown that enthusiastic supervision makes a dramatic difference in the degree of success that can be obtained by programs of pelvic muscle rehabilitation. Other workers have had similar results. Using an intensive program of physical therapy over 3 months with pre- and posttherapy urodynamic and radiographic evaluations, Benvenuti and colleagues cured 32% of their patients with genuine stress incontinence and brought about marked improvement in symptoms in the remaining 68%. A significant improvement in maximal urethral closure pressure and functional urethral length was seen after therapy. Both tonic and phasic contractility of the pubococcygeus muscle were improved, and clear-cut improvement of bladder neck support was seen on radiographic evaluation in 13 of 15 patients who underwent repeat studies. After 12–36 months of follow-up, 77% reported that they had maintained the functional level they had attained at the end of treatment.

Similarly, Peattie and coworkers trained 30 premen-opausal women with genuine stress incontinence in pelvic muscle rehabilitation using an ingenious form of resistive therapy using a set of weighted vaginal cones. These cones were of the same size but of increasing weight, from 20 to 100 g. The cones were retained in the vagina after insertion by contraction of the pelvic floor. As one cone was successfully retained for 15 minutes, the next heaviest cone was used, thus progressively increasing the weight retained. The feeling that the cone is slipping out of the vagina results in a form of sensory biofeedback that causes an increased contraction in the pelvic floor in an attempt to retain it. At the end of 1 month of therapy, 19 patients (70%) reported cure or significant improvement of symptoms and only 11 (37%) opted for subsequent surgical intervention. Other authors have reported similar results using similar methods.

This is not to suggest that physical therapy will cure or improve all cases of stress incontinence. A complete review of the literature on this subject is clearly beyond the scope of this chapter, but there is evidence to suggest that properly supervised and rigorously performed techniques for pelvic muscular rehabilitation can play a significant role in the treatment of genuine stress incontinence. Patients can expect improvement in their symptoms by tensing the musculature of the pelvic floor and holding these contractions for 5 seconds each, 15–20 times per session, three sessions per day. As this form of therapy is virtually without side-effects, involves the patient in her own care, and may prevent the development of subsequent pelvic relaxation if used regularly, gynecologists should make more use of it and should be encouraged to incorporate pelvic muscle exercises into routine health maintenance programs for women.

The tone of the urethra and bladder neck is maintained in large part by alpha-adrenergic activity from the sympathetic nervous system. For this reason many pharmacologic agents have been used to treat genuine stress incontinence, with varying degrees of success (Table 33-9). These drugs include imipramine, which has a concomitant relaxing effect on the detrusor;

TABLE 33–9
Drug Treatment of Genuine Stress Incontinence

DRUG	DOSE*
Ephedrine	15–30 mg po TID
Norephedrine	100 mg po BID
Norfenefrine	15–30 mg po TID
Phenylpropanolamine	50–75 mg po BID
Imipramine	10–25 mg po TID

*po = by mouth, BID = twice daily, TID = three times daily.

ephedrine; phenylpropanolamine; norfenefrine; and norephedrine. Unfortunately, many of these compounds also increase vascular tone and may therefore lead to problems with hypertension—a condition that afflicts many postmenopausal women with stress incontinence. These effects may preclude the use of alpha agonists in such patients. Of equal importance, however, is the role of alpha blockers such as prazosin in the development of stress incontinence. These drugs are commonly used in treating hypertension because of their relaxing effects on vascular smooth muscle. They may also relax the bladder neck and urethra to the point where incontinence develops. Patients who present with complaints of stress incontinence while taking this or a related drug should have their antihypertensive medication changed before surgery is considered, as their incontinence may resolve spontaneously with a change of medication.

Postmenopausal women with urogenital atrophy due to estrogen deprivation and concurrent urinary incontinence should be placed on hormone replacement therapy as part of their therapeutic regimen, unless such therapy is contraindicated for other reasons. Not only will many complaints of urgency, frequency, and irritation often disappear, but evidence suggests that estrogen replacement enhances the effectiveness of alpha-adrenergic receptors in the urethra.

Besides physical therapy and selected pharmacologic agents, electrical stimulation therapy has been used in an attempt to treat genuine stress incontinence. Passage of an electrical current through the muscles of the pelvic floor causes them to contract and simultaneously causes a reflex inhibition of detrusor activity. The stimulus can be applied transvaginally or transrectally in either continuous or intermittent fashion. Although many authors have reported good success rates using these devices, problems remain with poor patient acceptance of the technique and mechanical problems with device failure. While this mode of therapy remains an option for the patient with stress incontinence, it is unlikely to be used extensively at present outside of the research setting.

Selection of Operations for Genuine Stress Incontinence

When a patient presents herself as a candidate for operative management of genuine stress incontinence, the surgeon faces an enormous array of potential procedures from which to choose. Probably more than 100 operations can be found in the world medical literature as suggested surgical cures for this condition. This alone should alert the surgeon to the fact that the ideal operation has yet to be devised. The major operations can be grouped into seven categories (Table 33-10). Which of these many operations is best?

A review of the literature on the surgical treatment of genuine stress incontinence immediately reveals many problems. Many series have no urodynamic data, follow-up is short or shoddy, no objective criteria are used to define outcome, and most series represent the retrospective, personal experience of one surgeon with one procedure. Ideally, the answer to the question of which is the "best" operation should come from prospective studies where equivalent patients with urodynamically proven diagnoses are randomized to one of several operations done by one of several surgeons and followed for several years postoperatively. Out of the vast literature on stress incontinence, only a few studies come close to meeting these criteria. These are summarized in Table 33-11.

Review of these studies shows that anterior colporrhaphy is consistently inferior to the Burch colposuspension operation for the objective cure of genuine stress incontinence. Although it is obvious that anterior vaginal repair can produce a clinical cure in some patients that may be sustained over time, the available evidence strongly suggests that this operation should be used primarily for symptomatic cystocele without stress incontinence. Surgeons who routinely use anterior vaginal repair as their primary operation for genuine stress incontinence are doing their patients a disservice.

Review of the other surgical alternatives suggests that these may be divided into two broad groups: those for patients whose primary problem is incontinence due to hypermobility of the bladder neck and proximal ure-

TABLE 33-10
Surgical Procedures for Genuine Stress Incontinence

1. Anterior colporrhaphy
2. Needle suspension procedures
   a. Pereyra procdure
   b. Subsequent minor modifications
3. Retropubic bladder neck suspension
   a. Marshall-Marchetti-Krantz operation
   a. Burch colposuspension
   c. Paravaginal repair
4. Sling operations
   a. Organic materials
      1. Autologous tissues
      2. Hetereologous tissues
   b. Synthetic materials
5. Periurethral injections
   a. Teflon paste
   b. GAX collagen
6. Artificial urinary sphincter
7. Urinary diversion

TABLE 33–11
Comparative Surgical Studies of Operations for Genuine Stress Incontinence

| REFERENCE | NUMBER OF PATIENTS | OBJECTIVE CURE RATES BY OPERATION FOR PATIENTS WITH GENUINE STRESS INCONTINENCE | | | LENGTH OF FOLLOW-UP |
		Anterior Colporrhaphy	*Needle Suspension*	*Burch Colposuspension*	
Stanton and Cardozo	50	36%	—	84%	6 months +
Mundy	51	—	40%	89	12 months
Weil et al.	86	57	50	91	6 months +
Van Geelan et al.	90	45	—	85	1–2 years
Bergman et al.*	289	69	70	87	12 months
Bergman et al.†	107	65	72	91	12 months

* Patients with concurrent prolapse.
† Patients without concurrent prolapse.

thra and those whose incontinence is due to damage to the sphincteric unit itself. Although some disagreement in the literature exists, patients with genuine stress incontinence who have an associated defect of anatomic support leading to urethral and bladder neck hypermobility should be cured of their incontinence if the hypermobility is corrected. The best operations for this procedure appear to be retropubic bladder neck suspensions such as the Burch colposuspension. Needle suspension procedures such as the Pereyra procedure or one of its modifications work less well but seem to have a higher long-term success rate than anterior colporrhaphy. The vast majority of patients with genuine stress incontinence are patients whose incontinence is largely due to an anatomic defect leading to hypermobility of the bladder outlet with resultant "pressure equalization" incontinence.

Patients with complex stress incontinence rarely present as candidates for primary surgery. The patient with sphincteric damage almost always has some other problem at presentation—either a congenital abnormality of the lower urinary tract, previous failed incontinence surgery (often with multiple prior attempts at cure), incontinence developing after other pelvic surgery (eg, a radical hysterectomy or radical vulvectomy), or significant pelvic trauma. Evaluation of these patients requires special care, particularly in the face of failed incontinence surgery. If residual hypermobility is present, all that may be required for cure is adequate repositioning of the bladder neck in a retropubic position. This situation commonly occurs in patients who have had a failed anterior colporrhaphy, patients who have had a retropubic urethropexy that failed due to the use of chromic catgut suture, or patients who have had a needle suspension procedure that failed due to the permanent "guy wire" sutures breaking or pulling through the supporting fascia. However, if the urethra

and bladder neck are well supported and without excess mobility, further attempts to elevate them are unlikely to succeed. These patients require operations that compensate for sphincteric damage by supporting and partially occluding the urethra and bladder neck. These procedures are more difficult and may be plagued by considerable postoperative voiding difficulty.

At various times surgeons have attempted to inject material such as polytetrafluoroethylene (Teflon) paste around the urethral lumen to support it, narrow it, and restore some of its integrity. This procedure has been used with some success, but it requires both general anesthesia and a power injector. Furthermore, the Teflon particles have been shown to migrate to such distant locations as the brain and lungs. This has dampened enthusiasm for this procedure considerably. More recently, a glutaraldehyde cross-linked bovine collagen has been developed that can be injected under local anesthesia through small needles under cystoscopic guidance. This material is gradually replaced by host collagen and appears to be safe and nontoxic. The technique, which is still experimental, may require several collagen injections over time. Its place in the treatment of genuine stress incontinence remains to be established.

Sling procedures, of which there are many variations, are the most common operations performed on incontinent patients with sphincteric damage and bladder neck incompetence. All sling operations use a strap of some material to support and compress the bladder neck and proximal urethra. These operations require experience and a certain amount of surgical artistry to position the sling correctly and under the proper amount of tension. The tendency of the inexperienced surgeon is always to tighten the sling too much in an effort to cure the patient's incontinence. The result is often chronic urinary retention and significant voiding problems postoperatively. Sling procedures should be reserved for patients with a damaged sphincteric mechanism and should not be used as a primary operation except under rare circumstances. These operations should not be done by surgeons who do them rarely or who are unwilling to provide long-term follow-up and take care of the complications that can, and will, arise. Patients who are unwilling to embark on a long-term course of clean intermittent self-catheterization after surgery are high-risk patients for this operation.

Continuing advances in biomedical engineering and space-age plastics technology have made possible the creation of the artificial urinary sphincter. This device consists of a cuff that surrounds the bladder neck and proximal urethra, a reservoir for the medium that fills the device, and a pump that is implanted in the labium majus. When activated, the cuff maintains a constant circumferential pressure that occludes the urethra and the bladder neck. When the patient wishes to void, she deflates the cuff by pumping its contents into the reservoir balloon, opening the bladder neck and urethra. She is then able to void. The cuff automatically reinflates a minute or two after urination, reoccluding the bladder neck. The artificial urinary sphincter thereby allows the patient with a severely damaged urethra and truly debilitating incontinence to continue to use her own lower urinary tract without resorting to urinary diversion, which might be the only other alternative for restoring continence. These devices work especially well in men with postprostatectomy incontinence or neuropathic bladder disorders but have also been used successfully in women with scarred, functionless urethras. The short female urethra and the relatively thin amount of tissue between the bladder neck and vagina makes implantation of this device more difficult in females, however. As with all mechanical devices, there are still significant problems, including erosion through tissues, infection, and mechanical failure. Implantation of the artificial urinary sphincter belongs in the hands of a trained reconstructive urologist at a tertiary-care medical center who is prepared to create and sustain a sphincter-implant program, deal with its complications, and follow these patients for life. The same is true for the small number of patients requiring urinary diversion for management of their incontinence, a procedure that should rarely be required for women with genuine stress incontinence.

Management of Mixed Incontinence

Many patients present with urinary incontinence due to both detrusor instability and genuine stress incontinence. Although there is nearly universal agreement that a bladder neck suspension operation is contraindi-

cated in patients whose sole cause of incontinence is detrusor instability, the role of surgery in patients with mixed incontinence is more controversial. In general, the presence of preoperative detrusor instability is an unfavorable prognostic sign for the achievement of continence after an operation to cure coexistent genuine stress incontinence. Although the detrusor instability disappears in some patients postoperatively, some patients with previously stable cystometrograms will develop new-onset instability after surgery. Karram and Bhatia carried out a retrospective review of 52 patients with mixed incontinence, 27 of whom were treated with primary surgery (Burch colposuspension) and 25 of whom were treated with various pharmacologic regimens. There was no statistically significant difference in outcome between the two groups, and all the surgical failures were due to persistent detrusor instability rather than genuine stress incontinence. The prudent course of treatment would therefore appear to be an initial trial of behavioral and/or pharmacologic therapy for detrusor instability prior to surgery. If the patient remains unhappy with her situation after a trial of conservative management, she may be offered an attempt at surgical cure of her stress incontinence with the understanding that the outcome is unpredictable and the chances of complete success are probably diminished.

SELECTED OPERATIONS FOR GENUINE STRESS INCONTINENCE

JOHN D. THOMPSON

Almost 200 operations have been described for the surgical cure of genuine stress urinary incontinence, each of which has enthusiastic advocates. Each operation has variations. Some have withstood the test of time and careful scrutiny. Others have not but may not yet have been discarded completely. Some are new and not yet fully evaluated.

The editor for this chapter, Dr. Thompson, has chosen the four operations to be described in this chapter with full realization that the choices made will not satisfy everyone, especially those who are scholars of the subject. However, it is the editor's belief that the gynecologic surgeon can find relief for his incontinent patients among these four operations, given proper patient selection, clinical evaluation, and technical performance.

As stated by Hurt in a discussion of the vaginal versus the abdominal approach in the treatment of stress urinary incontinence:

Controversy continues as to the best surgical approach to treat stress urinary incontinence. It is unlikely that the necessary prospective, randomized studies with matched variables will ever be done to help resolve the matter. In the meantime, critical analysis of diagnostic methods, surgical techniques, and long-term results must continue.

Anterior Colporrhaphy

Anterior colporrhaphy is an operation to correct relaxation of the anterior vaginal wall—cystocele and urethrocele (Fig. 33-6). Its inclusion in this chapter is also an indication of its usefulness in curing mild to moderate degrees of genuine stress urinary incontinence. Properly performed in properly selected patients, anterior colporrhaphy is an effective primary operation for treating stress incontinence of urine, especially since it is well tolerated by most patients. The operating time is short and the postoperative morbidity

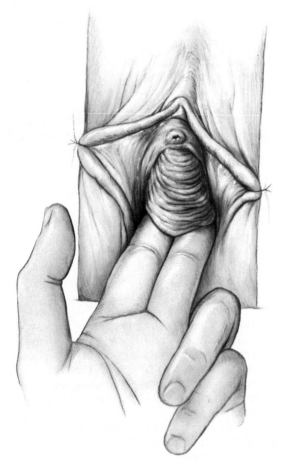

Figure 33–6. Anatomic relaxation of the bladder base (cystourethrocele) and fibromuscular floor of the urethra (urethrocele) with posterior rotation of the urethrovesical junction.

is minimal. It can even be done under local anesthesia and analgesia if absolutely necessary.

Anterior vaginal wall relaxation or prolapse consists of cystocele with or without urethrocele and represents one of the most common types of genital organ prolapse. Anterior vaginal wall prolapse may occur as an isolated defect. It is most commonly associated with other genital organ prolapse, such as rectocele, enterocele, and uterine descensus, however. When multiple defects are present in the same patient, the symptomatology and management of each one must be considered.

Relaxation of the anterior vaginal wall may involve the distal (anterior) half, distal to the interureteric ridge in the bladder, and is called an anterior cystocele. On the other hand, relaxations may involve the proximal (posterior) segment of the anterior vaginal wall proximal to the interureteric ridge and is called a posterior cystocele. Of course, both types of relaxations usually exist together. Recognition of these distinct and different relaxations of the anterior vaginal wall is important in understanding etiology, symptomatology, and management.

An anterior cystocele involves a defect in the support of the vesical neck, urethrovesical junction, and proximal urethra. Damage (stretching, tearing) or atrophy of the connective tissue and fascial supports of the lower anterior vaginal wall to the arcus tendineus and of the pubourethral ligaments is responsible for this defect. Straining as with a Valsalva maneuver causes a posterior rotational descent of the urethrovesical junction and proximal urethra. The lumen of the proximal urethra may be dilated if funneling or vesicalization has occurred. It is uncommon for the lumen of the distal urethra to be dilated; thus, a true urethrocele is uncommon. It is important to realize that anterior cystocele is more commonly associated with genuine stress urinary incontinence because of loss of the normal urethrovesical angle and loss of intra-abdominal pressure transmission to the proximal urethra with coughing, sneezing, and other causes of sudden increases in intra-abdominal pressure.

A posterior or true cystocele is one that occurs above the interureteric ridge and involves the proximal (posterior) vaginal wall. When it occurs without an anterior cystocele, it is generally asymptomatic unless it is noticed by the patient as a protrusion through the vaginal introitus. A true posterior cystocele is not usually associated with genuine stress urinary incontinence unless an anterior cystocele is also present. When a very large true posterior cystocele is present, the patient may have trouble emptying the bladder completely. Residual urine in the bladder may predispose to chronic cystitis. Digital replacement of the cystocele may be required to facilitate complete emptying.

Patients with advanced degrees of uterovaginal prolapse, including a large cystocele, seldom have genuine stress incontinence. This has been difficult to understand until the studies of Richardson and associates and Bump and associates demonstrated that urinary continence was related to physical kinking of the urethra as the prolapse is accentuated with sudden increases in intra-abdominal pressure. Since the proximal anterior vaginal wall is more mobile than the distal anterior vaginal wall, the urethra kinks with sudden stress.

As stated earlier, patients with cystocele may or may not complain of urinary incontinence. Those who are incontinent may have genuine stress incontinence or detrusor instability with incontinence or both. A meticulous recording of the degree of cystocele by urodynamic diagnosis was made by Thiede in 200 patients complaining of incontinence. Among 124 patients with genuine stress incontinence, 70 (56%) had second- or third-degree cystocele. Among 26 patients with detrusor instability, 10 (39%) had second- or third-degree cystocele. Among 35 patients with both genuine stress incontinence and detrusor instability, 14 (40%) had second- or third-degree cystocele. Clearly, the degree of anterior vaginal wall relaxation cannot be used to judge the presence or absence or type of associated urinary incontinence, as pointed out by this study and by Cardozo and Stanton. The findings on pelvic examination and the degree and type of anterior vaginal wall relaxation often do not correlate well with the presence or absence or type of bladder dysfunction. As pointed out by Thiede and others, there are a number of different reasons for stress incontinence that have no relationship to the anatomy of the anterior vaginal wall. Since symptomatology, physical findings, and bladder function do not always correlate well, urodynamic studies may be indicated to make a correct diagnosis in a patient with a cystocele who complains of and/or is demonstrated to have urinary incontinence.

Patients with cystocele who have detrusor instability do not require operation for relief. Patients with cystocele who have mild degrees of genuine stress incontinence may be improved or even cured by pelvic floor musculature exercises, as pointed out by Tchou and associates, Peattie and associates, and Olah and associates. The weighted vaginal cones may be especially useful in curing mild degrees of stress incontinence in patients with cystocele. Indeed, asymptomatic patients with cystocele may be advised to use weighted vaginal cones prophylactically, in the hope of preventing or delaying the onset of incontinence.

For minor degrees of stress urinary incontinence, Kegel's perineal exercises may be used to strengthen the urogenital diaphragm and to increase the voluntary muscular support to the proximal urethra. As described by Kegel, this technique not only exercises the bulbocavernosus muscle, but strengthens the superficial and deep transverse perineal and the levator ani muscles of the pelvic diaphragm. The exercise technique is beneficial for patients with minimal symptoms. Kegel was the first to emphasize that herniation of the bladder and urethra through a hiatus in the pelvic diaphragm would not be corrected by this exercise.

When surgery is contraindicated or must be deferred, a patient with cystourethrocele can be made comfortable with a vaginal pessary that provides support to the proximal urethra and bladder base.

A patient with an entirely asymptomatic cystocele will not require surgery for relief unless it is necessary as part of a complete operation for uterovaginal prolapse. Repair of an asymptomatic cystocele can cause trouble. Patients with a cystocele and no incontinence may develop stress urinary incontinence after anterior colporrhaphy. This fact has been well known to gynecologists for years. Patients with a posterior cystocele who have good support of the bladder neck and proximal urethra by ultrasonography or radiography do not develop urinary incontinence postoperatively following cystocele repair. When posterior cystocele is present and posterior descent of the bladder neck and proximal urethra is also demonstrated by ultrasonography or radiography, repair of the posterior cystocele is not enough. An additional anti-incontinence procedure, such as plication of the urethrovesical angle, bladder neck, and proximal urethra, must also be done. Otherwise, the patient may experience onset of stress incontinence after anterior colporrhaphy. One may try to simulate what will happen postoperatively following cystocele repair by replacing the anterior vaginal wall and holding it in a normal position with a pessary. It is most unfortunate when a patient develops bladder dysfunction, including incontinence, after an operation to correct an asymptomatic cystocele.

Bergman and associates evaluated 46 patients with a third-degree cystocele and no complaints of genuine stress urinary incontinence with urodynamic studies and ultrasonography. Twenty-four patients had a well-supported urethrovesical junction by ultrasound with mobility of <1 cm on straining. These patients had an anterior colporrhaphy only, and no patient became incontinent postoperatively. Twenty-two patients had an incompetent urethra and urethral mobility >1 cm by ultrasound in addition to the third-degree cystocele. These patients had an anterior colporrhaphy plus urethropexy, and no patient became incontinent postoperatively. This study shows clearly that careful evaluation of patients with a large cystocele and no incontinence is required to achieve good results with surgical repair.

Vaginal hysterectomy is not necessarily always indicated in a patient whose operation is done primarily to repair a cystocele. A cystocele can be repaired just as well without doing a hysterectomy. Although some believe that operations for stress urinary incontinence are more successful when a hysterectomy is also done, we believe that removing a normal uterus is not necessary to cure incontinence, and a cystocele can be repaired just as well without doing a hysterectomy. Occasionally, a Manchester operation with cervical amputation may be done rather than vaginal hysterectomy. Of course, most patients with significant anatomic relaxation of the anterior vaginal wall also have other evidence of uterovaginal prolapse for which vaginal hysterectomy, posterior culdoplasty, and appropriate colporrhaphies are desirable, or there even may be other indications for hysterectomy.

It has been said that vaginal hysterectomy with anterior colporrhaphy is responsible for producing a variety of disorders of bladder function, including stress incontinence, detrusor instability, and other voiding difficulties. Tanagho has suggested that anterior colporrhaphy dissection around the urethra and vesical neck damages the parasympathetic and sympathetic nerves, partially denervating the urethra and detrusor muscle and causing uninhibited contractions. Stanton and associates did clinical and urodynamic studies of 73 patients who had vaginal hysterectomy and anterior colporrhaphy. Pre- and postoperative urodynamic assessment continued for 2 years. Symptoms of urge incontinence, stress incontinence, and prolapse were significantly reduced; urodynamics showed no significant change; and the incidence of detrusor instability and voiding difficulties was not increased.

Most cases of stress incontinence are associated with cystourethrocele; fortunately, the operative results for this group of patients are quite successful if the operation is performed correctly. With loss of tone of the urethral wall and the loss of paraurethral support from the urogenital diaphragm, the circular fibers of the vesical sphincter and proximal urethra fail to remain closed when abdominal pressure is increased (Fig. 33-7). During surgery it is important to plicate the paraurethral and paravesical fascia carefully and to elevate the proximal urethra and urethrovesical junction to a high retropubic (intra-abdominal) position. To increase the total urethral closure pressure, the entire length of the functional urethra (except for the most distal 1 cm) should be plicated. By approximating the relaxed paraurethral fascia along the entire proximal and midportions of the urethra, the circular muscle fibers of the urethra are supported, and the total intraurethral pressure is increased.

Genuine stress urinary incontinence may have its onset after anterior colporrhaphy. Some believe that this is the result of overcorrection of the cystocele with elevation of the bladder base and straightening of the urethrovesical angle. We believe it is more likely the result of failure of permanent elevation of the urethrovesical angle high enough to allow kinking of the proximal urethra and transmission of pressure spikes from the abdomen to the proximal urethra. We believe the best results can be obtained in two ways.

First, permanent sutures must be used to keep the plicated fascia approximated beneath the vesical neck and proximal urethra for the several months required for proper healing. An important principle of surgery to repair hernias is to use permanent sutures to hold supporting tissue together long enough to allow secure healing. Relaxation of the vesical neck and proximal

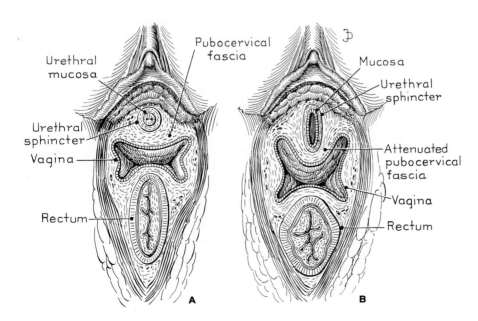

Figure 33–7. *A,* Schematic representation of camera-shutter-like action of normal urethral sphincter. *B,* Schematic representation of failure of urethral sphincter to close on straining after development of urethrocele.

urethra with posterior descent and rotation of the urethrovesical angle is very much like a hernia. Simply put, the tissues that provide their support have been damaged or have atrophied. These tissues must be repaired with permanent suture. Catgut or even delayed-absorbable sutures do not maintain their tensile strength long enough for secure healing, especially since some straining (and pulling against the new suture line) is necessary to initiate voiding after the catheter is removed postoperatively. Improvements in the results of operative procedures for stress urinary incontinence can be obtained by using permanent suture material, as pointed out by Baden and Walker and by Beck. We believe this applies to anterior colporrhaphy as well as other operative procedures.

Many surgeons are reluctant to use permanent suture material because of the possibility of placing the suture too deeply inside the bladder. A suture placed inside the bladder will cause chronic cystitis and urinary frequency and urgency until it is removed. To make this unlikely, dissection of the anterior vaginal wall for colporrhaphy should be done so that all fascia remains attached to the bladder and urethra. The proper plane of dissection is between the vaginal mucosa and the fascia rather than deeper between the fascia and bladder muscle. Injection of generous quantities of sterile saline just beneath the vaginal mucosa facilitates dissection in the proper plane. With the fascia left on the bladder, there is ample thickness of tissue beneath the vesical neck to place permanent sutures without danger of entering the bladder. To avoid infection, this first layer of permanent sutures must be covered over with a second layer of delayed-absorbable sutures before the vaginal mucosa is trimmed and approximated in the midline.

Second, dissection beneath the vesical neck and proximal urethra must be complete and taken as far laterally as possible. If these structures are mobilized adequately, then it should be possible to place the plicating sutures in good tissue laterally that will bring the pubourethral ligaments and the pubovesicocervical fascia into a better supporting position beneath the vesical neck and proximal urethra to elevate the proximal urethra behind the symphysis. If it is not possible to do this, then a Pereyra procedure may be done to supplement the vesical neck plication and to achieve appropriate elevation and kinking of the urethrovesical angle. When Riggs combined anterior colporrhaphy with a modified Pereyra procedure, the results were very satisfactory.

The results with properly done anterior colporrhaphy for mild to moderate genuine stress urinary incontinence are generally good in spite of some reports to the contrary. Cure or significant improvement in incontinence should be achieved in 85% to 90% of patients,

with a gradual reduction in satisfactory control to about 70% to 75% in 2 years. In a few patients, the anterior colporrhaphy will not be successful, and secondary attempts at restoration of continence with a repeat anterior colporrhaphy will generally be less successful, although Van Rooyen and Liebenberg have demonstrated an 89% long-term success rate with anterior colporrhaphy in a group of 150 patients, 60% of whom had documented evidence of periurethral fibrosis from previous surgery. However, if recurrent incontinence is marked following anterior colporrhaphy, treatment may be more successful by suprapubic colpourethropexy or by a Goebell-Stoeckel suburethral strap operation, presuming the incontinence is still genuine stress by repeat urodynamic studies. Generally, anterior colporrhaphy is not repeated for recurrent or persistent stress urinary incontinence following previous anterior colporrhaphy. Patients tolerate anterior colporrhaphy extremely well, especially if it can be done under local anesthesia. However, anterior colporrhaphy should not be chosen to cure genuine stress incontinence of urine when it is not the correct operation to perform. For example, we would not choose to do an anterior colporrhaphy on a patient with minimal relaxation of the anterior vaginal wall and marked genuine stress urinary incontinence. A suprapubic colpourethropexy would be more likely to give better results in such a patient.

Surgical correction of cystourethrocele is directed toward restoring the fascia and muscular support to the bladder neck and urethra. The Kelly urethral plication, originally described in 1911, remains one of the primary methods of surgical repair of this condition. Kelly deserves much credit for identifying the precise anatomic deficits in the urethral support mechanisms that result in stress urinary incontinence (Fig. 33-8). Although 20% of the patients on whom Kelly and Dumm reported in 1914 showed no improvement following the procedure, most of these had had previous surgery.

Historically, the Kelly method has been selected as the primary surgical treatment of choice in cases where there is demonstrable musculofascial relaxation of the levator hiatus as a result of childbearing. The success of the procedure is related to the thoroughness of the dissection and to the wide mobilization of the proximal urethra and the surrounding paraurethral fascia at the urethrovesical junction.

Two important reparative functions are required in addition to the Kelly plication sutures at the urethrovesical junction and along the urethra: (1) high, retropubic elevation of the urethrovesical junction from a dependent position to a position well above the urogenital diaphragm; and (2) restoration of the suburethral fascial support to strengthen the urethral musculature and consequently increase intraurethral pres-

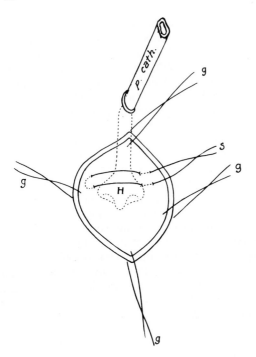

Figure 33–8. Original Kelly diagram of vesical sphincter plication. (*H*) Head of the catheter marking the neck of the bladder; (*G*) guy sutures holding the wound open; (*S*) suture at the neck of the bladder plicating the paraurethral fascia.

sure. For urinary continence to be achieved, the reparative procedure must increase the intraurethral pressure, but it cannot completely obstruct the urethra. Plication of the distal urethra to the region of the external meatus, as emphasized by Kennedy, is beneficial in restoring intraurethral and suburethral support, although the maximum surgical benefit is achieved in the region of the proximal urethra and urethrovesical junction. If mobilization of the proximal urethra is adequate, the basic plication sutures, which are strategically placed in the paraurethral fascia and anchored retropubically to the posterior pubourethral ligaments, will achieve the desired anatomic result. Excessive suturing in the region of the bladder neck should be avoided, since it does not ensure urinary continence

and may instead produce excessive scarring of the urethrovesical area. Urethral scarring can result in incomplete closure, shortening of the urethra, and further disturbance in the voiding process.

Urethral plication with urethrovesical repair is performed when the defect in the pelvic diaphragm is confined to the part of the vagina beneath the urethra and the base of the bladder (see Fig. 33-6).

Technique

Injection of generous quantities of sterile saline (without vasopressors added) just beneath the vaginal mucosa facilitates dissection in the proper plane. After a midline incision is made through the vaginal mucosa extending from the apex of the vagina to within a centimeter of the external urethral meatus (Fig. 33-9 *A–B*). The flaps are carefully dissected laterally, with sharp knife or scissors dissection (Fig. 33-9*C*). The electrosurgical unit may also be used. It is important that the dissection be made just beneath the vaginal mucosa so that all fascial tissue is left attached to the bladder (Fig. 33-9*D*). Entry into the white-appearing avascular plane just beneath the vaginal mucosa facilitates mobilization, which should be extended to the most lateral aspects of the urethra and bladder base. The fascial layer should be left intact. It should not be fragmented or developed into flaps. The correctness of this initial dissection has much to do with the success of the operation. Final separation of the fascial attachments of the urethra and bladder as far laterally as possible can be made by the operator's index finger dissecting beneath the pubic ramus.

The placement of permanent plication sutures in the fascia should begin at the bladder neck. In most cases, the urethrovesical junction can be identified without the use of a Foley catheter placed through the urethra. If necessary, a Foley urethral catheter can be inserted into the bladder and withdrawn to the point where it meets resistance at the vesical neck. Palpation of the inflated Foley catheter bulb at this point will identify the correct position for placement of plication sutures to elevate the urethrovesical junction and proximal urethra. The bladder neck suture begins with a firm bite in good fascial and pubourethral ligament tissue on the posterior aspect of the symphysis pubis on one side and then

(*text continues on page 913*)

Figure 33–9. *A, B,* Technique of anterior colporrhaphy. Scissor dissection of the vaginal mucosa to the region of the external urethral meatus. Traction must be maintained on the vagina along the course of the dissection to keep the wall of the bladder separate from the vaginal mucosa in order to avoid trauma to the bladder. *C,* Sharp dissection of the adherent fascia from the vaginal mucosa. The dissection should be deep enough to reach the white, relatively avascular plane just beneath the vaginal epithelium. *D,* Blunt finger dissection with a single thickness of a gauze sponge to provide sufficient traction against the fascia to free it from the mucosa beneath the urethra and bladder. (*Figure continued on page 910.*)

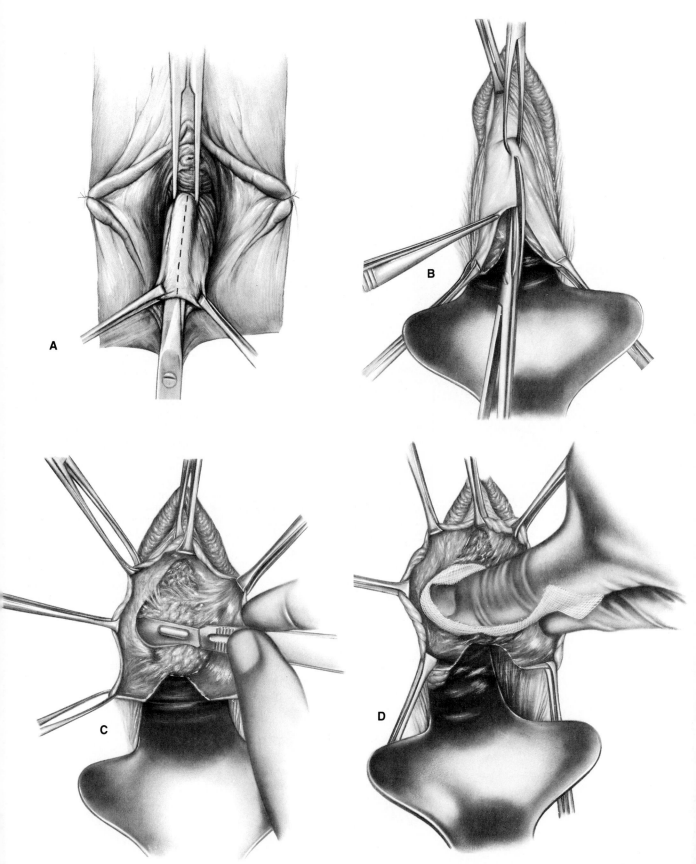

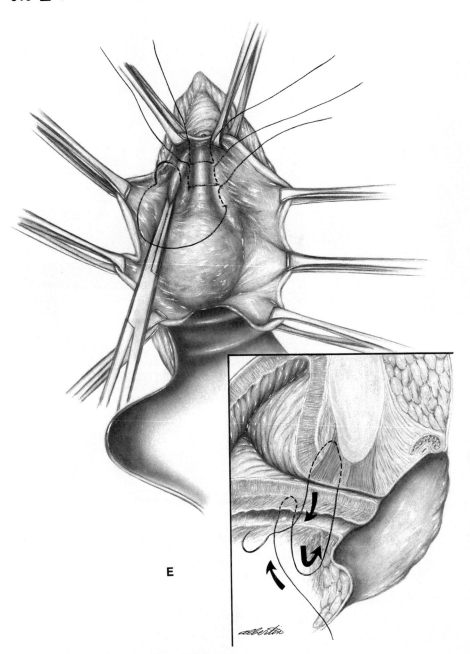

E

Figure 33–9. (continued) *E*, Beginning at the external meatus, successive vertical mattress stitches of No. 2-0 delayed-absorbable suture are placed in the mobilized paraurethral fascia. A Kelly clamp depresses the floor of the urethra as the sutures are tied to avoid necrosis of the wall of the urethra. The last suture at the bladder neck is anchored to the posterior pubourethral ligament using No. 2-0 permanent suture. The pubourethral ligament is grasped with a straight Ochsner clamp. The suture passes through the paraurethral fascia and is then firmly inserted through the pubourethral ligament on the posterior aspect of the symphysis pubis. A second suture is placed on the opposite side of the urethra where it incorporates the same anatomic structures. Both sutures are tied, drawing the paraurethral fascia beneath the urethra and elevating the posterior urethra to a high retropubic position.

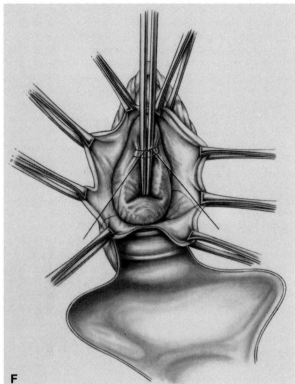

Figure 33–9. (continued) *F,* The posterior floor of the bladder and urethra should be inverted with an instrument as the sutures are tied. *G,* Another view of the suspension of the paraurethral fascia at the urethrovesical junction to the posterior pubourethral ligament, omitting the proximal urethral plication sutures for illustrative purposes. Insert shows the placement of permanent suture at the urethrovesical junction, firmly anchoring the suture to the opposite posterior pubourethral ligament at the tip of the Ochsner clamp and close to the lower one third of the posterior surface of the symphysis pubis. A similar suture is placed in the opposite paraurethral fascia and pubourethral ligament. *(Figure continued on next page.)*

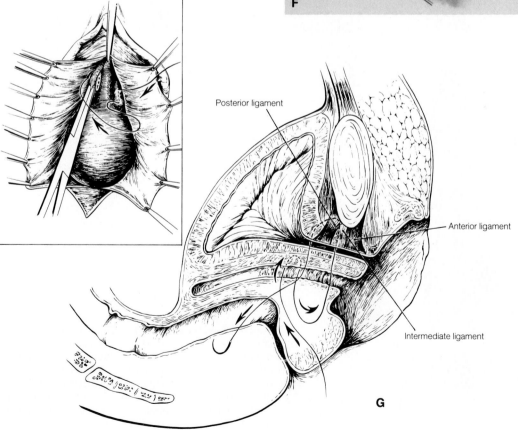

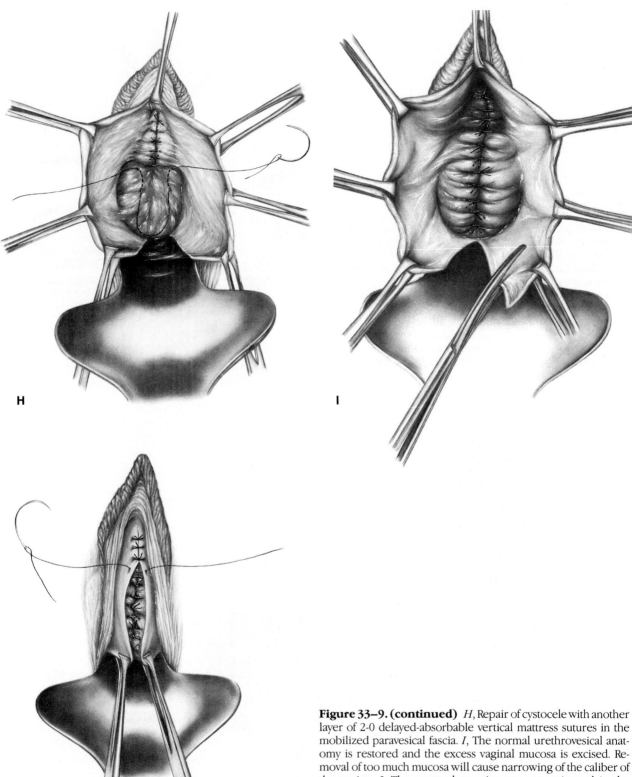

Figure 33–9. (continued) *H*, Repair of cystocele with another layer of 2-0 delayed-absorbable vertical mattress sutures in the mobilized paravesical fascia. *I*, The normal urethrovesical anatomy is restored and the excess vaginal mucosa is excised. Removal of too much mucosa will cause narrowing of the caliber of the vagina. *J*, The mucosal margins are approximated in the midline with interrupted, No. 3-0 delayed-absorbable sutures that include the underlying fascia.

crosses beneath the urethrovesical junction to pick up a firm bite of similar tissue on the opposite side (Fig. 33-9E). One to three sutures are placed proximal and distal to the initial suture. When the plication sutures are being tied along the course of the urethra and bladder neck, an assistant should invert the posterior floor of the bladder and urethra with a Kelly clamp (Fig. 33-9F, G). A permanent suture material (2-0 Tevdek or similar suture) should be used for this first layer and then covered over with another layer of 2-0 delayed-absorbable suture. The posterior cystocele is repaired by a similar series of 2-0 delayed-absorbable plication sutures placed in the mobilized subvesical fascia. Firm bites must be taken, but to avoid placement inside the bladder and kinking of the ureters, they must not be too deep (Fig. 33-9G).

One should avoid too high an elevation of the posterior cystocele to avoid a direct-run-off type of urinary incontinence following anterior colporrhaphy. As suggested by Beck, the basic surgical objective is to increase the cough pressure transmission to the urethra so that it equals or exceeds the cough pressure transmission to the bladder. This is done by creating differentially better support for the anterior cystocele (proximal urethra and vesical neck) than for the posterior cystocele (bladder base), so that effective urethral kinking occurs with cough, creating a urethral pressure spike that offsets the bladder pressure spike with coughing. To increase the support differential between the urethra and bladder base, we prefer to use permanent suture material to tighten and elevate the proximal urethra and bladder neck, while using delayed-absorbable suture material to correct (but not overcorrect) the posterior cystocele (bladder base) (Fig. 33-9H).

Although overcorrection of the posterior cystocele should be avoided, we believe that insufficient support and elevation of the urethrovesical angle is an even more common reason for an unsatisfactory result with anterior colporrhaphy. If properly placed, the suspension sutures at urethrovesical junction should restore the proximal urethra and vesical neck to their normal retropubic (intra-abdominal) position, above the pelvic diaphragm. Most vaginal procedures for the correction of stress incontinence fail to emphasize restoration of this intra-abdominal position, which may be the explanation for unsuccessful results. Permanent replacement requires the use of permanent suture material and placement of sutures in strong fascia on each side of the proximal urethra and vesical neck to create and elevate the urethrovesical angle that is securely anchored to the reflection of the posterior pubovesical ligament along the posterior surface of the pubic bone.

According to Low, there is a significant relationship between the degree of reduction of the posterior urethrovesical angle by surgical procedure and the improvement in bladder control. The average decrease in the urethrovesical angle of patients with good results was 34°; that for patients with surgical failures was only 15°. In the surgically successful case, this imbrication of periurethral fascia at the vesical neck causes an elevation of the urethrovesical junction behind the symphysis pubis of at least 1 cm, and much less in the unsuccessful case.

Low and Weil and associates state that unsuccessful anterior colporrhaphy is related to the severity of the anatomic defect and the presence of less favorable urodynamic features before the operation. Restoration of continence also depends on the quality of tissues, the mobility of the bladder neck and anterior vaginal wall, the characteristics of the posterior urethrovesical angle, and the presence of risk factors such as obesity, chronic bronchitis, neuropathies, hypertonic bladder, and low maximum urethral closure pressure. Most important, it depends on the ability of the surgeon to restore the cough spike pressure transmission ratio to its normal 100% and to create a urethral kinking mechanism, as described by Beck. If elevation of the vesical neck and proximal urethra has not been achieved by carefully placed plication sutures, further elevation usually can be achieved with a Pereyra procedure. Although this is not often necessary, it should be done without hesitation if the surgeon believes it will improve the likelihood of a successful result.

The excess vaginal mucosa is excised, taking care not to excise too much (Fig. 33-9I). The margins of the vaginal mucosa are approximated in the midline using interrupted No. 3-0 delayed-absorbable sutures. Including a bite of the fascia with each vaginal suture obliterates any dead space between the mucosa and the fascia (Fig. 33-9J).

As stated in Chapter 34, if a relaxed vaginal outlet exists with a symptomatic cystocele, with or without rectocele, the entire posterior vaginal wall and the perineum should be repaired, along with the cystocele if it can be done without constricting the vaginal caliber to the point of producing dyspareunia. Repairing a relaxed posterior vaginal wall, gapping vaginal outlet, and defective perineum may improve the complaint of stress incontinence of urine. Such a repair will elongate the posterior vaginal wall and bring it up beneath the anterior vaginal wall for better support. It will also bring the bulbocavernosus muscles attached beneath the labia minora closer together in the perineum and thereby improve the efficiency of the voluntary urethral sphincter. Although these mechanisms may be more theoretical than real, we have seen stress urinary incontinence improved by posterior colpoperineorrhaphy.

Ureteral integrity can be demonstrated by giving 5 cc of indigo carmine intravenously, filling the bladder with 200 cc of clear saline, and watching the efflux of the dye from each ureteral orifice with a cystoscope. The ureters are at risk of injury with anterior colporrhaphy, although actual injury is rare. The distance between anterior colporrhaphy sutures and the ureters can be as short as 0.9 cm, as measured by Hofmeister. The inside of the bladder can be examined with the same cystoscopy.

Continuous bladder drainage should be provided for several days following anterior colporrhaphy with plication of the vesicourethral angle. This can be done with suprapubic catheter placement at the beginning or the end of the procedure, provided one is willing to accept the risk of small intestinal perforation, although this risk is very low. Continuous bladder drainage can also be provided with a transurethral Foley catheter for several days. When it is removed, the patient must be carefully checked to be certain that the bladder does not become overdistended and must also be catheterized several times after voiding until the residual urine volume is lower than 50 cc. Patients are instructed to void frequently and to avoid straining with urination and defecation, even if stool softeners and intermittent self-catheterization are required.

Anterior colporrhaphy with plication of the vesicourethral angle has been used extensively with good results. When a meticulous preoperative urologic workup is done, when patients are selected properly, and when proper technique is employed, more than 85% of patients will achieve long-term urinary control, 5% to 10% have improved control, and only 5% are unimproved. In a recent series, Beck has obtained a 92% cure rate, a 3% improvement rate, and a 5% failure rate. Green, Hodgkinson, and Beck and McCormick also obtained excellent long-term results with anterior colporrhaphy. Van Geelen and associates reported unsatisfactory results with their technique of anterior colporrhaphy using No. 2-0 chromic catgut. Park and Miller found that the anterior colporrhaphy with Kelly plication and the Mars procedure gave equally good results more than 3 years after surgery. Bergman and associates, on the other hand, found similar cure rates for the anterior colporrhaphy, Burch procedure, and Pereyra procedure at 3 months, but at 1 year, the recurrence of incontinence was greater with anterior colporrhaphy. Permanent sutures were not used for plication. Finally, Everett reported on the results of anterior colporrhaphy with plication of the vesical sphincter in 109 patients with cystocele and stress incontinence followed for 2 or more years. Ninety-seven percent had complete relief of incontinence. Everett's report was from the Johns Hopkins Hospital, where plication of the vesical neck was done with permanent suture material since the operation first began at Johns Hopkins in about 1900.

Various special techniques of providing urethrovesi-cal angle support with anterior colporrhaphy have been described by Nichols and Randall. Ingelman-Sundberg has described a technique of supporting the urethrovesical angle with a pubococcygeus muscle transplant. Plastic mesh has been sewn beneath the bladder for added support by Moir, Moore and associates, and Nichols.

Suprapubic Colpourethropexy

With a basic understanding of the operative procedures discussed in this chapter, one should choose the method most suitable for each individual patient. It is difficult always to say with certainty which procedure is the best, and experience of the operator should influence the decision to some degree. Even the best-conceived and best-executed procedures for the correction of stress urinary incontinence have a certain percentage of failures, and analysis of these failures can teach the operator what to be aware of in future efforts to cure stress incontinence.

Failure of the operator to recognize urge incontinence or detrusor instability causes will result in a failure or a less satisfactory result with any surgical procedure to correct incontinence. Again, proper preoperative urodynamic study is emphasized. It has been pointed out in the discussion of preoperative studies of the patient and her bladder that much unnecessary trouble can be avoided if the neurologically impaired bladder is detected. This is most important because detrusor muscle dysfunction is only aggravated by an operative procedure that causes obstruction at the bladder neck, whether this obstruction is simply a constriction by vesical neck plication, a repositioning of the bladder neck and urethra by a suburethral sling procedure, or a retropubic or suprapubic urethral suspension. Careful preoperative study of bladder capacity and dynamics will eliminate this pitfall.

Scarring from previous injury, surgery, or disease can be another most important factor causing complete or partial failure. Scarring in the space of Retzius or around the urethra by previous surgery requires dissection and mobilization of the urethra for proper performance of any operative procedure to relieve incontinence.

Chronic pulmonary disease from chronic bronchitis, bronchiectasis, emphysema, asthma, or nicotine abuse resulting in an intractable cough may be a cause of failure of repair. Every effort should be made to treat the chronic pulmonary disease, improve the cough, and eliminate nicotine abuse. It is to be hoped that cough control measures will improve stress urinary incontinence, but too frequently this is not possible. Similarly, morbid obesity may be a relative contraindication to incontinence surgery. Since the pelvic floor is the target of orthostatic pressure created by the weight of the intra-abdominal viscera, obesity is one of the major high-risk factors that decreases the cure rate of operative procedures.

Because of simplicity, dependability, and paucity of complications, we have favored the anterior colporrhaphy with plication of the vesical neck for patients with mild to moderate stress urinary incontinence associated with anatomic defect of the anterior vaginal wall. On occasion, when a greater degree of retropubic vesical neck elevation is required, the anterior colporrhaphy with plication of the vesical neck can be combined with the Pereyra procedure.

The other preferred primary procedure for other patients is the suprapubic colpourethropexy to Cooper's ligament described originally by Burch of Nashville. It is indicated especially when the degree of incontinence is severe and when incontinence is present in the nulliparous patient or any other patient who has no significant relaxation of the anterior vaginal wall. It is more often chosen as the primary procedure when an abdominal incision is required to correct or remove pelvic pathology from above. For example, if a patient with stress incontinence requires abdominal hysterectomy for uterine leiomyomas, a suprapubic colpourethropexy is usually done at the same time. It is the preferred procedure in patients who are obese or in patients who have an intractable cough with chronic lung disease. When incontinence recurs after anterior colporrhaphy, we usually choose a suprapubic colpourethropexy rather than repeat anterior colporrhaphy. Of course, such patients must have repeat urodynamic studies to be certain that the incontinence is of the genuine stress variety before any operation is done. A repeat suprapubic colpourethropexy may be done to correct recurrent incontinence, especially if there is reason to believe that the initial operation was not done correctly. When abdominal sacral colpopexy is done for vaginal vault prolapse or enterocele, a suprapubic colpourethropexy should be done as a prophylactic measure to prevent, it is hoped, the postoperative development of urinary incontinence that may result from straightening the anterior vaginal wall and the urethrovesical angle.

Although anterior colporrhaphy is the preferred operation for cystocele, some improvement in anatomic relaxation of the anterior vaginal wall can be expected with a suprapubic colpourethropexy. This is especially true if a specific effort is made to place sutures in the upper anterior vaginal wall fascia for suspension to Cooper's ligament. Such sutures may stretch the vesical neck laterally and hold it open. For this reason, suspension sutures also should be routinely placed along the vesical neck and proximal urethra if an attempt is made to correct a posterior cystocele with a suprapubic colpourethropexy.

Stanton and associates reported on the effect of colposuspension on anterior vaginal wall prolapse. Either a cystocele or a cystourethrocele was found preoperatively in 32 patients. Only two of these patients showed no change in the relaxation of the anterior vaginal wall following colposuspension. Six enteroceles were found postoperatively, an incidence of 17%. Burch reported postoperative enterocele in 7.6% of his cases and recommended an operative technique for preventing its occurrence, especially in high-risk patients. Apparently, a suprapubic colpourethropexy to Cooper's ligament changes the upper axis of the vagina enough to expose the upper posterior vaginal wall to the pressure of intra-abdominal contents. In time, an enterocele may form. We have seen large enteroceles develop in only 3 months after colposuspension to Cooper's ligament in patients who did not have an enterocele preoperatively. For this reason, we usually open the peritoneal cavity first to close the cul-de-sac with a Moschcowitz or Halban technique. Plication of the uterosacral ligaments behind the upper posterior vaginal wall also protects against the development of an enterocele by bringing the vaginal apex toward the posterior pelvis. After this and any other indicated intra-abdominal procedure is completed, the peritoneum is closed and the suprapubic colpourethropexy is done.

There has been some controversy regarding the desirability of performing simultaneous hysterectomy with the Burch colposuspension for urinary stress incontinence. In 1975, Green strongly suggested that simultaneous hysterectomy had a beneficial effect. Others, including Stanton and Cardozo and Milani and associates, disagree. The effect of concomitant hysterectomy during colposuspension on the cure rate of genuine stress incontinence was reported by Langer and associates in 1988. Twenty-five months postoperatively, no differences were found in the cure rate between the two groups (95.5% and 95.7% for the no-hysterectomy and hysterectomy group, respectively). Interestingly, in the no-hysterectomy group, 13.6% of patients had enterocele formation after surgery. This complication did not occur postoperatively in the patients who had a hysterectomy with Moschcowitz obliteration of the cul-de-sac. In our opinion, the decision to perform hysterectomy should be a separate decision and depends on the presence of proper indications for hysterectomy. However, cul-de-sac obliteration can be done even though the hysterectomy is not done.

The suprapubic colpourethropexy to Cooper's ligament should eliminate the possibility of postoperative osteitis pubis. The Marshall-Marchetti-Krantz procedure, which suspends paraurethral fascia to the symphysis pubis, originally described in 1949, was followed in the late 1950s and 1960s with reports of postoperative osteitis pubis. Osteitis pubis is caused by trauma, infection, and impaired circulation of the symphysis. Symptoms include pain and tenderness in the symphysis, abductor muscle spasm, pain with walking, and waddling gait. Radiologic examination reveals rarefaction of bone. The condition may be chronic and last a year. It is an unusual complication of the Marshall-Marchetti-Krantz procedure, occurring in 3.2% of patients, according to Marchetti and associates in 1963, and 3.7%, according to Selim and Vasquez in 1979. However, it can cause significant disability. We believe permanent suture material should be used in operations to cure stress incontinence, but we prefer not to put permanent suture into the periosteum of the symphysis. This is an important reason we prefer to use Cooper's ligament for suspension rather than the symphysis. Permanent sutures can be placed in Cooper's ligament without causing problems. Therefore, we favor the suprapubic colpourethropexy to Cooper's ligament described by Burch over the Marshall-Marchetti-Krantz procedure.

In this original article, Burch made the following interesting comments:

One day, while we were doing a Marshall-Marchetti-Krantz operation, the sutures in the periosteum [of the symphysis pubis] continued to pull out and it was necessary to look for another point of attachment. An examination of the field revealed that the intravaginal finger was pushing the anterior vaginal wall up to a level as high as the origin of the levator muscle from the white line of the pelvis. Since the white line is the usually accepted origin of the so-called fascia surrounding the vagina, it seemed reasonable and anatomically correct to suture this perivaginal fascia to the white line and the underlying levator muscle with three interrupted sutures on each side. This maneuver produced a most satisfactory restoration of the normal anatomy of the bladder neck and, in addition, a surprising correction of most of the cystocele involving the base of the bladder. This demonstrated the possibilities of the operation not only in overcoming the anterior cystocele involving the neck of the bladder but also the posterior cystocele involving the base of the bladder.

Seven operations were performed with this technique. In all of these, an excellent anatomical result was obtained and the structures are holding well at this time. The white line, however, had the same disadvantage as the symphysis. It holds the sutures poorly. The final step in the development of the operation to be described was the utilization of Cooper's ligament as a point of fixation. This strong thick band of fibrous tissue runs along the superior surface of the superior ramus of the pubic bone and is ideal from the standpoint of both passing and holding a suture. Cooper's ligament is well known to surgeons and is used as a point of fixation for the conjoined tendon in the repair of inguinal and femoral hernia and in the repair following a radical groin dissection. From the inguinal approach, Cooper's ligament seems to be a rather short structure but when viewed from within the abdomen, the structure is several inches long and affords more than enough room for necessary sutures.

Thus was born a new and most effective operation for stress urinary incontinence. Several studies indicate that suprapubic colpourethropexy to Cooper's ligament results in objective cure in 85% to 95% of patients with good maintenance of these rates at 2 years.

As demonstrated by Peuttinen and associates and by others, a successful colposuspension reduces bladder neck mobility and increases the pressure transmission ratio to the urethra. In their patients, the posterior urethrovesical angle was reduced from an average value of 132° preoperatively to a postoperative normal value of 80°. The posterior urethrovesical angle on straining changed from 38° to 3°, indicating a greater stability of the urethrovesical junction after operation. More significantly, the pressure transmission ratio of the increased pressure in the bladder transmitted to the urethra on straining increased from 81.5% preoperatively to 105.9% postoperatively. Achieving a successful result may be due to other factors as well, including restoration of urethral length, elevation of the vesical neck, increased urethral closure pressure, or other factors; in failed suprapubic colposuspension many of these changes do not take place. According to Stanton and associates, other factors associated with failed suprapubic colpourethropexy surgery include increasing age, previous incontinence surgery, the presence of detrusor instability, and a postoperative rise of intrinsic bladder pressure. Bowen and associates found that the preoperative resting urethral closure pressure and functional urethral closure pressure and functional urethral length were significantly lower when a suprapubic colpourethropexy failed to cure stress incontinence. Accordingly, they suggest that identification of a low-pressure urethra by preoperative urethral profilometry suggests a greatly increased risk for failure with this operation. In these patients, a suburethral sling procedure may be a preferable operation, but this has not yet been investigated.

Sand and associates reported that 42% of 62 women who had previously undergone hysterectomy failed suprapubic colpourethropexy, despite anatomic correction in 95%. This finding was significantly different from the 17% failure rate in women without prior hysterectomy. This retrospective analysis suggests that prior hysterectomy may place women at increased risk of continued incontinence following suprapubic colpourethropexy, despite anatomic correction of the urethrovesical junction descent. Contrary to the results of other investigators, these authors found that women with a history of previous incontinence surgery were not at significantly greater risk of incontinence after suprapubic colpourethropexy.

Technique

A three-dose regime of perioperative antibiotics is used and has been shown by Bhatia and associates to be effective in reducing postoperative infectious morbidity in retropubic surgery.

The Burch suprapubic colpourethropexy suspension to Cooper's ligament begins after anesthesia induction by placing the patient in Allen Universal stirrups. The bladder is emptied with a catheter and careful pelvic examination is done, including a rectovaginal abdominal examination. Particular attention is given to the anterior vaginal wall, urethral length, relaxations, and posterior descent of the urethrovesical junction. The upper posterior vaginal wall should be examined for evidence of enterocele. After abdominal, perineal, and vaginal preparation, the patient is draped to include the vaginal introitus in the operative field. A No. 18 Foley catheter with a 5-cc bulb is inserted into the bladder and connected to a continuous drainage bag.

Because of the need for optimum exposure, a transverse Maylard incision is preferred unless contraindicated. A Pfannenstiel incision is rarely used. The abdominal cavity is entered and thoroughly explored. Adhesions are released in the pelvis. The bowel is placed in the upper abdomen and held there with packs. If an additional gynecologic operation is indicated, it is performed at this time. The appendix may or may not be removed. The surgeon then proceeds directly to close the cul-de-sac. The closure may be according to the Halban technique, the Moschcowitz technique, or a combination. There may be an advantage to using a bilateral hemi-Moschcowitz technique in order not to compromise the lumen of the rectum (Fig. 33-10). One may start a continuous suture of No. 2-0 polydioxanone at the very deepest point in the cul-de-sac on one side of the rectum. The suture is tied and then continued up in a spiral fashion, taking small bites in the peritoneum on one side of the cul-de-sac until an appropriate height has been reached. The suture is tied and the same technique is used to close the other side of the cul-de-sac. Great caution should be exercised in order not to occlude or kink the ureters. Sutures must not be placed into the lumen of the rectum. Additional support to the posterior vaginal fornix can be provided by plicating the uterosacral ligaments in the midline.

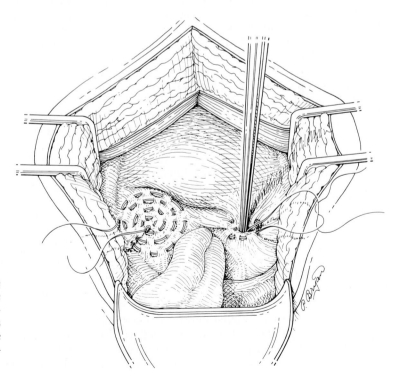

Figure 33–10. A continuous circular suture of No. 2-0 polydioxanone is used to obliterate the cul-de-sac on each side. This may be reinforced over the top by interrupted sutures from front to back and by sutures that plicate the uterosacral ligaments in the midline behind the vagina.

Carried out properly, the bilateral hemi-Moschcowitz and uterosacral ligament plication should reduce the risk of enterocele formation following suprapubic colpourethropexy. Following removal of all packs, the peritoneum is closed.

The space of Retzius is entered inferiorly by blunt dissection between the rectus muscles and the peritoneum. If no prior dissection has been made in this space, it is easy to develop completely. If prior dissection has been made, the space may be obliterated with dense fibrosis, and anatomic landmarks may be obscured. Careful scissors dissection will be required. The bladder is at risk of injury and may be entered. If so, the dissection should be completed and the colpourethropexy sutures should be placed before the cystotomy is closed. Lee and associates and others have recommended that a cystotomy be done deliberately in every case to facilitate accurate suture placement. Opening the anterior wall of the bladder carries minimal risk if it is closed properly in two layers with No. 3-0 delayed-absorbable sutures. We do not do a deliberate cystotomy in every case but would not hesitate to open the bladder when it was deemed necessary.

After the dissection is completed on each side and in the midline, proper illumination and retraction is needed for exposure of the paravesical spaces. A self-retaining retractor is helpful. The inflated Foley bulb above the urethrovesical junction is a landmark. Dissection close to the urethrovesical junction and proximal urethra is avoided, but fat, which may interfere with attachment of suspended structures in their new location, is carefully removed from the paravesical spaces. The large paravaginal venous sinuses cover the shiny white paravaginal fascia. Trauma to these large veins can cause troublesome bleeding. The lateral margins of the bladder attachments to the anterior vaginal wall are carefully dissected, mobilized, and rolled medially. Whatever bleeding is encountered can usually be controlled with pressure, individual ligatures, or careful fulguration.

The surgeon inserts one or two fingers into the vagina. With the aid of the Foley catheter as an anatomic marker, feeling from below and watching from above will allow identification of the urethra, urethrovesical junction, and anterior vaginal wall on each side of the urethra and bladder (Fig. 33-11A). A No. 2-0 permanent suture material (Tevdec, Ethibon, etc.) is used. A double-bite suture is placed through the full thickness of the vaginal wall at the level of and lateral to urethrovesical junction. Another double-bite suture is placed below the first one lateral to the proximal urethra (Fig. 33-11B). Unless it is necessary to control bleeding, these sutures are not tied. Similar sutures are placed on the opposite side again, facilitated by two fingers of the operator's hand in the vagina. If a posterior cystocele is present, another suture in the vaginal wall may be placed above the level of the urethrovesical junction. All sutures are held long. After removing his fingers from the vagina, the surgeon changes gloves.

Cooper's ligament is easily exposed as it comes off laterally from the posterior symphysis. Cooper's ligament must not be confused with the external iliac artery or the obturator nerve. The free ends of the sutures are passed through Cooper's ligament on each side (see Fig. 33-11B). With an assistant's finger in the vagina pushing the vaginal wall up toward Cooper's ligament, the sutures are snugged up and tied. It will not be possible to pull the vaginal wall all the way up to Cooper's ligament, nor should one try. A suture bridge will always be left, and this is as it should be. With the vaginal sling beneath the proximal urethra and vesicourethral junction elevated and held in position by permanent sutures, fibrosis in the paravesical space will secure the position permanently. The desired amount of elevation of the proximal urethra and vesical neck can be gauged by a Q-tip applicator inserted into the urethra just before the sutures are tied, as suggested by Goodno and Powers. Palpation of the anterior vaginal wall should also be done to determine the degree to which elevation of the proximal urethra and urethrovesical angle has occurred, and the degree to which a posterior cystocele has been corrected. Sutures can be removed, replaced, or added as needed. The anterior bladder wall is not plicated or suspended.

We do not routinely place drains in the space of Retzius. If bleeding is a problem, efforts to achieve hemostasis must continue until successful. If a drain is used, it should be a closed suction drain brought out through a separate stab wound. The incision is closed routinely. A posterior colpoperineorrhaphy can be done, if needed, without changing the patient's position in the stirrups. An extensive repair of a high rectocele may require repositioning in regular stirrups.

The Foley catheter is removed, the bladder is distended with 150–200 cc of clear saline, 5 cc of indigo carmine are given intravenously, and a cystoscope is passed to identify the ureteral orifices. In 3–5 minutes blue dye will efflux from both orifices, thus proving ureteral integrity. The Foley catheter is reinserted and connected to a bag for continuous drainage. Free urinary drainage is allowed for 4 days and the catheter is removed early in the morning of the fifth postoperative day. The bladder should not be allowed to overdistend if the patient is unable to void satisfactorily. Postvoid residual urine volumes must be checked twice each day until below 100 cc. If the surgeon chooses, a suprapubic catheter can be used for continuous bladder drainage. Of course, it is inserted into the bladder before the abdominal incision is closed. It may be clamped on the fifth postoperative day. The suprapubic catheter is unclamped to measure postvoid residual urine volumes.

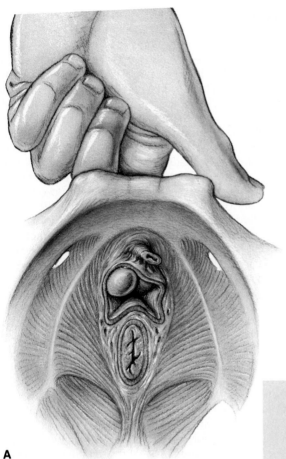

A

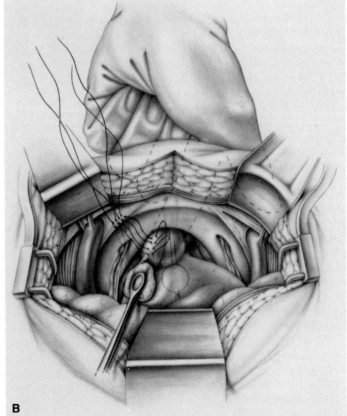

B

Figure 33–11. *A,* View of the pelvic floor showing the region of the urogenital diaphragm. The surgeon's fingers elevate the paraurethral tissue to demonstrate the anatomic placement for each paraurethral suture. *B,* Permanent suture (No. 2-0 Tevdec) is used. A double-bite is taken through the full thickness of the vaginal wall just beneath the vaginal mucosa. One suture is placed lateral to the proximal urethra, and another suture is placed lateral to the urethrovesical angle. A higher, third suture may be placed in the lateral vaginal fornix if correction of a cystocele is an objective. These stitches are anchored to Cooper's ligament and tied as the finger elevates the vaginal wall.

As soon as voiding is normal with less than 100 cc of residual on two occasions, the catheter may be removed and the patient discharged, provided her condition is satisfactory from other standpoints.

It is important to impress on the patient that at first she may be completely unable to void or may be able to void only in small amounts. If she is not reassured by this explanation, she may become apprehensive and her state of anxious tension may hamper prompt recovery. Prior to operation an explanation is given to her of just what the procedure sets out to accomplish and by what means this is done. Then she must be made to realize that a bladder weakened for such a time preoperatively will require some time to recover strength and function. In a few cases, the patient may have a protracted course in which voiding may be slow and difficult. This should not be too discouraging to the patient or the gynecologist. Such patients should be taught the technique of intermittent self-catheterization to avoid overdistention until voiding is satisfactory.

THE MODIFIED PEREYRA PROCEDURE

WILLIAM A. GROWDON

Although the "original" Pereyra procedure first reported in 1959 has been abandoned, this prototype retropubic needle suspension urethropexy procedure stimulated great interest in the development of modifications of instrumentation and technique that have become popular with surgeons preferring a vaginal approach in the surgical cure of incontinence. Many years of work and revision by Armand J. Pereyra, Thomas B. Lebherz, and their collaborators have produced a standard procedure using a new instrument and an open vaginal approach to the space of Retzius. The procedure allows for direct identification of the pubourethral ligaments, as demonstrated by Zacharin, which are sutured with nonabsorbable suture material and suspended by the anterior rectus sheath. This "modified Pereyra procedure" first reported in 1981 eliminated the dangerous blind passage of a needle ligature carrier through paraurethral supporting tissues as described in the original Pereyra procedure. Also, the addition of a helical suture of strong paraurethral supports with nonabsorbable suture decreased long-term failures.

The modified Pereyra procedure may be used alone or in conjunction with other procedures, such as vaginal hysterectomy, anterior/posterior colporrhaphy, the Le Fort procedure, colpocleisis, and sacrospinous fixation for vaginal vault prolapse when concomitant stress urinary incontinence must be remedied.

Technique

After prophylactic antibiotics are given, the patient is positioned in the dorsolithotomy position with care to avoid overflexion of the hips, since the anterior rectus sheath is used for suspension, and tension on this structure or the lack of it may later gain relative importance. The procedure may be performed under general, regional, or even local anesthesia if all that is performed is the procedure itself. If indications for vaginal hysterectomy exist, then that procedure is completed. If a cystocele is present, anterior colporrhaphy is begun by midline incision from the vaginal cuff to approximately 1 cm above the urethrovesical junction that may be identified by palpation of the 5-cc balloon of a 16 French Foley catheter under traction. The vaginal epithelium is reflected as previously described in cystocele repair in this chapter. If, however, a cystocele is not present, an inverted U-shaped incision described by Raz may be used such that the apex of the incision is at the urethrovesical junction.

A dilute solution of saline with epinephrine or Neo-Synephrine is injected in the subepithelial plane along the expected incision line and paravesically at the bladder neck toward the pubic rami to facilitate dissection. Allis Adar forceps are used to elevate the incised vaginal epithelium. Blunt dissection with the index finger at a 45° angle to the urethrovesical junction retropubically releases the musculofascial tissues of the inferior urogenital diaphragm from the pubic rami bilaterally. Release of this musculofascial attachment proceeds until the fingertip reaches a point of impasse. Ventral and cephalad pressure in this area allows the fingertip or, if necessary, the tips of scissors to pass into the retropubic space, a technique described by Studdiford. Once entered, the index finger should be used to explore the space of Retzius above the bladder neck to break down retropubic adhesions. Experience suggests that when previous procedures have been performed and failed, minimal retropubic adhesions are present in the face of descensus of the urethrovesical junction. Rarely, sharp dissection is necessary to release adhesions. Digital traction medially and caudad on the urethrovesical junction reveals the sharp bands of tissue attached to the urethra representing the lateral expansion of the posterior pillar of the pubourethral ligament and musculofascial tissues of the urogenital diaphragm. An Allis Adar forceps should be placed on the medial edge of these structures close to the urethrovesical junction. Number 0 or No. 1 polypropylene suture is then used to incorporate the posterior pillar of the pubourethral ligaments and paravesical musculofascial tissues in a continuous helical suture of three to five loops (Fig. 33-12). After both sides have been completed, sharp traction on the suture ends confirms the strength of

Transposition of the sutures is next accomplished by making a small suprapubic incision of approximately 3–4 cm in transverse length at the superior margin of the symphysis pubis down to the anterior rectus sheath. Adipose tissue should be bluntly dissected off of the anterior rectus sheath. The special Pereyra ligature carrier (Elway Industries; P.O. Box 791; Upland, Calif. 91786) is driven through the anterior rectus sheath lateral to the midline *only after* the surgeon's index finger is placed in the paravesical retropubic space abutting the undersurface of the rectus sheath from below. As the needle pierces the anterior rectus sheath onto the surgeon's finger, the sliding mechanism of the Pereyra needle is used to lengthen the ligature carrier needle, the tip of which is shrouded by the fingertip, while traveling through its course from the retropubic space, paravesically, and into direct view below. Both ends of the helical suture on one side are loaded into the ligature carrier and then simply withdrawn in a reverse manner through the previously described course (Fig. 33-13). Once this has been achieved on both sides, elevation of the urethrovesical junction can be achieved by traction on both sets of sutures simultaneously from above. The complete cystocele repair should take place at this time to avoid the problem of pulling the operative field out of the surgeon's view by premature elevation of the urethrovesical junction.

Once the cystocele repair is completed then, after 5 cc of IV indigo carmine is given to the patient, cystoscopy is performed for observation of the vesical neck, ureteral orifices, and bladder integrity.

The vaginal epithelium is trimmed and closed. Attention to the appropriate urethrovesical angle fixation is then made. Simultaneous urethroscopy, observing the closure of internal urethral meatus while elevation is occurring, is an excellent guide. Both visualization and palpation of the U–V junction from below are complementary methods that should be used to avoid overcorrection. Lateral mobility of the tissues of the urethra and U–V junction should be present. If the patient is awake with regional or local anesthesia, asking the patient to create a Valsalva effort with a full bladder will demonstrate incontinence with the sutures released and continence with traction from above on the sutures. This is an excellent method to assess the tension necessary to ensure continence. The optimal elevation having been achieved, the two suture ends from each side are simply tied in a surgeon's knot followed by six separate square knots. A surgical clip is placed above the last knot to decrease the incidence of unraveling. If the patient is thin, the pigtail of knots is pinned pointing cephalad against the anterior rectus sheath by a separate delayed-absorbable suture. This will prevent discomfort in the suprapubic area postoperatively. Another technique of suture fixation is to tie each side separately using an

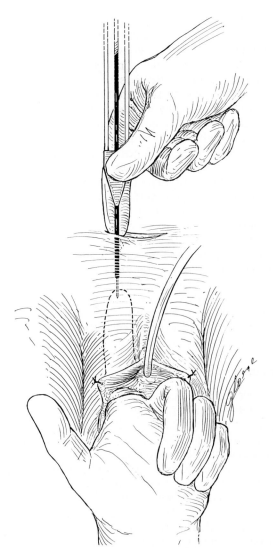

Figure 33–12. The surgeon's index finger enters the space of Retzius from below and abuts the rectus abdominus fascia, ready to accept and shroud the ligature carrier needle in its course paravesically to the sutured UVJ below. The ligature carrier pierces the anterior sheath 2–3 cm lateral to the midline onto the finger. Parallel support is desired rather than divergent or convergent support. The lateral entry point for the ligature carrier on the anterior rectus sheath will vary from patient to patient. The ligature carrier needle must never leave the guiding finger until in view below.

support as evidenced by the ability to move the patient slightly. In some patients the pubourethral ligament is either attenuated or surgically absent. In these cases a helical suture of the lateral edge of the prevesical musculofascial support previously released from the inferior margin of the pubic ramus at the urethrovesical junction may be connected with the vaginal epithelium, creating adequate support.

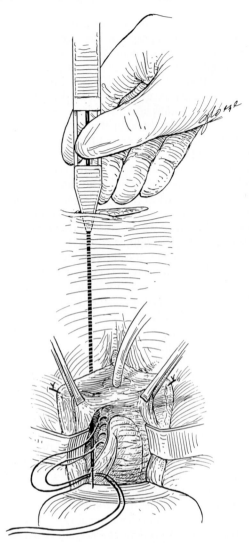

Figure 33–13. The two ends of the right helical suture are loaded into the needle and simply retracted in reverse course through the small transverse suprapubic wound. After the same procedure is completed contralaterally, pancystoscopy and cystocele repair are completed prior to elevation and fixation of the sutures.

aneurysm needle to move one end from the other on each side. This may be useful in a patient with a history of hernia, obesity, or "poor fascia." The suprapubic wound is lavaged and then closed with simple nylon sutures or subcuticular suture of delayed-absorbable material. A suprapubic catheter may be placed at this point in the procedure, although intermittent self-catheterization is preferred by many.

Postoperative Care

Whether a suprapubic catheter or intermittent self-catheterization is contemplated for postoperative blad-der drainage, a 16 French Foley catheter is used in the first 24 hours for dependent drainage and then discontinued. If a cystocele was not present, attempts at voiding may be encouraged in the second postoperative 24-hour period. Because of minimal dissection, most patients will be able to void 2–3 days after surgery without difficulty. Occasionally, elderly patients and patients in whom the surgeon desires some overcorrection (athletes, obese patients, and patients with chronic respiratory dysfunction) prolonged time to voiding of greater than 7 days occurs approximately 10% of the time. In those patients in whom only the Pereyra procedure was performed, discharge from the hospital may be anticipated in the second or third postoperative day, and occasionally on the first postoperative day in patients in whom the local anesthetic technique was used. Release of suprapubic catheter or intermittent self-catheterization at 4-hour intervals usually allows sufficient time for the patient to attempt to void. Interestingly, voiding difficulties seem less prominent once the patient is in her home environment. The patient may check for residual urine and report voiding and residual volumes.

Results

Pereyra, Lebherz, and Growdon and colleagues reported 94.5% success in patients undergoing this procedure primarily with 4 years or greater follow-up. Successful results of 89% were noted in 28 patients who had one to six previous unsuccessful repairs. In 1982, Pereyra and Lebherz reported 94.5% success in 162 patients followed for 1 year or more. Bhatia and Bergman reported 85% success in 20 patients with both primary and secondary repairs followed for 1 year. Roberts, Angel, Thomas et al. and Leach and Raz reported 94% and 97% success, respectively, in studies with minor variations of technique with 1- and 2-year follow-up.

Ease of surgical technique, shorter hospital stay and recovery, and minimal morbidity are notable attributes of this procedure as reported by Forneret and Leach. Dense retropubic scarring seems to be the only contraindication, and this is apparently rare. Prolonged catheter time (greater than fourth postoperative day) occurs in less than 15% of patients. Lower-urinary-tract injury occurs rarely (less than 1%) in these reports.

THE GOEBELL-STOECKEL SLING OPERATION

JOHN H. RIDLEY

Although a great majority of cases of stress incontinence of urine can be cured by a well-executed plication of the sphincter and the urethra, there are some failures, and one must look to another method for curing them. Failure is especially likely in those cases unrelated to childbirth injury in which the poor sphincter musculature has insufficient tone to control the urine when the intravesical pressure is raised to exceed intraurethral pressure. Failure with the plication operation, even in good hands, is often a consequence of previous bungling attempts in which the resulting scar tissue has made it impossible for the sphincter to contract adequately, regardless of how tightly it is plicated.

Other conditions, less frequently encountered, that are not amenable to the plication operation are congenital absence of the sphincter mechanism, which may occur as mentioned by Price in 1933. The absence of part or all of the urethra may be due to congenital deformity, such as hypospadias, or may be due to obstetrical or surgical accidents. In these latter cases, a urethra may be constructed, but lacking a sphincter mechanism, some procedure is required to ensure continence. In other, more common, instances, irradiation may render the urethra a virtually functionless "water tube." Finally, there is a group in which the incontinence depends upon faulty innervation, as may be seen in spina bifida, multiple sclerosis, and spine trauma.

One must be very careful in selecting cases for surgery that might have neurologic disease. Bladder hypotonia with possible ureteral reflux contraindicates any partially obstructive procedure, which may aggravate this underlying problem. In this condition, the bladder musculature would not be strengthened, and the reflux would be aggravated, leading to an ascending chronic urinary tract infection.

Hodgkinson has made us aware of detrusor dyssynergia dysfunction, which can be a primary cause of a type of incontinence that is not correctable by surgery. Although this condition may be suspected and diagnosed in a majority of cases by accurate history and simple tests, it requires sophisticated electronic equipment to be accurately evaluated.

Modern studies and work with highly specialized equipment have clarified some problems that heretofore have been less well understood, such as intraurethral and intravesical pressure gradients. This type of equipment is becoming available for more general use, despite its complexity and expense. Beck and Low have worked extensively in this field.

In all the preceding groups of cases, the surgeon must seek elsewhere than the vesical neck and the urethra to create a mechanism effective in the control of the urine. Many operations have been devised, none of which has been universally successful, although some can be used to advantage in certain cases. A short summary of these attempts may be useful to the student of incontinence of urine in women. The sling technique will be presented in more detail.

There are several basic surgical procedures for correcting stress urinary incontinence. This section deals with the Goebell-Stoeckel sling procedure, with a discussion of the indications for its use, the preoperative evaluation, the actual technique of the procedure, and the postoperative care. The other basic techniques have been discussed in detail earlier in this chapter.

Historical Development of the Sling Procedures

In 1907, Giordano utilized a portion of the gracilis muscle to encircle the urethra. This was done with enough success to encourage further efforts and modifications of this principle.

In 1910, Goebell described an operation in which he dissected free the pyramidalis muscles, brought them down posterior to the symphysis, and encircled the urethra near its junction with the bladder. He suggested crossing the muscles and the fascial components if their length permitted. He performed this procedure on both children and adults with encouraging success. An obvious difficulty with this operation lies in the fact that the pyramidalis muscles vary greatly in their development and may be too small or too short to encircle the urethra.

In 1914, Frangenheim used the pyramidalis muscle with an attached strap of fascia from the sheath of the rectus to encircle the male urethra. The strap was brought down retropubically around the urethra and then sutured to itself. This operation was also done for incontinent women.

In 1917, Stoeckel combined the use of the pyramidalis muscles and the fascial strap with plication of the sphincter region. He first dissected from the midline a strap of fascia with pyramidalis muscles attached, split the distal portion of the strap, and passed this retropubically to the urethral region. These split ends were then made to encircle the urethra and were sutured together below with the appropriate tension. He reported two cases treated successfully, and this type of procedure became one of those basics that could be depended upon in the carefully chosen cases.

In 1932, Norman Miller modified the Goebell-Frangenheim-Stoeckel operation by bringing the pyramidalis muscle with the attached fascia strap beneath the urethra but anterior to the symphysis. This was not adopted because of excessive dissection and bleeding and the wrong angle of the supporting sling beneath the urethra.

In 1933, Price reported the cure of urinary incontinence in a girl with congenital absence of the sacrum and the coccyx and without innervation of the sphincter. He used a sling of autogenous fascia lata, which he brought around the urethra retropubically and attached both ends to the rectus muscle. The principles of this technique with subsequent modification have been used as a most dependable procedure and will be described in more detail in this chapter.

In 1942, Aldridge devised a modification in which he combined some portions of the Goebell-Frangenheim-Stoeckel procedure with those of Price's procedure. Using a transverse lower abdominal incision, he developed straps of the aponeurosis from the rectus sheath parallel to Poupart's ligament, leaving the medial ends attached. The free ends of this fascia were then passed retropubically beneath the urethra and attached (Fig. 33-14).

Operators have used many types of material in search of the perfect material for this sling procedure, but none has yet been found that is completely satisfactory. Generally speaking, the autogenous materials, such as fascia, have functioned most dependably and with least tissue reaction. Foreign tissues, such as ox fascia or collagen, have not proven as satisfactory. Synthetic polyester fibers such as Dacron (Mersilene) or some similar product seemed at first to be the answer, because of the availability of the material and the facility with which it could be used. However, contrary to the success reported with its use in other areas of the body, Mersilene has proved to be unsatisfactory in the experience of this operator, and its use in the sling procedures was condemned. In 1962, Williams and Te Linde reported with guarded enthusiasm the use of Mersilene in the sling procedure, but they later condemned its use as longer periods of observation were made. In 1966, Ridley reported its use in 17 cases with four subsequent, rather serious complications involving erosion into the urethra; foreign-body reaction, necessitating its removal; and/or chronic infection with stone formation.

The original Goebell-Frangenheim-Stoeckel procedure is now rarely performed, because in many cases the abdominal fascia has been weakened by previous operative procedures, whether for pelvic pathology or for a previous surgical effort retropubically to correct the stress urinary incontinence.

The literature is replete with many modifications of the basic techniques for correction of stress urinary incontinence. Only time and experience will serve to evaluate them; however, the general principles of correction of stress urinary incontinence remain the same despite the passing parade of various procedures and modifications thereof. As the understanding of stress urinary incontinence increases, the likelihood of a much more successful procedure increases, but thus far there remains an apparently irreducible number of failures resulting from any procedure. Individual surgeons will select the type of procedure in which they are most proficient and successful and will use this specific procedure in the great majority of their cases. However, surgeons should not try to fit all cases into one particular type of operation to the exclusion of the others. The surgeon must be familiar enough with all the basic procedures to adapt the connective operation to the patient's problem.

More recent contributions have been made by Green, Ball, Ingelmann-Sundberg, Pereyra, Gunther, Low, Ostergard, and Beck. However, the percentage of failures and the incidence of complications remain about constant. In this chapter our recommendations will be based on our experience.

Choice of Operation

When the surgeon considers whether surgery is indicated and, if it is indicated, what the operation should be, many factors must be considered. In particular (and within the scope of this section, which is concerned primarily with cases in which stress urinary incontinence has not been cured by sphincter plication), consideration must be given to why the first efforts failed. Although the percentage of successful outcomes expected with the Kelly plication is high, the failures must be cared for by more sophisticated study and procedures. It is believed that the Kelly plication technique, with its simplicity, safety, and degree of success, should in the great majority of cases be the first effort. There is an exception to this rule, however, in cases of incontinence in women, often elderly, without anterior vaginal wall relaxation. In these cases the incontinence is apparently due to poor sphincter muscle tone and tissue weakness as a result of advancing years. Little or nothing can be expected from tightening these poor muscles. Hence, in cases of this kind that are severe enough to require correction, we have proceeded directly with the sling procedure.

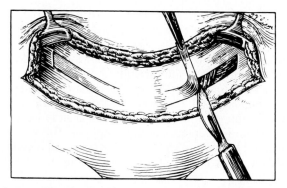

Figure 33–14. Aldridge modification of Goebell-Frangenheim-Stoeckel operation for urinary incontinence. The fascial strips are being separated through a Pfannenstiel incision.

When the Kelly plication is done, it has been found that using bold bites for suture placement in the paraurethral tissue is important. A semi-purse-string suture over the bladder neck has proven to be an excellent addition (Fig. 33-15).

Counsellor, Brewer, and others have noted that the rate of success in the plication procedure gradually declines as the years pass from the time of the plication, suggesting recurring tissue failure. This need not be true in the follow-up history of the Goebell-Stoeckel sling procedure or the Marshall-Marchetti-Krantz retropubic urethropexy. Green and others had stressed the importance of the urethrovesical angle in relation to incontinence. More recent studies by Greenwald, Thornbury, and Dunn have cast doubt on the importance of this factor. They found the same demonstrable deformities in 12 of 17 patients (71%) who had no stress urinary incontinence. Our own experience coincides more nearly with that of Greenwald, Thornbury, and Dunn. We have seen various types of angles in women with incontinence and with perfect control. The percentage of "normal" and "abnormal" angles in patients with and without control causes us to conclude that the angle is not the determining factor. It is true that the angle is changed by plication and by the sling, but we are convinced that this is incidental and that it is the suburethral support in the region of the urethrovesical junction that restores continence.

Our conclusions, however, do not mitigate the importance of and necessity for a thorough preoperative evaluation of the condition. The history is of the greatest importance in making certain that we are dealing with true stress urinary incontinence rather than incontinence due to excessive urge. A careful and detailed history can bring out other factors that may more clearly define the type of the patient's incontinence. This may include chronic urinary tract infection, previous surgery, previous irradiation, and neurogenic and psychogenic factors. We must remember that any of these conditions can coexist and must be clearly delineated before any surgery is undertaken. Preoperative urodynamic studies, excretory and retrograde urinary tract studies, urine cultures, and competent pelvic examinations must be done. It may be found that, to the surgeon's surprise and disappointment, although there has been a mechanical correction of the stress urinary incontinence by one of the previously mentioned basic procedures, a detrusor dyssynergia or some other more obscure factor may coexist that causes a less than satisfactory result.

In other instances it is well to combine the strap procedure with a cystocele repair and plication of the suburethral fascia. When this is done it is well to complete the placing of the fascial strap beneath the urethra first and then bury it beneath the suburethral fascia. The transplanted fascial strap is then less likely to cause any postoperative problems in the vagina. When the urethrovaginal tissue has been compromised by previous surgery or irradiation, one must avoid further trauma to this tissue, to avoid establishing a urethrovaginal fistula. Two other techniques are available—the *transected* or *exteriorized* sling techniques—and will be discussed more fully later.

Our experience and results with the Marshall-Marchetti-Krantz procedure have been very favorable, and in most instances in which concomitant intra-abdominal disease exists, it has been our first choice, since a combined abdominovaginal procedure is thereby avoided. If the Marshall-Marchetti-Krantz procedure fails, our choice for the "ultimate effort," regardless of what other procedures have failed previously, is the sling procedure. This conclusion has also been put forth by Marchetti and Green and more re-

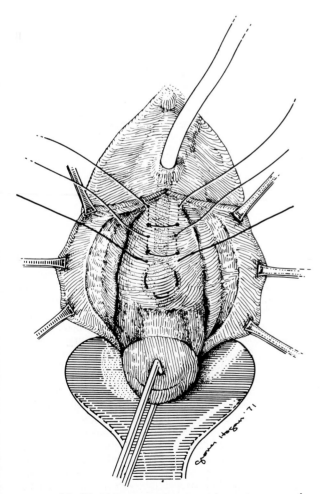

Figure 33–15. Using a semi-purse-string suture over the bladder neck has proven to be an excellent addition to the Kelly plication technique.

cently by Beck. We have had a great number of successes with the sling after the Marshall-Marchetti-Krantz procedure, or some modification thereof, but we should not like to give the impression that we consider only the sling procedure after Marshall-Marchetti-Krantz failures. Of the last 100 cases, from 1977 to 1987, in which we used the sling procedure, 72 were failed Marshall-Marchetti-Krantz procedures. This study also included the failures by the modified Pereyra, the Stamey, the Raz, or the Burch procedures. With the increasing experience and success with the fascia sling, we have favored the Goebell-Frangenheim-Stoeckel procedure more and more. Overall, except for earlier in our experience, when some of the concomitant conditions were not fully recognizable, our results have been successful.

Hodgkinson and Drukker have brought to our attention the important phenomenon of detrusor dyssynergia, in which a variable amount of urine may be lost insensibly by intrinsic neuromuscular dysfunction. Although rare, it is very important to recognize this, as it may coexist with other conditions mentioned earlier.

Preoperative Evaluation of the Bladder

Regardless of the chosen method of repair, an irreducible minimum number of cases of intractable stress urinary incontinence seem to defy correction. Some of these can be identified by careful screening, and operation upon these types is obviously contraindicated. The most serious condition can indeed be aggravated by the improper choice of procedure in the atonic or otherwise neurologically impaired bladder. In all cases of stress urinary incontinence in which any procedure other than the simple Kelly plication is contemplated, we routinely perform a cystometrogram to evaluate the bladder dynamics and capacity. In most cases this can be done as a simple office procedure. However, the use of more sophisticated and dependable urodynamics apparatus is more frequent in our modern clinics.

Except in the more complicated cases, dependable urodynamics studies can be done easily and without anesthesia in the gynecologist's office. Although a Lewis Recording Cystometer is desirable, it is not essential to evaluate the bladder properly. Again we emphasize that a careful history should be taken, particularly noting any previous surgery of the genitourinary tract and the exact subjective complaints of the patient.

Ridley has described a simple office procedure for evaluating the bladder: the patient is allowed to void and this specimen is saved for chemical analysis. With the patient on the examining table in dorsolithotomy position, the vulva and urethral meatus are properly prepared, using providone-iodine. A medium-sized straight metal catheter is carefully inserted into the urethra. The use of a cotton-tipped applicator for this test is discouraged, because even though covered with petroleum jelly, it is unnecessarily traumatic and frequently leaves lint fibers in the urethra. However, any straight, very smooth small metal rod can be used. With experience, the degree of inclination of the urethra to the axis of the symphysis can be noted. If the catheter passes into the bladder horizontally or with the inserted tip inclined upward, the relationship of the urethra to the symphysis axis is roughly normal and the urethra is probably continent. Conversely, if the inserted tip points downward and away from the horizontal, it can be assumed that the urethra has rotated downward from the axis of the symphysis, suggesting ineffectual urethral support (Fig 33-16). In this type of deformity we would expect improvement with proper supporting reconstruction, such as we have obtained

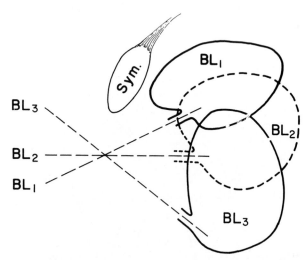

Figure 33–16. Schematic drawing showing composite of various positions and relationships of the bladder, urethra, and symphysis pubis. *BL₁*, the normal position of the bladder and urethra with acute posterior urethrovesical angle and relatively close normal relationships of the axis of the urethra and symphysis pubis. This patient usually has no stress urinary incontinence. *BL₂*, borderline loss of urethral support with posterior rotation of the axis of the urethra and straightening of the posterior urethrovesical angle. This patient usually has moderate stress urinary incontinence. *BL₃*, pronounced posterior rotation of the axis of the urethra with loss of the posterior urethrovesical angle. This patient usually has a marked amount of stress urinary incontinence.

In the lithotomy examining position the gynecologist will note the position of the rigid straight catheter placed in the bladder, which gives a good indication of the inclination of the angle that the urethra has with the perpendicular axis of the symphysis pubis. (After Ridley JH. Gynecologic surgery: errors, safeguards and salvage. Baltimore: Williams & Wilkins, 1974.)

with the sling procedure. This is only an approximation, but we find that it makes routine chain cystourethrograms less important. The amount of residual urine is measured as the catheterization is completed. This amount of urine—and there is usually a sufficient amount under any circumstances—is saved for microscopic examination, culture, and sensitivity tests. Next, a Foley No. 20 catheter with a 5-cc balloon is inserted for the tests of bladder capacity and dynamics. This catheter is connected to a graduated flask hanging about 90 cm (36 in) above the symphysis, and increments of 50 ml of normal saline lightly tinted with methylene blue are allowed to gravitate into the bladder. The patient is not apprehensive or uncomfortable if a detailed explanation of the planned procedure has been given to her. Allowing 10 seconds between influx of the increments of 50 cc of normal saline at body temperature, a careful record is kept of how much saline is allowed to flow in. The end result of this test comes when the patient has a true urgency and is just beginning to have spasms of micturition. A note is made of the amount of saline used. The bladder is promptly allowed to begin to drain. If the patient allows only 150 ml or less of the saline solution, we are dealing usually with urge incontinence or a bladder of chronic spasm (Hunner's ulcer) or of decreased capacity due to fibrosis. Any amount from 300 ml to 600 ml is classified as normal, and amounts over 600 ml suggest bladder atony or some neurologic impairment.

To test further for the amount of stress urinary incontinence, approximately 250 ml of the saline is allowed to remain in the bladder and the Foley catheter is removed. The patient is now asked to give a firm cough while the urethra is observed for evidence of leakage with the patient in the lithotomy position and in standing position. The Marchetti, or "stress," test of evaluation of the anterior vaginal wall without compression of the urethra is done. The vaginal mucosa in the region of the urethrovesical junction is infiltrated with a wheal of local anesthetic agent just lateral to the midline on either side. This area is grasped with an Allis clamp on either side of the urethra to avoid compression, and the structures are gently thrust upward and backward to a more retropubic position. A more practical procedure is to reposition the urethrovesical junction retropubically with the index and middle fingers without compression of the urethra to make the Marchetti test. The patient is now asked to cough firmly again. If there is no leakage with this strenuous effort, one may assume that repositioning the urethra by supporting it with a sling or by retropubic urethropexy should improve or cure the stress incontinence. All of this evaluation can be done easily and quickly at one appointment. If the patient has a history of chronic or recurring urinary tract infection or lithiasis, or if the bladder studies just completed are not within normal limits, the entire urinary tract should be further evaluated by excretory and retrograde urography and endoscopy.

If there is any question after this simple and dependable office test, the more sophisticated and refined techniques of urodynamic evaluation should be done. This can give both the differential pressure profiles of the bladder/urethra and the cystometric values.

The choice of operation for the correction of stress urinary incontinence must be even more refined if there is extraordinary scarring from previous surgery, neoplasm, or treatment thereof or congenital deformities. Search for irregularities of sphincter closure can be done easily through the air cystoscope, through the water cystoscope, or by indirect air cystoscopy. The latter technique, described by Ridley, may be helpful in determining the extent of the scarring and particularly the integrity of the trigone area. This is most helpful in evaluation of the vesicovaginal or urethrovaginal fistula.

Another instance in which the sling procedure is indicated is in the aged patient who has undergone previous colpocleisis for procidentia, in whom a suprapubic approach could not effectively elevate the urethra and bladder neck, but in whom the sling procedure could.

Still another example is that of a patient who has had previous surgery for construction of a congenitally or surgically absent urethra or in which there has been a successful repair of the vesicovaginal or vesicourethrovaginal fistula. Knowing that the weakened, compromised urethrovaginal membrane will tolerate no more trauma, we may use either a split fascia lata strap attached to the paraurethral tissues in the posterior third of the urethral area or the continuous fascia lata strap *exteriorized* beneath the urethra, as described by Ridley in 1974, thus not traumatizing the urethrovaginal membrane itself.

Operative Procedures

The Goebell-Frangenheim-Stoeckel Procedure Using the Fascia Lata Strap

The Goebell-Frangenheim-Stoeckel procedure using the fascia lata strap has become the most dependable, easy, and safe of the available procedures and thus is the one we have used most frequently. The sling procedure has an unwarranted reputation of difficulty.

Procurement of the fascia lata is quick and simple. The various materials used for the sling are numerous and all have been evaluated; for example: homologous abdominal fascia (Aldridge); the round ligament (Hodgkinson); synthetic materials (Marlex, Mersilene, Nylon), which are nonabsorbable; PGA mesh, which is absorbable; Lyodura; homologous dermis; porcine dermis; Gore-Tex; homologous tendon of the palmaris longus muscle; Teflon. Except for the use of a Mersilene strap in 17 cases in the early days of this series, the homologous fascia lata has been used exclusively in the 301 cases operated upon or under direction of this author (1947–1987). The use of this foreign-body material was abandoned after four complications developed with erosion into the urethra or bladder, with stone formation; erosion into the vagina, with a temporary urethrovaginal fistula; and the obvious foreign-body reaction. The Mersilene was necessarily removed in all these cases.

Technique. The patient is placed on the table in the supine position, with either thigh surgically prepared by shaving and cleansing. The site of the incision is optional, depending on the patient's desire for a less noticeable scar or the gynecologist's desire for the easiest approach to and procurement of the strap of fascia lata. The incision is made just above the lateral condyle of the femur, either transversely or longitudinally, over the distal insertion of the fascia lata near the femoral condyle. The fascia is easily identified (Fig. 33-17) and stripped of fat as well as possible with the gauzed finger. The fascia is split by two incisions 1 cm apart in the direction parallel to the course of the fibers. This strap is then transected 1 cm superior to the distal attachment and this free end is threaded through the Masson fascia stripper or a more recently developed Crawford fascia stripper (Storz). The fascia stripper is then thrust firmly and evenly cephalad beneath the skin until it can go no further (Fig. 33-18). The strap thus incised is cut then at its proximal end by sliding the sheath over the inner tube of the stripper. The strap is removed and put aside in sterile normal saline. An additional strap of fascia can be taken at the same time if there is any doubt about the sufficiency of the length or width of the first excision. Or the operator may elect to remove an auxiliary strap from the opposite thigh.

In some instances, if the length of the available fascia strap is insufficient, it may be lengthened by the simple plastic "turn-down" technique of hemisection (Fig. 33-19).

The fascial defect within sight beneath the incision is closed with two or three interrupted sutures of No. 3-0 delayed-absorbable material and the skin is closed. An elastic compression bandage is applied over the thigh to obviate any chance of bleeding or hematoma formation. This has been exceedingly rare.

It is again emphasized that the procurement of the fascia strap is easy and quick. It can be done through either the incision described earlier or just inferior to the greater trochanter of the femur. Because the fascia lata fibers fan out from below upward (Fig. 33-20), it is thought that the strap cut from below upward is more uniform in width and strength, thus facilitating its removal. Only rarely will the patient complain of any pain in the thigh postoperatively, and no complications have been encountered. However, the patient may develop an incisional hernia at the sites where the fascia straps have been developed from the anterior abdominal aponeurosis parallel to Poupart's ligament, although such an occurrence is relatively infrequent in the Aldridge technique.

The patient is now changed to a dorsolithotomy position and appropriately cleaned and draped so that the combined fields of the lower abdomen and the perineum are simultaneously accessible. A 7–10-cm transverse incision is made 3 cm above the symphysis down to the fibers of the anterior abdominal aponeurosis. If previous lower abdominal incisions have been made, which is frequently the case, the underlying fascia may be somewhat distorted by scarring, but with care the fascia can be identified. Two small, slitlike incisions about 1 cm in length are made 2 cm above the symphysis and 2 cm to either side of the midline and parallel to the direction of the aponeurotic fibers. The bladder is then partially filled and a suprapubic cystostomy is done routinely. (We use a Cystocath No. 12.) The bladder is then drained completely. We prefer to do the cystostomy at this time in order to observe any incidental hematuria that may result. However, this has never

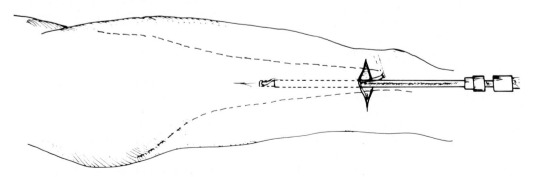

Figure 33–17. Method of obtaining fascial strap.

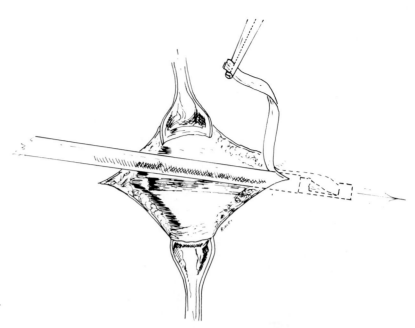

Figure 33–18. Method of action of Masson fascial stripper.

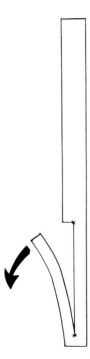

Figure 33–19. Schematic drawing showing splicing of fascia strap to lengthen without narrowing at midpoint.

been a significant problem. With finger dissection or blunt instrument dissection, the muscle bellies of the rectus abdominis are split or gently displaced to the midline. The finger is thrust into the space of Retzius on either side of the midline. This dissection is gently

performed, and even in the presence of scarring from previous retropubic surgery, the approach can be made to the inferior aspect of the pubic ramus. In some instances, however, the scarring may be so extensive that sharp or scissors dissection must be used. It is important to "stay on the periosteum" to lessen the chance for injury to the adherent bladder. There have been no instances of osteitis pubis in our series. Even with this careful dissection, the bladder may be entered, but this is no reason to change the operative plan. The bladder entry can be detected easily if a small amount of methylene blue has been injected into the bladder prior to this dissection. It is not feasible to attempt to repair this small rent in the bladder wall, and with the autogenous fascia lata and adequate bladder drainage, healing is usually prompt. However, the patient should be closely observed postoperatively, so that any retropubic extravasation or infection will be detected. These have not been a problem in our experience. After retropubic dissection has been carried out on either side and down to the inferior aspect of the pubic ramus (Fig. 33-21), the wound is lightly packed with a wet saline sponge. The operative site is shifted to the vagina.

The anterior vaginal wall is incised in the midline from about 1 cm posterior to the external urethral meatus and over the entire length of the urethra and to the cervix, or to the vaginal vault seam if previous hysterectomy has been performed. This allows adequate lateral dissection of the tissues of the posterior urethra and neck of the bladder as well as access for repair to any concomitant cystocele. The sphincter area

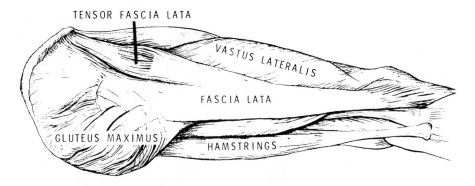

Figure 33–20. Anatomy of fascia lata.

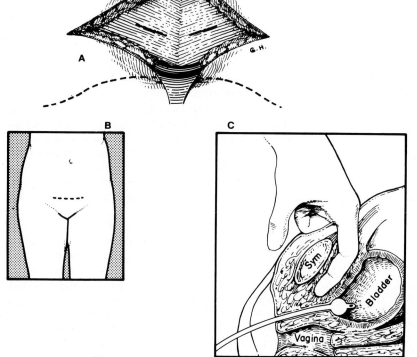

Figure 33–21. *A*, The anterior abdominal aponeurosis has been exposed and two 2-cm incisions made therein, parallel to the fibers of this fascia, 3 cm superior to level of Poupart's ligament. *B*, The site of the small suprapubic incision. *C*, Gentle finger dissection is done retropubically through the space of Retzius down to the level of the urogenital diaphragm and inferior aspect of the pubic ramus on either side. If the space of Retzius has been scarred by previous surgery, dissection may be performed with the blunt tip of uterine dressing forceps. (After Ridley JH. Gynecologic surgery: errors, safeguards and salvage. Baltimore: Williams & Wilkins, 1974.)

may be easily determined by an indwelling balloon catheter. The subjacent vaginal fascia is dissected and developed as described in the section on anterior colporrhaphy. Thus, one of the great advantages of the sling procedure is that any necessary vaginal surgery can be done in conjunction with the vaginal portion of the operation. In some cases, Kelly plication sutures are placed concomitantly. Again, by using gentle finger dissection upward, a shallow tunnel is developed on either side of the urethra, which is marked by the indwelling No. 16 French balloon catheter, beneath and posterior

to the inferior surface of the pubic ramus. Most of the potentially troublesome bleeding that may be encountered here is avoided by blunt dissection reflecting the tissues from lateral to medial toward the bladder neck.

A uterine dressing forceps with a medium blunt end is of a proper curvature for gently thrusting retropubically from above downward. The tip of the clamp (Fig. 33-22) with concave curve toward the symphysis is passed through the slitlike openings of the anterior aponeurosis retropubically downward until the instrument tip can be palpated in the shallow retropubic

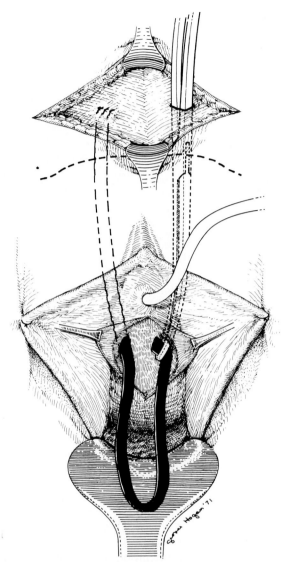

Figure 33–22. The passage of the fascia lata strap beneath the urethra and retropubically. The strap has been anchored to the anterior abdominal fascia on the patient's right side and drawn into the vagina. It is being grasped by the uterine dressing forceps to be drawn up to the left side and anchored with proper tension at the other slitlike incision in the fascia. Thus, a sling is formed beneath the urethra at the bladder neck. The retention catheter remains in place during the entire sling procedure. (After Ridley JH. Gynecologic surgery: errors, safeguards and salvage. Baltimore: Williams & Wilkins, 1974.)

tunnel on that side of the urethra. The tip of the retropubic instrument, still closed, is gently thrust through the resistant tissue of the urogenital diaphragm into the vaginal incision. If there is considerable scarring at this point, the thrust must be firm and under complete control, always being sure to be on the proper lateral side of the urethra with the indwelling catheter. A small slit made with a scalpel over the point of the clamp may be necessary to facilitate this passage.

Proper passage of the clamp retropubically is important. It is pressed gently against the posterior surface of the bone as it is passed downward, thus minimizing the chance of injuring the bladder or opening the venous sinuses that lie in the space of Retzius near the bladder neck. In other words, gently "scrape" the tip of the retropubic instrument over the periosteum downward. By using this technique and with gentle pressure, bleeding is unlikely. If it does, it is usually of venous origin and can be controlled by gentle pressure. The tip of the strap of fascia lata is grasped through the vaginal incision and drawn retropubically. It is attached firmly with two or three sutures of No. 3-0 silk to the anterior sheath of the rectus, thus also closing securely the slitlike incisions previously made.

The process of passing the uterine dressing forceps (or long Kelly clamp) retropubically into the vaginal field is repeated on the other side, and the other free end of the strap of fascia lata is drawn upward beneath the urethra without twisting, to be attached to the anterior abdominal aponeurosis at the contralateral incision previously made. Thus, a continuous sling is formed beneath the urethra; appropriate tension is applied before this strap of fascia lata is firmly attached to the abdominal fascia. Before fixation of the strap, the operator must check to be sure that the strap has been passed beneath the urethra near the junction with the bladder and that no injury has occurred. Two sutures may be placed to anchor and spread the fascia beneath the urethra.

Appropriate tension of the sling beneath the urethra must be more fully described, because this is a key to the success of this relatively simple procedure. The most frequent mistake of the less experienced operator is to suture the sling *too tight,* thus truly obstructing the urethra. It is necessary only to support the bladder neck at its posterior third. There can be no hard-and-fast rule about what tension to apply on the strap, but it can be safely said that a gentle support is desired rather than any obstructing or distorting force. The tip of a curved clamp (gallbladder clamp) can be passed freely between the urethra and the fascia sling (Fig. 33-23). This is one of the most important technical points in the proper placement and adjustment of the tension of the sling. Let the sling loosely support the posterior urethra. When the patient assumes the upright standing or sitting position, the force of gravity augments the support of the strap (Fig 33-24).

With the patient in the dorsolithotomy operating position, it may be valuable to note the relative inclination of the urethra to the horizontal. As has been mentioned, a rough estimate of correct anatomic position may be

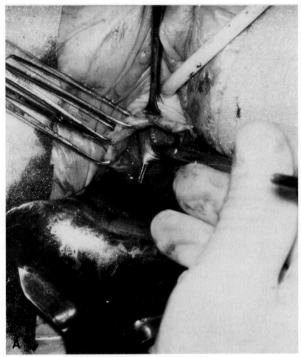
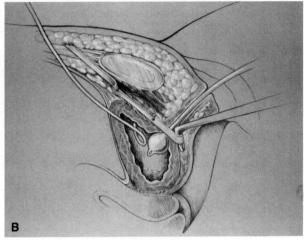

Figure 33–23. *A,* The curved clamp (gallbladder clamp) can be passed very easily between the urethra and the sling after appropriate tension has been applied on the fascia lata. *B,* The tension support of the fascia lata sling is adjusted with the curved clamp. The sling has been lengthened in this instance. (Photograph by Lester V. Bergman courtesy LTI Medica® and The Upjohn Company. Copyright 1987 by Learning Technology Incorporated. Drawing by Beverly Kessler courtesy LTI Medica® and The Upjohn Company. Copyright 1987 by Learning Technology Incorporated.)

demonstrated by insertion of a metal catheter into the bladder. It has been noted that proper supportive tension of the sling will bring the catheter tip to at least the horizontal with a retropubic inclination. A further test is made by filling the bladder with 300–400 ml sterile water and applying gentle suprapubic pressure. There should be no leakage. There is no obstruction to the passage of the metal catheter through the urethra after the sling is fastened. Again we say "gentle support" rather than obstructing force.

In rare instances, because of the dense scarring from previous surgical procedures, the bladder may be injured retropubically by entry into its lumen with a clamp tip. If the bladder wall has become firmly adherent to the periosteal surface retropubically, one should not discontinue the operation but should proceed to apply the strap. This rent in the bladder heals promptly if adequate drainage is assured from the bladder itself. No foreign-body reaction results if the fascia is used.

In 16 cases of a total of 301 procedures performed from 1947 through 1987, the patient was unable to void satisfactorily because too much tension had been applied to the supporting sling. In these cases, the fascia lata was transected vaginally. The incision was made 1 cm to either the right or the left of the midline of the urethra marked by an indwelling catheter. The fibers of the fascia lata could be easily identified and transected without injuring the urethra. No troublesome bleeding was encountered. Fourteen of the 16 cases had very satisfactory results, and there were two failures. If the operator waits for a least 8 weeks before transecting the sling, enough support by scar tissue will have formed to save the integrity of the original procedure.

The incision for this transection of the sling, of course, should *not* be made directly over the urethra for fear of causing a urethrovaginal fistula. No consideration of a transurethral resection should be considered in these cases because of irreparable damage!

The abdominal incision is closed, and after the necessary vaginal repair work is completed, the vaginal incision is closed. The balloon retention catheter is left in the bladder and the vagina is packed with Iodoform gauze for 24 hours as a gentle tamponade. The suprapubic tube is irrigated, is left in the bladder, but is clamped with the urethral catheter open and draining. The suprapubic cystostomy is used as a "safety valve"

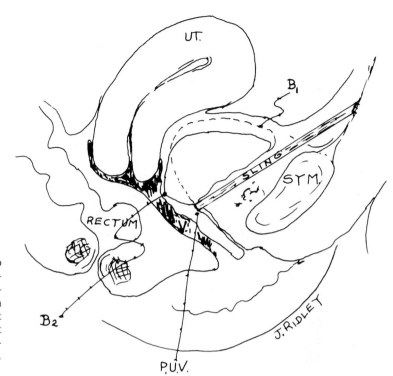

Figure 33–24. A composite illustration to show the difference in the posterior urethrovesical angle (PUV) with patient in the lithotomy position B_1 (dotted line) and patient in the upright position B_2 (solid line). The effect of gravity exaggerates and augments the effect of the sling. (From Ridley JH. Gynecologic surgery: errors, safeguards, and salvage. 2nd ed. Baltimore: Williams & Wilkins, 1981.)

and is a great help in educating the patient postoperatively about voiding. The presence of the suprapubic catheter also is for reassuring the patient. It can be removed in about 7 or 8 days or when the patient is voiding and having less than 50 cc residual.

Two modifications of the Goebell-Stoeckel sling procedure can be relied upon if, for some reason, the routine procedure is contraindicated.

The strap of fascia lata can be *exteriorized* beneath the urethra when the urethrovaginal tissues are unworkable because of previous surgical or irradiation scarring or in those cases where the urethra has been reconstructed or rebuilt.

In the placement of this *exteriorized* sling, two slitlike incisions, scarcely larger than the strap itself, are made within 1 cm on either side of the posterior third of the urethra. The fascia lata is brought downward and beneath the urethra, is exposed in the vagina, and is brought upward for similar attachment to the abdominal fascia lata on the contralateral side (Fig. 33-25).

The appropriate tension is adjusted in a similar manner as described for the routine placement of the sling discussed just previously in this chapter. The vagina is packed lightly with an Iodoform pack for 2 days. Upon its removal, a small amount of estrogen cream is placed in the vagina in the postmenopausal woman every other day and no further vaginal trauma is allowed. After approximately 4 weeks, the subtending segment of the *exteriorized* fascia is covered by new epithelialization. This, of course, would not be possible if a foreign material, other than homologous, is used.

A second modification of the treatment of the vaginal portion of the sling of attempting to bury the continuous sling beneath the urethra was described by Te Linde. An attempt would be made to tunnel beneath the urethra and between the urethral and vaginal membranes with a sharp knife and pass the fascia through this. However, this was not found to be dependable, particularly if the urethrovaginal membrane had been severely compromised by previous scarring or surgery.

A third modification was used briefly with transection of the sling but without passage of the new supporting ends beneath the urethra but sutured securely to the paraurethral and vaginal fascia approximately 1 cm to either side of the posterior third of the urethra. It was found that the tension was more difficult to adjust and the integrity of the vaginal fascia was unpredictable.

The use of the *exteriorized* treatment of the fascia subtending the urethra has replaced these last two procedures.

The Aldridge Modification of the Sling Operation

The Aldridge modification of the Goebell-Frangenheim-Stoeckel sling procedure has proven dependable and is widely used, although it has been used in only three cases in the present series of this author.

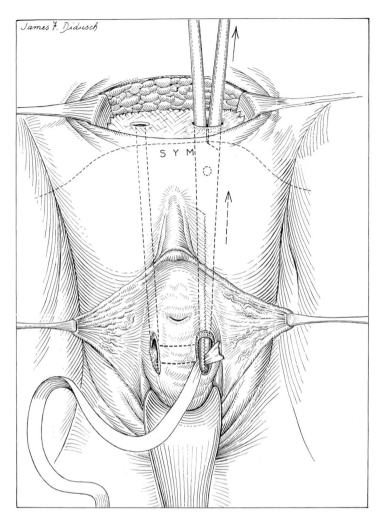

James F. Didusch

Figure 33–25. Modified Goebell-Frangenheim-Stoeckel operation. A retropubic tunnel has been made with a uterine dressing forceps and the fascia lata has been grasped. This end is drawn upward and sutured to the fascia of the anterior abdominal wall. The dotted line shows where the exteriorized segment of the fascia lata sling will lie.

Although the principles of the treatment of the fascia are essentially the same, the procurement of the fascia is different. It is of historic interest to describe the Aldridge modification of the Goebell-Frangenheim-Stoeckel sling procedure as a transition of the procedures of the original authors.

The fascia is procured from the abdominal aponeurosis through an adequate Pfannenstiel incision exposing the symphysis and the entire lengths of Poupart's ligament bilaterally. Incisions are made parallel to the fibers of the abdominal fascia 1 cm above Poupart's ligament and developing a band of fascia 1 cm in width. The strips are then transected near the area of the external iliac spine and the material is reflected medially. It is not detached at the medial end but is inverted retropubically and passed through the urogenital diaphragm in the same manner as that described in the use of the fascia lata. Great care is exercised to cause the least trauma to the bladder in what can be the previously scarred space of Retzius.

The free ends of the abdominal fascia are then led downward with a uterine dressing forceps or a similar gently curved clamp until these ends present into the vagina approximately 1 cm to either side of the posterior third of the urethra. The vaginal membrane and vaginal fascia already have been incised and dissected as a routine cystocele repair.

Now the loose ends of abdominal fascia are securely fastened beneath the urethra, forming the continuous sling. The ends are overlapped as appropriate tension is determined. Three or four sutures of 3-0 silk are used to join the fascial ends beneath the urethra. Here again it is emphasized that this sling must be supporting without obstructing the urethra. The remainder of the vaginal repair is done in routine manner.

Comment and Results

The Goebell-Stoeckel sling procedure used in the fascia lata strap has been found to be the easiest and most dependable technique for treating difficult cases where other techniques have failed. In some specific cases it has been used as the primary surgical attempt.

In using the Goebell-Stoeckel sling procedure from 1947 to 1987, the fascia lata was used almost exclusively, except for a temporary trial in 17 cases using Mersilene and in three cases where the Aldridge modification was used. Altogether, 301 cases have been done by this operator or under his supervision. If the case had not been evaluated for at least 6 months postoperatively, it was not considered for evaluation of final results. Many cases have been followed for months or even years after the original procedure, and a remarkably few late failures have been encountered. No problem directly attributable to the use of the fascia lata, either in its procurement or in its placement of the sling, has ever been encountered. The overall success rate is 88%.

The postoperative care of the sling procedures is important. The patient is made to understand the nature of the procedure fully and is told that the chances of success are good but not perfect. She must also be aware that a catheter must be used postoperatively for a given time to retrain micturition. The urethral catheter is removed on the second postoperative day but the suprapubic tube remains in place as a "safety-valve" until it is no longer needed. This time may be as brief as 3 or 4 days, but in some cases reeducation of the bladder and the act of micturition may require that it be kept in place for as long as 3 or 4 weeks. Good rapport must be established and kept with the patient. In rare instances, where the patient is unable to void satisfactorily or is subject to intermittent retention for 6 or 8 weeks, the strap must be divided as described earlier in this chapter. Although there is a risk of reestablishing the incontinence, this is fortunately rare. In 16 cases in which the sling was inappropriately tight and was transected, 14 had satisfactory results; there were two failures.

The patient might have to learn to assume variable positions to void, such as leaning forward or even, in emergency, voiding directly into a warm Sitz bath.

Intraoperative and postoperative antibiotics or sulfonamides are used routinely and/or appropriately according to the preoperative culture reports.

In cases in which the bladder may have intermittent urgency or retention, the patient is taught self-catheterization. This can be safely done with an unbreakable plastic or metal catheter. Basic antisepsis is taught.

Bibliography

Abrams P, Blaivas JG, Stanton SL, et al. Standardization of terminology of lower urinary tract function. Neurourol Urodynam 1988; 7:403.

Abrams P, Feneley R, Torrens M. Urodynamics. New York: Springer-Verlag, 1983.

Aldridge AH. Transplantation of fascia for relief of urinary stress incontinence. Am J Obstet Gynecol 1942;44:398.

Allen RE, Warrell DW. The role of pregnancy and childbirth in partial denervation of the pelvic floor. Neurourol Urodynam 1987; 6:183.

Anderson RE. A neurogenic element to urinary genuine stress incontinence. Br J Obstet Gynaecol 1984;91:41.

Appell RA, Goodman JR, McGuire EJ, et al. Multicenter study of periurethral and transurethral GAX-collagen injection for urinary incontinence. Neurourol Urodynam 1989;8:339.

Asmussen M. Aspects of continence, incontinence and micturition in women based on simultaneous urethral cystometry. In: Ostergard DR, ed. Gynecologic urology and urodynamics—theory and practice. Baltimore: Williams & Wilkins, 1980.

Award SA, Bryniak S, Downie JW, et al. The treatment of the uninhibited bladder with dicyclomine. J Urol 1977;117:161.

Award SA, McGinnis RH. Factors that influence the incidence of detrusor instability in women. J Urol 1983;130:114.

Baden WF, Walker T. Anterior vaginal reparative failures: why? Female Patient 1986;11:35.

Ball TL. Anterior and posterior cystocele revisited; of some antifascialists and fascialists as I knew them. Clin Obstet Gynecol 1964; 9:1062.

Ball TL, Knapp RC, Nathanson B, et al. Stress incontinence. Am J Obstet Gynecol 1966;94:997.

Ball TL, Wright KL. Stress incontinence, complications and sequelae of the Marshall-Marchetti operation. Pacif Med Surg 1965;73:290.

Barker G, Glenning PP. Treatment of the unstable bladder with propantheline and imipramine. Aus NZ J Obstet Gynecol 1987; 27:152.

Barrett DM. Evaluation of psychogenic urinary retention. J Urol 1978;120:191.

Bates CP, Loose H, Stanton SLR. The objective study of incontinence after repair operations. Surg Gynecol Obstet 1973;136:17.

Bates CP, Whiteside CG, Turner-Warwick RT. Synchronous cine/pressure/flow cystourethrography with special reference to stress and urge incontinence. Br J Urol 1970;42:714.

Bates P, Bradley WE, Glen E, et al. The standardization of terminology of lower urinary tract function. J Urol 1979;121:551.

Beck RP. Anterior colporrhaphy with and without stress incontinence. In: Surgical profiles, a publication of Merck Sharpe and Dohme, a Division of Merck and Company, September 15, 1988.

Beck RP, Armsch D, King C. Results in treating 210 patients with detrusor overactivity incontinence of urine. Am J Obstet Gynecol 1976;125:593.

Beck RP, Hsu N. Pregnancy, childbirth and the menopause related to the development of stress incontinence. Am J Obstet Gynecol 1965;91:820.

Beck RP, Maughan GB. Simultaneous intraurethral and intravesical pressure studies in normal women and those with stress incontinence. Am J Obstet Gynecol 1964;89:746.

Beck RP, McCormick S. Treatment of stress urinary incontinence with anterior colporrhaphy. Obstet Gynecol 1982;59:269.

Beck RP, McCormick S, Nordstrom L. Intraurethral-intravesical cough pressure spike difference in 267 patients surgically cured of stress incontinence of urine. Obstet Gynecol 1988;72:302.

Beck RP, McCormick S, Nordstrom L. The fascia lata sling procedure for treating recurrent genuine stress incontinence of urine. Obstet Gynecol 1988;72.

Bent AE, Richarson DA, Ostergard DR. Diagnosis of lower urinary tract disorders in postmenopausal patients. Am J Obstet Gynecol 1983;145:218.

Benvenuti F, Caputo GM, Sandinelli S, et al. Re-educative treatment of female genuine stress incontinence. Am J Phys Med 1987;66:155.

Bergman A, Ballard CA, Koonings PP. Comparison of three different surgical procedures for genuine stress incontinence: prospective randomized study. Am J Obstet Gynecol 1989;160:1102.

Bergman A, Bhatia NN. Pessary test: a simple prognostic test in women with stress urinary incontinence. Urology 1985;24:109.

Bergman A, Koonings PP, Ballard CA. Predicting postoperative urinary incontinence development in women undergoing operations for genitourinary prolapse. Am J Obstet Gynecol 1988;158:1171.

Bergman A, Koonings PP, Ballard CA. Negative Q-tip test as a risk factor for failed incontinence surgery in women. J Reprod Med 1989;34:193.

Bergman A, Koonings PP, Ballard CA. Primary stress urinary incontinence and pelvic relaxation: prospective randomized comparison of three different operations. Am J Obstet Gynecol 1989; 161:97.

Bergman A, Koonings P, Ballard CA, Platt LD. Ultrasonic prediction of stress urinary incontinence development in surgery for severe pelvic relaxation. Gynecol Obstet Invest 1988;26:66.

Bergman A, Mathews L, Ballard CA, Roy S. Suprapubic versus transurethral bladder drainage after surgery for stress incontinence. Obstet Gynecol 1987;69:546.

Bergman A, McCarthy TA, Ballard CA, et al. Role of the Q-tip test in evaluating stress urinary incontinence. J Reprod Med 1987; 32:273.

Bhatia NN, Bergman A. Modified Burch versus Pereyra retropubic urethropexy for stress urinary incontinence. Obstet Gynecol 1985;66:255.

Bhatia NN, Bergman A. Pessary test in women with urinary incontinence. Obstet Gynecol 1985;65:220.

Bhatia NN, Bergman A. Use of preoperative uroflowmetry and simultaneous urethrocystometry for predicting risk of prolonged postoperative bladder drainage. Urology 1986;28:440.

Bhatia NN, Karram MM, Bergman A. Role of antibiotic prophylaxis in retropubic surgery for stress urinary incontinence. Obstet Gynecol 1989;74:637.

Bhatia NN, Ostergard DR. Urodynamic effects of retropubic urethropexy in genuine stress incontinence. Am J Obstet Gynecol 1981;140:936.

Blaivas JG. The neurophysiology of micturition: a clinical study of 550 patients. J Urol 1982;127:958.

Blaivas JG. Multichannel urodynamic studies. Urology 1984;23:421.

Blaivas JG, Labib KB, Michalik SJ, et al. Cystometric response to propantheline in detrusor hyperreflexia: therapeutic implications. J Urol 1980;124:259.

Bo K, Hagen R, Jorgensen J, et al. The effect of two different pelvic floor muscle exercise programs in treatment of urinary stress incontinence in women. Neurourol Urodynam 1989;8:355.

Bowen LW, Sand PK, Ostergard DR, Franti CE. Unsuccessful Burch retropubic urethropexy: a case controlled urodynamic study. Am J Obstet Gynecol 1989;160:452.

Brack CB, Guild HG. Urethral obstruction in the female child. Am J Obstet Gynecol 1958;76:1105.

Bradley DV, Cozart RJ. Relief of bladder spasm by flavoxate: a comparative study. J Clin Pharmacol 1970;10:65.

Bradley WE, Scott FB. Physiology of the urinary bladder. Campbell's Urol 1978;1:87.

Brown ADG. The urodynamic management of female urinary incontinence. M.D. Thesis, Edinburgh, 1974, cited by Turner-Warwick.

Bump RC, Copeland WE Jr, Hurt WG, et al. Dynamic urethral pressure/profilometry pressure transmission ratio determinations in stress-incontinent and stress-continent subjects. Am J Obstet Gynecol 1988;159:749.

Bump RC, Fantl AJ, Hurt GW. The mechanism of urinary continence in women with severe uterovaginal prolapse: results of barrier studies. Obstet Gynecol 1988;72:291.

Burch JC. Urethrovaginal fixation to Cooper's ligament for correction of stress incontinence, cystocele, and prolapse. Am J Obstet Gynecol 1961;81:281.

Burch JC. Cooper's ligament urethrovesical suspension for stress urinary incontinence. Am J Obstet Gynecol 1968;100:764.

Burgio KL, Robinson JC, Engel BT. The role of biofeedback in Kegel exercise training for stress urinary incontinence. Am J Obstet Gynecol 1986;154:58.

Cardozo L, Stanton SL. Genuine stress incontinence and detrusor instability: a review of 200 patients. Br J Obstet Gynaecol 1980; 87:184.

Cardozo LD, Stanton SL, Williams JE. Detrusor instability following surgery for genuine stress incontinence. Br J Urol 1979;51:204.

Carson CC III, Segura JW, Greene LF. Clinical importance of microhematuria. J Am Med Assoc 1979;241:149.

Cole AT, Fried FA. Favorable experiences with imipramine in the treatment of neurogenic bladder. J Urol 1972;107:44.

Collste L, Lindskog M. Phenylpropanolamine in treatment of female stress urinary incontinence. Urology 1987;30:398.

Cramer H. Fundamental and technical facts concerning Goebell's operation for urinary incontinence. Zbl Gynaek 1929;53:342.

DeLancey JOL. Correlative study of paraurethral anatomy. Obstet Gynecol 1986;68:91.

DeLancey JOL. Structural aspects of the extrinsic continence mechanism. Obstet Gynecol 1988;72:296.

DeLancey JOL. Pubovesical ligament: a separate structure from the urethral supports ("pubo-urethral ligaments"). Neurourol Urodynam 1989;8:53.

Deming CL. Transplantation of the gracilis muscle for incontinence of urine. JAMA 1926;86:822.

Diokno AC, Taub M. Ephedrine in treatment of urinary incontinence. Urology 1975;5:624.

Eastwood HDH. Postural influences on urinary incontinence in the elderly. Gerontology 1986;32:207.

Ek A, Alm P, Andersson KE, et al. Adrenoceptor and cholinoceptor mediated responses of the isolated human urethra. Scand J Urol Nephrol 1977;11:97.

Ek A, Andersson KE, Gullberg B, et al. The effects of long-term treatment with norephedrine on stress incontinence and urethral closure pressure profile. Scand J Urol Nephrol 1978; 12:105.

Enhorning G. Simultaneous recording of intraurethral and intravesical pressure: a study on urethral closure in stress incontinent women. Acta Chir Scand 1961;276(suppl):1.

Eriksen BC, Bergmann S, Mjolnerod OK. Effect of anal electrostimulation with the "Incontan" device in women with urinary incontinence. Br J Obstet Gynaecol 1987;94:147.

Everett H. In discussion of Burch JC Cooper's ligament urethrovesical suspension for stress incontinence. Am J Obstet Gynecol 1968; 100:764.

Everett HS. A condemnation of resectoscopic procedures upon the female vesicle neck. Urol Cutan Rev 1948;52:80.

Everett HS, Ridley J. Gynecological and obstetrical urology. Baltimore: Williams & Wilkins, 1947.

Fall M, Erlandson BE, Ahlstrom K, et al. Contelle: pelvic floor stimulator for female stress-urge incontinence. Urology 1986;27:282.

Fantl JA. Urinary incontinence due to detrusor instability. Clin Obstet Gynecol 1984;27:474.

Fantl JA, Hurt WG, Bump RC, et al. Urethral axis and sphincteric function. Am J Obstet Gynecol 1986;155:554.

Fantl JA, Hurt WG, Dunn LJ. Detrusor instability syndrome: the use of bladder retraining drills with and without anticholinergics. Am J Obstet Gynecol 1981;140:885.

Fantl JA, Wyman JF, Anderson RL, et al. Postmenopausal urinary incontinence: comparison between non-estrogen-supplemented and estrogen-supplemented women. Obstet Gynecol 1988;71:823.

Farrar DJ, Osborne JL, Stephenson TP, et al. A urodynamic view of bladder outflow obstruction in the female: factors influencing the results of treatment. Br J Urol 1975;47:815.

Finkbeiner AE, Bissada NK, Welch LT. Uropharmacology VI. Parasympathetic depressants. Urology 1977;10:503.

Fisher AM, Gordon H. The gynecologic approach to the patient with urological symptoms. Clin Obstet Gynecol 1981;8:191.

Folsom AL, O'Brien HA. The female urethra. JAMA 1945;128:408.

Forneret E, Leach GE. Cost-effective treatment of female stress urinary incontinence: modified Pereyra bladder neck suspension. Urology 1985;25:365.

Frangenheim P. Zur Operativen Behandlung der Ankontinenz der Mannlichen Harnrohre. Verh Dsch Ges Chirurgie, 43rd Congress, 1914:149.

Frazer MI, Haylen BT, Sutherst JR. The severity of urinary incontinence in women: comparison of subjective and objective tests. Br J Urol 1989;63:14.

Freeman RM, Malvern J, eds. The unstable bladder. London: Wright, 1989.

Frewen WK. An objective assessment of the unstable bladder of psychosomatic origin. Br J Urol 1978;50:246.

Frewen WK. The significance of the psychosomatic factor in urge incontinence. Br J Urol 1984;56:330.

Friedman EA, Meltzer RN. Collagen mesh prosthesis for repair of endopelvic fascial defect. Am J Obstet Gynecol 1970;106:430.

Ghoneim MA, Rottembourg JL, Fretin J, et al. Urethral pressure profile: standardization of technique and study of reproducibility. Urology 1975;5:763.

Gilja, Radej M, Kovacic M, et al. Conservative treatment of female stress incontinence with imipramine. J Urol 1984;122:909.

Gilpin SA, Gosling JA, Smith ARB, et al. The pathogenesis of genitourinary prolapse and stress incontinence of urine. A histological and histochemical study. Br J Obstet Gynaecol 1989;96:24.

Giordano D. Vingtième Congrès Français de Chirurgie 1907:506.

Gleason DM, Reilly RJ, Bottaccini MR, et al. The urethral continence zone and its relation to stress incontinence. J Urol 1974;112:81.

Goebell R. Zur Operativen Beseitigung der angeborenen Incontinentia vesicae. Z Gynäk Urol 1910;2:187.

Goldberg S. The four-minute neurologic exam. Miami: Medmaster, 1987.

Golin AL, Howard RS. Asymptomatic microscopic hematuria. J Urol 1989;124:389.

Goodno JA Jr, Powers TW. Modified retropubic cystourethropexy. Am J Obstet Gynecol 1986;154:1211.

Gordon D, Pearce M, Norton P, Stanton S. Comparison of ultrasound and lateral chain urethrocystography in the determination of bladder neck descent. Am J Obstet Gynecol 1989;160:182.

Gosling J. The structure of the bladder and urethra in relation to function. Urol Clin North Am 1979;6:31.

Gosling JA. Why are women continent? Proc R Coll Obstet Gynecol 1981;Feb 13.

Gosling JA, Dixon JS, Critchley HOD, et al. A comparative study of the human external sphincter and periurethral levator ani muscles. Br J Urol 1981;53:35.

Green T. Urinary stress incontinence: differential diagnosis, pathophysiology, and management. Am J Obstet Gynecol 1975;122:368.

Green TH Jr. Development of a plan for diagnosis and treatment of urinary stress incontinence. Am J Obstet Gynecol 1962;83:632.

Green TH Jr. The problem of urinary stress incontinence in the female. Obstet Gynecol Surv 1968;23:603.

Green TH Jr. Vaginal repair. In: Stanton SL, Tanagho EA, eds. Surgery of female incontinence. New York: Springer-Verlag, 1980.

Greenwald SW, Thornbury JR, Dunn LJ. Cystourethrography as a diagnostic aid in stress incontinence: an evaluation. Obstet Gynecol 1967;29:324.

Griffiths DJ. Urodynamics: the mechanics and hydrodynamics of the lower urinary tract. Bristol: Adam Hilger, 1980.

Growdon WA, Lebherz TB. The modified Pereyra procedure: use of local anesthesia. Obstet Gynecol 1986;68:272.

Growdon WA, Lebherz TB. The modified Pereyra procedure for stress urinary incontinence. In: Sanz LE, ed. Gynecologic surgery. Oradell, N.J.: Medical Economics Books, 1988:220.

Halban J. Gynakologische Operationslihre. Berlin: Urban and Schwarzenberg, 1932.

Hald T, Bradley WE. The urinary bladder: neurology and dynamics. Baltimore: Williams & Wilkins, 1982.

Haylen BT, Sutherst JR, Frazer MI. Is the investigation of most stress incontinence really necessary? Br J Urol 1989;64:147.

Hertogs K, Stanton SL. Mechanism of urinary continence after colposuspension: barrier studies. Br J Obstet Gynaecol 1985;92:1184.

Hilton P. A clinical and urodynamic assessment of the Burch colposuspension for genuine stress incontinence. Br J Obstet Gynaecol 1983;90:934.

Hilton P. Surgery for urinary stress incontinence. In: Monaghan JM, ed. Operative surgery: gynaecology and obstetrics. 4th ed. London: Butterworths, 1987:105.

Hilton P, Stanton SL. The use of intravaginal oestrogen cream in genuine stress incontinence. Br J Obstet Gynaecol 1983;90:940.

Hilton P, Stanton SL. Urethral pressure measurement by microtransducer: the results in symptom-free women and in those with genuine stress incontinence. Br J Obstet Gynaecol 1983;90:919.

Hodgkinson CP. Stress urinary incontinence. Am J Obstet Gynecol 1970;108:1141.

Hodgkinson CP. Recurrent stress urinary incontinence. In: Slate WG, ed. Disorders of the female urethra and urinary incontinence. 2nd ed. Baltimore: Williams & Wilkins, 1982:213.

Hodgkinson CP, Ayers MA, Drukker BH. Dyssynergic detrusor dysfunction in the apparently normal female. Am J Obstet Gynecol 1963;87:717.

Hodgkinson CP, Cobert N. Direct urethrocystometry. Am J Obstet Gynecol 1960;79:648.

Horbach N, Blanco J, Ostergard D, Bent A, Cornella J. A suburethral sling procedure with polytetrafluoroethylene for the treatment of genuine stress incontinence in patients with low urethral closure pressure.

Hurt G. Personal communication, 1989.

Hutch JA, Kao MS. Anatomy and physiology of the bladder, trigone and urethra. New York: Meredith, 1972.

Ingelman-Sundberg A. Urinary incontinence in women excluding fistulas. Acta Obstet Gynecol Scand 1951;31:266.

Ingelman-Sundberg A. Stress incontinence of urine. J Obstet Gynaecol Br Emp 1952;59:699.

Iosif CS. Sling operation for urinary incontinence. Acta Obstet Gynecol Scand 1985;64:187.

Jarvis GJ, Hall S, Stamp S, et al. An assessment of urodynamic examination in incontinent women. Br J Obstet Gynecol 1980;87:893.

Jeffcoate TNA, Francis WJA. Urgency incontinence in the female. Am J Obstet Gynecol 1966;94:604.

Jonasson A, Larsson B, Pschera H. Testing and training of the pelvic floor muscles after childbirth. Acta Obstet Gynecol Scand 1989;68:301.

Jorgensen L, Lose G, Andersen JT. Cystometry: H_2O or CO_2 as filling medium? A literature survey of the influence of the filling medium on the qualitative and quantitative cystometric parameters. Neurourol Urodynam 1988;7:343.

Jorgensen L, Lose G, Molsted-Pedersen L. Vaginal repair in female motor urge incontinence. Eur Urol 1987;13:382.

Jorgensen L, Lose G, Mortensen SO, et al. The Burch colposuspension for urinary incontinence in patients with stable and unstable detrusor function. Neurourol Urodynam 1988;7:435.

Kadar N, Nelson JH Jr. Sling operation for total incontinence following radical vulvectomy. Obstet Gynecol 1984;64:85SS.

Kadar N, Nelson JH Jr. Treatment of urinary incontinence after radical hysterectomy. Obstet Gynecol 1984;64:400.

Karram MM, Bhatia NN. Management of coexistent stress and urge urinary incontinence. Obstet Gynecol 1989;73:4.

Kaufman J. Operative management of stress urinary incontinence. J Urol 1981;126:465.

Kegel AH. Progressive resistance exercise in the functional restoration of the perineal muscles. Am J Obstet Gynecol 1948;56:238.

Kegel AH. Physiologic therapy for urinary stress incontinence. JAMA 1951;146:915.

Kegel AH. Exercise in the treatment of genital relaxation, urinary stress incontinence and sexual dysfunction. In: Greenhill JP, ed. Office gynecology. 9th ed. Chicago: Year Book Medical Publishers, 1971.

Kegel AH, Powell TH. The physiologic treatment of stress incontinence. J Urol 1950;63:808.

Kelly HA. Operative gynecology. New York: Appleton, 1909.

Kelly HA. Incontinence of urine in women. Urol Cutan Rev 1913;17:291.

Kelly HA. History of redisplacement of the uterus. Surg Gynecol Obset 1915;20:598.

Kelly HA, Dumm WM. Urinary incontinence in women without manifest injury to the bladder. Surg Gynecol Obstet 1914;18:444.

Kennedy C. Stress incontinence of urine: a survey of 34 cases treated by the Milin/Sling operation. Br J Med J 1960;2:263.

Kennedy WT. Incontinence of urine in the female: some functional observations of the urethra illustrated by roentgenograms. Am J Obstet Gynecol 1937;33:19.

Kersey J, Martin MR, Mishra P. A further assessment of the gauze hammock sling operation in the treatment of stress incontinence. Br J Obstet Gynaecol 1988;95(April):382.

Kitzmiller JL, Manzer GA, Nebel WA, et al. Chain cystourethrogram for stress incontinence. Obstet Gynecol 1972;39:333.

Langer R, Ron-El R, Neuman M, et al. The value of simultaneous hysterectomy during Burch colposuspension for urinary stress incontinence. Obstet Gynecol 1988;72:866.

Langmade C, Oliver J Jr. Simplifying the management of stress urinary incontinence. Am J Obstet Gynecol 1984;149:25.

Leach GE, Bavendam TG. Prospective evaluation of the Incontan transrectal stimulator in women with urinary incontinence. Neurourol Urodynam 1989;8:231.

Leach GE, Raz S. Modified Pereyra bladder neck suspension after previously failed anti-incontinence surgery. Urology 1984; 23:359.

Lee LW, Davis Ed Jr. Gross urinary hemorrhage: a symptom, not a diagnosis. JAMA 1953;153:782.

Lee RA, Symmonds RE, Goldstein RA. Surgical complications and results of modified Marshall-Marchetti-Krantz procedure for urinary incontinence. Obstet Gynecol 1979;53:447.

Leight JK, Scott FB. Management of urinary incontinence in women with the artificial urinary sphincter. J Urol 1985;134:476.

Lindstrom S, Fall M, Carlsson CA, et al. The neurophysiological basis of bladder inhibition in response to intravaginal electrical stimulation. J Urol 1983;129:405.

Lockhart JL, Vorstman B, Politano VA. Anti-incontinence surgery in females with detrusor instability. Neurourol Urodynam 1984; 3:201.

Lose G, Diernaes E, Rix P. Does medical therapy cure female stress incontinence? Urol Int 1989;44:25.

Lose G, Jorgensen L, Johnsen A. Predictive value of detrusor instability in surgery for female urinary incontinence. Neurourol Urodynam 1988;7:141.

Lose G, Jorgensen L, Thunedborg P. Doxepin in the treatment of female detrusor overactivity: a randomized double-blind crossover study. J Urol 1989;142:1024.

Low JA. Management of anatomic urinary incontinence by vaginal repair. Am J Obstet Gynecol 1967;97:308.

Low JA. Management of severe anatomic deficiencies of urethral sphincter function by a combined procedure with a fascia lata sling. Am J Obstet Gynecol 1969;105:149.

Low JA. Patterns of urethral resistance in deficient urethral sphincter functions. Obstet Gynecol 1972;40:634.

Low JA, Kao MS. Intravesical and intraurethral pressure as a measure of urethral sphincter function. Obstet Gynecol 1972;40:627.

Malizia AA, Reiman HM, Myers RP, et al. Migration and granulomatous reaction after periurethral injection of polytef (teflon). JAMA 1984;251:3277.

Marchant DJ. Clinical evaluation of urinary incontinence, normal anatomy and pathophysiology. Clin Obstet Gynecol 1984;27:434.

Marchetti A, Marshall V, O'Leary J. Suprapubic vesicourethral suspension and urinary stress incontinence. Clin Obstet Gynecol 1963;6:195.

Markell R. Urine microscopy and culture in the selection of patients for urinary tract investigation. Br J Urol 1989;63:7.

Marshall VF, Marchetti AA, Krantz KE. The correction of stress incontinence by simple vesicourethral suspension. Surg Gynecol Obstet 1949;88:509.

Massey JA, Abrams P. Obstructed voiding in the female. Br J Urol 1988;61:36.

Mattingly RF, Davis LE. Primary treatment of anatomic stress urinary incontinence. Clin Obstet Gynecol 1984;27:445.

McGuire EJ. Bladder instability and stress incontinence. Neurourol Urodynam 1988;7:563.

McGuire EJ, Lytton B. Pubovaginal sling procedure for stress incontinence. J Urol 1978;119:82.

McGuire EJ, Lytton B, Kohorn EI, et al. Stress urinary incontinence. Obstet Gynecol 1976;47:225.

McGuire EJ, Lytton B, Kohorn E, et al. The value of urodynamic testing in stress urinary incontinence. J Urol 1980;124:256.

McGuire EJ, Lytton B, Pepe V, et al. Stress urinary incontinence. Obstet Gynecol 1976;47:255.

McGuire EJ, Wang CC, Vsitalo H, et al. Modified pubovaginal sling in girls with myelodysplasia. J Urol 1986;130:94.

Meyhoff HH, deNully MB, Olesen KP, et al. The effects of vaginal repair on anterior bladder suspension defects. A radiological and clinical evaluation. Acta Obstet Gynecol Scand 1985;64:433.

Milani R, Scalambrino S, Qadri G, et al. Marshall-Marchetti-Krantz procedure and Burch colposuspension in the surgical treatment of female urinary incontinence. Br J Obstet Gynaecol 1985; 92:1050.

Miller NF. Surgical treatment of urinary incontinence in the female. JAMA 1932;98:628.

Mitleman RE, Marraccini JV. Pulmonary Teflon granulomas following periurethral Teflon injection for urinary incontinence. Arch Pathol Lab Med 1983;107:611.

Moir JC. The gauze-hammock operation. J Obstet Gynaecol Br Commonw 1968;75:1.

Moisey CV, Stephenson TP, Brendler CB. The urodynamic and subjective results of treatment of detrusor instability with oxybutynin chloride. Br J Urol 1980;52:472.

Montz FJ, Stanton SL. Q-tip test in female urinary incontinence. Obstet Gynecol 1986;67:258.

Moore J, Armstrong JT, Will SH. The use of tantalum mesh in cystocele with critical report of ten cases. Am J Obstet Gynecol 1955; 69:1127.

Moschcowitz AV. The pathogenesis, anatomy and cure of prolapse of the rectum. Surg Gynecol Obstet 1912;15:7.

Muellner SR. The voluntary control of micturition in man. J Urol 1958;80:473.

Mundy AR. A trial comparing the Stamey bladder neck suspension procedure with colposuspension for the treatment of stress incontinence. Br J Urol 1983;55:687.

Mundy AR, Stephenson TP. Selection of patients for implantation of the Brantley Scott artificial urinary sphincter. Br J Urol 1984;56:717.

Mundy AR, Stephenson TP, Wein AJ, eds. Urodynamics: principles, practice, and applications. New York: Churchill Livingstone, 1984.

Muzsnai D, Carrillo E, Dubin C, et al. Retropubic vaginoplasty for correction of urinary stress incontinence. Obstet Gynecol 1982 ;59:113.

Neill ME, Swash M. Increased motor unit fibre density in the external anal sphincter muscle in anorectal incontinence: a single fibre EMG study. J Neurol Neurosurg Psychiatr 1980;43:343.

Nemir A, Middleton RP. Stress incontinence in young nulliparous women: a statistical study. Am J Obstet Gynecol 1954;68:1166.

Nichols DH. The Mersilene mesh gauze-hammock in repair of severe recurrent urinary stress incontinence. In: Taymor Ml, Green TH, eds. Progress in gynecology. Vol. 6. New York: Grune and Stratton, 1975.

Nichols DH. Vaginal prolapse affecting bladder function. Clin Obstet Gynecol 1985;12:449.

Nichols DH, Ponchak SF. Treating incontinence transvaginally. Contemp Obstet Gynecol 1986; (special issue: Update on surgery): 109.

Nichols DH, Randall CL. Vaginal surgery. Ch. 11. 3rd ed. Baltimore: Williams & Wilkins, 1989.

Nordling J, Meyhoff HH, Andersson JT, et al. Urinary incontinence in the female: the value of detrusor reflex activation procedures. Br J Urol 1979;51:110.

Norton PA, MacDonald LD, Sedgwick PM, et al. Distress and delay associated with urinary incontinence, frequency, and urgency in women. Br Med J 1988;297:1187.

Nurse DE, Mundy AR. One hundred artificial sphincters. Br J Urol 1988;61:318.

Nygaard I, DeLancey JOL, Arnsdorf L, et al. Exercise and incontinence. Obstet Gynecol 1990;75:848.

Olah KS, Bridges N, Denning J, Farrar DJ. The conservative management of patients with symptoms of stress incontinence: a randomized, prospective study comparing weighted vaginal cones and interferential therapy. Am J Obstet Gynecol 1990;162:87.

Ostergard DR. Gynecologic urology and urodynamics. Baltimore: Williams & Wilkins, 1980.

Park GS, Miller EJ. Surgical treatment of stress urinary incontinence: a comparison of the Kelly plication, Marshall-Marchetti-Krantz, and Pereyra procedure. Obstet Gynecol 1988;Ave71:575.

Parker RT, Ridley JH. Fascia lata urethrovesical suspension for stress urinary incontinence. Perspect Surg 1978;1(4):1.

Parnell JP, Marshall VM, Vaughn ED. Primary management of urinary stress incontinence by the Marshall-Marchetti-Krantz vesicourethropexy. J Urol 1982;127:679.

Peattie AB, Plevnik S, Stanton SL. Vaginal cones: a conservative method of treating genuine stress incontinence. Br J Obstet Gynaecol 1988;95:1049.

Penttinen J, Kaar K, Kauppila A. Colposuspension and transvaginal bladder neck suspension in the treatment of stress incontinence. Gynecol Obstet Invest 1989;28:101.

Penttinen J, Lindholm E.-L, Kaar K, Kauppila A. Successful colposuspension in stress urinary incontinence reduces bladder neck mobility and increases pressure transmission to the urethra. Acta Gynecol Obstet 1989;244:233.

Pereyra AJ. A simplified procedure for the correction of stress incontinence in women. West J Surg Obstet Gynecol 1959;67:223.

Pereyra AJ, Lebherz TB. Combined urethrovesical suspension and vaginourethroplasty for correction of urinary stress incontinence. Obstet Gynecol 1967;30:537.

Pereyra AJ, Lebherz TB. The modified Pereyra procedure. In: Buchsbaum HJ, Schmidt JD, eds. Gynecologic and obstetric urology. 2nd ed. Philadelphia: WB Saunders, 1982:259.

Pereyra AJ, Lebherz TB, Growdon WA, et al. Pubourethral supports in perspective: modified Pereyra procedure for urinary incontinence. Obstet Gynecol 1982;59:643.

Peters WA, Thornton WN. Selection of the primary operative procedure for stress urinary incontinence. Am J Obstet Gynecol 1980;137:923.

Politano VA. Periurethral polytetrafluoroethylene injections for urinary incontinence. J Urol 1982;127:439.

Preminger GM, Steinhardt GF, M al. Urinary incontinence in adults—National Institutes of Health Consensus Development Conference. JAMA 1989;261:2685.

Reed T, Anderson KE, Asmussen M, et al. Factors maintaining the intraurethral pressure in women. Invest Urol 1980;17:343.

Resnick NM. Voiding dysfunction in the elderly. In: Yalla SV, McGuire EJ, Elbadawi A, et al, eds. Neurourology and urodynamics: principles and practice. New York: Macmillan, 1988:303.

Richardson AC, Edmonds PB, Williams N. Treatment of stress urinary incontinence due to paravaginal fascial defect. Obstet Gynecol 1981;57:357.

Richardson DA, Bent AE, Ostergard DR. The effect of uterovaginal prolapse on urethral pressure dynamics. Am J Obstet Gynecol 1983;146:901.

Richelson E. Antimuscarinic and other receptor-blocking properties of antidepressants. Mayo Clin Proc 1983;58:40.

Ridley JH. Indirect air cystoscopy. South Med J 1951;44:114.

Ridley JH. Appraisal of the Goebell-Frangenheim-Stoeckel sling procedure. Am J Obstet Gynecol 1966;95:714.

Ridley JH. Gynecologic surgery: errors, safeguards and salvage. Baltimore: Williams & Wilkins, 1974.

Riggs JA. Retropubic cystourethropexy: a review of two operative procedures with long-term follow-up. Obstet Gynecol 1986; 68:98.

Roberts JA, Angel JR, McClung T, et al. Modified Pereyra procedure for stress incontinence. J Urol 1981;125:787.

Robertson JR. Endoscopic evaluation of the urethra and bladder. Clin Obstet Gynecol J 1983;26:347.

Rowe JW, Besdine RW, Ford AB, et al. Urinary incontinence in adults—National Institutes of Health Consensus Development Conference. JAMA 1989;261:2685.

Rud T, Andersson KE, Asmussen M, et al. Factors maintaining the intraurethral pressure in women. Invest Urol 1980;17:343.

Rydhstrom H, Isoif CS. Urodynamic studies before and after retropubic colpourethrocystopexy in fertile women with stress urinary incontinence. Arch Gynecol Obstet 1988;241:201.

Sand PK, Bowen LW, Ostergard DR, Nakanishi AM. Hysterectomy and prior incontinence surgery as risk factors for failed retropubic cystourethropexy. J Reprod Med 1988;33:171.

Schonauer S. Correction of stress incontinence in women by simple sling operation. Urology 1988;32:189.

Schreiter F, Fuchs P, Stockamp K. Estrogenic sensitivity of alpha-receptors in the urethral musculature. Urol Int 1976;31:13.

Scott FB. The artificial urinary sphincter: review and progress. Med Instrum 1988;22:174.

Selim MA, Vasquez HH. Modified Marshall-Marchetti-Krantz procedure. J Reprod Med 1979;22:271.

Shortliffe LMD, Freiha FS, Kessler R, et al. Treatment of urinary incontinence by the periurethral implantation of glutaraldehyde cross-linked collagen. J Urol 1989;141:538.

Smith ARB, Hosker GL, Warrell DW. The role of partial denervation of the pelvic floor in the aetiology of genitourinary prolapse and stress incontinence of urine. A neurophysiological study. Br J Obstet Gynaecol 1989;96:24.

Smith ARB, Hosker GL, Warrell DW. The role of pudendal nerve damage in the aetiology of genuine stress incontinence in women. Br J Obstet Gynaecol 1989;96:29.

Snooks SJ, Badenock DF, Tiptaft RC, et al. Perineal nerve damage in genuine stress urinary incontinence. An electrophysiological study. Br J Urol 1985;57:422.

Snooks SJ, Swash M. Abnormalities of the innervation of the urethral striated sphincter musculature in incontinence. Br J Urol 1984;56:401.

Snooks SJ, Swash M, Setchill M, et al. Injury to innervation of pelvic floor musculature in childbirth. Lancet 1984;2:546.

Sonda LP, Kogan BA, Koff S. Neurologic disease masquerading as genitourinary abnormality—the role of urodynamics in diagnosis. J Urol 1983;129:1175.

Stamey, TA. Endoscopic suspension of the vesical neck for urinary incontinence in females: report on 203 consecutive patients. Ann Surg 1980;192:465.

Stanton SL. Surgery of urinary incontinence. Clin Obstet Gynaecol 1979;5:83.

Stanton SL, Cardozo LD. A comparison of vaginal and suprapubic surgery in the correction of incontinence due to urethral correction of incompetence. Br J Urol 1979;51:497.

Stanton SL, Cardozo LD. Results of colposuspension operation for incontinence and prolapse. Br J Obstet Gynaecol 1979;86:693.

Stanton SL, Cardozo LD, Chaudhury N. Spontaneous voiding after surgery for urinary incontinence. Br J Obstet Gynaecol 1978;85:149.

Stanton SL, Cardozo L, Williams JE, et al. Clinical and urodynamic features of failed incontinence surgery in the female. Obstet Gynecol 1978;51:515.

Stanton SL, Norton C, Cardozo L. Clinical and urodynamic effects of anterior colporrhaphy and vaginal hysterectomy for prolapse with and without incontinence. Br J Obstet Gynaecol 1982; 89:459.

Stanton SL, Williams JE, Ritchie D. The colposuspension operation for urinary incontinence. Br J Obstet Gynecol 1976;83:890.

Steel SA, Cox C, Stanton SL. Long term follow-up of detrusor instability following colposuspension operation. Br J Urol 1986; 58:138.

Stoeckel W. Uber die Verwendung der Muculi Pyramidales bei der operativen Behandlung der Incontinentia urinae. Zbl Gynäk 1917;41:11.

Studdiford WE. The problem of stress incontinence and its surgical relief. Surg Obstet Gynecol 1946;83:742.

Swash M, Snooks SJ, Henry MM. Unifying concept of pelvic floor disorders and incontinence. J R Soc Med 1985;78:906.

Symmonds RE. Loss of urethral floor with total urinary incontinence. Am J Obstet Gynecol 1969;103:665.

Tanagho EA. Vesicourethral dynamics. In: Urodynamics. Berlin: Springer-Verlag, 1973.

Tanagho EA. Colpocystourethropexy: the way we do it. J Urol 1976; 116:751.

Tanagho EA. Effects of hysterectomy and paraurethral surgery on urethrovesical function. In: Ostergard DR, ed. Gynecologic urology and urodynamics. Baltimore: Williams & Wilkins, 1980:293.

Tapp A, Fall M, Norgaard J, et al. Terodiline: a dose-titrated, multicenter study of the treatment of idiopathic detrusor instability in women. J Urol 1989;142:1027.

Tchou DCH, Adams C, Varner RE, Benton B. Pelvic floor musculature exercises in treatment of anatomical urinary stress incontinence. Phys Ther 1988;68:652.

Teague C, Merrill DC. Electric pelvic floor stimulation: mechanism of action. Invest Urol 1977;15:65.

Thiede HA. Urogynecology: comments and caveats. Am J Obstet Gynecol 1987;157:536.

Torrens MJ. Neurophysiology. In: Stanton SL, ed. Clinical gynecologic urology. St Louis: CV Mosby, 1984:13.

Torrens MJ, Morrison JFB, eds. The physiology of the lower urinary tract. New York: Springer-Verlag, 1987.

Turner-Warwick R. Observations on the function and dysfunctions of the sphincter and detrusor mechanisms. Urol Clin North Am 1979;6(1):11.

Ulmsten U, Ekman G, Andersson KE. The effect of terodiline treatment in women with motor urge incontinence. Results from a double-blind study and long-term treatment. Am J Obstet Gynecol 1985;153:619.

Ulmsten U, Henriksson L, Iosif S. The unstable female urethra. Am J Obstet Gynecol 1982;144:93.

Van Geelen JM, Theeuwes AGM, Eskes TKAB, Martin CB. The clinical and urodynamic effects of anterior vaginal repair and Burch colposuspension. Am J Obstet Gynecol 1988;159:137.

Van Rooyen AJL, Liebenberg HC. A clinical approach to urinary incontinence in the female. Obstet Gynecol 1978;53:1.

Versi E. Discriminant analysis of urethral pressure profilometry data for the diagnosis of genuine stress incontinence. Br J Urol 1990;97:251.

Wall LL. The diagnosis and management of urinary incontinence due to detrusor instability. Obstet Gynecol Surv 1990(Suppl.);45:15.

Wall LL, Addison WA. Basic cystometry in gynecologic practice. Postgrad Obstet Gynecol 1988;8(26):1.

Wall LL, Addison WA. Prazosin-induced stress incontinence. Obstet Gynecol 1990;75:558.

Wall LL, Warrell DW. Detrusor instability associated with menstruation—case report. Br J Obstet Gynaecol 1989;96:737.

Walter S. Detrusor hyperreflexia in female urinary incontinence treated pharmacologically. Urol Int 1978;33:316.

Walter S, Olesen KD. Urinary incontinence and genital prolapse in the female: clinical, urodynamic and radiologic examinations. Br J Gynecol Obstet 1982;89:393.

Walters MD, Shields LE. The diagnostic value of history, physical examination, and the Q-tip cotton swab test in women with urinary incontinence. Am J Obstet Gynecol 1988;159:145.

Webster GD, Older RA. The value of subtracted bladder pressure measurements in routine urodynamic studies. Urology 1980; 16:656.

Webster GD, Sihelnik SA. Troubleshooting the malfunctioning Scott artificial urinary sphincter. J Urol 1984;131:269.

Webster GD, Sihelnik SA, Stone AR. Female urinary incontinence: the incidence, identification and characteristics of detrusor instability. Neurourol Urodynam 1984;3:235.

Weil A, Reyes H, Bischoff P, et al. Modifications of the urethral rest and stress profiles after different types of surgery for urinary stress incontinence. Br J Obstet Gynaecol 1984;91:46.

Wharton LR, Jr, Te Linde RW. An evaluation of fascial sling operation for urinary incontinence in female patients. J Urol 1959;82:76.

Williams TJ. Urinary incontinence in the female. Med Clin North Am 1974;58:729.

Williams TJ, Te Linde RW. The sling operation for urinary incontinence using Mersilene ribbon. Obstet Gynecol 1962;19:241.

Wolin LH. Stress incontinence in young, healthy nulliparous female subjects. J Urol 1969;101:545.

Woodside JR. Pubovaginal sling procedure for the management of urinary incontinence after urethral trauma in women. J Urol 1987;138:527.

Yalla SV, McGuire EJ, Elbadawi A, et al, eds. Neurourology and urodynamics: principles and practice. New York: Macmillan, 1988.

Yarnell JWG, Voyle GJ, Richards CJ, et al. The prevalence and severity of urinary incontinence in women. J Epidemiol Community Health 1981;35:71.

Zacharin RF. The suspensory mechanism of the female urethra. J Anat 1963;97:423.

Zacharin RF. Stress incontinence of urine. New York: Harper & Row, 1972.

Zacharin RF. Abdominal urethral suspension in the management of recurrent stress incontinence of urine: a 15-year experience. Obstet Gynecol 1983;62:644.

Zeegers AGM, Kieswetter H, Kramer AEJL, et al. Conservative therapy of frequency, urgency, and urge incontinence: a double-blind clinical trial of flavoxate hydrochloride, oxybutynin chloride, emepronium bromide, and placebo. World J Urol 1987;5:57.

34

Relaxed Vaginal Outlet, Rectocele, Fecal Incontinence, and Rectovaginal Fistula

JOHN D. THOMPSON

ANATOMY OF THE POSTERIOR VAGINAL WALL AND PERINEUM

The pelvic floor is formed chiefly by the levator ani muscles or crura, which create a broad muscular diaphragm, aided posteriorly by the coccygeus muscles (see Chapter 4). The levator ani consists of three distinct muscles: the iliococcygeus, the pubococcygeus, and the puborectalis. The iliococcygeal muscles arise from the posterior portion of the arcus tendineus and the ischial spine and insert along the lateral margin of the coccyx and lower sacral vertebrae, with a few fibers inserting into the levator plate. The pubococcygeus originates from the inner aspect of the pubic bone and the proximal portion of the arcus tendineus or white fascial line. The puborectalis muscle arises from the posterior portion of the pubic bone and the inferior ramus of the pubis.

The medial portion of the levator musculature is formed by the pubococcygeus, the largest of the three muscles. The muscle passes along each side of the levator or genital hiatus, near the urethra, vagina, and rectum. The fibers from both sides interdigitate between the rectum and the coccyx to form a median raphe, the levator plate. When this muscular portion of the pelvic diaphragm is contracted, it forms a horizontal plane supporting the rectum, vagina, and urethra.

The puborectalis lies beneath the point of origin of the pubococcygeus and the neighboring obturator fascia and deep fascia. It lies along the lateral aspect of the urethra, vagina, and rectum, inferior to the pubococcygeus. The U-shaped puborectalis muscle encircles the posterior aspect of the rectum, then returns along the opposite side of the levator hiatus to the posterior surface of the pubis. Besides providing support to the pelvic floor, vagina, and bladder neck, the puborectalis muscle also serves as a sling holding the rectum forward and providing continence control to the terminal colon.

Along with the pubococcygeus, the puborectalis muscle affixes firmly to the vagina and to the midportion of the urethra to provide support. Fibers from both the pubococcygeus and the puborectalis muscles send decussations to attach to the perineal body.

This pelvic diaphragm, then, is composed mainly of the pubococcygeus and coccygeus muscles, reinforced inferiorly by the puborectalis. The levator muscles contract in response to intra-abdominal pressure; the pelvic diaphragm acts as a trampoline to prevent descent of the intra-abdominal viscera. The musculature is penetrated by the urethra, vagina, and rectum, which form a central hiatus in the pelvic floor, weakening the muscular support to the pelvis.

The weakest external portion of the pelvic floor receives additional support from the urogenital diaphragm (Fig. 34-1). The musculofascial diaphragm, also known as the triangular ligament, is composed of two layers of fascia, deep and superficial. The fascial layers surround a number of supporting skeletal muscles lying within the triangular area formed by the ischial tuberosities and the inferior rami of the symphysis pubis. Within the deep fascial layer are fat, loose connective tissue, and thin, deep transverse perinei muscles.

Within the superficial layer lie the superficial transverse perinei muscles and the ischiocavernosus and bulbocavernosus muscles.

The superficial transverse perineal muscles arise from each ischial tuberosity and insert into the midline of the perineum, posterior to the vaginal introitus. The bulbocavernosus muscles arise from the midline of the perineal body, pass over the vestibular bulb and Bartholin's gland along each side of the vagina, and insert into the inferior crus of the clitoris.

The vaginal canal creates a central defect between the medial aspect of the levator muscles, and it separates the muscles of the urogenital diaphragm into

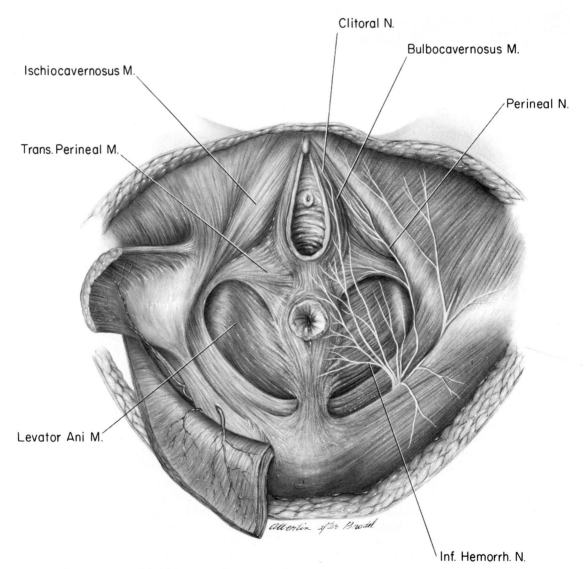

Figure 34–1. Urogenital diaphragm in relation to the levator ani muscles of the pelvic floor in the female.

pairs. The bulbocavernosus muscles may be considered as the superficial vaginal constrictors; the levator muscles are the deep constrictors. All the urogenital muscles are covered with fascia, which is visible during dissection in a perineal repair.

The vagina is a musculomembranous, tubal structure extending from the cervix to the vulva. The outer orifice, the introitus, has the smallest caliber; above this, the vagina is relatively roomy. The vaginal canal, which is approximately 8.5 cm long in the nulliparous patient, is covered with stratified squamous epithelium. The epithelial lining is quite thin before puberty and after the menopause and is referred to, erroneously, as a mucous membrane, because it is lubricated with mucus from the cervix and has a moist surface. During the menstrual life of a woman, the epithelial lining is much thicker and is thrown up into transverse folds, or rugae.

Beneath the epithelium of the vagina are two layers of smooth muscle, an outer longitudinal and an inner circular, that are surrounded externally by the perivaginal portion of the endopelvic fascia. The fascia extends from the symphysis pubis, passes beneath the bladder, and is inserted in the anterior surface of the cervix at the level of the internal os. The endopelvic fascia is the same pubovesicocervical fascia utilized in a cystocele repair. A posterior extension of the endopelvic fascia between the rectum and vagina is utilized in a rectocele repair, although it is more attenuated and less sturdy than the anterior fascia.

The upper posterior 2–3 cm of the vagina lie in close proximity to the cul-de-sac of Douglas. Studies by Kuhn and Hollyock demonstrated that the base of the cul-de-sac pouch could be extended with a probe to the junction of the upper and middle third of the vagina in 93% of the patients studied. The depth of the cul-de-sac measured more than 5 cm from the lower uterine segment to the upper third of the posterior vagina, where it separated the rectum from the vagina. If the peritoneal sac extends deeper into the rectovaginal space, it forms a peritoneal pouch, or enterocele, within which the small bowel may push against the upper posterior vaginal wall.

Below the level of the cul-de-sac, the fused peritoneal layers form the fascia of Denonvillier. The vagina is separated from the rectal wall by an attenuated layer of endopelvic fascia, which forms the rectovaginal septum. At this point, weakening of the levator muscle attachment may occur, making the middle one third of the posterior vaginal wall the most susceptible to rectocele formation should the rectum descend through the widened levator hiatus.

At the lower end of the vaginal canal, the rectum diverges posteriorly because of the interdigitating muscles of the external anal sphincter and the perineal body. The perineum is formed by the union of the levator ani muscles with the bulbocavernosus and superficial transverse perinei muscles. The lowermost portion of the rectum constitutes the anal canal, which is 2–3 cm long. The anal canal is supported in three ways: by the external, striated sphincter muscles, including the puborectalis; by both the superficial and the deep transverse perineal muscles; and by the inferior margins of the bulbocavernosus muscles.

When the musculofascial support between the rectum and vagina weakens (including the decussating fibers of the puborectalis and pubococcygeus muscles), the cul-de-sac of Douglas deepens, and widening of the levator hiatus permits both rectocele and enterocele formation (Fig. 34-2). Inadequate innervation and congenital weakness of the perineal muscle plus lacerations of the fascia of the rectovaginal septum (the "fascia" of Denonvillier) may also be important. One of the principal mechanisms of stretching, weakening, and often tearing of the fascia and muscles of the pelvic floor is trauma from the descent of the infant's head through the pelvic diaphragm. Prolonged pressure of the child's head between the muscles of the pelvic floor, particularly during a prolonged second stage of labor, weakens the rectovaginal and vesicovaginal septa. Strenuous work, straining at stool, multiple pregnancies, aging, and the orthostatic pressure of the pelvic viscera against the pelvic floor are other factors that may produce weakening of the musculofascial support, eventually causing rectocele and enterocele formation.

If an episiotomy or perineal laceration is not adequately repaired, the posterior part of the urogenital diaphragm, including the superficial transverse perinei and bulbocavernosus muscles, remains separated. Separation of the perineal attachment of the levator muscles produces a widening of the hiatus in the pelvic diaphragm and an elongation of the puborectalis sling that holds the rectum forward at the rectal neck. Since the puborectalis also serves as one of the voluntary (striated) muscles of the anal sphincter, weakening of the puborectalis muscle may cause subsequent anal incontinence.

Trauma to the perineal body may be either complete, extending through the underlying, multilayered anal sphincter and producing varying degrees of anal incontinence, or partial, in which case the damaged perineum may retain only a thin layer of weak connective tissue and muscle fibers. If the perineal tear extends through the rectovaginal septum and rectal mucosa, it is defined as a fourth-degree vaginal laceration.

When the levator ani muscles are seriously weakened and the levator hiatus is widened, shortening and posterior deflection of the levator plate (see Fig. 31-5) may cause the cul-de-sac of Douglas to deepen and permit the development of an enterocele between the rectum and the posterior vaginal wall. In severe cases, the

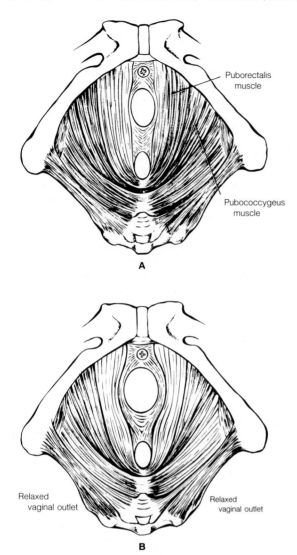

Figure 34–2. *A*, Perineal view of levator ani, showing the central hiatus in pelvic floor produced by penetration of urethra, vagina, and rectum. Note the decussations of levator fibers that pass between the rectum and vagina and support the hiatus. *B*, Schematic illustration of a widened levator hiatus, showing separation of decussating fibers of the levator ani from the perineal body and the margins of the pelvic portal and shortening of the levator plate between the rectum and coccyx.

enterocele may extend along the entire length of the rectovaginal septum between the vagina and the anterior rectal wall. With the passage of time, all physical activity that increases intra-abdominal pressure will contribute to the development of an enterocele by causing the peritoneal sac to dissect deeper into the area between the rectum and the vagina, where the fascia is anatomically thin and separates easily (see Fig. 31-7).

RELAXED VAGINAL OUTLET WITH RECTOCELE

Although the terms *relaxed vaginal outlet* and *rectocele* are frequently used synonymously, each condition represents a separate anatomic entity. The conditions usually occur together in patients with significant pelvic floor relaxation but may occur separately. Both a relaxed vaginal outlet and a rectocele may be entirely asymptomatic, requiring no treatment.

Simple relaxation of the vaginal outlet due to thinning and separation of the muscles of the perineal body is more often asymptomatic than is a rectocele. A relaxed outlet is often a contributing factor when increasing pelvic pressure is associated with uterine descensus. If either the relaxed outlet or uterine descensus requires surgical repair, both should be corrected. If a relaxed outlet exists with a symptomatic cystocele, with or without rectocele, the entire posterior vaginal wall and the perineum should be repaired along with the cystocele if it can be done without constricting the vaginal caliber to the point of producing dyspareunia. Repairing a relaxed posterior vaginal wall, gapping vaginal outlet, and defective perineum may improve the complaint of stress incontinence of urine. Such a repair will elongate the posterior vaginal wall and bring it up beneath the anterior vaginal wall for better support. It will also bring the bulbocavernosus muscle attached beneath the labia minora closer together in the perineum and thereby improve the efficiency of the voluntary urethral sphincter. Although these mechanisms may be more theoretical than real, we have seen stress urinary incontinence improved by posterior colpoperineorrhaphy.

Patients often blame unsatisfactory sexual relations on the relaxed conditions of the perineum and vagina, specifically the loss of support from the bulbocavernosus, the transverse perinei, and the levator ani muscles. Complaints may originate from the patient or from her husband. Coital inadequacy may depend on the degree of relaxation of the vaginal outlet and can be one of the secondary indications for perineorrhaphy, but it is rarely caused entirely by local anatomic conditions. More frequently, coital problems signal marital incompatibility or result from increasing age and stress. The entire marital relationship should be evaluated before sexual improvement from vaginal plastic surgery is promised. As emphasized by Jeffcate and others, dyspareunia is a frequent complication of an extensive posterior colporrhaphy and perineorrhaphy; such sexual complications could result in further deterioration of a tenuous sexual relationship.

One of the common complaints in women over the age of 50 is dyspareunia. This is a result of a reduction in plasma estrogen levels during the postmenopausal period that causes the vaginal epithelium to become thin and sensitive. Postmenopausal hormonal changes may lead to varying degrees of contracture of the vaginal outlet, particularly in nulliparous women and in women who have had previous perineal surgery. The eventual effects of estrogen depletion must always be considered when a vaginal repair is being planned. After the menopause, the vaginal caliber may be reduced by contracture due to hypoestrogenism.

Rectocele should not be considered a cause of constipation. It may be a cause of incomplete emptying of the rectum with defecation. Indeed, some women will learn to use digital pressure against the rectocele to initiate a bowel movement or finally to empty the rectum completely. Rectocele may be associated with an uncomfortable feeling of pressure and aching in the rectum. A rectocele may be a greater problem in a woman with constipation because of greater and less effective bearing-down efforts required to have a bowel movement. If stenosis of the anal canal is present, the straining necessary for defecation may aggravate a rectocele even more. Anal stenosis should be dilated and measures to relieve constipation should be instituted in any patient with a rectocele to keep it from enlarging or to prevent recurrence after repair.

Surgical Repair of Relaxed Vaginal Outlet with Rectocele

The repair of a relaxed vaginal outlet and the repair of a rectocele are two distinct operative procedures. If both conditions are present, they are usually repaired together. A perineal repair is often done when a rectocele is present. Occasionally a rectocele will require repair in a woman whose vaginal outlet has been well supported from a previous episiotomy repair.

The urogenital musculature is not visible during perineal surgery, because the muscles are ensheathed in fascia. The fascia is not dissected from the muscles because the firmest union is obtained by the healing of fascia to fascia.

Plastic surgery on the posterior vagina does not begin with a preconceived idea of the exact type of operation that will be done. Only after the vagina has been dissected, after the size and the position of the rectocele have been defined, and after the presence or the absence of an enterocele has been determined can the surgeon make a final decision about the type and extent of operation required. A few standard procedures are described here, with the understanding that variations in technique must be made to fit the individual case.

If the entire posterior vaginal wall is weak, then the entire posterior vaginal wall must be repaired. Unfor-

tunately, this important principle is frequently neglected. A simple posterior colpoperineorrhaphy to repair defects in the perineum, vaginal outlet, and lower one third of the vagina is simply not enough when weakness in the upper posterior vaginal wall is also present. In this circumstance, a high rectocele will eventually become larger and troublesome.

Technique of Simple Perineal Repair

The ultimate size of the vaginal orifice is determined by placing Allis clamps on the inner aspect of the labia minora, along both sides of the outlet, and approximating them in the midline. The clamps should be adjusted so that the final vaginal opening will admit three fingers easily, taking into account that the levator ani and perineal muscles are completely relaxed from the general anesthesia and that postmenopausal shrinkage may further contract the introitus.

A slightly curved, transverse incision is made posteriorly at the mucocutaneous junction connecting the two lateral Allis clamps (Fig. 34-3A). Making the incision over the perineal body toward the anus in a V-shaped fashion to a point on the perineum that is 1–2 cm from the anus provides better access to the perineal muscles by dissecting the skin overlying the posterior fourchette (Fig. 34-3B).

The mucosa of the vaginal introitus is dissected upward by blunt and sharp dissection (Fig. 34-3C). The dissection is carried only high enough and lateral enough to expose the fascia covering the levator muscles and to permit placement of the levator sutures, since the simple procedure does not include rectocele repair. The vaginal dissection is made vertically in the midline, placing an Allis clamp at the apex of the incision to elevate the vaginal wall. Injection of generous quantities of saline beneath the mucosa will facilitate dissection in the proper plane. The vaginal mucosa is incised in an inverted V-shaped manner, with traction placed on the apex clamp. As the vaginal mucosa is dissected free from the underlying fascia, it is opened in the midline, then the excess vaginal mucosa is excised. Excision of a V-shaped wedge prevents pouching of excessive tissue when the vaginal mucosa is sutured.

Interrupted stitches of No. 0 delayed-absorbable suture are placed through the pararectal fascia and levator ani muscles (Fig. 34-3D). The muscle fibers need not be exposed before placing these sutures; bold lateral stitches should include a large medial portion of the muscle mass in each bite. The number of stitches taken in the levator muscles varies, depending on the degree of relaxation and the amount of perineal support needed. In the average case, two or three sutures are sufficient.

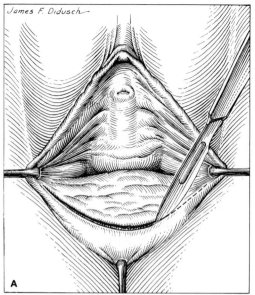

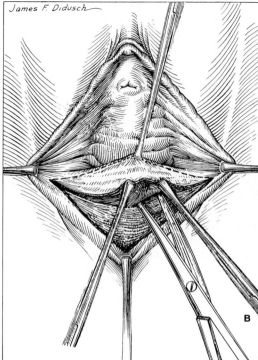

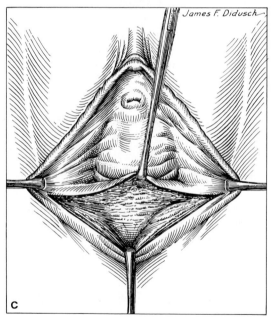

Figure 34–3. Simple perineal repair. *A*, An incision is made at the mucocutaneous border along the perineal body. *B*, A V-shaped incision is made over the perineal body toward the anus. The dotted line indicates the line of incision of the upper flap. *C*, The flap includes an inverted V-shaped piece of mucosa that has been excised.

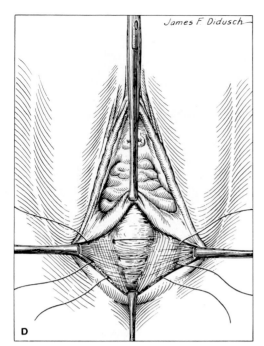 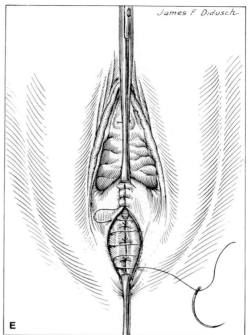

Figure 34–3 (continued) *D*, Three interrupted sutures have been placed in the levator ani muscles. *E*, The levator muscles have been approximated. The mucosa has been closed with a lock stitch of No. 2-0 delayed-absorbable suture, and the perineal skin is being approximated with a subcuticular stitch.

Starting at the top of the incision, the vaginal mucosa is closed in the midline, using a continuous lock-stitch of No. 2-0 delayed-absorbable suture. When the levator region is reached, the muscles are approximated by tying the previously placed sutures (Fig. 34-3*E*).

The diameter of the vaginal introitus must be evaluated carefully after the levator sutures are tied. If the introitus is found to be too small, the offending suture(s) should be removed or replaced until the diameter is satisfactory. Supporting sutures are then placed in the superficial fascia. Using a small cutting needle, the mucosa suture is continued over the perineal body as a subcuticular midline stitch.

Technique of Repair of Moderate-Sized Rectocele

As with a simple repair, the degree of closure of the relaxed outlet is determined before an incision is initiated at the lateral mucocutaneous border of the introitus and continued along the anterior surface of the perineal body in a V-shaped fashion to the region of the anal margin. The dissected perineal skin is excised horizontally along the vaginal outlet.

A midline vertical incision is initiated in the center of the mucosal edge by tunneling beneath the posterior mucosa with Metzenbaum scissors, incising the freed mucosa in the midline, and extending the dissection above the rectocele (Fig. 34-4*A*). In a manner similar to an anterior repair, traction is placed on the upper margin of each segment of the mucosal dissection using an Allis clamp. The lower margins of the incision are held under tension with additional clamps while the mucosa is separated with Metzenbaum scissors from the underlying fascia. When the midline incision is completed, the vaginal mucosa is separated laterally from the pararectal fascia and muscle attachments by sharp dissection, taking care to avoid penetrating the thin mucosa (Fig. 34-4*B*). The lateral dissection should be extended as far as possible to mobilize the pararectal fascia and to expose the medial margins of the levator ani muscles. The terminal ends of the bulbocavernosus and transverse perinei muscles are also freed from the adherent mucosa in the lower vagina.

The pararectal fascia is then drawn over the bulging rectocele, using as many vertical mattress sutures of No. 0 delayed-absorbable suture as are necessary to reinforce and completely close the hernial space over the rectal wall (Fig. 34-4*C*). Interrupted stitches of No. 0 delayed-absorbable suture are placed deeply in the medial margins of the levator muscles, approximating the muscles and fascia sufficiently over the lower rectal

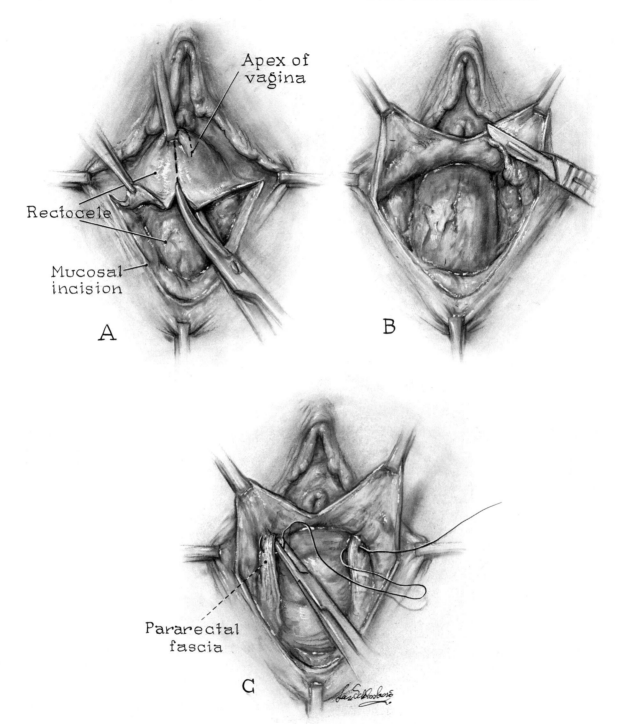

Figure 34–4. Repair of moderate-sized rectocele. *A*, A V-shaped incision is made from angles of introitus over perineal body; midline vertical incision extends to apex of vagina. *B*, Pararectal fascia is separated from mucosa by sharp dissection and (*C*) plicated over anterior wall of rectum.

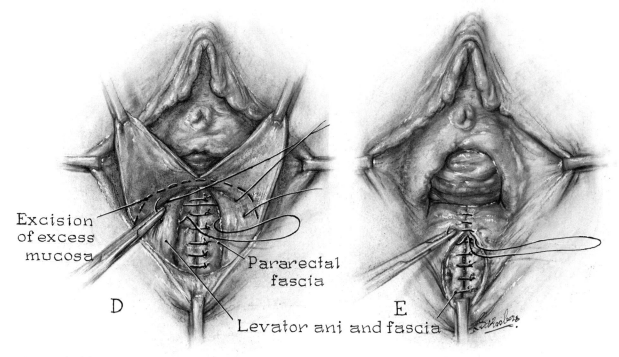

Figure 34–4 (continued) *D*, Levator ani muscles are approximated in the midline with deep sutures of No. 0 or 1 delayed-absorbable material. The excess vaginal mucosa is excised and the margins are closed (*E*) with either an interrupted or continuous suture.

wall to produce the desired support to the perineal body and lower posterior vaginal wall (Fig. 34-4*D*).

Although it is usually difficult to advance levators to the midline under the entire posterior vagina, the plicated pararectal fascia will provide firm fascial support over the upper portion of the rectocele. By plicating the levator muscles in the midline, the levator hiatus is narrowed, providing additional support to the relaxed pelvic floor.

After any excess vaginal mucosa has been excised, the margins are closed, beginning at the apex of the vagina. This is done with a continuous lock stitch of No. 2-0 delayed-absorbable suture, incorporating the underlying fascia with a running suture to obliterate the dead space between vaginal wall and rectum (Fig. 34-4*E*). When the continuous mucosal suture reaches the levator muscle sutures, these deep interrupted stitches are tied.

Excessive constriction of the vagina and introitus with the levator sutures must be avoided. If there is evidence that the diameter of the vagina or of the outlet is too small, the levator sutures should be removed and replaced until a satisfactory diameter is achieved.

After a few supporting plication sutures are placed in the fascia and underlying muscles of the perineal body, the mucosal suture is continued over the perineum as a subcuticular stitch, using a small, curved cutting needle.

The perineal muscle sutures, which include the lower margins of the bulbocavernosus and the transverse perinei muscles, give support to the levator hiatus and pelvic floor (Fig. 34-5).

Technique of Repair of High Rectocele

To make certain that a rectal hernia through the torn and stretched rectal and vaginal fascia and relaxed levator hiatus is adequately repaired, the full length of the rectovaginal wall should be dissected out and the musculofascial repair should be performed along the entire posterior vaginal wall, whether the rectocele is of moderate size or is more extensive. The upper portion of the rectovaginal fascia is the weakest, and failure to obtain a good restoration of the posterior vaginal wall usually results when an inherent musculofascial weakness in the upper aspect of the wall is not recognized. Differentiation between a high rectocele and enterocele may be difficult or even impossible until the entire posterior wall is dissected to the apex of the vagina.

The repair of a high rectocele should be approached like any other posterior colporrhaphy, with the midline mucosal incision extended to the apex of the vagina. In generous volumes, sterile saline is injected just beneath the vaginal mucosa to facilitate dissection in the proper

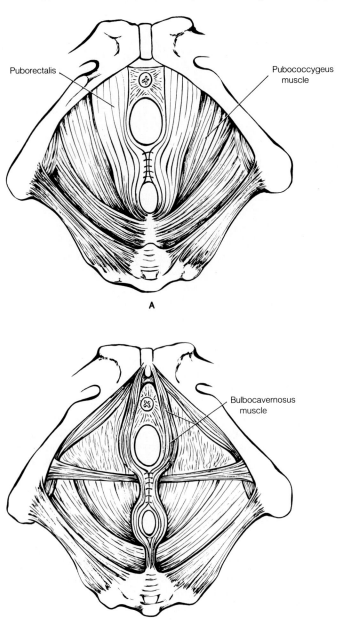

Puborectalis

Pubococcygeus muscle

A

Bulbocavernosus muscle

B

Figure 34–5. *A*, Schematic representation of the effect of plication of levator ani muscles in reducing the aperture of the levator hiatus, as viewed from the perineum. *B*, Plication of lower margins of bulbocavernosus and transverse perinei muscles strengthens the support of the urogenital diaphragm and the pelvic floor.

plane. The fascia of Denonvillier of the rectovaginal septum and the pararectal fascia are identified and separated from underneath the vaginal mucosa by sharp dissection and mobilized as far laterally as possible, avoiding the adjacent inferior hemorrhoidal vessels. From the vaginal apex, protrusion of an additional enterocele hernial sac can be determined easily. The small bowel usually fills an enterocele sac, providing a clear demarcation of the margins of the attenuated cul-de-sac peritoneum.

If no enterocele protrudes, the freed margins of the pararectal fascia are plicated with No. 0 delayed-absorbable interrupted vertical mattress sutures, making certain that the anterior rectal wall is displaced with a Kelly clamp while the sutures are tied in the midline. This series of plication sutures is best started at the apex of the vagina, where the initial suture may be anchored to the supporting tissues of the vaginal vault so that the entire hernial defect can be closed. The fascial sutures are placed in succession until the margins of the levator ani muscles can be approximated in the midline, adding further muscular support to the pelvic floor and the rectocele repair (see Fig. 31-11). The remainder of the repair follows the procedure for perineal closure.

Enterocele Associated with Rectocele

Although intestinal hernias protruding through the cul-de-sac of Douglas do not occur as often as either rectal or bladder hernias (rectocele or cystocele), they must be recognized and corrected surgically for treatment to be completed successfully. An enterocele that remains unrecognized usually becomes more obvious following a hysterectomy, causing pelvic pressure and discomfort.

An enterocele that follows a hysterectomy, known as a pulsion enterocele, may appear as a result of tissue weakness caused by ischemia and necrosis at the distal ends of excised ligaments tied *en masse* during vaginal or abdominal hysterectomy. In some cases, the patient has had a previous rectocele repair. Patients complain of a mass protruding from the vaginal outlet when they stand or strain. The mass, usually bowel or omentum, disappears when the patient lies down. The large neck of the cul-de-sac allows the bowel contents to slip in and out easily, usually without intestinal strangulation. Sometimes loops of small intestine adhere to the lining of the enterocele sac.

Like most hernias, the enterocele has an embryologic factor in its formation. During the development of the vagina, following the fusion of the mullerian ducts with the urogenital sinus, the cul-de-sac peritoneum is located deep between the rectum and the developing vagina. As the vaginal plate cannulates into the vaginal canal, the peritoneum regresses and the rectovaginal septum becomes fused into the fascia of Denonvillier. Although the cul-de-sac is commonly located posterior to the upper one third of the vagina, approximately 5 cm from the origin of the uterosacral ligament on the lower uterine segment, the embryologic attachment of the cul-de-sac peritoneum to the vaginal septum can, and does, occur at a lower level, producing a deep peritoneal pouch. A congenitally deep cul-de-sac can serve as a wedge by which the small bowel dissects down into the space between the posterior vaginal wall and the anterior surface of the rectum.

The most important acquired factor promoting the formation of an enterocele is attenuation of supporting tissues allowing prolapse of the uterus. With progressive descent of the uterus, the cul-de-sac is pulled through the levator hiatus, deep into the vaginal canal. Intra-abdominal pressure extends the herniation, called a traction enterocele, further down.

Enteroceles are frequently misdiagnosed as high rectoceles, in spite of basic differences. The contents of an enterocele are small bowel, not rectum. Attempting a cure by performing a rectocele operation at an unusually high level without separately identifying the enterocele will not provide adequate treatment.

When an enterocele occurs, as it commonly does, in association with a rectocele, the diagnosis can be made by inspection, since the division between the two types of herniation is indicated by a transverse furrow just above the rectocele (see Fig. 31-7). A finger inserted into the rectum will demonstrate the rectocele as distinct from the bulging sac that arises from a higher point. By compressing the enterocele on rectovaginal exam, it is usually possible to identify and displace small bowel in the hernial sac, unless the bowel is fixed to the sac with adhesions.

Diagnosis can be facilitated by examining the rectovaginal septum and cul-de-sac while the patient stands with one foot on a low stool, knees bent slightly, and straining by a Valsalva maneuver (see Fig. 32-9). Transillumination of the rectovaginal septum through the rectum does not provide enough information to warrant its use, especially since the procedure is intolerable for the patient. Transvaginal ultrasonography may be helpful.

After an enterocele has been diagnosed, surgical correction proceeds as for other types of hernia: isolation and complete dissection of the sac, upward displacement of the visceral contents, excision and high ligation of the sac, closure of the musculofascial defect through which the sac leaves the pelvic floor, and addition of fascial support to the closed anatomic defect. The choice of surgical technique depends upon what other conditions exist in association with the enterocele.

For example, an enterocele encountered while performing a pelvic laparotomy may be closed intra-abdominally by a succession of concentric purse-string sutures, starting at the bottom of the cul-de-sac, as described by Moschcowitz for cure of rectal prolapse (Fig. 34-6). An alternative to the classical Moschcowitz culdeplasty is illustrated in Figure 34-7. A 2-0 polydioxanone continuous purse-string suture is placed on each side of the rectum, beginning at the bottom of the pelvis and continuing up along the pelvic sidewalls, taking care not to incorporate the ureters in the sutures. A more complete closure of the cul-de-sac can be accomplished without constricting the rectum. When a small pulsion enterocele occurs through the vaginal vault after a vaginal or abdominal hysterectomy, the sac is dissected and completely excised through the vagina. High ligation of the sac is accomplished by placing No. 0 polydioxanone suture high on the inside of the circumference of the cul-de-sac peritoneum. All the available ligaments and the redundant cul-de-sac peritoneum are brought together and sutured to the vaginal vault to

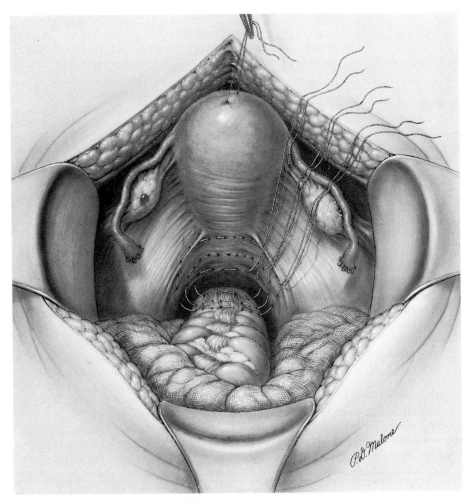

Figure 34–6. Transabdominal method of obliteration of deep cul-de-sac or enterocele, using multiple concentric purse strings (Moschcowitz procedure).

give it support and to secure closure of the hernial defect.

Repair of a small or medium-sized enterocele is often part of an extensive vaginal plastic procedure for a coexisting relaxed vaginal outlet that could also include rectocele, cystocele, and uterine descensus of varying degrees. The dissection and closure procedure is described as a posterior culdeplasty in Figure 27–47.

Usually, two or three deep bites through the uterosacral ligaments and into the cul-de-sac peritoneum suffice to obliterate completely the site of a small or medium-sized enterocele formation. The sutures may also include the vaginal mucosa of the posterior vaginal fornix in such a fashion that the vaginal apex is elevated at its deepest point. The procedure can be preventive or corrective when combined with a vaginal hysterectomy.

When a pulsion enterocele causes massive inversion of the vagina following a hysterectomy, there is insuffi-

cient ligamentous or fascial support within the levator ani diastasis to permit adequate repair by the usual vaginal approach. An abdominal sacral colpopexy provides a more permanent repair, using a mersilene gauze graft or an autogenous graft of rectus fascia to anchor the vault to the third or fourth sacral vertebra.

A very large traction enterocele accompanying total uterine procidentia requires a combined abdominoperineal procedure to place the prolapsed vagina over the levator plate and anchor the vault to the sacral vertebrae. An alternative method of repair is a sacrospinous ligament fixation of the vagina. The wide diastasis of the levator hiatus created by massive inversion of the vagina requires a surgical approach that is very different from that for the usual small enterocele. These additional procedures are discussed in Chapter 32.

A small to moderate-sized enterocele may be repaired vaginally at the time of posterior colporrhaphy,

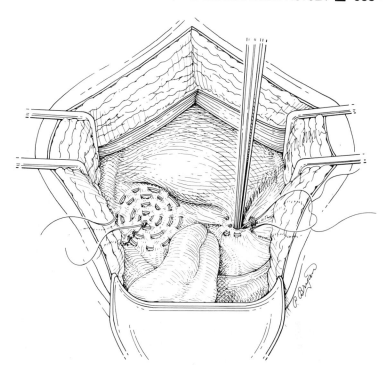

Figure 34–7. An alternative to the classical Moschcowitz procedure is illustrated. A continuous No. 2-0 polydioxanone suture closes the cul-de-sac on each side of the rectum.

vaginal hysterectomy, Manchester operation, or other vaginal procedures. A midline incision is made posteriorly as in a posterior colporrhaphy. A tunnel is made by inserting the curved Metzenbaum scissors beneath the vaginal mucosa and successively opening and closing the scissors, then incising the vagina in the midline. The process of tunneling and cutting is repeated until the apex of the vagina is reached. Injection of generous volumes of sterile saline just beneath the vaginal mucosa will facilitate dissection in the proper plane. The vaginal wall is dissected laterally on either side first to expose a rectocele, if one is present; then the enterocele sac is dissected free (see Fig. 31-11). The sac is opened. Any adherent bowel or omentum must be mobilized and displaced superiorly. A purse-string suture of No. 0 polydioxanone suture is placed on the inside of the sac at the neck. One or two additional purse-string sutures incorporating the uterosacral ligaments will provide support to the hernial repair, especially if the posterior vaginal fornix can be elevated to the uterosacral ligaments, as in the posterior culdeplasty. The sutures are tied and the excess peritoneum is trimmed away. If a rectocele or relaxed vaginal outlet is present, it is repaired before closure.

An advanced degree of relaxation of the upper posterior vaginal wall with rectocele and enterocele may require additional support from perirectal fascia described by Thornton and Peters or sacrospinous ligament fixation described by Nichols. A more complete discussion of this operation and of enteroceles will be found in Chapter 32.

ANATOMY OF THE ANAL CANAL AND LOWER RECTUM

The complete interrelated mechanisms of defecation and anal control are more easily visualized once the principal elements of the rectoanal musculature have been delineated.

The anal canal is approximately 2.5–4 cm in length and normally remains completely collapsed because of the tonic contractions of the sphincter mechanisms (Fig. 34-8). The canal is related posteriorly to the coccyx, from which it is separated by fibrofatty tissue and by the levator ani muscles until it opens onto the perineal skin. The levator ani muscles also separate the lateral boundary of the canal from the ischiorectal fossa, through which pass the important nerves, lymphatics, and blood supply of the terminal rectum, anal canal, and perineum. The canal is fused anteriorly with the lower portion of the rectovaginal septum and the perineal body.

The anal and rectal regions of the lower colon share a common embryologic origin. During their development, the terminal end of the alimentary canal is surrounded by muscular sphincters of somatic origin. The sphincter mechanism of the anal canal (see Fig. 34-8)

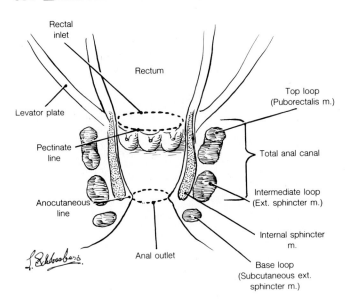

Figure 34–8. Diagrammatic illustration of the anal canal.

consists of two separate anatomic structures. The internal sphincter consists of circular smooth muscle from the rectal wall, which is innervated by the autonomic nervous system and is not under voluntary control. The internal sphincter plays no voluntary role in anal continence but provides continuous tone to the anal canal from autonomic innervation. The outer sphincter is composed of four separate external skeletal muscles surrounding the anal canal. These are voluntarily controlled. The external sphincter muscles lie in close approximation with the medial margin of the strong levator ani muscles, principally the pubococcygeus muscles. The tone of the levator ani is strengthened by the skeletal muscles of the anterior compartment of the urogenital diaphragm, the bulbocavernosus and transverse perinei muscles, which have a common insertion into the central perineal body between the anus and vaginal introitus.

The perineal body is an important anatomic landmark that is closely associated with the external sphincter and the anal canal. The perineal body itself includes two components of the transverse perineal muscles, a superficial and a deep muscle layer, both composed of striated muscle. The central tendon (raphe) of this transverse perineal musculature serves as a pivotal point where the external sphincter connects with the levator muscles, including the terminal end of the bulbocavernosus (see Fig. 34-1). Trauma or separation of the perineal raphe causes relaxation of the perineal body, which is attached to the base loop of the external anal sphincter. The resulting alteration of attachment generally causes loss of control of both liquid stool and gas.

Anatomic dissections and histologic sections of the anal canal show that the external anal sphincter is com-

posed of a triple-loop system: the top, intermediate, and base (see Fig. 34-8). The puborectalis muscle forms the top loop of the sphincter complex at the junction of the rectum and anus (rectal neck). This U-shaped muscle encircles the rectal neck, suspends the anal canal forward toward the symphysis pubis in a near right angle, and maintains anorectal continence by closure of the rectal inlet (Fig. 34-9). The puborectalis is a striated muscle, innervated by the inferior hemorrhoidal branch of the pudendal nerve. An extension of fibers from this muscle along the external surface of the anal canal forms the lateral external component of the longitudinal anal muscle.

The intermediate loop of the external sphincter pulls

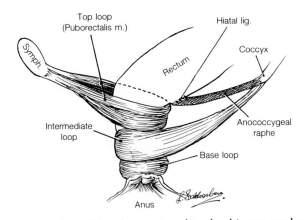

Figure 34–9. Triple-loop external anal sphincter mechanism. The top loop represents puborectalis muscles. The intermediate loop arises and inserts in the coccyx. The base loop attaches to the perianal skin and perineal body.

in the opposite direction from the top loop. The intermediate loop starts at the coccyx as a fibrous tendon, then evolves into a flat muscle bundle that encircles the middle segment of the anal canal and inserts into the same tendinous sheath on the coccyx (see Fig. 34-9). The intermediate segment of the sphincter is innervated by the perineal branch of the fourth sacral nerve.

The base loop is the smallest component of the external anal sphincter mechanism. The base loop, which lies beneath the anal mucosa in the same plane as the internal sphincter, circles the anal orifice and attaches to the perianal skin near the midline.

This concept of the anatomy of the external anal sphincter emphasizes the role of the levator ani as an ancillary mechanism for defecation and fecal control. From a functional viewpoint, the levator ani may be divided into two components, the pubococcygeus and iliococcygeus muscles. The anatomy of these muscles was described earlier. The major contribution of the levator ani in anorectal control is provided by the pubococcygeal muscles and the central (anococcygeal) raphe.

The raphe extends from the coccyx to the rectal angle and incorporates the fibers of each pubococcygeal muscle as they criss-cross the center of the pelvic floor and continue to the opposite pelvic wall. The pubococcygeus muscles include both a transverse segment (levator plate) and a longitudinal extension (anal suspensory sling) that serve specific functions in the entry and expulsion of gas and fecal content through the anal canal.

The transverse segment of the pubococcygeus (levator plate) surrounds the levator hiatus at the site of the rectal neck. Also surrounding the levator hiatus is the puborectalis muscle, located beneath the levator plate.

The levator plate is attached to the rectum by the hiatal ligament, an extension of the endopelvic fascia surrounding the levator ani. The fascia provides support by adhering the levator plate to the rectum, vagina, and urethra. The hiatal ligament permits a certain degree of mobility between the levator plate and the intrahiatal viscera during defecation and facilitates frequent changes in tonicity of the levator plate in response to such alterations of intra-abdominal pressure as coughing, laughing, or urination. The hiatal ligament provides the mechanism by which the rectal inlet is opened and closed by contraction or relaxation of the levator plate.

The musculature of the levator plate extends along the anal canal (anal suspensory ligament) and forms the intermediate layer of the longitudinal muscle of the canal wall. Ending in a central fibrous tendon, the suspensory ligament anchors to the base loop musculature and to the anal and perianal skin (Fig. 34-10). When the levator plate is voluntarily contracted, the anal canal is shortened, the rectal inlet is opened, the base loop is pulled upward and stretched open, and the anal and perianal skin is everted during the process of defecation.

The longitudinal muscle of the anal canal has three separate components: the inner smooth muscle, which blends with the wall of the anus; the intermediate striated muscular extension of the levator plate, the suspensory ligament; and the lateral striated muscular extension of the top loop of the external sphincter, the puborectalis. The major function of the striated components of the longitudinal muscle is to anchor the levator plate passively in a funnel-like fashion to the base loop of the sphincter and the perianal skin.

In the relaxed state, the funnel-shaped levator plate

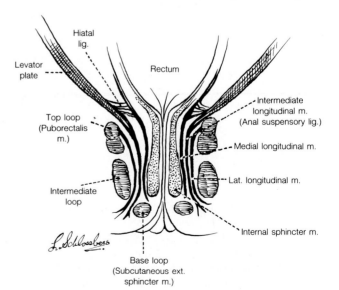

Figure 34–10. Coronal view of the three components of the longitudinal skeletal muscle, which is directly adjacent to the smooth muscle of the anal canal.

releases tension on the rectal neck, which permits the rectal inlet to be pulled forward and closed by the puborectalis muscle, thereby keeping the anal canal free of feces and gas. On voluntary contraction of the levator, the levator plate is flattened, the rectal neck is retracted posteriorly by the hiatal ligament, the rectal inlet is opened, the anal canal is shortened, and the basal loop is elevated and pulled open by the attachment of the suspensory sling. By this process, feces and gas may enter the anal canal, where they are aided in their expulsion by alternate contraction and relaxation of the three separate loops of the external anal sphincter (Fig. 34-11).

During defecation or following increased intra-abdominal pressure, the pubococcygeal muscles contract and the puborectalis muscle voluntarily relaxes. This muscular interaction causes widening of the levator hiatus and of the rectal angle. The levator plate changes from a funneled to a flattened position on contraction, opening and elevating the rectal inlet. Contraction of the levator plate produces contraction and shortening of the anal suspensory sling (longitudinal anal muscle), which elevates the base loop of the external sphincter, shortens and widens the rectal neck, and opens the anal outlet.

Relaxation of the levator muscles causes return of the funnel shape of the levator plate, closure of the rectal inlet with relaxation of the anal suspensory sling, descent of the base loop of the external sphincter, and finally, closure of the anal outlet. The base loop located adjacent to the anal mucosa closes the anal outlet with its resting tone. Voluntary contraction of the base loop firmly seals the anal orifice and prevents passage of gas or feces. Injury to this segment of the external sphincter by obstetric trauma, such as a third-degree tear, may cause anal incontinence of gas or liquid stool.

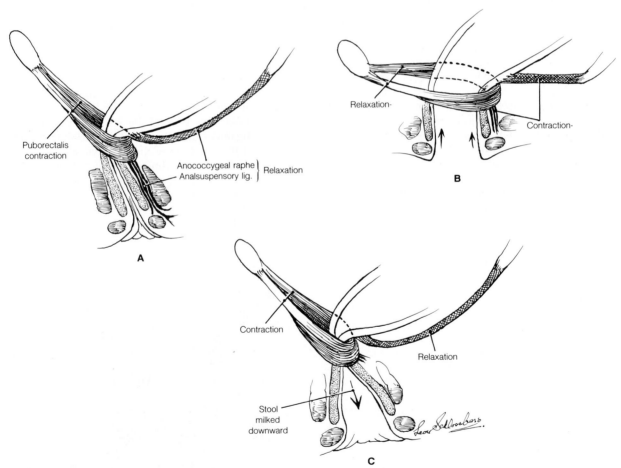

Figure 34–11. Function of the external anal sphincter. *A*, At rest, the rectal inlet is closed and pulled forward by contraction of puborectalis muscle. *B*, During defecation the rectal inlet is opened and the angle is straightened by relaxation of the puborectalis muscle and contraction and flattening of the rectal plate. *C*, Expulsion of feces from the canal is augmented by alternate contraction and relaxation of the three loops.

The top loop of the external sphincter, the puborectalis muscle, closes the rectal inlet as it draws the rectal neck toward the symphysis pubis, maintaining anal continence. Relaxation of the puborectalis in conjunction with contraction of the levator plate causes the rectal inlet to be elevated, opened, and drawn posteriorly, thereby allowing feces and gas to enter the anal canal during the process of defecation.

Anal continence is a function of both the external and internal sphincter. The external sphincter is responsible for voluntary continence, whereas the internal, smooth muscle sphincter maintains involuntary continence of the anal canal.

The lower half of the anal canal is lined with squamous epithelium, which is richly supplied with branches of the inferior hemorrhoidal nerves and is, therefore, very sensitive. The slightest stimulation of this squamous epithelium causes reflex contraction of the external sphincters and can be a powerful component of mechanisms responsible for maintaining fecal continence. Indeed, the anus is said to be one of the most sensitive parts of the human body, along with the synovial membrane and the conjunctiva.

Distention of the rectal ampulla by gas or feces causes an increase in the basal tone of external anal sphincter and the pelvic floor muscles. The receptors for this reflex lie in the levator ani muscles themselves.

Although the function of the levator ani muscles has caused dissension among researchers, most would agree to separating the puborectalis muscle from the functioning of the classic levator ani triad. The remaining levator ani muscles, principally the pubococcygeus, serve to dilate the rectal neck during the process of defecation. The opposing action of the puborectalis muscle causes obstruction and kinking of the rectal neck by contracting and displacing the rectal inlet forward toward the symphysis pubis. Defined in this way, the levator ani plays a limited role in anal continence and functions mainly during defecation. On contraction, the levator plate is straightened and tensed, which pulls the levator hiatal ligament laterally and posteriorly and opens the rectal neck inlet. Contraction of the anal suspensory ligament, the muscular extension of the levator plate, causes the anal canal to shorten, the rectal neck to open, and the external anal sphincter to be pulled open and the anus everted.

In contrast, the internal anal sphincter is responsible for the involuntary control of anal continence and is maintained in a continuous tonic state by autonomic innervation. The internal sphincter relaxes reflexly in response to a contraction of the smooth muscle of the rectum (detrusor) when stool or flatus enters the bowel lumen above the rectal inlet. As stool enters the rectal inlet, the rectal detrusor contracts, the internal sphincter relaxes, and the rectal inlet is opened by the action of the levator plate.

For defecation to occur, the external sphincter, principally the puborectalis muscle, must voluntarily relax while the levator plate contracts and pulls the rectal inlet into an open position. The rectal inlet will not open unless the top loop of the external sphincter is voluntarily relaxed. If defecation or passage of gas is inconvenient, the external sphincter remains firmly contracted and the levator plate remains relaxed, preventing relaxation of the internal sphincter. Failure of the internal sphincter to relax will inhibit further contraction of the rectal detrusor, and the rectum will dilate above the rectal inlet to accommodate the fecal contents.

Parks suggested some years ago the presence of an anal valve mechanism that assists in maintaining fecal continence. This flap valve mechanism is located at the anorectal junction at the point where the direction of the lower rectum is at right angles to the anal canal. The mucosa of the lower rectum actually lies across the anal canal and is kept in this position by intra-abdominal pressure. The greater the intra-abdominal pressure, the more secure the closure. This flap valve mechanism can be opened by increased intrarectal pressure. Voluntary relaxation of the sphincter then allows defecation.

Injury to the internal sphincter can permit the involuntary passage of liquid stool and gas due to loss of tonicity of the anal canal. Such an injury is particularly noticeable when the urge to defecate is persistent from a bolus of fecal content in the terminal rectum and when the voluntary contraction of the external sphincter wanes.

The triple-loop mechanism of the external sphincter provides an explanation for the varying degrees of anal incontinence that can result when the external sphincter is partially destroyed. If the lower portion of the external anal sphincter is traumatized, the top loop of the sphincter—the puborectalis muscle—may remain intact, in which case it will obstruct the rectal neck by forward displacement and closure of the rectal inlet. In this way, a defect to the lower portion of the internal and external sphincters can be partially compensated for by voluntary sphincter control. Damage to the entire external or internal sphincter would result in total incontinence.

Reconstructive surgery should restore the right-angle configuration of the rectal neck by appropriate plication of the puborectalis muscle. The important base and intermediate loops of the sphincter should be carefully identified and repaired to ensure anatomic control of gas and liquid stool. Although it is difficult to identify the anatomy of the internal sphincter, every effort should be made to restore continuity to both the internal and external sphincter when repair of the anal canal is performed.

The major effect of a disrupted and separated perineal musculature on anal continence is mediated through the severance of the fibers of the central tendon. Perineal trauma causes a separation of the fascial septa that anchors the levator plate and the lower segments of the top loop of the external sphincter into the perineum and perianal skin. With complete loss of the perineal body by an unrepaired second-degree laceration or episiotomy breakdown, the muscular tone of the canal wall is weakened and the contractile force of the base loop of the external sphincter system is diminished. As a result, the anal canal may be unable to control gas and liquid stool. To correct a perineal defect, the separated muscles of the perineal body and the supporting muscles of the pelvic diaphragm must be reapproximated.

Rectal continence and function depend on the maintenance of constant tone in the levator ani and external anal sphincter muscles. This is a special quality of these muscles that is different from other skeletal muscles in the body. The level of tone depends on the volume of feces and gas in the rectum and is normally maintained even during sleep. Function of the muscles depends on normal innervation through the pudendal nerves arising from S3 and S4. These nerves may be damaged with vaginal delivery and by constant straining. When incontinence is due to damaged innervation of muscles, rectal continence is difficult to restore with surgery. Normal defecation also depends on voluntary relaxation of muscle tone, increasing intra-abdominal pressure with Valsalva maneuver, the gastrocolic reflex, and the type of food ingested; it is also very much dependent on habit.

FECAL INCONTINENCE

Few problems seen in gynecology cause so much personal discomfort and social embarrassment to women as the problem of fecal incontinence. Both gas and fecal incontinence of some degree is a fairly common problem, especially among multiparous and older women. A surprisingly large number will not discuss it with their physician because of embarrassment and the feeling of being unclean. Many women conceal their symptoms until the problem becomes so troublesome that they withdraw from social contacts. For these reasons, multiparous and elderly women should always be asked specifically about fecal incontinence, and the gynecologic examination should always include careful inspection of the posterior vaginal wall, perineum, anal sphincter, anal canal, and rectum.

There are a variety of causes of fecal incontinence (Table 34-1). Rarely, fecal incontinence may be congenital, as seen usually in newborn females who have imperforated ani with associated fecal incontinence through a congenital rectovaginal or rectoperineal fistula. Hindgut duplication with congenital rectovaginal fistula was

TABLE 34-1
Etiology of Fecal Incontinence

I.	Obstetrical procedures
	a. Third- or fourth-degree perineal lacerations
	b. Episiotomy breakdown
	c. Forceps delivery
II.	Operative procedures
	a. Colpoperineorrhaphy
	b. Vulvectomy
	c. Difficult hysterectomy
	d. Colpotomy drainage of pelvic abscess
	e. Excision of Bartholin gland
	f. Hemorrhoidectomy
	g. Abdominoperineal resection
III.	Trauma
IV.	Inflammatory bowel disease
	a. Crohn's disease
	b. Tuberculosis
	c. Granulomatous veneral disease
	d. Ulcerative colitis
	e. Diverticulitis
	f. Perirectal abscess
V.	Malignancy
	a. Carcinoma of the cervix
	b. Carcinoma of the vagina
	c. Carcinoma of the vulva
	d. Carcinoma of the rectum
VI.	Radiation
VII.	Congenital causes
VIII.	Idiopathic causes
	a. With rectal prolapse
	b. Without rectal prolapse
IX.	Miscellaneous

reported by Paul and Lloyd. The etiology of most fecal incontinence, however, is acquired as the result of trauma or destruction of the tissues of the anus, rectum, perineum, and/or rectovaginal wall and their associated fascia and muscles.

Loss of anal sphincter and perineal fascia and musculature usually results from traumatic obstetric delivery. In Hibbard's series of 24 rectovaginal fistulas and 27 complete old perineal tears, 47 (92%) were due to obstetric trauma. Because of an excessively large fetus, a large fetal head, shoulder dystocia, precipitate and uncontrolled delivery, a rigid perineum, a narrow subpubic arch, abnormal presentations, or other factors, a perineal laceration may extend to involve the anterior fibers of the anal sphincter or even extend further up to cause a ragged-edged separation of the mucosa of the anterior rectal wall. Lacerations may occur in spite of a well-timed episiotomy. Every effort should be made to repair such lacerations properly and especially to recognize and repair associated defects in the anal sphincter and rectal mucosa. Unfortunately, even meticulously repaired lacerations occasionally break down, leaving the patient essentially with a cloaca. Fecal incontinence is usually a problem until the tissues are healed sufficiently for a secondary, hopefully successful, repair.

According to Hauth and associates, midline episiotomies extend to complete perineal lacerations in 4.6% to 8.0% of cases. Repair can be expected to result in healing in 99% of cases with no subsequent problem with fecal incontinence.

The advantages and disadvantages of midline episiotomy were investigated by Shiono and associates, using data from the Collaborative Perinatal Project. Midline episiotomy was associated with statistically significant 4.2-fold and 12.8-fold increases in the risk of lacerations among primiparous and multiparous women, respectively. Recent studies by Green and Soohoo, Wilcox and associates, and Thorp and associates all suggest that midline episiotomy is associated with an increased risk of injury to the anal sphincter. The suggested benefits of midline episiotomy include substitution of a routine straight surgical incision for an occasional ragged laceration; prevention of perineal, anal, and rectal trauma; prevention of pelvic relaxation; and reduction in the length of the second stage of labor. However, the Collaborative Perinatal Project data indicated that 10% of women who had a midline episiotomy had a severe laceration. Shiono and associates believe that the risks and benefits of midline episiotomy, as practiced in the United States, should be reevaluated, especially since midline episiotomy may cause rather than prevent lacerations.

Although anal incontinence from obstetric trauma is a relatively common problem in multiparous women, it is not always an easy problem to explain. A careful examination of the perineal body, the interdigitating perineal and levator muscles, the anal sphincter, and the rectum should be made in every patient. It is surprising how often one finds abnormalities if one looks carefully. For example, when there is a lack of anal sphincter tone, one very often finds no sphincter muscle fibers anteriorly but instead only the dimples of the laterally retracted ends of the anal sphincter muscles. In such cases, the anal sphincter was torn at delivery. The perineum was repaired and healed, but the anal sphincter beneath was either not repaired or did not heal when repaired. With modern obstetric care, the number of patients who are left with a problem of fecal incontinence after delivery should be greatly diminished.

In addition to obstetric trauma, fecal incontinence may result from the trauma of operative procedures. Entry into the rectum may occur during posterior colpoperineorrhaphy, especially when the anterior rectal wall and posterior vaginal walls are closely adherent, with very little or any septum between. Injection of sterile saline just beneath the vaginal mucosa facilitates dissection in the proper plane to avoid entry into the rectum. A difficult hysterectomy, either abdominal or vaginal, may result in injury to the rectum, especially when dissection behind the cervix is difficult because of dense adhesions, indurated tissue from infection, or

involvement of the cul-de-sac and anterior rectal wall with endometriosis. If the rectal defect does not heal properly or is not closed properly, a high rectovaginal fistula may develop through the vaginal apex. Partial excision of anal sphincter and other muscles involved in maintaining fecal continence may be required in extensive vulvectomy for cancer, and fecal incontinence may result, as reported by Berek and associates. Injury to the anterior rectal wall may occur during hemorrhoidectomy, excision of the Bartholin gland, and colpotomy for pelvic abscess drainage.

Traumatic injury, a side-straddle injury more often in young girls, may result in simple or extensive laceration of the perineum. The extent of the injury may be difficult to determine because of pain, fear, edema, hemorrhage, and hematoma formation. Examination under anesthesia is advisable so that appropriate repair can be made, looking carefully for lacerations of the anal sphincter and rectum as well as other structures. Hematoma dissection above the levator muscles must be ruled out.

Among a variety of inflammatory bowel diseases that may cause rectovaginal fistula, Crohn's disease is the most important. Among 138 patients with rectovaginal fistulas seen at Duke University Medical Center, Bandy and associates reported that 15 (11%) were caused by Crohn's disease. The diagnosis, perioperative management, and surgical technique chosen for these patients constitute a special challenge for the gynecologic surgeon. Crohn's disease must be considered as a possible cause of rectovaginal fistula in any patient in whom other etiologies are not clear.

Malignant tumors may erode through the tissues between the vagina and the rectum. When a patient with tumor involvement of the rectovaginal wall receives radiation, sloughing of the tumor may result in a rectovaginal fistula. Radiation may also cause a rectovaginal fistula without tumor erosion.

Finally, fecal incontinence may be idiopathic with or without associated rectal prolapse. It is usually associated with a patulous anal sphincter, passive stretching of the puborectalis muscles, and a long history of straining with constipation. Most of these patients will consult a proctologist for care.

CLASSIFICATION OF DEFECTS IN THE ANAL SPHINCTER, PERINEUM, AND RECTOVAGINAL WALL

According to Rosenshein and associates at the Johns Hopkins Hospital, a classification of defects of the perineum and rectovaginal wall should allow a better understanding of the anatomic components involved and a better result with repair. A modification of their classification is proposed here:

Type I defects. In this group are patients who have a more or less intact but thin perineum but in which there is a defect in anterior muscle fibers of the external anal sphincter, the lowest fibers of the puborectalis muscles and perirectal fascia, and the transverse perineal muscles. The anal sphincter tone is poor, dimples at 2 and 10 o'clock around the anal orifice represent retracted ends of the sphincter, the perineum feels thin because of retraction of the transverse perineal muscles, and the acute angulation of the anorectal juncture is lost. Although most of these patients have an obstetric etiology of their defect, some are related to other forms of trauma or to extensive surgery for anal or vulvar cancer. An operation to identify and unite the retracted ends of the muscle of the anal sphincter, the perirectal fascia, the puborectalis muscles, and the transverse perineal muscles and to restore the acute anorectal juncture should be done when fecal incontinence is present. Among 40 patients operated upon for fecal incontinence by Moore, this defect was found most frequently.

Type I defects of other etiologies may occur. For example, external anal sphincter damage and fecal incontinence may result from surgery for posterior vulvar carcinoma. In such cases, transposition of the levator ani muscle to replace partially obliterated anal sphincter muscles is a suitable procedure for patients who have insufficient sphincter tissue for simpler repairs, as reported by Berek and associates.

Type II defects. In this group are patients with total loss of the perineal body as a result of obstetric trauma, either a third-degree laceration (through the perineum and anal sphincter) or a fourth-degree laceration (through the perineum, anal sphincter, and rectal mucosa). The laceration either was not repaired at the time it occurred or was repaired and broke down.

Type III defects. In addition to a loss of the perineal body, a rectovaginal fistula in the lower rectovaginal wall is present. In the series of 57 patients reported by Rosenshein and associates, this type of defect was the most common, accounting for 37%. A history of obstetric trauma was almost always present.

Type IV defects. In this type of defect a fistula is present in the lower one third of the rectovaginal wall and the perineum is intact. In most patients, the etiology is obstetric trauma, usually a repaired fourth-degree laceration that heals except for a small defect in the most proximal (upper) end of the repair. Occasionally, a rectovaginal fistula in this location can be caused by operative trauma (posterior colporrhaphy, hemorrhoidectomy, etc.) or Crohn's disease.

Type V defects. A rectovaginal fistula involves the middle third of the rectovaginal wall. Fistulas in this region are unusual.

Type VI defects. A rectovaginal fistula involves the upper one third of the vagina and is usually caused by a difficult hysterectomy, although a variety of other etiologies may be seen.

The surgical procedures chosen to obtain an optimal result in repair depend on the etiology and the type of defect discovered in each patient.

COMPLETE PERINEAL LACERATION

Classic symptoms present in the majority of cases include the progressive loss of control of gas and feces from the anus. The severity of symptoms generally varies with the degree of perineal laceration and sphincter loss. A few remaining external sphincter fibers left intact can provide sufficient muscular contraction to permit control of feces when the patient is constipated or when the stool is of normal consistency. When the tear extends well above the external anal sphincter, gas and feces escape at all times (Fig. 34-12).

A complete perineal laceration through the anal sphincter and possibly through the anal mucosa can occur during vaginal delivery and should be repaired at that time. If complete anatomic reconstruction is not achieved, symptoms will usually develop within the first 7–10 days following delivery. With separation of the base and intermediate loops, symptoms are usually those of incontinence of intestinal gas. Fecal incontinence occurs more commonly with complete breakdown of the perineal body, separation of the entire sphincter, and extension of the tear through the rectal mucosa (a fourth-degree perineal tear).

Should repair at the time of delivery fail, a second attempt should be deferred for a minimum of 2–3 months, to provide sufficient time for return of an adequate blood supply to the margins of the defect and for return of optimum viability of the perineal tissues. A proctoscopic examination and barium enema should precede the second attempt so that the presence of an occult rectovaginal fistula can be excluded. If anatomic findings suggest a fistula, a fistulogram should be used to demonstrate whether or not a sinus tract has formed between the vagina and the previous repair.

The results of early repair of an external sphincter ani muscle and rectal mucosal dehiscence were reported in 1986 by Hauth and associates. Each patient presented within 10 days of delivery with dehiscence of a repaired fourth-degree laceration. Each patient underwent preoperative mechanical bowel preparation on admission and preoperative wound cleansing and debridement

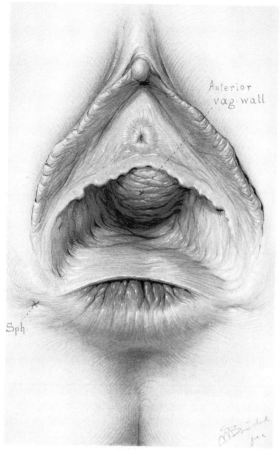

Figure 34–12. Old third-degree laceration with complete loss of anal sphincter and perineum. Note dimples on either side due to retraction of torn sphincter.

appropriate to the extent of superficial inflammation and necrosis. This ranged from 1 to 6 days before a layered closure was performed. The bowel was rested for 10 days after the repair. Seven of eight patients were successfully repaired with complete healing, normal external sphincter function, and no dyspareunia. Similar good results with early repair of dehiscence of fourth-degree episiotomy in 22 patients were reported by Hankins and associates in 1990, but two patients developed pinpoint rectovaginal fistulas after early repair. Secondary repair in both cases was successful. The results of early repair of dehiscence after mediolateral episiotomies was reported by Monberg and Hammen.

Three types of closure are recommended for repair of a complete perineal laceration: the layered method of repair, the Warren flap procedure, and the Noble operation.

The Warren flap method was devised to avoid a mucosal incision in the anus, to provide a pedicle graft of vaginal mucosa for enlargement of the perineal skin,

and to provide a more cosmetic result to the perineal body. However, the Warren technique offers no particular improvement in the results of the surgical correction of the muscular defect that produced the anal incontinence. The major advantage of the procedure is that a suture line is not created in the anal mucosa. With the Warren technique, the vaginal mucosa is turned backward and utilized as the new portion of the anterior wall of the end of the anal canal. The anal sphincter is then reapproximated over the inner portion of the vaginal flap, which is attached to the anal mucosa. The Warren flap procedure is still used today, but it is used less frequently than it was over a century ago when it was first described (1882).

The Noble operation, or anal pull-through procedure, as it is more commonly called, also avoids the presence of a suture line in the anal mucosa. The procedure was described originally in 1902 by Noble, but received little attention until redescribed independently by Mengert in 1955. Noble's original claims for the operation in the surgical era before the availability of antibiotics, blood banks, and modern advances in general anesthesia included (1) elimination of the danger of infection or fecal matter from the rectum in the surgical wound, (2) avoidance of the tediousness of dissecting a vaginal flap, (3) minimal blood loss, and (4) uniformly good results. The most important advantage is the absence of a suture line in the anterior rectal wall.

Layered Method of Repair of Complete Perineal Laceration

A transverse or crescent perineal incision is used at the junction of the posterior vaginal wall and anal mucosa. The lateral margins of the incision are extended to the region of the perineal dimple created by the retracted external sphincter, and a midline incision is made along the lower half of the posterior vaginal wall (Fig. 34-13A).

The edges of the vaginal and rectal mucosa are grasped separately with Allis clamps, and the rectal wall is separated in the midline from the anterior vaginal mucosa with careful Metzenbaum scissors dissection. The dissection is carried laterally by sharp dissection to the region of the external anal sphincter.

The external sphincter is identified by a fibrous band that is retracted against the lateral wall of the anal canal (Fig. 34-13B). The exact anatomic margins of the external sphincter are frequently difficult to ascertain. Usually, the base and intermediate loops of the external sphincter are disrupted in a complete perineal laceration; the top loop (puborectalis muscle) is attached to the inferior rami of the symphysis pubis.

To test the function of the retracted sphincter, the Allis clamps containing the muscle bundles are brought

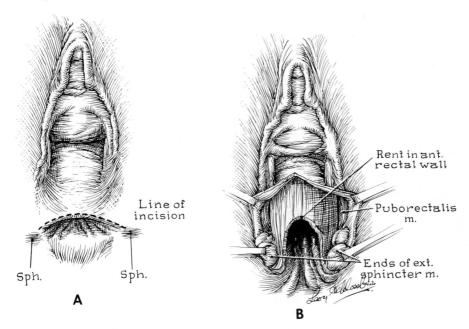

Figure 34–13. Layered closure of a complete third-degree perineal laceration with anal extension. *A,* A small transverse incision is made at the junction of the vaginal and rectal mucosa. A midline incision is made in the mucosa of the lower one-half of the posterior vaginal wall. *B,* The ends of the lower portion of the anal sphincter have been identified and grasped with Allis clamps.

together in the midline, and the sphincter action is tested by inserting a double-gloved index finger into the rectum. If necessary, the clamps should be readjusted to incorporate more of the retracted muscle bundles, until the constricted effect of the reapproximated sphincter can be demonstrated.

Any scar tissue is excised from the margins of the rectal mucosa, and the defect in the anal mucosa is closed using a continuous suture of No. 3-0 delayed-absorbable material (Fig. 34-13C). If interrupted sutures are used as the initial layer, a small opening can be left in the mucosa through which colon bacteria and feces can enter and interfere with tissue healing. A submucosal suture would be ideal, but because of the friability of the tissue, residual tearing could occur. Complete approximation of the anal mucosa by full-thickness suturing of the mucosa is the safest method. As the mucosa margins are approximated, the initial mucosal suture line is inverted by a second supporting suture that is placed into the muscle layer of the anal canal, using interrupted sutures through the submucosa and muscularis.

The sphincter ends are then united in the midline with interrupted delayed-absorbable or permanent sutures (Fig. 34-13D). Number 0 or No. 1 delayed-absorbable suture material has the advantage of excellent tensile strength while avoiding a permanent foreign-body reaction should the operative site become infected with colon bacilli. Some surgeons prefer a permanent suture, preferably medium-strength silk or braided silicone-treated polyester (Tycron). Three or four sutures are used to approximate the sphincter

muscle. Then the dissection is continued laterally along the anal canal and rectal wall to free the medial borders of the puborectalis muscles.

An important component of this procedure is careful identification and adequate plication of the puborectalis muscle, which serves as the top loop of the external sphincter. A series of interrupted, delayed-absorbable sutures should be placed to bring the muscle to the midline as high as possible without constricting the diameter of the vaginal canal. Extending this procedure to the midportion of the vagina can produce excellent anatomic support for the underlying anal canal and rectal neck. Because the hiatus of the puborectalis sling requires so much support, the preferred procedure is to approximate the medial margins of these muscles along the lower half of the vagina, until the sutures produce narrowing of the vaginal lumen. Delayed-absorbable sutures of No. 0 or No. 1 strength are used and provide excellent support to the underlying anorectal canal.

Further support and elevation of the perineal body are provided by plicating the transverse perineal muscle separately. Following this step, the redundant vaginal mucosa is excised, and the remaining mucosa is approximated in the midline with a continuous running No. 2-0 suture. One further effort is made to reestablish and elevate the perineal body by making a wide plication of the fascia of the perineal body followed by a subcuticular closure of the perineal skin (Fig. 34-13E). Excessive narrowing of the vaginal introitus should be avoided because it can produce a painful midline scar and troublesome dyspareunia.

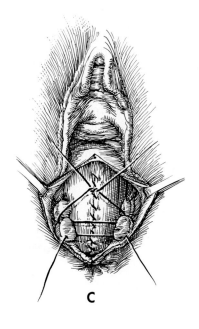

C

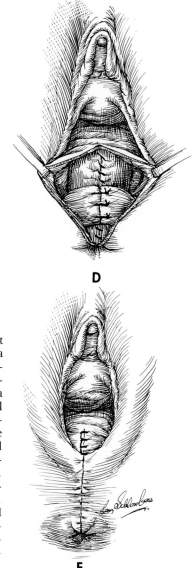

D

E

Figure 34–13 (continued) *C,* The rent in the anal mucosa has been closed with a continuous No. 3-0 delayed-absorbable suture. A second, supporting layer of interrupted sutures is placed in the submucosa and inner muscularis to invert the mucosal edges into the bowel lumen. *D,* After approximating the base loop and possibly the intermediate loop of the external anal sphincter with two or three delayed-absorbable or permanent sutures as shown in *C,* the puborectalis muscles are brought together with deep interrupted No. 0 or No. 1 sutures. *E,* The vaginal mucosa is closed with a continuous lock stitch of No. 2-0 delayed-absorbable suture, which is continued subcuticularly to approximate the perineal skin.

Paradoxical Relaxing Incision

In 1937, Miller and Brown proposed making a paradoxical incision in the inferior portion of the anal sphincter at 5 or 7 o'clock to relax the tension on the suture line. The modern method of anatomic dissection and repair of the entire external sphincter adds enough support to the sphincter muscles to make a paradoxical relaxing incision unnecessary. The procedure is fraught with physiologic risk, such as poor healing of the base loop of the sphincter, with the potential for postoperative anal incontinence of gas and liquid feces.

Preoperative Care

Preparation of the entire gastrointestinal tract with antibiotics is unnecessary. Four days prior to surgery, patients should begin using a laxative. During the 48-hour preoperative period, patients should be placed on a clear liquid diet, and stool softeners and laxatives should be continued to empty the colon completely of fecal material. Alternatively, an oral bowel slush preparation (Golytely) may be given on the day before surgery is scheduled. The bowel is then emptied prior to surgery, with enemas repeated until the return is clear.

The last enema given should be a retention enema of 2% neomycin in 200 ml normal saline.

Postoperative Feeding

Oral feedings should not begin postoperatively for approximately 48 hours, during which time intravenous fluid replacement is maintained and bowel function is gradually restored. Patients should begin with clear liquids for 24 hours, with progression to a soft, low-residue diet for an additional 48 hours. A regular diet may be started when patients can intentionally pass gas or following the first soft bowel movement. To keep the terminal rectum and anal canal free of fecal material for as long as possible following surgery, the use of laxatives should be avoided for 4 or 5 days, until the mucosal suture line has healed adequately and the reparative process is well established. Stool softeners are advisable.

Warren Flap Operation for Complete Third-Degree Tear

An inverted V-shaped incision is made in the posterior vaginal mucosa, outlining the flap that is to be turned down. The lower ends of the incision should be just lateral to the dimples caused by retracted sphincter ends (Fig. 34-14A). The length of the flap should measure a minimum of 3 cm to provide sufficient vaginal mucosa to be incorporated into the anal canal and to cover the reconstructed perineal body.

Taking care to avoid injuring the bowel wall, the flap of mucosa is dissected free from the top downward (Fig. 34-14B), stopping short of the margin between the vaginal and the anal mucosa. If this margin is perforated, the blood supply to the mucosal flap would be compromised, thereby nullifying the advantage of the flap technique. The properly demarcated flap allows the areas overlying the sphincter ends to be denuded. The flap is grasped with two mucosal Allis clamps and is turned down to hang over the anus.

The sphincter ends are then dissected free, using Allis clamps for traction. The ends are sutured together with three or four interrupted stitches of No. 1 delayed-absorbable or Tycron sutures (Fig. 34-14C). Sphincter tone should be tested using a double-gloved finger. If the tone is not satisfactory, a further attempt should be made to find and approximate more sphincter fibers.

The lateral aspects of the puborectalis muscle are identified, and the medial margins are brought together with a series of interrupted sutures of No. 1 delayed-absorbable material for reinforcement (Fig. 34-14D). Then the muscles are plicated in the midline as high as possible, in the manner described for the layered technique, using No. 0 or No. 1 delayed-absorbable sutures.

Closure of the vaginal mucosa is carried out as in an ordinary perineal repair. Interrupted plication stitches of No. 0 delayed-absorbable suture are used to advance the fascia and shorten the muscle fibers of the perineal body, which strengthens the external sphincter as well. The margins of the vaginal mucosa and graft are approximated in the midline by a continuous lock stitch of No. 2-0 delayed-absorbable suture. The tip end of the vaginal mucosal flap should not be trimmed too closely, even though it protrudes somewhat from the repaired perineal body; it will retract as healing is completed (Fig. 34-14E).

Noble Procedure for Complete Perineal Laceration

The initial incision is made near the dimple in the lateral aspect of the perineum caused by the retracted external anal sphincter musculature. The incision follows the margin of the anal mucosa, along the anatomic defect in the rectovaginal septum. A small margin of vaginal mucosa is left attached to the anal wall for traction because the anal mucosa is so friable (Fig. 34-15A).

Allis clamps are placed along the margin of the anal canal, and sharp dissection with fine Metzenbaum scissors is used to separate carefully the anal wall from the overlying vaginal mucosa. Any remnants of the lower loops of the external anal sphincter, particularly the base loop, should be preserved and separated from the underlying anal wall (Fig. 34-15B). The lateral wall of the anal canal should not be extensively mobilized, because doing so would cause bleeding from the inferior hemorrhoidal vessels. Using a midline incision, the vaginal mucosa is separated from the anal and lower rectal wall to the areas of the lateral vagina and underlying levator muscles. The dissection must extend into the middle or upper one third of the vagina to permit adequate mobilization of the rectum and lower end of the anal canal without undue tension, and to prevent retraction of the reconstructed wall of the anal canal.

Mobilization of the anterior anorectal wall allows the wall to be withdrawn outside the margin of the anal orifice without difficulty (see Fig. 34-15B). Then the retracted and obscured margins of the lower loops of the external anal sphincter are dissected from the lateral margins of the anal wall, with careful attention to the base loop located directly beneath the anal mucosa and perianal skin. With an Allis clamp placed on the attenuated muscle and its capsule, sharp dissection is continued to free both ends of the external sphincter muscle with its surrounding fascial capsule.

Once the ends meet in the midline with traction on the Allis clamps, the sphincter is approximated with at

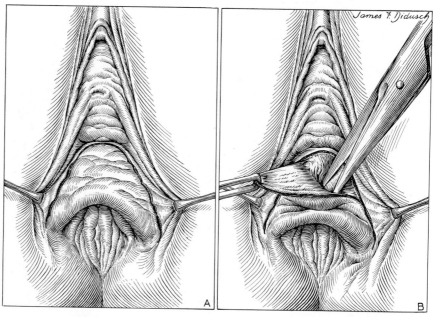

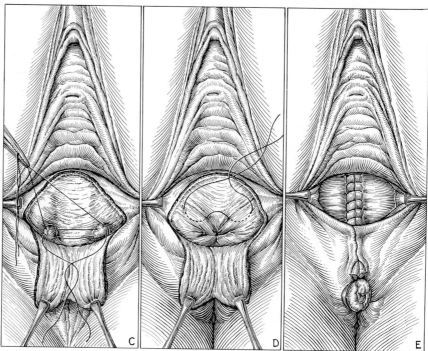

Figure 34–14. Warren flap operation for complete third-degree tear. *A*, Line of incision, outlining flap of vaginal mucosa. *B*, The flap is dissected free and turned back. *C*, The flap is retracted downward. The ends of the sphincter are delivered and are sutured with delayed-absorbable sutures. *D*, The sphincter ends have been united, and the puborectalis muscles are approximated in the midline with No. 0 delayed-absorbable sutures. *E*, The vaginal incision has been closed with a continuous lock stitch that is continued subcuticularly over the perineum. The margins of the flap are included in the continuous suture, which may create a peaked appearance, temporarily, to the perineal skin. If redundant, it may be trimmed.

least three or four interrupted No. 0 delayed-absorbable or polydioxanone sutures (Fig. 34-15*C*).

Although the upper loop of the sphincter is rarely traumatized by a complete perineal tear, plication of the puborectalis muscle high in the midline provides additional support to the rectal inlet and reestablishes the 90° angle of the rectal neck with the terminal portion of the rectal colon. The suture plication of the puborectalis is continued until there is anatomic evidence of narrowing or constriction of the vaginal canal (Fig. 34-15*D*). If constriction is noticed when the vagina is palpated, the uppermost suture(s) should be removed until a smooth posterior vaginal wall is reestablished.

The transverse perineal muscles and the inferior margins of the bulbocavernosus muscles are reapproximated in the midline with interrupted sutures of No. 0 delayed-absorbable material (Fig. 34-15*E*). Building a high perineal body must not cause narrowing of the

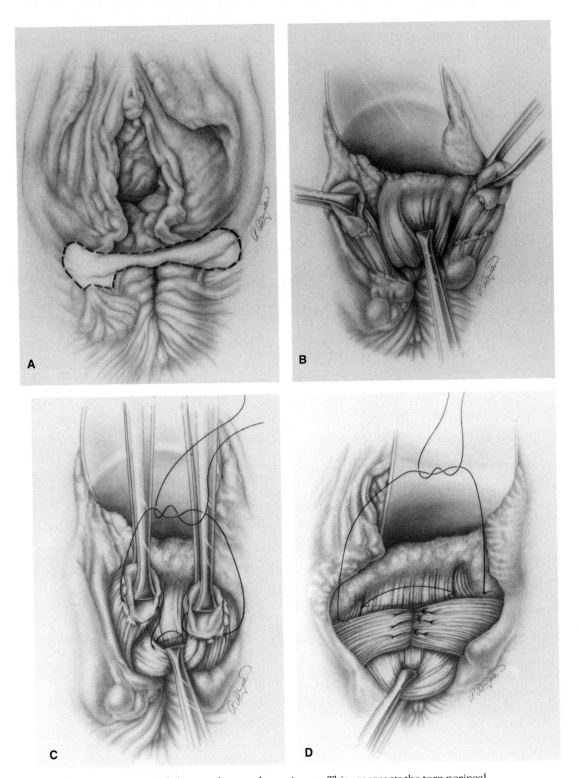

Figure 34–15. *A,* A "butterfly" is noted across the perineum. This represents the torn perineal, anal, and rectal tissue. The ends of the anal sphincter are attached beneath each "butterfly wing." An incision is made at the dotted line. *B,* The "wings" of the "butterfly" are left attached to facilitate dissection of the retracted ends of the anal sphincter. The anterior rectal wall must be mobilized extensively from the posterior vaginal wall to allow it to be pulled down without tension. *C,* Ends of the anal sphincter are trimmed and sutured together and to the fascia of the advanced anterior rectal wall.

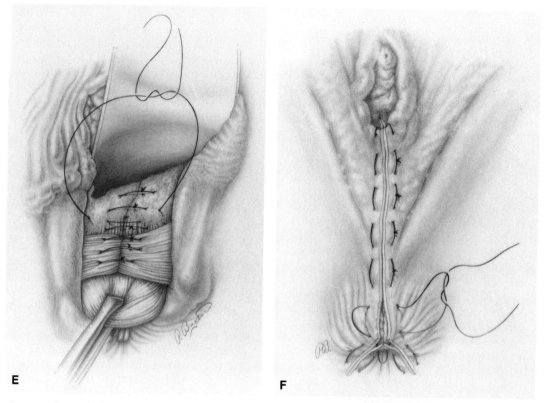

E   F

Figure 34–15 (continued) Several No. 0 polydioxanone sutures are used. *D*, The levator muscles and perirectal fascia are sutured together in the midline. *E*, The transverse perineal muscles and inferior margins of the bulbocavernosus muscles are reapproximated with No. 0 delayed-absorbable sutures. *F*, The vaginal mucosa and perineal skin are closed. No suture line is exposed to the rectal lumen.

vaginal introitus, which would result in introital dyspareunia.

The vaginal mucosa is trimmed, if necessary, and the margins of the posterior vaginal wall are approximated with a continuous lock stitch of No. 2-0 delayed-absorbable suture. The fascia of the perineal body is approximated with vertical mattress sutures that support the perineal repair. The continuous suture is carried over the perineal body as a subcuticular stitch, and the perianal skin is approximated at the midline.

The mobilized anterior wall of the anal canal is now drawn outside the reconstructed anal orifice and sutured without tension to the perianal skin (Fig. 34-15*F*). Then the excess anal mucosa is trimmed. Vertical mattress sutures of No. 0 or No. 2-0 delayed-absorbable suture are used to approximate the broad surface of the anal submucosa to the perianal skin. Any residual separation of the margins of the anal mucosa and perianal skin can be approximated with interrupted sutures.

To avoid the development of a hematoma in the rectovaginal wall, the vagina may be packed firmly with gauze for a period of 24 hours following surgery. Other postoperative procedures are identical with those described for the layered closure and the Warren flap operations.

RECTOVAGINAL FISTULAS

Rectovaginal and anovaginal fistulas result from several different causes. A fistula occurring adjacent to the external sphincter is classified as anovaginal, whereas defects more than 3 cm from the anal orifice are rectovaginal. Considered together, these fistulas occur with sufficient frequency that the operating gynecologist must understand them completely.

Many fistulas occur after an unsuccessful attempt to repair a fourth-degree tear that extends through the anal and lower rectal mucosa. A bridge of tissue or the complete sphincter heals while the previous suture line in the anal canal above the sphincter breaks down. A low rectovaginal or anovaginal fistula of variable size results. Small and moderate-sized fistulas can follow rectal injury during a posterior vaginal repair. A perirectal abscess, when opened spontaneously or surgically, may result in a fistula that opens into the vagina. The unsuccessful repair of a fistula can result in other fistulas with more scar tissue. Some uncommon causes of rectovaginal fistulas are inflammatory bowel disorders such as Crohn's disease and systemic lupus erythematosus, a collagen-vascular disorder that produces ulceration in the vagina and rectum, with subsequent breakdown of the rectovaginal septum.

When surgery and chronic pelvic disease are combined, the risk of rectovaginal fistula is increased. For example, if the cul-de-sac has become involved in an obliterative disease process such as endometriosis, chronic inflammation, or pelvic abscess, the chances of injuring the rectum during a total hysterectomy are increased and a fistula may form at the very top of the vagina. The risk of rectal injury is also greater when hysterectomy follows external or intracavitary irradiation in patients with uterine cancer and obliterative cul-de-sac disease. High rectovaginal fistulas also result from irradiation treatment for cervical or endometrial cancer. The fistulas are caused by radiation injury to the rectum adjacent to the posterior vaginal fornix. Rarely, destruction of carcinomatous tissue that has invaded the rectovaginal septum may result in a fistulous tract.

A small rectovaginal fistula may be entirely asymptomatic. A slight leakage of gas and seepage of feces may not be detected in the vaginal discharge. When the fistula is a bit larger, the escape of gas may be the only complaint, or there may be the complaint of fecal odor in the vaginal discharge. When the fistula is large, the entire bowel content may be evacuated through the vagina, an extremely distressing condition. As occurs with a fourth-degree perineal laceration, voluntary constipation may reduce the amount of leakage.

The diagnosis of a rectovaginal fistula is usually very simple. By spreading the labia, a low fistula can be disclosed; a high fistula can be seen using a duckbill speculum. The opening in the vagina may be filled with feces, or, if the bowel has been emptied recently, the dark red rectal mucosa may be seen at the fistulous opening, contrasting with the lighter vaginal mucosa.

When the fistula is small, it may be difficult to locate the opening between the rectum and the vagina, but the location of both orifices is essential for complete care. A small probe can be pushed through the fistula from the vaginal side, and the tip may be felt on rectal examination. Instillation of methylene blue through the vaginal orifice may aid in proctoscopic visualization of the rectal orifice.

A very special challenge exists when Crohn's disease causes a rectovaginal fistula. The patient is often a young adult with mucoid or bloody diarrhea, abdominal tenderness, sepsis, and weight loss when the disease is active. Multiple fistulas between loops of intestine or between the intestine and abdominal wall may develop. Fistulas between the ileum and vagina may occur. Although most commonly found in the small intestine, the large bowel and rectum can also be involved. Rectal and anal lesions are more common when the colon is involved. Multiple perianal, perirectal, and rectovaginal fistulas with or without perirectal abscess may develop. Among 266 patients with regional enteritis of Crohn's disease, Van Patter and associates from the Mayo Clinic found 10 patients with rectovaginal fistulas. In other reports, the incidence has been higher. Although the disease is usually clinically evident before the fistula is diagnosed, on occasion the fistula may develop first, with other manifestations of the disease developing later.

Rectovaginal fistulas are usually tender and may be multiple or single in Crohn's disease. A single vaginal orifice may be connected by many circuitous tracts to multiple anal or rectal orifices, with microabscesses along the tracts. Sometimes multiple sinuses in the perineum can be outlined with methylene blue injection of an orifice in the vagina or on the perineum. Excision of all perineal sinuses and closure of all rectal orifices requires tedious and meticulous dissection and magnification provided by surgical loupes. A transverse transperineal approach should be used to preserve the external anal sphincter muscle. A labial fat pad may be used to bring in new blood supply and fill the defect. A drain should not be used. Preoperative diversion of the fecal stream with a colostomy is not usually necessary unless the fistula is located high in the vagina.

There has been a generally pessimistic view regarding repair of rectovaginal fistulas whose etiology is Crohn's disease. However, the experience at Duke University Medical Center, reported by Bandy and associates, indicates good results in 9 of 10 patients with primary repair. These authors emphasize that the selection of patients, the proper timing of repair, and the participation of an interested gastroenterologist are the most important factors in achieving a successful result. Only patients in clinical remission, with favorable sigmoidoscopic findings, should be considered for repair of fistulas.

In general, colostomy for diversion of the fecal stream is not necessary before repairing a simple rectovaginal fistula in the lower vagina, especially one resulting from obstetric trauma. A colostomy may be necessary if the fistula is large, located high in the vagina, or due to irradiation. Before a colostomy is done, one must be certain that the fistula communicates between the vagina and the lower large bowel. A colostomy is of no value in a patient with an enterovaginal fistula. A fistula between the ileum and the vagina usually causes intense excoriation and redness of vaginal and vulvar tissues because of irritation by secretions from the small intestine. A barium enema, gastrointestinal series with small bowel followthrough, colonoscopy, and/or injection of radiopaque dye through the vaginal orifice of the fistula may be needed to identify the intestinal segment involved. Some intestinal fistulas in the upper vagina may not be rectovaginal fistulas.

Surgical Repair of Rectovaginal Fistulas

The surgical cure of a rectovaginal fistula may be exceedingly simple or quite complicated. Small fistulas may be closed by two or more purse-string sutures (see Fig. 34-16). Regardless of the exact technique of closure, it is desirable to approximate broad tissue surfaces without tension for healing. A standard technique for closure of a typical fistula is layer-for-layer closure (see Fig. 34-17). When the fistula is fairly large and lies just above the sphincter or the perineal bridge, some prefer to cut the bridge, thus converting the fistula into a complete third-degree perineal tear. The complete perineal tear is then repaired by the layered method described in Figure 34-13. The transverse transperineal approach can be used to repair the fistula and preserve an intact anal sphincter (see Fig. 34-19).

A fistula that occurs after irradiation or a fistula with scar tissue from previous surgical attempts often requires a more complicated operation. First, feces should be diverted from the field of operation by performing a temporary sigmoid colostomy, such as the modified Mikulicz procedure (see Chapter 37). A transverse colostomy may also be used, utilizing essentially the same technique. A transverse colostomy is indicated especially in patients who have had heavy pelvic radiation. The bowel is completely transected to ensure complete diversion of feces, and subsequent closure is simple.

After the colostomy, a delay of at least 8 weeks is required before the vaginal repair of the fistula should be attempted, so that the cellulitis accompanying this type of fistula will have sufficient time to heal. The process of tissue revascularization and healing cannot begin until bacterial contamination from feces passing through the fistulous tract is eliminated by a colostomy. Only when there is complete regression of the cellulitis around the fistula and when the adjacent rectovaginal septum is soft and pliable should closure of the fistula be performed.

Most high rectovaginal or sigmoidovaginal fistulas can be repaired using the Latzko technique (Fig. 34-18), but occasionally such a fistula, usually resulting from bowel injury at the time of total hysterectomy, may require transabdominal closure. Rectal fistulas induced by radiation treatment are notoriously resistant to healing after surgical repair, as a result of obliterative endarteritis and limitation of blood supply. The use of the Martius bulbocavernosus muscle or labial fat pad procedure as described for urethrovaginal fistula repair (see Chapter 30) has improved the success rate in the closure of these difficult fistulas by transplanting a vascular graft to the operative site.

Boronow reported excellent results in the management of radiation-induced vaginal fistulas with the labial fat pad (bulbocavernosus fat pad) method of Martius. In 10 patients with radiation-induced rectovaginal fistulas, two of whom also had urethrovesicovaginal fistulas, closure was successful in eight with the first closure. Boronow emphasized five essential steps in the management of radiation-induced rectovaginal fistulas to assure the best results: (1) recurrent or persistent cancer should be excluded with multiple biopsies of the fistula margin; (2) one must wait at least 6 months or longer for the radiation effect of the fistula to become quiescent; (3) the fecal stream should always be diverted by colostomy; (4) a technique to bring in a new source of blood supply into the fistula repair area (bulbocavernosus muscle or labial fat pad, rectus abdominus muscle, omentum, gracilis muscle, sartorius muscle, adductor muscle, gluteus maximus muscle) should be used; (5) finally, a proper repair of the fistula and closure broad surface to broad surface without tension is essential. If these principles are followed closely, even large radiation-induced rectovaginal fistulas can be closed.

To enhance healing by reducing the number of bacteria in the colon and anal canal, patients should be given a rapid bowel preparation before rectovaginal fistula repair. Recently, we have used an oral bowel slush preparation (Golytely) that is much simpler than a 3-day preparation with laxative and antibiotics. The Golytely solution is started about 18–20 hours before the operation is scheduled, say about 12 noon on the day before surgery. Erythromycin 100 mg and neomycin 100 mg are given by mouth at 1 PM, 2 PM, and 10 PM. Rectal irrigations with 200 ml 2% neomycin solution may be given in the early morning of surgery until the fluid returns clear. Obviously, if a colostomy has been done prior to rectovaginal fistula repair, oral bowel preparation is not needed, but neomycin solution should be used to irrigate the lower colon and the rectum.

Postoperatively, the patient's diet is restricted to clear liquids for 3 days followed by a low-residue diet and stool softeners for 3 weeks. For added comfort, the perineum may be exposed to a heat lamp for several days, but hot sitz baths are not used.

Closure of Small Rectovaginal Fistula

An incision is made in the vagina, encircling the small fistulous opening (Fig. 34-16*A*). With fine-pointed scissors, enough vaginal mucosa is dissected free to allow mobilization of the bowel wall and closure of the opening in the bowel by two or three purse-string sutures without tension (Fig. 34-16*B*). The first suture is placed in the submucosal opening, a few millimeters from the mucosal edge, using No. 3-0 delayed-absorbable suture (Fig. 34-16*C*), taking care to avoid perforating the bowel mucosa. The edges of the fistula are inverted into the lumen of the bowel as the purse string is tied. A second purse-string suture is placed around the first in the muscularis (Fig. 34-16*D*). If a third purse-string can be placed without tension, it is used (Fig. 34-16*E*). The perirectal fascia is then approximated in the midline, using interrupted sutures of No. 2-0 delayed-absorbable material (Fig. 34-16*F*). Excess vaginal mucosa is excised, and the mucosa is closed with a continuous lock stitch of No. 2-0 suture (Fig. 34-16*G*).

Another technique of repairing a rectovaginal fistula is illustrated in Figure 34-17. An incision is made around the fistulous opening through the vaginal mucous membrane (Fig. 34-17*A*). The vaginal mucosa is dissected back far enough to permit mobilization of the bowel wall for closure without tension (Fig. 34-17*B*). Since the fistulous opening into the bowel is too large

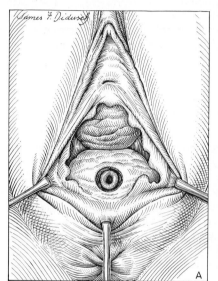
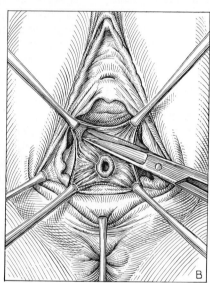
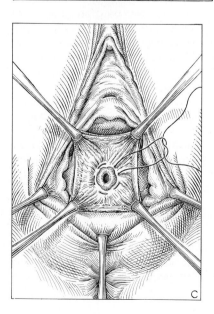
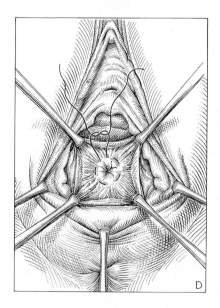

Figure 34–16. Repair of small rectovaginal fistula. *A*, A circular incision through the vaginal mucosa is made about the fistulous opening. *B*, Flaps of vaginal mucosa are dissected free for about 2 cm from the margin of the fistulous opening. *C*, A No. 3-0 delayed-absorbable material purse-string is placed about the fistulous opening. *D*, The first purse-string has been tied, inverting the fistulous opening. The second purse-string has been placed and is about to be tied.

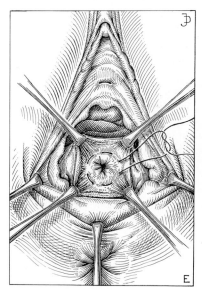
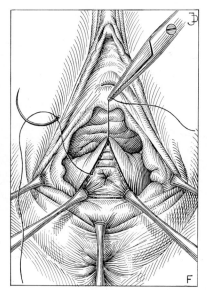
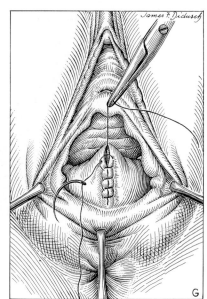

Figure 34–16 (continued) *E*, The second purse-string has been tied, and a third has been placed. *F*, Submucosal–muscularis tissues are approximated with No. 2-0 continuous or interrupted delayed-absorbable sutures. *G*, The mucosa is closed with a continuous lock stitch of No. 2-0 suture.

to be closed by a purse-string, a series of vertical mattress sutures are used (Fig. 34-17C). The bites in the tissue are taken parallel with the edges of the fistula and ideally do not enter the lumen of the bowel. Either No. 3-0 or No. 4-0 delayed-absorbable suture is most suitable for the first layer, which is reinforced by a second layer of deeper interrupted sutures into the muscular wall of the rectum. The second layer of sutures should be approximated gently, using No. 2-0 delayed-absorbable material to bring broad surface of tissue to broad surface for proper healing, and to avoid necrosis.

As an alternative to using vertical mattress sutures, the initial layer can be made with continuous sutures, inverting the edges into the bowel lumen. The second, supporting layer is then made with interrupted mattress sutures, which invert the first layer.

After the second layer of stitches has been tied, the pararectal fascia is approximated over the fistula with No. 2-0 interrupted delayed-absorbable sutures. The puborectalis muscle may also be plicated to add further support to the closure and to correct any significant anal incontinence from damage to the external sphincter. The vaginal mucosa is closed with a continuous No. 2-0 suture. As the midline mucosal suture is placed, the subjacent fascia is picked up with each bite, thus closing all potential dead space.

If several previous operations have been performed without success, or if the fistula has developed because of irradiation, new and healthy tissue with good blood supply should be transposed to the repair site. A labial fat pad can be used, as suggested by Elkins and associates, by Boronow, and by others (see Chapter 30).

Latzko Closure of Rectovaginal Fistula

The Latzko technique of using both the anterior and posterior vaginal walls in the closure of a vesicovaginal fistula is an effective method of closing a high rectovaginal fistula located at the apex of the vagina (Fig. 34-18).

A sufficient area around the fistula must be denuded so that broad surfaces of well-vascularized tissues can be approximated. Incisions are made around the margins of the fistula (Fig. 34-18A). Mucosa from both the anterior and the posterior vaginal walls are removed for a 2–3-cm margin (Fig. 34-18B).

With the first layer of the closure, the edges are inverted into the bowel lumen, using No. 3-0 delayed-absorbable suture (Fig. 34-18C). An alternate and frequently preferable technique for beginning closure is to use a continuous inverting suture for the first layer to assure complete closure of the rectal defect. When a colostomy has preceded the fistula repair, closure may be made by using a continuous suture and not inverting the mucosa into the bowel lumen.

In the second line, the sutures are of the horizontal mattress type; the bite of the needle is taken parallel with the suture line into the rectal musculature and fascia (Fig. 34-18D). In the last step the vaginal mucosal edges are brought together with mattress sutures of No.

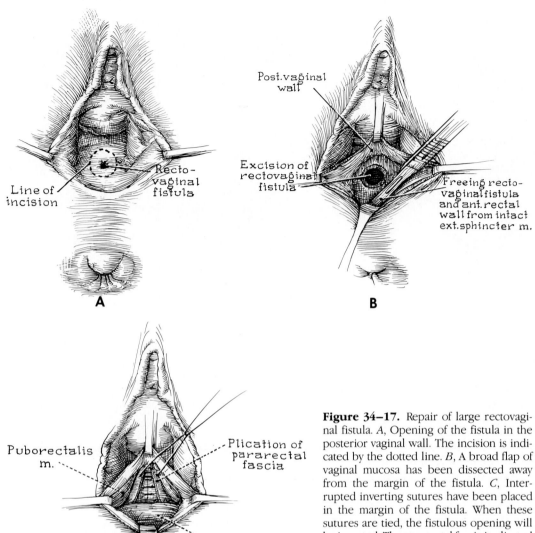

Figure 34–17. Repair of large rectovaginal fistula. *A*, Opening of the fistula in the posterior vaginal wall. The incision is indicated by the dotted line. *B*, A broad flap of vaginal mucosa has been dissected away from the margin of the fistula. *C*, Interrupted inverting sutures have been placed in the margin of the fistula. When these sutures are tied, the fistulous opening will be inverted. The pararectal fascia is plicated over the rectal wall to support the initial suture layers. The puborectalis muscle should be plicated to add further support to the anal canal and perineal body.

2-0 delayed-absorbable material (Fig. 34-18*E*). Delayed-absorbable sutures are now used instead of silver wire. The nonreactive delayed-absorbable suture material has proven to be as effective as silver wire and produces less necrosis of the vaginal mucosa and no discomfort to the patient.

Technique of Transverse Transperineal Repair of Low Rectovaginal Fistulas

In 1886, Lawson Tait adapted his technique of complete perineorrhaphy to repair of rectovaginal fistulas

with satisfactory results. The perineum was incised transversely midway between the anus and vulva. The vaginal wall was separated from the rectal wall well above the upper limit of the fistula. The fistula openings in the vaginal and rectal wall were sutured separately and the perineum was reconstructed.

Although the Tait operation was used with success at the turn of the century, it has been almost forgotten in recent years. The most common method of repair at present is by an episioproctotomy followed by a layered closure similar to the repair of a fourth-degree perineal laceration. A major disadvantage of this procedure is

(*text continues on page 976*)

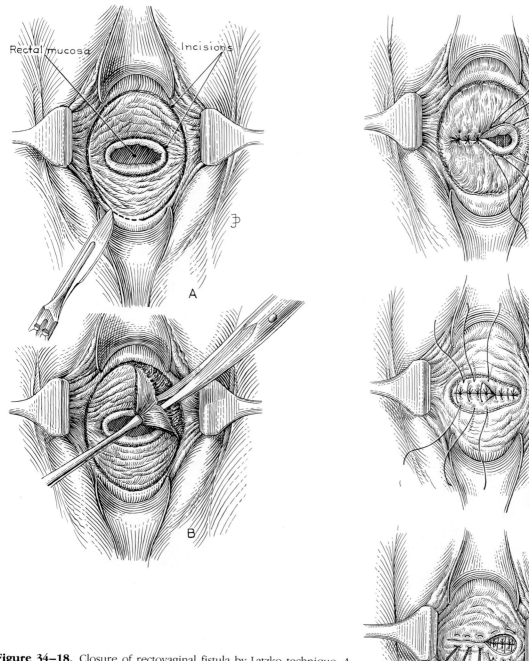

Figure 34–18. Closure of rectovaginal fistula by Latzko technique. *A*, Incisions around margins of fistula. *B*, Excision of mucosa from anterior and posterior vaginal walls. *C*, The first line of sutures is placed, inverting the edge into the rectal lumen. *D*, The first line of sutures has been placed and tied. The second line of sutures is being placed into the rectal musculature and fascia. Note horizontal mattress sutures in the second layer. *E*, Vertical or horizontal mattress sutures of delayed-absorbable suture form the third layer of closure.

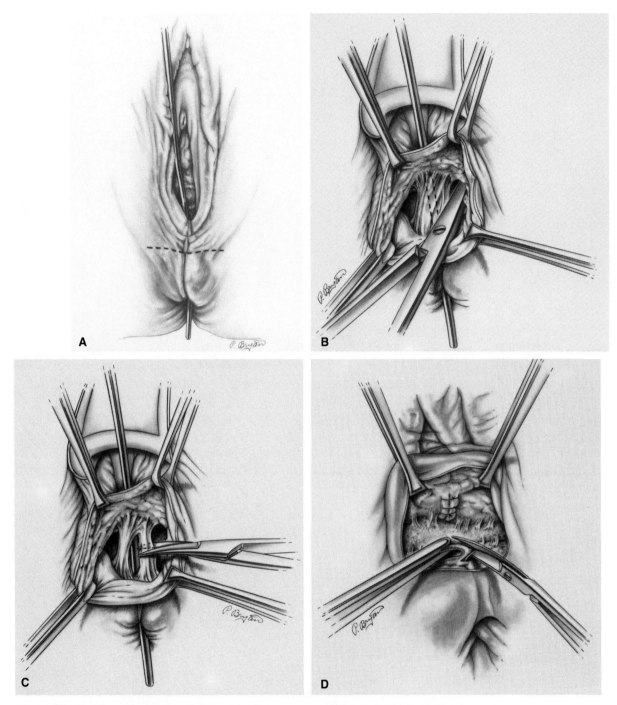

Figure 34–19. Transverse transperineal repair of low rectovaginal fistula. *A*, The fistula tract has been identified with a wire probe. The dotted line indicates where the transverse perineal incision should be made. Injection of the perineal tissues with sterile saline prior to making the incision will facilitate the dissection. *B*, Dissection between the anterior rectal wall and posterior vaginal wall is carried laterally well around the fistula with the scissors. Wide mobilization is necessary. *C*, The fistula tract is completely transected by sharp dissection. The posterior vaginal wall and anterior rectal wall are widely mobilized, especially superior and lateral to the fistula. *D*, The vaginal mucosa and subvaginal fascia have been closed longitudinally. Scar tissue from the margin of the rectal orifice of the fistula is being removed sharply.

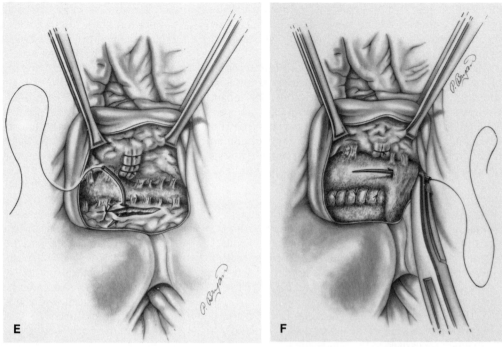

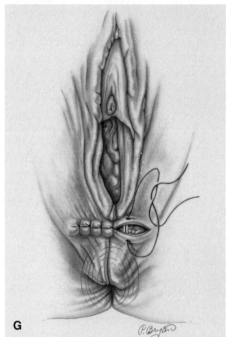

Figure 34–19. (continued) *E*, The anterior rectal wall defect is closed transversely with interrupted sutures of 3-0 vicryl. The first suture is placed beyond the lateral margin of the fistula orifice. Because of the wide mobilization of tissues, the margins of the defect are clearly visible. *F*, Tissues of the perineal body, including the puborectalis muscle, are approximated in the midline with mattress sutures of 2-0 Vicryl, reinforcing the closure of the fistula. *G*, The perineal skin is closed with interrupted sutures of 4-0 Vicryl.

the requirement that an intact anal sphincter, usually present, be transected and then repaired, which may result in improper healing and scarring with impairment of sphincter function.

The transverse transperineal approach to the repair of low rectovaginal fistulas, which preserves the anal sphincter, is superior to episioproctotomy for repair. Goligher used the transperineal approach for rectovaginal fistula repair in five patients, with successful results in all patients. There is merit in preserving an intact and properly functioning anal sphincter, as evidenced by the description of Bornemeier in distinctive prose:

> You can damage, deform, ruin, remove, abuse, amputate, maim, or mutilate every structure in and around the anus except one. That structure is the sphincter ani. There is not a muscle or structure in the body that has a more keenly developed sense of alertness and ability to accommodate itself to varying situations.
>
> They say that man has succeeded where the animals fail because of the clever use of his hands, yet when compared to the hands, the sphincter ani is far superior. If you place into your cupped hands a mixture of fluid, solid, and gas and then through an opening at the bottom try to let only the gas escape, you will fail. Yet the sphincter ani can do it! The sphincter apparently can differentiate between solid, fluid, and gas. It apparently can tell whether its owner is alone or with someone; whether standing up or sitting down; whether its owner has his [her] pants off or on. No other muscle in the body is such a protector of the dignity of man, yet so ready to come to his relief. A muscle like this is worth protecting.

After careful pelvic examination in which the fistula tract is delineated, the patient is prepared and draped in the dorsal lithotomy position. The perineal tissues are injected with sterile normal saline solution to facilitate dissection. We do not recommend adding a vasoconstricting agent (epinephrine, vasopressin) to the injection solution, because such agents can produce tissue ischemia and interfere with local host defense mechanisms against infection.

A transverse incision is made across the perineal body above the anal sphincter with the scalpel (Fig. 34-19A). The perineal skin is mobilized superiorly by sharp dissection. Dissection between the anterior rectal wall and posterior vaginal wall is carried laterally well around the fistula and continued superiorly several centimeters above the fistula (Fig. 34-19B). Sterile normal saline is injected repeatedly as the dissection is continued superiorly to facilitate dissection in the appropriate

tissue planes. Operating through the transverse perineal incision, the fistula tract is completely transected by sharp dissection (Fig. 34-19C). The posterior vaginal wall and anterior rectal wall are widely mobilized, especially above the fistula, where the vagina and rectum are loosely connected.

Scar tissue from the margin of the vaginal orifice of the fistula is removed and the vaginal mucosa is approximated longitudinally with interrupted 3-0 delayed-absorbable sutures. Interrupted sutures are then placed on the undersurface of the posterior vaginal wall to reinforce the closure with a second layer.

Scar tissue from the margin of the fistula orifice in the anterior rectal wall is removed sharply (Fig. 34-19D). The anterior rectal wall defect is closed transversely with interrupted 3-0 delayed-absorbable sutures, with the first suture placed beyond the lateral margin of the fistula orifice (Fig. 34-19E). These sutures should invert the rectal mucosa without tension. A second layer of interrupted sutures is placed in the anterior rectal wall transversely, imbricating the first line of sutures and reinforcing the closure.

Tissues of the perineal body, including the puborectalis muscle, are next approximated in the midline with 2-0 delayed-absorbable sutures (Fig. 34-19F). This provides an additional layer of tissue between the anterior rectal wall and posterior vaginal wall and reinforces the closure of the fistula. If needed, a bulbocavernosus flap can be mobilized and transposed beneath the posterior vaginal wall. This provides another layer of tissue between the vagina and rectum and introduces additional blood supply, should these tissues be poorly vascularized because of previous scarring, irradiation, or inflammatory bowel disease. Any necessary external anal sphincter repair can also be done at this time.

The subcutaneous tissue of the perineum is approximated with interrupted sutures of 3-0 Vicryl. The skin is closed with interrupted sutures of 4-0 Vicryl (Fig. 34-19G).

Postoperatively, the patient's diet is restricted to clear liquids for 3 days, followed by a low-residue diet and stool softeners for 3 weeks. The perineum is exposed to a heat lamp three times a day for several days.

Transverse transperineal repair of low rectovaginal fistulas of various etiologies was done in 20 patients in our department at Emory University. In all, including two patients with Crohn's disease, the repair was successful.

The transverse transperineal approach for rectovaginal fistula repair has many advantages over more conventional methods of repair. Adequate dissection of the posterior vaginal wall and anterior rectal wall with wide mobilization of tissue and transection of the fistula tract is facilitated with this technique. At least five layers of tissue are interposed during the repair for a secure closure. Initially, the vaginal mucosa is closed followed by the subvaginal fascia. The margins of the rectal orifice are clearly visible for a meticulous closure. Adequate mobilization allows the anterior rectal wall to be folded over to reinforce the first row of sutures, approximating broad surface to broad surface of the rectal wall and perirectal fascia in at least two layers. The medial margins of the puborectalis muscles can be reapproximated in the midline over the repair, making it even more secure. If the anal sphincter is torn or weak, it can be repaired through the same incision. If the anal sphincter is intact, it can be preserved and not be subjected to injury and scarring caused by transection and subsequent repair.

Bibliography

Aartsen EJ, Sindram IS. Repair of the radiation induced rectovaginal fistula without or with interposition of the bulbocavernosus muscle (Martius procedure). Eur J Surg Oncol 1988;14:171.

Amreich J. Aetiologie und Operation des Scheidenstumpf prolpases. Wien Klin Wochenschr 1951;63:74.

Ayoub SF. Anatomy of the external anal sphincter in man. Acta Anat 1979;105:25.

Bandy LC, Addison A, Parker RT. Surgical management of rectovaginal fistulas in Crohn's disease. Am J Obstet Gynecol 1983;147:359.

Barton JR. A rectovaginal fistula—cured. Am J Med Sci 1840;26:305.

Bastiaanse MA. Bastiaanse's method for surgical closure of very large irradiated fistulae of the bladder and rectum. In: Youssef AF, ed. Gynecological urology. Springfield, Ill.: Charles C Thomas, 1960.

Bastiaanse MA, Sindram IS. Surgical closure of very large fistulae of the bladder and rectum due to radium therapy. Virginia Med Monthly 1960;87:547.

Berek JS, Lagasse LD, Nacker NF, et al. Levator ani transposition for anal incompetence secondary to sphincter damage. Obstet Gynecol 1982;59:108.

Berglas G, Rubin IC. Study of the supportive structures of the uterus by levator myography. Surg Gynecol Obstet 1953;76:677.

Birnbaum W. A method of repair for a common type of traumatic incontinence of the anal sphincter. Surg Gynecol Obstet 1948;87:716.

Bornemeier WC. Sphincter protecting hemorrhoidectomy. Am J Proctol 1960;11:48.

Boronow RC. Management of radiation-induced vaginal fistulas. Am J Obstet Gynecol 1971;100:1.

Byron RL, Ostergard DR. Sartorius muscle interposition for the treatment of the radiation-induced vaginal fistula. Am J Obstet Gynecol 1969;104:104.

Denny-Brown D, Robertson EG. An investigation of the nervous control of defecation. Brain 1935;58:256.

Elkins TE, DeLancey JOL, McGuire EJ. The use of modified Martius graft as an adjunctive technique in vesicovaginal and rectovaginal fistula repair. Obstet Gynecol 1990;75:727.

Emge LA, Durfee RB. Pelvic organ prolapse—4000 years of treatment. Clin Obstet Gynecol 1966;9:997.

Funt MI, Thompson JD, Birch H. Normal vaginal axis. South Med J 1978;71:1534.

Gabriel WB. The principles and practice of rectal surgery. 5th ed. London: HK Lewis, 1963.

Garlock JG. The care of an intractable vesicovaginal fistula by the use of a pedicled muscle flap. Surg Gynecol Obstet 1928;47:255.

Garry RC. Responses to stimulation of the caudal end of the large bowel in the cat. J Physiol 1933;78:208.

Gaston EA. Physiology of faecal continence. Surg Gynaecol Obstet 1948;87:280.

Goligher J. Surgery of the anus, rectum and colon. 5th ed. London: Baillier Tindall, 1984:208.

Goligher JC, Leacock AG, Brossy JJ. Surgical anatomy of anal canal. Br J Surg 1955;43:51.

Graham JB. Vaginal fistulas following radiotherapy. Surg Gynecol Obstet 1965;120:1019.

Green JR, Soohoo SL. Factors associated with rectal injury in spontaneous deliveries. Obstet Gynecol 1989;73:732.

Greenwald JC, Hoexter B. Repair of rectovaginal fistulas. Surg Gynecol Obstet 1978;146:443.

Hankins GDV, Hauth JVC, Gilstrap LC, et al. Early repair of episiotomy dehiscence. Obstet Gynecol 1990;75:48.

Hankins J, ed. Shaw's textbook of operative gynecology. 3rd ed. London: E & S Livingstone, 1968.

Hauth JC, Gilstrap LC, Ward SC, Hankins GDV. Early repair of an external sphincter ani muscle and rectal mucosal dehiscence. Obstet Gynecol 1986;67:806.

Henry MM, Swash M. Coloproctology and the pelvic floor. London: Butterworths, 1985.

Hibbart LT. Surgical management of rectovaginal fistulas and complete perineal tears. Am J Obstet Gynecol 1978;130:139.

Hudson CH. Acquired fistulae between the intestine and the vagina. Ann R Coll Surg Engl 1970;46:20.

Hughes ESR, Johnson WR. Abdominoperineal levator ani repair for rectal prolapse: technique. Aust NZ J Surg 1980;50:117.

Ingleman-Sundberg A. Transplantation of the levator muscles in the repair of complete tear and rectovaginal fistula. Acta Chir Scand 1947;96:313.

Ingleman-Sundberg A. Pathogenesis and operative treatment of urinary fistulae in irradiated tissue. In: Youssef AF, ed. Gynecological urology. Springfield, Ill.: Charles C Thomas, 1960.

Jeffcoate TNA. Posterior colporrhaphy. Am J Obstet Gynecol 1959;77:490.

Kottmeier PK. A physiological approach to the problem of anal incontinence through use of the levator ani as a sling. Surgery 1966;60:1262.

Kuhn RJP, Hollyock VE. Observations on the anatomy of the rectovaginal pouch and septum. Obstet Gynecol 1982;59:445.

Landeen JM, Habal MB. The rejuvenation of the anal sphincteroplasty. Surg Gynecol Obstet 1979;149:78.

Latzko W. Postoperative vesicovaginal fistulas. Am J Surg 1942;58:211.

Leacher TC, Pratt JH. Vaginal repair of the simple rectovaginal fistula. Surg Gynecol Obstet 1967;124:1317.

Mahfouz-Bey N. A new technique in dealing with superior rectovaginal fistulae. J Obstet Gynaecol Br Emp 1934;41:579.

Martius H. Die operative Wiederherstel-lung der vollkommen fehlenden. Harnrohare und des Schliessmuskels derselben. Zentralb Gynakol 1928;52:480.

Martius H. Gebrutsh v Frauenth 1940;2:453.

Martius H. Operative gynecology. In: McCall ML, Bolten KA, eds. Boston: Little, Brown, 1956.

McCall ML. Posterior culdeplasty: surgical correction of enterocele during vaginal hysterectomy. A preliminary report. Obstet Gynecol 1957;10:595.

McCall ML, Bolten KA, ed., trans. Martius gynecological operations with emphasis on topographic anatomy. Boston: Little, Brown, 1956.

Mengert WF, Fish SA. Anterior rectal wall advancement. Obstet Gynecol 1955;5:262.

Miller NF, Brown W. The surgical treatment of complete perineal tears in the female. Am J Obstet Gynecol 1937;34:196.

Milligan ETC, Morgan CN. Surgical anatomy of the anal canal, with special reference to anorectal fistulae. Lancet 1934;2:1150.

Moore FA. Anal incontinence: a reappraisal. Obstet Gynecol 1973;41:483.

Moschcowitz AV. The pathogenesis, anatomy and cure of prolapse of the rectum. Surg Gynecol Obstet 1912;15:7.

Munde P. My experience with the flap-splitting operation for lacerated perineum. Am J Obstet Gynecol 1889;22:673.

Nichols DH. Effects of pelvic relaxation on gynecologic and urologic problems. Clin Obstet Gynecol 1978;21:770.

Nichols DH. Transvaginal sacrospinous fixation. The Pelvic Surgeon 1981;1:10.

Nichols DH. Sacrospinous fixation for massive eversion of the vagina. Am J Obstet Gynecol 1982;142:901.

Nichols DH, Milley PS, Randall CL. Significance of restoration of normal vaginal depth and axis. Obstet Gynecol 1970;36:251.

Nichols DH, Randall CL. Vaginal surgery. 3rd ed. Baltimore: Williams and Wilkins, 1989.

Noble GH. A new technique for complete laceration of the perineum designed for the purpose of eliminating infection from the rectum. Trans Am Gynecol Soc 1902;27:357.

Parks AG. Anorectal incontinence. Proc R Soc Med 1975;68:21.

Parks AG. The biological basis of modern surgical practice. In: Sabiston DC Jr, ed. Davis-Christopher textbook of surgery. 10th ed. Philadelphia: WB Saunders, 1982.

Paul DJ, Lloyd TV. Hindgut duplication with rectovaginal fistula. Obstet Gynecol 1979;54:390.

Pepe F, Panella M, Arihian S, Panella P, Pepe G. Low rectovaginal fistulas. Aust NZ J Obstet Gynecol 1987;27:61.

Richter K. Massive eversion of the vagina: pathogenesis, diagnosis and therapy of the "true" prolapse of the vaginal stump. Clin Obstet Gynecol 1982;25:897.

Rock JA, Woodruff JD. Surgical correction of a rectovaginal fistula. Int J Gynecol Obstet 1982;20:413.

Rosenshein NB, Genadry RR, Woodruff JD. An anatomic classification of rectovaginal septal defects. Am J Obstet Gynecol 1980;137:439.

Rothenbergr DA, Goldberg SM. The management of rectovaginal fistulae. Surg Clin N Am 1983;63:61.

Russell TR, Gallagher DM. Low rectovaginal fistulas. Am J Surg 1977;134:13.

Shafik A. A new concept of the anatomy of the anal sphincter mechanism and the physiology of defaecation. I. The external anal sphincter: a triple-loop system. Invest Urol 1975;12:412.

Shafik A. A new concept of the anatomy of the anal sphincter mechanism and the physiology of defaecation. II. Anatomy of the levator ani muscle with special reference to puborectalis. Invest Urol 1975;13:175.

Shafik A. A new concept of the anatomy of the anal sphincter mechanism and the physiology of defaecation. III. The longitudinal anal muscle: anatomy and role in anal sphincter mechanism. Invest Urol 1976;13:271.

Shafik A. A new concept of the anatomy of the anal sphincter mechanism and the physiology of defaecation. IV. Anatomy of the perianal spaces. Invest Urol 1976;13:424.

Shiono P, Klebanoff MA, Carey JC. Midline episiotomies: more harm than good? Obstet Gynecol 1990;75:765.

Smout CFV, Jacoby F, Lillie EW. Gynaecological and obstetrical anatomy. London: Lewis Publishers, 1969.

Stern HS, Dreznik Z. Rectovaginal fistula. Adv Surg 1987;21:245.

Stirnemann H. Treatment of recurrent rectovaginal fistula. Am J Proctol 1969;20:52.

Symmonds RE, Williams TJ, Lee RA, et al. Posthysterectomy, enterocele, and vaginal vault prolapse. Obstet Gynecol 1981;140:852.

Te Linde RW. Prolapse of the uterus and allied conditions. Am J Obstet Gynecol 1966;94:444.

Thompson JD. Transperineal repair of a rectovaginal fistula. Ob-Gyn Illustrated, New Scotland, N.Y.: Learning Technology, 1985.

Thorp JM, Bowes WA, Brame RG, Cefalo R. Selected use of midline episiotomy: effect on perineal trauma. Obstet Gynecol 1987; 70:260.

Uhlenhuth E, Nolley GW. Vaginal fascia, a myth? Obstet Gynecol 1957;10:349.

Uhlenhuth E, Wolfe WM, Smith EM, et al. The rectogenital septum. Surg Gynecol Obstet 1948;76:148.

Ulfelder H. Entrocele. In: Meigs JV, Sturgis SH, eds. Progress in gynecology. New York: Grune and Stratton, 1970.

Van Patter WN, Bargen JA, Dockerty MB, et al. Regional enteritis. Gastroenterology 1954;26:347.

Ward GG. Operative technique for repair of enterocele and injury to the pelvic floor. Surg Gynecol Obstet 1929;48:399.

Warren JC. A new method of operation for the relief of rupture of the perineum through the sphincter and rectum. Trans Am Gynecol Soc 1882;7:322.

White AJ, Buchsbaum HJ, Blythe JG, Lifshitz S. Use of bulbocavernosus muscle (Martius procedure) for repair of radiation-induced rectovaginal fistulas. Obstet Gynecol 1982;60:114.

Wilcox LS, Strobino DM, Baruffi G, Dellinger WS. Episiotomy and its role in the incidence of perineal lacerations in a maternity center and a tertiary hospital obstetric service. Am J Obstet Gynecol 1989;160:1047.

Zacharin RF. Pulsion enterocele: review of functional anatomy of the pelvic floor. Obstet Gynecol 1980;55:135.

Zacharin RF, Hamilton NT. Pulsion enterocele: long-term results of an abdominoperineal technique. Obstet Gynecol 1980;55:141.

35

Benign and Malignant Diseases of the Breast

GEORGE W. MITCHELL

ANATOMY

The breast occupies the space between the second or third and the sixth or seventh ribs and between the sternum and the midaxillary line (Fig. 35-1). Breast tissue may also extend into the anterior axillary fold along the margin of the insertion of the pectoralis major muscle. Beneath the breast is a thin layer of fibrous connective tissue through which lymphatic extensions pervade the underlying muscles. The glandular tissue lies upon this pectoral fascia and, to a lesser extent, upon a similar layer overlying the serratus anterior muscle. Both the ducts and the acini are enveloped in a rich interlocking network of lymphatic channels that communicate with the larger interlobular channels. Major lymphatic channels from the outer quadrants of the breast extend along the course of the axillary vein and, from the inner, descend through the intercostal spaces to the chain accompanying the internal mammary vessels. Supraclavicular extensions are present but are relatively minor. In the axilla, palpable lymph nodes are characterized as being at levels 1, 2, or 3, depending upon whether they are located just medial to the latissimus dorsi, at the level of the pectoralis minor, or at the sternoclavicular junction (Fig. 35-2). The blood supply is from three sources: the anterior aortic intercostals, the internal mammary artery, and the thoracoacromial trunk of the axillary artery. These considerations are important in the clinical examination of the breast and in understanding the spread of infection or carcinoma.

The areola is a circular pigmented patch of skin, 3–5 cm in diameter, overlying the center of the breast and surrounding the nipple. On its surface are many small, rounded elevations indicating the presence of sebaceous glands, which lubricate the nipple during lactation. Infection in these glands is common, especially during nursing, when the superficial integument is liable to abrasions. The nipple consists of erectile tissue surrounding the ductal network that delivers milk at the time of lactation. Both nipple and areola are rich in blood vessels and lymphatics. Beneath the skin is a fatty subcutaneous tissue investing the glandular parenchyma of the breast and dividing it into partitions, which assist in supporting both glandular and fatty elements. This connective tissue also forms a network for blood vessels and lymphatics and maintains breast contour. The parenchyma consists of 15 or 20 lobes of varying size and roughly pyramidal shape, radiating from the nipple and lying close to the under surface of the corium throughout the breast. The lobes are enclosed in fatty envelopes, which provide a smooth contour. Their close proximity to the skin makes it difficult to excise all breast tissue while leaving the skin intact. Each lobe has its own excretory duct that converges toward a main channel close to the surface of the nipple. The lobes are subdivided further by connective tissue into lobules, and the lobules are subdivided into alveoli, the functional secreting units. As the ducts approach the nipple, they enlarge, forming a sinus or reservoir, which temporarily holds the secretions of the gland (Fig. 35-3). Each duct is surrounded by a column of connective tissue that connects directly with the over-

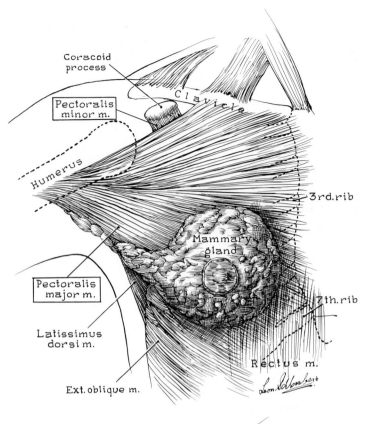

Figure 35–1. Topography of the breast. The breast lies approximately over the midportion of the hemithorax with the tail extending toward the axilla. Ramifications also penetrate the interstices of the underlying muscle. These extensions and the close adherence of the skin to subcutaneous breast tissue make complete subcutaneous mastectomy nearly impossible.

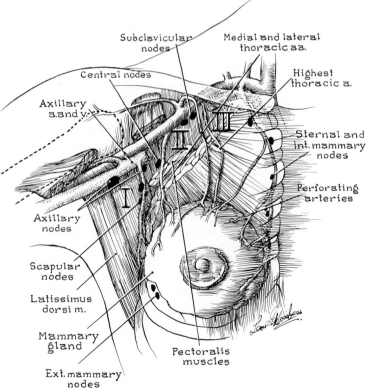

Figure 35–2. Lymphatics and blood supply of the breast. Lymphatic drainage from the outer half of the breast is first to the axillary nodes shown here at Levels 1, 2, and 3. Medial lesions are more likely to metastasize first to the internal mammary chain.

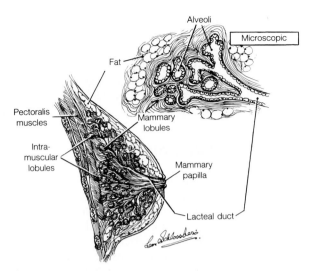

Figure 35–3. Internal structure of the breast. The breast is a large apocrine gland. The secreting parenchyma is composed of lobules containing acini, fat, and fibrous tissue. The ducts drain centrally toward large lacunae located directly beneath the nipple. These act as reservoirs until they receive the impetus for ejection.

lying skin. Enlarging tumors within the lobules exert downward pressure on this relatively rigid periductal connective tissue, causing localized skin retraction.

Fatty tissue comprises a large part of the bulk of the breast, and for this reason breast size may bear little relation to function. A shriveled breast with redundant skin may still contain adequate glandular tissue in a woman in the reproductive age group. Conversely, very large breasts offer no assurance of good function.

The breasts of prepubertal children consist entirely of ducts and connective tissue. At puberty, rudimentary gland buds increase in size and proliferate, the first manifestation of which is a symmetrical palpable enlargement or bud beneath the nipple. Full development requires about 4 years.

During the reproductive years, the amount of fatty tissue increases, along with the development of the lobular structure, and the proportion of fat to glandular tissue has a significant effect on the size and consistency of the breast and the clarity of mammographic studies. Fat offers a translucent background against which abnormal x-ray images can be seen to better advantage. After menopause the lobules and ducts atrophy, leading to sagging, and the size of the breast depends almost solely on the amount of adipose tissue.

At puberty, the development of glandular tissue, the growth of the duct system, and the pigmentation of the areola and nipple are influenced by the rise in estrogen levels. Progesterone affects the growth of the alveolar portion of the breast lobule. Prolactin also makes a

contribution to this process, but the specific nature of its activity is not well understood. During pregnancy the breasts undergo a very active increase in size because of the secretion of large amounts of estrogen, progesterone, and lactogen by the placenta. Prolactin levels increase sharply, possibly a result of the increase in estrogen. Prolactin-inhibiting factor (PIF), produced by the hypothalamus, depresses prolactin secretion and consequent lactation, but suckling suppresses its formation and allows prolactin to remain at a functional level until nursing stops. Suckling also causes release of oxytocin from the posterior pituitary, which, by contraction of perialveolar myoepithelial cells, moves the milk along into the large ductal lacunae from which it is ejected through the nipple.

THE BREAST EXAMINATION

Examination of the female breast should be a routine part of the physical examination of gynecologic patients. Previous examinations by family practitioners, internists, or surgeons in no way alters this obligation or obviates the need to be thorough. The gynecologist has both a professional obligation to the patient and an obligation to protect himself legally by avoiding errors of omission. Sufficient time, not less than 3 minutes, depending upon the size of the breasts, should be set aside for this purpose. Pregnant women are not exempt from this examination.

The breasts are first inspected while the patient is seated on the edge of the table without encumbering clothes or drapes and with her hands clasped behind her head and her shoulders retracted. The presence of skin lesions, striae, erythema, increased vascularity, or abnormal development is noted. Inverted nipples are significant only when they have developed secondarily, and this change is usually unilateral. Secondary inversion of the nipple or dimpling of the skin over any part of the breast suggests the possibility of an underlying malignancy even if no mass is palpable.

The skin of the breast is subject to the same types of disease as the skin elsewhere on the body. Small lesions such as nevi, warts, papillomas, hemangiomas, keratoses, and furuncles, which seem obviously minor, may have a more serious connotation to the patient and should be noted in the record on a breast diagram. More serious lesions like melanoma and Paget's disease, which has a characteristic eczematoid appearance, must be biopsied, as must every abnormality when there is a reasonable doubt about the diagnosis.

Pendulous breasts often conceal beneath their inferior margins an erythematous reaction to chafing, referred to as intertrigo, which may become widespread, indurated, and even ulcerated. Chafe marks along the inner and outer sides of the breast or deep strap marks on the shoulders indicate the use of a bra that does not fit properly or is drawn too tight.

The left breast is often slightly larger than the right, but marked asymmetry sometimes occurs. Anomalies of this type can cause reclusive behavior and distressing neuroses, and appropriate counseling and plastic surgery are indicated in such cases. Variations in the size of normal breasts are a cause of concern to many women and should not be treated casually. Women whose breasts are seriously underdeveloped are candidates for augmentation mammoplasty. Women whose breasts are within the normal range should be discouraged from having surgery.

Breast growth depends upon the presence of adequate numbers of steroid receptors as well as normal cyclic estrogen and progesterone production and is difficult to predict in any individual case. The mammary hypertrophy of adolescents or women in early adult life and the fatty, heavy breasts of the perimenopausal or postmenopausal years may cause distressing psychological problems as well as discomfort in neck, back, and shoulders from the abnormal weight. Reduction mammoplasties afford great relief to these women.

The seated patient next places her hands on her hips and assumes a more relaxed position. The breasts are palpated by gently squeezing them between the examiner's hands, with the fingers perpendicular to the rib cage and with outward traction on the breast to permit accurate evaluation of the tissue close to the chest wall and by pressing the breast tissue against the underlying muscle with the flats of the second, third, and fourth fingers.

With the patient still in the seated position, the lymph nodes in the anterior cervical and supraclavicular and infraclavicular areas are palpated. The examiner then takes the patient's left hand in his left hand and brings her left arm across the front of her chest to relax the pectoralis major muscle while he feels beneath its insertion, in the high axilla and midaxilla, and along the border of the latissimus dorsi for enlarged nodes. A similar examination is done on the right side, and palpable nodes are charted according to estimated level.

The patient is then placed supine on the examining table with a pillow under the shoulder on the side to be examined. First one arm and then the other is extended above her head while the breast tissue is pressed against the chest wall with the flats of the examiner's middle fingers, proceeding clockwise around the full circumference of the breast at its perimeter and gradually moving inward toward the areola. The major ductal system beneath the nipple is reached last. The examination is repeated after the patient has lowered her arms to her sides (Fig. 35-4 *A–E*). Some experts recommend routine "milking" of the breasts from each quadrant

toward the nipple in an attempt to express secretion, but others feel that this is unnecessary in the absence of a history of nipple discharge. When there is such a history, an attempt should be made to determine from which part of the breast the discharge originates or whether it is general and based on a systemic etiology rather than a local lesion.

NIPPLE DISCHARGE

Lactation may persist for many months following the cessation of nursing, and in these individuals prolactin levels tend to remain above normal. In instances unrelated to pregnancy, lactation is referred to as galactorrhea and may be due to a variety of causes, many of which have in common high-normal or elevated prolactin levels. The causes of galactorrhea and nipple discharge due to local conditions are listed in Table 35-1.

Among the more common causes of galactorrhea are breast manipulation, sucking, or some form of athletic activity such as jogging. Improperly fitting garments may compress or inadequately support the breasts, causing discharge. Reflex stimulation of thoracic nerves 2–6 as a result of surgical procedures or trauma may signal the hypothalamus to release prolactin into the blood. The possibility that pituitary micro- or macroadenomas (Forbes-Albright syndrome) may be secreting elevated levels of prolactin must be ruled out, and a serum prolactin level and CT scan of the brain should be obtained for this purpose. The pressure of extrasellar tumors may produce similar effects.

Some women with galactorrhea may have normal ovulatory function, but the abnormal secretion may be associated with other manifestations of an endocrine disorder, including postpartum amenorrhea (Chiari-Frommel syndrome) and non-pregnancy-related amenorrhea (Ahumada-Del Castillo syndrome). Galactorrhea has also been known to occur following hysterectomy and myomectomy and as a result of psychic stimuli. Its cause in these cases is unclear.

Since PIF is thought to be dopamine or a dopamine analogue, it is to be expected that dopamine antagonists would increase prolactin secretion and occasionally produce lactation. A broad range of drugs used for diverse medical conditions may have this effect. Defects in the synthesis of PIF or in receptor binding may also be caused by drug administration. Chronic renal disease and hypothyroidism are associated with elevated prolactin levels that may be mediated through the PIF system.

Other nipple secretions occur in a wide variety of colors and consistencies and are usually due to local disease. From a surgical viewpoint, a frankly bloody or brownish discharge, especially one that is unilateral, is

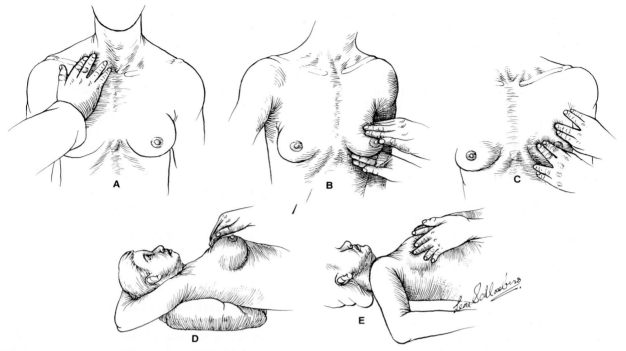

Figure 35–4. *A*, With the patient seated the examiner palpates the supra- and infraclavicular areas and the anterior cervical chain for enlarged nodes. *B*, With the patient seated the examiner squeezes the breast between the fingers of both hands while pulling it outward in order to palpate lesions close to the chest wall. *C*, With the patient seated the examiner palpates the breast tissue with the flats of the fingers of both hands in a clockwise direction, leaving no area untouched. *D*, With the patient supine and the arm extended in order to flatten the breast, the tissue is palpated with the fingers by pressing it gently against the chest wall, again using a plan that will cover the entire breast, including the axillary tail. *E*, The procedure is repeated with the patient's arm at her side to relax the pectoral muscles.

TABLE 35–1
Causes of Nipple Discharge

GALACTORRHEA	OTHER TYPES
Pregnancy and childbirth	Cancer
Neonatal	Intraductal papilloma
Breast manipulation	Ductal ectasia
Surgery	Gross cystic change
Stress	Infection
Drugs*	
Sellar tumors	
Hypothyroidism	
Chronic renal disease	

* Phenothiazines, rauwolfia alkaloids, tricyclic antidepressants, methyldopa, oral contraceptives.

the most significant. A discharge of this type is often first noted by the patient and should be confirmed at the time of examination. A sample should be checked microscopically for red blood cells. Cytologic evaluation of the fluid is often unsatisfactory because of its rela-tively acellular composition, but specimens should initially be sent to the cytology laboratory. They should be taken directly from the nipple on a frosted or albumin-coated slide and fixed carefully to avoid washing away the cells. In the diagnosis of cancer the incidence of false negative cytologic reports is between 15% and 20%, and, if atypical changes are included, the incidence of false positive reports is approximately 20%. Because of this inaccuracy, the presence of a discharge containing blood necessitates surgical exploration of the breast ductal system with biopsy or resection of suspicious lesions regardless of the absence of a palpable mass. Usually an intraductal papilloma is found, and in about 30% of cases atypical cells or malignant changes are present.

The breast may be the site of acute or chronic infection. Abscesses are rare and usually develop during the puerperium or as a result of trauma and hematoma formation. Occasionally, bacterial flora, particularly *Staphylococcus aureus,* may be introduced through the nipple and give rise to disseminated breast disease. Collections of pearly or yellow pus may drain through the duct system to the nipple, but such drainage is often inadequate, and incision and drainage are required. Because of the possibility of an associated carcinoma, biopsy of the abscess wall should be done at this time. In cases of widely disseminated acute infection, subcutaneous excision of all or large portions of the breast tissue under antibiotic coverage may be necessary, preserving the skin for the insertion of a prosthesis later.

Chronic infection is present in ductal ectasia, a common condition during the perimenopausal and menopausal years. The ductal changes are caused by the inspissation of secreted material, with the development of intraductal and interstitial infiltration of plasma cells and atrophy of the epithelium. The nipple discharge is characteristically pale yellow, sticky, and bilateral. Usually there is no mass or tenderness present, but the breast feels lumpy. Conservative management is indicated, and it is important to advise the patient to wear a carefully fitted garment and to avoid undue constraint or friction.

Women should be instructed to perform monthly examinations of their breasts postmenstrually, when the breast is least engorged. Patience, repetition, reassurance, and visual aids are required to indoctrinate many fearful patients, and often these can best be offered by female office attendants. The office examination previously described should be repeated yearly or more often, depending upon the assessed degree of risk for breast cancer. Factors affecting risk are listed in Table 35-2. The differential diagnosis between benign and malignant disease depends upon the patient's age, the symptoms, and the findings on palpation. Although no absolute generalizations can be made, carcinomas tend to be irregular, firm, nontender, and occasionally fixed to the skin or underlying muscle. Pain is seldom a feature except in the very late stages. Benign lesions, such as cysts and fibroadenomas, are more likely to be smooth, well defined, and relatively mobile. The breasts of women with fibrocystic change are often lumpy and tender, especially in the upper outer quadrants, and the changes tend to vary with the menstrual cycle. Degrees of discomfort up to severe pain may be present. One or more enlarged firm lymph nodes in the axilla associated with an ipsilateral breast mass strongly suggest the likelihood of carcinoma, but axillary lymphadenopathy may also be caused by lesions of the hand, arm, and adjacent thorax, especially those due to trauma. The breasts of pregnant women are swollen, tender, and difficult to palpate, but pregnancy does not confer immunity from breast cancer.

DIAGNOSTIC AIDS

Diagnostic aids available to the clinician are listed in Table 35-3. Of these, x-ray mammography is by far the most accurate and best able to diagnose breast cancer before it is palpable. Evaluation of the breast by x-ray techniques, both for screening and for diagnosis, is now well established. Because of concern about the theoretical carcinogenic effect of cumulative diagnostic x-rays on the breast and the knowledge that the danger is inherently greater the earlier in life the exposure occurs, opinions differ about the age at which screening of asymptomatic women should begin. However, most authorities agree that women over the age of 35 should have one or two baseline mammograms, or more in the presence of risk factors, and that those over 50 should be screened yearly. Table 35-4 lists recent

---

TABLE 35–2
Risk Factors Predisposing to Breast Carcinoma

Data Good

Family history: first degree premenopausal relative
Advancing age
Carcinoma in other breast
Precancerous mastopathy
Early puberty
Late age at first childbirth
Late menopause
Western culture
Irradiation
Other carcinoma (colon, uterus, ovary)

Data Doubtful

Exogenous estrogens
Nutrition
Obesity
Breastfeeding
High parity

TABLE 35–3
**Diagnostic Aids in the Management
of Breast Disease**

1. Mammography
    Standard
        Magnification
    Xeroradiography
    Duct injection
2. Thermography
    Tele (infrared)
    Brachy (liquid crystal)
3. Ultrasonography
    B scan
    Real time
4. Diaphanography
5. Nuclear magnetic resonance

TABLE 35–4
Recommendations for Screening Mammography

Baseline at age 35–40 years
Every 1–2 years at ages 40–50
Annually for those over age 50

(American College of Surgeons, American College of Radiology, and American Medical Association)

(After DeVita VT, Hellman S, Rosenberg SA. Cancer: principles and practice of oncology. 3rd ed. Philadelphia: JB Lippincott, 1989:446.)

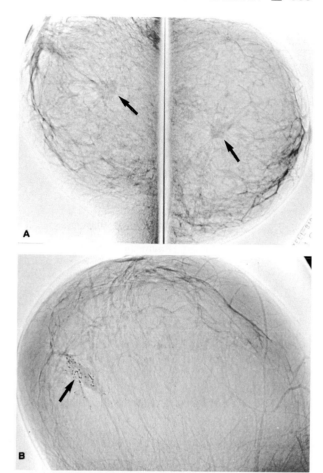

Figure 35–5. *A,* Xeroradiogram showing a dense irregular lesion in the upper outer quadrant with projections into the surrounding breast tissue characteristic of carcinoma. *B,* Xeroradiogram showing the translucent breast of a postmenopausal woman with a cluster of calcifications in the lower inner quadrant characteristic of carcinoma.

guidelines for screening mammography. Xeroradiography, a later extension of the standard technique, also utilizes x-rays but has the advantage that vascular markings and microcalcifications stand out more clearly for the amateur. To the radiologist who is expert in the interpretation of film screen breast mammograms, however, it is inferior to the older method. Moreover, xeroradiography requires higher doses of radiation. Experience is of the utmost importance in the accurate interpretation of breast x-rays, and high-intensity light sources and magnification have been used to refine the technique further. On balance, the estimated carcinogenic effect of x-ray exposure is less important than the potential for saving lives by early diagnosis. This is particularly true of older women, since the benefit of early diagnosis in this age group is better demonstrated than for younger women and since their shorter actuarial life expectancy provides less time for the development of cancer due to the x-ray exposure. Modern equipment utilizes dosages of less than 0.5 rad tissue dose for the superior and lateral views ordinarily obtained for screening, and patients should be instructed to obtain their films in institutions where the equipment is dedicated to mammography and where radiologists specializing in mammography are available.

Mammographic screening is highly accurate, with a false negative rate of less than 10%. In screening, 45% of all cancers are detected only by mammography; about 55% are discovered on physical examination, but physical examination alone is positive in only 10% of cases. For this reason accurate screening requires both mammography and palpation of the breast, and biopsies must be done if either of these examinations is positive. Mammography should always precede biopsy to sharpen diagnostic accuracy and to rule out the possibility of other disease in the same or contralateral breast. The diagnosis is made on the presence of a mass with specific characteristics suggesting cancer (Fig. 35-5*A*), on the basis of a localized cluster of microcalcifications (Fig. 35-5*B*), or on the more controversial variations in breast architecture.

For the diagnosis of specific breast problems, mammography is indicated in many different situations (Table 35-5). When cancer is suspected, mammography should be done regardless of the patient's age or pregnancy. Questionable but probably benign shadows should be rechecked in 3 to 6 months to determine whether there has been any progression of the process. A change in the diameter or contour of such a shadow or a further separation of microcalcifications is an indication for biopsy. A thermogram suggesting malignant change should be followed by the more definitive mammography before biopsy is performed. Whenever a patient believes that she has felt a lump in her breast, it is advisable to order a mammogram even if the lump cannot be palpated by the examining physician. Differences in opinion by two or more physicians regarding

TABLE 35–5
Indications for Mammography, by Age

AGE	INDICATION
Screening Mammography	
<25	None
25–35	Baseline if high risk
35–49	Baseline and biannual examination
	Annual examination if high risk
>50	Annual examination
Diagnostic Mammography	
<25	Suspected cancer
>25	Dominant mass
	Discrete thickening
	Undiagnosed symptoms
	Change in previous lesion
	Positive thermography
	Patient request
	Large breasts
	Discrepancy in opinions
	Prebiopsy evaluation

what can or cannot be felt should be resolved by mammography. Patients with large or very dense breasts that are difficult to palpate should have spaced sequential mammograms to detect subtle changes in shadow patterns. The fact that dense breasts are relatively difficult to interpret by x-ray, as they are by physical examination, does not obviate the need to obtain regular films.

In recent years, radiologists have attempted to classify the parenchymal patterns noted on breast x-rays according to the likelihood that cancer will develop in those breasts. The term *dysplasia* has been used increasingly to denote deviations from the normal that have serious implications for the future. It is important to understand that *dysplasia* in this context covers a broad range of histopathologic entities, particularly in the realm of so-called fibrocystic disease, and cannot be equated with a specific cellular change. Many of the studies contributing to the development of a premalignant taxonomy for mammographic patterns have been retrospective and on selected populations, but they indicate the possible presence of a high-risk category that must be closely followed.

The search for a screening technique for breast cancer that is noninvasive and cost effective has led to significant advances in the technique of thermography. The basic principle upon which this type of assessment depends is that disease states, and cancer in particular, tend to generate relatively increased amounts of heat, presumably because of intensified cellular metabolism. Beginning about 30 years ago, the patterns of heat waves emanating from the breast were detected by sensors that were hand-held about the skin and recorded variations in the infrared range. This method,

referred to as telethermometry, has undergone many technical improvements since its inception, and efforts have been made to reduce background interference by lowering the patient's temperature prior to the test. Electronic imaging of this type is reasonably reliable but requires elaborate apparatus and experienced interpretation, usually available only in large institutions.

More recently, many thermographers have resorted to an innovation known as liquid crystal thermography, a type of brachythermometry, in the course of which the breasts are pressed directly against a thermosensitive plate lined with cholesteric crystals. The resulting thermographic film depicts the skin of the breast in contrasting colors that represent the underlying thermal pattern. The equipment with which this is accomplished is relatively less expensive and has been widely advertised for use in free-standing breast clinics and private offices. It appears to be a helpful tool, but much remains to be learned about the range of its reliability, especially in the category of nonpalpable or minimal breast cancer.

Thermography, in general, has the disadvantage of a higher degree of inaccuracy than mammography, particularly in the false positive range, leading to overdiagnosis and unnecessary biopsies in some instances. New modifications offer hope of improved specificity, but the criteria for accuracy comparable to mammography have not been met to date in any long-range, well-controlled prospective studies.

Ultrasonography accurately depicts the difference between solid and cystic masses and is being subjected to extensive trials of its accuracy in diagnosing early malignant disease in the breast. It is used as an adjunct to mammography, since combinations of the two modalities have been shown in some reports to be better than either alone, and it is available for this purpose in many institutions.

Fiberoptic transillumination to map the breast (diaphanography) is increasing in popularity, but prospective randomized, controlled studies proving its efficacy have not been published. The delineation of soft tissue lesions by nuclear magnetic resonance holds hope for the future, but this technique has not been widely tested for efficacy in the diagnosis of breast disease. Before great reliance can be placed on screening techniques other than mammography, rigid clinical trials will be necessary. For screening or diagnosis, mammography is the essential adjunct to physical examination.

PATHOLOGY

The term *fibrocystic disease,* formerly referred to as chronic cystic mastitis, includes a spectrum of conditions in which may be listed microcysts (less than 2 mm), macrocysts (greater than 2 mm) (Fig. 35-6), fibroadenomas, papillomas, and adenosis, all of which may be subject to hyperplastic epithelial changes with or without atypical cells. The universality of occurrence of microcystic disease (60%–90% of the female population) and the fact that both it and its macrocystic counterpart are subject to the cyclic changes of ovarian hormone production suggest that, at least in the subclinical variants, the process is physiologic rather than pathologic. Approximately 60% of all breast biopsies will be diagnosed in one of these categories. There would be no real significance to the term *fibrocystic disease* were it not for the anxiety-provoking discomfort and lumpiness imparted to the breast, especially premenstrually, the difficulty in distinguishing it from a so-called dominant mass, and the alleged positive relationship to the future development of cancer. The evidence that all fibrocystic changes constitute precancerous mastopathy consists largely of retrospective data of questionable statistical validity, especially since it has been shown that these changes will appear in up to 90% of all biopsies, if those in which cancer is also present are included. When biopsied material shows epithelial hyperplasia, however, the evidence indicates that the risk of future cancer is increased, and if atypical cellular changes are present in addition, the risk is even greater. Proliferative intraductal lesions may also have greater potential for the development of subsequent malignancy. Papillomas tend to develop in the larger subareolar ducts, whereas papillomatosis occurs in the medium-sized or smaller ductal ramifications. The nonproliferating forms of fibrocystic change, the micro- and macrocysts, arise in the terminal lobules and ducts. In younger women with fibrocystic change, there may

be proliferation of both glandular and stromal tissue, forming firm masses that on biopsy are referred to as sclerosing adenosis. Histologically, this variant may be confused with carcinoma by the inexperienced, but it has little malignant propensity. In older women there may be a tendency for an increase in the fibrous elements at the expense of the glands, which can impart a feeling of firmness to the breast and occasionally suggest discrete masses.

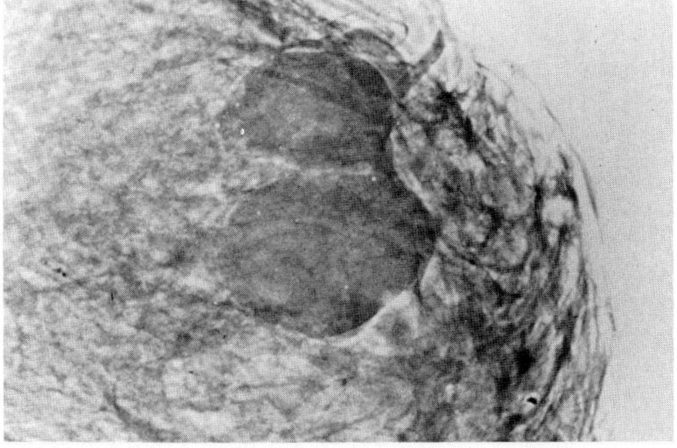

Atypical hyperplasias, both lobular and ductal, may be difficult to separate histologically from carcinoma in situ and even from early invasive carcinoma. It seems likely that in some cases there is a progressive linear relationship between these changes and the eventual development of malignant disease. A diagnosis of atypical hyperplasia or carcinoma in situ by the pathologist necessitates careful study of the biopsy specimen and serious consideration of the risk factors involved in allowing such patients to continue without more definitive treatment. In some series, the progression of lobular carcinoma in situ to invasive carcinoma is as high as 20%, and since the duration of the follow-up is critical in this assessment, the figure may be higher. Because it is impossible to predict which woman with in situ lobular neoplasia will eventually develop invasive carcinoma, prophylactic mastectomy is sometimes advised. A policy of professional observation and regularly repeated mammography for patients with this disease process is usually indicated, unless other serious risk factors are present or the level of anxiety of the patient is high.

Carcinoma in situ in ductal epithelium is a matter of even greater concern, and consideration should be given to wide local resection or even mastectomy. If conservative management is elected, the breasts should be reexamined two or three times yearly and mammograms ordered.

MEDICAL TREATMENT

Breast symptoms, other than nipple secretion, consist chiefly of lumpiness and discomfort related to swelling and vascular engorgement, especially premenstrually. Since in most women these complaints are not caused by disease and are endurable, reassurance is the most important form of therapy. For those with more severe or unduly prolonged pain, a variety of medical regimens is available.

For years it has been known that small doses of androgens by mouth or by injection relieve breast pain and soreness. Not only do these drugs have an undesirable virilizing effect in some women if taken over a long period of time, but the idea of taking male hormones, regardless of side-effects, is abhorrent to many. More recently, it has been shown that small doses of an

Figure 35–6. Xeroradiogram showing two smooth, rounded shadows in the relatively dense breast of a premenopausal woman. These are characteristic of cysts but could be mistaken for fibroadenomas.

impeded androgen, Danocrine, inhibit the development of fibrocystic changes that produce breast discomfort. Dosages in the range of 100–400 mg/day for 6 months are usually effective and do not cause amenorrhea, hirsutism, or acne in most women. The favorable result is often maintained for months to years after discontinuance of the drug.

Oral contraceptives have been used to create a balanced menstrual cycle with relatively lower amounts of circulating estrogen and progesterone and, consequently, less stimulation of breast tissue. For those who wish to avoid pregnancy and who are not at risk for the possible undesirable side-effects of oral contraceptives, this is an acceptable method of treatment of cyclic mastalgia. No cause-and-effect relationship between the use of oral contraceptives and the subsequent development of carcinoma of the breast has been established, nor is it clear that the use of these drugs is protective against subsequent disease.

Studies attempting to equate the histologic changes of fibrocystic disease with an increase in estrogen and progesterone receptors have been inconclusive, but Minton and associates have stated that there is a buildup of cyclic AMP and GMP in fibrocystic breast tissue, presumably as a result of an enzymatic failure to permit proper metabolic clearance. He postulated that this enzyme, phosphodiesterase, is inhibited by high levels of circulating methyl xanthines, which are commonly ingested in coffee, tea, and cocoa. Abstention from these beverages should permit free action of the enzyme, the reduction of cyclic AMP and GMP, and amelioration of breast swelling and soreness. Clinical trials of this theory have been conducted with largely favorable results, but the lack of prospective randomized studies makes the statistics questionable. Nevertheless, dietary regimens restricting coffee, tea, and cocoa have been adopted by many women with subjectively satisfactory effects.

Vitamin E has been recommended for the relief of breast symptoms, first by Abrams and more recently by London and associates. Neither the clinical trials that have been conducted nor the scientific explanation—which postulates that the vitamin alters the metabolic pathway from pregnenolone to pregnanediol so that a 17-keto steroid with androgenic action is produced—is convincing, but the possible placebo effect cannot be discounted.

Of great importance in the control of breast symptoms is the support, or lack of it, in the everyday garments used. The weight of heavy breasts not properly supported exacerbates discomfort, and constriction, which interferes with proper circulation, increases disability. Advice about this factor is best given by female office personnel familiar with the problems of fitting and with the manufacturers of special clothing.

OFFICE SURGERY

Palpable discrete or dominant lumps in the breast must be surgically investigated after mammography, even if the latter is negative. When the mass is rounded, well circumscribed, smooth and 1 cm or greater in diameter, it is probably a cyst or fibroadenoma, and ultrasound can usually differentiate between the two. Aspiration should be attempted first (Fig. 35-7). With the patient lying supine in a relaxed position, well prepared by prior instruction, the mass is stabilized with the thumb and first two fingers of the left hand (Fig. 35-7A). Local anesthesia is undesirable in the tissue to be aspirated because it disrupts the parenchyma and dilutes the specimen, but it may be used intradermally in very sensitive patients. A No. 22 needle attached to a 20-cc syringe is passed tangentially into the mass while suction is maintained. If the lesion is cystic, the fluid obtained usually flows freely into the syringe and is light brown. All this fluid should be sent to the laboratory for cytologic evaluation, although it is often acellular and nondiagnostic. If no fluid is obtained after several attempts, the needle is withdrawn and whatever material is available should be blown onto a clean slide and fixed for cytologic analysis. Cysts smaller than 1 cm are difficult to aspirate, and if one of these is the first such lesion, it should be treated by open biopsy. Insertion of the needle perpendicular to the chest wall, rather than at an angle of 30° or 40°, or the use of needles longer than an inch and a half may lead to inadvertent perforation of the pleural cavity and pneumothorax.

When a solid mass is present, a multiple-aspiration technique is attempted, preferably without local anesthesia. A No. 22 needle attached to a 20-cc syringe fitted with a specially designed handle that permits the maintenance of a constant vacuum within the syringe is passed rapidly through the mass in several different planes to sample all its ramifications (Fig. 35-8). Once through the skin and into the suspicious area, the needle is advanced and withdrawn rapidly four or five times, like the action of a sewing machine. To avoid bringing the aspirated material into the syringe, suction is discontinued before the needle is pulled back through the skin. The syringe is then separated from the needle and 5 cc of air are aspirated. Reattached to the needle, the syringe is used to blow its contents on a clean glass slide. The material on the slide is spread evenly across its surface with another slide in the manner of preparing a blood smear. The services of a good technician are helpful in producing a smooth preparation. The procedure is repeated five or six times, and aspirates are deposited on separate slides. Each of these aspirations should be done quickly to avoid contamination of the specimens with gross blood, which makes

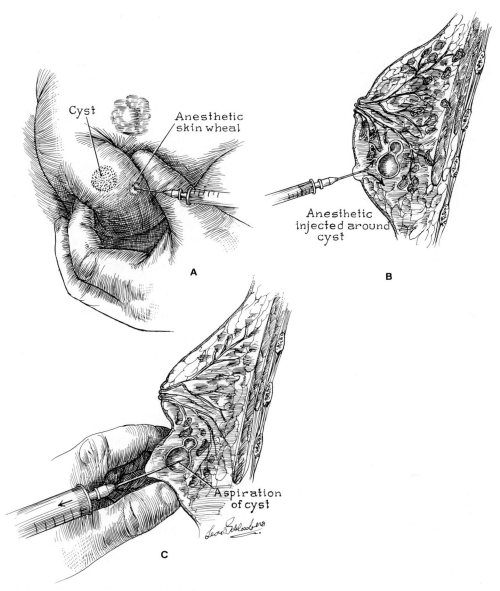

Figure 35–7. Aspiration of cyst. In many cases local anesthesia is not necessary. *A,* When it is used, a small intradermal wheal is raised over the cyst. *B,* From this area the anesthesia is injected along the estimated path of the aspirating needle. *C,* The portion of the breast containing the cyst is stabilized with the left hand while a No. 18 or No. 20 needle is passed into the cyst along a line tangential to the surface of the thorax in order to avoid penetration of the pleura. Fluid obtained is sent for cytologic interpretation.

them difficult to evaluate. Experience is essential to acquire the expertise necessary to obtain good specimens.

When Papanicolaou stains are to be used, as they are in most laboratories, the specimens are fixed with 95% alcohol, either by spray or immersion, and this fixative is appropriate for hematoxylin and eosin. If a Romanovsky stain is used, the specimens should be air-dried.

The predictive value of this technique for both positive and negative findings is above 90% when sufficient material is obtained, and the specificity is equally high. False negative findings are usually due to poor technique, insufficient or poorly prepared material, or

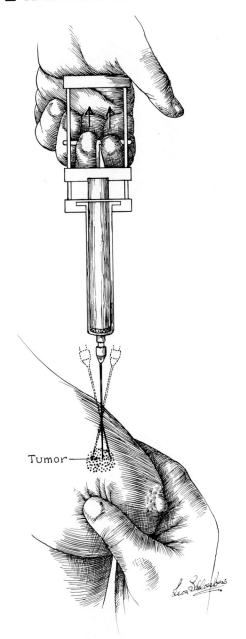

Figure 35–8. Percutaneous needle aspiration of solid tumors. Using local anesthesia, a skinny needle (No. 22) is passed repeatedly through the lesion in different planes and directions while constant suction is maintained by means of the attached syringe holder. The aspirate is ejected on a slide and sent for cytologic analysis. A high degree of accuracy in diagnosis is possible, but the result is not definitive.

specimens heavily contaminated with blood. Because the false negative value of this technique is higher than that of open biopsy, a negative report on a suspicious lesion necessitates biopsy. In institutions where cytologic evaluation of aspirates is not of the highest quality,

tissue biopsy is essential. Although in certain situations it is possible to follow patients whose needle aspirations are negative without biopsy, the lump will remain a source of concern to the patient. In a few institutions positive aspiration findings may be considered justification for initiating definitive surgery. Fine needle aspirates may also be used for the analysis of estrogen receptors by immunocytochemistry, for the determination of ploidy by flow cytometry, and for electron microscopy.

Small biopsy specimens can be obtained by the percutaneous passage of a trocar containing a cutting needle (Fig. 35-9). Because of the size of the sheath and the necessity of pushing the cutting edge of the trocar into the breast tissue, local anesthesia is desirable. Specimens so obtained are examined histologically, but because of their small size, they may not be representative; therefore, a negative report cannot be relied upon. A positive report, however, is definitive.

When aspiration techniques are not available or cytologic findings from aspirations are inconclusive or negative for malignancy, open biopsy is indicated in the case of a mass, a secondarily retracted nipple or skin area, a bloody nipple discharge, a dominant projection from an area of fibrocystic change, or a positive mammogram. Before surgery, mammograms should always be obtained to improve the accuracy of diagnosis and localization of the lesion and to rule out other lesions in the same or other breast. Biopsies can be done under local anesthesia in an office or clinic surgical suite or the ambulatory surgery area of a hospital. The evidence indicates that a delay of a few days between diagnostic biopsy and subsequent definitive surgical procedures does not adversely affect the prognosis, and patient acceptance of ambulatory surgery, which permits full discussion of the problem before major surgery, is much greater. Counseling the patient and the patient's spouse or other member of the family is most important in securing the understanding that leads to good cooperation during the procedure. Each step of the operation is outlined and the patient is reassured that nothing further will be done without consultation.

The patient should come to the minor surgical operating room having had nothing by mouth since the night before and accompanied by an interested second party. She is placed supine on the operating table with the arm on the affected side at right angles to the body or above the head, which stretches the pectoral muscles and helps to make the lesion more accessible. A pillow under the shoulder has a similar effect. If the patient is nervous, analgesic drugs such as meperidine 50 mg and diazepam 5 mg may be given intravenously a few minutes before starting.

The location of the incision is important—for cosmetic reasons (if the lesion is benign) and to keep it out

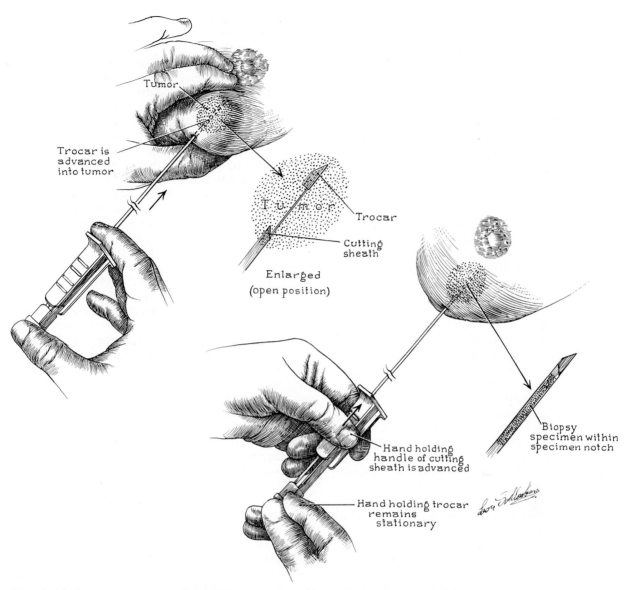

Figure 35–9. Percutaneous needle biopsy. Because of the large caliber of the sheath to be passed, local anesthesia is usually necessary. A number of instruments are available for this purpose. The sheath is passed tangentially to the surface of the solid lesion and then directly engaged. The trocar is pushed well into the lesion and then withdrawn into the sheath, bringing a small core of tumor tissue. Bleeding following this procedure can usually be controlled by pressure.

of the line of a later mastectomy incision (if the lesion is malignant). When the lesion is beneath the areola or within 3 or 4 cm of its outer margin, the incision is made along its edge, not including more than one half the circumference, to avoid compromising its blood and nerve supply. For lesions further toward the periphery or deep in a large breast, a curved incision 3 or 4 cm long is made parallel to the areolar margin and just over

the lesion to permit its being more easily encompassed in any subsequent dissection, thus avoiding possible dissemination of tumor cells from the biopsy site. An intradermal wheal is made with 1% Lidocaine just below the inferior pole of the proposed incision and is carried upward along the areolar margin to a point above the upper pole. Using a longer needle at several points along the wheal, the area around the lesion is infiltrated with anesthetic solution. Too much solution distends the tissue and interferes with localization of the lesion; too little can always be supplemented later. If a nonpalpable intraductal papilloma is suspected, the major ductal system beneath the nipple is infiltrated. When the lesion is further out, it is best to delineate the proposed incision with a marking pen after careful palpation has indicated proper placement.

Using a No. 15 blade, the 3–5-cm incision is carried down through the dermis and the subcutaneous fat to the lobular tissue of the breast. The skin margins are slightly undercut and held back on fine hooks to facilitate exposure. Hemostasis is provided by the electrocautery except in the case of large arteries. An assistant is helpful for this purpose and to provide retraction. The surgeon explores the location of the lesion with his or her forefinger. If the lesion is not directly beneath the incision, it is necessary to tunnel toward it with scissors, pushing, spreading, and cutting toward the desired location while upward and lateral traction is maintained on the margins of the dissection. With his finger on the lesion the surgeon will usually have a better understanding of its size, consistency, and mobility and will be able to assess its nature with a high degree of accuracy. Lesions less than 4 cm in diameter and probably malignant should be sharply excised with a surrounding margin of normal tissue (Fig. 35-10 A–B). Larger, probably malignant, tumors should be sampled by a representative V-shaped wedge of tissue, since total excision might require a difficult operation, significant blood loss, and a poorer prognosis (Fig. 35-11 A–B). Should the original biopsy prove negative on frozen section, additional biopsies, either with the knife or with a cutting needle, must be taken. Large cysts are often dark blue, and these may be aspirated and a piece of the wall taken for histologic verification. Smaller cysts and fibroadenomas in adolescence and early adult life are completely excised in the primary procedure but can be treated conservatively secondarily.

Since the results of the National Surgical Adjuvant Breast and Bowel Project were published in 1985, showing that in carefully selected cases of tumors 4 cm in size or less, tylectomy or segmental resection, with or without irradiation, was equal or superior to total mastectomy, the trend toward more conservative operations for breast cancer has accelerated. When the workup, the needle aspiration, or the gross findings at the beginning of the biopsy operation suggest the presence of malignancy and the lesion is less than 5 cm in diameter, the possibility that the biopsy might also be the definitive surgery must be kept clearly in mind, and a margin of at least 4–5 mm of tissue around the lesion must be removed with it. It is often possible to tell grossly whether the tumor extends to the margin of resection, and frozen section histologic diagnosis of this

condition is highly accurate. When this occurs, further removal of tissue in the area is obviously necessary. Pregnancy does not obviate the necessity to adhere to standard principles of breast cancer therapy.

Conservative surgery of breast cancer makes staging by evaluation of axillary lymph node metastases impossible and, since in many institutions the use of adjunctive chemotherapy depends upon lymph node involvement, axillary dissection necessarily follows local excision of a malignant lesion. Provided permission has been obtained, this step can be taken following primary resection and frozen section, in which case general anesthesia is usually required, or it can be done secondarily later. Thorough removal of all lymph nodes at levels 1 and 2 (see Fig. 35-2) is required, and there should be 12–15 nodes in the specimen. Level 3 nodes are technically more difficult to obtain and are seldom positive when levels 1 and 2 are negative. When adjunctive chemotherapy is used regardless of lymphatic involvement, axillary lymph nodes resection is still essential for determining prognosis and result of treatment.

Once the decision has been made to excise the lesion, the surgeon places a self-retaining retractor in the wound and grasps the tissue immediately overlying the lesion with an Allis clamp or tooth forceps. Minor bleeding, which can obscure the field, must be controlled at each step, usually by cautery. Although it is possible to perform the operation alone, an assistant is very helpful in keeping the field clear and providing countertraction. Maintaining traction on the tissue to be resected, the surgeon enucleates it with small curved scissors (see Fig. 35-10 C–E). Blunt dissection is of little help, since there are no well-defined tissue planes. Frequent pauses are necessary to evaluate the scope of the dissection and to avoid cutting into the lesion or removing too much normal lobular tissue. The instrument elevating the lesion is shifted around its periphery as the dissection progresses to provide better exposure of the underside.

After removal of the tumor, the defect is closed with fine absorbable suture material, taking care that these sutures do not cause retraction or dimpling of the overlying skin. (Some surgeons prefer to drain the area, and some do not appose the deeper tissues.) If any part of the closure involves tension on the sutures, it is best to omit it. All bleeding must be controlled before closure. When there is a large residual defect, as after segmental resection, a plastic type of closure is necessary for a satisfactory cosmetic result, and suction drainage may be used to avoid the postoperative accumulation of fluid. The skin is closed with either a subcuticular stitch of fine absorbable suture material or interrupted 5.0 nylon. A pressure dressing for the first 24 hours is desirable but may not be necessary in relatively minor cases. The sutures should be removed

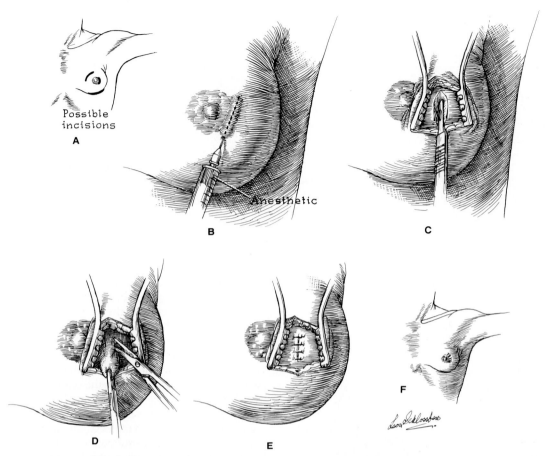

Figure 35–10. Open biopsy. *A,* For cosmetic reasons circumareolar incisions are preferable when the lesion is thought to be within 2 or 3 cm of the areola. Not more than one half of the areolar margin should be incised. A curved incision parallel to the areola is made over lesions further out from the center. When malignant disease is strongly suspected, the surgeon should attempt to avoid the probable path of the subsequent mastectomy incision. *B,* An intradermal wheal is raised along the path of the proposed incision using 1% lidocaine and a hypodermic (No. 25) needle. From the wheal, deeper injections of anesthetic are made around the circumference of the lesion and beneath it. *C,* The incision is carried down through the dense subcutaneous tissue and into the lobule containing the lesion. Self-retaining retractors are helpful when an assistant is not available. *D,* If the lesion is small or easily mobilized, it should be sharply dissected and excised with a thin margin of adjacent tissue. *E,* The lobular defect is sutured with fine absorbable suture material if the closure places no tension on the overlying skin. Bleeding is controlled with absorbable ligatures or electrocoagulation. Absolute hemostasis is essential. *F,* The skin is closed with interrupted No. 5-0 silk or nylon sutures. Drainage is seldom necessary. A pressure dressing for 24 hours is desirable if a significant amount of dead space has been left behind.

in not more than 6 days to prevent scarring, and steristrips are applied as necessary.

When a bloody nipple discharge suggests the likelihood of an intraductal papilloma, sharp dissection is carried medially from a circumareolar incision placed in the breast quadrant that pressure tests have indicated is most likely to be the source of bleeding. Directly beneath the nipple, the main ducts are encountered

and placed on traction with a small hook. The ducts are followed downward until the lesion is found, usually not more than 3 or 4 cm from the surface. Papillomas are dark red and soft and may be multiple. A generous portion of the duct system around the diseased area is resected, and the severed ends are ligated (Fig. 35-12). Usually there is a relatively small defect that need not be closed, and care must be taken not to cause retraction of

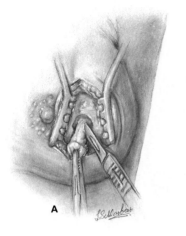

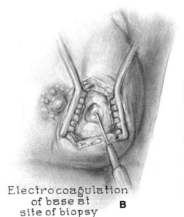

Electrocoagulation
of base at
site of biopsy

Figure 35–11. Incisional biopsy. *A,* When a large (greater than 5 cm) or very adherent lesion is encountered, especially when carcinoma is strongly suspected, a wedge of tissue of approximately 1 cc in volume is excised from the exposed surface of the tumor and sent for frozen section. If the first pathology report is negative, additional biopsies may be necessary. *B,* The base of the incision is usually coagulated to control bleeding.

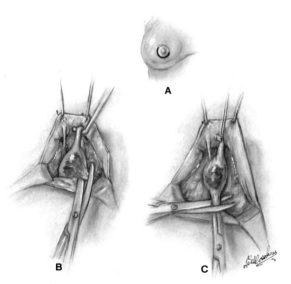

Figure 35–12. Ductal exploration and resection of papilloma. *A,* The incision is circumareolar and toward the quadrant most likely to be the site of the lesion. *B,* With traction on the main duct, peripheral branches are dissected out until lesion is identified. *C,* The duct system above and below the lesion is clamped, and the portion containing the lesion is excised.

the nipple by suturing. Inverting the nipple and scraping all ductal tissue from the undersurface has been advocated but seems unnecessary in most cases.

Nonpalpable lesions noted on mammograms must be investigated. Often these consist of clusters of tiny calcifications or distortions of the breast architecture, which may represent the earliest stage of a malignant process and which may, therefore, have the best possible prognosis if resected early. The procedure must be done in cooperation with a diagnostic radiologist inter-

ested in breast disease. Under continuous x-ray visualization, the radiologist inserts a special needle until its tip is in close proximity to the lesion. A fine wire with a memory reverse hook on the leading end is passed beyond the needlepoint and then pulled back until the hook engages near the lesion. The needle is withdrawn. The wire is stabilized at the skin level with tape, and the patient is carefully removed to the operating room on a stretcher. Under these circumstances, some surgeons prefer general anesthesia, but in most instances the operation can be done with local. The incision is made as previously noted, but subcutaneously the dissection is directed toward the wire and carried down toward the hook. A block of tissue 3 cm or more in diameter is resected from the area under suspicion and sent back to the radiologist to determine by x-ray whether the suspicious area is present (Fig. 35-13). If so, the tissue is sent to the pathologist, but if not, the surgeon must do a wider resection until successful.

All the removed tissue, including fat, must be sent to the pathologist. It is his duty to see that a portion of the specimen is sent to the laboratory for assay of estrogen and progesterone receptors, but it is not safe to assume that this will happen. Until recently, estrogen receptors alone were considered sufficient, but recent evidence indicates that progesterone receptors are also important markers of hormone dependence and indicators of prognosis. The remaining tissue is divided into blocks so that representative frozen sections can be taken from each area. The report should be available within 20 minutes once it has reached the laboratory, and should be above the 99th percentile in accuracy as compared with the permanent sections.

After receiving the report, the surgeon can discuss modalities of future treatment and their pros and cons with the patient and her spouse or counselor. The possible complications of the biopsy procedure are

Figure 35–13. Directed biopsy of nonpalpable lesions. *A,* The incision has been directed downward to the insertion of the flexible hook in the vicinity of the lesion, and an appropriate volume of tissue around it is being undermined. *B,* The lesion with at least 1 cc of surrounding tissue is resected and verified radiologically and pathologically. If the lesion is not identified in the specimen by x-ray, an additional volume of tissue must be resected.

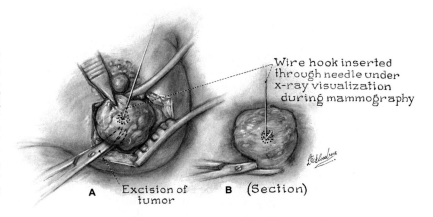

Wire hook inserted through needle under x-ray visualization during mammography

A Excision of tumor   **B** (Section)

also discussed. These include skin ecchymoses, hemorrhage, seromas, and infection. Ecchymoses clear within a few days, but acute hemorrhage requires immediate reopening of the wound. Chronic accumulation of serous fluid, forming an enlarging pocket, may require repetitive needle evacuation or occasionally constant suction drainage. Pain is seldom a factor postoperatively, and no convalescence or loss of working time is usually necessary.

HOSPITAL PROCEDURES

Axillary lymph node dissection should be attempted only by surgeons with adequate training in the method or under the direct supervision of surgeons so trained. As previously stated, it can be done as a second-stage operation following conservative resection of the primary tumor, or it can be postponed pending the availability of general anesthesia or a surgeon familiar with the technique. Separate permission must be obtained from the patient.

A diagonal incision is made across the base of the axilla from the edge of the pectoralis major to the latissimus dorsi. This incision should be separate from the incision in the breast. The axillary vein is exposed by incising the costocoracoid fascia. The fatty tissue and enclosed lymphatics beneath the vein are carefully dissected free, dividing the inferior veins traversing the fat pad as necessary (Fig. 35-14). Sampling of individual lymph nodes is unsatisfactory; complete resection of the lymphatics at levels I and II is mandatory. Because of the possibility of fluid collection in the resulting dead space, it is advisable to place a small suction drain before closure.

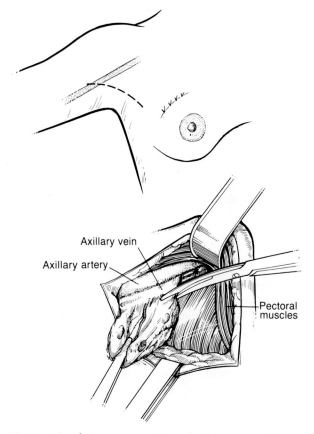

Axillary vein

Axillary artery

Pectoral muscles

Figure 35–14. *Top,* Breast incision has been closed following excision of lump that showed carcinoma. Line of axillary incision for lymphadenectomy has been marked. *Bottom,* With the pectoral muscles retracted, the axillary vein is exposed medially. Dissection of lymphatic tissue and fat proceeds along the course of the vein.

Several different approaches to *augmentation mammoplasty* are currently used. The incision may be made beneath the breast along the skin attachment to the chest wall or in a circumareolar position at the pigmented border. The latter provides limited exposure but leaves a nearly invisible scar; both are cosmetically satisfactory. The prosthesis, usually a nonreactive plastic envelope filled with silicone gel, may be placed between the breast and the superior surface of the pectoralis major muscle. This location provides a good contour for the breast but has the disadvantage in some cases of the late development of a fibrotic periprosthetic capsule, which gradually puckers the external outline of the breast and causes discomfort. To avoid this long-term complication, some surgeons split the muscle fibers of the pectoralis major and insert the prosthesis beneath it. This provides better long-term stability, but the protrusion of the breast above it is less accentuated and therefore less natural in appearance. All modifications of technique are subject to the short-term risks of hemorrhage and infection, which may require removal of the prosthesis, and the long-term risk of displacement. Sensation is usually preserved and lactation occurs following pregnancy.

Women at risk for the development of breast cancer as a result of a positive family history or the presence of precancerous mastopathy and those with dense breasts that make both physical examination and mammography less accurate may have *subcutaneous mastectomies* and the insertion of a prosthesis recommended for prophylaxis. Because of the close attachment of the breast to the skin, the presence of the axillary tail, and the possibility that there are extensions of breast tissue beyond its observed perimeter and into the pectoral muscle, the operation is often incomplete, and carcinomas have been reported in the residual breast parenchyma. The gel-filled silicone implant is most commonly used following resection, but subcutaneous Dacron screens or shields have also been employed. Postoperatively, there is often loss of sensation as well as loss of function, and complications include infection, skin necrosis, and migration of the prosthesis. Indications for this procedure remain poorly defined but lately have been extended to include patients with severe breast pain and those with a high level of anxiety concerning cancer. It seems reasonable at present to restrict the operation to women in the very-high-risk group.

Reduction mammoplasties must be carefully tailored to the size and degree of ptosis of the breast to be reconstructed, and for this reason many different types of plastic procedures have been devised to fit the various special circumstances. Some have the disadvantage of a clearly visible scar on the remodeled breast, and because of the necessity of resecting large areas of skin with resultant tension on the closure, these scars are likely to stretch with time and to form keloid. Various ingeniously placed incisions have been devised to hide and reduce the scarring, some of which require relocation of the nipple–areola complex. In some instances, it has been possible to resect pie-shaped sections of breast tissue without affecting function in young people afflicted with severe mammary hypertrophy. The goal of forming a saucer-shaped or conical breast of normal volume is usually realized, and complications during the healing process are uncommon. The operations are done in the hospital under general anesthesia and require several days of convalescence. The results of reduction mammoplasty are uniformly excellent in terms of relief of symptoms and improved appearance.

Until about 15 years ago, the Halsted type of *radical mastectomy* was the standard treatment for breast cancer against which all other modalities were measured, and it still has its adherents. The gradual realization that local control of the disease is only one factor in determining the success of treatment and that systemic spread accounts for a preponderance of the failures has led to a step-by-step reduction in the extent of surgery to the point where some surgeons feel that the pendulum has swung too far in the other direction. A broad spectrum of operations is being performed by surgeons with widely divergent opinions about the scope of surgery necessary for different stages of disease. The TNM staging taxonomy recommended by the American Joint Committee for Cancer Staging and End Results Reporting in 1988 is now used by all cancer centers. T1 tumors, less than 5 cm in diameter, are usually selected for lesser procedures such as *lumpectomy* (tylectomy) and segmental resection. The removal of a large wedge of breast tissue provides a wider tumor-free margin around the primary lesion than can be obtained by a simple lumpectomy and the defect can often be closed with a reasonable cosmetic effect; however, the final appearance depends upon the original size of the breast and how much of it was resected. Operations less than total mastectomy are usually followed by local irradiation, which produces fibrosis and a certain amount of contraction but permits the retention of a fairly normal breast contour.

Lesser operations, in which *simple mastectomy* may be included, followed by irradiation, are often appropriate for very elderly patients and those with life-threatening medical problems. For women with a reasonable life expectancy whose tumors are 5 cm or greater, *modified radical mastectomy* is indicated. The modified radical mastectomy differs from the Halsted type in that the pectoralis major and minor muscles can be preserved, providing better arm motion and thoracic outline and reducing the incidence of postoperative lymphedema of the arm. It is probably the procedure most frequently used today for breast cancer. The Madden variant severs the insertion but retains the pectoralis minor and, by retracting the pectoral muscles medially, permits the resection of lymph nodes at all levels. In the Patey operation the arm on the affected side is fully extended above the head rather than at a right angle to the body, and the pectoralis minor is resected for better exposure, facilitating resection of the level III lymph nodes. The available data do not indicate that radical resection of positive lymph nodes improves the prognosis.

Following modified radical mastectomy, radiotherapy to the chest wall, internal mammary lymph nodes, and the dissected axilla was customary for patients whose final pathologic report indicated the presence of lymph node metastases, but this approach has been superseded because radiotherapy has not been effective in controlling lymph node metastases or hematogenous spread. It is now designed to treat only the primary lesion after local resection, and either external or interstitial sources may be used for this purpose.

Reconstruction procedures following modified radical and simple mastectomies have become increasingly common. These are done either at the time of mastectomy or after healing. The original line of incision about the breast, which is either oblique from the axilla to the origin of the rectus muscle or, more often, transverse from axilla to sternum, may be modified if it is known beforehand that reconstruction is desired, so long as the modification does not compromise adequate envelopment of the tumor. The plastic surgeon should be involved in planning such operations and may be present at the time of resection if immediate reconstruction is desired. Because of variations in anatomy and physical condition, the type of reconstruction must be individualized. Subcutaneous fat, muscle flaps developed from latissimus dorsi or rectus muscles, or expansible prostheses may be utilized. For those who feel that an external prosthesis is adequate for their self-image, many different types of garments are available in medical supply and department stores.

Since the radical mastectomy and its extensions—designed to remove tumor-bearing lymph nodes in the chest, neck, and clavicular areas, followed by external irradiation—failed to improve survival rates during an entire generation, it became evident that a better prognosis would have to be achieved by a systemic attack on micrometastases, presumed to exist at the time of surgery but not definable by current x-ray or laboratory studies. Before the advent of modern chemotherapy, it was well known that breast cancers were sensitive to changes in their hormonal environment, and the first attempt at systemic control was combined radical mastectomy and prophylactic oophorectomy. Although imperfect in their planning by today's standards, early reports suggested that oophorectomy prolonged the time to first recurrence but did not affect long-term survival. Another school of thought advocated therapeutic oophorectomy at the time of first recurrence, and the estrogen sensitivity of the tumor was assessed by the administration of estrogens to determine whether the patient's symptoms improved or became worse. A beneficial response to oophorectomy was often followed by adrenalectomy or hypophysectomy, and these surgical procedures, either singly or in combination, were given extensive clinical trials, often with conflicting interpretation of results.

Beginning with the alkylating agents, chemotherapy was used prophylactically following mastectomy in the late 1950s without discernible benefit. From that time, new drugs, as they became available, have been tried both prophylactically and therapeutically in various combinations, with some improvement in results in the latter group but no breakthrough in the former until well-controlled studies here and abroad demonstrated that a relatively prolonged disease-free interval could be achieved in premenopausal patients having one or more positive axillary lymph nodes. Single agents did not prove as effective as combinations in high dosage administered early. There was no similar advantage for postmenopausal women.

Many questions remain to be answered regarding the routine use of adjuvant chemotherapy for breast cancer, not the least of which is whether women should be treated whether or not they have positive lymph nodes. The optimum combination of drugs has yet to be determined, as well as the size of the dose and the duration of treatment. The role of estrogens, androgens, progestins, and antiestrogens is not clearly defined, nor is the relationship of hormonal to cytotoxic treatment. Oophorectomy is likely to be most effective in patients with known positive receptor sites who are premenopausal or postmenopausal for less than 5 years. Antiestrogens such as Tamoxifen are used for both prophylaxis and the treatment of persistent disease in the postmenopausal years, and in some instances in the premenopause. Hormonal therapy should not be used alone either prophylactically or therapeutically just because it is well tolerated. Combination cytotoxic therapy is superior in most instances. Stem cell assays have not provided the key to the selection of chemotherapeutic agents, but at present regimens based on doxorubicin, an alkylating agent, and an antimetabolite are in vogue.

Bibliography

Abrams AA. Use of vitamin E in chronic cystic mastitis. N Engl J Med 1965;272:1080.

Baker LH. Breast Cancer Detection Demonstration Project: five year summary report. Cancer 1982;32:194.

Barnes AB. Current concepts: diagnosis and treatment of abnormal breast secretions. N Engl J Med 1966;275:1184.

Beahrs OH, Henson DE, Hutter RVP, Myers MH. Manual for staging of cancer. 3rd ed. Philadelphia: JB Lippincott, 1988.

Beale S, Lisper H, Palm B. A psychological study of patients seeking augmentation mammaplasty. Br J Psychiatry 1980;136:133.

Bergkvist L, Adami H-O, Persson I, et al. The risk of breast cancer after estrogen and estrogen-progestin replacement. N Engl J Med 1989;321:293.

Biggs RM, Cukier J, Worthing LF. Augmentation mammoplasty: a review of 18 years. Plast Reconstr Surg 1982;69:445.

Bonadonna G, Valagussa P. Dose-response effect of adjuvant chemotherapy in breast cancer. N Engl J Med 1981;304:10.

Brinton LA, Hoover R, Fraumeni JF, Jr. Epidemiology of minimal breast cancer. JAMA 1983;249:483.

Carter SK. Adjuvant chemotherapy of breast cancer. N Engl J Med 1981;304:45.

Centers for Disease Control. Original contributions. Cancer and steroid hormone study: long-term oral contraceptive use and the risk of breast cancer. JAMA 1983;249:1591.

Clark GM, McGuire WL, Hubay CA, et al. Progesterone receptors as a prognostic factor in stage II breast cancer. N Engl J Med 1983;309:1343.

Conference on Breast Disease. The American Board of Obstetrics and Gynecology. Northwestern University Medical School Alumni Center for Continuing Education, Chicago, September 1987.

Consensus Conference. Adjuvant chemotherapy for breast cancer. JAMA 1985;254:3461.

Dash N, Lupetin AR, Daffner RH, et al. Magnetic resonance imaging in the diagnosis of breast cancer. AJR 1986;146:119.

Elston CW, Cotton RE, Davies CJ. A comparative use of the "Tru-cut" needle and fine needle aspiration cytology in the pre-operative diagnosis of carcinoma of the breast. Histopathology 1978;2:239.

Ernster VL, Cummings SR. Progesterone and breast cancer. Obstet Gynecol 1986;68(5):715.

Fisher B. Commentary. Reappraisal of breast biopsy prompted by the use of lumpectomy. Surgical Strategy. JAMA 1985;253:3585.

Fisher B, Bauer M, Poisson R, et al. Five-year results from the NSABP trial comparing total mastectomy to segmental mastectomy with and without radiation in the treatment of breast cancer. N Engl J Med 1985;312:665.

Fisher B, Redmond C, Poisson R, et al. Eight-year results of a randomized clinical trial comparing total mastectomy and lumpectomy with or without irradiation in the treatment of breast cancer. N Engl J Med 1989;320:822.

Foster RS, Costanza MC. Breast self-examination practices and breast cancer survival. Cancer 1984;53:999.

Frable WJ. Needle aspiration of the breast. Cancer 1984;53:671.

Goldwyn RM. Subcutaneous mastectomy. N Engl J Med 1977;297:503.

Goldwyn RM. Breast reconstruction after mastectomy. N Engl J Med 1987;317:1711.

Goodson WH, Mailman R, Miller TH. Three year follow-up of benign fine needle aspiration biopsies of the breast. Am J Surg 1987;154:58.

Greenspan EM. Toward the chemoprevention of breast cancer. The Female Patient 1989;14:103.

Griffith CN, Kern WH, Middleson WP. Needle aspiration cytologic examination in the management of suspicious lesions of the breast. Surg Gynecol Obstet 1986;162:142.

Gruber RP, Friedman GD. Periareolar subpectoral augmentation mammoplasty. Plast Reconstr Surg 1981;67:453.

Haagensen CD, Bodian C, Haagensen DE, Jr. Breast carcinoma. Risk and detection. Philadelphia: WB Saunders, 1981.

Hall FM. Screening mammography—potential problems on the horizon. N Engl J Med 1986;314:53.

Handley RS. The conservative radical mastectomy of Patey: 10-year results in 425 patients. Breast Dis 1976;2:16.

Harvey JC, Rosen PP, Ashikari R, et al. The effect of pregnancy on the prognosis of carcinoma of the breast following radical mastectomy. Surg Gynecol Obstet 1981;153:723.

Henderson IC. Breast cancer management progress and prospects. Wayne, N.J.: Lederle Laboratories, 1982:3.

Himel HN, Liberati A, Gelber RD, Chalmers TC. Adjuvant chemotherapy for breast cancer. JAMA 1986;256:1148.

Hindle WH, Navin J. Breast aspiration cytology: a neglected gynecologic procedure. Am J Obstet Gynecol 1983;146:482.

Homer MJ. The mammography report. (Editorials) AJR 1984;142:643.

Homer MJ, Smith TJ, Marchant DJ. Outpatient needle localization and biopsy for nonpalpable breast lesions. JAMA 1984;252:2452.

Hutter RVP. Goodbye to "Fibrocystic Disease." N Engl J Med 1985;312:179.

Hutter RVP. Is "Fibrocystic Disease" of the breast precancerous? Consensus Meeting, Oct 3–5, 1985, New York, Arch Pathol Lab Med 1986;110:171.

Jewell WR, Krishnan L, Reddy EK, et al. Intraoperative implantation radiation therapy plus lumpectomy for carcinoma of the breast. Arch Surg 1987;122:687.

Jones WD, III, Reed ML. What you should know about reconstructive breast surgery. Contemp Obstet Gynecol 1983;22:177.

Kleinberg DL, Noel GL, Frantz AG. Galactorrhea: a study of 235 cases, including 48 with pituitary tumors. N Engl J Med 1977; 296:589.

Leis HP, Jr, Cammarata A, LaRaja RD, Higgins H. Breast biopsy and guidance for occult lesions. Int Surg 1985;70(2):115.

Letterman G, Schurter M. The effects of mammary hypertrophy on the skeletal system. Ann Plast Surg 1980;5:425.

London RS, Solomon DM, London ED, et al. Mammary dysplasia: clinical response and urinary excretions of 11-deoxy-17-ketosteroids and pregnanediol following a-tocopherol therapy. Breast Dis Breast 1976;4:19.

Love SM, Gelman RS, Silen W. Fibrocystic "disease" of the breast—a nondisease? N Engl J Med 1982;307:1010.

Mahler D and Hauber DJ. Retromammary versus retropectoral breast augmentation—a comparative study. Ann Plast Surg 1982;8:370.

Manni A. Hormone receptors and breast cancer. N Engl J Med 1983;309:1383.

Marchac D, de Olarte G. Reduction mammaplasty and correction of ptosis with a short inframammary scar. Plast Reconstr Surg 1982;69:45.

McGuire WL. Adjuvant therapy of node-negative breast cancer. N Engl J Med 1989;320:525.

McGuire WL, De La Garza M, Chamness GC. Evaluation of estrogen receptor assays in human breast cancer tissue. Cancer Res 1977;37:637.

McSwain GR, Valicenti JF, Jr, O'Brien PH. Cytologic evaluation of breast cysts. Surg Gynecol Obstet 1978;146:921.

Mitchell GW. Benign breast disease and cancer. Clin Obstet Gynecol 1986;29(3):705.

Mitchell GW, Jr, Homer MJ. Outpatient breast biopsies on a gynecologic service. Am J Obstet Gynecol 1982;144:127.

Minton JP, Abou-Issa H, Reiches N, and Roseman JM. Clinical and biochemical studies on methylxanthine-related fibrocystic breast disease. Surgery 1981;90:299.

Moskowitz M. Clinical examination of the breasts by nonphysicians: a viable screening option? Cancer 1979;44:311.

Moskowitz M, Fig SA, Cole-Beuglet C, et al. Evaluation of new imaging procedures for breast cancer: proper process. AJR 1983;149:591.

Moskowitz M, Fox SH, Brun del Re R, et al. The potential value of liquid-crystal thermography in detecting significant mastopathy. Radiology 1981;140:659.

Mueller CB. Surgery for breast cancer: less may be as good as more. N Engl J Med 1985;312:712.

Mushlin AI. The use of diagnostic tests for screening and evaluating breast lesions. Ann Intern Med 1985;103:143.

Nezhat C, Asch RH, Greenblatt RB. Danazol for benign breast disease. Am J Obstet Gynecol 1980;137:604.

Parkes D. Drug therapy—Bromocriptine. N Engl J Med 1979;301:873.

Paulus DD. Imaging in breast cancer. CA 1987;37(3):133.

Poole GV, Jr, Choplin RH, Stershi JM, et al. Occult lesions of the breast. Surg Gynecol Obstet 1986;163:107.

Puga FJ, Welch JS, Bisel HF. Therapeutic oophorectomy in disseminated carcinoma of the breast. Arch Surg 1976;111:877.

Reiner A, Spona J, Reiner G, et al. Estrogen receptor analysis on biopsies and fine-needle aspirates from human breast carcinoma. Correlation of biochemical and immunohistochemical methods using monoclonal antireceptor antibodies. Am J Pathol 1986;125:443.

Remvikos Y, Magdelenat H, Zajdela A. DNA flow cytometry applied to fine needle sampling of human breast cancer. Cancer 1988;61:1629.

Ribeiro G, Jones DA. Carcinoma of the breast associated with pregnancy. Br J Surg 1986;73:607.

Rosenthal DL. Breast lesions diagnosed by fine needle aspiration. Pathol Res Pract 1986;181:645.

Rosner D, Blaird D. What ultrasonography can tell in breast masses that mammography and physical examination cannot. J Surg Oncol 1985;28:308.

Saltzstein SL. Potential limits of physical examination and breast self-examination in detecting small cancers of the breast. Cancer 1984;54:1443.

Sattin RW, Rubin GL, Wingo PA, et al. Oral-contraceptive use and the risk of breast cancer. N Engl J Med 1986;315:405.

Schwartz GF, D'Ugo DM, Rosenberg AL. Extent of axillary dissection preceding irradiation for carcinoma of the breast. Arch Surg 1986;121:1395.

Schwartz GJ, Marchant D, eds. Breast disease diagnosis and treatment. Miami: Symposia Specialists, 1981.

Schwartz GJ, D'Ugo D, Rosenberg AL. Extent of axillary dissection preceding irradiation for carcinoma of the breast. Arch Surg 1986;121:1395.

Seidman H, Geb SK, Silverberg E, LaVerda N, Lubera JA. The Breast Cancer Detection Demonstration Project end results. CA 1987;37(5):258.

Senn HJ. Current status and indications for adjuvant therapy in breast cancer. Cancer Chemother Pharmacol 1982;8:139.

Sickles EA. Mammographic features of 300 consecutive nonpalpable breast cancers. AJR 1986;146:661.

Tengrup I, Nittby LT, Landberg T. Prophylactic oophorectomy in the treatment of carcinoma of the breast. Surg Gynecol Obstet 1986;162:209.

Townsend CM, Jr. Management of breast cancer. Clinical Symposia 1987;39(4).

Walker GM, Foster RS, Jr, McKegney CP, McKegney FP. Breast biopsy. Arch Surg 1978;113:942.

Wallberg H, Alveryd A, Carlsson K. Breast carcinoma and benign breast lesions. Acta Radiol (Diagn) 1985;26:535.

Weintraub J, Weintraub D, Redard M, Vassilakos P. Evaluation of estrogen receptors by immunocytochemistry on fine-needle aspiration biopsy specimens from breast tumors. Cancer 1987;60:1163.

Whitehead J, Carlile T, Kopecky KJ, et al. Wolfe mammographic parenchymal patterns. Cancer 1985;56:1280.

Willett WC, MacMahon B. Diet and cancer—an overview. Part II. N Engl J Med 1984;310:697.

Wolfe JN. Breast patterns as an index of risk for developing breast cancer. Am J Roentgenol 1976;126:1130.

The Vermiform Appendix in Relation to Gynecology

36

JOHN D. THOMPSON

That the appendix is the site of significant disease is exemplified by the approximately 1500 deaths that occur each year in the United States from appendicitis. Although the mortality from acute appendicitis is now below 1% as reported in large series, untold thousands suffer from complicated septic illnesses caused by appendicitis.

The differential diagnosis between acute conditions in the pelvis and acute appendicitis is one of the most frequent that the gynecologist is called upon to make. It is a serious undertaking and one in which a mistake could be fatal to the patient. The diagnosis of appendicitis may be especially difficult in the elderly, in children, and in pregnant women. Acute inflammation of the appendix commonly extends to the right adnexa (Fig. 36-1) and may involve the left as well when a periappendiceal abscess develops in the pelvis. When appendiceal rupture takes place, bilateral tubal involvement is common, and complete or partial tubal closure may result, with sterility or tubal pregnancy as sequelae. Even when the appendix is normal, the gynecologist and the obstetrician must decide whether it should be removed during operations done for other reasons as prophylaxis against future disease of the appendix.

A thorough and interesting recitation of the history of appendicitis was published by Williams in 1983. According to Williams, the first known surgical removal of the appendix occurred in December, 1735, when Claudius Amyand operated on an 11-year-old boy with a long-standing scrotal hernia and fecal fistula. He found a perforated appendix in the hernia sac and removed it.

The fistula closed and the lad recovered. The first known successful appendectomy for a diagnosis of appendicitis was done in 1880 by Lawson Tait, the renowned British abdominal and gynecologic surgeon who was also the first to operate successfully for a ruptured tubal pregnancy.

In 1905, Howard A. Kelly coauthored with Hurdon a beautifully illustrated book entitled *The Vermiform Appendix and Its Diseases.* In its depiction of the pathology, clinical manifestations, and natural history of appendicitis and its complications, the book is unexcelled. An excellent current review of appendicitis by Condon was published in 1986.

INCIDENTAL APPENDECTOMY IN GYNECOLOGIC AND OBSTETRIC SURGERY

An appeal for appendectomy was made by Fischer in 1909 and by Goldspohn in 1911. Subsequent experience and evidence in the literature support our belief and recommendation that incidental or elective or prophylactic appendectomy in gynecologic and obstetric surgery is a safe procedure and should be performed in younger women unless the appendix is not conveniently available or the patient's condition is such that her well-being might be placed in jeopardy by the removal of the appendix. In other words, we believe that incidental appendectomy should be done unless there are contraindications.

There has been much controversy concerning the

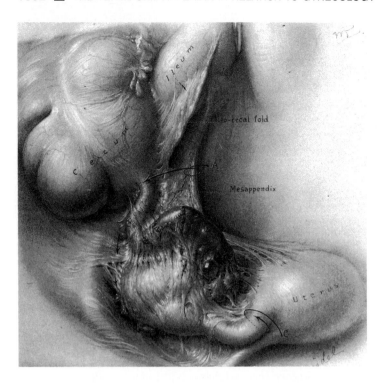

Figure 36–1. As illustrated in this original Max Broedel drawing, inflammatory disease of the appendix may involve the fallopian tube or vice versa. Extensive adhesions may form. The tube and the appendix may be removed as a single mass.

routine performance of this procedure. Today some of the most frequently done operations are hysterectomy, cesarean section, salpingectomy, oophorectomy, and tubal ligation. In these operations, the appendix is usually available for removal if the operator decides to do so and the patient agrees. That the controversy still exists is apparent from reports indicating that most gynecologic and obstetric operations are still done without incidental removal of the appendix. For example, in 1967, Loeffler and Stearn reported that only 26.5% of 555 patients had appendectomy at the time of total hysterectomy. In 1977, Hays found that most training programs recommended the performance of incidental appendectomy with uncomplicated abdominal hysterectomy. But the percentages were 66% in favor and 27% against. In 1986, Westermann and associates reported that the appendix was removed electively in 93% of 250 patients during the course of even extensive gynecologic operations. The pendulum may be swinging in favor of a more frequent performance of incidental appendectomy. We hope that it will not swing too far.

There are three main reasons to do incidental appendectomy:

1. To reduce future mortality and morbidity from appendicitis, including possible infertility following perforated appendix.
2. To eliminate undiagnosed incidental pathology in the appendix.

3. To eliminate the appendix from diagnostic consideration when the patient has abdominal or pelvic complaints in the immediate postoperative period and in future years.

The incidence of appendicitis has decreased markedly in recent decades, possibly due to a more frequent use of antibiotics and to an increase in the fiber content of the American diet. Although the mortality rate from appendicitis has improved tremendously, morbidity from this disease is still an important public health problem. Further improvement in morbidity and mortality from appendicitis will involve all major medical specialists, especially internists, surgeons, pediatricians, family practitioners, emergency medicine specialists, and gynecologists-obstetricians.

The incidence of appendicitis is high among teenagers and very low in elderly women. The incidence in women over 20 and under 50 years of age is still significant. The annual incidence is about 1.9 per thousand for females of ages 17–64. The overall lifetime risk of females developing appendicitis is about 1 in 6 at birth and 1 in 50 at 50 years of age. The risk of females developing appendicitis within the next year of life is greatest in the 15–19-year-old age group, where it is about 1 in 99. Of special concern to the obstetrician is the difficulty in diagnosing appendicitis in pregnancy and the resultant increase in fetal loss. Hewitt and associates have estimated that for women the death rate secondary to acute appendicitis is 1 in 1100 for all ages up to 80 years of age. Of course, although appendicitis is less common among elderly women, it is more difficult to diagnose in this group. Because of a frequently noncharacteristic and confusing clinical presentation, the diagnosis is delayed, perforation is more common, and the mortality rate is increased. Nevertheless, pointing out that 80% of cases of appendicitis in Wisconsin occur in patients between the ages of 5 and 30, with a rapid fall in subsequent years, Nockerts and associates feel that incidental appendectomy cannot be justified in the elderly. Unless epidemiologic data prove to the contrary, however, we shall continue to offer incidental appendectomy to patients up to 50 years of age, believing that the hazards of acute appendicitis following pelvic operations without appendectomy are great enough to warrant routine removal of the appendix in these younger patients. Routinely, the appendix of an older patient should be inspected, and it should be removed if an abnormality is discovered. According to Morrow, at age 60 in women, about 125 incidental appendectomies need to be done to prevent 1 case of appendicitis, 250 to prevent a ruptured appendix, and 5000 to prevent 1 death.

Although Puri and associates do not agree, acute perforated appendicitis, especially when associated with pelvic abscess and peritonitis, has been associated with subsequent infertility by other investigators. In the study by Wiig and associates, of 48 patients under 25 years of age who developed appendicitis with simple perforation, 19% were infertile; of 16 patients with appendiceal pelvic abscess, 31% were infertile. In the control group of 58 patients, 12% could not have children. A study by Powley also found an increased incidence of infertility following appendicitis. Forsell and Pieper found that 25% of the patients with perforated appendicitis in their study were involuntarily infertile compared with 4% in the control group. It may be advisable, therefore, for young girls to have an incidental appendectomy whenever this can be performed conveniently during abdominal or pelvic operations done for other reasons.

In addition to preventing appendicitis in future years, incidental appendectomy offers the advantage of removing unsuspected pathology. In the series of 532 cases reported by Taniguchi and Kilkenny, a relatively high incidence of acute inflammation was found in appendixes removed incidental to pelvic laparotomies: 9.6% showed catarrhal appendicitis and 0.9% showed subacute or early acute appendicitis. In a study of 45 incidental appendectomy specimens, Melcher found only 12 to be normal. Among the pathologic findings in the abnormal appendixes were acute, subacute, and chronic appendicitis; carcinoid tumors; and endometriosis. Others have confirmed that approximately 10% of incidental appendectomy specimens show significant pathology. The incidence will obviously depend on how carefully the appendix is examined by the pathologist.

Ectopic pregnancy and endometriosis have been reported in association with appendicitis. Indeed, the appendix is a frequent site of involvement in patients with pelvic endometriosis, although endometriosis is rarely confined only to the appendix. Pittaway found endometriosis in 13% of appendixes removed from patients with pelvic endometriosis at the Johns Hopkins Hospital. In 38%, the appendix was grossly normal when histologic evidence of endometriosis was found. The author concluded from the study that:

1. Appendectomy is warranted in patients who are not interested in having children and are undergoing definitive surgery for endometriosis.
2. Appendectomy should be done when the appendix is abnormal even in patients with endometriosis who are undergoing surgery to restore fertility.
3. In this latter group, routine appendectomy to remove occult appendiceal endometriosis is probably unnecessary.

We agree with these recommendations.

The appendix is the most common site for carcinoid tumors, with an incidence of 0.03% of all appendixes removed. Almost all appendiceal carcinoids are benign. It is rare for the carcinoid syndrome to be present. In a collected series of 1173 appendiceal carcinoid tumors, Sanders and Axtell reported that only 2.9% showed evidence of metastasis. Of two carcinoid tumors found by Melcher among 45 incidental appendectomies, one had spread into the surrounding adipose tissue. In Waters's series of 830 patients in whom elective appendectomy was performed, six appendiceal carcinoid tumors were suspected or diagnosed on gross surgical appearance.

One of the main reasons to perform incidental appendectomy is to eliminate the appendix from consideration when a patient presents subsequently with perplexing pelvic or abdominal pain. In spite of medical progress in many other areas, the diagnosis of appendicitis still remains difficult in many cases. The complication of acute appendicitis in the first several weeks after pelvic laparotomy or cesarean section is admittedly rare but could have serious consequences because of the difficulty of interpreting physical signs and laboratory data in the postoperative patient. Howkins reported four cases in which appendicitis occurred within a week of hysterectomy. However, in many other large series of abdominal hysterectomies without appendectomy there are no recognized cases of appendicitis in the postoperative recovery period, but over and over again the appendix does cause considerable confusion in the diagnosis of obscure abdominal and pelvic disease. An excellent example is the study by Isaacs and Knaus of nongenital pelvic tumors that mimicked gynecologic disease. Of 470 patients operated on for suspected tubo-ovarian pathology, 27 were found to have unsuspected nongenital pelvic tumors at the time of laparotomy. Chronic appendiceal infection was found most often. Of course, acute appendicitis is often confused with acute salpingitis, ectopic pregnancy, twisted or ruptured ovarian cysts, and other conditions within the abdomen and female pelvis. When such conditions arise, it is a significant diagnostic advantage to know that the patient has had a previous incidental appendectomy. However, in this situation the history of appendectomy must be certain. For example, one cannot assume that an appendectomy has been performed previously simply because the patient has an old incision in the lower abdomen.

There are no data on whether incidental appendectomy has a deleterious effect on fertility when done at the time of an operation whose purpose is to restore or enhance fertility. In other words, should an incidental appendectomy be done in conjunction with a microsurgical tubal reconstruction operation or a myomectomy or a uterine unification operation? The fact that there is no significant difference in postoperative febrile morbidity does not preclude the possibility of a mild, subclinical, localized peritonitis that might cause pelvic and peritubal adhesions, with the possibility of affecting fertility adversely. For this reason we usually do not remove the appendix when the operation is done for the primary purpose of restoring or enhancing fertility. The appendix is inspected at the end of the operation and is removed only if there is significant gross pathology.

Until recently, the removal of the appendix incidentally at cesarean section or at tubal ligation in the postpartum period was considered ill advised. Larsson was one of the first to advocate incidental appendectomy with cesarean section. Since then there have been other proponents of this procedure. Sweeney compared the results for 230 cesarean section patients on whom appendectomy was performed with the results for a control group of 230 cesarean section patients without appendectomy. Except for a 16-minute increase in operative time for those with appendectomy, there were no significant differences between the groups: there was no increase in operative risk, no difference in postoperative febrile morbidity, and no increase in the duration of hospitalization among the patients in the appendectomy group. Douglas and Stromme reported no significant complications in more than 500 selected cases of cesarean section where incidental appendec-

tomy was performed. Waters electively removed the appendix at the time of cesarean section during a personal experience of 40 years. Wilson and associates found no increase in morbidity when appendectomy was combined with cesarean section, cesarean tubal ligation, cesarean hysterectomy, postpartum tubal ligation, or postpartum hysterectomy. Incidental appendectomy should be done with caution when cesarean section is done for prolonged labor, prolonged rupture of the membranes, or amnionitis and is most acceptable in patients who are having an elective cesarean section. Good results from performance of incidental appendectomy at the time of elective cesarean section were reported by Parsons and associates. These authors also point out that a significant decrease in appendiceal disease in women could result from frequent removal of the appendix during this procedure since 20% to 25% of all deliveries are now by cesarean section.

The practice of incidental appendectomy at the time of operation for tubal ectopic gestation is more controversial. We agree with Pelosi and associates that the prognosis for subsequent pregnancy is so dismal after operation for ectopic pregnancy that any additional insult should be avoided. Bacterial contamination of free blood in the peritoneal cavity has been a primary concern. However, according to Schreier and Meyers, among 264 laparotomies for ectopic pregnancy, incidental appendectomy was done in 86%. The incidence of postoperative febrile morbidity was the same in both groups.

Incidental appendectomy could not be justified if it could not be done safely. Elective surgery must always be safe. There is ample evidence that, provided good judgment is used, no increase in morbidity or mortality occurs when incidental appendectomy is performed at the time of routine abdominal hysterectomy, salpingectomy, tubal ligation, or cesarean section. The studies of Pittaway, Waters, Loeffler and Stearn, Wilson and associates, Voitk and Lowry, and others confirm this. Of course, it cannot be denied that there are complications of incidental appendectomy, just as with any operative procedure. These include bleeding and hematoma formation; adhesion formation with subsequent intestinal obstruction; blow-out of the appendiceal stump with abscess or fecal fistula or both; and others. These complications, in fact, have been reported in patients who have had an incidental appendectomy, as one might expect. One cannot have a zero complication rate with any operative procedure done in great numbers. The complication rate is not negligible, but we believe that it is low enough to justify incidental appendectomy under proper circumstances. These include care in performance of the procedure; satisfactory condition of the patient during the operation, including satisfactory tolerance of the anesthetic; and easy exposure of the appendix. If the patient has lost a great deal of blood or the operation has been unusually prolonged, incidental appendectomy should be performed only when significant pathology of the appendix is found. Incidental appendectomy should not be performed in the presence of bowel obstruction or when severe postoperative ileus is likely.

Incidental appendectomy is uncommonly performed during vaginal surgery. In 1949, Bueno of Spain reported three cases of incidental appendectomy at the time of vaginal hysterectomy. Subsequently, McGowan reported the incidental vaginal removal of the appendix in 10 patients (eight following vaginal hysterectomy and two through posterior colpotomy incisions) without complications. Reiner reported 100 consecutive patients who underwent incidental appendectomy at the time of vaginal surgery with no significant alteration in postoperative morbidity. The appendiceal stump was buried beneath a purse string suture in all cases. During the same study period, there were 25 cases in which the appendix could not be removed because of technical difficulties in mobilization and visualization. The largest series of 225 vaginal appendectomies was reported by Massoudnia in 1975. Although incidental appendectomy at the time of vaginal hysterectomy is not considered acceptable practice in our clinic, it may not be absolutely contraindicated when adequate exposure and mobility of the appendix and its base are possible. Obviously, impeccable surgical judgment must be exercised so that the safe performance of the vaginal hysterectomy is not jeopardized.

A statistically significant higher appendectomy rate has been found among cancer patients than among matched controls by McVay, by Bierman, and by others. Studies by Moertel and associates, by Berndt, and by others do not confirm this association. Indeed, Cassimos found that appendectomy was less frequent in cancer patients than among controls. Current evaluation of these studies suggests no increased risk of cancer from performance of appendectomy.

ACUTE APPENDICITIS

Acute appendicitis is initiated by an obstruction of the appendiceal lumen. The obstruction may be caused by hyperplasia of lymphoid follicles of the appendix as part of a generalized response of lymphoid tissue to a systemic infectious disease; by bacterial enterocolitis; or by a fecalith, foreign body, or intestinal parasites in the appendix. An increase in intralumenal pressure distal to the obstruction from increased mucus secretion is followed by an increase in bacteria and finally the production of frank pus. The appendix becomes swollen and the appendiceal wall becomes edematous

from obstruction of lymphatic and venous drainage. Ulceration of the mucosa allows invasion of the wall by bacteria. Further progression causes venous thrombosis and obstruction of blood flow through the appendiceal artery. Since this is an end-artery, no collateral circulation is available to prevent ischemic necrosis and gangrene with eventual rupture of the wall. Escape of bacteria through the perforation causes peritonitis. Unless necrosis of the base of the appendix occurs, continued fecal contamination of the peritoneal cavity is prevented by the initial blockage of the appendiceal lumen. The infection in the right lower quadrant may be walled off efficiently in young, healthy patients. In females, it will usually involve the right adnexal organs to a greater or lesser extent. In advanced age or in the presence of reduced host resistance from other illnesses or immunosuppression, generalized peritonitis may ensue. A correlation between the clinical course and the pathologic progress of appendicitis is illustrated in Figure 36-2.

The diagnosis of acute appendicitis is based primarily on history and physical examination. Pain is present in 95% of patients and is the most consistent symptom. The typical pain of acute appendicitis is diffuse and mild and initially located in the epigastrium and periumbilical region, subsequently to become more severe and localized in the right lower quadrant. Anorexia, nausea, and occasional vomiting are usually present. This classic sequence may be found in 50% of patients. However, it should be emphasized that the typical presentation is absent in the remaining 50%. Atypically, pain may be localized in the right lower quadrant in the beginning, or it may remain diffuse throughout the abdomen. It should be remembered that, although the location of the cecum is constant, the inflamed appendiceal tip may be located in the right upper quadrant, in the cul-de-sac, and anywhere in between. The location and magnitude of the pain may vary with the position of the appendix and the age of the patient. Elderly patients may have less severe pain and delayed localization in the right lower quadrant. Indeed, appendicitis in the elderly presents a real challenge to early diagnosis, since very few abnormal clinical findings may be present in early stages of the disease and even in the presence of advanced disease. This is the reason for the higher incidence of appendiceal perforation and consequently morbidity and mortality rates in older patients as confirmed by the report of Lau and associates in 1985. The diagnosis is more difficult and the incidence of appendiceal perforation is also higher in infants and children. Improvement in the results for these two age groups will depend on a higher index of suspicion and a lower threshold for intervention, which will inevitably result in the removal of a larger number of normal appendixes. But removal of a normal appendix in a

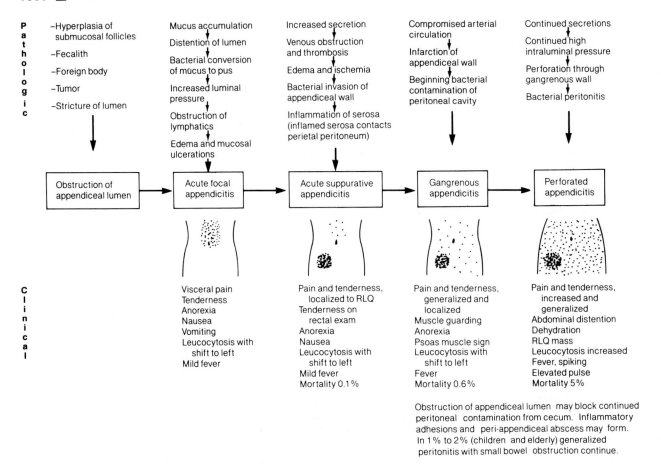

Figure 36–2. Some pathologic and clinical correlations in appendicitis. (Modified from Condon, 1981; DeVore, 1980.)

patient who is thought to have appendicitis, a potentially lethal disease, should not be considered an unnecessary operation. More elderly patients and children die of appendicitis because of failure to operate early enough when the diagnosis is in doubt than die from removal of a normal appendix. The morbidity of negative laparotomy is about 15% and is much more acceptable than the much higher morbidity of perforated appendix. Unfortunately, after age 60 about 50% of patients will be found to have a ruptured appendix when the operation is finally done. The mortality rate in these patients is 5%.

Usually 12–48 hours will elapse from the onset of symptoms until the patient consults her physician. On physical examination, patients with appendicitis will have tenderness to direct palpation, rebound tenderness, and muscle guarding in the right lower quadrant over the point where the inflamed appendiceal serosa is in contact with the parietal peritoneum, usually at McBurney's point. Rovsing's sign (pain in the right lower quadrant when pressure is applied in the left

lower quadrant) as well as psoas and obturator muscle signs may be positive. Rectal and pelvic examinations should always be done and often reveal tenderness high on the right side of the pelvis. Indeed, a pelvic mass from an inflamed appendix can sometimes be felt on pelvic examination. The appendix is located at the pelvic brim or lower in the pelvis in 30% of patients. The rectovaginal-abdominal examination is also necessary to rule out gynecologic and other problems. As the disease progresses to gangrene and appendiceal rupture occurs, a mass consisting of inflammatory adhesions, omentum, indurated bowel, mesentery, and pockets of purulent exudate can usually be felt in the right lower quadrant or by pelvic examination. Tenderness and muscle rigidity are more pronounced. If the infection fails to localize, generalized peritonitis ensues, with diffuse tenderness, guarding, distention, ileus, dehydration, tachycardia, and spiking fever. All these signs may be less apparent in the elderly.

Most would agree that the frequency of appendicitis does not vary with phases of the menstrual cycle. However, Arnbjornsson did find the frequency of acute appendicitis was highest in the luteal phase, almost twice the frequency of occurrence of the disease in the remaining half of the cycle.

Routine laboratory determinations and special diagnostic procedures are not especially helpful except to rule out other diseases that cause a similar clinical picture. A detailed analysis of laboratory findings has been published by Andersen and associates. The white cell count is usually elevated and the differential count shows a shift to the left in most patients with appendicitis. In elderly patients, on the other hand, the white cell count may be elevated only slightly or not at all, even though the differential count is abnormal. The erythrocyte sedimentation rate is elevated when the appendix is severely inflamed. Some white cells and red cells may be present in the urine with appendicitis, although with concomitant bacteriuria a urinary tract infection is a more likely diagnosis. Abdominal x-rays, barium enema, and ultrasonography are usually not helpful. A calcified fecalith may be seen on abdominal x-ray in the right lower quadrant, but this is a rare finding. When the infection is advanced, abdominal x-ray may show an indistinct right psoas muscle shadow, a sentinel loop ileus, and a soft tissue mass with or without gas bubbles. Occasionally, a barium edema will be helpful in ruling out appendicitis if the lumen of the appendix fills with barium. It may be possible to locate an appendiceal abscess with ultrasonography or CT scan, and once located, its progress and response to therapy may be followed by repeat studies.

The diagnostic error for acute appendicitis in all adults is 15% to 20%, and this figure has been acceptable. The diagnostic error in young adult females in the reproductive years is higher (35%–40%) because of the frequent occurrence of nearby gynecologic disease that may confuse the clinical picture. Although appendectomy with removal of a normal appendix carries a very minimal mortality risk, there is some morbidity to be considered. Therefore, efforts should be made to improve diagnostic accuracy. Laparoscopy has been used in recent years to define more accurately the cause of pelvic pain and to eliminate an appendectomy when the appendix is normal. According to Leape and Ramenofsky, and Deutsch and associates, approximately one third of selected patients suspected of having appendicitis did not require appendectomy after laparoscopy was performed. A few false positive and false negative examinations were reported, however. The plan of operation (eg, different incision) was altered in some patients who were found to have another condition. In doubtful cases of suspected early appendicitis, diagnostic accuracy will be improved by laparoscopy.

Since there is no single generally applicable and accurate diagnostic test for acute appendicitis, most would agree with Levine and associates that a decrease in the number of negative explorations is most likely to be achieved by a generous application of sound clinical judgment supplemented by basic laboratory and x-ray studies. Using this standard classical approach assiduously, these authors reported negative laparotomy in only 7.4% of 282 patients with a preoperative diagnosis of suspected appendicitis. Most patients with the classic pattern of migratory abdominal pain, direct and rebound tenderness in the right lower abdominal quadrant, and increased metamyelocytes in the peripheral blood smear will most likely require prompt operation, as advised by Nauta and Magnant and many others. However, when there is an atypical presentation in a young adult female, close in-hospital observation may be indicated instead to follow carefully the progression of the clinical picture, the signs, the symptoms, the fever, and the laboratory data. A brief period of observation for 12–24 hours will also allow time for x-ray studies. Nakhgevany and Clarke studied 108 female patients between the ages of 15 and 45 years who had undergone appendectomy for a preoperative diagnosis of acute appendicitis. Twenty-two percent of the patients between the ages of 36 and 45 years had a negative laparotomy as compared with 59% of the patients between the ages of 15 and 25 years. In-hospital observation with frequent examinations and reevaluations has been studied and advised by White and associates, by Neutra, and by Nase and associates, and may be especially valuable in these younger patients with an atypical presentation. Simultaneous evaluation by the general surgeon and gynecologist will also be of benefit in improving diagnostic accuracy. It must be understood and emphasized, however, that one cannot expect to achieve a preoperative diagnostic accuracy of 100%. To achieve a perfect score, it probably would be necessary to allow most appendixes to rupture before deciding to operate. Without question, in almost all circumstances a laparotomy with negative findings is to be preferred over expectantly watching the natural progression of the disease to its late stage of rupture and peritonitis. An unnecessary delay increases the likelihood of perforation. When operation is performed within 24 hours of the onset of symptoms, less than 20% of appendixes will be perforated, compared with over 70% when operation is delayed more than 48 hours after symptoms began. A delay in diagnosis in pregnant patients will have especially devastating effects on the outcome. A proper evaluation of the clinical presentation will allow the "index of suspicion" to be set at the proper level so that a "threshold for intervention" can be reached before the appendix ruptures. According to Condon, "The removal of a normal appendix in appropriate clinical circumstances never constitutes an unnecessary appendectomy. A policy of active surgical intervention on the basis of minimal clinical suspicion has been demonstrated to reduce both the morbidity and mortality of appendicitis. Watching and waiting, however careful it may be, runs the risk of increasing both morbidity and mortality."

Treatment of Acute Appendicitis

There is general agreement that the treatment of acute appendicitis in the nonperforated stage is immediate appendectomy. Clinical experience and numerous reports on mortality show clearly the advantage of early operation. The current operative mortality for appendicitis without perforation is essentially nil, and only 5% of patients have postoperative complications. Following perforation, the overall mortality is less than 5%, but over 30% of patients have postoperative complications. Obviously, antibiotics and earlier surgical intervention have contributed to the improvement in these statistics.

Thus, there is no controversy concerning the treatment of the acute appendicitis per se, but there is considerable difference of opinion concerning the treatment of the principal complication, namely, abscess. We believe that, as a general policy, an immediate operation should be performed when the diagnosis is made, regardless of the stage of the disease.

In almost all patients, 2 or 3 hours should be spent in intensive preoperative preparation with fluid replacement. Nasogastric suction may be necessary. All patients receive antibiotics preoperatively, although administration of antibiotics may not benefit those without appendiceal perforation and peritonitis. After satisfactory anesthesia is established, an indwelling transurethral Foley catheter is inserted and a careful examination of the pelvis and lower abdomen is performed. The findings of this examination may influence the diagnosis or the choice of incision.

Our general rule is to operate immediately through a McBurney or Rockey-Davis incision in cases of acute appendicitis. A transverse incision made just below McBurney's point usually provides adequate exposure, can be extended into the lateral rectus sheath if necessary, and is more cosmetically acceptable when healed. When the diagnosis is uncertain and there is a possibility that other surgery may be required, either a low midline or a right paramedian incision may be used.

Occasionally, one may diagnose a well-walled-off abscess that is palpable abdominally in a patient whose history suggests strongly that she is improving. It may be apparent from her history that she is not as ill as she was previously and that the walled-off abscess is subsiding. Such a patient should be kept under close observation, with frequent white blood counts, differential counts, and repeated radiologic evaluation of the dilated bowel pattern for documented evidence of clinical improvement. Serial ultrasonography examinations of CT scans are helpful. Operation should be deferred as long as improvement continues. During the period of observation, the patient should have the advantage of intensive antibiotic therapy. If there is evidence of spread of infection, or if the patient's general condition becomes worse, surgical intervention is carried out immediately. Our reason for making this exception to the rule of immediate operation is that, in our experience with cases of this kind, patients who were treated conservatively responded better than those who were operated upon immediately. Reports by Bradley and Isaacs from Emory University and from others suggest a high rate of complications when such patients are managed with aggressive surgery. Some of the latter patients died of obstruction or peritonitis with septic shock. In retrospect, it appears that such patients probably would have continued to improve if surgical intervention had been omitted at that stage. Such a conservative approach to the management of certain cases of appendiceal peritonitis was originally advocated by Ochsner in 1906. In 1982, Skoubo-Kristensen and Hvid reported the results of their experience with the conservative management of 193 patients with an appendiceal inflammatory mass. The course was uneventful in 88%.

When appendiceal abscesses are operated upon, it is our custom to make a transverse incision (Rockey-Davis) directly over the abscess. The abscess cavity is entered with the greatest of care to avoid breaking up the adhesions that are responsible for the walling off of the abscess, especially those located on the medial side. If the appendix can be removed readily without danger of injury to the bowel wall or of dissemination of the infection, appendectomy is done; if appendectomy is not feasible, the abscess is simply drained. Intensive antibiotic therapy is continued. When the abscess is localized in the cul-de-sac, it may be drained by colpotomy, with drains placed in the cavity. Generally, we perform an interval appendectomy 6 or 8 weeks after the abscess has ceased to drain. In a few patients who have responded well, have no evidence of active infection, and have medical contraindications to operation, interval appendectomy may be postponed indefinitely as long as the patient remains well.

Perhaps the term *immediate operation* should be defined. In the usual case of unruptured appendicitis, the operation is done as soon as preoperative preparation is completed and the operating room can be made ready. On the other hand, very ill patients with abscess or generalized peritonitis often are dehydrated, have abnormal serum electrolytes, have marked gastric and intestinal distention, and may have circulatory collapse from gram-negative shock. Often more intensive preoperative treatment is required for the patient's condition to improve, so that she is stable enough to tolerate general anesthesia. Unnecessary delay in surgery is one of the major factors in the very high mortality associated with ruptured appendix in the elderly patient. Such patients are admitted to the hospital and placed in Fowler's position. A nasogastric tube is passed and suction is started. High-dose, intravenous antibiotics are administered in an effort to produce adequate blood levels and tissue perfusion of the antibiotics rapidly. These antibiotics include 20–40 million units of penicillin and 1–1.5 g of the aminoglycoside kanamycin per day or other appropriate agents (eg, clindamycin) that are effective against coliform bacteria. One of the newer cephalosporins or metronidazole may be indicated if an agent effective against *Bacteroides fragilis* is needed. The question of antibiotics for appendicitis—when they should be used, which ones to give, in what dosage, and for how long—is an area of active clinical research. Antibiotic coverage with a second-generation cephalosporin such as cefoxitin is currently our first choice with metronidazole with or without an aminoglycoside added for significant peritoneal contamination or abscess.

Postoperatively, supportive treatment is continued in the ill patient. All food and fluids by mouth are forbidden. Nasogastric suction is continued until distention has disappeared and there is clinical evidence of intestinal activity. Intensive antibiotic therapy is continued until the patient is well on her way to recovery. Continued use of antibiotics in the postoperative period can reduce the wound infection rates.

If a normal appendix is found at laparotomy, the surgeon may or may not elect to remove it, depending on circumstances. Careful exploration of the abdomen and pelvis should be carried out to determine the cause of the patient's signs, symptoms, and abnormal lab values. If necessary, the incision should be extended. A careful search should be made for Meckel's diverticulitis, regional enteritis, mesenteric adenitis, ectopic pregnancy, pelvic inflammatory disease, ovarian pathology, endometriosis, ruptured sigmoid diverticulum, gall bladder disease, and cancer of the cecum (especially in older women).

TECHNIQUE OF APPENDECTOMY

The appendix and the cecum are delivered through the incision. Usually this is a simple matter, but in some instances an immobile cecum, adhesions, or retrocecal position of the appendix may make it difficult. Adhesions around the appendix and cecum should be cut,

and sometimes it is necessary to incise the lateral peritoneal attachment of the cecum to bring it and the appendix into the operative field. When the appendix is mobile, the mesoappendix may be conveniently grasped near the tip of the appendix with a Kelly clamp and the appendix supported with a Babcock clamp near its base. Clean lap pads should be placed around the base of the appendix in such a way that it is isolated from the remainder of the operative field.

The mesoappendix can then be ligated en masse with No. 3-0 delayed-absorbable suture, if it is sufficiently mobile (Fig. 36-3A). Often ligation of the mesoappendix en masse is not feasible, and if this is the case, it is clamped with Kelly clamps in a succession of small bites; each segment of the clamped mesoappendix is ligated individually. It may be appropriate to pass one suture into the musculature of the cecal wall and mesoappendix at the base of the appendix to ligate the appendiceal artery securely. Packs are then placed around the appendix to isolate it from the operative field.

A purse-string suture of medium silk is placed about the base of the appendix (Fig. 36-3B). The circumference of the purse string should be large enough to permit easy inversion of the stump. A half-knot is placed in the silk. A cuff of peritoneum is turned back after a circular incision is made about the base of the appendix (Fig. 36-3C) to permit complete occlusion of the appendiceal lumen when the stump is ligated. The appendix is crushed at the point of denudation with a Kelly or Halsted clamp and ligated with No. 3-0 delayed-absorbable suture (Fig. 36-3D). A Kelly clamp is placed across the appendix a short distance distal to the ligature, leaving sufficient space between the ligature and the clamp to permit the passage of the cautery or scalpel.

The appendix is amputated with the scalpel, although amputation with a cautery is an equally good technique. The appendix and the attached clamps are dropped into a small basin kept on the operating table for receiving the appendix and the instruments that might be contaminated in doing the appendectomy. The peritoneal edge of the appendix stump is grasped by the assistant with a mosquito clamp, and the ligature about the base of the appendix is cut short. The stump is inverted (Fig. 36-3E) and the purse string is drawn tight (Fig. 36-3F). The mosquito clamp is dropped into the appendix basin, and the basin is passed from the operating table.

The site of inversion of the appendiceal stump into the cecum should be covered over with the mesoappendix or any convenient flap of fat located around the terminal ileum (Fig. 36-3 G–H). If the appendiceal stump has not been inverted but has been left exposed, it is especially important that it be covered. If the appendix was retrocecal, this step may not be necessary.

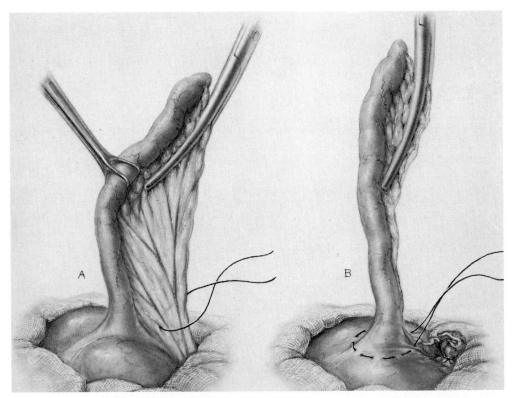

Figure 36–3. Technique of appendectomy. *A,* Appendix is delivered and supported with Kelly and Babcock clamps as the mesoappendix is ligated. Often this can be done with a single ligature of No. 3-0 delayed-absorbable suture as illustrated. *B,* A purse-string of medium silk has been placed about the base of the appendix.

(Figure continued on next page.)

We are aware that there are criticisms of a technique of appendectomy that includes burying a ligated appendiceal stump (Fig. 36-4). An abscess may form in the cecal wall leading to blow-out of the cecum. A space-occupying mass in the cecum may be found on barium enema and lead to diagnostic confusion. However, these problems are rare. We still prefer to bury the appendiceal stump and have it isolated completely rather than run the risk of localized infection and adhesion formation or even intestinal obstruction from adhesions to an exposed stump. Admittedly, inversion of the stump is more applicable when a normal appendix is being removed, as in incidental appendectomy. It is less feasible when an inflamed appendix is being removed. Further discussion of this subject may be found in Chapter 38.

If the appendix is inflamed, gangrenous, or perforated, its removal may be much more difficult. An unruptured appendix should be handled very gently, to avoid rupture if at all possible. If pus is already present, the dissection should be careful and meticulous to avoid spreading the infection. The omentum and other tissues will be found adherent to the appendix in an attempt to isolate and contain the infection. The appendix, mesoappendix, and enveloping tissues will be thickened and edematous. Adhesions may be freed with gentle finger dissection. Pus should be removed with suction and should be collected for anaerobic and aerobic cultures and antimicrobial sensitivity studies. If the appendix is gangrenous or perforated, the stump generally should not be buried but should be doubly ligated and covered if possible.

If drains are required for residual abscess material in the pelvis, we prefer a separate stab-wound incision rather than a drain placed in one end of the incision. This will decrease the incidence of secondary infection of the incision. Infection of the wound occurs in 5% to 10% of the reported cases of acute appendicitis, depending on the severity of the infection and the virulence of the offending organism. Incisional infection occurs in 34% to 50% of the cases where the appendix has ruptured. The important points in surgical technique to assist primary wound healing in these infected cases include minimal tissue trauma, meticulous hemostasis, and use of the least possible amount of absorbable suture buried in the wound. Nonabsorbable suture

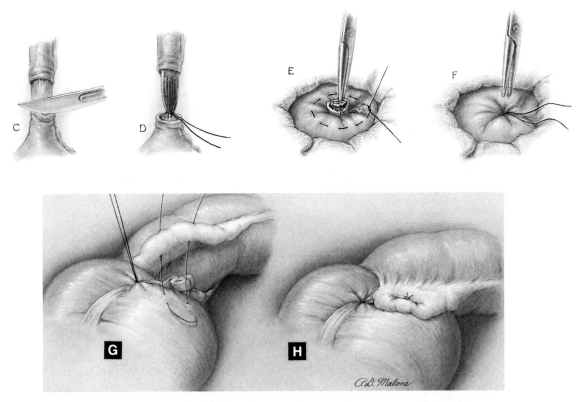

Figure 36–3. (continued) *C*, An incision through the serosa is made about the appendix near its base and the serosa is pushed down. *D*, The appendix has been crushed at the point where it has been freed of serosa and ligated with No. 3-0 delayed-absorbable suture. *E*, The stump is inverted as the purse-string is drawn tight. *F*, The mosquito clamp is withdrawn as the purse-string suture is tied. *G*, A simple method of peritonizing the mesoappendix stump. Fine silk is used for this. *H*, Completed appendectomy.

material should not be used in this incision closure. We are convinced, as are Ackerman and others, that the use of subcutaneous drains and subcutaneous antibiotic irrigations is important in reducing wound infection if primary closure is used in cases with a ruptured appendix.

Occasionally, it may be advisable to omit primary closure of the subcutaneous fat and skin and rely on secondary healing from the base of the incision. Skin mattress sutures may be placed and left untied. The open incision may be irrigated or sprayed with an antibiotic solution (Neosporin) and packed with sterile gauze. The wound should be inspected, irrigated, sprayed, and repacked twice each day. On the third to fifth postoperative day, if the wound is clean, the skin sutures are tied. Sterile adhesive strips may also be applied. A wound that does not appear healthy should not be closed. It should be allowed to granulate from the bottom until healing is complete in approximately 1 month. It has been our experience that primary wound closure results in fewer postoperative incisional hernias.

APPENDICITIS IN PREGNANCY

In 1848, Hancock reported the first case of appendicitis complicating pregnancy. Ten days after premature delivery, an appendiceal abscess was drained and the patient recovered. Our active knowledge of appendicitis complicating pregnancy dates from a 1892 monograph by Wiggins.

During pregnancy, acute appendicitis—and especially its sequelae—present serious dangers for both mother and fetus. It is the most common acute surgical emergency in pregnancy. Brant noted an incidence of acute appendicitis of 1 in 1789 pregnancies (0.06%), and Finch and Lee reported the same incidence in the Oxford region in England. Taylor reported an increase in the frequency of this complication of pregnancy to 1 in 704 cases. Babaknia and associates found the incidence of appendicitis to be 1 in 1500 pregnancies (0.07%) over a 12-year period. Earlier reports by Baer, Reis, and Arens recorded the incidence as approximately 0.17%. The incidence of acute appendicitis does not seem to be increased during pregnancy above

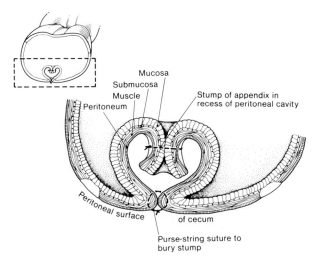

Figure 36–4. Diagrammatic representation of inversion of the ligated appendiceal stump into the cecal wall.

that of the nonpregnant state, but the diagnosis is often delayed. In our clinics and in others, acute appendicitis occurs more frequently during the second trimester (50%) than in the first trimester (10%) or third trimester (35%). Five percent of cases occur during labor or in the puerperium. Because of the difficulty in diagnosis and consequent delay in operation, the number of patients with appendiceal rupture is highest in the third trimester.

Appendicitis is responsible for approximately 75% of all cases of an acute abdomen during pregnancy. Errors in the clinical diagnosis of acute appendicitis are quite common during pregnancy, with a normal appendix being found in between 20% and 30% of the cases at removal, as recently reported by Mohammed and Oxorn. Although this removal rate of an uninflamed appendix may seem high, this diagnostic error is far more acceptable than a delay in surgery in the case of an acute abdomen during pregnancy, which could result in appendiceal rupture and an increased risk of maternal mortality and morbidity, as well as fetal mortality.

Delay in diagnosis is consistently the reason for gangrenous and perforated appendix with associated increased risk of maternal mortality and morbidity and perinatal mortality. The incidence of gangrenous and perforated appendix has been reported to be twice as high in pregnant patients as in women who are not pregnant and is highest in advanced pregnancy. Patient delay or a policy of observation before operating allows the inflamed appendix time to become gangrenous and to perforate. In a pregnant patient, the omentum may not be able to reach the site of infection and perform its walling-off function efficiently. If rupture is followed by abscess formation, the uterus is always a part of the

abscess wall, because of its proximity. Generalized peritonitis without abscess is more common in advanced pregnancy and is a serious threat to the expectant mother and her unborn child. The speed of onset and spread of peritonitis in pregnant patients may be strikingly and insidiously rapid. The patient may become seriously ill and appear moribund within 24 hours. Appendiceal perforation and involvement of the uterus in peritonitis cause uterine irritability and increase the risk of preterm labor.

In addition to difficult and delayed diagnosis, there are other reasons that mortality and morbidity from appendicitis are higher in pregnant patients. When the appendix is displaced high in the abdomen, inflammation is more difficult to isolate. The omentum is prevented from performing its function. The intermittent movement of the uterus keeps adhesions from forming to wall off the infection. Higher levels of adrenocorticoids in pregnancy may interfere with the natural host response to infection. To avoid these consequences, every attempt should be made to intervene early in the course of the disease.

Diagnosis of Appendicitis in Pregnancy

Babler's statement written in 1908 is unfortunately still pertinent today: "The mortality of appendicitis complicating pregnancy and the puerperium is the mortality of delay." Several factors cause a delay in the diagnosis of acute appendicitis in pregnant patients. Consider first that a normal pregnancy may cause some of the same symptoms as acute appendicitis and may be confusing. For example, the classic symptoms of abdominal pain, nausea, vomiting, and constipation are common to both pregnancy and appendicitis. Lower abdominal discomfort, a common symptom of normal pregnancy, is frequently attributed to round ligament stretching. The evaluation of the abdomen by physical examination is more difficult in the presence of an enlarging uterus, especially since only 50% of the patients with acute appendicitis have peritoneal irritation with rebound tenderness. Alder described a useful clinical sign to differentiate appendiceal from uterine pain. If the pain is localized in the right lower abdominal quadrant with the patient lying supine but shifts to the left when she rolls to her left side, the pain is most likely of uterine or adnexal origin. On the other hand, if the pain remains localized to the right lower quadrant after she rolls to the left, then appendicitis should be suspected.

The change in the position of the appendix during pregnancy makes the interpretation of abdominal pain and tenderness more difficult than in the nonpregnant woman. One can interpret pain and tenderness much more intelligently if one bears in mind these changes. Baer, Reis, and Arens showed by repeat roentgenographic studies throughout pregnancy and the puerperium that the appendix rotated in a counterclockwise direction, with the tip displaced near the right kidney at term. The base of the appendix underwent upward and outward displacement after the third month, caused by the enlarging uterus, reaching the level of the iliac crest at the end of the sixth month. After the seventh month of pregnancy, in 88% of their cases, the appendix was found above the iliac crest (Fig. 36-5). However, in interpreting these findings in relation to abdominal pain and tenderness, one must remember that in dealing with the abnormal appendix, in which previous attacks of appendicitis are frequent, adhesions may fix it in a low position and do not permit its upward displacement. Because the appendix is embryologically a midline structure, the afferent sensory fibers to this vestigial organ register pain more frequently in the periumbilical region, as well as on both sides of the abdomen. Once local peritonitis occurs, however, the maximum tenderness is usually located in the region of the appendix.

The organ that most often leads to a mistaken diagnosis of appendicitis in pregnancy is the kidney. An acute urinary tract infection is frequently misdiag-

nosed. Since urinary tract symptoms occur in more than 50% of the cases of appendicitis in pregnancy, the patient is frequently treated initially for pyelitis of the right kidney. Acute torsion of an ovarian cyst also mimics the clinical signs of appendicitis in pregnancy, but in general this entity has fewer intestinal symptoms and the onset is more abrupt. Torsion of an ovarian cyst can be traced in many cases to strenuous physical activity, such as dancing, swimming, coitus, or the like. Dysmenorrhea, ovulation, dysfunctional ovarian cysts, salpingitis, and ectopic pregnancy are common problems that mimic appendicitis in nonpregnant patients. These problems do not need to be considered in the differential diagnosis of appendicitis in late pregnancy.

Although a mild leukocytosis is common in pregnancy, one should observe the white count frequently for a gradual or rapid increase and particularly for a shift in the differential leukocyte count. A white count above 16,000 per cubic millimeter and a differential count of more than 80% polymorphonuclear leukocytes suggest an acute inflammatory process, but these are not specific for appendicitis. One must always be aware of the occasional case in which the white blood count remains normal throughout the acute phase of the disease. Fever is usually mild and sometimes absent.

All the preceding factors tend to make the diagnosis of appendicitis more difficult in pregnancy; hence, a tendency to delay operation is common. The important thing for the clinician to bear in mind is the possibility of appendicitis, remembering that the symptoms of acute appendicitis are generally the same in a pregnant as in a nonpregnant patient. The clinician should have no concern about the possibility of removing a normal appendix during pregnancy but should remember that this operation is a small price to pay to avoid the increased risk to the life of the mother and fetus that accompanies a prolonged delay in the diagnosis of this disease. Although the laparoscope is beneficial in establishing the diagnosis in suspected cases in early pregnancy, its use is limited by the size of the uterus in late pregnancy.

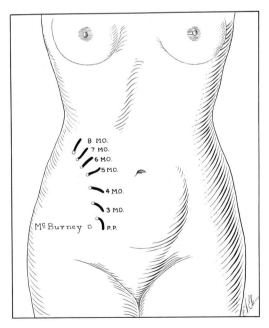

Figure 36–5. Change of position of appendix during pregnancy (Baer JL, Reis RA, Arens RA. Appendicitis in pregnancy, with changes in position and axis of normal appendix in pregnancy. JAMA 1932; 98:1359. Copyright 1932, American Medical Association.)

Treatment of Appendicitis in Pregnancy

Immediate operation is the treatment for acute appendicitis in pregnancy, regardless of the duration of pregnancy. Preoperative measures to improve the patient's condition should be brief and intensive. Although antibiotics may not be needed in simple acute appendicitis, antibiotic therapy should be initiated as soon as possible in all cases of suspected appendicitis so that an adequate level can be present in the tissues before the incision is made. Where a gangrenous or perforated appendix is found, antibiotics with broad-spectrum bacterial coverage should be continued or initiated immediately in both the pregnant and non-pregnant state. One may choose to give cefoxitin and metronidazole. In the more serious cases, triple antibiotic therapy with ampicillin, gentamycin, and Cleocin should be used. Ritodrine, a beta-mimetic tocolytic agent, or terbutaline, should be given prophylactically to all patients beyond 16 weeks to prevent uterine contractions and premature labor. It should be continued as long as there is evidence of active infection. In this inflammatory environment, some suggest the use of nonsteroidal anti-inflammatory agents such as indomethacin or ibuprofen for tocolysis. Although it is controversial, we also administer progesterone intramuscularly, especially to patients who are earlier in pregnancy than 16 weeks. Spontaneous premature termination of pregnancy is more likely when the appendix has ruptured. Delay in operating can also stem from concern about what harm the operation will do to the pregnancy, with the consequent desire to operate only when acute appendicitis is definitely present. Such a delay will result in a larger number of perforated appendixes being found and a far greater harm to the pregnancy. Proper removal of a normal appendix found at operation for suspected appendicitis is rarely associated with preterm labor, especially with the prophylactic use of modern tocolytic agents.

If the pregnancy is 3 months or less in duration, the appendix may be removed through the usual gridiron McBurney or Rockey-Davis incision. The more advanced the pregnancy, the higher should be the incision. If a midline incision is not used, it is important to center the incision over the point of maximum tenderness, which usually means using a high transverse muscle-cutting or a right paramedian incision. Turning the patient on her left side minimizes displacement and handling of the uterus and relieves the compression of the vena cava by the gravid uterus. The appendectomy should be done as quickly and atraumatically as possible, and the patient should be given intensive antibiotic therapy. In the case of appendiceal rupture with or without frank abscess formation, the patient should be treated immediately, in the same way as in the nonpregnant state, with the understanding that premature labor will usually occur as a result of the infection. Cesarean section should not be performed at the time of appendectomy with or without rupture in order to avoid infection in the newborn and postoperative endometritis and parametritis. Cesarean section in the third-trimester patient with appendicitis is indicated only for strict obstetric reasons. When cesarean section is indicated for obstetric reasons, the fetus is near term size, and an advanced infection is present, some authors have advised that a cesarean section hysterectomy may be indicated to control the spread of the infection into the uterus and broad ligaments.

Maternal and Perinatal Mortality

In his 1908 collection series of 735 cases of appendicitis complicating pregnancy, labor, and the puerperium, Babler reported that the perinatal mortality was 66% and the maternal mortality was 48.5% when the appendix ruptured.

Significant progress has been made in reducing maternal and perinatal mortality from appendicitis in recent decades. The maternal mortality in the first trimester has usually been comparatively low, since diagnosis is less difficult at that stage. Black reported in 1960 that the mortality rate was 4% in the second trimester, 11% in the third trimester, and 16.7% if labor had begun. However, this high maternal mortality rate is considered to be due to the occurrence of many deaths prior to the use of antibiotics. In 1967, Brant reported an overall maternal mortality rate of 2%, with a mortality rate of 7.3% in the last trimester. In a 1977 review of 333 cases reported since 1963, Babaknia found only three maternal deaths (1.0%), all three of which occurred among 70 cases with a ruptured appendix (4%). Cunningham and McCubbin reported no maternal deaths among 34 pregnant patients with documented appendicitis at Parkland Memorial Hospital between 1960 and 1975. Between 1949 and 1988, two maternal deaths from appendicitis in the antepartum period occurred at Grady Memorial Hospital. Both deaths occurred more than 31 years ago. During this period of 39 years, approximately 250,000 deliveries occurred in this hospital. Most reports of appendicitis complicating pregnancy since 1980 show no maternal deaths. When this is compared with the nonpregnant mortality of an unruptured acute appendicitis of 0.1%, it is evident that progress has been made in reducing maternal mortality from appendicitis. That it continues to represent a significant problem today is clear from the 1985 report of Horowitz and associates in which 12 patients underwent appendectomy during pregnancy or the puerperium. Six patients were found to have a perforated appendix; one mother and three fetuses were lost.

There has also been considerable improvement in the combined fetal and neonatal (perinatal) mortality associated with appendicitis during the past two decades. Perinatal mortality is related to the duration of pregnancy and the severity of the infection. During the first trimester, spontaneous abortion may occur postoperatively in as many as 20% of cases. Midtrimester fetal loss is less common, but in the third trimester, perinatal mortality may reach as high as 15%, primarily because of prematurity. In the presence of perforation of the appendix and peritonitis, the perinatal mortality increases. In 1980, McComb and Laimon reviewed a collected series of 171 cases of appendicitis complicating pregnancy and found that the overall perinatal mortality was 10%. The perinatal mortality was 7% when the appendix was not perforated and 30% when it was perforated. More than 20% of patients with appendicitis occurring in the third trimester will develop premature labor postoperatively. It is clear that early diagnosis and operative intervention, proper antibiotic administration, and prophylactic use of tocolytic agents to prevent preterm labor are the keys to further reduction in perinatal and maternal mortality from this disease.

Bibliography

Ackerman NB. The continuing problems of perforated appendicitis. Surg Gynecol Obstet 1974;139:29.

Adler N. A sign for differentiating uterine from extrauterine complications of pregnancy and puerperium. Br Med J 1951;2:1194.

Allen NJW, Heringer R. Coincident acute appendicitis and tubal pregnancy. Can Med Assoc J 1970;103:531.

Andersen M, Lilja T, Lundell L, Thulin A. Clinical and laboratory findings in patients subjected to laparotomy for suspected acute appendicitis. Acta Chir Scand 1980;146:55.

Arnbjornsson E. Varying frequency of acute appendicitis in different phases of the menstrual cycle. Surg Gynecol Obstet 1982;155:709.

Ashley JSA, Morris JN. Deaths from appendicitis. Lancet 1967;1:217.

Babaknia A, Parsa H, Woodruff JD. Appendicitis during pregnancy. Obstet Gynecol 1977;50:40.

Babler EA. Perforative appendicitis complicating pregnancy. JAMA 1908;51:1310.

Baer JL, Reis RA, Arens RA. Appendicitis in pregnancy with changes in position and axis of normal appendix in pregnancy. JAMA 1932;98:1359.

Barber HRK, Graber EA. Surgical diseases in pregnancy. Philadelphia: WB Saunders, 1974.

Berndt H. Is appendectomy followed by increased cancer risk? Digestion 1970;3:187.

Bierman HR. Human appendix and neoplasia. Cancer 1968;21:109.

Black WP. Acute appendicitis in pregnancy. Br Med J 1960;1:1938.

Boyd A, Hoffmeister FJ. Cesarean section and associated surgery. Obstet Gynecol 1964;24:533.

Bradley EL, Isaacs J. Appendiceal abscess revisited. Arch Surg 1978;113:130.

Brant H. Acute appendicitis in pregnancy. Obstet Gynecol 1967;29:130.

Brumer M. Appendicitis. Seasonal incidence and postoperative wound infection. Br J Surg 1970;57:93.

Bueno B. Primer caso de apendicetomia por via vaginal. Tokoginec Pract (Madrid) 1949;8:152.

Cassimos Chr, Sklavunu-Zurukzoglu S, et al. The frequency of tonsillectomy and appendectomy in cancer patients. Obstet Gynecol Survey 1974;29:569.

Champion P, Doolittle J. Appendectomy at the time of cesarean section. Obstet Gynecol 1964;24:533.

Christhilf SM, Jr. Simplified incidental appendectomy. Surg Gynecol Obstet 1966;122:607.

Condon RE. Appendicitis. In: Sabiston DC, Jr, ed. Davis-Christopher textbook of surgery. Philadelphia: WB Saunders, 1986.

Cunningham FG, McCubbin JH. Appendicitis complicating pregnancy. Obstet Gynecol 1975;45:415.

Deutsch AA, Zelikovsky A, Reiss R. Laparoscopy in the prevention of unnecessary appendectomies: a prospective study. Br J Surg 1982;69:336.

DeVore GR. Acute abdominal pain in the pregnant patient due to pancreatitis, acute appendicitis, cholecystitis, or peptic ulcer disease. Clin Perinatol 1980;7:349.

Douglas RG, Stromme W. Operative obstetrics. 3rd ed. New York: Appleton-Century-Crofts, 1976.

Farquharson RG. Acute appendicitis in pregnancy. Scot Med J 1980;25:36.

Finch DRA, Lee E. Acute appendicitis complicating pregnancy in the Oxford region. Br J Surg 1974;61:129.

Fischer LC. Should the appendix be removed in all cases where the abdomen is opened for other causes? Atlanta J—Rec Med 1908–1909;10:410.

Forsell P, Pieper R. Infertility in young women due to perforated appendicitis? Acta Chir Scand 1986;530 (suppl):59.

Foster JH, Morgan CV, Therikell JB, et al. Vascular malformation of the appendiceal stump. A rare cause of massive hemorrhage. JAMA 1971;215:636.

Geerdsen J, Hansen JB. Incidence of sterility in women operated on in childhood for perforated appendicitis. Acta Obstet Gynecol Scand 1977;56:523.

Gilmore OJA, et al. Appendicitis and mimicking conditions. Lancet 1975;2:421.

Goldspohn A. Why the vermiform appendix should usually be removed when an abdominal incision made for other causes is available and the condition of the patient admits of the additional operating. Illinois Med J 1911;19:593.

Gomez A, Wood M. Acute appendicitis during pregnancy. Am J Surg 1979;137:180.

Greenwald JC, Fenton APN. Ovarian abscess secondary to incidental appendectomy at cesarean section. Obstet Gynecol 1959;14:593.

Grosfeld JL, Solit RWP. Prevention of wound infection in perforated appendicitis: experience with delayed primary wound closure. Am Ann Surg 1968;168:891.

Hancock H. Disease of the appendix caeci cured by operation. Lancet 1848;2:381.

Hays, RJ. Incidental appendectomy: current teaching. JAMA 1977;238:31.

Hewitt D, Milner J, LeRiche WH. Incidental appendectomy: a statistical appraisal. Can Med Assoc J 1969;100:1075.

Holtz G, Tucker E, Holtz F. Primary pure insular ovarian carcinoids. Obstet Gynecol 1979;53:85S.

Horowitz MD, Gomez GA, Santiesteban R, et al. Acute appendicitis during pregnancy. Arch Surg 1985;120:1362.

Howkins J. Appendicectomy during gynaecological operations. Lancet 1956;1:1016.

Howkins J, Williams D. Total abdominal hysterectomy: 1,000 consecutive, unselected operations. J Obstet Gynaecol Br Commonw 1963;70:20.

Isaacs JH, Knaus JV. The detection of nongenital pelvic tumors mimicking gynecologic disease. Surg Gynecol Obstet 1981;153:74.

Israel SL, Roitman HB. Cesarean section and prophylactic appendectomy: the passing of a prejudice. Obstet Gynecol 1957;10:102.

Kazarian KK, Roeder WJ, Merscheimer WL. Decreasing mortality and increasing morbidity from acute appendicitis. Am J Surg 1970;119:681.

Kelly HA, Hurdon E. The vermiform appendix and its diseases. Philadelphia: WB Saunders, 1905.

Kocsard-Varo G. Physiologic role of tonsils, adenoids and the appendix in immunity. Med J Aust 1964;2:873.

Langman J, Rowland R, Vernon-Roberts B. Endometriosis of the appendix. Br J Surg 1981;68:121.

Larsson E. Elective appendectomy at time of cesarean section. JAMA 1954;154:549.

Lau WY, Fan ST, Yiu TF, et al. Acute appendicitis in the elderly. In: Schwartz SI, ed. The year book of surgery. Chicago: Year Book Medical Publishers, 1986:380.

Leape LL, Ramenofsky ML. Laparoscopy for questionable appendicitis. Ann Surg 1980;191:410.

Levine JS, Gomez GA, Dove DB, et al. Negative appendix with suspected appendicitis: an update. South Med J 1986;79:177.

Loeffler F, Stearn R. Abdominal hysterectomy with appendectomy. Acta Obstet Gynecol Scand 1967;46:435.

MacLeod D, Howkins J. Bonney's gynaecological surgery. 7th ed. London: Hoeber Medical Div, Harper & Row, 1964.

Maier WP, Rosemond GP. A late complication of inversion of the appendiceal stump. Am J Surg 1969;118:467.

Massoudnia N. Incidental appendectomy in vaginal surgery. Int Surg 1975;60:89.

McComb P, Laimon H. Appendicitis complicating pregnancy. Can J Surg 1980;23:92.

McGowan L. Incidental appendectomy during vaginal surgery. Am J Obstet Gynecol 1966;95:588.

McVay JR, Jr. The appendix in relation to neoplastic disease. Cancer 1964;17:929.

Melcher DH. Appendicectomy with abdominal hysterectomy. Lancet 1971;1:810.

Moertel CG, Dockerty MB, Baggenstoss AH, et al. Multiple primary malignant neoplasms. Cancer 1961;14:221.

Mohammed JA, Oxorn H. Appendicitis in pregnancy. Can Med Assoc J 1975;112:1187.

Morrow CP. In: Mishell DR, ed. The year book of obstetrics and gynecology. Chicago: Year Book Medical Publishers, 1990:235.

Nakhgevany KB, Clarke, LE. Acute appendicitis in women in childbearing age. Arch Surg 1986;121:1053.

Nase HW, Kovalcik PJ, Cross GH. The diagnosis of appendicitis. Am Surg 1980;46:504.

Nauta RJ, Magnant C. Observation versus operation for abdominal pain in the right lower quadrant. Am J Surg 1986;151:746.

Neutra RR. Appendicitis: decreasing normal removal without increasing perforation. Med Care 1978;16:956.

Nockerts SR, Detmer DE, Fryback DG. Incidental appendectomy in the elderly? No. Surgery 1980;88:301.

Ochsner AJ. A handbook of appendicitis. 2nd ed. Chicago: GP Engelhard & Company, 1906.

Parsons AK, et al. Appendectomy at cesarean section: a prospective study. Obstet Gynecol 1986;68:479.

Pelosi MA, Apuzzio J, Iffy L. Ectopic pregnancy as an etiologic agent in appendicitis. Obstet Gynecol 1979;53:45.

Pittaway DE. Appendectomy in the surgical treatment of endometriosis. Obstet Gynecol 1983;61:421.

Powley PH. Infertility due to pelvic abscess and pelvic peritonitis in appendicitis. Lancet 1965;1:27.

Punnonen R, Aho AJ, Gronroos M, et al. Appendicectomy during pregnancy. Acta Chir Scand 1979;145:555.

Puri P, Guiney EJ, O'Donnell B, et al. Effects of perforated appendicitis in girls on subsequent fertility. Br Med J 1984;288:25.

Reiner IJ. Incidental appendectomy at the time of vaginal surgery. Tex Med 1980;76:46.

Rubio PA, Farrell EM, Alvarez BA, et al. Endometriosis presenting as acute appendicitis. Int J Gynaecol Obstet 1978;15:559.

Sanders RJ, Axtell K. Carcinoids of the gastrointestinal tract. Surg Obstet Gynecol 1964;119:369.

Schreier PC, Meyers JD. Appendectomy incidental to cesarean section, postpartum sterilization, or ectopic pregnancy. South Med J 1960;53:359.

Silvert MA, Meares EUM, Jr. Rationale of incidental appendectomy. Urology 1976;7:129.

Skoubo-Kristensen E, Hvid I. The appendiceal mass: results of conservation management. Ann Surg 1982;196:584.

Sweeney WJ, III. Incidental appendectomy at the time of cesarean section. Obstet Gynecol 1959;14:588.

Taniguchi T, Kilkenny G. Prophylactic appendectomy in gynecological surgery. Am J Obstet Gynecol 1950;60:1359.

Taylor JD. Acute appendicitis in pregnancy and the puerperium. Aust NZ J Obstet Gynaecol 1972;12:202.

Thompson WT, Lynn HB. The possible relationship of appendicitis with perforation in childhood to infertility in women. J Ped Surg 1971;6:458.

Voitk AJ, Lowry JB. Is incidental appendectomy a safe procedure? Can J Surg 1988;31:1988.

Waters EG. Elective appendectomy concurrent with abdominal and pelvic surgery. Obstet Gynecol 1977;50:511.

Westermann C, Mann WJ, et al. Routine appendectomy in extensive gynecologic operations. Surg Gynecol Obstet 1986;162:307.

White JJ, Santillana M, Haller JA. Intensive in-hospital observation: a safe way to decrease unnecessary appendectomy. Am Surg 1975;41:793.

Wiig JN, Janssen CW, Jr, Fuglesang P, et al. Infertility as a complication of perforated appendicitis. Acta Chir Scand 1979;145:409.

Williams GR. Presidential address: a history of appendicitis. Ann Surg 1983;197:495.

Wilson EA, Dilts PV, Jr, et al. Appendectomy incidental to postpartum sterilization. Am J Obstet Gynecol 1973;116:76.

Wound infection after appendectomy. Lancet 1970;1:930. Editorial.

37

The Intestinal Tract in Relation to Gynecology

LARRY C. CAREY
PETER J. FABRI

The gynecologist may encounter disease of the gastrointestinal tract in four ways. First, postoperative complications of gynecologic surgery frequently involve the intestinal tract; intestinal obstruction, adynamic ileus, and fistula formation may be imposing problems. Second, primary gastrointestinal disease may mimic pelvic disease. Acute intra-abdominal and intrapelvic disorders may be difficult to differentiate preoperatively; appendicitis, Meckel's diverticulum, colon diverticulitis, and volvulus may appear to be acute gynecologic disorders. Third, primary gastrointestinal disease may be encountered during pelvic surgery. Such disease includes regional enteritis, occult colon carcinoma, and colon diverticulitis. Fourth, primary gynecologic disorders may involve the gastrointestinal tract. These disorders include intestinal obstruction from tubo-ovarian abscess, endometriosis, and pelvic cancer.

The following discussion outlines the diagnosis and treatment of the more common gastrointestinal diseases that the gynecologic surgeon is likely to encounter.

POSTOPERATIVE COMPLICATIONS THAT INVOLVE THE GASTROINTESTINAL TRACT

Intestinal Obstruction

Etiologically, adhesive bands, groin hernias, and neoplasms of the bowel account for more than 80% of all intestinal obstructions. Other causes, such as intra-abdominal abscess, volvulus, intussusception, gallstone ileus, and congenital disorders, occur less frequently.

Review of the recent literature shows small-bowel obstruction from adhesions to be increasing, whereas small-bowel obstruction from hernias is decreasing. Undoubtedly the increasing enthusiasm for hernia repair is in part responsible for this trend, as is the increasing frequency of pelvic surgery. Intestinal obstruction caused by adhesions often follows gynecologic surgery, in which the dependent position of the female reproductive tract provides a favorable operative site for bowel adherence and possible obstruction.

Pathophysiology

Increased understanding of the pathophysiology of intestinal obstruction has led to great improvement in survival rate. Forty years ago mortality of 40% to 60% was not uncommon. There currently is a mortality rate between 10% and 20% for all patients with obstruction of the small intestine. If we could choose a single factor to alter to further reduce mortality, it would be to lessen the delay between onset of symptoms and surgical intervention. Few diseases that do not involve overt hemorrhage are as adversely influenced by delays in treatment as intestinal obstruction. The difference between simply dividing an adhesive band to relieve an early obstruction and resecting 2 ft of black, gangrenous, perforated ileum in the presence of extensive peritonitis and gram-negative shock may be as little as 12 hours.

Older patients have a greater tendency to ignore the discomfort of intestinal obstruction and to delay seeking medical advice. The need for prompt action by the physician dealing with intestinal obstruction is clear. If inordinate patient delay has occurred, the need for physician haste is even greater. The adage "One never goes to bed on intestinal obstruction" is well conceived.

Obstruction of the small intestine causes distention, which occurs as a result of fluid collection proximal to the obstruction. But of much greater importance is swallowed air. Well over 70% of the air in the gastrointestinal tract is swallowed. In their classic experiments Wangensteen and Rea showed that animals could survive for long periods with complete small-bowel obstruction if the esophagus was simultaneously ligated to prevent air-swallowing. The tension on the surface of a cylinder is proportional to the diameter and intraluminal pressure (Laplace's law). Because the veins and arteries enter the intestinal wall tangentially, the tension on them increases rapidly with distention. The veins, having the lower pressure of the two, show the effect of the increase in tension first. As they are stretched, resistance in them increases, and flow slows. Fluid rich in protein and salt begins to exude from the capillaries. Edema is the result. Intraluminal fluid accumulation increases from both decreased absorption and active secretion. Blood cells begin to escape from the capillaries, venous flow finally stops, arterial flow continues, blood accumulates in the wall and in the lumen of the bowel, gangrene occurs, intestinal integrity is lost, and peritonitis quickly follows.

The effect of increased intraluminal pressure on absorption and secretion from the human ileum was measured in volunteers who had ileostomies. Absorption of test solution increased at moderate elevation of intraluminal pressures, but at pressures three or four times normal the absorption began to decrease. Conversely, secretion of fluids into the lumen steadily increased as the pressure rose. These findings indicate that increased secretion is the primary cause of vascular fluid loss, and that decreased absorption plays a lesser role.

The total volume of daily secretions into the normal gastrointestinal tract is estimated to be about 10 l. As much as 7–8 l of fluid can easily be sequestered in the bowel with intestinal obstruction.

The important effects of nonstrangulating obstruction and its progression to peritonitis have been studied in detail by both Wangensteen and Rea, and Sperling. Stagnant bowel contents in a distended loop of ileum show an increase in the number of bacteria. As long as the mucosa is intact and viable, the bacteria are harmless; however, increased intraluminal pressure for a sustained period will produce patchy areas of necrosis that allow some of the intestinal contents to escape into the peritoneal cavity. The main avenue of sepsis from intestinal obstruction is absorption from the peritoneal cavity and not the venous and lymphatic drainage system.

Diagnosis

Intestinal obstruction is characterized by sudden onset of crampy abdominal pain. Vomiting may be associated with the first symptoms and then may stop, only to start again as the obstruction persists. The pain is periodic, with pain-free intervals longer than the periods of pain. The pain is classically periumbilical for a midgut obstruction.

Initial inspection of the abdomen may show little abnormality. As obstruction persists, distention will occur. In the very thin patient loops of intestine can be seen beneath the abdominal wall, and peristalsis may be visible. The characteristic bowel sounds of obstruction are high-pitched, tinkling, or metallic and occasionally may be heard without a stethoscope. These sounds reflect the existence of the air–fluid interface. Motility with violent bursts of peristalsis occurs proximal to the obstruction. The duration of quiet intervals between bursts of peristalsis may suggest the level of obstruction; in high obstruction the time may be 3 to 5 minutes, whereas in low obstruction it may be 10 to 15 minutes.

Palpation in the early stage of the disease may disclose no tenderness. As distention progresses it is usual to find tenderness over the point of obstruction. One must remember that distended loops of bowel are painful when disturbed, so vigorous examination may produce misleading signs. The intraluminal pressure, normally 2 mm Hg to 4 mm Hg in the small bowel, may reach 30 mm Hg with vigorous peristalsis. Pressures of more than 30 mm Hg cause lymphatic and capillary stasis. Any evidence of peritoneal irritation should sound the alarm to consider impending strangulation, and plans for operative intervention should begin. Strangulation occurs secondary to adhesive bands (60%), strangulated hernia (25%), volvulus (12%), and mesenteric thrombosis (2%).

Laboratory tests are helpful, and frequently indicate hypovolemia and, specifically, plasma volume loss. An increase in the hematocrit level, with high urine osmolality and normal serum osmolality, is a common finding. The presence of leukocytosis is distressing, and levels of more than 15,000/mm^3 after hydration suggest strangulation. Metabolic acidosis is an ominous sign, and may indicate dead bowel, as may thrombocytopenia or hyponatremia.

Radiographic evidence of small-bowel obstruction must be interpreted in light of clinical findings. If clinical evidence points toward intestinal obstruction and radiographic examination shows distended bowel with air–fluid levels, the diagnosis is confirmed. Early in the course of the disease the roentgenograms may be of little diagnostic assistance. Lo and coworkers reported in their Milwaukee series that in only 60% of their cases was the conclusive diagnosis made preoperatively by abdominal radiographic examination. Late in intestinal obstruction, as the bowel becomes filled with fluid, air–fluid levels may be few or even absent. The importance of an upright or lateral decubitus film cannot be overstressed. Supine films of the abdomen may be of no benefit and indeed may be misleading. Contrast material may be helpful in distinguishing adynamic ileus from obstruction. Recent reports advocate the use of thin barium suspensions rather than the more irritating water-soluble media. If the contrast material has not reached the cecum within 6 hours, small-bowel obstruction, rather than ileus, is likely.

Preoperative Preparation

Correction of existing hypovolemia is the keystone of preoperative preparation for surgery for small-bowel obstruction. It has been shown that nearly 50% of the plasma volume and 30% of the blood volume may be sequestered in the bowel in intestinal obstruction. Blood pressure, pulse rate, clinical appearance, central venous pressure, hematocrit, urine output, and urine and plasma osmolality are all helpful in evaluating the degree of hypovolemia. Central venous pressure and hematocrit, along with pulse and urine output, should be monitored as fluid replacement is accomplished with balanced salt solution, whole blood, and solutions that contain protein. If a specific electrolyte disturbance exists (eg, hypochloremic alkalosis in high intestinal obstruction), it should be corrected. The loss of extracellular fluid with normal electrolyte concentration usually does not result in electrolyte disturbance. As soon as central venous pressure, pulse rate, and urine output indicate that intravascular volume is adequately replaced, surgery should be begun.

Preoperative antibiotics are useful, especially when strangulated obstruction is suspected. Significant advances in antibiotic therapy have resulted in dramatic change in the first-line antibiotics for this situation. Any agent chosen should have a wide bacteriostatic or bactericidal spectrum of activity for both aerobic and anaerobic organisms. Recent data suggest that the parenteral administration of antibiotics with a spectrum that covers aerobic as well as anaerobic organisms increases the tolerance of the intestine to ischemia and may delay the onset of full-thickness necrosis of the intestinal wall. On the basis of this observation most authorities would recommend preoperative broad-spectrum antibiotics for all patients as soon as a diagnosis of intestinal obstruction is made. To date no specific antibiotic or combination has proved superior.

Operative Procedure

The incision should allow exploration of the entire abdomen. If possible, the incision should not be made over a previous one because the obstructing adhesion may be directly under a previous incision, and injury to the bowel may be difficult to avoid.

After the peritoneum has been opened, a loop of collapsed bowel should be located and followed until the point of obstruction is found. Nondistended bowel is much easier to handle and less susceptible to injury, and the point of obstruction is more easily identified in this manner. Unless the patient's condition is grave, all adhesions should be taken down and loops of bowel returned to the peritoneal cavity. Great care should be used in taking down the adhesions. Only the gloved hand should handle the intestine, and the use of sponges or laparotomy pads should be avoided. Sharp dissection is the only safe method of dispensing with adhesions. The ease with which distended bowel can be torn may come as a disastrous surprise to the neophyte. If the bowel is injured, it should be repaired with interrupted No. 4-0 silk sutures. Rents in the serosa are not dangerous, and there is no need to repair serosal tears unless the mucosa is injured. In fact, current evidence suggests that repaired serosal injuries actually enhance the likelihood of postoperative adhesion formation.

Distinguishing between viable and nonviable bowel may be extremely difficult. All obviously necrotic bowel should be resected. If areas of questionable viability remain, reexploration after 24 hours may be necessary to ascertain that no necrotic intestine has been overlooked. Clinical factors such as color, peristalsis, serosal appearance, and consistency are not reliable, although brisk bleeding from the cut end of the bowel may help in determining viability. Several intraoperative adjuncts may be helpful in identifying safe margins of intestine with blood supply adequate to support an anastomosis. Doppler apparatus and intravenous fluorescein have received the greatest attention. Intraoperative use of a hand-held Doppler instrument along the antimesenteric border of the intestine will identify the sounds of characteristic arterial pulsatile flow. Areas of bowel with intact antimesenteric pulsations will have a blood supply adequate to support an intestinal anastomosis. Some areas of bowel without audible Doppler signals may still be suitable. For this reason the use of intravenous fluorescein is recommended in patients in whom major segments of bowel must be removed. One thousand milligrams of sterile fluorescein (1500 mg in dark-complected patients) is administered intravenously. After about 10 minutes the lights in the operating room are extinguished and a Wood's lamp is used to induce fluorescence of the bowel. Patches less than 2 cm in diameter that do not demonstrate fluorescence can safely be left in place but should not be included in the areas of anastomosis. By using the fluorescein technique the minimum amount of bowel is resected, which may make the difference in preventing a short bowel syndrome. Even with the use of Doppler and fluorescein there should be a high index of suspicion for reinfarction. A second-look operation within 24 hours should be used when there is clinical suspicion of intestinal necrosis.

Nonoperative Treatment

There are three circumstances in which nonoperative treatment for intestinal obstruction should be considered. Patients with known widespread intra-abdominal cancer may be successfully treated by using intestinal intubation (Miller-Abbott or Cantor tube). Some patients who have had several operative procedures for intestinal obstruction and who are known to have dense intra-abdominal adhesions also may be treated best nonoperatively. Last, patients who develop obstructions in the early postoperative period are candidates for a trial of nonsurgical treatment.

If nonoperative treatment is chosen, one of the long, small intestinal tubes should be used. Our preference is the Miller-Abbott tube with a balloon containing 2 mL of mercury. A nasogastric tube is passed simultaneously and connected to intermittent suction to avoid continued distention from air-swallowing. The long tube is not connected to suction, since this often interferes with its passage. Frequent roentgenograms demonstrate the progress of the tube through the pylorus. The mercury bag often remains in the stomach even when the patient is optimally positioned. In this circumstance it is desirable to bring the patient to the radiology department for directed advancement of the tube with fluoroscopic control. Once the mercury has passed the pylorus, appropriate positioning of the patient should result in continued passage through the duodenum into the small intestine. After passing the ligament of Treitz the tube may be attached to intermittent suction. Continued use of the nasogastric tube may be beneficial, but it may be discontinued if adequate bowel decompensation is being accomplished with the long tube.

Careful surveillance must be maintained for the previously described signs of strangulation (ie, leukocytosis, metabolic acidosis, loss of pain, and loss of bowel sounds). If they are discovered, operative intervention must proceed immediately.

Adynamic Ileus

Some degree of adynamic ileus occurs after every intra-abdominal operation and with any intra-abdominal inflammation. The rate of recovery of motor function depends on many factors, including the extent of handling of bowel, the length of operation, the extent of chemical or bacterial peritonitis, and the underlying disease. After abdominal operations the patient usually becomes hungry and begins to pass flatus on about the third postoperative day. If the patient is not interested in eating, denies flatus, and the abdomen is distended, further diagnostic studies may be in order. Radiographic evidence of adynamic ileus shows distention of both small and large bowel with scattered air–fluid levels. The treatment consists of correction of electrolyte imbalance, if present. Both low potassium and low sodium can cause bowel atony, as can hypomagnesemia or severe protein depletion. The possibility of intra-abdominal localized inflammation or a leaking anastomosis must be considered. Otherwise, nasogastric decompression, ambulation, and, occasionally, localized intestinal stimulation by rectal suppositories may be helpful. Postoperative ileus seldom fails to respond to appropriate nonoperative measures.

Intestinal Fistulas

Fistula formation, one of the more difficult problems associated with intra-abdominal surgery, often is associated with a technical error in intestinal anastomosis, para-anastomotic abscess, or an anastomosis incorporating diseased bowel. Broadening the scope of gynecologic surgery to include radical pelvic dissection has greatly increased the frequency with which the gynecologist encounters fistulas of the intestinal tract. Previous irradiation damage to the intestine compounds the problem, greatly increasing the risk of fistula development.

The priority in the management of a patient with a suspected fistula is to evaluate and control the underlying septic process. Patients with uncontrolled sepsis should undergo early operation after appropriate fluid and electrolyte replacement. Adequate drainage of abscesses and control of ongoing peritoneal soilage are essential components of the early treatment of intestinal fistulas. Although nonoperative management of intestinal fistulas has become widely accepted, only when sepsis is well controlled by antibiotics or operation can expectant management of a fistula be used.

The severity of physiologic disturbance resulting from an intestinal fistula varies with the location of the fistula. Fistulas of the stomach, duodenum, or high jejunum may be devastating. The volume of electrolyte and protein-rich fluids lost from such a fistula may cause life-threatening imbalance in a very short time. Distal ileal or colonic fistulas may be well tolerated and cause no greater electrolyte disturbance than would an ileostomy or a colostomy.

In some cases diagnosing a fistula may be difficult. If the intestinal opening is small, drainage may be intermittent. Some abdominal wounds infected with enteric organisms discharge material that resembles intestinal contents. In these instances the oral administration of a dye, such as brilliant blue or carmine red, may readily establish the diagnosis. Alternatively, a radiographic contrast material may be injected into the cutaneous opening through a small rubber catheter to determine whether a fistula exists. Caution should be exercised when injecting contrast material. Vigorous injection may separate the bowel from its adherence to the abdominal wall, with peritonitis resulting.

Fistulas tend to close spontaneously, but some circumstances prevent closure. The most common is the presence of some degree of obstruction distal to the fistula, a factor that also may play a role in the genesis of most fistulas. Malignant growth in the fistulous tract also inhibits spontaneous closure. The presence of a foreign body in the fistulous tract prevents healing. Chronic fistulas may remain patent because of epithelialization of the tract. Previous radiation to the involved bowel is a notorious cause for failure of fistulas to heal and may be one of the more absolute negative factors in fistula closure. If none of these conditions pertain, intestinal fistula closure can be anticipated. When fistulas do not close after an appropriate time interval, surgical closure becomes necessary and must be associated with correction of the factors that have prevented spontaneous closure.

The more proximal the fistula, the more urgent is the need for closure. There are measures, however, that enable control of even the most difficult fistulas. As in intestinal obstruction, the consideration of prime concern is restoration of fluid and electrolyte balance. This, on a rare occasion, may be nearly impossible without performing an enterostomy distal to the fistula. A jejunostomy distal to the duodenal fistula allows the fistula drainage to be instilled into the gastrointestinal tract and greatly facilitates the fluid and electrolyte management. Proximal suction by intestinal intubation may lessen fistulous drainage and encourage healing.

The development of intravenous nutritional support (total parenteral nutrition) has clearly emerged as a cornerstone in the management of intestinal fistulas. Whether parenteral nutrition actually hastens closure of intestinal fistulas is a matter of some debate. Most authorities, however, agree that appropriate use of parenteral nutrition maintains positive nitrogen balance in fistula patients and encourages wound healing. The improvement in nutrition with concomitant improvement in collagen synthesis may allow closure that might not otherwise occur. Even when fistulas do not close, appropriate nutritional support during the management period results in a well-nourished patient who is capable of withstanding additional operations (see Ch. 6).

A major problem in fistula management is the care of the skin about the fistula. Gastrointestinal content, especially from the upper tract, has an ulcerative effect on skin. Enterostomal therapists have become skillful at constructing collection and drainage devices to facilitate control of the fistula drainage. A well-trained enterostomal therapist can assist in minimizing skin breakdown around the area of the cutaneous opening. When an enterostomal therapist is not available, techniques should be developed to allow adequate control of drainage and prevent puddling in dependent areas. The great variety of methods used to protect the skin suggests that in fact no good method is available. Most effective is the total isolation of the skin from the effluent. If it is technically possible, the following procedure is used. The skin is washed and carefully dried; a square of peristomal covering (Stomadhesive) is cut so that the opening in the square approximates the opening of the fistula; the backing of the Stomadhesive is removed and, when the skin is perfectly dry, pressed into place. Any postoperative pouch can be applied to this square, so that the skin surrounding the fistula is protected. The dressing needs to be changed every 3 to 4 days, depending on the level of the fistula and the volume of drainage from the tract. The bag can be connected to a drainage system to assist collection and further protect the skin. The indication to change the peristomal square is leakage underneath the edge. Many of the bags are odorproofed, and various tablets and liquids can be put into the pouch to neutralize undesirable odor.

If the fistulous opening does not permit placement of such a bag, other methods may be used. The drainage may be partially controlled by insertion of a commercial or fabricated sump drain. The skin may be further protected by such agents as karaya powder or a paste made of zinc oxide ointment and castor oil. If severe corrosive dermatitis has occurred, use of a heat lamp and local measures will succeed in controlling the problem, but only with great effort and constant attention. Like many problems in medicine, prevention of skin irritation from an intestinal fistula is infinitely easier and more successful than treatment. Early studies suggest a role for parenteral somatostatin in decreasing the volume of intestinal secretions and facilitating or hastening fistula closure.

The operative management of an intestinal fistula

requires superb timing and judgment as well as great technical facility. By and large, intestinal fistulas usually are attacked too soon. Unless large volumes of fluid are being lost or severe skin problems supervene, a fistula is fairly well tolerated. Most fistulas can be expected to close in 4 to 6 weeks if sepsis has been controlled and appropriate nutritional support is instituted. If a fistula has not closed by 6 weeks, the likelihood of spontaneous closure is small. Waiting an additional 4 to 6 weeks to allow complete resolution of the intra-abdominal inflammatory response, however, will make the subsequent surgical procedure considerably easier. Abdominal adhesions will become much easier to dissect and the possibility of intestinal injury will be minimized. The actual optimum time for surgical intervention is variable and should be individualized for each patient.

If possible, the fistula should be excised and the bowel resected. The involved bowel occasionally may be excluded from the gastrointestinal tract but not removed. This is particularly helpful in the presence of radiation enteritis or recurrent carcinoma, when attempts to resect the diseased area with primary anastomosis may be associated with major postoperative complications in a patient whose ability to tolerate the complications is poor. Bypassing the area of disease may accomplish the objective of intestinal decompression without instigating uncontrolled bleeding or multiple accidental enterostomies with recurrent postoperative fistula. Careful surgical technique is required in reconstructing the gastrointestinal tract if recurrence of the fistula is to be avoided.

PRIMARY GASTROINTESTINAL DISEASE THAT MIMICS ACUTE GYNECOLOGIC DISORDERS

Meckel's Diverticulum

Meckel's diverticulum, a remnant of the vitelline duct, is a congenital abnormality of the small bowel. The diverticulum occurs in the terminal 24 to 48 in of the ileum. Sometimes gastric mucosa is found in the sac, and perforation or hemorrhage may result from ulceration. These diverticula should be resected if they have caused difficulty or have a narrow neck. The technique consists simply of clamping the base and excising the pouch. Closure of the resulting defect is best accomplished with interrupted No. 3-0 catgut. Lembert sutures supported by a seromuscular layer of interrupted silk (No. 2-0) sutures. Care must be taken to avoid narrowing the bowel lumen. If encountered in an asymptomatic patient, Meckel's diverticulum need not

be removed. Most complications occur in young children, and the likelihood of difficulty with a Meckel's diverticulum in an adult is extremely small.

Colon Diverticulitis

Perforated diverticulitis of the sigmoid colon occasionally may be mistaken for pelvic inflammatory disease. Ordinarily these two processes occur in different age groups, but acute diverticulitis does occur in patients under 40 years of age. Discovery of acute diverticulitis of the sigmoid colon with perforation warrants special consideration. If the perforation has occurred into the free peritoneal cavity and generalized peritonitis is present, drainage of the area of perforation with several soft Penrose drains is necessary. In addition, a proximal diverting colostomy is indicated. If possible, the colostomy should be placed in the descending colon proximal to the perforation. This shortens the segment of bowel between the colostomy and the perforation. The disease may then be managed with only one subsequent procedure. If the colostomy is placed in the right colon, resection and colostomy closure must be done as separate procedures. Sometimes an area of diverticulitis is mobile enough that the diseased segment may be exteriorized or resected primarily with construction of an end sigmoid colostomy. When this can be done without extensive dissection in the presence of acute inflammation, it is the ideal approach; extensive dissection should be avoided when it is difficult or hazardous.

If the perforation is localized and an abscess has formed, the abscess should be drained extraperitoneally, if possible. This may require a separate flank incision, which should be done without hesitation, or can be done percutaneously. Proximal colostomy is necessary. Perforated diverticulitis is life-threatening if generalized peritonitis supervenes, and patients with this condition require constant attention postoperatively.

Volvulus

Sigmoid volvulus is of interest to the gynecologist only as it pertains to differential diagnosis. Although the sudden onset of pain may resemble ovarian torsion, the presence of obstipation, abdominal distention, and the characteristic radiographic appearance (massively distended sigmoid colon, "bird-beak" in appearance on barium enema) should establish the correct diagnosis. Sigmoid volvulus is radiographically characterized by a massively dilated, gas-filled sigmoid colon that resembles an inverted horseshoe, extending up from the pelvis into the upper abdomen. In the mentally deficient patient the colon may be distended and full of stool. But the characteristic radiographic picture is not present, which differentiates the two entities.

Although volvulus usually is seen in people over 60 years of age, two cases have been encountered in women under 25 in our clinic. When sigmoid volvulus is diagnosed preoperatively, the problem usually can be remedied nonoperatively by careful and expeditious sigmoidoscopy or low-pressure barium enema. When the diagnosis is discovered at the time of a pelvic laparotomy, the surgical treatment usually consists of untwisting the loop of bowel. Colostomy may be necessary, particularly when the viability of the segment is doubtful. Use of intravenous fluorescein or Doppler apparatus, as described previously, may be helpful. Primary resection should never be used unless gangrene or nonviability is documented. Furthermore, primary anastomosis is never justified in the presence of an unprepared distended colon.

Volvulus of the cecum is quite rare. It usually occurs in very elderly people and is managed by simple derotation. Fixation of the cecum to the posterolateral peritoneum (cecopexy) or resection may prevent recurrence. Right colon resection should be performed if the cecum is nonviable.

PRIMARY GASTROINTESTINAL DISEASE ENCOUNTERED DURING GYNECOLOGIC SURGERY

Among the primary gastrointestinal diseases found during the course of gynecologic surgery, colon diverticulitis has already been discussed.

Regional Enteritis (Crohn's Disease)

Regional enteritis is a granulomatous inflammatory process that usually involves the small intestine. It occasionally is encountered by the gynecologic surgeon and usually is unexpected. This disease may occur in all age groups but is most frequent in young adults. The usual age at onset of symptoms is late teens.

Clinically, the disease usually causes diarrhea, weight loss, and abdominal pain. Surgery is most often necessitated by either acute exacerbation of the inflammatory process or intestinal obstruction from edema and cicatrix. Fistula formation is common and in women may involve the bladder or vagina. Fistulas also may develop between the terminal ileum and the site of a previous appendectomy. When the disease is encountered unex-

pectedly, resection should not be performed unless obstruction is present, since medical treatment may be successful and disease recurrence is frequent. The diseased segments appear beefy, dull purple-red, and thickened and are covered with strands of thick, gray-white exudate. The mesenteric fat creeps over the serosa, so that it nearly encompasses the bowel. Because skip areas are common, the extent of the disease should be thoroughly documented by examining the entire length of the bowel. Extensive clinical and laboratory investigations have been directed at identifying the cause of this disease. Initial enthusiasm about a possible viral cause has been dampened by failure to reproduce experimental results. Consequently regional enteritis is still an enigma, and medical treatment is less than optimal.

Definitive procedures should, when possible, be directed at resection of the diseased bowel. The terminal ileum and right colon usually are removed and an ileotransverse colostomy performed. A bypass procedure has been recommended but seems less satisfactory than resection in most cases, since it is attended by a higher recurrence rate and may be associated with late malignant transformation.

In doing a small-bowel resection for regional enteritis, there is no advantage in removing the enlarged mesenteric lymph nodes. If a dilated ureter is found near the area of the terminal ileum, no attempt should be made to free it. This condition will resolve with successful treatment of the small bowel. When the disease is encountered, the rule of thumb is to avoid resection unless there is perforation or obstruction. The patient should be given a trial of medical management. Only when there is no improvement with expectant management or when a surgical complication develops should surgical intervention be entertained. If operation is performed, the appendix may be resected if the base of the cecum is not involved with disease. This eliminates any future diagnostic concern about appendicitis if right lower quadrant pain recurs. Several recent reports suggest that the incidence of enterocutaneous fistulas increases if the appendix has been removed, but most patients probably can safely undergo appendectomy. This complication may be avoided by omitting an appendectomy in any case where the terminal ileum or cecum is involved with regional enteritis.

Special mention must be made of the treatment of fistulas. Enterocutaneous, enterovesical, and enterovaginal fistulas are common, and present an extreme challenge to the physician or surgeon. Treatment by traditional surgical approaches is fraught with a high complication rate and almost certain recurrence. When a fistula to the vagina is identified in a patient with a history compatible with inflammatory bowel disease, careful and extensive preoperative evaluation is necessary. If regional enteritis can be diagnosed preoperatively, intense nutritional support and medical therapy should be attempted. Initial experience with parenteral nutrition support in the cure of regional enteritis has been followed by a more realistic understanding of the role of nutrition in the disease. Nutritional support is clearly essential in preparing these patients for surgery and in maintaining their general nutritional status. Operation often can be delayed or postponed, and occasionally even avoided, by the use of aggressive parenteral nutrition support.

Sulfasalazine and corticosteroids are the mainstay of therapy. Sulfasalazine is administered in 1-g doses four times a day, and appears to have some benefit both in the treatment of acute disease and in maintaining remission. It is not free of gastrointestinal adverse effects, however, and patient compliance may be poor. Steroids have been used in acute exacerbations of the disease and, in refractory patients, for long-term maintenance. Most commonly prednisone is given in a dosage of 30 to 60 mg/24 h, tapered to the lowest possible dosage that will control the symptoms. Adrenocorticotropic hormone (ACTH) has been used by some experts with comparable results. This is no good evidence, however, that ACTH is superior to prednisone. Whether prednisone or ACTH is given, the dose should be decreased to the minimum amount possible to prevent the serious and frequently irreversible consequences of long-term corticosteroid therapy.

Demonstration of high recurrence rates after surgical resection of regional enteritis has dampened enthusiasm for prophylactic resections. Virtually all patients develop at least radiographic recurrence of the disease if follow-up is long enough. Medical therapy is the mainstay of treatment unless complications (perforation, obstruction, bleeding, or fistula) occur.

Definite treatment of an enterovaginal fistula must include treatment of intra-abdominal disease. Perineal approaches to closure of the fistula are uniformly unsuccessful. As previously indicated, preoperative evaluation, optimum nutritional support, and attempts at medical management with sulfasalazine and steroids are essential. If surgical intervention becomes necessary, the intra-abdominal disease must be resected. The area of resection should include only the section of bowel that is grossly involved, with its sequela of short bowel syndrome. Considerable judgment is required in any surgical undertaking because of the chronicity and high recurrence rate. Because long-term follow-up is essential and complications frequent, it is preferable to enlist the help of a specialist in treating inflammatory bowel disease.

Colon Operations

If elective surgery that may involve colostomy is planned, the question of bowel preparation is raised. The traditional approach to mechanical cleansing of the bowel includes clear liquids for 48 to 72 hours preoperatively, combined with citrate of magnesia and, possibly, saline enemas the evening before operation. Recently, the efficacy and practicality of a brief (12 hours) preparation, beginning the afternoon before surgery and using an oral "lavage" with 4–6 l of a specially formulated mannitol and electrolyte solution has become popular. This preparation is self-administered by the patient at a rate of 1–2 l/h by mouth until the rectal effluent is clear. For patients who cannot consume the large amounts required, a nasogastric tube can be placed to administer the solution.

Colon Obstruction

Etiologically, obstruction of the large intestine differs from that of the small bowel, in that adhesions and hernia are uncommon causes, and tumor and inflammation are quite common. The gynecologist may encounter obstruction of the large intestine as a result of contiguous or metastatic cancer, irradiation changes in the intestine, pelvic abscess, or primary intestinal inflammatory disease. The general principles for management of large-bowel obstruction are the same as those for small-bowel obstruction, but there are some differences. In the presence of a competent ileocecal valve, an obstructed large bowel becomes a closed loop. A closed loop is the most dangerous of all types of intestinal obstruction. When the large bowel is involved, the most likely site of complication is the cecum, which may perforate if overdistended. For this reason obstruction of the colon with a competent ileocecal valve is a matter of great surgical urgency. If the ileocecal valve is incompetent, large-bowel obstruction becomes, in effect, a total small-bowel obstruction.

A major difference between large- and small-bowel obstruction is the operative management. In the large intestine, obstruction may be relieved with a relatively minor operation and the causative problem may be dealt with electively. Any part of the large bowel, including the cecum, may be exteriorized proximal to the point of obstruction. Before operation, sigmoidoscopy and barium enema under fluoroscopic observation are needed to clearly define the point of obstruction. The exception to this rule is acute obstructed or perforated diverticulitis, in which case a barium enema may be dangerous, even in experienced hands.

Sigmoid colon cancer or severe diverticulitis should

be managed by transverse colostomy in the right upper abdomen. If the disease is encountered through an incision that does not permit the colostomy to be done easily, the incision should be closed. A separate muscle-splitting incision is made in the right upper quadrant, and a loop of bowel exteriorized. The bowel can be opened later. If immediate decompression is required, it is best done by insertion of a large tube into the colostomy, thus avoiding soilage of the peritoneal cavity. After the incision is sealed, in 24 to 48 hours, the colostomy can be safely opened.

Radiation Injury to Large and Small Intestines

Radiation therapy for malignant pelvic tumors, particularly carcinoma of the cervix, occasionally causes complications in the colon or small intestine. Although the radiation complications of colitis, proctitis, or enteritis are not common, they are definite complications. In a series of 777 patients treated for pelvic malignant disease in the radiation department of Hahnemann Medical College and Hospital in Philadelphia from January 1969 to June 1973, 47 (6.1%) such complications occurred. The average dose was 6000 rad of external radiation and 2000 rad from radium insertion. Colcock and Hume indicated that bowel symptoms began to be produced at total radiation doses of about 4800 rad. Symptoms during or directly after irradiation therapy are common but usually short-lived and present no significant long-term problems. Persistence of symptoms beyond 1 month after the termination of therapy strongly suggests that permanent bowel damage may have occurred. The most common bowel symptoms include diarrhea, abdominal pain, rectal bleeding, vomiting, and weight loss. In the analysis of the 47 patients Colcock and Hume found the following complications: small-bowel obstruction in 15, large-bowel stenosis in 5, rectal bleeding in 36, and proctitis in 31.

Radiation enteritis can be characterized as acute, subacute, or chronic. Acute radiation enteritis occurs during and immediately after a course of therapeutic radiation. It is caused by suppression of mucosal regeneration in the exposed area of intestine, and results in malabsorption with diarrhea and occasional bleeding. This usually is a self-resolving problem and is not correlated with the subsequent occurrence of chronic symptoms.

Subacute and chronic radiation enteritis is distinguished by the delay between treatment and the onset of symptoms. Symptoms of subacute radiation damage usually occur within 3 to 6 months of radiation treatment, whereas chronic radiation enteritis may not be obvious until years after the therapy. Both abnormalities are characterized pathologically by fibrosis and endarteritis. The fibrosis results in areas of stricture and may lead to intestinal obstruction. Another finding is dense interloop adhesions that defy surgical separation. The pathologic manifestation that requires an attitude of extreme caution is the endarteritis, which causes obliteration of the native blood vessels of the intestine, even in areas of bowel that appear grossly normal. The characteristic appearance of chronic radiation enteritis, a marblelike bowel with telangiectatic blood vessels, is by no means a reliable indicator of radiation damage. Adjacent, grossly normal appearing segments of intestine also may show microscopic damage. It is important to recognize that the endarteritis of radiation results in a poor blood supply for the support of intestinal anastomosis or closure of enterotomies.

Operation should be avoided in the patient with abdominal complaints after radiation treatment unless definitive indications are present. The wary clinician will recognize the high risk associated with operation and advise his patient to use caution. When operation is necessary, however, several principles are important. First, the surgeon must recognize the significance of the endarteritis and its effect on healing of intestinal suture lines. Extreme caution should be taken to avoid injury to the bowel because of the subsequent hazards of closure. Second, the surgeon should remember that radiation damage occurs only within the area of the radiation portal. Incisions can be safely placed out of the radiated field in many cases. Extensive lysis of adhesions should be avoided, and dissection should be confined to those areas where it is necessary. Intestinal anastomosis should be performed with at least one and preferably two segments of grossly normal bowel. These can be reinforced with a tongue of omentum over the suture line to provide additional exogenous blood supply. Intestinal bypass with side-to-side anastomosis in normal bowel frequently is preferable to extensive mobilization of irradiated intestine from the pelvis. Irradiated bowel should be regarded warily. Such an approach will be rewarded by a decrease in the incidence of intra-abdominal abscess and enterocutaneous fistula.

Rectovaginal and vesicovaginal fistulas after radiation to the pelvis are not trivial problems and should be managed by experienced personnel. Simple mobilization and closure usually are attended by major complications and are seldom successful.

When operation is necessary in the patient who has previously undergone radiation therapy, careful postoperative monitoring for signs of peritonitis is essential. When peritoneal irritation is apparent, reexploration is essential because of the high likelihood of a failed suture line.

PRIMARY GYNECOLOGIC DISEASES THAT AFFECT THE GASTROINTESTINAL TRACT

Techniques of Treatment for Tubo-ovarian Abscess, Endometriosis, and Pelvic Cancer

Tubo-ovarian abscess, endometriosis, and pelvic cancer are discussed in other chapters. Each of these entities occasionally causes small-bowel obstruction. It should be remembered that although endometriosis is a frequent finding in women, it seldom causes obstruction of the small bowel. Endometriosis of the small bowel tends to be limited to the serosal and muscular coats and usually does not penetrate to the mucosa. Obstruction is due to fibrosis and kinking of the bowel. When obstruction from endometriosis of the small bowel is encountered, the involved segment should be resected. As a general rule, the postoperative course is uneventful.

Open End-to-End Anastomosis

Open end-to-end anastomosis follows intestinal resection (Fig. 37-1). Crushing clamps are placed obliquely on the intestine, with the apex on the mesenteric side. This gives some advantage in providing a large lumen at the anastomotic site and favors a good blood supply to the antimesenteric margin. With fine needles (French eye or "pop-off" gastrointestinal needles), a row of No. 3-0 silk mattress sutures is used to approximate the serosal surface. The crushing clamps are then removed, the crushed ends of the bowel are trimmed, and a mucosal layer of No. 3-0 or No. 4-0 silk sutures is placed. At the angles the sutures become interrupted Connell sutures, with the knots on the luminal aspect. The serosal suture line is then completed with mattress or Lembert sutures. The use of continuous absorbable suture on the mucosal layer is quite acceptable. When the lumen is small, however, continuous sutures are more likely to narrow the anastomotic stoma. After the anastomosis is completed the mesenteric rent is repaired with fine sutures. Care must be taken not to injure the blood supply to the suture line during mesentery closure.

Closed Anastomosis

Closed anastomosis is particularly useful in ileocolostomy construction with unprepared bowel (Fig. 37-2). Four noncrushing clamps, such as Allen clamps, are placed across the unopened bowel to isolate the segment to be removed. As with all anastomoses, moist pads are used to carefully isolate the gut from the peritoneal cavity. The mesentery of the segment to be resected is divided in a wedge.

Careful placement of hemostats on the mesenteric vessels is critical. Suture ligation of these vessels is much safer than simple ligation. If a vessel is lost and retracts into the mesentery, attempts to find and control it may result in vascular damage, necessitating a greater bowel resection. The time spent carefully isolating and ligating these vessels will be well rewarded.

After the bowel to be resected has been removed the clamps on the cut ends are approximated, and No. 3-0 silk Lembert sutures are placed through the bowel wall to include the mucosa, about 3 mm apart, around the entire circumference. The clamps are then removed and the cut, compressed ends of bowel separated to ensure that no suture has been placed across the lumen, possibly occluding the anastomosis. The sutures are then tied. As they are tied, any needed additional stitches are placed. Patency of the lumen is assured and the mesenteric defect repaired. This anastomosis, carefully performed, is quick and safe and assures maximum patency. For the surgeon who only occasionally performs an anastomosis, it is an excellent method. The area of greatest difficulty is at the site of mesenteric attachment to the bowel wall; by carefully dissecting the mesentery off the bowel for 5 mm, trouble can be avoided. If this is not done, the bowel wall may be missed and the sutures placed in the mesenteric fat, with disastrous results.

Side-to-Side Anastomosis

The side-to-side method of anastomosis is less popular than the end-to-end method (Fig. 37-3). It may be quite useful in excluding a segment of the intestinal tract, as in regional enteritis. The two segments of bowel to be anastomosed are approximated with stay sutures. A distance of about 4 in between these sutures is ideal. Serosal mattress sutures of No. 3-0 silk are placed. With noncrushing clamps, the segments to be connected are isolated. This aids in controlling bleeding and also in avoiding contamination. Both segments of bowel are then opened with a parallel incision about 3 mm from the suture line. Mucosal sutures may be either continuous or interrupted. The larger lumen in this method makes continuous suture less hazardous. The serosal suture line is then completed as before.

An important aspect of this technique is to place the initial suture line in a perfectly straight line parallel to the long axis of the bowel. Angulation may interfere with stomal function.

(text continues on page 1034)

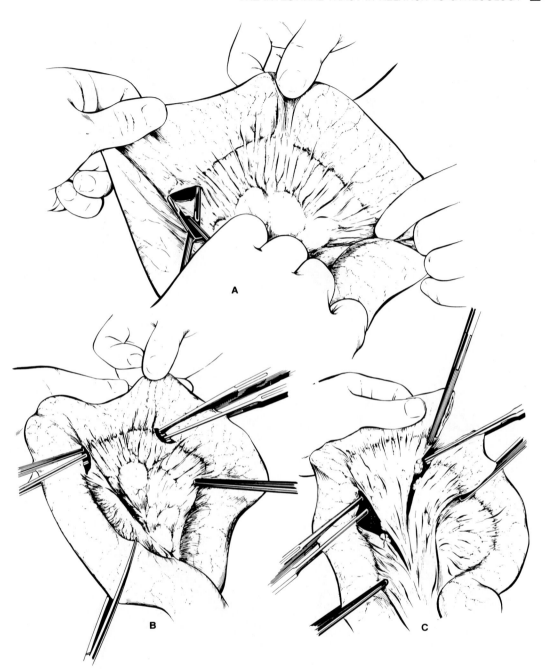

Figure 37–1. Open end-to-end anastomosis. *A*, The mesentery is carefully dissected from the intestine. *B*, The resected segment is defined by clamps. Note the noncrushing clamps proximally placed to control spill. *C*, Note the individual ligatures on the mesentery. Suture ligation of these vessels is important. (*Figure continued on next page.*)

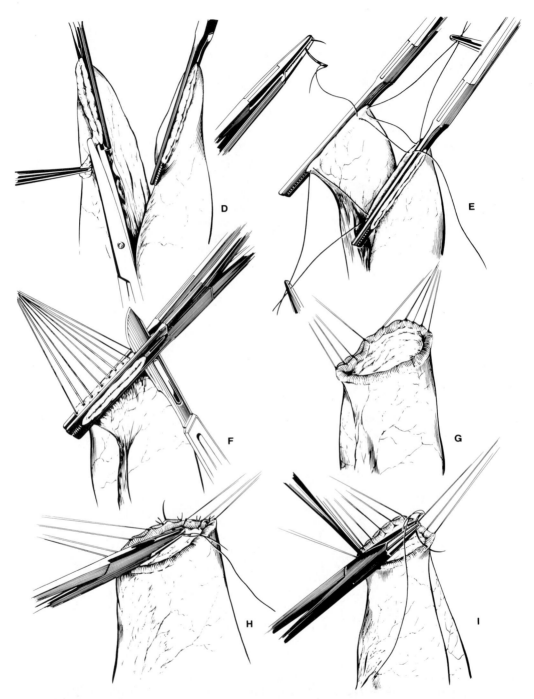

Figure 37–1. (continued) *D*, Careful dissection of the mesentery from the intestine is essential. *E*, Posterior interrupted sutures are about 5 mm apart. *F*, The crushed end of the bowel is trimmed away. *G, H,* Note that the posterior serosal sutures are not cut until the first mucosal suture has been placed. *I*, Beginning to "turn the corner."

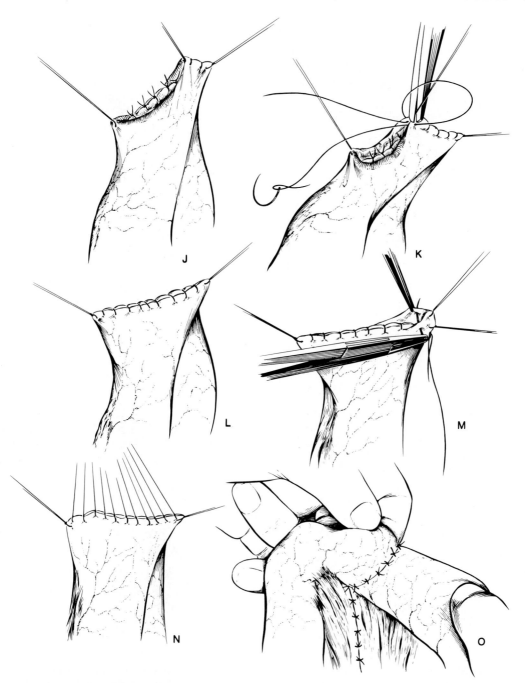

Figure 37–1. (continued) *J,* The inverting suture is continued anteriorly. *K,* Note the placement of each suture before cutting the previous one. *L, M,* Completion of the anterior mucosal suture line and beginning the anterior serosal one. *N, O,* The anastomosis is complete and the mesenteric defect closed.

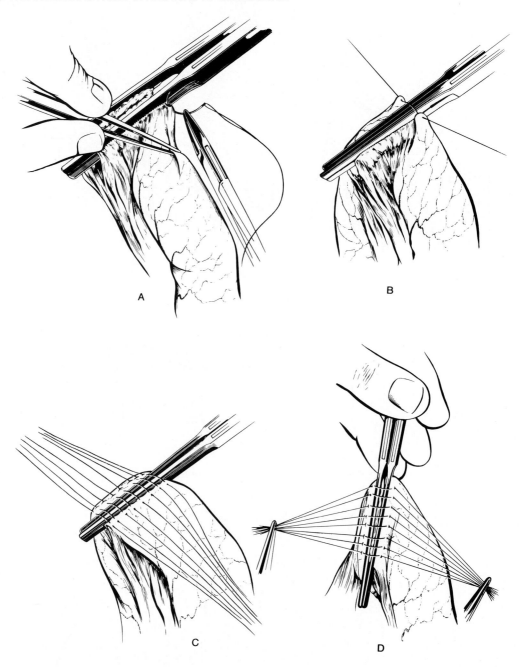

Figure 37–2. Closed anastomosis. *A*, Note the placement of the suture very close to the clamp. *B*, The first suture is completed. *C*, The row of sutures has now been placed. *D*, The clamp on the intestine is rotated 180 degrees.

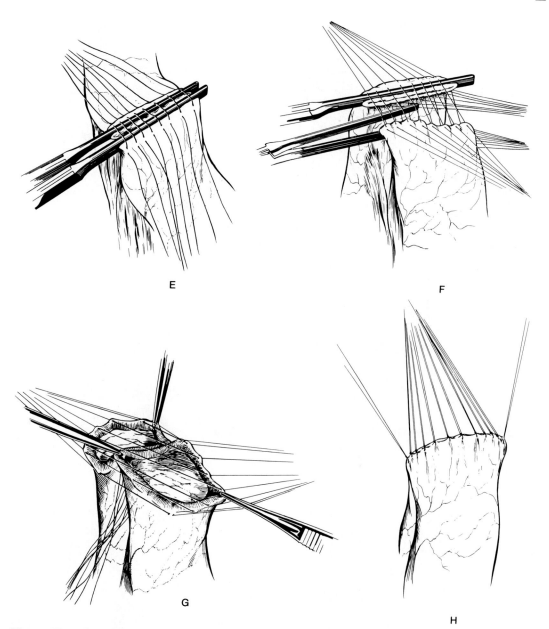

E

F

G

H

Figure 37–2. (continued) *E*, After rotation of the clamp the suturing is completed. *F*, Clamps are removed before tying the sutures. *G*, The lumen is inspected to assure that no sutures have been placed across the lumen. *H*, Sutures tied. One layer is adequate. The mesenteric defect is closed as in Figure 37–1 *N* and *O*.

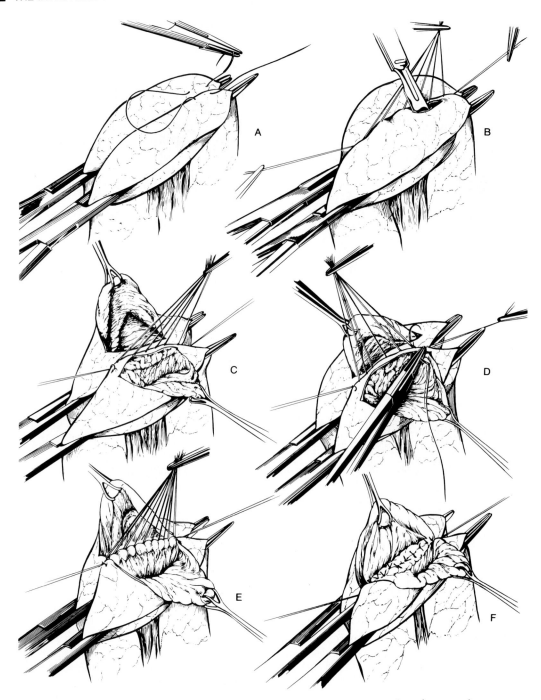

Figure 37–3. Side-to-side anastomosis. *A,* Horizontal mattress sutures are used on the posterior row. *B,* The noncrushing clamps avoid spill as the bowel is opened. *C, D,* The posterior serosal suture line is completed and the first mucosal suture is placed before cutting the serosal ones. *E, F,* Completion of the posterior mucosal sutures.

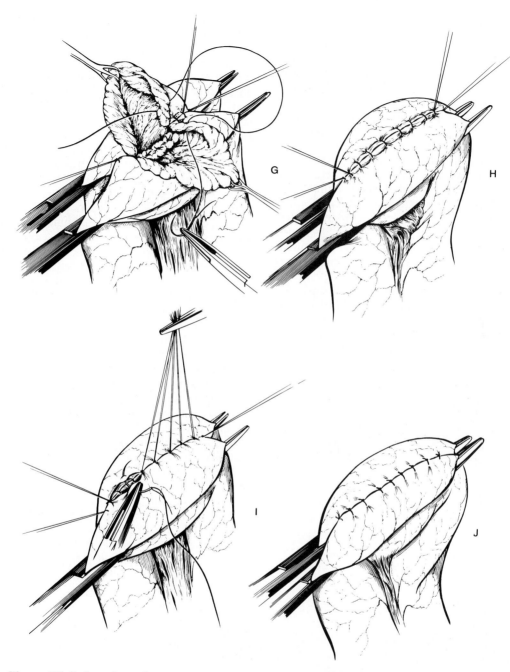

Figure 37–3. (continued) *G, H*, Completion of the anterior mucosal suture line. Continuous suture can be used more safely in side-to-side than in end-to-end anastomosis. *I, J*, Completion of the anterior serosal suture line.

Stapled Anastomosis

The development of intestinal staples has simplified the performance of anastomoses, particularly for the person who infrequently operates on the bowel. The three most commonly used instruments are the GIA stapler, the TA 55 or TA 90 stapler, and the EEA stapler. Each instrument is designed to perform a different function, and they frequently are used in combination.

The GIA instrument is designed to place two double parallel rows of metallic staples over a length of about 5 cm and simultaneously cut between them (Fig. 37-4). This instrument can be used in various settings. The most common use is in dividing the intestine. Applied across the bowel, it effectively closes both ends of the divided bowel and prevents peritoneal spillage. It also can be used in conjunction with the TA 55 instrument for constructing a side-to-side (functional end-to-end) anastomosis.

The TA 55 and TA 90 instruments apply two parallel rows of staples, and most commonly are used for permanently closing the end of a segment of bowel (Fig. 37-5). The two instruments differ in width of the staple line. Care must be exercised that the entire width of bowel is included within the instrument and that the open end of the instrument is effectively closed by

placement of the retaining pin. After placement and firing of the TA instrument, the bowel is divided with a knife.

The EEA instrument performs an inverting end-to-end anastomosis (Fig. 37-6). It requires an opening in an adjacent portion of bowel (enterotomy, colotomy, or anus), which usually must be closed subsequently with sutures or with a single application of a TA stapler. Purse-string sutures of polypropylene or nylon are applied over the ends of the bowel to be anastomosed. This can be accomplished with a purse-string instrument or by a simple over-and-over baseball stitch around the circumference of the intestine. After both ends of the bowel have been placed and secured around the center rod of the instrument and the purse-string sutures tied, the instrument is closed and fired. This effectively staples the two ends together and removes the excess intraluminal tissue with a circular blade. After removal of the apparatus, security of the anastomosis can be tested by removing the two circular "doughnuts" of tissue contained within the instrument. If either remnant is not a complete circle, a secure anastomosis is unlikely. The anastomosis may be reinforced, if desired, with a row of Lembert sutures.

Stapled Side-to-Side Anastomosis. A side-to-side anastomosis (which has been popularized as a functional end-to-end anastomosis) can be performed by a single application of the GIA instrument followed by an application of the TA 55 or TA 90 instrument. After removal (or clamping) of the appropriate section of intestine the two ends of intestine are placed side to side and secured with stay sutures (Fig. 37-7A). The two arms of the GIA instrument are inserted into the open ends of the intestine, and traction is applied on the open end to seat the instrument to its maximum depth (Fig. 37-7B and C). The instrument should be applied on the

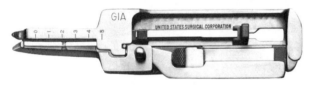

Figure 37-4. The GIA instrument applies two double rows of staples and cuts between them. It is available in only one size.

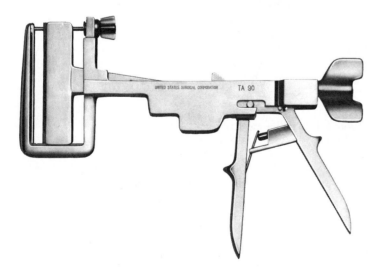

Figure 37-5. The TA 90 is wider than the TA 55 (not shown). This instrument crushes the tissue while applying a double row of staples. It is best suited for an end closure of the intestine and is frequently reinforced with an external row of sutures.

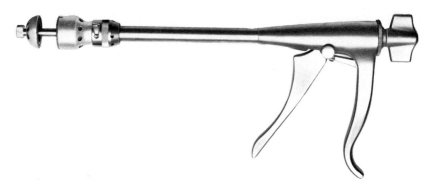

Figure 37–6. The EEA performs an end-to-end anastomosis by applying two circular concentric rows of staples and cuts away the central redundant tissue. The distal end (opposite the pistol grip) is disposable and is available in three sizes—25 mm, 28 mm, and 31 mm. The appropriate size is determined with the assistance of the sizers that are provided with the instrument. In general, the largest size should be used.

antimesenteric border of both segments of intestine. The instrument is closed by squeezing the locking lever into the instrument. Before firing the instrument, location of application should be rechecked to ensure that the instrument is fully seated and does not include the mesentery. The instrument is fired by sliding the push bar forward, stapling and dividing the tissue between the two double rows of staples. The TA 55 or TA 90 instrument is then applied to the combined ends, closed by tightening the wing nut, and fired (Fig. 37-7*D* and *E*). After the redundant tissue is trimmed with a scalpel, patency of the anastomosis can be confirmed by palpation (Fig. 37-7*F*). A row of Lembert sutures exterior to the staple line is optional but preferred by many surgeons to take the tension off the staples.

Stapled End-to-End Anastomosis. An end-to-end anastomosis can be constructed quite easily with the use of the EEA instrument, and an end-to-side anastomosis can be done with the EEA and the TA 55 or TA 90 instrument. After the bowel is resected the EEA instrument, with the end cone (anvil) removed, is inserted through a small colotomy made with a knife, about 5 cm from the transected end of the bowel (Fig. 37-8*A*). The free end of the bowel is secured around the rod with a purse-string suture. The cone (anvil) is then securely attached to the center rod. A purse-string suture of No. 3-0 polypropylene is placed on the opposite loop of intestine with the provided clamp (Fig. 37-8*B*). The intestine is then brought over the anvil with the aid of Allis clamps. The polypropylene suture is tied and the instrument closed by tightening the wing nut (Fig. 37-8*C*). The instrument is fired, which cuts out a round segment of tissue and simultaneously anastomoses the two segments of bowel. The instrument is carefully removed by turning the wing nut two or three turns and carefully extracting the instrument with a back-and-forth rotary motion (Fig. 37-8*D*). The colotomy site can be closed with a single application of the TA 55 or TA 90 instrument (Fig. 37-8*E*). Both staple lines can be reinforced with Lembert sutures if desired.

An end-to-side anastomosis can be performed in an analogous manner by inserting the EEA instrument into the open end of the colon, passing the center rod (without the anvil) through a small colotomy in the antimesenteric taenia, and securing this with a purse-string suture around the rod. The small intestine or colon is treated as in Figure 37-8*A* through *C*. After the instrument is closed and fired the open end of the colon can be closed with a single application of the TA 90 instrument.

Enterostomy

The safest method for performing an enterostomy is shown in Figure 37-9. Two concentric purse-string sutures of No. 3-0 silk are placed in the bowel wall. A stab wound is made and a catheter inserted. The sutures are tied, and the bowel is sutured to the anterior abdominal wall. Omentum may be pulled up to the catheter to assist in controlling any leakage.

Colostomy

Although ideally gastrointestinal continuity should be restored with an appropriate anastomosis whenever possible, there are many circumstances in which a colostomy is either essential or unavoidable. Examples of an essential colostomy include an end sigmoid colostomy after a standard proctectomy or pelvic exenteration, an ileostomy after a total proctocolectomy, and an end colostomy and oversewing of the rectum (Hartmann pouch) for an urgent sigmoid resection with unprepared bowel. A colostomy may be undesirable yet unavoidable when an injury has occurred to the colon without prior mechanical and antibiotic preparation, when incontinuity resection of the colon for pelvic disease is required, or for proximal decompression when obstruction or perforation is discovered (Fig. 37-10). Although a colostomy may be protective when it is placed proximal to an anastomosis or a perforation, and thus decreases the risk of complications, it offers an advantage only if it is performed correctly and free of its own complications. For that reason the technical per-

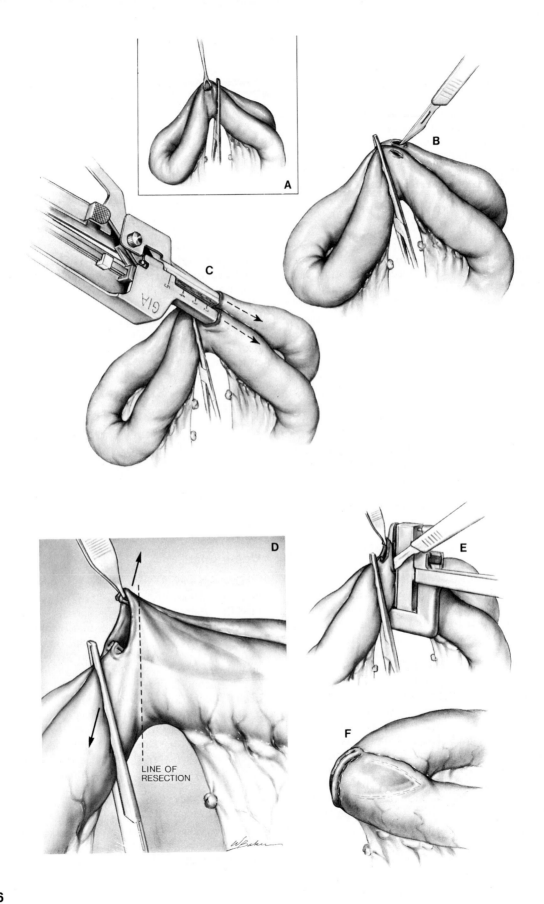

D

LINE OF
RESECTION

formance of a colostomy must be exact and must protect the blood supply of the colon as well.

Colostomies traditionally are considered as either temporary or permanent. Classically, a loop colostomy is considered temporary and an end colostomy permanent, although a loop colostomy can be permanent and an end colostomy temporary. Loop colostomies usually are performed in areas of the colon that have a free mesentery, that is, the sigmoid colon or the right transverse colon. Although the colon can be adequately mobilized to bring it to the abdominal wall for performance of an end colostomy in almost any portion of the colon, an end colostomy most commonly is performed in the sigmoid colon, left or right transverse colon, or (rarely) the ascending colon or cecum.

Loop Colostomy. A loop colostomy usually is performed as a proximal diverting procedure for a distal obstruction or perforation. It is considered temporary, and is closed after successful management of the distal problem. A loop colostomy normally is performed in the sigmoid colon or right transverse colon. It can be performed as a separate surgical procedure or as a complement to a definitive surgical procedure. If done as a primary procedure, the surgical incision typically is placed over the rectus muscle in the right upper quadrant for a right transverse colostomy. The incision for a sigmoid colostomy also can be oblique, transverse, or vertical (paramedian) in the left lower quadrant. When the procedure is performed as a complement to a laparotomy, a small transverse incision can be made in either area centered over the lateral border of the rectus sheath.

The colon is freed from any secondary attachments to the peritoneum and elevated through the incision. In the case of a sigmoid colostomy, a rod that can later fit into a specially designed appliance is inserted through a small defect created in the mesentery at the mesenteric margin of the colon (Fig. 37-11A). A piece of rubber tubing is connected to both ends to keep it in place. A No. 20 plastic chest tube also works well. In the case of

a right transverse colostomy, the omentum should be freed up from the inferior margin of the colon for a short distance. The serosa of the colon can be attached to the peritoneum and posterior fascia. Reapproximation of the fascia under the rod may help to minimize the risk of colostomy prolapse.

After the loop of colon has been brought through the fascia and secured with the rod or sutures, it can be left closed for 24 to 72 hours to prevent contamination, or the colostomy can be opened immediately in the operating room by making a longitudinal incision along the tinea (Fig. 37-11B). Alternatively, after the longitudinal incision is made, the edges of the open colon can be sutured to the margin of the surgical defect (allowing the rod to protrude on either side), which results in a primarily matured colostomy (Fig. 37-11C). This primarily matured colostomy has been reported by Turnbull and Weakley to be totally diverting, as long as the rod is left in place, yet without separation or closure of the distal colon.

End Colostomy. When the sigmoid colon must be resected without preoperative bowel preparation, a primary anastomosis usually is inappropriate. In such a setting an end colostomy with either a Hartmann procedure (closure of the distal rectum) or a mucous fistula (attaching the distal end of the open bowel to the abdominal wall like a colostomy) can be performed. After resection of the bowel, sigmoid colostomy is performed by excising a circular defect of skin at the appropriate point. It is helpful to have the site of an end sigmoid colostomy identified by an enterostomal therapist preoperatively to minimize the likelihood of placing the colostomy in a fold of the abdominal wall or too close to the anterior superior iliac spine or groin crease, which could cause difficulties in the fitting of the appliance. This prior identification is seldom possible, however, in an emergency setting, whereupon an estimate of the location of the colostomy should be made. An end sigmoid colostomy traditionally is placed at the midpoint of a line connecting the umbilicus to the

---

Figure 37–7. A side-to-side anastomosis (functional end-to-end) can be constructed with the GIA and the TA 55 or TA 90. *A,* Both segments of intestine are freed up at the appropriate locations by dividing the mesentery. Bowel to be anastomosed may be approximated with interrupted seromuscular sutures. *B,* Small enterotomies are made on the antimesenteric border of both limbs. *C,* The arms of the GIA are inserted into the enterotomies. The instrument is closed and the push bar is advanced. This simultaneously approximates the two limbs of intestine by parallel double rows of staples and opens the intestine between the rows. *D,* The line of transection of bowel is identified so as to resect the area containing the enterotomies. The lumen between the two limbs is indicated by the shaded area. The TA 55 or TA 90 is applied along this line and closed until the vernier lines on the handle line up, indicating complete closure. *E,* The resected bowel is amputated using the groove in the instrument as a guide for the knife. *F,* The completed functional end-to-end anastomosis. The staple line can be reinforced with sutures if desired.

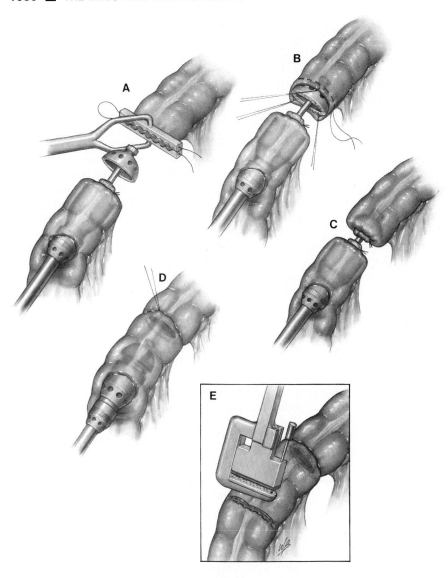

Figure 37–8. The technique of end-to-end anastomosis is demonstrated with the EEA. *A*, The EEA instrument is inserted through a colotomy in the anti-mesenteric taenia, the cone (anvil) is reattached, and the free end of the bowel is secured around the rod with a purse-string suture. *B*, Intestine is advanced on the anvil after placement of purse-string suture near the free margin. *C*, The purse-string suture is tied and the instrument is closed, drawing free margins of bowel together. *D*, The instrument is fired and free margins of bowel are severed, removing a round segment of mucosa and anastomosing the two segments of bowel. *E*, The colotomy site is closed with a single application of the TA 55 or TA 90 instrument. Staple lines are reinforced with Lembert sutures of No. 3-0 silk.

anterior superior iliac spine (Fig. 37-12*A*). This point is acceptable except in obese or elderly patients. In these patients it is helpful to place the colostomy as high as possible to facilitate colostomy care.

When the site for the colostomy has been chosen and the circle of skin and underlying soft tissue has been removed, either a cruciate incision is made in the anterior rectus fascia along the lateral edge of the rectus muscle or a circular defect can be excised (Fig. 37-12*B*). The rectus muscle is not divided, but the external and internal oblique muscles are bluntly separated. An opening that will accommodate three fingers is made in the underlying posterior sheath and transversalis fascia (Fig. 37-12*C*). The end of the colon is brought through the defect, taking care not to twist the colon on its mesentery. It often is helpful during an emergency

resection to use the GIA stapler to simultaneously divide the bowel and close the ends to prevent contamination. In patients with a fatty mesentery it is helpful to divide the mesentery from its point of attachment to the bowel over a distance of several centimeters from the end of the cut colon. In a less fatty mesentery this may not be necessary. The colon is attached to the posterior fascia and peritoneum with several interrupted fine sutures placed at intervals around the circumference of the bowel. The defect created between the edge of the mesentery and the lateral abdominal wall is eliminated by suturing the free mesenteric margin to the peritoneum of the lateral abdominal wall with interrupted or continuous suture. The abdominal incision is closed before the colostomy is opened and matured. After the abdominal skin has been reapproximated and an occlu-

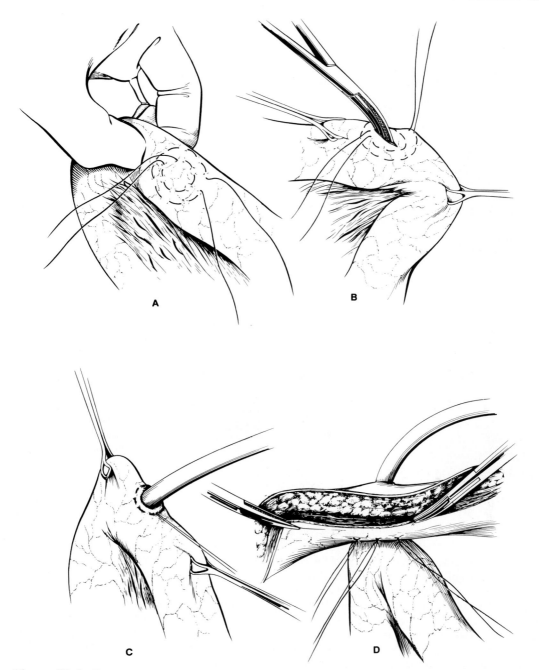

Figure 37–9. Enterostomy. *A,* Note the concentric purse-string sutures with the free ends opposite each other. *B,* After a stab wound is made with a scalpel, the patency of the musosal wound is established with a clamp. *C,* After introducing the tube, the purse-string sutures are both tied. *D,* The intestine is tacked to the peritoneum.

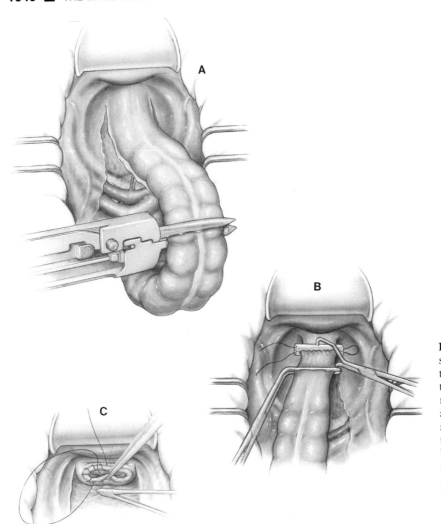

Figure 37–10. *A,* In preparation for a sigmoid colostomy, the colon can be transected to avoid spillage by using the GIA instrument. *B,* Resection of the rectosigmoid colon is done with a right-angle clamp applied to the proximal side of bowel and a polypropylene suture placed around the distal end of the bowel, using a purse-string instrument and a straight needle. *C,* If the terminal rectum is to be used as a site for drainage of the pelvis, a continuous suture is placed around the circumference of the open end of the bowel.

sive dressing applied, the clamp on the end of the colon is removed or the staple line effectively closing the end of the colon is excised. The colostomy is matured primarily by placing four quadrant delayed absorbable No. 2-0 sutures initially (Fig. 37-13*A*). These sutures are placed by taking a bite of dermis, a seromuscular bite of colon about 3 cm from the edge of the colon, and a third bite through the full thickness of the end of the colon from the outside in (Fig. 37-13*B*). After all four sutures are placed they are tied, which primarily everts the mucosa and matures the colostomy (Fig. 37-13*C*). One or two sutures can be taken between each of these quadrant sutures, again beginning with a bite of the dermis but following with a full-thickness bite of the end of the colon. After all sutures have been placed a temporary colostomy appliance is applied. A Hartmann pouch can be created in the distal bowel segment by oversewing a previously placed staple line or by closing

the end of the bowel in two layers. A mucous fistula can be created by primary attachment of the distal segment to the skin of the inferior portion of the wound or, preferably, to a separate lower quadrant incision, after the seromuscular surface of the bowel is tacked to the surrounding fascia. Alternatively, a Stone clamp or similar crushing clamp can be left on the end of the bowel for 5 to 7 days and then removed.

A colostomy, whether temporary or permanent, will markedly alter a person's self-perception and life-style. Although psychological adjustment can easily be made and reinforced with the help of enterostomal therapists and ostomy clubs, one should not assume that a patient's life will not be changed materially by the addition of a colostomy. With that in mind, one can appreciate the overwhelming importance of the location of a colostomy. Modern enterostomal therapists can cope with a stoma that does not protrude adequately by using

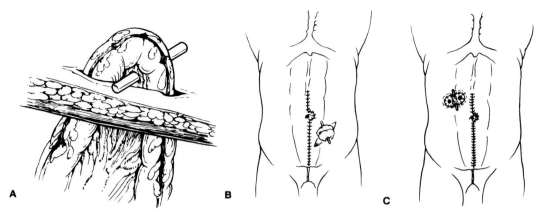

Figure 37–11. Loop colostomy. *A*, A rod or segment of vinyl tubing is inserted through an opening at the edge of the mesentery. *B*, The abdominal incision is closed. The loop sigmoid colostomy is shown, with rod in place, before opening the colon with the electrocautery along the tinea. The rod can be secured with an applicance (Hollister), or a segment of rubber tubing attached to both ends. *C*, Alternatively, as shown with this right transverse colostomy, the stoma can be matured primarily over the rod.

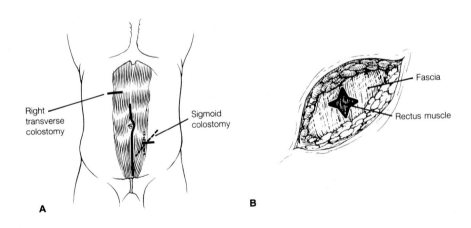

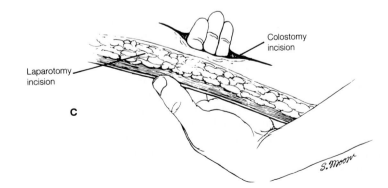

Figure 37–12. End colostomy. *A*, A midline abdominal incision is indicated. Sites for sigmoid colostomy (transverse, oblique, or vertical paramedian incisions) are indicated overlying the lateral border of the rectus muscle. *B*, The incision is extended to the rectus fascia, where a cruciate incision is made. *C*, The rectus muscle is bluntly separated and the peritoneum is opened to allow passage of three fingers.

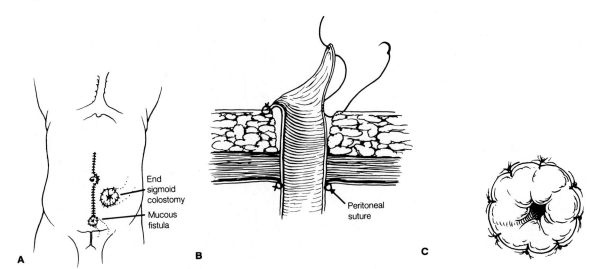

Figure 37–13. End sigmoid colostomy. *A*, A left lower quadrant, end sigmoid colostomy with a mucous fistula at the base of the wound. *B*, Details of the end colostomy. Peritoneal sutures secure the colon to the abdominal wall circumferentially. A simple suture between skin edge and colon has been placed and tied. An everting suture is being placed with a bite of dermis, a seromuscular bite in the colon at skin level, and the edge of the colon. Four such sutures, one in each quadrant, will evert the stoma. *C*, The completed end-colostomy "rosebud."

newer appliances and adhesives. Even the most ingenious enterostomal therapist, however, cannot improve on a poorly placed colostomy.

Surgery of the Anus and Rectum

Although there is no occasion that requires the gynecologic surgeon to perform major rectal surgery electively, there are many occasions when gynecologists performing vaginal plastic operations can conveniently remove a symptomatic hemorrhoid and provide relief to the patient. This section, however, deals primarily with the nonoperative management of rectal disorders.

Hemorrhoids

Human beings have paid several rather dear premiums for having assumed an upright posture, not the least of which is hemorrhoids. Few human afflictions cause more discomfort without posing any threat to life.

The pathophysiology of hemorrhoids is quite simple. Increased pressure in the perianal and rectal veins causes distention, with dilatation of the veins (Fig. 37-14). The distention may be favored by spasm in the internal sphincter and resistance to outflow. It is assumed that as the vein walls become chronically distended, varices develop. Internal hemorrhoids are covered with mucous membrane and protrude into the

rectal lumen (Fig. 37-15). They usually are painless, and the primary symptom is bleeding, which may be severe enough to require transfusion. As the hemorrhoids enlarge they may protrude through the anal opening. When this occurs the mucocutaneous junction becomes exposed, and itching and burning may be severe. As a hemorrhoid prolapses through the anal opening, the external sphincter may go into spasm, and the hemorrhoids may be strangulated, with gangrene resulting. This is an excruciatingly painful process. Rupture of a perianal vessel, with hemorrhage into the perianal subcutaneous tissue, also is quite painful, and is identified clinically as a thrombosed hemorrhoid.

One of the more common conditions associated with hemorrhoids in women is pregnancy. Several theories have been proposed. Possibly the increased blood volume, plus pelvic venous congestion, is a factor; arteriovenous fistulas may be of importance. If symptoms can be managed until parturition, operation may not be necessary.

Local treatment often is quite beneficial. Relief of constipation by the administration of a bulk laxative (eg, Metamucil) is important. Sitz baths, two to four times daily, are helpful. Suppositories with local antiinflammatory agents may be of benefit. Topical anesthetic ointments should be avoided because of a high incidence of hypersensitivity, with resultant burning and itching. In the case of prolapse or acute thrombosis, cold compresses of saturated magnesium sulfate solution may bring great relief. Perianal injections of local

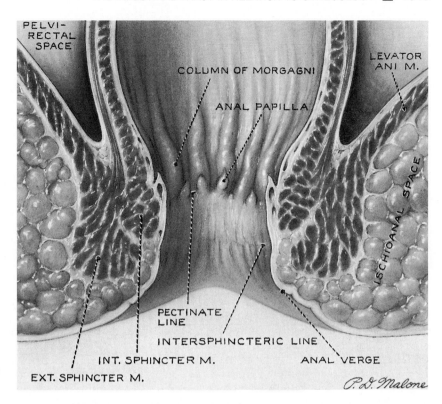

Figure 37–14. Normal anatomy of the anus and lower rectum.

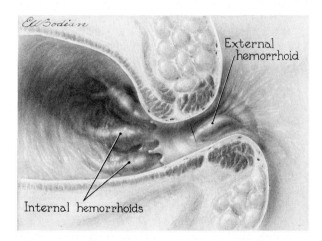

Figure 37–15. Position of external and internal hemorrhoids.

anesthetic agents may be required, to relieve sphincter spasm.

Symptomatic protruding hemorrhoids occasionally are excised at the time of vaginal surgery by the radial technique shown in Figure 37-16. Care should be exercised to avoid removing excessive anoderm, which could result in anal stenosis. Hemorrhoidectomy at this time ensures that a second operative procedure will not

be needed. At the end of a week a gentle digital examination is made. This is painful but prevents adhesion formation and constriction. It is advisable to have the patient return to the office about 2 weeks after leaving the hospital for another digital examination. If there is any tendency to stricture formation, the patient should return at weekly intervals as long as necessary. Continued use of a bulk laxative allows continued regular dilatation of the anus during defecation. This prophylactic attention often prevents the formation of a troublesome stricture later.

The gynecologist may have a patient with acutely thrombosed external hemorrhoids. It is important to recognize that these are in fact perianal hematomas and not thrombosed blood vessels. These subcutaneous blood clots increase in size as the osmotic activity of the clot draws water into the elastic perianal skin. If encountered during the first 3 days of onset, incision and drainage or excision with primary closure is an appropriate method of treatment. Many authorities favor excision over incision and drainage because excision precludes recurrence, postoperative bleeding, and the otherwise universal formation of skin tags. Lesions seen after 72 hours are probably best treated nonoperatively with sitz baths, bulk-forming agents, and topical magnesium sulfate.

In 1954 Blaisdell presented a new technique for

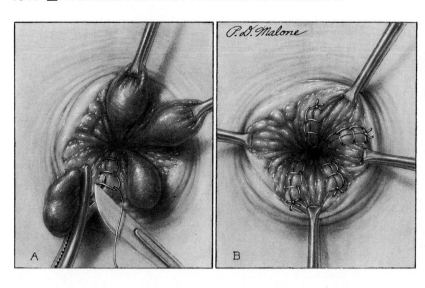

Figure 37–16. Typical radial operation for internal hemorrhoid. *A*, Groups of hemorrhoids are retracted with mucosa clips, and one mass of hemorrhoids is being excised. *B*, The wounds have been sutured with continuous lock stitch of No. 0 delayed-absorbable suture.

ligation of hemorrhoids using an instrument that employed a silk ligature, but premature loosening of the suture sometimes led to bleeding. In 1963 Barron modified Blaisdell's instrument, using a cone for loading the ligating drum and substituting an elastic latex rubber ring for the silk suture. Subsequently the McGivney hemorrhoid ligator was developed from modifications of those of Blaisdell and Barron. Results in large series from the Cleveland Clinic, the Lahey Clinic, and others led to the conclusion that, in selected patients, elastic ligation is an acceptable form of treatment for internal hemorrhoids. Absolute contraindications are the presence of associated anorectal disease that might require operation, and thrombosed hemorrhoids.

The technique of elastic ligation is quite simple (Fig. 37-17). The anoscope is inserted, and the largest hemorrhoid is selected for treatment. The cylindrical drum is placed over the hemorrhoid, and the long-handled forceps is used to draw the hemorrhoid through the drum. The point at which the hemorrhoid is grasped should be at least 5 mm above the anorectal line. The handle is then closed, and two rubber bands are ejected around the neck of the hemorrhoid. The patient may experience a dull ache but no significant pain. Any appreciable pain suggests the inclusion of sensitive anoderm into the ligature. This necessitates urgent removal of the rubber band through an anoscope with a scalpel. Some patients experience a sense of fullness and the desire to defecate later in the day, and this should be discouraged for 12 to 24 hours. No more than one to two hemorrhoids should be ligated at a time; subsequent ligation should not be done for at least 3 weeks. Sloughing usually is complete in 8 days, and may be associated with the passage of a small amount of red blood. Laxatives and stool softeners usually are given to

avoid constipation, prevent excessive straining, and passively dilate the anal canal.

Complications are rare but include delayed hemorrhage, anal ulceration, pain, and slipping of the ligature. Recent reports of serious infection, often with *Clostridium* organisms, occasionally resulting in death have moderated the original enthusiasm for hemorrhoidal banding. To minimize the risk of such devastating soft-tissue infections, one or no more than two sites should be banded at one session. The role of prophylactic antibiotics in this setting is unclear.

Anal Fissure

An anal fissure seldom requires surgical treatment unless it becomes chronic with scar formation. The problem usually is created by hard stool tearing the mucous membrane during defecation. Once the tear occurs, sphincter spasm follows. Each subsequent bowel movement aggravates the problem.

Management is the same as for hemorrhoids. Constipation must be alleviated and sphincter spasm relieved. A palpable abnormality, usually in the posterior midline, suggests chronicity and may necessitate surgical intervention.

Fistula in Ano

Fistula in ano most often makes its presence known by the development of a perirectal abscess. The fistula usually begins in the anal crypt (Fig. 37-18). It is preceded by an inflammatory process in the crypt, which then extends through the rectal wall to contaminate the

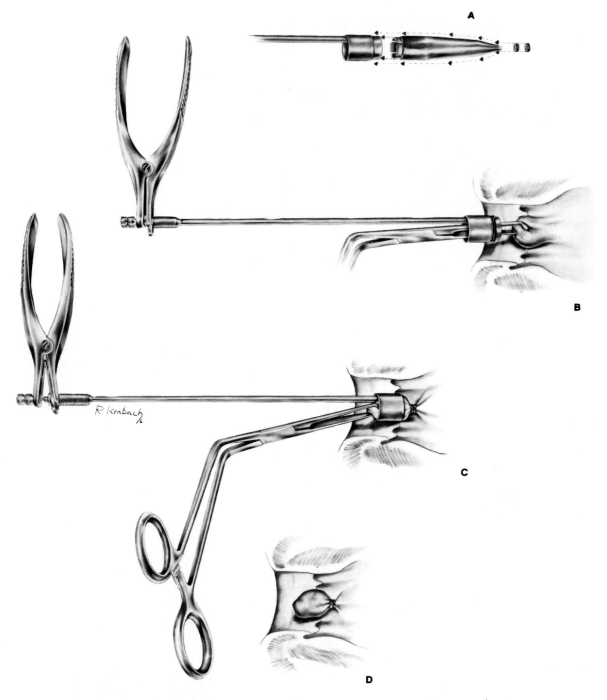

Figure 37–17. Rubber band ligation of internal hemorrhoid. *A,* Two rubber bands are loaded on the cylindrical drum. *B,* The anoscope is inserted and the largest internal hemorrhoid is grasped after placing the Allis clamp *through* the cylindical end drum. The drum is then advanced over the hemorrhoid. This must be at least 5 mm above the anorectal line. *C,* The handle of the applicator is closed, ejecting the two bands at the base of the hemorrhoid. *D,* Appearance of the ligated hemorrhoid with the rubber bands in place.

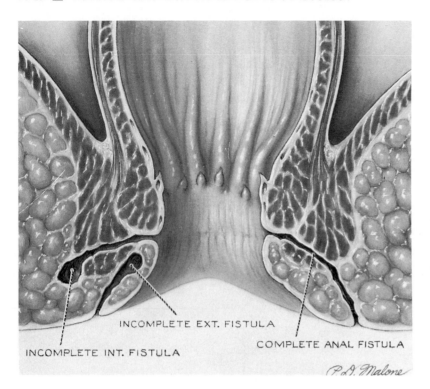

INCOMPLETE INT. FISTULA

INCOMPLETE EXT. FISTULA

COMPLETE ANAL FISTULA

P. D. Malone

Figure 37–18. Schematic illustration of three types of fistulas.

fat-containing perirectal spaces. The poor blood supply of this space makes it extremely vulnerable to infection. Fistula development is complete when the abscess drains spontaneously or is drained surgically. In the acute stage, management is aimed at the control of sepsis. Basic to the control of sepsis is the provision of adequate drainage. Because the ischiorectal space is traversed by fibrous septa, a perirectal abscess may be multiloculated. Because of the need for sigmoidoscopy through a painful anus to define the abnormality, as well as the possibility of multiloculation, perirectal abscesses are most appropriately drained in the operating room, with the patient under general anesthesia. Systemic antibiotics should be given if evidence of systemic reaction, such as leukocytosis, fever, or tachycardia, is present. Special attention should be given to very elderly patients, debilitated patients, and those with associated illnesses, such as diabetes, because of the increased likelihood of a supralevator component of the abscess. A supralevator abscess may require diversion of the fecal stream by colostomy.

After a perirectal abscess is drained a persistent fistula is common. This fistula connects the initial crypt abscess with the perianal skin. The external opening of the fistula in ano often gives a clue to the location of the internal opening. It is shown in Figure 37-19. Knowledge of this principle can be of assistance in probing a fistula, to find the internal opening. There is little need for the gynecologic surgeon to perform definitive sur-

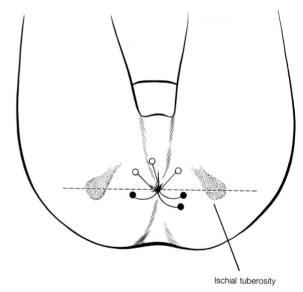

Ischial tuberosity

Figure 37–19. Goodsall's rule of the fistula. This rule usually is valid, and provides a clue to the site of the internal (mucosal) opening of a fistula-in-ano. External openings posterior to the line between ischial tuberosites enter in the posterior midline; those anterior to this line tend to have a radial course.

gery for a chronic fistula in ano. The need is to drain or to improve spontaneous drainage of a perirectal abscess.

Bibliography

Arnold FJ, Nance RC. Volvulus of the sigmoid colon. Ann Surg 1973;77:527.

Barnett WO, Truett G, Williams B, et al. Shock in strangulation obstruction: mechanisms and management. Ann Surg 1963;157:747.

Barron J. Office ligation of internal hemorrhoids. Am J Surg 1963;105:563.

Billig DM, Jordan PJ. Hemodynamic abnormalities in intestinal obstruction. Surg Gynecol Obstet 1969;128:1274.

Blaisdell PC. Scientific exhibit. American Medical Association, San Francisco, 1954.

Bricker EA, Johnston WD. Repair of postirradiation rectovaginal fistula and stricture. Surg Gynecol Obstet 1979;148:499.

Campbell CD, Carey LC. Shock: differential diagnosis and immediate treatment. Postgrad Med 1974;55:85.

Classen JN, Bonardi R, O'Mara CS, et al. Surgical treatment of acute diverticulitis by staged procedures. Ann Surg 1976;184:582.

Colcock BJ, Hume A. Radiation injury to the sigmoid and rectum. Surg Gynecol Obstet 1959;108:306.

Corman ML, Veidenheimer MS: The new hemorrhoidectomy. Surg Clin North Am 1973;53:417.

Delancy HM. Prognostic factors in infraction of the intestine. Surg Gynecol Obstet 1972;135:253.

Dirksen PK, Matalo NM, Trelford JD. Complications following operation in the previously irradiated abdomino-pelvic cavity. Am Surg 1987;(April):234.

Edmunds LJ Jr, Williams GM, Welch CE. External fistulas arising from the gastrointestinal tract. Ann Surg 1960;152:445.

Fabri PJ. Intestinal ischemia in radiation enteritis. In: Cooperman M, ed. Intestinal ischemia. Mt. Kisco, New York, Futura Publishing Co, 1983;325.

Gallagher DM, Russell TM. Surgical management of diverticular disease. Surg Clin North Am 1978;58:563.

Gehamy RA, Weakly FL. Internal hemorrhoidectomy by elastic ligation. Dis Colon Rectum 1974;16:347.

Green WW. Bowel obstruction in the aged patient. Am J Surg 1969;118:541.

Greenwald JC, Hoexter B. Repair of recto-vaginal fistulas. Surg Gynecol Obstet 1978;146:443.

Hines JR. Method of transverse loop colostomy. Surg Gynecol Obstet 1975;141:426.

Horwitz A, Smith DF, Rosesweig J. The acutely obstructed colon. Am J Surg 1962;104:474.

Kawarda Y, Brady L, Matsumoto T. Radiation injury to the large and small intestines. Am J Proctol 1974;24:49.

Leffall LO, Syphax B. Clinical aids in strangulation intestinal obstruction. Am J Surg 1970;120:756.

Lo AM, Evans WE, Carey LC. Review of small bowel obstruction at Milwaukee County General Hospital. Am J Surg 1966;111:884.

Localio SA, Stone A, Friedman M. Surgical aspects of radiation enteritis. Surg Gynecol Obstet 1969;129:1163.

McGivney JQ. The ligation treatment of internal hemorrhoids. Tex Med 1967;63:56.

Martimbeau P, Pratt JH, Gaffey TA. Small bowel obstruction secondary to endometriosis. Mayo Clin Proc 1975;50:239.

Miller TG, Abbott WO. Intestinal intubation: practical technique. Am J Med Sci 1934;187:595.

Mortensen E, Nilsson T, Vesterhauge S. Treatment of intestinal obstruction. Dis Colon Rectum 1974;17:638.

Nadrowski LF. Pathophysiology and current treatment of intestinal obstruction. Rev Surg 1974;31:381.

Neff CC, Van Sonnenberg E, Casola G, et al. Diverticular abscesses: percutaneous drainage. Radiology 1987;163(1):15.

Nelson SW, Christoforidis AJ, Roenigk WJ. Dangers and fallibilities of iodinated radiopaque media in obstruction of the small bowel. Am J Surg 1965;109:546.

Parks AG, Gordon PJ, Hardcastle JD. A classification of fistula in ano. Br J Surg 1976;63:1.

Perry EP, Peel AL. The treatment of obstructing intestinal endometriosis. J R Soc Med 1988;81(3):172.

Plyforth RH, Holloway JB, Griffin WO. Mechanical small bowel obstruction: A plea for earlier surgical intervention. Ann Surg 1970;1:783.

Preston FW. The intestine and rectum. In Preston FW, Beal JM, eds. Basic surgical physiology. Chicago, Year Book Medical Publishers, 1969.

Romsdahl MM, Cole WH. Diverticulitis of the colon. Arch Surg 1963;86:751.

Russel JC, Welch JP. Operative management of radiation injuries of the intestinal tract. Am J Surg 1979;137:433.

Schmitt EG, Symmonds RE. Surgical treatment of radiation-induced injuries of the small intestine. Surg Gynecol Obstet 1981;153:896.

Seyfer AE, Mologne LA, Morris RL, et al. Endometriosis causing acute small bowel obstruction: report of a case and review of the literature. Am Surg 1975;41:168.

Smith GA, Perry JF Jr, Yonehiro EG. Mechanical intestinal obstructions: study of 1,252 cases. Surg Gynecol Obstet 1955;100:651.

Smith JS, Milford HE. Management of colitis caused by irradiation. Surg Gynecol Obstet 1976;142:569.

Snyder EN, McCranie D. Closed loop obstruction of the small bowel. Am J Surg 1966;111:398.

Steichern RM, Ravitch MM. History of mechanical devices and instruments for suturing. Curr Prob Surg 1982;19:1.

Steinberg DM, Liegois H, Alexander-Williams J. Long term review of the results of rubber band ligation of haemorrhoids. Br J Surg 1975;62:144.

SuFian S, Matsumoto T. Intestinal obstruction. Am J Surg 1975;130:9.

Tejler G, Jiborn H. Volvulus of the cecum. Report of 26 cases and review of the literature. Dis Colon Rectum 1988;31:455.

Turnbull RB, Weakley FL. Atlas of intestinal stomas. St. Louis, CV Mosby, 1967.

US Surgical Corporation. Stapling techniques, general surgery. 2nd ed. 1980.

Wangensteen OH, Rea CE. The distention factor in simple intestinal obstruction: an experimental study with exclusion of swallowed air by cervical esophagostomy. Surgery 1939;5:327.

Nongynecologic Conditions Encountered by the Gynecologic Surgeon

38

JOHN H. ISAACS

Eventually, with enough time and a reasonable patient load, the gynecologic surgeon will unexpectedly encounter a nongynecologic disorder when the contemplated surgery was supposedly for gynecologic pathology. Indeed, it is unlikely that any pelvic surgeon, whether a gynecologist, urologist, colorectal surgeon, or a general surgeon, has not encountered an intraoperative lesion entirely unsuspected before surgery. As Symmonds has pointed out, only those who do not operate often (or who have short memories) will fail to unexpectedly encounter pelvic pathology with which they are unfamiliar.

The gynecologist must constantly bear in mind that women of all ages look to their gynecologist to diagnose, treat, or triage any problem that arises within the pelvis. A pain or mass in the pelvis may arise primarily from the reproductive organs, but may just as easily arise from the urinary tract, the gastrointestinal tract, the retroperitoneal space, or the bony pelvis. It also is important to remember that double lesions are not uncommon. For example, an ovarian cancer and a colon cancer present at the same time is always a possibility. It is extremely important, therefore, that the gynecologic surgeon be aware of the various conditions that may be present in the pelvis, and search for them preoperatively. If this caveat is not heeded, the gynecologic surgeon may be faced with the unenviable position of attempting to manage unfamiliar disease intraoperatively. The gynecologist will then realize that the

patient has had an inadequate preoperative evaluation, possibly an inappropriate surgical incision, unprepared bowel, an uninformed patient and family, and the need for a major change in the surgical procedure. This chapter discusses the various diagnostic tools available that may help to circumvent these sometimes disastrous situations.

PREOPERATIVE DIAGNOSTIC EVALUATION

A careful history and physical examination combined with routine laboratory data remain the cornerstone of the preliminary evaluation. Although nongynecologic pelvic disorders can occur at any age, they most often are found in the obese or elderly patient with an ill-defined pelvic mass. The symptoms often are vague and, particularly in the elderly patient, minimized, since most elderly patients do not want to be any trouble or burden to their spouses or families. Most elderly patients have a high threshold for pain.

Gastrointestinal Disease

Complaints such as pelvic pain, low-grade fever, change in bowel habits, hematochezia, or melena should arouse suspicions of intestinal pathology. In such instances a gastrointestinal evaluation is essential before laparotomy.

A pelvic examination may reveal a right or left adnexal mass that may seem to be an inflammatory or neoplastic disorder of the tube or ovary, or both. Figure 38-1 shows the various intestinal disorders that may easily be mistaken for ovarian or tubal pathology. Although the guaiac test (Hemoccult slide) is a helpful screening test for asymptomatic patients, it is not reliable in symptomatic patients and, if negative, may give the physician a false sense of security.

Preoperative evaluation should include lower gastrointestinal radiologic studies and possibly a colonoscopic examination. The gynecologic surgeon should be aware, however, that radiologic studies of the colon can be in error from 10% of the time in cooperative and well-prepared patients to as high as 50% in uncooperative or improperly prepared patients. A large number of colon lesions are missed on x-ray examination because they are mistaken for fecal material or are hidden by fecal material. This is particularly true when the solid column barium enema is used. For this reason it is vital that the gynecologic surgeon make certain that the patient is properly prepared for the x-ray studies and that they are of the air contrast type. Without air contrast study the colonic mucosa cannot be adequately outlined. Even if the air contrast barium enema is performed, a conscientious gynecologist should carefully

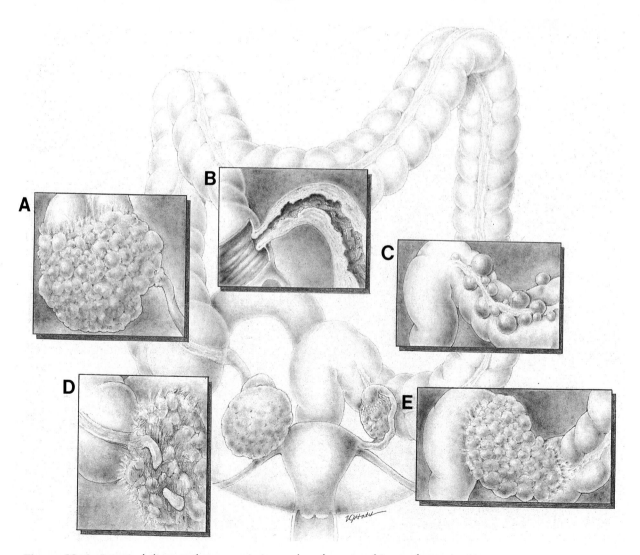

Figure 38–1. Intestinal diseases that may mimic an adnexal mass on bimanual examination. *A*, Cecal carcinoma. *B*, Crohn's disease at terminal ileum. *C*, Sigmoid colon diverticulitis. *D*, Appendiceal abscess. *E*, Rectosigmoid carcinoma.

and critically review the films with the radiologist. Without this precaution grave error may result (Fig. 38-2).

To ensure a properly prepared colon, the patient should be given instructions on colon cleansing before the x-ray studies. On the day before the test a regular breakfast is advised, but only clear liquids for lunch and dinner. Although cathartics and cleansing enemas are acceptable, the colon is best prepared by using an electrolyte-balanced liquid (Colyte), which washes the colon clean. The Colyte is begun at noon on the day before the test, with the patient drinking 8 to 16 oz every 10 to 15 minutes until the rectal discharge is clear. This usually requires 2 to 4 qt of Colyte. After midnight the patient should not have anything to eat or drink. Early on the morning of the test a 10-mg bisacodyl suppository (Dulcolax) should be inserted into the rectum. If such a preparation is not done, unsatisfactory x-ray studies may be the result, and the error only discovered in the operating room.

In addition to being an invaluable aid in the detection of colon cancer and diverticulitis, the barium enema may detect an appendicitis or an appendiceal abscess. Nonvisualization of the appendiceal lumen or the presence of secondary signs of irritability of the cecum may be of extraordinary diagnostic assistance in establishing the diagnosis of appendiceal disease. Figures 38-3, 38-4, and 38-5 are examples of the value of the barium enema in detecting appendiceal pathology.

Although the value of digital rectal examination and sigmoidoscopy in detecting lesions of the rectum and

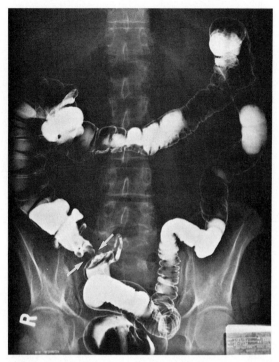

Figure 38–2. Barium enema reported as normal performed 6 months before surgery for a large ovarian tumor mass. At the time of surgery an ovarian carcinoma was found, but in addition a carcinoma of the cecum was found that required a right colectomy. Arrows reveal the deformed cecum that was overlooked by the radiologist.

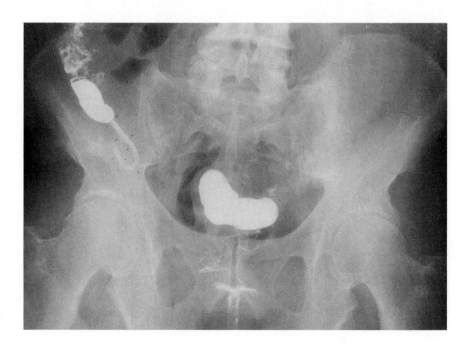

Figure 38–3. Filling of normal appendix.

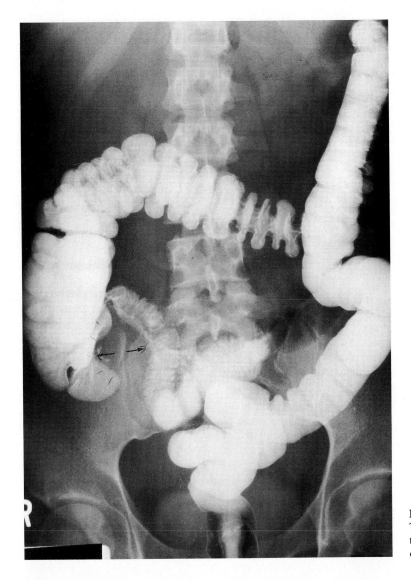

Figure 38–4. Pressure effect on the cecum. There is nonfilling of the appendix and separation of the cecum and terminal ileum because of an appendiceal abscess.

sigmoid cannot be overemphasized, the changing distribution of colon cancer makes colonoscopy more important in the diagnostic workup. Cohn and Nance have noted that the incidence of left-sided colon and rectal cancer in their 1950–1954 series was 78.6% and right-sided colon and rectal cancer was 21.4%. In their 1975–1979 series the incidence of left colon and rectal cancer had dropped to 68.4%, and the incidence of right-sided colon cancers had increased to 31.6%. Because almost 75% of colon cancers arise in the rectosigmoid or cecum, the gynecologist should not mistake a palpable pelvic mass for ovarian pathology rather than colon cancer. Thus, if the symptoms suggest colon pathology—even if the barium enema is reported normal—colonoscopy is indicated.

Unusual small-bowel lesions may present as a pelvic mass; thus small-bowel barium contrast x-ray studies often are helpful. Such studies are particularly useful in delineating mesenteric cysts, volvulus of the small bowel, or Crohn's disease of the ileum, any one of which may prolapse into the pelvis and be mistaken for gynecologic pathology.

Urologic Tumors

Urinary pathology concomitant with or mimicking gynecologic disease includes pelvic kidney, carcinoma of the distal ureter, paraganglioma of the bladder wall, hemangiopericytoma posterior to the bladder, and bladder cancer. A routine urinalysis that reveals hematuria should alert the gynecologist to the possibility of urinary tract disease.

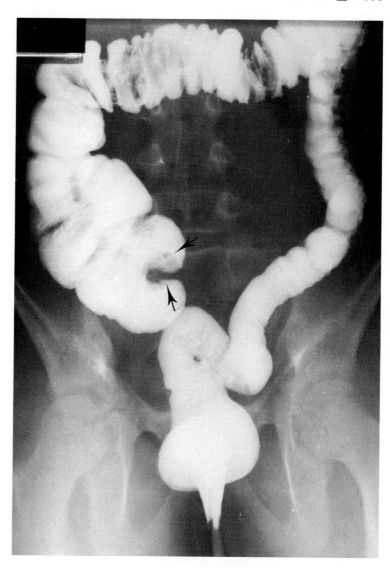

Figure 38–5. Defect in the cecum at the origin of the appendix and nonfilling of the appendix because of appendicitis.

Excretory urography before laparotomy is almost always indicated in a patient with a pelvic mass. It establishes the function of the kidneys and determines the presence of a pelvic kidney or a partially obstructed distal ureter. When performing a bimanual examination bear in mind that a large tumor of the distal ureter may be confused with an intraligamentous leiomyoma. Cystoscopy and retrograde pyelography are indicated in patients in whom suspicion of urinary tract disease is high and in patients who are allergic to the iodine used for excretory urography.

Retroperitoneal Tumors

Although gastrointestinal tract disease is the most frequent pathology mistaken for gynecologic disease, retroperitoneal tumors occur often enough within the pelvis that the gynecologic surgeon must keep such tumors in mind, especially when dealing with vague or unusual pelvic symptoms and physical findings. Beck reported on seven collected series of retroperitoneal tumors, and noted that the major symptoms include abdominal pain, abdominal mass or swelling, and weight loss or anorexia, or both. The symptoms depend on the location of the tumor in the retroperitoneal space. Retroperitoneal tumors in the pelvis may become manifest earlier than those in the abdomen because the bony confines of the pelvis cause pressure on adjacent organs to occur earlier than in the upper abdomen.

Abnormal findings noted on an excretory urogram and on upper and lower gastrointestinal x-ray studies may be secondary to extrinsic involvement and not caused by intrinsic pathology. The most reliable tool for diagnosing retroperitoneal tumors is computed tomography (CT) scanning. It is ideal for the obese patient who has not undergone previous pelvic surgery. If the patient has been operated on previously, if there is only scant retroperitoneal fat, or if there are metallic clips present from previous surgery, the CT scan is more difficult to interpret (see Chapter 12).

If the tumor is a lymphoma, a careful history will elicit complaints of fever, night sweats, pruritus, and weight loss. On physical examination, patients with a lymphoma may have skin nodules, enlarged lymph nodes, liver and spleen enlargement, and areas of joint or bone tenderness. A biopsy of a peripheral lymph node or skin nodule may establish the diagnosis of lymphoma. Additionally, a core needle biopsy of the bone marrow can be helpful, since it is positive in many patients with a lymphoma. The gallium 67 scan is quite accurate in identifying a lymphoma above the diaphragm, but it is of little value in detecting abdominal or pelvic lymphomas because gallium excretion into the bowel may cause a false-positive interpretation.

The anterior meningocele is rare, and may be mistaken for an ovarian cyst. The pelvic findings reveal a cystic mass in midline resting high on the sacrum. Compression by the examining hand on the mass may produce a sudden and rather severe headache or cough that disappears as soon as the compression is released. A radiograph of the sacrum in a patient with an anterior meningocele reveals a large sacral defect (occult spina bifida). Myelography confirms the diagnosis.

In addition to the anterior meningocele, there is a group of rare neurogenic tumors that arise in the pelvis. The largest group has been reported by Lee. Those arising from the nerve sheath of the obturator or sacral nerve complex are the neurofibromas (often associated with Recklinghausen's disease) and the neurilemmomas. Tumors also may develop from the sympathetic nervous system of the pelvis, and include ganglioneuroma, sympathicoblastoma, and neuroblastoma. Soft-tissue sarcomas may occur anywhere in the retroperitoneal space. According to Adam and colleagues, these tumors are diagnosed most easily by CT scan, but ultrasonography, arteriography, and venography may be useful.

Orthopedic Disorders

Disorders to be considered that may arise from the bony pelvis include those that are congenital, iatrogenic, metabolic, or septic, as well as fractures and tumors. The congenital or developmental abnormalities include anterior sacral meningocele (discussed above), spondylolisthesis, and sacrococcygeal teratomas. Spondylolisthesis is a slow, forward displacement of the lumbar spine over the sacrum. The degree of slip usually is not severe enough to cause significant impairment. If the entire fifth lumbar is displaced forward of the sacrum (spondyloptosis), however, severe narrowing of the anteroposterior diameter of the pelvis and displacement of the pelvic viscera are noted. Pelvic examination is significantly abnormal. A pelvic radiograph defines the problem.

Sacrococcygeal teratomas usually are diagnosed by age 2 or 3, but occasionally the dermoid forms are present in early adulthood. These anomalies are four times more common in women, and malignant forms are more common in adults. Such lesions usually can be defined by ultrasonography and CT scanning.

Total hip arthroplasty has become commonplace since it was introduced in the 1960s. In some earlier cases the orthopedic surgeon penetrated the inner wall of the acetabulum, allowing the cement (methyl methacrylate) to flow into the pelvis to improve fixation. The cement produces a bony, hard mass fixed to the pelvic wall that varies in size, shape, and convolution. If such a mass is encountered on pelvic examination, it may well represent a challenging diagnostic problem. Only a high degree of suspicion can warn the examining gynecologist that the hard, nodular fixed pelvic mass is indeed a cementing substance that should not be disturbed.

The gynecologist also should be aware that an intrapelvic protrusion of the acetabular cup owing to trauma or weakness of the inner wall may occur in patients with total hip arthroplasty. This protrusion may present as a pelvic mass fixed to the side of the pelvic wall, causing considerable confusion and difficulty in diagnosis. A good plan is to order x-ray studies of the pelvis of any patient with a history of total hip arthroplasty or with a telltale scar over the lateral aspect of the involved hip before considering pelvic surgery for a lateral sidewall mass.

Certain metabolic disorders of the skeletal system can cause gradual development of pelvic deformities that may be confusing on pelvic examination. With bone deficiency sometimes there is inward protrusion of the femoral head through the inner acetabular wall (protrusio acetabuli). Other causes of protrusio acetabuli include Marfan's syndrome, Paget's disease of the bone, rheumatoid arthritis, and osteomalacia.

Fungal, parasitic, and pyogenic afflictions of the bony pelvis can cause the development of soft-tissue masses that may be difficult to diagnose. Fungal and parasitic disorders are extremely rare, but pyogenic osteomyelitis of the pelvis and sacroiliac joints is not uncommon. Most of these cases present as acute, painful infectious processes, but some develop as subacute or chronic pyogenic infections. Pelvic examination may cause severe discomfort and produce findings suggestive of a deep fullness or mass on either pelvic sidewall. Sometimes such infections present as a presacral abscess. There usually is an associated tenderness over the sacroiliac joints and both buttocks. Orthopedic consultation is essential.

A rather common cause of intrapelvic distortion is residual bony deformities caused by pelvic fractures. These are fairly common occurrences in automobile accidents. X-ray examination of the pelvis reveals the cause of the unusual findings.

Primary bone tumors that involve the pelvis are quite rare except for those on the anterior sacrum. The sacrum is the primary site of more than 50% of chordomas (malignant) and 6% of giant cell tumors (benign). These tumors usually are found on pelvic or rectal examination. Urinary frequency and constipation are common presenting symptoms. X-ray studies of the pelvis usually are sufficient for diagnosis, and a technetium 99 bone scan demonstrates bone destruction not apparent on the x-ray films.

Vascular Considerations

The two vascular lesions of significance to the gynecologic surgeon are iliac aneurysms and arteriovenous fistulas. Isolated iliac aneurysms are rare, but many patients with abdominal aortic aneurysms have associated iliac aneurysms. This lesion is 10 times more common in men than in women. They are more common on the common iliac and hypogastric arteries and very rare on the external iliac artery. Most iliac aneurysms remain asymptomatic until rupture unless they impinge on adjacent structures. Diagnosis of iliac artery aneurysms is difficult, but ultrasonography and CT scanning occasionally detect these aneurysms. Contrast angiography is necessary to formulate the therapeutic plan.

Pelvic arteriography is a valuable part of preoperative evaluation of unusual pelvic tumors or findings. The technique involves a percutaneous puncture of the femoral artery; a wire is introduced into the femoral artery through the needle. The wire serves as a guide for a catheter threaded over the wire. Under fluoroscopic control the catheter tip is advanced to the desired level and a contrast medium injected. Although pelvic arteriography is not often necessary, it helps to delineate a highly vascular tumor. Hasty exploration without knowledge of the source of a tumor's blood supply could lead to uncontrollable hemorrhage, with disastrous results (Fig. 38-6).

Aneurysms that are symptomatic because of local factors or because of distal emboli should be carefully evaluated. Growing aneurysms should almost always

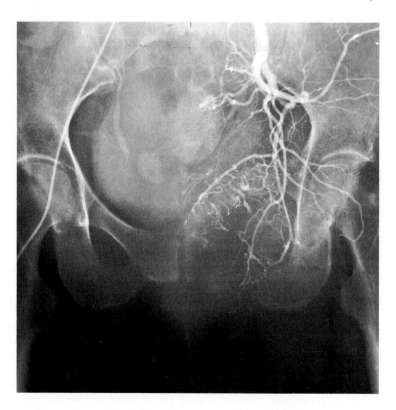

Figure 38–6. Pelvic arteriogram obtained on a patient with an unusual pelvic mass resting on the medial aspect of the left pubic arch. The tumor was receiving its blood supply from vessels from both the anterior and posterior divisions of the left hypogastric artery.

be resected. Internal iliac aneurysms, however, usually are not resected, but are treated by simple ligation.

Metastatic Lesions to the Pelvis

The ovary is a frequent recipient of metastases from numerous primary sites. In comparison with the ovary, solitary extragenital metastases to the fallopian tubes or uterus are rare. Although statistics vary, probably 10% to 25% of all ovarian tumors are metastatic in origin. The most common metastases to the ovary are from the gastrointestinal tract, the breast, and the uterus. The functional ovary seems particularly prone to extragenital metastatic disease. When the ovarian metastasis is from the gastrointestinal tract, it is almost always bilateral. As the ovaries enlarge from gastrointestinal cancer, both ovaries usually become symmetrically enlarged while retaining their shape and capsule integrity.

When a pelvic mass is detected and preoperative evaluation is being carried out, the possibility of a retroperitoneal metastatic cancer must always be considered. If metastasis is suspected, CT-guided percutaneous needle aspiration or biopsy may prevent unnecessary laparotomy by revealing the true nature of the suspicious mass.

Magnetic resonance imaging (MRI) promises to make solid contributions to the detection, management, and follow-up of metastatic ovarian disease. Although not yet commonly used, MRI has advantages over existing diagnostic techniques. In imaging the pelvis MRI complements sonography and CT in refining anatomic details and displaying pelvic pathology more accurately. Pelvic imaging lends itself to better quality compared with MRI studies of the abdomen because respiratory and intestinal motion are at a minimum in the pelvis. As pointed out by Hricak, MRI is emerging as an important imaging technique in studying the pelvis. It offers more precise localization and tissue differentiation. Although many applications of MRI are already established, clinical experience is still limited, and the full potential of MRI for evaluation of diseases of the pelvis has not yet been determined (see Chapter 12).

Nonsurgical Acute Abdomen

There are a number of nonsurgical causes of acute abdominal pain that may be mistaken for a gynecologic problem. Sickle cell anemia is one of these conditions. Such patients may have attacks of bone and joint pain but also may suffer abdominal pain. A careful history and laboratory testing for sickle cells usually establish the diagnosis.

Recurrent attacks of abdominal pain occur with acute porphyria. This disease is most common in women in the third and fourth decades of life. Abdominal tenderness is much less than would be expected, considering the severity of pain. Fever and leukocytosis may be present, and abdominal x-rays studies show distended loops of bowel. Diagnosis is made by a history of similar attacks and by detection of excessive porphobilinogen in the urine.

Other nonsurgical causes of abdominal pain include familial Mediterranean fever, lower-lobe pneumonia, rectus sheath hematoma (frequently preceded by a paroxysm of coughing), pyelonephritis, and acute gastroenteritis.

Laparoscopy

Diagnostic laparoscopy has been of inestimable value in gynecology. Although its use is common, the gynecologist should bear in mind that it is not an entirely innocuous procedure, and he or she should know what to do in the event of an accident during this procedure. If the Veres needle is inserted and a sudden gush of blood results, immediate laparotomy to repair the vascular rent is lifesaving. If the needle is inserted and bowel gas flows out of the needle, the abdomen should be opened, leaving the needle in place to more easily identify the puncture site in the bowel. It also is possible to perforate the stomach with the Veres needle. This will not become apparent until the carbon dioxide insufflation begins, at which time the gas is expelled from the stomach in the form of a loud belch. In such instances the needle should be repositioned, and the abdomen filled with carbon dioxide. After the laparoscope is in place a nasogastric tube is placed in the stomach and the stomach filled with saline solution that has been colored with methylene blue. If there is a significant leak in the stomach from the puncture, it will be seen with the laparoscope. If no leak is noted, a laparotomy is not necessary, but the nasogastric tube should be left in place for 2 to 3 days (see Chapter 16).

Preoperative Preparation

Preparation of the patient for pelvic surgery begins with the establishment of as accurate a diagnosis as possible. Because an absolute diagnosis is not always possible, the extent of the surgery is difficult and sometimes impossible to determine. Thus, when major pelvic surgery is anticipated, it is imperative that the patient (and often the family) be as well informed as possible. If the patient understands that bowel or bladder resection may be needed, requiring a colostomy, ileostomy, or urinary conduit, she will be much better prepared to cope with these problems postoperatively. It cannot be overemphasized that despite extensive diagnostic strides, it is not always possible to know what the findings might be until the abdomen is opened. It is prudent to advise the patient and the family that intraoperative consultation may be necessary. If possible, the patient should have the opportunity to meet the specialists before the contemplated surgery.

Preoperative Bowel Preparation

If there is the slightest possibility that the surgery might involve opening or resecting a portion of the colon, bowel preparation should be carried out. Although opinions vary as to what type of bowel preparation is best, everyone agrees that preoperative preparation of the colon should include adequate mechanical cleansing. In addition to mechanical cleansing, almost everyone believes that intestinal antisepsis is indicated. A high-protein, low-residue diet is a major aid to preparation of the colon, since it provides protein supplements while eliminating bulk from the colon. The single 24-hour period of mechanical cleansing using a continuous lavage of the entire gastrointestinal tract with large quantities of a saline preparation is acceptable, but the 3-day mechanical preparation is preferred. On the first day the patient is given a laxative (usually magnesium citrate), and a clear-liquid diet is begun and continued throughout the period of preparation. Enemas are given each night throughout the period. Erythromycin base (1 g) and neomycin (1 g) are given four times a day for 48 hours before surgery. Additionally, intravenous antibiotics are given preoperatively, intraoperatively, and in the recovery room.

Additional Preoperative Preparation

If the patient is chemically depleted, nutritional support is indicated, usually by instituting total parenteral nutrition. Dehydrated patients undergoing bowel preparation should be given intravenous fluids for 16 to 24 hours before major pelvic surgery. This is particularly important in the older patient.

Any question of bleeding problems in the past must be investigated (see Chapter 8). Patients on broad-spectrum antibiotics and bowel preparations may have prolonged prothrombin time secondary to depressed vitamin K production. Such patients usually respond well to vitamin K in doses of 10 mg/day for a couple of days preoperatively. Some medications, such as aspirin and coumarin, may be forgotten by the patient, and the physician should ask specifically about medications.

Patients receiving corticosteroids will need additional corticosteroids during surgery. Postoperatively,

they are tapered down over 4 to 5 days to their usual maintenance dose.

Patients with cardiopulmonary problems should have maximum pulmonary preparation. Smoking should be stopped several days before surgery. If possible, pulmonary toilet with chest physiotherapy can begin when preoperative workup takes place.

INTRAOPERATIVE MANAGEMENT OF NONGYNECOLOGIC PELVIC DISORDERS

After a thorough history and physical examination and a meticulous diagnostic laboratory workup, most nongynecologic conditions should have been diagnosed, or at least highly suspected, before laparotomy. Despite all effort, situations may arise that are outside the purview of the gynecologic surgeon, and intraoperative consultation is indicated. In certain circumstances, however, such consultation is not available. In that situation the gynecologist may need to close the abdomen before undue damage is done. On the other hand, the gynecologic surgeon may have enough experience and surgical skill that the problem encountered can be managed without difficulty.

Once the abdomen has been opened, a thorough evaluation of first the upper abdomen and then the pelvis is necessary. If the upper abdomen is normal, the upper abdominal contents should be packed away with laparotomy pads. Next, the pelvic findings are assessed and the problem sorted out, with things being put in as near an anatomically normal position as possible. If dense adhesions are present, these should be lysed by sharp dissection. If the pathology involves the uterus or the tubes and ovaries with extension into the surrounding organs, the appropriate surgery to remove the diseased organs should be carried out. If, for example, this involves removing a portion of the bowel or urinary bladder, this should be done by the gynecologist, if his or her surgical experience permits this, or in conjunction with some other surgical specialist, depending on what pathology is present.

If the findings are not gynecologic in nature, then a determination of the problem is essential. The most common nongynecologic disease is pathology of the gastrointestinal tract. If the colon and small bowel are normal, the gynecologic surgeon must consider retroperitoneal tumors or pathology of the distal ureter or urinary bladder. Assuming that the patient has had an adequate bowel preparation and has been apprised of the various possibilities (ie, colostomy, bowel resection, urinary diversion, excessive blood loss, and, possibly, prolonged hospital stay), definitive surgery should be carried out. Clearly, if these precautions have not been taken preoperatively, the gynecologic surgeon has no choice but to close the abdomen and explain to the patient and family that the patient was not initially prepared for the surgery that is required and that further surgery will be necessary at a later date. This is not an ideal situation for the gynecologic surgeon. If, on the other hand, preoperative preparation has been properly carried out, the indicated surgery can be performed.

Gastrointestinal Disease

Appendicitis

If the abdomen has been opened for a presumed acute gynecologic problem, such as a twisted or ruptured ovarian cyst, a tubo-ovarian inflammatory mass, or an ectopic pregnancy, and acute appendicitis is found instead, an appendectomy should be carried out. Once the appendix has been removed, the stump can be left uninverted after cleaning the exposed mucosa with phenol and alcohol. Condon has cautioned, however, that if it is elected to invert the stump, the distal end should not be tied, but rather inverted and a purse-string suture closed over the appendiceal stump. The appendiceal stump that is ligated and then inverted may lead to an intramucosal abscess or mucocele (Fig. 38-7). If a mucocele is found at celiotomy, it should be excised, even if this necessitates removing a small portion of the base of the cecum.

If an appendiceal abscess is found, it may rupture spontaneously at laparotomy. If not, a finger should be introduced into the abscess and its loculations broken down by blunt dissection. If the appendix is readily accessible, appendectomy can be performed. Often, however, it cannot even be found. If the appendix is not removed, either because it is not easily accessible or because it cannot be found, an interval appendectomy should be performed 6 to 8 weeks after drainage from the abscess has ceased and the wound has healed. A sump drainage tube should be inserted into the abscess cavity and extracted through a stab wound in the flank. The sump tube should be left undisturbed until it is draining less than 60 ml/d. The tube should then be rotated but not advanced. If drainage does not resume, a sinogram should be obtained. When the abscess cavity has been obliterated, the drain should be progressively advanced and removed (see Chapter 36).

Diverticulitis

The usual therapy for diverticulitis is medical. The gynecologist, however, may find himself or herself in a situation where he or she is operating on a patient for what was presumed to be recurring attacks of pelvic inflammatory disease or an ovarian mass and comes on a portion of the rectosigmoid involved with diverticulitis. These patients may undergo elective resection of the involved segment of colon and a primary anastomosis with a very low operative risk. If, on the other hand, there is acute inflammation with evidence of perforation, fistula, obstruction, or bleeding, the diseased colon must be mobilized and resected. The proximal colon is brought out as an end colostomy, and the distal rectal segment is closed (Hartmann procedure). The colon may be reanastomosed 1 to 3 months after recovery.

Cancer of the Colon and Rectum

Cancer of the colon is predominantly a disease of older people, but it can occur at any age. It is important to remember that the incidence of right-sided colon cancer is steadily increasing. Surgical removal of the primary lesion is the only acceptable curative therapy. If a colon cancer is found unexpectedly and the bowel has had both mechanical and antibiotic preparation, an appropriate resection should be carried out by a colorectal surgeon. A carcinoembryonic (CEA) blood sample should be obtained in the operating room before the colon resection. This is helpful when follow-up CEAs are obtained. If the patient has not had suitable bowel preparation, or if a surgeon experienced in colorectal surgery is not available, the abdomen should be closed and definitive surgery performed at a later date. Proper preoperative planning would prevent such an unfortunate happening. If the patient has been adequately prepared and a pelvic surgeon competent in performing colon surgery is available, then surgery can be carried out. The resection includes the entire segment of the involved portion of the colon and its associated lymphovascular pedicle up to the level of its takeoff from the aorta for left colon lesions or to the mesenteric vessels for right colon lesions. Primary resection and anastomosis of right colon lesions may be carried out even in the absence of prior bowel preparation because of the more liquid nature of the bowel contents at this level.

Crohn's Disease (Regional Enteritis)

Crohn's disease is a chronic inflammatory disorder of the gastrointestinal tract of unknown cause. Because it usually involves the terminal ileum and proximal colon, it may easily be mistaken by history and pelvic examination as an inflammatory process of the fallopian tube and ovary. The most common complaint is right lower quadrant pain that usually is associated with a tender, palpable abdominal mass. The disease most commonly has its onset in the young, but there appears

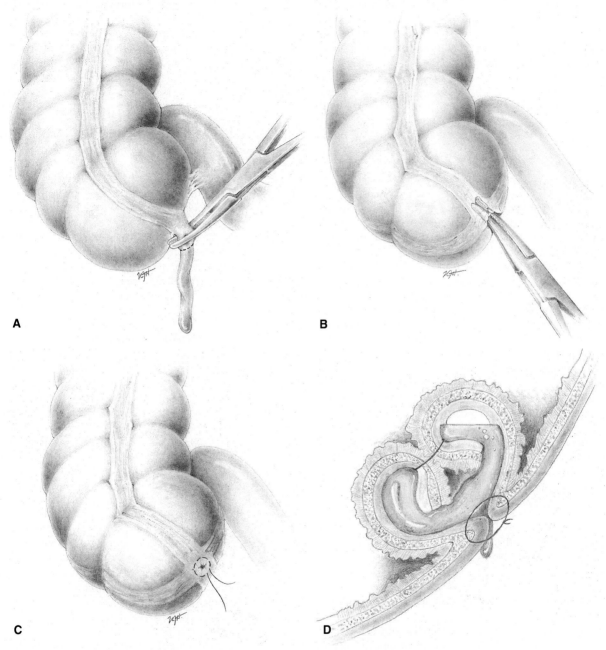

Figure 38–7. *A*, The base of the appendix is grasped with a forceps and the appendix excised. *B*, The appendiceal stump is inverted into the cecum and the clamp removed. *C*, The purse-string stitch is drawn up and tied over the stump of the appendix. *D*, If the stump is ligated and inverted, there is a closed space, creating the possibility of an intramucosal abscess or mucocele.

to be an increased incidence in people after age 60. The findings at laparotomy of thickened mesentery with growth of mesenteric fat around the circumference of leathery fibrotic bowel is almost always pathognomonic of Crohn's disease.

The long-term care of a patient suffering from Crohn's disease usually involves medical management, possibly including total parenteral nutrition. Eventually these patients will need surgery, and it should be within the domain of the gastrointestinal surgeon. If the gynecologic surgeon encounters a patient with Crohn's disease who has had the abdomen opened for what was believed to be a gynecologic problem, the surgeon should have some concept of what is to be done. Surgeons no longer expect to cure the disease by excision of grossly diseased bowel area, since the process is systemic, probably involving the entire gut and varying in intensity only along the course of the bowel. Consequently surgical procedures currently are more conservative, designed to treat complications of the disease rather than pursue the unrealistic goal of curing it.

The gynecologist should know that the primary indication for surgery continues to be partial small-bowel obstruction owing to the disease process. Limited resection of a grossly involved area of bowel or a short-segment enteroenteric bypass is acceptable. If an isolated segment of Crohn's disease is encountered when a gynecologic disease was expected, the treatment of choice is to resect the grossly involved segments of bowel when possible. A simple bypass procedure or a short-circuiting procedure, such as an ileotransverse colostomy with closure of the proximal end of the bypassed bowel, is not used today. Such procedures often result in such complications as stagnant loop syndrome, cancer developing in the bypassed bowel, or closed-loop obstruction with possible perforation. Properly performed conservative surgery often results in complete relief of symptoms and a prolonged restoration of normal activity.

Metastatic Carcinoma of the Ovaries

Metastatic carcinoma to the endometrium or fallopian tube from distant sites may occur, but this is relatively rare and does not present a surgical dilemma to the gynecologist. The uterus, tubes, and ovaries are removed, and the presence of metastatic lesions most often is discovered in the pathology laboratory.

The ovaries, on the other hand, are a frequent site of metastases from cancer originating in many different organs, including the breast, stomach, pancreas, and colon. It has been reported by Israel and colleagues and by Webb and coworkers that young women are more prone to metastatic carcinoma than to primary ovarian cancer and that half of all women with ovarian metastases are premenopausal.

In most situations ovarian metastases can be regarded as a local manifestation of generalized carcinomatosis, and extensive resection is not indicated.

On the other hand, ovarian metastases from the colon may have a better prognosis if aggressive resection is undertaken, providing all gross tumor can be extirpated. Morrow and Enker have noted that the most important discriminant of survival in patients with metastatic ovarian disease from colorectal cancer was whether the patient could be surgically rendered free of gross disease. In their series the mean survival rate for patients rendered free of gross disease was 48 months compared with 8 months for all other patients. Thus significant palliation is achieved by removing large tumor masses in and around the ovaries. Aggressive resection seems justified if such a lesion is encountered by the gynecologic surgeon, particularly if the metastases represents a late recurrence of colon cancer.

Urologic Disease

If, at the time of surgery, the retroperitoneal pelvic mass appears to be a kidney, an attempt should be made to identify a renal pelvis or ureter. Aspiration with a 22-gauge needle may reveal the presence of urine within the mass. Excretory urography can be performed during surgery by injecting 50 to 100 ml of contrast material and taking a 10- to 20-minute film. An alternative is to inject 5 to 10 ml of indigo carmine intravenously and obtain an aspirate from the suspected renal pelvis 5 to 10 minutes later. The presence of blue or green urine confirms that the mass is a functioning kidney. One cannot rely on palpation of the same or opposite side to ascertain that a kidney is present. According to Schuster, palpating the "kidney" was done in almost all the reported cases of removing a solitary pelvic kidney, and the surgeon thought a kidney was present in its proper position.

If by chance the unwary surgeon unwittingly attempts to remove a pelvic kidney, when the "tumor mass" is entered, bleeding will become profuse. If the "tumor mass" is recognized as a kidney, the injured kidney usually can be repaired. Packing the wound will stop some of the small bleeders and control massive bleeding until the situation can be evaluated. If the vascular pedicle can be located, vascular or bulldog clamps can be placed across the vessels and left for about 30 minutes without harm to the kidney. The intrarenal blood vessels need to be individually ligated. Electrocautery will not stop parenchymal bleeding and may increase it. If defects in the collecting system are noted, these defects should be repaired with fine absorbable suture.

Tumors of the lower third of the ureter are five times more frequent than ureteral tumors of the upper third of the ureter. Although ureteral tumors normally are quite small, they may be large and infiltrate the surrounding tissue. When they infiltrate the surrounding tissues and are firm, they theoretically may be palpated on bimanual examination and mistaken for an adnexal or pelvic mass. The treatment of ureteral tumors traditionally has been nephroureterectomy with removal of the entire renal unit and ureter. Some authors believe that a more conservative approach, involving local resection of the tumor with preservation of the renal unit, is acceptable.

If an adequate preoperative workup has been carried out, it is unlikely that a cancer of the bladder will be encountered. The surgeon may encounter a paraganglioma of the bladder wall invading adjacent loops of small bowel that had been mistaken for a leiomyoma or an adnexal mass. These tumors usually are benign, and can be managed by resection of the involved portion of the bladder wall and small bowel. Hemangiopericytomas posterior to the bladder require total resection of the tumor mass.

Retroperitoneal Tumors

Although retroperitoneal tumors are relatively rare, the pelvic surgeon should be prepared to deal with them. Primary retroperitoneal tumors arise from retroperitoneal tissue that does not represent growth from another body organ in the retroperitoneum. Ackerman has compiled and classified a lengthy list of all the possible retroperitoneal tumors. Interested readers are referred to *Atlas of Tumor Pathology* published by the Armed Forces Institute of Pathology.

The retroperitoneal tumor most often unexpectedly encountered if a careful preoperative workup is not carried out is a lymphoma. If a pelvic mass is found to be enlarged retroperitoneal nodes, a biopsy should be taken. If, on frozen section, this is found to be a lymphoma, no further surgery is indicated; there is no role for surgical debulking of this tumor. The abdomen should be closed and appropriate medical management undertaken.

There are a group of retroperitoneal tumors that are amenable to surgical removal. These may be congenital, neurogenic, osseous, or soft-tissue tumors. These tumors have no classic signs or symptoms. It is vital that as accurate a diagnosis as possible be made before surgery. Clinically, an anterior sacral meningocele presents as a midline mass and, as mentioned previously, may produce a cough or headache when pressure is applied on the meningocele at pelvic examination. Sacral chordomas are solid and usually fixed to the sacrum. Neurogenic tumors lie unilaterally on the posterior rectal wall and are firm, smooth, semifixed, and nontender.

If the gynecologic surgeon encounters a cystic structure on the anterior surface of the sacrum that is filled with fluid, the possibility of an anterior meningocele must be considered. The structure should not be aspirated, nor should drainage be attempted. If such is done, there is a strong possibility of the patient's developing an ascending meningitis with resultant mortality. If such a cyst is encountered, it should be left alone and the abdomen closed. The surgery of choice at a later date is a neurologic decision; usually a transsacral approach is used, and the neck of the meningocele sac is ligated.

Aside from a meningocele, once a retroperitoneal tumor is diagnosed, the treatment of choice is surgical resection. Potential complications, such as seeding of a malignant tumor, presacral abscess, or fistulas, usually preclude needle biopsy. Because these tumors may infiltrate the areas of several surgical specialists, the gynecologic surgeon contemplating surgery should have other surgical specialties, such as orthopedists or neurosurgeons, participate. Many of these tumors are best managed by a transsacral approach.

The abdominal approach, however, presents the advantage of a thorough evaluation of the pelvis and the upper abdomen. The ureters and rectum also must be mobilized from the superior and anterior surfaces of the tumor. Neurofibroma or neurilemmoma tumors usually arise from the sciatic or obturator nerve (Figs. 38-8 and 38-9). In such cases the entire hypogastric vascular supply lies anterior to these tumors. These vessels must be ligated before resection, otherwise uncontrollable hemorrhage will result. Complete en bloc excision should be performed, if possible, to eliminate the possibility of recurrence or persistent tumor.

Hunter and associates have reported on neurilemmomas and neurofibromas. They caution that neurilemmomas usually are encapsulated solitary tumors and fairly easy to resect from the nerve itself. Neurofibromas, on the other hand, are nonencapsulated tumors and, therefore, more difficult to resect. If the gynecologic surgeon plans on resecting such retroperitoneal pelvic tumors, it is advisable to have a neurosurgeon available, especially to measure the somatosensory evoked potential above and below the area of dissection.

The tumor most likely to be seen is a presacral teratoma. Its removal requires careful exposure of the ureters and dissection of the rectosigmoid off the anterior surface of the tumor. The vascular supply must be controlled by meticulous ligation of all surrounding

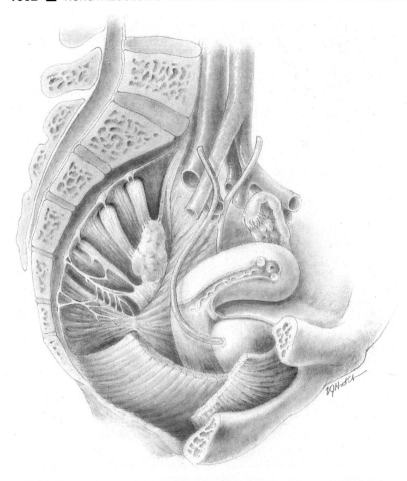

Figure 38–8. Neural tumor arising from the sciatic nerve.

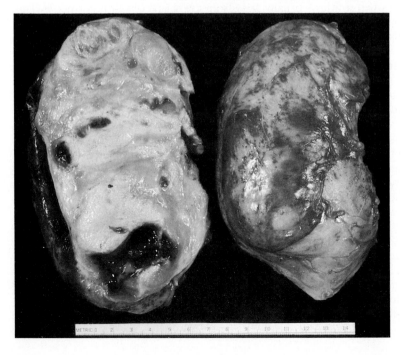

Figure 38–9. Gross specimen of a resected retroperitoneal neurilemmoma. (Courtesy of Raymond A. Lee, M.D., Mayo Clinic)

blood vessels. Disruption of the presacral venous complex presents a real danger of hemorrhage. If this occurs, the tumor should be removed as quickly as possible and pressure applied to the area. These vessels are difficult, if not impossible, to control by ligature, hemoclips, or cautery. It is best to place a pack firmly over the bleeding area for 20 to 30 minutes (see Chapter 8).

SUMMARY

A thorough history, physical examination, and appropriate laboratory and imaging procedures usually detect an unsuspected pathology before laparotomy. Even if a thorough workup suggests gynecologic pathology, bowel preparation and a thorough discussion with the patient of problems that may be encountered will prevent many otherwise difficult, if not impossible, situations. Because gastrointestinal disease most often is the unexpected pathology, the gynecologist should be aware of the correct management of these disorders. Urinary tract pathology and retroperitoneal tumors require a thorough knowledge of the retroperitoneal space, if successful surgery is to be carried out.

Bibliography

Ackerman LV. Tumors of the retroperitoneum mesentery and peritoneum. In: Atlas of tumor pathology, Section VI, Fascicles 23 & 24. Washington, D.C.: Armed Forces Institute of Pathology, 1954.

Adam YG, Halevy A, Reif R. Primary retroperitoneal soft-tissue sarcomas. J Surg Oncol 1984;25:8.

Aufses AH. The surgery of granulomatous inflammatory bowel disease. In: Current problems in surgery. Chicago: Year Book Publishers, 1983.

Beck HH. Retroperitoneal tumors: diagnosis and treatment. In: Isaacs JH, Byrne MP, eds. Pelvic surgery—a multidisciplinary approach. Mt Kisco, NY: Futura Publishing Co, 1987:91.

Cohn I, Nance JC. The colon and rectum. In: Sabiston DC Jr, ed. Textbook of surgery. Philadelphia: WB Saunders, 1986:1004.

Condon RE. Appendicitis. In: Sabiston DC Jr, ed. Textbook of surgery. Philadelphia: WB Saunders, 1986:967.

Drennan DB. Orthopedic lesions. In: Isaacs JH, Byrne MP, eds. Pelvic surgery—a multidisciplinary approach. Mt Kisco, NY: Futura Publishing Co, 1987:173.

Drucker WR. Crohn's disease (regional enteritis). In: Sabiston DC Jr, ed. Textbook of surgery. Philadelphia: WB Saunders, 1986:914.

Hricak H. MRI of the female pelvis: a review. AJR 1986;146:1115.

Hunter VP, Burke TW, Crooks LA. Retroperitoneal nerve sheath tumors: an unusual cause of pelvic mass. Obstet Gynecol 1988;71:1050.

Israel SL, Helsel EV, Hansman DH. The challenge of metastatic ovarian carcinoma. Am J Obstet Gynecol 1965;93:1094.

Knaus JV, Barber HRK. Metastatic lesions presenting as pelvic mass. In: Isaacs JH, Byrne MP, eds. Pelvic surgery—a multidisciplinary approach. Mt Kisco, NY: Futura Publishing Co, 1987:69.

Lee RA. Presacral tumors in gynecologic oncology. Personal communication 1988.

Miller RE. Detection of colon carcinoma and the barium enema. JAMA 1974;230:1195.

Miller RE. The clean colon. Gastroenterology 1976;70:289.

Morrow W, Enker WE. Late ovarian metastases in carcinoma of the colon and rectum. Arch Surg 1984;119:1385.

Paulson DF. The urinary system. In: Sabiston DC Jr, ed. Textbook of surgery. Philadelphia: WB Saunders, 1986:1658.

Pickelman J. Gastrointestinal pathology. In: Isaacs JH, Byrne MP, eds. Pelvic surgery—a multidisciplinary approach. Mt Kisco, NY: Futura Publishing Co, 1987:57.

Rajagopalon AE, Mason JH, Kennedy M, et al. The value of the barium enema in the diagnosis of acute appendicitis. Arch Surg 1977;112:531.

Schuster G. Urologic disease. In: Isaacs JH, Byrne MP, eds. Pelvic surgery—a multidisciplinary approach. Mt Kisco, NY: Futura Publishing Co, 1987:150.

Symmonds RE. Preface. In: Isaacs JH, Byrne MP, eds. Pelvic surgery—a multidisciplinary approach. Mt Kisco, NY: Futura Publishing Co, 1987:vi.

Webb MJ, Decker DG, Mussey E. Cancer metastatic to the ovary, factors influencing survival. Obstet Gynecol 1975;45:391.

39

Surgical Conditions of the Vulva

J. DONALD WOODRUFF
JOSEPH BUSCEMA

The vulva and the adjacent perianal skin are designated the anogenital area. The ectoderm of this area must be considered separately from the vagina and the cervix, the latter of mesodermal origin. Nevertheless multifocal genital diseases, particularly the human papillomavirus (HPV), often affect all of these epithelia.

DERMATOLOGIC CONDITIONS OF THE VULVA

Dermatitis is the most common affliction of the vulva. It causes major diagnostic and therapeutic problems for the dermatologist, the generalist, and the gynecologist.

The vulvar epithelium is subject to all of the dermatologic irritants that occur elsewhere on the body. Although some of the dermatitides are seldom seen on the external genitalia (eg, psoriasis), others, particularly those of reactive origin, are extremely common and produce major problems for the patient and the physician.

Local reactions to many otherwise simple dermatologic lesions are exacerbated by seborrheic, eccrine, and apocrine secretions; by vaginal and cervical discharges; by menstrual blood; and by urine and fecal contamination. The frequently irritating discharges from common vaginal infections may be added to the normal vulvar excretions and secretions. Other irritants are deodorants, hygiene sprays, perfumed soaps and powders, local anesthetic agents, and colored toilet tissue. Tight-fitting pants and underclothing, particularly those made of nonabsorbent synthetic fabrics, aggravate the local problems because they retain moisture and are conducive to fissuring of the skin.

In the acute phase most dermatitides require only local therapy. When such a dermatologic process persists, the vulvar epithelium and subcutaneous tissues become altered, with deep-seated perineural inflammation and pruritus. These may be resistant to the usual local forms of therapy, such as the hydrocortisones.

The antiquated term *leukoplakia* has been used to denote vulvar skin that has become thick and dystrophic, with elongated rete pegs (acanthosis), surface hyperkeratosis, and underlying chronic inflammatory infiltrate. The term has been used to describe any white plaque, varying from "leukoderma" to cancer. Because these terms are unrelated, in 1976 the International Society for the Study of Vulvar Disease (ISSVD) published new nomenclature identifying the condition as hyperplastic dystrophy, with and without atypia. More recently, in 1987, the ISSVD proposed further revision in terminology, abandoning the term *hyperplastic dystrophy* in favor of "squamous cell hyperplasia NOS (not otherwise specified)." In instances in which atypia is present, lesions are classified as vulvar intraepithelial neoplasia. The availability of more realistic terminology should simplify the diagnosis of vulvar disease and, more important, should prevent unnecessary vulvectomy to remove benign white lesions. The new terminology does not clarify the issue but may be accepted.

Treatment of Intractable Pruritus

Before any therapy for vulvar lesions caused by chronic irritation is begun, an accurate tissue diagnosis must be established. The epidermis may be thickened and the skin markings accentuated (lichenification), but the extent of the epithelial proliferation cannot be assessed without biopsy. All patients should be given detailed instruction to eliminate local irritants; associated vaginitis should be treated vigorously; a thorough investigation for any systemic disease such as diabetes should be completed; and local medication for control of the symptoms must be given satisfactory trial. Vulvectomy *should not be performed* for chronic dermatitis or for the benign dystrophies, including lichen sclerosus, without careful histologic evaluation. Only in the presence of neoplasia is vulvectomy indicated.

Topical Agents

Topical agents should be tried first, although they often are ineffective because they cannot penetrate the thickened hyperkeratotic surface. Injection of the topical agent into the subepithelial dermis circumvents the problem of absorption through the thickened skin. The injection of 20 to 30 mg of triamcinolone acetonide (Kenalog, 10mg/ml) in a localized area of 2 × 6 cm has proved to be effective. The most commonly involved region is the outer surface of the labium majus. The injected solution should be rubbed thoroughly into the tissues to prevent focal distribution. Relief of symptoms usually occurs within 48 hours, and remission lasts about 4 to 6 months (Fig. 39-1). The procedure can be repeated as the symptoms demand.

The efficacy of intradermal steroid injection is attested to by the virtual elimination of the need to perform local alcohol injection. Nevertheless the occasional recalcitrant case is seen that warrants this approach. Unremitting vulvar pruritus leads to inevitable trauma secondary to fingernail excoriation. It would appear that the latter is important in the development of neoplasia at this site. For recalcitrant pruritus, local injection of absolute alcohol produces immediate relief by

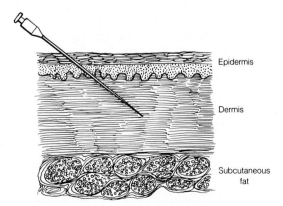

Figure 39–1. Insertion of a needle into the subepithelial dermis for the injection of steroid for the relief of chronic pruritus.

compromising nerve endings. Relief continues for at least 12 months in 90% of cases. Elimination of pruritus and subsequent scratch-induced epidermal injury may alleviate the stimulus for epithelial proliferation.

Technique of Administration. Although local alcohol injection may be performed as an outpatient procedure, general or regional anesthesia is necessary. The anogenital area should be shaved, cleaned, and draped. The region is marked into 1-cm squares with either an autoclaved felt-tipped marker or a dye such as brilliant green (Fig. 39-2*A*). Then 0.2 ml of absolute alcohol is injected into the subcutaneous tissues at each point where the lines intersect (Fig. 39-2*B*). Most important, the alcohol must not be injected into the epithelium or the deep subcutaneous tissues, to avoid slough.

The procedure should begin at the lowest level to prevent the alcohol from leaking from the needle point and destroying the pattern. After all the points have been injected the whole area should be thoroughly massaged to prevent localization of the alcohol, and the patient should be instructed to use cold packs or cool sitz baths for 1 week. Numbness and swelling persist for about 2 to 3 weeks.

Mering Procedure

When all forms of local treatment fail to relieve a patient's symptoms, the Mering procedure should be considered as a last resort. Although surgery is required, the vulvar skin must be protected from the trauma produced by scratching.

The Mering procedure requires hospitalization for the patient and careful surgical technique by the physician (Fig. 39-3). The skin is thoroughly cleaned after being shaved, and the incision is outlined with a marking pencil. The incision is made on the outer surface of the labium majus. It extends to the fascia of the urogenital diaphragm from the level of the clitoris to slightly beyond the fourchette and may continue inferiorly to the level of the anal orifice, depending on the extent of the pruritus. The nerves in the adjacent tissue are severed using a finger on each side, moving from the lateral aspect of the clitoris toward the midline, over the clitoris, where the fingers meet. The procedure interrupts branches of the ilioinguinal and genitofemoral nerves (Fig. 39-4). Blunt dissection extends posteriorly to the lateral side of the rectum, outside of the external anal sphincter. If the perianal area is involved, blunt dissection may extend to the posterior limit of the anal orifice, where the two fingers meet behind the anus in the midline, breaking up the branches of the pudendal nerve.

It is important that hemostasis be meticulously maintained because the accumulation of blood and fluid may

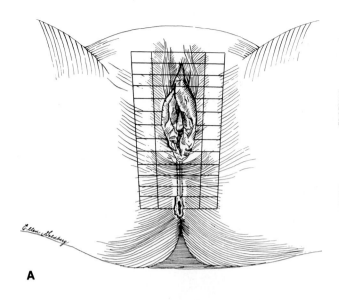

A

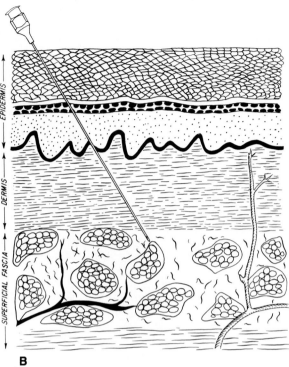

B

Figure 39–2. *A,* Marking of external genitalia into 1-cm squares in preparation for alcohol injection. *B,* Depth of penetration of 25-gauge needle into the subcutaneous tissue. (From Woodruff JD, Thompson B: Local alcohol injection in the treatment of vulvar pruritus. Obstet Gynecol 1972; 40:18)

produce local cellulitis, which would delay recovery. A small drain should be placed at the dependent portion of the incision. The underlying tissue is approximated with absorbable sutures, and the skin is sutured with polyglycolic acid or polyglactin 910 sutures. The area must be packed tightly for 24 hours, and then the patient should use ice packs or cool tub baths. Domeboro sitz baths (Burow's solution) may help to relieve edema.

Specific Infections

Treatment of viral infections of the vulva depends on the specific entity present. HPV, which is responsible for benign condylomatous growths and strongly associated with vulvar intraepithelial neoplasia (VIN), typically requires surgery, and is discussed under solid tumors. Molluscum contagiosum, a member of the pox virus family, requires accurate identification; evacuation of the umbilicated lesions, facilitated by use of a dermal curette, followed by chemical cauterization of the bases typically leads to control. The treatment of herpes simplex virus, conversely, is medical. Acyclovir, 200-mg tablets, administered during an acute episode up to six times per day for 10 to 14 days, limits the duration of viral shedding; this is especially true for the primary outbreak. It also helps to control symptoms of pain and shortens the time to healing. For patients afflicted with frequent recurrences, Jeffries has re-

ported that acyclovir may be administered for long periods of time to reduce the chronicity of outbreaks.

The number of diseases transmitted by sexual contact has increased; the basic group of syphilis and gonorrhea is treated with systemic therapy. Rarely seen in the United States today are the granulomatous diseases. Nevertheless, in the chronic stages of lymphogranuloma venereum and granuloma inguinale, the lymphedematous distortion of the vulva does not respond to local or systemic treatment. Chronic granulomatous lesions must be evaluated by biopsy to differentiate benign from malignant lesions, since chronic granulomatous lesions often have been reported to undergo malignant degeneration. A vulvectomy with wide excision of affected tissues should be performed if local and systemic therapies fail to produce satisfactory healing.

Hidradenitis

An infectious process commonly demanding extensive local surgery is suppurative hidradenitis. This pustular disease begins as an infection in the apocrine sweat glands. The early manifestations frequently are cyclic, since the secretory activity of the apocrine glands corresponds to the progestational phase of the menstrual cycle. Consequently, in the early stages of the disease or in the chronic pruritic phase (Fox-Fordyce

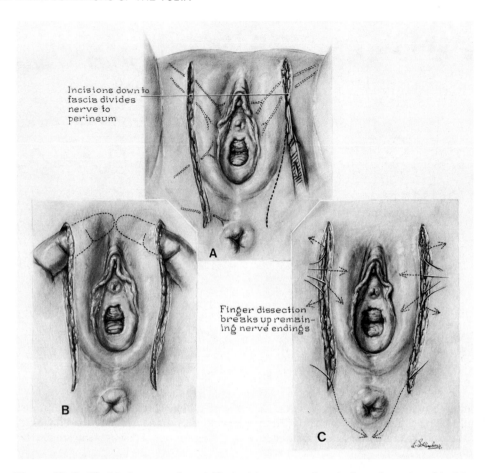

Figure 39–3. The Mering procedure. *A*, The incisions are made at the lateral margins of the labia majora, extending to the level of the clitoris superiorly and the anal orifice inferiorly. The depth of dissection is the deep fascia, to incise the adipose tissue and the nerves. *B*, The finger dissects the underlying tissue, breaking up the fibers of the pudendal, ilioinguinal, and genitofemoral nerves. *C*, The underlying tissues are carefully approximated to attain good hemostasis. A small drain should be inserted at the most dependent aspect of the incision to avoid the accumulation of blood in the operative sites.

disease), the use of hormonal therapy, such as oral contraceptives, may help to modify the secretory activity of the glands. Once the disease extensively involves the deeper tissues, local and systemic agents usually are ineffective. Isotretinoin (Accutane) has been effective in some cases, but care must be taken in prescribing this agent, since it is a powerful teratogen. The pustules often infect the entire area, so that pressure at one point may produce an exudation of purulent material from sinus tracts (Fig. 39-5A). Because the entire anogenital area is honeycombed by the underlying infection, simple incision into a few of the pustules is useless. Extensive debridement must be carried out to allow healing from the base.

The incision extends into the underlying fat, and the involved skin is removed in segments, leaving bridges of normal skin between the excised pustules. Loose approximation of the skin edges may be carried out using polyglycolic acid or polyglactin 910 suture material, but more commonly the entire area is left open and treated locally to promote granulations (Fig. 39–5B). Results of therapy are rewarding in most cases, and skin grafting usually is unnecessary. The patient must be treated with antibiotics both before and after surgery. Ampicillin usually is used, but cultures should be taken from the draining sinuses to check for organisms that are sensitive to other antibiotic agents. Vulvectomy has been used with success in some cases, but it is more traumatic to the patient both physically and psychologically.

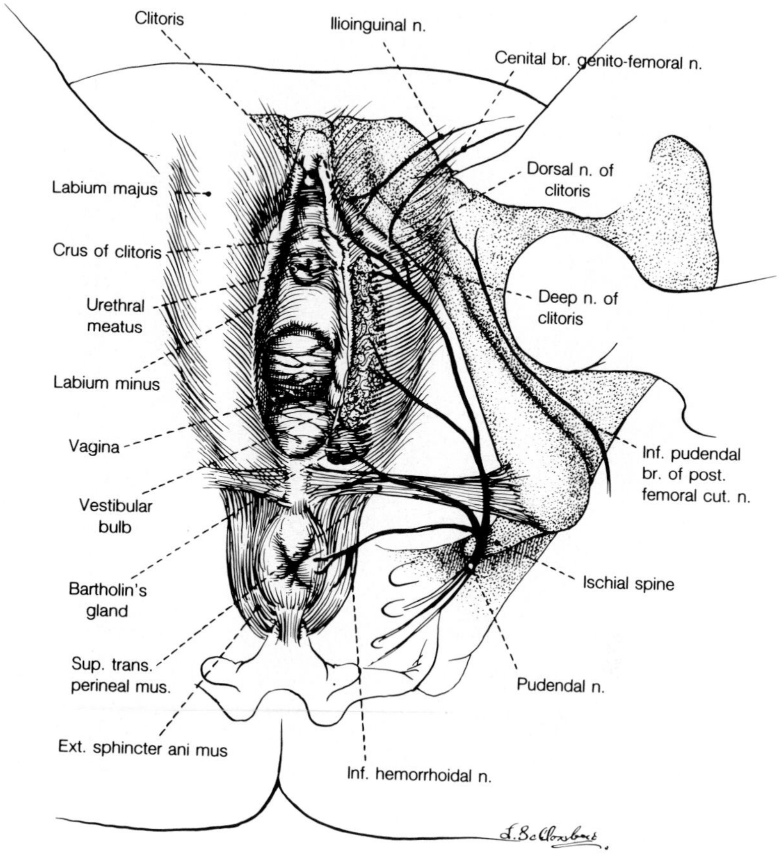

Figure 39–4. Nerve supply to anogenital region. (From Woodruff JD, Julian CG. In: Ridley JH, ed. Gynecologic surgery: errors, safeguards and salvage. Baltimore: Williams & Wilkins, 1974)

Crohn's Disease

Crohn's disease, a chronic inflammatory disease of the bowel, affects the vulva and perianal area in about 25% to 30% of the cases in which there is the classic intestinal involvement. The draining sinuses often communicate with the vagina or the rectum, thus resulting in formation of fistulous tracts. On rare occasions the vulva may be involved even though the small and large bowel apparently are not affected.

Before any surgical therapy is begun, diagnosis can be confirmed by studying the bowel or by obtaining a biopsy of the affected tissues in the perineum. The presence of noncaseating granulomas is characteristic of Crohn's disease. Further deterioration of the tissue may result from attempts to excise a draining sinus produced by Crohn's disease. Rectal incontinence may result from destruction of the anal sphincter or the development of a rectovaginal fistula.

The preferred treatment is prednisone, 20 mg daily, in addition to metronidazole, 1 to 2 g daily in four divided doses for a minimum of 4 to 6 weeks. Treatment must be continued for a longer period of time if surgery is considered necessary.

In addition to pharmacotherapy, a submucosal anal pull-through procedure may bring relief. A layered surgical repair of a fistula caused by Crohn's disease usually is unsuccessful, particularly without appropriate medical management. Nevertheless, after appropriate medical therapy, surgical excision or incision of the tract is classically effective (see Ch. 34). Results are difficult to predict because multiple areas of the terminal colon may be affected, and any affected area may involve the vagina or perineum. Medical therapy, noted above, should always be given during this type of surgical procedure, and continued postoperatively for at least 2 months.

Trauma

Major trauma to the vulva most often occurs when young girls experience injuries as a result of sledding or bicycling accidents. Hematomas, and occasionally lacerations, can develop from falls astride the crossbar of a bicycle or from being thrown from a sled against an obstacle such as a tree or fence (Fig. 39-6). Trauma also may result from sexual assault.

Most traumatic injuries do not require surgical atten-

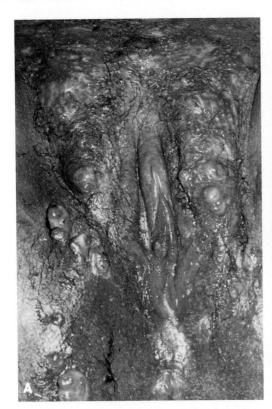 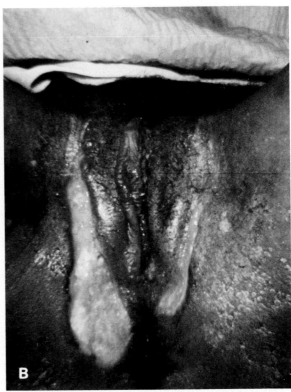

Figure 39–5. *A*, Extensive suppurative hidradenitis with numerous communicating sinuses. *B*, Same vulva 4 weeks after debridement with exuberant granulations (complete healing in 2 months).

tion. Patients should be treated conservatively with activity restriction and immediate and continued use of Burow's solution (aluminum sulfate, calcium acetate; available as Domeboro tablets or powder) added to the sitz bath to reduce edema. Antibiotics may be used to prophylax against superinfection in damaged tissues. If a hematoma should increase in size and extend well into the perineum or over the lower abdominal wall, incising the vulvar skin, evacuating the hematoma, and ligating the bleeding vessels may reduce the period of convalescence. When a hematoma produces urethral obstruction, evacuation may reduce the time an indwelling urethral catheter is needed. Lacerations into the rectum or urethra should be repaired expeditiously.

Necrotizing Fasciitis

Necrotizing fasciitis of the vulva represents an uncommon invasive infection characterized by rapid progression and high mortality ranging from 12% to 60%. Multiple bacterial pathogens are implicated, including staphylococci, streptococci, and gram-negative bacilli.

Associated vessel thrombosis leads to skin and subcutaneous tissue necrosis. Fisher's criteria have been emphasized in diagnosis, and help to exclude clostridial infections. Diabetes mellitis has been the most frequent associated predisposing condition, although other factors, such as radiation, have been identified.

Devascularization of the skin proceeds with sparing of underlying muscle and bone. Early skin changes include hemorrhagic bullus formation. Typically the underlying fascial necrosis exceeds the boundaries of visible skin involvement. Inflammatory alterations and edema usually are present. Most patients present with fever, tachycardia, and signs of systemic toxic reaction. Prompt diagnosis is important, as this disorder progresses rapidly.

Treatment combines expeditious surgery, antibiotics, and maintenance of circulation and tissue oxygenation. Surgical treatment should include aggressive excision of nonviable skin, subcutaneous tissue, and avascular fascia. Debridement must be carried out until viable, well-vascularized tissue margins are identified. Wounds are packed, not primarily closed. Broad-spectrum anti-

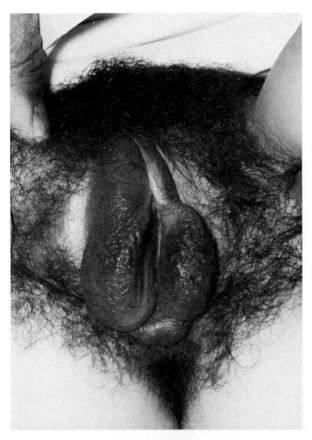

Figure 39–6. Hematoma of the vulva. (From Woodruff JD, Julian CG. In: Ridley JH, ed. Gynecologic surgery: errors: safeguards and salvage. Baltimore: Williams & Wilkins, 1974)

which may precede the actual cyst formation, an abscess often develops with symptoms of tenderness, swelling, and erythema.

Incision and drainage bring almost immediate relief to the patient, and may be accomplished under local anesthesia. A small wick may be left in the cavity to maintain adequate drainage. Marsupialization seldom can be accomplished during the acute stage, but the procedure is useful for chronic or recurrent abscesses. Injection of an antibiotic into the abscess has been tried as treatment for the acute infection, but has proved to be less effective than systemic antibiotic therapy.

Most Bartholin's duct cysts are asymptomatic, and usually are found during routine pelvic examinations. Patients may even be unaware of larger cysts. When symptoms do occur most patients complain of discomfort during coitus or pain while sitting or walking.

Most symptomatic Bartholin's duct cysts can be treated by the insertion of a Word catheter (Fig. 39-7). A small incision (2 cm) is made in the area of the normal duct orifice. A catheter is inserted, and the bulb inflated with 2 to 3 ml of saline solution. If the catheter remains in place for 3 to 4 weeks, the tract will become epithelialized, and the catheter may subsequently be removed.

Technique of Excision

It seldom is necessary to excise a Bartholin's duct cyst, particularly in the younger patient, unless there is

biotic coverage is advisable, and where applicable, control of diabetes is advantageous to infectious management.

CYSTS OF THE VULVA

Bartholin's Duct Cysts

Obstruction of Bartholin's duct, usually near the orifice, is common. Depending on the cause, secretion from the cyst may be mucoid or cloudy. Although such obstructions can result from gonococcal infection, other infections and trauma more commonly explain the occlusion. During a mediolateral episiotomy or a posterior colporrhaphy, for example, sutures easily can injure or even ligate the duct. The lining of the main cyst is transitional epithelium. The mucus-secreting glands are not affected by the obstruction, but may be distorted by the infectious process. During the acute infection,

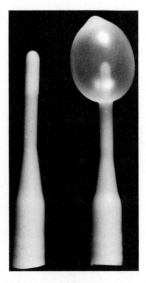

Figure 39–7. The Word catheter *left* is inserted into Bartholin's duct cyst through a vaginal incision. *Right,* The bulb is inflated with saline solution and the end of the catheter is placed in the vagina.

induration at the base. The latter may signify deep-seated infection that is inaccessible to marsupialization. Conversely, this may represent neoplasm in the base of the gland, an issue of greater concern in the patient over the age of 40. An elliptical incision in the vaginal mucosa is made as close as possible to the site of the gland orifice (Fig. 39-8A–E). An incision on the mucosal side is preferable because an incision through the vulvar skin makes it difficult to dissect the cyst wall from the skin without incising or tearing it. If an opening is accidentally made through the skin, a permanent fenestration may result. No difficulty usually is encountered in dissecting the cyst from the inner surface of the vulvar skin when the incision is made on the mucosal side. Excising a small ellipse of mucosa with the cyst allows the surgeon to have a site for traction and reduces the risk of rupturing the cyst.

Because cyst formation usually is preceded by in-flammation, the wall is adherent and cannot be easily enucleated with blunt dissection only. The blunt-pointed Mayo scissors serves admirably for sharp dissection of the cyst from its bed (Fig. 39-8C). The cyst can be mobilized further with the handle of the scalpel. A large cyst may develop posteriorly, and approximate the rectum. The rectal wall can easily be distinguished from the cyst by inserting a finger into the rectum during dissection.

Complete removal of the gland tissue adherent to the cyst wall is essential, for residual glandular tissue may result in the formation of a tender nodule or a recurrent cyst. If the margins of the cyst have become obscured, the cyst may be opened and the wall dissected from the surrounding tissue.

Directly beneath Bartholin's duct is the vestibular bulb, which is composed of anastomosing venous channels. In the dissection of the gland from the vestibular

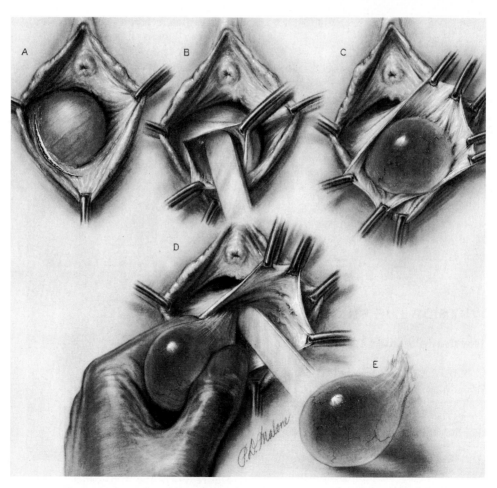

Figure 39–8. Excision of Bartholin's gland cyst. *A*, An incision is made in the mucosa over the cyst. *B*, Dissection is begun, using the handle of the scalpel. *C*, Dissection has been continued by sharp and blunt dissection. *D*, Dissection is almost complete. *E*, Intact cyst after removal.

bulb additional care must be taken to avoid troublesome bleeding. To ensure permanent hemostasis, the entire cavity must be obliterated by approximating the walls with fine delayed absorbable suture material after excising the cyst.

Approximation of the vaginal mucosa is best accomplished with a continuous mucosal suture of No. 1-0 delayed absorbable material. Bleeding from the labia or vestibular bulb usually causes a postoperative hematoma of the labia, which can progress to include the mons pubis and the abdominal wall beneath Scarpa's fascia. Bed rest, ice packs, and a pressure dressing to the vulva are the methods of treatment for a hematoma; attempts to ligate the venous bleeding points will prove futile. Although the blood usually reabsorbs with time, sometimes evacuation and drainage are necessary.

If the bleeding deep in the bed of the gland seems uncontrollable, deep mattress sutures may be placed from the skin through the bleeding bed into the vagina. The sutures should not be tied too tightly because necrosis may result, with fenestration of the vaginal outlet. A small drain should be stitched into the bed with fine absorbable sutures to avoid the accumulation of blood and serous fluid.

Technique of Marsupialization

Drainage of a Bartholin's duct cyst by marsupialization is a less involved procedure technically than exci-sion and eliminates many complications. The procedure makes it possible to avoid excising the gland with the cyst and to preserve the secretory function of the gland for lubrication.

The procedure may be performed under local, regional, or general anesthesia. A wedged-shaped, vertical incision is made in the vaginal mucosa over the center of the cyst, outside the hymenal ring (Fig. 39-9A). The incision should be as wide as possible to enhance the postoperative patency of the stoma. After the cyst wall is opened and drained of its contents the lining of the cyst is everted and approximated to the vaginal mucosa with interrupted sutures of No. 2-0 delayed absorbable material (Fig. 39-9B). Drains and packs are not necessary, but the patient's postoperative care should include daily sitz baths beginning on the 3rd or 4th postoperative day.

As a result of closure and secondary fibrosis of the orifice after marsupialization, 10% to 15% of cysts recur. Abscess formation is another occasional sequela of marsupialization.

Marsupialization has had limited use since the Word catheter was introduced. The catheter accomplishes the same result as surgery with minimal or no trauma. The nipple of the catheter may be inserted into the vagina. There essentially is no discomfort associated with the procedure, and coitus may be resumed normally. Because this procedure can be performed with local analgesia in the office setting and yields results

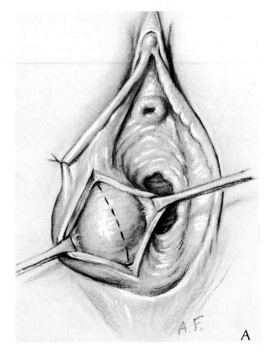
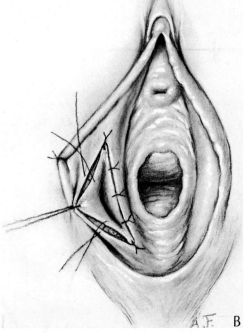

Figure 39–9. *A*, Incision for marsupialization. *B*, Marsupialization. (From Tancer ML, Rosenberg M, Fernandez D. Cysts of the vulvovaginal [Bartholin's] gland. Obstet Gynecol 1956; 7:609)

comparable to marsupialization, its use should be encouraged.

Minor Vestibular Glands

Numerous minor glands encircle the vaginal outlet immediately outside the hymenal ring, located superficially in comparison to the Bartholin or the major vestibular glands. Nonspecific infection in the small vestibular glands, termed vestibular adenitis or vestibulitis, produces constriction of the hymen with associated dyspareunia and tenderness to motion or touch (Fig. 39-10A–C). Local procedures, antibiotics, and cortisone have been used unsuccessfully to treat such lesions. Laser therapy usually has resulted in more constriction.

Excision of the hymen along with the adjacent infected glands has produced relief of symptoms in about 75% to 90% of cases. The incision begins at the lower margin of the labia minora, includes the hymen and the 0.5 to 1.0 cm of tissue containing the glands, and proceeds posteriorly toward the anal orifice, where it meets the incision from the opposite side, laterally and medially to the anal outlet. As in a perineoplasty, the

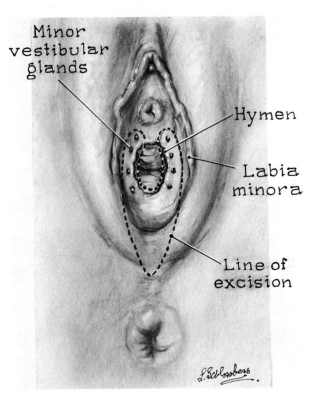

Figure 39–10. The minor vestibular glands exit lateral to the hymenal ring. They are very superficial, and thus seldom produce definable "nodules" even when chronically infected.

vaginal mucosa is undermined and approximated to the skin edges with delayed absorbable suture (see Fig. 39-21). Postoperative treatment also is the same as for perineoplasty. Results are obtained in 2 to 3 months. The contribution of a significant psychologic overlay commonly prevents observation of more definitive results.

Vulvodynia

Vulvodynia refers to chronic vulvar discomfort of which burning is a major component. One expression of this entity, originally termed the "burning vulva syndrome," was investigated by the ISSVD, and gave rise to the newer terminology. Vulvodynia may well represent a confusing group of disparate conditions that affect the introital epithelium, vestibule, and inner labia minora, unified by symptoms of chronic burning, irritation, and dyspareunia. Typically, patients have received numerous topical antiinflammatory, antifungal, and antibacterial agents, prescribed by numerous physicians, for symptoms lasting longer than 6 months.

McKay has defined five subsets of vulvodynia after evaluating 52 patients. These include vulvar dermatoses, cyclic candidiasis, squamous papillomatosis, vulvar vestibulitis, and essential vulvodynia. McKay states that these subsets may not be mutually exclusive, and stresses individualized therapeutic modalities.

Despite claims that lesions of increased papillation present in this region are secondary to HPV, the histologic findings are unimpressive and viral hybridization studies have been negative or inconclusive. Others contend that squamous papillomatosis is a congenital condition. Many such patients have been aggressively treated with laser vaporization. This often has led to no improvement and too frequently to a worsening of local discomfort, coupled with protracted healing.

Vulvodynia remains enigmatic. Certain cases with vestibular gland processes, "vestibulitis," may best be treated by excision, as described above. Careful evaluation should be conducted in each patient to identify a cause of the discomfort, and conservative approaches should be encouraged when diagnostic uncertainty prevails.

Hydrocele or Cyst of the Canal of Nuck

Hydrocele is an uncommon vulvar cyst. The cyst appears as a dilatation in the labium majus and adjacent labium minus, and must be differentiated from a Bartholin's duct cyst. Figure 39-11 shows a hydrocele. The patient had received two procedures for drainage of Bartholin's duct cysts, but the mass recurred after each procedure.

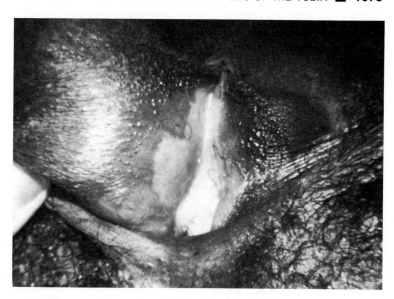

Figure 39–11. A hydrocele is caused by the extension of a peritoneal sac with the round ligament from the inguinal canal into the vulva.

The hydrocele is a dilatation of the peritoneum that accompanies the round ligament and extends from the inguinal canal into the vulva. Dilatation in the inguinal canal is known as a cyst of the canal of Nuck. Because the peritoneum may remain in the inguinal canal without close attachment to the round ligament, fluid may accumulate in this peritoneal sac. On rare occasions a loop of intestine may follow the pathway of the round ligament, forming a hernia in the vulva. When a hydrocele is treated as a Bartholin's duct cyst, peritoneal fluid reaccumulates and the hydrocele recurs.

Surgical treatment for a hydrocele begins with an incision into the mass. The external inguinal ring is identified by inserting a finger along the round ligament to the inguinal canal. The peritoneal lining is then excised from the cyst cavity, and the external inguinal ring is closed along with the subjacent tissue in the vulva. If a hernia is present, inguinal herniorrhaphy should be performed along with excision of the peritoneal covering of the round ligament.

SOLID TUMORS

Fibromas, fibromyomas, and lipomas seldom affect the vulva, although combinations of these elements frequently appear as mesodermal tumors, originating in the fibromusculature of the vulvar area, in the round ligament, or in the fatty tissues of the labia majora. Hyaline degeneration often occurs with the larger fibromyomas. Lipomas often are mistaken for cystic lesions because of their consistency, whereas hernias and hydrocele of the canal of Nuck must be differentiated from tumors because they require different surgical approaches.

Most solid tumors should be excised, both to ascertain diagnosis and to relieve the patient's discomfort. Small pedunculated tumors can be removed by simple ligation of the stalk; the more deeply situated lesions require more extensive local dissection.

The boundaries of such mesodermal tumors are difficult to delineate, but most of the tumors are benign. Even recurrence does not signify malignant alteration; the fibromyoma may recur even when the original specimen had no histologic evidence of malignancy. Although a fibrosarcoma rarely may arise in the vulva, histologic studies must be carefully made because the lesion can be confused with a tumor caused by degenerating multinucleate cells.

As in any vulvar surgery, hemostasis is important, since compression is difficult to obtain in these soft tissues. Extravasation of blood can dissect the fascial planes well out to the abdominal wall.

Sarcoma

Vulva sarcomas constitute a diverse group of lesions unified by their relative rarity, accounting for less than 1% of primary neoplasms at this site. Patients afflicted with sarcomas range in age from prepuberty to senescence; however, typically they are considerably younger than those with epithelial vulvar neoplasms. In a collected series of 17 patients reported by McLellan and colleagues from the authors' clinic, the mean age was 34. Most presented with a mass as the leading complaint. Histopathology disclosed a number of entities, although leiomyosarcoma was the most frequently seen pattern. In the authors' series leiomyosarcomas accounted for 40%. Embryonal rhabdomyosarcomas represented nearly 30%, and were noted among the youngest patients (Fig. 39-12).

Treatment for vulvar sarcomas has not been uniform. Surgery has been the primary approach. Most patients have undergone vulvectomy; however, inguinal node dissections are not a consistent feature. Wide radical excision should be emphasized as the key feature in surgical therapy. Groin dissections do not necessarily confer survival benefit. Embryonal sarcomas should ostensibly receive consideration of adjuvant multiagent chemotherapy. Survivorship appears to be related to tumor histology and grade, tumor volume, and stage at presentation. Statements about appropriate therapy must be tempered by the relative rarity of such lesions and their propensity for hematogenous dissemination.

Condyloma Acuminatum

Condyloma acuminatum is one morphologic manifestation of HPV infection in the lower genital tract. These lesions have an incubation period ranging from several weeks to 8 months; however, clinical infection usually is apparent in 3 months. Transmission of the virus is attributed to coitus, and the process is efficient, as most sexual partners are affected. The disease process is clearly increasing in prevalence; between 1966 and 1984 Becker and coworkers reported an increase in private office consultations in the United States by 670%. Interestingly, clinically apparent condylomas may constitute only a fraction of HPV infections, with the majority left undetected without application of DNA probes for the virus in asymptomatic patients. Such hybridation technology, which became readily available in the 1980s, has identified 57 related HPV types. Among these, a dozen have a predilection to infect the genital tract. The HPV genome in all types is a double-stranded DNA molecule with about 8000 base pairs.

HPV genome types 6, 11, 16, 18, and 31 account for most genital tract infections. Careful histopathologic and virologic study of vulvar lesions has demonstrated an association of HPV-6 and HPV-11 with the majority of exophytic condylomas, as well as flat cervical condylomas and low-grade cervical dysplasias. HPV-16 and HPV-18 infrequently are identified in benign lesions: Reid and associates demonstrated that these are the typical viral types found in association with high-grade dysplasia and invasive carcinomas. From the authors' clinic Buscema, Naghashfar, Sawada, and others recently reported a study of vulvar lesions including condylomas, VIN, and invasive cancers. HPV-16 was identified in 12% of condylomas and 81% of VIN III; this study supported the concept of HPV-16 as the dominant oncogenic virus in vulvar neoplasms.

Condylomata acuminata that manifest on the vulva also may be associated with cervical, vaginal, and perianal HPV infection. Careful clinical evaluation mandates vaginocervical cytology and colposcopy in patients who present with vulvar warts. This is appropriate not only to exclude cervical and vaginal dysplasia, but also to define the extent of condylomatous involvement and permit appropriate tailoring of regional therapy.

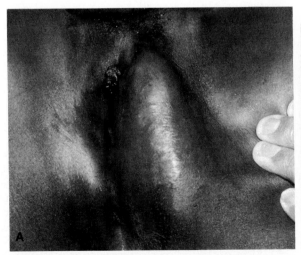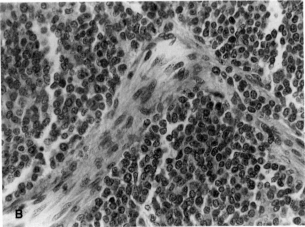

Figure 39–12. *A,* Vulvar sarcoma—gross. Vulvar mass presenting in a 13-year-old. Note absence of epidermal alterations and distortion of left labium majus. *B,* Vulvar sarcoma—microscopic. Originally described as "round cell sarcoma." Electron microscopy demonstrated muscle elements and led to designation as rhabdomyosarcoma. Patient died of metastatic disease in 9 months despite multiagent chemotherapy. (× 350)

Warts initially may be reddish-brown because of parakeratosis; however, with time and exposure to local trauma, they become gray or white. The latter appears to be associated with hyperkeratosis and the generalized keratin disturbance associated with viral infection (Fig. 39-13).

Condylomata acuminata are small and usually multifocal lesions. They may be attended by pruritic discomfort or irritation. Unless traumatized, bleeding is not a typical feature. In pregnancy, however, owing to marked vascular alterations, condylomas of the vagina and perineum can be a source of abundant bleeding if laceration occurs. Massive vulvar and perianal condylomata may occur in certain circumstances, preventing identification of the introitus and anal orifice; conditions that foster this growth potential include immunosuppression and, less frequently, pregnancy (Fig. 39-14).

Various treatment approaches are available to the clinician, and are characterized by their inability to eliminate the offending agent, the virus. Perhaps only 5-fluorouracil and interferon afford specific antiviral therapy (see below). Decisions to use certain ablative approaches should be individualized with consideration of prior treatment, volume and location of disease, the presence or absence of associated dysplasia, and other idiosyncratic patient factors.

The most common approach to vulvar condylomata is local application of 25% podophyllin resin, often prepared in benzoin. This method, although reasonably well tolerated in the office setting, often requires numerous applications. Burning discomfort ensues after sustained contact, which is necessary for efficacy. Most recommend that the agent be left in place for 6 hours before tub baths, so compliance may be problematic. Podophyllin appears to be more effective on exophytic, rather than flat, condylomata. Use is restricted to the vulva in nonpregnant patients; vaginal application may lead to undesirable absorption and neurotoxicity. An alternative is halogenated acetic acid, either bichloroacetic or trichloroacetic (TCA). The authors' preference is for 90% TCA. This agent rapidly interacts with cellular proteins, inducing a coagulative effect, and rapidly turns lesions white. Advantages include the ability to sustain a prompt chemical effect on the condyloma, its availability for intravaginal use as well as during pregnancy, and the potential to rapidly neutralize the acid with sodium bicarbonate, which may be dissolved in water and applied as a cooling paste.

Surgical excision, destruction, or ablation are reserved for certain patients. Criteria for selection may include the following: (a) extensive volume of condylomas exceeding what may be resolved with chemi-

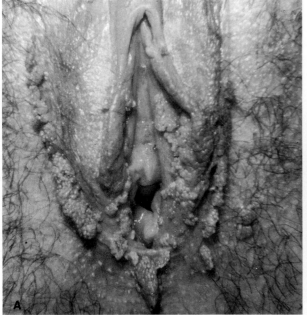
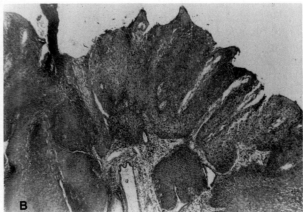

Figure 39–13. *A*, Condylomata acuminata—gross. Condylomata acuminata involving labia majora and minora. Note exophytic quality and lack of pigmentation. *B*, Condylomata acuminata—microscopic. Epidermal hyperplasia featuring acanthosis and elongated, distorted rete pegs is evident. Keratin disturbances present. (×225)

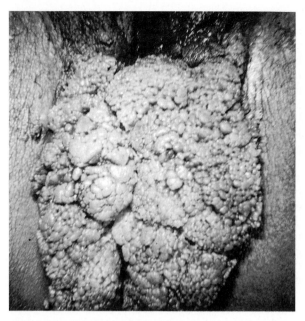

Figure 39–14. Massive condylomata acuminata. Note abundant exophytic lesions producing confluent, cauliflowerlike growth. Lesion is present on perineum and totally obscures anal orifice. Patient is 23 years old and maintained on prednisone because of neurosarcoidosis.

cal agents; (b) multicentric HPV infections, particularly with involvement of the vagina, urethra, or anus; (c) failure of concerted office therapy with topical chemical agents; (d) presence of significant associated intraepithelial neoplasia; and (e) some immunocompromised hosts. One should certainly liberally use biopsy to evaluate presumed condylomas that are refractory to topical treatment or that have an atypical appearance. This will help to prevent sustained, ineffective chemical treatment of high-grade VIN, often presenting as a flat and pigmented verrucous lesion in the younger patient, and to exclude a frank tumor with warty features.

Cryotherapy has been used on the vulva to eradicate warts. The freezing induces localized tissue necrosis. Although healing usually is satisfactory, and numbing effects induce analgesia, application is limited by delivery systems and probe-tip sizes. Larger condylomatous masses are more difficult to treat, as are vaginal lesions. Depth of apparent tissue destruction can be difficult to assess.

Electrocautery with a loop has been used effectively, particularly with massive lesions. Analgesic needs are definitely a factor in this approach. Smaller lesions may be fulgurated. Buildup of charred tissue can be removed by abrasion to identify residual warty tissue. Precision and depth of tissue injury can be problematic.

Colposcopically directed laser ablation in appropriately selected cases and performed by trained personnel may afford effective treatment. Smaller condylomatous lesions may be vaporized; starting at the center of the lesion causes the wart to collapse inward toward the beam. The level of the adjacent normal skin should be selected as a landmark. In treating condylomata there is no need for deep laser vaporization into the dermis, exceeding the so-called first laser surgical plane. Issues of appropriate power density may be debated; however, the inexperienced laser surgeon will need to use lower power densities (larger spot size or lower laser output) to protect against unnecessarily deep laser injury. In experienced hands higher laser output may be feasible, which speeds the procedure. Power densities of 500 to 800 W/cm^2 normally are used for vaporization. Lower power densities are associated with undesirable thermal injury to adjacent tissues. Sites of laser vaporization should be wiped with moistened gauze sponges to remove carbon and thermally coagulated tissue and to permit accurate assessment of depth and remaining disease. Large lesions may be dealt with by combined excision using the laser followed by vaporization at the base (see Ch. 21).

Brush laser vaporization of the normal epithelium surrounding warty lesions usually has been adopted. This technique uses lower power densities (200 to 300 W/cm^2) to superficially denude 1 to 2 cm of adjacent epidermis. The rationale for this approach is the presence of HPV in tissue proximal to the condyloma, demonstrated by Ferenczy and colleagues. Brush vaporization and laser treatment of so-called subclinical HPV infection that may be appreciated with the colposcope has been proposed to lessen viral reservoir and reduce recurrence rates.

Nevertheless, recurrences must be anticipated in 25% to 50% of patients with extensive disease treated with the laser, particularly if immunocompromise is operative. These patients require further treatment with either laser or chemical approaches such as 5-fluorouracil topically.

Patients subjected to extensive laser treatment require considerable local care until healing proceeds. Cool tub or sitz baths with Burow's solution followed by application of silver sulfadiazine (Silvadene) cream often afford relief and protect against bacterial superinfection. Narcotics for pain management are appropriate short term. Systemic antibiotics do not appear to be indicated prophylactically. Office follow-up weekly is advised for 2 to 3 weeks to assess tissue healing, prevent undesirable areas of tissue agglutination, and allow potential early identification of recurrences, which may be managed with chemical ablation. Patients should be followed carefully for several months after treatment, to monitor for recurrences.

Topical application of 5-fluorouracil cream (Efudex 5%) has been used to treat warts. The agent offers a more specific antiviral therapy by interfering with HPV DNA and RNA polymerases. Although effective for vaginal condylomata and dysplasia, intense burning of the vulvar epithelium may ensue, which, understandably, lessens compliance.

Natural interferon alfa, derived from leukocytes, has been used intralesionally for refractory condylomas, as reported by Friedman-Kien and coworkers. Studies have cited use two to three times weekly, and flulike effects should be anticipated for at least several weeks. Efficacy has been demonstrated with this technique, although treatment is cumbersome, can be costly, and remains investigational. Its primary role has not been defined but may be refractory HPV infection.

Regardless of selected approaches to therapy, all patients should be advised to have their consorts examined to lessen risk of reexposure to lesions with a large viral burden. This theoretically will help to diminish treatment failures.

Hidradenoma (Sweat Gland Tumor) of the Vulva

A rare benign tumor of the vulva, hidradenoma was first described by Schickele in 1902. The tumor is characterized by its intricate papillary adenomatous pattern, which may be readily mistaken for cancer.

Clinically, a hidradenoma is small, rarely more than 1 cm in diameter (Fig. 39-15A). Its consistency can range from firm to as soft as a sebaceous cyst, with which it often is confused. Most of these lesions are found in the interlabial folds, in the labia majora, or in the perineum. Because these tumors are apocrine in origin, labia minora location is unusual. The occasional occurrence of reddish-brown pulpy material on the surface results when the tumor is evulsed through the duct of the gland.

These lesions have been carefully studied in numerous laboratories, and the complex microscopic patterns have been repeatedly stressed (Fig. 39-15B). The superficial papillary adenomatous pattern appears aggressive, but careful inspection shows that the glandular structures are lined by a single layer of well-organized cuboidal cells. In some parts of the tumor the pink-staining secretory elements can be identified superficial to the basal layer. Beneath the epithelium is an indefinite layer of flattened myoepithelial cells. When the clear cell variant of the myoepithelium proliferates, an ominous picture is created, yet this clear cell hidradenoma also behaves in a benign manner. Although occasionally hidradenocarcinoma does occur, a finding of distinct adenocarcinoma in the vulva probably indicates a metastatic lesion, most commonly from the endometrium.

Hidradenomas are classically asymptomatic, and most lesions are discovered during a routine pelvic examination. Curative treatment consists of local excision; recurrences only result from incomplete excision.

Hemangioma

Hemangiomas are common vulvar lesions that usually do not require treatment. The lesions normally are small, often multiple, and may bleed with trauma. On occasion keratinization causes the superficial surface to appear white or gray-white (angiokeratoma). Hemangiomas should be differentiated from small varicosities, which commonly are seen in the postmenopausal patient.

An accurate diagnosis is imperative because a malignant melanoma may be misinterpreted as a hemangioma. The abrupt appearance of any pigmented lesion demands biopsy. In 2 of 11 melanomas seen in our clinic the lesions were diagnosed as hematoma or angioma, and a correct diagnosis was provided only by histologic study (Fig. 39-16).

The best treatment for congenital hemangioma is careful observation. The lesions regress spontaneously in almost all cases, and attempts at excision may be mutilating. If bleeding is a problem, the troublesome vascular channels may be treated by surgical ligation.

Granular Cell Myoblastoma (Schwannoma)

Granular cell myoblastoma is an uncommon lesion that presents two major problems for the clinician and surgeon: its gross appearance is nondescript, and its diagnosis is seldom made preoperatively. During the excisional process most surgeons realize that the tumor is not localized and that because it has spread into the underlying tissues, total removal may not be possible. Although the tumor may recur, it usually is benign. Further excision is unnecessary unless a subsequent mass develops, suggesting increased growth.

Sometimes the overlying pseudoepitheliomatous changes are misinterpreted as carcinoma in situ (CIS) or early invasive cancer (Fig. 39-17). Identification is possible with recognition of the granular cells dispersed within the underlying stroma of the tumor. The epithelial atypicality results because the "myoblasts" are actually cells arising from the nerve sheath (thus the more correct term *schwannoma*). In a few patients granular cell myoblastoma has been reported to be malignant, but the appearance of a second lesion at a site outside the vulva usually indicates multiple disease processes, not metastasis.

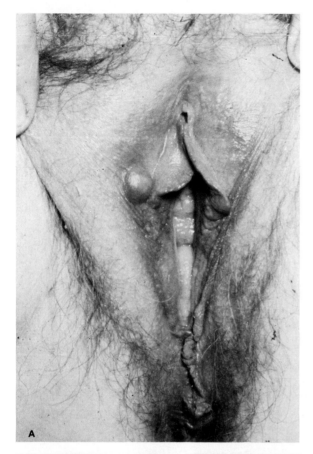

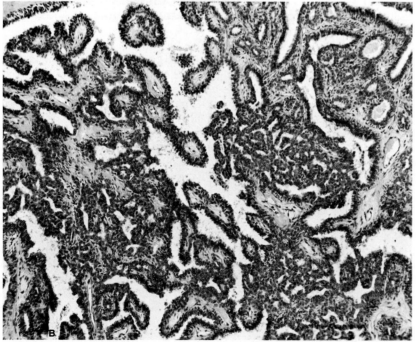

Figure 39–15. *A*, Hidradenoma of the vulva. *B*, Low-power magnification section of hidradenoma of the vulva. (*A*, from Novak E, Woodruff JD. Obstetric and gynecologic pathology. 7th ed. Philadelphia: WB Saunders, 1974)

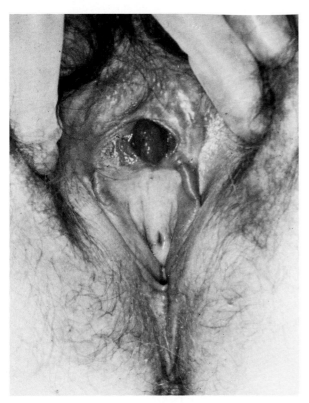

Figure 39–16. Hemangioma of the clitoris misdiagnosed grossly as melanoma.

VARICOCELE AND VARICES

Varices are common on the vulva, and the larger lesions are almost routinely unilateral. As with most varicosities, treatment depends on size and symptoms. Whereas varicoceles in the scrotum arise from dilatation of the veins in the pampiniform plexus of the inguinal canal, the lesions on the vulva are related to the pudendal veins (Fig. 39-18). Careful evaluation usually demonstrates more extensive involvement of the tributaries of the hypogastric vein, with varicosities of the gluteal vessels over the buttock.

If the patient experiences discomfort from the engorgement that follows exercise or standing for long periods, ligation is indicated with excision of the segment of vulvar skin that contains the varices. Knowledge of the intricate vascular system that supplies the external genitalia is necessary to ensure that surgery will result in long-term success and would prevent recurrences.

WHITE LESIONS OF THE VULVA

The terms *kraurosis* and *leukoplakia* suffer from overuse. In 1877 Schwimmer reported that leukoplakia

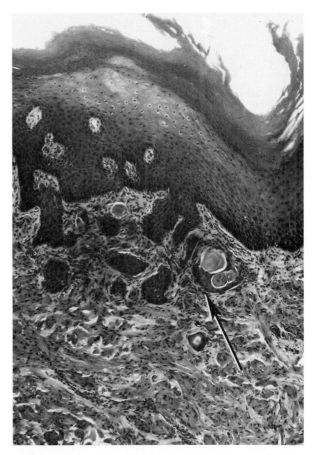

Figure 39–17. Granular cell myoblastoma. Note the pseudoepitheliomatous hyperplasia, nests of large, pale "myoblasts" beneath the epithelium.

on the buccal surfaces of the mouth was a premalignant lesion, and Beisky later described kraurosis as an atrophic lesion similar to lichen sclerosus. Because of these early reports, every lesion on the vulva that appeared white and constricted the vaginal outlet was called kraurosis. Moreover, conditions as varied as leukoderma and invasive cancer have been called leukoplakia. Other terms, such as *primary senile atrophy* and *atrophic leukoplakia,* are used interchangeably and should be eliminated.

Although some physicians have suggested that they have different histopathologies, the microscopic appearance of lichen sclerosus and kraurosis is similar. A safe approach would be for surgeons to describe the anatomic appearance (ie, whether the vulva is shrunken and constricted or thickened and leathery), leaving the pathologist, who is familiar with both histology and anatomy, to define the cellular abnormalities.

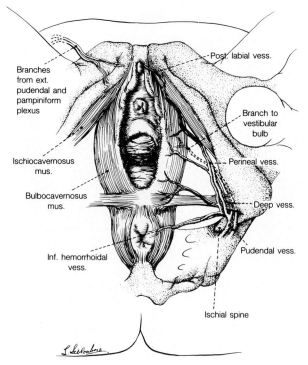

Figure 39–18. Vascular supply of the vulva.

Depigmentation Lesions

Leukoderma and *vitiligo* are terms that are used interchangeably. Treatment is not required unless the symptoms of the commonly associated chronic dermatitis cannot be controlled by local medications. The hyperkeratotic lesions comprise a number of diverse entities that share a white to grayish white appearance in a moist environment. Biopsy is the only reliable criterion for accurate assessment.

The most adequate biopsy instrument is the dermatologic, or Keyes, punch. This simple procedure can be performed under local anesthesia, directed to the most suspicious area, and allows for proper histologic orientation (Fig. 39-19). The 4- or 6-mm instrument allows for the removal of an adequate sample that can be positioned on a filter paper or a small fragment of cucumber so that the epithelial surface will lay flat. A full-thickness section can then be more readily prepared, averting tangential cuts.

Hyperkeratosis

Both chronic infections and benign tumors, most commonly condylomata acuminata, appear white because keratin absorbs moisture, which reflects light back to the observer.

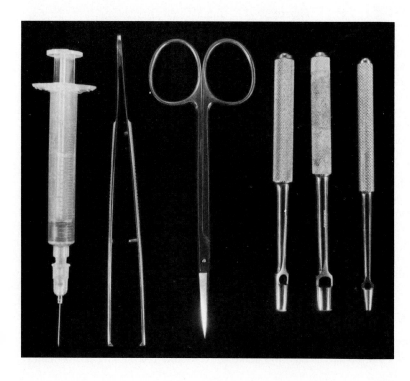

Figure 39–19. Biopsy instruments (dermatologic punch).

To avoid the ambiguous term *leukoplakia,* Jeffcoate, in 1966, introduced the term *dystrophy* into the nomenclature of benign epithelial lesions of the vulva. Predictions about the malignant potential of vulvar dystrophy vary, but of all types of dystrophy, the one most often benign is lichen sclerosus. As noted above, the terminology for "vulvar dystrophies" has been altered.

Lichen sclerosus is characterized by hyperkeratosis, thinning of the epidermis, loss of rete peg architecture, homogenization of the underlying tissue, and associated inflammatory infiltrate dispersed throughout the dermis (Fig. 39-20).

Typical hyperplasia (hyperplastic dystrophy) is characterized by a thickened epithelium, elongated rete pegs, and infiltration of the underlying tissue with chronic inflammatory cells. Practically, typical hyperplasia is a benign form of chronic dermatitis with hyperkeratosis and acanthosis; thus the designation "dystrophy" should be eliminated.

In contrast to typical hyperplasia, atypical hyperplasia is largely related to prolonged, chronic irritation. There is cellular atypia characterized by abnormal maturation in the acanthotic epithelium. The most important feature is the very mature, abnormally keratinized cells in the basal layer of the epithelium. The significance of this alteration is demonstrated in the histopathologic study of invasive cancer. It has been repeatedly noted that atypical keratinization, not mitotic activity, is the most classic histologic feature adjacent to cancer.

Clinical Features, Diagnosis, and Treatment

Lichen sclerosus may occur at any age. The disease has been noted in the prepubertal child, and it also occurs during the menstrual years. Nevertheless, it most frequently is seen in the postmenopausal era, when the lesions more commonly are symptomatic, perhaps owing to the additional epithelial compromise caused by atrophy. The genetic aspects of lichen sclerosus have not been clearly identified, but the finding of the lesions in mother and child has been clearly documented.

If biopsies reveal lichen sclerosus, testosterone ointment (2%), topically applied, is the most successful agent in improving the nutrition of the dermis, thicken-

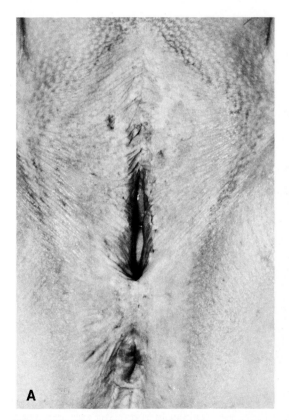

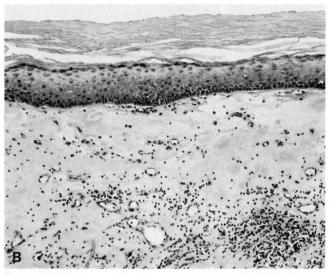

Figure 39–20. Vulvar dystrophy. *A,* Distorted vulva with superficial ulcerations and extensive hyperkeratosis and loss of normal architecture. *B,* Microscopic picture of lichen sclerosus.

ing the epithelium, and alleviating the symptomatology. More potent preparations (5%) seldom are indicated. Nevertheless, testosterone should not be used if there is an associated phimosis. Enlargement of the clitoris occurs in about 20% to 25% of patients who receive the topical agent; if the clitoris is covered by the prepuce, paraphimosis will occur and the patient subsequently will have major local discomfort. Under these circumstances a 2% progesterone preparation will alleviate the symptoms in most cases and will not be accompanied by the paraphimosis. If the latter does occur, a circumcision may be necessary. If such is contemplated, it should be appreciated that the incision should not be made to the base of the clitoris; a small cuff of skin should be maintained at the clitoral base so that the adjacent skin after circumcision may be approximated without tension to this base. Finally, neither testosterone nor progesterone will eliminate the pruritus, and thus the patient should be given a topical cortisone preparation; in our opinion, fluorinated corticosteroids are preferable for control of itching. These agents

should not be mixed with testosterone or progesterone, since the latter must be continued over a long period, whereas the fluorinated corticosteroid should be used only for pruritus, not on a routine basis.

Many patients with chronic vulvar dermatitis, stenosis of the outlet specifically related to lichen sclerosus, or vestibular adenitis have an associated constriction of the vaginal outlet with resultant dyspareunia. Local intravaginal or vulvar applications of estrogen do not improve this condition, although every conservative effort should be made before any surgical approach.

Plastic surgery to the outlet (Fig. 39-21) may be helpful. By excising a triangular area of skin beneath the fourchette, the surgeon can undermine and evert the adjacent vaginal epithelium, incise the transverse perineal muscle and fascia, and cover the denuded area with a flap of vaginal mucosa. Although the suture line often lies at the anal orifice, postoperative retraction will eliminate any difficulty that might accrue from scarring near the anal orifice. The procedure is simple, and the use of delayed absorbable suture material lessens the

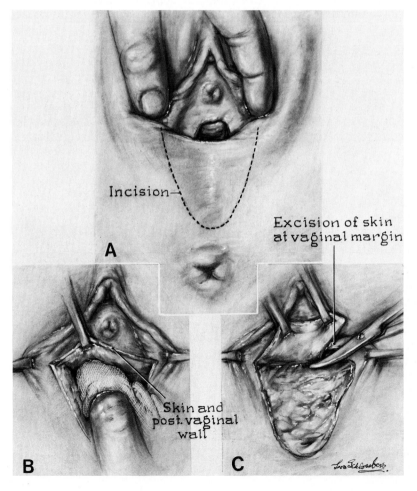

Figure 39–21. Perineoplasty. *A*, The incisional line is identified. The incision must be sufficiently extensive to allow for postoperative retraction and subsequent constriction of the outlet. *B*, The vagina is undermined to allow for exteriorization without tension. *C*, The scarred skin of the fourchette is excised. The vaginal epithelium is preserved for exteriorization.

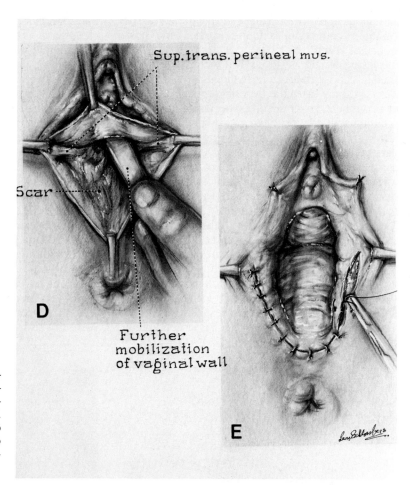

Sup. trans. perineal mus.

Scar

D

Further
mobilization
of vaginal wall

E

Figure 39–21. (continued) *D*, The vaginal epithelium is sufficiently undermined for the margins to be approximated to the skin (*E*) without tension. Occasionally a small incision is made into the midline of the exteriorized mucosa to allow for an adequate outlet without tension.

incidence of wound breakdown, which commonly occurs when absorbable suture is used. The results of this procedure have been most satisfactory; about 95% of patients are greatly relieved of dyspareunia.

PAGET'S DISEASE

The lesion originally described by Sir James Paget in 1874 has been a cause of confusion and controversy over the years, but particularly in the past few decades. The disease most commonly is described as an eczematous lesion of the areola that reflects an underlying neoplasm in the ductile system. Many have considered the alterations in the vulvar skin to represent an invasion of the epithelium by cells from the underlying neoplasm in the ductile system. Recent studies of vulvar Paget's disease, as well as those of the breast, indicate that there are two forms of the neoplasm: an intraepithelial and an invasive variety. Although some cases undoubtedly are associated with an underlying apo-

crine adenocarcinoma, the invasive characteristics of Paget's disease more commonly are demonstrated by foci of neoplastic cells directly invading from the basal layer, as in most skin neoplasms. The invading epithelial nests contain not only the Paget's, but also the basal cells; the invasive and metastatic foci similarly contain both cellular elements.

In more than 70% of the cases the vulvar disease is representative of in situ neoplasia and tends to remain so even though the local disease may recur frequently. One patient in our clinic had 10 local excisions of recurrences over a period of 23 years, without invasive neoplasia. Even though the appendages, particularly the hair follicles, usually are involved, the lesions are still representative of in situ neoplasia, and the survival rate is unchanged. Electron microscopic studies have confirmed that Paget's tumor is of apocrine origin, substantiating the clinical features of the lesion.

The primary symptoms of extramammary Paget's disease are itching and burning, although some patients have discomfort and some even recognize asymptomatic alterations in the color of the external genitalia. The lesion most commonly is found in the early postmenopausal years.

The lesion usually is velvety red with dotted white epithelial islands that are grossly suggestive of CIS (Fig. 39-22A). In some cases the hyperkeratotic foci are the most prominent gross feature. The lesion seldom is well circumscribed, and often can involve both labia majora without being grossly apparent. Multiple biopsies are mandatory to exclude the presence of invasive disease. Because the basic treatment of Paget's disease is conservative vulvectomy, the final opinion can be made only after careful examination of many representative sections from the most grossly involved areas.

The Paget's cell is identified with the use of special histochemical studies. The cell reacts positively with the mucicarmine stain, in contrast to the elements of the junctional nevus. Periodic acid–Shiff stains also are positive. Attempts to determine histologic differences between the invasive and the in situ form of the neoplasm have not provided definite results to date.

Histologically, the vulvar Paget's cell is large, contain-ing abundant, almost clear cytoplasm and a pale nucleus with a prominent nucleolus (Fig. 39-22B). This cell originally appears in the basal layer of the epithelium, although the basal cells themselves are intact and simply distorted by the presence of the Paget's cell. Metabolic studies have shown that the epithelium surrounding the Paget's cell is more active than the Paget's cell. Even the most superficial layers of epithelium and the appendages, particularly the hair follicle, are involved in 75% to 90% of cases.

Vulvectomy is justified if the lesions are multicentric or if the entire lesion is too extensive to be evaluated by biopsy. It is necessary to exclude, as thoroughly as possible, the rarely encountered underlying carcinoma. Because the tumor is of apocrine origin, the gland-bearing areas have to be removed to eliminate the commonly involved appendages. Frozen section diagnosis may be used to assess surgical margins of excision, as Paget cell alterations identifiable histologically often exceed the recognized limits of the gross lesion. A recent study by Bergen and associates confirms this and supports the use of intraoperative frozen

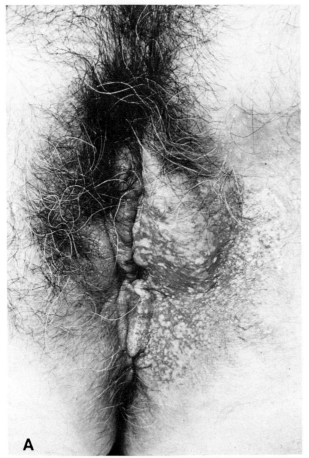

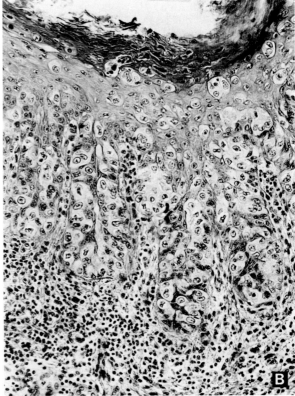

Figure 39–22. Paget's disease of the vulva. *A,* Gross appearance. *B,* Microscopic appearance: note the large, clear apocrine cells.

section assessment, especially in the setting of conservative surgery. Nevertheless, local recurrences may be seen despite histologically clear margins. Friedrich and Wilkinson have reported instances of frequent local recurrences and associated breast neoplasia, an important relation to understand during follow-up of the patient with Paget's disease.

If the lesion is invasive, radical vulvectomy and groin dissection should be performed. Although the prognosis is poor for the patient with invasive disease, by adding radiation therapy, two of seven patients in our clinic survived, one for more than 5 years without evidence of recurrence. In the treatment of recurrent in situ neoplasia topical 5-fluorouracil has not been used satisfactorily in our experience, although Fetherston and Friedrich have reported some initial favorable results. Watring and colleagues have used topical bleomycin. Reexcision and laser vaporization are the preferred treatments; in 20 years of experience none of the lesions that were originally in situ have progressed to invasive cancer.

CARCINOMA IN SITU

The first two cases of CIS of the skin were described by Bowen in 1912. Bowen also stated that although stromal invasion had not developed in patients observed over periods of 12 to 16 years, curettage and cauterization did not eliminate recurrence of the lesions. Since that time the name *Bowen's disease* has been used to describe a clinically indolent, intraepithelial lesion that seldom, if ever, progresses to invasive cancer. In the past Bowen's in situ neoplasm was considered to be extremely uncommon in the vulva. In 1943 Knight reported 6 patients from his experience along with another 26 he had collected from the literature. In several of the cases Knight described the in situ changes occurred next to invasive cancer. Other isolated examples of these uncommon neoplasms have been reported by DeLima, Peterson, Robinson, and Gardner.

In 1958 Woodruff and Hildebrandt reported 13 cases of vulvar intraepithelial neoplasia and suggested that since the histology varied from one area to another in the same section, the general term *carcinoma in situ* should be used to designate the lesion if certain microscopic criteria were fulfilled. Although the concept was not accepted wholeheartedly, clinicians are now recognizing the importance of the lesion and treating each case on an individual basis.

An increase in the incidence of CIS was noted by Woodruff and associates in 1973. Whereas only 13 cases of CIS were recorded in 1958, at the authors' clinic, representing less than 20% of all vulvar neoplasia, the current incidence of vulvar CIS has markedly surpassed that of invasive cancer. These increases could be artificial, stemming from heightened awareness of pathologists. More likely the upward trend is due to an increased incidence of the disease process and appears to be associated with a regional phenomenon often involving the cervix, vulva, and vagina. This concept is tenable and perhaps best explained by postulating that these increases are related to viral proliferative activity in the lower genital tract. HPV has certainly been the viral agent most often implicated. Recent research studies have depicted HPV-16 as the predominant papillomavirus operative here, found recently in 81% of VIN III lesions in the authors' clinic.

Epidemiology

Age. Previous studies suggested that most patients with in situ vulvar neoplasia were in the early sixth decade of life. Recent investigations have uncovered a much younger age group at risk, so that the disease occasionally affects a patient in the early third decade of life, and the average age is in the mid–fourth decade.

Race. In situ vulvar lesions occur in all racial groups; Charleswood and Shippel recorded cases in Bantu women. Nevertheless, good epidemiologic studies have not been carried out, possibly because of a paucity of material.

Parity. Parity does not seem to play a role in the development of CIS of the vulva; both nulliparous and multiparous patients are susceptible to local irritants that may promote the disease.

Clinical Features

Symptoms. Pruritus is the predominant symptom of most vulvar disease, including cancer, yet itching was the primary symptom in only 50% of patients with in situ cancer in a series reported by Buscema, Woodruff, Parmley, and associates. Other presenting complaints were the presence of a lump, bleeding, and pain. In a small percentage of the cases the lesion was discovered on routine examination, but in others diagnosis commonly was made in patients seen in follow-up of cervical neoplasia.

Diagnosis. The best technique for early diagnosis is careful inspection of the external genitalia under a bright light, and if suspicion is aroused either by history of preexisting neoplasia in the lower genital canal or by the suggestion of an abnormal configuration, magnification should be used. An experienced colposcopist can describe white lesions and areas of abnormal vasculature, but as a screening procedure, colposcopy has not

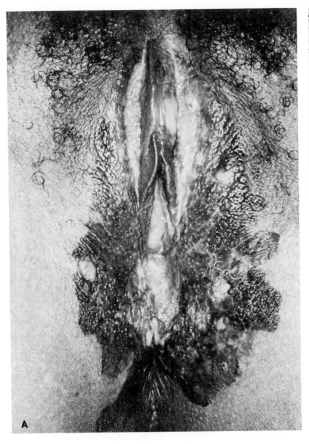

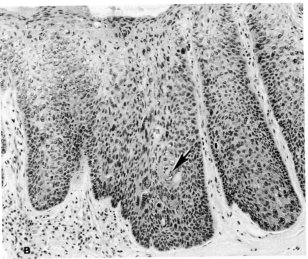

Figure 39–23. *A,* Carcinoma in situ of vulva showing multiple patterns, particularly atypical pigmentation. *B,* Carcinoma in situ of the vulva. There is full-thickness alteration in the architecture with elongation and distortion of the rete pegs. At *arrow,* there is intraepithelial pearl formation. (× 160)

contributed to the early detection of vulvar neoplasia. The use of nuclear staining, specifically 1% toluidine blue and tetracycline fluorescence, has delineated foci of increased metabolic activity, but the false-negative and false-positive rates are high enough to make the results unpredictable.

Careful visual evaluation of the vulvar region should be directed at the focally white, hyperkeratotic areas, and at the more important, slightly elevated areas of skin. Atypical pigmentation, most significantly associated with gray-white areas that are even minimally ulcerated or slightly elevated above the surrounding skin, should be viewed with suspicion (Fig. 39-23A). Biopsy provides the final diagnosis.

Microscopic Features

Biopsy with a Keyes (dermatologic) punch can be performed in the office using local anesthesia. Knife biopsies often are tangential and contain only the superficial layers, not allowing for the most accurate histo-

logic interpretation. Correct orientation of the tissue in the fixative is mandatory if accurate evaluation of the specimen is to be rendered. Such orientation may be obtained by placing the biopsy on filter paper and toweling with the epithelial surface exposed, so that the pathologist may embed the specimen accurately. Tangential cutting may result in the erroneous diagnosis of invasive disease.

Cytology has not proved to be a satisfactory screening technique in the evaluation of the precursory cellular atypias in vulvar neoplasia. Suspicious lesions can be sampled by scraping with a saline-moistened applicator to screen for microscopic aberrations. The classic bowenoid changes vary from one microscopic section to another, but typical sections show individual cell keratinization, corps ronds, nuclear graining, and clumping. Other gross variations include the erythroblastic lesion (erythroplasia of Queyrat) with immature cells extending from base to surface (Fig. 39-23B) and lesions that appear almost normal, being marked only by intraepithelial pearl formation at the rete tips (marked atypical hyperplasia) and appearing in the older age group.

Multicentricity

Multifocal areas of neoplasia that involve the external genitalia and the epithelium of the lower genital canal are common; in fact more than half the patients with intraepithelial disease in the lower genital tract have multifocal lesions, which suggests an infectious, possibly viral origin for the neoplasia. In contrast, patients over age 60 with invasive or in situ cancer more commonly have unifocal disease. When the vulva is the primary site of the lesion, the cervix, vagina, and perianal areas are frequent sites for associated neoplastic alterations. The combination of vulvar and cervical cancer makes up about 20% of all multicentric neoplasia in the lower genital tract.

The most pressing question about multifocal disease is whether invasive disease that develops from in situ lesions will arise in many foci or only in one. Only two of our cases of in situ neoplasia in patients under age 40 have developed invasive cancer, and both cases appeared as solitary perianal lesions. Because the vulva and the cervix are of different embryologic origins, the tendency to correlate the histopathology of one area with that of the other can be hazardous. For example, the full-thickness changes that signal cervical intraepithelial neoplasia are not as serious when they occur on the vulva, but keratinization at the rete tips with marked atypical hyperplasia is the most ominous preinvasive vulvar alteration (see Fig. 39-23A).

Treatment and Results

Although the treatment of in situ vulvar neoplasia is basically surgical, not all patients require total vulvectomy. Except for the patient older than 50 or the patient with Paget's disease, total vulvectomy usually is unnecessary with in situ neoplasia. Wide local excision usually is successful, provided no other foci have been found in the area. The adjacent area can provide sufficient extra skin to cover minor defects. The incidence of recurrence is no greater with local excision than with total vulvectomy, but still approaches 30% to 40%. Thus careful follow-up is mandatory.

A skinning vulvectomy, in which the epidermis and underlying dermis are removed, has been proposed for the treatment of multifocal vulvar in situ disease, but because the recurrence rate is comparable to careful local excision, there is no justification for the procedure. The skinning vulvectomy requires surgery at a donor site, which produces an additional scar in a patient who usually is young. Furthermore, it imposes prolonged bed rest, near complete immobilization of the lower extremities, and indwelling bladder catheterization.

The carbon dioxide laser has been successfully used in treatment of in situ vulvar neoplasia. This approach is of particular appeal in treatment of the younger patient with multifocal, viral proliferative disease. This subset with VIN would undoubtedly be at lower risk for occult invasion. Emphasis in therapy should be directed toward preservation of maximum tissue and vulvar function. Given these considerations and the reality of recurrences, laser ablation provides an effective medium. Pretreatment requirements include liberal use of biopsies to exclude occult invasion and careful examination of the lower genital tract, preferably colposcopically, to define possible multicentric disease.

Bornstein and Kaufman have proposed combining laser ablation with surgical excision in the treatment of selected patients with VIN. Laser is used particularly in areas where excision hampers preservation of anatomy, such as in the clitoral region.

The laser itself is directed colposcopically after examination of tissues prepared by application of dilute acetic acid. The latter may enhance detection of minimal viral changes not readily seen with the naked eye. Although benign condylomata may be adequately treated by superficial vaporization (so-called first and second plane), laser treatment of VIN must address the extension of disease into the hair follicles (pilosebaceous ducts). This mandates deeper laser vaporization beyond the papillary dermis and into the upper reticular dermis (third plane). The colposcope permits recognition of landmarks that characterize these levels. Baggish and coworkers identified skin appendage involvement in 36% of vulvar in situ carcinoma and predicted that laser vaporization to a depth of 2.5 mm would effectively treat involved appendages in 95% of cases. Shatz and associates advocated ablation of VIN to a depth of 1 and 2 mm in nonhairy and hairy skin to achieve similar success.

In laser treatment of VIN, use of appropriate power densities should be emphasized. Low power densities lead to thermal conduction injury in adjacent and underlying normal tissue. The latter increases the risk of scarring. Power densities of greater than 750 W/cm^2 are recommended.

Laser ablation also may be used to treat perianal VIN. In this setting two concerns should be kept in mind. This location appears to be at greater risk for development of invasive squamous cancer, and the likelihood of fibrosis, scarring, and stricture is heightened.

As with all treatments for VIN, the potential of recurrence and the need for further follow-up must be appreciated. With ablative approaches such as laser, diligence must be exercised to exclude invasion.

Topical agents have been used in the treatment of VIN with inconsistent results. Most notable among these topical treatments has been 5-fluorouracil (Efudex 5%).

The mechanism of action appears to be related to inhibition of DNA and RNA synthesis—the latter is not specific to dysplastic or HPV-infected cells. Normal epithelium is susceptible to the agent, and a component of hypersensitivity reaction appears operative in its mode of action. Among young patients with erythroplastic VIN a 50% to 60% complete response rate is observed. The hyperkeratotic VIN lesion has not proved to be as responsive to 5-fluorouracil. In instances where treatment is effective, denudation of the epithelium is a requisite finding. This understandably leads to localized discomfort, often reported as intense burning.

Treatment regimens with topical 5-fluorouracil are diverse, and no standardized administration protocol has been widely adopted, even for intravaginal use. One technique is topical application on an alternate-night basis for as long as 6 weeks; patient compliance problems typically lead to earlier curtailment.

The theoretical benefits of 5-fluorouracil are its adaptability to diffuse areas of skin involvement and possible specific antiviral activity. The latter is an important treatment consideration in the younger patient with viral proliferative lesions, as the agent may prophylax against recurrences.

TECHNIQUE OF CONSERVATIVE (SIMPLE) VULVECTOMY

Conservative (simple) vulvectomy is performed when premalignant lesions, such as granulomatous diseases, do not respond to medical therapy or wide local excision. Other patients who require simple vulvectomy are those with marked atypical hyperplasia who are 60 to 70 years of age; these women are at risk for developing invasive carcinoma. Patients over age 50 with extensive CIN may benefit from such a procedure, as do some patients with Paget's disease of the vulva.

An outline of the surgical margins is made using a coloring agent, such as brilliant green. The initial incision should be made at the vaginal outlet so that the urethral borders can be well demarcated and the vaginal epithelium undermined for a short distance (Fig. 39-24A and B). If the incision is begun at the lateral skin margins, bleeding can mask the area, making the incision at the outlet more difficult to define. When the first incision is at the outlet, a small pack can be placed into the vagina to control the bleeding while the elliptical incision at the outer skin margins of the lesion is made.

The skin incision usually encompasses most of the labia majora, depending on the extent of the lesion. The incision through the skin is made with a knife to avoid tissue necrosis that occurs at the skin margins when an electrosurgical instrument is used. Minor vessels can be coagulated.

Major bleeding concerns may arise at the clitoris, particularly from the dorsal vein. Hemostatic sutures must be used to control the bleeding. A second point of concern are the pudendal vessels, which enter at the lower one-third of the vulva, about at the opening of the Bartholin's duct. Branches of the pudendal vessels extend down to the anus as the external hemorrhoidals, and bleeding may be rather profuse in this area (see Fig. 39-18).

Because the lesions for which conservative vulvectomy is performed are superficial, dissection need not extend down to the deep fascia or to the muscles of the urogenital diaphragm. Although it is unnecessary to remove the bulbocavernosus and ischiocavernosus muscles, they may be difficult to avoid when the vulva is quite atrophic.

Removal of some of the adipose tissue, particularly in the obese patient, allows for better approximation of the skin edge to the vaginal mucosa. The incision may be carried almost to the anal orifice; careful dissection here is important, so that the external anal sphincter is not damaged. If the disease extends onto the anal mucosa or protruding hemorrhoidal tissue, the mucosa should first be carefully dissected from the underlying external sphincter and then excised with the tumor-free margins and sutured to the perianal skin with No. 3-0 delayed absorbable suture. When hemostasis is achieved the underlying tissues are approximated with No. 2-0 delayed absorbable suture and the skin edges with No. 0 suture (Fig. 39-24C). With the use of No. 0 suture material troublesome tissue breakdown is avoided, particularly in the area around the anal orifice, because the No. 0 suture usually resorbs slowly for a month or more. If bleeding is a problem, a small drain may be placed at the lower end of the incision, but it is better to achieve meticulous hemostasis and then use a firm pack against the area for 24 hours.

In the closure of the perineal defect above the anal orifice, it is important to evert the vaginal epithelium over the perineum in approximation to the anal orifice, rather than to suture the lateral skin edges snugly across the perineum and fourchette. Everting the vaginal mucosa allows for satisfactory coitus. Conversely, tightly approximated skin at the fourchette may constrict the vaginal introitus and predispose to pain and fissuring.

After the tight packing has been removed in 24 hours, the entire area should be exposed. Initial application of ice packs to the operative site for 24 to 48 hours seems to provide more comfort to the patient than heat. Warm air blown across the perineum is both comforting and therapeutic because it helps to keep the operative site dry, enhancing the healing process. An indwelling urethral catheter or a suprapubic catheter is used while the suture line undergoes initial healing of the skin edges. The suprapubic catheter may be maintained for

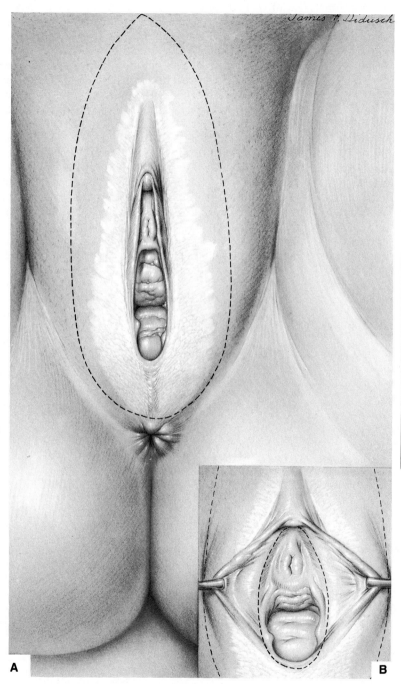

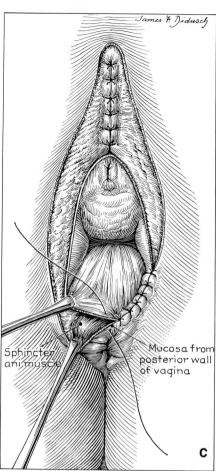

Figure 39–24. *A–C,* Conservative vulvectomy for vulvar carcinoma in situ.

4 to 5 days, if desired. Antibiotics are not necessary for the average simple vulvectomy. Infrequently a local cellulitis may develop, necessitating antibiotic therapy; extruded-spectrum cephalosporins and semisynthetic penicillins have proved effective.

Vulvar Reconstruction

Procedures performed for extensive VIN or atypical hyperplasia include total or partial vulvectomy, skinning vulvectomy, and multiple wide excisions. These may engender large denuded regions, creating challenges for reconstruction. Fortunately, with the advent of laser ablation, fewer procedures such as skinning vulvectomy are performed for VIN.

Reconstructive efforts for superficial excisions typically require split-thickness grafts. These usually are ill-suited for reconstruction after radical excision because the depth of tissue defect is too great, and poor cosmetic and functional results ensue. A buttocks donor site is selected. Perioperative antibiotics are used. Bowel preparation and slow postoperative feeding minimize contamination of the graft site.

Split-thickness skin grafts may be procured with an air-driven dermatome. The size of the vulvar defect helps to determine donor site excision. Meticulous hemostasis should be sought before application of the graft. Fine absorbable sutures are used to secure the skin edges of the graft. The donor site should be covered with an occlusive dressing such as OpSite or Tegaderm until significant healing proceeds. A soft pressure dressing may be applied to the vulva for 3 to 5 days, accompanied by an indwelling catheter for urinary drainage.

BASAL CELL CARCINOMA OF THE VULVA

Basal cell carcinoma of the vulva differs from other forms of vulvar cancer in both treatment and prognosis. Although the tumor occurs infrequently, representing only 2% to 3% of all vulvar cancers, the slow-growing, local in situ neoplasm presents a variety of confusing histopathologic patterns, suggesting more aggressive disease. Basal cell carcinoma, formerly called basal cell epithelioma, appears much like adenoid-basal (not to be confused with adenoid-cystic cancer) or keratotic basal cell lesions. Although giving the histologic appearance of invasion, the basal cells maintain continuity with the overlying epithelium, demonstrated by palisading of the basal cells.

The gross lesion is characterized by a slightly elevated rolled edge surrounding a superficial ulcer, commonly called rodent ulcer when it appears on other parts of the skin (Fig. 39-25A). The microscopic picture shows the deeply stained basal cells extending into the stroma from the overlying epithelium (Fig. 39-25B).

Basal cell tumors are quite radiosensitive, but the vulva is a difficult area to treat because of skin folds that predispose to dosing problems and chronic moisture that fosters mucositis and breakdown. Although simple vulvectomy has been recommended by Marcus and by others who found the origin of the lesion to be multicentric, wide local excision is adequate. The local recurrences of basal cell lesions can be repeatedly excised with essentially 100% cure rate. Because multifocal disease is common, recurrences in other sites are to be expected. On rare occasions the regional lymph nodes may be involved, but more distant metastasis has not been reported. Topical Efudex has been successfully used, but it requires sustained application and should be reserved for patients who refuse excision.

INVASIVE CARCINOMA OF THE VULVA

Carcinoma of the vulva is one of the more uncommon cancers of the genital tract, accounting for only 3% to 4% of all gynecologic cancers. Although the vulva is the fourth most frequently affected site in the female genital tract—after the endometrium, ovary, and cervix—the occurrence of vulvar cancer varies widely throughout the world. For example, vulvar cancer seldom occurs in strict Muslim women who shave the pubic area frequently and who are extremely meticulous about vaginal cleansing. Vulvar cancer most often is seen in women with poor vulvar hygiene and in patients who have a history of chronic vulvar irritation.

For the most part, vulvar cancer affects women of advanced years; more than two-thirds of the cases occur in women between the ages of 61 and 80, with the average age being 65. Only rarely does invasive disease occur in younger patients; Hay and Cole reported a study of 52 cases of invasive cancer with an age range from 29 to 39 years. Of interest was the fact that in the Hay and Cole series, 65% of the young women (34 patients) also had granulomatous disease. In general, the cancer develops in the postmenopausal years and is associated with a prolonged period of vulvar irritation. A current concern relates to the increasing incidence of VIN in younger patients and the potential impact on the incidence of invasive neoplasia.

Symptoms and Diagnosis

The most frequent symptom of vulvar cancer is pruritus that often has been present for months or even

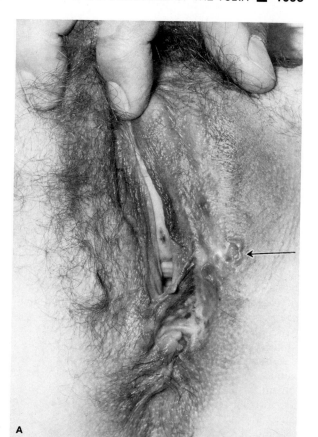

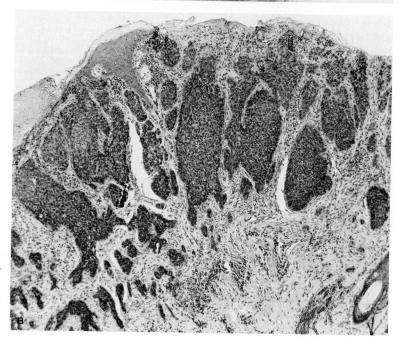

Figure 39–25. *A,* Basal cell carcinoma of the vulva. Note the elevated edge of the localized lesion. *B,* Basal cell carcinoma of the vulva with deeply stained basal cells extending well into the stroma.

years before the diagnosis of the cancer. The cancer often is a source of pain, and when locally advanced, the discomfort may be extreme. Sometimes the appearance of a lump, an ulcer, or a bloody discharge first draws the patient's attention to the vulvar region. When a patient complains of any or all of these symptoms, diagnosis is simple after inspection of the vulva. A nodule or raised ulceration, often on a white background, is a characteristic picture, but lymphogranuloma venereum, tuberculosis, chronic herpetic vulvitis, and other ulcerative lesions may simulate carcinoma. In all cases a biopsy must be taken when a suspicious lesion appears on the vulva.

A question frequently asked about the diagnosis of carcinoma of the vulva is where on the diffusely abnormal vulvar skin the biopsy should be taken. Invasive carcinoma commonly is associated with dystrophic vulvar epithelial lesions; therefore, concern about missing the cancer is valid. Biopsy may be targeted to areas of increased palpable thickness or deeper ulceration, denoting potential dermal involvement.

As noted in the discussion of CIN, Collins reported on the use of 1% solution of toluidine blue as a method of staining the abnormal epithelium. After the vulva is painted with toluidine blue, the stain is allowed to remain for 2 or 3 minutes and then removed with a decolorizing solution of 1% aqueous acetic acid. Because toluidine blue is a nuclear stain, the abnormal epithelium, particularly in areas of parakeratosis, retains the stain and identifies the suspicious areas for biopsy. False-positive results occurred in 16% of Collins' cases, but others have experienced less success in diagnosing cancer with this stain. The most prudent method requires obtaining multiple biopsies of areas that appear clinically to be the most abnormal until the entire vulva has been thoroughly evaluated.

Carcinoma of the vulva is typically indolent in growth, but despite the long time period and the fact that the growth is external, many patients do not seek evaluation until lesions are advanced. Among 136 patients treated at the Medical College of Wisconsin between 1960 and 1977, 32% of the cases presented as stage III and stage IV disease, whereas 68% were diagnosed as stage I or stage II disease. The reasons for delay are several, but they usually are related to the fact that elderly women are reluctant to consult a physician. The disease also occurs at a time in the patient's life when financial constraints are of great importance. Taussig's warning that "not only the women but the *medical profession* is at fault in delayed diagnosis and treatment" is still, unfortunately, not heeded.

Clinical Staging

In 1967 the International Union Against Cancer proposed a preoperative classification of the stages of vulvar cancer based on the size and location of the primary tumor (T), the spread of tumor to the regional (inguinal-femoral) nodes (N), and metastasis (M) of disease outside the regional area. This TNM classification has been in clinical use since January 1971; the system was proposed as a more accurate method of defining the clinical status of disease before treatment.

TNM CLASSIFICATION OF VULVAR CARCINOMA

CLASSIFICATION	DESCRIPTION
T—Primary Tumor	
T1	Tumor confined to the vulva, 2 cm or less in largest diameter
T2	Tumor confined to the vulva, more than 2 cm in largest diameter
T3	Tumor of any size with adjacent spread to the urethra, vagina, perineum, or anus
T4	Tumor of any size infiltrating the bladder mucosa, the rectal mucosa, or both, including the upper part of the urethral mucosa, or fixed to the bone
N—Regional Lymph Nodes	
N0	No lymph node metastasis
N1	Nodes palpable in one or both groins, not enlarged, mobile (not clinically suspicious of neoplasm). Proved by biopsy.
N2	Nodes palpable in one or both groins, enlarged, firm, and mobile (clinically suspicious of neoplasm). Proved by biopsy.
N3	Fixed or ulcerated nodes
M—Distant Metastases	
M0	No clinical metastases
M1a	Palpable deep pelvic lymph nodes
M1b	Other distant metastases

The TNM classification has proved to be too cumbersome for practical use. The Cancer Committee of the International Federation of Gynecology and Obstetrics (FIGO) adopted a revised clinical classification of vulvar carcinoma in 1976 that had actually been in use since July 1, 1974. This classification is a more useful and practical method of staging vulvar carcinoma. A comparison of the two methods of staging vulvar carcinoma shows the complexities of the TNM classification.

The clinical assessment of the status of the groin lymph nodes is used as a major indicator in individualizing treatment and in establishing a prognosis for invasive carcinoma of the vulva. The accuracy of the assessment of whether inguinal-femoral nodes are positive or negative for metastatic tumor has been summarized by Plentl and Friedman. They noted a 39% false-negative clinical error with histologically proven posi-

FIGO CLASSIFICATION OF VULVAR CARCINOMA

CLASSIFICATION	DESCRIPTION
Stage 0	Carcinoma in situ (eg, Bowen's disease, noninvasive Paget's disease)
Stage I	Tumor confined to the vulva, 2 cm or less in largest diameter. Nodes are not palpable or are palpable in either groin, not enlarged, mobile (not clinically suspicious of neoplasm).
Stage II	Tumor confined to the vulva, more than 2 cm in largest diameter. Nodes are not palpable or are palpable in either groin, not enlarged, mobile (not clinically suspicious of neoplasm). Proved by biopsy.
Stage III	Tumor of any size with (a) adjacent spread to the urethra, all of the vagina, perineum, or anus, or (b) nodes palpable in either or both groins (enlarged, firm, and mobile, not fixed but clinically suspicious of neoplasm) Proved by biopsy.
Stage IV	Tumor of any size (a) infiltrating the bladder mucosa, the rectal mucosa, or both, including the upper part of the urethral mucosa, or (b) fixed or ulcerated nodes in either or both groins, or distant metastases

tive nodes and a 35% false-positive clinical error with histologically proven negative nodes. In general, clinical assessment accurately predicts positive or negative regional lymph nodes in only about 66% of the cases, even when performed by experienced surgeons. The experience of Way is somewhat better than that of other investigators. In comparing histological with clinical assessments, Way reports a 25% rate for false-positive clinical assessments.

The large error in clinical assessment of vulvar carcinoma means that the preoperative staging may be inaccurate in 20% to 40% of the cases that are initially classified as stage I or stage II lesions. The clinical error rate should be given serious consideration whenever the treatment of invasive carcinoma is planned. Friedrich has proposed a postoperative staging of vulvar cancer that is much more accurate, but it is not applicable when patients are not surgical candidates.

Recently FIGO has again proposed amendments in staging of vulvar neoplasia. The essence of the alterations is to incorporate surgical pathologic information obtained from lymph node biopsies in final staging assessment. Unilateral regional lymph node metastasis would allot cases to stage III and bilateral regional node involvement to stage IVa. Pelvic lymph node extension would represent stage IVB disease. Although the overall staging system remains clinical, lymph node status must be ascertained by biopsy. This staging modification has been broadly adopted.

Prognostic Factors for Invasive Carcinoma of the Vulva

Patterns of Lymphatic Spread

Since Mayer wrote the earliest clinicopathologic treatise on vulvar carcinoma in 1866, views have differed on the extent and type of surgical treatment advisable

COMPARISON OF CLINICAL STAGING

FIGO	TNM	DESCRIPTION
Stage 0		Carcinoma in situ, intraepithelial carcinoma
Stage I	T1 N0 M0 T1 N1 M0	Tumor confined to the vulva, 2 cm or less in diameter. Nodes are not palpable, or are palpable in either groin, not enlarged, mobile (not clinically suspicious of neoplasm)
Stage II	T2 N0 M0 T2 N1 M0	Tumor confined to the vulva, more than 2 cm in diameter. Nodes are not palpable, or are palpable in either groin, not enlarged, mobile (not clinically suspicious of neoplasm). Proved by biopsy.
Stage III	T3 N0 M0 T3 N1 M0 T3 N2 M0 T1 N2 M0 T2 N2 M0	Tumor of any size with adjacent spread to the lower urethra, vagina, perineum, and anus. Nodes palpable in either or both groins, enlarged, firm, and mobile, not fixed (but clinically suspicious of neoplasm). Proved by biopsy.
Stage IV	T4 N0 M0 T4 N1 M0 T4 N2 M0	Tumor of any size that is infiltrating the bladder mucosa, the upper part of urethra mucosa, or the rectal mucosa, or is fixed to the bone or other distant metastases. Fixed or ulcerated nodes in either or both groins.
	All conditions containing N3 or M1a or M1b	

for the disease. The basis for recommending a lymphadenectomy of the groin originated in 1874, when the anatomist Sappey first demonstrated that the lymphatic drainage of the vulva flowed to the inguinal and femoral nodes en route to the iliac and other pelvic nodes. Groin dissection was another early treatment, based on reports from several European physicians, including Rupprecht (1893) and Schauta, Kustner, and Mauchaire (1903), who advocated bilateral groin lymphadenectomy.

In his description of the treatment of malignant melanoma in 1908, Pringle was the first to recommend a monobloc excision of the vulvar tumor, including the groin lymphatics. Basset made an important contribution in his graduation thesis of 1912, recommending en bloc excision of the groin lymphatics for the primary treatment of carcinoma of the clitoris. Basset reported 147 cases of clitoral carcinoma, but an indeterminate number of these cases were obtained from autopsy studies and others were surgical cases. Interest in the en bloc surgical approach was continued by Taussig of St. Louis, who reported his initial experience in 1929 and was responsible for developing the technique in the United States. In the United Kingdom, Way achieved considerable personal experience with treatment of vulvar disease, and his description of the lymphatic drainage of the vulva (1948) was one of the important anatomic contributions influencing the treatment of vulvar carcinoma.

The use of bilateral extraperitoneal pelvic lymphadenectomy in conjunction with radical vulvectomy and groin dissection was initially suggested by Kehrer in 1918. Kehrer preferred to use two independent, low oblique groin incisions. Stoeckel, a few years before, had recommended the same surgical approach but advocated preliminary exploratory laparotomy to determine the extent of the intrapelvic and abdominal spread. Williams and Butcher revived the exploratory approach for pelvic lymphadenectomy in 1961, and the method was reported by Byron and colleagues in 1962 and by Hacker and associates in 1981. With localized vulvar disease, involvement of the paraaortic lymph nodes is regarded as particularly uncommon and the intraperitoneal approach does not appear justified.

In 1963 Parry-Jones made an important contribution to our understanding of the lymphatic drainage of the vulva by extending the previous work of Way. Parry-Jones studied the pathways of lymphatic drainage by injecting patent-blue dye and colloidal iron subcutaneously into the vulva to demonstrate that the vulvar lymphatics were confined within the labiocrural folds and do not spread laterally onto the thigh. Only from the perineum were the lymphatics demonstrated to skirt the vulva onto the adjacent thigh, rather than to travel exclusively along the labia majora to the inguinal-femoral nodes (Fig. 39-26). The studies also suggested that the lymphatic communication to the deep pelvic nodes occurred from channels along the urethra, outer

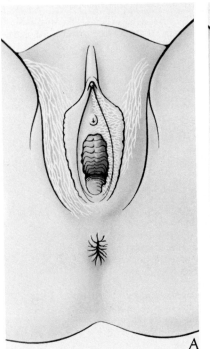
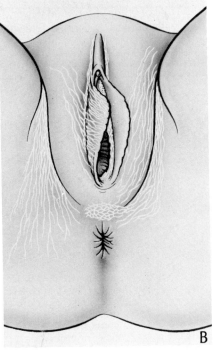

Figure 39–26. *A*, Lymphatic drainage of vulva demonstrating the discrete margin of lymphatic channels of the labia majora at the labiocrural fold. Periurethral and labia minora (medial surface) lymphatics may communicate with drainage of outer vagina. *B*, Lymphatic drainage of inner aspect of thigh and perineal body of superficial inguinal and femoral nodes. (From Parry-Jones E. Lymphatics of the vulva. J. Obstet Gynaecol Br Comm 1963; 70:751.)

vagina, and perineum, primarily through the internal pudendal lymphatics.

Studies by Iversen and Aas, using preoperative injection of radioactive technetium (^{99m}Tc colloid) into the anterior and posterior regions of the labia majora and minora and into the clitoris and perineum, showed that there are no specific differences in lymphatic drainage from any vulvar site, either to the external groin nodes or to the deep pelvic nodes. Only the clitoris and the perineum were found to have a bilateral lymph flow. Based on the understanding of the lymphatic drainage of the vulva from these studies, radical vulvectomy with groin dissection is the preferred method for treating invasive carcinoma of the vulva.

The Iversen and Aas studies showed that 28 of the 42 patients injected with ^{99m}Tc colloid showed very low, but detectable radioactivity in the pelvic nodes removed from the side opposite their lesion, confirming the fact that a bilateral lymph flow does exist between both sides of the vulva and the deep pelvic nodes. The data also explain the occurrence of bilateral groin metastasis (15%) in patients with unilateral tumors and ipsilateral groin metastasis. The work confirms the absence of contralateral metastases in the absence of tumor spread to ipsilateral groin nodes; only 1 out of 54 studied patients had this unusual metastasis.

Depth of Stromal Invasion

The term *microinvasive* is used to describe vulvar carcinoma with tumor invasion of less than 5 mm beneath the basement epithelial membrane, but the term is misleading, and treatment cannot be equated with that of microinvasive carcinoma of the cervix. A separate FIGO classification has not been defined for microinvasive carcinoma of the vulva. Typically lesion size has

been limited to 2 cm; hence these cases have been alloted to FIGO stage I. Patients with these tumors are being treated by more conservative excision, as with simple vulvectomy or wide local excision. Nevertheless, numerous studies suggest that this approach may be inadequate because lymph node metastasis occurs in 10% to 12% of such cases (Table 39-1). Although individualized treatment of vulvar cancer is highly recommended, the potential for metastatic disease must be recognized. Microinvasive carcinoma, like clinically invasive vulvar carcinoma, has the potential for groin metastasis, and many believe that both lesions should be treated similarly. However, some individualization of treatment for microinvasion is appropriate. If the disease is confined to one side of the vulva and does not present as a midline lesion or involve the clitoris or anus, appropriate treatment is hemivulvectomy and ipsilateral groin dissection. Midline lesions have the potential for bilateral metastasis, so both groins must be dissected, as is necessary with clinically invasive carcinoma.

In an attempt to define the microinvasive lesion, which may be treated more conservatively, particularly in the younger patient, the following criteria have been suggested: (a) small lesion size, up to 2 cm; (b) early stromal invasion (Fig. 39-27) characterized by a single focus of neoplasia traversing basement membrane; (c) absence of lymph vascular space involvement; (d) absence of confluent or multifocal invasion demonstrating coalescence; and (e) good health of remaining vulvar tissue. These patients may be considered for wide radical excision without node sampling. A prerequisite to this decision is complete histopathologic evaluation of the lesion, which can only be afforded by prior excisional biopsy. Patients with small lesions that exceed the criteria above should receive appropriate excision of the neoplasm and lymph node sampling.

TABLE 39-1
Frequency of Lymph Node Metastasis in Microinvasive Carcinoma of the Vulva

STUDY (YR)	NO. OF PATIENTS	NO. OF LYMPHADENECTOMIES	NODES INVOLVED	FREQUENCY (%)
Wharton et al. (1974)	25	10	0	0.0
Parker et al. (1975)	58	37	3	8.1
DiPaola et al. (1975)	12	11	4	36.4
Kunschner et al. (1978)	17	13	0	0.0
Kabulski, Franklin (1978)	23	23	5	21.7
MaGrina et al. (1979)	96	71	9	12.7
Buscema et al. (1982)	58	40	6	15.0
Kneale et al. (1982)	86	56	5	8.9
Wilkinson et al. (1982)	30	27	2	6.7
Total	405	288	34	11.8

(Wilkinson EJ, Rico MJ, Pierson KK. Microinvasive carcinoma of the vulva. J Gynecol Pathol 1982;1:30.)

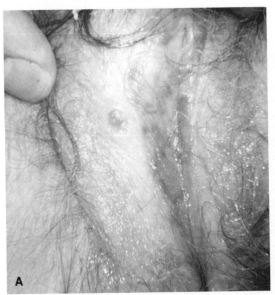
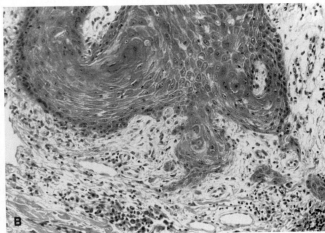

Figure 39–27. *A*, "Microinvasive" squamous carcinoma (gross). Small erythematous lesion right labium majus. Superficial ulceration is apparent. Lesion is 1 cm in diameter. *B*, "Microinvasive" squamous carcinoma (microscopic). Minimal invasion is evidenced by nest of pale staining cells dropping off basement membrane. Note atypical keratinization in overlying epithelium. (×120)

The histologic type and differentiation of tumor significantly influence the incidence of lymph node involvement and the 5-year survival rate. In Way's 1982 data patients with a well-differentiated squamous carcinoma had one-third as many positive groin nodes as patients with more anaplastic tumors and a 30% improvement in 5-year survival. Moran and Parry-Jones found a 32% incidence of lymph node involvement in cases with well-differentiated carcinoma and a 71% incidence with poorly differentiated tumors. The experience of Podratz and associates at the Mayo Clinic was similar. The poorly differentiated carcinoma is a rare entity, accounting for only 2% to 4% of all cancers. Well-differentiated and moderately well differentiated lesions have similar prognoses.

Invasive carcinoma originates primarily from the squamous epithelium (Table 39-2). Tumors of the Bartholin's gland or the Bartholin's duct are included with carcinoma of the vulva because the gland is located beneath the labium majus. These account for 1% to 2% of vulvar cancers. Malignant melanoma is the second most common primary vulvar neoplasm, accounting for 4% to 5%. Sarcomas are reported in 2% of patients with vulvar neoplasia.

Tumor Size

Tumor volume is the major criterion on which all classification systems are based. The FIGO and TNM classifications use a 2-cm diameter as the upper limit of the earliest stage of vulvar cancer because the size of primary lesion is known to correlate with the frequency of lymph node metastasis. Krupp and coworkers have recommended that the critical upper limit distinguishing stage I from stage II lesions be increased to 3 cm because in their data, regional lymph node metastasis infrequently occurs in 2-cm lesions (3.8% of their cases) as compared with 3-cm lesions (9.7% of their cases). Although many clinics use a 3-cm limit between stage I and stage II, the international classification continues to use the 2-cm diameter of a vulvar tumor as the criterion for dividing stage I and stage II lesions.

TABLE 39–2
Histologic Types of Vulvar Cancer and Frequency of Occurrence

TYPE	FREQUENCY (%)
Epidermal (squamous) lesions	90
Differentiated	75–85
Anaplastic	10–15
Basal cell	2–3
Verrucous carcinoma	2
Melanoma	4–5
Sarcoma	2
Bartholin's carcinoma	1–2

Treatment of Invasive Carcinoma of the Vulva

En bloc dissection of the inguinal-femoral regions and the vulva is the time-honored treatment for frank, invasive vulvar carcinoma, and the procedure is described here in detail. The general surgical approach to the treatment of vulvar carcinoma became more individualized in the late 1960s than it had been since Basset made the initial description in 1912. Before 1968 all patients received a radical vulvectomy, groin dissection, and routine extraperitoneal pelvic lymphadenectomy, if surgery was feasible. Now radical vulvectomy and groin dissection are performed without a preoperative decision to perform a pelvic node dissection.

During surgery a frozen section study of suspicious groin nodes, particularly of the superficial sentinal nodes or deepest femoral (Cloquet's) nodes, is performed. If metastatic tumor is found, the pelvic nodes may be dissected or the dissection may be deferred in lieu of pelvic radiotherapy. Deep-node dissection commonly is omitted from the current surgical treatment of vulvar cancer to reduce the incidence of operative and postoperative complications. Removing positive pelvic nodes does not confer any clear therapeutic benefit, so as an alternative, megavoltage pelvic irradiation is used as adjunctive therapy (5000 cGy, midpelvic dose) if the inguinal-femoral lymph nodes are positive.

In a study by Curry and associates in 1980 none of their patients with three or less unilaterally positive groin nodes had positive pelvic nodes. In addition, no patients had positive pelvic nodes if the ipsilateral groin nodes were negative. In a study by Hacker and associates (1983) two of three patients with three positive unilateral groin nodes had positive pelvic nodes, and five of six patients with four or more positive groin nodes had metastases to the pelvic nodes.

The change in treatment reflects the new understanding that pelvic node metastasis almost never occurs unless there is metastasis to the groin nodes. Although Krupp and Bohm found positive pelvic nodes in 4.6% of 195 patients treated with pelvic node dissection, only 1 patient in their series had pelvic lymph node metastasis in the absence of positive groin nodes. Studies from the University of California, Los Angeles (Hacker and associates, 1983), and from the Mayo Clinic (Podratz and associates, 1983) reaffirm this important therapeutic point. Whether or not postoperative irradiation is used, fewer than 20% of the patients with proven positive lymph nodes will survive for 5 years.

A still controversial issue in treating vulvar carcinoma is whether or not a contralateral groin dissection should be performed in patients with unilateral, localized vulvar carcinoma. Morris (1977) first questioned the procedure because few of his patients had contralateral metastasis to groin nodes when there was only ipsilateral disease. Historically, Way's findings of a 20% incidence of bilateral groin metastasis in unilateral tumors provided support for the bilateral procedure. A review of Way's total clinical experience shows that only 5% of the patients who had negative ipsilateral nodes had contralateral nodal spread. Iversen and Aas demonstrated a low incidence of flow of radioactive technetium to contralateral groin or pelvic nodes, but concluded that the main pathway for lymph node metastasis from a unilateral tumor is to the ipsilateral groin. Our own findings in 92 cases of vulvar cancer similarly indicated that if the tumor did not cross the midline or involve the clitoris, the contralateral nodes were never involved. Conversely, in bilateral lesions the nodes were positive on both sides equally. Finally, there is no direct pathway from the vulva to the deep pelvic nodes without involvement of the superficial inguinal nodes. Because the removal of deep pelvic lymph nodes with metastasis does not increase the survival rate, most current treatment protocols concentrate on the inguinal-femoral lymph nodes and not on pelvic lymph node spread.

Feasibility of Surgery

The feasibility of surgery for patients with vulvar carcinoma is seldom limited by the extent of the lesion or the presence of metastasis to the lymph nodes of the groin. More crucial is the patient's cardiovascular-pulmonary-renal reserve. Among 136 patients treated for invasive vulvar carcinoma at the Medical College of Wisconsin, all but one were able to undergo primary surgical treatment. Podratz and coworkers at the Mayo Clinic have a comparable rate of 91%. The availability of careful postoperative cardiopulmonary and renal monitoring in intensive care units has increased the rate of operability for elderly or medically infirm patients.

En Bloc Technique of Radical Vulvectomy with Groin Dissection

The conventional treatment for carcinoma of the vulva consists of one-stage en bloc dissection of the inguinal and femoral lymph node regions and a total radical vulvectomy that includes wide surgical margins beyond the tumor and depth of excision to the urogenital diaphragm. The groin incision extends in an arcuate manner from each anterior iliac superior crest and passes 2 cm above the symphysis and inguinal ligament. The groin dissection includes the adjacent skin, underlying fat, and lymphatic channels, which lie directly over the inguinal ligament and mons pubis.

The superior and lateral incisions include the area of primary lymphatic drainage from the vulva and mons pubis to the inguinal and femoral lymphatics (Fig. 39-28). The butterfly vulvar incision of Marshall and Parry-Jones includes the skin over the region of the fossa ovalis and excludes the skin of the inner thigh. The incision extends inferiorly along the lateral aspect of the labia majora to remove all of the perineal body and the tissue around the superior aspect of the anus. The dissection avoids the necessity of undermining and skeletonizing the skin margins, which subsequently may undergo necrosis owing to compromised blood supply. The skin and subcutaneous fat, including both Camper's and Scarpa's fascia, must be dissected to remove the superficial lymphatic channels and to avoid necrosis of skin margins.

The vulvar incision depends on the location and extent of the primary lesion. Parry-Jones has demonstrated that contrary to Sappey's original description, the vulvar lymphatics drain through the labia majora and do not leave the vulva during their course to the inguinal and femoral nodes. Only from the perineum do the lymphatics extend beyond the vulva and communicate with lymphatics in the inner thigh to reach the groin nodes. The incision is confined inside the labiocrural folds and extends for 2 cm or more beyond the tumor margins; when the tumor extends laterally into or beyond the crural fold, the vulvar incision must be modified accordingly.

As shown in Figure 39-29, the gross lesion is in the region of the clitoris, whereas the extensive dystrophy is confined to the boundaries of the labium majus. All of the lesion must be removed in the dissection with a wide skin margin (at least 2 cm) from the tumor. The

boundaries of the incision are marked on the skin (see Fig. 39-28), with the upper incision extending 2 cm above the inguinal ligament and about 2 cm above the symphysis pubis. The dimensions are particularly important when vulvar lesions are in the region of the clitoris because the lymphatics of the mons frequently are involved.

The groin dissection is accomplished with two teams. This has reduced the operating time of this portion of the procedure by more than 50%. The groins are periodically irrigated with antibiotic-containing solutions during the dissection. The lateral incision extends to the fascia lata, while the superior incision removes all the lymphatic and areolar tissue down to the aponeurosis of the external oblique and anterior rectus fascia. The dissection extends from the lateral aspect of the inguinal ligament to the region of the mons pubis (Fig. 39-29A).

The femoral sheath is incised along the medial margin of the sartorius muscle (Fig. 39-29B) and along the lateral side of the artery, adjacent to the femoral nerve, using palpation of the femoral artery for identification. The artery is thoroughly cleaned of its sheath, the cribriform fascia. The external pudendal artery must be carefully identified and ligated because it marks the entrance of the saphenous vein into the fossa ovale, a major tributary of the femoral vein. The proximal end of the saphenous vein is transfixed and doubly ligated with nonabsorbable suture material (Fig. 39-29C), and the femoral sheath is dissected medially as an en bloc procedure. Later the distal segment of the saphenous vein is ligated and excised as the dissection continues toward the inner thigh.

A particular effort is made to identify and remove Cloquet's nodes (Fig. 39-30) as the deep femoral lymph chain is dissected from the surrounding artery and vein and from the tissue in the femoral canal (Fig. 39-31A). Cloquet's nodes, also called Rosenmüller's nodes, are the nodes at the femoral ring beneath the inguinal ligament, filtering the lymphatic channels that surround the vessels in the femoral triangle. If Cloquet's nodes are found by frozen section to be negative for metastatic tumor, extraperitoneal gland dissection of the iliac, obturator, and hypogastric nodes is not necessary.

The deep inguinal chain is dissected by opening the inguinal canal from the external inguinal ring (Fig. 39-31B). The internal ring begins where the round ligament passes into the canal from the peritoneal cavity. The round ligament is excised, and the deep inguinal lymphatic tissue is removed.

If an extraperitoneal pelvic lymphadenectomy is performed at the time of the initial groin operation, a procedure *largely abandoned in favor of radiotherapy to the pelvis* for positive superficial nodes, the procedure is initiated by opening the external oblique

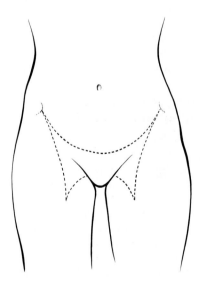

Figure 39–28. Radical vulvectomy and groin dissection. Skin incision of Marshall and Parry-Jones, removing the area of femoral nodes without the skin of the inner thigh.

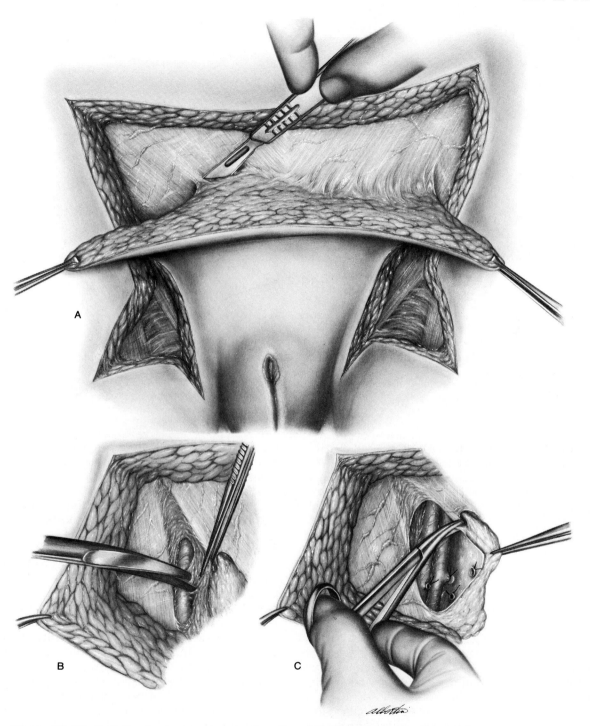

Figure 39–29. Radical vulvectomy and groin dissection. *A*, En bloc dissection of the groin lymphatics with attached skin and subcutaneous fat to the region of the mons pubis. *B*, Opening of femoral sheath along medial border of sartorius muscle and the lateral side of the femoral artery. Femoral artery is cleaned of adherent fascia. Inguinal lymphatics are seen entering external inguinal ring. *C*, Dissection of femoral sheath medially after ligation of the saphenous vein and external pudendal artery. Superficial inguinal lymph chain is seen entering inguinal canal.

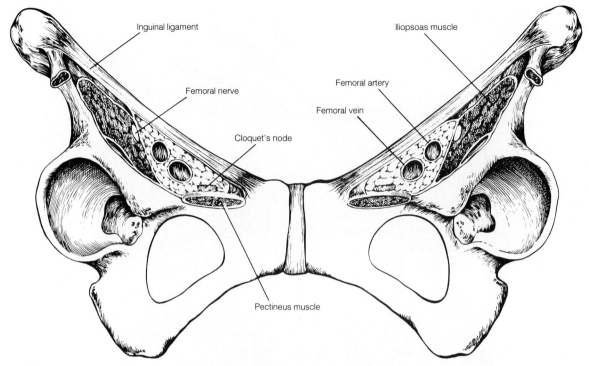

Figure 39–30. Cloquet's node in the femoral triangle. The femoral triangle is bounded superiorly by the inguinal ligament, medially by the pectineus muscle, and laterally by the iliopsoas muscle.

muscle 2 cm above the inguinal ligament (Fig. 39-31*C*). The round ligament has been divided to facilitate dissection. The incision can be extended as far laterally as necessary and is continued through the internal oblique and transversalis muscles, and the iliac vessels are exposed by retracting the peritoneum medially.

Extraperitoneal lymphadenectomy includes the external iliac, common iliac, and, if accessible, the upper part of the hypogastric vessels (Fig 39-32*A*, see Figs. 42-39 to 42-45). The obturator space is thoroughly cleaned. The position of the obturator nerve should be sought before aggressive dissection of the space, to avoid inadvertent injury. The inferior epigastric artery and vein should be ligated where they originate from the external iliac vessels, just inside the inguinal ligament, as they course upward to supply the abdominal wall. An anomalous obturator artery or vein may arise from the external iliac vessels and enter the obturator fossa along the lateral pelvic wall. The ureter is easily identified as it enters the pelvis at the bifurcation of the common iliac artery, and it should be displaced medially with the parietal peritoneum to avoid injury (Fig. 39-32*A*).

Although cleaning the deep lymphatic channels along the pelvic vessels is important, more essential is avoiding trauma to the vessel walls by excessive skeletonization. Leaving a loose layer of adventitia attached to the vessel wall can help to prevent injury, thrombosis, and bleeding. The retroperitoneal space is routinely drained abdominally through separate stab wounds. This is best achieved with closed-suction drain systems such as the Jackson-Pratt, which ensure adequate removal of fluid from the retroperitoneal spaces. The latter should probably be used routinely, since fluid accumulation is unavoidable after such extensive dissection and its removal decreases risk of lymphocyst, infection, and deep venous thrombosis.

The external oblique, internal oblique, and transversalis muscles are closed in a two-layer manner, with obliteration of the inguinal canal by the second suture layer. A double-layer, vest-over-pants closure of the inguinal canal also may be used. No. 1 delayed absorbable suture is used for muscle closure.

An important step in radical vulvectomy was introduced by Baronofsky in 1948 and popularized by Way. The procedure includes transposing the sartorius muscle over the femoral neurovascular trunk to protect the femoral vessels from postoperative infection, thrombophlebitis, and, possibly, hemorrhage, but now that prophylactic antibiotics are used, many surgeons do not perform this procedure. The origin of the sartorius muscle is excised from the anterior superior iliac spine and adjacent inguinal ligament. The muscle is freed

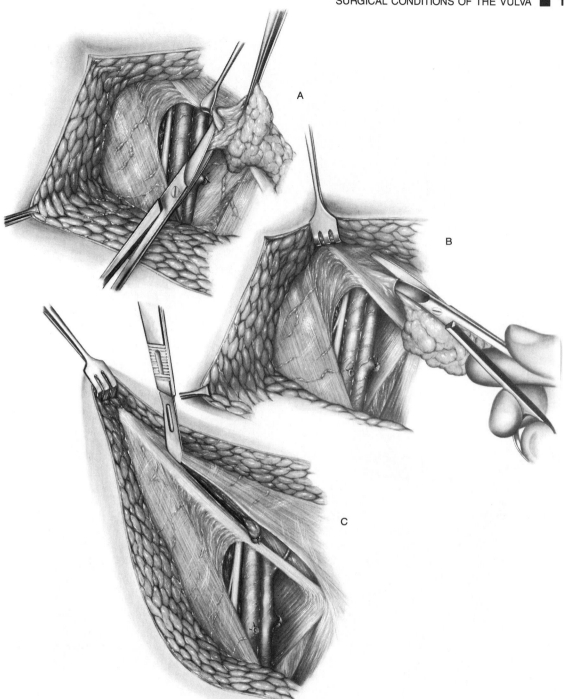

Figure 39–31. Radical vulvectomy and groin dissection. *A,* Dissection of femoral canal and Cloquet's node. The artery, vein, and nerve in the femoral triangle are completely dissected. The inguinal ligament is elevated for dissection of deep femoral lymphatics from the femoral canal. *B,* Opening the inguinal canal for dissection of deep inguinal lymph chain. Scissors are placed in the external inguinal ring to open the roof of the canal. *C,* Incision of external oblique muscle from inguinal canal for extraperitoneal node dissection. The round ligament protrudes from the internal inguinal ring. The inferior epigastric artery and vein (vein only shown) arise from the external iliac artery and vein above the medial border of the inguinal ligament.

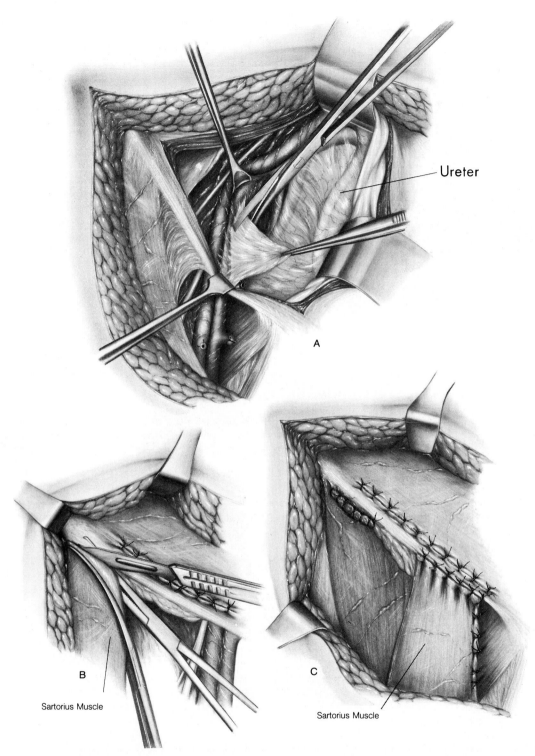

Ureter

Sartorius Muscle

Sartorius Muscle

Figure 39–32. Radical vulvectomy and groin dissection. *A*, Extraperitoneal pelvic lymph-adenectomy. Dissection includes the external iliac, common iliac, hypogastric, and obturator lymph nodes. Ureter is reflected medially, attached to parietal peritoneum. *B*, Excision of proximal portion of sartorius muscle at origin from anterosuperior iliac spine. *C*, Transposed sartorius muscle over femoral vessels with suture of muscles to medial border of inguinal ligament and pectineus muscle. Abdominal musculature is closed after extraperitoneal pelvic lymphadenectomy.

from its fascial attachments and is sutured to the medial border of the inguinal ligament with interrupted delayed absorbable sutures (Fig. 39-32B). The medial border of the sartorius muscle is sutured to the pectineus fascia to avoid collection of serum and exudate in the femoral space (Fig. 39-32C). Closed-suction drains, such as Jackson-Pratt, are sutured in place above or below the inguinal ligament for drainage. The inguinal incision is then approximated by sufficiently mobilizing the upper and lower skin flaps to permit closure without tension (Fig. 39-33A). The groin specimen is wrapped in a sterile towel, and the patient is placed in the lithotomy position for the vulvectomy.

The vulvar incision is continued along the labiocrural folds or by maintaining a 2-cm margin of the vulvar tumor. The vulvar incision includes the perineal skin along the lateral side of the anus. Some conservation of uninvolved skin is acceptable, but the major portion of each side of the labia should be excised to remove the microlymphatic channels that may contain tumor emboli (Fig. 39-33A). Dissection is continued along the periosteum of the symphysis at the level of fascia of the deep musculature of the urogenital diaphragm. The bulbocavernosus, ischiocavernosus, and superficial transverse perinei muscles are removed in the vulvar dissection (Fig. 39-33B).

The internal pudendal vessels, which provide the major blood supply to the vulva, are ligated as they are identified in the dissection (Fig. 39-33C). The pudendal vessels emerge from Alcock's canal at about the 4 o'clock and 8 o'clock positions.

The vaginal incision is made proximal to the external urethral meatus and circumscribes the introitus adjacent to the carunculae hymenales (Fig. 39-34A). The mucosa of the lateral and posterior vaginal walls is undermined for 3 to 4 cm to form a mucosal flap for anastomosis to the perianal and vulvar skin, to avoid tension on the suture line as well as introital stricture. The vulva is removed after careful ligation of the blood supply to the clitoris, which can be difficult because these vessels tend to retract beneath the inferior pubic ligament. Identification and ligation of the clitoral vessels frequently can be more effectively accomplished from above after completing the groin dissections by mobilizing the specimen off the mons pubis in a caudal direction. If tumor is present on the medial aspect of the labia minora near the urethra, the outer one-third of the urethra should be excised to obtain adequate tumor-free surgical margins because the lymphatics of the labia drain to the periurethral region. The outer one-third of the urethra can be removed without serious risk of urinary incontinence unless there is a prominent cystourethrocele. In such cases plication and retropubic elevation of the urethrovesical angle are necessary.

If the outer urethra has been removed, care must be taken in approximating the skin near the excised urethra. Retraction of the urethra beneath the vulvar suture line can be avoided by anchoring the periurethral fascia to the subcutaneous fat at the lateral skin margins. The urethra should be securely sutured to the skin margins beneath the symphysis pubis to avoid retraction or formation of a hood of scar tissue over the meatus. If a hood is formed, spraying of urine may occur with voiding, which may necessitate a secondary plastic procedure to remove the hood.

Closure of the vulvar incision is accomplished by slightly undermining the thigh skin flaps and the outer vaginal mucosa (Fig. 39-34B). The vaginal mucosa is approximated to the mobilized skin flaps of the lateral vulva or thigh with a series of vertical mattress sutures of No. 0 delayed absorbable material, bringing broad surface to broad surface (Fig. 39-34C). Tension on the skin margins should be avoided if at all possible. Extensive mobilization of the vaginal mucosa occasionally is required. Under certain circumstances reconstruction is better accomplished with full-thickness or myocutaneous flaps. This is discussed below. Figure 39-35 shows the specimen after en bloc dissection.

Radical Vulvectomy with Groin Dissection Through Separate Incisions

One of the recent modifications of the en bloc dissection of the vulva and inguinal-femoral regions has been the use of a three-incision technique with separate incisions for each groin and for the vulva (Fig. 39-36). This three-incision procedure, described originally by Kehrer in 1918 and again by Byron and associates in 1962, has significantly improved the rate of primary wound healing and also has reduced the length of hospital stay. Evaluation of the technique by Hacker and colleagues showed that none of the 100 patients in their study had recurrence of tumor in the inguinal skin bridge above the symphysis pubis. Major breakdown of the groin incision occurred in only 14% of the cases, a significant improvement over the 40% to 80% incidence of wound infection and breakdown observed with the traditional en bloc procedure.

We have used the three-incision method with therapeutic success equivalent to the en bloc procedure. Primary wound healing also has been favorable with this technique in our clinic. Lymphedema of the lower extremities has not been ameliorated with the separate groin dissections, but some lymphedema is to be expected if the inguinal-femoral node dissection has been thoroughly performed.

Technique. The patient is prepared for the groin (text continues on page 1109)

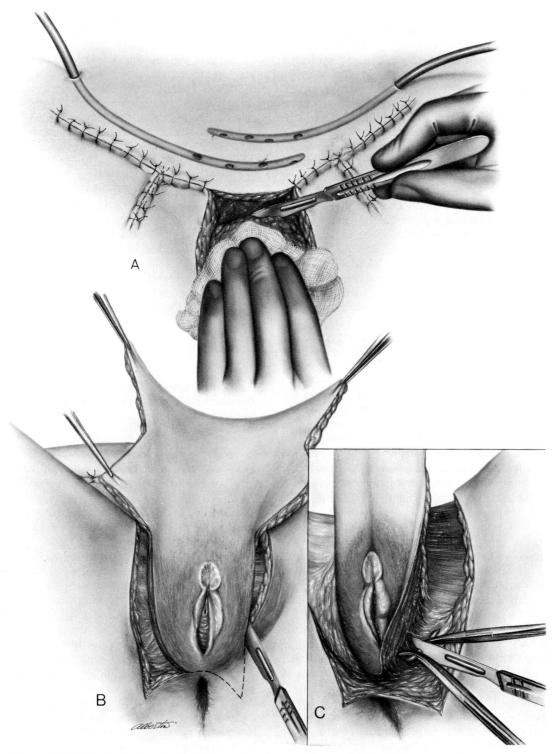

Figure 39–33. Radical vulvectomy and groin dissection. *A,* Closure of skin margins over groin with rubber catheter drains sutured beneath skin flap. *B* and *C,* Clamping and incision of internal pudendal vessels at posterior lateral margin of vulvar incision.

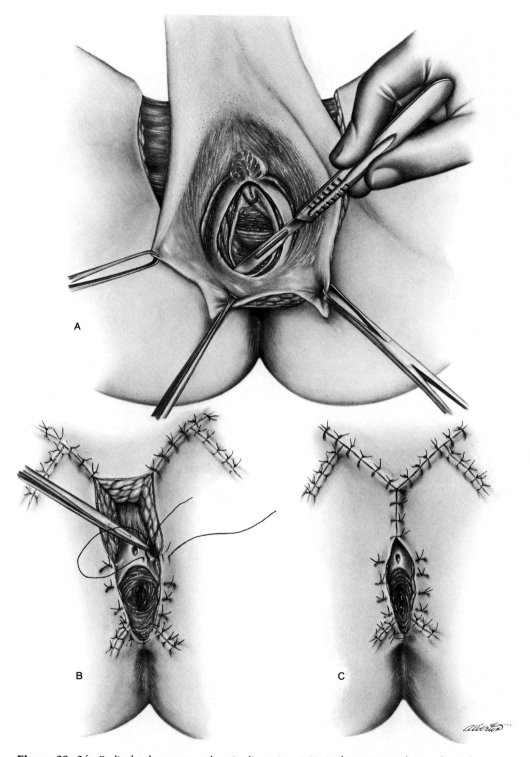

Figure 39–34. Radical vulvectomy and groin dissection. *A,* Vaginal incision made just above the meatus and circumscribing the introitus. *B,* Closure of undermined vaginal mucosa to thigh skin flaps. *C,* Complete closure of vaginal suprapubic and inguinal incision with vertical mattress sutures.

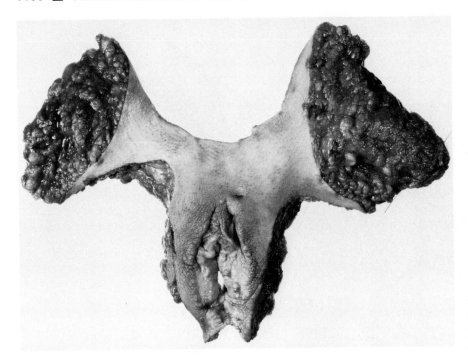

Figure 39–35. Radical vulvectomy specimen in fresh state. (Courtesy of Eduard G. Friedrich, Jr., MD)

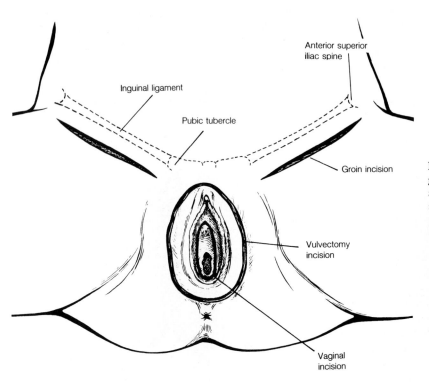

Anterior superior iliac spine

Inguinal ligament

Pubic tubercle

Groin incision

Vulvectomy incision

Vaginal incision

Figure 39–36. Radical vulvectomy and groin dissection through separate incisions. The vulvectomy incision is placed along the lateral margin of the labia majora in the labiocrural folds. The vaginal incision encircles the introitus at a position that provides a tumor-free margin of 2 cm or more. The introital incision should provide a 1-cm margin from the urethral meatus unless an adjacent tumor requires the removal of the outer one-third of the urethra. Separate groin incisions are placed 2 cm below and parallel with the inguinal ligament, extending from the anterior superior iliac spine to the pubic tubercle.

and vulvar dissections in the same manner as for the en bloc procedure, using two operating teams. The lateral margin of each groin incision begins at the region of the anterior superior iliac spine, about 2 cm below the inguinal ligament. Each incision passes medially and obliquely along the inferior course of the inguinal ligament and terminates at a position just below the pubic tubercle, passing over the region of the fossa ovale of the femoral triangle. The inguinal and femoral regions are isolated and dissected, including Cloquet's nodes. If an extraperitoneal pelvic lymph node dissection should be warranted, the lateral margins of the incision can be extended vertically in a cephalad direction, along the lateral aspect of the lower abdominal wall.

Closure of the groin incisions is done with a two-layer technique, using No. 3-0 delayed absorbable suture to approximate the subcutaneous fat and to obliterate the underlying dead space. A large suction drain should be placed over the femoral triangle and brought out through a separate stab wound above the incision. A Jackson-Pratt closed-suction drain may be used for proper drainage of each groin. To ensure a good blood supply to the skin margins, the skin edges may be trimmed from both the medial and lateral aspects for about 0.5 to 1.0 cm each.

Perioperative broad-spectrum antibiotics are given for 24 hours and may be extended for a longer period if clinically indicated. Prophylactic low-dose heparin, 5000 units, is given subcutaneously 2 hours preoperatively and every 12 hours postoperatively for about 7 to 10 days. In addition, sequential calf and thigh compression of both legs may be used during and after surgery to prevent venous thrombosis, as an adjunct in prevention of deep venous thrombosis.

Unilateral Radical Vulvectomy and Groin Dissection

The traditional ultraradical treatment of all stages of vulvar cancer with bilateral vulvectomy and groin dissection has been questioned for many years by serious students in this field. DiSaia and colleagues (1975) have treated patients with superficially invasive lesions (to 1 mm beneath the basement membrane) by wide local excision of the primary lesion and bilateral superficial inguinal-femoral lymphadenectomy. Only if positive superficial nodes were found by frozen section study would the cribriform fascia be opened and the deep femoral nodes be dissected. This would be accompanied by radical vulvectomy. The modified procedure was used in an effort to reduce the morbidity, disfigurement, and sexual dysfunction of younger patients. None of the 60 patients treated had evidence of metastatic disease to the superficial groin nodes.

Iversen and associates and other investigators also have challenged the conventional radical treatment of patients with early, nonmidline unilateral stage I lesions. Iversen and coworkers remain cautious in recommending hemivulvectomy and ipsilateral groin dissection but have used this procedure for patients with stage I disease in whom tumor invasion is 1 mm or less with no vessel invasion. This conservative treatment is based on anatomic studies that show that the major pathway of vulvar metastasis is to ipsilateral inguinal-femoral nodes. This experience of ipsilateral groin metastasis from unilateral lesions also has been documented in 92 cases of vulvar cancer treated at the Johns Hopkins Hospital from 1970 to 1980. In all of these patients contralateral metastases were not found without positive ipsilateral groin nodes.

In an effort to individualize the treatment of patients with vulvar cancer, we have carefully selected patients with midlabial, nonmidline invasive cancer of 2 cm or less for unilateral surgery. Hemivulvectomy and bilateral groin dissection are performed by a three-incision technique that separates the vulvar incision from the inguinal-femoral dissection (Fig. 39-37). It seems prudent at this time to continue to do a bilateral groin dissection despite the infrequency of a positive contralateral groin metastasis in the absence of metastasis to the ipsilateral groin nodes. Deep pelvic node dissection is no longer performed, and pelvic irradiation is used as adjunctive treatment when there are two or more posi-

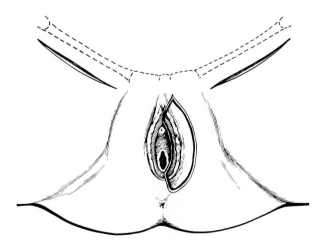

Figure 39–37. Radical hemivulvectomy with bilateral groin dissection through separate incisions. The vulvar incision begins at the lateral side of clitoris. It continues along the labiocrural fold, laterally, and the vaginal introitus, medially, to include a 2-cm tumor-free margin, and extends to the medial aspect of the perineum. Separate groin incisions begin at the anterior superior iliac spine, 2 cm below the inguinal ligament, and extend to the pelvic tubercle.

tive groin nodes. When clinical evaluation of the procedure is more complete, unilateral radical vulvectomy may become the treatment of choice for early unilateral disease. Nevertheless, it must be appreciated that the anatomic configuration after the unilateral procedure is not well accepted by many patients (ie, the differential in appearance is somewhat disturbing).

Pelvic Exenteration for Advanced Carcinoma of the Vulva

In the infrequent case when vulvar cancer extends beyond the boundaries of the vulva to include the adjacent urinary tract or rectum, ultraradical surgery, including anterior, posterior, or total pelvic exenteration, has been performed. The initial experience with advanced vulvar carcinoma was reported by Brunschwig and Daniel in 1956; from 27 cases the operative mortality was 47%. In a survey of the literature from 1960 to 1973 Boronow found that the operative mortality had declined to 10.7%, with a 5-year survival of 16%. Cavanagh and Shepherd reviewed their experience along with five other reports from the 1970s to find a collective cure rate of 47% in patients treated with exenteration and vulvectomy. In all of these cases there were no cures among patients with positive node metastases.

Boronow has advocated alternatives to exenteration for advanced stage IVa lesions. One such approach uses surgical extirpation of lymph nodes in conjunction with external beam radiotherapy and brachytherapy to control the central lesion. The latter has been difficult to perform for vulvar cancer owing to features of this region. Skin moisture and tissue redundancy can lead to problems of intense mucositis and vulvitis; frequent breaks in therapy ensue. Another option proposed consists of preoperative radiotherapy to lymph nodes and central lesion followed 6 weeks later by radical vulvectomy after tumor regression occurs. Among 26 primary cases and 7 recurrent cases this combined therapy resulted in 17 patients (65%) who were free of disease for 1 to 11 years after therapy.

In general, the cure rate from Boronow's combined therapy is similar to that from pelvic exenteration, as reviewed by Phillips and associates. Among 78 cases of pelvic exenteration for advanced vulvar cancer, including the authors' cases and those reported from the literature, there was a 48% cumulative 5-year survival rate, ranging from 20% to 66%. Because exenteration is associated with about 5% surgical mortality resulting from intraoperative or postoperative complications, and considerable morbidity, and because the extensive exenterative procedure is contraindicated when there are bony or extrapelvic metastases and in debilitated patients, Boronow's combination therapy is a welcome substitute. Wharton at M.D. Anderson Hospital and

Tumor Institute recently has advocated a similar approach to the large bulky lesion.

More recent attempts to address the challenges of locally advanced disease have used combination therapy consisting of chemotherapy, radiation, and radical surgery. Example has been drawn from treatment of head and neck as well as anal squamous cancers. Meeker and colleagues have reported a regimen of multiagent chemotherapy using mitomycin and 5-fluorouracil and simultaneous external beam radiation in anal cancers to achieve tumor regression. This approach has been proposed for advanced vulvar lesions to permit less radical surgery, sometimes permitting preservation of bladder or rectum. The increased hazards of groin dissection after radiation should be mentioned. Results from studies are preliminary, and this approach remains investigational.

Complications of Radical Vulvar Surgery

Necrosis and Infection of Skin Flaps

The incidence of wound separation and breakdown has been improved remarkably with the use of separate groin incisions. With the three-incision technique the incidence of significant wound breakdown has decreased from the usual 40% to 80% to less than 15% of all cases. The reduction of tension on the skin incision and the improvement in blood supply to the skin margins, coupled with suction drainage beneath the incision, have greatly reduced the problem of incision breakdown. The routine use of broad-spectrum antibiotics perioperatively also has decreased the incidence of wound infection. If incisions breakdown despite utilization of these advanced methods, total healing time can be shortened by using debridement and secondary closure or by making a split-thickness skin graft. This may be preferable to enforcing a long period of hospitalization to allow the wound to close slowly by secondary granulation. The method above may be considered only if active infection has been excluded.

Serum and Lymph Collection

Copious amounts of serum and lymph collect beneath the skin flaps in the operative site. Suction drainage is imperative, and may extract as much as 200 to 300 ml/day, depending on the amount of adipose tissue in the groin and the degree of secondary infection after the operation. Large rubber or polyethylene drainage catheters are connected to low Gomco or Hemovac suction pumps and left in place as long as there is drainage beneath the skin flaps. Alternatively, a Jackson-Pratt closed-suction drain placed in each groin and exited through a separate stab wound provides excellent drainage to this region. As a rule, the drains or catheters may be advanced on the 4th or 5th day and removed within the 1st postoperative week. However, if appreciable amounts of fluid are continuing to drain, it is important to maintain the evacuation to obviate breakdown of the incision.

Lymphedema

The lymphedema that normally results from vulvectomy and groin dissection usually is temporary, lasting only until secondary lymphatic drainage channels from the leg are reestablished. Nevertheless, about 25% to 30% of patients have significant residual lymphedema, which is improved somewhat by the continuous use of fitted elastic stockings and by elevation of the legs to a horizontal position when sitting.

Postoperative Hemorrhage and Venous Thrombosis

Although hemorrhage from infection and necrosis of the denuded femoral vessels was formerly a serious postoperative problem, this has been virtually eliminated by the procedure of transposing the sartorius muscle over the femoral vessels and liberally using antibiotics. The formation of a retroperitoneal hematoma from deep pelvic gland dissection remains a problem. The hematoma may localize in the cul-de-sac, where vaginal drainage can be carried out. If venous bleeding from obturator or pelvic floor veins is a problem at the time of surgery, retroperitoneal polyethylene catheter drains may be inserted and connected to low suction to avoid a pelvic hematoma. This complication is infrequently seen, since dissection of the pelvic nodes is not readily performed.

The prophylactic use of low-dose heparin or mechanical calf and thigh compression—both during and after surgery—has reduced the incidence of venous thrombosis and thromboembolism from the lower extremities. If thrombophlebitis or pulmonary embolism should occur, vigorous anticoagulation therapy, initially with heparin, is required.

Hernia

An inguinal or femoral hernia may occur postoperatively unless both canals are appropriately closed at the completion of the femoral and inguinal dissection. Nonabsorbable or delayed absorbable suture is preferable to catgut suture in approximating the inferior border of the inguinal ligament to the Cooper's ligament and the pectineus fascia. The inguinal ligament should not be transected by the deep pelvic node

dissection because a postoperative hernia may result from secondary infection or from poor healing of the inguinal region.

Introital Stenosis and Dyspareunia

More than 50% of the elderly patients with carcinoma of the vulva who are sexually active at the time of radical vulvectomy confide that dyspareunia becomes a serious problem after surgery. Their husbands also attest that coitus often is abandoned because of painful intercourse, while others have a psychological barrier of touching the genitalia where cancer had been present. Dyspareunia has been greatly reduced by advanced methods of mobilization and exteriorization of the outer vaginal mucosa. Such techniques minimize the rigid circular scar at the introitus (see perineoplasty).

Even when intercourse remains possible patients experience a marked reduction in sexual activity as a result of the negative body image that attends this type of radical surgery. Sexual responsiveness may be compromised by clitoral resection. Reconstruction of the vulva and perineum with the use of gracilis myocutaneous grafts and rotational flaps after radical resection may help to improve the functional and sometimes cosmetic appearance of the external genitalia. Although the grafting procedure increases the length of the primary surgery, the excellent functional and anatomic results are worthwhile for patients in whom large defects in the vulvar skin preclude primary closure. Postoperative constriction and scarring of the perineum and the vulvar skin can be eliminated by using such techniques at the time of primary surgery.

Reconstruction After Radical Vulvar Surgery

The pursuit of the primary goal of radical vulvar surgery—the removal of neoplasm with adequate margins—can create challenges in reconstruction inadequately addressed by primary closure. Important considerations in the reconstructive aspect include maintenance of sexual function, preservation of the distal urinary and gastrointestinal tracts, and restoration of cosmetically desirable anatomy. The last issue, although primarily a cosmetic concern, may be of vital psychological significance to the patient.

Three reconstructive approaches used in association with radical vulvar surgery are depicted. Split-thickness skin grafts are described above. They are of limited value in radical vulvar reconstruction because of the typical need for full-thickness skin replacement. They may be used in circumstances of wound breakdown; in this scenario an adequate base of granulation tissue must be present before grafting. Alternatively, split-thickness skin may be applied to reepithelialize sites of full-thickness flap failure. The considerations of importance in using these grafts are discussed above.

Full-thickness skin flaps are cutaneous pedicle grafts. They may be used to reconstruct large defects of the vulva, perineum, and perianal region. Skin and underlying subcutaneous tissue may be mobilized from the inner thigh, buttocks, mons pubis, and, occasionally, anterior abdominal wall to serve as the donor site. The mobilized tissue is not entirely severed from the point of origin, and represents a rotational flap that remains attached to its base. These may be either random flaps or a flap rotated with a designated arterial supply. The typical random flap has been used to repair a circular defect by creating an equilateral rhomboid defect (Fig.

39-38*A* through *C*). In this approach, also called a Z-plasty, the following considerations are of importance:

1. A careful assessment of defect size is required to permit accurate designation of "requisite" flap size.
2. The incision should be carried down to the fascia to maintain blood supply.
3. The rhomboid defect created should have equilateral sides, 60-degree angles, and the length of the flap should not exceed the width of its pedicle (Fig. 39-39*A* and *B*).
4. Hemostasis must be maintained.
5. The flap should be attached to the underlying fascia to reduce dead space.
6. Suction drains should be used to reduce fluid accumulations that can undermine flaps.

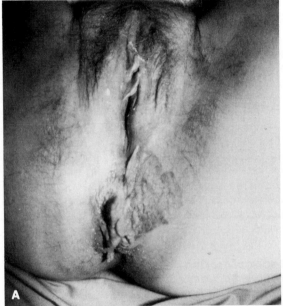

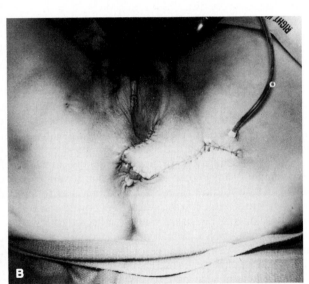

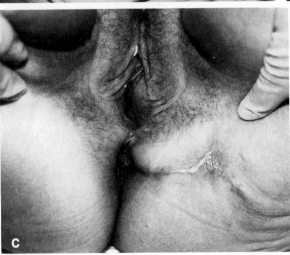

Figure 39–38. *A*, Large recurrence of VIN III with involvement of perineum and perianal region. *B*, Full-thickness rotational flap performed after wide excision. Suction drain in place. *C*, Appearance of vulva and perineum 2 months after rotational flap. (Courtesy of Jeffrey L. Stern, MD, and Conley Lacey, MD)

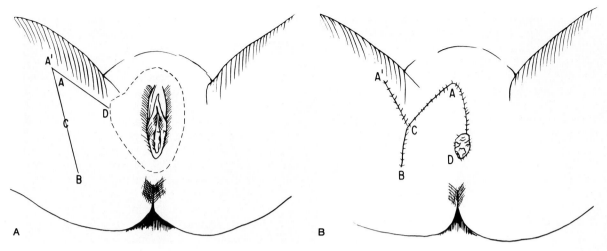

Figure 39–39. Full-thickness rotational flap for large defect after radical vulvectomy. *A*, Outline of inner thigh graft site made up of triangle ABD. C represents the midpoint of the long incision. *B*, Diagrammatic rotational flap closure of vulvar defect. A' to C represents the line of closure of the apex of the triangle.

7. Fine delayed absorbable suture material should be used on the skin to prevent early incision line breakdown.
8. Pressure dressings that compromise the blood supply should be avoided.

Arterial rotational flaps may be performed that utilize the superficial circumflex iliac, inferior epigastric, or branches of the deep external pudendal. Outcome depends on preservation of the arterial blood supply and venous return.

The technique of myocutaneous flaps for gynecologic reconstruction was described by McCraw and Massey in 1976. It originally was depicted as a means of vaginal reconstruction and remains so. In addition, several muscle groups with overlying cutaneous tissue have been used in vulvar and groin reconstruction. The concept central to this flap is the identification of a nonvital muscle that may be sacrificed for mobilization with a single dominant artery that can sustain the muscle and overlying subcutaneous tissue and skin. The principle muscle groups used are the gracilis, the tensor fascia lata, and the rectus abdominus. The gracilis muscle flap is probably the most versatile, and may be performed unilaterally or bilaterally, depending on the size and location of the defect (Fig. 39-40A through *C*). The tensor fascia lata approach may be more adaptable to certain groin reconstructions.

A major advantage of this technique is the feature of bringing a new and independent blood supply to the surgical site. This may promote healing, especially in circumstances such as post radiation, in which vascular insufficiency ensues.

The performance of successful myocutaneous flaps

depends on many factors similar to those described above for full-thickness flaps. In addition, maintenance of good hydrational status is important to prevent intravascular depletion and vasoconstriction. Oxygen delivery also can be enhanced by adequate hemoglobin levels and supplemental inhaled oxygen.

Hypercalcemia Complicating Carcinoma of the Vulva

Hypercalcemia complicating squamous cell carcinoma of the vulva was initially reported by Schatten and associates in 1958. Since that time five additional cases have been reported in which hypercalcemia was noted without clinical evidence of osseous metastasis, renal disease, or parathyroid malfunction. The most common symptoms of this condition affect the gastrointestinal tract, and include anorexia, nausea, vomiting, and constipation. Many patients are disoriented because of central nervous system disturbance from high free calcium ion concentrations in their serum. Parathormone levels are normal, and there is no pathophysiologic evidence of primary hyperparathyroidism.

Several theories of the cause of this uncommon paraneoplastic disorder have been advanced. A general belief ascribes the hypercalcemia to the production of a parathormone-like substance by the larger neoplasms. A number of tumors have been found to produce a polypeptide hormone with immunologic reactivity similar to that of parathormone, producing hypercalcemia. Neuroendocrine small cell carcinoma of the lung has been the primary cancer most frequently associated

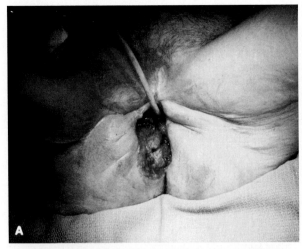

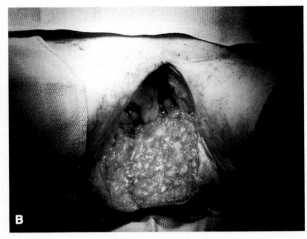

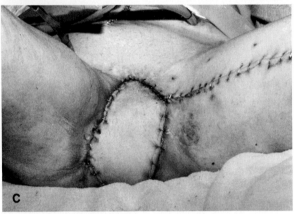

Figure 39–40. Gracilis myocutaneous flap. *A*, Recurrent squamous carcinoma after radical vulvectomy. Tumor involves urethra, anterior and posterior vagina. *B*, Massive defect resulting from ultraradical resection; closure mandates unilateral gracilis flap. *C*, Closure of defect achieved with left gracilis myocutaneous flap. Urine and fecal streams diverted. (Courtesy of Conley Lacey, MD, and Jeffrey L. Stern, MD)

with this condition; other, less common tumors include hypernephroma, reticulum cell sarcoma, lymphoma, and carcinoma of the head, neck, and skin.

Niebyl and associates have reported that vulvar carcinoma is the second most common gynecologic tumor to produce hypercalcemia; ovarian carcinoma is the cancer most frequently associated with this disorder.

The hypercalcemia is abruptly resolved with removal of the parent tumor, after which the serum calcium level returns to normal, the sensorium improves, and the metabolic derangements of hypercalcemia rapidly improve. Recurrence of hypercalcemia cannot be used as a marker for recurrent disease.

Operative Mortality Associated with Invasive Carcinoma of the Vulva

A significant mortality rate still attends treatment of vulvar carcinoma, mainly because of pulmonary emboli and the fact that the older patient group has a high incidence of generalized cardiovascular disease, including myocardial infarction and cerebrovascular acci-

dent. Morley reports a surgical mortality rate of 1.8% and a hospital mortality rate of 2.1% over 40 years of experience at the University of Michigan. Since 1955 the overall operative mortality for the first 60 days after radical vulvar surgery at the Mayo Clinic was 2.2%, as reported by Podratz and colleagues. The five deaths among 223 surgical cases at the Mayo Clinic were related to pulmonary emboli, respiratory failure, myocardial infarction, and intraoperative cardiac arrest. The mortality rate at the Medical College of Wisconsin also was 2.2%, with 3 postoperative deaths among 136 operated cases within a 30-day period after surgery.

The use of low-dose heparin has decreased the incidence of fatal postoperative pulmonary emboli and improved the mortality rate from thromboembolism. The dosage is 5000 I.U. given 2 hours before surgery and every 12 hours after surgery for a period of at least 5 to 7 days and until the patient is ambulatory. Another prophylactic method, external pneumatic calf and thigh compression, also has demonstrated a reduction of deep vein thrombosis of the lower extremities. When used during surgery and for the first 5 days postoperatively, pneumatic calf compression reduced the incidence of deep venous thrombosis from 34.6% to 12.7%, according to Clark-Pearson and associates. No postoperative deaths from pulmonary emboli occurred during their study. Venous thrombosis and pulmonary emboli also have decreased with the use of early ambulation and vigorous exercise of the lower extremities during bed rest, and with decreased cellulitis of wounds.

Cure Rate of Invasive Carcinoma of the Vulva

Many factors affect the possibility of curing vulvar cancer. Of the various prognostic factors, those that influence the spread of the disease beyond the vulva and the frequency of metastases to the regional lymph nodes are most important. Tumor size and location are critical. Centrally located tumors that involve the urethra, vagina, perineum, anus, and rectum are known to have the highest incidence of regional lymphatic metastases. In contrast to previous reports, experience has shown that clitoral lesions do not have a preferential lymph drainage to the deep pelvic lymph nodes or a lower cure rate.

Although cure rates for vulvar carcinoma have improved, most of the favorable data are related to the treatment of patients with early disease and an absence of regional lymph node metastases. In a 20-year period at the Mayo Clinic between 1955 and 1975, Podratz and associates reported an overall absolute 5-year cure rate of 75%, compared with an expected survival of 89% based on life table analysis of control subjects matched for sex and age. When corrected for intercurrent disease the 5-year survival rate was 90%, 81%, 68%, and 20% for stage I, II, III, and IV, respectively. Local recurrences were noted in 12% of patients with stage I and 10% with stage II disease, despite the fact that the surgical margins were reportedly negative for residual tumor.

The incidence of regional node metastasis profoundly affected the Mayo Clinic survival statistics. Among the 175 patients who underwent inguinal-femoral lymphadenectomy, 59 (34%) demonstrated metastatic involvement in one or more nodes. The 5-year survival rate fell precipitously from 90% in patients with no node involvement to 57% for patients with a single regional node involved. A further decline in the cure rate to 37% occurred when two or more regional nodes were positive for metastatic tumor. Among the 25% of cases with bilateral groin node metastasis, the 5-year survival rate was only 29%.

Experience from 136 cases treated at the Medical College of Wisconsin shows similar cure rates. The incidence of positive groin metastases increased with the stage of the disease: 5% in stage I, 18.5% in stage II,

60% in stage III, and 84% in stage IV, for an overall incidence of 30% of positive groin nodes among the 136 cases (Table 39-3). There was a 14% incidence of deep pelvic node metastases. The corrected 5-year survival rate with negative regional and pelvic nodes was 91%, whereas the cure rate fell to 30% in cases with positive inguinal-femoral nodes. Only 2 of 19 cases with positive pelvic nodes survived 5 years (11%), and there was no case of metastasis of pelvic nodes in the absence of positive inguinal-femoral nodes.

Nearly identical data have been published by Iversen and associates from the Norwegian Radium Hospital for the period between 1956 and 1974. Among 424 patients with squamous cell carcinoma of the vulva followed for 3 to 21 years, there was an incidence of 10.5% of lymph node metastases in stage I, 29.8% in stage II, 66.0% in stage III, and 100% in stage IV lesions. Using the life table analysis, the 5-year survival rate for the entire series was 67%, with 93% in stage I, 75% in stage II, 50% in stage III, and 15% in stage IV. Only 1 of 53 patients with unilateral inguinal-femoral node metastasis was found to have contralateral lymph node involvement.

The survival rates of 4531 cases reported to FIGO after treatment of vulvar cancer from 120 collaborators in the 10-year period from 1966 through 1975 are shown in Table 39-4. When analyzed by the life table method the survival data of 3953 cases of vulvar cancer reported to FIGO during this 10-year period are similar to current cure rates from North American clinics (Fig. 39-41).

In summary, the survival of patients with carcinoma of the vulva depends on many prognostic factors, including lesion size, tumor location, histologic features of differentiation, degree of cellular anaplasia, lymph vascular space involvement, and lymph node metastasis. In general, there is nearly uniform agreement that metastasis to the deep pelvic nodes does not occur

TABLE 39–3
Incidence of Regional Node Metastases

| STAGE | INCIDENCE (%) | | |
	UCLA* (n = 104)	Oslo† (n = 175)	MCW‡ (n = 136)
I	10.7	10	5
II	25	29.8	18.5
III	71.4	66	60
IV	100	100	84
Total	25	34	30

* University of California, Los Angeles: Hacker et al. Management of regional lymph nodes and their prognostic influence in vulvar cancer. Obstet Gynecol 1983;61:408.

† Oslo: Iverson et al., 1981.

‡ Medical College of Wisconsin, unpublished data.

TABLE 39–4
Survival Rates for Vulvar Cancer

STAGE	NO. OF CASES (%)	5-YEAR SURVIVAL (%)
I	1382 (30.5)	70.0
II	1367 (30.2)	49.1
III	1361 (30.0)	29.8
IV	388 (8.6)	8.2
Not Staged	33 (0.7)	30.3
Total	4531 (100)	46

(FIGO. Annual report on the results of treatment in cancer. Vol 18. Stockholm: Radiumhemmet, 1982.)

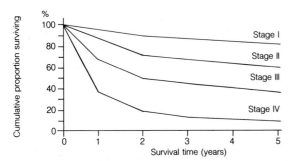

Figure 39–41. Life-table analysis of survival rates among 3953 cases of carcinoma of the vulva by stage of disease. (From FIGO Annual Report, vol 18, 1982)

in the absence of groin node metastases. Because the 5-year survival rate of 15% to 20% is not influenced by the dissection of positive pelvic nodes, there is no longer any rationale for performing this procedure. Instead, the currently preferred adjunctive treatment for the 25% to 35% of patients with positive groin nodes is whole pelvic radiotherapy with inclusion of the groins.

Recurrent Carcinoma of the Vulva

Recurrent carcinoma of the vulva is among the most difficult of all types of genital cancer to treat.

Way treated 39 patients with recurrent cancer by a variety of techniques: diathermy coagulation (10 cases), local excision (3 cases), and radical vulvectomy and node dissection (26 cases). Only 10 of the 26 patients treated by radical vulvectomy survived 5 years or more, whereas 2 of the 3 patients who had local excision of the recurrent tumor survived 5 years.

Buchler and colleagues treated 29 patients with recurrent vulvar carcinoma. Most of the tumors were

confined to the perineum (18 cases) or the groin and perineum (7 cases). Recurrent perineal disease was treated mainly by wide local excision (five patients), while three patients had radical vulvectomy with lymphadenectomy, one patient had a simple vulvectomy, and two patients required posterior exenteration. Irradiation treatment was provided by either external beam therapy or interstitial implants. Although the results were not ideal, 18 patients with perineal recurrence had an average survival of 43 months after surgery and an additional 26 months after irradiation. Two patients had no evidence of disease at 4 and 13 years.

Boronow (1982) treated seven patients with recurrent vulvar cancer with preoperative irradiation followed by vulvectomy. Five of the seven cases were alive from 1 to 3 years after therapy. Boronow's procedure is the preferred method of managing recurrent vulvar cancer, with wide local excision of perineal lesions and radiation therapy to recurrences in the groin or pelvis. It must be recognized that carcinoma of the vulva is characterized by local recurrence. In a large autopsy series of patients dying of vulvar cancer, it was noted that less than 10% died of extrapelvic disease; thus continued treatment of the local recurrences is of major importance.

UNCOMMON VULVAR CANCERS

Carcinoma of Bartholin's Gland

Lying in the vestibule, the only endodermal vestige of the urogenital sinus, is Bartholin's gland, nestled beneath the bulbocavernosus muscle, inferior to the vestibular bulb. The gland lies within the fascia that separates the superficial and deep perineal compartments of the urogenital diaphragm. The duct of the gland is lined by transitional epithelium, the minor ducts by low flat cuboidal epithelium, and the gland by mucus-secreting acini. The duct opens into the lateral wall of the vestibule just outside the hymenal ring and slightly below the midplane of the introitus. Most authorities consider Bartholin's gland and its duct to be components of the vulva because of their location.

Primary carcinoma of Bartholin's gland accounts for about 1% to 2% of vulvar cancers. Histologically, the lesions are divided into three groups: squamous cell carcinoma arising at the orifice, transitional cell carcinoma developing in the main duct, and adenoid cystic tumor arising in the glandular acini. Basically, the squamous cell carcinoma is a "vulvar" lesion and should be treated as such. There is no actual squamous component to the gland, and thus the nomenclature is erroneous. Furthermore, statistics that include all three varieties noted above are not realistic. Each of the variants has a definable genesis and demands a specific therapy.

Diagnostic Criteria

The original criteria for diagnosing a primary cancer of Bartholin's gland were established by Homan in 1897 and included (a) correct anatomic position of the tumor; (b) location deep in the labium; (c) intact overlying skin; and (d) presence of some elements of glandular epithelium.

Although all of these criteria may not be met by a single tumor, the anatomic site of the lesion is important, particularly if the remnants of the normal glandular epithelium are replaced by the tumor. It is particularly easy to misidentify an undifferentiated tumor as a lesion arising in the vulva.

Clinical Features

Patients with Bartholin's gland carcinoma are, on average, about 10 years younger than patients with other epithelial cancers of the vulva. The mean age is 57 years, and the range is from 14 to 85 years. The most common symptom is the presence of a vulvar mass or the occurrence of perineal discomfort, which frequently is treated as a Bartholin's gland cyst or abscess without initially establishing a correct diagnosis.

The clinical diagnosis of Bartholin's gland carcinoma frequently is delayed because the tumor is located beneath the bulbocavernosus muscle; vulvar ulceration and bleeding are absent. Only when the tumor erodes through the overlying vulvar skin does bleeding occur and the symptoms become more acute. In the report by Leuchter and colleagues 23% of their cases were incorrectly diagnosed as having a Bartholin's gland cyst or abscess and were inappropriately treated by incision and drainage or with the use of antibiotics for prolonged periods before the final diagnosis. The Leuchter series is typical of other reports, with a mean time of 10.8 months before the establishment of an accurate diagnosis.

Pathway of Spread and Treatment

The lymphatic drainage of Bartholin's gland parallels that of the vulva and outer portions of the vagina. As anticipated, primary lymphatic drainage is to the inguinal-femoral lymph nodes and secondary drainage is by way of the internal pudendal lymphatics to the pelvic lymph nodes. The incidence of inguinal-femoral node involvement with Bartholin's gland carcinomas is about one in three and twice the observed frequency of pelvic node extension. As with squamous carcinomas, pelvic node involvement in the absence of groin node metastasis occurs only in the exceptional case. The somewhat higher incidence of node involvement with neoplasms of Bartholin's gland probably reflects increased tumor volume, as diagnosis is delayed owing to the absence of symptoms early on.

Treatment of Bartholin's gland carcinoma does not differ substantially from the treatment outlined for typical squamous cancer. Radical vulvectomy and groin dissection remain the mainstay; however, owing to the histologic varieties of lesions that make up this entity, some individualization is appropriate.

Squamous carcinoma identified as Bartholin's gland tumors clearly should be dealt with as outlined above. The transitional cell carcinoma, arising within the duct, is rare but rather aggressive. Again, treatment parallels that of squamous cancers, but anticipated survivorship should be lower.

Adenoid-cystic tumors arising within the gland are unique and behave similarly to these lesions at other sites in the body, specifically tumors of the salivary glands. Local recurrences may be observed over a period of years, as well as late pulmonary metastasis. Vulvar dissection for adenoid-cystic tumors should be aggressive and extend to the level of the deep transverse perineal muscle. Frozen section analysis intraoperatively may be important to establish tumor-free deep margins, since the gland is anatomically close to the deep compartment of the urogenital diaphragm. Positive deep margins may be managed with reexcision or radiotherapy. Occasionally vaginectomy or partial rectal resection may be required to affect complete tumor extirpation. Regional node dissection is standardly performed, especially if tumor volume is large and lesions extend to involve skin, vagina, or rectum. Although the prognosis for adenoid-cystic carcinomas usually is more favorable, diligent surveillance for local recurrence should be emphasized. The latter should be addressed by wide excision and possibly localized radiation.

More conservative treatment may be considered for small Bartholin's gland carcinomas that lateralize to one labium. In such instances radical hemivulvectomy with bilateral groin dissection is undertaken; substantial tumor-free margins are sought.

Lymph node involvement patterns do not differ from squamous cell lesions. Contralateral nodes typically are negative unless ipsilateral node metastasis is present. Among 90 cases reviewed by Leuchter, only 1 patient out of 59 who underwent bilateral inguinal-femoral node dissection was found to have a contralateral lymph node involvement without metastasis of the ipsilateral groin. This may justify ipsilateral lymph node dissection; or irradiation of the opposite groin may be reserved for instances in which ipsilateral nodes are positive.

Pelvic lymphadenectomy has been proposed by Barclay and associates because of the acknowledged internal pudendal lymphatic pathway. Leuchter reviewed 25 cases in which both inguinal-femoral and pelvic node dissections were performed. In no instance were pelvic lymph nodes positive in the absence of inguinal-femoral involvement. As with squamous lesions, positive groin nodes are probably best addressed with groin and pelvic irradiation.

Survivorship and treatment modalities for Bartholin's gland carcinoma have been reported for 90 patients in Leuchter's series. A summary of this series is shown in Table 39-5.

Melanoma

Malignant melanoma, although allegedly uncommon, is the second leading primary vulvar neoplasm, behind squamous cell cancer. It usually accounts for up to 4% to 5% of vulvar cancers, or about 0.1% to 0.5% of all primary neoplasms of the female genital tract. The concept that most melanomas develop from melanocytic nevi (moles) is incorrect. Although some melanomas do arise from nevi, most arise as de novo lesions that clinically resemble nevi during early phases of their development. An extensive discussion of the dermal pathology of melanoma is not included here; the interested reader is referred to reports by Silvers and Halperin and Balch and Milton.

Melanomas may occur in any age group, most commonly in patients aged 27 to 75 years. The lesions must be distinguished from the deep brown pattern of seborrheic keratosis and from any chronically infected lesion; the latter often show pigment in the underlying tissue.

Focal lesions that are hyperpigmented should be studied by excisional biopsy, not by sampling a segment of the lesion. Most primary melanomas (80%) are located on the central vulvar structures and on the labia minora, clitoris, and introital mucosa, whereas most squamous carcinomas are located on the labia majora.

An understanding of the pathogenesis of melanoma has evolved from the microanatomy of the skin. The skin of the vulva, like the skin of the body, is composed of three distinct layers; epidermis, dermis, and subcutis. Two principal epidermal cell types are related to the development of melanoma: keratinocyte and melanocyte. The keratinocyte (squamous cell) is of ectodermal origin, and gives rise to the stratified squamous epithelium and the overlying keratin layer on the vulva. The melanocyte is the pigment-producing cell in the basal layer of the vulvar epithelium and is derived from the neural crest. The melanocyte produces pigment granules in the skin and transfers them to neighboring keratinocytes. As described by Silvers and Halperin, the melanocyte is the site of pigment production, whereas the keratinocyte serves as a reservoir for the pigment.

The dermis lies between the epidermis and the underlying subcutis. The upper portion of the dermis contains collagen bundles and is called the *papillary dermis*. The lower two-thirds of the dermis, which contains collagen fibers that are tightly bound together, is termed the *reticular dermis*.

Conventional staging systems for vulvar squamous carcinoma have limited application to prediction of biologic behavior for melanomas. Consequently Clark

TABLE 39–5
Treatment Modalities and 5-Year Survival for Bartholin's Gland Carcinoma

TREATMENT	PATIENTS TREATED		5-YEAR SURVIVORS FREE OF DISEASE	
	Number	*Percent*	*Number*	*Percent*
Local excision	12	13.3	1	3.8
Local excision + radiation therapy	8	8.9	2	7.7
Radical vulvectomy	4	4.5	2	7.7
Radical vulvectomy + nodes	51	56.7	20	77.0
Radical vulvectomy, nodes,* + radiation therapy	7	7.8	1	3.8
Exenteration	2	2.2	0	
Radiation therapy only	2	2.2	0	
Chemotherapy	1	1.1	0	
Biopsy only	2	1.1	0	
Unknown	1	1.1	0	
Total	90	100	26	100

* Inguinal-femoral nodes only.
(Leuchter RS, Hacker NS, Vote RL, et al. Primary carcinoma of the Bartholin's gland: a report of 14 cases and review of the literature. Obstet Gynecol 1982;60:361.)

and associates and McGovern have proposed a classification for primary cutaneous melanomas that is related to the microanatomy of the skin. Utilizing this approach, these investigators divide primary cutaneous melanomas into three basic types: lentigo maligna melanoma, superficial spreading melanoma, and nodular melanoma. Each type has a relatively distinct clinical and histologic appearance.

Superficial spreading melanoma is the most common type, accounting for about 80% of melanoma cases. Nodular melanoma, unlike the other two types, does not have a clinically identifiable in situ phase. The nodular lesion apparently rises from a proliferation of melanocytes within the epidermis and rapidly extends vertically into the underlying dermis and connective tissues. Nodular melanoma has a poor prognosis, but fortunately it represents only 10% of all melanomas. Lenitgo maligna melanoma, which accounts for the remaining 10%, and superficial spreading melanoma have a relatively long in situ phase characterized by a spread in a radial or centrifugal manner before significant dermal invasion occurs. The in situ phase of melanomas may persist as long as 5 or more years.

The prognosis of the patient with melanoma is largely related to the histology of the lesion and the level of involvement of the underlying dermal tissues.

CLARK'S CLASSIFICATION OF LEVELS OF INVOLVEMENT	
CLASSIFICATION	*DESCRIPTION*
Level I	Intraepithelial
Level II	Extending into papillary layer of dermis
Level III	Filling dermal papillae
Level IV	Invading bundles of collagen in reticular dermis
Level V	Invading subcutaneous fat

When the subcutaneous fat has been invaded, as in the level V lesion, the potential for regional and pelvic node involvement is high and the survival rate is low. Clark reported an 8.3% mortality rate in level II melanoma, 35.2% in level III lesions, 46.1% in level IV lesions, and 52% in level V tumors.

As stated above, most melanomas arise in central vulvar locations and subsequently involve the mucous membrane. Clark's microstaging system, which relies on delineation of the upper and lower papillary dermis and the interface with the deeper reticular dermis, is not as applicable here compared with cutaneous sites. An alternative microstaging system, proposed by Breslow, has been successfully applied and widely adopted. This system assesses lesions by measured vertical thickness from the top of the granular layer to the point of deepest invasion. In cutaneous melanomas the Breslow system of vertical thickness appears to be more prognostic of recurrence risk and regional node involvement than Clark's levels of invasion. Whichever microstaging system is used, in the absence of clinically evident metastasis, more predictive information is obtained than by using conventional FIGO staging methods for vulvar cancer. Chung, Woodruff, and coworkers has combined principles from Clark and Breslow classifications (Fig. 39-42).

Treatment

Treatment of vulvar melanoma is almost exclusively surgical. Radical vulvectomy with bilateral inguinal-femoral lymphadenectomy has traditionally been advocated; however, it is clear that this treatment is excessive in many patients and inadequate in others. Data derived from treatment of patients evaluated by microstaging have permitted modification in the surgical approach. These include patients with genital and extragenital melanomas. Lesion thickness has been used to tailor surgical procedures. The melanoma should be excised, and if on thorough sectioning it demonstrates less than 0.76-mm thickness, wide excision with 2-cm margins is adequate therapy. For cutaneous lesions the risk of node involvement is 1%; hence regional node dissection is unnecessary. Similar behavior can be assumed for vulvar lesions. Lesions that exceed 0.76 mm should be excised more radically, with attention to deep tissue planes, wider margins of resection, and lymph node status. Margins of 3 to 4 cm are probably adequate, and the extent of regional node dissection may be tempered by melanoma thickness. Lesions up to 1.49 mm may warrant a less aggressive groin node sampling, whereas greater thickness should mandate thorough dissection.

For localized lesions wide excision is preferred to radical vulvectomy. The latter does not confer additional therapeutic benefit by removal of uninvolved, particularly contralateral aspects of the vulva. The major objective in the surgical treatment is the need to secure adequate tumor-free margins of resection. A recent report from Rose and associates supports conservative surgical approaches. The primary concern for suboptimal therapy is at the vulvovaginal and vulvourethral regions. Standard vulvectomy does not yield adequate margins centrally. The disease has a predilection for clitoral and introital structures, and the central recurrence rate of 30% or greater attests to difficulty in attaining adequate margins (Fig. 39-43). When the vagina or distal urethra are involved, particularly for a thick lesion, consideration should be given to vaginectomy and anterior exenteration.

Controversy exists regarding the role of regional

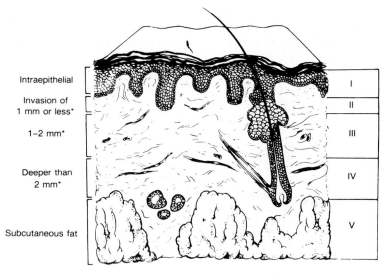

Intraepithelial

Invasion of
1 mm or less*

1–2 mm*

Deeper than
2 mm*

Subcutaneous fat

I
II
III
IV
V

*As measured from the granular layer of surface
epithelium

Figure 39–42. Levels of invasion of vulvar melanoma. Level I (melanoma confined to the surface epithelium and pilar sheath) and level V (tumor extension into the underlying adipose tissue) are the same as Clark's levels I and V. Levels II, III, and IV are determined by measurements from the granular layer of the vulvar skin or outermost epithelial layer of the squamous mucosa. (From Chung AF, Woodruff JM, Lewis JL Jr. Malignant melanoma of the vulva: A report of 44 cases. Obstet Gynecol 1975; 45:638)

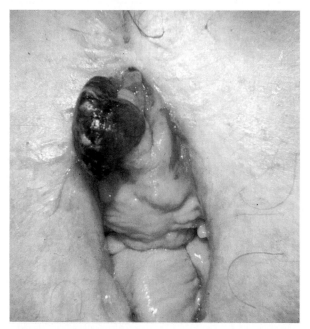

Figure 39–43. Central recurrence of malignant melanoma. Primary lesion involved right labium minus with invasion to Clark's level V. Despite radical vulvectomy, lesion recurred centrally at vulvovaginal junction and urethral meatus.

lymphadenectomy. Groin node metastasis occurs in 20% to 45% of cases in which lymphadenectomy is performed. Not infrequently the nodal involvement is clinically apparent. Excluding the lesion of less than 0.76-mm thickness, nodal involvement is substantial. The problematic issue is defining clinical benefit from

performing lymphadenectomy. There is little doubt that nodal status is of prognostic importance, but lymphadenectomy is unlikely to be curative. If groin lymph nodes are positive, irradiation may be offered, but responses are much less likely compared with squamous lesions. Further confusion exists regarding the role of pelvic lymph node dissection. Although probably not indicated on a routine basis, Chung, Woodruff, and coworkers has reported long-term survivors with positive pelvic nodes. It would appear that groin nodes should be done through separate incisions to minimize morbidity.

The use of the chemotherapeutic agent dimethyl-triazene-imidazole-carboxamide (DTIC; dacarbazine) has produced tumor regression in 20% to 25% of patients with disseminated disease. Immunotherapy also is used in some clinics, although the treatment has been used in only a limited number of patients with only limited success as a temporary control of the disease. Nevertheless, such treatment appears to be the therapy of choice for the future.

Survival

Data on the survival of patients with malignant melanoma of the vulva are difficult to accumulate because the lesion occurs infrequently. In a collected series of 155 patients reported by Morrow and Rutledge in 1981 the overall survival rate for all stages of the disease was 34% (Table 39-6). Among 129 cases of vulvar melanoma presented in the annual report of FIGO during the 10-year period from 1966 to 1975, the 5-year survival rate was 31.8%.

TABLE 39–6
Vulvar Melanoma: 5-Year Survival

STUDY	NO. OF CASES	NO. ELIGIBLE FOR 5-YEAR FOLLOW-UP	ALIVE AT 5 YEARS	
			Number	*Percent*
Pack and Oropeza (1967)	31*	20	7	35
Yackel et al. (1970)	27	20	7	35
Morrow and Rutledge (1972)	30	14	7	50
Chung et al. (1975)	44	33	10	30
Karlen et al. (1975)	23	20	5	25
Total	155	107	36	(34)

*Includes three vaginal melanomas.
(Morrow CP. Gynecologic oncology: fundamental principles and clinical practice. Vol 2. New York: Churchill Livingstone, 1981.)

TABLE 39–7
Vulvar Melanoma: Survival and Microstaging

CLARK MICROSTAGING			BRESLOW MICROSTAGING		
Level	*No. of Patients*	*Percentage Alive*	*Lesion Thickness (mm)*	*No. of Patients*	*Percentage Alive*
II	16	100	<0.76	17	100
III	18	72	0.76–1.49	14	72
IV	31	50	1.50–3.0	33	55
V	30	27	>3.0	32	22

(Chung AF et al. Malignant melanoma of the vulva: a report of 44 cases. Obstet Gynecol 1975;45:638; Jaramillo BA et al. Malignant melanoma of the vulva. Obstet Gynecol 1985;66:398; Podratz KC et al. Melanoma of the vulva. An update. Gynecol Oncol 1983;16:153.)

A number of investigators have evaluated survival as a function of level of invasion and tumor thickness. These data are summarized in Table 39-7. Chung, Woodruff, and coworkers reported no tumor-related deaths or nodal metastasis for level II disease, contrasted with 60% mortality in levels III and IV. Podratz and colleagues reported similar trends, but overall better survival with level III and IV lesions and lesions less than 3-mm thickness. More recently Jaramillo and coworkers confirmed these findings. All studies demonstrated the superior predictive value of microstaging. The rationale of more limited surgery for early invasive vulvar melanomas is sustained by these studies.

Bibliography

Addison A, Parker RT. Adenoid cystic carcinoma of Bartholin's gland: a review of the literature and report of a patient. Gynecol Oncol 1977;5:196.

Andersen BL, Hacker NF. Psychosocial adjustment following vulvectomy. Obstet Gynecol 1983;62:457.

Aquinaga A. Cancer de glandula de Bartholin. Obstet Ginecol Latinoam 1944;2:178.

Baggish MS, Sze EH, Adelson MD, et al. Quantitative evaluation of the skin and accessory appendages in vulvar carcinoma in situ. Obstet Gynecol 1989;74:169.

Balch CM, Milton GW. Cutaneous melanoma. Philadelphia: JB Lippincott, 1985.

Ballon SC, Lagasse LD, Change NH, et al. Primary adenocarcinoma of the vagina. Cancer 1977;40:101.

Barclay DL, Collins CR, Macey HB. Cancer of the Bartholin gland: a review and report of 8 cases. Obstet Gynecol 1964;24:329.

Baronofsky ID. Technique of inguinal node dissection. Surgery 1964;24:329.

Basset A. Traitement chirurgical operatoire de l'epithelioma primiftif du clitoris. Rev Chir 1912;46:546.

Becker TM, Stone KM, Alexander RE. Genital human papillomavirus infection: a growing concern. Clin Obstet Gynecol 1987;14:389.

Beisky A. Über kraurosis vulvae. Z Heik (Prague) 1885;6:69.

Bergen S, Di Saia PJ, Liao SY, et al. Conservative management of extramammary Paget's disease of the vulva. Gynecol Oncol 1989;33, 151.

Bornstein J, Kaufman RH. Combination of surgical excision and carbon dioxide laser vaporization for multifocal vulvar intraepithelial neoplasia. Am J Obstet Gynecol 1988;158:459.

Boronow RC. Therapeutic alternative to primary exenteration for advanced vulvovaginal cancer. Gynecol Oncol 1973;1:233.

Boronow RC. Combined therapy as an alternative to exenteration for locally advanced vulvovaginal cancer. Cancer 1982;49:1083.

Bowen JD. Precancerous dermatoses. J Cutan Dis 1912;30:241.

Breen JL, Neubecker RD, Greenwald E, et al. Basal cell carcinoma of the vulva. Obstet Gynecol 1975;46:122.

Breslow A. Thickness, cross-sectional areas, and depth of invasion in the prognosis of cutaneous melanoma. Ann Surg 1970;172:902.

Breslow A. Tumor thickness, level of invasion and node dissection in Stage I cutaneous melanoma. Ann Surg 1975;182:572.

Brunschwig A, Daniel W. Pelvic exenteration for advanced carcinoma of the vulva. Am J Obstet Gynecol 1956;72:489.

Buchler DA, Cline JC, Tunca JC, et al. Treatment of recurrent carcinoma of the vulva. Gynecol Oncol 1979;8:180.

Buscema J, Naghashfar Z, Sawada E, et al. The predominance of human papillomavirus type 16 in vulvar neoplasia. Obstet Gynecol 1988;71:601.

Buscema J, Stern J, Woodruff JD. The significance of histologic alterations adjacent to invasive vulvar carcinoma. Am J Obstet Gynecol 1980;137:902.

Buscema J, Woodruff JD, Parmley TH, et al. Carcinoma in situ of the vulva. Obstet Gynecol 1980;55:225.

Byron RL, Lamb EJ, Yonemoto RH, et al. Radical inguinal node dissection in the treatment of cancer. Surg Gynecol Obstet 1962;114:401.

Calame RJ. Pelvic relaxation as a complication of radical vulvectomy. Obstet Gynecol 1980;55:716.

Cavanagh D, Shepherd JH. The place of pelvic exenteration in the primary management of advanced carcinoma of the vulva. Gynecol Oncol 1982;13:318.

Chamlian DL, Taylor HB. Primary carcinoma of Bartholin's gland: a report of 24 patients. Obstet Gynecol 1972;39:489.

Charleswood GP, Shippel S. Vulva and condylomata acuminata as a premalignant lesion in the Bantu. S Afr Med J 1953;27:149.

Chung AF, Krumerman M. Hypercalcemia complicating vulvar carcinoma. NY State J Med 1977;84:1763.

Chung AF, Woodruff JM, Lewis JL. Malignant melanoma of the vulva: a report of cases. Obstet Gynecol 1975;45:638.

Clark WH, From L, Bernardino EA, et al. The histogenesis and biologic behavior of primary human malignant melanomas of the skin. Cancer Res 1969;29:705.

Clark-Pearson DL, Synan IS, Hinshaw WM, et al. Prevention of postoperative venous thrombo-embolism by external pneumatic catheter compression in patients with gynecologic malignancy. Obstet Gynecol 1984;63:92.

Collins CG, Hansen LH, Theriot EA. Clinical stain for use in selecting biopsy sites in patients with vulvar disease. Obstet Gynecol 1966;28:158.

Crocker HR. Paget's disease, affecting the scrotum and penis. Trans Pathol Soc Lond 1889;40:187.

Curry SL, Wharton JT, Rutledge F. Positive lymph nodes in vulvar squamous carcinoma. Gynecol Oncol 1980;9:63.

Daly JW, Million RI. Radical vulvectomy combined with elective node irradiation for squamous carcinoma of the vulva. Cancer 1974;34:161.

Davis BL, Robinson DG. Diverticula of the female urethra: assay of 120 cases. J Urol 1970;104:850.

DiPaola GR, Gomez-Rueda N, Arrighi L. Relevance of microinvasion in carcinoma of the vulva. Obstet Gynecol 1975;45:647.

DiSaia PJ, Creasman WT, Rich WH. An alternate approach to early cancer of the vulva. Am J Obstet Gynecol 1979;133:825.

DiSaia PJ, Morrow CP, Townsend DE, eds. Synopsis of gynecologic oncology. New York: John Wiley & Sons, 1975.

Dodson DL, Collins CG, Macey HB. Cancer of Bartholin's gland. Obstet Gynecol 1970;35:578.

Donaldson ES, Powell DE, Hanson MB, et al. Prognostic parameters in invasive vulvar cancer. Gynecol Oncol 1981;11:184.

Dubreuilh W. Paget's disease of the vulva. Br J Dermatol 1901;13:497.

Ferenczy A, Mitao M, Nagai N, et al. Latent papillomavirus and recurring genital warts. N Engl J Med 1985;313:784.

Fetherston WC, Friedrich EG Jr. Origin and significance of vulvar Paget's disease. Obstet Gynecol 1972;39:735.

FIGO. Annual report on the results of treatment in cancer. Vol 18. Stockholm: Radiumhemmet, 1982.

Fisher JR, Conway MJ, Takeshita RT, et al. Necrotizing fasciitis. Importance of roentgenographic studies for soft-tissue gas. JAMA 1979;241:803.

Franklin EW III, Rutledge F. Prognostic factors in epidermoid carcinoma of the vulva. Obstet Gynecol 1971;37:892.

Friedman-Kien AE, Eron LJ, Conaut M, et al. Natural interferon alfa for treatment of condylomata acuminata. JAMA 1988;259:533.

Friedrich EG Jr. Vulvar disease: diagnosis and management. 2nd ed. Philadelphia: WB Saunders, 1983.

Friedrich EG Jr, Wilkinson EJ. Mucous cyst of the vulvar vestibule. Obstet Gynecol 1973;42:407.

Friedrich EG, Wilkinson EJ, Steingraeber PH, Lewis JD. Paget's disease of the vulva and carcinoma of the breast. Obstet Gynecol 1975;46:130.

Gardiner J. Modified technic of inguinal lymphadenectomy. Obstet Gynecol 1966;28:147.

Green TH Jr. Radical vulvectomy. Clin Obstet Gynecol 1965;8:642.

Green TH Jr. Carcinoma of the vulva: a reassessment. Obstet Gynecol 1978;52:462.

Hacker NF, Berek JS, Lagasse LD. Management of regional lymph nodes and their prognostic influence in vulvar cancer. Obstet Gynecol 1983;61:408.

Hacker NF, Berek JS, Lagasse LD, et al. Individualization of treatment for stage I squamous cell vulvar carcinoma. Obstet Gynecol 1984;13:155.

Hacker NF, Leuchter RS, Berek JS, et al. Radical vulvectomy and bilateral inguinal lymphadenectomy through separate groin incisions. Obstet Gynecol 1981;58:574.

Hay DM, Cole FM. Primary invasive carcinoma of the vulva in Jamaica. J Obstet Gynecol Br Commonw 1961;67:821.

Helwig EB. Cited by Koss LG, Ladinsky S, Brockunier A Jr. Paget's disease of the vulva: a report of 10 cases. Obstet Gynecol 1968;31:513.

Hey W. Practical observations in surgery. Philadelphia: James Humphreys, 1805.

Homan JH. Uber die Carciome der gladulae Bartholini. Inaugural dissertation, Berlin, 1897.

Homesley HD, Bundy BN, Sedlis A, et al. Radiation therapy versus pelvic node dissection for carcinoma of the vulva with positive groin nodes. Obstet Gynecol 1986;68:733.

International Society for the Study of Vulvar Disease, Committee on Terminology. New nomenclature for vulvar disease. Obstet Gynecol 1976;47:122.

International Society for the Study of Vulvar Disease, Committee on Terminology. New nomenclature for vulvar disease. Am J Obstet Gynecol 1989;160:769.

Iversen T, Aalders JG, et al. Squamous cell carcinoma of the vulva: a review of 424 patients, 1956–1974. Gynecol Oncol 1980;9:271.

Iversen T, Aas M. Pelvic lymphoscintigraphy with ^{99m}Tc-colloid in lymph node metastases. Eur J Nucl Med 1982;7:455.

Iversen T, Abeler D, Aalders JG. Individualized treatment of Stage I carcinoma of the vulva. Obstet Gynecol 1981;57:85.

Jafari K, Cartnick EN. Microinvasive squamous cell carcinoma of the vulva. Gynecol Oncol 1976;4:158.

Japaze H, Dinh T, Woodruff JD. Verrucous carcinoma of the vulva: study of 24 cases. Obstet Gynecol 1982;60:462.

Jaramillo BA, Ganjei P, Averette HE. Malignant melanoma of the vulva. Obstet Gynecol 1985;66:398.

Jeffcoate TNA. Chronic vulvar dystrophies. Am J Obstet Gynecol 1966;95:61.

Jeffries DJ. Acyclovir update. Br Med J 1986;293:1523.

Julian CG, Callison J, Woodruff JD. Plastic management of extensive vulvar defects. Obstet Gynecol 1971;38:193.

Kakar VV. Prevention of fatal postoperative pulmonary embolism by low dose heparin: an international multicenter trial. Lancet 1975;2:45.

Karlen JR, Piver MS, Barlow JJ. Melanoma of the vulva. Obstet Gynecol 1975;45:181.

Kaufman RH, Gardner HL, Brown D Jr, et al. Vulvar dystrophies: an evaluation. Am J Obstet 1974;120:363.

Kehrer E. Soll das Vulvakarzinom operiert oder bestrahlt werden? Geburtsh & Franuenk 1918;48:346.

Knight RV. Bowen's disease. Am J Obstet Gynecol 1943;6:514.

Koss LG, Ladinsky S, Brockunier A Jr. Paget's disease of the vulva. Obstet Gynecol 1968;31:513.

Krupp PJ, Bohm JW. Lymph gland metastases in invasive squamous cell cancer of the vulva. Am J Obstet Gynecol 1978;130:943.

Krupp PJ, Lee FYL, Bohm JW, et al. Prognostic parameters and clinical staging criteria in epidermoid carcinoma of the vulva. Obstet Gynecol 1975;46:84.

Leuchter RS, Hacker NF, Vote RL, et al. Primary carcinoma of the Bartholin's gland: a report of 14 cases and review of the literature. Obstet Gynecol 1982;60:361.

McCraw JB, Massey FM. Vaginal reconstruction with gracilis myocutaneous flaps. Plast Reconstr Surg 1976;58:176.

McGovern VJ. The classification of melanoma and its relationship with prognosis. Pathology 1970;2:85.

McKay M. Subsets of vulvodynia. J Reprod Med 1988;3308:695.

McLellan R, Buscema J, Anasti J, et al. Vulvar sarcoma: a clinicopathologic review. (in press).

MaGrina JF, Webb MJ, Gaffey TA, et al. Stage I squamous cell cancer of the vulva. Am J Obstet Gynecol 1979;134:453.

Marcus SL. Multiple squamous cell carcinomas involving the cervix, vagina and vulva: the theory of multicentric origin. Am J Obstet Gynecol 1960;80:802.

Masterson JG, Goss AS. Carcinoma of the Bartholin's gland: review of the literature and report of a new case in an elderly patient treated by radical operation. Am J Obstet Gynecol 1955;69:1323.

Matthews D. Marsupialization in the treatment of Bartholin's cyst and abscesses. J Obstet Gynecol Br Commonw 1966;73:1010.

Meeker WR, Sickle-Santanello BJ, Philpott G, et al. Combined chemotherapy, radiation, and surgery for epithelial cancer of the anal canal. Cancer 1986;57:525.

Mering JH. A surgical approach to intractable pruritus vulvae. Am J Obstet Gynecol 1952;64:619.

Moran AJ, Parry-Jones E. The surgical treatment of invasive squamous carcinoma of the vulva using a modified incision. Ir Med J 1950;73:426.

Moran AJ, Parry-Jones E. Cancer of the vulva: a review. Cancer 1981;48(suppl 2):597.

Morley GW. Infiltrative carcinoma of the vulva: results of surgical treatment. Am J Obstet Gynecol 1976;124:874.

Morris JM. A formula for selective lymphadenectomy: its application to cancer of the vulva. Obstet Gynecol 1977;50:152.

Morrow CP, Rutledge FN. Melanoma of the vulva. Obstet Gynecol 1971;39:745.

Nakao CY, Nolan JF, DiSaia PJ, et al. "Microinvasive" epidermoid carcinoma of the vulva with an unexpected natural history. Am J Obstet Gynecol 1974;120:1122.

Niebyl JR, Genadry R, Friedrich EG, et al. Vulvar carcinoma with hypercalcemia. Obstet Gynecol 1975;45:343.

Novak ER, Woodruff JD. Gynecologic and obstetric pathology. 8th ed. Philadelphia: WB Saunders, 1979.

Oriel JD. Genital warts. In: KK Holmes, PA Mardh, PF Sparling, PJ Wiesner, eds. Sexually transmitted diseases. New York: McGraw-Hill, 1984:496.

Pack GT, Oropeza R. A comparative study of melanomas and epider-

moid carcinomas of the vulva: a review of 44 melanomas and 58 epidermoid carcinomas (1930–1965). Rev Surg 1967;24:305.

Paget J. Disease of the mammary areola, preceding cancer of the mammary gland. St. Bartholomew's Hospital Rep 1874;10:87.

Parmley T, Woodruff JD, Julian CG. Invasive vulvar Paget's disease. Obstet Gynecol 1975;46:341.

Parry-Jones E. Lymphatics of the vulva. J Obstet Gynecol Br Commonw 1963;70:751.

Phillips B, Buchsbaum HJ, Lifshitz S. Pelvic exenteration for vulvovaginal carcinoma. Am J Obstet Gynecol 1981;141:1038.

Plentl AA, Friedman EA. Lymphatic system of the female genitalia. Philadelphia: WB Saunders, 1971.

Podratz KC, Symmonds RE, O'Brien PC, et al. Melanoma of the vulva: an update. Gynecol Oncol 1983;16:153.

Podratz KC, Symmonds RE, Taylor WF, et al. Carcinoma of the vulva: analysis of treatment and survival. Obstet Gynecol 1983;61:63.

Pringle JH. A method of operation in cases of melanotic tumours of the skin. Edinburgh Med J 1908;23:496.

Purola E, Widholm O. Primary carcinoma of the Bartholin's gland: report on two cases. Acta Obstet Gynecol Scand 1966;45:205.

Reid R, Greenberg M, Jenson AB, et al. Sexually transmitted papillomaviral infections. I. The anatomic distribution and pathologic grade of neoplastic lesions associated with different viral types. Am J Obstet Gynecol 1987;156:212.

Rose PG, Piver MS, Tsukada Y, et al. Conservative therapy for melanoma of the vulva. Am J Obstet Gynecol 1988;159:52.

Rutledge FN, Boronow RC, Wharton JT. Gynecologic oncology. New York: John Wiley & Sons, 1976.

Sappy C. Traite d'Anatomie, Physiologie et Pathologie des Vaisseaux Lymphatiques, Consideres Chez l'Homme et les Vertebres. Paris: Delahaye, 1874.

Schatten WE, Ship AG, Pieper WJ, et al. Syndrome resembling hyperparathyroidism associated with squamous cell carcinoma. Ann Surg 1958;148:890.

Schueller EF. Basal cell cancer of the vulva. Am J Obstet Gynecol 1965;93:199.

Schwimmer E. Die idiopathischen schlim haut der mundhohle, Vrljscher Dermatol Syph 1877;9-10-510.

Shatz P, Bergeron C, Wilkinson EJ, et al. Vulvar intraepithelial neoplasia and skin appendage involvement. Obstet Gynecol 1989;74:769.

Silvers DN, Halperin AJ. Cutaneous and vulvar melanoma: an update. Clin Obstet Gynecol 1978;21:1117.

Stoeckel W. Wie lassen sich die Dauerresultate bei der Operation des Vulvakarzinoms verbessern. Zbl Gynak 1912;36:1102.

Tancer ML. Bartholin's cysts paraurethral lesions. Clin Obstet Gynecol 1965;8:982.

Tashjian AH, Levine L, Munson PL. Immunochemical identification of parathyroid hormone in non-parathyroid neoplasms associated with hypercalcemia. J Exp Med 1964;119:467.

Taussig FJH. Leukoplakic vulvitis and cancer of the vulva (etiology, histopathology, treatment, five-year results). Trans Am Gynecol Soc 1929;54:60.

Taussig FJH. Diseases of the vulva. New York: Appleton-Century-Crofts, 1931.

Trelford JD, Deos PH. Bartholin's gland carcinomas: five cases. Gynecol Oncol 1976;4:212.

Tsukada Y, Lopez RG, Pickren JW. Paget's disease of the vulva. Obstet Gynecol 1975;45:73.

Wahlstrom T, Vesterinen E, Saksela E. Primary carcinoma of Bartholin's gland: a morphological and clinical study of 6 cases including a transitional cell carcinoma. Gynecol Oncol 1978;6:354.

Watring WG, Roberts JA, Lagasse LD, et al. Treatment of recurrent Paget's disease of the vulva with topical bleomycin. Cancer 1978;41:10.

Way S. The anatomy of the lymphatic drainage of the vulva and its influence on the radical operation for carcinoma. Ann R Coll Surg Engl 1948;3:187.

Way S. Carcinoma of the vulva. In: Deeley TJ, ed. Modern radiotherapy: gynecological cancer. London: Butterworths, 1971.

Way S. Malignant diseases of the vulva. New York: Churchill Livingston, 1982.

Way S, Benedet MD. Involvement of inguinal lymph nodes in carcinoma of the vulva. Gynecol Oncol 1973;119:119.

Wharton JT. Carcinoma of the vagina. In: Rutledge F, Boronow RC, Wharton JT, eds. Gynecologic oncology. New York: John Wiley & Sons, 1976.

Wharton JT, Gallager S, Rutledge FN. Microinvasive carcinoma of the vulva. Am J Obstet Gynecol 1974;118:159.

Wharton LR, Kearnes W. Diverticulum of the female urethra. J Urol 1950;63:1063.

Wharton LR Jr, Everett HS. Primary malignant Bartholin gland tumors. Obstet Gynecol Surv 1951;6:1.

Wheeless CR Jr, McGibbon B, Dorsey JH, et al. Gracilis myocutaneous flap in reconstruction of the vulva and female perineum. Obstet Gynecol 1979;54:97.

Wilkinson EJ, Rico MJ, Pierson KK. Microinvasive carcinoma of the vulva. Int J Gynecol Pathol 1982;1:30.

Williams K, Butcher HR Jr. A technique for inguinal and iliac lymphadenectomy. Am Surg 1961;27:55.

Woodruff JD, Genadry R, Poliakoff S. Treatment of dyspareunia and vaginal outlet distortions by perineoplasty. Obstet Gynecol 1981;57:750.

Woodruff JD, Hildebrandt EE. Carcinoma in situ of the vulva. Obstet Gynecol 1958;12:414.

Woodruff JD, Julian C, Paray T, et al. The contemporary challenge of carcinoma in situ of the vulva. Am J Obstet Gynecol 1973;115:677.

Woodruff JD, Richardson EH Jr. Malignant vulvar Paget's disease. Obstet Gynecol 1957;10:10.

Woodruff JD, Thompson B. Local alcohol injection in the treatment of vulvar pruritus. Obstet Gynecol 1972;40:18.

Yackel DB, Symmonds RE, Kempers RD. Melanoma of the vulva. Obstet Gynecol 1970;35:625.

Surgical Conditions of the Vagina and Urethra

40

JOHN A. ROCK

THE VAGINA

Imperforate Hymen and Its Complications

The hymen represents a junction of the sinovaginal bulbs with the urogenital sinus. The hymen is composed of endoderm from the urogenital sinus epithelium. It is perforated during embryonic life to establish a connection between the lumen of the vaginal canal and the vestibule. The hymen may be cribriform in appearance. If there are no perforations through this membrane, the hymen is imperforate. Figure 40-1 shows a hymen that is almost imperforate. An opening the size of a pinhead was sufficient to permit the entrance of sperm, and pregnancy ensued.

Although variations in hymen development occur, complete failure to form an orifice is rare. Pokorny and Kozinetz recently presented the various configurations and anatomic details of the prepubertal hymen. In a case series of 265 children with known genital problems, there were three main hymenal configurations: fimbriated, circumferential, and posterior rim. Interestingly, bleeding without a history of trauma was associated with hymenal bumps or breaks suggestive of trauma (31%) or with other hemorrhagic vulvar lesions (40%).

Symptoms

If an imperforate hymen is noticed before puberty, the condition can be treated before symptoms develop.

Some observant mothers notice the absence of an orifice in their daughters' hymens before puberty, when the condition is entirely asymptomatic. When the hymen is incised, the vagina is found to contain mucoid fluid, which results from accumulated cervical secretion.

Most patients are brought to the gynecologist at 13 to 15 years of age when their mothers begin to notice symptoms and the girls appear not to have begun menstruating. The symptoms that appear after the onset of puberty are due to the accumulation of menstrual blood. The blood of the first period or two is collected in the vagina. The vagina can hold blood from one or two cycles without undue stretching and with no other symptoms. Accumulation of menstrual blood in the vagina is termed *hematocolpos*. The patient may feel a little fatigue and have crampy discomfort suggesting menstruation, but no blood appears at the vaginal outlet.

As menstruation recurs the vagina becomes greatly overdistended, and the cervical canal also dilates. *Hematometra,* which is the accumulation of menstrual blood in the uterine cavity, may occur. When the intrauterine pressure reaches a certain point, there is retrograde passage of blood into the tubes, forming *hematosalpinx.* Adhesion formation within or at the fimbriated end of the tubes can seal them, and little or no blood may enter the peritoneal cavity. In some cases blood passes freely into the peritoneal cavity, forming *hematoperitoneum* (Fig. 40-2).

The most common symptoms caused by vaginal overdistention are lower abdominal pain, discomfort in

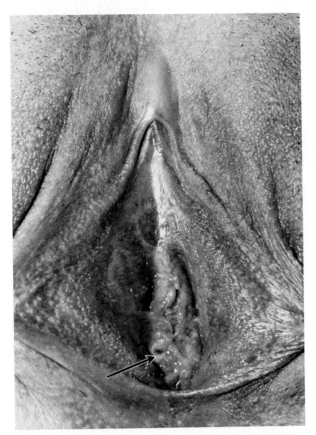

Figure 40–1. Hymen that is almost imperforate. The pinhead-sized opening was sufficient to permit pregnancy.

the pelvis, and pain in the lower back. Pain often is aggravated on defecation. Urination also can be difficult because pressure of the distended vagina on the urethra may compress the urethra and prevent emptying of the bladder. Cramplike pains recur in the suprapubic region, along with the common urologic symptoms of dysuria, frequency, and urgency. Overflow incontinence may eventually develop.

When the patient is examined a tender mass often is palpable suprapubically, the result of uterine enlargement and upward displacement, or bladder distention, or both. If hematoperitoneum occurs, the irritation of the free blood may cause the patient to experience all the symptoms and demonstrate signs of peritonitis. Protrusion of the hymen usually is visible; in some instances the protrusion is massive and dark in color because the occult blood shows through the stretched mucous membrane.

At the Johns Hopkins Hospital 22 patients with an imperforate hymen were operated on between 1945 and 1981. The mean age at surgical correction was 14.7 years. Associated anomalies, including urinary tract anomalies, were rare. Thirteen patients subsequently conceived and 10 patients were noted to have living children at the time of the report. The greater distensibility of the vagina in adolescence probably protects patients with imperforate hymen from retrograde menstruation and subsequent development of pelvic endometriosis as long as the diagnosis is made reasonably early.

Treatment

When an imperforate hymen is discovered before puberty, the hymenal membrane is simply incised, preferably at the 2, 4, 8, and 10 o'clock positions. The quadrants of the hymen are then excised and the mucosal margins are approximated with fine delayed absorbable suture (Fig. 40-3). If hematocolpos has already developed (see Fig. 40-2), all unnecessary intrauterine instrumentation should be avoided because of the risk of perforating the thin overstretched uterine wall. To prevent scarring and stenosis, which could result in dyspareunia, the hymenal tissue should not be excised too close to the vaginal mucosa.

Nothing more is needed surgically unless the uterine mass does not regress within 2 to 3 weeks. Then inspection and dilatation of the cervix should be performed to make certain that drainage from the uterus is satisfactory.

Carcinoma of the Vagina

Carcinoma of the vagina is uncommon, occurring in only 2% of all patients with gynecologic cancer, and usually appearing between the ages of 55 and 65. Vaginal carcinoma results more frequently from metastases of tumors in the cervix and vulva than from conditions originating in the vagina, so differentiation is important. Lesions that encroach on the outer vagina from the vulva also must be separated from lesions that originate in the vaginal canal.

The International Federation of Obstetrics and Gynecology (FIGO) has agreed on the following criteria for the classification of vaginal cancer: a vaginal growth that has extended to the portio of the cervix and has reached the area of the external os should always be considered the result of carcinoma of the cervix. A vulvar growth that has extended to the vagina should be classified as carcinoma of the vulva. A vaginal growth that is limited to the urethra should be classified separately as carcinoma of the urethra. The criteria for the definition of primary carcinoma of the vagina were established after many clinicians reported the recurrence of vaginal lesions after treatment of carcinoma in situ of the cervix. Tumors recurred in 1% to 6% of cases.

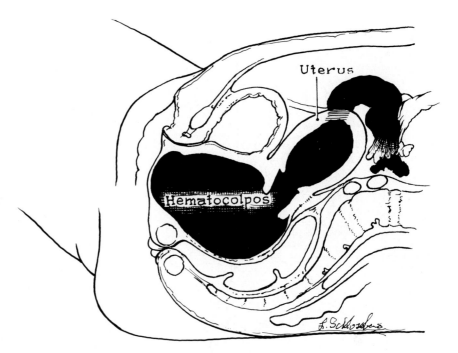

Figure 40–2. Hematocolpos, hematometra, hematosalpinx, and hematoperitoneum consequent to an imperforate hymen.

Today the extension of carcinoma in situ and invasive carcinoma of the cervix to the vaginal fornices or upper vagina can be easily excluded with the use of colposcopy. Clinicians now satisfy the staging criteria for the diagnosis of primary carcinoma of the vagina by showing a histologically negative cervix, urethra, vulva, and endometrium.

The clinical stages of carcinoma of the vagina agreed on by FIGO are listed in Table 40-1. In 1973 Perez and coworkers proposed that stage II be divided into stage IIa and IIb to provide a more accurate definition of the extent of the lesion. In the proposed modified FIGO classification stage IIa includes subvaginal infiltration not extending into the parametrial or paravaginal regions, while stage IIb includes parametrial or paravaginal infiltration not extending to the pelvic wall.

Symptoms

Unfortunately the diagnosis of vaginal tumors frequently is delayed because of the lack of early symptoms. Progressive vaginal discharge and postmenopausal bleeding are the most frequent symptoms. Postcoital bleeding usually is not a common clinical feature of this tumor in the early stages, possibly because sexual activity is decreased in the population in which the tumor occurs, and bleeding does not occur until the surface epithelium has become ulcerated. The tumor is detected in the early stages only if vaginal cytology is routinely performed for patients between the ages of 60 and 70.

The symptoms of vaginal carcinoma resemble those of cervical carcinoma, except that obvious bleeding occurs later than with neoplasms on the cervix. The overt bleeding eventually forces the patient to see her physician for diagnosis. Pain is an uncommon symp-

TABLE 40–1
FIGO Classification of Vaginal Carcinoma

CLASSIFICATION	DESCRIPTION
Preinvasive Carcinoma	
Stage 0	Carcinoma in situ, intraepithelial carcinoma
Invasive Carcinoma	
Stage I	Carcinoma limited to the vaginal wall
Stage II	Carcinoma involving the subvaginal tissue, but not extending onto the pelvic wall
Stage III	Carcinoma extending onto the pelvic wall
Stage IV	Carcinoma extending beyond the true pelvis or involving the mucosa of the bladder or rectum. Bullous edema such as does not permit a case to be allotted to stage IV.
Stage IVa	Spread of the growth to adjacent organs
Stage IVb	Spread to distant organs

(Pettersson F, ed. Annual report on the results of treatment in gynecologic cancer. Stockholm: FIGO, 1988:174)

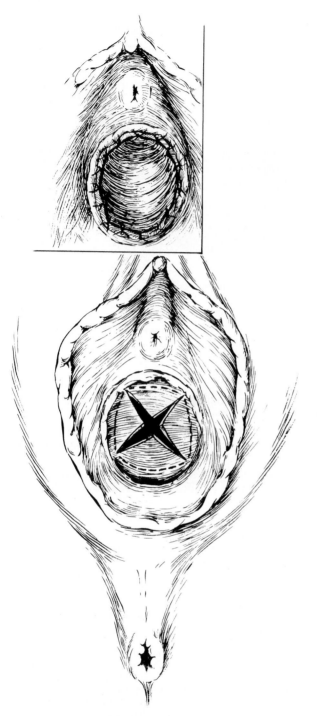

Figure 40–3. Excision of imperforate hymen. Stellate incisions are made through the hymenal membrane at the 2, 4, 8, and 10 o'clock positions. The individual quadrants are excised along the lateral wall of the vagina, avoiding excision of vagina. *Inset* Margins of vaginal mucosa are approximated with fine delayed-absorbable suture.

tom, associated only with advanced stages. Bladder symptoms occur late in the disease, when the tumor has involved the anterior vaginal septum and has encroached on or invaded the base of the bladder or urethra.

Histopathology

Histologic types of vaginal cancer are listed in Table 40-2.

Squamous carcinoma is the most common histologic type of vaginal tumor; 88% to 90% of all primary vaginal cancers are of this type. Adenocarcinoma, including diethylstilbestrol (DES)-related cases, represents about 4% to 5% of vaginal cancers. Uncommon lesions such as sarcoma, including leiomyosarcoma and sarcoma botryoides, account for 2% to 3% of vaginal lesions, whereas melanoma is an infrequent neoplasm of the vagina. Such rare tumors as endodermal sinus tumors or neoplasms originating in embryologic cloacal remnants may form a transitional cell neoplasm that involves the vagina.

The fact that squamous carcinoma of the vagina occurs in 10% to 15% of cases after the finding of squamous cancer in other parts of the lower genital tract, such as the vulva or cervix, has led to the theory of multicentric origin of squamous cancer in the lower genital tract. Woodruff and Parmley and others emphasize this correlation and have recommended that patients with squamous cancer in one area be categorized as high risk for the development of squamous carcinoma in other sites of the lower genital tract.

Carcinoma may arise in the neovagina lined with a split-thickness graft from the buttock or lateral thigh. Carcinoma of the neovagina is a rare cancer, with only nine patients reported. The primary carcinoma seems to be related to the transplanted tissue. In three cases adenocarcinoma was associated with the use of a large- or small-bowel intestinal graft for vaginal reconstruc-

TABLE 40–2
Histologic Types of Vaginal Cancer
and Frequency of Occurrence

TYPE	FREQUENCY (%)
Squamous carcinoma	88–90
Adenocarcinoma (including DES-related)	4–5
Sarcoma	2–3
Leiomyosarcoma	
Sarcoma botryoides	
Melanoma	1
Other	1–2

tion. Five patients with squamous cell cancer arising from the graft have been documented. The transplanted epithelium in the vagina may be exposed to an unidentified carcinogen or mutagen, as has been documented with the vulva, and can undergo malignant transformation in this environment. These observations underscore the need for regular pelvic examinations for patients who have undergone an operative vaginoplasty with either a bowel graft or a split-thickness graft.

Vaginal neoplasia may result from the use of DES during the first trimester of pregnancy. Women who had a history of previous spontaneous abortions or other problems with early loss of pregnancy were given DES, a nonsteroidal estrogenic hormone thought to enhance embryo implantation and placental development. DES was introduced into clinical obstetrics in 1944 in Boston and became popular and widely used during the next two decades. Only when a cluster of cases of adenocarcinoma appeared in the offspring of these patients, in young women under the age of 25 in the late 1960s, did Herbst and colleagues connect the result with the unusual coincidence.

From 1944 to 1970 from one-half to two million female offspring were exposed to DES. Fortunately the incidence of vaginal adenocarcinoma in these young women has been quite low, ranging from 0.14 to 1.4 per 1000 exposed women. More than 500 documented cases have been reported to the DES registry to date.

Observing the development of vaginal adenosis and adenocarcinoma in teenage girls whose mothers were given DES before the 18th week of pregnancy started a new approach to the study of squamous tumor cells in the lower genital tract. This drug's effect provided a histologic foundation for the development of an uncommon vaginal adenocarcinoma in women under age 29. The strange experience also increased our understanding of the embryologic development of the vagina.

The DES-associated adenocarcinoma originally was thought to arise from mesonephric remnants in the vagina, and consequently the disease was mislabeled as a clear cell carcinoma. After making an electron microscopic analysis of the ultrastructure of both the adenocarcinoma and the vaginal adenosis, Richart clearly defined these lesions to be composed of columnar epithelium, similar in all respects to endocervical epithelium and of paramesonephric (müllerian) origin. The colposcopic studies of Stafl and Mattingly, as well as others, confirmed these observations.

Vaginal adenosis has been found by colposcopic examination to occur in between 34% and 90% of the exposed women and in 50% of those with DES-associated vaginal adenocarcinoma. To date, the transition of the benign disease to frank adenocarcinoma has been observed in 10 women. Although the hypothesis is still unproven, a strong possibility exists that the benign vaginal lesion is the cell of origin for vaginal adenocarcinoma. The risk that clear cell adenocarcinoma will develop in an exposed female from birth through age 34 is 1 case per 1000 women.

Etiology

During embryologic development the vagina is formed from the columnar epithelium of the müllerian ducts and urogenital sinus. The tissue then transforms into squamous epithelium, so that the vaginal and cervical epithelia have a common embryologic origin. Squamous metaplasia has been observed with a colposcope within the vaginal adenosis; transformation of the metaplastic tissue also has been demonstrated in the development of intraepithelial neoplasia. Although many agents have been postulated as carcinogenic factors, none have been positively demonstrated. It is quite possible that squamous carcinoma arises from the effects of an oncogenic agent on the transformation zone within the foci of vaginal adenosis. The studies now being done on the effects of DES may find some interesting causative factors that influence vaginal carcinoma.

Carcinoma of the vagina also may share a common causative denominator with cervical carcinoma. Because slightly more than 50% of the cases occur in the posterior wall of the upper one-third of the vagina, which is the end point of vaginal coitus, vaginal carcinoma could be venereally induced. As with cervical carcinoma, primary carcinoma of the vagina usually occurs in sexually active women. Except for the cases of adenocarcinoma in young women exposed to DES, squamous carcinoma of the vagina is unquestionably associated with sexual activity.

Site of Lesion

Plentl and Friedman found that 51% of vaginal carcinoma lesions occur in the upper one-third of the vagina, 30% in the lower one-third, and 19% in the middle. In the lower one-third, lesions most often occur in the anterior wall, whereas in the upper one-third most cases appear in the posterior vaginal wall. Although the location is noted on diagnosis, the precise site of origin is difficult to identify because the tumors usually have spread to various parts of the vagina by that time.

Pathways of Spread

The lymphatic drainage of the vagina takes place through different pathways. The upper one-third drains by way of the cervical lymphatics, the lower one-third passes by way of the vulvar lymphatics, and the middle one-third communicates with both the upper and the lower lymphatic channels. The vaginal vault and the anterior wall of the upper vagina drain to the interiliac pelvic lymph nodes, where they communicate with the external iliac, the hypogastric, and the common iliac nodes. The lymphatic drainage of the posterior vagina communicates directly with the deep pelvic nodes, including the inferior gluteal, sacral, and rectal nodes.

Because the major pathways of lymphatic drainage are to the superior and inferior gluteals and the common iliac lymph nodes, the potential for extrapelvic spread of vaginal carcinoma is great. When extrapelvic spread occurs, prognosis usually is poor. The primary site of origin of the tumor is an important indicator of lymph node metastases, whether the tumor will metastasize to the inguinal-femoral chain or to the deep pelvic lymph nodes. When the disease involves the lower one-third of the vagina, 6% to 7% of patients have metastases to the inguinal-femoral lymph nodes.

Diagnosis

In general, invasive carcinoma of the vagina appears as either a raised exophytic lesion or an ulcerative, depressed lesion in the vaginal wall. Both types of lesion can be biopsied easily, and diagnosis can be established without difficulty. Vaginal cytology usually is positive if an adequate cell sample is obtained from the exfoliated lesion, although, as often happens with cervical carcinoma, many cases of false-negative cytology occur even when an invasive lesion is present. Lugol's solution can be used to demarcate the areas for biopsy, although iodine staining usually is unnecessary if the lesion is clearly visible.

Identifying vaginal carcinoma at an early stage can be a major problem because the first lesions appear within the epithelial cells, frequently indistinguishable from the remainder of the vaginal epithelium. Only by colposcopic examination or with iodine staining can alterations in the surface epithelium of the vagina be identified. Ng and associates have achieved an accuracy of 88% to 90% in detecting dysplastic lesions in DES-exposed patients with adenosis, but their technique requires separate, four-quadrant vaginal smears from the walls of the vagina. Herbst and coworkers emphasize the advantage of iodine staining of the vagina to demonstrate occult lesions that may be associated with adenosis. Stafl and Mattingly have reported an accuracy of 96% in detecting abnormal epithelial lesions of the vagina in DES-exposed females by careful examination and colposcopy.

Because the vaginal speculum can obscure surface lesions and delay early diagnosis, the instrument should be rotated during the examination, so that the entire canal can be inspected. With iodine staining, the clinician can detect multifocal lesions, but the entire vagina also should be cytologically tested. A thorough colposcopic examination can be used to detect vaginal carcinoma, if the clinician has that expertise.

Treatment

Primary vaginal carcinoma is treated either with surgery or with radiotherapy. The choice of treatment depends on three factors: the size of the lesion, the location of the tumor in the vagina, and the clinical stage of the disease.

Stage 0 Lesions. Intraepithelial carcinoma of the vagina is by far the easiest to treat and offers the most hopeful prognosis. Either surgery or radiotherapy can be used, depending on the location of the lesion. If the disease is located in the upper vagina and the margins of the disease are distinct, a partial vaginectomy, with or without hysterectomy, is a practical and successful method of treatment.

When an epithelial lesion is multicentric, the entire vagina could require treatment, which would render the surgical approach impractical. A vaginal cylinder, such as the Bloedorn applicator, can be used for radiotherapeutic treatment to deliver 7000 rad to the vaginal surface over a period of about 72 hours. If the lesion is confined to the vaginal fornices, vaginal colpostats can be used to deliver a similar dosage. Lesions in the lower one-third of the vagina may be treated by partial vaginectomy or by intravaginal irradiation, using a variety of brachytherapy techniques.

The use of the carbon dioxide laser has proved to be a simple, effective method of treatment for noninvasive vaginal carcinoma. Laser therapy offers a conservative treatment for both focal and multicentric lesions without impairment of normal coital function. Because there is a risk of residual disease in 10% of laser-treated patients, careful colposcopic and cytologic follow-up are critical. Histologic study is difficult after the treated lesions are vaporized by the carbon dioxide laser.

Stage I Lesions. Radical surgery, including hysterectomy, vaginectomy, and pelvic lymphadenectomy, can be used in stage I carcinoma of the vagina. Surgical evaluation of the paraaortic nodes should be included if lesions are bulky or extensive. Before initiating a radical procedure, the surgeon must establish that the disease is confined to the pelvis, as is done with stage I carcinoma of the cervix.

Radical surgery is used infrequently for the treatment of invasive carcinoma of the vagina, except with very early lesions for which the margins of the disease can be clearly defined and confidently removed. Radical surgery is difficult because the bladder and rectum are closely attached to the vaginal walls, limiting the surgical margins. When the disease occurs, as it does most commonly, in the upper posterior vaginal wall, the tumor must be completely freed from the underlying rectum. Radical surgery also may require the replacement of the upper vagina with a split-thickness skin graft to reestablish normal vaginal length for a sexually active woman. Irradiation therapy is an alternative treatment for this stage of disease.

The radical Wertheim hysterectomy has been quite successful in treating stage I adenocarcinoma in young women who were exposed to DES in utero. More than 75% of patients are cured. When the disease extends beyond a stage I lesion, the preferable treatment is to follow external beam megavoltage therapy with intravaginal irradiation.

Stage II and Stage III Lesions. More extensive lesions of the vagina pose an extremely difficult therapeutic problem for the gynecologist. Because the vagina is surrounded by the levator ani muscles of the pelvic diaphragm, penetration of the lateral wall of the vagina by the invasive tumor frequently is associated with fixation of the disease to the adjacent pelvic musculature. Even radical surgery cannot effectively control the disease when it extends beyond the confines of the vagina into the paravaginal tissues. Instead, the major method of treatment for stage II and stage III lesions is radiotherapy.

When stage II lesions involve the anterior or posterior wall of the vaginal septum, an anterior or posterior exenteration with pelvic node dissection may be required. When the disease includes the lower one-third of the vagina, a groin dissection is necessary as well. Because surgery must be so extensive, its use has been limited when the disease affects the paravaginal region (stage IIb) or the lateral vaginal wall (stage III).

Stage IV Lesions. When advanced lesions involve only the bladder or the rectum, exenteration may be required to control the disease effectively. Unfortunately pelvic exenteration, either anterior or posterior, can be used only when there is no other extension of the disease, and it is rare for the bladder and rectum to be involved without involvement of the adjacent paravaginal tissues. If the patient is not an acceptable surgical risk for exenteration, external beam megavoltage irradiation therapy, followed by intravaginal or interstitial irradiation, can be used to control the local disease and to offer palliation. If the tumor does not respond after 5000 rad of irradiation treatment to the whole pelvis, an exenteration may be required to control the disease in properly selected patients.

Irradiation Therapy

Irradiation treatment of vaginal carcinoma is easily divided between lesions in the upper and middle and the lower thirds of the vagina.

Upper and Middle Thirds of the Vagina. Because the lymphatic drainage of the upper and middle vagina extends through the hypogastric and pelvic nodes, full pelvic irradiation is necessary. Treatment usually includes a combination of techniques.

External beam megavoltage therapy using 4500 to 5000 rad focused on the midplane of the pelvis is used to treat the full pelvis and to encompass the vagina. A vaginal implant of radium, cesium, or iridium follows, delivering an additional 3000 to 4000 rad to a depth of 0.5 to 1.0 cm or more, depending on the thickness of the lesion.

At the M.D. Anderson Hospital, Brown and coworkers have demonstrated the efficacy of using a radium needle implant for localized lesions. When the implant is used, high doses of radiation to the entire vagina, bladder, and rectum are avoided. Interstitial needles and iridium wires have been used as a primary treatment for localized vaginal lesions, and they also can be used for persistent disease.

Lower One-third of the Vagina. Lesions in the lower one-third of the vagina frequently metastasize to the inguinal-femoral lymphatics, and must be treated with full external and intravaginal irradiation followed by external beam irradiation treatment to the inguinal-femoral lymph nodes. The inguinal-femoral regions require either a surgical groin dissection or the application of 5000 to 6000 rad of electron beam teletherapy in addition to full pelvic irradiation. When vaginal lesions have metastasized to the groin lymph nodes, the cure rate is equally poor for both methods. In general, the presence of tumor in the groin nodes is a poor prognostic sign, suggesting that the deep pelvic nodes also may be involved in about 6% to 7% of cases. Because the incidence of vaginal cancer is so low, the exact frequency with which the deep pelvic nodes are involved has not been documented.

Cure Rates

In all, 547 patients with vaginal carcinoma were reported by international clinics to the FIGO registry between 1979 and 1981. Of these patients, the majority were treated by radiation (78%). Only 38.6% of these patients were alive at 5 years.

Results from other institutions that have primarily followed radiation therapy show that only stage I lesions have an adequate 5-year survival rate (Table 40-3).

Overall survival rates for stages I through IV from published reports are outlined in Table 40-4. The highest survival rates are noted in stage I disease, whereas few patients survive for 5 years after the diagnosis of stage IV disease.

In a retrospective analysis of 134 patients with carcinoma of the vagina treated at Washington University, Perez and Camel report an actuarial disease-free, 5-year survival rate of 85% for stage I lesions, 51% for stage IIa lesions, 33% for stage IIb lesions, 33% for stage III

TABLE 40–3
Absolute 5-Year Survival After Irradiation Therapy
for Carcinoma of the Vagina

FIGO STAGE	PROPORTION SURVIVING*		
	M.D. Anderson Hospital (1948–1967)	*University of Maryland (1957–1970)*	*Washington University (1950–1977)*
I	11/16 (69%)	5/6 (83%)	33/39 (85%)
II	13/19 (68%)	20/31 (64%)	28/60 (47%)
IIa	— —	13/20 (65%)	21/39 (51%)
IIb	— —	7/11 (63%)	7/21 (33%)
III	4/15 (27%)	8/20 (40%)	4/12 (33%)
IV	0/11 (0%)	0/7 (0%)	1/8 (19%)
I–IV	28/61 (46%)	33/64 (52%)	66/119 (53%)

*Percentage figures are in parentheses.
(Adapted from Hilgers RD. Squamous cell carcinoma of the vagina. Surg Clin North Am 1978;58:25; Perez CA, Camel HM. Long-term follow-up in radiation therapy of carcinoma of the vagina. Cancer 1982;49:1308)

lesions, and 19% for stage IV lesions. The actuarial study demonstrates that beyond stage I of the disease, control is poor. For stage IIa lesions, local control of the disease was achieved in only 65% of cases at the University of Maryland because external irradiation was not used in all cases. Pelvic control was achieved in 48% of stage IIb and stage III lesions, but in none of the seven patients (0%) with stage IV disease.

THE URETHRA

The female urethra develops from the caudal end of the urogenital sinus after it separates from the vaginal canal between the 8th and 12th week of embryologic life. Because they are so closely integrated, the urethra shares many common disease processes and anatomic defects with the vagina. Bacteria in the lower genital tract frequently colonize in the outer urethra, harbor in the paraurethral glands, and enter the bladder to produce acute infections. A bacterial infection in the lower genital tract may not become clinically manifest for several years, until a Skene's duct cyst or a urethral diverticulum develops.

Estrogen deficiency, which causes atrophic changes of the vaginal mucosa, can have a similar effect on the urethral mucosa. Thinning of the epithelium and irritation of the sensory nerve fibers can cause urinary frequency and dysuria. Prolapse at the external meatus also may result from atrophic changes of the urethra.

Diverticulum of the Urethra

Despite the many documented cases of urethral diverticula, the condition has not been well recognized by the medical profession. Anderson observed a urethral diverticulum in 3% of a group of 300 women who were undergoing treatment for cervical carcinoma. The condition occurs more frequently than it is diagnosed; whenever an article about urethral diverticulum appears in the literature, there is an upsurge in the number of cases diagnosed.

Etiology

In 1941 Parmenter suggested several congenital factors that could develop into a urethral diverticulum, including Gartner's duct, a faulty union of primal folds, cell nets, and wolffian ducts, or vaginal cysts that rupture into the urethra. Other possible causes include trauma from childbirth, instrumentation, urethral stone, urethral stricture, and infection of the urethral glands.

Of the many possible causes of urethral diverticula that have been considered, none have been proved. Two of the most probable causes are neisserial infection, although the gonococcus is seldom cultured, and infection of the suburethral tissue resulting from vaginal flora. Huffman's experiments support the concept of a suburethral infection developing into an abscess that becomes lined with epithelium. Huffman showed periurethral openings by constructing wax models of infected urethras. The usual organisms cultured are *Escherichia coli, Aerobacter aerogenes,* and other gram-negative bacilli; *Staphylococcus aureus*; and *Streptococcus faecalis.*

Symptoms

Dysuria, urgency, frequency, and hematuria occurred together in 85% to 90% of 32 cases reviewed by Peters and Vaughn. Other frequently occurring symptoms are a lump in the vagina, dyspareunia, intermittent

TABLE 40–4
Carcinoma of the Vagina: Comparison of Survival

STUDY	STAGE				
	I	*II*	*III*	*IV*	*Total*
Puthawala et al. (1976–1979)	1/1 (100%)	12/16 (75%)	2/9 (22%)	0/1 (0%)	15/27 (56%)
Gallup and Morley (1971–1984)	4/4 (100%)	6/12 (50%)	0/4 (0%)	2/8 (25%)	12/28 (43%)
Brown et al. (1948–1967)	11/16 (69%)	13/19 (68%)	4/15 (27%)	0/11 (0%)	28/61 (46%)
Nori et al. (1950–1974)	10/14 (71%)	4/6 (61%)	1/3 (33%)	0/13 (0%)	15/36 (42%)
Perez (1965–1981)	26/32 (81%)	22/52 (42%)	3/10 (30%)	1/11 (9%)	52/105 (50%)
Prempree (1957–1975)	7/9 (78%)	21/37 (57%)	10/26 (39%)	0/8 (0%)	38/80 (48%)
Benedet et al. (1950–1980)	20/28 (71%)	12/24 (50%)	2/13 (15%)	0/10 (0%)	34/75 (45%)
Manetta et al. (1976–1986)	5/7 (71%)	7/15 (47%)	1/3 (33%)	1/4 (33%)	14/29 (48%)

(Adapted from Manetta A, Perito JL, Larson JE, et al. Primary invasive carcinoma of the vagina. Obstet Gynecol 1988;72:77. Reprinted with permission from The American College of Obstetricians and Gynecologists)

discharge from the urethra, and pain on walking. Pyuria and cystitis also occur, depending on the location of the diverticular orifice. If the opening is sufficiently close to the outer end of the urethra, there may be no leakage of purulent exudate back into the bladder, which may explain the absence of symptoms of cystitis in 5% of cases. If the diverticulum is located in the posterior urethra near the urethrovesical junction, stress urinary incontinence may be a significant symptom. In a review of 70 cases from the Johns Hopkins Hospital, Ginsberg and Genadry found that 17% of the diverticula were located in the proximal (outer) urethra, 43% in the midurethra, and 31% in the distal (posterior) urethra; in the remaining cases the site was not specifically identified.

Not only are urinary tract symptoms the most common clinical expression of this urethral lesion, but a history of recurrent refractory cystitis is a clue that a diverticulum is the source of the infection.

Diagnosis

Urethral diverticula usually are small, varying from 3 mm to 3 cm in diameter. Some of the larger sacs cover the entire length of the urethra. On palpation a suburethral mass or tenderness commonly is found. Pressure on the mass may cause the escape of urine or exudate from the urethral meatus.

An examination of the floor of the urethra through the water cystoscope while suburethral pressure is being applied reveals an opening in 50% to 70% of cases. The pressure may force contents of the diverticulum into the urethra while it is being viewed. Some of the openings are extremely small and may be missed. Inflammatory swelling can result in edema of the orifice, which makes visualization difficult or impossible.

The diagnosis of urethral diverticulum is firmly established by means of positive pressure urethrography. A special catheter is used to block the urethra at both ends and fill it and the diverticulum under pressure with water-soluble contrast medium (Figs. 40-4 and 40-5). The diverticulum then shows up clearly on a roentgenogram (Fig. 40-6). If the urethral orifice to the diverticulum is quite large, a voiding cystourethrogram together with a positive pelvic film may demonstrate the diverticulum.

Occasionally a diverticulum occurs with no clinical evidence of inflammation. If the diverticulum is diagnosed during a careful pelvic examination, and if the patient is completely asymptomatic except for a previous history of urinary tract problems, surgery is not necessary. With a complication rate of 15% to 20%, diverticulectomy should not be considered a quick and easy procedure. Removal of an asymptomatic urethral diverticulum may create more problems than it prevents, particularly if the sac is small or located in the floor of the posterior urethra. Only if a patient experiences acute or recurrent symptoms should urethral surgery be performed.

Treatment

A diverticulum that requires treatment must be completely excised before the defect in the urethra can be closed. Failure to remove the entire diverticulum only results in recurrence of the problem.

Many techniques have been used to identify the anatomic boundaries of the diverticulum. A popular method is to pass a sound into the diverticulum through the urethral orifice. The diverticulum also can be distended by injecting it with fibrinogen and thrombin mixed in a syringe to form a firm fibrin clot. Direct anatomic dissection of the diverticulum from the paraurethral fascia and vaginal wall offers a better success rate. The smooth covering of a diverticulum protruding into the vagina can be easily distinguished from the rugal folds of the vaginal mucosa.

If the wall of the diverticulum is left unopened until the dissection has reached the base of the sac, the neck of the diverticulum can be seen directly when it is removed. A common error is the inadvertent removal of a portion of the urethral floor along the base of the diverticulum. If the mucosa is closed with too much

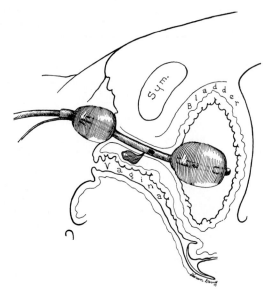

Figure 40–5. Double-ballooned catheter in use for positive-pressure urethrography. (From Davis HJ, Cian LG. Positive-pressure urethrography: A new diagnostic method. J Urol 1958; 80:34)

tension, a urethral stricture or a postoperative fistula may result.

Surgical Technique. EXCISION AND LAYERED CLOSURE. A midline incision is made through the vaginal mucosa, which is then separated from the wall of the diverticulum (Fig. 40-7A). The wall of the diverticulum also is dissected from the paraurethral fascia in as wide a circumference as can be developed.

The diverticulum is opened and the interior of the cavity inspected. If the orifice of the diverticulum is large, the opening of the urethra can easily be seen, especially if a catheter has been placed in the urethra and bladder (Fig. 40-7B). The rest of the thin, friable mucosa of the diverticulum is separated from the vaginal mucosa and fascia, before the neck of the diverticulum is trimmed near the urethral orifice. The lining of the diverticulum becomes friable as a result of inflammatory changes, and the thin layer fragments during the dissection. Meticulous sharp dissection is required to separate the lining completely from the vagina and from the floor of the urethra. The neck of the diverticulum should be carefully resected to avoid eversion and to prevent removal of the mucosa from the urethral floor.

The urethral defect is closed with interrupted No. 3-0 delayed absorbable sutures so that the edges can be inverted (Fig. 40-7C). After the interrupted sutures are tied the paraurethral fascia is closed in a double-layer, vest-over-pants technique. The layer of fascia from one side of the urethra is sutured beneath the opposite,

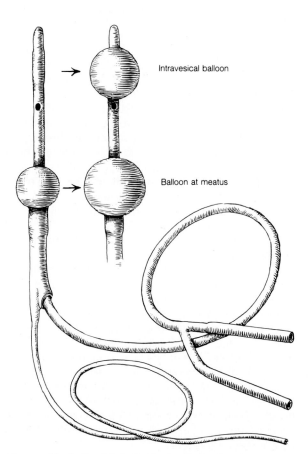

Intravesical balloon

Balloon at meatus

Figure 40–4. Double-ballooned catheter for positive-pressure urethrography. (From Davis HJ, Cian LG. Positive-pressure urethrography: A new diagnostic method. J Urol 1958; 80:34)

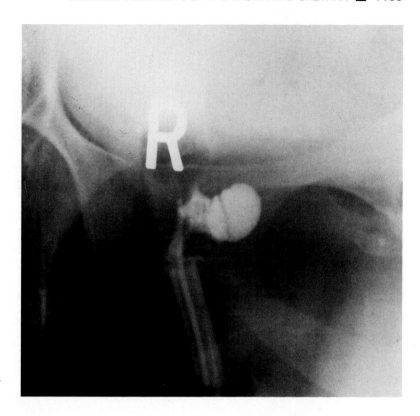

Figure 40–6. A large urethral diverticulum filled with contrast medium.

overlapping fascia and fastened to the urethral wall on that opposite side. The top layer of fascia is then sutured to the underlying fascial layer. A more durable No. 2-0 delayed absorbable suture is used to suture the fascial margins (Fig. 40-7*D* and *E*). Finally, the vaginal mucosa is trimmed and closed with interrupted No. 2-0 delayed absorbable sutures.

The bladder is filled with 300 ml of distilled water, and a suprapubic Silastic catheter is inserted and left in place until the morning of the 5th postoperative day. A suprapubic catheter is used in preference to a urethral catheter for three major reasons: to avoid trauma to the operative site; to avoid the necessity for transurethral catheterization during attempts to initiate voiding; and to avoid the discomfort of a urethral catheter. On the 5th day after surgery the patient should attempt to void by closing the three-way stopcock of the suprapubic catheter, which allows the bladder to fill.

URETHROTOMY AND MARSUPIALIZATION. Urethrotomy has been used by Edwards and Beebe, and more recently by Kropp, to treat diverticula. By splitting the floor of the urethra from the meatus down its full length to the site of the orifice of the diverticulum, the sac can be well visualized during excision. Most cases of urethral diverticula can be successfully repaired without the added risk involved with such an extensive incision. The floor

of the urethra must heal along the entire length, and healing is particularly a problem if there has been recent infection in the diverticulum.

In 1970 Spence and Duckett recommended marsupializing the diverticulum to prevent recurrence, to minimize operating time, and to reduce blood loss. This procedure has been endorsed by Lichtman and Robertson and more recently by Ginsberg and Genadry. Although stress urinary incontinence has not been reported as a complication, the incidence would probably increase if marsupialization were used to treat lesions in the posterior urethra near the bladder base. Marsupialization is a useful procedure when diverticula occur in the outer one-third of the urethra because a permanent opening in the outer floor of the urethra would not adversely influence intraurethral pressure.

Results of Diverticulectomy. Complications arise in about 20% of patients treated for diverticula of the urethra (Table 40-5). Urethral stricture may result when too much urethral mucosa is removed, but strictures usually can be resolved by urethral dilatations. Urethral fistula, a serious and troublesome complication of diverticulectomy, occurs in about 5% of treated patients.

Postoperatively, fistulas frequently result when acute or subacute infection in the walls of the diverticulum cause the urethral mucosa to become friable. The uri-

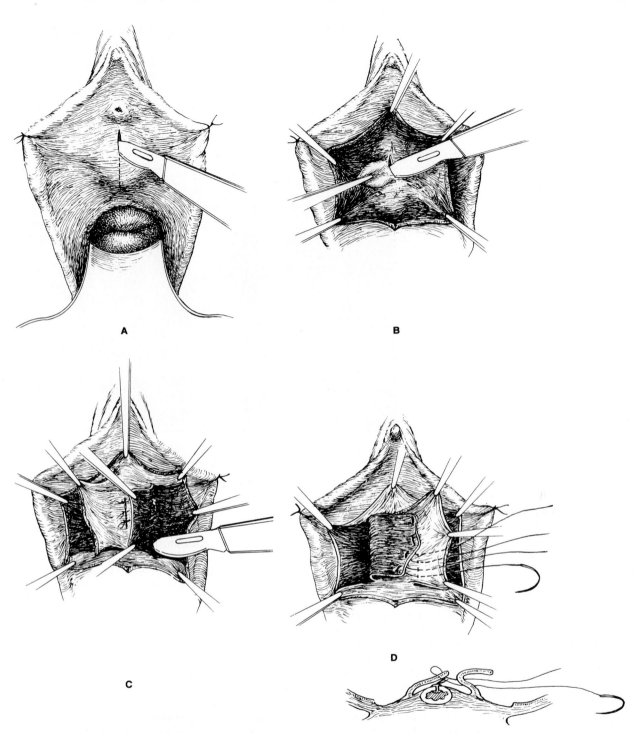

Figure 40–7. Suburethral diverticulum. *A*, A midline vaginal incision is made over the diverticulum. *B*, The diverticulum is dissected from the vaginal mucosa and surrounding fascia. Freed diverticulum is excised from the floor of the urethra, avoiding removal of an excessive amount of urethral wall. *C*, The urethra is closed with interrupted No. 3-0 delayed absorbable sutures placed through the muscularis and mucosa to ensure mucosa-to-mucosa approximation. The paraurethral fascia is mobilized with sharp dissection from the vaginal mucosa. *D*, The paraurethral fascia is plicated beneath urethral incision, using the vest-over-pants technique. Note suture of the inner layer of fascia to the undersurface of the outer layer, using horizontal mattress sutures of No. 2-0 delayed absorbable material. Inset shows cross-sectional view of suture placement.

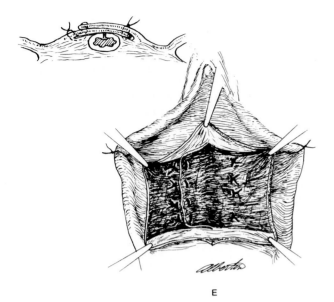

E

Figure 40–7. (continued) *E*, Completion of vest-over-pants plication of paraurethral fascia over the floor of the urethra. Note that the free margin of the outer fascia is sutured to the inner fascial layer. Inset shows cross-sectional view of suture placement.

nary incontinence that develops from a urethral fistula is far more troublesome to the patient than the initial symptoms of the diverticulum.

Closure of a urethral fistula is quite difficult because the blood supply to the floor of the urethra is delicate, and scarring and infection often result from repeated efforts to close the urethra. A fistula in the outer part of the urethra may be asymptomatic and may not need to be repaired. Most patients with an outer fistula complain of spraying urine when voiding.

Urethral Prolapse

Although there have been few recent reports of urethral prolapse, nearly 400 cases have appeared in the English literature since 1732. More than half the cases occurred in infants and children; the remainder occurred in elderly patients.

Urethral prolapse is characterized by a sliding outward of the urethral mucosa around the entire urethral meatus. The urethra may become cyanotic, edematous, and infracted (Fig. 40-8). Symptoms vary greatly. Prolapse may cause no discomfort, in which case it is detected only when bloody discharge results from the breaking down of the congested tissues. Some patients complain of severe and continuous pain, with urinary frequency and tenesmus. Occasionally, in a small child, the edema and tissue reaction of the outer urethra produce urinary retention.

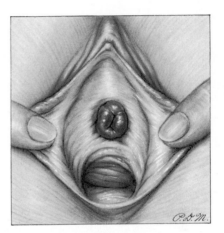

Figure 40–8. Prolapsed urethra.

TABLE 40–5
Complications of Urethral Diverticulectomy

OPERATIVE SERIES	NO. OF CASES	FISTULA	RECURRENCE	STRESS INCONTINENCE	STRICTURE	RECURRENT URINARY TRACT INFECTION	COMPLICATION RATE (%)
Wharton, Te Linde	58	4	—	1	3	5	22
Ward et al.	24	2	7	3	—	—	50
Boatwright, Moore	48	4	—	2	1	—	15
Pathak, House	42	—	—	—	—	3	7
Davis, Te Linde	84	—	10	—	—	11	26
Hoffman, Adams	60	1	—	4	1	—	10
Davis, Robinson	98	4	1	—	—	—	6
Lee	108	1	10	16	—	1	—
Ginsberg, Genadry	70	1	20	6	—	—	39
Total	592	17 (3%)	48 (8%)	32 (5%)	5 (1%)	20 (3%)	21 (avg.)

(Adapted from Ginsberg DS, Genadry R: Suburethral diverticulum in the female. Obstet Gynecol Surv 1984;39:1)

Urethral prolapse is thought to result from a lack of development of or atrophic changes in the collagen and elastic tissues of the submucosa. In infants, prolapse usually follows a severe coughing or crying spell. In some older patients, too, prolapse has followed paroxysms of coughing. In older patients diminished tone and elasticity of tissue are considered to be causative factors in some cases of urethral prolapse.

Treatment of urethral prolapse may be palliative or surgical. Hot, moist compresses provide temporary comfort. Sometimes a small mass of tissue can be reduced, but recurrence is common.

Several surgical procedures have been suggested, including the one advocated by Kelly and Burnam. The prolapsed mucosa is excised by a circular incision (Fig. 40-9A). The cut edges are then sutured with No. 3-0 delayed absorbable suture material, avoiding an excessive number of stitches, which can result in stricture of the urethral meatus (Fig. 40-9B). In most cases circumcision has proved to be the preferred method of correction.

Cryosurgery also has been used to treat urethral prolapse. The method is extremely effective in producing complete annular necrosis and healing of the prolapsed tissue (Fig. 40-10). The cryosurgical procedure can be performed without anesthesia; for a young child

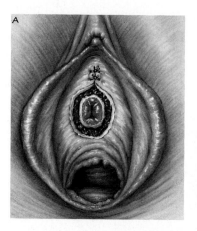
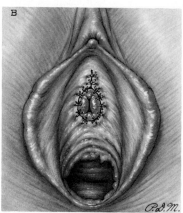

Figure 40–9. Operation for urethral prolapse. A, The prolapsed mucosa has been excised. B, Completed operation; cut edges of urethral and vaginal mucosa are sutured with No. 3-0 delayed absorbable suture material.

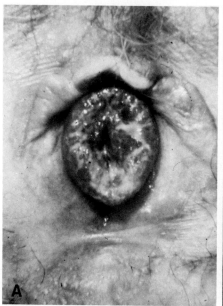
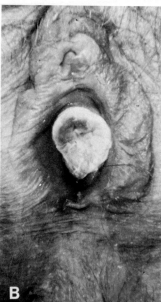
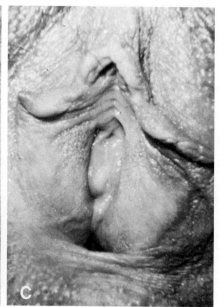

Figure 40–10. Cryosurgery in the treatment of urethral prolapse. A, Urethral prolapse in an elderly female. B, Regression of urethral prolapse after cryosurgery. C, Repeat cryosurgery of urethral prolapse resulted in complete regression and healing of urethral meatus within 8 weeks.

a local anesthetic is advisable. A suprapubic Silastic catheter is inserted to permit bladder drainage until complete, spontaneous voiding occurs. The catheter also helps to prevent postoperative trauma to the suture line around the meatus.

Bibliography

Anderson MJF. The incidence of diverticula of the female urethra. J Urol 1967;98:96.

Benedet JL, Murphy KJ, Fairey RN, et al. Primary invasive carcinoma of the vagina. Obstet Gynecol 1983;62:715.

Benjamin J, Elliott L, Cooper JF, et al. Urethral diverticulum in adult female: clinical aspects, operative procedure, and pathology. Urology 1974;3:1.

Blaikley JB, Dewhurst CJ, Ferreira HP, et al. Vaginal adenosis: clinical and pathological features with special reference to malignant change. J Obstet Gynaecol Br Commonw 1971;78:1115.

Breslow A. Thickness, cross-sectional areas, and depths of invasion in the prognosis of cutaneous melanoma. Ann Surg 1970;172:902.

Brown GR, Fletcher GH, Rutledge FN. Irradiation of in situ and invasive squamous cell carcinoma of the vagina. Cancer 1971;28:1278.

Curran JW, Rendtorff RC, Chandler RW, et al. Female gonorrhea: its relationship to abnormal uterine bleeding, urinary tract symptoms and cervicitis. Obstet Gynecol 1975;45:195.

Davis BL, Robinson DG. Diverticula of the female urethra: assay of 120 cases. J Urol 1970;104:850.

Davis HJ, Cian LG. Positive pressure urethrography. A new diagnostic method. J Urol 1958;80:34.

Davis HJ, Te Linde RW. Urethral diverticula: an assay of 121 cases. J Urol 1956;75:753.

DiSaia PJ, Morrow CP, Townsend DE, eds. Synopsis of gynecologic oncology. New York: John Wiley & Sons, 1975.

Edwards E, Beebe RA. Diverticula of female urethra. Review: New procedure for treatment: report of 5 cases. Obstet Gynecol 1955;5:729.

Fenoglio C, Ferenczy A, Richard RM, et al. Scanning and transmission electron microscopic studies of vaginal adenosis and the cervical transformation zone in progeny exposed in utero to diethylstilbestrol. Am J Obstet Gynecol 1976;126:170.

Frick HC. Primary carcinoma of the vagina. Am J Obstet Gynecol 1968;101:695.

Gallup DG, Morley GW. Carcinoma in situ of the vagina: a study and review. Obstet Gynecol 1975;46:334.

Ginsberg DS, Genadry R. Suburethral diverticulum: classification and therapeutic considerations. Obstet Gynecol 1983;61:685.

Hamilton WJ, Boyd JD, Mossman HW. Human embryology. 3rd ed. Cambridge: W Heffer & Sons, 1962.

Herbst AL, Scully RE, Robboy SJ. The significance of adenosis and clear-cell adenocarcinoma of the genital tract in young females. J Reprod Med 1975;14:5.

Herbst AL, Ulfelder H, Poskanzer EC. Adenocarcinoma of the vagina: association of maternal stilbestrol therapy with tumor appearing in young women. N Engl J Med 1971;284:878.

Hilgers RD. Squamous cell carcinoma of the vagina. Surg Clin North Am 1978;58:25.

Hoffman MJ, Adams WE. Recognition and repair of urethral diverticula. Am J Obstet Gynecol 1965;92:106.

Hopkins MP, Morley GW. Squamous cell carcinoma of the neovagina. Obstet Gynecol 1987;69:525.

Huffman JW. The detailed anatomy of the paraurethral ducts in the adult human female. Am J Obstet Gynecol 1948;55:86.

Hutch JA. Anatomy and physiology of the bladder, trigone and urethra. New York: Appleton-Century-Crofts, 1972.

International Federation of Obstetrics and Gynecology. Annual report on the results of treatment of carcinoma of the uterus, vagina, and ovary. Vol 18. Stockholm: Norestedt, 1982.

Kamat MH, DelGaiso A, Seebode JJ. Urethral prolapse in female children. Am J Dis Child 1969;118:691.

Kanbour AE, Klionsky BK, Murphy Al. Carcinoma of the vagina following cervical cancer. Cancer 1974;34:1838.

Kelly HA, Burnam CF. Malfunctions of the urethra. In: Kelly HA, ed. Diseases of the kidneys, ureters, and bladder. New York: D. Appleton & Co., 1922:564.

Klaus H, Stein RT. Urethral prolapse in young girls. Pediatrics 1973;52:645.

Klobe JM. Pathologische Anatomieder Weiblichen Sexualorgane. Vien, 1864.

Kropp KA. The female urethra. In: Glenn JF, ed. Urologic surgery. Hagerstown, Md: Harper & Row, 1975.

Lee RA. Diverticulum of the urethra: clinical presentation, diagnosis and management. Clin Obstet Gynecol 1984;27:490.

Lichtman A, Robertson J. Suburethral diverticula treated by marsupialization. Obstet Gynecol 1976;47:203.

Lintgen C, Herbert P. Clinical-pathological study of 100 female urethras. J Urol 1946;55:298.

Livermore GR. Treatment of prolapse of the urethra. Surg Gynecol Obstet 1921;32:557.

Manetta A, Perito JL, Larson JE, et al. Primary invasive carcinoma of the vagina. Obstet Gynecol 1988;72:77.

Marcus SL. Multiple squamous cell carcinoma involving the cervix, vagina and vulva: the theory of multicentric origin. Am J Obstet Gynecol 1960;80:802.

Melneck S, Cole P, Anderson D, Herbst A. Rates and risks of DES-related clear cell adenocarcinoma of the vagina and cervix. N Engl J Med 1987;316:514.

Ng ABP, Reagan JW, Hawliczek S, et al. Cellular detection of vaginal adenosis. Obstet Gynecol 1975;46:323.

Nori D, Hilaris B, Stanimir G, et al. Radiation therapy of primary vaginal carcinoma. Int J Radiat Oncol Biol Phys 1983;8:1471.

Parmenter FJ. Diverticulum of the urethra. J Urol 1941;45:749.

Pathak UN, House MJ. Diverticulum of the female urethra. Obstet Gynecol 1970;36:789.

Perez CA. Definitive radiotherapy for carcinoma of the vagina. Int J Radiat Oncol Biol Phys 1981;7:20.

Perez CA, Arneson AN, Dehner LP, et al. Radiation therapy in carcinoma of the vagina. Obstet Gynecol 1974;44:862.

Perez CA, Arneson AN, Galakatos A, et al. Malignant tumors of the vagina. Cancer 1973;31:36.

Perez CA, Arneson AN, Galakatos A, et al. Treatment of carcinoma of the vagina. Cancer 1973;31:36.

Perez CA, Camel HM. Long-term follow-up in radiation therapy of carcinoma of the vagina. Cancer 1982;49:1308.

Peters WA, Vaughn EJ Jr. Urethral diverticula in the female: etiologic factors and postoperative results. Obstet Gynecol 1976;47:549.

Pettersson F, ed. Annual report on the results of treatment in gynecological cancer. Stockholm: FIGO, 1988:174.

Plentl AA, Friedman EA. Lymphatic system of the female genital tract. Philadelphia: WB Saunders, 1971.

Pokorny SF, Kozinetz CA. Configuration and other anatomic details of the prepubertal hymen. Adolesc Pediatr Gynecol 1988;1:97.

Prempree T. Role of radiation therapy in the management of primary carcinoma of the vagina. Acta Radiol [Oncol] 1982;21:195.

Prempree T, Viravathana T, Slawson RG, et al. Radiation management of primary carcinoma of the vagina. Cancer 1977;40:101.

Pride GL, Schultz AE, Chuprevich TW, et al. Primary invasive carcinoma of the vagina. Clin Obstet Gynecol 1979;53:218.

Puthawala A, Syed AMN, Nalick R, et al. Integrated external and interstitial radiation therapy for primary carcinoma of the vagina. Obstet Gynecol 1983;62:367.

Rock JA, Zacur HA, Dlugi AM, et al. Pregnancy success following the surgical correction of imperforate hymen as compared to the complete transverse vaginal septum. Obstet Gynecol 1982; 59:448.

Rutledge FN, Boronow RC, Wharton JT. Gynecologic oncology. New York: John Wiley & Sons, 1976.

Sander R, Nuss RC, Rhatigan RM. DES-associated vaginal adenosis followed by clear-cell adenocarcinoma. Int J Gynecol Pathol 1986;5:362.

Schubert G. Uber Scheidenbildung bei Angeborenem Vaginaldefekt. Zbl Gynak 1911;45:1017.

Sholem SL, Wechsler M, Roberts M. Management of the urethral diverticulum in women: a modified operative technique. J Urol 1974;112:485.

Smith WG. Invasive carcinoma of the vagina. Clin Obstet Gynecol 1981;24:503.

Spence H, Duckett J. Diverticulum of the female urethra: clinical aspects and presentation of simple operative technique for cure. J Urol 1970;104:432.

Stafl A, Mattingly RF. Vaginal adenosis: a precancerous lesion? Am J Obstet Gynecol 1974;120:666.

Stern A, Patel S. Diverticulum of the female urethra: value of the post-void bladder film during excretory urography. Radiology 1976;121:22.

Tait L. Saccular dilatation of the urethra: removal, cure. Lancet 1875;2:625.

Wharton JT. Carcinoma of the vagina and urethra. In: Rovinsky JJ, ed. Obstetrics and gynecology. Hagerstown, Md: Harper & Row, 1972.

Wharton JT. Carcinoma of the vagina. In: Rutledge F, Boronow RC, Wharton JT, eds. Gynecologic oncology. New York: John Wiley & Sons, 1976;259.

Wharton JT, Kearns W. Diverticulum of the female urethra. J Urol 1950;63:1063.

Wheeles CR Jr, McGibbon B, Dorsey JH, et al. Gracilis myocutaneous flap in reconstruction of the vulva and female perineum. Obstet Gynecol 1979;54:97.

Woodruff JD, Parmley TH. Epidermoid carcinoma of the vagina. In: Hafez ECE, Evans TN, eds. The human vagina. New York: Elsevier North Holland, 1979.

41

Cervical Intraepithelial Neoplasia

ADOLF STAFL

In the past five decades the age-adjusted incidence rate for cervical carcinoma has steadily decreased. Cervical cancer was the most common cancer of female reproductive organs after breast cancer. The incidence of cervical cancer currently is lower than the incidence of endometrial or ovarian cancer. In 1986 14,000 women in the United States developed cervical carcinoma and 7000 women died of this disease. Squamous cell carcinoma of the cervix arises from noninvasive forms. Detection and destruction of these forms prevents the development of the often fatal invasive cancer. There is no doubt that exfoliative cytology, introduced to gynecologic practice in 1943 by Papanicolaou and Traut, had the greatest impact on lowering the death rate of cervical cancer. This was documented by Boyes and coworkers, who reported that the refined death rate from invasive cancer declined in cytologically screened population in British Columbia from 11.4 per 100,000 women in 1958 to 3.8 per 100,000 in 1976. The death rate from cervical cancer was decreasing steadily years before cytologic screening was introduced, and therefore, in the declining death rates from cervical cancer, other factors also must be considered, such as the increased number of hysterectomies.

EPIDEMIOLOGY OF CERVICAL CANCER

In the middle of the 19th century Italian scholar Demenico Rigoni-Stern noticed that the frequency of cervical cancer varied in different groups of women. His conclusion, based on review of mortality records, showed that more uterine cancers were found in married than in unmarried women and that cervical cancer was most prevalent in women between the ages of 30 and 40. Cervical cancer also was rare among unmarried women and almost absent in certain orders of nuns.

In the 1930s Gagnon substantiated these findings in studies of Canadian nuns. The study involved a 20-year follow-up with a fully documented cohort. Also, a retrospective study was done by Nix, who reviewed hospital records and autopsy records of 100,000 Catholic nuns and found only one death caused by cervical carcinoma. Celibacy would, therefore, seem to confer protection from cervical cancer.

In the 1950s there were a number of reviews of the epidemiology of cancer of the cervix, and the findings included the following: (1) there appeared to be an increased incidence of cervical cancer in married women, but even more if the woman married before age 20; (2) there appeared to be an increased incidence of cervical cancer if marital instability was present (divorce); (3) there was a high association between carcinoma of the cervix and syphilis; (4) there was an extremely high incidence of cervical cancer among prostitutes.

In 1967 Martin identified the low-risk group of women for development of cervical cancer. In this group he included Muslim women, Amish women, Jewish women, Seventh-Day Adventist women, Irish immigrant women, Italian immigrant women, Protestant and Catholic women who regularly attend religious services, women of high economic status, and rural women. In the high-risk group of women for cervical cancer development he included Puerto Rican women, Mexican immigrant women, Negro women, inmates of women's prisons, prostitutes, venereal disease clinic patients, women of low economic status, and urban women. It is obvious that socioeconomic status, race, and education have only an indirect role in epidemiology of cervical cancer. The conclusion from all current epidemiologic investigations is that the incidence of cervical cancer is related just to three factors:

1. *Age of first intercourse.* Rotkin and King found that the age of first intercourse is the variable of greatest clinical correlation. In their study it was reported that patients who began coitus between the ages of 15 and 17 have twice the incidence of cervical cancer as in the control group. Furthermore, in contrast to rates of matched controls, comparatively few cervical cancers developed in patients who began coitus after the age of 21. There were almost none when the first coitus was as late as age 37.
2. *Number of sexual partners.* The number of sexual partners is another factor that is closely related to the incidence of cervical neoplasia. Although it is difficult to obtain exact data, it is well established that women with multiple sexual partners have a higher frequency of cervical cancer than matched controls.
3. *Parity.* Cervical cancer is more frequent in parous women than in nulliparous women, but total number of pregnancies is not directly related to the frequency of cervical cancer. Women with a high number of pregnancies usually start sexual life early, and the early age of first intercourse might be etiologically more important than the actual number of pregnancies.

The epidemiologic data correlate well with the current understanding of the pathogenesis of cervical neoplasia. The period of early squamous metaplasia is the time of greatest risk for cellular transformation and development of cervical neoplasia (Fig. 41-1). In this period young metaplastic cells have phagocytic properties, and if some potential mutagen is present in the vagina during this time, the epithelium might undergo the cellular transformation. The early squamous metaplasia occurs almost exclusively in puberty and early adolescence and in the first pregnancy. Therefore, women who begin sexual activity at an early age, when the metaplastic process is most active, have a greater chance of developing cervical cancer. Women who have multiple sexual partners have a higher possibility that some potential mutagen might be introduced into the vagina. Also, women who have at least one pregnancy in which columnar epithelium is everted to the portio because of hypertrophy of the cervix and undergoes early squamous metaplasia would have a higher frequency of cervical neoplasia than nulliparous women.

ROLE OF POSSIBLE MUTAGENS

Epidemiologic data suggest that venereally transmitted agents may act as mutagens. Syphylis, gonorrhea, trichomonas, and fungus have been related to a higher frequency of cervical neoplasia. There is no substantiating evidence, however, that any of these are causative in nature, and they appear to be only circumstantial. The role of viruses as potential causative agents has been investigated in depth. Viruses are obligate intracellular parasites and are likely, therefore, to interfere with DNA replication of the host. Several viruses (adenovirus, papovaviruses, SV 40 virus) are unequivocally oncogenic for certain rodent species. Several other herpesviruses have induced tumors in monkeys, rabbits, chickens, and frogs. There is evidence implicating the herpesvirus as oncogenic in a variety of animal species, and strong, but not conclusive, evidence implicating the

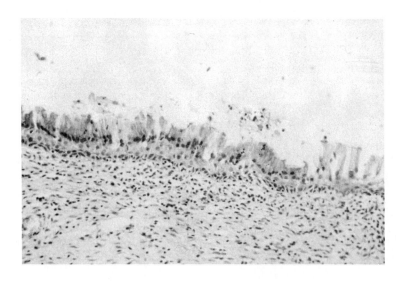

Figure 41–1. Early squamous metaplasia. Young metaplastic cells form three to four cell layers, columnar cell still on top. (Courtesy of Dr. A. Sedlis)

Epstein-Barr virus as the causative agent of Burkitt's lymphoma in humans. Herpes simplex virus type II has been suggested as an causative agent based initially on circumstantial evidence. Naib and associates have shown that women of low socioeconomic status have a high incidence of exposure to the type II herpesvirus, as confirmed by positive serum antibody titers. The incidence of type II neutralizing antibody titers was found to be significantly higher in women with preinvasive or invasive cervical carcinoma than in a control group of similar-aged gynecologic patients without cervical cancer or in patients attending venereal disease clinics. Although differences in incidence of positive type II antibody titers have not been noted universally in women with cervical cancer (exceptions include Caucasian women in New Zealand, mestizo women in Colombia, Oriental women in Taiwan, and Jewish women in Israel, where control groups have a higher incidence of positive antibody titers), there is almost complete agreement that Caucasian and black women in the western hemisphere who have cervical cancer have an increased incidence of positive antibody titers to herpes type II infection. Royston and Aurelian reported that 31% of dyskaryotic cells from patients with invasive carcinoma showed evidence of herpesvirus antigens by immunofluorescent studies. There was no evidence, however, of virus antigens in frozen section biopsies from cervical tumors, which raises questions about the significance of these observations. The best evidence regarding the oncogenic role of the herpes type II virus currently is indirect, and does not confirm that the association of a herpesvirus infection in patients with cervical cancer is one of cause-and-effect relationship.

The role of the human papillomavirus (HPV) in cervical carcinogenesis was not recognized until 1976. Papillomaviruses are found in a variety of human warty lesions: condylomata acuminata, oral and laryngeal papillomas, and skin warts. For a long time it was believed that these lesions were caused by the same virus. Biochemical and immunologic studies, however, have revealed that there are several serotypes of HPV. HPV 6 and 11 infections are sexually transmitted diseases that may be associated with cervical intraepithelial neoplasia (CIN). HPV 16 and 18 are two principal HPV types found in in situ and invasive cervical carcinoma.

Warty lesions of the vulva and vagina had been recognized and described as far back as ancient times. Cervical condylomata also occur but are less readily diagnosed. They may occur in the original ectocervical squamous epithelium as well as in the metaplastic epithelium located in the colposcopic transformation zone. The stratified squamous epithelium covering the condyloma is characterized by parakeratosis and hyperkeratosis as well as by atypical cells in the outer intermediate cell layers, which show perinuclear cytoplasmic clearing or ballooning. These cells have been referred to as koilocytotic cells. The nuclei usually are round and rather uniform, with frequent binucleation. Meisels and associates, in a review of previously diagnosed cases of dysplasia, found that more than 70% were actually condylomata. In a correlative study of colposcopy and histology they also demonstrated that cervical condylomata occur more frequently than previously suspected.

To differentiate clinically HPV lesions from CIN lesions is difficult. The diagnosis of exophytic condylomatous lesions with typical fingerlike projections is easy. To differentiate flat papillomas from CIN I lesions, however, is colposcopically very hard or even impossible. Colposcopically, HPV lesions produce three typical appearances: (1) a flat, acetowhite epithelium with no vessel pattern; (2) a microvillus appearance; and (3) a mosaic-type lesion with large lacuna in the center of the mosaic. Many HPV lesions are multifocal with so-called satellite lesions (small lesions around the main lesion, often in original squamous epithelium).

The humoral antibody response to HPV particles may be important in preventing or spreading infection, whereas the events surrounding regression of warts and condylomas appear to be primarily associated with specific cell-mediated immunity. Local cell-mediated immune responses, particularly cell-associated soluble mediators and stationary macrophagelike cells, may be particularly important in the host immune response to mucosal infections.

The spontaneous remission of wart virus infections may explain the well-known regression of mild dysplasia. It is premature to suggest that noncondylomatous wart virus lesions are actually precursors of cervical neoplasia. The epidemiologic behavior of the HPV lesion is similar to that of cervical neoplasia. HPV lesions often coexist on the cervix with dysplasia or neoplasia, can be seen in adjacent or distant areas of the squamous epithelium, or are sometimes intermingled. In terms of therapy, it does not matter if a patient has histologically proven CIN alone, or intraepithelial neoplasia along with wart virus changes. The management of all these lesions is identical, and depends on the severity of intraepithelial neoplasia.

Papillomavirus infection might play an important role in the pathogenesis of cervical neoplasia; however, only association between HPV infection and cervical neoplasia was demonstrated, but not causal relationship. Only in the transformation zone is HPV infection perhaps associated with CIN. HPV infection is prevalent outside the transformation zone or in the vagina, but seldom does neoplasia develop in these anatomic sites. It seems that the HPV virus might be only one of the cofactors in cervical neoplasia.

NATURAL HISTORY OF CERVICAL NEOPLASIA

The cervix is readily available for visual or colposcopic inspection. Tissue samples can be obtained in colposcopically directed biopsy, and today more is known about the natural history of cervical cancer than that of many other cancers. The current concepts about the pathogenesis of cervical neoplasia are summarized in Figure 41-2.

All changes that might lead to cervical neoplasia develop in the area originally covered with columnar epithelium. The columnar epithelium is established on the ectocervix during the fetal development in 70% of newborns or can be everted to the ectocervix during the first pregnancy. The columnar epithelium on the ectocervix is exposed to the vaginal environment, which, after puberty, is acid. The low pH of the vagina is the main stimulus for squamous metaplasia. In the beginning of squamous metaplasia the young metaplastic cells have phagocytic properties and phagocytize whatever is present in the vagina. The period of early squamous metaplasia is the most critical event for the potential risk of cellular transformation and for the development of cervical neoplasia. If some potential mutagen is present in the vagina during this early process of squamous metaplasia, transformation of the epithelium toward premalignant changes may occur. This altered metaplastic process can be recognized colposcopically by the presence of abnormal colposcopic lesions (white epithelium, mosaic, punctation). Although the causative agent remains undetermined, the important aspect is that the mutagenic agent must be present at a specific time in the life cycle of a specific cell to produce neoplastic transformation.

The specific time for this biologic event is during the beginning of squamous metaplasia, when the active columnar cells are susceptible for the transformation process. The transformed pathologic epithelium, by its own growth, will compress the vessels in the grapelike structures of the columnar epithelium, and on the mode and degree of the capillary constriction either mosaic, punctation, or acetowhite epithelium will develop. The transformation to premalignant changes is a rapid process that lasts for days or weeks at most. The promotion of these changes, however, is a long-term process. Some lesions can stay on the cervix indefinitely without change, and some can progress quickly to carcinoma in situ or invasive carcinoma. The progression rate is unpredictable and perhaps is related to immunologic host response. If the host response is normal, the lesion will stay without change. If the host

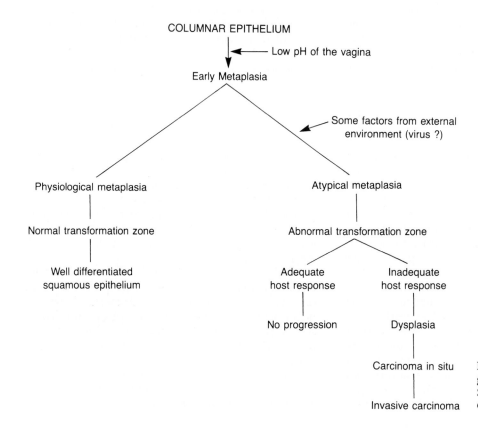

Figure 41–2. Schema of pathogenesis of cervical neoplasia (From Stafl A, Mattingly RF. Am J Obstet Gynecol 1974; 120:666)

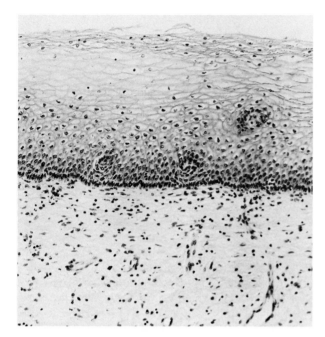

Figure 41–3. Normal cervical epithelium. Note the stratification from deepest layer of basal cells to superficial flattened spinal cells.

response, for any reason, decreases, then there is a possibility of progression to more significant changes. Current data based on observations of immunosuppressed patients seem to support this hypothesis.

Clinically important is that after these two periods of early squamous metaplasia are completed (after puberty and after the first pregnancy), it is possible to divide a patient population into two groups: (1) Patients who have, after the first pregnancy, normal transformation zone with components of the normal transformation zone (tongues of squamous metaplasia, gland openings, and nabothian cysts). In these patients the metaplastic epithelium is well differentiated. Only the biologically active cells are at the basal membrane, and they are separated from the vaginal environment by 20 or 30 layers of differentiated or cornified cells (Fig. 41-3). Therefore, the possibility that some mutagen from the external environment might interfere with these biologically active cells is minimal. Thus these patients are at low risk for developing cervical neoplasia in the future. (2) The second group are patients with an abnormal colposcopical lesion (acetowhite epithelium, punctation, mosaic). On the average about 8% of colposcopically or cervicographically screened patients belong to this group. The percentage also depends on low-risk and high-risk populations concerning the development of cervical neoplasia. Many abnormal colposcopical lesions that can be clearly col-

poscopically documented do not show any abnormal histopathologic changes. Still these patients are considered at higher risk for development of cervical neoplasia because these lesions might represent subclinical HPV infections.

PATHOLOGY OF CERVICAL CANCER

Two histologic classifications for premalignant changes of cervical neoplasia are used. The traditional classification described mild, moderate, or severe dysplasia, and carcinoma in situ. Mild dysplasia is used for lesions in which abnormal cells involve the lower one-third of the epithelium (Fig. 41-4); moderate dysplasia, one-half of the epithelium (Fig. 41-5); and severe dysplasia for lesions with almost full-thickness involvement, but still with some differentiated cells on the surface of the epithelium. Carcinoma in situ is diagnosed when complete undifferentiation of the entire thickness of the epithelium is present (Figs. 41-6 and 41-7). Richart introduced a new concept in which dysplasia and in situ carcinoma form a biologic continuum. In any particular case of dysplasia or carcinoma in situ potential for invasion cannot be predicted by histologic or cytologic analysis. All dysplasias, from mild through severe, have the capacity to persist or to progress to a higher rate of abnormality or directly to invasive carcinoma (Figs. 41-8 and 41-9). Burghardt demonstrated that even mild dysplasia can directly progress to invasive cancer. This seldom happens, but it can happen. It is not necessary for a lesion compatible with mild dysplasia always to progress up to in situ carcinoma before it has a potential for invasion.

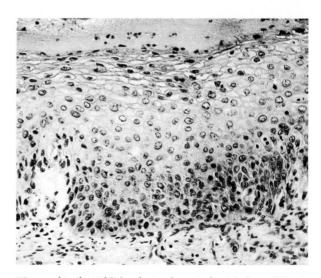

Figure 41–4. Mild dysplasia of cervical epithelium (CIN I).

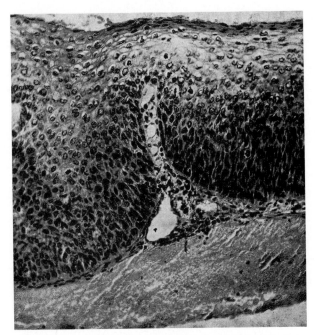

Figure 41–5. Moderate dysplasia of cervical epithelium (CIN II).

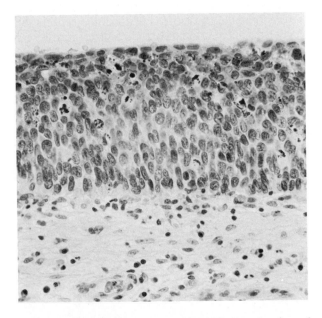

Figure 41–6. Carcinoma in situ (CIN III). Complete loss of stratification and distribution of atypical cells and mitotic figures through full thickness of epithelium. Note that there is no penetration or breakthrough of the basement membrane.

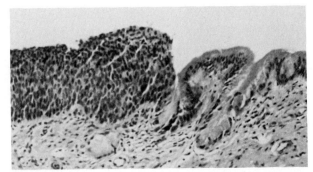

Figure 41–7. Abrupt margin between *left* CIN III, and *right* normal columnar epithelium.

All degrees of intraepithelial lesions represent a spectrum of the same disease; therefore, Richart proposed that the term *cervical intraepithelial neoplasia* be divided into three grades: CIN I correlates to mild dysplasia; CIN II, to moderate dysplasia; and CIN III, to severe dysplasia or carcinoma in situ.

DETECTION OF CERVICAL CANCER

CIN has no clinical signs or symptoms, and therefore routine surveillance is required to detect these early lesions. Several diagnostic methods are available, and include cytology, colposcopy, cervicography, cervical biopsy, endocervical curettage (ECC), and conization.

Cytology

Cytology was introduced into gynecologic practice by George Papanicolaou in 1943. Screening by cytology (Pap smear) resulted in the increased detection of preinvasive cervical cancer and the decrease in the incidence of invasive carcinoma and in the mortality rate from this disease. The classic demonstration of the benefits of cytologic screening was the study of Boyes and Worth, with supporting data from the British Columbia screening program. This program, started in 1949, was designed to test the hypothesis that screening for cervical cancer was of value in reducing the incidence of invasive cervical cancer. A registry was maintained in British Columbia for the prevalence and incidence of invasive cervical carcinoma as well as a registry for mortality from this disease. It was considered essential to keep the cases of preclinical invasive carcinoma separate from the cases of clinical carcinoma. The only accurate index, therefore, that can be used for evaluation of the morbidity from this disease is

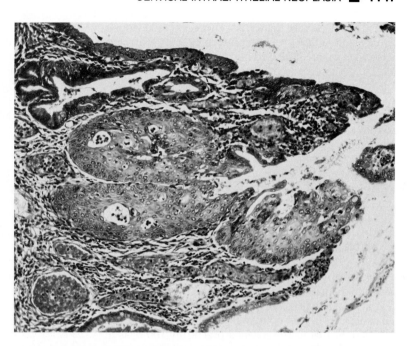

Figure 41–8. Squamous metastasis displacing cervical glands well into cervix.

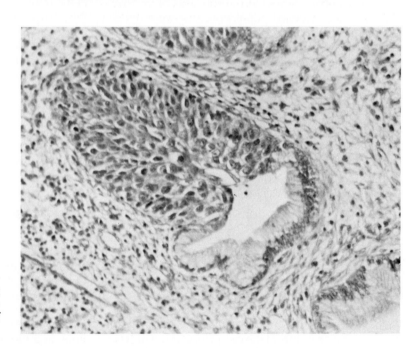

Figure 41–9. Carcinoma in situ with involvement of endocervical clefts showing neoplastic epithelium "snowplowing" beneath glandular epithelium and filling of the gland-like lumen.

the incidence of clinical invasive carcinoma. The incidence of invasive cancer decreased from 28.4 per 100,000 women in 1955 to 7.6 per 100,000 in 1977. The second index used in evaluating the program was the mortality from invasive carcinoma. The refined death rate from invasive cervical cancer declined from 11.4 per 100,000 women in 1958 to 3.8 per 100,000 in 1976.

Mortality from cervical carcinoma decreased by about 60% during the period of the study.

Because of the financial resources required for mass population screening, screening programs may be more appropriately aimed at populations with the highest risk for cervical cancer. There is no doubt that the highest-risk group can be identified among women with certain sexual patterns. These include those women with a history of first intercourse or marriage before age 21, an increased number of sexual partners, and an increased rate of sexually transmitted diseases.

Concerning the optimum time for initiation of cytologic screening and for rescreening, there is agreement that a woman should have regular vaginal cytologic examinations when she becomes sexually active. According to the report of Fidler and coworkers, the number of cases that progress from negative to positive cytology after age 55 is extremely small, such that it is possible to consider decreasing the frequency of cytology screening at the age of 55 in women who have had regular cervical-vaginal cytologic smears. The data clearly demonstrate that cytology can significantly decrease the morbidity and mortality from cervical cancer.

When cytology was introduced there was an idealistic opinion that with screening every woman once a year it would be possible to eliminate all cases of cervical cancer. This goal never was accomplished, even in populations that were screened practically 100%, as in British Columbia. Always there were cases of invasive cancers in the screened populations that were undetected. The false-negative rate of cytology is difficult to establish because if the cytology is negative and the cervix is clinically not suspicious, no further procedures are done. Using mathematical models, Coppleson and Brown estimated the false-negative rate of a single Pap smear to be between 20% and 42% (20% in detection of in situ lesions, 42% in detection of invasive lesions). The reasons for false-negative Pap smears are numerous, for example:

Improper cell collections
Absence of endocervical cells
Smears too thin
Smears too thick
Bloody smears
Improper fixation
Incorrect staining
Mistakes in screening by cytotechnicians
Mistakes in diagnosis by cytopathologists.

The lowest contribution to the false-negative rate of cytology is probably from the cytopathologist. This was demonstrated by Richart, who, by reviewing all slides in his study by himself, achieved a false-negative rate of cytology as low as 2.8%. In a clinical situation it is humanly impossible for the cytopathologist to screen all slides. The screening of a single slide is time-consuming, and therefore the cytopathologist depends on the quality of screening by cytotechnicians. By current standards 10% of all negative smears must be reviewed by the pathologist; therefore, 90% of all negative smears

are not seen by the cytopathologist. How high the false-negative rate is depends on the quality of the laboratory. With new detection methods, colposcopy and cervicography, it was demonstrated that the false-negative rate of cytology is much higher than was expected.

Colposcopy

Whereas cytology is a laboratory method of detection, colposcopy is a clinical method. Each method deals with a different aspect of neoplasia. Cytology evaluates the morphologic changes in exfoliated cells, whereas colposcopy mainly evaluates changes in the terminal vascular network of the cervix that reflect the biochemical and metabolic changes in the tissue.

The colposcope is basically a stereoscopic microscope by which the cervix may be visualized in bright light under 6× to 40× magnification. The examination is rapid, requiring almost the same time as the inspection of the cervix with the unaided eye.

Colposcopy is based on the stereoscopic evaluation of the transformation zone. The transformation zone is the portion of the cervix that was originally covered by columnar epithelium that, through a process of squamous metaplasia, has been transformed to squamous epithelium. The transformation zone extends between the original squamocolumnar junction (border between original squamous epithelium and endocervical epithelium) and the physiologic squamocolumnar junction (border between metaplastic epithelium and columnar epithelium). Colposcopically, it has been shown that cervical neoplasia develops almost exclusively within the transformation zone as a result of atypical metaplasia.

Colposcopic Terminology

Based on the concept of the changes in the transformation zone, a revision of colposcopic terminology was adopted during the Fourth International Congress of Cervical Pathology and Colposcopy in London, England, in 1981. Colposcopic findings are divided as follows.

Normal colposcopic findings include the original squamous epithelium, the normal columnar epithelium, and the transformation zone.

Abnormal colposcopic findings include an atypical transformation zone in which there are colposcopic findings suggestive of cervical neoplasia: mosaic, punctation, acetowhite epithelium, leukoplakia, (elevated whitened plaque of hyperkeratosis or parakeratosis), or atypical blood vessels.

Suspect frank invasive cancer includes those cases with colposcopically obvious invasive cancer that are not evident on clinical examination.

Unsatisfactory colposcopic findings are those cases in which the squamocolumnar junction cannot be visualized.

Other colposcopic findings include inflammatory changes, atrophic epithelium, true erosion, and condyloma or papilloma.

Diagnostic Features with Colposcopy

Cervical neoplasia does not develop in patients with normal colposcopic findings. In patients with abnormal colposcopic findings a colposcopic biopsy should be taken from the most suspicious lesion for histopathologic diagnosis. The histopathologic changes associated with mosaic, punctation, and acetowhite epithelium range from immature squamous metaplasia to carcinoma in situ. When atypical vessels are present there is already a suspicion of invasion. To predict the type of histopathologic changes that will be found in a colposcopically directed biopsy, extensive clinical experience is required in the evaluation of vascular pattern, intercapillary distance, surface contour, color tone, and clarity of demarcation of the focal lesion.

The *vascular pattern* is one of the most important diagnostic features. Changes in the vascular pattern correspond closely to the histologic picture. It usually is accepted that the first changes in carcinogenesis occur biochemically at the cellular level, and can be detected only by sophisticated laboratory methods, which are not clinically applicable. During the earliest stages of carcinogenesis the morphology of the tissue may not yet be changed. The blood vessels, however, do react to these changes in tissue metabolism, and such vascular alterations constitute the first morphologic features in the development of cervical neoplasia. These vascular changes are not detectable in 5-µm histologic sections, but they are clearly visible through the colposcope. For a detailed description of the different patterns of vascular change and their diagnostic significance, the reader is referred to the colposcopic literature.

Intercapillary distance refers to the space between corresponding parts of two adjacent vessels or to the diameter delineated by a network of mosaiclike vessels. During actual colposcopy an estimation of the intercapillary distance in abnormal areas can best be made by comparing it with that of the capillaries found in the adjacent normal epithelium. In preinvasive and invasive carcinoma of the cervix the intercapillary distance increases as the stage of the disease advances.

The colposcope provides stereoscopic magnification, which greatly facilitates the study of the *surface contour.* This may be described as smooth, uneven, granular, papillomatous, or nodular. Normal squamous epithelium has a smooth surface, whereas carcinoma in situ and early invasive cancer may have an uneven,

slightly elevated surface. Different colposcopic lesions show different *colors,* varying from white to deep red. The difference between the color before and the color after the acetic acid test is important; if there is a marked change from deep red to white, a more serious histologic lesion may be expected.

The *border between the lesion and the adjacent normal tissue* is an important feature concerned with the colposcopic diagnosis of cervical neoplasia. The borderline between normal squamous epithelium and inflammatory lesions or mild dysplasia is diffuse. On the other hand, severe dysplasia and carcinoma in situ usually produce sharp-bordered lesions, distinctly demarcated from the adjacent epithelium.

Unsatisfactory colposcopic findings mean that the squamocolumnar junction is not visible, a condition that occurs more often in postmenopausal women. Unsatisfactory colposcopy is present in less than 15% of patients under 45 years of age. In patients with unsatisfactory colposcopic findings one cannot rely on colposcopy for a clinical diagnosis, since the pathologic changes may be high in the endocervical canal, and other diagnostic methods (ECC or conization) are required.

The main value of colposcopy is in the evaluation of patients with abnormal cytologic findings. With colposcopy it is possible to localize the lesion, evaluate its extent, and obtain a directed biopsy whereby the histopathologic diagnosis can be established. Colposcopy is accurate in differentiating between invasive and noninvasive lesions and in the differential diagnosis between inflammatory atypia and neoplasia. The limitation of colposcopy lies in its inability to detect lesions deep in the endocervical canal in cases where the squamocolumnar junction is not visible. In these cases colposcopy is not negative, but unsatisfactory, and further diagnostic steps, mainly ECC or conization, are necessary in evaluating a patient with abnormal cytology.

The term *unsatisfactory colposcopy* was not recognized in original German terminology, which explains the high false-negative rate of colposcopy reported in the German literature. When cases of unsatisfactory colposcopic findings are excluded, the true false-negative rate of colposcopy is very low.

Colposcopic Evaluation of Patients with Suspicious or Positive Pap Smears

After review of the patient's medical history a bivalve speculum is inserted. The mucus is carefully removed from the cervix, using a cotton swab or dry gauze. The colposcope is then focused on the cervix. During the inspection the surface of the cervix should be moistened with normal saline solution. A dry epithelial surface is insufficiently transparent and allows an incomplete view of the underlying vascular pattern. In a routine colposcopic examination a magnification of 16 × is used. Optimal contrast of the vessels is achieved by the insertion of a green filter. After inspection of the cervix moistened with saline solution a generous amount of 5% acetic acid is applied to the cervix. The acetic acid helps to coagulate the mucus, which can then be easily removed from the clefts and folds of columnar epithelium. Acetic acid also temporarily removes the water from the cells, and in areas where there is a high nuclear density (immature squamous epithelium, dysplasia, or carcinoma in situ) the epithelium becomes white over a fairly well demarcated area. The effect of acetic acid is transient, lasting for only a few minutes, but the acetic acid test can be repeated several times. Abnormal colposcopic lesions are then sampled by colposcopically directed biopsies. When the squamocolumnar junction is not visible or the lesion extends into the endocervical canal, ECC is performed.

Cervicography

In 1956 Navratil and associates demonstrated that the accuracy of cancer detection can be significantly increased by the combination of two detection methods—cytology and colposcopy. Their data showed that although both cytology and colposcopy used alone will miss some cases, by combining the two methods it is possible to increase the accuracy to 98.8%.

This was known already in 1956, but still almost nowhere in the world were cytology and colposcopy used simultaneously in cervical cancer screening. There are two reasons for this. First, the colposcope is an expensive instrument, and not every examination room can be equipped with the colposcope. Second, perhaps more important, few gynecologists are sufficiently trained in colposcopy to do the colposcopy screening. To overcome these problems, cervicography was invented in 1981 by Stafl.

The cervicograph is an optical instrument, a kind of photo camera. With this instrument a macroscopic picture of the cervix can be taken (Fig. 41-10). Everything on the instrument is locked (eg, f-stop, exposure time, and focusing), and therefore the instrument is practically foolproof. The focusing is done by the moving of the entire instrument. After a short period of instruction (1–2 hours) anyone (physician, nurse, technician) can take a picture of the cervix, which can then be sent to an expert for evaluation. Thus the principle of cervicography is similar to the principle of cytology. In cytology also the physician does not need to be an expert in cytopathology to take a cytologic smear, and he or she just sends the slide to a cytologic laboratory. Similarly in cervicography, the person taking the picture does not need to have colposcopic expertise. Just a picture of the cervix is taken that is then sent to an expert for evaluation (Figs. 41-11 and 41-12). Cervicography is a noninvasive procedure. The instrument does not come in contact with the body of the patient and, therefore, no risk is involved.

With colposcopy and with cervicography exactly the same parameters are observed, only the instrument is

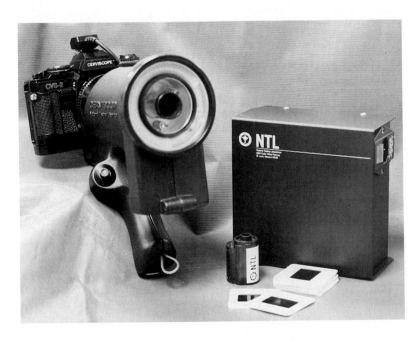

Figure 41–10. Cerviscope with power pack. Instrument has a bright light for focusing and flash light for taking pictures. (Courtesy of National Testing Laboratories, St. Louis)

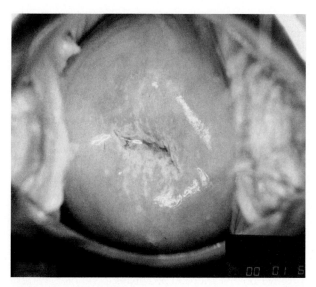

Figure 41–11. Negative cervigram. Normal transformation zone with gland openings visible, but no abnormal lesion present.

different. It is therefore not surprising that in the original study published in 1981, it was found that the diagnostic accuracy of colposcopy and cervicography was identical. Therefore, the results of cervicography and colposcopy screening also should be identical.

In a pilot cervicography screening study involving 404 patients six cases of CIN I, two cases of CIN II, and one case of CIN III were detected that were missed by cytology.

A much larger study was published in 1988 from Kaiser Permanente in California by Tawa and associates. This study involved 3271 patients between ages 18 and 50, in whom 81 cases of CIN were detected. Pap smear and cervicography were done during the same visit. It was a prospective study with blind evaluation of Pap smear and cervicography. If the cervigram or Pap smear was positive, colposcopically directed biopsy was obtained. Fourteen cases of CIN were detected with cytology; 72 cases were detected with cervicography. The conclusion from this study was that the sensitivity of cervicography is 5.1 times higher than cytology. Also of significance is that the cervigram is 3.7 times more cost-effective than cytology when all the costs related to screening are combined.

Although the sensitivity of cervicography in cancer detection is higher than cytology, the specificity of cervicography is lower. It is well known from colposcopy research that there are well-established colposcopic (or cervicographic) lesions, but still, if a biopsy is taken on the border between a normal tissue and the lesion, the normal light microscope cannot differentiate be-

tween the normal epithelium and the lesion. These cases are considered false positive for cervicography. Hypothetically it is possible that these lesions represent an abnormal cervical lesion that can be detected by colposcopy or cervicography, but not yet by light microscopy in a histologic specimen. With the HPV infections and the possible relation of this infection to cervical neoplasia, these lesions might represent subclinical HPV infection and precursors to cervical neoplasia.

Reid studied 1400 patients for the prevalence of HPV infection. Patients were screened by cytology, cervicography, and DNA hybridication. In this study the false-negative rate for cytology was 64%, for cervicography 20%, and for DNA hybridization 81%.

Spitzer and coworkers compared the utility of repeat Pap smear, cervicography, and colposcopy in the evaluation of patients with atypical Pap smear. The sensitivity of cervicography was much better than that of Pap smear for both referral (89% compared with 58%) and detection (78% compared with 18%). Pap smears were more specific than cervicography (55% compared with 29%).

Cervicography represents a natural development of colposcopy and replaces subjective colposcopic evaluation with objective cervicography assessment and permanent documentation.

If cervicography could always be used in combination with cytology, the cancer detection rate could be close to 100%. Cervicography will never replace colposcopy. If a lesion is found, expert colposcopy evalua-

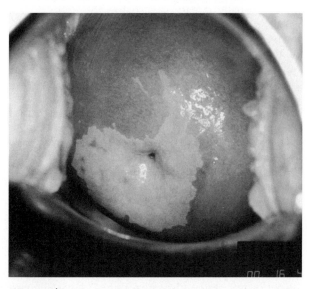

Figure 41–12. Suspicious cervigram. Acetowhite epithelium both on anterior and posterior lip with irregular borders. Lesion compatible with mild dysplasia (CIN I), but satellite lesion also suggests herpesvirus infection.

tion is necessary, and a colposcopically directed biopsy should be taken.

Current studies demonstrate that cervicography can effectively detect cases of precancer and cancer missed by cytology, and thus play an important role in cervical cancer detection.

Biopsy Technique

There are several biopsy instruments on the market. In our clinic we mainly use Kevorkian biopsy forceps. When the lesion is close to the cervical os, the teeth of the biopsy forceps can be angled in the external os and, with the movable jaw of the biopsy forceps, a relatively shallow biopsy can be obtained. The biopsy should contain stroma; 1 to 2 mm is sufficient. With deeper biopsies there is more potential for bleeding. After a 2- to 3-mm deep biopsy the bleeding usually is minimal, and just contact pressure from a vaginal tampon is sufficient to stop the bleeding. When the lesion is located more on the periphery of the cervix, the biopsy forceps often slip and only a strip of epithelium without the stroma is obtained. In this situation it is easier to grasp the cervix just lateral to the lesion with a tenaculum. This will produce a fold that can then be easily biopsied.

In pregnant patients the cervix is soft and hypertrophic, and there usually is some eversion of columnar epithelium to the portio. It is unusual to have an unsatisfactory colposcopy in pregnancy. When the squamocolumnar junction is not visible in a pregnant patient, it usually is easy to visualize the endocervical canal. An endocervical speculum should not be used. It is a pointed instrument that can cause bleeding or even rupture of membranes in later stages of pregnancy. It is better to use ring forceps, and with the ring forceps it is possible to visualize the entire endocervical canal.

Cervical biopsies in pregnant patients often are associated with significant bleeding, mainly in the second half of the pregnancy. Before the biopsy in a pregnant patient is obtained the physician should have ready swabs soaked in Monsel's solution (ferrous subsulfate) that can be applied to the biopsy site immediately after the biopsy. Monsel's solution should significantly reduce the danger of bleeding in pregnant patients.

Endocervical Curettage

Experts vary in their opinion as to when ECC should be performed. Some advocate routine ECC to safeguard against missing occult cancer within the canal and strongly recommend ECC before any outpatient methods of therapy, even if the squamocolumnar junction is fully visible. Others reserve its use for triage of women with suspicious or positive cytology and unsatisfactory colposcopy. Less experienced colposcopists lose nothing by performing routine ECC as a fail-safe measure and as a potential aid for medicolegal defense. When a physician is certain that he or she has seen the entire squamocolumnar junction and can see a ring of columnar epithelium within the lower cervical canal, omission of the routine ECC is justified. Before outpatient methods of therapy are initiated there should be some permanent documentation that the endocervical canal is negative; however, ECC is not the only way of documentation. Confirmation that the squamocolumnar junction is visible can be done without discomfort of the ECC to the patient with a simple cervigram. ECC should be done before performing ectocervical biopsies under colposcopic control so as not to inadvertently contaminate the curettings with fragments of ectocervical lesion. Otherwise, ECC will produce false-positive results, thereby provoking cone biopsies that are otherwise not indicated. For ECC a sharp, narrow Kevorkian curette is used. ECC is done without anesthesia and without holding the cervix with a tenaculum. The endocervical curette is inserted to the level of the internal os, and then with short, firm strokes the entire endocervical canal is curetted two times around, making sure not to pull the curette out through the external os. After the endocervical canal is curetted twice around, the curette still inside the endocervical canal is turned several times around so that the majority of curettings will remain in the curette. The ECC material is then deposited on a small square of Telfa and placed into fixative. Any fragments that remain around the external os are picked up with sponge forceps.

Because the material from the ECC is fragmented, often tangentially cut, and maloriented, it is impossible to get exact histopathologic diagnosis. From the histopathologist just three diagnoses are expected: (1) Negative—only fragments of normal squamous or columnar epithelium are found. (2) Frank invasive cancer—in this case a large chunk of tissue that has created suspicion of cancer usually is obtained during the ECC. From this large piece of tissue it usually is possible to establish a definite diagnosis of invasive cancer. (3) Fragments from ECC show some degree of CIN lesion. In this situation it is impossible to distinguish between CIN I, II, and III, and conization is required for definite diagnosis.

Conization of the Cervix

Cold-knife conization of the cervix consists of the annular removal of a cone-shaped wedge of tissue from the cervix uteri. To be considered adequate for diagnostic purposes, the operative specimen must include uninvolved endocervical epithelium above the lesion and uninvolved ectocervix below and lateral to any lesion on the portio. Just how much tissue such a specimen should encompass must vary with the individual case. During the reproductive years most lesions are found on the portio, so that the cone usually has a broad base and the top has a wide angle. In older women, in whom the squamocolumnar junction has shifted to a location higher in the endocervical canal, the cone specimen is long and narrow with a sharp endocervical angle at the top of the cone. The width of the base is best determined by including all Schiller light areas of the portio within the cone margins. The cervix is exposed, and a Lugol's stain is performed. Tenaculae or holding sutures are placed into the cervix laterally at the 3 and 9 o'clock positions beyond the margins of Schiller light epithelium. With traction on the cervix, the cervical stroma is infiltrated with 40 to 60 ml of 1:200,000 solution of phenylephrine (Neo-Synephrine) in a circumferential manner. If the injection is correctly placed into the stroma, a significant amount of pressure will be required on the syringe plunger. The cervix will blanch and increase in size.

The uterine canal is gently sounded, and the sound is left in place to mark the course of the endocervical canal. A circular incision is then made outside the Schiller light margin beginning posteriorly with the tip of the blade directed against the metal probe in the cervical canal. The specimen should be excised in a single piece. It is our custom to identify the 12 o'clock position on the specimen with a single suture placed into the cervical stroma. The excised tissue should not be placed in fixative at this time. The uterine canal is then curetted with a small Kevorkian curette to rule out pathology above the upper margins of the cone.

At this point the cervix may be treated in one of two ways: the cone site may be left open or Sturmdorf sutures may be used to close the raw areas. If the Sturmdorf suture is used, it should be placed in the posterior lip first. No. 1 delayed absorbable sutures are used on a large cutting needle. The suture initially picks up the posterior flap of mucosa in the midline near the edge (Fig. 41-13). Then the suture is directed high into the endocervical canal, passing through the wall of the cervical canal and out through the portio of the posterior cervical lip near the fornix, about 2 cm from the site of the initial suture. As the mucosal flap is pulled forward, the other end of the suture is threaded into the cutting needle and the process of suturing through the cervical canal is repeated. The two ends of the suture should emerge on the posterior surface of the cervix about 0.5 cm apart. Firm traction on this suture will pull the posterior mucosal flap well into the newly made cervical canal. The suture is tied, and the procedure is repeated on the anterior lip.

If the cone site is left open, a superficial electrocoagulation of the bleeding points in the cervical stroma is performed, followed by application of a piece of Gelfoam sponge to the cervical defect. This is held in place with a vaginal pack that is removed in 24 hours. The cosmetic results of this method are better compared with those obtained with the Sturmdorf suture technique, and there is the added theoretical advantage that one is not covering up deep residual nests of tumor that may be unable to reveal their presence by exfoliation. Because the Sturmdorf suture is gradually released with the dissolution of the suture material, its only advantage has been in the immediate control of bleeding. Comparing these two methods of closure, Chao and colleagues found no significant difference in operative blood loss or incidence of postoperative hemorrhage.

When the conization specimen is received in the laboratory it should be opened lengthwise with a sharp knife blade at the 12 o'clock position and spread flat. The margins of the cone are pinned to a large paraffin block, care being taken not to pierce the epithelium with the holding pins. Then the entire block is placed in fixative solution. After fixation the cone is cut lengthwise into as many sections as possible, again using a sharp, thin blade. The average cone specimen can easily be divided into 15 or more tissue slices. Each slice is separately imbedded, and multiple sections are cut from each block. If five sections are obtained from each tissue slice, 75 slides will be available for histologic examination. The number of sections examined is crucial. As reported by Burghardt, diagnostic errors will increase by 22% if only 15 histologic sections are examined from each cone instead of 80 sections. Most investigators have reported a fairly consistent diagnostic error rate for conization of 3.5%, with a range varying between 0.5% and 9.0%.

Conization is not an innocuous procedure; it is associated with such serious complications as hemorrhage, requiring transfusion in 5% to 10% of cases; cervical stenosis; uterine perforation; pelvic cellulitis; and even injury to the bladder and rectum. Bladder and rectal complications usually are seen in cases in which there is a significant atrophy with shallow vaginal fornices. Of all the complications of sharp conization of the cervix for diagnostic purposes, none is more significant than the morbidity that occurs in the pregnant patient. After cervical conization during pregnancy the average fetal loss is about 10% and the incidence of postoperative hemorrhage is 30%.

TREATMENT OF CERVICAL INTRAEPITHELIAL NEOPLASIA

The basic philosophy in the treatment of CIN is that pathologic cells in CIN will not involve the lymphatic channels and the lymph nodes; therefore, any type of

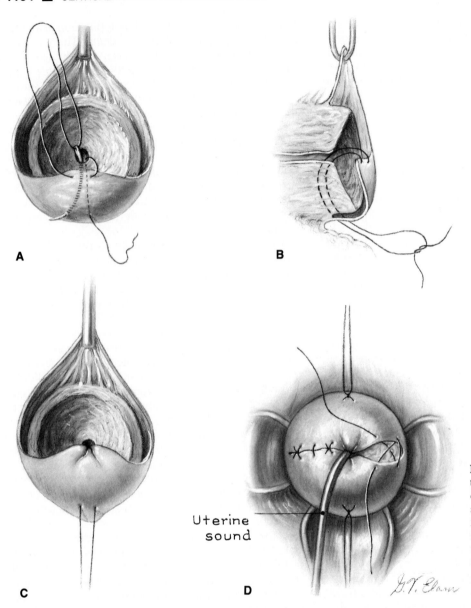

Uterine
sound

Figure 41–13. *A,* Mattress suture is being placed as in Sturmdorf tracheloplasty. *B,* Method of action of suture in drawing the flap into the canal. *C,* The lower flap has been pulled into position. *D,* Anterior and posterior flaps have been drawn into the canal. Lateral mucosa wounds are being sutured.

complete local destruction is a satisfactory treatment. For treatment results, more important is the size and distribution of the lesion than the actual degree of CIN. The pretreatment evaluation of the patient is the most important part of the management. It is imperative to use outpatient methods of treatment only by a colposcopist who can positively rule out invasive carcinoma; otherwise, significant mistakes can occur. In 1978 Townsend and associates established a registry of invasive cervical cancers diagnosed after outpatient evaluation for abnormal Pap smear or after therapy for benign or premalignant cervical disease. Ninety-nine such cases were evaluated. Forty-five of

them had outpatient therapy for benign cervical disease. Of the remaining 54 cases, 16 had colposcopy only, and the remaining 38 had colposcopy followed by outpatient therapy such as cryosurgery, hot cautery, or carbon dioxide laser therapy. Most patients had stage Ib cervical cancer. The interval from outpatient procedure to the definite therapy of cancers showed a wide dispersion. Most patients had the invasive lesion diagnosed and managed within 12 months of the outpatient procedure. It is therefore obvious that the cancer was present at the time of outpatient procedure but was not recognized. This report is retrospective, based on questionnaires, and the extent of the problem cannot be evaluated because the denominator is unknown.

Common Mistakes in Patient Evaluation

The most common mistakes in evaluation of patients before outpatient methods of therapy are as follows.

Nonrecognition of Atypical Vessels. Although the recognition of a colposcopic pattern compatible with intraepithelial lesion (mosaic, punctation, or acetowhite epithelium) is relatively easy, the recognition of atypical vessels requires expertise. A lesion with atypical vessels is much less impressive than mosaic or punctation compatible with CIN. Failure to recognize atypical vessels results in failure to recognize invasive cancer.

The training of a colposcopist in the recognition of atypical vessels is difficult or almost impossible because the number of patients with microinvasive or preclinical cervical cancer is limited unless the physician worked in a cancer referral center. With the current use of cervicography, teaching the colposcopist how to recognize atypical vessels is much easier. The instructor can include a few cases of microinvasive or small invasive cancers in a larger number of other cervigrams, and the trainee is then required to identify these cases. When this procedure is repeated several times accuracy in the recognition of atypical vessels increases significantly.

Nonrecognition of Unsatisfactory Colposcopy. Before beginning outpatient methods of treatment, the physician must be sure that the squamocolumnar junction is fully visible and that the lesion does not extend into the invisible portion of the cervical canal. If one of these conditions is not fulfilled, outpatient methods of treatment are contraindicated.

Role of ECC. Some colposcopists require ECC before every outpatient method of treatment, even when the squamocolumnar junction is fully visible. The reason for ECC is that the physician will have a permanent histologic documentation that the endocervical canal was negative. Although we agree basically with this philosophy, we still believe that ECC is not the only way to document that the endocervical canal was negative and the squamocolumnar junction fully visible. Permanent documentation of this condition can be achieved by a simple cervigram, which will eliminate the need for the patient to have an uncomfortable ECC.

Number of Biopsies. During outpatient methods of treatment the entire cervix will not be available for histologic examination (like after conization); therefore, the diagnosis in the colposcopically directed biopsy is crucial. In the biopsy the most suspicious area on the cervix should be sampled. The number of biopsies will depend on the expertise of the examiner. In some cases experts in colposcopy take just one biopsy; for a beginner in colposcopy several biopsies and ECC are recommended, especially if the colposcopic lesion is complex.

Outpatient Methods of Treatment in Patients with Positive ECC. When the ECC shows any type of tissue abnormality, the patient is not suitable for outpatient methods of treatment and either cold-knife conization or laser conization is indicated. To perform outpatient methods of treatment can result in significant mistake.

Quality of Follow-up. Outpatient methods of treatment should be done only in patients in whom we can expect reasonably good follow-up. All outpatient treatment methods have some failure rate; however, in patients who return for follow-up visits they do not represent a danger. In patients who have failure of primary treatment and do not return for follow-up examination for several years they can represent a significant danger.

Methods of Therapy

The following methods can be used in the management of CIN.

Electrocautery

Electocauterization has been used in the management of cervical lesions for several decades. Peyton and Rosen reported absence of cervical cancer in 10,500 patients who were cauterized before age 45. Bouda and Dohnal reported that they had found only two new cases of cervical carcinoma in 94,072 patients who had been treated by cervical electrocoagulation. Richart and Sciarra treated 170 patients with mild to severe dysplasia by electrocautery, and in 89% of the patients the lesions was eradicated by the first course of electrocautery.

Cryosurgery

Cryosurgery has gained popularity in the treatment of cervical dysplasia and carcinoma in situ. It is an outpatient procedure that is done without anesthesia, and the discomfort to the patient is minimal. The refrigerants used in cryosurgery include freon ($-60°$ C), carbon dioxide ($-60°$ C), nitrous oxide ($-80°$ C), and liquid nitrogen ($-90°$ C). Townsend and Ostergaard have treated more than 500 patients with CIN by cryosurgery. Of this group, more than 200 patients had either severe dysplasia or carcinoma in situ. Their method of evaluation of the patients before cryosurgery included repeat cytology, colposcopic examination, directed biopsies from the most suspicious areas, and ECC. They selected only those patients for cryosurgery in whom the entire limits of the lesion were seen and in whom the ECC revealed no abnormal tissue. Cryosurgery was effective in 90% of the patients treated. Of the freeze failure, about 35% occurred in patients in whom the lesion was so extensive that the initial freezing was inadequate. Fifteen patients have been retreated, and all but one have been free of disease after the second treatment session.

In 1980 Creasman and Weed reported on 557 patients with CIN who were treated by cryosurgery. Treatment failures were 9% in CIN I, 5% in CIN II, and 12% in CIN III.

The risk of recurring disease after cryosurgery was studied by Richart and associates. From nine institutions, 2839 patients were treated by cryosurgery for CIN and were followed longitudinally after three negative Pap smears to ascertain the risk of recurrence. The cumulative risk of developing CIN after successful cryosurgical treatment was 0.41% at year 5, 0.44% at year 10, and 0.44% at year 14. There was no significant difference in risk between patients originally treated for CIN I, CIN II, or CIN III.

In his initial report (1973) Creasman demonstrated in a group of 27 patients who had received a single freeze that cervical dysplasia persisted in 48%. In 48 patients undergoing a "double freeze" technique 18% had severe dysplasia or carcinoma in situ in the surgical specimen. After this report most authors have favored the freeze-thaw-freeze technique. Benedet and associates produced results that compared favorably with any obtained to date by using only the standard 7-minute freeze. With new cryosurgical equipment using nitrous oxide, a double freeze is not necessary and will not produce better results.

Radical Electrodiathermocautery

Developed in Australia, radical electrodiathermocautery achieved better results than simple electrocoagulation. Chanen and Rome selected a group of 1864 nonpregnant patients in whom the margins of a noninvasive lesion were fully visible and located entirely within view of the colposcope. These patients were treated by electrocoagulation diathermy. Needle and ball electrodes were used with the standard Bovie electrosurgical unit. The needle electrodes were inserted into the cervix to a depth of 1.5 cm, and multiple punctures were made over the entire abnormal transformation zone and the adjacent area of the columnar epithelium.

The aim of the treatment was the destruction of the lesion and any involvement of deep glandular spaces. A ball electrode was then used to coagulate the surface of the area that had been subjected to the needle diathermy electrode. The coagulation extended into the lower endocervical canal, which had previously been dilated. The procedure was performed under general or regional anesthesia. The duration of follow-up was from 1 to 15 years. Of the 1734 patients who returned for follow-up examination after electrocoagulation diathermy treatment, 47 were found to have persistent disease. This represented an apparent primary cure rate of 97.3% for this method of treatment.

Carbon Dioxide Laser Therapy

See Chapter 21.

Conization

Conization is considered as definitive treatment of cervical carcinoma in situ when the exact limits of the lesion are defined by colposcopy, or when the histopathologic specimen has completely free margins after careful evaluation of the cone.

Creasman and Rutledge found that 18% of 261 patients treated for cervical in situ carcinoma developed a second malignant or premalignant lesion elsewhere in the body and that half of these second cancers were found in the genital tract. This high incidence of second primaries is significant, and requires a diligent and continued search for other lesions in patients with carcinoma in situ. The same authors also agree that the recurrence of carcinoma in situ does not depend on the amount of vaginal cuff removed. The same recurrence rate (2.6%) was found if the length of removed cuff was less than 1 cm, between 1 and 3 cm, or more than 3 cm.

Cure rates with conization are higher in series in which colposcopy was used in the preoperative evaluation, as reported by Ahlgren and associates. The importance of long-term follow-up is evident from a report by Kolstad and Klem. Their series of 1121 patients with carcinoma in situ represents both the largest and the longest follow-up experience available with this disease. These patients were followed from 5 to 25 years. Therapeutic conization was performed in 795 patients, of which 19 patients (2.3%) developed recurrent carcinoma in situ and 7 patients (0.9%) developed invasive cancer. Of particular interest was the finding in 238 patients with carcinoma in situ who were treated with hysterectomy, of which 3 patients (1.2%) developed invasive cancer. This large series indicates that the recurrence rate after conization is not higher than after a conventional hysterectomy, provided the conization is performed after colposcopic evaluation of the size and localization of the lesion. It is stressed that women who have once had carcinoma in situ of the cervix will always be at some risk for recurrent disease or a second primary and, therefore, should be carefully followed for a much longer time than the conventional 5 years.

Hysterectomy

Hysterectomy is seldom justified for initial treatment of carcinoma in situ. A hysterectomy is indicated after initial treatment of carcinoma in situ by conization when the margins of the cone specimen are not free of disease, when there is persistent abnormal cervicovaginal cytology after cone, or for other gynecologic indications.

TREATMENT OF RECURRENCE OF CARCINOMA IN SITU

After the treatment of cervical carcinoma in situ a recurrent carcinoma in situ develops in about 2% of patients, either in the vaginal cuff or as isolated islands in the vagina. It is our opinion that most cases of carcinoma in situ in the vaginal cuff represent residual disease that was not removed at the time of primary treatment. These cases might have been avoided if a Schiller test or colposcopic examination of the cervix and upper vagina had been performed preoperatively to ascertain the extent of the lesion.

Controversy persists as to whether isolated islands of carcinoma in situ of the vagina found after treatment of the cervix represent a recurrent disease or a new primary lesion. It is well recognized that a woman who developed carcinoma in situ of the cervix has a higher chance of developing carcinoma in the lower genital canal, including the vagina and vulva.

In the management of recurrent carcinoma in situ of the vagina a colposcopic evaluation is important to assess the extent and location of the lesions. Depending on the location and extent of the lesion and the age and parity of the patient, one of the following modalities of treatment can be used: excisional biopsy, carbon dioxide laser vaporization, partial vaginectomy, total vaginectomy, topical 5-fluorouracil treatment, and irradiation therapy.

Excisional biopsy can be used only in very small, isolated lesions in the vagina. When colposcopic examination 3 months after the excisional biopsy reveals that the lesion was completely removed, the patient can be followed with cytology.

Carbon dioxide laser vaporization provides an ideal modality of treatment of vaginal carcinoma in situ. After laser vaporization therapy little granulation tissue develops; therefore, large areas of the vagina can be treated without narrowing or scarring of the vagina. Carcinoma in situ of the vagina usually is a superficial lesion and, unlike cervical lesions, involves only squamous epithelium. A relatively superficial vaporization of the vaginal mucosa (2–3-mm depth) can completely evaporate all the pathologic tissue. The risk of injury to the bladder or rectum is, therefore, minimal. Laser treatment of the upper one-third of the vagina can be tolerated by most patients without anesthesia. For treatment of the lower portion of the vagina, anesthesia is necessary. Capen and associates reported on the treatment of 15 unselected patients with vaginal intraepithelial neoplasia, primarily with carbon dioxide laser; there were two failures. The follow-up time, however, was short. More failures occur after the laser treatment if there is a carcinoma in situ of the vaginal cuff after hysterectomy. In this situation carcinoma in situ usually is buried deeper in the suture line and is not destroyed by the laser beam. Therefore, recurrences are more common in this location.

Partial vaginectomy is used for the treatment of lesions in the vaginal cuff after hysterectomy, mainly in patients in whom there was a previous failure of laser vaporization. The margins of the resection should extend at least 5 mm from a colposcopically visible lesion. The margins of the vaginal mucosa are grasped with Allis clamps and the vaginal mucosa is incised around the lesion and separated from the underlining tissue with sharp and blunt dissection. In the suture line the vaginal mucosa must be sharply separated by scissors, carefully avoiding injury to the bladder or rectum. After the removal of the operative specimen it is necessary for the pathologist to carefully examine the resected margins to make sure they are free of disease. Lee and Symmonds reported 43 patients with recurrent carcinoma in situ treated by partial vaginectomy. There were no bladder or rectal injuries and no recurrence in follow-up in these cases. Our experience has been similar.

Total vaginectomy with or without skin graft is a formidable procedure, and is necessary only in patients who have multicentric areas of recurrence. Lee and Symmonds prefer to delay the placement of the split-thickness skin graft for 3 or 4 days after the total vaginectomy to ensure a dry bed for the graft and a good graft take. More commonly the vaginal canal is replaced with a split-thickness skin graft from the thigh at the time of the vaginectomy.

Topical 5-fluorouracil (5-FU) treatment of in situ carcinoma of the vagina was first reported by Woodruff and associates, who treated nine patients and had only one failure. They advise frequent examination and repeat applications of the agent. Daly and Ellis treated 17 patients with 5% 5-FU applied twice daily for 14 days with a vaginal applicator. Zinc oxide ointment was placed on the vulva and perineum to minimize external irritation. Of the 17 patients treated in this study, two were unable to complete the full 14-day course because of ulceration in the vaginal vestibule. The remaining 15 patients were followed for 2 to 4 years, and no recurrence was detected.

Irradiation therapy usually is used in patients who have complicated medical diseases, are elderly, and are unable to tolerate any of the other modalities of treatment. Intravaginal radium or cesium usually is contained in a vaginal cylinder 3.5 cm in diameter. The radium sources are arranged so as to deliver an average dose of 7000 rad to the surface of the vagina in a single application. The depth of the effective dose is limited to the vaginal membranes and the immediate 5 mm of underlining subcutaneous tissues. Rutledge treated 31 patients with in situ vaginal cancer with irradiation therapy and no recurrence was diagnosed. The sequelae of the irradiated vagina usually are greater than those of surgical treatment of vaginal recurrences; vaginal atrophy, contracture, fibrosis, and synechiae can result unless specific efforts are taken to maintain vaginal patency with a dilator or frequent coitus. The use of estrogen vaginal suppositories or cream also is important in maintaining a functional vaginal canal after intravaginal irradiation.

Bibliography

Ahlgren M, Ingemarsson I, Lindberg L, et al. Conization as treatment of carcinoma in situ of the uterine cervix. Obstet Gynecol 1975;46:135.

Anderson SG, Linton EB. The diagnostic accuracy of cervical biopsy and cervical conization. Am J Obstet Gynecol 1967;99:113.

Benedet JL, Nickerson KG, Anderson GH. Cryotherapy in the treatment of cervical intraepithelial neoplasia. Obstet Gynecol 1981;57:5.

Beral V. Cancer of the cervix: a sexually transmitted disease. Lancet 1975;1:1037.

Bouda VJ, Dohnal V. Geburtschilfe Frauenheilkd 1965;25:1186.

Boyes DA, Worth AJ. Cytological screening for cervical cancer. In: Jordan JA, Singer A, eds. The cervix. Philadelphia: WB Saunders, 1976.

Boyes DA, Worth AJ, Anderson GH. Experience with cervical screening in British Columbia. Gynecol Oncol 1981;12:143.

Burghardt E. Die diagnostische Konisation der Portio Vaginalis Uteri. Geburtschilfe Frauenheilkd 1963;23:1.

Capen CV, Masterson BJ, Magrina JF, et al. Laser therapy of vaginal intraepithelial neoplasia. Am J Obstet Gynecol 1982;142:973.

Chanen W, Rome R. Electrocoagulation diathermy for cervical dysplasia and carcinoma in situ: a 15-year survey. Am J Obstet Gynecol 1983;61:673.

Chao S, McCaffrey RM, Todd WD. Conization in evaluation and management of cervical neoplasm. Am J Obstet Gynecol 1969; 103:574.

Coppleson LW, Brown B. Estimation of the screening error rate from observed detection rates in repeated cervical cytology. Am J Obstet Gynecol 1974;119:953.

Coppleson M, Pixley E, Reid B. Colposcopy. Springfield, IL: Charles C. Thomas, 1971.

Coppleson M, Reid B. Preclinical carcinoma of the cervix uteri. London: Pergamon Press, 1967.

Creasman WT, Rutledge F. Carcinoma in situ of the cervix: an analysis of 861 patients. Obstet Gynecol 1972;39:373.

Creasman WT, Weed JC Jr. Conservative management of cervical intraepithelial neoplasia. Clin Obstet Gynecol 1980;23:281.

Daly JW, Ellis GF. Treatment of vaginal dysplasia and carcinoma in situ with topical 5-fluorouracil. Obstet Gynecol 1980;55:350.

Fenoglio CM, Ferencyz A. Etiological factors in cervical neoplasia. Semin Oncol 1982;9:349.

Fidler HK, Boyes DA, Worth AJ. Cervical cancer detection in British Columbia. J Obstet Gynecol Br Commonw 1968;75:392.

Frenkel N, et al. A herpes simplex 2 DNA fragment and its transcription in human cervical cancer tissue. Proc Natl Acad Sci USA 1972;69:3784.

Gagnon F. Contributions to the study of the etiology and prevention of cancer of the cervix and uterus. Am J Obstet Gynecol 1950;60:516.

Griffiths CT, Younge PA. The clinical diagnosis of early cervical cancer. Obstet Gynecol Surv 1969;24:967.

Kaufman RH, Strama T, Norton PK, et al. Cryosurgical treatment of cervical intraepithelial neoplasias. Am J Obstet Gynecol 1973;42:881.

Kessler II. Human cervical cancer as a venereal disease. Cancer Res 1976;36:783.

Kivlahan C, Ingram E. Pap smear without endocervical cells. Obstet Gynecol 1985;65:000.

Kolstad P, Klem V. Long term follow-up of 1,121 cases of carcinoma in situ. Obstet Gynecol 1976;48:125.

Kolstad P, Stafl A. Atlas of colposcopy. Baltimore: University Park Press, 1982.

Kurihara S. Study of premalignant lesions of the uterine cervix—benign to malignant lesions. Tokyo: Keio Gijuku University School of Medicine, 1972.

Lange P. Clinical and histological studies on cervical carcinoma; precancerous, early metastasis, and tubular structures in the lymph nodes. Copenhagen: Munksgaard, 1960:40.

Laverty C, Russel P, Hills E, et al. The significance of noncondylomatous wart virus infection of the cervical transformation zone. A review with discussion of two illustrative cases. Acta Cytol 1978;22:195.

Lee RA, Symmonds RE. Recurrent carcinoma in situ of the vagina in patients previously treated for in situ carcinoma of the cervix. Obstet Gynecol 1976;48:61.

Linhartova A. Comparative study of the morphology and evolution of congenital and adult ectopy of the uterine cervix. Plzen Lek Sborn 1972;37:85.

Lohe KJ. Early squamous cell carcinoma of the uterine cervix. Gynecol Oncol 1978;6:10.

McIndoe WA, McLean MR, Jones RW, et al. The invasive potential of carcinoma in situ of the cervix. Am J Obstet Gynecol 1984;61:000.

Martin CE. Marital and coital factors in cervical cancer. Am J Public Health 1967;57:803.

Meisels A, Fortin R. Condylomatous lesions of the cervix and vagina. I. Cytologic patterns. Acta Cytol 1976;20:505.

Meisels A, Fortin R, Roy M. Condylomatous lesions of the cervix. II. Cytologic, colposcopic and histopathologic study. Acta Cytol 1977;21:379.

Naib ZM, et al. Genital herpetic infection—association with cervical dysplasia and carcinoma. Cancer 1969;23:940.

Navratil E, Burghardt E, Bajardi F, et al. Simultaneous colposcopy and cytology used in the screening for carcinoma of the cervix. Am J Obstet Gynecol 1958;75:1292.

Nelson JH, Avarette HE, Richart RM. Detection, diagnostic evaluation and treatment of dysplasia and early carcinoma of the cervix. CA 1975;25:134.

Peyton FW, Rosen NA. Am J Obstet Gynecol 1963;86:111.

Reid DL, French PB, Singer A, et al. Sperm, basic proteins and cervical carcinogenesis: correlation with socio-economical class. Lancet 1978;12:60.

Reid R. Personal communication, 1986.

Reid R, Stanhope R, Herschman BR, et al. Genital warts in cervical cancer. Cancer 1982;50:377.

Richart RM. Natural history of cervical intraepithelial neoplasm. Clin Obstet Gynecol 1967;10:748.

Richart RM. Cervical intraepithelial neoplasia. Pathol Annu 1973;8:301.

Richart RM, Sciarra JJ. Treatment of cervical dysplasia by outpatient electrocauterization. Am J Obstet Gynecol 1968;101:200.

Richart RM, Townsend DE, Crisp W. An analysis of "long-term" follow-up results in patients with cervical intraepithelial neoplasia treated by cryotherapy. Am J Obstet Gynecol 1980;137:823.

Rotkin EK, King R. Environmental variables related to cervical cancer. Am J Obstet Gynecol 1962;83:720.

Rotkin ID. Adolescent coitus and cervical cancer: associations of related events and increased risk. Cancer Res 1967;27:603.

Rotkin ID. A comparison review of key epidemiological studies in cervical cancer related to current searches for transmissible agents. Cancer Res 1973;33:1353.

Royston I, Aurelian L. The association of genital herpes virus with cervical atypia and carcinoma in situ. Am J Epidemiol 1970;91:531.

Sabatelle R, et al. Cervical biopsy versus conization. Cancer 1969;23:663.

Silbar EL, Woodruff JD. Evaluation of biopsy, cone, and hysterectomy sequence in intraepithelial carcinoma of the cervix. Obstet Gynecol 1966;27:89.

Silverberg E, Lubera J. Cancer statistics 1986. CA 1986;36:9.

Singleton WP, Rutledge F. To cone or not to cone the cervix. Obstet Gynecol 1968;31:430.

Spitzer M, Krumholz BA, Chernys AE, et al. Comparative utility of repeat Papanicolaou smears, cervicography and colposcopy in the evaluation of atypical Papanicolaou smears. Obstet Gynecol 1987;69:731.

Stafl A. Cervicography: a new method for cervical cancer detection. Am J Obstet Gynecol 1981;139:815.

Stafl A. Cervicography. Clin Obstet Gynecol 1983;26:1007.

Stafl A, Friedrich EG Jr, Mattingly RF. Detection of cervical neoplasia: reducing the risk of error. Clin Obstet Gynecol 1973;16:238.

Stafl A, Mattingly RF. Colposcopic diagnosis of cervical neoplasia. Obstet Gynecol 1973;41:168.

Stafl A, Mattingly RF. Vaginal adenosis: a precancerous lesion. Am J Obstet Gynecol 1974;120:666.

Starreveld AA, Romanowski B, et al. The latency period of carcinoma in situ of the cervix. Obstet Gynecol 1983;62:348.

Stenkvist B, Bergstrom R, Eckland G, et al. Papanicolaou smear screening and cervical cancer: what can you expect? JAMA 1984;252:1423.

Tawa K, Forsythe A, Cove K, et al. A comparison of the Papanicolaou smear and the cervigram: sensitivity, specificity, and cost analysis. Obstet Gynecol 1988;71:229.

Townsend DE, Ostergaard DR. Cryocauterization for preinvasive cervical neoplasia. J Repro Med 1977;6:55.

Townsend DE, Richart RM, Marks E, Nielsen J. Invasive cancer following outpatient evaluation and therapy for cervical disease. Obstet Gynecol 1981;57:145.

Trevathan A, et al. Cigarette smoking and dysplasia and carcinoma in situ of the uterine cervix. JAMA 1983;250:499.

Weiner I, Burke L, Goldberger MA. Carcinoma of the cervix in Jewish women. Am J Obstet Gynecol 1951;61:418.

Woodruff JD, Parmley TH, Julian CG. Topical 5-fluorouracil in the treatment of vaginal carcinoma in situ. Gynecol Oncol 1975;3:125.

42

Cancer of the Cervix

JOHN D. THOMPSON

In the first half of the 20th century invasive cervical cancer was the most common cancer of the female reproductive tract in the United States. Since 1950 both the incidence and the death rate have decreased, so that the disease now ranks second in incidence to endometrial cancer and second in mortality to ovarian cancer in the total female population. There has been a 5% decrease in the incidence and death rate of cervical cancer since 1950. The incidence has been consistently two to three times higher in nonwhite women as compared with white women. For white women the incidence is about 10 per 100,000 women; for nonwhite women the incidence is 20 to 30 per 100,000 women. In some inner-city hospitals that serve a predominantly indigent and black population (eg, Grady Memorial Hospital in Atlanta, Georgia) cervical cancer is the most frequent primary malignant disease seen. Carcinoma of the cervix occurs more frequently in women of lower income and educational levels; this accounts for much of the observed racial difference in incidence, according to Devesa. In the United States the death rate is highest in the South, among elderly women and among black women (Fig. 42-1).

From 1984 through 1986 cervical cancer was the underlying cause of death in a mean of 4543 women per year in the United States. Cervical cancer accounted for less 3% of U.S. cancer deaths among women and was the 11th most common cause of cancer mortality. Worldwide, however, cervical cancer follows breast cancer as the second most common cause of cancer mortality among women. For 1974 through 1985 the National Cancer Institute reported an overall 5-year survival rate of 67% for women with cervical cancer. Of course, survival rates vary with stage of disease at diagnosis. Survival was 88% for women whose disease was diagnosed at the local stage; 51%, at the regional stage; and 14%, at the distant stage. From 1979 to 1986 age-

adjusted death rates for cervical cancer declined by 18% for all women.

Progress in reducing mortality from cervical cancer is primarily attributed to the introduction of cervical cancer screening as part of regular gynecologic examinations. Regular testing with a Papanicolaou (Pap) smear started in the 1950s and has become the standard of care in most developed countries. It has resulted in an increase in the number of cases of cervical intraepithelial neoplasia detected and treated, which has prevented the subsequent development of invasive cervical cancer in many women. In 1985 only 5% of U.S. women 20 to 80 years of age reported never having had a Pap smear. An estimated 37% of cervical cancer deaths occur among these women. According to Day, mass screening programs for cancer of the cervix in Scandinavian countries were followed by marked reductions in the incidence and mortality from invasive cervical cancer within 10 years. In many countries, also as a result of screening, from 35% to 50% of cases of cervical cancer are being detected in stage I disease, a marvelous improvement over the past 30 years. Fewer women die when treatment is given in the earliest stages. There has been a corresponding decrease in the number of cervical cancers diagnosed in stages II, III, and IV. This is confirmed by the 1988 International Federation of Gynecology and Obstetrics (FIGO) Annual Report on the Results of Treatment in Gynecological Cancer. In the 1950–1954 period 23% of cases were diagnosed in stage I; in the 1979–1981 period 36.4% were diagnosed in stage I and 31.9% were diagnosed in stage II. Unfortunately 31.1% were still diagnosed in stages III and IV.

Worldwide, cervical cancer continues to be a major public health concern. Incidence and death rates for cervical cancer vary widely among countries of the world. Chile has the highest death rate and Egypt has the lowest (15.7 and 0.3 per 100,000 women, respec-

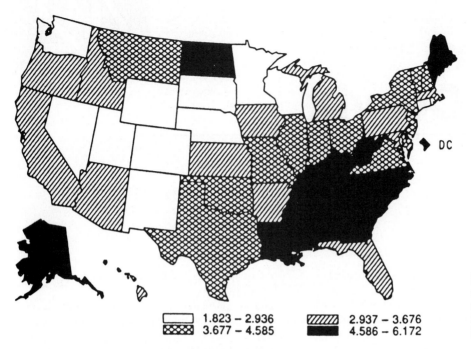

Figure 42–1. Chronic disease reports: Deaths from cervical cancer in the United States from 1984 to 1986. (MMWR 1989; 38:650)

1.823 – 2.936	2.937 – 3.676
3.677 – 4.585	4.586 – 6.172

tively). There may be substantial underreporting of cases in many countries, including eastern Mediterranean countries. In some developing countries cervical cancer is the leading cause of death among adult women because of a high prevalence rate and inadequate early detection and treatment programs. In other countries, such as China, great strides have been made in reducing mortality from cervical cancer, primarily through a national commitment to early detection through mass population screening with cervical cytology. In the United States there has been a dramatic decrease in the number of deaths each year from cervical cancer compared with previous decades. Because it can be said that each death could be prevented if cervical cancer detection programs were universally available and utilized by all adult women in the country, 4543 deaths annually is, regrettably, a large number. Thus, in the United States, this potentially curable cancer has not been eliminated and remains an important and potentially lethal disease. In the absence of universal early detection it is still necessary to treat women for advanced invasive cervical cancer with complicated methods that provide the best hope of cure with as little interference with function as possible; inevitably, these methods can cause significant complications.

In 1984 Lunt reported on data (described as incomplete and fragmentary) available to the World Health Organization on the frequency of cancers of the cervix in developing countries. He states:

There are many indications that cancers of the cervix represent problems of a public health di-

mension in these countries. With a few exceptions, screening efforts are low-volume institution based cytology services reaching limited segments of the female population. On the other hand, the recognized risk factors for cancer of the cervix are widely prevalent in developing countries. Cultural and educational constraints often bar women from seeking medical attention. Diagnostic and treatment facilities, particularly radiotherapy, and all levels of trained staff have been insufficient to permit screening programs for cancers of the cervix.

FACTORS ASSOCIATED WITH CERVICAL CANCER DEVELOPMENT

A number of factors have been associated with cervical cancer development, as reviewed by Devesa. Racial differences and differences related to income and educational status were previously mentioned. Certain religious groups have a low risk (Jewish, Amish, Mormon, and Seventh-Day Adventist women, and nuns). Women with increased risk include prostitutes, prison inmates, and female attendants in clinics that treat patients with sexually transmitted diseases. Other factors associated with increased risk include multiple marriages, early age at first intercourse and first marriage, poor personal hygiene, noncircumcision of partner, and multiple sexual partners. The number of sexual partners of the husband has been associated with an increased risk of cervical cancer in the wife, as has carcinoma of the penis, although this latter association has been denied by some authors. Corbett and Crompton reported a patient who developed invasive squamous cell carcinoma in only one cervix of a didelphic uterus. A longitudinal septum divided the vagina into two sides. The cancer was found on the side where the vagina was of normal caliber. No cancer was found on the side where the vagina was too small to permit intercourse. This case and other information suggest that the development of cervical cancer is related to the sexual transmission of one or more agents, possibly herpesvirus or papillomavirus. Changes in the patterns of sexual behavior of men and women in future years may change the risk of developing cervical cancer. Cervical cancer mortality also has been attributed to cigarette smoking.

According to Walker and coworkers, human papillomavirus (HPV) is the most likely to cause cervical cancer by sexual transmission. Their review of the evidence includes the following observations: (a) cattle and rabbit papillomaviruses induce malignant transformation of virally infected squamous epithelium in their natural hosts; (b) HPV DNA persists and is expressed in human cervical tumors; and (c) HPV DNA can morphologically transform rat and mouse cells in vitro. More than 55 HPV types have been described to date, and Walker and her group analyzed 100 women with cervical cancers for the presence of HPV types 6, 11, 16, 18, and 31. More aggressive clinical behavior was demonstrated for tumors that contained HPV type 18. Also, evidence in the study suggested that HPV type 18–containing tumors might progress to invasion without a prolonged preinvasive phase. Large cell keratinizing squamous cell carcinomas were more likely to contain HPV type 16, whereas tumors that were anaplastic were significantly more likely to contain HPV type 18. Adenocarcinomas of the cervix have also been closely associated with HPV type 18. In the future, depending on the results of additional studies, HPV status of cervical tumors may be useful in treatment plans and may be used to identify women at greater risk for cervical cancer.

Women with acquired immunodeficiency syndrome have a higher frequency of malignant disease. In immunosuppressed patients the incidence of squamous cell carcinoma of the cervix is increased. With human immunodeficiency virus I (HIV) infection, the incidence of cervical intraepithelial neoplasia is increased. Rellihan and coworkers have reported a patient with HIV infection and stage IIb poorly differentiated cervical cancer whose disease progressed rapidly to death despite aggressive therapy. These authors warn that this pattern of aggressive tumor behavior may occur more frequently as HIV infection spreads into the heterosexual population.

The risk of cervical cancer is significantly increased in women who have not been regularly screened with a Pap smear. For example, Shy and coworkers found that the risk of squamous cell cervical cancer was increased 3.9 times for women who had Pap smears at 3-year intervals compared with women who had annual screening. For women who had not had a smear in the preceding 10 years, the risk increased 12.3 times. The presence of well-known risk factors for cervical cancer did not modify these results.

CLASSIFICATION OF CERVICAL CANCER

In 1937 the Health Organization of the League of Nations adopted a clinical classification of cervical cancer. The cervix was the first cancer to be so classified. In 1950 this classification was modified to include preinvasive (in situ) cervical cancer, which was designated stage 0. New recommendations for the clinical classification of carcinoma of the cervix were adopted by the General Assembly of FIGO in 1961, and several other modifications have been made since then. The general use of this classification abroad and in the United States has been extremely helpful in reporting and comparing results of various modalities of therapy. Descriptions of the clinical stages in carcinoma of the cervix uteri published in the FIGO Annual Report for 1988 are listed in Table 42-1.

Stages II, III, and IV have remained essentially unchanged through the various modifications (Fig. 42-2). The major redefinition and refinements have occurred in stage I, especially as regards early microinvasive stage Ia carcinoma, which has been further subdivided into stage Ia1 and stage Ia2.

HISTOPATHOLOGY

The principal histologic type of invasive cervical cancer, occurring in about 80% to 90% of cases, is the squamous (epidermoid) lesion. In 1923 Martzloff classified these squamous tumors into three main histologic subtypes and grades. Grade 1 tumors contain well-differentiated spinal cells, keratin, and squamous pearls (Fig. 42-3). Grade 2 tumors, the most common, are predominantly composed of transitional cells of the large cell nonkeratinizing type (Fig. 42-4). Grade 3 tumors, the least common, are poorly differentiated small basal cell–type tumors (Fig. 42-5). The classification of Martzloff did not prove to be clinically useful, mainly because it was not known that biopsies taken from different areas of the same tumor often show different degrees of differentiation and different predominant cell types. Martzloff's work did stimulate Broders, Wentz and Reagan, and others to continue to categorize the histologic types and degree of differentiation of squamous cell cervical tumors and to study

TABLE 42–1
FIGO Classification of Carcinoma of the Cervix

CLASSIFICATION	DESCRIPTION
Stage 0	Carcinoma in situ, intraepithelial carcinoma. (Cases of stage 0 should not be included in any therapeutic statistics for invasive carcinoma.)
Stage I	The carcinoma is strictly confined to the cervix. (Extension to the corpus should be disregarded.)
Stage Ia	Preclinical carcinomas of the cervix, that is, those diagnosed only by microscopy.
Stage Ia1	Mimimal microscopically evident stromal invasion.
Stage Ia2	Lesions detected microscopically that can be measured. The upper limit of the measurement should not show a depth of invasion of more than 5 mm taken from the base of the epithelium, either surface or glandular, from which it originates. A second dimension, the horizontal spread, must not exceed 7 mm. Larger lesions should be staged as Ib.
Stage Ib	Lesions of greater dimensions than stage Ia2 whether seen clinically or not. Preformed space involvement should not alter the staging but should be specifically recorded so as to determine whether it should affect treatment decisions in the future.
Stage II	The carcinoma extends beyond the cervix but has not extended on to the pelvic wall. The carcinoma involves the vagina but not as far as the lower third.
Stage IIa	No obvious parametrial involvement.
Stage IIb	Obvious parametrial involvement.
Stage III	The carcinoma has extended on to the pelvic wall. On rectal examination there is no cancer-free space between the tumor and the pelvic wall. The tumor involves the lower third of the vagina. All cases with a hydronephrosis or nonfunctioning kidney should be included, unless they are known to be due to other cause.
Stage IIIa	No extension to the pelvic wall, but involvement of the lower third of the vagina.
Stage IIIb	Extension on to the pelvic wall and/or hydronephrosis or nonfunctioning kidney.
Stage IV	The carcinoma has extended beyond the true pelvis or has clinically involved the mucosa of the bladder or rectum.
Stage IVa	Spread of the growth to adjacent organs.
Stage IVb	Spread to distant organs.

their clinical behavior and response to treatment. There is some evidence that well-differentiated tumors respond poorly to radiation therapy. A histologic classification of squamous cell tumor types introduced in 1959 by Wentz and Reagan sometimes is used in pathology reports. Willen and coworkers were unable to confirm a predictive value for survival from the Wentz-Reagan classification, however. Cellular differentiation in the advancing margins of the squamous cell tumor correlates better with survival than does cellular differentiation in the center of the tumor, according to Baltzer and coworkers.

The small basal cell–type tumor has been found to be more aggressive by van Nagell and coworkers, Silva and coworkers, and others. Indeed, this histologic type may not be a squamous cancer, since many have been shown to contain the same argyrophilic cells seen in carcinoids. Sheets and coworkers, in 1988, reported on 14 cases of neuroendocrine undifferentiated small cell

cervical cancer in stages Ib and IIa. Cytologically, the tumor cells were small, round, and often oat shaped, with a high nuclear-cytoplasmic ratio. By electron microscopy, neurosecretory granules were found in all tumors examined. Despite complete treatment, 12 of 14 patients died of their disease and the remaining 2 were treated for recurrence. Usual methods of therapy are not adequate for this histologic type.

A rare form of squamous cell cancer of the cervix is a verrucous carcinoma. It is a well-differentiated papillary squamous cell neoplasm with extensive keratinization that usually presents as a large bulky tumor of the cervix and often is confused with giant condylomata such as those seen on the vulva. There is a sharp line between the tumor and underlying cervical stroma. Verrucous carcinoma has been shown to be associated with HPV infection. Although metastatic disease is rare, this tumor may become more virulent if treated with irradiation. Goldberger and coworkers reported an un-

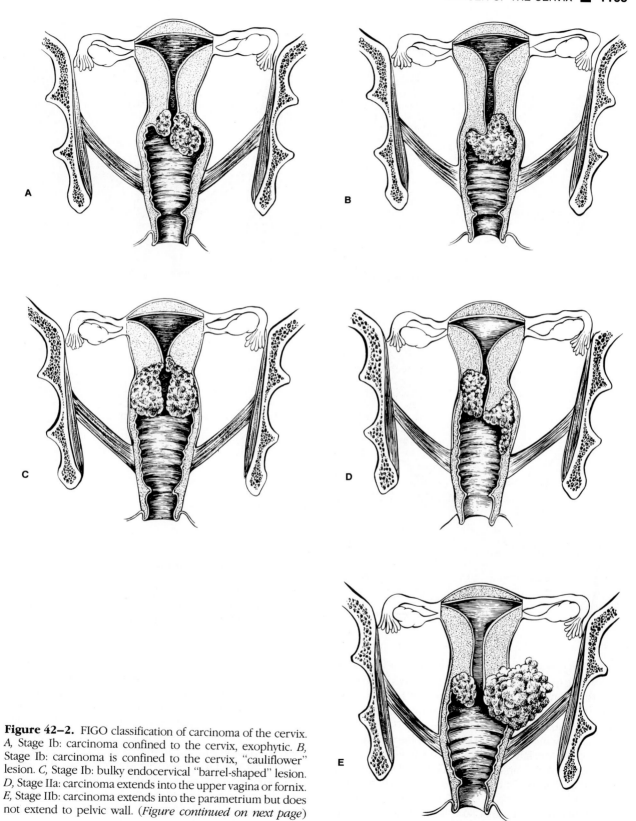

Figure 42–2. FIGO classification of carcinoma of the cervix. *A*, Stage Ib: carcinoma confined to the cervix, exophytic. *B*, Stage Ib: carcinoma is confined to the cervix, "cauliflower" lesion. *C*, Stage Ib: bulky endocervical "barrel-shaped" lesion. *D*, Stage IIa: carcinoma extends into the upper vagina or fornix. *E*, Stage IIb: carcinoma extends into the parametrium but does not extend to pelvic wall. (*Figure continued on next page*)

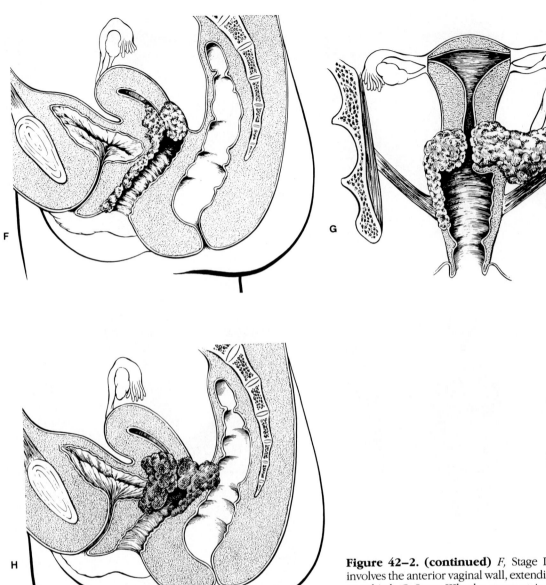

Figure 42–2. (continued) *F,* Stage IIIa: carcinoma involves the anterior vaginal wall, extending to the lower one-third. *G,* Stage IIIb: the parametrium is infiltrated and the carcinoma extends to the pelvic wall. *H,* Stage IVa: the bladder base or rectum is involved.

usually aggressive verrucous carcinoma of the cervix. According to deJesus and coworkers, at least 49 cases of this tumor have been reported in the female genital tract, sometimes as verrucous carcinoma and sometimes as squamous papillary tumor.

Adenocarcinomas of the cervix are becoming more common, especially in younger women. They constitute between 5% and 30% of all cervical cancers in various series. The increased frequency has occurred worldwide. For example, of 520 new cases of cervical carcinoma treated at Helsinki University Central Hospi-

tal, 1976 through 1980, 95 (18.3%) were pure adenocarcinomas and 17 (3.3%) were adenosquamous tumors, according to Vesterinen and coworkers. Although it is possible to recognize adenocarcinoma of the cervix as an in situ stage, relatively few cases are seen or described. Kashimura and coworkers were able to find only 278 cases of in situ adenocarcinoma reported, 150 of which (54%) were associated with squamous intraepithelial neoplasias. Many in situ adenocarcinomas are discovered as incidental findings in hysterectomy specimens. Only two cases of in situ adenocarcinoma of

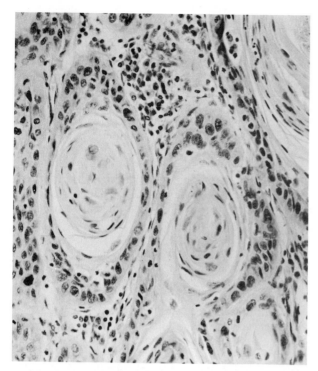

Figure 42–3. Grade 1, well-differentiated epidermoid carcinoma of the cervix. High-power view of spinal cell type. The tumor cells contain abundant keratin that forms epithelial pearls.

the cervix are known to have developed into invasive cancer. The authors point out that the natural history of early cervical adenocarcinoma is not known.

In addition to ordinary adenocarcinoma (Fig. 42-6), a variety of other histologic patterns are described, including adenoma malignum, adenoacanthoma, adenoid cystic, endometrioid, mesometanephric, clear cell, and adenosquamous. Not infrequently an adenocarcinoma and squamous cell carcinoma coexist in the same cervix. Glassy cell adenocarcinoma of the cervix is rare, and probably represents a variant of poorly differentiated adenosquamous carcinoma. It is known to be especially aggressive, with frequent early distant spread. Clear cell adenocarcinoma of the cervix may occur in the presence or absence of intrauterine exposure to diethylstilbestrol. Saigo and coworkers found that the endometrioid pattern was associated with a more favorable prognosis than any other histologic type of adenocarcinoma of the cervix.

Various cervical sarcomas have been described by Rotmensch and coworkers. These tumors constitute less than 0.5% of all cervical cancers, and include adenosarcomas, leiomyosarcomas, carcinosarcomas, and rhabdomyosarcomas. It is extremely rare for a lym-

phoma to develop primarily in the cervix, although undoubted cases have been reported. Lymphoma in the cervix is more likely to represent evidence of generalized lymphomatous disease.

CLINICAL PRESENTATION

Patients with cervical intraepithelial neoplasia usually are asymptomatic. When symptoms are present they usually are caused by some associated gynecologic pathology. Invasive cervical cancer is more likely to cause such symptoms as abnormal vaginal bleeding (menorrhagia, metrorrhagia, postcoital bleeding, or postmenopausal bleeding). Many patients have a profuse and often malodorous discharge, especially when the disease is advanced. Any patient with abnormal vaginal bleeding or discharge should have a complete pelvic examination, including a speculum examination with visualization of the cervix. Failure to examine the cervix in a patient with abnormal vaginal bleeding or discharge may result in failure to diagnose cervical cancer.

Pain is not a common complaint in patients with cervical cancer unless the disease is advanced. In the late stages patients complain of bladder and rectal

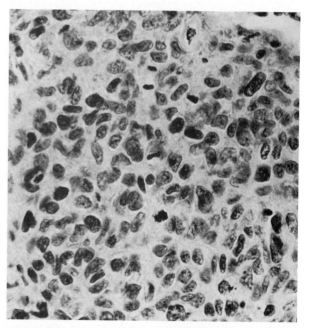

Figure 42–4. Grade 2, moderately differentiated epidermoid carcinoma of the cervix, transitional cell type. The tumor cells are characterized by a moderate amount of cytoplasm but are without pearl formation. Extensive pleomorphism and mitosis are evident. The tumor is frequently classified as being of large cell, nonkeratinizing type.

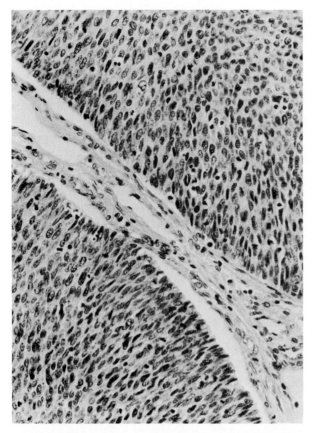

Figure 42–5. Grade 3, poorly differentiated epidermoid carcinoma of the cervix, fat spindle or basal cell type. The tumor cells have little cytoplasm, numerous mitoses, and no keratin or epithelial pearls.

symptoms. When the disease involves lumbosacral and sciatic nerve roots and the lateral pelvic sidewall, chronic boring pelvic bone pain radiating down the leg can be excruciating and indicative of advanced disease. Edema of the lower extremities likewise indicates tumor obstruction of lymphatic drainage. Ascites is uncommon in cervical cancer.

Unfortunately one cannot rely on the presence of symptoms to lead to a diagnosis of early carcinoma of the cervix. Many women remain asymptomatic for many months. It is known that one-third of patients with advanced stage III and stage IV disease have had symptoms for less than 3 months. We have seen a patient whose first symptom was anuria caused by parametrial invasion and complete bilateral ureteral obstruction before a lesion appeared on the exocervix. The only way to diagnose cervical cancer in the earliest possible stages is to routinely apply special diagnostic procedures to large groups of gynecologically asymptomatic as well as symptomatic women. This means screening the adult female population with Pap smears.

Invasive cervical lesions may be exophytic, infiltrative, ulcerative, or occult. The size of the lesion on the cervix may not correlate well with the extent or depth of invasion (Fig. 42-7).

An everted exophytic carcinomatous growth may feel friable. Bits of tissue may break off on the examining hand. On inspection the friable exophytic cancer shows a rough, granular bleeding surface that may be sloughing and infected, with a foul-smelling discharge.

A tumor that develops beneath the mucosa of the exocervix and infiltrates the cervical stroma causes cervical enlargement. The surface of the cervix may feel smooth, but the cervical consistency to palpation is hard. It is characteristic of cervical cancers that develop in the endocervical canal to cause cervical enlargement and a hard cervical consistency before breaking through the mucosa of the exocervix to cause a lesion. This also is characteristic of cervical cancers that develop in postmenopausal women. In fact, it is possible for a cervical cancer that is developing high in the endocervical canal to invade the parametrial tissue and even obstruct the ureters before causing a visible cervical lesion. An ulcerative lesion may look like a fairly clean punched-out ulcer, but more commonly it is an irregular crater with a necrotic bleeding base and a foul-smelling discharge.

Any gross lesion of the cervix should be considered suspicious for cancer, and biopsied. Good visualization with a speculum and adequate illumination is essential. A Pap smear should be taken even though it is less accurate in the presence of a gross cervical lesion.

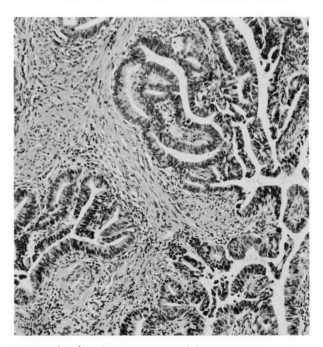

Figure 42–6. Adenocarcinoma of the cervix.

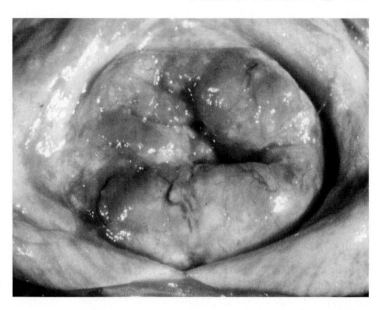

Figure 42–7. Squamous cell carcinoma, cervix uteri, FIGO stage IIa.

Colposcopic examination is not needed for a gross cervical lesion, but may be helpful when there is a minimal lesion to identify the colposcopically most abnormal area for directed rather than random biopsies. The primary benefit of colposcopy is in visualizing a noninvasive or minimally invasive lesion that cannot be visualized without magnification.

Cervical biopsy techniques are discussed in Chapter 41. Biopsies can be taken with any of a number of special instruments; the Kevorkian (Fig. 42-8), Younge, or Gaylor biopsy forceps are particularly good for taking an adequate biopsy specimen. Conization is unnecessary when a gross lesion is present. Indeed, it is contraindicated in the presence of a gross lesion, since it may delay the initiation of irradiation or surgical treatment. Iodine (Schiller) staining may be used to outline the vaginal margins of the lesion. All of these procedures can be done in the office. It usually is not necessary to take the patient to the operating room to diagnose cervical cancer. If an anesthetic is necessary for some other reason, such as cystoscopy or vaginal biopsy, a careful pelvic examination under anesthesia, biopsy of vaginal lesions, cervical and uterine sounding, and even uterine curettage may be done. Useful information to plan treatment may be obtained.

PROGNOSTIC FACTORS

The spread of cervical cancer has been studied more intensively than that of any other gynecologic cancer. Several factors have been shown to be related to prognosis, and some are important in planning therapy. These factors are as follows:

Tumor volume
Gross tumor configuration (exophytic, endophytic, barrel shaped)

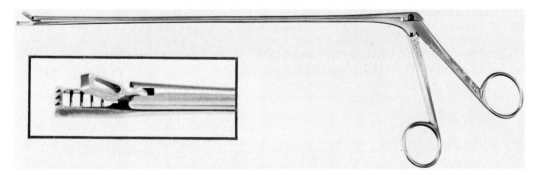

Figure 42–8. Kevorkian square-jawed cervical biopsy forceps.

Vaginal or endometrial cavity extension
Histologic grade of tumor
Depth of tumor invasion
Vascular invasion
Regional (pelvic) and distant (paraaortic) lymph node metastases
Distant metastases

Although the methods available for the clinical staging of cervical cancer have improved since the 1960s, inaccuracies in defining the precise extent of the disease occur in 15% to 25% of each clinical stage. Despite this inaccuracy, the selection of a specific method and plan of therapy is still based on the stage of disease mainly determined on palpable pelvic findings from the initial examination. An experienced pelvic examiner can be expected to make fewer mistakes in staging. The use of new radiologic imaging techniques can be helpful in evaluating the extent of the central disease (cervix, corpus, vagina, and parametrium) and lymph node involvement, but these techniques also have inaccuracies.

In all stages of invasive cervical carcinoma, *tumor volume* is an important factor in predicting the spread of disease and in determining the best method of therapy. Burghardt and others studied tumor volume as a factor in the treatment of microcarcinoma of the cervix (stage Ia). They found that when microcarcinoma was accurately measured by serial step-sectioning and the maximum tumor volume was less than 400 mm^3, a variety of conservative treatment programs could control the disease. When conization was the only therapy, only 1 of 44 cases was found to progress. Piver and coworkers, van Nagell and coworkers, Shingleton, and others found that invasive carcinoma lesions less than 2 or 3 cm in diameter were less likely to metastasize to the pelvic lymph nodes than larger lesions (Table 42-2). The 5-year survival rate for patients with stage Ib cervical lesions less than 3 cm in diameter ranges from 85%

to 90%, whereas for patients with lesions greater than 3 cm the cure rate is around 65%.

The *gross tumor configuration* also has a bearing on prognosis. Bulky exophytic and endophytic lesions, especially those that are barrel shaped, have a poor clinical prognosis because of large tumor volumes. As tumors become larger, the neovascularity is quite tortuous, with numerous arteriovenous shunts causing a quite vascular and bloody appearance. Despite an increased vascularity, gases exchange poorly. As cervical tumors grow, they exceed their blood supply and become necrotic. In fact, it has been estimated that in tumors in excess of 2 cm in diameter, 99% of the cells in the center are hypoxic. As tumor cells extend away from the vascular source they become more hypoxic. Because oxygen plays a central role in the chain of events leading to cellular death after irradiation, such hypoxic cells may require more than twice the dose of irradiation for cytotoxic effect as compared with fully oxygenated cells (so-called oxygen enhancement ratio). Because the effect of megavoltage irradiation on a tumor is mainly determined by blood supply and oxygenation, larger doses of irradiation are necessary to kill tumor cells in the hypoxic, central portions of a tumor mass. The more peripheral parts of the tumor may be quite radioresponsive, but the more central parts quite resistant. This explains the rationale of combined irradiation and less extensive surgery in some large barrel-shaped cervical tumors, since the central part of a large cervical tumor may be readily excisable without compromising adjacent structures. The negative effect of oxygenation enhancement ratio is also the reason numerous procedures have been tried to make the central portions of the tumor more radiosensitive, such as the use of proton or neutron beams with high linear transfer energy, which overcome oxygen dependency. Other measures that have been tried include hyperthermia, hyperbaric oxy-

TABLE 42–2
Correlation of Tumor Size with Incidence of Positive Nodes and Survival Rates in Cervical Cancer (Stage Ib)

STUDY (YR)	NO. OF PATIENTS	TUMOR SIZE (cm)	POSITIVE NODES (%)	SURVIVAL (%)
Piver (1975)	96	≤3	21.2	85.5*
	52	>3	35.2	65.4
van Nagell (1977)	46	≤2	9.0	94.0†
	36	>2	31.0	40.0
Shingleton (1982)	117	≤2	12.0	91.4*
	64	>2	37.5	63.9

* 5-year survival.
† 1- to 10-year survival.

gen, and electron-affinic compounds such as misonidazole. Unfortunately, in most instances, these measures have proved to be borderline effective. The ability of irradiation to cure a squamous or glandular tumor is directly related to tumor volume. As the tumor volume increases to more than 2 cm in diameter, irradiation doses of more than 6000 rad are necessary to attain 90% control. Only by combining central brachytherapy with external beam megavoltage therapy can a dose of this magnitude be achieved.

When *vaginal extension* of cervical cancer occurs, even with no parametrial involvement, the incidence of pelvic lymph node metastases will be higher. Piver and Chung noted a 42% incidence of pelvic node spread in stage IIa lesions. Averette found two of nine such cases to have occult paraaortic lymph node metastases. Most lesions that extend onto the vagina from the cervix are larger than 3 cm in diameter, a factor that, by itself, increases the frequency of regional and distant metastases.

Uterine corpus and endometrial cavity extension from primary cervical cancer was originally thought to be a poor prognostic factor. The original League of Nations classification of 1937 included such lesions in the stage II category. Over the years classification of the disease based on extension to the uterine corpus or endometrial cavity has gradually been discounted. These lesions, classified as stage Ic in 1950, were included in the broad category of stage Ib in 1961.

Despite the change in classification, we still have greater concern about patients whose tumor extends into the corpus of the uterus. Evidence from Washington University reported by Perez and coworkers and by others shows that tumor extension into the endometrial cavity lowers the 5-year survival rate of stage Ib and IIa lesions by 10% to 20%. Lesions that involve the corpus also have a twofold greater incidence of distant metastases when compared with lesions without corpus extension. Similar observations have been reported by Prempee and coworkers from 82 cases of stage I and stage II disease with endometrial extension. The absolute 5-year cure rate of 68% for stage I and 62% for stage II disease reflects the higher risk of metastases: 20% for stage I cases and 24% for stage II cases.

Establishing a diagnosis of endometrial extension by using microscopic study of endometrial curettings admittedly can be difficult. Frequently the curettage specimen is contaminated by the cervical tumor, making it difficult to be certain about endometrial extension. Any finding that indicates endometrial involvement should be given serious consideration, and the information should be used in planning treatment.

Lymph node metastases, either regional (pelvic) or to the distant (paraaortic) lymph nodes, have proved to be one of the most reliable prognostic factors for patients with cervical cancer (Fig. 42-9). The frequency of metastases to pelvic lymph nodes is about 0% to 0.5% for patients with stage Ia1; 1% to 2% for stage Ia2; 10% to 15% for stage Ib; 20% to 25% for stage IIb; greater than 35% for stage III; and greater than 50% for stage IV. The detection of positive pelvic and paraaortic lymph nodes is difficult, even with newer radiologic imaging techniques. Detection of positive lymph nodes is greatly facilitated when lymphadenectomy is used in preoperative staging or treatment. Kolstad has shown that when intraoperative lymphography is used, 15% to 25% more

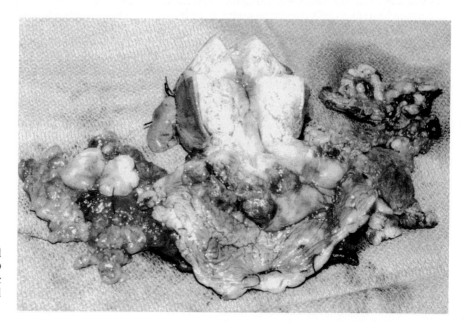

Figure 42–9. Squamous cell carcinoma, cervix uteri, FIGO stage IIa, with gross metastatic tumor in a right parametrial lymph node.

patients with stage Ib disease are found to have positive regional lymph nodes.

When patients with stage Ib cervical cancer are primarily treated with extensive hysterectomy and pelvic lymphadenectomy, the 5-year cure rate is about 90%, if there are no lymph node metastases. If metastatic disease to lymph nodes is found, the 5-year cure rate is about 65%. The number of positive nodes also influences prognosis. In Masterson's study, with one positive node there was a 74% 5-year survival; with four or five positive nodes there was only a 29% 5-year survival. Prognosis is better when lymph node metastases are microscopic; prognosis is worse when lymph nodes are grossly involved with tumor. In a retrospective study of 51 patients with cervical carcinoma with lymph node metastases, Tinga and associates found an 87% survival with single node metastasis and 24% survival in patients with multiple node involvement. All patients were treated with adjuvant postoperative irradiation.

Metastatic disease to paraaortic lymph nodes occurs in less than 5% of patients with stage I disease, 10% to 15% with stage II disease, 25% to 30% with stage III disease, and more than 40% with stage IVa disease. Most studies confirm that metastases to paraaortic nodes occur more frequently when positive pelvic nodes also are present. Rarely are patients found to have positive paraaortic nodes when pelvic nodes are negative. When pelvic nodes are positive the risk of positive paraaortic nodes is increased. When paraaortic node metastasis has progressed beyond the microscopic stage, there is little chance of control using current methods of treatment with irradiation alone. Long-term survivals have occurred only sporadically with chemotherapy.

Histologic grade of the tumor can affect prognosis. Squamous tumors usually are categorized as well differentiated, grade 1 (see Fig. 42-3); moderately differentiated, grade 2 (see Fig. 42-4); or poorly differentiated, grade 3 (see Fig. 42-5). Because a mixture of cell types is common in the same tumor, cell type alone cannot be used as an indicator of the outcome of treatment for most squamous tumors. Data presented by Chung and coworkers, Gilmore and coworkers, and Sedlacek show that a higher incidence of lymph node metastases and a lower cure rate occur among patients with poorly differentiated tumors.

Small cell grade 3 carcinomas show a higher incidence of pelvic node metastasis (53%), of focal recurrence (25%), and of distant metastases (20%) than do grade I, stage Ib and IIa lesions, according to studies by Chung and coworkers. Van Nagell and coworkers presented a similar finding. Patients with small cell grade 3 tumors had lymph–vascular space involvement in 93% of the cases, compared with 20% and 24% involvement in patients with grade 1 and grade 2 lesions, respectively.

Tumor differentiation has a greater prognostic role for adenocarcinoma of the cervix because the cellular patterns can be correlated with the curability of the disease. As with endometrial carcinoma, well-differentiated grade 1 lesions have the best 5-year survival rate and the lowest incidence of pelvic node metastases. Berek and coworkers studied 51 patients with stage I adenocarcinoma of the cervix and found a 5-year cure rate of 50.0% for those who had poorly differentiated grade 3 tumors, whereas patients with grade 1 and grade 2 tumors had 84.2% and 77.8% cure rates, respectively. In Berek's study patients with grade 3 tumors who had more advanced stages of cervical cancer had similar poor cure rates. In the report by Fu and coworkers 67% of patients with well-differentiated tumors were alive after 5 years, whereas only 19% of patients with poorly differentiated adenocarcinoma survived that long. Shingleton considers the lower cure rate of cervical adenocarcinoma to result from the bulky tumor volume rather than from tumor grade.

Berek also studied lesion size, depth of invasion, and tumor grade in patients with adenocarcinoma of the cervix to determine whether these factors influenced the status of lymph node metastases or patient survival. No positive pelvic lymph nodes were found in patients with lesions that were less than 2 cm in greatest diameter. Positive lymph nodes were found in 16.7% of patients with 2- to 4-cm lesions and in 82.3% of patients with lesions greater than 4 cm. Berek's study also found that pelvic lymph node metastases did not occur in adenocarcinoma patients who had a depth of tumor invasion of less than 2 mm, whereas positive nodes were found in 12.5% of patients with 2- to 2.5-mm invasion, 37.5% with 5- to 10-mm invasion, and 50% of patients with greater than 10 mm of stromal invasion.

Several investigators, including Swan and Rutledge, Wheeless and Graham, and Julian and coworkers, have drawn attention to the fact that when there is a mixture of adenocarcinomatous and squamous elements—so-called adenosquamous tumors—the prognosis is poor and the incidence of pelvic lymph node metastases is high. Histologic combinations should be considered when comparing the prognoses of adenocarcinoma and squamous cancers of the cervix.

An aspect of cervical cancer that can be considered with tumor volume in making a prognosis is *depth of stromal invasion*. In a study of 139 patients with stage I squamous carcinoma of the cervix Boyce and coworkers clearly demonstrated that the depth of invasion was positively correlated with the involvement of pelvic lymph nodes and with pelvic recurrence. When the tumor had extended more than 10 mm beneath the basement membrane, 34% of the patients had positive pelvic lymph nodes, and the 5-year cure rate was only 63%. One third of the patients had recurrences of disease in other pelvic tissue when the depth of invasion of the original tumor exceeded 10 mm.

Although the depth of cervical stromal invasion frequently is not analyzed as a prognostic factor, Abdulhayoglu and coworkers included stromal invasion in an analysis of prognostic factors in 35 patients with stage Ib cervical cancer. These researchers categorized stromal invasion as involving the inner, middle, or outer one-third of the cervix. Of 11 patients with metastases to pelvic nodes, 9 had tumor extending to the outer one-third of the cervix, whereas the remaining 2 cases had tumor limited to the middle one-third of the cervix. In addition to an increased risk of pelvic node metastases, advanced depth of stromal invasion was correlated with a recurrence of disease in the pelvis, even when the lymph nodes were negative. These investigators concluded that patients who had stage Ib cervical cancer extending to the outer one-third of the cervix with vascular invasion and little differentiation would probably benefit from adjuvant pelvic irradiation after extensive hysterectomy and pelvic lymphadenectomy.

Although frequently overlooked, the presence of *vascular invasion* by tumor emboli can influence the prognosis in cervical cancer. Chung and coworkers reported that 63% of the patients with either stage Ib or IIa carcinoma who had vascular invasion also had positive pelvic lymph nodes. Boyce and coworkers noted positive pelvic lymph nodes in 32% of 41 cases with vascular invasion. The incidence of vascular invasion with stage I and stage IIa lesions varies widely, depending on the number of sections of the cervix prepared and the depth of stromal invasion. Vascular invasion has been reported in as few as 9% and as many as 34% of stage I lesions.

The finding of tumor in capillary-like microlymphatic spaces is another ominous sign, portending pelvic node involvement and a generally poor prognosis. In many instances the lymph nodes are inadequately sampled, so that small microemboli associated with microlymphatic invasion are not detected. Tumor found in capillary-like spaces within the cervix represents the earliest stage of invasion of the lymphatic system and metastatic disease, and should be considered as a possible indication of pelvic lymph node metastases when making treatment plans.

PRETREATMENT CLINICAL EVALUATION

When a diagnosis of invasive cervical cancer has been established histologically, patients require an evaluation of all pelvic organs to determine whether the tumor is confined to the cervix or has extended to the adjacent parametrium, vagina, and endometrial cavity or to the bladder, ureters, or rectum. A thorough assessment requires excretory urography, cystoscopic examination of the bladder and urethra, a proctosigmoidoscopic study, a barium enema, and a thorough colposcopic study of the vagina and vaginal fornices. Colposcopic findings may be used for assigning a stage to the tumor, but the results must be confirmed by biopsy. Chest radiographs and electrocardiographic studies are used to determine cardiopulmonary disease, particularly in the older patient. Pulmonary function studies also are important, especially for evaluating patients who are candidates for extensive surgery.

When urographic studies detect ureteral obstruction, a tumor is classified as a stage IIIb lesion. Ureteral obstruction, either hydronephrosis or nonfunction of the kidney, has become well established as an indicator of poor prognosis, and is recognized in the FIGO classification. Retrograde pyelography may be performed after the ureteral obstruction is located, for further evaluation. Kidney function studies provide important baseline information before treatment; serum creatinine and creatinine clearance studies as well as complete urinalysis are useful for detecting the presence of albumin or white and red blood cells and renal tubular casts.

The bladder mucosa also should be inspected for possible bullous edema, which indicates lymphatic obstruction within the bladder wall. Evidence of disease in the bladder must be confirmed by biopsy before the lesion can be classified as stage IV. Rectal lesions require a similar examination because they may be related to an inflammatory process rather than to the cervical tumor.

Pretreatment pedal lymphangiography has been used by many clinics to detect pelvic and paraaortic lymph node metastases (Fig. 42-10), but the procedure is tedious and associated with many false-negative and false-positive findings. When compared with lymphadenectomy, positive lymphangiograms have an accuracy rate less than 75%. Unfortunately a lymphangiogram only detects metastatic lesions when the parenchyma of the lymph node has become distorted, by which time the lesions are larger than 3 mm. In many clinics, including our own, a false-negative rate of 50% is not uncommon.

Lymphangiography is more appropriate for fine needle aspiration studies and determining the completeness of lymphadenectomy during surgery than for specific diagnosis of metastatic disease. In a study of 275 patients with stage Ib cervical carcinoma, Kolbenstvedt and Kolstad increased their surgical findings of positive pelvic lymph nodes from 15% to 25% using preoperative and intraoperative lymphangiography. The technique also is helpful for directing lymph node dissection to suspicious lesions and for planning the extent of the radiation field at the time of irradiation therapy.

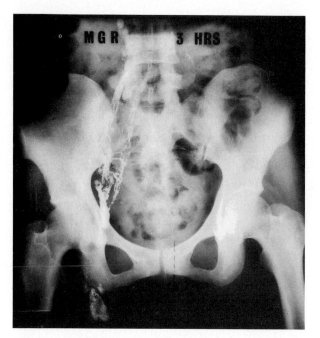

Figure 42–10. Pelvic lymphangiogram outlining the right external iliac, common iliac, and para-aortic lymph nodes shows metastatic disease. The obturator and hypogastric nodes are not seen with this technique.

Isotope scanning of the long bones, liver, and lungs has not proved useful for evaluating the clinical extent of early cervical cancer, although the technique is good for detecting distant metastases from stage IIIb or stage IV lesions or from recurrent disease. Radionucleotide scans, once used preoperatively to identify metastases in liver or other viscera, have been replaced by computed tomography (CT). The CT scan also may show retroperitoneal node enlargement and other intraabdominal masses. In experienced hands fine needle aspiration of retroperitoneal nodes with CT scan or sonographic direction has an accuracy rate of 75% to 85%. When the aspiration study shows cytologic evidence of neoplastic cells, a surgical biopsy need not be performed.

A pelvic examination must be performed as part of the staging process, and the procedure may be done with the patient completely relaxed by general anesthesia. In 20% of patients, in our experience, the initial classification of the disease has proved to be incorrect on pelvic examination with general anesthesia. A careful examination may reveal a more advanced stage of the disease than was originally found. At the time of pelvic examination under anesthesia fractional curettage may be useful in identifying extension of the disease to the endometrium.

The pelvic examination should provide a complete evaluation of the reproductive tract, so that the location and extent of the tumor can be clearly defined. Surgical experience from pelvic lymphadenectomy has confirmed an error rate of 15% to 25% in the clinical staging of patients with stage Ib or II lesions. In 10% to 30% of cases with stage II or III tumors, in addition to positive findings of occult pelvic lymph nodes, other metastases may be found in the paraaortic nodes.

Brodman and coworkers found that the clinical determination of disease extent was correct in 62.5% of patients who underwent extensive surgery for early invasive cervical cancer. In none of their cases did the CT scan indicate disease more extensive than predicted by clinical staging. CT did not detect macroscopic parametrial disease in two of three patients, and did not detect enlarged pelvic lymph nodes in six cases. Magnetic resonance imaging (MRI) predicted parametrial disease in two cases that could not be confirmed with histopathology, and only one of four patients with pelvic nodal metastases was detected.

TREATMENT OF INVASIVE CERVICAL CANCER

Based on the pretreatment evaluation of the patient, including the prognostic factors of tumor size, clinical stage of the disease, and risk of pelvic node metastases, a treatment schema may be developed for invasive cervical cancer as shown in Table 42-3. Almost all patients are treated with either primary irradiation therapy or primary surgery. Some patients are appropriately treated with combinations of irradiation and surgery. Chemotherapy is not effective as primary treatment for invasive cervical cancer but may be used as adjuvant therapy and when the disease is recurrent or persistent. In three investigations of the Gynecologic Oncology Group the response rate of cervical cancer for cisplatin was 23% (183 responses among 791 patients). Further discussion of chemotherapy for cervical cancer can found in Chapter 46.

The surgical treatment of invasive carcinoma of the cervix is primarily limited to those patients in whom the disease is confined to the cervix or vaginal fornix (stage Ia, stage Ib, or stage IIa disease) and who are good surgical risks. Because only 35% to 40% of patients with invasive cervical cancer have disease treatable with primary surgery (a stage Ib or IIa lesion less than 3 cm in diameter), irradiation therapy remains the major method of treatment in most cases. Stage Ib or IIa lesions with a diameter greater than 3 cm are associated with a high incidence of pelvic lymph node metastasis. For example, in Piver's study patients with a tumor size of 3 cm or less had a 21.2% incidence of pelvic node metastasis, a finding that has been confirmed by other

TABLE 42–3
General Treatment Schema for Invasive Cervical Carcinoma*

DISEASE STAGE	TREATMENT
Stage Ia1	Cervical conization or total hysterectomy, abdominal or vaginal.
Stage Ia2	Extensive abdominal hysterectomy, bilateral pelvic lymphadenectomy.
Stage Ib and IIa	
Lesions ≤3 cm and good surgical risk	Extensive abdominal hysterectomy, bilateral pelvic lymphadenectomy with postoperative irradiation in selected patients.
Lesions >3 cm or poor surgical risk	Full external and intracavitary pelvic irradiation.
Large bulky "barrel-shaped" lesions	Full external and intracavitary pelvic irradiation plus extrafasical abdominal hysterectomy with paraaortic node biopsy.
Stage IIb Stage IIIa and IIIB } Stage IVa and IVb	Full external and intracavitary pelvic irradiation.

*For individual patients, recommendations for treatment may vary, depending on circumstances. For example, a patient with a stage IVa lesion that extends only in the anterior or posterior direction may be a candidate for pelvic exenteration. Also, adjuvant chemotherapy and/or para-aortic node irradiation may be given to some patients with extensive or undifferentiated tumors.

investigators. When the lesion size was greater than 3 cm a 35.2% incidence of positive nodes was found, and the 5-year cure rate declined from 85.5% to 65.4% (see Table 42-2). When a high risk for pelvic node metastasis exists most clinicians in the United States prefer to treat the patient with full pelvic irradiation, since the cure rates in this country for stage Ib or IIa disease are comparable for extensive surgery and irradiation therapy. Although surgery is much more thorough today, in terms of the extent and completeness of pelvic node dissection, than when described by Wertheim at the turn of the century, some tumor emboli in the pelvic microlymphatic channels are impossible to remove surgically and remain even after the most extensive operation. If adjunctive pelvic irradiation is used for patients with positive pelvic lymph nodes, it is preferable to give the irradiation treatment to the tumor-bearing area with an intact blood supply, so that tissue oxygenation can be used to enhance the radiobiologic effect of the treatment.

It has been recognized for many years that simple hysterectomy is not adequate treatment for stage Ib cervical cancer. In 1943 Jones and Jones reported a 5-year survival of only 41.6% in patients who had been treated for early stage I cervical cancer with simple hysterectomy only. Such poor results also have been reported by Schmidt and others. When more than stage Ia1 invasive cervical cancer is a surprise finding in a simple hysterectomy specimen, additional therapy, usually irradiation therapy, should be given. Current

survival rates in these patients has improved with the advent of megavoltage irradiation, as reported by Andras and coworkers, Davy and coworkers, and Papavasilou and coworkers. Heller and coworkers reported 35 patients with invasive cervical carcinoma discovered in a uterus removed for benign conditions. All patients received radiation therapy. Patients with presumed stage Ib disease had a corrected 5-year survival of 78%, and those with presumed stage IIb disease had a corrected 5-year survival of 67%.

The management of cervical cancer has gradually evolved into a team approach in which the best minds available in surgery, radiotherapy, and cellular biology are utilized. With increasing frequency medical oncologists also are being called on to use chemotherapy to treat special problems presented by patients with cervical cancer, as discussed in Chapter 46.

IRRADIATION TREATMENT

Initially, several methods of intracavitary therapy were developed, including the Stockholm technique from the Radiumhemmet; the Paris technique, designed at the Curie Foundation; and the Manchester technique from England. The Stockholm radium technique consisted of high-intensity central irradiation, repeated two or three times in 3 weeks, whereas the Paris technique used low-intensity central irradiation continuously delivered over 1 week. The Manchester technique, derived from the Paris method, used low, hourly dosage rates that required at least two insertions of radiation sources. The use of radium therapy peaked in the United States between 1920 and 1940. Other radioactive elements, including cesium and iridium, are now more commonly used in central brachytherapy.

With the establishment of the roentgen as a defined unit of radiation exposure (Stockholm, 1921) it became possible to measure the quantity of irradiation delivered by an x-ray unit. High-energy nuclear radiation sources, ranging to 25 mV for the betatron and linear accelerator, have significantly improved the complications rates after irradiation therapy, and possibly improved the cure rates. An intracavitary dose can be combined with external irradiation to best achieve the high central irradiation derived from the gamma rays of radium or cesium in addition to uniform megavoltage external irradiation with penetration of the cervix, broad ligament, and lateral pelvic walls.

To compare the survival rates of irradiation and primary surgery, Delgado analyzed the reports from patients treated for stage I cervical cancer. The 1995 patients treated by irradiation had an average 5-year survival rate of 85.6%, which was essentially identical to the survival rate with radical surgery (Table 42-4). Patients treated with both surgery and irradiation had a similar survival rate of 86.6%.

Einhorn reported a favorable 5-year cure rate for stages I and II cervical cancer treated with irradiation alone (Table 42-5). When Einhorn compared different types of tumors by volume he found the cure rate for adenocarcinoma to be comparable, stage for stage, with that for epidermoid cancer whether patients were treated with irradiation alone or with a combination of irradiation plus surgery. A simple total hysterectomy was used in some cases to remove the parent tumor in the endocervix if it was bulky or barrel shaped, but lymph node dissection was not performed.

Complications

Ionizing irradiation interrupts the biochemical and metabolic processes of the human cell, causing mitotic inhibition or reproductive failure of the cell, which results in cell death. Even cells that have received lethal doses may show no visible damage initially, but eventually they degenerate, owing to their inability to undergo continued cell division. Some cells undergo an immediate interruption of viability and rapid cellular death.

Tissue tolerance depends not only on the dose, but also on the volume of tissue irradiated and the interval between fractions of therapy. Modern irradiation therapy exploits the penetrability of the photon beams

TABLE 42–4
5-Year Survival of Patients with Stage I Squamous Cancer of Cervix by Treatment Modality

STUDY	NO. OF PATIENTS	5-YEAR SURVIVAL (%)
Surgery		
Liu, Meigs, 1955	116	78.4
Brunschwig, Daniel, 1958	127	78.7
Carter et al, 1958	119	81.5
Mitra, 1959	25	64.0
Brunschwig, 1960	138	81.9
Welch et al, 1961	95	85.7
Green et al, 1962	315	83.0
Dobrotin, Bicheikina, 1963	349	76.2
		(8 year)
Masterson, 1963	100	80.0
Christensen et al, 1964	168	82.7
Brunschwig, Barber, 1966	173	81.5
Masterson, 1967	120	87.5
Masubuchi et al, 1969	296	90.5
Crisp, 1969	98	90.0
Ketcham et al, 1971	28	86.0
Park et al, 1973	126	91.0
Newton, 1975	58	81.0
Morley, Seski, 1976	149	91.3
Total	2600	83.4
Radiation		
Makowski et al, 1962	442	81.3
Kottmeier, 1964	611	89.5
Crawford et al, 1965	63	46.0
Masubuchi et al, 1969	152	88.2
Marcial, 1970	41	87.0
Neinminen, Pollanen, 1970	77	70.0
Fletcher, 1971	549	91.5
Newton, 1975	61	74.0
Welander et al, 1975	19	89.5
		(2 year)
Total	1995	85.6
Combination Therapy		
Welch et al, 1961: RT and hyst.	78	90.4
Currie, 1963: RT and lymph.	123	81.3
Gorton, 1964: RT and lymph.	166	86.0
Kottmeier, 1964: RT and lymph.	53	79.0
Crawford et al, 1964: RT and rad. hyst.	74	90.0
Rutledge et al, 1965: RT and lymph.	30	86.1
Decker et al, 1965 RT and lymph.	44	88.6
Burch, Chalfant, 1970: RT and hyst.	138	85.5
Nienminen, Pollanen, 1970: lymph. and RT	114	87.0
Rampone et al, 1973: RT and lymph.	537	88.3
Lagasse et al, 1974: RT and lymph.	60	88.3
Lagasse et al, 1974: lymph. and RT	58	74.1
Quigley et al, 1975: RT and lymph.	136	89.4
Total	1611	86.6

(Adapted from Delgado G. Stage Ib cancer of the cervix: the choice of treatment. Obstet Gynecol Survey 1978;33:174.)

TABLE 42–5
Cervical Cancer 5-Year Survival Rates with
Irradiation Therapy Only

CLINICAL STAGE	NO. OF PATIENTS	5-YEAR SURVIVAL	
		Number	*Percentage*
Ia	35	35	100
Ib	60	53	88
IIa	60	39	65
IIb	53	21	40
III	38	6	16
IV	19	2	11
Total	265	156	59

(Einhorn N: Frequency of severe complications after radiation therapy for cervical carcinoma. Acta Radiol Ther 1975;14:42.)

emitted by megavoltage machines. The skin is no longer a barrier; 80% of an emitted irradiation dose can be delivered to a tumor 10 cm below the surface. With this sophisticated technology more procedures are feasible, such as whole-pelvic irradiation. Unfortunately, megavoltage rays also can irreversibly destroy adjacent pelvic structures. But it is true that with high-energy accelerators, the beam of external irradiation can be better defined and the doses to intervening tissues between the skin and target tissues can be reduced. The volume of tissues that receive irradiation unnecessarily is reduced. The treatment is more precise, and therefore can be expected to be more effective with fewer complications.

The ideal irradiation treatment achieves the delicate balance of a dosage that can be tolerated by normal tissue while providing permanent arrest of the tumor cell. Complications occur when the ionization tolerance of the nonmalignant cell is exceeded. During the treatment course for cervical cancer the bladder and rectum are constantly at risk of receiving excessive irradiation.

One of the most frequent and most distressing complications of irradiation treatment is its effect on the vagina. The vagina may become narrowed in caliber throughout its entire length. Constriction of the upper one-third to one-half is almost inevitable, and obliteration from synechiae formation is common. These changes frequently result in dyspareunia and cessation of coitus. The prophylactic use of vaginal dilators after treatment and the generous use of estrogen creams are recommended to minimize these effects.

Kottmeier reported that the complication rates for the bladder and the rectum are directly related to the dosage received. The glandular mucosa of the bowel is more radiosensitive than the transitional epithelium of the bladder. At the Radiumhemmet rectal injuries oc-

curred with intracavitary brachytherapy when the dosage was more than 6000 rad. When the dosage exceeded 8000 rad to the vaginal wall serious injuries of the rectum occurred in 26.1% of the patients. By using high-energy accelerators that produce well-defined beams, and better brachytherapy computerized dosimetry, we have gradually increased the accepted tolerance to the posterior wall of the bladder and the anterior wall of the rectum from 5000 rad to almost 6000 rad.*

Although local relief may be obtained with hydrocortisone enemas and analgesic rectal suppositories, the radiobiologic effect of the ischemic endarteritis is progressive and irreversible. Rectal wall dosages of greater than 6000 rad produce a high incidence of proctosigmoiditis, which frequently progresses to rectal ulcers and stricture, requiring a colostomy even years after the original treatment. Even with standard treatment a high incidence of serious rectal injuries can occur. Einhorn reported an incidence of 11% in patients treated with 5000 rad to the midplane of the pelvis.

Serious intestinal injuries from irradiation therapy should not exceed 2% to 3% of the treated cases. An increased incidence of injury to the small bowel has followed the use of high-energy megavoltage therapy, particularly in cases of fixation of the bowel in the pelvis. When adhesions cause fixation of the bowel the total tumor dose also is delivered to the immobilized segment. Piver reported 12 cases of enterovaginal and enterocutaneous fistulas after irradiation. Two-thirds of the patients had undergone a pretherapy laparotomy for surgical staging and lymph node sampling. Fixation of the small bowel into the pelvis is a frequent complication of surgical staging. The use of a retroperitoneal approach to the paraaortic and common iliac nodes should reduce this intestinal complication.

Irradiation injuries of the bladder occur less frequently, and the symptoms usually are delayed. In Kottmeier's report 1.4% of the patients developed serious bladder injuries after standard irradiation therapy of 6000 rad to the outer bladder wall. When irradiation dosages exceeded 6000 rad to the internal surface of the bladder wall, injuries, including fistulas, occurred in 31.2% of the patients. The incidence of fistulas alone was only 0.8%. Ureteral damage caused by irradiation treatment is uncommon. In Underwood's review less than 0.5% of the patients who received irradiation had this rare injury, which usually is caused by displacement of intracavitary radium or cesium sources, producing ureteral fibrosis and obstruction. Monitoring

---

*Gynecologic oncology is currently in a transitional state regarding the manner in which radiation dose is expressed. The unit "rad" is being changed to the new unit "gray." For those who are interested: 1 gray = 100 rad; 1 gray = 100 centigray (cGy); 5000 cGy = 5000 rad.

with excretory urograms at yearly intervals will keep the incidence of unrecognized ureteral complications low, while providing an opportunity to examine the pelvic walls for possible neoplasia. Patients who develop ureteral obstruction after radiation therapy for cervical cancer almost always are found to have recurrent or persistent cancer.

When intracavitary radium or cesium is combined with megavoltage external therapy the dosage received at the lateral pelvic wall can easily exceed 6000 rad. With these high megavoltage dosages increased incidence of pelvic cellulitis, ureteral and rectal strictures, and fistula formation can be expected. Greiss and coworkers found a 55% complication rate with various degrees of severity when the combined midpelvic irradiation dose exceeded 7000 rad. Meticulous monitoring of the irradiation dosage at the rectovaginal and vesicovaginal septa is crucial for maintaining the condition of the bladder and rectum. The combined irradiation dosage from external therapy and intracavitary radiation should not exceed 6000 rad to large volumes of the anterior rectal wall or posterior bladder wall, but there will be situations in which the dosage of smaller volumes may reach 7000 rad.

Correlating the total dosages of intracavitary and external beam irradiation can be extremely difficult. Buchler discovered that even with the advantages of a wide clinical experience assisted by computerized dosimetry curves, a high frequency of serious bowel and bladder complications occurred, including stricture and fistula. The problems were found to result from the use of an unrestricted amount of intracavitary irradiation. The only controlling limitation in Buchler's work was the total irradiation dose to the bladder and rectum of 8000 rad, measured by scintillation probe reading.

Montana and coworkers analyzed their results of radiotherapy for 197 patients with stage Ib squamous cell carcinoma of the cervix. Their treatment consisted of external beam and intracavitary brachytherapy designed to deliver 7000 to 8000 rad to point A and 5000 to 5500 rad to the pelvic lymph nodes. The 5-year disease-free survival rate was 83%. Only 15 patients developed moderate to severe complications of treatment. The mean dose to point A, to the bladder, and to the rectum in patients without complications was 7453 rad, 5590 rad, and 5837 rad, respectively. For patients with complications the corresponding doses were 7737 rad, 6335 rad, and 6810 rad.

It should be recognized that radiation damage to normal tissue comes in two distinct phases. The acute damage occurs in the first several months after treatment is given. Many years later symptoms may again develop from interference with function of the urinary or intestinal tract. This is thought to result primarily from gradually increasing ischemia and fibrosis owing to progressive obliterative endarteritis caused by chronic effects of irradiation on tissues. Intestinal strictures, chronic radiation cystitis, and ureteral stricture with chronic pyelonephritis and impairment of renal function may occur many years after irradiation therapy for cervical cancer (Fig. 42-11).

Technique

The basic method of treating cervical carcinoma combines high-dosage gamma ray irradiation from intracavitary sources with external irradiation using high-energy megavoltage photon beams to the midplane of the pelvis, including the uterus, broad ligament, and lateral pelvic wall.

The modern intracavitary brachytherapy treatment programs have evolved from the Stockholm, Paris, and Manchester techniques. The principle involved is that a radiation dose from a central point decreases inversely as the square of the distance from the source of radiation. This is known as the *inverse square law,* which states that the amount of radiation delivered varies inversely with the square of the distance from the source to the point treated. For example, an area that is 2 cm distant from a cesium source in the cervical canal

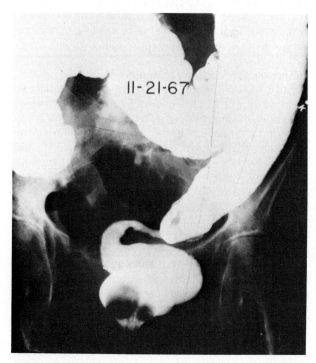

Figure 42–11. Barium enema study showing rectosigmoid obstruction secondary to irradiation stenosis 16 years after therapy for carcinoma of the cervix.

would receive only one-fourth the dose emitted at the source. At a distance of 4 cm the dose would be only one-sixteenth the central dose. The number of gamma rays that penetrate to the full depth of the tumor is controlled by the use of large colpostats, which increase the distance between the radium or cesium source and the tumor surface, and thus decrease the dose to the vaginal mucosa. By increasing the diameter of the colpostat a longer exposure time would be necessary, but a relatively larger dose would be delivered to the tumor as compared with the dose delivered to the vaginal mucosa.

All methods of combined intracavitary radium or cesium (brachytherapy) and external irradiation therapy are designed to provide a dose of ionizing irradiation that is tumoricidal for both squamous cell carcinoma and adenocarcinoma of the cervix. About 5500 to 6000 rad are applied to the midplane of the pelvis, the horizontal plane equidistant between the symphysis pubis and the sacrum, presumed to include the broad ligament and the lymphatics extending from the uterus to the lateral pelvic wall. Tissues adjacent to the cervical canal (point A) receive a much higher combined irradiation dosage (about 8000 rad) than the 4500 to 5500 rad that are given near the lateral pelvic wall (point B). In more precise terminology, point A refers to the paracervical area located on a horizontal plane that is 2 cm lateral to the cervical canal at a level 2 cm above the external cervical os. Point B is arbitrarily located on the same horizontal plane, but 5 cm from the endocervical canal. For practical purposes, many clinics consider point B to represent the location of the obturator nodes on the lateral pelvic wall.

The 25-mV betatron unit or linear accelerator is used for external irradiation, providing a dose rate of 900 rad per week given in 180-rad daily fractions. The Fletcher-Suit afterloading system (Fig. 42-12) provides a convenient, safe, and efficient method of administering intracavitary irradiation. Of the many convenient isotope sources available for intracavitary irradiation, radium and cesium are used most often.

Treatment can begin with either external or intracavitary irradiation. For the more advanced lesions (stages IIb, III, and IV) or large exophytic lesions, external irradiation is preferable initially, using opposing anterior and posterior pelvic fields (15 × 15 cm) until a midpelvic dose of 4500 to 5000 rad has been attained. At an appropriate dose level in external therapy a midline shield may be used to protect those areas in the central pelvis that will be heavily irradiated with brachytherapy. Intracavitary cesium is then applied. The tissue dosages obtained by intracavitary gamma irradiation and external megavoltage x-ray therapy are dissimilar on a rad-for-rad basis, varying with the geometry of the tumor and the accuracy of the application. Nonetheless, the rad

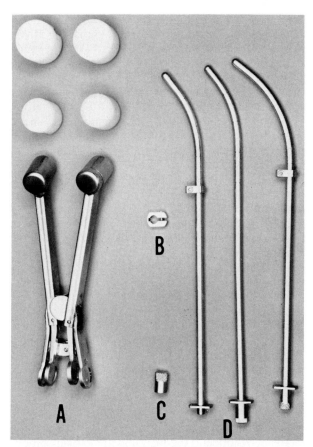

Figure 42–12. Fletcher-Suit Afterloading System. *A,* Afterloading colpostat (2 cm in diameter) and plastic jackets used to increase the colpostat size to medium (2.5 cm in diameter) or large (3 cm in diameter). *B,* Keel. *C,* Cap. *D,* Uterine afterloading tandems (the three most useful curvatures) with metal keel to stabilize the tandem against the cervix by proper packing around it.

(*r*adiation *a*bsorbed *d*ose) dosages obtained from the isodose curves of the radium or cesium implantation are combined, for practical purposes, with the dosage from the external beam therapy to determine the amount of total midpelvic irradiation. Only a fraction of the total dose needed for the lateral pelvic wall (point B) comes from the central intrauterine, intracervical, and contracervical radium or cesium sources. If the applicator is not in the center of the pelvis, the dose to each side of the pelvis will be unequal. The dose can be equalized with external therapy.

The amount of cesium applied and the number of sources used depend on the volume of the tumor and the vaginal and uterine size. The duration of each application is based on the size of the uterus, the location of the lesion, the amount of external irradiation given, and the analysis of the isodose curves from a computer program. The bladder and rectum doses are calculated from computerized isodose curves, so that the maximum dosage does not exceed 7000 rad to the rectum.

The biologic effectiveness of a radiation treatment program can only be determined by analyzing several factors. It is essential to know the tumor volume, the overall treatment time, the number of fractions given each week, and the amount of irradiation in each fraction to compare treatments given by different treatment centers. The following conclusions have been drawn from a survey of the current data on irradiation therapy.

In the treatment of stage Ib and stage IIa epidermoid carcinoma of the cervix, surgery and irradiation produce similar results; the cure rate for stage IIa lesions is somewhat lower but, again, is similar for both methods. Stages IIb, III, and IV are more effectively treated by irradiation therapy.

The incidence of serious bowel or bladder complications is slightly higher (2%–6%) with megavoltage irradiation than with surgery, and radiation injuries are far more debilitating and more difficult to correct surgically. The overall incidence of surgical fistulas usually is no more than 2%, and most injuries are correctable.

Primary extensive surgery is particularly useful in the young patient with early invasive cervical cancer because conservation of the ovaries is possible and the sclerosing effects of irradiation on the vagina and pelvis are avoided.

With either irradiation or surgery the major emphasis in treatment is the inclusion in the plan of therapy of the pathways of tumor spread, including the cervix, vaginal fornices, parametria, and pelvic lymph nodes.

When an exophytic tumor protrudes into the vagina from the portio of the cervix, the entire exocervix may be encompassed. The treatment program can then be modified to exploit the advantages of external beam teletherapy before using intracavitary irradiation. Because exophytic tumors have a highly vascular base, the lesions respond rapidly to external irradiation, which produces necrobiosis from ischemia and cell death.

A tumor—particularly a stage II tumor—that has enlarged sufficiently to produce distortion of the cervical canal or of the lower uterine segment usually is bulky and barrel shaped. Treatment with irradiation therapy alone has an unfavorable prognosis. In the central portion of these bulky tumors one finds poorly perfused hypoxic tissue containing neoplastic cells that are noncycling and resistant to radiation. Because of their growth pattern, bulky endophytic lesions extend beyond the therapeutic reaches of currently available intracavitary irradiation systems. The extended growth pattern is particularly evident in adenocarcinomas of the cervix. Consequently these lesions require a more

aggressive form of treatment, including external and intracavitary irradiation plus surgery. Rutledge used a simple extrafascial hysterectomy after full irradiation treatment to achieve a 5-year survival rate of 54% for these patients with difficult stage II lesions. When irradiation alone was used as treatment the 5-year survival rate for patients with stage II tumors decreased to 42%. In Rutledge's experience patients with stage I lesions had a satisfactory survival rate of 85% whether irradiation treatment was used alone or in combination with hysterectomy. In comparing the international (FIGO) statistics for bulky stage I and stage II adenocarcinomas, however, when either surgery alone or surgery combined with irradiation therapy was used, the 5-year cure rate was 20% higher than when irradiation alone was used.

Gallion and coworkers studied 75 patients with bulky barrel-shaped stage Ib cervical cancers. Thirty-two patients were treated with irradiation therapy alone and 43 were treated with irradiation followed by extrafascial hysterectomy. Recurrent cancer was noted in 47% of patients treated by irradiation alone as compared with 16% of those treated with combined therapy. The incidence of pelvic recurrence was reduced from 19% to 2%, and extrapelvic recurrence from 16% to 7% in patients treated with combination therapy. There was no significant increase in treatment-related complications. Histologic examination of the hysterectomy specimen revealed residual tumor in 14 of 43 patients. These authors emphasize that patients undergoing hysterectomy received only 4000 rad whole-pelvis plus 1000 rad sidewall dose irradiation and one intracavitary implant providing an additional 2000 rad to point A.

The treatment of lymph node metastasis is a major source of controversy. Clinical evidence to date indicates that only 50% to 60% of the patients with involvement of the pelvic lymph nodes will survive 5 years, whether they receive full pelvic irradiation or no irradiation therapy following lymphadenectomy.

A review of the results of postoperative irradiation for patients with stage Ib carcinoma of the cervix and pelvic node metastasis after extensive hysterectomy and lymphadenectomy was done by Morrow in 1980. The study found no statistically significant difference in the 5-year cure rates between those who received adjuvant pelvic irradiation and those who did not.

A large individual study in Morrow's review was reported by Masterson, who operated on 600 patients with stage Ib cervical cancer. For 103 patients (17%) with pelvic node metastases who did not receive postoperative irradiation the 5-year cure rate was 55%. This rate was similar to that reported from other clinics for patients with comparable disease who had received irradiation.

Once a patient has been found to have pelvic node metastases, the risk of having paraaortic disease is quite high, which explains the causes of treatment failure in 148 cases of stage III disease compiled by Fletcher and Rutledge: In only 25% of the cases was residual tumor confined to the irradiated pelvis; in 75% the disease recurred outside the pelvic treatment field.

The control of metastatic tumor in lymph nodes is based on the same relation of irradiation dose and tumor volume as in irradiation treatment of cervical tumors. Over the years tumor diameter as a measure of tumor volume has been carefully correlated with the required treatment dosage to control the tumor. If a tumor-bearing node in the pelvic or paraaortic region is 2 cm in diameter, an irradiation dose of 6000 rad is required to control 90% of the disease. If the tumor mass is larger than 2 cm but less than 4 cm in diameter, a 7000-rad dose is needed to achieve 90% control, whereas a 4- to 6-cm lesion will require 7500 to 8000 rad (Table 42-6).

Except for lesions confined to the cervix or immediate parametrium, it is difficult to achieve complete control of tumor masses larger than 2 cm in diameter without producing serious risk of irradiation injury to the intestinal or urinary tract. When the dose is raised to more than 6000 rad at the lateral pelvic wall, a prohibitive incidence of serious complications ensues. Because a high rate of serious bowel injury followed a paraaortic irradiation dose of 5500 rad, the total treatment dose for positive paraaortic nodes in most clinics today has been reduced to 4500 to 5000 rad, given through four fields over five to five and one-half weeks.

The major problem for survival, however, is not whether the regional nodes respond to irradiation therapy. Many studies have shown that current methods of irradiation provide reasonable control of local disease less than 2 cm in diameter within the cervix, parametrium, and pelvic lymph nodes. But large, bulky cervical lesions and disease spread beyond the pelvis do not respond to current methods of treatment.

Although some tumors are radioresistant even though more than adequate megavoltage irradiation dosage is used, recent studies have confirmed that lateral pelvic wall recurrence of cervical carcinoma more often is caused by inadequate irradiation dosage. Fletcher and coworkers showed that postirradiation recurrences are more common in extrapelvic sites than in the central or lateral pelvis.

As described above, the standard radiotherapeutic management of carcinoma of the cervix consists of a combination of external irradiation and low-dose rate brachytherapy usually utilizing cesium sources placed in afterloading uterovaginal applicators. Recent technology has allowed the development of high-dose rate afterloader equipment using iridium-192 high-activity sources and offering new possibilities for irradiation treatment of invasive cervical cancer and other gynecologic cancers. High-dose rate brachytherapy combined with external beam irradiation has been tested and used in Europe, Japan, and some developing countries, but there is as yet little experience in the United States except in selected clinics. Our own experience is limited and just beginning. The advantages of high-dose rate brachytherapy include better dosimetry, more constant source positioning during applications, increased ability to retract the adjacent rectum and bladder away from the active sources, and better integration with the irradiation given through pelvic ports from external sources. The treatment can be given in the outpatient clinic without admission to the hospital, thus avoiding prolonged bed rest with attendant risks of thrombophlebitis, pulmonary emboli, and indwelling catheter drainage. Although various treatment techniques have been used in a number of centers throughout the world, the overall results suggest an equivalent local control rate and 5-year survival with comparable and acceptable complication rates. Initially, there was a high rate of rectal complications. With adjustment of the dose and frequency of treatments the complication rate is now comparable to that of low-dose rate brachytherapy.

A variety of efforts have been made to enhance the effectiveness of therapy with irradiation. These include using hyperbaric oxygen, hypoxic sensitizers, hyperthermia, and chemotherapy in combination with irradiation. To date, no clear advantages in disease control have been achieved. Symonds and coworkers did show a favorable response to chemotherapy (cisplatin, bleomycin, vincristin) given before radiotherapy to patients with advanced cervical cancer. Patients with stage III or IV disease who showed evidence of response to chemo-

TABLE 42-6
Relation Between Dose and Tumor Volume in Squamous Cell Carcinoma of the Cervix*

TUMOR VOLUME	DOSE
<2 cm	5000 rad
2 cm	6000 rad
2–4 cm	7000 rad
4–6 cm	7500–8000 rad
>6 cm	8000–10,000 rad

*Average irradiation dose required to obtain 90% tumor control in area treated.

(Modified from Fletcher GH: Clinical dose–response curves of human malignant epithelial tumors. Br J Radiol 1973;46:1.)

therapy had a 69% 2-year disease-free survival compared with 35% for those patients who showed no evidence of response.

STAGING LAPAROTOMY AND EXTENDED-FIELD IRRADIATION

In a reasonably orderly manner invasive cancer spreads from its primary site in the cervix through the lymphatic system, first to primary pelvic nodes and then to common iliac and paraaortic nodes. Although it can happen, it is unlikely for a tumor to metastasize to the upper common iliac and paraaortic nodes without first involving the primary pelvic nodes. In a significant percentage of patients with positive pelvic nodes, lymph nodes along the proximal common iliac vessels, aorta, and vena cava are positive. If treatment is confined to the cervix, parametrium, and primary pelvic nodes in these patients, the disease will not be cured.

Lagasse and coworkers reported the results of a Gynecologic Oncology Group study of operative staging in 290 patients. Of 125 patients with stage IIb through IVa disease, 39 (31%) were found to have positive paraaortic nodes. Patients with adenocarcinoma of the cervix were more likely to have positive paraaortic nodes than patients with squamous cell carcinoma. As stated by Nelson and coworkers, the high incidence of paraaortic node involvement in stages IIb and III cervical carcinoma can no longer be ignored, especially if results of treatment in these stages are to be improved.

Current nonoperative methods of detecting metastases to the pelvic and paraaortic nodes are inaccurate. Fewer than 30% of positive pelvic nodes are detected by lymphangiography, and the technique is especially inadequate for detecting microscopic involvement of lymph nodes. CT scanning also is unreliable unless the lymph node is grossly involved with tumor. If lymphangiography or CT scanning demonstrates suspicion of paraaortic node metastasis, a CT-directed fine needle aspiration may be done. If tumor is found in the aspirant, a surgical procedure to sample the paraaortic nodes is not necessary. However, because these diagnostic procedures are not dependable, staging laparotomy with paraaortic node sampling usually is required.

Unfortunately severe intestinal and other complications may occur when staging laparotomy is followed by postoperative extended-field radiation therapy to treat positive paraaortic lymph nodes. To avoid the occurrence of these problems, assessment of the pelvis with surgical staging should be limited to inspection and palpation. The development of pelvic planes and spaces should be avoided. The detection of metastases in proximal common iliac and paraaortic nodes should be the major objective of the operation. If possible, the opera-

tion should be done extraperitoneally, an approach that has been shown to reduce the serious intestinal complications that may follow postoperative irradiation therapy. Lapolla and coworkers used three extraperitoneal approaches for surgical staging to accomplish bilateral paraaortic lymphadenectomy, selective pelvic nodal sampling, intraperitoneal cytology, and selected biopsies in 96 patients. Significant late postoperative small-bowel complications after radiation therapy was not a problem. Berman and coworkers did surgical staging through a transperitoneal approach in 31 patients and through an extraperitoneal approach in 39 patients. The group of patients operated on through a *transperitoneal approach* experienced a 30% complication rate secondary to small-bowel damage after irradiation therapy (two patients died). The group of patients operated on through an *extraperitoneal approach* had only a 2.5% morbidity secondary to small-bowel complications (no patients died). These authors advise using an incision on the left side parallel to Poupart's ligament but extended laterally and vertically above the iliac crest. A different technique of extraperitoneal paraaortic lymph node sampling utilizing a right midrectus upper abdominal incision is described by Schellhas. Good results were obtained in 20 patients, 9 of whom received extended-field postoperative irradiation.

Besides late intestinal complications after staging laparotomy and irradiation, complications (intraoperative and postoperative) include vascular injuries, hematomata, thromboembolism, ureteral injury, fistulas, and lymphocysts. Moore and coworkers found the morbidity of staging laparotomy acceptable, but suggested that "these procedures should be done only by those skilled in the surgical management of vascular, intestinal, and genitourinary complications."

Staging laparotomy and extended-field irradiation are inexorably tied together. An operation to discover positive paraaortic lymph nodes only to give the patient a more accurate prognosis cannot be justified. However, if surgical staging results in improved salvage by extending the field of irradiation in patients with positive paraaortic nodes, it can be justified. Unfortunately experience reported to date has been mixed regarding the likelihood of benefit. In 1977 Wharton and coworkers reported the M. D. Anderson Hospital and Tumor Institute experience between 1971 and 1974 with preirradiation celiotomy and extended-field irradiation for invasive carcinoma of the cervix. Of 89 patients with stage IIb, III, or IV cancer treated by exploratory celiotomy followed by irradiation, 24 were found to have positive common iliac and paraaortic lymph nodes. Irradiation to extended fields (using 5500 rad at 850 rad per week) controlled the cancer satisfactorily within the treated area, but the incidence of bowel complications was high. Forty-four patients died of cancer and 15 patients died of complications of the treatment. Only three patients were reported to survive for 2 or more years. These authors believe that many of their patients had distant metastases before treatment was started. When a bulky cervical cancer is associated with metastatic disease in lymph nodes, systemic cancer may already be present. After this experience the treatment program was altered to include a more conservative node-sampling technique, a lower dose of irradiation to extended fields, and chemotherapy or immunotherapy, or both.

In 1981 Welander and coworkers described the 1971 to 1979 experience at Memorial Sloan-Kettering Cancer Center. Pretreatment laparotomy was done in 127 patients, 91 of whom had stages IIb, III, and IVa disease. Twenty-two (24.2%) of these patients had positive paraaortic nodes. Standard radiation therapy to the pelvis was supplemented with paraaortic irradiation in those patients with positive paraaortic nodes. Of patients with positive paraaortic nodal metastases, 25.8% remained clinically free of disease in follow-up observation periods greater than 2 years. Survival was more likely in patients whose disease in paraaortic nodes was only microscopic. Although the most frequent complication was intestinal obstruction, no patient died as a result of treatment, probably because the dose (4400 rad) to the paraaortic region was lower.

Hughes and coworkers performed surgical staging in 355 patients with carcinoma of the cervix. Forty-one patients received extended-field irradiation. Three of 22 patients with metastatic cancer in paraaortic nodes and no peritoneal involvement survived longer than 5 years. Nelson and coworkers performed paraaortic node biopsies in 104 patients with stage II and stage III cervical cancer. Patients with positive paraaortic nodes subsequently received 6000 rad to the paraaortic area in addition to standard pelvic irradiation. The complication rate was high, and only 1 of 13 patients with positive paraaortic nodes was alive at the end of 4 years. Sixteen of 25 patients demonstrating common iliac or paraaortic nodal metastases were given extended-field irradiation by Lapolla and coworkers. A 30% 5-year survival was observed.

There are several important reasons why survival of patients with positive proximal common iliac and paraaortic nodes is not improved by extended-field irradiation. They are as follows:

When metastatic disease is present in paraaortic nodes, the pelvic disease usually is more extensive and difficult to control. The incidence of central pelvic recurrence is, therefore, high.

Metastatic disease in these nodes often is associated with disease within the peritoneal cavity.

The percentage of patients who die of treatment complications is high.

When metastatic disease is present in these nodes, systemic disease may already be present, especially if tumor in the paraaortic nodes is grossly apparent. Buchsbaum found 8 patients with positive scalene nodes in 23 patients with positive paraaortic nodes. Lee and coworkers found that three of seven patients (43%) with positive paraaortic nodes had metastases to clinically negative scalene nodes.

To consider a condition hopeless is likely to render it so. It is true that a significant number of patients with invasive cervical cancer thought to be contained within the pelvis have lymphatic extension beyond the pelvis. Unfortunately pretreatment surgical staging and extended-field irradiation currently does not result in significant improvement in survival in these patients and should remain investigational until more effective chemotherapy, immunotherapy, or radiation enhancers are available.

MICROINVASIVE CARCINOMA OF THE CERVIX

In 1961 FIGO officially subdivided stage I cervical carcinoma into stages Ia and Ib. The new stage Ia classification was made to include preclinical or early stromal invasion, which is now termed *microinvasive carcinoma*. In 1971 stage Ia was further subdivided by FIGO into early stromal invasion and occult cancer. The 1976 modification of the international classification of carcinoma of the cervix redefined stage Ib as either occult or clinically invasive cancer, restricting Ia to microinvasive carcinoma. Because occult invasive tumors cannot be diagnosed by routine clinical evaluation, they should be classified as *stage Ib* when identified by conization of the cervix. The term "Ib occult" has been omitted from the FIGO classification.

Diagnosis is based on microscopic examination of the tissue removed by biopsy, conization, portio amputation, or hysterectomy. Microinvasive disease includes unambiguous cases of epithelial anaplastic abnormalities with early stromal invasion. According to FIGO notes to the staging,

Stage Ia carcinoma should include minimal microscopically evident stromal invasion as well as small cancerous tumors of measurable size. Stage Ia should be divided into those lesions with minute foci of invasion visible only microscopically as stage Ia1, and the macroscopically measurable microcarcinomas as stage Ia2 in order to gain further knowledge of the behavior of these lesions.

The diagnosis of both stage Ia1 and Ia2 should be based on microscopic examination of removed tissue, preferably a cone, which must include the entire lesion. As noted above, the lower limit of stage Ia2 should be that it can be measured macroscopically (even if dots need to be placed on the slide prior to measurement) and the upper limit of Ia2 is given by measurement of the two largest dimensions in any given section. The depth of invasion should not be more than 5 mm taken from the base of the epithelium, either surface or glandular, from which it originates. The second dimension, the horizontal spread, must not exceed 7 mm. Vascular space involvement, either venous or lymphatic, should not alter the staging, but should be specifically recorded as it may affect treatment decisions in the future. The remaining stage I cases should be allotted to stage Ib. As a rule these cases can be diagnosed by routine clinical examination.

Up until the statement above was published by FIGO in 1988 there was a major debate among pathologists and gynecologists concerning the depth of stromal invasion that should separate stage Ia and stage Ib lesions. Most clinics divided stage Ia from stage Ib somewhere between 3 and 5 mm of stromal invasion beneath the basement membrane, when there was no microlymphatic involvement. Formerly, many authorities, including the Armed Forces Institute of Pathology, agreed that stromal penetration to a depth of no more than 3 mm from the basement membrane constituted the limits of stromal extension for microinvasive disease (Fig. 42-13). The Armed Forces Institute of Pathology also measured the depth of invasion from the surface of the epithelium rather than from the basement membrane. Many clinics considered confluent tongues of tumor cells to represent a more advanced degree of invasion (Fig. 42-14), but this factor was not accepted universally as indicating frank invasive carcinoma. Most clinicians defined stage Ia disease to exclude microlymphatic or vascular involvement because of a presumed greater risk of pelvic lymph node metastases in such cases (Fig. 42-15). The study of Roche and Norris found no evidence of pelvic lymph node metastases after primary extensive hysterectomy and pelvic lymphadenectomy for microinvasive lesions in 30 patients, 17 (57%) of whom had microlymphatic involvement in the cervical stroma.

There has been difficulty getting consensus agreement to an exact definition of microinvasive cervical cancer. Now, however, it is hoped that the uniform use of the FIGO definition in future years will allow accumulation of a sufficient number of accurately described and staged patients to decide how extensive their treatment needs to be.

Lymph Node Metastases

The question of lymph node metastases remains a major point of debate in discussions of the treatment of microinvasive carcinoma. Averette and Nelson restricted the definition of microinvasion to penetration of less than 1 mm beneath the basement membrane with no invasion of microlymphatic or vascular spaces, and they found no lymph node metastases in 162 patients whose treatment included lymphadenectomy. Van Nagell and coworkers made detailed studies of the pelvic lymph nodes of patients with microinvasive disease. In a group of 52 patients with stromal invasion of 3 mm or less a total of 984 lymph nodes were examined, and none had evidence of metastases. Of 32 patients with stromal invasion of 3.1 to 5.0 mm, 3 (9.3%) had metastases to the pelvic nodes.

Van Nagell's work has been supported by several others. Seski and coworkers reported no evidence of regional node metastases among 37 patients with microinvasive carcinoma after pelvic lymphadenectomy when tumor invasion was 3 mm or less. Benson and Norris reviewed reports of 57 cases with stromal invasion of 3 mm or less, with no biasing factors, and found that none had nodal metastases. Van Nagell collected 397 cases with stromal microinvasion of 3 mm or less from the literature. Of these, one patient (0.25%) with 1 mm of tumor invasion did have lymph node metastasis. Of 98 patients with stromal invasion of 3.1 to 5.0 mm, 8

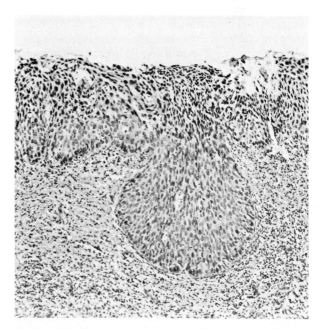

Figure 42–13. Microinvasive carcinoma of the cervix with stromal invasion of tumor to a depth of 3 mm below the base of the epithelium in the absence of lymphatic or vascular involvement.

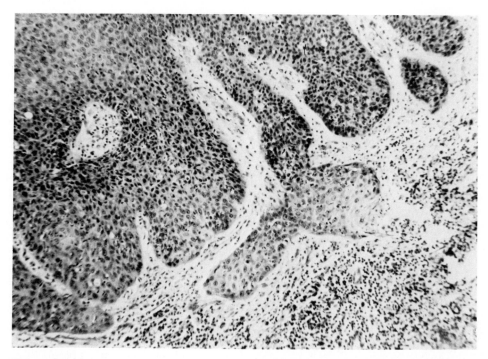

Figure 42–14. Microinvasive carcinoma of the cervix with infiltration of confluent tongues of tumor within 5 mm from the basement membrane.

patients (8%) had positive pelvic lymph nodes (Table 42-7). It is better to base recommendations for therapy on the findings of large series of patients rather than individual case reports. For example, Collins and co-workers described a patient with maximum stromal invasion of 0.8 mm who had extensive pelvic and para-aortic nodal metastases. Despite combined modality therapy she died with progressive disease.

A more accurate but tedious method of predicting lymph node metastases uses a three-dimensional evaluation of the volume of microinvasive carcinoma. Burghardt and Pickel demonstrated the importance of tumor volume in a meticulous study of 282 patients with microinvasive disease. They showed that patients who had less than 420 mm³ of tumor had no pelvic lymph node extension, and only one patient had pelvic recur-

TABLE 42–7
Frequency of Lymph Node Metastasis in Microinvasive Carcinoma of the Cervix

STUDY (YR)	STROMAL INVASION ≤3.0 MM		STROMAL INVASION 3.1 TO 5.0 MM	
	No. of Cases	Cases with Positive Nodes	No. of Cases	Cases with Positive Nodes
Smith et al (1969)	16	0	13	1
Roche, Norris (1975)	9	0	21	0
Leman et al (1976)	32	0	3	0
Seski et al (1977)	37	0	—	—
Taki et al (1979)	55	0	—	—
Yajima, Noda (1979)	90	0	—	—
Hasumi et al (1980)	106	1	29	4
van Nagell (1983)	52	0	32	3
Total	397	1 (0.25%)	98	8 (8%)

(Van Nagell JR Jr, Greenwell N, Powell DF, et al. Microinvasive carcinoma of the cervix. Am J Obstet Gynecol 1983; 145:981.)

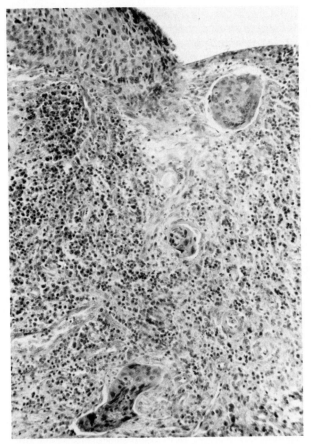

Figure 42–15. Microlymphatic or vascular involvement of cervical carcinoma with early stromal invasion within 5 mm from basement membrane.

rence of the tumor. Lohe used an upper limit of 500 mm³ to define microcarcinoma. Although this technique of analyzing tumor volume requires the time-consuming and laborious study of many large sections from a cone specimen, the three-dimensional approach provides the most accurate method of evaluation and allows a greater degree of confidence in recommending more conservative treatment for some patients with microcarcinoma.

Diagnosis

Because stage Ia lesions in asymptomatic women usually are detected by vaginal cytology, and because few gross clinical features separate this microinvasive lesion from carcinoma in situ, differential diagnosis is best made by an experienced colposcopist in conjunction with a colposcopically directed biopsy. If the question of microinvasion is raised from the colposcopic

findings, from the biopsy, or from a scrape of the endo-cervical canal, a conization of the cervix is mandatory to rule out the presence of deeply invasive cancer. Colposcopy cannot be used to make a final diagnosis, but it is used most appropriately to identify the most suspect areas of the cervix, so that they can be studied more closely. When the suspicious lesion extends into the endocervical canal and cannot be entirely seen colposcopically, then the examination is not satisfactory in defining the entire extent of the lesion. In this situation and when pathologic findings include any possibility of microinvasive carcinoma, a cervical conization is required. Microinvasive carcinoma cannot be diagnosed from a random punch biopsy, or from the colposcopic findings of superficial horizontal vessels. Conization is required for definitive diagnosis. The accuracy of the diagnosis depends on the adequacy of the cone and the adequacy of the pathologic examination of the cone. The entire cone should be blocked, so that an adequate number of histologic sections can be taken from each block. If the diagnosis is still not certain, more sections should be made.

Treatment

Although not clearly stated in the FIGO definition, we define stage Ia1 as invasive cervical carcinoma that penetrates the stroma to a depth of 3 mm or less beneath the basement membrane and does not involve the capillary lymph–vascular spaces. Such patients who are good surgical candidates can be treated with a total hysterectomy, either abdominal or vaginal. Because a pelvic lymphadenectomy will not be done as part of the surgical management of this stage of disease, vaginal hysterectomy is preferred because of the lower postoperative morbidity. Although some gynecologists restrict such conservative surgery to patients with stromal invasion of 1 mm or less, current data support a more liberal policy. The diagnosis of limited invasion, however, must be absolutely certain from adequate examination of an adequate cone.

When colposcopic examination demonstrates no evidence of extension of the tumor onto the portio or adjacent vaginal fornices, an extensive partial vaginectomy with removal of a wide vaginal cuff need not be done, since vaginal lymphatics are not involved. Recurrence in the vaginal vault usually is the result of failing to accurately define the extent of the lesion and the presence of involvement of adjacent vaginal mucosa. This usually can be prevented with a careful colposcopic examination before hysterectomy. If vaginal fornices are involved, partial vaginectomy is easier to perform with hysterectomy if the operation is done vaginally (Fig. 42-16). Alternatively, if the hysterectomy

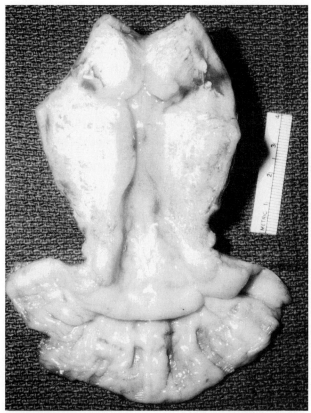

Figure 42–16. Vaginal hysterectomy and partial vaginectomy specimen from patient with squamous cell carcinoma, cervix uteri, FIGO stage Ia1 with extension to adjacent vaginal fornix. Note uniform width of vaginal cuff.

must be done abdominally, the vaginal cuff can first be developed vaginally. If Schiller's stain is applied, all nonstaining vaginal mucosa around the cervix can be removed. The technique of partial vaginectomy is shown in Figure 42-17.

The hysterectomy specimen must be subjected to the most careful examination the main purpose of which is to confirm that deeper stromal invasion does not exist. It is to be expected that the hysterectomy specimen will show no tumor or, at the most, persistent intraepithelial neoplasia high in the endocervical canal. If deeper than expected invasive cancer persists in the uterus, additional treatment may be needed.

Te Linde developed an extrafascial "modified Wertheim hysterectomy" that included a conservative resection of the most medial parametrium and upper vagina (Fig. 42-18). Although originally designed for patients with carcinoma in situ of the cervix, it is no longer used for this purpose. It is still used for patients with microinvasive cervical cancer with less than 3 mm of invasion into the stroma. It also is used in patients with bulky barrel-shaped tumors of the cervix who have

been treated with irradiation. Because clamps are placed close to the ureters but the ureters are not dissected sufficiently to allow their identification, it is advisable to place ureteral catheters preoperatively to facilitate dissection without ureteral injuries. Otherwise, an alternative method of proving ureteral integrity should be used before the operation is completed (see Chapter 29).

In our judgment, only rarely and under extraordinary circumstances should one treat stage Ia1 invasive cervical cancer with cervical conization. In a young patient who strongly desires to preserve fertility one may consider doing cervical conization only. If an adequate conization has been done and is thoroughly examined in such a patient, if the pathologist finds only the most minimal and limited superficial invasion, and if the margins of the cone are free of disease, one may consider postponing hysterectomy and doing only the cervical conization. The patient must return for regular follow-up examinations, and the postcone endocervical scrape and cytology must be negative. Because stage Ia1 invasive cervical cancer is potentially curable with simple hysterectomy in 100% of patients, one must be cautious in recommending cervical conization except under the most optimal circumstances. Brown and coworkers recently identified 8 patients with invasive cervical cancer whose cervical intraepithelial neoplasia was treated with cervical conization. The mean interval from cone biopsy to diagnosis of invasive cervical cancer was 6.7 years (range 1.5–16.5 years).

A patient who has a stage Ia2 invasive cancer should not be treated with cervical conization or simple hysterectomy. If the cervical conization shows invasion to a depth greater than 3 mm beneath the basement membrane, lymph-vascular involvement, or confluence of tumor in the stroma, extensive abdominal hysterectomy and pelvic lymphadenectomy should be recommended, just as in patients who have a stage Ib lesion less than 3 cm in diameter. One can expect about 8% of patients with stage Ia2 to have positive pelvic lymph nodes. In managing microinvasive disease it is better to overtreat than to undertreat a borderline lesion, especially one that has the potential to extend into the lymphatic system with a lethal outcome.

Patients who are not good surgical risks can be treated effectively with intracavitary irradiation. One or two intracavitary applications of cesium, using the Fletcher-Suite applicator, should be used to deliver a total dose of 15,000 rad to the cervical canal and portio. Lateral pelvic wall irradiation is not given. Kottmeier has stressed the use of intracavitary irradiation therapy for microinvasive carcinoma. He has reported 5-year cure rates equal to the rates for surgery (98%–99%). One should be extremely cautious about giving less than

(text continues on page 1190)

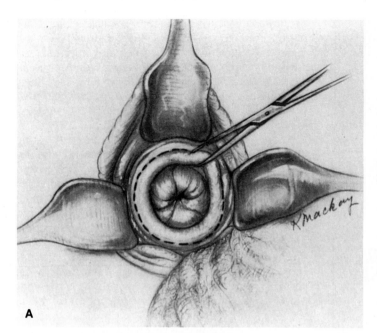

A

Figure 42–17. Technique of partial vaginectomy. This is an essential part of vaginal hysterectomy when the operation is done for carcinoma in situ or stage Ia1 with extension to adjacent vaginal fornices. *A,* The margin of the vaginal cuff to be removed is identified by placing single-toothed tenaculae through the vaginal mucosa only, being certain by Schiller's stain or colposcopy examination that the entire lesion on the vaginal mucosa will be removed. *B,* Using the electrosurgical unit, traction, and countertraction, the vaginal mucosa is incised posteriorly. This dissection is facilitated if sterile saline is injected submucosally. *C,* The incision is continued anteriorly around the entire circumference of the vagina, taking care not to injure the bladder.

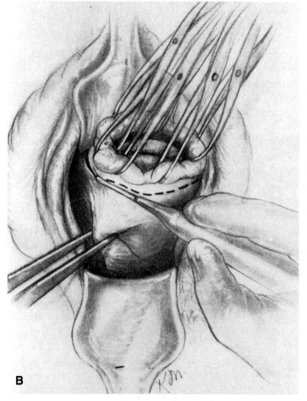

B

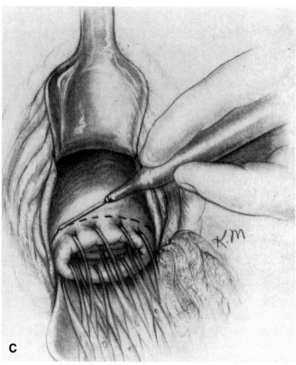

C

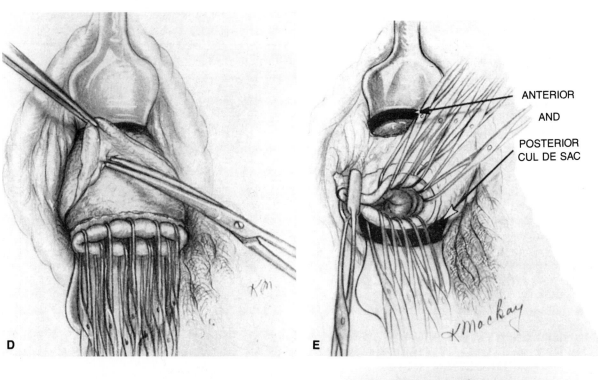

D

E

ANTERIOR

AND

POSTERIOR
CUL DE SAC

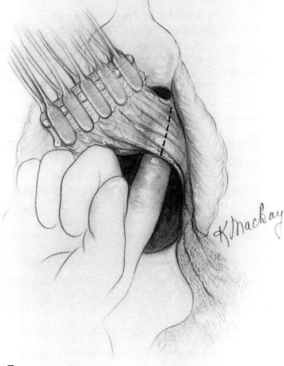

Figure 42–17. (continued) *D,* The bladder is dissected free of the cervix. *E,* The anterior and posterior cul-de-sac is entered. The vaginal cuff margins are clamped together below the cervix, using special broad clamps with double teeth. These clamps are used as tenaculae for traction. *F,* After the vaginal cuff is developed, the operation continues by clamping the paravaginal tissue close to the lateral vaginal wall.

F

total pelvic irradiation to patients unless microinvasive cervical cancer has been confirmed by cervical conization. Also, one must be aware of an increased morbidity with intracavitary irradiation application to a recently coned cervix. The cervix must be allowed to heal completely before intrauterine, intracervical, and contracervical irradiation is given. The survival rates for microinvasive disease should reach 98% to 99% if patients are adequately studied and properly treated.

Few studies of microinvasive adenocarcinoma of the cervix have been done; therefore, data on which to make recommendations for treatment of microinvasive adenocarcinoma do not exist. In most clinics early invasive adenocarcinoma of the cervix is managed as stage Ib disease. Teshima and coworkers studied 30 patients with microinvasive (5 mm or less) adenocarcinoma of the cervix. All patients were treated with extensive hysterectomy, and only one developed a recurrence. More information is needed about microinvasive adenocarcinoma of the cervix.

EXTENSIVE ABDOMINAL HYSTERECTOMY WITH PELVIC LYMPHADENECTOMY

Historical Points in the Development of Extensive Surgery for Cervical Cancer

Surgical removal of cervical cancer was suggested by Osiander and Wrisberg in the 18th century. In 1821 Sauter did a vaginal hysterectomy on a patient with a "six months bleeding tumor." This was a remarkable achievement, in that the patient survived the operation but died of intercurrent disease 4 months later, as reported by Zweifel. Little could be done for patients with this dreadful disease until basic discoveries had been made in medical and surgical therapy (eg, anesthesia). The primary surgical treatment of carcinoma of the cervix had its beginning in Europe more than 100 years ago when Freund (1878), in Germany, developed a technique for removal of the uterus in patients with cervical cancer. This operative procedure was not adequate for cervical cancer, and the operative mortality was 50%. A more extensive operation was proposed by Reis of Chicago, who, in 1895, demonstrated the technique of lymph gland removal at the autopsy table, although he apparently never performed lymphadenectomy with extensive hysterectomy. J. G. Clark, while still a resident trainee at the Johns Hopkins Hospital in 1895, performed extensive abdominal operations for cancer of the cervix. His operations did not include lymphadenectomy, but did include removal of the broad ligament to the lateral pelvic wall and removal of the upper vagina with the surgical specimen.

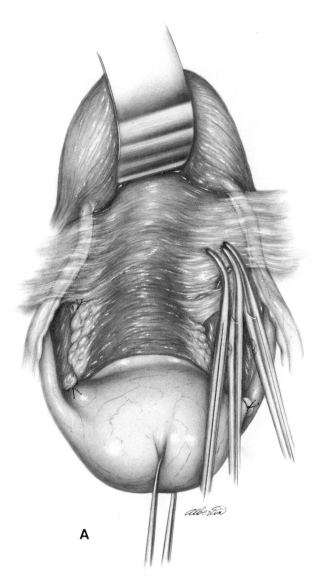

A

Figure 42–18. Modified Wertheim hysterectomy. *A,* Round ligaments and infundibulopelvic ligaments have been cut and ligated as in the usual hysterectomy. The broad ligament has been dissected widely by deep displacement of the bladder and terminal ureter. The right uterine vessels are clamped medial to the ureter, removing the medial one-third of the cardinal ligament with the uterus.

In the late 19th century (1898) Wertheim of Vienna performed his first radical extended abdominal hysterectomy and partial lymphadenectomy, and thereby began his monumental work of systematically investigating the surgical treatment of cervical cancer. His initial operative mortality was 30%. In 1911, when Wertheim reported his series of 500 cases, the operative mortality was reduced to 10%.

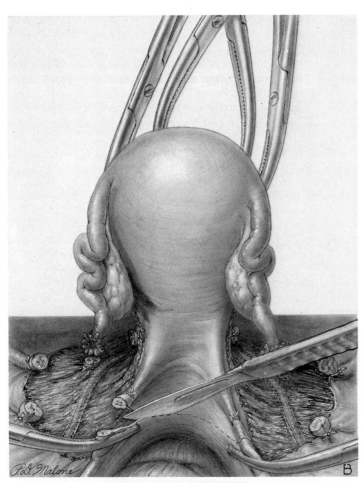

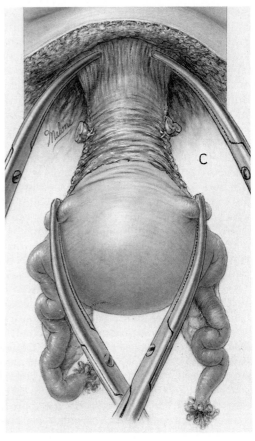

Figure 42–18. (continued) *B,* Uterosacral ligaments are clamped close to the rectum, and are being cut. The peritoneum between the two ligaments is cut as indicated by the dotted line. *C,* The bladder is dissected down from the pubocervical fascia, well below the tip of the cervix. The pubocervical fascia is not dissected from the cervix, and the vaginal wall is grasped on both sides with curved Ochsner clamps.

Because of the high mortality associated with the abdominal approach, Schauta, also of Vienna, developed an extensive vaginal operation in 1902. The surgical mortality was about 10% with a 5-year survival rate of 40%.

In the several decades that followed, the technique of the original Schauta operation was modified and further developed by Amreich, Navratil, Mitra, Van Bastiaanse, and others. The technique of Wertheim's original operation was modified and further extended by Wertheim's pupil, Werner, and by other outstanding pelvic surgeons in Europe. Latzko and Schiffmann offered important modifications to extend the abdominal approach. Okabayashi (Japan) described his radical abdominal hysterectomy in 1921, and this operation was

further developed by technically skilled Japanese surgeons to include a more extensive dissection of the parametrium. Competition developed between the abdominal (Wertheim) and vaginal (Schauta) approaches that has continued almost to the present.

Extensive pelvic surgery in the early 20th century by either the vaginal or the abdominal route before the advent of antibiotics and blood transfusions was accompanied by an unacceptably high surgical mortality in the hands of even the most skillful surgeons. Also, operability by either method was less than satisfactory. The original enthusiasm for surgery waned because of these problems and because of the discovery of radium by the Curies in Paris in 1898. In 1907 Klein irradiated carcinoma of the cervix. In the United States during the first half of the 20th century more attention was given to irradiation as the primary therapy in carcinoma of the cervix because of greater applicability, lower mortality rates, and good survival rates with irradiation treatment. Patients were treated with central radium applications according to the Paris, Stockholm, or Manchester technique, plus additional external pelvic irradiation with 200- or 400-kV x-ray machines. It was soon realized that the 5-year cure rate for all cases treated with irradiation therapy was only about 40%. As the dose of irradiation therapy was increased in an attempt to achieve a better cure, the rate of complications also increased. In 1949 Morton and Kerner reported complications in 90.5% of patients treated with irradiation therapy, including colitis, proctitis, bowel obstruction, and even death. Despite the popularity of irradiation therapy, fortunately interest in surgery as primary treatment for invasive cervical cancer had continued, mostly in Europe and by pupils of Wertheim and Schauta.

Victor Bonney (England) was another advocate of the Wertheim hysterectomy. In 1941 Bonney reported his series of 500 patients who received primary surgical treatment for invasive cervical cancer. The 5-year cure was 42%, comparable to cure rates achieved with irradiation therapy. The operative mortality, however, was 14%. Stallworthy, a disciple of Bonney, continued to use the Wertheim hysterectomy and pelvic lymphadenectomy. Although Stallworthy modified the approach with the use of preoperative central radium treatment, the extensive parametrial and lymph node dissection remained an integral part of his operative technique, with good results.

Full credit for the American renaissance of extensive pelvic surgery belongs to Joe V. Meigs. In the early 1930s Meigs, a surgeon from Boston, visited Vienna and was impressed with the logic of Wertheim's original operative procedure and the potential for surgical control of cervical cancer by this technique. Meigs returned to Boston and championed the Wertheim operation as primary treatment of cervical cancer. To the Wertheim operation he added a more extensive pelvic lymphadenectomy. The Wertheim-Meigs procedure resulted in an estimated increase in survival of 30%. The first report of his primary surgical treatment of invasive cervical cancer appeared in 1944 and included 344 cases. It set the stage for the subsequent use of this operative procedure by others. Many outstanding gynecologic surgeons in the United States (Parsons, Ulfelder, Green, Brunschwig, Barber, Morton, Pratt, Symmonds, Rutledge, Morley, Nelson, Averette, Shingleton, and many others) have made contributions and modifications in an attempt to decrease the incidence of urinary tract and other complications while preserving the necessity of extensive parametrial dissection and complete pelvic lymphadenectomy. Some gynecologic surgeons have extended the lymphadenectomy to include the paraaortic nodes. Despite obvious advances in the surgical treatment of cervical cancer, radiation has remained the mainstay of treatment for most patients. After all, advances and improvements in the technique of irradiation therapy also have been made, especially the availability of new megavoltage equipment. Admittedly, most patients who are cured with primary surgery also could be cured with irradiation. By and large, the gynecologic surgeon is privileged to treat the most favorable patients. In some clinics this may constitute as many as 50% of all patients referred with invasive cervical cancer, since, thankfully, a larger and larger percentage of patients are being diagnosed in the earliest stages of the disease.

Patient Selection for Extensive Hysterectomy*

Extensive hysterectomy and pelvic lymphadenectomy occasionally is used to treat patients with adenocarcinoma of the endometrium with involvement of the endocervical canal and also patients who have a small cervical cancer that persists or recurs in the cervix after primary irradiation therapy. In this chapter emphasis is given to the use of extensive abdominal hysterectomy and pelvic lymphadenectomy as primary treatment for invasive cervical cancer.

In most clinics throughout the United States most patients with stage Ib and stage IIa cervical cancer are offered extensive abdominal hysterectomy and bilateral pelvic lymphadenectomy as primary treatment. Patients with stage IIb invasive cervical cancer usually are excluded from primary treatment with surgery and treated instead with radiation therapy. Admittedly, it is somewhat difficult to be certain about extension of disease into the parametrium based on pelvic examination alone.

The clinical significance of parametrial involvement dates from the early studies of Kundrat and of Sampson. Kundrat, working in Wertheim's clinic, found in a careful study of more than 21,000 serial microscopic sections of the parametrium that in 44 of 80 patients, the parametrium of one or both sides was involved. In a similar study at the Johns Hopkins Hospital, Sampson pointed out that the parametrium may feel indurated and yet show no evidence of cancer. Also, the parametrium may feel normal and yet contain cancer. Sampson emphasized that only by the microscope can one ex-

---

*I have a preference for the word *extensive* rather than the word *radical* when referring to this operation. There are unfortunate and undesirable connotations in using the word radical that may be disturbing to the patient and to others. An operation that needs to be extensive to cure the disease is not a radical operation, in the sense of being an extreme measure, nor is it necessary that it be done by a radical surgeon.

clude cancer from the parametrium. More recently Inoue and Okumura found parametrial extension in 7% of stage Ib patients and only 34% of stage IIb patients. Burghardt and Pickel found true parametrial involvement in only 19% of stage IIb patients. Matsuyama and coworkers found no parametrial cancer in 58% of stage IIb patients. These studies were based on careful examination of microscopic sections, and emphasize again the difficulty of being certain about parametrial extension from pelvic examination alone. If there is reasonable suspicion of spread into the parametrial tissues by examination, CT scan, or MRI (stage IIb), we prefer to offer irradiation therapy as primary treatment, sometimes following initial laparotomy with selective pelvic lymphadenectomy for staging. When tumor has broken through the fibrous "capsule" within which it is contained in the cervix, the percentage of lymph nodes involved with metastatic disease more than doubles and rates of persistent disease after surgery, with or without postoperative radiation, increase. Inoue and Okumura studied 628 operative specimens from patients treated with radical hysterectomy and lymphadenectomy and found that parametrial extension is an important factor in the number of positive lymph nodes found and in patient survival.

We also are somewhat reluctant to treat patients with primary extensive surgery who have large bulky (more than 4 cm in diameter) endophytic tumors invading the cervix and lower uterine segment. Such patients are probably best treated with radiation therapy plus extrafascial hysterectomy, as suggested by Fletcher in 1979. Gallion and coworkers and others have reported good results with combined irradiation therapy and extrafascial hysterectomy in the treatment of stage Ib barrel-shaped cervical cancer. We occasionally have been successful in shrinking large predominantly exophytic cervical lesions with preoperative transvaginal irradiation, thus rendering such patients more acceptable candidates for extensive surgery. Six patients in our series at Emory University received planned preoperative, transvaginal irradiation in variable doses to control bleeding or to shrink large, bulky tumors. None of these patients had extensive disease in their surgical specimen and required no further irradiation therapy postoperatively. None of the patients in this small group has developed a recurrence. We have had no experience in using preoperative chemotherapy, as suggested by Kim and coworkers and by others, especially in patients with large lesions limited to the cervix, to reduce the size of the central tumor mass so that operability is facilitated and possibly survival improved. Preliminary results of these studies sound promising, however.

The major point to be emphasized is that the gynecologic surgeon should not attempt to treat a patient with a large cervical tumor with primary extensive surgery unless there is reasonable assurance that the operation will result in the complete removal of the central tumor with an adequate margin of tumor-free tissue around it. One should not operate on patients with the idea that irradiation can be used postoperatively to eliminate residual fragments of tumor tissue left behind after incomplete resection. Such patients are better treated with primary complete irradiation therapy from the beginning, possibly after staging laparotomy has been done.

Primary extensive surgical treatment is not contraindicated in any histologic type of cervical cancer. Indeed, there is some evidence that the survival of patients with stage I adenocarcinoma of the cervix is better with surgery than with irradiation, as suggested by Brand and coworkers. Patients with stage I adenosquamous cancer, clear cell cancer, and undifferentiated adenocarcinoma have a poorer prognosis, regardless of the method of treatment chosen, and should be considered for adjuvant irradiation therapy or chemotherapy after primary surgery. Experience in the management of 203 patients with gland cell carcinoma of the cervix at the University of Michigan Medical Center indicated no difference in survival according to histologic type, but considerable difference in survival according to degree of differentiation (well-differentiated 57%, poorly differentiated 29%). Another study from the same clinic compared the pattern of metastatic spread of squamous cell cancer and adenocarcinoma of the cervix as determined by autopsy findings of 21 patients with each tumor type. Patients dying of adenocarcinoma were found to have a higher incidence of tumor involvement of paraaortic nodes, uterine corpus, and adrenal glands. Ascites and hydrothorax also were significantly more common. The findings imply that adenocarcinoma of the cervix does behave differently in regard to pattern of metastatic spread and response to treatment, according to the authors.

Patients must be acceptable candidates for operation and free of serious medical problems that might contraindicate extensive surgery. In former years we limited extensive surgery as primary treatment to premenopausal women so that ovarian function might be conserved. As experience accumulated it was apparent that the operation also was well tolerated by older women, but patients older than age 70 usually are treated with radiation therapy. In 1988 Kinney and coworkers from the Mayo Clinic reported their experience with the Wertheim operation in a geriatric population. Thirty-eight selected patients between ages 65 and 89 (median age 69 years) were compared with 320 patients younger than age 65. The survival rates were almost identical in the two groups. Perioperative morbidity was minimally increased in the geriatric group. To achieve such excellent results in older women, the authors point out that "meticulous surgical technique, high quality ancillary services, and support from internal medicine and anesthesia services" are required. Such high-quality care is not available in every hospital.

Extreme obesity (especially morbid obesity) presents especially difficult technical problems when extensive surgery is chosen for primary treatment. Not only is the performance of the operation less satisfactory, but there is an increased risk of wound dehiscence and evisceration, postoperative infection, intraoperative hemorrhage, pulmonary embolus, pulmonary atelectasis, and anesthesia and other problems. Unfortunately, primary treatment with irradiation therapy also is less satisfactory in extremely obese patients. Quite honestly, the result of treatment for the extremely obese patient is likely to be poor, regardless of the method of treatment chosen.

In our experience, primary treatment with extensive surgery is, paradoxically, also riskier in very thin patients. The incidence of fistula formation is higher. Perhaps in his or her enthusiasm for curing the cancer and removing the usual adequate specimen from an operative field with superb exposure, the gynecologic surgeon may strip the ureters, the bladder, the rectum, and the major blood vessels too cleanly, thereby removing essential vasculature from essential tissues. Ischemic necrosis may result. A thin patient has less fat around the pelvic vessels and in the lymph fields; thus the gynecologic surgeon should be satisfied to remove less tissue in an operation that will still be adequate in a thin patient. Special care must be taken to leave vital circulation intact, especially around the ureters.

Pregnancy is not a contraindication to primary treatment of stage Ib or IIa carcinoma of the cervix with extensive surgery, as experience reported from our clinic indicates (Fig. 42-19). Extensive abdominal hysterectomy and pelvic lymphadenectomy was performed in 26 selected obstetric patients in the antepartum (22), intrapartum (1), and postpartum period (3) with no operative deaths, five major complications, and a good survival rate. A larger series was reported by Sall and and coworkers in 1974. Twenty-nine patients with stage Ib invasive carcinoma of the cervix in pregnancy were treated with extensive abdominal hysterectomy and pelvic lymphadenectomy. Twenty-eight patients were alive and well, and 23 patients had been followed for more than 5 years. There were no fistulas or major complications. In our experience, it is difficult to accurately judge the tolerance of pelvic tissue to radiation during or after a recent pregnancy. Fifty percent of our pregnant patients irradiated for stage Ib and IIa cancer of the cervix had major complications of treatment. On the other hand, extensive hysterectomy and pelvic lymphadenectomy are only slightly more difficult and associated with only slightly greater blood loss in pregnant patients.

In select obstetric patients desiring to maintain their pregnancy, Greer and coworkers also recommend a delay in delivery until fetal lung maturity can be definitively documented. We subscribe to the dictum that once invasive carcinoma of the cervix is diagnosed in a pregnant patient, a decision should be made to either go for the pregnancy or go for the cancer, and regardless of which way it is, one should go all the way. A

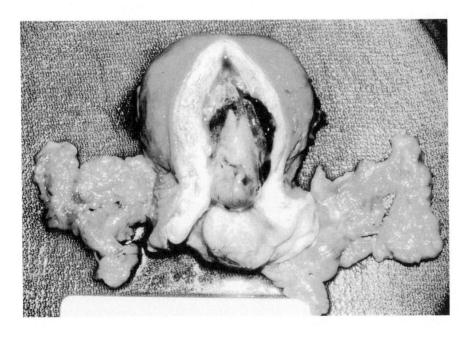

Figure 42–19. Squamous cell carcinoma, cervix uteri, FIGO stage Ib with intrauterine pregnancy, 16 weeks (lymphadenectomy specimen not included).

compromise could yield tragic results, possibly losing the mother because of delaying treatment for several weeks or months or losing the baby from premature delivery by cesarean section, or both. We have made an exception to this dictum only in some carefully selected patients with stage Ia carcinoma of the cervix. It should be emphasized that such an exception is made only if an adequate examination of an adequate cervical conization specimen shows only minimal microscopic stromal invasion limited to the superficial 3 mm of stroma beneath the surface. In such patients a planned delay in definitive treatment until delivery at term may be recommended without undue risk. Our experience with this carefully selected group of pregnant patients has been uniformly satisfactory. All other patients should either be treated promptly in an attempt to cure the cancer or be allowed to continue their pregnancy to term in an attempt to deliver by cesarean section a mature infant whose chance of survival is optimal. The patient makes the final decision whether to go for the cancer now or delay treatment and go for the baby with delivery at term. She will need to be carefully informed of the risks involved to make a proper choice.

Advantages of Extensive Surgery as Primary Treatment for Invasive Cervical Cancer

The most important considerations in choosing a method of therapy for any cancer are, first, effectiveness of the treatment in curing the disease and, second, mortality and morbidity rates associated with the treatment plan. For the indications listed previously the cure rates of primary radiotherapy and primary extensive surgery are about equal. The modern mortality rates also are about equal. Both modalities of therapy have a list of complications unique to each that seem about equal with the potential to be serious complications when they occur. There are, however, important major and minor advantages of primary extensive surgery over irradiation, some of which are discussed.

1. The findings at operation and from careful pathologic examination of the surgical specimen can be immensely helpful in selecting patients for adjuvant postoperation irradiation therapy or chemotherapy, or both. Most patients who are operated on will not need either, but some (about 20%) will.
2. The findings at operation and by careful pathologic examination of the surgical specimen can be helpful in prognosis and in identifying those patients who are at greatest risk for persistence of disease. Such high-risk patients may require spe-

cial diagnostic procedures and follow-up examinations at more frequent intervals.
3. When primary irradiation therapy is used to treat invasive cervical cancer in premenopausal women, premature loss of ovarian function is an unfortunate and inevitable result. When primary surgery is used instead the function of normal ovaries can be conserved. In 1981 Zander and coworkers reported that 53% of 1092 patients operated on for invasive cervical cancer had one or both ovaries conserved. As pointed out by McCall and coworkers, conservation of ovaries does not interfere with the completeness of an extensive operation. Ovarian function, including cyclic production of estrogen *and* progesterone, will continue until the usual age of the menopause in most patients, even when an extensive operation has been done, as indicated by Thompson and coworkers, Webb, and Ellsworth and coworkers. There is no evidence that continued ovarian function will interfere with the rate of cancer cure in such patients. The adnexal organs (the tube and ovary usually are conserved together so as not to interfere with ovarian blood supply) are an infrequent site of metastasis from primary carcinoma of the cervix, even in late stages of the disease, and rarely are involved in patients with stages I and II, as pointed out by Henriksen. And finally, the "residual adnexal syndrome" seems to be reasonably infrequent in patients who have had ovaries conserved at the time of extensive hysterectomy. Reoperation for pathologic conditions of the adnexa was necessary in 1 of 20 patients reported by Ellsworth and coworkers (peritoneal inclusion cyst adherent to an ovary), in 10 of 183 patients reported by Langley and coworkers (9 for "cystic degeneration" and 1 for ovarian carcinoma), and 2 of 61 patients in our series at Emory University (1 for benign cystic teratoma and 1 for benign cystadenoma of the ovary).

Podczaski and coworkers transposed ovaries into the paracolic gutters in 30 patients who had pretreatment laparotomy. Some patients experienced periodic cysts that could be felt by abdominal palpation. No patient required reexploration for a persistent mass, but four patients had vasomotor symptoms and elevated levels of gonadotropins after irradiation therapy. The technique used for ovarian transposition was described by Husseinzadeh and coworkers. In the series reported by Owens and coworkers 8 of 14 patients who had transposition of their ovaries at the time of extensive hysterectomy also received postoperative radiation therapy. Only one of these patients required estrogen replacement therapy for estrogen deficiency symptoms. There were no complications in the transposed ovary group. Chambers and coworkers found a threefold increase in symptomatic benign ovarian cyst formation with lateral ovarian transposition, but no additional surgery was necessary.

Mann has warned that the incidence of ovarian metastasis may be higher in women with adenocarcinoma of the cervix as compared with squamous cell carcinoma, and has advised that ovarian conservation is not indicated in these young women. Nahhas and coworkers reported ovarian metastases in a postmenopausal patient whose deeply invasive glassy cell carcinoma was treated with extensive surgery, including bilateral salpingo-oophorectomy. A glassy cell cancer is the most undifferentiated form of adenosquamous cancer with a greater risk for metastases and poor survival rates. Most patients with ovarian metastases from cervical adenocarcinoma also have metastases to pelvic lymph nodes, as reported by Tabata and coworkers. On the other hand, Berek and Brand report no ovarian metastases in more than 60 patients with adenocarcinoma of the cervix treated with extensive surgery. Greer and coworkers treated 55 patients with stage Ib adenocarcinoma of the cervix with radical hysterectomy and pelvic lymphadenectomy. Ninety-one percent had ovarian preservation, and there was no evidence that this contributed to tumor recurrence. Hopkins and coworkers found the best cumulative 5-year survival (93%) with cervical adenocarcinoma was in those patients treated by radical hysterectomy without bilateral salpingo-oophorectomy, and concluded that "ovarian conservation seems to be an acceptable alternative to bilateral salpingo-oophorectomy" in young patients.

The Gynecological Oncology Group studied ovarian metastases in stage Ib carcinoma of the cervix. Ovarian spread was found in 4 of 770 patients (0.5%) with squamous carcinoma and in 2 of 121 patients (1.7%) with adenocarcinoma. The difference was not statistically significant. All six patients with ovarian metastases had other evidence of extracervical disease. This study confirms that ovarian metastasis is rare in patients with stage Ib cervical cancer and extremely rare in the absence of other evidence of extracervical disease.

Although we have no hesitation about ovarian conservation in a young women with a small, well-differentiated adenocarcinoma limited to the cervix, there may be a reason for concern about spread to the ovaries in the presence of large or undifferentiated gland cell tumors or when positive pelvic lymph nodes or parametrial extension is found at operation.

All patients who are postmenopausal should have tubes and ovaries removed when extensive hysterectomy and pelvic lymphadenectomy are done for cervical cancer. But in premenopausal patients ovarian conservation has important health benefits, especially in protection against osteoporosis and heart disease and maintenance of healthy vaginal tissues (see Chapter 27). In addition, there is the important psychological benefit derived to the young patient who has just learned that she has cervical cancer when she also is told that it may be possible to conserve ovarian function. As gynecologic surgeons strive to eradicate cervical cancer with extensive surgery, they also should strive to modify their treatment so that as many as possible of those cured may live with bodies more nearly normal, as advised by Randall.

4. Studies of the effect of surgical and radiation treatment for cervical carcinoma on sexual function have been published by Seibel and coworkers from Emory University and by others. Among patients treated with irradiation, there is decrease in sexual enjoyment, ability to attain orgasm, frequency of intercourse, and desire for intercourse. Marked alterations can be seen and felt in the upper vagina and paravaginal tissues. The vagina usually is shorter from stenosis. The upper vagina is less pliable. Tissues are fixed and firm. The vaginal mucosa is thin, smooth, and dry with a tendency to split and bleed with slight trauma. Some of these changes are made more pronounced in young women because of hypoestrogenism from irradiation-induced premature menopause. They are not completely reversed by intravaginal or oral administration of estrogen. These functional and anatomic changes are not seen nearly as frequently in patients treated with primary extensive surgery. Even if the vagina has been shortened by several centimeters with primary surgery, it remains soft, pliable, healthy, and functional. Unfortunately, in those patients who must receive postoperative adjuvant pelvic irradiation some of this advantage is lost.

5. Primary surgical treatment allows, first and foremost, an accurate assessment of the extent of the cervical cancer. It also allows discovery of the other intra-abdominal incidental conditions and diseases entirely unrelated, which may or may not be important to the overall health of the patient. For example, in the last 100 patients in our series significant pelvic pathology in addition to primary disease was found in 4 patients (stage Ia cys-

tadenocarcinoma in 1 patient, early endometrial carcinoma in 2 patients, and pelvic tuberculosis in 1 patient). Any number of other patients are found to have sigmoid diverticulitis, cholelithiasis, and other conditions.

6. Late recurrences after treatment for cervical cancer are almost never seen after primary extensive surgery. They occur more often when patients are treated with primary irradiation therapy. The same can be said for complications of treatment. Because of the gradual and progressive obliterative endarteritis produced by radiating tissue, complications resulting from ischemic changes (eg, cystitis, proctitis, enteritis, colpocliesis, pyelonephritis) can be seen many years after the treatment was given. Late onset of complications after primary extensive surgery are unusual. These points are especially important when selecting a method of primary treatment for young patients.

7. There are probably important psychological benefits of primary treatment with extensive surgery compared with radiation. Most patients prefer to have the tumor removed and are especially encouraged when the surgeon can report that no evidence of metastatic disease was found at operation. Irradiation therapy carries an unfortunate connotation to some patients who feel that it is the treatment of last resort, that the treatments are actually "cooking" the tissues in the pelvis, or that irradiation can cause other cancers. All gynecologic surgeons have heard the disappointment patients express when they are told that they cannot be treated with an operation. Some patients continue to request an operation even after they have completed irradiation.

Justification for Pelvic Lymphadenectomy

For many years there was competition between gynecologic surgeons who advocated extensive vaginal hysterectomy without lymphadenectomy and those who advocated extensive abdominal hysterectomy with lymphadenectomy. The advocates of extensive vaginal hysterectomy without lymphadenectomy (the Schauta-Americh-Navratil operation) argued that their patients had fewer postoperative complications (especially urinary fistulas), a lower operative mortality rate, and a cure rate that was almost equal to that achieved by an abdominal operation that included lymphadenectomy. Furthermore, they pointed out that pelvic lymphadenectomy is an incomplete operation at best in that removal of all pelvic lymph nodes that may possibly be involved with metastatic tumor is technically impos-

sible. This is especially true of those inferior gluteal nodes that are located in the region of the ischial spine, as pointed out by Reiffenstuhl. It also has been known since Henriksen's work that involvement of paraaortic lymph nodes also may be present in a significant number of patients with metastasis to pelvic nodes, and paraaortic nodes cannot be completely removed and are not routinely sampled by gynecologic surgeons in abdominal operations for cervical cancer. Even Navratil, however, stated in 1965 that "indications for the Schauta operation must take the lymph node problem into account." Later he performed extraperitoneal pelvic lymphadenectomy with the Schauta operation in all cases of stage I and II that were locally advanced. So did Mitra.

In recent years the operative mortality and rate of complications in patients with extensive abdominal hysterectomy and bilateral pelvic lymphadenectomy have significantly decreased. Operative mortality and fistulas currently occur in only 1% of patients. Therefore, this disadvantage of lymphadenectomy has essentially been removed, and one can now concentrate on the question of whether or not lymphadenectomy adds anything to the possibility of cure.

It is the opinion of some that pelvic lymphadenectomy is of no value in those 80% to 90% of patients who have negative lymph nodes. We disagree with this view. We believe that lymphadenectomy is helpful in achieving an adequate central dissection around the cervical tumor, the most important part of the operation. This is especially true of that part of the lymphadenectomy that involves removal of tissue from around the hypogastric vessels, from the obturator fossa, and from the lower presacral region. Admittedly, dissection of lymph nodes from the common iliac vessels and from the paraaortic region does not add to the completeness of the central dissection. Removal of these and other nodes, however, is helpful in prognosis and in identifying those patients at greater risk for persistent disease who should receive adjuvant postoperative irradiation therapy to the pelvis and perhaps to extended fields along the aorta. Although we seldom dissect and remove the highest paraaortic lymph nodes, the lowest paraaortic nodes around and just above the aortic bifurcation may be removed. If pelvic lymph nodes involved with tumor are found during the operation, a concerted effort is made to do a more complete paraaortic dissection. Although it is possible for paraaortic nodes to be directly involved without involvement of pelvic nodes, this does not happen very often. For the group of patients who usually would be chosen for treatment with primary extensive surgery, routine paraaortic lymph node dissection would not result in therapeutic benefit very often. Podczaski and coworkers found positive paraaortic lymph nodes in 7 of 52 patients (13.4%) with stages Ib and IIa disease. Twenty-eight of the 52 patients, however, had bulky tumors greater than 5 cm in greatest diameter. Such patients are not considered by us to be appropriate candidates for treatment with primary extensive surgery. It is our estimate that few patients who are appropriate candidates for treatment with primary extensive surgery would benefit from routine paraaortic node dissection; therefore, it is not done routinely, but selectively in patients who appear to have positive pelvic nodes at operation. The paraaortic region should be carefully palpated and any enlarged or firm nodes removed, but the gynecologic surgeon should be aware of the added morbidity attendant on routine paraaortic lymphadenectomy.

A contrary view of the value of paraaortic lymphadenectomy has been expressed by Lovecchio and coworkers from the University of Miami. Three hundred forty patients with clinical stage Ib and stage IIa cervical cancer were explored for probable radical hysterectomy. A complete paraaortic lymphadenectomy in all patients showed histologically documented metastatic disease in 10.6% (36 patients). In all cases clinically suspicious pelvic lymph nodes were histologically positive for carcinoma. Irradiation therapy was extended to the paraaortic region with no increase in complications. The 5-year actuarial survival rate was 50%, with a median survival of 29 months. Cancer recurred in 80% of patients, two of whom remained clinically free of disease after chemotherapy. Thus paraaortic lymphadenectomy in 340 patients with early invasive cervical cancer benefitted 9 patients (2.6%). The authors believe that "these data demonstrate that survival may be favorably influenced by employing extended-field radiotherapy in those patients with early clinical stage cervical cancer and paraaortic nodal metastases."

If pelvic lymphadenectomy is not done in patients who have extensive hysterectomy for invasive cervical cancer, about 15% to 20% of patients with positive nodes will be inadequately treated for their disease (unless perhaps all patients received postoperative pelvic irradiation). In our judgment it is better to do pelvic lymphadenectomy in all patients and give postoperative irradiation selectively than to avoid lymphadenectomy and give postoperative irradiation to all patients.

In 1978 Tulzer and Kupka of the First University Women's Clinic in Vienna discussed the effectiveness of obligatory lymphadenectomy in treating carcinoma of the cervix. They reported a significant reduction in mortality from persistent disease when complete lymphadenectomy was made an obligatory part of extensive hysterectomy. When lymphadenectomy was selective (only suspicious nodes were removed) there was a 71% mortality rate in patients with positive nodes. When lymphadenectomy was made obligatory and complete the mortality rate in patients with positive nodes was reduced to 39%.

If one does extensive hysterectomy and bilateral pelvic lymphadenectomy in 100 patients with stages I and IIa cervical cancer, theoretically one might find positive nodes in 20 patients and negative nodes in 80. Of the 80 patients without positive nodes, maybe 74 (93%) will be cured. Of the 20 patients with positive nodes, about 12 (60%) will be cured by a combination of extensive hysterectomy and pelvic lymphadenectomy plus postoperative pelvic irradiation. In other words, pelvic lymphadenectomy is done in 100 patients to cure an additional 12 patients in this theoretical exercise. We believe that the risk of doing the lymphadenectomy in all patients is worth the benefit of additional cures. One must presume that all patients with untreated positive pelvic lymph nodes would eventually die of their disease.

A recent study from the University of Minnesota Hospital and clinics provides indirect evidence that postoperative pelvic irradiation is more effective in controlling disease after pelvic lymphadenectomy has removed lymph nodes that contain metastatic tumor. The amount of irradiation required to eliminate tumor in lymph nodes is directly related to the volume of tumor present (see Table 42-6). Thus removing the larger nodes involved with tumor increases the probability of control of tumor with irradiation. Despite a 44% rate of paraaortic metastases, patients in this study who underwent resection of large positive pelvic nodes followed by postoperative extended-field irradiation had a surprisingly high 5-year survival rate (51%) without evidence of persistent disease. The advantages of surgical debulking of positive lymph nodes also was discussed by Potish and coworkers in a later study from the same center. No patient with unresectable pelvic nodes was cured. Eighty-four percent (49/58) of grossly positive nodes could be debulked. The 5-year actuarial relapse-free survival rates were the same for patients with only microscopically involved pelvic node metastases (56%) and for patients with grossly involved but surgically resected pelvic node metatases (57%). All patients with positive pelvic nodes received postoperative irradiation to the pelvis and to paraaortic nodes. These authors believe that surgical debulking of grossly involved pelvic lymph nodes to microscopic residual disease may improve the chance of control with postoperative irradiation.

Adjuvant Therapy in Combination with Extensive Surgery

Experience has shown that a planned treatment program consisting of complete pelvic irradiation followed by extensive abdominal hysterectomy and pelvic lymphadenectomy yields a prohibitively high rate of complications, especially as regards fistulas and urinary tract difficulties. Such a combination has been abandoned in almost all clinics. Routine preoperative treatment with central radium followed by extensive surgery followed by selective external irradiation therapy is still used in some clinics. The good results of such a program in 612 patients with stage Ib cancer of the cervix treated at the Norwegian Radium Hospital were reported in 1983. The crude 5-year survival was 81%. The authors concluded that no significant increase in complications could be attributed to the use of preoperative intracavitary irradiation. Because there has been no clinical trial that conclusively proves that preoperative central radium treatments improve the cure rates (and results seem equally good without it), we have chosen to use it in only a few selected patients, as described above, to shrink large, bulky exophytic or bleeding cervical tumors.

Irradiation therapy is used in the postoperative period as an adjunct to extensive abdominal hysterectomy and bilateral pelvic lymphadenectomy. It is given selectively to patients considered to be at high risk for persistent disease based on operative findings and a careful study of the surgical specimen. If only one or two lymph nodes show micrometastases, postoperative irradiation may not be given. When several nodes are involved, the risk of persistent disease is greater. In such cases postoperative irradiation is given, and may be extended as high as T12 if proximal common iliac or paraaortic nodes are involved with metastatic disease.

In a retrospective study conducted at the University of Alabama at Birmingham, the University of Michigan, and the Mayo Clinic, reported by Alvarez and coworkers, 185 patients with previously untreated FIGO stage Ib and stage IIa squamous cell carcinoma of the cervix were found to have nodal metastases at the time of extensive hysterectomy and pelvic lymphadenectomy. Patients with small tumor dimensions (diameter less than 1 cm) and one or two involved nodes had an excellent prognosis (92% 10-year survival). The authors believe that adjuvant radiotherapy is not indicated in this group. Conversely, patients with large tumor dimensions (diameter more than 4 cm) and more than two involved nodes were at high risk for tumor recurrence and had compromised survival (13% 10-year survival). The authors state that this high-risk group warrants aggressive adjuvant treatment with systemic therapy in the presence or absence of pelvic radiotherapy. In another analysis of the same patients Kinney and coworkers found that the survival rates from irradiated patients matched with nonirradiated controls were not significantly different. Adjuvant radiotherapy did decrease the proportion of recurrences that occurred in the pelvis—27% compared with 67% in the surgery only group.

Justification for selectively using postoperative pelvic irradiation in high-risk patients is difficult to find. In 1989 Barter and coworkers reported on 50 patients who were treated with extensive hysterectomy and lymphadenectomy followed by postoperative irradiation therapy for high-risk factors (nodal metastases, lymph-vascular space invasion, close or involved margins) at the University of Alabama at Birmingham Medical Center. Thirty percent of patients had serious complications, some requiring reoperation, and one patient died as a result of the combined treatment. The overall 5-year survival for the group was 66%. These authors reviewed a list of studies that show no evidence that survival rates are improved by administering postoperative pelvic irradiation to patients at high risk for persistent disease (Rutledge and coworkers, 1965; Baltzer and coworkers, 1985; Zander and coworkers, 1981; Fuller and coworkers, 1982; Hogan and coworkers, 1982). Russell and coworkers reported on 37 patients who received combined therapy. Fourteen patients (38%) demonstrated persistent disease, ten of whom showed persistent tumor within the field of irradiation treatment. In a matched, controlled study Kinney and coworkers reported no survival benefit to adjuvant radiation therapy. According to Soisson and coworkers, adjuvant radiotherapy appeared to be well tolerated in their series of 72 patients who received it. Although there was no significant increase in serious complications, the extent to which local control rates and survival in high-risk patients were improved appeared to be limited.

In a collected series Morrow reported a 50% 5-year survival in patients with positive nodes treated with surgery alone and a 61.5% 5-year survival in patients treated with adjuvant irradiation therapy. The difference approached but did not attain statistical significance. In a more recent report from the University of Texas M. D. Anderson Hospital Larson and coworkers suggest that adjuvant postoperative radiotherapy may reduce pelvic recurrences and improve survival in patients with pelvic node metastases treated with extensive abdominal hysterectomy and lymphadenectomy. Five of 20 patients who received adjuvant radiotherapy had persistent disease, compared with 5 of 10 patients who did not receive radiotherapy. The irradiation therapy–treated group contained all the patients with four or more metastases. Postoperative irradiation therapy caused only one serious complication.

The morbidity and survival patterns in 50 patients after extensive hysterectomy and postoperative adjuvant pelvic radiotherapy was reported by Fiorica and coworkers. Ninety percent of patients were FIGO stage Ib and 10% were stage IIa or IIb. Indications for adjuvant radiotherapy included pelvic node metastasis, large tumor volume, deep stromal invasion, lower uterine segment involvement, or capillary space involvement. An average of 4700 cGy of whole-pelvic radiotherapy was administered. Ten percent of patients suffered major gastrointestinal complications and others experienced minor problems. Actuarial survival was 90% and disease-free survival 87% at 70 months. From this study it appears that postoperative adjuvant radiotherapy is advantageous in such a high-risk population.

In our modest series 15 patients had invasive lesions close to the margins of resection, or extensive involvement of lymphatic or vascular channels in the cervical stroma, or positive pelvic nodes, and were, therefore, treated with 4500 to 5800 rad from combined vaginal ovoids and whole-pelvis irradiation. Two patients died of persistent disease, but 13 patients are living without evidence of tumor. Most have been followed for 5 years. Irradiation therapy was well tolerated by all 15 patients. The only complaints were temporary diarrhea and gastroenteritis. One patient did develop a progressive hydronephrosis owing to ureteral stenosis beginning 6 months postoperatively. This patient had required complete pelvic irradiation after her surgical procedure because of extensive tumor in the cervix and positive pelvic nodes. She underwent a ureteroneocystotomy and lymphocyst removal.

Because of this favorable experience, we continue to give postoperative pelvic irradiation to patients at greater risk for persistent disease. As reported by Hatch, most gynecologic oncologists in the United States use adjuvant postoperative irradiation therapy in high-risk patients.

More and more often patients are selectively treated with extended-field irradiation to include the paraaortic lymph chain, especially in patients who have several positive pelvic nodes. To numerous previous studies can be added two recent studies from Japan that describe the results of paraaortic node irradiation in the treatment of cervical cancer. Inoue and Morita administered extended-field irradiation after extensive surgery to 76 patients with nodal metastases. The 5-year disease-free survival rates were 95% for 27 patients with one positive node, 64% for 37 patients with multiple positive nodes, and 44% for 12 patients with unresectable nodes. Two patients developed severe intestinal complications that required reoperation. Postoperative extended-field irradiation improved the survival of patients with four or more positive nodes from 39% to 69% as well as the survival of patients with unresectable nodes from 0% to 44%. The authors concluded that postoperative extended-field irradiation can control the distant spread by way of lymphatic routes and can increase the survival time of patients with nodal metastases from cervical carcinoma in stages Ib to IIb.

Eighty-six patients with cervical cancer were treated with paraaortic node irradiation by Horii and coworkers. None of the patients developed severe complications of the treatment, although this is certainly not the usual experience. Based on their selection criteria for paraaortic node irradiation, the authors found a statistically significant improvement in the prognosis for the treated group. If complications of paraaortic irradiation can be kept to a minimum by further refinements in technique, lymphadenectomy will be essential in the management of patients with cervical cancer.

In 1987 Jones reported a collected series of 332 patients with paraaortic lymph node metastases who received extended-field irradiation. Twenty-six percent were long-term survivors. Although it is true that the majority of patients with positive paraaortic lymph nodes will die of their disease (probably because systemic disease is already present), it also is clear that some patients are curable with extended-field irradiation, especially if the nodes are involved with only microscopic disease. One must anticipate a 10% incidence of enteric complications even with doses limited to 5000 rad. Again, micrometastatic disease is more likely to be eradicated by a dose of paraaortic irradiation that can be tolerated by the patient. Patients with paraaortic nodes that contain a large volume of tumor are not likely to be cured even with a dose of paraaortic irradiation that exceeds 5000 rad.

Few studies of adjuvant chemotherapy with extensive hysterectomy have been done. Kim and coworkers used vinblastine, bleomycin, and cisplatin before extensive hysterectomy in 35 patients. They found an 89% response rate in seven patients in whom all evidence of invasive cancer had disappeared. Lai and coworkers used the same chemotherapy combination to treat patients who were at high risk for recurrence after extensive hysterectomy. The 3-year disease-free survival rate was 75% for patients treated with adjuvant chemotherapy compared with 46.8% for those not treated.

Dottino and coworkers at Mount Sinai Medical Center in New York evaluated the therapeutic potential of cytotoxic therapy in 28 patients with squamous cell carcinoma of the cervix limited to the pelvis. Treatment consisted of preoperative cisplatin, mitomycin C, vincristine, and bleomycin induction chemotherapy followed by radical hysterectomy and pelvic and paraaortic lymphadenectomy in 26 patients and total pelvic exenteration in 2 patients. All patients achieved a clinical and histologic response to chemotherapy. There were 35% complete and 65% partial responses. Four patients were found to be histologically free of disease at the time of surgery. The induction chemotherapy was well tolerated. These authors believe that such treatment may be beneficial in the management of some patients with cervical cancer who are at high risk for failure with conventional treatment.

Preoperative Evaluation and Preparation

After the initial history and physical examination have indicated the possibility of primary treatment with extensive hysterectomy and pelvic lymphadenectomy, there are a number of additional tests and procedures that may be appropriate before the operation is actually performed. The list may include the following:

Medical evaluation and treatment
Anesthesia consultation
CT scan of chest, abdomen, and pelvis
Excretory urography
MRI of the abdomen and pelvis
Cystoscopy
Sigmoidoscopy or barium enema
Pelvic examination under anesthesia

Contrary to the frequent practice of doing all possible tests on every patient, it is my practice to be selective and to do only those tests and procedures that are expected to yield useful information. It is not necessary (and indeed may be inappropriate) to subject every patient to a long list of preoperative procedures that are expensive and exhausting and have little, if any, expectation of providing useful information. Indeed, it is most unfortunate when a test or procedure yields "questionable" or "suspicious" findings that require that the test be repeated over and over before a "negative" or "indeterminant" answer is finally given, when the test or procedure was not indicated or needed to begin with. A young, healthy patient with a small cervical lesion will need an admission history and physical examination, chest radiograph and routine laboratory studies, and anesthesia consultation on the day of admission. In the evening she receives a bath and vaginal douches with hexachlorophene and preparation for excretory urography. The excretory urography is done early the next morning, with the operation to begin shortly after it is completed. A careful pelvic examination is done as the initial step after anesthesia is induced. Cystoscopy and whatever shaving is necessary also may be done. Then the operation begins. If the patient is older, has medical complications, or has a larger or undifferentiated cervical lesion, the preoperative workup and preparation may be more involved and thorough. As much as possible should be done on an outpatient basis before admission to the hospital.

If the patient has a large or undifferentiated cervical cancer, CT studies of the chest may be more valuable than simple chest radiographs. CT scans may be used to look for enlarged paraaortic lymph nodes, which may need further study with fine needle aspiration. Matsukuma and coworkers evaluated the accuracy of abdominopelvic CT scans in the diagnosis of paraaortic and pelvic lymph node metastases from carcinoma of the cervix. CT scans were positive in 71.4% of patients with paraaortic lymph node metastases. In two patients the CT scan was falsely positive. These authors found the CT scan more useful in evaluating paraaortic than pelvic lymph nodes. Only a small number of metastatic

pelvic nodes were diagnosed by CT scan as enlarged nodes. Vercamer and coworkers studied CT and bipedal lymphangiography in 62 patients, and concluded that only limited information was added to the routine presurgical staging of patients with cancer of the cervix. Bandy and coworkers used CT for detecting metastatic tumor in the common iliac and paraaortic lymph nodes in 44 patients with cervical carcinoma. The sensitivity for detection of metastatic nodes was 75%, the specificity was 91%, the negative predictive value was 91%, and the positive predictive value was 75%. Fine needle aspiration of nodes 1.5 cm or greater in size detected 67% of metastatic nodes. Camilien and coworkers studied the preoperative abdominopelvic CT scans of 61 patients and compared the findings with gross and microscopic surgical findings. For paraaortic nodes the CT scan had a specificity of 100% and a sensitivity of 67%. Histologically positive pelvic nodes often were missed by CT scan. Parker and coworkers concluded that routine use of CT scan in patients with clinical stage Ib cervical carcinoma is not warranted unless the patient's body habitus precludes accurate physical examination. Our clinical experience would agree with these findings. Because CT scanning is a noninvasive procedure with no significant contraindications, it often is done as a part of the preoperative evaluation of stage Ib and IIa patients with larger or undifferentiated cervical tumors. If a double urinary collecting system can be ruled out by a combination of CT scan and cystoscopy (finding only one ureteral orifice on each side), then excretory urography may not be needed in the preoperative evaluation.

MRI can be helpful in the preoperative evaluation of patients with cervical cancer. Burghardt and coworkers have used MRI to determine exactly the *in vivo* measurements of the volume of the tumor in the cervix. The measurements of tumor volume correlated extremely well ($r = 0.983$) with those obtained by histomorphometric analysis of surgical specimens. On the contrary, the correlation with clinical examination was poor. The authors concluded that MRI in the future could provide a basis for more precise classification of cervical cancer than the current staging system based on clinical examination. It also might provide a more accurate means of predicting the likelihood of parametrial spread and metastatic tumor in pelvic and paraaortic nodes. It is to be expected in the future that further advances in imaging techniques will be able to provide additional useful information to the gynecologic surgeon in selecting the best primary treatment for patients with cervical cancer.

In 1979 Zaritsky and coworkers reported on their first use of transrectal ultrasonography in evaluation of cervical carcinoma. In 1990 Aoki and coworkers attempted to assess parametrial involvement by cervical cancer in 23 patients (46 parametria) using transrectal ultrasonography. They found transrectal ultrasonography significantly more sensitive than rectal examination in diagnosing parametrial extension. Transvaginal ultrasonography, well accepted for evaluation of other gynecologic diseases, is not suitable for assessment of the parametria. Sclerotic changes in parametrial vessels and parametritis may interfere with interpretation of findings. These authors suggest that a high level of expertise is necessary to accurately perform transrectal ultrasonography.

To evaluate the extent of a very early lesion, cervical conization occasionally is required. If simple extrafascial hysterectomy is subsequently chosen as the correct surgical treatment, the operation should be done within 48 hours of the conization or delayed until the cervix has healed, usually about 4 to 6 weeks later. If the hysterectomy is done after 48 hours and before the cervix has healed, the risk of serious postoperative infectious morbidity is increased. We have found, however, that an extensive abdominal hysterectomy and bilateral pelvic lymphadenectomy can be done at almost anytime after cervical conization, even before the cervix is completely healed, without increasing the risk of serious postoperative infectious morbidity. The reason for this difference is not clear but may be related to the fact that indurated and possibly infected paracervical and parametrial tissue is actually removed when an extensive hysterectomy is done. Whenever possible one should avoid doing diagnostic cervical conization in a patient with deeply invasive cervical cancer. Cervical conization is unavoidable in some patients to confirm a depth of invasion limited to the superficial 3 mm of cervical stroma, so that a more conservative extrafascial hysterectomy may be correctly chosen as adequate primary treatment.

Patients are asked to start a liquid diet 48 hours before surgery. Bowel preparation ordinarily required for intestinal resection usually is not needed for extensive abdominal hysterectomy. The usual preparation for excretory urography or CT scan (without oral contrast) usually is sufficient preoperative bowel preparation. An intestinal tube for suction also usually is not necessary.

Pertinent Pelvic Anatomy

Arterial and Venous Anatomy

Although the lower portions of the aorta and vena cava are frequently incorporated into the operative field of the pelvic lymphadenectomy, the major operative dissection includes the common iliac, external iliac, and hypogastric arteries and veins and their various branches and tributaries. The abdominal aorta emerges

through the aortic hiatus of the diaphragm at the lower border of the last thoracic vertebra and descends along the ventral surface of the vertebral column where it bifurcates into the left and right common iliac artery at the fourth lumbar vertebra (Fig. 42-20). This is an important anatomic landmark, as the bifurcation at L4 lies directly beneath the umbilicus in most cases. Therefore, an abdominal midline incision that would provide surgical exposure to the lower aorta would need to be extended somewhat above the umbilicus. As shown in Figure 42-20, the right common iliac artery crosses the upper portion of the left common iliac vein at the aortic bifurcation. This segment of the venous drainage of the left side of the pelvis joins with the right common iliac vein to form the vena cava, which lies directly along the right side of the aorta and on the right lateral side of the bodies of the lumbar vertebrae in its retroperitoneal course through the abdomen.

Both common iliac arteries continue along the medial border of the psoas muscle to the pelvic brim where they divide into external iliac and hypogastric vessels. As shown in Figure 42-20, this important vascular division marks the site where the ureters enter the pelvis from the abdomen, usually overlying the terminal end of the common iliac artery on the left and commonly crossing the actual bifurcation of the artery on the right. Both external iliac arteries pass beneath the inguinal ligament to proceed into the leg as the femoral artery. The external iliac artery makes no direct vascular contribution to the pelvis, although there is a fairly consistent arterial branch to the ureter from the midportion of the common iliac artery.

The external iliac vein emerges from beneath the inguinal ligament where it courses along the lateral pelvic brim on the medial side of the artery until it reaches the proximal segment. Here the vein passes directly beneath the artery at the bifurcation of the common iliac artery and then passes along the lateral side of the upper half of the artery. It then joins the left common iliac vein to become the inferior vena cava at the fifth lumbar vertebra. In dissecting the lymph nodes along the external iliac vessels, these anatomic landmarks are important to avoid trauma to the wall of the vein as it deviates from the medial to the lateral side of the arterial tree.

The hypogastric artery provides the major blood supply to the pelvic viscera. For descriptive purposes, it is conveniently divided into an anterior and a posterior division. The important branches of the hypogastric artery are shown in Figures 42-21 and 42-22 and are outlined in Table 42-8.

A fairly consistent arterial branch to the ureter arises from the hypogastric artery near the common iliac bifurcation. This vessel passes medially to the ureter, and should be preserved, if possible, during the dissec-

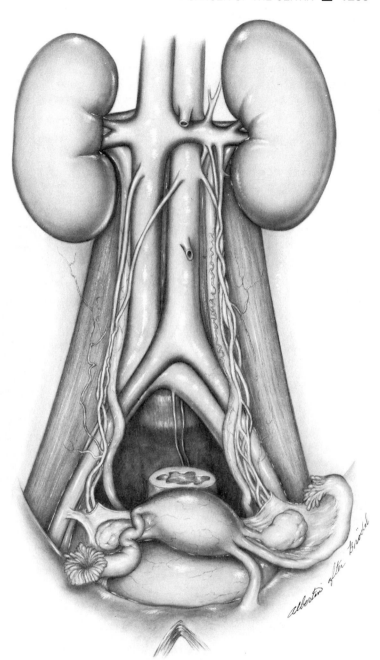

Figure 42–20. Abdominal and pelvic anatomy, showing the anatomic relations of the aorta, vena cava, iliac vessels, and ureters. Note the arterial-venous crossing of the right common iliac artery·and the left iliac vein.

tion of the hypogastric vessels. The hypogastric artery continues beneath the coccygeus muscle through the ischiorectal fossa, where it becomes the internal pudendal artery to supply the perineum and vulva.

It is important to understand that the major blood supply to the pelvic viscera is derived from the anterior division of the hypogastric artery. As shown in Figure 42-21, the anterior division gives off the uterine artery before continuing along the posterolateral pelvic wall

to give off the superior and inferior vesical branches to the bladder. The anterior division then continues as the obliterated umbilical artery as it passes cephalad along the inferior surface of the rectus muscle to the umbilicus. In dissecting along the hypogastric artery in a caudad direction the uterine artery is the first vessel that one encounters; it emanates from the medial side of the vessel. Passing more inferiorly and medially is the middle hemorrhoidal artery, which supplies a major

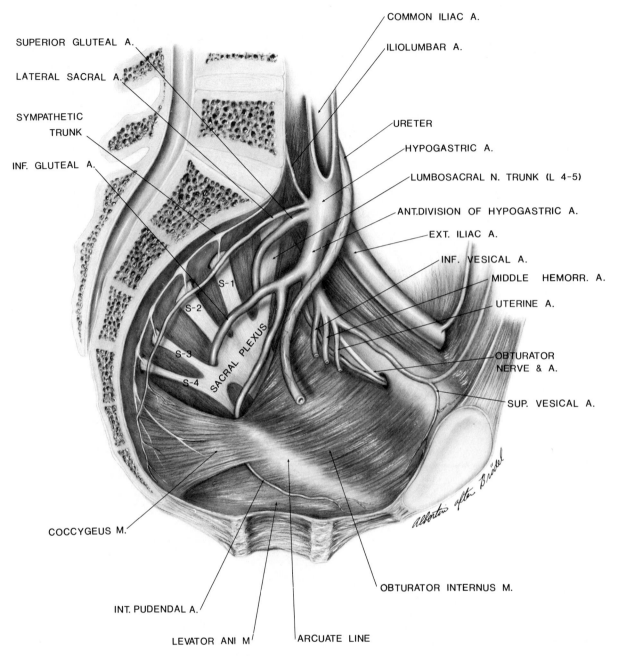

Figure 42–21. Anatomy of the arterial blood supply to the female pelvis showing relations of pelvic musculature, divisions of hypogastric artery, and lumbosacral and sacral nerve plexes. Note that the anterior division of the hypogastric artery provides the blood supply to the pelvic viscera.

segment of the rectum and communicates with the superior hemorrhoidal (from the inferior mesenteric) and the inferior hemorrhoidal (from the internal pudendal) arteries.

The hypogastric vein and its tributaries course along the pelvic floor and medial side of the artery to drain

the pelvis in close relation to the arterial blood supply. Its extensive anatomic variations and its location along the pelvic sidewall and floor place these tortuous, thin-walled veins in a precarious and vulnerable position for trauma during deep dissection of the pelvis. As shown in Figure 42-22, the delicate tributaries of the trunk of

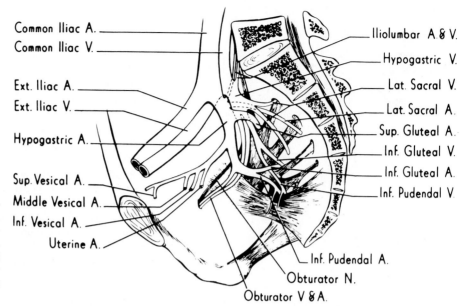

Common Iliac A.
Common Iliac V.
Ext. Iliac A.
Ext. Iliac V.
Hypogastric A.
Sup. Vesical A.
Middle Vesical A.
Inf. Vesical A.
Uterine A.

Iliolumbar A. & V.
Hypogastric V.
Lat. Sacral V.
Lat. Sacral A.
Sup. Gluteal A.
Inf. Gluteal V.
Inf. Gluteal A.
Inf. Pudendal V.
Inf. Pudendal A.
Obturator N.
Obturator V & A.

Figure 42–22. Anatomy of hypogastric vein. (Thompson JD. Extensive hysterectomy and bilateral pelvic lymphadenectomy. In: Coppleson M, ed. Gynecologic oncology. 2nd ed. Fig 4. New York: Churchill Livingstone. With permission.)

TABLE 42–8
Branches of the Hypogastric Artery

ANTERIOR DIVISION	POSTERIOR DIVISION
Visceral Branches	*Parietal Branches*
Uterine	Iliolumbar
Superior vesical	Lateral sacral
Middle vesical	Superior gluteal
Inferior vesical	
Middle hemorrhoidal	
Inferior hemorrhoidal	
Vaginal	
Parietal Branches	
Obturator	
Inferior gluteal	
Internal pudendal	

the hypogastric vein extend into sacral foramina and pass beneath nerve fibers and muscles within the pelvis such that their identity during the dissection of the pelvis frequently is obscured. The continuation of the hypogastric vein, in association with the artery, beneath the coccygeus muscle is a frequent site of bleeding when dissection is undertaken along the pelvic floor. When this occurs it is difficult to identify the vessel as it retracts beneath the margins of the muscle.

The profuse collateral blood supply to the ureter is an important anatomic safeguard that protects its pelvic segment from ischemic necrosis as a result of extensive hysterectomy. As shown in Figure 42-23, the ureter has the advantage of a multiple-source blood supply. This favorable collateral circulation permits interruption of small arteries and veins deep in the pelvis during extensive dissection of the base of the broad ligament without producing a significant incidence of ischemic necrosis and fistula formation. The freely anastomosing arterial and venous network that courses along the longitudinal surface of the ureter in its adventitial layer is supplied in its superior segment by branches from the renal and ovarian arteries. The middle segment of the ureter derives its blood supply directly from aortic branches and from a vessel from the common iliac artery. As the ureter enters the pelvis and courses along the lateral pelvic wall it receives arterial branches from the uterine, vaginal, middle hemorrhoidal, and vesical arteries. As it approaches the trigone of the bladder it has a rich arterial and venous collateral circulation from the arterial branches to the vagina and base of the bladder. Protection of this important vascular network is important for the integrity of the terminal ureter during extensive dissection of the cardinal ligament. Preservation of the lateral aspect of the posterior segment of the vesicouterine ligament has been recommended to ensure adequate vascularity to the terminal segment of the ureter, but we have encountered no difficulty in removing this tissue and have no hesitation in doing so to enhance the adequacy of the central dissection.

Lymphatic Anatomy

The lymphatic drainage of the pelvis follows the course of the arterial and venous blood supply. Although there are multiple variations in the lymphatic

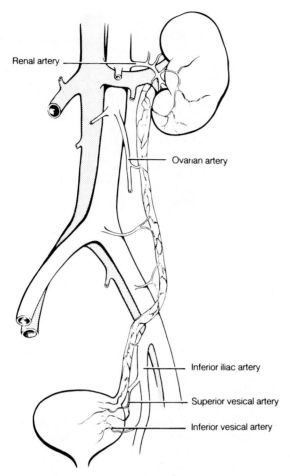

Figure 42–23. Blood supply of the ureter showing multiple source of collateral arterial circulation.

anatomy of the pelvis, in general there are lateral, superior, medial, and inferior lymph nodes and communicating lymphatic channels that surround the common iliac, external iliac, and hypogastric vessels. One of the important pathways of the pelvic nodes and thin-walled lymphatics that drain the upper vagina, cervix, and uterus courses along the posterior aspect of the endopelvic fascia. Here they pass through the uterosacral ligament area and terminate in lymph nodes along the lateral aspect of the sacrum. These nodes communicate freely with lymphatic channels from the bifurcation of the common iliac artery near the lateral sacral and ischiosacral fossae. These may be difficult nodes to resect, as they are closely attached to the thin-walled tributaries of the hypogastric vein. In dissecting the nodes from the bifurcation of the common iliac vessels care must be taken to avoid injury to the hypogastric vein, which extends from beneath the artery on the medial side in this area.

The most direct lymphatic drainage of the cervix and upper vagina is through the lateral parametrium (cardi-

nal ligament) to the hypogastric and obturator lymphatics. Because of the presence of obscure obturator veins and multiple venous tributaries from the hypogastric vein along the pelvic floor, the obturator dissection may be associated with troublesome venous bleeding. Injury also may occur to the obturator nerve, which arises from the anterior division of the second, third, and fourth lumbar nerves; enters the pelvis through the psoas muscle; and runs along the lateral pelvic wall in the obturator fossa to exit the pelvis through the obturator foramen along with the obturator vessels. It is a motor nerve to the adductor muscles of the thigh and the only motor nerve that arises from the lumbar plexus without innervating any of the pelvic structures. Damage to the obturator nerve produces not only motor impairment to the adductor muscles, but also sensory loss along the medial aspect of the thigh (Fig. 42-24). Deep dissection beneath the obturator nerve may be complicated by bleeding from the tributaries of the hypogastric and obturator veins. Many clinics omit this portion of the pelvic lymph node dissection along the floor of the obturator space to avoid this complication. It is our position, however, that such a conservative dissection provides a sanctuary for occult metastatic tumor and can give false assurance of the absence of tumor spread from the cervical cancer. It is on this point that gynecologic surgeons can be divided into two groups: those who do a rather timid removal of pelvic lymph nodes, taking counsel from Wertheim's own modifications to limit the procedure; and those who do an extensive lymphadenectomy, insisting that all removable pelvic nodes that are potential sites for tumor metastasis be removed.

Reiffenstuhl, in his classic study of the lymphatics of the female genital organs, describes efferent lymph channels from the cervix to the interiliac lymph nodes, to the lateral and medial external iliac lymph nodes, to the lateral and medial common iliac lymph nodes, to the sacral lymph nodes, to the subaortic lymph nodes, to the aortic lymph nodes, to the superior gluteal lymph nodes, to the inferior gluteal lymph nodes, and to the rectal lymph nodes. Of these, the inferior gluteal nodes are not technically possible to remove. This is because the nodes lie around the ischial spine in proximity to the inferior gluteal artery and pudendal artery and nerve. An imposing network of veins also surrounds the inferior gluteal nodes. They are thin-walled, easy to damage, difficult to expose, and difficult to control when damaged. Admittedly, this is a weak point in the performance of pelvic lymphadenectomy and in attempting to remove all nodes that represent a primary station to which cancer from the cervix may metastasize.

Reiffenstuhl's concepts of the lymphatic drainage of the cervix are partially shown in Figures 42-25 to 42-28.

(text continues on page 1211)

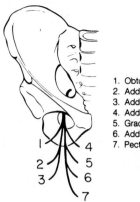
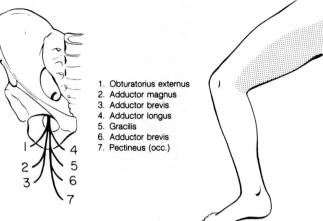

1. Obturatorius externus
2. Adductor magnus
3. Adductor brevis
4. Adductor longus
5. Gracilis
6. Adductor brevis
7. Pectineus (occ.)

Figure 42–24. Obturator nerve (L2-3-4): motor and sensory innervation.

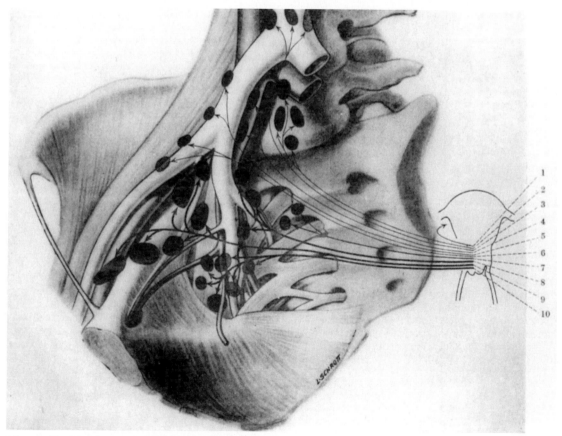

Figure 42–25. The regional lymph node stations of the uterine cervix. Channels 8, 9, and 10 (indicated by especially heavy lines) lead to those regional lymph node stations most frequently reached by the efferent lymph vessels of the cervix. Nonetheless, it is necessary to remember that carcinoma cells also can reach the pelvic lymph nodes by way of channels 1 to 7, without previous interruption. To (1) rectal, (2) sub-aortic (promontorial), (3) aortic, (4) medial common iliac, (5) lateral common iliac, (6) lateral external iliac, (7) sacral, (8) superior gluteal, (9) interiliac, and (10) inferior gluteal lymph nodes. (Reiffenstuhl G. The lymphatics of the female genital organs. Philadelphia: JB Lippincott, 1964.)

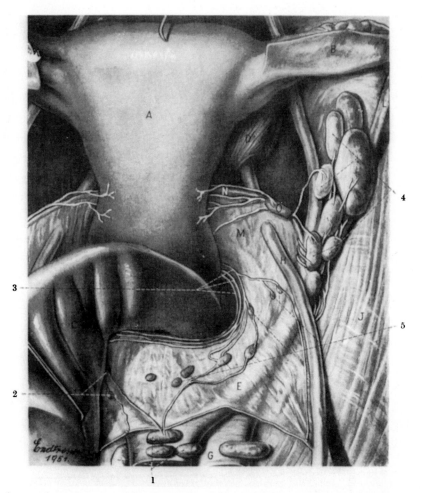

Figure 42–26. Lymphatic drainage of the cervix along the uterine artery and the sagittal rectal pillar (recto-uterine ligament). The uterus is drawn markedly upward. View of the posterior surface of the uterus (A). Several lymph vessels from the cervix twine about the uterine artery (N), pass the uterine-ureteral module (O), which is located on the right side of the specimen at the lateral edge of the ureter (H), and, after crossing over the lateral umbilical ligament (K), empty into the uppermost interiliac lymph nodes (4). A few lymph channels from the cervix (3) run dorsally at the base of Mackenrodt's ligament (M) in the sagittal rectal pillar and reach the superior rectal lymph nodes (2) that lie along the like-named artery on the posterior surface of the rectum. The lymph vessels in the ureteral leaf, coming from the cervix, first run dorsally in the sagittal rectal pillar for some distance and then, before reaching the rectum, turn upward to the nodes in the ureteral leaf (5). The ureteral leaf is a continuation of the sagittal rectal pillar cranially. The lymph channels then empty directly into the lowest aortic lymph nodes (1). One lymph vessel from the cervix runs upward on the medial edge of the right ureter (variant). (A) Uterus (intestinal surface); (B) right ovary; (C) rectum; (D) urinary bladder (posterior surface); (E) common iliac artery; (F) aorta; (G) inferior vena cava; (H) ureter; (j) psoas muscle; (K) lateral umbilical ligament; (L) external iliac artery; (M) Mackenrodt's ligament; (N) uterine artery; (O) lymph node. (1) Aortic lymph nodes; (2) rectal lymph nodes; (3) lymphatic vessels; (4) interiliac lymph nodes; (5) lymph nodes. (Reiffenstuhl G. The lymphatics of the female genital organs. Philadelphia: JB Lippincott, 1964.)

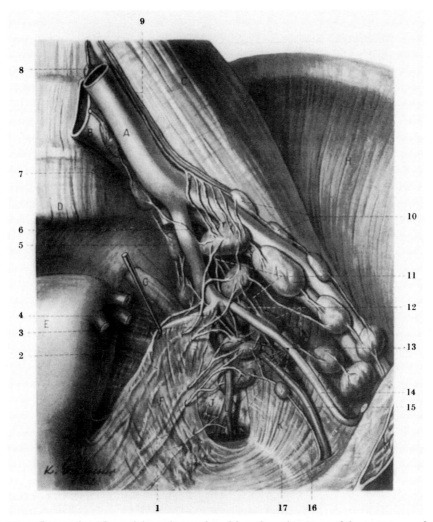

Figure 42–27. Inflow and outflow of the inferior gluteal lymph nodes. View of the anterior surface of Mackenrodt's ligament (F). The uterine artery is drawn upward by means of a hook. The lateral portion of the pelvic origin of Mackenrodt's ligament was removed to bring the deep nodes of the group on the sacral plexus (J) into view. Furthermore, the veins of the vesico-utero-vaginal plexus, which hide the nodes, were not drawn in. The lateral umbilical ligament (14) was left in place. Cervical lymphatic channels (1), which run to the pelvic wall in the basal portions of the parametrium and then empty into the inferior gluteal lymph nodes (13), predominate. These nodes extend along the inferior gluteal–internal pudendal artery down as far as the infrapiriform foramen and, in part, lie behind the parietal blood vessels. From the inferior gluteal lymph nodes (a) efferent vessels (3) run to the superior gluteal lymph nodes (5), (b) vessels turn as deep channels (4, then 11) to the posterior side of the parietal blood vessels, and (c) connections run to those interiliac lymph nodes on the obturator artery (12), which on their part, send their deep channels (11) upward to the deep lateral common iliac lymph nodes. From the uppermost interiliac lymph nodes lying in the hypogastric angle, 1 lymph channel (6) reaches the medial common iliac lymph nodes (7) by crossing over the stem of the internal iliac artery. Note also the numerous efferent vessels of the uppermost interiliac nodes that cross over the initial portion of the external iliac artery and then run upward on the lateral edge of the common iliac artery as a cable (9). (A) Common iliac artery; (B) common iliac vein; (C) psoas muscle; (D) promontory; (E) uterus; (F) Mackenrodt's ligament; (G) 1st sacral nerve; (H) iliac muscle; (J) sacral plexus; (K) internal obturator muscle; (L) internal pudendal-inferior gluteal artery; (M) internal oblique and transverse abdominal muscles. (1 & 2) Cervical lymph vessels; (3 & 4) efferent vessels; (5) superior gluteal lymph nodes; (6) efferent vessel; (7) medial common iliac and (8) deep lateral common iliac lymph nodes; (9) lymphatic vessels; (10) lateral external iliac lymph nodes; (11) efferent vessels; (12) interiliac (obturator) and (13) inferior gluteal efferent vessels; (12) interiliac (obturator) and (13) inferior gluteal lymph nodes; (14) lateral umbilical ligament; (15) obturator artery; (16) lymphatic vessel; (17) tendinous arch of the levator ani muscle. (Reiffenstuhl G. The lymphatics of the female genital organs. Philadelphia: JB Lippincott, 1964.)

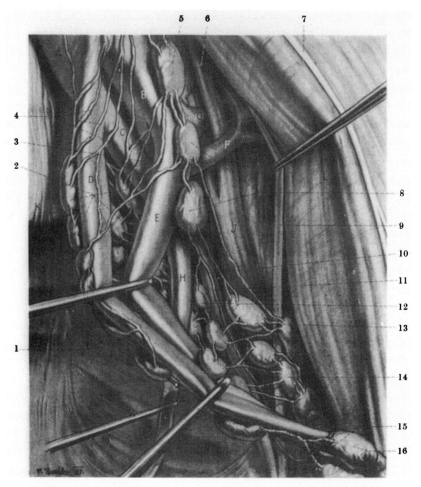

Figure 42–28. View into the niche between the psoas muscle and the external iliac vessels, down to the femoral ring. The blood vessels (C, D, E, H) were drawn medially by a hook (view of their posterior side!), and the psoas muscle (L) with the obturator nerve (9) was forced laterally. The lumbosacral trunk (J) appears at the bottom of the niche. The efferent channels of the uppermost interiliac lymph nodes climb over (4) the outer edge of the external and the common iliac arteries and reach the deep lateral common iliac lymph nodes (see Fig. 45). However, the deep efferent channels (3) of the uppermost interiliac lymph nodes also open into the deep nodes located on the posterior side of the parietal blood vessels, after crossing under the internal iliac artery (C). The nodes (12) lying at the cranial edge of the obturator artery (13) and the nodes (14) of this group (interiliac lymph nodes) found laterally to the obturator nerve (9) send efferent vessels to the deep lateral external iliac lymph nodes (8). From the great nodes on the femoral ring (16) two primary lymphatic paths lead upward. One path (15) runs along the outer edge of the external iliac artery, where several superficial lateral external iliac lymph nodes (1) are located. The other, in the form of numerous lymph nodes (14, 12), which in part lie lateral and in part medial to the obturator nerve, and their connecting lymph vessels lead upward. (A) Common iliac artery; (B) common iliac vein; (C) internal iliac artery (posterior aspect); (D) external iliac artery (posterior aspect); (E) external iliac vein (posterior aspect); (F) iliolumbar artery; (G) iliolumbar vein; (H) lateral umbilical ligament; (J) lumbosacral trunk; (K) promontory; (L) psoas muscle. (1) Lateral external iliac and (2) interiliac lymph nodes; (3) deep efferent vessels; (4) efferent vessels; (5) deep lateral common iliac lymph node; (6) half of 4th lumbar nerve; (7) genitofemoral nerve; (8) deep lateral external iliac lymph nodes; (9) obturator nerve; (10 & 11) efferent vessels; (12) interiliac lymph nodes; (13) obturator artery; (14) interiliac lymph nodes; (15) efferent vessels; (16) femoral ring lymph nodes. (Reiffenstuhl G. The lymphatics of the female genital organs. Philadelphia: JB Lippincott, 1964.)

Concept of Extensive Abdominal Hysterectomy and Bilateral Pelvic Lymphadenectomy

Various modifications of the extensive hysterectomy and pelvic node dissection are practiced at the M. D. Anderson Hospital in Houston, where five classes of extended hysterectomy are used for the treatment of cervical cancer. The class I hysterectomy is a slight extension of the total hysterectomy with removal of a small amount of parametrium. It is primarily used for microinvasive carcinoma and for removal of the uterus with a barrel-shaped endocervical adenocarcinoma after preoperative irradiation. The class II extended hysterectomy (Te Linde–modified Wertheim) removes a more generous parametrial cuff, ligates the uterine artery on the medial side of the ureter, but does not dissect the ureter from the vesicouterine ligament. The class III operation is the classic Meigs' procedure, with removal of all of the parametrium and paravaginal tissue in addition to some of the pelvic lymph nodes. A more extensive procedure is performed in the class IV radical hysterectomy, whereby the ureter is completely dissected from the cardinal and vesicouterine ligaments; the superior vesical artery is sacrificed and three-fourths of the vagina is removed as well as the uterus and parametria, along with a complete lymphadenectomy. A far more extensive procedure is done with the class V radical hysterectomy, whereby the terminal ureter or a segment of the bladder or rectum is removed along with the uterus, parametria, adnexa, and pelvic lymph nodes.

Although many techniques emphasize a more or less extensive dissection in one phase of the operation or another, the management of the parametria and the dissection of the pelvic lymph nodes appear relatively uniform. Because the most serious complication of this procedure is related to ureteral fistulas and stenosis, many modifications have been undertaken in recent years to assure an adequate blood supply to the terminal ureter. We agree that the terminal ureter must have a good blood supply, and believe that this can be accomplished without jeopardizing the adequacy of the central dissection. The classic extensive hysterectomy with wide resection of the parametrium, dissection of the terminal ureter from the vesicouterine ligament, and wide resection of the uterosacral ligaments, upper 2 to 3 cm of vagina, and paravaginal tissues, along with a thorough pelvic lymphadenectomy, constitutes the traditional procedure that is used in this clinic.

The major focus of the operation is the adequacy of the central dissection. The central cervical tumor must be removed with an adequate margin of uninvolved normal tissue around it. This is the most crucial point in the success of the operation and has been emphasized

by many of the famous pelvic surgeons of former years, especially Parsons and Navratil. The central dissection can be facilitated by developing the pelvic spaces and utilizing proper planes for dissection. Correct dissection along natural rather than artificial connective tissue planes, and correct development of the pelvic spaces (paravesical, pararectal, vesicocervical, and rectovaginal) avoid unnecessary injury to pelvic vessels, keep blood loss to a minimum, and facilitate an adequate central dissection (see Fig. 42-29). These connective tissue planes and pelvic spaces are beautifully described by Reiffenstuhl. The central dissection also is facilitated by a complete removal of the contents of the obturator fossa (except the obturator nerve), so that branches of the hypogastric artery and vein in the cardinal ligament are clearly visible and can be dissected away from their attachment to the lateral pelvic sidewall.

The importance of an adequate central dissection also was emphasized by Girardi and coworkers. By studying surgical specimens processed according to the giant section technique of Burghardt and Pickel, parametrial lymph nodes were found in 280 (78%) of the 359 surgical specimens from extensive hysterectomies. Metastatically involved parametrial nodes were found in 63 (22.5%) of these 280. The lymphatic drainage from the cervix to the pelvic lymph nodes runs through the parametrium, and deposits of tumor often are found there. An adequate central dissection must include removal of a wide margin of parametrial tissue around the central tumor and total removal of the parametria from the bladder, the rectum, and the lateral pelvic wall, since positive lymph nodes can be found in the lateral as well as medial parametrium.

When a large vaginal cuff must be removed because of a bulky cervical tumor or involvement of adjacent vaginal mucosa, starting the operation from below will facilitate the central dissection. Sometimes a bulky lesion is excised and fulgurated transvaginally. The formation of the vaginal cuff is done in a manner similar to that in the Schauta-Amreich procedure. The vaginal incision is made around the entire circumference of the vagina, mobilizing the vaginal cuff from paravaginal tissue. Further dissection into the paravesical space, vesicocervical space, and rectovaginal space from below may be easier than from above.

Above the mid-common iliac arteries and in the para-aortic region lymph nodes are sampled and a special effort is made to remove any nodes that look or feel suspicious. A serious effort is made to do a complete lymphadenectomy below the level of the mid-common iliac artery; this includes the tissue around the major vessels down to the inguinal ligament. Special attention is given to removal of lymph nodes that are located between the lower common iliac vessels and the psoas muscle (lateral common iliac nodes) at the point where the obturator nerve enters the obturator fossa through the belly of the psoas muscle. Complete removal of these nodes will expose the roots of the lumbosacral nerve plexus. The obturator nerve is dissected free from its entrance into the superior obturator fossa through the psoas muscle to its exit through the obturator foramen inferiorly. The anterior division of the hypogastric artery is routinely ligated at a point just distal to the origin of the posterior trunk. According to Roberts and coworkers, it cannot be proved that ligation of the anterior division of the hypogastric artery increases the risks of urinary tract fistulas. We agree with this. The dissection leaves the hypogastric vein and its branches exposed and intact. The various vessels that compose the cardinal ligament are individually clipped or ligated at the lateral pelvic sidewall, and an attempt is made to remove as much of the cardinal ligament as possible. No attempt is made to do an *en bloc* removal of the nodes. Suspicious nodes may be sent for frozen section, and various parts of the specimen are marked for identification. The ureters are left intact until the lymphadenectomy is completed. The surgeon is cognizant of the closeness of the dissection to the central tumor throughout the remainder of the operation. The plane of dissection usually comes closest to the cervix in development of the vesicocervical space. The ureter is freed from its passage through the "tunnel," and the anterior and posterior parts of the vesicouterine ligament are ligated as close to the bladder as possible without injury. The periureteral sheath is carefully preserved, but the ureter usually is completely detached for a distance of 4 to 5 cm above its entrance into the bladder wall. The development of the posterior rectovaginal space allows identification of the posterior parametrium, including the uterosacral ligaments. This tissue is clamped and dissected away as close to the rectum as possible. The only remaining tissue to be clamped and removed is paravaginal, after which the specimen is removed by an incision in the vaginal wall at an appropriate distance from the cervix. Several biopsies are taken from the margin of the vaginal apex left remaining to be certain that the inferior margin of the dissection below the tumor is uninvolved.

Two approaches to performing an extensive abdominal hysterectomy and bilateral pelvic lymphadenectomy are described. The traditional transperitoneal approach has been used in our clinic for many years with satisfactory results. The transverse Maylard incision is preferred for this approach, but lower midline incisions also have been used in selected patients. In recent years, encouraged by the previous experience of doing extraperitoneal lymphadenectomies after the Schauta-Amreich extensive vaginal hysterectomy and by the experience of Breen and others, our preferred technique is to first perform the bilateral pelvic lymphadenectomy extraperitoneally through an elliptical transverse Maylard incision across the lower abdominal wall that is extended upward and laterally to the level of the anterior superior iliac spine or above if necessary. Exposure of the pelvic sidewall is superb, and removal of lower paraaortic lymph nodes can be accomplished with proper retraction. Reflection of the intact peritoneum away from the pelvic sidewalls greatly assists in retraction of the bowel with less trauma to the serosa. Unnecessary and prolonged exposure of intraperitoneal organs is avoided during the time it takes to perform the extraperitoneal lymphadenectomy. It is our impression that intestinal function returns more promptly in the postoperative recovery period. There also may be fewer intestinal problems when postoperative irradiation is necessary.

There are a few disadvantages of this approach related to the fact that exploration of the abdomen and pelvis, ordinarily done first, is delayed. The transperitoneal central dissection is delayed until the extraperitoneal lymphadenectomy is completed, and is the last stage of the operation. Theoretically, there could be findings from exploration that might alter the treatment plan, but we have thus far not encountered a situation in which we regretted having done the bilateral extraperitoneal lymphadenectomy before exploring the abdomen and pelvis transperitoneally.

In a study of 284 patients from Gynecologic Oncology Group institutions a comparison of extraperitoneal and transperitoneal selective paraaortic lymphadenectomy was made. Although the difference in the two approaches was not great, the authors concluded that selective paraaortic lymphadenectomy should be performed by the extraperitoneal approach rather than the transperitoneal approach to minimize certain postirradiation enteric complications. Gallup and coworkers have favored extraperitoneal pelvic lymphadenectomy for preradiation surgical staging and also extensive hysterectomy, although their preference is for a midline incision. Extraperitoneal pelvic lymphadenectomy has been done for many years in patients with advanced vulvar cancer, for urologically related cancers, and after the Schauta-Amreich extensive vaginal hysterectomy for cervical cancer. It is a familiar technique to most gynecologic surgeons.

We currently use the combined extraperitoneal-transperitoneal extensive hysterectomy and pelvic lymphadenectomy technique for all patients selected for primary surgical treatment with few exceptions. If, in addition to cancer of the cervix, there exists a large pelvic tumor (eg, leiomyomata uteri, ovarian cysts, intrauterine pregnancy), the removal of which will improve exposure, then the entire operation is done through a transperitoneal approach using the extended Maylard incision. If there is good reason to suspect paraaortic node metastases or other significant upper abdominal or intraperitoneal disease, the entire operation is done through a transperitoneal approach. Otherwise, we believe that there is an advantage to performing the bilateral lymphadenectomy extraperitoneally and the extensive hysterectomy transperitoneally through the same extended transverse Maylard incision.

Teamwork is needed to do the operation correctly, and no member of the team is more important than the anesthesiologist. With prior planning and cooperation between the surgeon and the anesthesiologist, a safe and effective technique of anesthesia can be chosen that will not only provide pain relief and relaxation, but also deliberately induce hypotension and reduce circulation to the operative field. A reduction in arteriolar resistance will lower blood pressure and reduce, to a certain degree, bleeding in the operative field. The main mechanism for control of operative field bleeding by anesthesia, however, lies in reduction of venous tone, which reduces ventricular filling and cardiac output, the major determinant of blood pressure. The desired reduction in venous tone is achieved by one or more of the following anesthetic techniques: ganglionic blockage; spinal or epidural anesthesia; specific venodilating agents, such as sodium nitroprusside or glyceryl trinitrate; and the effect of some anesthetic agents. The use of induced hypotension is more effective if the operative field is raised above the level of the heart to encourage local venous emptying by gravity. Therefore, a modest Trendelenburg position should be used.

Deliberate hypotension is now an established practice, although some anesthesiologists are more enthusiastic about its use than others, and all must be trained in the technique to use it safely. Our experience with its use in extensive pelvic dissections for malignant disease has been uniformly favorable. The blood loss in extensive hysterectomy can be reduced by 50% and more, and the need for blood replacement reduced by a corresponding amount. In a report by Powell and coworkers a deliberate hypotensive anesthetic technique utilizing nitroglycerin and general anesthesia decreased the blood loss in extensive abdominal hysterectomy with pelvic lymphadenectomy by 70% when compared with a control group. The percentage of patients who required blood transfusion was reduced from 81% to 11.5%. Favorable experience with induced hypotensive anesthetic techniques to reduce blood loss during extensive hysterectomy and pelvic lymphadenectomy also was reported by Bithal and coworkers and Wong and coworkers. Eisenkop and coworkers suggest that among patients who undergo extensive hysterectomy and retroperitoneal lymphadenectomy with clear surgical margins, negative lymph nodes, and no lymph–vascular space involve-

ment, blood transfusion appears to be an independent variable predictive of earlier recurrence and diminished survival possibly because transfusion is immunosuppressive.

Unnecessary bleeding in the area of dissection stains tissues, obscures visibility, restricts technical freedom, increases the possibility of unnecessary injury to other structures, and gradually adds up to a significant amount of blood loss that may require replacement. We have no doubt that deliberate hypotension is a valuable technique, but it cannot substitute for a lack of technical skill or careful surgical hemostasis. Reactionary hemorrhage, bleeding after blood pressure returns to normal, occurs until hemostasis is meticulous.

After anesthesia is induced the patient is placed comfortably in Allen Universal stirrups with the buttocks brought to the edge of the "broken" table. The knees are separated about 90 degrees. The thighs are elevated only 15 to 20 degrees relative to the abdomen. Care is taken to avoid pressure on the peroneal nerves in the legs. This position has several advantages. There is less strain on the patient's lumbosacral spine when the thighs are slightly flexed. This is especially important for patients with lumbosacral back problems. It is possible to have a second assistant stand at the foot of the table between the patient's legs. His or her participation in the operation is greatly facilitated by being closer to the operative field. Lastly, in this position the urethral orifice, vaginal introitus, and anal orifice are all available for instrumentation in case this is necessary to clarify anatomy.

After the patient is positioned on the operating table the bladder is emptied with a catheter and a careful rectovaginal-abdominal pelvic examination is done. This may be followed by cystoscopy or sigmoidoscopy if desired. It may be necessary to shave a small amount of the escutcheon, but vulvar hair is not shaved completely. The skin is prepared from the rib margin to the midthigh, with special attention given to the umbilicus, perineum, and vagina. The patient is draped, a transurethral Foley catheter is inserted into the bladder, and the operation begins.

When operating abdominally the exposure achieved depends on the choice of incision, the method of retracting, the placement and intensity of overhead lights, and the participation of willing and skillful assistants. Suction should be available to keep the field as dry as possible and is preferred over sponges for two reasons. First, sponges are more traumatic to delicate serosal surfaces and other tissues. And second, a determination of the amount of blood lost can be more accurate if the largest percentage has been suctioned from the operative field into a calibrated bottle and measured. Unfortunately, patients undergoing extensive hysterectomy and lymphadenectomy are not considered appropriate candidates for intraoperative autologous transfusion unless the need is desperate.

It usually is possible (and always desirable) to keep the number of clamps in the operative field to an absolute minimum. If the field is cluttered with clamps, the operator cannot see as well to operate. There is an unfortunate tendency for gynecologic surgeons to use instruments that are too short. Pedicle clamps, tissue forceps, dissecting scissors, needle holders, and all other instruments must be longer when operating deep in the pelvis and when operating on obese patients. The handles of the instruments must come all the way out and above the level of the incision, so as not to interfere with the operator's vision.

After the incision is made the lymphadenectomy is done first. The surgeon usually stands on the patient's right side to dissect the left pelvic sidewall. He or she usually changes positions several times during the course of the operation. One should chose to dissect the side of the pelvis first that corresponds to the side of the cervix with the greatest tumor involvement.

Surgical Technique of Transperitoneal Approach

Evaluation at Laparotomy

The operation is initiated through an extended Maylard or low midline incision. In most cases the umbilicus identifies the location of the bifurcation of the aorta; therefore, extension of the incision about 2 to 3 cm above the umbilicus is recommended for adequate exposure if a lower midline incision is used. The midline incision is protected by a moist pack beneath each arm of the self-retaining retractor to avoid excessive compression of the epigastric vessels that course beneath the rectus muscles. In case of a lengthy operative procedure the mechanical retractors are released at periodic intervals to improve circulation through the abdominal musculature. The bladder is decompressed by an indwelling catheter throughout the procedure to facilitate exposure and to maintain an accurate record of urine output.

Before initiating the pelvic procedure the abdominal viscera and parietal peritoneum of the abdominal cavity are evaluated meticulously for possible evidence of metastatic tumor. The superior and inferior surfaces of the liver are carefully palpated, as well as the region of the coeliac plexus. The undersurface of the diaphragm is particularly vulnerable for metastases, especially the right hemidiaphragm, where the paraaortic lymphatics pass from the abdominal cavity into the mediastinum. The mesentery of the large and small bowel and the serosal surface of the bowel along with the omentum should be carefully examined for evidence of metastatic tumor. The kidneys are examined and the retroperitoneal space along the aorta and vena cava is palpated assiduously, as these are the major sites of extrapelvic spread of cervical cancer. It is well known that 15% or more of paraaortic node metastases are occult; therefore, even the most unsuspecting node should be removed and evaluated histologically by frozen section study for possible metastatic tumor. It is our practice, therefore, to sample any paracaval or paraaortic node that is identifiable before initiating the procedure. If there should be histopathologic evidence of unsuspected, metastatic tumor in a paraaortic lymph node, the operation is abandoned and the disease usually is considered technically inoperable. In such cases the patient usually is treated with full pelvic and paraaortic irradiation. Only if one believes that removing gross disease enhances the effectiveness of pelvic and aortic radiation, and is willing to use aggressive chemotherapy for the likely probability of already existing systemic disease, can full extensive hysterectomy and lymphadenectomy be justified in technically operable cases.

Although considered unnecessary by some, we take peritoneal washings routinely for cytologic examination. The significance of a positive result may be difficult to determine.

At this point in the procedure any adhesions in the pelvis are lysed and the intestines are placed in the upper abdomen and held there with packs. A suitable self-retaining retractor may be used. If Bookwalter, Turner-Warwick, or Balfour retractors are used in a lower midline incision, care must be taken to avoid compression of the femoral nerves by the lateral blades. Lateral blades are not necessary with a transverse incision.

Evaluation of the extent of the pelvic tumor is carried out at this time by examining the course of the lymphatic drainage of the pelvis, which is carefully palpated along the pelvic vessels. When enlarged or clinically suspicious nodes are found they are removed and immediately sent for frozen section study while further evaluation of the pelvis is undertaken. The paravesical and pararectal spaces are important anatomic landmarks. When developed they provide an opportunity for thorough exploration of the intervening base of the broad ligament (Fig. 42-29). Tumor will extend into the base of the broad ligament without anatomic evidence of disease being detected before operation. This step is, therefore, a safeguard in determining the possible extension of tumor beyond the cervix and into the immediate paracervical tissues. When there is evidence of extracervical disease we may abandon the surgical procedure unless there is clear evidence that the disease

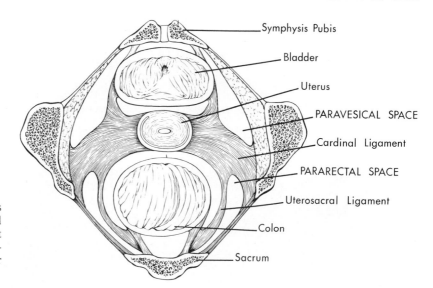

Figure 42–29. Cross section of pelvis showing paravesical and pararectal space. The base of the broad ligament (cardinal ligament) extends to the lateral pelvic wall and contains the major lymphatics draining the cervix.

can be cleanly removed. In either case, full pelvic irradiation is indicated. Certainly, the lateral pelvic wall must be free of tumor. When the central tumor is clearly resectable we do not hesitate to complete the operation, even if there is evidence of metastatic disease in the pelvic lymph nodes.

Before the pelvic planes and spaces are developed a decision must be made about conservation or removal of the tubes and ovaries. If normal ovaries are conserved in premenopausal patients, the tubes usually are also left in. After the round ligaments are clamped, cut, and ligated the utero-ovarian ligaments and medial fallopian tubes are clamped and doubly ligated. The infundibulopelvic ligaments are carefully mobilized and the adnexal organs are packed out of the operative field with the intestines.

Development of Paravesical Space

The anterior leaf of the broad ligament forms the roof of the paravesical space and blends with the bladder peritoneum medially and the parietal peritoneum laterally. This deep fossa beneath the peritoneal covering is composed of loose connective tissue and fat. It occupies the area between the bladder and the retropubic space medially, with the pelvic sidewall and obturator muscle forming the lateral boundaries. The superior boundary is formed by the cardinal ligament, while the floor is composed of the levator ani muscle. After clamping and ligating the round ligament about midway along its course the anterior leaf of the broad ligament is opened in an inferior direction, passing well into the pelvis before diverting the incision medially to reflect the bladder peritoneum from the lower uterine segment (Fig. 42-30). With gentle digital pressure the

paravesical space can be entered without difficulty, making certain that the dissection is initiated on the lateral side of the obliterated hypogastric artery (lateral umbilical ligament) and carried all the way down to the levator ani muscle (Fig. 42-31). The hypogastric artery gives off the superior vesical artery in this area and continues onto the undersurface of the rectus muscle, where it becomes the obliterated umbilical artery. There are no major blood vessels in this potential space, although occasionally an aberrant obturator vessel may emerge from the inferior epigastric artery and course along the posterior aspect of the pubic bone to the obturator space. With gentle digital dissection the pelvic floor can be palpated and the posterior aspect of the space can be identified, including the anterior margin of the cardinal ligament.

Development of Pararectal Space

The pararectal space lies beneath the pelvic peritoneum and extends between the cardinal ligament laterally and the uterosacral ligament medially. It can be entered by extending the incision in the anterior leaf of the broad ligament in a cephalic direction along the lateral margin of the infundibulopelvic ligament (Fig. 42-32A). By retracting the infundibulopelvic ligament and displacing the uterus medially, the uterosacral ligament is placed on a stretch and the pararectal space is widened. Dissection of this space is much more precarious than that of the paravesical space. Unskilled dissection in this area frequently is associated with troublesome bleeding. The medial border of the fossa is bounded by the uterosacral ligament and rectum, and the lateral border is formed superiorly by the piriformis muscle and inferiorly by the levator muscle. The sacrum

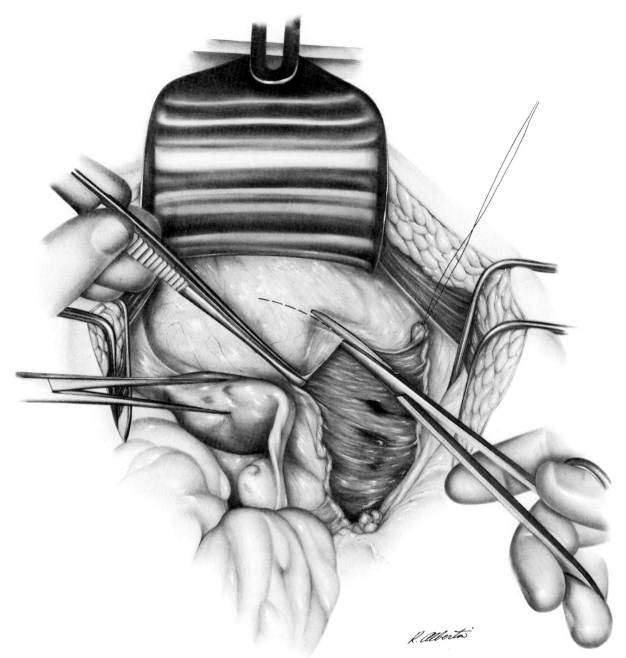

Figure 42–30. Opening the anterior leaf of the broad ligament after ligating the round ligament and infundibulopelvic ligament.

forms the posterior margin of the space, and the ureter is attached to the peritoneum along the roof of the space before entering the medial aspect of the cardinal ligament.

The hypogastric artery and vein are located in the deeper aspect of the pararectal space along the levator ani muscle. The cardinal ligament forms the caudal and lateral borders of this important area. Entry into the pararectal space must be made cautiously (Fig. 42-32A) with medial displacement of the ureter and its attached peritoneum. A point between the ureter, which is attached to the medial leaf of peritoneum, and the hypogastric artery is selected. Blunt dissection should be used in this area, and careful handling of tissue is

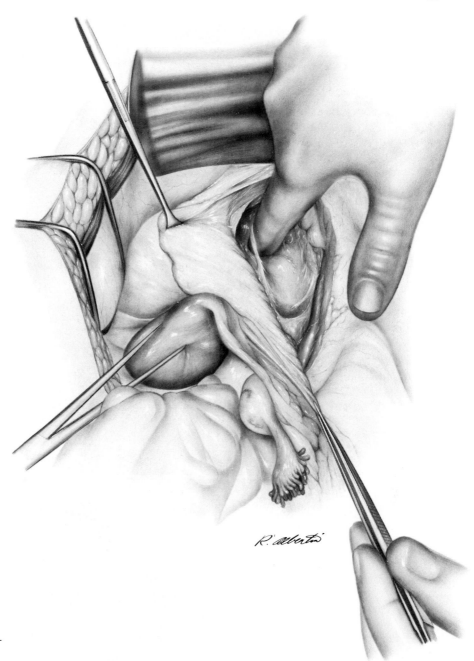

Figure 42–31. Development of paravesical space.

imperative to avoid unnecessary damage to small veins deep in this fossa. When the examining finger reaches the pelvic floor and levator ani muscle the fossa narrows, and care must be taken to avoid damage to the lateral sacral and hemorrhoidal vessels. The dissection is carried vertically downward for a short distance. The further development of the space then changes to an inferior and caudad direction lateral to the rectum. If the development of the space is difficult, it should be delayed until a later time in the operation. When the paravesical and pararectal spaces have been dissected (Fig. 42-32B) the pelvic floor and cardinal ligament can be easily identified and palpated. In the absence of demonstrable tumor extension the case is considered operable and the lymph node dissection is initiated at this time.

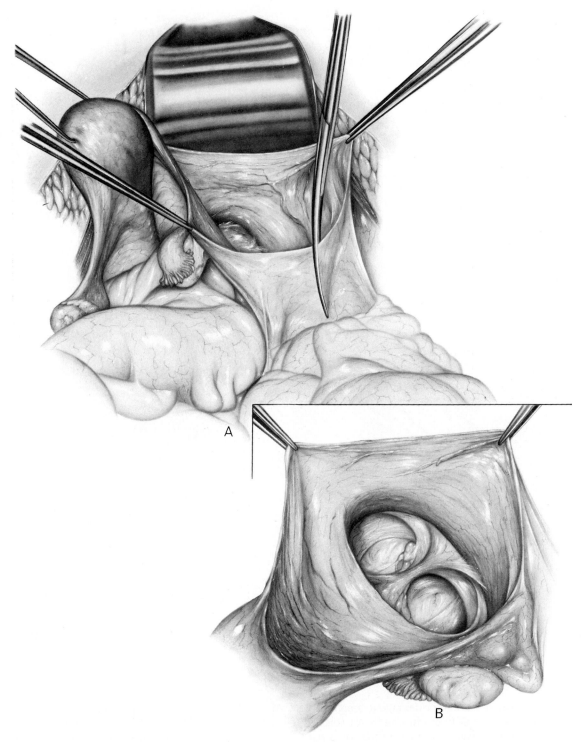

Figure 42–32. *A,* Extending the incision in the anterior leaf of the broad ligament in a cephalic direction along the lateral margin of the right infundibulopelvic ligament. *B,* Paravesical and pararectal fossae with intervening base of broad ligament attached to pelvic floor and lateral pelvic wall.

Pelvic Lymphadenectomy

Dissection of the lymphatic tissue along the iliac vessels may begin in the region of the bifurcation of the common iliac artery and extend superiorly to the bifurcation of the aorta and inferiorly to the inguinal ligament, or it may begin at another point along the course of the iliac vessels. The opening of the posterior peritoneal leaf of the broad ligament must be extended to the area of the pelvic brim, where the ureter is easily identified as it enters the pelvis at the bifurcation of the common iliac artery. This dissection is made easier if the infundibulopelvic ligament has been ligated and divided; however, the ligament and ovarian vessels can be retracted medially if the adnexa are preserved. The ovary and tube can also be detached from the uterine corpus and gently tucked beneath the retractor above. In dissecting the presacral area in the angle of the bifurcation of the aorta, care must be taken to avoid bleeding from the middle sacral vessels, as well as from the proximal part of the left external iliac vein, which courses through this retroperitoneal space. It is best to occlude the middle sacral vessels with smaller vascular clips as they are identified, and if traumatized, the venous bleeding can be controlled with positive pressure against the sacrum and with vascular clips. The lymphatic tissue along the common iliac vessels is removed by sharp dissection with the points of the Metzenbaum scissors directed upward, while special care is taken to avoid trauma to the ureter (Fig. 42-33).

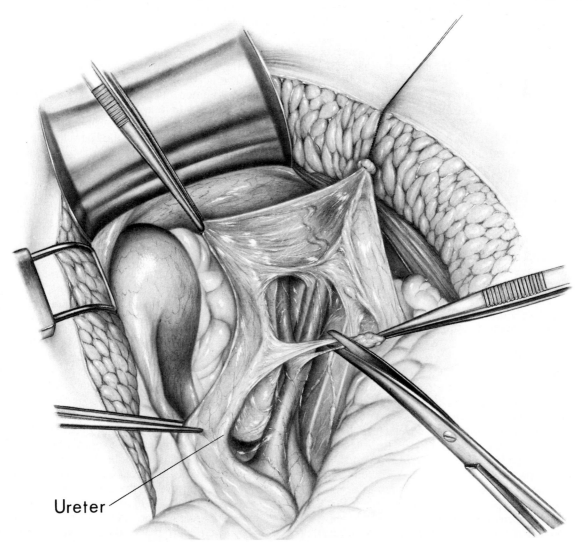

Ureter

Figure 42–33. Pelvic lymphadenectomy with dissection of right common iliac vessels and their branches, including the external iliac and hypogastric artery and vein. Note attachment of ureter to parietal peritoneum. Genitofemoral nerve courses along psoas muscle.

The ureter is reflected medially during the dissection of the common iliac vessels and left attached to the parietal peritoneum to maintain its blood supply.

It is important to remove the loose areolar tissue and fascial sheath from the iliac vessels, but to avoid trauma to the intima or wall of the vessels (particularly the veins), one should not attempt to skeletonize the pelvic vessels to the point of producing a pearl-white vascular tree. If there is tumor in the adventitia of the vessel wall, the patient will probably not be cured by this procedure; consequently such compulsive surgical efforts produce far more complications than benefits. It is important to rotate the vessels medially and laterally with a vein retractor during the dissection of the common and external iliac trunks to obtain the posterior lymphatic chain behind the vessels along the psoas muscle. The genitofemoral nerve, which is seen lateral to the external iliac vessels, should be preserved, as damage to this peripheral nerve will produce postoperative discomfort in the groin and medial aspect of the thigh.

The external iliac vessels are carefully dissected until they are seen to pass beneath the inguinal ligament. At this point care must be taken to avoid injury to the inferior epigastric artery and vein, which arise from the anterior and medial side of the iliac vessels and course along the anterior peritoneum onto the lower abdominal wall. One also must be cognizant of the anomalous obturator artery and vein, which may arise from the lower portion of the external iliac or inferior epigastric vessels and course over the pelvic sidewall into the obturator space. If accidentally traumatized, they should be ligated at their point of origin from the artery or vein. To avoid bleeding in the obturator space, these vessels are frequently occluded with small vascular clips as they pass through the obturator space, regardless of their origin. The clips also can be used to occlude the lymphatic channels coming into the pelvis from the leg.

The obturator space is entered by reflecting the external iliac vessels medially away from the psoas muscle and freeing the areolar tissue that lies directly between these vessels and the lateral pelvic wall (Fig. 42-34A), usually with the index finger. Once the space has been entered and the adjacent tissue cleaned from the external iliac vessels, the artery and vein are released and gently retracted laterally with a vein retractor, and the obturator space is clearly exposed. The lymphatic and areolar tissue are dissected from the obturator space to the region of the pelvic floor, with particular care taken to avoid trauma to the obturator nerve and vessels (Fig. 42-34B). The dissection is continued by removing all of the nodes below the bifurcation of the iliac vessels, including the hypogastric nodes and the nodes in the obturator fossa. A lymph node may be encountered in the angle formed by the external iliac and hypogastric arteries and must be carefully dissected out, avoiding trauma to the adjacent hypogastric vein.

Retraction of the common iliac artery and vein medially will expose a group of lymph nodes that should be carefully removed. These lymph nodes are the lateral common iliac nodes. There is danger of venous bleeding in this area. When this area has been cleared one can see the obturator nerve entering the obturator fossa through the body of the psoas muscle. The nerve roots of the lumbosacral plexus also will be exposed. Particular care must be exercised in the dissection of the lateral sacral and sacroiliac plexus, just medial to the hypogastric artery and vein, near their origin. The rich arcade of small arteries and veins increases the risk of bleeding in this area. When the vessels retract into the sacral foramen control of bleeding becomes quite difficult.

The obturator artery can be identified as it courses along the lateral pelvic wall adjacent to the obturator nerve. The nerve, artery, and vein advance toward the obturator foramen, through which they leave the pelvis. Care must be taken to avoid trauma to all of the structures, particularly the obturator veins, which have a rich anastomotic network against the lateral pelvic wall and communicate freely with the adjacent hypogastric veins. It is best to ligate or clip the obturator vessels, but in the event that uncontrolled bleeding should occur in this area, hemostasis is best obtained by packing the space tightly with a hot pack and providing adequate time for a fibrin clot to develop. If excessive bleeding occurs on one side of the pelvis, dissection may continue on the opposite side in the interim after pressure packing.

Dissection of Hypogastric Artery, Bladder, and Ureter

The hypogastric artery is dissected with identification of the visceral branches of the anterior trunk, which include the uterine, superior, middle, and inferior vesical, vaginal, and middle hemorrhoidal arteries. The anterior division of the hypogastric artery continues along the paravesical fossa to become the obliterated lateral umbilical ligament beneath the anterior abdominal wall. If the superior vesical artery should be damaged, it can be ligated without serious compromise to the blood supply of the bladder. In patients who have a small-volume tumor in the cervix the uterine artery may be ligated at its origin from the hypogastric artery. Rather than ligating the uterine artery individually, however, we believe that a more adequate central dissection is achieved by ligating the anterior division of the hypogastric artery just distal to the point of origin of its posterior division. The vessel is doubly ligated. The

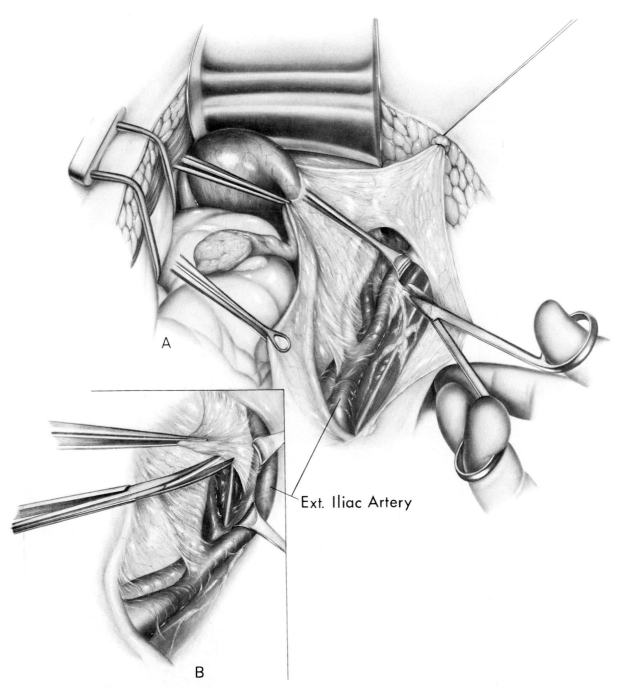

Figure 42–34. *A,* Entry into obturator space by medial reflection of external iliac vessels. *B,* Dissection of obturator fossa demonstrating obturator nerve with areolar tissue attached superiorly to external iliac vessels.

distal branches traversing the cardinal ligament are removed with the specimen or are ligated again distally. No attempt is made to remove the hypogastric vein. The other, adjacent veins should be ligated to avoid brisk bleeding in this area.

The bladder is now reflected off the lower uterine segment by incising the bladder peritoneum from its attachment to the uterus. The fascial adhesions of the base of the bladder are released from the cervix and upper vagina by sharp scissor dissection and the ves-

icocervical space is developed inferiorly and laterally. The ureter tunnels between the anterior fascial bundles of the base of the broad ligament, commonly called the vesicouterine ligament. This fascial tunnel is carefully opened by sliding the Metzenbaum scissors, with concave surface pointed upward, along the anterior and medial surface of the ureter and by gently spreading the blades, as shown in Figure 42-35*A*. The uterine artery and vein course along the fascial roof of this ligament. Adson clamps are used in dissecting the tunnel, as these

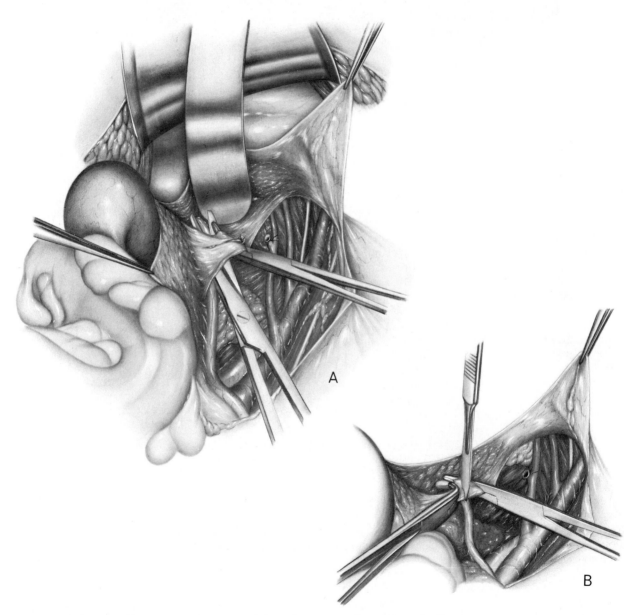

Figure 42–35. *A,* Metzenbaum scissors inserted above the ureter in the vesicouterine ligament or ureteral tunnel of the broad ligament. Note ligated uterine artery in anterior fascial sheath of tunnel. *B,* Roof of tunnel is opened between clamps.

long-handled instruments have delicate points that are relatively atraumatic when placed adjacent to the ureter and bladder. As shown in Figure 42-35B, the anterior sheath of the vesicouterine ligament is opened by doubly clamping and incising this tissue. Each of the fascial bundles is suture ligated for control of bleeding, and the ureter is dissected free of its attachment to the posterior leaf of the vesicouterine ligament. Care must be taken to prevent damage to the adventitia and muscular wall of the ureter, which contain nutrient vessels from the collateral circulation. In the event that the blood supply to the ureter is compromised by thrombosis or trauma to the veins, fistula formation is a serious and frequent complication. The ureter is gently retracted with an umbilical tape or vein retractor. Forceps should not be used in handling the ureter.

Dissection of Cardinal Ligament

The base of the broad ligament (the cardinal ligament) may now be excised from its attachment at the lateral pelvic wall. The technique of clamping and ligating the vascular cardinal ligament varies, depending on the circumstances. Sometimes part of the ligament can be included in a single clamp. Sometimes it is better to ligate or clip individual vessels. The ligament is excised with sharp scissor dissection and ligated with No. 1 delayed absorbable suture. A series of clamps are placed until the dissection is completed to the pelvic floor and along the paravaginal tissues (Fig. 42-36). If serious bleeding should occur in this region owing to trauma to the pelvic floor veins, hemostatic control is best obtained by firm packing of the pelvis and shifting the dissection temporarily to the opposite side.

The uterosacral ligaments, commonly called the pararectal stalks, are placed on a stretch by sharply withdrawing the uterus forward. The peritoneal reflection of the cul-de-sac of Douglas is now incised, leaving a small segment of peritoneum attached to the anterior surface of the rectum. Care must be taken to avoid injury to the ureters, which are attached to the peritoneum just lateral to the uterosacral ligament (Fig. 42-37A). The rectovaginal space is opened by sharp scissor dissection and deepened by blunt and sharp dissection (Fig. 42-37B). This procedure separates the posterior reflection of the endopelvic fascia from the lateral wall of the rectum, which includes the more superficial uterosacral ligaments. The entire fascial bundle of the uterosacral ligament is identified, clamped as far posteriorly and close to the rectum as possible, and cut and ligated (Fig. 42-37C). Continuation of this plane of dissection along the posterior endopelvic fascia will free the posterior aspect of the cervix from the pelvic floor. It is important to dissect the paravaginal fascia to obtain all of the microlymphatic

channels that communicate between the cervix and upper vagina (Fig. 42-38A). The bladder is then dissected further from the upper portion of the vagina by sharp and blunt dissection, making certain to avoid trauma to the blood supply of this organ. It is important, therefore, that sharp dissection, rather than blunt trauma, be used to free the base of the bladder from the anterior vagina to avoid forceful tearing of the blood vessels and musculature of the bladder. The specimen is removed by the open technique, as shown in Figure 42-38B, applying long right-angle clamps in front of the cervix (not shown) along the proximal surgical margins of the vagina to avoid gross spillage of tumor cells into the pelvis.

Closure

Several biopsies are taken from the margin of the vaginal apex. The vaginal margins are sutured with a continuous locking No. 2-0 delayed absorbable suture, and the vagina is left open to obtain adequate pelvic drainage (Fig. 42-38C). No additional attempt is made to support the vaginal vault, since all of the fascial support of the uterus and vagina has been removed. The remaining vagina, which has been shortened by about 3 cm, is well supported by its attachments to the levator ani muscles and urogenital diaphragm and mainly by the effects of postoperative fibrosis during the healing phase. Suction catheters are placed in the obturator fossae and along the lateral pelvic walls and brought out through stab wounds in the lower abdomen. These catheters are later connected to intermittent, low-suction drainage units and are effective in preventing lymphocyst formation and ureteral damage.

No attempt is made to suspend the ureters to the hypogastric artery, as suggested by Green and coworkers, or to place the terminal ureter on the inside of the peritoneal surface, as recommended by Novak. In view of the fact that the pelvis is well drained and the blood supply of the terminal ureter is preserved, we have had little difficulty with stenosis or fistula formation of the terminal ureter. In contrast to the method of Novak from Yugoslavia, Green and coworkers from Boston, and Ohkawa from Japan, our technique, adopted from Symmonds and Pratt, is to leave the pelvic ureters in their normal retroperitoneal position, and to place retroperitoneal suction drains along the pelvic walls. If the operative field remains dry postoperatively, it has been our experience that pelvic cellulitis and lymphocysts can be avoided and ureteral complications are infrequent (1%).

Before reperitonizing the pelvis the free margin of the bladder peritoneum is sutured to the anterior cuff of the vagina for additional protection to the denuded bladder

(*text continues on page 1227*)

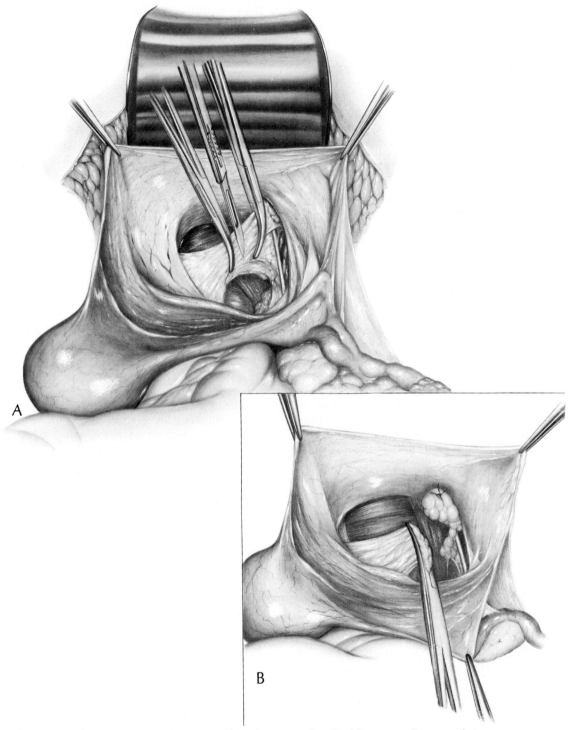

Figure 42–36. *A,* Clamping and incision of lateral portion of cardinal ligament adjacent to the lateral pelvic wall. *B,* Excised ligament showing pelvic floor and levator muscles. Dissected obturator nerve is seen in obturator space.

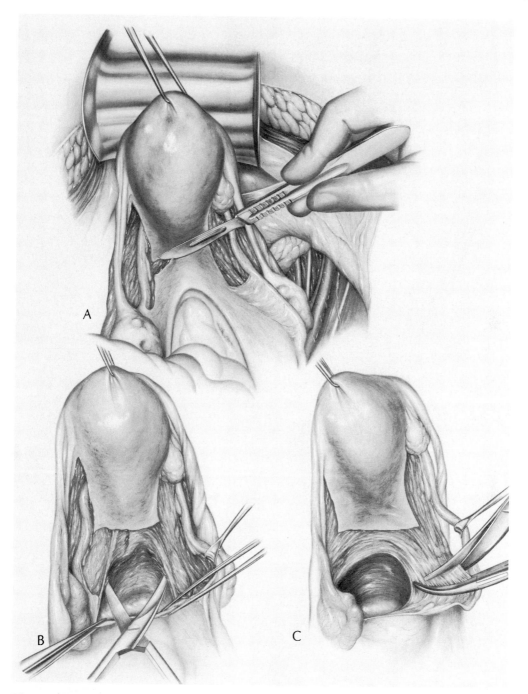

Figure 42–37. *A,* Cutting the cul-de-sac peritoneum as it reflects onto the rectum. Ureters course laterally, devoid of peritoneum. *B,* Dissection of the rectovaginal septum with development of rectal stalks (uterosacral ligaments) laterally. *C,* Clamping the uterosacral ligament. Ureter is gently retracted to avoid trauma.

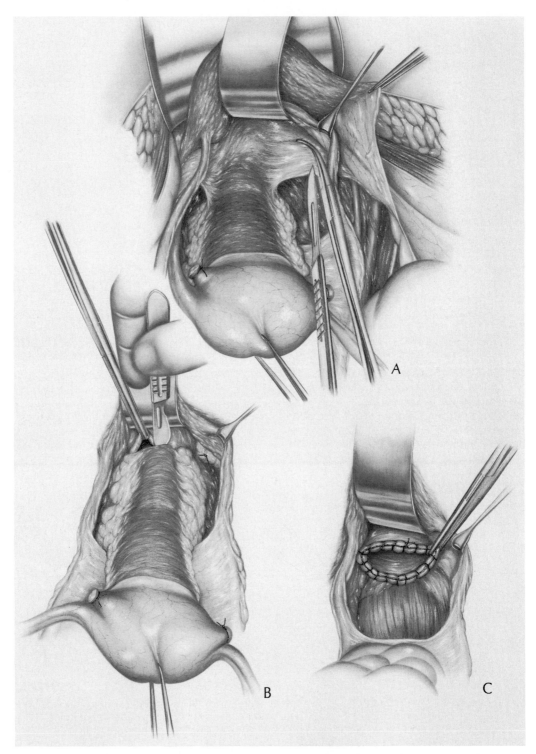

Figure 42–38. *A*, Dissection and retraction of bladder and terminal ureter from vagina and excising the paravaginal fascia from the lateral pelvic wall. *B*, Opening of vagina and securing lower vaginal cuff. Upper 3 cm of vagina are removed with surgical specimen. *C*, Closure of open vaginal cuff with continuous locking suture for hemostasis. Ureters are seen laterally and denuded rectum posteriorly.

base. In essence, this provides an extra layer of tissue between the denuded pelvis and the base of the bladder and terminal ureters. This added step is useful in decreasing both vesicovaginal and ureterovaginal fistulas. The edge of peritoneum over the rectum is sutured to the posterior vaginal cuff. The peritoneum is then closed across from one side to the other with a continuous suture. This method of closure was first described by Symmonds and Pratt and has been helpful in preventing fistulas and lymphocysts (see Fig. 42-57).

If the tubes and ovaries are to be preserved, a tunnel is dissected beneath the peritoneum laterally and superiorly toward each lateral gutter. An incision in the peritoneum is made as high as possible at the top of the tunnel. The adnexal structures are guided through the tunnel and through the incision at the top of the tunnel, making absolutely certain that the ovarian vessels in the infundibulopelvic ligament are not twisted. Permanent suture material is used to suture the tubo-ovarian pedicle as high as possible to the peritoneum and underlying muscle. Two large metal clips also are placed across the pedicle to later identify the location of the ovaries with an abdominal radiograph. This ovarian suspension is done when there is a reasonable chance that a patient will need postoperative pelvic irradiation (see Figs. 42-59 and 42-60). Otherwise, the tubes and ovaries may be left in their natural position in the pelvis.

Before closure of the peritoneum over the pelvis a careful inspection for bleeding points should be made, preferably after the patient's blood pressure has been returned to normal. In closing the peritoneum one should carefully avoid constriction, compression, or kinking of the ureter beneath.

Description of Technique of Extraperitoneal–Transperitoneal Approach

The preparation of the patient is the same as for the previously described approach. After preparation and draping an operator standing on the patient's right side makes a transverse elliptical incision that begins just above the left anterior superior iliac spine and continues medially about 2 cm above the inguinal ligament, across the midline about 3 cm above the symphysis pubis, turning upward on the right side toward the right anterior superior iliac spine (Fig. 42-39). Only about two-thirds of the length of the incision need be made at this point. The rectus muscles are transected transversely. The incision is extended laterally and superiorly on the left through the external abdominus, transverse abdominus, and internal abdominus muscles. With sharp and blunt dissection beneath the inferior edge of the muscles the peritoneum is carefully reflected superiorly and medially. Three structures must be clamped and ligated to accomplish this: the inferior epigastric artery and vein, the round ligament, and the obliterated hypogastric artery. Once these have been ligated, dissection usually proceeds without difficulty, attempting to preserve the integrity of the peritoneum. The psoas muscle, the external iliac artery and vein, and

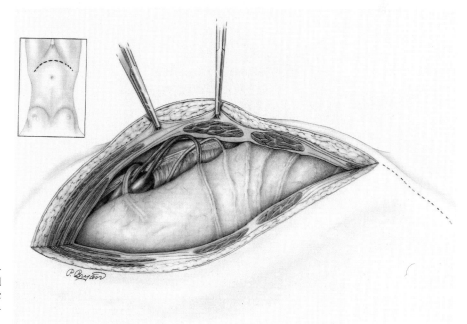

Figure 42–39. Transverse incision demonstrating the round ligament, the inferior epigastric artery and vein, and the obliterated hypogastric artery.

the lateral bladder wall come easily into view. The left paravesical space is developed down to the levator muscle (Fig. 42-40). The peritoneum is peeled away from the vessels. After identification of the lateral femoral cutaneous and genitofemoral nerves, dissection of the lymphatic and fatty tissue may begin at any point along the external iliac artery and vein (Fig. 42-41). Further reflection of the peritoneum identifies the ureter attached to the peritoneum as it is peeled away and identifies the uterine artery crossing over the ureter. Between the bifurcation of the common iliac artery and vein and the reflected peritoneum a point to begin the dissection of the pararectal space is selected. The space is developed by sharp and blunt dissection posteriorly and then changed to an inferior direction. The development of the pararectal space usually goes easily, but it should not be forced if difficulty is encountered. The tissue between the paravesical space and the pararectal space is the cardinal ligament, or "web" (Fig. 42-42). As dissection proceeds the tissue must be removed from the peritoneal attachments medially and from the pelvic sidewall. The obturator fossa can be entered between the psoas muscle and the external iliac artery and vein, or medially and beneath these vessels. The small lateral perforating vessels are clipped. The obturator nerve can be identified along with the obturator artery and vein (Fig. 42-43). These vessels must be securely ligated before they traverse the obturator foramen. All lymph nodes and fat are removed from the obturator fossa

(Fig. 42-44). After the retroperitoneal reflection of the rectum and sigmoid further medially it usually is helpful to put a self-retaining retractor in place. A Bookwalter retractor has multiple blades of various sizes and configurations that can be assembled around the operative field to provide optimum exposure. A retractor blade should not be placed beneath the inguinal ligament just lateral to the external iliac vessels pressing against the psoas muscle. Although not visible without further dissection, the femoral nerve is located here, and can be damaged by pressure from a retractor.

With the excellent exposure provided by the incision, the retractor, and the extraperitoneal approach, the dissection continues. Lymphatic tissue is removed from the presacral area between the sigmoid medially and the common iliac vein. A small artery to the ureter can be seen and usually can be sacrificed to accomplish a clean dissection. Lymphatic tissue is then removed up to the level of the mid-common iliac vessels, but if necessary, the dissection can be extended to the lower paraaortic nodes with proper retraction and lighting (Fig. 42-45). The anterior division of the hypogastric artery is identified just distal to the origin of the posterior trunk. Thorough cleaning of this vessel will allow its safe ligation, usually first with a free tie followed by a transfixation suture distally. One must be careful to avoid injury to the hypogastric vein (Fig. 42-46). In the dissection of the cardinal ligament that follows, the

(text continues on page 1232)

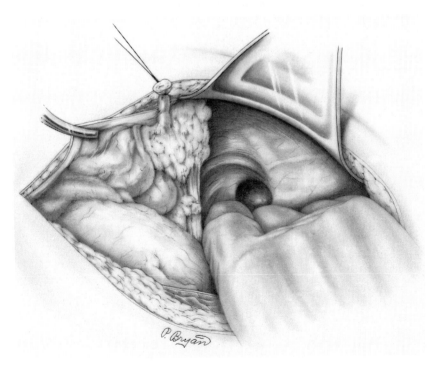

P. Bryan

Figure 42–40. The peritoneum is reflected from the left lateral pelvic sidewall, and the left paravesical space is entered.

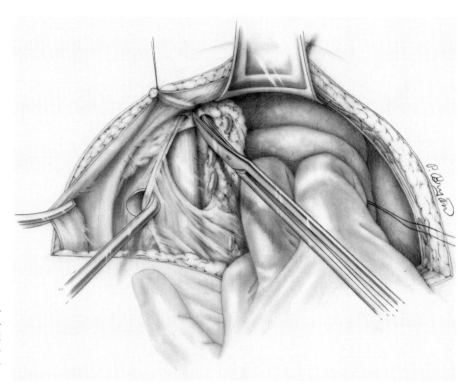

Figure 42–41. After identification and retraction of the genitofemoral and lateral femoral cutaneous nerves, the lymphadenectomy begins along the external iliac artery and nerves.

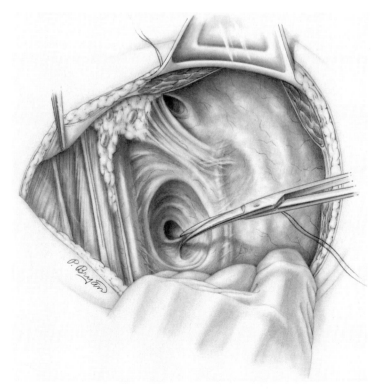

Figure 42–42. The ureter is peeled away from the lateral pelvic wall with the peritoneum. The pararectal space is developed.

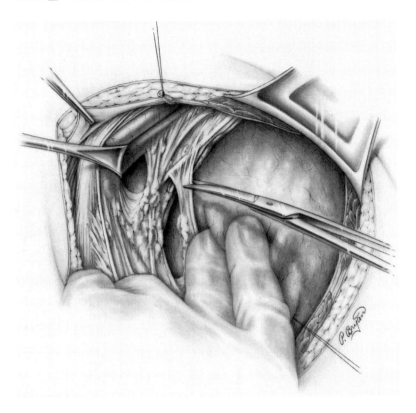

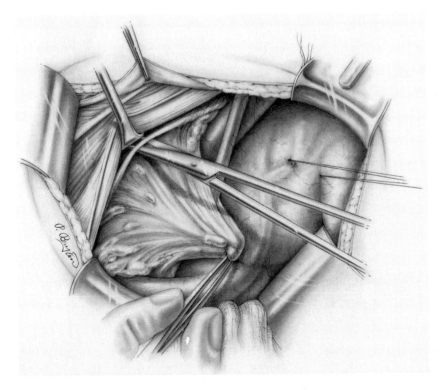

Figure 42–44. With careful identification of the obturator nerve, the contents of the obturator fossa are removed.

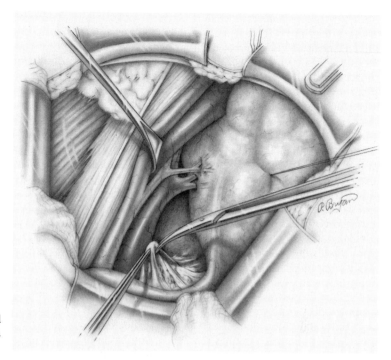

Figure 42–45. Lymphatic tissue is removed from the presacral area and from the common iliac artery and veins.

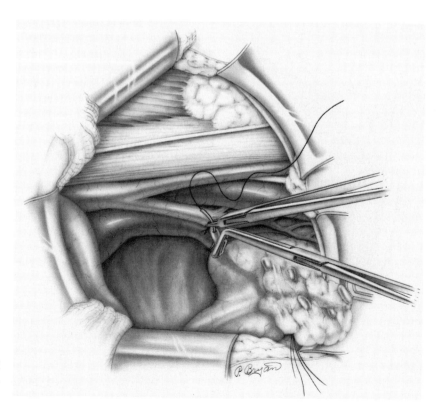

Figure 42–46. The anterior trunk of the hypogastric artery is first ligated with a free tie and then suture ligated.

branches of the anterior division of the hypogastric artery are removed and ligated distally. For example, the uterine artery is traced to its point of crossing over the ureter and is secured with a clip. Ligation or clipping individual arteries and veins in the cardinal ligament involves a meticulous and tedious dissection to avoid unnecessary bleeding that may be difficult to control (Fig. 42-47). Removal of some superior gluteal nodes usually is accomplished if the most inferior portion of the cardinal ligament is removed. It is not possible to remove the inferior gluteal nodes, as this is an extremely dangerous and inaccessible area for dissection in the region of the ischial spine. This is probably the weakest point in performing pelvic lymphadenectomy for cervical cancer, since superior and inferior gluteal nodes are among those most frequently involved with metastatic disease from cervical cancer.

Dissection of the ureters from the tunnel is done in the transperitoneal phase of the operation.

Finally, the extraperitoneal lymphadenectomy is completed by removing all tissue around the bifurcation of the common iliac artery and vein, the region called the "axilla of the pelvis" by Leitch. Retraction of the distal common iliac artery and vein medially away from the psoas muscle exposes the lateral common iliac lymph nodes. We insist that these nodes be completely removed (Fig. 42-48). Dissection must be done carefully to avoid injury to the common iliac vein and its branches and the iliac branches of the iliolumbar artery and vein. Clean removal of the lipolymph node tissue exposes the obturator nerve as it enters the obturator fossa through the psoas muscle and also the fourth and fifth lumbar nerves and nerve roots of the lumbosacral plexus. It has been suggested that the lateral common iliac nodes should be preserved to reduce the incidence of postoperative edema of the lower extremities. We insist that they be removed in an effort to do as complete a lymphadenectomy as possible.

The operative field is carefully inspected for bleeding. When hemostasis is achieved the retractor is removed, the abdominal incision is extended to the right anterior superior iliac spine, and the right extraperitoneal pelvic lymphadenectomy is done in a similar manner. On completion of the bilateral pelvic lymphadenectomy the remainder of the operation, the central dissection, is carried out through a transverse incision in the peritoneum (Fig. 42-49). Exploration of the upper abdomen is followed by placement of the self-retaining retractor. Peritoneal washings are taken for cytologic study. The round ligaments have already been ligated extraperitoneally; their medial portions still attached to the uterus can be easily retrieved into

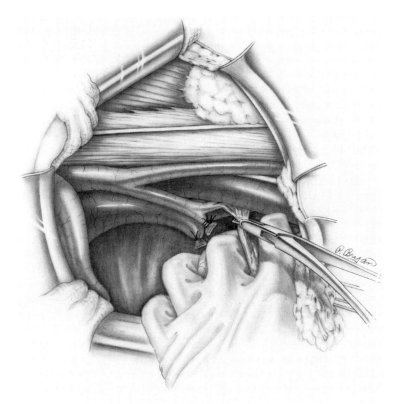

Figure 42–47. Cardinal ligament vessels along the lateral pelvic wall are clipped or ligated.

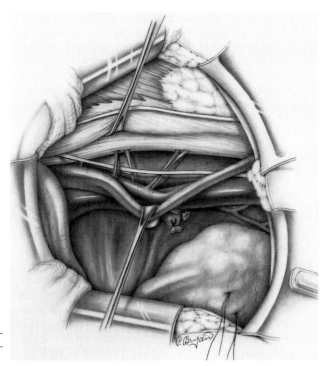

Figure 42–48. The lateral common iliac nodes are completely removed, thus exposing the entire course of the obturator nerve.

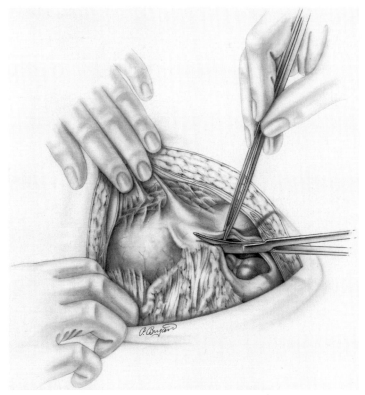

Figure 42–49. After bilateral extraperitoneal lymphadenectomy, a transverse incision is made in the peritoneum.

the peritoneal cavity. Depending on whether the tubes and ovaries are conserved or removed, the clamps are placed across the infundibulopelvic ligaments or the utero-ovarian ligaments. The remainder of the central dissection is carried out as previously described and illustrated. The exposure provided by the incision described is unsurpassed. The suction catheters are placed, the ovaries are suspended (if appropriate), and the peritoneum is closed in the manner previously described (Figs. 42-50 to 42-60).

Pathologic Examination of the Operative Specimen

Considerable useful information about the extent of the disease can be obtained by a careful pathologic examination of the operative specimen. This is helpful in determining prognosis, but is also absolutely essential to the identification of patients at greater risk for persistent disease, so that additional therapy and close surveillance can be provided. Even though the operator may be exhausted at the end of the operation, he or she should accompany the specimen to the pathology laboratory, where it should be examined with the pathologist before it is placed in fixative and sectioned. The gynecologic surgeon can point to worrisome parts of the specimen; such information will assist the patholo-

gist in taking sections. Critical margins of dissection can be pointed out and stained with india ink, so that they can be seen on the microscopic slides. The primary cervical tumor should be measured as accurately as possible, so that at least an estimate of its size and volume can be recorded. Numerous microscopic sections of the cervix with adjacent vaginal cuff, lower uterine segment, and paravaginal, paracervical, and parametrial tissue should be examined to show the cell type, the degree of differentiation, the depth of stromal invasion, the presence or absence of invasion of lymphatic and vascular spaces, and the stromal reaction to the tumor. It is important to know not only the depth of invasion, but also the thickness of the uninvolved fibromuscular stroma of the cervix, as pointed out by Kishi and coworkers. These authors found that the nodal metastasis and 5-year cancer death rates were 7% and 8%, respectively, in patients with uninvolved fibromuscular stroma thickness above 3 mm, and 37% and 26%, respectively, in patients with the thickness below 3 mm. The thickness of the cancer-unaffected cervical fibromuscular stroma may be as useful as other parameters in determining the biologic behavior of invasive cervical cancer.

Unfortunately the exquisite giant section technique of pathologic examination used by Burghardt and coworkers is not available in all laboratories. These au-

(text continues on page 1240)

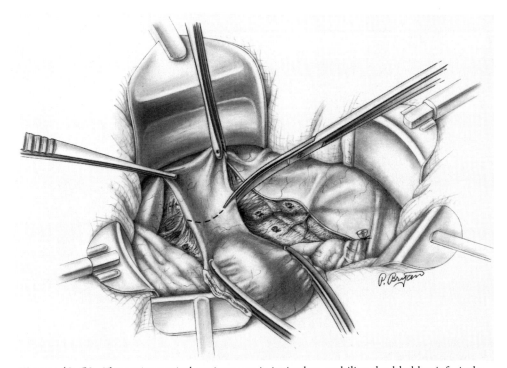

Figure 42–50. The vesicocervical peritoneum is incised to mobilize the bladder inferiorly.

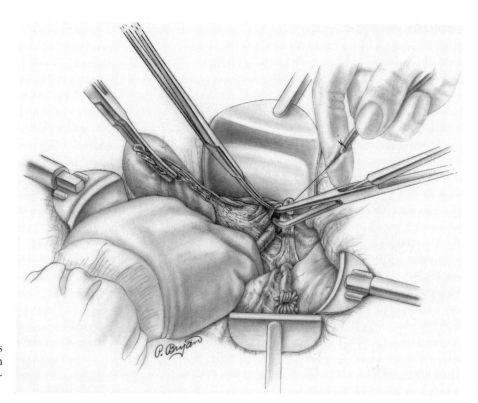

Figure 42–51. The ureter is dissected completely free from its tunnel in the cardinal ligament.

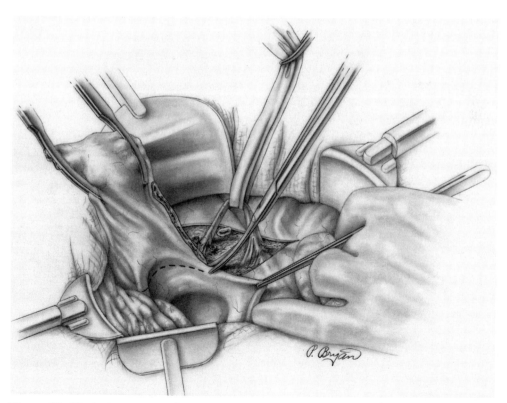

Figure 42–52. An incision is made in the cul-de-sac peritoneum below the cervix, if possible, to allow development of the rectovaginal space.

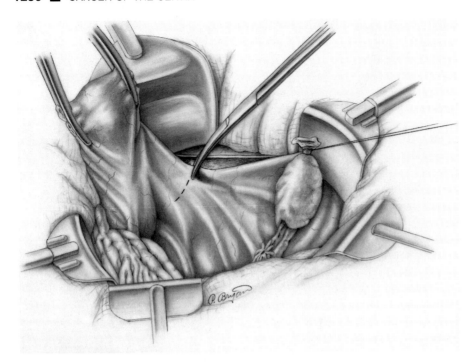

Figure 42–53. An incision is made in the anterior and posterior leaves of the right broad ligament. The round ligament was previously ligated extraperitoneally.

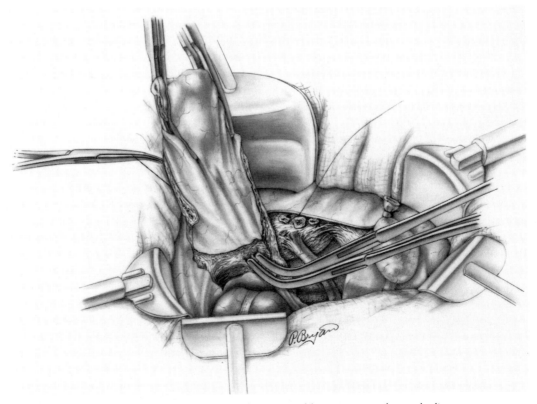

Figure 42–54. The posterior parametrium and uterosacral ligaments are clamped adjacent to the rectum.

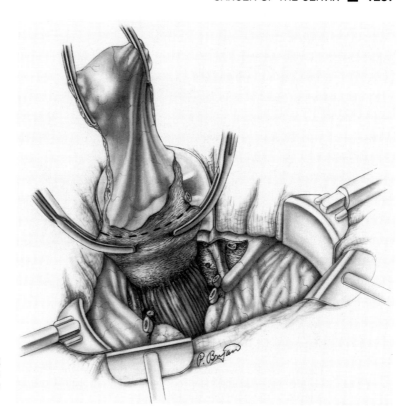

Figure 42–55. After clamping and ligating paravaginal tissue laterally, an incision is made in the vagina several centimeters below the cervix.

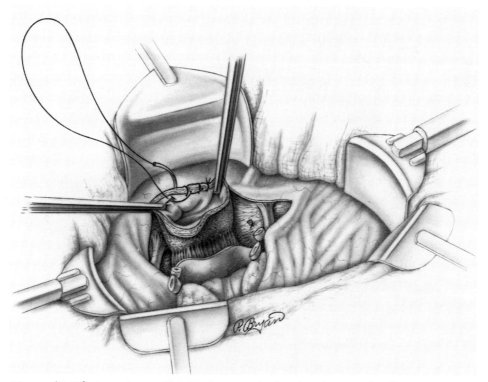

Figure 42–56. A continuous hemostatic suture is placed in the vaginal cuff.

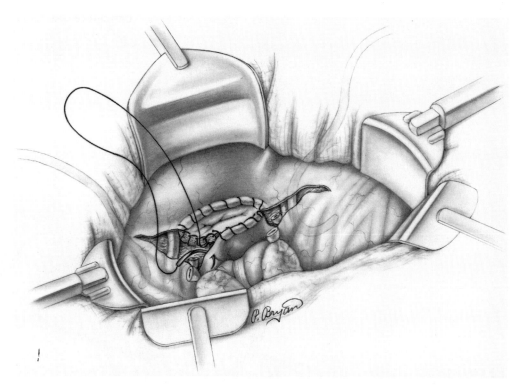

Figure 42–57. Suction catheters are placed in the retroperitoneal spaces bilaterally. The bladder peritoneum is sutured to the anterior vaginal cuff and the cul-de-sac peritoneum is sutured to the posterior vaginal cuff.

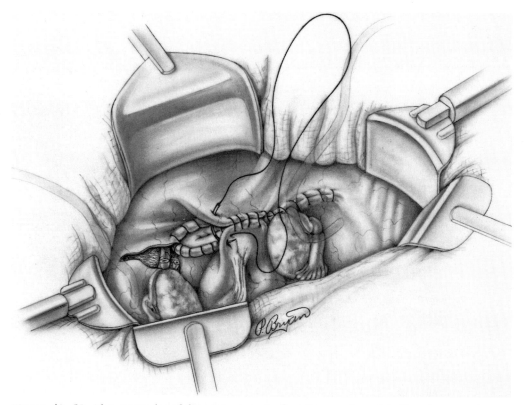

Figure 42–58. The remainder of the peritoneum is closed across the pelvic floor.

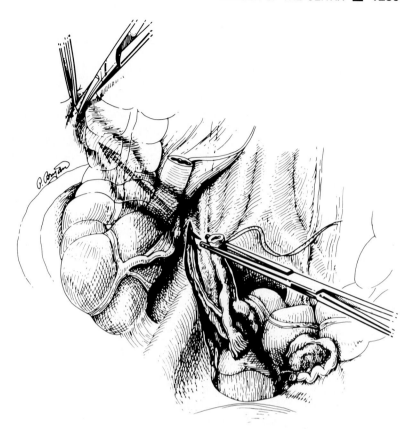

Figure 42–59. If the ovaries are to be suspended, a tunnel can be made under the peritoneum and the cecum on the right. The tube and ovary are guided through the tunnel to the new position in the right colic gutter above the pelvis.

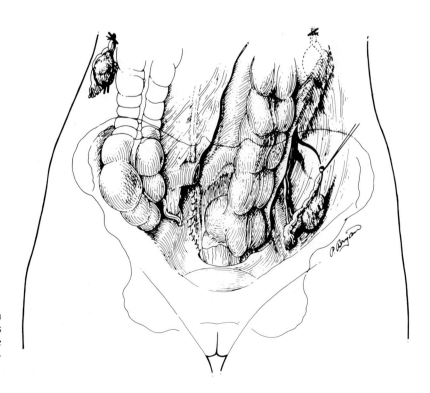

Figure 42–60. A similar procedure can be done on the left. The ovarian vessels should not be twisted. Metal clips are placed on the pedicles to allow later identification with abdominal radiograph.

thors measured ratio of tumor size to the size of the cervix. The incidence of lymph node involvement increased with tumor size, reaching a maximum of 68.3% in the group with a ratio from 70% to 80%. Surprisingly, direct spread into the parametrium was seldom found, even when large tumors were found to occupy the entire cervix. This finding is contrary to that of Bleker and coworkers, who found 16.8% unrecognized parametrial tumor involvement in patients with stage Ib and IIa lesions. The 5-year survival fell with parametrial involvement.

Thorough examination of the lymphadenectomy specimens must be done. Tumor metastasis to lymph nodes affects patient survival adversely and may suggest postoperative adjuvant therapy. In patients with positive nodes the pathologic examination should report whether the metastatic disease is microscopic or macroscopic, single or multiple, unilateral or bilateral. The location of lymph nodes positive for tumor also should be reported, since the prognosis is especially poor in patients with positive common iliac or paraaortic nodes. The usual standard technique of pathologic examination of lymphadenectomy specimens involves removal of visible and palpable nodes from fatty tissue with bisection of each node for microscopic examination. This standard technique may not be adequate for an accurate assessment of lymph node metastases. A significant increase in positive findings can be obtained if special pathologic examination techniques are used, as demonstrated by To and coworkers, Ahrens and Tschoke, and Wilkinson and Hause. With their technique of dissection of lymph nodes at multiple levels before paraffin embedding, To and coworkers showed that 9% of patients originally reported to have negative nodes actually had positive nodes.

An accurate assessment of the extent of disease by a careful pathology examination of the operative specimen is imperative in deciding whether or not additional treatment is needed. Indeed, it is such an important component in the surgical management of patients with cervical cancer that such patients should be operated on only in hospitals where expert pathologists also work.

Postoperative Complications

Bladder

Fistula. In the absence of prior pelvic irradiation, bladder ischemia and vesicovaginal fistula are infrequent complications of this procedure. In our experience, suture of the bladder peritoneum to the margins of the anterior vaginal wall has protected the bladder and terminal ureter from secondary infection and subsequent fistula formation. It is our view that this has significantly decreased the incidence of vesicovaginal and ureterovaginal fistula. The management of vesicovaginal fistulas is discussed in Chapter 30. The management of ureterovaginal fistulas is discussed in Chapter 29.

Neurogenic Bladder Dysfunction. An extensive abdominal hysterectomy effectively denervates the bladder and upper urethra. The more extensive the dissection, the greater the degree of interference with their function. Parasympathetic and sympathetic nerve fibers to and from the bladder and urethra are removed along with paracervical, paravaginal, cardinal ligament tissues, and pelvic lymph nodes. All patients have some degree of bladder dysfunction; the incidence of significant bladder dysfunction may be as high as 50%.

Mundy, and Sasaki and coworkers have suggested that the posterior part of the cardinal ligament (pars nervosa) contains the major part of the parasympathetic and sympathetic nerve supply to the bladder and urethra, and that its removal is responsible for postoperative bladder dysfunction. Sasaki and coworkers demonstrated that removal of the anterior cardinal ligament (pars vasculosa) with preservation of the pars nervosa reduces the incidence of postoperative bladder dysfunction. The work of Kadar and coworkers and of Asmussen and Ulmsten suggests that the nerve supply to the bladder and urethra can be spared without compromising the necessary extensive dissection and tissue removal around the central disease, thus sparing many patients the loss of urethrovesical function. This suggestion has not been widely adopted by gynecologic surgeons, presumably because of a concern that this same cardinal ligament tissue also carries lymph channels draining the cervix and should be removed in a complete central dissection. It would seem to us, therefore, that some degree of bladder dysfunction is inevitable with a technique of extensive hysterectomy that emphasizes adequacy of the central dissection and complete lymphadenectomy.

Studies have demonstrated that the bladder may initially be hypertonic, with decreased bladder capacity, increased resting pressure, and increased residual urine volume. Many patients have difficulty initiating micturition and a loss of sensation of bladder fullness. Using sensitive urodynamic instrumentation, Scotti and coworkers found a variety of abnormalities, including obstructive voiding patterns, immediate and delayed loss of compliance, sensory losses, and genuine stress incontinence. Some patients had complete absence of bladder contractions during voiding.

Techniques of managing the postoperative bladder have varied widely. Duration of catheter drainage, suprapubic versus transurethral drainage, the value of self-catheterization, and the value of cystometric studies have all been debated, as described by Bandy and co-workers. These authors also found that patients receiving postoperative adjunctive pelvic radiation had significantly more contracted and unstable bladders than patients treated with surgery alone. Proper management of the bladder in the first several weeks after operation is essential to avoid overdistension. Our preference is for continuous catheter drainage, either transurethral or suprapubic, for 7 days, followed by intermittent

clamping and release of the catheter for several more days. Postoperative intravenous pyelography is performed on the 10th postoperative day. If only the usual mild ureteral dilatation is seen, the catheter is removed and the patient is taught intermittent self-catheterization. She must be thoroughly schooled in the importance of not allowing her bladder to become overdistended. Allowing the bladder to overdistend, especially in the early postoperative recovery period, may result in a flaccid bladder from stretching and decompensation of the detrusor muscle, prolongation of bladder dysfunction with high residual urine volumes, and the likelihood of urinary infections. Patients are asked to void by the clock and to catheterize themselves three times each day after voiding. When bladder sensations return and residual urine volumes are consistently below 50 to 75 ml, then self-catheterization can be cautiously discontinued, to be reinstituted at anytime there is a suggestion of incomplete bladder emptying. Those patients who are unwilling or unable to perform these tasks assiduously are best managed with prolonged indwelling catheter drainage for several weeks before attempting to remove it. If a serious episode of overdistension of the bladder ever occurs, continuous indwelling catheter drainage should be reinstituted, sometimes for several weeks, with the hope that permanent impairment of bladder function can be avoided. Urinary tract infections may occur in conjunction with bladder dysfunction, and should be looked for with periodic urinalysis and culture and treated with appropriate antibiotics. Patients should be encouraged to maintain a urine output above 2000 ml/day to avoid urinary tract infection.

In most patients a satisfactory voiding pattern can be established within several months. Urodynamic studies, however, may show some evidence of slight and persistent chronic bladder dysfunction for several years. Fraser stated that 20% of his patients continued to report changes in bladder sensation as long as 5 to 15 years after operation. In many patients who have had properly performed extensive abdominal hysterectomy and pelvic lymphadenectomy it is inevitable that bladder function will never be completely normal again. With proper postoperative bladder care and rehabilitation, however, function should be satisfactory in

most patients at the end of the first year. According to Fishman and coworkers, 35% of patients continued to express unhappiness at the extent and effect of their postoperative urinary dysfunction.

Ureter

Clark, working at the Johns Hopkins Hospital, published one of the first descriptions of extensive hysterectomy for cervical cancer in 1895. Sampson, working in the same institution during the same time, recognized that injury to the ureter was the most serious problem associated with primary extensive surgery for this disease. His publications on ureteral anatomy and blood supply, and the relation between the ureter and gynecologic disease are classic and pertinent today. Devascularization and ischemic necrosis of the wall of the terminal ureter has proved to be one of the more serious complications of this operation. Wertheim himself found this complication to be one of the more serious sequelae. In Meigs' clinic there was a 12.5% significant ureteral complication rate, including an 8.5% incidence of ureterovaginal fistulas and a 4% incidence of ureteral stricture. As recently as 1965 Talbert and coworkers reported that 9 of 112 patients (8%) who had extensive hysterectomy developed ureterovaginal fistulas, two of which were bilateral. Seven kidneys were lost. The incidence of ureteral stricture also was high. The high percentage of ureteral complications may have been related to a large number of patients with pelvic cellulitis and also a large number of patients (71%) who received preoperative irradiation. It is well known that these two factors increase the risk of ureteral complications. In a recent report of 111 patients undergoing extensive hysterectomy and lymphadenectomy for cervical cancer in the same institution, only two minor ureteral injuries and no fistulas occurred.

For many years gynecologic surgeons have attempted to lower the rate of ureteral complications with special techniques. Novak, from Yugoslavia, reduced the incidence of ureteral fistula to 2% after primary extensive surgery by placing the dissected pelvic ureter on the inside (peritoneal surface) of the pelvic peritoneum and by preserving the lateral mesentery to the terminal ureter. Green and coworkers suggested that the terminal ureter should be lifted out of the accumulated fluid in the retroperitoneal space by suturing it to the obliterated hypogastric artery. Ohkawa developed a procedure that attempted to elevate and isolate the ureter from the infected retroperitoneal fluid and also to develop a new blood supply to the terminal ureter by placing it in a peritoneal envelope from the pelvic brim to the bladder. Blythe and coworkers compared this technique with simple retroperitoneal suction drainage first advised by Symmonds and Pratt. They found that ureteral obstruction and ureterovaginal fistulas occurred twice as often and the operative time was extended 45 minutes to 1 hour with the Ohkawa technique.

Given a normal unirradiated ureter, we believe that the incidence of ureteral fistula and permanent stenosis can be kept below 1% with meticulous intraoperative management of the ureter by a technically skillful operator who can prevent vascular trauma to the periureteral sheath and injury to the muscularis of the ureter, and by postoperative removal of retroperitoneal space fluid by constant suction.

Some temporary postoperative changes in ureteral function are an almost inevitable result of extensive hysterectomy, as pointed out by Gal and Buchsbaum. Using special static and cinefluoroscopic intravenous pyelography techniques, these authors found ureteral dilatation in 87% of patients in the 1st week after surgery. In most cases by 6 weeks after surgery the dilatation had regressed and the pyelograms had returned to normal. Peristalsis was altered in the distal ureter, which appeared as a rigid conduit during the 1st postoperative week. Peristalsis had returned 1 month later. These changes may explain the increased frequency of urinary tract infections after extensive hysterectomy, and the possibility of permanent ureteral stenosis if radiation, serious infection, or lymphocyst formation is superimposed.

A compilation of the frequency of urinary fistulas and operative mortality in a collected series of 4716 nonir-

radiated patients treated by extensive hysterectomy is presented by Shingleton and Orr in Table 42-9.

Retroperitoneal Spaces

A closed system of constant suction must be used in the retroperitoneal spaces on each side. The purpose is to remove the potentially enormous accumulation of fluid that normally collects in these spaces after a complete and thorough lymphadenectomy. The fluid composition is similar to that which exudes from the surface of a third-degree burn. It consists of blood components, lymph, and tissue fluid, and contains a high percentage of protein. The drains should be irrigated with sterile saline solution as often as necessary to ensure their patency and continued function. The amount of drainage varies but may be as much as several hundred milliliters per day for as long as a week before the amount begins to decrease. Such a large amount of fluid loss must be replaced intravenously until the patient is able to take adequate oral fluids and food. A drain may be removed if it produces less than 50 ml in a 24-hour period for 2 consecutive days.

Prolonged closed drainage of the retroperitoneal spaces is probably responsible for a reduction in the incidence of ureterovaginal fistulas. The lower ureter, which has been dissected free of its surrounding attachments, is not constantly bathed in a large accumulation of retroperitoneal fluid under pressure and probably heals better. Likewise, the incidence of lymphocyst formation has been reduced by suction drainage of retro-

TABLE 42–9
Urinary Fistulas and Operative Deaths in Nonirradiated Patients Treated by Extensive Hysterectomy

STUDY (YR)	NO. OF PATIENTS	URETERAL FISTULAS (%)	VESICAL FISTULAS (%)	OPERATIVE DEATHS (%)
Käser (1973)	717	3.3	0.6	NS
Park (1973)	156	0	0	0.64
Hoskins (1976)	224	1.3	0.45	0.89
Morley (1976)	208	4.8	0.5	1.4
Sall (1979)	349	2.0	0.8	0
Webb (1979)	423	1.4	0.7	0.3
Benedet (1980)	241	1.2	0.4	0.4
Langley (1980)	284	5.6	1.4	0
Lerner (1980)	108	0.9	0	0
Bostofte (1981)*	479	3.8	1.4	0.2
Powell (1981)	135	1.5	0	0.74
Zander (1981)	1092	1.4	0.3	1.0
Shingleton (1982)	300	1.3	0	0.3
Total	4716	2.3	0.57	0.55

*Okabayashi technique.
(Shingleton HM, Orr JW, Jr. Cancer of the cervix. New York: Churchill Livingstone, 1983.)

peritoneal spaces to less than 5% of patients. The use of antibiotics and attempts to ligate or clip lymphatic channels also may contribute to a reduced incidence of postoperative lymphocysts. The few patients who develop lymphocysts today usually are those whose retroperitoneal suction catheters did not function properly to provide adequate drainage.

A lymphocyst will become obvious by symptoms and examination several months after extensive hysterectomy and pelvic lymphadenectomy. It may be small and asymptomatic. Most patients with large lymphocysts complain of lower abdominal discomfort on the same side with radiation to the back, hip, or thigh. Some edema of the lower extremity on the same side may be present. Evidence of ureteral obstruction may be found on excretory urography.

Small symptomatic lymphocysts that do not cause ureteral obstruction may be observed. Large symptomatic lymphocysts that cause ureteral obstruction should be aspirated either vaginally or abdominally with a needle. As much as 500 ml of clear yellow fluid may be obtained. CT-directed needle aspiration may be done with local anesthesia, and may be repeated as needed. The fluid should be submitted for cytologic examination. It is seldom necessary to perform open drainage of a lymphocyst. Mann and coworkers have reported successful sclerosis of a recurrent lymphocyst by injection of a solution of tetracycline.

Infection

The occurrence of pelvic cellulitis has been greatly diminished after radical pelvic surgery with the use of adequate abdominal drainage of the operative site. Further, the prophylactic use of broad-spectrum antibiotics, including both aerobic and anaerobic coverage, has proved to be a useful addition to the surgical armamentarium. Previously patients were treated with antibiotics only if postoperative infection occurred. It currently is our practice to initiate broad-spectrum antibiotic coverage for both aerobic (gram-positive and gram-negative) and anaerobic bacteriologic coverage immediately before surgery. This treatment is maintained for 72 hours postoperatively, and has resulted in a markedly reduced incidence of pelvic cellulitis to less than 5% of the cases. When secondary infection does occur despite the use of prophylactic antibiotics, the vaginal vault is cultured; drainage from the abdominal suction catheters is cultured; and bacteria-specific, high-dose antibiotic therapy is used. Seldom is it necessary to drain a pelvic abscess when there has been accumulation of serum and blood with secondary infection. In our experience, this has occurred in less than 0.5% of cases.

Admittedly, only a few studies have been done on the use of perioperative prophylactic antibiotics in extensive hysterectomy patients. The rates of postoperative infectious morbidity appeared to be reduced in studies by Orr and coworkers, Rosenshein and coworkers, and Sevin and coworkers. Bendvold and Kjorstad, however, were unable to find justification for prophylactic antibiotics, since patients undergoing extensive hysterectomy in the Norwegian Radium Hospital had a very low incidence of postoperative infectious morbidity. Indeed, there were no instances of surgical site–related infections observed among 35 patients who had extensive abdominal hysterectomy.

Venous Thrombosis and Pulmonary Embolus

The patient who undergoes extensive pelvic surgery is at the highest risk for the development of venous thrombosis of the lower extremity, as compared with patients who have other types of gynecologic surgery. Virchow's classic triad of causative factors, as described more than one and a quarter centuries ago, is relevant today in the patient who has undergone extensive pelvic surgery. Such factors as postoperative alteration of blood coagulation, trauma to the vein wall, and venous stasis are recognizable features of this type of surgery. In particular, pelvic lymphadenectomy invariably produces some trauma to the vein wall during the mobilization of the vessel and resection of the adherent lymphatic tissue. One of the biologic effects of extensive surgery is the occurrence of local tissue necrosis during healing. This results in the release of tissue thromboplastin into the circulation, which contributes to venous thrombosis by acceleration of the clotting mechanism. The release of thromboplastin from the intima of the vein wall itself also provides an excellent nidus for the formation of fibrin, particularly in an area of the venous system where there is alteration in venous flow with stagnation of blood. This is frequently seen behind the valves of the veins of the lower extremity, where silent thrombosis is common. In studies using iodine-125–labeled fibrinogen scanning of the lower extremity, as many as 20% of gynecologic patients having a hysterectomy have been found to have venous thrombosis by this technique. Prolonged immobilization of the lower extremities during a lengthy operative procedure is responsible for intraoperative venous stasis and clot formation. There is now good evidence to document the fact that patients who develop postoperative thrombosis of the lower extremity have the origin of this complication during the surgical procedure in more than 50% of cases. Efforts to decrease the frequency of this complication include prophylactic low-dose heparin, using 2500 to 5000 units subcutaneously, three times daily, beginning 2 hours before surgery and given every 8 hours thereafter for the subsequent 5 postoperative days. By using perioperative heparin alone the incidence of deep vein thrombosis in Kakkar's study was decreased from 24.6% in the untreated control group to 7.7% in the heparin-treated group of surgical cases. More impressive was the observation in the latter study that 16 patients in the control group, as compared with only 2 patients in the heparin-treated group, were found on autopsy study to have died of acute, massive pulmonary embolism. Clarke-Pearson and coworkers believe that the most effective pharmacologic thromboembolism prophylaxis for gynecologic cancer patients is several doses of heparin preoperatively and continuing doses every 8 hours postoperatively. Each dose of heparin is 5000 units subcutaneously. According to these authors, this regimen is well tolerated and is not associated with clinically significant bleeding complications. We currently are using perioperative minidose heparin for selected high-risk patients. We also use intermittent compression hose on the lower extremities, beginning in the operating room or recovery room, as also advocated by Clarke-Pearson.

Recent clinical evidence, as shown by iodine-125 fibrinogen scans, demonstrates that 3% to 5% of patients with occult venous thrombosis of the lower extremities will develop a pulmonary embolus. Unfortunately more than 50% of the cases of fatal pulmonary embolism occur in patients with silent venous thrombosis and without any clinical evidence of this complication before the acute pulmonary catastrophe. When evidence of venous thrombosis of the lower extremity is verified, full anticoagulation therapy is required for prevention of pulmonary embolism. If a pulmonary embolus should occur after full anticoagulation has been achieved, it is necessary in such rare cases to prevent further migration of clot to the lung by either inferior vena cava ligation or the use of an intracaval Silastic umbrella. Such complications are rare, but the sinister effects of thromboembolism must be carefully evaluated on a daily basis in this high-risk group of patients.

Hemorrhage

Intraoperative and postoperative pelvic hemorrhage are also discussed in Chapter 8.

Intraoperative Bleeding. Despite the surgeon's adequate technical skills and careful dissection, serious hemorrhage may suddenly appear, especially during retroperitoneal dissections on the lateral pelvic sidewalls and around the sacrum. When it happens, it is hoped that the operative field will not be cluttered with clamps, exposure will be adequate, the patient's condition will be stable, and anesthesia will be sufficient to maintain good relaxation. If the bleeding vessel cannot be clamped quickly, the simplest and most effective method of controlling the bleeding is provided by pressure applied by the index finger of the gloved hand. With cessation of bleeding the operative site can be cleared of accumulated blood by suctioning, exposure of the area can be improved, and the surgeon can gain a few moments to evaluate the situation and choose the best possible course of action. Arterial bleeding is easy to identify and control with clips, clamps, and ligatures. The difficult problem with hemorrhage in the pelvis comes from lacerations of deep pelvic veins that are fragile, tortuous, distended, sometimes hidden or retracted from view, and sometimes held open by attachment of the vein wall to surrounding tissue. Blood returning through the lacerated vein may come from multiple sources unavailable for ligation. Placing clamps or sutures blindly is dangerous and may even make the problem worse. Sometimes digital pressure for at least 7 minutes is the most effective procedure to control venous bleeding. Sometimes additional careful dissection in the area is required to free the vessel above and below the bleeding point to allow more precise clipping or suture ligation. A cardinal rule in dissecting in the pelvis is to avoid creating a deep hole the bottom of which cannot be exposed in case a deep vein is lacerated. This is the reason dissection of the pararectal space should not be forced if it does not develop easily.

Whenever an extensive pelvic dissection is anticipated preparations should be made in advance just in case severe intraoperative bleeding is suddenly encountered. Adequate quantities of blood should be available to replace lost volume. More blood should be requested in advance of its need. A responsible member of the operating team or anesthesia team should be assigned the task of monitoring blood loss, blood replacement, and urine output. When bleeding is profuse, in the excitement of the moment it is possible to lose count of the number of units of whole blood, blood components, crystalloids, and other fluids that have been given, and how much blood has been lost. A dependable route for administering blood must be maintained. Without it rapid blood replacement is not possible. If massive hemorrhage occurs or even a possibility of its occurrence exists, a Swan-Ganz or similar catheter should be placed for better monitoring of physiologic functions and blood replacement. In extreme cases where no other vessels are available for rapid intraoperative blood volume replacement, transfusions may be given under pressure directly into the common iliac artery with the needle pointed in the direction of the heart.

The most frequent site of troublesome intraoperative bleeding during extensive hysterectomy occurs from the pelvic floor veins in the dissection of the cardinal ligament and the hypogastric vessels. The collateral venous circulation of the hypogastric veins is an ever-present source of troublesome bleeding owing to difficulty in identification of these vessels as they course among muscle bundles and fascial planes on the pelvic floor. The pararectal fossa, cardinal ligament, and pre-sacral and paraaortic areas are frequent sites of venous bleeding. Therefore, meticulous dissection is important to avoid such complications. When venous bleeding does occur it may be difficult to identify the site of the lacerated vein. In such circumstances it is important to use compression of the pelvic floor veins by either a sponge stick or finger held in place for no less than 7 minutes, or the use of an abdominal pack placed firmly against the site of bleeding for a similar length of time. In such cases it is advisable to keep pressure on the vein until full control of the bleeding has been established, in the meantime dissecting in other places in the pelvis. Only when the wall of a major pelvic vein has been severely traumatized and has retracted out of the operative field is there a serious problem in reestablishing hemostasis. In contrast to arterial bleeding, hemorrhage from deep pelvic veins is seldom benefitted by hypogastric artery ligation owing to the extensive collateral venous circulation to the pelvis from the lower extremity and vena cava. It occasionally is beneficial to ligate the anterior division of both hypogastric arteries to determine if interruption of the major arterial blood supply to the pelvis will reduce the venous bleeding. When more extensive trauma to the wall of the external or common iliac vein has occurred, it is necessary to place vascular clamps above and below the area of injury and to repair the defect with fine vascular sutures.

Postoperative Hemorrhage. This condition is a rare complication of extensive pelvic surgery. Because all of the blood supply to the pelvis has been skeletonized as part of the operative procedure, it is exceedingly rare for secondary hemorrhage to occur unless there has been uncontrolled bleeding at the completion of the operation. In such cases the pelvis usually is packed with multiple gauze packs with one end exteriorized through the open vagina. Tamponade of the pelvis by means of an umbrella (Logothetopolis) gauze pack and external ring (see Fig. 8-9) has been used in many clinics where there has been persistent venous oozing in the pelvis at the completion of the operation. Pelvic packs should be advanced within 24 to 48 hours and removed shortly thereafter, to avoid ascending infection from the vagina by aerobic and anaerobic bacteria.

Neuropathies

Nerve injury with extensive hysterectomy was reviewed by Hoffman and coworkers, who reported its infrequent occurrence. The most important injuries are to the femoral, obturator, peroneal, sciatic, genitofemoral, ilioinguinal, iliohypogastric, lateral femoral cutaneous, and pudendal nerves. An awareness of the anatomic location of these nerves in the operative field, careful surgical technique in dissection and securing hemostasis, careful placement of self-retaining retractors, and careful positioning of patients in stirrups will prevent most nerve injuries. Fortunately most nerve injuries are not associated with serious or permanent disability, but a few are.

Follow-up After Extensive Surgery for Cervical Cancer

Despite carefully planned and executed extensive surgery for stage I and stage IIa cervical cancer, 5% to 20% of patients in various series show evidence of recurrent or persistent tumor. About one-half occur in the 1st year after treatment. Almost all occur within the first 3 years. Few occur later. Very, very late recurrences are extremely rare after primary surgical treatment, and are more likely to be seen in patients treated with primary radiotherapy.

Persistent or recurrent disease after primary extensive surgery may represent incomplete resection of the central tumor undetected at operation or by the pathologist's examination of the surgical specimen. Microscopic metastatic involvement of lymph nodes may be undetected by incomplete pathology examination or left behind by incomplete lymphadenectomy. Viable tumor cells in small numbers may escape by way of lymphatics or vascular channels to distant sites and overcome host resistance. Probably in as many as 10% of patients with persistent disease it may result from continued growth of unrecognized intraperitoneal spread of tumor. Cytologic study of peritoneal fluid and washings may have been overlooked or may have been falsely negative.

After the immediate postoperative recovery is completed patients are scheduled for regular follow-up examinations, which will vary, depending on circumstances. Patients who are at greater risk for recurrence should be followed especially closely at frequent intervals. These usually are the same patients who have been given postoperative radiotherapy and include patients with metastatic disease in lymph nodes, close surgical margins, large-volume cervical tumors, lymph-vascular channel involvement, highly undifferentiated tumors, adenosquamous and glassy cell tumors, and positive peritoneal cytology. The frequency of examination varies somewhat from patient to patient. Most patients are seen every 2 to 3 months during the 1st and 2nd years after primary treatment, every 3 to 4 months during the 3rd and 4th years, and every 6 months to a year thereafter. Patients are instructed to report unusual signs or symptoms (eg, vaginal bleeding or discharge, leg swelling, discomfort in the pelvis, discomfort or swelling in the legs, difficulty with urination or defecation, enlarged nodes) at any time they appear. Krebs and coworkers, however, reported that 25% of their patients were asymptomatic when persistent disease was diagnosed. In the study reported by Larson and coworkers 37% were asymptomatic.

A follow-up examination should include palpation of the neck for enlarged lymph nodes, abdominal and leg examination, and a speculum and bimanual rectovaginal abdominal examination. A vaginal cytology smear is performed with each visit. CT scan of the abdomen and pelvis, proctosigmoidoscopy, cystoscopy, excretory urography, and biopsy (needle or punch, or both) of any suspicious lesions may be required, depending on the patient's symptoms and examination findings. These special diagnostic procedures are not done routinely as part of postoperative follow-up surveillance in asymptomatic patients. Positive findings are rare unless the patient is symptomatic. For example, excretory urography seldom shows ureteral obstruction in a patient who does not also have symptoms of pelvic sidewall persistent disease, and is, therefore, not routinely done at specific intervals. It is in the patient's best interest to have follow-up examinations done in the same center in which her treatment was administered. Current findings at each visit must be compared with previous information all the way back to her original presentation.

Soisson and coworkers reported a comparison of symptoms, physical examination, and vaginal cytology in the detection of recurrent cervical carcinoma after extensive hysterectomy. The study group consisted of 203 women with stage Ib and IIa cervical cancer followed at the Duke University Medical Center. Thirty-one (15%) developed recurrence. For the detection of recurrent tumor, vaginal cytology had a sensitivity and specificity of 13% and 100%, pelvic or general physical examination 58% and 96%, and the presence of suspicious symptoms 71% and 95%, respectively. Ninety-four percent of all patients with recurrent tumor had at least one abnormal surveillance index.

Of 817 patients with cervical cancer treated and followed, 50 (6.1%) developed pulmonary metastases, according to Imachi and coworkers. The percentage ranged from 3.2 in stage I to 20.9 in stage IV. The percentage was higher in patients with adenocarcinoma and undifferentiated carcinoma. Ninety-six percent occurred within 2 years of treatment, and local recurrence or other distant metastases were present in 81%. Chest radiographs should be done every 3 to 4 months during the first 2 years after treatment and every 6 to 12 months thereafter. Patients with pulmonary metastases may be offered chemotherapy or, occasionally, segmental lung resection for solitary lesions.

Regular pelvic examinations and vaginal cytology smears may detect a central pelvic recurrence early. This may be a great advantage. Just as it is important to detect the original cancer in the earliest stage possible, so that the patient may have the best possible chance of cure, so also is it important to detect persistent disease at the earliest possible moment, and for the same reason. For example, Jobsen and coworkers have recently reported on the use of radiotherapy to treat "locoregional recurrence" of carcinoma of the cervix after primary surgery. The overall 5-year survival was 44%. Response to radiotherapy was strongly correlated with tumor volume, providing additional supportive evidence to the idea that persistent disease should be diagnosed as early as possible and, it is hoped, when the volume of persistent tumor is still small and responsive.

Patients with recurrent or persistent cancer of the uterine cervix following initial radiation therapy can have extensive surgery provided the disease is limited and judged to be surgically resectable. Depending on the circumstances, an extensive hysterectomy and pelvic lymphadenectomy or some type of pelvic exenteration may be done. Ibsen and coworkers achieved a 31% 5-year survival among 47 women with postirradiation recurrent tumor.

Tumor ulceration in the upper vagina may produce vaginal discharge and spotting, a palpable tumor mass, and induration and nodularity of tissue extending to the pelvic sidewalls. Pain may not be present unless the tumor involves nerve roots. Symptoms related to urination and defecation may result from pressure, infection, or tumor involvement of the bladder and rectum. Either unilateral or bilateral edema of the lower extremities or unilateral or bilateral hydroureter and hydronephrosis may be an ominous sign of persistent disease, but also may be the result of a combination of the effects of extensive surgery and postoperative irradiation treatment. When initially diagnosed, recurrences may be central in about one-fourth of patients, may involve the pelvic sidewall in one-fourth, may involve distant sites in one-fourth, with the remaining one-fourth of patients showing multiple sites of involvement.

About 20% to 25% of patients with recurrence after primary extensive surgery may still be cured. The best chance of cure is in patients who had no postoperative radiation treatment and no metastatic disease to pelvic lymph nodes, and whose persistent disease is limited to the central pelvis. A combination of total pelvic irradiation to 5000 rad central pelvis plus vaginal brachytherapy may be effective in controlling the disease. When there is evidence of unresectable persistent disease in the pelvis in patients who have already received postoperative pelvic radiation, or there is persistent disease in distant sites, chemotherapy may be given for palliation but is not often effective in eradication of the disease. Fuller and coworkers analyzed the experience at the Memorial Sloan-Kettering Cancer Center, and reported that "none of the 29 patients with recurrent carcinoma and positive nodes at the time of their initial lymphadenectomy was successfully treated."

Because recurrence or persistence of cervical cancer after treatment is difficult but important to detect as early as possible, attempts have been made to use a serum marker that would monitor the course of the disease. Kato and Torigoe isolated a squamous cell carcinoma antigen from cervical carcinoma tissue. A squamous cell carcinoma antigen radioimmunoassay kit, developed by Abbott Laboratories, has been tested by Senekjian and coworkers and by Holloway and coworkers. In both studies serial serum levels of this antigen provided a fairly accurate means of monitoring regression and progression of disease after therapy. The test can be used as an adjunct to the other tests and follow-up examinations. When levels are elevated a more thorough search for persistent or recurrent disease can be carried out.

Although the early detection of persistence is the primary purpose of and justification for follow-up visits, assessment of urinary tract function also is important. Particular attention should be paid to bladder function and maintaining a satisfactory voiding pattern. Urinary tract infection should be diagnosed and treated promptly. If ureteral stenosis impairs renal function, early intervention may be successful in avoiding nephrectomy. This is more likely to be seen in patients who receive a combination of extensive surgery and irradiation as primary treatment.

Rehabilitation of sexual function after surgical therapy for cervical cancer usually is easily done by the patient and her partner, but is more difficult if the vagina and paravaginal tissues have received heavy doses of radiation or if the patient has lost ovarian function as a result of treatment. The gynecologic surgeon should inquire about sexual problems and should give advice and permission when needed. Counseling, including instruction in the technique of alternative means of sexual gratification (eg, interfemoral intercourse), may be needed (see Ch. 2). If ovarian function has been lost as a result of treatment, estrogen replacement therapy should be provided, even though symptoms of hypoestrogenism are not present. If normal

ovaries were conserved, their function should be monitored with periodic follicle-stimulating hormone and estrogen levels, so that estrogen replacement may be provided when ovaries cease functioning in future years. There may be other contraindications to estrogen replacement therapy in patients treated for cervical cancer, but a history of treatment for cervical cancer is not one of them.

And finally, patients who have been treated for cervical cancer are at greater risk for developing other primary cancers at different sites, especially if the treatment included irradiation. Detection of other primary cancers should be part of posttreatment follow-up. This subject has been studied by Hoffman and coworkers, Buchler, and others. Axelrod and coworkers reported that 3.9% of patients with invasive cervical cancer had second primaries. In 1987 Arneson and Kao reported that 61 new primary cancers were detected among 718 patients with invasive cervical cancer who had been studied from 1955 to 1979.

Summary

There have been many improvements in the operative technique of the extensive hysterectomy and lymphadenectomy since its original description. The incidence of complications after this procedure has decreased during the past three-quarters of a century and the survival rates have increased. The operation has achieved its peak of clinical usefulness during this period and is now considered to be the principal method of treatment of early invasive carcinoma of the cervix. Among the better surgical clinics the meticulous execution of this operative procedure has reduced the incidence of complications to an acceptable and infrequent occurrence. The operation affords little additional surgical risk to the patient than a hysterectomy performed for benign disease. In surgical clinics where the operation is performed well the 5-year cure rate of stage Ib carcinoma of the cervix varies between 85% and 90% of cases. When its use is extended for the treatment of stage IIa lesions the 5-year cure rate varies between 70% and 75%. Comparative studies with primary radiation therapy demonstrate an equal cure rate with primary radical surgery, although the complications of irradiation are far more difficult to manage than are those of primary surgery. In young women, when preservation of ovarian function is important, primary surgery is a preferable choice of treatment.

The major limiting factor in the long-term surgical cure of this tumor is related to the spread of the disease at the time of initiation of treatment. In cases where pelvic lymph nodes are positive for metastatic tumor the 5-year cure rate is reduced to about 60%. The use of postoperative irradiation in these cases is controversial, as there seems to be difficulty in showing statistically significant improvement of cure rates in long-term follow-up studies, as compared with control studies, in those cases where supplemental pelvic irradiation therapy is given. Because this question remains unanswered, it is our preference to give megavoltage irradiation therapy postoperatively to cases that have histologic evidence of pelvic lymph node metastases or close surgical margins, or both, since this additional treatment usually is well tolerated. The indications for extended-field postoperative irradiation to include paraaortic lymph nodes have not been firmly established.

It is important to understand that it is the individual surgical expertise that offers the highest cure rate and lowest incidence of complications to the patient with invasive carcinoma of the cervix. One of the greatest errors in clinical judgment is made by the gynecologist who attempts an extensive hysterectomy and pelvic lymph node dissection without adequate surgical experience. Unless the pelvic surgeon is performing this type of surgery regularly in a well-staffed medical center with trained assistants, he or she would be well advised to refer the patient to an established oncology center. From the patient's point of view, the initial treatment, whether primary surgery or irradiation, provides the best chance for long-term cure of this disease. It would be to her advantage to have the treatment conducted in the most expert hands, since secondary treatment for recurrent disease offers only limited long-term cure.

The gynecologic surgeon who becomes thoroughly familiar with the pathology and natural history of cervical cancer, who appreciates the history of the development of extensive hysterectomy and pelvic lymphadenectomy as primary treatment of the disease, and who then thoroughly masters the technical details of performing the operation can feel enormous pride in his or her achievement, for there is no greater challenge in gynecologic surgery and no greater personal satisfaction than that which comes to those who are able to perform the operation correctly and save a woman from the intense suffering and undignified death that cervical cancer can cause.

Bibliography

Ahrens CA, Tschoke S. Lymphknotenbefunde nach Wertheim-Meigscher operation. Geburtshilfe Frauenheilkd 1961;21:219.

Alvarez RD, Soong S-J, Kinney WK, et al. Identification of prognostic factors and risk groups in patients found to have nodal metastasis at the time of radical hysterectomy for early-stage squamous carcinoma of the cervix. Gynecol Oncol 1989;35:130.

Andras EJ, Fletcher GH, Rutledge F. Radiotherapy of carcinoma of the cervix following simple hysterectomy. Am J Obstet Gynecol 1973;115:647.

Anonymous. Deaths from cervical cancer, United States, 1984–1986. MMWR 1989;38:650.

Aoki S, Hata T, Senoh D, et al. Parametrial invasion of uterine cervical cancer assessed by transrectal ultrasonography: preliminary report. Gynecol Oncol 1990;36:82.

Arneson A, Kao MS. Long-term observations of cervical cancer. Am J Obstet Gynecol 1987;156:614.

Asmussen M, Ulmsten U. Simultaneous urethrocystometry and urethra pressure profile measurement with a new technique. Acta Obstet Gynecol Scand 1975;54:385.

Axelrod JH, Fruchter R, Boyce JG. Multiple primaries among gynecologic malignancies. Gynecol Oncol 1984;18:359.

Baltzer J, Kopcke W, Lohe KJ, et al. Die operative behandlung des zervixkarzinoms. Geburtshilfe Frauenheilkd 1984;44:279.

Baltzer J, Lohe KJ, Kopcke W, Zander J. Histologic criteria for the prognosis in patients with operated squamous cell carcinoma of the cervix. Gynecol Oncol 1982;13:184.

Bandy LC, Clarke-Pearson DL, Silverman PM, Creasman WT. Computed tomography in evaluation of extrapelvic lymphadenopathy in carcinoma of the cervix. Obstet Gynecol 1985;65:73.

Bandy LC, Clarke-Pearson DL, Soper JT, et al. Long-term effects on bladder function of radical hysterectomy with and without postoperative radiation. Gynecol Oncol 1987;26:160.

Barter JF, Soong S-J, Shingleton HM, et al. Complications of combined radical hysterectomy–postoperative radiation. Gynecol Oncol 1989;32:292.

Bendvold E, Kjorstad KE. Antibiotic prophylaxis for radical abdominal hysterectomy. Gynecol Oncol 1987;28:201.

Berek JS, Brand E. Controversies in the management of cervical adenocarcinoma [Reply to letter to the editor]. Obstet Gynecol 1988;72:289.

Berek JS, Hacker NF, Fu Y, et al. Adenocarcinoma of the uterine cervix: histologic variables associated with lymph node metastasis and survival. Obstet Gynecol 1985;65:46.

Berman ML, Lagassee LD, Watring WG, et al. The operative evaluation of patients with cervical carcinoma by an extraperitoneal approach. Obstet Gynecol 1977;50:658.

Bithal PK, Vijayaraghavan S, Shahani JM, Oberoi GS. Bold loss in Wertheim's hysterectomy: comparison of three anaesthetic techniques. Indian J Med Sci 1987;41:78.

Bleker OP, Ketting BW, van Wayjen-Eecen B, Kloosterman GJ. The significance of microscopic involvement of the parametrium and/or pelvic lymph nodes in cervical cancer stages IB and IIA. Gynecol Oncol 1983;6:56.

Blythe JG, Hodel KA, Wahl TP. A comparison between peritoneal sheathing of the ureters (Ohkawa technique) and retroperitoneal pelvic suction drainage in the prevention of ureteral damage during radical abdominal hysterectomy. Gynecol Oncol 1988;30:222.

Bonney V. The results of 500 cases of Wertheim's operation for carcinoma of the cervix. J Obstet Gynaecol Br Emp 1941;48:421.

Bonney V. Wertheim's operation in retrospect. Lancet 1949;1:637.

Bradbeer C. Is infection with HIV a risk factor for cervical intraepithelial neoplasia? Lancet 1987;2:1277.

Brand E, Berek JS, Hacker NF. Controversies in the management of cervical adenocarcinoma. Obstet Gynecol 1988;71:261.

Breen JA. Personal communication. 1989.

Brodman M, Friedman F, Dottino P, et al. A comparative study of computerized tomography, magnetic resonance imaging, and clinical staging for the detection of early cervix cancer. Gynecol Oncol 1990;36:409.

Brown JV, Peters WA, Corwin DJ. Invasive carcinoma after cone biopsy for cervical intraepithelial neoplasia. Gynecol Oncol 1991;40:25.

Buchler DA. Multiple primaries and gynecologic malignancies. Am J Obstet Gynecol 1975;123:376.

Buchsbaum HJ. Extrapelvic lymph node metastases in cervical carcinoma. Am J Obstet Gynecol 1979;133:814.

Burghardt E, Pickel H. Local spread and lymph node involvement in cervical cancer. Obstet Gynecol 1978;52:138.

Burghardt E, Hofmann HMH, Ebner F, et al. Magnetic resonance imaging in cervical cancer: a basis for objective classification. Gynecol Oncol 1989;33:61.

Burghardt E, Pickel H, Haas J, Lahousen M. Prognostic factors and operative treatment of stages IB to IIB cervical cancer. Am J Obstet Gynecol 1987;156:988.

Camilien L, Gordon D, Fruchter RG, et al. Predictive value of computerized tomography in the presurgical evaluation of primary carcinoma of the cervix. Gynecol Oncol 1988;30:209.

Chambers SK, Chambers JT, Holm C, et al. Sequelae of lateral ovarian transposition in unirradiated cervical cancer patients. Gynecol Oncol 1990;39:155.

Clark JG. A more radical method of performing hysterectomy for cancer of the uterus. Bull Johns Hopkins Hosp 1895;6:120.

Clarke-Pearson DL, DeLong E, Synan IS, et al. A controlled trial of two low-dose heparin regimens for the prevention of postoperative deep vein thrombosis. Obset Gynecol 1990;75:684.

Clarke-Pearson DL, Jelovsek FR, Creasman WT. Thromboembolism complicating surgery for cervical and uterine malignancy: incidence, risk factors, and prophylaxis. Obstet Gynecol 1983;61:87.

Collins HS, Burke TW, Woodward JE, et al. Widespread lymph node metastases in a patient with microinvasive cervical carcinoma. Gynecol Oncol 1989;34:219.

Corbett PJ, Crompton AC. Invasive carcinoma of one cervix in a uterus didelphys. Br J Obstet Gynaecol 1982;89:171.

Crawford JS, Harisiadis L, McDowan L, Rogers CC. Para-aortic lymph node irradiation in cervical carcinoma without prior lymphadenectomy. Radiology 1987;164:255.

Creasman WT, Fetter BF, Clarke-Pearson DL, et al. Management of stage IA carcinoma of the cervix. Am J Obstet Gynecol 1985;153:164.

Day NE. Effect of cervical cancer screening in Scandinavia. Obstet Gynecol 1984;63:714.

DeJesus M, Tang W, Sadjadi M, et al. Carcinoma of the cervix with extensive endometrial and myometrial involvement. Gynecology 1990;36:263.

Devesa SS. Descriptive epidemiology of cancer of the uterine cervix. Obstet Gynecol 1984;63:605.

Dottino PR, Plaxe SC, Beddoe AM, et al. Induction chemotherapy followed by radical surgery in cervical cancer. Gynecol Oncol 1991;40:7.

Downey GO, Potish RA, Adcock LL, et al. Pretreatment surgical staging in cervical carcinoma: therapeutic efficacy of pelvic lymph node resection. Am J Obstet Gynecol 1989;160:1055.

Drescher CW, Hopkins MP, Roberts JA. Comparison of the pattern of metastatic spread of squamous cell cancer and adenocarcinoma of the uterine cervix. Gynecol Oncol 1989;33:340.

Durrance FY, Fletcher GH, Rutledge FN. Analysis of central recurrent disease in stages I and II squamous cell carcinomas of the cervix on intact uterus. Am J Roentgenol Radiat Ther Nucl Med 1969;106:831.

Eisenkop SM, Spirtos NM, Montag TW, et al. The clinical significance of blood transfusion at the time of radical hysterectomy. Obstet Gynecol 1990;76:110.

Ellsworth LR, Allen HH, Nisker JA. Ovarian function after radical hysterectomy for stage IB carcinoma of the cervix. Am J Obstet Gynecol 1983;145:185.

Fiorica JV, Roberts WS, Greenberg H, et al. Morbidity and survival patterns after radical hysterectomy and postoperative adjuvant pelvic radiotherapy. Gynecol Oncol 1990;36:343.

Fishman IJ, Shabsigh R, Kaplan AL. Lower urinary tract dysfunction after radial hysterectomy for carcinoma of the cervix. Urology 1986;28:462.

Fletcher GH. Predominant parameters in the planning of radiation therapy of carcinoma of the cervix. Bull Cancer 1979;66:561.

Fraser AC. Late effects of Wertheim's hysterectomy on the urinary tract. J Obstet Gynaecol Br Comm 1966;73:1002.

Freund WA. Eine neue methode der exstirpation des ganzen uterus. Zentralbl Gynakol 1878;10:222.

Freund WA. Method of complete removal of the uterus. Am J Obstet Gynecol 1879;7:200.

Fuller AF Jr, Elliott N, Kosloff C, Lewis JL Jr. Lymph node metastases from carcinoma of the cervix, stage Ib and IIa: implications for prognosis and treatment. Gynecol Oncol 1982;13:165.

Fuller AF Jr, Elliott N, Kosloff C, et al. Determinants of increased risk for recurrence in patients undergoing radical hysterectomy for stage IB and IIA carcinoma of the cervix. Gynecol Oncol 1989;33:34.

Gal D, Buchsbaum HJ. A cinefluoroscopic study of ureteral function following radical hysterectomy. Obstet Gynecol 1983;61:82.

Gallion HH, van Nagell JR Jr, Donaldson ES, et al. Combined radiation therapy and extrafascial hysterectomy in the treatment of stage IB barrel-shaped cervical cancer. Cancer 1985;56:262.

Gallup DG, Jordan GH, Talledo OE. Extraperitoneal lymph node dissections with use of a midline incision on patients with female genital cancer. Am J Obstet Gynecol 1986;155:559.

Gallus AS, Hirsh J, Tuttle RJ, et al. Small subcutaneous doses of heparin in prevention of venous thrombosis. N Engl J Med 1973;228:545.

Girardi F, Lichtenegger W, Tamussino K, Haas J. The importance of parametrial lymph nodes in the treatment of cervical cancer. Gynecol Oncol 1989;34:206.

Goldberger SB, Rosen DJD, Fejgin MD, et al. An unusually aggressive verrucose carcinoma of the uterine cervix. Acta Obstet Gynecol Scand 1988;67:369.

Goodman HM, Buttlar CA, Niloff JM, et al. Adenocarcinoma of the uterine cervix: prognostic factors and patterns of recurrence. Gynecol Oncol 1989;33:241.

Gordon-Smith IC, Grundy DJ, LeQuesne LP, et al. Controlled trial of two regimens of subcutaneous heparin in prevention of postoperative deep vein thrombosis. Lancet 1972;1:1133.

Green TH Jr, Meigs JV, Ulfelder H, Curtin RR. Urologic complications of radical Wertheim hysterectomy: incidence, etiology, management and prevention. Obstet Gynecol 1962;20:293.

Greer BE, Easterling TR, McLennan DA, et al. Fetal and maternal considerations in the management of stage I-B cervical cancer during pregnancy. Gynecol Oncol 1989;34:61.

Greer BE, Figge DC, Tamimi HK, Cain JM. Stage IB adenocarcinoma of the cervix treated by radical hysterectomy and pelvic lymph node dissection. Am J Obstet Gynecol 1989;160:1509.

Heller PB, Barnhill DR, Mayer AR, et al. Cervical carcinoma found incidentally in an uterus removed for benign conditions. Obstet Gynecol 1986;67:187.

Henriksen E. Lymphatic spread of carcinoma of the cervix and of body of uterus. Study of 420 necropsies. Am J Obstet Gynecol 1949;58:924.

Hoffman MS, Roberts WS, Cavanagh D. Second pelvic malignancies following radiation therapy for cervical cancer. Obstet Gynecol Surv 1985;40:611.

Hoffman MS, Roberts WS, Cavanagh D. Neuropathies associated with radical pelvic surgery for gynecologic cancer. Gynecol Oncol 1988;31:462.

Hogan WM, Littman P, Griner L, et al. Results of radiation therapy given after radical hysterectomy. Cancer 1982;49:1278.

Holloway RW, To A, Moradi M, et al. Monitoring the course of cervical carcinoma with the squamous cell carcinoma serum radioimmunoassay. Obstet Gynecol 1989;74:944.

Hopkins MP, Schmidt RW, Roberts JA, Morley GW. Gland cell carcinoma (adenocarcinoma) of the cervix. Obstet Gynecol 1988;72:789.

Hopkins MP, Schmidt RW, Roberts JA, Morley GW. The prognosis and treatment of stage I adenocarcinoma of the cervix. Obstet Gynecol 1988;72:915.

Horii T, Mitsumoto T, Noda K. Significance of para-aortic node irradiation in the treatment of cervical cancer. Gynecol Oncol 1988;31:371.

Hughes RR, Brewington KC, Hanjani P, et al. Extended field irradiation for cervical cancer based on surgical staging. Gynecol Oncol 1980;9:153.

Husseinzadeh N, Nahhas WA, Velkley DE, et al. The preservation of ovarian function in young women undergoing pelvic radiation therapy. Gynecol Oncol 1984:18:373.

Ibsen TB, Sorensen BL, Knudsen JB, Sorensen HM. Operative treatment of recurrent cancer of the uterine cervix after radiotherapy. Acta Obstet Gynecol Scand 1988;67:389.

Imachi M, Tsukamoto N, Matsuyama T, Nakano H. Pulmonary metastasis from carcinoma of the uterine cervix. Gynecol Oncol 1989;33:189.

Inoue T, Morita K. 5-Year results of postoperative extended-field irradiation of 76 patients with nodal metastases from cervical carcinoma stages Ib to IIIb. Cancer 1988;61:2009.

Inoue T, Okumura M. Prognostic significance of parametrial extension in patients with cervical carcinoma stages Ib, IIa, and IIb: a study of 628 cases treated by radical hysterectomy and lymphadenectomy with or without postoperative irradiation. Cancer 1984;4:1714.

International Federation of Gynecology and Obstetrics. Annual report of the results of treatment in gynecological cancer. Vol 20. Stockholm: 1988.

Jobsen JJ, Leer JWH, Cleton FJ, Hermans J. Treatment of locoregional recurrence of carcinoma of the cervix by radiotherapy after primary surgery. Gynecol Oncol 1989;33:368.

Jones HW, Jones GES. Panhysterectomy versus irradiation in early cancer of the cervix. JAMA 1943;122:930.

Jones WB. Surgical approaches for advanced or recurrent cancer of the cervix. Cancer 1987;60:2094.

Kadar N, Saliba N, Nelson JH. The frequency, causes, and prevention of severe urinary dysfunction after radical hysterectomy. Br J Obstet Gynaecol 1983;90:858.

Kakkar VV, Corrigan TP, Fossard DP. Prevention of fetal postoperative pulmonary embolism by low dose heparin. Lancet 1975;2:45.

Kakkar VV, Corrigan T, Spindler J, et al. Efficacy of low doses of heparin in prevention of deep-vein thrombosis after major surgery. Lancet 1972;2:101.

Kakkar VV, Field ES, Nicholaides AN, Flute PT. Low dose of heparin in prevention of deep-vein thrombosis. Lancet 1971;2:669.

Kashimura M, Shinohara M, Oikawa K, et al. An adenocarcinoma *in situ* of the uterine cervix that developed into invasive adenocarcinoma after 5 years. Gynecol Oncol 1990;36:128.

Kato H, Torigoe T. Radioimmunoassay for tumor antigen of human cervical squamous cell carcinoma. Cancer 1977;40:1621.

Kim DS, Moon H, Kim KT, et al. Two-year survival: preoperative adjuvant chemotherapy in the treatment of cervical cancer stages Ib and II with bulky tumor. Gynecol Oncol 1989;33:225.

Kim DS, Moon H, Hwang YY, Cho SH. Preoperative adjuvant chemotherapy in the treatment of cervical cancer stage Ib, IIa, IIb with bulky tumor. Gynecol Oncol 1988;29:321.

Kinney WK, Alvarez RD, Reid GC, et al. Value of adjuvant whole pelvic irradiation after Wertheim hysterectomy for early-stage squamous carcinoma of the cervix with pelvic nodal metastasis: a matched controlled study. Gynecol Oncol 1989;34:258.

Kinney WK, Egorshin EV, Podratz KC. Wertheim hysterectomy in the geriatric population. Gynecol Oncol 1988;31:227.

Kishi Y, Hashimoto Y, Sakamoto Y, Inui S. Thickness of uninvolved fibromuscular stroma and extrauterine spread of carcinoma of the uterine cervix. Cancer 1987;60:2331.

Kjorstad KE, Martimbeau PW, Iverson T. Stage IB carcinoma of the cervix, the Norwegian Radium Hospital: results and complications. Gynecol Oncol 1983;15:42.

Knapp RC, Donahue VC, Friedman EA. Dissection of paravesical and pararectal spaces in pelvic operations. Surg Gynecol Obstet 1973;137:758.

Kolstad P. Follow-up study of 232 patients with stage Ia1 and 411 patients with stage Ia2 squamous cell carcinoma of the cervix (microinvasive carcinoma). Gynecol Oncol 1989;33:265.

Krebs HB, Helmkamp BF, Sevin B-U, et al. Recurrent cancer of the cervix following radical hysterectomy and pelvic node dissection. Obstet Gynecol 1982;59:422.

Kundrat R. Uber die ausbreitung des karzinoms in parametranen gewebe beim krebs des collum uteri. Arch Gynakol 1903;69:355.

Lagasse LD, Creasman WT, Shingleton HM, et al. Results and complications of operative staging in cervical cancer: experience of the gynecologic oncology group. Gynecol Oncol 1980;9:90.

Lai C-H, Lin T-S, Soong Y-K, et al. Adjuvant chemotherapy after radical hysterectomy for cervical carcinoma. Gynecol Oncol 1989;35:193.

Langley II, Moore DW, Tarnasky JW, Roberts PHR. Radical hysterectomy and pelvic lymph node dissection. Gynecol Oncol 1980;9:37.

Lapolla JP, Schlaerth JB, Gaddis O, Morrow CP. The influence of surgical staging on the evaluation and treatment of patients with cervical carcinoma. Gynecol Oncol 1986;24:194.

Larson DM, Copeland LJ, Malone JM Jr, et al. Diagnosis of recurrent cervical carcinoma after radical hysterectomy. Obstet Gynecol 1988;71:6.

Larson DM, Stringer CA, Copeland LJ, et al. Stage IB cervical carcinoma treated with radical hysterectomy and pelvic lymphadenectomy: role of adjuvant radiotherapy. Obstet Gynecol 1987;69:378.

Latzko W, Schiffmann J. Klinisches und anatomisches zur radikaloperation des gebarmutterkrebses. Zentralbl Gynakol 1919;43:715.

Lee RB, Weisbaum GS, Heller PB, Park RC. Scalene node biopsy in primary and recurrent invasive carcinoma of the cervix. Gynecol Oncol 1981;11:200.

Leitch A. On the pathological bases of operations for cancer of the uterus. Trans R Soc Med, London, Obstet Gynecol 1910;4:69.

Lovecchio JL, Averette HE, Donato D, Bell J. 5-Year survival of patients with periaortic nodal metastases in clinical stage IB and IIA cervical carcinoma. Gynecol Oncol 1989;34:43.

Low JA, Mauger GM, Carmichael JA. The effect of Wertheim hysterectomy upon bladder and urethral function. Am J Obstet Gynecol 1981;139:826.

Lunt R. Worldwide early detection of cervical cancer. Obstet Gynecol 1984;63:708.

McCall ML, Keaty EC, Thompson JD. Conservation of ovarian tissue in the treatment of carcinoma of the cervix with radical surgery. Am J Obstet Gynecol 1958;75:590.

Maiman MA, Fruchter RG, DiMaio TM, Boyce JG. Superficially invasive squamous cell carcinoma of the cervix. Obstet Gynecol 1988;72:399.

Mann WJ. Controversies in the management of cervical adenocarcinoma [Letter to the editor]. Obstet Gynecol 1988;72:289.

Mann WJ, Chumas J, Amalfitano T, et al. Ovarian metastases from stage Ib adenocarcinoma of the cervix. Cancer 1987;60:1123.

Mann WJ, Vogel F, Patsner B, Chalas E. Management of lymphocysts after radical gynecologic surgery. Gynecol Oncol 1989;33:248.

Matsukuma K, Tsukamoto N, Matsuyama T, et al. Preoperative CT study of lymph nodes in cervical cancer—its correlation with histological findings. Gynecol Oncol 1989;33:168.

Matsuyama T, Inoue I, Tsukamoto N, et al. Stage Ib, IIa, and IIb cervical cancer, postsurgical staging and prognosis. Cancer 1984;54:3072.

Mattingly RF, Thompson JD, eds. Te Linde's operative gynecology. 6th ed. Philadelphia: JB Lippincott, 1985.

Meigs JV. Carcinoma of the cervix: the Wertheim operation. Surg Gynecol Obstet 1944;78:195.

Meigs JV. The Wertheim operation for carcinoma of the cervix. Am J Obstet Gynecol 1945;49:542.

Mitra S. Radikale vaginale hysterektomie and extraperitoneale lymphadenektomie bei zervixkrebs. Zentralbl Gynakol 1951;73(5a):574.

Moore DH, Fowler WC, Walton LA, Droegemueller W. Morbidity of lymph node sampling in cancers of the uterine corpus and cervix. Obstet Gynecol 1989;74:180.

Morley GW, Seski JC. Radical pelvic surgery vs. radiation therapy for stage I carcinoma of the cervix (exclusive of microcarcinoma). Am J Obstet Gynecol 1976;126:785.

Morrow CP. Panel report: Is pelvic radiation beneficial in the post-operative management of stage Ib squamous cell carcinoma of the cervix with pelvic node metastases treated by radical hysterectomy and pelvic lymphadenectomy? Gynecol Oncol 1980;10:105.

Morton DG, Kerner JA. Reactions to x-ray and radium therapy in the treatment of cancer of the uterine cervix. Am J Obstet Gynecol 1949;57:625.

Mundy AR. An anatomical explanation of bladder dysfunction following rectal and uterine surgery. Br J Urol 1982;54:501.

Nahhas WA, Abt AB, Mortel R. Stage Ib glassy cell carcinoma of the cervic with ovarian metastases. Gynecol Oncol 1977;5:87.

National Cancer Institute. Cancer statistics review, 1973–1986. Bethesda, Maryland: National Institutes of Health, 1989; DHHS publication no. 2789.

Natsume M. Systematic radical surgery for carcinoma of uterine cervix. Tokyo: NanKodo, 1973.

Navratil E. Indications and results of the vaginal and abdominal radical operation in the treatment of carcinoma of the cervix. J Int Coll Surg 1965;43:82.

Nelson JH, Boyce J, Macasaet M, et al. Incidence, significance and follow-up of para-aortic lymph node metastases in late invasive carcinoma of the cervix. Am J Obstet Gynecol 1977;128:336.

Novak F. Gynakologische operationstechnik. Piccin Editore-Padova. Berlin: Springer-Verlag, 1978.

O'Quinn AG, Fletcher GH, Wharton JT. Guidelines for conservative hysterectomy after irradiation. Gynecol Oncol 1980;9:68.

Okabayashi H. Radical abdominal hysterectomy for cancer of the cervix uteri. Surg Gynecol Obstet 1921;33:335.

Orr JW, Shingleton HM, Hatch KD, et al. Correlation of perioperative morbidity and conization to radical hysterectomy interval. Obstet Gynecol 1982;59:726.

Owens S, Roberts WS, Fiorica JV, et al. Ovarian management at the time of radical hysterectomy for cancer of the cervix. Gynecol Oncol 1989;35:349.

Papavasilou C, Yiagarakis D, Pappas J, Keramopoulos A. Treatment of cervical carcinoma by total hysterectomy and postoperative external irradiation. Int J Radiat Oncol Biol Phys 1980;6:871.

Parker LA, McPhail AH, Yankaska BC, Mauro MA. Computed tomography in the evaluation of clinical stage Ib carcinoma of the cervix. Gynecol Oncol 1990;37:332.

Parsons L, Cesare F, Friedell GH. Primary surgical treatment of invasive cancer of the cervix. Surg Gynecol Obstet 1959;109:279.

Piver MS, Rutledge F, Smith JP. Five classes of extended hysterectomy for women with cervical cancer. Obstet Gynecol 1974;44:265.

Plentl AA, Friedman EA. Lymphatic system of the female genitalia. Philadelphia: WB Saunders, 1974.

Podczaski ES, Palombo C, Manetta A, et al. Assessment of pretreatment laparotomy in patients with cervical carcinoma prior to radiotherapy. Gynecol Oncol 1980;33:71.

Potish RA, Downey GO, Adcock LL, et al. The role of surgical debulking in cancer of the uterine cervix. Int J Radiat Oncol Biol Phys 1989;17:979.

Powell JL, Mogelnicki SR, Franklin EW III, et al. A deliberate hypotensive technique for decreasing blood loss during radical hysterectomy and pelvic lymphadenectomy. Am J Obstet Gynecol 1983;147:196.

Rampone JF, Klem FV, Kolstad P. Combined treatment of stage IB carcinoma of the cervix. Obstet Gynecol 1973;41:163.

Reiffenstuhl G. The lymphatics of the female genital organs. Philadelphia: JB Lippincott, 1964.

Reiffenstuhl G. The clinical significance of the connective tissue planes and spaces. Clin Obstet Gynecol 1982;25:811.

Reis E. Modern treatment of carcinoma of the uterus. Chicago Med Res 1895;9:284.

Rellihan MA, Dooley DP, Curke TW, et al. Rapidly progressing cervical cancer in a patient with human immunodeficiency virus infection. Gynecol Oncol 1990;36:435.

Roberts WS, Cavanagh D, Marsden DE, Roberts VC. Urinary tract fistulas following ligation of the internal iliac artery during radical hysterectomy. Gynecol Oncol 1985;21:359.

Rosenshein NB, Ruth JC, Villar J, et al. A prospective randomized study of doxycycline as a prophylactic antibiotic in patients undergoing radical hysterectomy. Gynecol Oncol 1983;15:201.

Rotmensch J, Rosenshein NB, Woodruff JD. Cervical sarcoma: a review. Obstet Gynecol Surv 1983;38:456.

Rubin SC, Brookland R, Mikuta JJ, et al. Para-aortic nodal metastases in early cervical carcinoma: long-term survival following extended field radiotherapy. Gynecol Oncol 1984;18:213.

Russell AH, Tong DY, Figge DC, et al. Adjuvant postoperative pelvic radiation for carcinoma of the uterine cervix: pattern of cancer recurrence in patients undergoing elective radiation following radical hysterectomy and pelvic lymphadenectomy. Int J Radiat Oncol Biol Phys 1984;10:211.

Rutledge FN, Fletcher GH, MacDonald RJ. Pelvic lymphadenectomy as an adjunct to radiation therapy in treatment for cancer of the cervix. Am J Roentgenol Radium Ther Nucl Med 1965;93:607.

Saigo PE, Cain JM, Kim WS, et al. Prognostic factors in adenocarcinoma of the uterine cervix. Cancer 1986;57:1584.

Sall S, Rini S, Pineda A. Surgical management of invasive carcinoma of the cervix in pregnancy. Am J Obstet Gynecol 1974;118:1.

Sampson JA. A careful study of the parametrium in twenty-seven cases of carcinoma cervicis uteri and its clinical significance. Am J Obstet 1906;54:433.

Sardi J, Sananes C, Giaroli A, et al. Is subradical surgical treatment for carcinoma of the cervix uteri stage Ib logical? Gynecol Oncol 1989;32:360.

Sasaki H, Yoshida T, Noda K, et al. Urethral pressure profiles following radical hysterectomy. Obstet Gynecol 1982;59:101.

Sauter JN. Die ganzlich exstirpation der carcinomatosen. Gebarmutter ohne Vorfall Konstanz. 1822.

Schellhas HF. Extraperitoneal para-aortic node dissection through an upper abdominal incision. Obstet Gynecol 1975;46:444.

Schmidt RTF. Panhysterectomy in the treatment of carcinoma of the uterine cervix: evaluation of results. JAMA 1951;146:1310.

Scotti RJ, Bergman A, Bhatia NN, Ostergard DR. Urodynamic changes in urethrovesical function after radical hysterectomy. Obstet Gynecol 1986;68:111.

Seibel MM, Freeman MG, Graves WL. Carcinoma of the cervix and sexual function. Obstet Gynecol 1980;55:484.

Seibel MM, Freeman MG, Graves WL. The effect of surgical and radiation treatment for cervical carcinoma on sexual function. South Med J 1982;75:1195.

Senekjian EK, Young JM, Weiser PA, et al. An evaluation of squamous cell carcinoma antigen in patients with cervical squamous cell carcinoma. Am J Obstet Gynecol 1987;157:433.

Sevin B-U, Ramos R, Lichtinger M, et al. Antibiotic prevention of infections complicating radical abdominal hysterectomy. Obstet Gynecol 1984;64:539.

Sheets EE, Berman ML, Hrountas CK, et al. Surgically treated, early-stage neuroendocrine small-cell cervical carcinoma. Obstet Gynecol 1988;71:10.

Shy K, Chu J, Mandelson M, et al. Papanicolaou smear screening interval and risk of cervical cancer. Obstet Gynecol 1989;74:838.

Silva EG, Kott MM, Ordonez NG. Endocrine carcinoma intermediate cell type of the uterine cervix. Cancer 1984;54:1705.

Silverberg E, Lubera JA. Cancer statistics, 1989. CA 1980;39:3.

Slattery ML, Overall JC, Abbott TM, et al. Sexual activity, contraception, genital infections, and cervical cancer: support for a sexually transmitted disease hypothesis. Am J Epidemiol 1989;130:248.

Soisson AP, Geszler G, Soper JT, et al. A comparison of symptomatology, physical examination, and vaginal cytology in the detection of recurrent cervical carcinoma after radical hysterectomy. Obstet Gynecol 1990;76:106.

Soisson AP, Soper JT, Clarke-Pearson DL, et al. Adjuvant radiotherapy following radical hysterectomy for patients with stage Ib and IIa cervical cancer. Gynecol Oncol 1990;37:390.

Speert H. Obstetrical-gynecological eponyms: Ernst Wertheim and his operation for uterine cancer. Cancer 1956;9:859.

Spurett B, Jones DS, Stewart G. Cervical dysplasia and HIV infection. Lancet 1988;1:237.

Stallworthy J. Radical surgery following radiation treatment for cervical carcinoma. Ann R Coll Surg Engl 1964;34:161.

Stallworthy J. Pelvic cancer priorities. Am J Obstet Gynecol 1976;126:777.

Sutton G, Bundy B, Delgado G, et al. Ovarian metastases in stage IB carcinoma of the cervix. Presented at the Annual Clinical Meeting of the American College of Obstetricians and Gynecologists, San Francisco, May 5-10, 1990.

Symmonds RE. Morbidity and complications of radical hysterectomy with pelvic lymph node dissection. Am J Obstet Gynecol 1966;94:663.

Symmonds RE. Some surgical aspects of gynecological cancer. Cancer 1975;36:646.

Symmonds RE, Pratt JH. Prevention of fistulas and lymphocysts in radical hysterectomy: preliminary report of a new technic. Obstet Gynecol 1961;17:57.

Symonds RP, Burnett RA, Habeshaw T, et al. The prognostic value of a response to chemotherapy given before radiotherapy in advanced cancer of the cervix. Br J Cancer 1989;59:473.

Tabata M, Ichinoe K, Sakuragi N, et al. Incidence of ovarian metastases in patients with cancer of the uterine cervix. Gynecol Oncol 1987;28:255.

Talbert LM, Palumbo L, Shingleton H, et al. Urologic complications of radical hysterectomy for carcinoma of the cervix. South Med J 1965;58:11.

Teshima S, Shimosato Y, Kishi K, et al. Early stage adenocarcinoma of the uterine cervix. Histopathologic analysis with consideration of histogenesis. Cancer 1985;56:167.

Thigpen JT, Blessing JA, DiSaia PJ, et al. A randomized comparison of a rapid versus prolonged (24 hr) infusion of cisplatin in therapy of squamous cell carcinoma of the uterine cervix: a Gynecologic Oncology Group Study. Gynecol Oncol 1989;32:198.

Thompson JD, Caputo TA, Franklin EW III, Dale E. The surgical management of invasive cancer of the cervix in pregnancy. Am J Obstet Gynecol 1975;121:853.

Tinga DJ, Timmer PR, Bouma J, Aalders JG. Prognostic significance of single versus multiple lymph node metastases in cervical carcinoma stage Ib. Gynecol Oncol 1990;39:175.

To ACW, Gore H, Shingleton HM, et al. Lymph node metastasis in cancer of the cervix: a preliminary report. Am J Obstet Gynecol 1986;155:388.

Tulzer H, Kupka S. The effectiveness of obligatory lymphadenectomy in treating carcinoma of the cervix. Int J Gynaecol Obstet 1978;16:197.

Uyttenbroeck F. Verleden en heden van de radicale chirurgie in de gynecologische oncologie. Verh K Acad Geneeskd Belg 1987;49(1):5.

van Nagell JR Jr, Donaldson ES, Parker JC, et al. The prognostic significance of pelvic lymph node morphology in carcinoma of the uterine cervix. Cancer 1977;39:2624.

van Nagell JR Jr, Greenwell N, Powell DF, et al. Microinvasive carcinoma of the cervix. Am J Obstet Gynecol 1983;145:981.

Vercamer R, Janssens J, Usewils R, et al. Computed tomography and lymphography in the presurgical staging of early carcinoma of the uterine cervix. Cancer 1987;60:1745.

Vesterinen E, Forss M, Nieminen V. Increase of cervical adenocarcinoma: a report of 520 cases of cervical carcinoma including 112 tumors with glandular elements. Gynecol Oncol 1989;33:49.

Walker J, Bloss JD, Liao S, et al. Human papillomavirus genotype as a prognostic indicator in carcinoma of the uterine cervix. Obstet Gynecol 1989;74:781.

Webb GA. The role of ovarian conservation in the treatment of carcinoma of the cervix with radical surgery. Am J Obstet Gynecol 1975;122:476.

Webb MJ, Symmonds RE. Wertheim hysterectomy: a reappraisal. Obstet Gynecol 1979;54:140.

Weiser EB, Bundy BN, Hoskins WJ, et al. Extraperitoneal versus transperitoneal selective para-aortic lymphadenectomy in the pretreatment surgical staging of advanced cervical carcinoma (a Gynecologic Oncology Group Study). Gynecol Oncol 1989;33:283.

Welander CE, Pierce VK, Nori D, et al. Pretreatment laparotomy in carcinoma of the cervix. Gynecol Oncol 1981;12:336.

Wentz WB, Reagan JW. Survival in cervical cancer with respect to cell type. Cancer 1959;12:384.

Wertheim E. Zur frag der radikaloperation beim uteruskrebs. Arch Gynakol 1900;61:627.

Wertheim E. Discussion on the diagnosis and treatment of carcinoma of the uterus. Br Med J 1905;2:689.

Wertheim E. Die erweiterte abdominale operation bei carcinoma colli uteri (auf grund von 500 fallen). Berlin: Urban, 1911.

Wertheim E. The extended abdominal operation for carcinoma of the cervix. Am J Obstet Gynecol 1912;66:169.

Wharton JT, Jones HW III, Day TG, et al. Preirradiation celiotomy and extended field irradiation for invasive carcinoma of the cervix. Obstet Gynecol 1977;49:333.

Wilkinson EJ, Hause L. Probability in lymph node sectioning. Cancer 1974;33:1269.

Willen H, Willen R, Stendahl U: Invasive squamous cell carcinoma of the uterine cervix. VI. Prediction value of non-keratinizing, para-keratotic and orthokeratotic cell forms and clinical staging. Acta Radiol (Oncol) 1982;21:401.

Williams HT. Prevention of postoperative deep-vein thrombosis with perioperative subcutaneous heparin. Lancet 1971;2:950.

Wong C-H, Tso H-S, Ho ES, Mok MS. Induced hypotension during radical hysterectomy and bilateral pelvic lymphadenectomy. Anesth Sinica 1985;23:181.

Zander J, Baltzer J, Lohe KJ, et al. Carcinoma of the cervix: an attempt to individualize treatment. Results of a 20 year cooperative study. Am J Obstet Gynecol 1981;139:752.

Zaritzky D, Blake D, Willard J, Resnick M. Transrectal ultrasonography in the evaluation of cervical carcinoma. Obstet Gynecol 1979;53:105.

Zweifel P. Zum Ancleken an die erste Totalexstirpation des Karzinomaatosen uterus. (Ausgefuhrt von Dr. John Neb Sauter in konstanz) Much Med Wochem 1922;69:19.

Malignant Tumors of the Uterine Corpus

43

JOHN L. CURRIE

Cancer of the uterine corpus is the most common cancer in the female lower reproductive tract. The vast majority of these tumors are endometrial in origin, accounting for more than 95% of cases, while tumors of the uterine mesenchyme and mixed tumors, termed uterine sarcomas, account for a much smaller percentage of cases. Uterine cancer occurs in about 1 to 2 cases per 1000 postmenopausal women per year in the general population and is one of the most common cancers in the female, exceeded in frequency only by carcinoma of the breast, bowel, and lung. Thus the importance of these neoplasms and their management to the gynecologic surgeon is obvious because of the frequency with which they are encountered.

Further, two additional factors emanating in the next decade emphasize this importance: First, data accumulated during the 1980s have propelled the return of endometrial cancer to the surgical arena for primary treatment, as the current International Federation of Gynecology and Obstetrics (FIGO) staging is *surgical*; second, the continued increase in the older segment of the population—by the year 2000 more than 13% of U.S. citizens will be over age 65—suggests that the prominence of this cancer will be maintained. Concomitantly, advances in preoperative and postoperative care make surgical therapy available to virtually every woman diagnosed with the disease.

The rather monumental changes brought about by new surgical staging, coupled with the new economics of practicing surgery with reviews of hospital stay, permitted diagnostic tests, and limitations on treatment locations and facilities, have introduced new controversies into the management of patients with corpus tumors. The ensuing discussion reflects the impact of these and other changes in the diagnosis and treatment of endometrial cancers.

INCIDENCE

Despite the increase in the older segment of the population, it is apparent that the actual incidence of cancer of the uterine corpus is, overall, decreasing.

Although the third National Cancer Survey in the United States in 1969 and 1970, as reported by Cramer and coworkers, showed no evidence of an increase in the incidence of endometrial cancer from the time of the previous survey in 1947, there was a consistent increase in the incidence between 1970 and 1975, as shown by case studies from the Connecticut Tumor Registry (Fig. 43-1), followed by a gradual decline since that time. Data collected by Walker and Jick from hospital discharge summaries in the United States show that between 1970 and 1975, the incidence of endometrial carcinoma in women aged 50 to 59 increased by 85%, from 72 to 133 cases per 100,000 women-years. From 1975 to 1979 rates declined in this age group, returning to the starting level of 72 per 100,000 women-years in 1979. In the same period among women aged 60 to 69 there was an 83% increase in the incidence of endometrial cancer, from 82 to 150 cases per 100,000 women-years. After age 70 the risk increased by 83%, from an incidence of 45 cases per 100,000 women-years in 1970 to a peak in 1978 of 83 cases per 100,000 women-years. Premenopausal women between the ages of 25 and 44 showed no increased risk, and the incidence was low: 5 or fewer cases per 100,000 women.

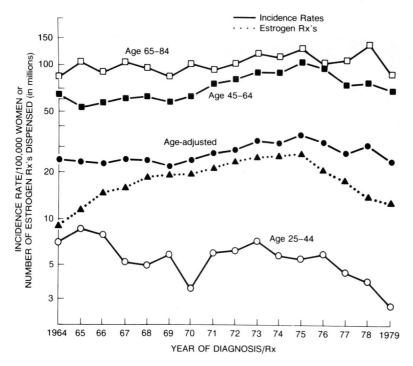

Figure 43–1. Annual age-adjusted (1970 standard population) and age-specific incidence rates for localized cancer of the uterine corpus, corrected for women in Connecticut who have had hysterectomies, and annual numbers of noncontraceptive oral estrogen prescriptions dispensed in the United States, 1964–1979. (Marrett LD, Meigs JW, Flannery JT. Trends in the incidence of cancer of the corpus uteri in Connecticut, 1964–1979, in relation to consumption of exogenous estrogens. Am J Epidemiol 1982;116:62)

Data reported by the American Cancer Society (ACS) in its annual cancer statistics suggested that endometrial cancer in the United States reached a high of 39,000 estimated cases in 1984. Since that time the ACS annual estimates have steadily decreased to 34,000 new cases of endometrial cancer in 1989 and 33,000 in 1990 (Fig. 43-2).

Gusberg recently termed this phenomena "the rise and fall of endometrial cancer," and suggested that careful analysis of data allowed a less enigmatic interpretation of the apparent decline in incidence. He points out a 23.2 per 100,000 rate in 1950 as being not significantly different from the 23.4 per 100,000 rate in 1985, with the precipitous 43% rise to 33.2 cases per 100,000 women in 1975 alarming the oncology community into anticipating an epidemic of new cases.

Gusberg and others indict the estrogen–tumor relation as the culprit; surely the widespread use of unopposed estrogens contributed to this rise culminated by the ACS estimates in 1984. Data from the Connecticut Tumor Registry (see Fig. 43-1) attempted to correlate the incidence of endometrial cancer with the annual number of oral estrogen prescriptions dispensed in the United States. Although these trends suggested a relation, they were by no means conclusive. But aggressive treatment of precursors as well as pathologists' recent discrimination between the relation of the hyperplasia and the actual invasive disease (eg, what may have been called cancer in the 1970s may now be termed complex hyperplasia with atypia) have perhaps triggered the

decreased incidence. The role of screening, prevention, and earlier detection in the decline of endometrial cancer is uncertain.

The older population of women in the United States have, for the most part, become a sophisticated and highly informed group. The vast press coverage of the use of exogenous estrogens has led to the almost universal awareness that unopposed estrogens are not in the patient's best interest, and when an intact uterus is present, most clinicians appropriately utilize progestin compounds to offset the effects of estrogen. Thus the number of estrogen-induced tumors appears to be decreasing. Yet, at the same time, the increased occurrence of these tumors in older women, at a time of increasing life expectancy and vigorous health, makes appropriate awareness of the problem of uterine cancer even more important.

The earlier apparent increase in endometrial cancer might be linked to the increasing age of the population. Data suggest that not only has incidence increased as the age of the patients increased, but also the degree of differentiation and incidence of other poor prognostic factors has increased as women become older. Nevertheless, despite the apparent leveling off of the incidence of endometrial cancer, and an apparent stabilization of occurrence rate in younger and premenopausal women, the increased age of the population and the incidence of endometrial cancer in this age group still portend the serious nature of this disease in older women.

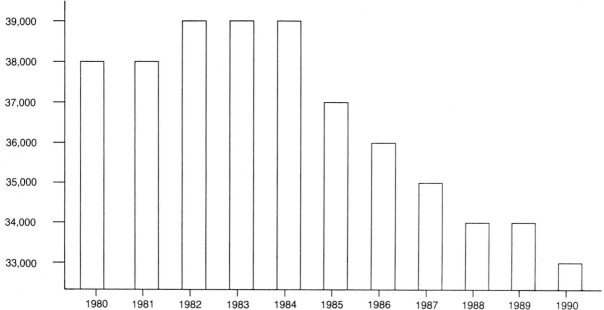

Figure 43–2. Estimated cases of endometrial cancer, 1980–1990. These estimates, projected by the American Cancer Society in their Annual Cancer Statistics, reflect the continued rise in the suspected number of cases of endometrial cancer to a high of 39,000 in 1982 through 1984. Since that time the numbers predicted have gradually fallen to about 33,000 new cases anticipated in 1990. Whether this reflects an actual decrease in the number of new cases, more accurate interpretation of atypical neoplasias, or a combination of the two remains to be answered. (Silverberg E, Boring CC, Squire TS. Cancer statistics, 1990. CA 1990; 40, and previous issues, 1980–1989)

As the population ages, the grade and stage at diagnosis appear to increase. Thus, in the 20th FIGO Annual report, the mean age for 12,119 cases of corpus cancer diagnosed in 1979–1987 was 60.9 years for grade 1, stage I patients, gradually increasing by grade and stage to 65.7 years for grade 3, stage IV patients.

CAUSE AND RISK FACTORS

Risk Factors Associated with Endometrial Cancer

The "corpus cancer syndrome," a triad consisting of obesity, diabetes mellitus, and hypertension, has long been associated with an increased risk of endometrial cancer. More modern analysis of epidemiologic data concludes that the existence of this triad in women without endometrial cancer is the same as in women who have the disease, and is more appropriately called a "postmenopausal syndrome." The overwhelming evidence at this time implicates factors that have one common thread: estrogen stimulation of the uterine lining. Thus major risk factors, such as obesity, late meno-

pause, and exogenous estrogen use, as well as minor risk factors, such as infertility, anovulatory cycles, and the syndromes of polycystic ovarian disease, all have one link: a theoretical, if not apparent, increase in estrogen stimulation of the endometrial cavity.

Obesity

Obesity is the major risk factor associated with endometrial carcinoma. In fact, multivariate analysis reveals that among all risk factors, only exogenous obesity can be implicated in the actual cause of endometrial cancer.

Again, a suggested link with estrogens is incontrovertible. Circulating androgens at extraglandular sites, principally in fatty tissue, can be converted to estrone, which supposedly will create a more favorable milieu for the formation of endometrial cancer. Siiteri and coworkers documented the conversion rate of androstenedione to estrone, which was directly increased with the weight of the patients. In a series of patients with endometrial cancer reported by Kottmeier, 29% weighed more than 180 lb; another 7% weighed more than 220 lb. In Peterson's series a total of 81% weighed more than 150 lb, while 63% of the group weighed more than 200 lb. Wynder and coworkers concluded that in women 21 to 50 lb overweight, the risk of endometrial carcinoma is increased threefold; in women 50 lb or more over ideal weight, the risk is nine times greater than in women of normal weight.

Obesity also is associated with an increase in the serum level of free, unbound estrogen because the levels of sex hormone–binding globulin, which inactivates the estrogen molecule, are decreased. Thus, in obese patients, there is an increased bioavailability of estrogen that appears to parallel the degree of obesity.

Not only is obesity associated with a high risk of developing endometrial cancer, but the association of other disorders, including diabetes, hypertension, and arteriosclerotic disease, makes treatment planning for this group of patients more difficult. Although modern preoperative and postoperative care techniques have minimized the risk of surgical therapy in this group of patients, nonetheless a more elderly population with these disorders portends a higher operative risk.

Onsrud and coworkers showed that the prognosis in patients with endometrial cancer who were more than 30% above ideal weight was poorer than that in patients of normal weight. Although these data were not corrected for the more currently known poor prognostic indicators, it is known that obese patients with endometrial cancer are more likely to die of an intercurrent disease than are patients of normal weight.

Additionally, with the advent of surgical staging, technical factors associated with obesity may adversely affect the patient's outcome. Hence obesity not only is a potent risk factor etiologically, but also looms as a potential poor prognostic factor for reasons of relative operative risk.

Diabetes Mellitus

The data regarding diabetes mellitus as having a causative effect on endometrial cancer is inconclusive. Several investigators have addressed the question of whether or not an altered carbohydrate metabolism affects or is affected by endometrial carcinoma, but most of the reports are retrospective surveys that provide poor data for critical evaluation. Dunn and coworkers conducted one of the earliest controlled studies using oral glucose tolerance tests, taking into consideration the age and weight of patients. Although patients with endometrial cancer had significantly less tolerance to the glucose test than did normal women, the data did not show a relation between altered metabolism of carbohydrates and endometrial carcinoma. Dunn estimated that 7.7% of the patients were also diabetic, an incidence similar to that for a random sample of women of the same age without cancer. Fox and Sen also were unable to show any statistically signif-

icant increase in diabetes among patients with endometrial cancer.

Although Kaplan and Cole reported the risk of abnormal glucose tolerance to be 2.4 times higher in the presence of endometrial cancer, it has not been convincingly demonstrated that a true increase in the incidence of insulin-dependent diabetes is associated with endometrial cancer.

Thus the association of diabetes mellitus with endometrial cancer has more importance in the preoperative and postoperative care of patients than as a causative factor. The clinician treating a patient with endometrial cancer must always be aware that the possibility of diabetes mellitus exists, and appropriately monitor glucose levels.

Hypertension

As with diabetes mellitus, when multivariate analysis is performed on patients with endometrial cancer, hypertension appears to be more related to body weight than to an increased incidence of endometrial cancer. Wynder and Dunn correlated blood pressure with body weight. Using a controlled comparison, these researchers found no statistical difference between the incidence of hypertension in patients with endometrial carcinoma and that in women without cancer. Again, the implication of risk for hypertension lies in the preoperative and postoperative care of patients with endometrial cancer, as hypertension and arteriosclerotic vascular disease mandate vigorous monitoring and fastidious management if surgery is to be successful.

Syndromes of Increased Endogenous Estrogen Stimulation

In addition to the apparent endogenous estrogen stimulation that occurs in obese postmenopausal women, several syndromes are associated with the production of endogenous estrogens in excess of progestins, and such patients carry a higher relative risk of endometrial cancer.

It is well documented that the age at menopause for American women is gradually and steadily increasing. By implication, late onset of menopause suggests longer stimulation of the endometrial cavity by estrogens. Antunes and coworkers compared 179 patients with endometrial cancer with 155 hospitalized controls. Among all the factors studied, only excess weight, late menopause, and estrogen use were found to be associated with a statistically significant increase in the risk of this disease. Their findings showed that, compared with controls, patients with excess weight had 2.4 times greater risk; those with a late menopause, a 2.5 times greater risk; and those using estrogen, an 8.6

times greater risk of endometrial carcinoma. Late menopause has long been a recognized risk factor among women who develop endometrial carcinoma. In an epidemiologic study by Kaplan and Cole the relative risk was 2.4 times greater among women with a menopause delayed until after age 52 than among women in whom menopause occurred before age 49. Patients in the perimenopausal age group frequently assume that irregular bleeding is physiologic, which delays the diagnosis and treatment of this disease. Thus, as populations increase in age, and as menopause occurs later and later, it is expected that this factor will become more important in the incidence of endometrial cancer.

Similarly, syndromes related to infertility and low parity also suggest long periods of potentially unopposed estrogen stimulation. Patients with polycystic ovarian disease have an increased incidence of endometrial cancer, as demonstrated by Coulam and coworkers and numerous case reports; this presumably is because of long anovulatory cycles. The risk is increased in younger women, and suggests a higher awareness of this possibility in women who have chronic anovulation and who also are obese. In Coulam's study a cohort of 1270 patients with chronic anovulation syndrome developed 20 cancers; the endometrium was the only site at increased risk. The authors determined a relative risk of 3.1 of developing carcinoma of the endometrium in women with chronic anovulation.

Relative infertility, as exhibited by low parity, also has been associated with increased risk of endometrial carcinoma. Women who are nulligravida have a five times greater incidence of endometrial cancer than women of high parity (five or more children). The incidence might be even higher for nulligravidas who are involuntarily childless, and again suggests the association with prolonged anovulation.

Since 1922, when Schroeder first described it, the association of endometrial cancer with estrogen-producing ovarian neoplasms has become more clinically evident. Estrogen-secreting granulosa cell and theca cell tumors of the ovary have been associated with endometrial carcinoma in an incidence ranging from 3.5% to 27%. Most commonly, the association is found to be present in less than 5% of cases. If endometrial cancer is associated with these functioning ovarian tumors in about 3.5% of the cases—that is, if there are 35 cases of endometrial cancer per 1000 women with such ovarian tumors—the risk of endometrial cancer is 10 to 50 times greater for women with estrogen-producing ovarian neoplasms than for women with normal ovaries. It also should be remembered that virtually any tumor, primary or metastatic, can stimulate ovarian stroma to produce hormones. Such production may be responsible for such phenomena as synchronous tumors of the ovary and endometrium or endometrial hyperplasias in women with non–hormone-producing tumors metastatic to the ovary.

Other Factors

Smoking is implicated as a cofactor in many cancers, but the association of smoking and endometrial cancer is unclear. Lesko and coworkers, reporting on a hospital-based, case-control study of 510 women with endometrial cancer, estimated that current postmenopausal smokers actually had a lowered risk of developing endometrial cancer (relative risk 0.5). This apparent protective effect of smoking was not evident in premenopausal women. The mechanism of this phenomenon is apparently due to the known reduction in circulating estrogens among smokers, rather than molecular protection by nicotine. Clearly, these observations should not incite smoking to prevent endometrial cancer; the deadly consequences of smoking clearly outweigh the apparent advantage. A subset of younger smoking patients had more aggressive cancers, but this observation's significance is unknown.

Prior radiation to the pelvis has long been implicated as a causative risk factor in the later development of uterine sarcomas, but an association with epithelial corpus cancers has not been established. However, as demonstrated by Barnhill and coworkers, endometrial activity can persist after therapeutic irradiation for cervical cancer. They studied the endometria from 16 previously irradiated patients who underwent sampling because of uterine bleeding: 9 patients had proliferative endometrium or hyperplasia and 1 patient had frank adenocarcinoma. Although there is no suggestion that irradiation is a risk factor for development of endometrial cancer, neither is it totally protective. Thus caution should be used in administering estrogen replacement therapy, and prompt sampling, when indicated, is essential.

For unknown reasons blacks are less likely to be diagnosed with endometrial cancer than whites of the same age group; a white woman at birth is almost twice as likely to develop endometrial cancer in her lifetime. Women of high socioeconomic class are at increased risk for endometrial cancer over those in a lower socioeconomic class. Both of these risk factors are probably related to the availability of exogenous estrogens.

Exogenous Estrogens and Endometrial Cancer

Out of the flood of literature in the medical and lay press since the mid-1970s regarding the use of exogenous estrogens and the increased risk of endometrial cancer have come four relatively incontrovertible facts: (1) prolonged use of unopposed estrogens is associated with a high risk of endometrial cancer; (2) the use of concomitant or cyclic progestins will greatly reduce this risk; (3) prior usage of combination oral contraceptives reduces the risk of endometrial cancer; and (4) endometrial carcinomas that are associated with exogenous estrogen use may behave differently biologically from their non–estrogen-associated counterparts.

Role of Exogenous Estrogen. As early as 1936 Novak and other medical pioneers noted that many women with estrogen excess or estrogen stimulation developed endometrial adenocarcinoma. Gusberg in 1947 warned about the carcinogenic potential and established a causal relation with the precursor lesions of adenomatous hyperplasia.

Although the role of endogenous estrogens in the etiology of endometrial cancer is inferred from epidemiologic data, as outlined above, the role of exogenous estrogens in the etiology of endometrial cancer, while still somewhat controversial, has been more firmly established. The popularity of administration of exogenous estrogen in postmenopausal women increased markedly in the 1960s, resulting in the highly publicized reports in 1975 and 1976 by Ziel, Smith, Mack, and their respective coworkers showing an up to eightfold increase in endometrial cancer relative risk in women who took unopposed estrogen (Table 43-1). Although these studies have been subject to intense epidemiologic scrutiny since that time, and the risks have declined with reevaluation of these and other studies, nevertheless, these landmark papers brought the awareness of the problem to the popular forefront, and have subsequently led to marked alteration in the prescribing of exogenous estrogen.

It is known that patients with primary ovarian failure have been singularly devoid of endometrial carcinoma. Thus the untimely occurrence of endometrial cancer in patients with gonadal dysgenesis who were treated with nonsteroidal estrogens firmly points to exogenous estrogen as the causative agent in this disease. As shown in Table 43-2, the estrogen replacement most commonly given to patients with gonadal dysgenesis who developed a well-differentiated adenocarcinoma or adenosquamous carcinoma was diethylstilbestrol (DES). Other types of estrogen were given in 7 of 14 reported cases, indicating that a variety of estrogen compounds can produce neoplastic changes. One case, reported by Rosenwaks and coworkers, shows that the patient was treated regularly with medroxyprogesterone, and this combination did not prevent the development of adenocarcinoma. As discussed below,

TABLE 43–1
Risk of Endometrial Cancer with Estrogen Replacement Therapy

STUDY (YR)	PERIOD OF ESTROGEN USE	WOMEN WITH CANCER		CONTROLS WITHOUT CANCER	ODDS RATIO OR CALCULATED RELATIVE RISK
		Cases of Cancer	Percentage Using Estrogens	Percentage Using Estrogens	
Jensen et al (1954)	1.5–15 yr	105	33	21	1.9
Wynder et al (1966)	Any use	112	2	4	0.6
Dunn, Bradley (1967)	Any use	56	29	28	1.0
Smith et al (1975)	>6 mo	317	48	17	7.5
Ziel, Finkel (1975)	>1 yr	94	57	15	7.6
Mack et al (1976)	Any use	63	89	50	8.0
McDonald et al (1976)	>6 mo	145	17	8	2.3
Gray et al (1977)	>3 mo	205	27	15	2.2
Horwitz, Feinstein (1978)	>6 mo	149	30	15	2.3

(Drill VA. Relationship of estrogens and oral contraceptives to endometrial cancer in animals and women. J Reprod Med 1980; 24:5)

TABLE 43–2
Endometrial Carcinoma in Patients with Gonadal Dysgenesis and Estrogen Replacement

STUDY (YR)	NO. OF PATIENT	AGE AT DETECTION (YR)	KARYOTYPE	DURATION OF ESTROGEN USE (YR)		TOTAL DOSE (g)	TYPE OF CARCINOMA
				DES	Other		
Lewis et al (1963)	1	45	45, X/46, XY				Adeno
Dowsett (1963)	2	28	45, X	6		5	Adenosquamous
Scott (1963)	3	31	45, X	4	2	9	Adenosquamous
Canlorbe et al (1967)	4	32	45, X	6	3	3	Adeno
Cutler et al (1972)	5*	29	45, X	9	1	2.8	? Adenosquamous
	6	35	45, X/46, XY	20	0	5	Adenosquamous
	7†	35	46, XXqi§	17	1	6.2	? Adeno
Wilkinson et al (1963)	8	26	45, X	9	0	2.6	Adeno
Roberts and Wells (1975)	9*	28	45, X	4	0	1.5	? Adenosquamous
McCarroll et al (1975)	10‡	35	45, X	13	0	3.7	Adeno
Sirota et al (1975)	11	27	45, X	8		15	Adeno
Ostor et al (1978)	12	34	45, X/47, XXX				Adenosquamous
	13‡	27	45, X/46, XX		3	15 mg	Adeno
Louka et al (1978)	14	36	45, X	0		0.2	Adenosquamous
Rosenwaks et al (1979)	15‡	24	45, X		4.2	2.5	Adeno

*Uncertain if squamous component is malignant.
† Uncertain about presence of true carcinoma.
‡ Patient also treated with progesterone.
§ Isochromosome for the long arm of X.
(Ostor AG, Fortune DW, Evans JH, et al. Endometrial carcinoma in gonadal dysgenesis with and without estrogen therapy. Gynecol Oncol 1978; 6:316)

it is clinically established that such a dual regimen will most probably prevent estrogen-induced carcinoma in postmenopausal women. Despite the isolated reports of cases of patients with gonadal dysgenesis who developed endometrial carcinoma and who also were treated with progestins, the strongest evidence to date for an association between long-term estrogen use and endometrial carcinoma rests with the estrogen-treated cases of gonadal dysgenesis. Unfortunately there are no case controls in these cases, and a cause-and-effect relation is not secure.

As with other carcinogens, the duration of hormone use appears to be one of the most important factors in the development of adenocarcinoma. In the case of gonadal dysgenesis, adenocarcinoma developed after periods of estrogen use ranging from 4 to 20 years.

The work of multiple investigators supports the hypothesis of the association between estrogen use and the development of endometrial carcinoma; however, a direct relation has still not been conclusively proven. Numerous epidemiologic studies designed to investigate this hypothesis have been published; the wide range of associated risks leads to the conclusion that the studies are not conclusive, yet the trend is obvious, and few clinicians would consider unopposed estrogens in a woman with an intact uterus. As previously stated, this relation has even been shown to exist in women who

have been irradiated for cervical cancer, indicating that the biologic activity of estrogen, even on an irradiated endometrium, is potent. The Food and Drug Administration has responded to this epidemiologic information by clearly stating in package inserts and in drug company informational systems that the use of unopposed estrogen is associated with the risk of endometrial carcinoma.

Knab summarized the reports on prolonged postmenopausal use of estrogen, and emphasized that it was associated with an increased incidence of endometrial cancer. These studies, which are retrospective and not randomized, show that women taking estrogens for 1 to 5 years have a four to five times greater risk of developing endometrial cancer than untreated women. Women who take the hormones for 7 or more years have a 13 times greater risk. Silverberg estimates that a 55-year-old woman with a life expectancy of 20 years who received estrogen therapy for all 20 years has a 3% chance of developing endometrial carcinoma, which is nearly 40 times the normal risk of this disease for a 75-year-old woman.

Thomas recently reviewed the association of steroid hormones that could modify the risk of cancer. He cited several reviews that cumulatively estimated the increased risk for estrogen users to be between 5 and over 11 times that of women not taking unopposed estrogens. This was demonstrated by both case-control and cohort studies, and again suggested increase in risk with longer duration of use and higher dosages. Thomas also noted the marked delayed parallel in the rise and fall of the prescribing practices for estrogens and the subsequent increase and later decrease in the incidence of endometrial cancer.

Although the evidence is not conclusive, the data suggest that prolonged use of estrogen can have a neoplastic effect on DNA metabolism in sensitive endometrial tissue. Even without conclusive evidence, the data provide a strong warning against high-dose and continuous estrogen therapy in high-risk patients. On the other hand, the rate of endometrial cell mitoses does not appear to be increased over the basal levels seen in the early follicular phase as circulating levels of estrogen increase dramatically. Thus, as suggested by Sutton, the increased risk of endometrial cancer seen with unopposed estrogen therapy may be related to progesterone deficiency rather than to estrogen overexposure.

Gelfand and Ferenczy studied the endometrial response in 95 postmenopausal women who were administered oral, cyclic conjugated equine estrogens with and without progesterone, and evaluated morphology and bleeding patterns. They found that up to 57% of patients taking unopposed estrogen developed hyperplasia in a dose–response pattern and 54% experienced breakthrough bleeding. This clearly demonstrated that the endometrium of older women can proliferate in response to oral estrogens.

It appears that the stimulating effects of estrogen occur despite the route of administration. Thus Chetkowski and coworkers demonstrated that the biologic effects of transdermal estradiol mimicked that of oral conjugated estrogens. Similarly, the absorption of estrogens from the vagina mirrors that from the gut; thus the clinician should never administer vaginal estrogen cream without (a) assuming that it will be readily absorbed and (b) considering the status of the endometrial cavity in a woman with an intact uterus.

Synthetic, nonsteroidal estrogens, as shown above in patients with Turner's syndrome, can induce endometrial stimulation. In 1971 Herbst and coworkers showed that there was an association between the use of nonsteroidal estrogens during the first trimester of pregnancy and the occurrence of adenocarcinoma in the vagina and cervix of female offspring. Although this cohort of offspring has not reached the age of maximum risk for adenocarcinomas of the endometrium, they should be carefully watched.

Similarly, the nonsteroidal tamoxifen may possess a dual role in its relation to endometrial cancer. Rutzvizt and coworkers recently demonstrated a rather high rate of new endometrial cancers among 1846 post-menopausal women who underwent surgery for carcinoma of the breast and subsequently took tamoxifen as prophylaxis against recurrence. With a median exposure of 3.8 years to 40 mg of tamoxifen daily, there was a sixfold increase in the number of endometrial cancers that would be expected for this group. Tamoxifen's primary mode of action is antiestrogenic, although it is in actuality a very weak estrogen. Thus, unopposed in therapeutic doses, it can stimulate the endometrium.

Despite the many reports suggesting that the risk of endometrial carcinoma is significantly increased in postmenopausal women who are given replacement estrogen therapy, there are those who contend that this strong association is the result of detection bias. It is well known that estrogen replacement therapy can induce endometrial proliferation and that endometrial bleeding frequently results from proliferation. It is suggested that estrogen-induced proliferation and bleeding lead to the discovery of preexisting endometrial carcinomas, which may then erroneously be described as estrogen-related. Horowitz and Feinstein, two noted biostatisticians who are the major protagonists of this opposing theory, remain firm in their conviction that the estrogen genesis of endometrial carcinoma is, as yet, unproven.

In a prospective screening program of 2586 asymptomatic women aged 45 years or older, Koss and coworkers have attempted to answer the question of whether estrogen-induced proliferative bleeding leads to the early detection of endometrial carcinoma. Endometrial biopsy failed to confirm that endometrial hyperplasia preceded adenocarcinoma. Furthermore, no significant association between estrogen medication and endometrial adenocarcinoma could be shown. These investigators conclude that endometrial cancer in postmenopausal women may develop as a focal event rather than from existing diffuse endometrial hyperplasia.

Although other drugs, such as digitalis, can have an estrogen-like effect on the endometrium, there are no known proven cases of endometrial cancer caused by such drugs. Thus the risk of developing cancer of the uterus from exogenous drugs appears to be confined to unopposed estrogens and nonsteroidal estrogenic compounds.

Progesterone Protection. Since the first indication of the association between endometrial carcinoma and exogenous estrogen use, numerous studies have appeared in the literature supporting the concept that progestins given concomitantly greatly reduced the risk of development of endometrial carcinoma. Hammond and coworkers demonstrated in a careful retrospective study that progestin cyclically reduced the risk of endometrial carcinoma. No cases of endometrial cancer developed in 72 women using the combination, whereas 11 of 1967 women who used unopposed estrogens developed corpus cancer.

In a 10-year prospective study by Nachtigall and coworkers, 84 institutionalized women were given high doses of conjugated estrogen plus medroxyprogesterone acetate while 84 control cases were treated with a placebo. The groups were carefully matched for age and associated disease after 10 years of hormone use. Among the postmenopausal women receiving the estrogen-progestin replacement therapy there were no cases of endometrial carcinoma, although an estimated 3.8 cases of endometrial carcinoma should have developed. In these cases the use of a progestin, as recommended by Gambrell, showed a definite protective benefit.

There is ample physiologic and laboratory evidence to prove the inhibitory effects of progesterone against the proliferative action of estrogen. Progesterone inhibits synthesis of both estrogen and progesterone receptors. Within the endometrial cell progesterone stimulates the estradiol-17β dehydrogenase enzyme, which allows conversion of estradiol to the less potent estrone. It appears that these effects hold true regardless of the progestin used.

Nisker and coworkers recently demonstrated that the synthetic progestin levonorgestrel could reduce the incidence of endometrial neoplasia in rabbits, which occurs in this species as they age, similar to human females. In their experimental model Silastic capsules of levonorgestrel were implanted into one uterine horn and the animals' uteri were serially examined. Not only did their results show a significant reduction of tumors in the treated group, but a definite dose–response of the protective effect was demonstrated, with no animals developing neoplasia when serum concentrations of levonorgestrel were satisfactorily therapeutic.

Thus current accepted prescription practices mandate the addition of a progestin to any regimen of estrogen replacement therapy in women with an intact uterus. To date, no one regimen for estrogen replacement with progestin has been conclusively demonstrated to be superior to any other, with many clinicians forced to choose the regimen that apparently best fits their patient population. The most popular regimen— 0.625 mg of conjugated estrogens 25 days a month, with 10 mg of medroxyprogesterone on days 15 to 25—is associated with a low incidence of side effects, probably offers adequate protection against adenocarcinoma of the endometrium, and enjoys the endorsement of an American College of Obstetricians and Gynecologists (ACOG) technical bulletin (#70, June 1983). Gelfand demonstrated that 5 mg of medroxyprogesterone for the last 11 days of the cycle was associated with no hyperplasia when used with 0.625 mg of conjugated estrogens 25 days a month in women followed for 1 year. This lower dosage of progesterone may not be totally protective for long-term use. For women using the transdermal estrogen or continuous vaginal estrogen, similar cyclical progestin is necessary to avoid undesirable endometrial stimulation.

In addition to progesterone "protection," appropriate clinical investigation of irregular withdrawal, good historical and laboratory information to document the need for estrogen replacement therapy, and aggressive use of endometrial sampling can help to avoid untimely administration of estrogen and increase early diagnosis of an existing endometrial cancer. Further, it should be noted that progesterone augmentation of exogenous estrogen will not prevent endometrial carcinoma from occurring. In some women moderately to poorly differentiated adenocarcinomas may arise despite the use of progestins, and women who are begun on such replacement regimens should be warned that although progesterone may be preventive, there is no guarantee that endometrial carcinoma will not develop.

Oral Contraceptives. An unexpected benefit of combination oral contraceptives has been a sharp reduction in the relative risk of endometrial cancer in women who have used these medications. At least five case-control studies have shown a 50% reduction in the endometrial carcinoma risk of women who have ever used combination oral contraceptives, but it appears that this protection can be reversed by unopposed postmenopausal estrogens. Thomas claims that this apparent protection is secondary to the net progestational effect that results in a virtually inactive endometrium with long-term usage.

On the other hand, the older sequential contraceptives were implicated in endometrial cancer. Studies by Silverberg and Makowski demonstrated that 11 of 21 young women with endometrial carcinoma had used sequential estrogen-progestin combinations as birth control pills. Because of these and similar studies by Lyon and others, this contraceptive agent was removed from the marketplace. The long-term effects of the tricyclic oral contraceptives remain to be elucidated as far as corpus cancer is concerned.

Virulence of Estrogen-induced Cancer. It appears that adenocarcinomas of the endometrium that develop after prolonged unopposed estrogen use are, for the most part, well-differentiated tumors with minimal myometrial invasion. When these cancers are diagnosed at the time of the onset of first irregular postmenopausal bleeding or at the time of routine surveillance, immediate treatment is effective and the prognosis is excellent. Many of these cases are diagnosed as carcinoma in situ. In fact, part of the controversy occurs because some clinicians consider many of the lesions in question to be atypical endometrial hyperplasia, not invasive carcinoma. This potential detection bias was studied by Gordon and coworkers, who found that three pathology reviewers agreed on the diagnosis of endometrial cancer in 66 (74%) of the original 89 cases reported by Ziel and Finkel, and at least two reviewers agreed on 82 of the cases (92%).

In a 1981 study of 28 cases of endometrial carcinoma Horowitz and coworkers found that three pathology reviewers concurred with the original diagnosis of adenocarcinoma in 82% of the cases reviewed. Most of the disagreements were about whether particular lesions should be designated as markedly atypical adenomatous hyperplasia or as grade 1 endometrial cancer. Therefore, there appears to be a relatively accurate diagnosis in these lesions in some 75% to 80% of cases. It is thus optimal to obtain second pathology opinions before embarking on definite treatment, especially in younger women who might want to preserve fertility.

DIAGNOSIS OF ENDOMETRIAL CANCER

Screening. According to the 1989 ACOG bulletin on screening for gynecologic cancers, routine screening for endometrial cancer is neither cost effective nor warranted. Unfortunately, for corpus cancer there are no effective methods to satisfy the standard criteria for a good screening test, which include a painless, low-cost screen of masses of asymptomatic patients. The uterine cavity is barricaded from screening detection by the oft-sclerotic postmenopausal endocervical canal, which impedes the flow of exfoliated cells from an early cancer to allow a reliable cytology screen and also obstructs an easy, painless effort to sample the endometrial lining. Attempts have been made to initiate broad screening for endometrial cancer, but the routine Papanicolaou (Pap) smear is notoriously unreliable in detecting endometrial cancer, and poor patient compliance with intrauterine sample techniques led clinicians to abandon these methods of screening.

The Pap smear usually detects only 50% to 60% of endometrial carcinomas. Aspiration or scraping of the endocervical canal usually is 70% to 85% effective. Reagan and Ng reported 85% accuracy for all types of endometrial cancer, using both endocervical aspiration and vaginal cytology, but vaginal cytology alone detected abnormal cells in only 50% of the patients with known endometrial carcinoma.

Frost suggested sampling the cytologic material from the posterior fornix in combination with an endocervical scraping. The problem with this method is that the postmenopausal cervix does not always allow insertion of the tip of the spatula, so an endocervical specimen may not always be obtained. Even with the recent popularity of the endocervical brush, the Pap smear cannot be reliably used to detect endometrial cancer.

Certain Pap smear findings, however, may be useful in detecting endometrial carcinoma. Zucker and coworkers evaluated 102 women with clinical pathologic correlation, using six parameters found on their Pap smears: (1) histiocytes, (2) multinucleated histiocytes, (3) nonspecific inflammation, (4) bleeding, (5) elevated squamous maturation index, and (6) the degree of cytologic atypicality of endometrial glandular cells. Using multivariate analysis, he determined that only cytologically scored endometrial glandular cells were predictive of an endometrial lesion.

Thus screening in the routine sense is not appropriate for detecting endometrial cancer. However, surveillance and sampling of women at high risk is appropriate.

Evaluation of Symptomatic Women. Abnormal uterine bleeding is the harbinger of endometrial cancer and should alert the clinician to rule out corpus cancer, regardless of the age of the patient. In fact, 5% to 10% of endometrial carcinomas occur in women under the age of 40, and irregular heavy bleeding in this age group should not afford the complacency of hormonal manipulation without appropriate endometrial sampling. In the perimenopausal age group it becomes even more mandatory to histologically sample endometrium in situations of abnormal bleeding. Finally, any episode of postmenopausal bleeding represents endometrial cancer until proved otherwise.

The traditional inpatient dilatation and curettage has long since been abandoned as the premier means of endometrial sampling, but in its outpatient version still must be considered the gold standard of histologic diagnosis of endometrial pathology. Today numerous devices are available for the physician to obtain endometrial samples in the office or clinic, and choice should be determined by the age of the patient, the experience of the clinician, anatomic considerations (eg, stenosis), and the emotional milieu of the individual patient. Thus four basic categories of instruments are available to sample the endometrial cavity, as listed in Table 43-3. In addition to dilatation and curettage, cytologic procedures, endometrial biopsy by Novak curette, and various aspiration techniques currently are used to evaluate abnormal bleeding.

A dilatation and fractional curettage can provide definitive results, even though a thorough curettage may fail to encompass the entire intrauterine cavity in 50% to 60% of patients.

Even with the newer surgical staging (see below), a separate endocervical scraping should be considered, especially if there is a suspicion of primary endocervical cancer, or if existing medical conditions might preclude any surgical intervention. Most women can undergo dilatation and curettage in the office; premedication with ibuprofen followed by paracervical block allows a comfortable dilation and gentle curet-

TABLE 43–3
Diagnosis of Endometrial Cancer

Definitive technique
    Dilatation and (fractional) curettage
Cytologic evaluation
    Cervicovaginal Pap
    Endometrial jet washing
    Endometrial brush
Traditional four-quadrant biopsy
    Novak curette
Histologic suction devices
    VABRA aspirator
    Tis-U-trap
    Pipelle

tage in all but the most apprehensive patients. Those with severe cervical stenosis, the very elderly, and those with high-risk cardiovascular or pulmonary disease should have the procedure performed in the operating room with concomitant monitoring as appropriate. In circumstances where cervical stenosis is apparent either from prior radiation, sclerosing atrophy, advanced age, or multiple previous manipulations, real-time ultrasonography in the operating room can guide the fine-curve probe to the cavity and help prevent false passages or perforation.

As far as intrauterine cytology is concerned, many attempts have been made to brush, wash, or aspirate the endometrial cavity. The endometrial lavage technique introduced by Gravlee has been used with both good and bad results. Twiggs and coworkers found that endometrial lavage failed to demonstrate carcinoma in 14 of 25 proven cases of endometrial cancer. Even with adequate samples, the investigators had a 27% false-negative rate. Other clinics, however, have reported a 90% accuracy rate using endometrial lavage.

Among 93 patients referred to the Duke Medical Center with a histologic diagnosis of endometrial cancer, Creasman found a poor correlation with clinical diagnostic techniques. Among this group of patients with endometrial cancer, only 67% were identified by a Pap smear and 76% by an endometrial biopsy. When the brush technique was combined with any other method, including jet wash, VABRA aspirator, or endometrial biopsy, the accuracy rate improved to 91%. If any of these diagnostic techniques is negative or obtains an inadequate sample, a complete dilatation and fractional curettage is required to properly evaluate the patient. These mixed results with cytologic techniques has led to their virtual abandonment as routine diagnostic and screening tools.

The traditional Novak curette, long the standard tool of endometrial dating, can be useful in sampling the endometrium to detect endometrial carcinoma. How-

ever, because of the discomfort associated with its use, as well as its limited sampling of the cavity, it is recommended that this device alone not be used to rule out endometrial carcinoma in highly suspicious cases. Hofmeister has used the endometrial biopsy in more than 30,000 patients since 1949. Of all the patients, 187 cases of endometrial cancer were diagnosed. Of the women found to have endometrial cancer, 17% had no symptoms but had the biopsy as part of a routine examination during the perimenopausal years. Vaginal smears taken at the time of the biopsy were positive in only 25% of the cancer cases. Because of all of the negative factors, the Novak curette seldom is used for diagnosis of endometrium cancer.

Histologic tissue diagnosis of endometrial cancer most often is rendered on material obtained on an outpatient basis by one of various aspiration devices. The VABRA aspirator (Berkeley Medures, Berkeley, California) and the Tis-U-trap (Milex Products, Chicago) are two popular aspiration devices that use a pump as a vacuum source connected to a rigid metal or plastic cannula, usually 3 to 4 mm in diameter. The former has been shown by Grimes to compare favorably with the traditional dilatation and curettage.

Recently the Pipelle (Unimar, Inc., Wilton, Conn.), a softer, more flexible endometrial suction curette developed in France, has been introduced in the United States, and in a randomized clinical trial by Koonings and coworkers was shown to obtain a sample comparable to Tis-U-trap in both adequacy and quality. In my experience this device is extremely well tolerated by patients while producing a satisfactory sample. By using a tenaculum on the cervix for traction, all but the most stenotic cervices can be transversed, leading to prompt sampling.

Despite the apparent usefulness of any of the techniques above, an important clinical caveat in using these devices is to recall three basic facts: First, none of the devices provide 100% sensitive results, and failure to detect abnormal endometrium in high-risk patients should prompt a more thorough curettage. Second, a close relationship must exist between the clinician and the cytopathologist or histopathologist who is interpreting these results. Concomitantly, careful historical documentation must be made on the requisition, so that the pathologist interpreting the results knows the patient's age, menstrual history, and hormonal status. Third, anatomic variation in the uterine cervix, such as stenosis or presence of polyps, must warn the clinician against relying on these office-based devices to render the diagnosis in every situation.

The usefulness of hysteroscopy in the diagnosis of corpus cancer has yet to be determined. Certainly, in puzzling episodes of postmenopausal bleeding or when there is persistence of symptoms despite negative histology, hysteroscopy may offer definitive diagnosis.

Precursors of Endometrial Cancer. Various architectural distortions and epithelial proliferations as well as stratification of the endometrium—collectively known as the endometrial hyperplasias—frequently are encountered when evaluating patients for endometrial cancer. Although never proved to be premalignant, these lesions certainly can appear to evolve into frank cancer. In addition, multiple classifications of hyperplasias have served to confuse gynecologists who often remain uncertain of the malignant potential of these lesions but at the same time are faced with clinical decisions after their discovery.

Kurman and coworkers evaluated endometrial hyperplasia in 170 patients followed for 1 to 26.7 years (mean 13.4 years) by analyzing separately cytologic and architectural alterations. When atypia alone was used to subdivide patients, 1.6% of those without cytologic atypia developed endometrial cancer, whereas 23% of those with cytologic atypia progressed to cancer, a highly significant ($p = .001$) difference. Further attempts to subdivide patients on the basis of structural features resulted in defining complex hyperplasias, such as those displaying marked glandular complexity and back-to-back glands, and simple hyperplasias, such as those with proliferations but lacking the back-to-back glands and complexities. When these features were combined with atypia to form four groups, they found 1 of 93 patients with simple hyperplasia but no atypia developed cancer; however, cancer occurred in 29% of patients with complex atypical hyperplasias.

Similarly, Ferenczy and Gelfand divided 85 patients with endometrial hyperplasia treated with oral medroxyprogesterone acetate therapy into two groups: those without (group 1) and those with (group 2) cytologic atypia. No patients in group 1 developed cancer, although 20% had persistence or recurrence of hyperplasia. Seventy-five percent of those in group 2 had persistence or recurrence, and 25% developed cancer, despite progesterone treatment, within 2 to 7 years after starting hormonal therapy.

Data from these and other studies confirm the importance of cytologic atypia as being the prime factor to consider when making therapeutic choices, although certainly the degree of complexity should be considered. Thus, for a woman with complex hyperplasia with cytologic atypia, hysterectomy is the treatment of choice, not only because of the high likelihood that these lesions will progress despite hormonal treatment, but also because the risk of an occult frank carcinoma may be as high as 10% to 15% in these patients. Those who have documented simple hyperplasia with or without atypia and those with complex hyperplasia without atypia can be considered for hormonal therapy.

Choosing conservative therapy (ie, hormonal, not surgical) for endometrial hyperplasias should always be accompanied by informed consent as well as information about risks and side effects of the medications. Further, the immediate overall physical condition of the patient with some long-range projection of possible deterioration of operative status in the future must likewise enter the therapeutic decision. For instance, a 65-year-old woman with insulin-dependent diabetes and well-controlled hypertension who is a moderate surgical and anesthetic risk and who is diagnosed with endometrial hyperplasia might be an even poorer risk at age 70 if conservative treatment failed. Therefore, the gynecologic surgeon should consider endometrial hyperplasia as a long-term problem that usually is best served by short-term definitive surgery.

STAGING OF ENDOMETRIAL CANCER

Although the revised FIGO staging of 1988 converted endometrial cancer into a surgically staged disease, the clinical staging adopted in 1976 still must be used when patients are inoperable or when completion of the entire surgical staging is not possible. Thus the gynecologic surgeon should be familiar with both staging systems.

Clinical Staging of Endometrial Cancer

Since Kelly first discussed endometrial carcinoma in 1900, many attempts have been made to define and categorize the clinical stages of the lesions. The depth of myometrial involvement and the extension of the disease were considered, but additional criteria were needed for patients who could not undergo surgery.

The four-stage clinical classification (Table 43-4) was developed in 1958, revised by the FIGO Cancer Committee in 1961 and 1970, and officially adopted by the FIGO General Assembly in 1976.

The older FIGO classification of the stage of the disease is based on a standard of uterine cavity length and the extension of the disease beyond the uterus and pelvis. Lesions that do not enlarge the size of the uterus (8 cm or less) are considered stage Ia, whereas lesions that result in enlargement of the uterine cavity to more than 8 cm are categorized as stage Ib disease. It is presumed that the increase in uterine size to more than 8 cm is related to myometrial extension of tumor.

If it is anticipated that clinical staging alone will be used, it is imperative that endocervical curettage be performed during patient evaluation. Further, if clinical stage III or IV is suspected, the surgeon may elect to use the clinical system to initiate radiation therapy before any surgical intervention (see later).

TABLE 43–4
FIGO Clinical Staging of Endometrial Carcinoma

CLASSIFICATION	DESCRIPTION
Stage 0	Carcinoma in situ. Histologic findings suspicious of cancer. (Cases of stage 0 should not be included in statistics on invasive disease.)
Stage I	Carcinoma confined to the corpus, including the isthmus
Ia	The length of the uterine cavity is 8 cm or less
Ib	The length of the uterine cavity is more than 8 cm
	Stage I cases should be subgrouped with regard to the histologic type of adenocarcinoma as follows:
	Grade 1: Highly differentiated adenomatous carcinoma
	Grade 2: Differentiated adenomatous carcinoma with partly solid areas
	Grade 3: Predominantly solid or entirely undifferentiated carcinoma
Stage II	Carcinoma involving the corpus and cervix but not extending outside the uterus
Stage III	Carcinoma extending outside the uterus but not outside the true pelvis
Stage IV	Carcinoma extending outside the true pelvis or obviously involving the mucosa of the bladder or rectum (Bullous edema alone does not permit a lesion to be considered stage IV.)
IVa	Spread to the growth of bladder or intestine
IVb	Spread to distant organs

Staging and Preoperative Assessment Studies in Endometrial Cancer

Regardless of the planned usage of clinical or surgical staging, thorough evaluation of the patient with endometrial cancer is essential. A detailed history and a complete general physical examination are the foundation of evaluation. Special attention should be paid in the history to details of family history of cancer, which may provide clues to the risk of concomitant cancers and suggest additional evaluation studies, such as colonoscopy. In addition to queries about the cardinal symptom of corpus cancer—abnormal uterine bleeding—the history should include such pertinent negatives as pelvic pain or referred leg pain, leg edema or swelling, disturbances in bowel function, abdominal swelling, pelvic pressure, excessive flatulence, and early satiety. All may be indicative of more advanced disease than otherwise suspected. When doing the general physical examination, attention should be paid to careful palpation of axillary, supraclavicular, and inguinal lymph nodes. Table 43-5 details staging and preoperative studies for patients with corpus cancer.

The staging or preoperative pelvic examination is critical for patients with cancer of the uterus. After inspection of the vulva, palpation of Bartholin glands, and speculum evaluation of the vagina and cervix with Pap smear, careful bimanual examination should discover any vaginal metastasis, adnexal masses, or extension of the tumor anteriorly and establish a clinical estimate of the size of the uterus. Sounding of the uterus and endocervical curettage can be performed if the patient is deemed inoperable or if primary radiation therapy will be used. Rectovaginal examination is essential for determining possible extension into the parametria or into the uterosacral ligaments.

Certain laboratory tests are useful in preoperative assessment. Complete hematologic profile, liver and kidney function tests, serum electrolyte determinations, urinalysis, and, if indicated, urine culture, pulmonary function tests, thyroid parameters, and clotting profile, although not essential to staging, form part of a thorough preoperative assessment of the patient with corpus cancer.

There is no highly specific marker for endometrial cancer but the ovarian cancer antigen CA-125 may be useful in the assessment of patients with endometrial cancer. In a retrospective study of 121 patients with endometrial cancer, Duk and coworkers in the Netherlands found that the incidence of elevated CA-125 increased with the increased stage of disease. Before treatment CA-125 levels correlated with tumor outside the corpus found at surgery as well as with vessel invasion of malignant cells; after treatment CA-125 paralleled the clinical course of disease, with elevated CA-125 levels preceding clinical evidence of intra-abdominal recurrence. Patsner and coworkers measured preoperative levels of CA-125 in 89 patients before surgical staging and found that 98% of patients with clinical or surgical stage I or II disease had normal preoperative values, whereas 28 of 31 patients (90.3%) with surgically proven extrauterine disease had elevated values. Kukura and coworkers, in a recent study from Yugoslavia, reported a significantly higher CA-125 value

TABLE 43–5
Staging and Preoperative Assessment Studies in Endometrial Cancer

History and complete physical examination
  Include careful evaluation of axillary, supraclavicular, and inguinal nodes.
Pelvic examination
  Careful inspection of vaginal vault
  Papanicolaou smear
  Endocervical curettage (for clinical staging)
  Sounding of endometrial cavity (for clinical staging)
  Palpation of fundal size, adnexa
  Rectovaginal to assess parametria, rectum, and cul-de-sac
Blood tests
  Complete hematology profile
  Chemistry screening panel, including liver and kidney function studies, electrolytes
  CA-125
  Optional: Thyroid function tests, clotting profile
Urinalysis and urine culture
Imaging studies
  Chest x-ray (computed tomography of chest, if indicated)
  Computed tomography of pelvis and abdomen
  Magnetic resonance imaging (optional)
  Pelvic ultrasonography (optional) [abdominal or vaginal technique]
  Barium enema (optional)
  Intravenous pyelography (optional)
Pulmonary function tests (for markedly obese patients or those with respiratory compromise) and arterial blood gas analysis
Proctosigmoidoscopy (colonoscopy if indicated)
Cystoscopy (if clinical stage II, III, or IV suspected)
Needle aspiration of suspicious nodes or masses
Indicated medical consultations

when tumor had invaded more than one third of the myometrium. Therefore, it appears that CA-125 levels have a useful predictive value in the preoperative assessment of patients with endometrial cancer, in that a higher than normal value should alert the surgeon to search for signs of extrauterine tumor.

Radiographic assessment of the patient with endometrial cancer should certainly include chest radiography, not only to look for metastatic disease, but also for preoperative assessment. For most patients the only other necessary study is a computed tomography scan of the pelvis and abdomen. Because of wide availability and the high ratio of information gained to cost, this study has supplanted the old duo of barium enema and excretory urography, except in instances where the specificity of those two studies is required. Cancer of the colon is more prevalent than endometrial cancer; thus the workup of patients with the latter must include some screening for the former. In asymptomatic patients I prefer several stool examinations for occult blood; a colonoscopy may be more sensitive but is not performed routinely in most clinics. Rectovaginal ex-

amination may suggest the necessity of proctosigmoidoscopy to document invasion into the rectum.

Other imaging studies are less essential in the routine evaluation of these patients, but in certain circumstances hysterography, ultrasonography, or magnetic resonance imaging (MRI) may provide useful information.

Hysterography has been used to provide additional information once a diagnosis of endometrial cancer is made. Using a water-soluble medium, the extent, size, and precise location of the tumor can be defined. Long-term follow-up studies conducted in Sweden dispelled the initial concern that hysterography could cause retrograde dissemination of tumor cells. Devore and coworkers noted abnormal hysterography findings in 40% of the patients they studied. Information about the size and contour of the uterine cavity, uterine preformation, and the location of the endometrial cancer helped in planning treatment for the patients. Tak and coworkers reported that pretreatment hysterography provided enough new information to cause them to alter their treatment plans for 28% of the patients tested. For the most part, however, the sophistication of other imaging techniques makes hysterography almost anachronistic.

Ultrasonography has a well-entrenched role in imaging adnexal disease, and may prove useful in the preoperative assessment of patients with corpus cancer. Delineation of adnexal enlargement may differentiate myomas from ovarian metastasis from endometrial cancer, or suggest the uncommon double primary. Ultrasonography also may be useful in identifying myometrial invasion. Cacciatore and coworkers in Helsinki found that myometrial invasion was correctly predicted by ultrasonography in 80% of 93 patients, with polypoid growth being the most common reason for inaccuracy. Gordon and coworkers found similar accuracy figures in a smaller number of patients in a study using both MRI and ultrasonography. Thus the overall usefulness of ultrasonography is unquestioned in evaluation of the adnexal areas, but its ability to accurately detect and define myometrial invasion has yet to be proved.

On the other hand, MRI shows promise of providing the surgeon with greater resolution of depth of myometrial invasion. A recent study conducted in Italy by Beloni and coworkers found diagnostic accuracy for MRI to be about 90% in predicting cervical involvement and myometrial invasion. Chen studied 50 consecutive patients with clinical stage I endometrial cancer and found that MRI accurately predicted deep myometrial invasion in 94% of cases and suggested an increase in clinical staging in 18%. This apparent ability to predict myometrial invasion might further assist the surgeon in preoperative planning (see Ch. 12).

The inclusion of cystoscopy in the preoperative

workup of patients with endometrial cancer depends on the index of suspicion that bladder invasion might be present. A negative urinalysis and an apparent stage I clinical examination makes bladder invasion a remote possibility, and cystoscopy would be unnecessary. Either microscopic or certainly gross hematuria mandates cystoscopy before surgery, and even a hint on examination or imaging that anterior extension has occurred should prompt visualization of the lower urinary tract. Urinary cytology may prove useful in occasional circumstances.

Fine needle aspiration of suspicious nodes or palpable cutaneous masses may provide documentation of distant metastasis and greatly alter surgical plans; appropriate, timely utilization of this technique is important. Fine needle aspiration of pelvic masses before definitive surgery usually is unwise.

Sound clinical judgment will dictate which of the extensive staging and preoperative evaluations in Table 43-5 are indicated for the individual patient. Suffice it to say that the wise surgeon is well prepared before surgery, and surgical staging of endometrial cancer is most proficiently accomplished after thoughtful and thorough preoperative evaluation.

Surgical Staging of Endometrial Carcinoma

Since the early textbook by Cullen, which stated that treatment of cancer of the endometrium was total abdominal hysterectomy and bilateral salpingo-oophorectomy, the cornerstone of the treatment of endometrial cancer has been surgical therapy. In the mid-1930s the use of preoperative radiation was popularized, and this remained the standard of care for many years. Beginning in the early 1970s attention was refocused on early surgical staging of endometrial cancer; this was first shown to be prognostically significant by the pilot staging studies conducted by the Gynecologic Oncology Group. Subsequently this cooperative group has helped to firmly establish the principle of surgical staging by continued analysis of a cohort of about 1000 patients who underwent a standard staging operation. Even without their impetus, numerous prominent groups have long considered that initial surgical therapy was appropriate, and the recent FIGO decision has rendered this approach the modern choice.

Surgical Staging Technique

The patient is brought to the operating suite after appropriate bowel preparation. It is important in the perioperative period to pay particular attention to the risk of thrombophlebitis. Clarke-Pearson has con-

clusively shown that patients undergoing radical gynecologic surgery, including lymphadenectomy and staging of endometrial cancer, are at a high risk for thrombophlebitis; in the age group at risk for corpus cancer these problems are likewise important to recognize. Thus all patients who are undergoing exploratory surgery for staging or therapy of endometrial cancer should receive prophylactic heparin or be fitted with intermittent pneumatic compression stocking devices, or a combination of both should be used if the risk is extremely high. Preoperative antibiotics usually are recommended, and I prefer to use a broad-spectrum antibiotic with good anaerobic coverage. Positioning the patient for surgery in the operating room is done according to the surgeon's preference. Some gynecologic oncologists prefer to have the patient's legs elevated in a modified lithotomy position when doing radical surgery, and indeed, this does assist technically in performing the paraaortic lymph node dissection, if the operator stands between the patient's legs. Most surgeons, however, prefer to have the patient in the supine position. If the former is chosen, care should be taken to appropriately pad vulnerable pressure points to avoid neuropathy.

A lower midline incision should be used, except in extremely obese patients, in whom a paramedian incision adjacent to the umbilicus works well and avoids the problems of the panniculus.

After entering the abdomen, peritoneal washings are obtained by injecting 50 to 100 ml of cool saline or other physiologic solution into the pelvis. By holding the intestines away and gently lifting the uterus forward, fluid can be collected after admixture with peritoneal fluid already present. It is important not to agitate or squeeze the uterus, as malignant cells may be dislodged and cause a spurious reading. Also, it is important not to use overly warm irrigating saline, as this may cause coagulation and shrinkage of cytoplasm of mesothelial cells, rendering them difficult to interpret. After washings are aspirated they are placed in a sterile container with dilute heparin and processed by standard cytologic techniques.

Next the peritoneal cavity is thoroughly explored. The uterus, tubes, and ovaries are palpated, and the retroperitoneal spaces are palpated for obviously suspicious lymph nodes. Care is taken to palpate the paraaortic area up to the level of the renal vessels. Thorough palpation of the hemidiaphragms, omentum, liver, kidneys, and peritoneal gutter is essential. After meticulous evaluation of the upper abdomen, the intestines are packed away and the pelvis is exposed, carefully dividing adhesions as necessary; suspicious adhesions or suspected implants should be preserved and submitted for analysis.

Old techniques suggest suturing the ends of the fallopian tubes shut at this juncture, but I believe that merely grasping each side of the fundus with long Kelly clamps, which serve the double purpose of being elevators, is sufficient.

After ligation and division of the round ligaments the retroperitoneal spaces are exposed. It is important to open the paravesical and pararectal spaces before initiating the hysterectomy. This not only allows discovery of obviously positive lymph nodes, but also more clearly defines the anatomy and circumvents distortion that can accompany hysterectomy. Sometimes extension of uterine cancer to the lower segment can balloon out the isthmus, and opening the spaces will allow identification of the ureter down to its entry into the vesicouterine tunnel, where it may be necessary to ligate the uterine artery. The infundibulopelvic ligaments and ovarian vessels are divided and ligated with direct visualization of the ureter. At this point appropriate dissection of the uterine vessels can be performed, but it is important not to dissect to the body of the cervix itself. Rather, after ureteral identification, the uterine vessels should be cross-clamped at the level just below the internal os. One cardinal point needs to be continually emphasized: To accomplish an appropriate extrafascial hysterectomy, the technique of "bouncing off" the cervix when placing clamps on the uterine vessels and parametria should be avoided (see Fig. 43-13 A–C). Likewise, after the clamps are appropriately placed, taking a wedge of the lower uterine segment or cervix to assure more voluminous pedicle is, in essence, leaving a portion of uterus in the patient. Therefore, after the appropriate tissues are clamped both the uterine vessels and the broad ligaments can be incised directly adjacent to the clamps with careful tying of the pedicle. Many gynecologists make the mistake of attempting large bites of tissue (the "gyn hog" technique) and thus necessitate a bulkier pedicle; bites of no more than 1 cm will allow tying of the pedicles with appropriate approximation and also fulfill extrafascial total abdominal hysterectomy criteria. In circumstances where the lower segment is ballooned out, such as discussed in the section on uterine sarcoma, it is even more mandatory that the "bouncing off" technique not be used (see Fig. 43-13 A–C), as the cervix at this point can rupture and allow tumor to be extruded into the operative field and traction on the cervix to be compromised.

After the parametrium has been divided dissection should continue along the upper vagina, after sharply dissecting the bladder away from the lower uterine segment and upper vagina. It is important at this point not to incise the endopelvic fascia in order to avoid the bladder. Paravaginal bites should be taken at least 1 cm below the fornix to allow a full cuff vaginal specimen, but it is not necessary to remove the upper third of the vagina, as is appropriate for a radical hysterectomy. The vaginal cuff should be closed with interrupted sutures after thorough irrigation of the peritoneal cavity. Irrigation should be repeated after the cuff is closed; use of an antibiotic solution for irrigation is per the surgeon's preference.

In certain circumstances a more radical hysterectomy may be necessary. When there is occult invasion outside the lower segment, where operative discovery of induration of the parametria occurs, or if gross disease is evident on the uterosacral ligaments, individualized wider margins must be taken according to the anatomic abnormality. Thus the anterior vesicouterine ligament may be dissected away from the anterior surface of the ureter, the bladder dissected further down the vagina, or the uterosacral ligament excised more radically. The posterior vesicouterine ligament does not need extensive dissection, and indeed, preservation of the posterior and inferior portions of the ureteral blood supply may prevent subsequent ureteral fistula or stenosis if postoperative radiation is necessary.

After hysterectomy the uterus is opened and evaluated intraoperatively. This must be done according to the preference of the department of pathology, as some pathologists prefer to open the uterus in the laboratory and others come to the operating room and open the uterus with the surgeon. The latter method is the most preferred, with direct communication between the surgeon and the pathologist. When this is not feasible, clear written instructions should accompany the specimen. In either circumstance preoperative consultation with the pathologist can speed the process and improve the quality of the evaluation.

In situations where the tumor is moderately to poorly differentiated, and the surgical staging system will most certainly be chosen, the pathologist will not need to determine depth of invasion. In well-differentiated tumors, however, surgical staging may not necessarily be advised or may not be the surgeon's choice; thus determination of depth of invasion is important. It often is impossible to tell from gross examination how much uterine invasion is present, and in certain circumstances it may be difficult to tell exactly where the uterine tumor is located. Accordingly, frozen sections should be performed for such patients. If depth of invasion is greater than the inner third in a well-differentiated tumor, complete surgical staging, including lymph node sampling, should be performed.

The actual method of determining the depth of myometrial invasion intraoperatively should be agreed on preoperatively by surgeon and pathologist. Doering and coworkers prospectively studied 148 patients with clinical stage I endometrial cancer, and found that gross visual examination of the cut surface of the tumor at the time of hysterectomy accurately determined the depth of myometrial invasion in 135 patients (91%), for a calculated sensitivity of 0.72, a specificity of 0.96, and a positive predictive value of 0.80. Malviya and coworkers in Detroit tested the reliability of intraoperative frozen section in 55 patients with clinical stage I corpus cancer. By comparing the results of gross examination with selected frozen section at the time of surgery with the results obtained from extensive sampling and subsequent observation of permanent microscopic sections they found that the depth of myometrial invasion was accurately predicted in 96.5% and the histologic grade, in 94.5%. Further, they found occult cervical invasion on frozen section in two thirds of patients who were later determined to have extension to the cervix. It would appear, therefore, that together, gross inspection and frozen sections intraoperatively offer reliable evaluation of the operative specimen.

After removal of the uterus, with intraoperative evaluation for myometrial invasion and grade and search for intraperitoneal disease, a decision must be made whether or not to proceed with lymph node sampling to complete the surgical staging. Three issues are of paramount importance: First, is the safety of lymph node sampling and its use on a routine basis sufficiently high to justify the additional operation time and possible complications? The second issue is whether the experience of the operator warrants lymph node sampling. Finally, the extent of the lymphadenectomy is an unsettled parameter.

Moore and coworkers clearly demonstrated that surgical morbidity in situations where lymph node sampling was performed supported its inclusion in the operative evaluation. This retrospective series included 292 patients with endometrial cancer and 262 patients with cervical cancer. All of the sampling was performed by residents and fellows in training under the direct supervision of certified gynecologic oncologists. In this clinical setting blood loss, transfusion requirements, operative time, and length of hospital stay were not significantly increased ($p > .05$) compared with those of similar patients who had surgical care without lymph node sampling. Although vascular injuries, hematomas, and lymphocysts were more common after lymph node sampling, there was no significant increase in mortality or long-term sequelae. Thus, based on the expected incidence of lymph node involvement versus the low complication rate, lymph node sampling is relatively safe and worthwhile.

Certain medical problems may alter the safety of the procedure. In patients with severe arteriosclerosis—not an unlikely occurrence in the age subject to risk of endometrial cancer—lymph node dissection may be associated with difficulty in establishing hemostasis; thus extensive lymph node sampling of nonsuspicious nodes probably should be avoided. It is not uncommon to encounter medical problems intraoperatively that require termination of an operation; hence the surgical procedure should always begin with a total abdominal hysterectomy and bilateral salpingo-oophorectomy in case the operation must be prematurely terminated. If excessive blood loss occurs with a hysterectomy, for whatever reason, it might be wise to forego the lymph node dissection, especially if the patient is unstable. Additionally, in very obese patients, retraction may be compromised, and no attempt at lymph node sampling—especially in the paraaortic area—should be undertaken if adequate exposure is not available.

In general, I believe that surgical therapy for endometrial cancer should not be undertaken by gynecologic surgeons who are not prepared to do a thorough staging procedure. For gynecologists not trained in lymph node sampling, gynecologic oncologists are widely available to assist in these procedures; or if a gynecologic oncologist is not available, a general surgeon, a vascular surgeon, or a trained urologist may assist in lymph node sampling. It is hoped that those who finish modern training programs would be able to perform adequate sampling.

The extent of the sampling will determine its actual worth in establishing the spread pattern of the disease. Thus lymph node sampling and evaluation of all the major lymph node areas should be performed. For example, obtaining one easy-to-dissect external iliac node and referring to this as lymph node sampling is inadequate. When the Gynecologic Oncology Group was conducting the endometrial surgical staging protocol, many such cases were encountered in the early years; subsequent protocol revisions required at least 10 lymph nodes cumulatively from each patient to qualify for staging. Thus, for lymph node sampling to be meaningful, all the major node-bearing areas, as shown later in Figure 43-6, should be sampled, removing all palpable and enlarged nodes. I do not, however, advocate a meticulous, complete lymphadenectomy such as indicated for cervical cancer.

Lymph node sampling should begin with removal of the external iliac nodes down to the level of the circumflex femoral vein and removal of the interiliac or obturator nodes down to the level of the obturator nerve. Care should be taken not to disrupt the superior vesical artery. Dissection of the hypogastric and common iliac nodes should then be performed.

Removal of paraaortic nodes may be the most important prognostically; some authors recommend removal of these nodes before or in lieu of pelvic node removal, using other prognostic factors in circumstances where the procedure must be aborted. Equally important is the issue of whether or not to perform the paraaortic dissection through the same peritoneal incision used for the pelvic nodes.

I prefer to mobilize and pack away the colon and small intestine and make an incision in the retroperitoneal space alongside the right common iliac artery and lower aorta. Using hemaclips or electrocautery for hemostasis, the common iliac artery is exposed and lymph nodes are removed from the right precaval chains, up to about the level of the renal or ovarian vessels. Although not required for surgical staging, evaluation of the middle aortic nodes as well as left paraaortic nodes may be accomplished, especially if these are enlarged. The latter may be difficult to expose without mobilizing the left colon along its peritoneal reflection and reflecting the descending and sigmoid colon medially. Thus, for complete paraaortic dissection, both approaches may be necessary, unless the inferior mesenteric artery is sacrificed or carefully retracted.

It is customary when complete lymph node dissection is performed to close the retroperitoneal space and use closed-suction drains, which may be removed in 5 days. Photopulos recently described leaving the retroperitoneal space open in a group of patients who underwent radical hysterectomy and node dissection without any increased morbidity. It has hence been my custom not to routinely use closed-suction drainage after lymph node sampling unless specifically indicated.

Postoperatively, early ambulation and attention to fluid and electrolyte balance in this patient group are important. Many patients are elderly and may be in precarious fluid balance preoperatively; thus the use of a standing fluid order is contraindicated. Additionally, node dissection may cause slow return of bowel function, and nasogastric suction might be helpful.

Although the surgical staging procedure just described has gained wide acceptance, the role of surgical debulking in endometrial cancer is not well established. Most investigators believe that when endometrial cancer extends into the peritoneal cavity, the disease is incurable and further surgical risks are unwarranted. The recent use of whole abdominal radiation and combination chemotherapy, however, has suggested that debulking might be of benefit. Thus omentectomy, resection of visible tumor, and appropriate biopsies should accompany the standard surgical procedure. At this time no effective chemotherapy for endometrial cancer is available (see below). Thus the maximum debulking effort that usually is expended in ovarian cancer is not recommended. Still, when there is pelvic extrauterine disease (such as with the cul-de-sac seeding), every effort should be made to remove the tumor en bloc with the uterus, as pelvic irradiation may be of benefit.

The surgical staging procedure should not greatly prolong the operative time, and with its completeness, accurate staging is afforded. After the operative procedure and appropriate postoperative recovery the pathologic findings should be discussed and the surgical staging system as outlined in Table 43-6 should be applied in treatment planning. It is best that such planning be performed by a tumor board or similar mechanism with multidisciplinary attendance, including pathologist, gynecologist, gynecologic oncologist, radiation therapist, and medical oncologist. Such a group allows definite opinions as to options of adjunctive

TABLE 43–6
Surgical Staging of Corpus Cancer

Stage

IA	G123	Tumor limited to endometrium
IB	G123	Invasion to $<1/2$ myometrium
IC	G123	Invasion to $>1/2$ myometrium
IIA	G123	Endocervical glandular involvement only
IIB	G123	Cervical stromal invasion
IIIA	G123	Tumor invades serosa and/or adnexae and/or positive peritoneal cytology
IIIB	G123	Vaginal metastases
IIIC	G123	Metastases to pelvic and/or paraaortic lymph nodes
IVA	G123	Tumor invasion of bladder and/or bowel mucosa
IVB	G123	Distant metastases, including intraabdominal and/or inguinal lymph nodes

Histopathology: Degree of Differentiation

Cases of carcinoma of the corpus should be grouped with regard to the degree of differentiation of the adenocarcinoma as follows:

G1 = 5% or less of a nonsquamous or nonmorular solid growth pattern

G2 = 6%–50% of a nonsquamous or nonmorular solid growth pattern

G3 = more than 50% of a nonsquamous or nonmorular solid growth pattern

Notes on Pathologic Grading

(1) Notable nuclear atypia, inappropriate for the architectural grade, raises the grade of a grade 1 or grade 2 tumor by 1.
(2) In serous adenocarcinomas, clear cell adenocarcinomas, and squamous cell carcinomas, nuclear grading takes precedent.
(3) Adenocarcinomas with squamous differentiation are graded according to the nuclear grade of the glandular component.

Rules Related to Staging

(1) Because corpus cancer is now surgically staged, procedures previously used for differentiation of stages are no longer applicable, such as the finding of D&C to differentiate between stage I and stage II.
  (a) It is appreciated that there may be a small number of patients with corpus cancer who will be treated primarily with radiation therapy. If that is the case, the clinical staging adopted by FIGO in 1971 would still apply, but designation of that staging system would be noted.
(2) Ideally, the width of the myometrium should be measured along with the width of tumor invasion.

(International Federation of Gynecologists and Obstetricians. Annual report on the results of treatment in gynecologic cancer. Int J Gynaecol Obstet 1989;28:189.)

treatment available. Thus the surgicopathologic findings are used to assign the patient a surgical stage, and treatment plans are formulated.

PROGNOSTIC FACTORS

The surgical staging system allows for evaluation of multiple significant prognostic factors (Table 43-7). All may be important individually in a given clinical situation, although ferreting them out with multivariate analysis to create independent factors to determine treatment has proved to be more difficult. Again, the results of the Gynecologic Oncology Group's surgical staging studies has proved to be a reliable source for analysis of prognostic factors, as each of the patients entered underwent the standard surgical staging procedure. Exact reporting and quality control were used throughout so that the individual prognostic factors could be analyzed both singly and with multivariate analysis. Much of the data has matured, so that in general, the prognostic variables substantiate uncontrolled observations about the same characteristics in previous studies. Virtually all older studies were not prospective, and the surgical procedure was not standardized. Although Gynecologic Oncology Group data may not be representative because of the group's referral center base, it appears that these data can be analyzed for their own merit and applied to clinical situations in any patient population, using the prognostic characteristics individually and as a group.

Histologic Grade

It comes as no surprise that grade is a highly important prognostic variable in endometrial cancer, and the degree of histologic differentiation of endometrial carcinoma has become a reliable indicator of the prognosis of the disease. The rating system introduced by Broders in 1941 included four categories that have correlated well with patient survival rates over many years of analysis. Mahle used the system to categorize

TABLE 43–7
Prognostic and Staging Factors Determined by Surgical Staging in Endometrial Cancer

Histologic grade of tumor
Depth of myometrial invasion
Status of pelvic and paraaortic nodes
Presence of malignant cells in peritoneal washings
Histologic type
Lymph-vascular invasion
Cervical invasion
Adnexal spread
Intraperitoneal disease
Estrogen and progesterone receptors

cellular differentiation in the endometrial cancer of 186 patients at the Mayo Clinic, and demonstrated a direct relation between histologic pattern and clinical results.

Both FIGO systems of staging include only three gradations of histopathologic differentiation of endometrial carcinoma, including well differentiated, grade 1 (Fig. 43-3); moderately differentiated, grade 2 (Fig. 43-4); and poorly differentiated, grade 3 (Fig. 43-5) tumors.

The FIGO classification is a modification in which Broders' grades 3 and 4 are combined into the FIGO grade 3. The FIGO classification was correlated with patient survival rates in a comprehensive review in an older paper by Jones (Table 43-8), which showed that a decrease in tumor differentiation was accompanied by a decrease in survival. Histologic differentiation also is related to lymph node metastasis, as Lewis, Cowdell, and Stallworthy found in a series of 107 patients who were treated by radical hysterectomy and lymph node dissection. Only 5% of the patients with well-differentiated tumors had positive pelvic lymph nodes, whereas 25% of the patients with poorly differentiated tumor had lymph node metastases. This early observation is supported by the data collated from the FIGO annual report (1988), in which 106 collaborating institutions provided information on age, histology of disease, type of treatment, and 5-year survival in cases of endometrial

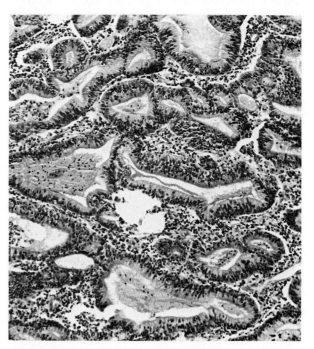

Figure 43–3. Well-differentiated adenocarcinoma (grade 1). The distinct glandular pattern is preserved with minimal stroma. Nuclear atypia, palisading, and cribriforming usually are present.

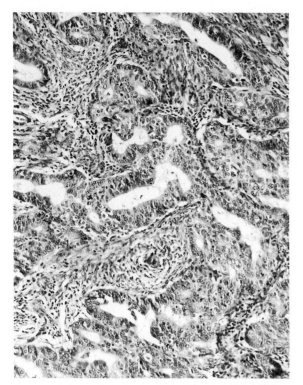

Figure 43–4. Moderately differentiated adenocarcinoma (grade 2). Well-formed glands are mixed with solid sheets of malignant cells. Although present, there is only moderate pleomorphism and chromatin clumping.

carcinoma treated between 1979 and 1981. In this report the mean age and clinical stage were higher among patients with a grade 3 tumor than among those with grade 1 and grade 2 lesions.

It has long been held that higher grade is a risk factor that can alone increase the chance of recurrence. Attempts to establish the relative risk by multivariate analysis are fraught with difficulties because of the nuances

of grading that some aggressive histologic types present. Yet for endometrial carcinoma the relative risk for recurrence of grade 3 may be three times that of grade 1 when grade is the only poor-risk factor.

Data from the FIGO annual report (volume 20) reflect a similar assigned risk for grade when large groups of patients are reported. As shown in Table 43-9, survival for 4476 clinical stage I patients with grade 1 tumors was 77.7%, but survival for 1192 patients with grade 3 tumors was 58.5%.

Histologic Type

About 70% to 75% of epithelial tumors of the endometrium are of the pure standard endometrioid histologic type and another 20% to 25% have mixed squamous elements. Less frequent are the more virulent clear cell and papillary serous subtypes, while mucinous and pure squamous carcinomas are relatively rare. It appears that among the endometrioid tumors, with or without squamous differentiation, the glandular grade is most important, but the uncommon types

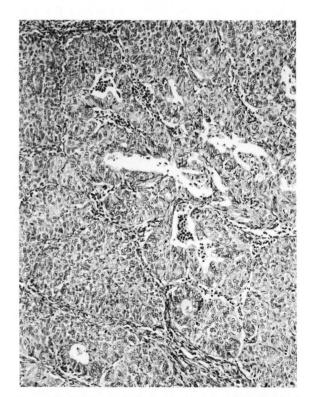

Figure 43–5. Poorly differentiated or undifferentiated adenocarcinoma (grade 3). The tumor is virtually all solid and has lost most glandular organization with shells of atypical cells and prominent mitotic activity, pleomorphism, and chromatin clumping.

TABLE 43–8
Correlation of Tumor Differentiation and 5-Year Survival Rates

TUMOR TYPE	NO. OF PATIENTS	5-YEAR SURVIVAL	
		Number	*Percentage*
Grade 1	1558	1267	81
Grade 2	1515	1124	74
Grade 3	917	462	50

(Adapted from Jones HW III. Treatment of adenocarcinoma of the endometrium. Obstet Gynecol Surv 1975; 30:147)

TABLE 43-9
Five-Year Survival Rates by Histologic Grade and Stage of Disease

HISTOLOGIC GRADE	STAGE I		STAGE II		STAGE III		STAGE IV	
	No. Treated	No. 5-yr Survival (%)	No. Treated	No. 5-yr Survival (%)	No. Treated	No. 5-yrSurvival (%)	No. Treated	No. 5-yr Survival (%)
Grade 1	4476	3480 (77.7)	564	364 (64.5)	191	80 (41.9)	74	13 (17.6)
Grade 2	3068	2257 (73.6)	625	374 (59.8)	256	95 (37.1)	85	10 (11.8)
Grade 3	1192	697 (58.5)	377	148 (39.3)	226	34 (15.0)	133	9 (6.8)
Not graded	907	568 (62.6)	211	107 (50.7)	103	34 (33.0)	57	6 (10.5)
Total	9643	7002 (72.6)	1777	993 (55.9)	776	243 (31.3)	349	38 (10.9)

(Adapted from FIGO. Statements of results obtained in patients treated in 1979 to 1981. In: Pettersson F, ed. Annual report on the results of treatment in gynecological cancer. Stockholm: Panorama Press, 1988.)

present special problems in management, risk of recurrence, and overall prognosis.

The term adenoacanthoma is probably entrenched in the minds of generations of pathologists and clinicians, yet the preferred expression, endometrioid carcinoma with benign squamous metaplasia, is more modern and less confusing. It is clear, however, that the prognosis for patients with adenoacanthoma is not worse. Fanning and coworkers reported 418 cases of clinical stage I corpus cancer and found absolute survival for adenocarcinoma (endometrioid) to be 88% and that for adenoacanthoma to be 91%. This corroborates with Connelly and coworkers' data, which showed that adenoacanthomas still had a somewhat better prognosis, grade for grade.

As shown in Table 43-10, adenosquamous carcinoma has been noted more commonly as part of this disease in recent years. In my experience this type constitutes less than 10% of all cases of endometrial carcinoma and represents a mixed tumor of glandular and squamous carcinoma. This tumor originally was considered to be a highly virulent tumor that metastasized rapidly. Salazar and coworkers conducted a clinicopathologic study by comparing the clinical behavior and cure rates of 87 patients with mixed adenosquamous carcinoma with those of 260 patients with pure adenocarcinoma and 29 patients with adenoacanthoma. As shown by this study, the prognosis is now considered to be similar, on a stage-for-stage basis, to that of a pure adenocarcinoma. Many gynecologists and pathologists have historically considered the degree of malignancy of adenosquamous carcinoma to be comparable to that of a poorly differentiated (grade 3) adenocarcinoma. Adenosquamous carcinoma occurs in an older age group than adenocarcinoma and is more frequently associated with a poorly differentiated glandular component. Based on these characteristics, it has been considered to carry a poorer prognosis. These beliefs have been challenged by the Salazar group. They found no basic difference in incidence, clinical history, response to

TABLE 43-10
Relative Frequency of Cell Subtypes

STUDY (YR)	FREQUENCY (%)					
	Adenocarcinoma	Adenocanthoma	Adenosquamous	Clear Cell	Papillary	Secretory
Christopherson et al (1982)	59.6	21.7	6.9	5.7	4.7	1.5
Underwood et al (1977)	70.0	14.0	7.0	1.0	8.0	
Wentz (1982)	56.3	18.9	24.8			
Salazar et al (1977)	69.0	8.0	23.0			
Boronow et al (1984)	82.9	6.7	10.4			
Fanning et al (1989)	66.0	16.0	5.0	3.0	8.0	2.0

irradiation therapy, or prognosis among adenosquamous carcinoma, adenoacanthoma, and pure adenocarcinoma.

These findings are not shared by Boronow and his colleagues in the Gynecologic Oncology Group, who had a different experience with 21 patients with adenosquamous carcinoma. In this group three patients (14%) had pelvic node metastases and five patients (23.8%) had aortic node metastases. The clinical behavior of this tumor was similar to a grade 3 lesion or a tumor with deep myometrial invasion.

Similarly, Fanning and coworkers found survival of patients with adenosquamous carcinoma to be much poorer than that of patients with adenocarcinoma (88% vs. 62%). This is apparently due to the greater predilection of adenosquamous carcinoma to have a grade 3 glandular component (52%) and deep myometrial invasion (36%).

As emphasized by Connelly and coworkers, the precise separation between adenoacanthoma and adenocarcinoma is, at times, difficult. They found in their overall group of 537 patients 30 whose squamous component was atypical but not frankly malignant. Those patients' survival was similar to that for the adenocanthoma group. Thus, when evaluating such patients, other risk factors must be used to determine postoperative treatment and establish prognosis.

More intense pathologic review has firmly established other histologic variants as distinct entities. Papillary serous adenocarcinoma has been subclassified from the epithelial tumors of the endometrium in recent years. Christopherson and coworkers reported 46 patients with papillary serous carcinoma, and described this lesion as a more aggressive type of papillary lesion. They found it to have a more anaplastic cellular pattern, to be associated with a more advanced stage of disease, and to have a 5-year cure rate of 51%, which is typical for extrauterine spread of tumor. Clinically, the spread pattern is more typical of ovarian carcinoma, and intraperitoneal disease is common even with clinical stage I disease. The Gynecologic Oncology Group finds this variant sufficiently virulent to include even early-stage cases in high-risk treatment protocols on the basis of histology alone.

Similarly, clear cell carcinoma is associated with a more aggressive clinical course. Fanning and coworkers found clear cell tumors to have deep myometrial invasion in 36% of their cases, and only 43% of their patients with stage I disease survived for 5 years. Several other histologic types have been described, but cases are few and analysis difficult. The secretory or mucinous adenocarcinoma has an appearance similar to that of other mucinous tumors of the lower genital tract, but its behavior appears to mimic adenocarcinoma of the endometrioid variety when grade and myometrial invasion are considered. Glassy cell carcinoma of the endometrium has been reported, but most pathologists consider this a poorly differentiated adenosquamous carcinoma, as is the case for its counterpart in the cervix. Pure squamous cell carcinoma of the endometrium seldom occurs, and appears to be moderately aggressive.

Again, when such rare histologic types are encountered, the use of other prognostic features is essential in treatment planning.

Depth of Myometrial Invasion

The inclusion of depth of myometrial invasion as the primary substaging mechanism for surgical stage I endometrial cancer emphasizes the paramount importance of this parameter. Although the grade of the tumor accurately reflects the aggressiveness and nuclear distortion, depth of invasion is the most reliable indicator of tumor volume. Careful analysis has shown that this histologic measurement is decidedly more predictive than the clinical staging's depth of the uterus as determined by preoperative sounding.

The extent of tumor invasion in the myometrium has been studied for correlations with the size of the uterine cavity, the frequency of pelvic node metastases, and the 5-year survival rate. In an older study Lewis, Cowdell, and Stallworthy reported that no pelvic nodes were found to be positive when the tumor involved only the endometrium or when the tumor extended only to the superficial layer of the myometrium. The 5-year survival rate was 93.7% among patients with no myometrial involvement and 88.1% among those with superficial myometrial involvement. Among patients who had tumors that extended within 2 mm or less from the serosal surface, 36.2% were found to have positive pelvic nodes and only 33% survived for 5 years even though they received irradiation therapy after surgery. These early data correlate well with the published pilot study of the Gynecologic Oncology Group, as reported by Boronow and coworkers. In this multi-institutional study involving 222 patients with stage I endometrial carcinoma there was an overall 10% incidence of positive pelvic lymph nodes (Table 43-11), which is similar to the 12% finding in the Oxford study. Deep myometrial tumor invasion of grade 3 tumors was associated with a 43.7% incidence of pelvic lymph node metastasis among the 222 cases in which pelvic lymph nodes were resected. In all degrees of myometrial invasion, including superficial, intermediate, and deep myometrial extension, pelvic node metastasis was more common in patients with grade 3 tumors. The later update of the groupwide study involving 621 patients, as reported by Creasman, substantiated the im-

TABLE 43–11
Node Metastasis in Patients with Clinical Stage I Endometrial Carcinoma by Invasion and Grade*

INVASION AND GRADE	NO. OF PATIENTS	PELVIC NODE METASTASIS		AORTIC NODE METASTASIS IN SAMPLED PATIENTS		AORTIC NODE METASTASIS OVERALL	
		Number	*Percentage*	*Number*	*Percentage*	*Number*	*Percentage*
Endometrium G1	58	1	1.7	1/47	2.1	1/58	1.7
Endometrium G2	27	1	3.7	0/15	0.0	0/27	0.0
Endometrium G3	7	0	0.0	0/06	0.0	0/07	0.0
Superficial G1	27	0	0.0	0/18	0.0	0/27	0.0
Superficial G2	40	1	2.5	0/26	0.0	0/40	0.0
Superficial G3	13	3	23.1	5/11	45.5	5/13	38.5
Intermediate G1	4	0	0.0	0/02	0.0	0/04	0.0
Intermediate G2	8	2	25.0	1/04	25.0	1/08	12.5
Intermediate G3	5	1	20.0	0/03	0.0	0/05	0.0
Deep G1	4	1	25.0	0/03	0.0	0/04	0.0
Deep G2	13	6	46.2	5/09	55.5	5/13	38.5
Deep G3	16	7	43.7	5/14	35.7	5/16	31.3
Total	222	23	10.3	17/158	10.08	17/222	7.7

* It should be noted that patients were clinically staged and many would be up-staged on the new system. Also, depth of invasion is calculated by thirds of muscle thickness.

(Boronow RC, Morrow CP, Crasman WT, et al. Surgical staging in endometrial cancer: clinical pathologic findings of a prospective study. Obstet Gynecol 1984; 63:825)

portance of deep myometrial invasion in predicting spread patterns and, hence, prognosis.

The three grades of stage I lesions have been correlated with the extent of tumor invasion. Holmesly and coworkers observed 539 patients with carcinoma confined to the corpus (stage I), and found that only 1 of 93 patients with deep myometrial invasion had a grade 1 lesion. Of the other 92 patients with deep myometrial extension, 48 had grade 2 lesions, 32 had grade 3 lesions, and 12 were not recorded. Deep myometrial invasion resulted in a 5-year survival of only 61%.

Many investigators have analyzed clinical stage I adenocarcinoma for correlations between myometrial involvement and pelvic node metastasis. By collecting data from many reports Morrow and coworkers reviewed 193 patients who were treated with radical hysterectomy and pelvic lymphadenectomy. They found metastases in only 3.4% of the patients with no myometrial invasion, whereas in the patients with deep myometrial involvement 14.4% had positive pelvic nodes. The data confirmed the earlier report of Lewis and coworkers.

In the 1988 FIGO report on endometrial cancer, data on depth of myometrial invasion was available in 6584 operated cases. Of these, there were 3224 patients with clinical stage I cancer who showed a 82.4% 5-year survival when less than one third of the myometrium was invaded, but in 1144 patients with more than 50% myometrial invasion survival was 66.8%. For stage II patients depth of myometrial invasion affected survival

similarly, with survival 73.8% and 50.3%, respectively, for these subgroups.

Despite the importance of myometrial invasion when taken as a single independent variable and prognostic factor, it is less impressive than would be anticipated when subjected to multivariable analysis. It appears that as a single risk factor, myometrial invasion carries a medium risk when it is superficial or mid-muscle, but carries a higher risk when it is deep. Clearly, the patient with deep myometrial invasion also is more than likely to demonstrate one or more other poor prognostic factors. The Gynecologic Oncology Group currently has an ongoing study that is prospectively analyzing patients with medium-risk disease as determined by myometrial invasion.

Lymph Node Metastasis

It was not until the early 1970s, when the pendulum of treatment began to swing away from requisite preoperative radiation, that pelvic lymph node involvement in endometrial carcinomas began to be more appreciated. This prompted collaborative attempts by the Gynecologic Oncology Group and others to more accurately determine patterns of spread.

Endometrial carcinoma spreads through three separate lymphatic pathways: paracervical and parametrial lymphatics, ovarian lymphatics, and round ligament lymphatics (Fig. 43-6). Although the lymphatic drainage

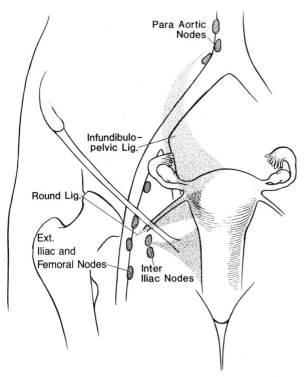

Figure 43–6. Lymphatic pathways of tumor spread of endometrial carcinoma to pelvic and extrapelvic nodes.

of the uterine fundus and cervix directs most of the metastases to the pelvic lymph nodes, the paraaortic nodes also are within the pathway of metastatic spread through the ovarian (infundibulopelvic ligament) lymphatic vessels. Because the left ovarian vein drains into the left renal vein, it is understandable that distant metastases may occur directly into the upper abdomen. Although an infrequent site of lymph node metastasis, the lymphatic vessels adjacent to the round ligament provide an anatomic explanation for the uncommon occurrence of tumor involvement of the external iliac and femoral lymph nodes. The liver may be involved in tumor metastases, either from the interchange from paraaortic and portal vein lymphatics or more directly by hematogenous spread. Bone and lung metastases are more commonly the result of bloodstream dissemination of tumor cells, and these are more common when lymph nodes are involved.

In the Gynecologic Oncology Group collaborative pilot study Boronow and coworkers made a clinicopathologic study of the uterus, fallopian tubes, ovaries, and pelvic lymph nodes of 222 patients and the aortic nodes of 158 patients with clinical stage I endometrial carcinoma. As shown in Table 43-11, among 222 patients operated on for stage I endometrial cancer, both the grade of the tumor and the extent of myo-

metrial invasion were important determinants of the frequency of pelvic node metastases. Pelvic nodes were involved in 10.3% of the patients, with a 2.2% incidence for grade 1, 11.4% for grade 2, and 26.8% for grade 3 tumors. Pathologic examination of surgical specimens showed that the risk of pelvic lymph node metastasis was negligible when the cancer was confined to the endometrium, regardless of the grade of the tumor. When superficial invasion to the inner one third of the myometrium had occurred, only grade 3 lesions showed a significant incidence of pelvic node metastasis (23.1%). However, when the middle (intermediate) one third of the myometrium had been invaded by tumor, the incidence of pelvic node metastasis for grade 2 and grade 3 tumors was 25% and 20%, respectively. When deep myometrial invasion had occurred with extension of tumor to the outer one third of the uterine wall, all grades of tumor showed a high incidence of pelvic node metastases: 25.0%, 46.2%, and 43.7%, respectively, for grade 1, 2, and 3 lesions.

Paraaortic node metastases were detected in 10% of the 158 patients in the Gynecologic Oncology Group study in whom lymph nodes were sampled and in 7.7% of the entire 222 cases. The pelvic nodes provide a valid indicator of the risk of paraaortic node metastasis. In Boronow's study, when pelvic nodes were negative, only 1.5% of paraaortic nodes were found to be positive for metastatic tumor. When pelvic node metastases occurred, the paraaortic nodes also were involved in 60% of the cases. Further, this study found that 80% of stage I tumors were grade 1 and grade 2 lesions (40% each), and 20% were poorly differentiated, grade 3 lesions. About 40% of the tumors were confined to the endometrium, and 20% showed deep myometrial invasion. As noted in Table 43-11, when deep myometrial invasion occurs, between 25% and 46% of cases will have pelvic lymph node metastases. Also, when deep myometrial invasion occurs, more than 30% of the cases with grade 2 or grade 3 lesions will have paraaortic lymph node metastases. Again, the data on these 222 patients were substantiated in the extended group-wide study as reported by Creasman. The estimated true risk for lymph node metastasis for clinical stage I endometrial cancer varies between 7.7% and 10.8%.

Metastasis to the pelvic lymph nodes also is related to tumor extension into the cervical canal (stage II). Because of the rich concentration of lymphatics in the paracervical tissues (cardinal ligaments), cervical involvement increases the potential for dissemination of tumor cells to pelvic lymph nodes. The frequency of extension of endometrial carcinoma to the isthmus and cervical canal increases with the extent of myometrial invasion. As reported by Lewis and Bundy, endocervical involvement (occult stage II) increases from 7.3% of cases with tumor in the endometrium only to 9.3% with superficial myometrial invasion, to 10.8% with intermediate invasion, and to 25% with deep myometrial invasion. About 15% of all cases of endometrial cancer will have either occult or clinical extension of tumor to the cervix. The incidence of pelvic node metastases in stage II disease approximates 30% and increases to nearly 45% with grade 3 lesions. Thus to the classic triad of stage of disease, grade of tumor, and myometrial extension must be added histologic type of tumor, all of which appear to be independent variables that influence the frequency of pelvic and extrapelvic lymph node metastases and the hematogenous spread of the tumor. In addition, tumor permeation of lymphatic channels that drain the uterus and cervix is interrelated with the extent and location of the disease. Regardless of the stage of the disease, the overall 5-year cure rate is reduced to 50% to 55% when pelvic lymph nodes are found to contain metastatic tumor.

Similarly, when these factors are further analyzed, intraperitoneal disease is markedly increased when any of these variables are more advanced, as documented by Creasman's analysis of the spread patterns of the 621 patients in the Gynecologic Oncology Group study, which were all surgically staged.

Other Prognostic Variables

To the dominant prognostic variables detailed above—histologic grade and type, depth of myometrial invasion, and status of target lymph nodes—must be added other factors that are somewhat less pivotal in making treatment decisions. These factors may not only alter final surgical stage, but also portend a statistically worse prognosis.

Increasing age of the patient continues to play an important role in predicting outcome. As stated earlier, the mean age at diagnosis continues to rise and other poor prognostic factors tend to accelerate as age increases. The data from the 20th FIGO report were subjected to intense multivariate analysis; in each subgroup increasing age appears to portend a worse prognosis. For instance, among 8495 clinical stage I and stage II patients who underwent surgery as part of their therapy there was 88.9% survival in the age group 30 to 69 years, but only 71.8% survival in those over 70. When no surgery was used in treatment, an assumed higher-risk group medically, survival was 64.9% for those aged 40 to 69 and 41.0% for those over 70. Bonham and Bonham collected a 24-year follow-up study of 535 patients with endometrial carcinoma in New Zealand and found that of the survivors, 27.7% had been diagnosed before menopause. The group diagnosed before menopause had an 88.8% survival rate for more than 5 years. The postmenopausal patients had a lower sur-

vival rate, which continued to decline until it stabilized after 15 years at 58.3%.

Preliminary analysis of data from the Gynecologic Oncology Group larger-group reports suggests that age greater than 55 would impact a three times greater relative risk of recurrence, but this must be weighed against the extended FIGO multivariate analysis, which suggests that in those women with good outlooks from other risk factors, age becomes less a factor in survival. For example, in the most favorable clinical stage I group treated with surgery or surgery and intracavitary radiation, 92.6% of 1017 patients aged 60 to 69 survived 5 years, whereas 97% of 1594 similarly treated women aged 30 to 59 survived the 5-year benchmark. Therefore, age appears to be an independent variable of uncertain significance in treatment planning; the surgeon must discount the chronologic age of the patient and plan treatment according to the apparent biologic and physiologic age.

Steroid receptors from endometrial cancer specimens are clearly less well established as indicators for making therapeutic decisions, as are their receptor counterparts in breast cancer. However, accumulated data have shown the information useful for predicting outcome as well as for suggesting initial therapy if disease recurs. Ehrlich and coworkers reported the relation of clinical outcome to steroid receptor content as determined by the dextran-charcoal method in 175 patients with endometrial adenocarcinoma. Progesterone receptor content appeared to be more useful than estradiol receptors, and the former correlated well with grade, histology, adnexal spread, age, and, more important, recurrence. The latter in those with stage I disease was significantly more common if tumors were negative for progesterone receptor than if they were positive (37.2% vs. 7%). Although a similar relation in recurrence was noted for estradiol receptor content (41.2% recurrence for negative vs. 12.7% for positive), overall survival correlated only with progesterone receptor content, with those patients positive for progesterone receptor showing overall superior survival ($p < .001$). The usefulness of receptors may be limited by available methods, as it has been clearly shown that the contribution of varying amounts of receptor-positive benign tissue components, such as stroma, myometrium, and adjacent normal glandular epithelium, is significant and may skew results of analysis. Segreti and coworkers, using monoclonal antireceptor antibodies, immunohistochemically demonstrated significant levels of both receptors in nonmalignant elements surrounding the tumor cells. These and other conflicting reports regarding quality control of receptor assays have made interinstitutional studies virtually impossible; hence the overall utility of steroid receptors in endometrial cancer has yet to be established. Still, obtaining this information from surgical specimens remains part of the prognostic portfolio and should be accomplished at the time of intraoperative specimen evaluation.

Peritoneal cytology has been thrust into the surgical staging system with a degree of importance that perhaps belies its somewhat controversial role as a high-risk indicator. In a comprehensive review of the existing literature McLellan and coworkers combined 15 studies to establish an incidence of 11.4% positive peritoneal cytology among 3091 patients with clinical stage I adenocarcinoma. Their review clearly indicated that patients with positive cytology are at higher risk for recurrent disease, and that the presence of malignant cells is predictive of other poor prognostic factors, including advanced histologic grade, depth of myometrial invasion, and lymph node metastasis. Their cumulative data suggests that the importance of peritoneal cytology, a rather easy maneuver to accomplish, might rest in its predictive value for presence of lymph node metastasis. Thus the incidence of positive lymph nodes in patients with positive cytology was 35%, but only 8.7% in those with negative cytology ($p < .001$). Sutton confirmed the importance of peritoneal cytology in a series of 615 patients, in which survival in clinical stage I with negative cytology was superior to that when there were malignant cells in the washings. He correctly pointed out, however, that the proper assessment of peritoneal cytology as an *independent* risk factor is not possible without a prospective study, which has been deemed by statisticians as virtually impossible. Therefore, surgical staging mandates obtaining cytologic evaluation of the peritoneal cavity; if the results are positive, the prognosis for patients clearly is guarded.

Cervical invasion, lymph-vascular space invasion, adnexal spread, and *presence of intraperitoneal disease* are clear indicators of aggressive disease. All correlate well with other poor prognostic factors, and seldom is their presence isolated, requiring therapeutic decisions on that information alone. Boronow and coworkers' report of the Gynecologic Oncology Group pilot study confirmed that any of these factors portend a higher risk for lymph node metastasis, which was confirmed by Creasman and coworkers' report of the expanded series. Three of the four factors increase the actual surgical stage, but the individual clinician must assign the prognostic weight of lymph-vascular invasion. In the Gynecologic Oncology Group study, however, lymph-vascular invasion portended a much worse prognosis, and including this histologic observation in the pathology report is useful.

POSTOPERATIVE TREATMENT

After the comprehensive operation the gynecologic surgeon can accurately assess the prognostic factors above (summarized in Table 43-12), assign the appropriate surgical stage, and plan postoperative treatment with full knowledge of disease extent as well as prognostic variables. By this method it is estimated that 50% to 60% of

TABLE 43–12
Postoperative Treatment Plan for Endometrial Carcinoma

STAGE		TREATMENT
IA	G1, G2, G3	Close follow-up
IB	G1	Close follow-up
IB	G2	Consider radiation
IB	G3	Postoperative radiation
IC	G1, G2, G3	Postoperative radiation
IIA	G1	Consider radiation
IIA	G2, G3	Radiation
IIB	G1, G2, G3	Radiaton therapy
IIIA	G1, G2, G3 (positive washings only)	Intraperitoneal ^{32}P
IIIA	G1, G2, G3 (adnexal spread)	Radiation
IIIA	G1, G2, G3 (serosal spread)	Radiation
IIIB	G1, G2, G3	Pelvic radiation; Groin irradiation if lower 1/3 of vagina involved
IIIC	G1, G2, G3	High-risk protocol treatment; if not available, pelvic radiation; consider whole abdomen radiation
IVA	G1, G2, G3	Radiation
IVB	G1, G2, G3	Whole-abdomen radiation or chemotherapy

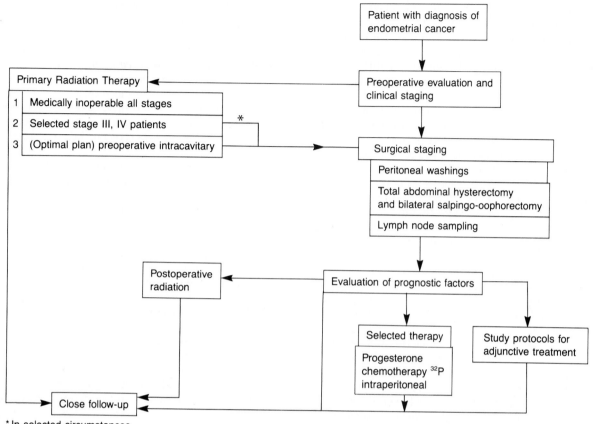

Figure 43–7. Algorithm for the overall treatment of endometrial cancer.

patients may need no further therapy, but those with proven risk factors can have treatment tailored to actual disease parameters.

For patients who are thought to need additional therapy after definitive surgery, three basic modalities are available: radiation therapy, chemotherapy, and hormonal treatment, all of which are incorporated into Table 43-12. The latter two are primarily used for advanced disease or in palliative situations, but the use of irradiation in corpus cancer is time honored and should be considered part of the therapeutic plan, not mere adjunctive treatment. Further, as discussed later, there is still a role for primary or preoperative radiation, and the wise clinician must keep all options open in planning therapy. The overall treatment plan for endometrial cancer is schematically depicted in Figure 43-7.

Irradiation Therapy

The potential options for the use of radiation therapy in endometrial carcinoma are summarized in Table 43-13. These should be selectively used after tumor

TABLE 43–13
Radiation Therapy in Endometrial Cancer

1. After surgical staging
   Vault radiation
   Whole-pelvic radiation
   Extended-field radiation
   (to paraaortic nodes)
   Whole-abdomen radiation with pelvic boost
2. Preoperatively
   Intracavitary and vault brachytherapy
   Whole-pelvis external therapy
3. As sole therapy
   Intracavitary
   Heymon packing
   Standard tandem with ovoids
   Whole pelvis with or without extended field
   Whole abdomen with pelvic boost
4. For recurrent disease
   Whole pelvis, with or without vault brachytherapy
   Spot irradiation for symptomatic metastasis
5. Special applications
   Intraperitoneal ^{32}P
   Template interstitial brachytherapy
   Intraoperative radiotherapy

board conference with close interaction and cooperation between the gynecologist and radiation therapist.

Radiation After Surgical Staging. Vault irradiation alone can be used to help prevent vaginal recurrence in selected cases. The benefit of this method alone has never been proved in a randomized trial, but numerous studies have advocated its use. In a randomized study of 540 patients from the Norwegian Radium Hospital by Aalders and coworkers 6000 rad was given to the vaginal mucosa postoperatively, and the patients were then randomized to receiving either no further therapy or additional whole-pelvis external therapy (4000 rad). The patients who received only vault radiation had a 6.9% vaginal recurrence rate, whereas in the combination group only 1.9% suffered vault occurrences. These data clearly indicate that postoperative vaginal radiation alone is ineffective in *eliminating* local recurrence, and hence it should probably be used only when high-risk factors are present, and then as part of a whole-field radiation plan. Additionally, the proximity of adhered bowel in the postoperative pelvis should be considered when advocating vault brachytherapy.

The use of whole-pelvis radiation therapy postoperatively is a realistic option for patients with endometrial cancer, although no randomized prospective trial with stratification for risk factors has ever been reported. Raw survival data suggest benefit of the combination, but when analyzed in multivariate analysis the differences are small or insignificant. Jones' review of more than 6000 clinical stage I cases showed 5-year survival of 75% for those treated with surgery alone and 78% for those treated with surgery and irradiation. Although many clinicians believe that the cure rate of patients with advanced endometrial cancer can be improved with the adjunctive use of irradiation, patients with a well-differentiated tumor in a small uterus without myometrial invasion have an equally high survival rate without preoperative or postoperative irradiation. Some physicians continue to debate the issue, but Aalders and coworkers from the Norwegian Radium Hospital in Oslo have somewhat clarified this matter in the aforementioned study of 540 patients with clinical stage I endometrial carcinoma. In their prospective randomized study that compared vault postoperative irradiation therapy with or without whole-pelvis irradiation therapy, there was no difference in survival among patients with grade 1 and grade 2 disease. This study recommended that external therapy was advisable, primarily for patients with grade 3 lesions or those with deep myometrial invasion. This conclusion also has been supported by Piver and coworkers.

The Gynecologic Oncology Group currently is conducting a randomized study (GOG #99) to attempt to scientifically predict the benefit of postoperative irradia-

tion in a medium-risk group of patients. The study design excludes patients with nodal metastasis, intraperitoneal disease, positive cytology, adnexal spread, or cervical stromal invasion, and hence makes eligible virtually many surgical stage I patients. Postoperatively, patients are randomized to receive either no further treatment or 5040 centigray (cGy) whole-pelvis irradiation to begin no later than 8 weeks after surgery. It is hoped that future editions of this textbook can report the preliminary results of that study to guide the surgeon in recommending postoperative treatment.

Until firm scientific information is available, clinicians must use local treatment patterns and time-honored clinical practices. The schema shown (Fig. 43-8) can be used in patients with clinical or surgical stage I as a rough guide to postoperative treatment, realizing that the middle- or gray-zone patients should be informed that there is no proven benefit from radiation treatment except perhaps a decrease in pelvic recurrence.

Postoperative extended-field radiation should be considered for patients with nodal metastasis. The poor survival rate of patients with metastases to the paraaortic nodes has led to the practice of extending postsurgical irradiation to include the entire paraaortic lymph node chain. Only recently has this aggressive irradiation approach proved to be effective in controlling metastatic disease, with 5-year actuarial survival rates approaching 60% in some studies. Such radical and

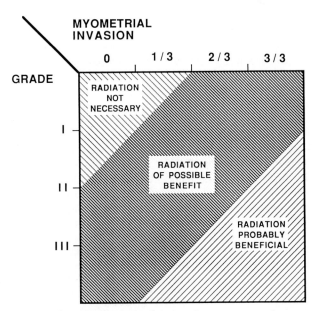

Figure 43–8. Schematic diagram for treatment planning postoperatively when depth of myometrial invasion and grade are the principal prognostic indicators that can be established.

somewhat risky techniques need to be continually evaluated in clinical trials.

Whole-abdomen radiation may offer benefit to high-risk groups, such as those with intraperitoneal disease or positive paraaortic nodes. Greer and Hamberger from M. D. Anderson Hospital reported that for 31 patients who had intraperitoneal endometrial cancer treated by the whole-abdomen moving strip technique with residual disease equal to or less than 2 cm, the corrected 5-year survival was 80%. Only one patient required operative intervention for a radiation complication. Although these results seem overly optimistic, they do suggest that aggressive irradiation therapy may be of benefit to patients with advanced disease. The Gynecologic Oncology Group currently is conducting a nonrandomized study of patients with ultra high-risk disease using a different whole-abdomen technique. This method calls for megavoltage with two pairs of parallel opposed fields, the whole abdomen being treated to a total dose of 3000 cGy in 20 fractions of 150 cGy each. This treatment is followed by a pelvic boost with a midplane dose of 1980 cGy at 180 cGy per fraction for 11 treatments. This combined treatment takes about 6 to 7 weeks. Those patients with positive paraaortic nodes resected can receive an additional boost of 1500 cGy to the paraaortic chain. Such intense therapy can be expected to be accompanied by a relatively high frequency of both minor and major bowel complications, but most should be manageable. This aggressive approach should be viewed as investigational, but may be necessary to salvage high-risk patients.

Preoperative Radiation. Preoperative radiation treatment is still the standard of practice in many institutions, although it is clear that for many patients with clinical stage I disease, it is unnecessary. If used, about 5000 cGy is given to the whole pelvis followed by intracavitary treatment.

The use of intracavity radiation alone preoperatively still has many advocates, even among those who are champions of surgical staging. In 1916 Howard Kelly suggested using intrauterine radium before surgery to sterilize the endometrium. Kelly, a pioneer in the use of radium, had noticed that treatment with intrauterine radium before a dilatation and curettage had resulted in sterilization of the endometrium in several cases.

Although the benefits of preoperative irradiation treatment are still argued, one positive effect has been relatively well documented. A definite decrease in the incidence of vaginal recurrence for certain risk groups results when either intracavitary or external irradiation is used in addition to surgery. In a collective review of 2264 patients Jones showed that when surgery was used without prior irradiation, the vaginal recurrence rate was 10.3%. When postoperative vaginal radium or ces-

ium was used, the rate of vaginal recurrence decreased to 5.2%, and the rate decreased further, to 4.6%, when preoperative radium or cesium was given. These data, however, were neither randomized nor prospective, and certainly not stratified for risk factors.

If the decision is made to use preoperative intracavitary therapy, the ideal brachytherapy dose is 6000 cGy given by Fletcher-Suit applicator to a depth of 1.0 to 1.5 cm beneath the endometrial surface, while 7000 cGy is applied to the vaginal surface with colpostats. The dosage should be delivered over 48 to 72 hours, and the rectum and bladder should be carefully displaced from the vaginal sources to avoid irradiation damage. Computer programming of the isodose curves can be used to check the dosage at the wall of the uterus and of contiguous organs.

With modern irradiation techniques the vesicovaginal and the rectovaginal septa can be monitored while irradiation is applied. Intracavitary doses can be programmed with computerized isodose curves so that the precise irradiation dose to the bladder base, the rectum, and the entire broad ligament can be recorded. These improved techniques have increased the effectiveness of irradiation therapy while decreasing the incidence of injury to the bowel and bladder.

Radiation Therapy Alone. In many cases surgery is performed 48 to 72 hours after central irradiation treatment. Immediate surgery has several advantages for both physician and patient. The patient can be treated completely during one hospital admission. The surgeon benefits because the pelvic tissues will not show long-term irradiation effects, so that the surgical specimen can be studied to determine both histologic grade and extent of myometrial invasion.

When patients are medically inoperable irradiation only may be used for definitive treatment. Despite general agreement that without surgery survival rates are lowered by 10% to 20%, amazingly good results have been provided with sophisticated radiotherapeutic techniques.

The M. D. Anderson Hospital and other expert radiotherapeutic centers have now achieved favorable results for the treatment of patients with serious medical complications or advanced disease, with cure rates that equal those of primary surgery and combined irradiation and surgery. As reported by Landgren and coinvestigators, a 5-year survival rate of 68% was achieved in the M. D. Anderson study, and a 10-year survival rate of 57% was achieved for patients with medical contraindications for surgery. Patients with an unresectable tumor treated with megavoltage irradiation had a 26% survival rate at both 5 and 10 years.

Varia and coworkers from the University of North Carolina reported on 73 patients with clinical stage I and stage II disease who were poor operative risks and were treated with radiation only. Their data were broken down to show the impact of grade on survival, with the 5-year survival for grade 1, 72%; for grade 2, 59%; and for grade 3 only 31%, a profound and significant variance. In addition, they pointed out the limitations of using radiation only, as 83% of the recurrences had a local or pelvic component, and suggested aggressive techniques, including chemoradiation, to improve local control.

The M. D. Anderson series stressed the use of intrauterine and intravaginal radiation sources combined with high-voltage external irradiation, when possible, to control the central tumor and any extension to the parametrium and pelvic wall. Autopsy reports from the medically inoperable patients showed that pelvic control of the disease had been obtained in 89% of stage Ia, 78% of stage Ib, 82% of stage II, and 62% of stage III lesions.

Recurrence Disease. Radiation is the treatment of choice for pelvic recurrent disease if the patient has not received the maximum adjuvant radiation previously. Both intravaginal and external techniques can be used. Irradiation therapy is most effective for local recurrences confined to the central pelvis. The poor cure rates reported by Columbia-Presbyterian Hospital indicate the grave prognosis for recurrent endometrial carcinoma. Even when lesions recurred in the vagina, the survival rates were only 15% to 20%. Brown and coworkers from the Mayo Clinic reported a much more favorable survival rate of 50% for 30 patients with vaginal recurrences treated with irradiation.

When preoperative intracavitary irradiation was used before the initial surgical treatment, the secondary treatment should be limited to 5000 cGy of betatron or linear accelerator megavoltage delivered to the midpelvis. If no irradiation had been used during the initial treatment, 5500 cGy of megavoltage irradiation may be given to the whole pelvis followed by an additional 4000 cGy given to the vaginal surface with vaginal ovoids. Normal tissue tolerance must be carefully observed. The total irradiation dose to the vesicovaginal wall should not exceed 8000 cGy delivered to a depth of 0.5 cm. The rectovaginal wall should not be treated with doses higher than 7000 cGy delivered to a depth of 0.5 cm.

When endometrial cancer metastasizes to bone or peripheral nodal areas, spot irradiation can be used for pain control and to reduce unsightly and frightening lesions. The tolerance of adjacent tissues usually allows relatively high fractions, so that therapy can be completed quickly.

Special Applications. Customized radiation applications may be necessary in treating endometrial cancer. Interstitial therapy is often necessary in advanced disease when vaginal, parametrial, or pelvic disease needs higher doses than can be delivered by standard applicators. Similarly, the use of intraoperative radiation, when available, may be useful for isolated, unresectable metastasis. Although neither of these techniques can be relied on alone, they could be part of a comprehensive, customized therapy for advanced disease.

Intraperitoneal radioactive phosphorus (^{32}P) is a specialized intracavity treatment used for patients with positive peritoneal cytology, but such treatment cannot yet be termed standard care for all centers. Soper and coworkers at Duke University reported on 65 women with malignant cytology from endometrial cancer who were treated with intraperitoneal radioactive chromic phosphate suspension. Disease-free survival was 94% for surgical stage I (older staging system adaptation), and the incidence of intraperitoneal recurrences was low, as only 1 of 11 patients who recurred did so solely in the peritoneal cavity. None of the 48 patients who received ^{32}P alone suffered chronic intestinal morbidity requiring surgery, but 5 of 17 patients who received adjuvant pelvic irradiation in addition to ^{32}P had complications necessitating surgical intervention. It was the authors' conclusion that when peritoneal cytology was the only increased risk factor present, ^{32}P was the treatment of choice. I concur, but this is by no means a universal opinion. Further, as previously pointed out, malignant cytology frequently is accompanied by other poor prognosis factors, and such patients might better be treated with whole-abdomen radiation and certainly, if possible, with advanced protocols in an oncology center.

TREATMENT OF ADVANCED DISEASE

Clinical Stage II

Most patients with stage II disease should enter the surgical staging protocol and be evaluated operatively. Many clinicians, however, prefer to treat stage II patients as an entirely separate group.

When the cervix is involved with endometrial cancer the incidence of pelvic lymph node metastasis is 36.5%, as shown in a review by Morrow and coworkers. Some clinicians believe that the patient should, therefore, be treated with preoperative irradiation. First, a midpelvic dose of 5400 cGy is given over 5 to 6 weeks by megavoltage external irradiation, followed by a single intracavitary application of cesium using the Fletcher-Suit afterloading method and vaginal colpostats. The dose of irradiation to the vaginal surface should be adjusted appropriately. Four weeks after irradiation therapy a total abdominal hysterectomy and a bilateral salpingo-oophorectomy are performed to remove the tumor in the uterus. Surgery should include an examination of the pelvic and paraaortic lymph nodes, removing all palpable nodes from the bifurcation of the aorta to the level of the inferior mesenteric artery because of the high incidence of extrapelvic node metastasis. Patients who are not able to undergo surgery should be treated with full external and intracavitary irradiation, as noted above.

In 1989 Boothby and coworkers reported on 42 patients with stage II disease treated at the Hospital of the University of Pennsylvania. Their results showed the best 5-year survival in patients treated only with radical hysterectomy with pelvic lymphadenectomy (68.5%) over combined surgery and radiation (46.1%) or radiation alone (36.5%), but the small numbers did not allow statistical significance. In a more recent report Andersen in Denmark reviewed 54 patients with clinical stage II corpus cancer and found a higher survival in patients treated with postoperative external and vaginal radiation after simple hysterectomy than in patients treated with radiation alone (70.6% vs. 50%).

For practical purposes, therefore, patients with stage II disease clinically should undergo surgery first, unless there are technical problems, such as extreme ballooning of the cervix, which suggests the benefit of preoperative irradiation to reduce the overall size. After surgery postoperative radiation treatment can be tailored to the individual patient according to the surgical findings. There is no apparent decrease in survival with this approach.

Clinical Stage III

The cure rate for endometrial adenocarcinoma that extends outside the uterus depends on control of the disease within the pelvis. Most clinical stage III tumors are found with an enlarged uterus, which should be removed, if surgery is possible.

Preoperative radiation treatment is similar to that for stage II lesions (if used). The initial approach is to deliver 5400 cGy of megavoltage external radiation to the midplane of the pelvis over 5 to 6 weeks. Intracavitary irradiation follows, with vaginal surface dosage limited to 4000 cGy. Depending on the extent of the parametrial lesion, a second course of intracavitary brachytherapy may be required. Some clinics use a second intracavitary dose, whereas others eliminate the intracavitary therapy completely but increase the external beam therapy.

Four weeks after irradiation an exploratory laparotomy should be performed if the patient is able to withstand surgery. During laparotomy any extrauterine masses should be carefully examined. Unrelated benign adnexal masses may cause errors of diagnosis and treatment. Any suspicious pelvic or paraaortic lymph nodes should be removed and evaluated, and the liver, bowel, omentum, and upper diaphragm should be examined for metastatic growths. Peritoneal washings are probably superfluous if the patient has received whole-pelvis irradiation.

After the abdominal evaluation a total hysterectomy with bilateral salpingo-oophorectomy should be performed if the uterus and most of the tumor can be removed without damaging the other pelvic organs. It may be preferable to perform a subtotal hysterectomy, if good intracavitary radiation was delivered, to decrease the chance of bladder or bowel fistula.

Clinical Stage IV

The advanced endometrial tumor that has extended to the rectum or bladder is difficult to treat effectively. Because the tumor has extended so far, a hysterectomy alone is not effective, although removing the bulk of tumor in the enlarged uterus may be beneficial to irradiation therapy of the pelvis. Because clinical stage IVa disease usually involves metastasis beyond the pelvic cavity, exenteration is not appropriate. Brunschwig used exenteration in such cases, but results were poor and the complication rate was so high that the procedure was determined unsuitable even for palliative treatment.

Preoperative irradiation therapy should be structured to each patient's needs. A basic approach is to give 5400 to 6000 cGy of external teletherapy to the midplane of the pelvis. For tumors in the vesicovaginal or rectovaginal septum, additional irradiation can be applied locally with interstitial radium or cesium needles, iridium wire, or vaginal cylinders.

Some patients may need a colostomy if a rectovaginal fistula should result from irradiation and tumor regression. Aggressive local treatment of tumor in the bladder wall also may cause a fistula, but a urinary diversion seldom is indicated for palliative therapy. When endometrial carcinoma involves the upper abdomen or organs outside the abdomen, pelvic surgery should only be used to removed bulk cancer tissue. Although full irradiation normally is given to the abdomen and pelvis, it usually is not able to control the extrapelvic spread of the disease. Localized irradiation may help to control pain and bleeding. An individual patient also may benefit from irradiation treatment of a lesion in the bladder or rectal wall.

After irradiation therapy high doses of progestins, such as 17α-hydroxyprogesterone caproate (Delalutin), medroxyprogesterone acetate (Depo-Provera), or megestrol acetate (Megace), may be given, although the hormones provide only temporary control for about one third of the patients. Other chemotherapeutic agents, including the combination of doxorubicin (Adriamycin) and cyclophosphamide (Cytoxan) with cisplatin, have not been effective in giving long-term control of this tumor, but short-term survival in patients adequately debulked may make such combinations worth trying. Certainly, each of these cases must be considered individually (see Ch. 46).

SPECIAL CONSIDERATIONS IN ENDOMETRIAL CANCER

The Role of Radical (Clark-Wertheim) Hysterectomy

Because radical hysterectomy and lymphadenectomy were used for cervical cancer, surgeons naturally extended the use of the procedure to the treatment of endometrial carcinoma. First the disciples of Bonney from London and then the Oxford school of pelvic surgeons, including Stallworthy and Hawksworth, practiced the radical method until statistical evaluations clearly showed that a radical procedure offered no improvement in patient survival. The best 5-year survival rate reported by Lewis and coworkers and by other investigators using radical hysterectomy and lymphadenectomy to treat stage I tumors was 71%. Better survival rates were achieved with less aggressive surgery with or without irradiation.

Endometrial carcinoma spreads through the regional lymphatics and bloodstream to recur at the lateral pelvic wall or outside the pelvis. It is obvious, therefore, that parametrial dissection is not useful for controlling the disease. Lymphadenectomy by the most experienced surgeon is not a complete anatomic dissection. It is no more useful than irradiation used alone for controlling spread of disease through the pelvic lymph nodes, although removing suspicious lymph nodes during the surgical procedure allows the surgeon to distinguish which patients require irradiation after surgery.

Even though Park and coworkers were able to report an excellent cure rate of 91% for stage I endometrial adenocarcinoma treated with the modified Wertheim procedure at the Walter Reed Hospital, patients had a high complication rate of 24%. Evaluation of the removed pelvic nodes showed that only 1.6% had been positive for metastatic tumor. Rutledge also has reevaluated the role of radical hysterectomy for stage I disease and has concluded that this procedure has a limited role, if any, in the treatment of endometrial carcinoma.

As previously indicated, the surgeon must be prepared to customize the surgical procedure to mimic portions of the radical dissection to fit anatomic, concurrent disease (eg, endometriosis) or cancer spread circumstances. Because Onsrud and coworkers have shown that removing all the nodes associated with endometrial carcinoma is not feasible, even with a radical lymphadenectomy, the adjunctive use of irradiation is obviously the better method for controlling the local spread of the disease at the side walls.

Many patients with endometrial carcinoma are elderly, obese, and fraught with multiple coexisting medical problems. Radical surgical procedures in these high-risk patients are all the more traumatic and the complication rate naturally is increased; thus the surgeon must exercise good judgment in treating such patients.

Vaginal Hysterectomy

Although vaginal hysterectomy occasionally has been used for treatment of endometrial tumors, use of the procedure should be limited. For instance, when a patient is so obese that abdominal surgery would be extremely difficult, performing vaginal surgery is better than not removing the tumor. The patient will tolerate vaginal surgery better, but the surgeon will have difficulty assessing the extent of the disease in the pelvis and abdomen. Examining the lateral pelvic walls and upper abdomen is virtually impossible from the vaginal route, but peritoneal washings can be obtained when entering the posterior cul-de-sac.

Butler and coworkers from the Mayo Clinic have reported more than 40 years of positive experience with the use of vaginal hysterectomy for many selective cases, mainly those with well-differentiated endometrial carcinoma and a small uterus. These patients with stage Ia tumors had an 84% survival rate, with only one vaginal recurrence. Peters and coworkers' report of 56 patients with stage I disease treated by vaginal hysterectomy, with or without adjunctive therapy, showed a 94% survival, but both of these studies should be viewed with extreme caution, as undoubtedly candidates were carefully chosen.

Vaginal hysterectomy may be ideal for very elderly, frail patients confined to nursing homes for multiple reasons. Surgically, these cases may be difficult, but by using Schuchardt incisions, proceeding slowly with small tissue bites, and having adequate retraction, the cases can proceed smoothly with a striking difference in postoperative care requirements. Removal of the ovaries is almost always possible, is an important part of the treatment, and should be performed if technically feasible during a vaginal procedure.

When the vaginal approach is required for the treatment of a patient who is not a candidate for abdominal surgery, postoperative irradiation treatment should be guided by the grade of the tumor and the extent of myometrial invasion, using Figure 43-8. Only in cases with a well-differentiated lesion and either superficial or no myometrial invasion should the vaginal hysterectomy and adnexectomy alone be considered the final treatment without carefully weighing options.

Unsuspected Endometrial Carcinoma

On rare occasions an endometrial carcinoma has been discovered during surgery for a supposedly benign disease. Although not originally planned, the ovaries and fallopian tubes also must be removed and, if possible, the full staging procedure should be done if intraoperative evaluation of the uterus suggests poor prognostic factors. In a case where the uterus has been removed for benign disease and the ovaries and tubes have been left in place, histologic study occasionally discloses unsuspected endometrial carcinoma. If there is no evidence of myometrial invasion and the lesion is a well-differentiated, grade 1 tumor, the adnexa need not be removed. If the uterine disease is grade 3 or shows deep myometrial invasion, the adnexa may be effectively treated with postoperative irradiation. Alternatively, the adnexa should be removed surgically, not only to exclude a potential site of tumor metastasis, but also to decrease the serum estrogen level if the patient is premenopausal. In postmenopausal patients the small risk of ovarian metastasis alone should be compared with the stage of the disease and the grade of the tumor before an additional laparotomy is recommended for the specific purpose of removing the tubes and ovaries and completing the surgical staging.

In either case the decision to reexplore the patient rests with the likelihood of the need for additional therapy. Even though a good estimate can be made on examination of the specimen, clear informed consent after patient appraisal of the facts is essential. For healthy women with moderate risk factors, I usually recommend the complete operation rather than blindly choosing either no further therapy or adjunctive radiation.

Concomitant Independent Ovarian Cancer

The coexistence of primary tumors in the ovary and uterus is not rare but causes considerable clinical pondering when it occurs. First, metastatic disease from either site or a remote primary from a distant organ (eg, breast) must be ruled out. In the former case this can be quite difficult, as most synchronous tumors are endometrioid and differentiation can be troublesome. Albright and Rath discussed 34 cases of simultaneous cancers of the uterus and ovary and found that 21 could be classified as endometrial primary with ovarian metastasis. They established both major and minor criteria

in reaching this decision: a multinodular ovarian pattern was a major criterion; minor criteria included small (less than 5 cm) ovaries, bilateral ovarian involvement, deep myometrial or vascular invasion, and tubal lumen involvement. Twelve of their patients had none of these criteria and were thought to have independent tumors.

When this eventuality is encountered, the surgical staging procedure is virtually identical, except evaluation of the diaphragm, omentum, and random peritoneal sites is indicated to properly assess the spread patterns of ovarian cancer. If full staging information is available, postoperative treatment usually is tailored to the disease with the worst prognosis or the most high-risk factors. Many times treatment can be consolidated to cover both primary sites and their spread patterns. When exact staging has not been accomplished, the surgeon must surmise risk factors from available data and either plan treatment or reexplore surgically for definitive information.

Variable-Level Invasion Limited to Adenomyosis

Adenomyosis is a common occurrence in women at risk for endometrial cancer, and the presence of cancer deep in the uterine muscle may be solely due to adenomyotic involvement. It is clear that myometrial invasion limited to foci of adenomyosis offers a better prognosis than true invasion to that depth. Jacques and Lawrence in Detroit recently provided more data supporting this concept in their clinicopathologic review of 23 cases. Their criteria included presence of stroma, adjacent benign glands, expansion patterns of the tumor, contour of myometrial lesions, and absence of peritumoral desmoplasia. When these criteria were properly identified, the data supported the earlier literature, and also suggested that endometrial adenocarcinoma may arise de novo in adenomyosis. This may explain the occasional presentation of a patient with stage III or IV disease who never exhibits a classic bleeding pattern. Thus, patients who demonstrate this entity after careful review should be treated according to the grade of tumor and other surgical staging factors rather than myometrial invasion.

Simultaneous Cancers in Other Organs

A small percentage of patients with endometrial cancer may be found to have simultaneous cancers in other organs, discovered at the time of workup for corpus disease or in the immediate posttreatment period. In a review of 456 cases of endometrial cancer from the Johns Hopkins Tumor Registry, Abbas found 12 cases

(2.5%) of nonovarian cancers that were diagnosed either at the time of workup or within 6 months of treatment. In almost all patients who subsequently died the other primary tumor was responsible for their demise. Therapy, therefore, should be complete for the corpus cancer, but treatment of the second primary mandates vigorous regimens, considering the corpus disease to be no deterrent.

RESULTS OF TREATMENT AND PROGNOSIS

Traditional 5-year survival rates, the yardstick of cancer cure, are reasonably impressive for endometrial cancer, but the numerous subsets of patient groups makes interpretation of survival data somewhat difficult. The annual report compiled by FIGO reveals the most comprehensive worldwide data, with the 20th volume, published in 1988, representing the most recent analysis of solid 5-year survival data on 14,906 cases treated in the years 1979 to 1981 by 115 collaborating institutions (Table 43-14). These additions raise the total of reported cases to 66,042, of which 98.7% (65,214) were treated. The most striking aspect of this report, which can be seen pictorially in Figure 43-9, is that the overall cure rate for endometrical cancer has remained essentially unchanged with the cumulative cure rate for 1979–1981 cases being 65.1%, compared with the 1982 report of 11,501 cases treated in 1973–1975 with a cure rate of 66.6%. In a study of the literature Morrow collected reports on 2342 patients and found that the 5-year survival rate for all stages was similar (68%). A comparison of Morrow's data with the two FIGO reports shows the similarity of the survival rates for each stage of endometrial carcinoma (Fig. 43-9).

These data quickly dispel the designation of endometrial cancer as a "good" cancer, viewing the relatively unfavorable results in stage-per-stage subsets provides a more realistic opportunity to predict the outcome in individual cases. For instance, subdividing cases on grade alone, as seen in Table 43-9, can more accurately estimate survival with FIGO's report of 4476 clinical stage I patients showing a 77.7% 5-year survival compared with the 58.5% survival of a similar clinical stage but with poorly differentiated tumors. Similarly, the report reveals that when depth of myometrial invasion is considered, the 5-year survival of 3224 clinical stage I patients with less than one third of the myometrium invaded by cancer had a survival of 82.4%, whereas a similar stage cohort of 1144 patients with greater than half the myometrium invaded had a 66.8% survival. Even more dramatic is the difference in outcome when lymph nodes are invaded. FIGO reports 3286 stage I cases with no nodal involvement to have a 81.3% survival of 5 years, whereas the 110 clinical stage I cases with histologically proven cancer in regional nodes suffered a dismal 36.4% 5-year cure.

It is theoretically possible, therefore, to comprehensively analyze data to create all-inclusive categories for predicting survival, based on shown prognostic characteristics, and this is the foundation of the surgical staging system. Thus a patient with a well-differentiated tumor, surgical stage Ia, can be shown by analysis of FIGO data to expect to have more than a 95% chance of surviving her disease, whereas her counterpart with a poorly differentiated lesion with deep invasion has less than a 65% chance of living 5 years. When viewed in subsets the FIGO data become more applicable to modern comprehensive treatment practices, and more closely approximate the detailed, evenly staged data compiled by the huge Gynecologic Oncology Group staging study of endometrial cancer. Morrow and colleagues' more recent analysis of the Gynecologic Oncology Group survival data on the almost 1000 cases similarly staged and evaluated suggests that the survival predictions based on prognostic factors are highly accurate, and clearly gives the gynecologic surgeon sound basis for not only choosing adjunctive surgery, but also allows judicious prognostication for the individual patient.

FOLLOW-UP AND RECURRENCE

After definitive treatment patients should be carefully followed according to the outline in Table 43-15. Emphasis should be placed not only on detection of recurrent disease, but also on screening for other cancers or health problems. The follow-up outlined should allow detection of the most common sites of recurrence.

TABLE 43–14
Five-Year Survival Rates by Clinical Stage of Disease, 1979–1981

CLINICAL STAGE	NO. TREATED	NO. 5-YR SURVIVAL (%)
I	11,035	7,976 (72.3)
II	2,014	1,135 (56.4)
III	921	290 (31.5)
IV	409	43 (10.5)
Unstaged	527	253 (47.8)
Totals	14,906	9.697 (65.1)

(Adapted from FIGO. Statements of results obtained in patients treated in 1979 to 1981. In: Pettersson F, ed. Annual report on the results of treatment in gynecological cancer. Stockholm: Panorama Press, 1988.)

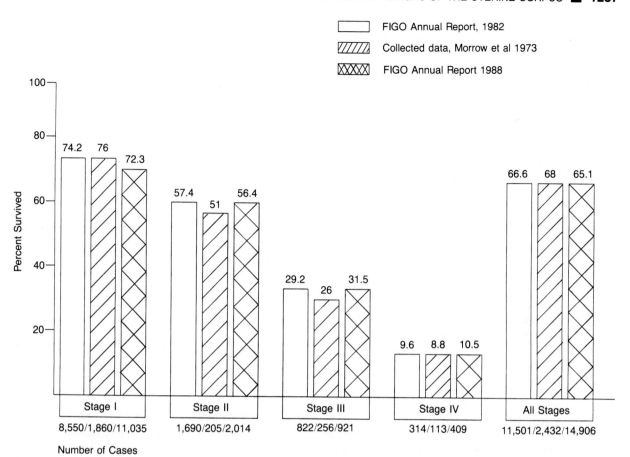

Figure 43–9. Combined survival data from three different periods. These graphs clearly illustrate that, stage for stage, survival from endometrial cancer has changed very little in the past two decades.

Whether or not to give estrogen replacement therapy during follow-up to patients with corpus cancer is an unsettled issue. Creasman audaciously addressed this previously taboo approach at a national presentation that was subsequently modified for publication. Although widely criticized by some, many clinicians surveyed recently secretly admitted giving low-risk patients estrogens; fortunately this problem is being studied in an ongoing randomized study. I believe that physicians should use extreme caution with the prescribing practice until definite information is available, as it appears that other medications undergoing trials may be beneficial for the postmenopausal patient. The 1990 ACOG committee opinion on estrogen replacement therapy and endometrial cancer reflects a similar view, and can be used as a guide for the clinician.

The factors that influence the recurrence of endometrial carcinoma are the extent of disease at time of initial treatment, the degree of differentiation of the tumor, the adequacy of the primary treatment, individ-

ual host response, and the presence of other high-risk factors, including the patient's age. More than two thirds of all recurrent tumors develop within 2 years of initial therapy.

Flow cytometry of cell nuclei from endometrial cancers for DNA content and index has recently been shown to be a reliable prognosticator of treatment failure and recurrent disease. Iversen performed DNA indexing in a prospective study of 52 cases of cancer of the corpus and found 27% to be aneuploid, which was correlated to tumor grade but not to the other prognostic variables such as stage, degree of invasion, or age. He found higher recurrence rates, shorter disease-free intervals, and higher death rates in the aneuploid group. Newbury and coworkers at Geisinger Medical Center reported 233 cases of endometrial cancer, with a median follow-up time of 8.7 years, from which flow cytometry of archival paraffin blocks was used to determine DNA content. Aneuploidy was not detected in low-grade tumors and, similar to Iversen's work, was

TABLE 43–15
Follow-up After Treatment for Endometrial Cancer

EXAMINATION OR TEST	INTERVAL
History and physical examination, including pelvic examination, cuff Pap smear, and rectal examination	Every 3 months for 2 years, then every 6 months for 3 years, and then yearly for life
Chest radiography	Every 6 months for 5 years and then yearly
Mammography	Yearly for life
Computed tomography scan, magnetic resonance imaging, and ultrasonography	Only if clinically indicated
Screening for colon cancer	Every other year

strongly predictive of death from disease when the DNA index was greater than 1.5. Thus more sophisticated techniques on the horizon may assist standard staging methods to predict recurrence, including current ongoing oncogene studies.

The most frequent sites of recurrence of endometrial carcinoma are the upper vagina, uterus, pelvic lymph nodes, paraaortic nodes, and lungs. Dede and coworkers reported that in 75% of their patients with recurrent endometrial carcinoma, the secondary lesion developed outside the pelvis. This is in agreement with results in a current multi-institutional study by DiSaia and coworkers in the Gynecologic Oncology Group, in which 222 patients with clinical stage I carcinoma of the endometrium were studied. During the 36- to 72-month follow-up of this study 79% of the recurrences were located outside the pelvis. When definable extrauterine disease was absent at the time of the original surgery, the recurrence rate was only 7%, whereas if disease was found anywhere outside the uterus, the recurrence rate was 43%. In this study the undifferentiated grade 3 tumors, the tumors with deep myometrial invasion, and the tumors with either pelvic or aortic node involvement showed the highest incidence of recurrence. Curiously, of the 34 patients with recurrence among the 222 studied cases, local and distant recurrence was present in 3% of patients treated by primary surgery with radium treatment and in 5% of those treated by primary surgery alone.

Among 171 cases in studies by Malkasian, by Salazar, and by Aalders the failure rate in the pelvis with surgery alone was 16.4%. In the abdomen or other sites the rate was 11%. In contrast, among 198 patients treated with radiotherapy and surgery with stage I, grade 3 tumors reported by Aalders, by Salazar, and by Komaki, the rate of failure in the pelvis was only 5.6% and in either the abdomen or distant sites the rate was 15%. This large study gives clear evidence that the more advanced tumors that require surgery and external irradiation are more likely to recur. When such recurrences are found they usually are in distant, extrapelvic sites.

Specific information about the original tumor and its treatment is needed to determine whether or not secondary treatment is possible. If secondary treatment is to be given, irradiation and chemotherapy are the primary methods used in an attempt to arrest recurrent growth.

Additional surgery is only a palliative effort, and rarely can ultraradical surgery be of benefit. Sometimes a vaginal cuff recurrence in a patient who has previously been irradiated can be treated with radical vaginectomy with good results, but such cases are unusual. Exenteration for recurrent endometrial cancer is almost anecdotal. In a series of 100 patients at the University of Michigan who underwent pelvic exenteration, Morley and coworkers performed only four such procedures for adenocarcinoma of the endometrium and only one patient survived for 5 years. Thus, before embarking on radical surgery, a meticulous search for extant disease outside the pelvis must be accomplished preoperatively.

SYSTEMIC TREATMENT OF RECURRENT DISEASE

Hormonal Therapy

Progestins are among the main systemic agents used in the treatment of advanced endometrial cancer that have produced a measurable response (Table 43-16). Objective remission occurs in about one third of the patients treated with progestin. Response to the hormone is best when a long, tumor-free period existed before recurrence of a well-differentiated, slow-growing tumor with positive receptor activity.

TABLE 43–16
Response to Hormonal Agents

DRUG	NO. OF PATIENTS	RESPONSE (%)
Hydroxyprogesterone caproate	384	32
Medrogestone	56	49
Medroxyprogesterone acetate	195	41
Megestrol acetate	125	47
Tamoxifen	59	20

(Modified from Deppe G. Chemotherapeutic treatment of endometrial cancer. Clin Obstet Gynecol 1982;25:93.)

Progestins appear to work at the cellular level by slowing both DNA and RNA replication. They also have a modulating effect on estrogen stimulation. The intracellular effects of hormonal therapy are mediated by the interaction of the steroid and its receptor. Estrogen and progesterone cytoplasmic receptors have been shown to be markedly involved in the tumor response to hormonal therapy. Tumors that lack receptors are presumably unresponsive to a specific hormone. Therefore, in the treatment of patients with recurrent endometrial carcinoma, one might expect a good response to progesterone therapy in patients who had a high concentration of progesterone receptors in the primary tumor. Also, progestins are known to effect a reduction in available estrogen receptors, thereby decreasing the response of tumors to circulating estrogens. Progesterone also stimulates the production of 17β-estradiol dehydrogenase, which converts the active form of estradiol to a weaker estrogen, estrone. Both of these physiologic events—decreasing the number of estrogen receptors and decreasing the concentration of intracellular estradiol—have an antiestrogenic effect on the tumor. Therefore, progesterone receptors commonly are measured at the time of initial treatment to determine the likely biologic effect of the hormone on a recurrent neoplasm. Ehrlich and coworkers have shown a strong correlation between the responsiveness of progestins in recurrent endometrial cancer and the presence of progesterone receptors. In their study, patients with high concentrations of progesterone receptors in the tumor responded more frequently to progesterone treatment. Many investigators have shown that levels of progesterone receptors are higher in well-differentiated than in poorly differentiated endometrial carcinoma.

Limited experience to date suggests a greater than 90% correlation between receptor status and response to progestin therapy. In 1961 Kelley and Baker reported the initial results of using Delalutin for the treatment of metastatic endometrial carcinoma. Objective remission occurred in 6 of 21 patients who had pulmonary metastasis and lasted from 9 months to 4.5 years. A more recent report listed a 32% remission rate. Kistner also reported a 30% remission rate.

In a collaborative study reported by Reifenstein the average duration of tumor regression was 30 months. The dosage of Delalutin used was 1 g or more each week for 12 or more weeks. Most patients showed a better response when treated for longer than 12 weeks. Of 314 women studied, 21 had complete arrest of the disease. Cure could not be considered the specific result of progestin therapy because the women in Reifenstein's study also received ancillary treatment. No correlations have been made between survival rates and the amount of drug given each week, the patient's age, or the type of concomitant anticancer therapy provided.

About 15% of all poorly differentiated tumors that were treated by Reifenstein responded to progestin therapy, indicating that a hormonal trial is warranted, even with less than favorable conditions. At one time researchers believed that pulmonary and osseous lesions responded better than pelvic or abdominal tumors, but an analysis of new data shows that pelvic metastases have a similar rate of response to progestins.

Other progestational agents have provided similar results. Deppe analyzed various reports of the treatment of advanced or recurrent endometrial carcinoma with various hormonal agents and found that response rates varied between 30% and 49% (Table 43-16). Megace showed a 47% objective response rate in a combined series of studies when oral doses of 80 mg/day were given. Higher doses resulted in similar rates. Depo-Provera has been tried in doses of 400 to 800 mg three times a week for a month, then once a week for a second month, and then once a month for maintenance. The results currently available show a 42% response rate, but the drug appears to given results similar to those for the other progestins used. Preliminary Gynecologic Oncology Group data suggest that increasing the dose of progestin above those mentioned above adds nothing to the efficacy.

The activity of tamoxifen, an antiestrogen nonsteroidal agent that blocks the estrogen receptor, was reported by Swenerton in 1980. Unfortunately only 3 of 10 patients showed objective response when given an oral dose of 10 mg twice daily on a continuous basis for the treatment of recurrent endometrial carcinoma. Quinn and Campbell reported on 49 patients treated with tamoxifen, 20 mg twice daily, and noted 10 responses, 6 of which were complete. Significantly, median survival of responders was 34 months compared with only 6 months for those who did not respond.

The toxicity of tamoxifen is minimal, and it is worth trying in patients who fail progestins. Quinn suggests concomitant tamoxifen therapy with progestins because in tumors that prove to be unresponsive to progestin, the antiestrogen tamoxifen can be used to block estrogen receptors in an effort to affect specific steroid receptor mechanisms.

Cytotoxic Chemotherapy

Various chemotherapeutic agents have been used in limited trials. In an earlier collaborative study by the Gynecologic Oncology Group, Cohen and coworkers observed the response of 358 patients with advanced (stage III and stage IV) or recurrent endometrial cancer when treated with one of two multiagent regimens: (1) melphalan and 5-fluorouracil daily for 4 days, repeated every 4 weeks with Megace daily for 8 weeks and (2) adriamycin, 5-fluorouracil, and cyclophosphamide, intravenous bolus every 21 days with Megace daily for 8 weeks. The objective response rate in patients with measurable disease was 36.8% in both groups; 36.8% of each group had stable disease and 26.4% progressed on treatment. Response was not affected by age, site of recurrence, time to first recurrence, and presence or absence of previous treatment by progestational or irradiation therapy. Grade of the tumor, however, and performance status did affect response, although 44 of 57 objective responders had undifferentiated tumors. The median survival for complete responders of both groups was only 18.3 months, compared with 12.9 months for partial responders and 8.8 months for patients with stable disease. The overall objective response rate of 36.8% for the multidrug regimens is no higher than the objective response rate for Adriamycin alone, which was reported by the Gynecologic Oncology Group headed by Thigpen in 1979 as showing an observed response role of 37%, with a median duration of response of 7.4 months for complete responders and survival for this group at a median of 14 months.

Thigpen and coworkers more recently reported on cisplatin as first-line chemotherapy in a Phase II Gynecologic Oncology Group trial for advanced or recurrent disease in 49 evaluable patients. There were only two complete responses, with eight partial responses, but 45% of patients exhibited stable disease for at least 2 months. The authors believed that this limited activity warranted further trials. Cisplatin chemotherapy has been used for advanced or recurrent endometrial carcinoma by Seski and coworkers at the M. D. Anderson Hospital in 26 women, using doses at 50, 70, and 100 mg/m^2 every 4 weeks. An objective response was obtained in 42% of the patients, but the median duration of the remission was only 5 months with a range from 2 to 11 months. Although cisplatin was found to be definitely active against endometrial cancer, the high rate of toxicity (31%) limited the use of this agent in high doses on an outpatient basis.

The newer platinum analog, carboplatin, was studied by the Southwest Oncology Group for activity in endometrial cancer. They found two complete and five partial responses in 23 evaluable patients for an overall response rate of 30%. Four responders showed significant (839+ days) duration of response, which suggests that this newer drug may prove to be a promising drug for corpus cancer. Similar results have been found with Adriamycin, Cytoxan, and cisplatin, but the toxicity of this regimen has been significant and durations of response disappointing. Although many ongoing studies appear promising, the preferential combination of therapeutic agents has not yet been defined.

Based on all these studies, progestational agents alone should be used primarily in patients with well-differentiated tumors or high levels of progesterone receptors. Cytotoxic chemotherapy should be reserved for patients with less favorable prognoses—those with poor tumor differentiation, absent progesterone receptors, and reduced performance status—and then only after failed trials with progestins. If available, all patients with recurrent disease not amenable to radiation therapy should be considered for cooperative chemotherapy trials.

Unfortunately chemical control of recurrent endometrial carcinoma currently is limited and temporary, but newer agents, such as ifosfamide and etoposide (VP-16), in combination with other agents, are being studied in hopes of gaining control over recurrent disease.

The advent of standardized surgical staging along with detection of early disease may preclude or decrease the current need for advanced disease treatment in most patients.

UTERINE SARCOMAS

The uterine sarcomas constitute only about 3% of corpus cancers. Nevertheless, they are important neoplasms for multiple reasons: First, they are the most rapidly growing of the uterine tumors, reputedly having a tumor cell doubling time as short as 4 weeks; second, although a unifying theme is that all arise from mesoderm, their histologic diversity has made them interesting and intriguing; third, because they appear most commonly in the older age group, the incidence appears to be increasing; and finally, because of the virulent nature of these aggressive tumors, the clinical management is challenging.

Unlike the pure epithelial tumors, uterine sarcomas can occur in perplexing sarcoma-like states, presenting a spectrum of clinical behaviors for each individual category, often confusing not only the clinician, but also the pathologist. Distinguishing between the benign variants can be difficult, as overall treatment and prognosis vary markedly. Consultation, therefore, is advised when planning treatment.

There is no known cause for sarcomas of the uterus, but there has been a long association with prior pelvic irradiation. This relationship appears to be more commonly linked to the mixed mesodermal tumors, but on occasion has been remotely present in all histologic varieties. The incidence of this association varies, lending some doubt as to whether or not there is a causative factor. Podczaski and coworkers, in a retrospective review of 42 patients with mixed mesodermal tumors seen at Hershey, found that 6 had a history of prior radiation, for a incidence of 14%. This figure is consistent with the median of several series relating a prior exposure. Thus historical information about previous radiation in an older woman with a pelvic mass or bleeding should raise suspicion of uterine sarcoma.

Staging and Classification

Because there is no official FIGO staging for uterine sarcoma, most clinicians use a modification of the clinical staging system outlined in Table 43-17. It is important to designate for documentation whether this staging is merely clinical or has been substantiated by surgical staging. I prefer to perform the same basic surgical staging operation used for epithelial tumors in assigning stage, and admix the surgical findings into a rough parallel of the clinical staging system. Because extension of disease outside the uterus portends such a poor outcome for patients with sarcoma, the basic staging without subgroups is adequate for postoperative treatment planning.

Most systems of classification that are purely pathologic can become overly verbose and clumsy; a much more practical system reflects the observed frequency of the different sarcomas and is detailed in Table 43-18. The system revolves around the three basic tissues in the uterus derived from mesoderm: myometrium, stroma, and mixed patterns, including both epithelial and mesodermal elements, which are most often termed mixed mesodermal tumors, although the term mixed müllerian tumor and the more specific carcinosarcoma also have been used. Included in this classification are the sarcoma-like entities associated with each tissue of origin.

The relative frequency of sarcoma type more often depends on referral patterns and practice type than on pure epidemiologic data, mainly because of the rela-

TABLE 43–18
Classification of Uterine Sarcomas

Mixed mesodermal tumors
  Homologous
  Heterologous
  Adenosarcoma
Leiomyosarcoma
Stromal sarcoma
Others (hemangiopericytoma, angiosarcoma, etc.)

tively rare occurrence of sarcomas. The Gynecologic Oncology Group recently closed a comprehensive long-term staging study of uterine sarcomas that was presented by Major and coauthors. Of 447 evaluable cases, most were mixed mesodermal tumors (337, or 75%), but a more realistic distribution of cases as judged by literature search (Fig. 43-10) would suggest that 50% of uterine sarcomas are mixed, mostly heterologous or homologous with a lesser number of adenosarcomas, with about one third of cases leiomyosarcomas, about one sixth of stromal origin, and the rarer types occurring much less frequently.

Overall Surgical Management

Preoperative assessment of uterine sarcomas parallels that of the more common epithelial cell type. Indeed, as many as 15% to 25% of poorly differentiated endometrial cancers in elderly women prove to have sarcomatous changes on final pathology, thus, the surgical staging procedure should be virtually identical. Data from the recent Gynecologic Oncology Group staging study suggests that lymph node metastasis may be less important prognostically than previously suspected in sarcomas, especially leiomyosarcoma. Therefore, during the initial surgical procedure, total extrafascial hysterectomy with bilateral salpingo-oophorectomy is the basis of treatment, accompanied by lymph node sampling of suspicious nodes, with pelvic washings done on entry to the abdomen. A total lymph node dissection is not recommended merely for staging purposes. Although previous staging studies have recommended omentectomy, this procedure has proved not to be worthwhile unless there is gross evidence of intraperitoneal disease.

Some surgical aspects of uterine sarcoma are unique. Figure 43-11 shows a surgical specimen from an older woman with mixed mesodermal tumor of the uterus, which has extended into the left broad ligament and adnexa. Because of cervical stenosis, there was no symptomatic bleeding until disease was advanced, and

TABLE 43–17
Staging for Uterine Sarcoma

CLASSIFICATION	DESCRIPTION
Stage I	Sarcoma confined to the endometrium
Ia	The length of the uterine cavity is 8 cm or less
Ib	The length of the uterine cavity is more than 8 cm
Stage II	Sarcoma involving the fundus and endocervix or cervix but not extending outside the uterus
Stage III	Sarcoma extending outside the uterus but confined to the pelvis
Stage IV	Sarcoma spread outside the pelvis or invading the bladder or rectum

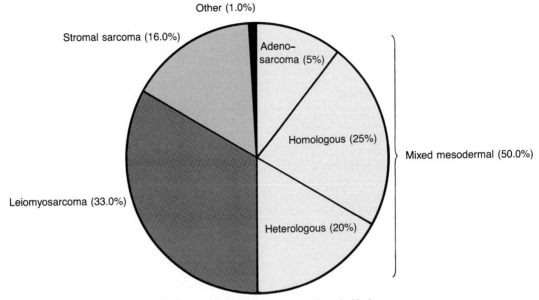

Figure 43–10. Distribution of cell types in uterine sarcoma. At least half of uterine sarcomas are mixed mesodermal tumors.

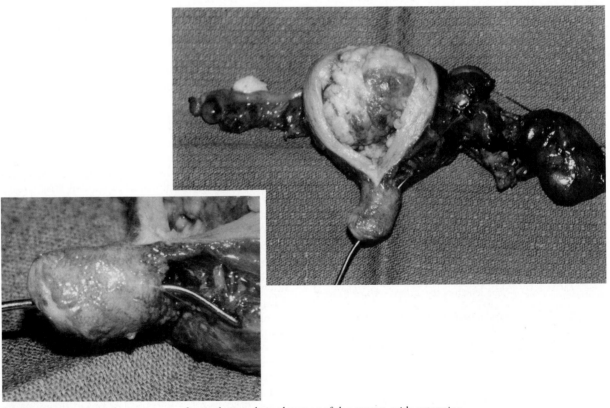

Figure 43–11. Typical appearance of mixed mesodermal tumor of the uterus, with extension into the left adnexa. The *inset* reveals how the preoperative D&C created a false passage in the stenotic cervix.

then curettage was thwarted by the false passage created (inset, Fig. 43-11). Thus the gynecologist must take caution when attempting to sound the uterus in such patients; we have found ultrasonography useful intraoperatively to guide the surgeon to the uterine cavity.

More commonly, sarcomas tend to be polypoid masses that dilate and balloon out the cervix and lower uterine segment (Fig. 43-12). This is a surgical challenge, and dissection of the parametria must be done in a more radical manner if complete removal of the uterus is to be accomplished; failure to do so may mean tumor extruded into the peritoneal cavity or a portion of tumor-laden cervix left behind, virtually assuring a vaginal recurrence. In Figure 43-13 this technique is demonstrated, showing a dissection of the ureter more laterally, crossclamping the uterine vessels away from the cervix, and avoiding the "bounce off the cervix" maneuver when clamping the lower broad ligament and parametria. This also requires lower dissection of the bladder away from the upper vagina, and allows a more complete vaginal cuff. If there is suspicion that the tumor actually invades the lower cervix, additional vaginal cuff may be removed, with frozen section guidance of free margins. The vaginal cuff should be closed with interrupted sutures. If closed-suction drainage is necessary, it should be accomplished transabdominally.

Postoperatively, there is no proven benefit to radiation therapy. Some authors claim a reduction in local failure rate if radiation therapy is given, but there is clearly no increase in overall survival. Salazar and coworkers suggested, in their review of radiation after surgery, a significant improvement in local control, but

Spanos and coworkers found a local failure rate of 11% with combined treatment. Kohorn and coworkers, using both teletherapy and brachytherapy postoperatively, found a 18% failure rate in the pelvis, while Podczaski's series reported a 14% local persistence or recurrence with adjunctive radiation.

I believe that postoperative treatment must be tailored to the surgical findings, but adjunctive treatment for advanced disease is mandatory. As recommended by Peters and others, I first administer vigorous chemotherapy systemically, using agents that are protocol specified, if possible; the histologic type appears to most influence choice of drugs. Pelvic radiotherapy can then be given for local control, if indicated.

Ultraradical surgical therapy seldom is indicated for uterine sarcomas. In a series of nine patients with pelvic sarcomas treated with pelvic exenteration, as reported by Reid and coworkers, four had primary uterine tumors. Two patients, one with stromal sarcoma and the other with leiomyosarcoma, were long-term survivors, but both patients with mixed mesodermal tumors succumbed to disease within a few months. As discussed below, I believe that extended surgical therapy plays an important role in the overall management of leiomyosarcomas, but in general, exenerative procedures and other ultraradical surgical maneuvers must be approached with caution in patients with uterine sarcomas.

Clinical Presentation and Management

Mixed Mesodermal Tumors

Mixed mesodermal tumors are the most common of the uterine sarcomas, and constitute about 2% of all corpus cancers. This diverse group of tumors usually occur in postmenopausal women aged 55 to 65, and the incidence of the tumor appears to be increasing. These patients do not have the characteristics associated with endometrial carcinoma, such as prolonged estrogen stimulation or obesity, and commonly present with uterine bleeding. Speculum examination often reveals polypoid masses extruding through the cervix. Diagnosis is rendered by histologic sampling of the endometrium, and the cellular patterns vary from one field to another. Further subdivision of these tumors depends on cellular elements present (Figs. 43-14 and 43-15).

A more benign acting variant is *adenofibroma and adenosarcoma,* which can be defined histologically as showing a benign epithelial component intimately admixed with a benign or malignant mesenchymal component. Zaloudek and Norris presented a clinicopathologic study of 35 cases and found that ade-

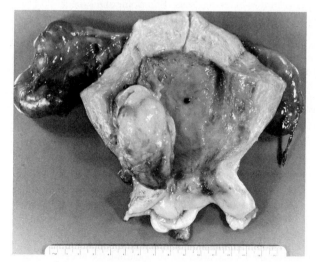

Figure 43–12. Characteristic polypoid pattern of a mixed mesodermal tumor of the uterus in an elderly woman. This tumor may appear grossly as a large endometrial polyp or an aborting submucous leiomyoma.

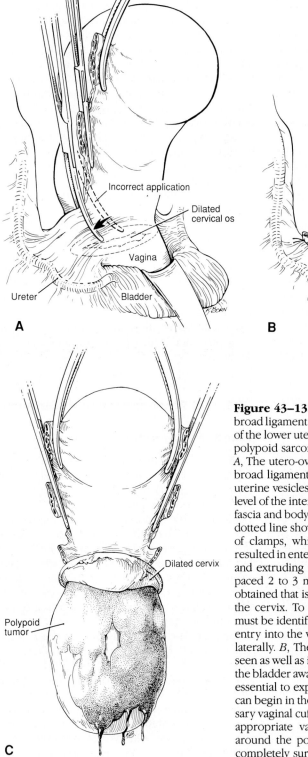

Figure 43–13. Correct technique for dissecting the lower broad ligament in parametria in patients with a ballooning out of the lower uterine segment and dilatation of the cervix from polypoid sarcoma, or extended stage II endometrial cancer. *A,* The utero-ovarian ligaments, round ligaments, and upper broad ligaments have been cross-clamped and divided. The uterine vesicles have been cross-clamped and divided at the level of the internal os, without extending into the endopelvic fascia and body of the lower uterine segment and cervix. The dotted line shows the incorrect application of the next series of clamps, which, in this schematic diagram, would have resulted in entering in cervix above the level of the external os and extruding tumor into the wound. Instead, the clamp is paced 2 to 3 mm lateral to the cervix, so that a pedicle is obtained that is sufficient for hemotasis but without entering the cervix. To accomplish this maneuver safely, the ureter must be identified and dissected at a point just superior to its entry into the vesicouterine ligament (tunnel) and retracted laterally. *B,* The outline of the ureter through the tunnel is seen as well as its entry into the bladder. Careful dissection of the bladder away from the lower ureter segment and vagina is essential to expose this area. The next application of clamps can begin in the paravaginal area before obtaining the necessary vaginal cuff. *C,* The removed specimen is shown with an appropriate vaginal cuff and a dilated cervix extending around the polypoid tumor. For a uterine sarcoma to be completely surgically excised, this technique must be used.

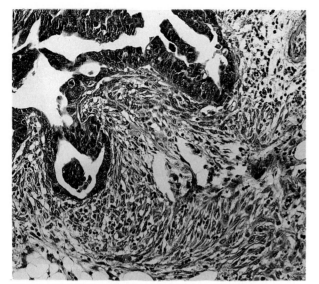

Figure 43–14. Homologous mixed mesodermal tumor. Malignant epithelial elements and malignant stromal sarcoma are admixed in this rather poorly differentiated tumor.

nofibromas had fewer than four mitotic figures per 10 high-power fields and behaved almost as benign tumors. On the other hand, the more malignant adenosarcoma, with more than four mitotic figures per 10 high-power fields histologically, behaved like other sarcomas, with a 40% recurrence rate and a median interval to recurrence of 5 years. These authors found that the deeper the invasion of the myometrium, the worse the prognosis. About 11% of the mixed müllerian tumors in the Gynecologic Oncology Group study were adenosarcomas, and their clinical behavior was less malignant when no heterologous elements were found. This supports our view that adenosarcoma as an entity must be closely examined with multiple pathologic samples to allow a prediction of a low incidence of recurrence.

Most mixed mesodermal sarcomas contain both malignant epithelial and mesenchymal components. The stromal component is basically an stromal sarcoma that contains rhabdomyoblasts, and the epithelial component demonstrates a wide variety of patterns from well-differentiated carcinoma to adenosquamous carcinoma. When the cell types are confined to these varieties only, the tumor is termed *homologous* mixed müllerian tumor, or the older term *carcinosarcoma*. In about half the cases these cancers contain tissues foreign to the endometrium, such as striated muscle, bone, cartilage, or adipose tissue, and are termed *heterologous* mixed mesodermal tumors. Heterologous tumors originally were thought to have a worse prognosis than the homologous variety, but all types have proved to have similar outcomes when extent of disease is the

basis of comparison. This was borne out in the Gynecologic Oncology Group study, in which 42% of homologous tumors and 58% of heterologous tumors recurred. The group found presence of lymph node metastasis, adnexal spread, tumor size, lymph-vascular space involvement, and histologic grade to be more predictive of recurrence than was cell type or mitotic index.

Postoperatively, patients with disease confined to the uterus should be closely followed, as there appears to be no proven benefit to adjunctive chemotherapy. In a randomized trial Omura and coworkers from the Gynecologic Oncology Group showed no benefit of adjuvant Adriamycin in preventing recurrence, although Adriamycin as a single agent and in combination with dacarbazine (DTIC) had shown activity in these sarcomas. Thigpen and coworkers from the Gynecologic Oncology Group demonstrated activity of cisplatin in these tumors. It currently appears that ifosfamide is the most active single agent, and trials using ifosfamide in all uterine sarcomas, both as a single agent and in combination with cisplatin, are ongoing. Because none of these agents, alone or in combination, have been

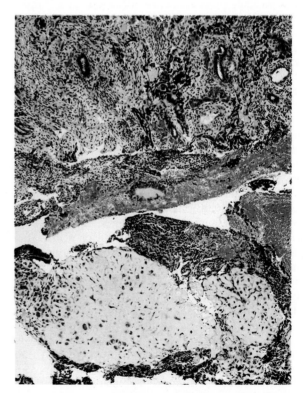

Figure 43–15. Heterologous mixed mesodermal tumor. The presence of sarcomatous elements ordinarily foreign to the uterus characterizes this variant of mixed mesodermal tumor.

shown in a randomized study to prevent recurrence in early-stage patients, they should be used with caution in patients who have not demonstrated extrauterine disease. I believe, however, that patients with known disease outside the uterus or with recurrence should be vigorously treated with chemotherapy, preferably on groupwide protocols. Choice of agents should be done in consultation with gynecologic oncologists or medical oncologists with experience in treating mixed mesodermal tumors.

Leiomyosarcoma

Leiomyosarcomas arise from the myometrium and account for roughly one third of uterine sarcomas. Like their counterparts in the endometrium, these lesions demonstrate a spectrum of clinical diseases, from absolutely benign to highly malignant. Often there is great concern when a rapidly growing leiomyoma is excised and found to be a *cellular myoma*. These are characterized as showing dense cellularity but with rare mitotic activity and no pleomorphism. Thus their behavior is benign, and surgical excision is the treatment of choice, either with myomectomy or hysterectomy. There are three variants of sarcoma-like conditions of the myometrium that can be mistaken for frank leiomyosarcoma: *intravenous leiomyomatosis, benign metastasizing leiomyoma,* and *leiomyomatosis peritonealis disseminata.* Although all have distinct clinical presentations, they are similar in their benign histologic appearance, and all appear to have sensitivity to progesterone treatment.

Intravenous leiomyomatosis involves vascular channels and often extends from the uterus into the veins of the broad ligament, and even into the major vasculature of the pelvis and upper abdomen. Grossly, it has a wormlike appearance, with sworls of tissue extruding from vessels that are cross-clamped and divided. The lesion may arise from adjacent myometrium and extend into the vessels, or develop de novo from the muscle of blood vessel walls. Surgically, care must be taken to remove all extension of disease into the pelvic vasculature, but otherwise, a simple hysterectomy is sufficient. The adnexa should be removed, and postoperative treatment with long-term progesterone is indicated.

Benign metastasizing leiomyoma is a rare condition in which apparently benign-appearing myomas can spread to the lungs and, occasionally, regional lymph nodes. In postmenopausal women such nodules usually remain stable, but in premenopausal women they can enlarge enough to cause pulmonary insufficiency. Treatment with progesterone can cause remission or stabilization, but surgical excision occasionally is required. Lesions that continue to grow despite hormonal

therapy must be treated with systemic chemotherapy or excised; this behavior is associated with a poor outcome.

Leiomyomatosis peritonealis disseminata is a diffuse, multifocal lesion in the peritoneal cavity that consists of benign-appearing leiomyomatas that can reach several centimeters in size. Two thirds of the cases appear in black women, and most patients are diagnosed during the postpartum period or after taking oral contraceptives on a long-term basis. The origin of this entity is controversial, but Woodruff believes that it may be a consequence of fibrosis of the peritoneal decidua, or have some other multifocal cause. Treatment revolves around removing the estrogenic stimulus, either with delivery or discontinuation of oral contraceptives. With no apparent source of estrogen evident, postoperative treatment with progesterone is indicated.

Frank *leiomyosarcoma* is a highly malignant tumor associated with a poor outcome, unless it develops in a preexisting benign leiomyoma. Sarcomatous lesions of this kind are found in about 0.1% to 0.2% of all removed leiomyomata (Fig. 43-16). When the lesion is present in a preexisting encapsulated tumor, the prognosis is ex-

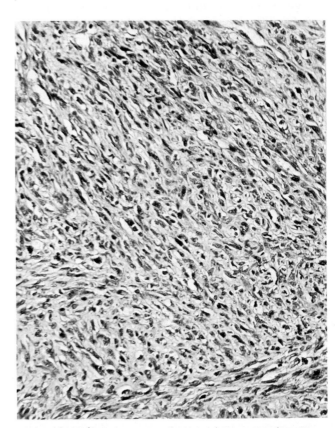

Figure 43–16. Sarcomatous change in leiomyoma showing frequent mitoses.

cellent, even when there is a high mitotic count. Thus simple surgical excision, preferably with total hysterectomy, is sufficient therapy.

The classic approach to determining cancer in a leiomyomatous lesion is to count the number of mitoses per 10 high-power fields. Unless the lesion in question is completely encapsulated in a benign leiomyoma, this approach appears to poorly predict clinical behavior until the mitotic count exceeds 20 mitoses per 10 high-power fields. Thus the traditional approach of designating as low grade those sarcomas with between 5 and 10 mitoses per 10 high-power fields must be used with caution, as the extent of disease at the time of surgery offers a much better prediction of recurrence and, hence, survival. Interestingly, the propensity for these tumors to metastasize to regional nodes is surprisingly low—only 4% in the large Gynecologic Oncology Group study.

Surgical treatment involves total hysterectomy with removal of the adnexa and any suspicious regional nodes or metastatic nodules. Adjunctive treatment with radiation appears to offer no benefit, and may indeed impede future chemotherapy or surgical treatment.

In contrast to sarcoma arising in a leiomyoma, sarcoma developing de novo in the myometrium has an extremely poor prognosis. These lesions metastasize early and often to the lungs, and overall survival is rather dismal. In the Gynecologic Oncology Group study, 36 of 56 patients with leiomyosarcomas had recurrence within 4 years of the original therapy, and similar results are reported elsewhere. Size of tumor, vascular invasion, and extrauterine spread are poor prognostic factors.

Recurrent disease should be treated with chemotherapy. Currie and coworkers presented encouraging data using a combination of hydroxyurea, DTIC, and etoposide in recurrent leiomyosarcomas, and noted several complete responses. This combination is now being tested in a group-wide Gynecologic Oncology Group Phase II study. Currie and Rosenshein recently presented a group of seven patients with recurrent leiomyosarcoma who underwent surgical excision of abdominal disease followed by combination chemotherapy with subsequent long disease-free intervals. Thus it appears that selected patients can benefit from aggressive surgical intervention, especially if chemotherapy can be effective in controlling small-volume disease (see Ch. 46).

Primary Stromal Tumors

An isolated *stromal nodule* occasionally is encountered, and raises the question of true sarcoma. These behave as a benign counterpart of malignant stromal disease and need no further therapy other than hyster-

ectomy. If there is a possibility of extrauterine extension, postoperative progesterone is indicated. The most common stromal tumor usually is classified as *stromatosis*, or *endolymphatic stromal myosis* (Fig. 43-17). The typical patient is aged 35 to 45. Although stromatosis normally is asymptomatic, some cases produce the same complaints as adenomyosis. Stromatosis is considered an adenomyosis without glandular involvement.

Because the lesions are primarily composed of proliferative stroma, mitoses occur frequently, and mitotic count is not a criterion of malignant potential. Although tumors with less than 10 mitoses per 10 high-power fields are considered low-grade stromal sarcomas, the 10-year survival rate is almost 100% when lesions are confined to the uterus.

As with all uterine tumors, the adnexa should be

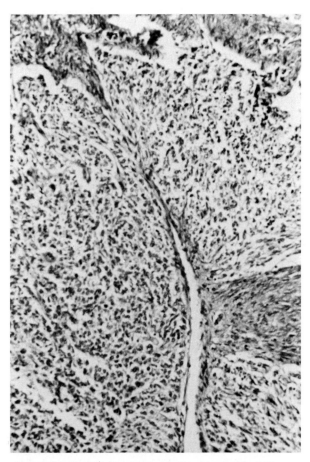

Figure 43–17. High-power microscopic view of stromatosis uteri or endolymphatic stromal myosis. The tumor is composed of proliferating endometrial stromal cells with many mitotic figures. Although relatively benign, it infiltrates the myometrium like adenomyosis without glands.

evaluated during surgery. If a diagnosis of stromatosis is made by frozen section of the uterine tumor, the tubes and ovaries should be removed, regardless of the patient's age. The lesions tend to spread without gross clinical evidence of the disease. Lesions extend through the myometrium, invade the adjacent tissues, and eventually metastasize.

Surgical evaluation of this entity is important because local recurrences are common and can lead to death by ureteral obstruction, intestinal obstruction, and massive intravascular involvement. When removing the uterus the characteristic wormy extensions into the parametria can be obvious, and the cut surface of the freshly removed uterus virtually exudes low-grade sarcoma. Obtaining receptor data is vital to future therapy, as these lesions have high progesterone receptor content, as demonstrated by Baker and coworkers and others.

In a follow-up study of 33 patients reported by Thatcher and Woodruff adjunctive progesterone treatment resulted in a high 10-year survival rate even when lesions had extended into adjacent tissue. Patients treated with irradiation had recurrences and eventually metastases. If more than 50% of the myometrium is involved, postoperative therapy with progestational agents (40 to 160 mg megestrol acetate daily) should be started. In a long-term follow-up of nine cases similarly treated no recurrence was found in 10 years.

Montag and Manart recently reported on a patient with extensive venous recurrence treated with extirpation of intravascular disease extending up the inferior vena cava as well as removal of pelvic tumor. Postoperative treatment with progesterone resulted in good long-term follow-up. I have recently encountered a similar case that presented with venous thrombosis and unilateral leg edema. Both of these recurrences probably could have been prevented with initial postoperative progesterone treatment, but both also demonstrate not only the ability of this disease to recur dramatically in vessels, but also that aggressive surgical therapy is warranted.

The true stromal sarcoma is characterized by rapid mitotic activity, a loss of stromal cell differentiation, and frequent appearances of "strap cells" or rhabdomyoblasts (Fig. 43-18). The tumor is aggressive, and the adjacent myometrium frequently is destroyed by invasion and infiltration with inflammatory cells.

The treatment for the true stromal sarcoma should be total abdominal hysterectomy and adnexectomy. A careful histologic search should be made for epithelial elements. One area of the uterus can be invaded by stromal sarcoma, whereas mixed mesodermal tumor may exist in another area. Adjunctive chemotherapy should be used in most cases.

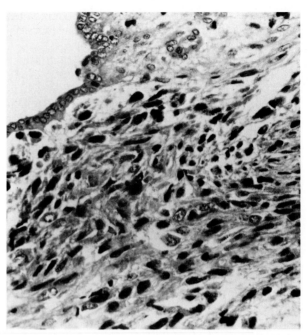

Figure 43–18. Endometrial stromal sarcoma. High-power microscopic view, showing spindle cell pattern of stromal sarcoma cells. Bizarre nuclear changes of pleomorphism, hyperchromasia, and frequent mitoses are the features of this lesion (× 250).

Other Uterine Sarcomas

Other pure heterologous sarcomas can arise from the uterus, but they, with other rare variants, constitute only a fraction of mesodermal tumors. Buscema and coworkers recently reported a series of hemangiopericytoma, which is an extremely uncommon lesion that can occur at any site, in any age group, and in either sex. In female patients the preoperative diagnosis usually is leiomyoma; the fundus is the most common site of origin. Although hemangiopericytomas are reported in many sizes, most are less than 10 cm in diameter. The surface of the tumor appears yellowish brown and greasy. When analyzed histologically the lesion is characterized by a proliferation of the cells surrounding small blood vessels. The proliferating cells are known as the pericyte of Zimmerman, but it was identified more than 100 years ago by Rouget.

Although of vascular origin, the tumor is not as hemorrhagic as an angioma or an angiosarcoma. Because solitary tumors usually extend into the adjacent tissue, complete removal may be difficult, but surgery reported to date, including a total abdominal hysterectomy and adnexectomy, has resulted in a 5-year survival rate of almost 100% for uterine hemangiopericytomas.

Tumors in other parts of the body tend to recur, to extend into adjacent tissue, and to metastasize to the lungs. No adjunctive therapy is used for treatment of a hemangiopericytoma.

Bibliography

Aalders J, Abeler V, Kolstad P, Onsrud M. Postoperative external irradiation and prognostic parameters in stage I endometrial carcinoma. Obstet Gynecol 1980;56:419.

Abbas F. Personal communication.

American College of Obstetricians and Gynecologists. Report of Task Force on Routine Cancer Screening. ACOG Committee Opinion 1989;68.

Andersen ES. Stage II endometrial carcinoma: prognostic factors and the results of treatment. Gynecol Oncol 1990;38:220.

Anderson B, Marchant DJ, Munzenrider JE. Routine noninvasive hysterography in the evaluation and treatment of endometrial carcinoma. Gynecol Oncol 1976;4:354.

Annegers JF, Malkasian GD. Patterns of other neoplasia in patients with endometrial carcinoma. Cancer 1981;48:856.

Antunes CMF, Stolley PD, Rosenshein NB, et al. Endometrial cancer and estrogen use: report of a large cancer-control study. N Engl J Med 1979;30:9.

Barnhill D, Heller P, Dames J, et al. Persistence of endometrial activity after radiation therapy for cervical carcinoma. Obstet Gynecol 1985;66:805.

Bean HA, Bryant AJ, Carmichael JA, Mallik A. Carcinoma of the endometrium in Saskatchewan: 1966 to 1971. Gynecol Oncol 1978;6:503.

Bonham DG, Donham RJC. Cancer of the endometrium, an improved epidemiological assessment. Aust NZ J Obstet Gynecol 1973;13:172.

Bonte J, Decoster JM, Ide P, Billiet G. Hormonoprophylaxis and hormonotherapy in the treatment of endometrial adenocarcinoma by means of medroxyprogesterone acetate. Gynecol Oncol 1978;6:60.

Boothby RA, Carlson JA, Neiman W, et al. Treatment of stage II endometrial carcinoma. Gynecol Oncol 1989;33:204.

Boronow RC, Morrow CP, Creasman WT, et al. Surgical staging in endometrial cancer: clinical pathologic findings of a prospective study. Obstet Gynecol 1984;63:825.

Broders AC. Microscopic grading of cancer. In: Pack GT, Livingston EM, eds. Treatment of cancer and allied diseases. Vol 1. New York: Hoeber & Harper, 1941.

Brown JM, Dockerty MD, Symmonds RE, et al. Vaginal recurrence of endometrial carcinoma. Am J Obstet Gynecol 1968;100:544.

Brown R. Clinical features associated with endometrial carcinoma. J Obstet Gynaecol Br Commonw 1974;81:933.

Burke TW, Heller PB, Woodward JE, et al. Treatment failure in endometrial carcinoma. Obstet Gynecol 1990;75:96.

Buscema J, Klein V, Rotmensch J, et al. Uterine hemangiopericytoma. Obstet Gynecol 1987;69:104.

Butler CF, Pratt JH. Vaginal hysterectomy for carcinoma of the endometrium: forty years' experience at the Mayo Clinic. In: Gray LA, ed. Endometrial carcinoma and its treatment. Springfield, Ill: Charles C Thomas, 1976.

Cacciatore B, Lehtovirta P, Wahlstrom T, Ylostalo P. Preoperative sonographic evaluation of endometrial cancer. Am J Obstet Gynecol 1989;160:133.

Charpin C, Andrac L, Habib MC, et al. Immunocytochemical assays in human endometrial carcinoma: a multiparametric comput-

erized analysis and comparison with nonmalignant changes. Gynecol Oncol 1989;33:9.

Chen SS. Propensity of retroperitoneal lymph node metastasis in patients with stage I sarcoma of the uterus. Gynecol Oncol 1989;32:215.

Chen SS, Rumancik WM, Spiegel G. Magnetic resonance imaging in stage I endometrial carcinoma. Obstet Gynecol 1990;75:274.

Chetkowski RJ, Meldrum DR, Steingold KA, et al. Biologic effects of transdermal estradiol. N Engl J Med 1986;314:1615.

Christopherson WA, Alberhasky RC, Connelly PJ. Carcinoma of the endometrium. II. Papillary adenocarcinoma: a clinical pathological study of 46 cases. Am J Clin Pathol 1982;77:534.

Clarke-Pearson D, DeLong E, Synan I, Coleman R, Creasman W. Variables associated with postoperative deep venous thrombosis. A prospective study of 411 gynecology patients with creation of a prognostic model. Obstet Gynecol 1987;69:152.

Clement PB, Scully RE. Müllerian adenosarcoma of the uterus. A clinicopathologic analysis of ten cases of a distinctive type of müllerian mixed tumor. Cancer 1974;34:1138.

Cohen CJ, Brukner HW, Deppe G, et al. Multi-drug treatment of advanced and recurrent endometrial carcinoma: a gynecological oncology group study. Obstet Gynecol 1984;63:719.

Connelly PJ, Alberhasky RC, Christopherson WN. Carcinoma of the endometrium. III. Analysis of 865 cases of adenocarcinoma and adenoacanthoma. Obstet Gynecol 1982;59:569.

Coulam CB, Annegers JF, Kranz JS. Chronic anovulation syndrome and associated neoplasia. Obstet Gynecol 1983;61:403.

Cramer DW, Cutler SJ, Christine D. Trends in the incidence of endometrial cancer in the U.S. Gynecol Oncol 1974;2:130.

Creasman WT. Estogen replacement therapy: is previously treated cancer a contraindication? Obstet Gynecol 1991;77:308.

Creasman WT. New gynecologic cancer staging. Obstet Gynecol 1990;75:287.

Creasman WT, DiSaia PF, Blessing J. Prognostic significance of peritoneal cytology in patients with endometrial cancer and preliminary data concerning therapy with intraperitoneal radiopharmaceuticals. Am J Obstet Gynecol 1981;141:921.

Creasman WT, Morrow CP, Bundy BN, et al. Surgical pathologic spread patterns of endometrial cancer. Cancer 1987;60:2035.

Cullen TS. Cancer of the uterus. Philadelphia: WB Saunders, 1900.

Currie JL, Swiger T, Dudzinski M, Walton LA, Fowler WC. Combination chemotherapy for patients with recurrent or advanced uterine sarcomas. Gynecol Oncol 1985;20:254.

Currie JL, Rosenshein NB. Surgical resection of recurrent leiomyosarcoma: aggressive intervention can result in long-term survival. Gynecol Oncol 1990;36:2.

Dede JA, Plentl AA, Moore JG. Recurrent endometrial carcinoma. Surg Gynecol Obstet 1968;126:553.

Devore GR, Schwartz PE, Morris JM. Hysterography: a 5-year followup in patients with endometrial carcinoma. Obstet Gynecol 1982;60:369.

Dinh TV, Slavin RE, Bhagavan BS, et al. Mixed müllerian tumors of the uterus: a clinicopathologic study. Obstet Gynecol 1989;74:388.

DiSaia PJ, Creasman WT, Boronow RC, Blessing JA. Risk factors and recurrent patterns in stage I endometrial cancer. Am J Obstet Gynecol 1985;151:1009.

Doering DL, Barnhill DR, Weiser EB, et al. Intraoperative evaluation of depth of invasion in stage I endometrial adenocarcinoma. Obstet Gynecol 1989;74:930.

Duk JM, Aalders JG, Fleuren GJ, de Bruijin AWA. CA-125: a useful marker in endometrial cancer. Am J Obstet Gynecol 1986;155:1097.

Dunn LJ, Bradbury JT. Endocrine factors in endometrial carcinoma. Am J Obstet Gynecol 1967;97:465.

Dunn LJ, Merchant JA, Bradbury JT, et al. Glucose tolerance and endometrial carcinoma. Arch Intern Med 1968;121:236.

Ehrlich CE, Young PCM, Stechman FB, et al. Steroid receptors and clinical outcome in patients with adenocarcinoma of the endometrium. Am J Obstet Gynecol 1988;158:796.

Enriori CL, Vico CM, Calandra RS, Charreau EH. Cytoplasmic steroid receptors in tumoral and "normal" endometrial samples from symmetrical uterine zones. Gynecol Oncol 1989;33:40.

Fanning J, Evans MC, Peters AJ, et al. Endometrial adenocarcinoma histologic subtypes: clinical and pathologic profile. Gynecol Oncol 1989;32:288.

Ferenczy A, Gelfand M. The biologic significance of cytologic atypia in progestogen-treated endometrial hyperplasia. Am J Obstet Gynecol 1989;160:126.

FIGO. Annual report on the results of treatment in gynecological cancer. Int J Gynecol Obstet 1989;28:189.

FIGO. Statements of results obtained in patients treated in 1979 to 1981. In: Pettersson F, ed. Annual report on the results of treatment in gynecological cancer. Stockholm: Panorama Press, 1988.

Fox H, Sen DK. A controlled study of the constitutional stigmata of endometrial adenocarcinoma. Br J Cancer 1970;24:30.

Friedl A, Gottardis JP, Buchler A, Jordan VC. Enhanced growth of an estrogen receptor-negative endometrial adenocarcinoma by estradiol in athymic mice. Cancer Res 1989;49:4758.

Frost JF. Gynecologic clinical cytopathology. In: Noval ER, Jones GS, Jones HW, eds. Novak's textbook of gynecology. 9th ed. Baltimore: Williams & Wilkins, 1975:782.

Gambrell DR Jr. Role of hormones in the etiology and prevention of endometrial and breast cancer. Acta Obstet Gynecol Scand (Suppl) 1982;106:337.

Gelfand MM, Ferenczy A. A prospective 1-year study of estrogen and progestin in postmenopausal women: effects on the endometrium. Osbtet Gynecol 1989;74:398.

Gordon AN, Fleischer AC, Dudley BS, et al. Preoperative assessment of myometrial invasion of endometrial adenocarcinoma by sonography (US) and magnetic resonance imaging (MRI). Gynecol Oncol 1989;34:175.

Green JB III, Green S, Alberts DS, et al. Carboplatin therapy in advanced endometrial cancer. Obstet Gynecol 1990;75:696.

Greer B, Hamberger AD. Treatment of intraperitoneal metastatic adenocarcinoma of the endometrium by whole abdomen moving strip technique and pelvic boost irradiation. Gynecol Oncol 1983;16:365.

Gusberg SB. Precursors of corpus carcinoma: estrogen in adenomatous hyperplasia. Am J Obstet Gynecol 1947;54:905.

Gusberg SB, Chen SY, Cohen CJ. Endometrial cancer: factors influencing the choice of therapy. Gynecol Oncol 1974;2:308.

Gusberg SB, Kaplan AL. Precursors of corpus cancer: adenomatous hyperplasia as stage 0 carcinoma of the endometrium. Am J Obstet Gynecol 1963;87:662.

Hachsug T, Sugimori H, Kaku T, et al. Case report: glassy cell carcinoma of the endometrium. Gynecol Oncol 1990;36:134.

Hammond CB, Jelovsek FR, Lee KL, et al. Effects of long-term estrogen replacement therapy. Am J Obstet Gynecol 1979;133:537.

Haqqani MT, Fox H. Adenosquamous carcinoma of the endometrium. J Clin Pathol 1976;29:959.

Herbst AL, Robboy SJ, Scully RE. Clear-cell adenocarcinoma of the vagina and cervix in girls: analysis of 170 registry cases. Am J Obstet Gynecol 1974;119:713.

Herbst AL, Scully RE. Adenocarcinoma of the vagina in adolescence. A report of 7 cases including 6 clear cell carcinoma (so-called mesonephromas). Cancer 1970;25:745.

Herbst AL, Ulfelder H, Poskanzer EC. Adenocarcinoma. Association of maternal stilbestrol therapy with tumor appearing in young women. N Engl J Med 1971;284:878.

Hoffman MS, Roberts WS, Cavanagh D, et al. Treatment of recurrent and metastatic endometrial cancer with cisplatin, doxorubicin, cyclophosphamide, and megestrol acetate. Gynecol Oncol 1989;35:75.

Hofmeister EJ. Endometrial biopsy: another look. Am J Obstet Gynecol 1974;228:773.

Holmesly HD, Boronow RC, Lewis JL. Treatment of adenocarcinoma of the endometrium at Memorial-James Ewing Hospitals, 1949–1965. Obstet Gynecol 1984;47:200.

Hoogerland DL, Buchler DA, Crowley JJ, Carr WF. Estrogen use—risk of endometrial carcinoma. Gynecol Oncol 1978;6:451.

Horowitz RI, Feinstein AR. Alternative analytic methods for case-control studies of estrogens and endometrial cancer. N Engl J Med 1978;299:1089.

Iversen OE. Flow cytometric deoxyribonucleic acid index: a prognostic factor in endometrial carcinoma. Am J Obstet Gynecol 1986;155:770.

Iversen OE, Laerum OD. Ploidy disturbances in endometrial and ovarian carcinomas. Anal Quant Cytol Histol 1985;7:327.

Iwamori M, Sakayori M, Nozawa S, et al. Monoclonal antibody-defined antigen of human uterine endometrial carcinomas is Le$^\beta$. J Biochem 1989;105:718.

Jones HW. Treatment of adenocarcinoma of the endometrium. Obstet Gynecol Surv 1975;30:147.

Kaplan SD, Cole P. Epidemiology of cancer of the endometrium, 1980.

Kelley RM, Baker WH. Progestational agents in the treatment of carcinoma of the endometrium. N Engl J Med 1961;264:216.

Kennedy AW, Flagg JS, Webster KD. Gynecologic cancer in the very elderly. Gynecol Oncol 1989;32:49.

Kistner RW. Endometrial hyperplasia and carcinoma in situ. In: Stall BA, ed. Endocrine therapy in malignant disease. Philadelphia: WB Saunders, 1972.

Knab DR. Estrogen and endometrial carcinoma. Obstet Gynecol Surv 1977;32:267.

Kohorn EI, Schwartz PE, Chambers JT, et al. Adjuvant therapy in mixed müllerian tumors of the uterus. Gynecol Oncol 1986;23:212.

Komaki R, Cox JD, Hartz A, et al. influence of preoperative irradiation on failures carcinoma with high risk of lymph node metastases. Am J Clin Oncol 1984;7:661.

Komaki R, Mattingly RF, Hoffman RG, et al. Irradiation of paraaortic lymph node metastases from carcinoma of the cervix or endometrium. Radiology 1983;147:245.

Koonings PP, Moyer DL, Grimes DA. A randomized clinical trial comparing Pipelle and Tis-U-Trap for endometrial biopsy. Obstet Gynecol 1990;75:293.

Koss LG, Schreiber K, Oberlander SG, et al. Detection of endometrial carcinoma and hyperplasia in asymptomatic women. Obstet Gynecol 1984;64:1.

Kottmeier H. Individualization of therapy in carcinoma of the corpus. In: Carcinoma of the uterus and ovary. Chicago: Year Book Medical Publishers, 1969:102.

Kukura V, Zaninovic I, Hrdina B. Concentrations of CA-125 tumor marker in endometrial carcinoma. Gynecol Oncol 1990;37:388.

Kurman RJ, Kaminski PF, Norris HJ. The behavior of endometrial hyperplasia. Cancer 1985;56:403.

Landgren RC, Fletcher GH, Delclos L, et al. Irradiation of endometrial cancer in patients with medical contraindication to surgery or with unresectable lesions. Am J Roentgenol Rad Ther Nucl Med 1976;126:148.

Lawrence C, Tessaro I, Durgerian S, et al. Advanced-stage endometrial cancer: contributions of estrogen use, smoking, and other risk factors. Gynecol Oncol 1989;32:41.

Lesko SM, Rosenberg L, Kaufman DW, et al. Cigarette smoking and risk of endometrial cancer. N Engl J Med 1985;313:593.

Lewis B, Cowdell R, Stallworthy JA. Adenocarcinoma of the body of the uterus. J Obstet Gynaecol Br Commonw 1970;77:343.

Lewis GC Jr, Bundy B. Surgery for endometrial cancer. Cancer 1981;48:568.

Lewis GC Jr, Slack NH, Mortel R, Bross IDJ. Adjuvant progestogen therapy in the primary definitive therapy of endometrial cancer. Gynecol Oncol 1974;2:368.

Long CA, O'Brien TJ, Sanders M, et al. ras Oncogene is expressed in adenocarcinoma of the endometrium. Am J Obstet Gynecol 1988;159:1512.

Lurain JR, Runsey NK, Schink JC, et al. Prognostic significance of positive peritoneal cytology in clinical stage I adenocarcinoma of the endometrium. Obstet Gynecol 1989;74:175.

Lyon FA. The development of adenocarcinoma of the endometrium in young women receiving long-term sequential oral contraception. Am J Obstet Gynecol 1975;123:299.

McLellan R, Dillon MB, Currie JL, Rosenshein NB. Peritoneal cytology in endometrial cancer: a review. Obstet Gynecol Surv 1989;44:711.

Mach TM, Pike MC, Henderson BE, et al. Estrogens and endometrial cancer in a retirement community. N Engl J Med 1976;294:1262.

Mahle AE. The morphological history of adenocarcinoma of the body of the uterus in relation to longevity. Surg Gynecol Obstet 1923;36:385.

Major F, Silverberg S, Morrow P, Blessing J, Creasman W, Currie J. A preliminary analysis of prognostic factors in uterine sarcoma: a Gynecology Oncology Group study (abstract). Gynecol Oncol 1987;26:411.

Malfetano JH, Hussain M. A uterine tumor that resembled ovarian sex-cord tumors: a low-grade sarcoma. Obstet Gynecol 1989; 74:489.

Malkasian GD Jr, Annegers JS, Fountain KS. Carcinoma of the endometrium, stage I. Am J Obstet Gynecol 1980;136:872.

Malviya VK, Deppe G, Malone J Jr, et al. Reliability of frozen section examination in identifying poor prognostic indicators in stage I endometrial adenocarcinoma. Gynecol Oncol 1989;34:299.

Marrett LD, Elwood JM, Epid SM, et al. Recent trends in the incidence and mortality of cancer of the uterine corpus in Connecticut. Gynecol Oncol 1978;6:193.

Marziale P, Atlante G, Pozzi M, et al. 426 cases of stage I endometrial carcinoma: a clinicopathologic analysis. Gynecol Oncol 1989; 32:278.

Mazurka JL, Krepart GV, Lotocki RJ. Prognostic significance of positive peritoneal cytology in endometrial carcinoma. Am J Obstet Gynecol 1988;158:303.

Meyer WR, Mayer AR, Diamond MP, et al. Unsuspected leiomyosarcoma: treatment with a gonadotropin-releasing hormone analogue. Obstet Gynecol 1990;75:529.

Montag TW, Manart FD. Endolymphatic stromal myosis: surgical and hormonal therapy for extensive venous recurrence. Gynecol Oncol 1989;33:255.

Moore DH, Fower WC Jr, Walton LA, Droegemueller W. Morbidity of lymph node sampling in cancers of the uterine corpus and cervix. Obstet Gynecol 1989;74:180.

Morley GW, Hopkins MP, Lindenauer SM, Roberts JA. Pelvic exenteration, University of Michigan: 100 patients at 5 years. Obstet Gynecol 1989;74:934.

Morrow CP, DiSaia PJ, Townsend DE. Current management of endometrial cancer. Obstet Gynecol 1973;42:399.

Nachtigall LE, Nachtigall RH, Nachtigall RD, et al. Estrogen replacement therapy. II. A prospective study in the relationship to carcinoma and cardiovascular metabolic problems. Obstet Gynecol 1979;54:74.

Nardone FD, Benedetto T, Rossiella F, et al. Hormone receptor status in human endometrial adenocarcinoma. Cancer 1989;64:2572.

Newbury R, Schuerch C, Goodspeed N, et al. DNA content as a prognostic factor in endometrial cancer. Obstet Gynecol 1990;76:251.

Niloff JM, Klug TL, Schaetzl E, et al. Elevation of serum CA-125 in carcinomas of the fallopian tube, endometrium, and endocervix. Am J Obstet Gynecol 1984;148:1057.

Nisker JA, Kirk ME, Nunez-Troconis JT. Reduced incidence of rabbit endometrial neoplasia with levonorgestrel implant. Am J Obstet Gynecol 1988;158:300.

Novak E, Anderson DF. Sarcoma of uterus. Am J Obstet Gynecol 1937;34:740.

Novak E, Woodruff JD. Gynecologic and obstetric pathology. 8th ed. Philadelphia: WB Saunders, 1979.

Novak E, Yui E. Relation of endometrial hyperplasia to adenocarcinoma of the uterus. Am J Obstet Gynecol 1936;32:674.

Omura GA, Blessing JA, Major FJ, et al. A randomized trial of adjuvant Adriamycin in uterine sarcomas: a Gynecologic Oncology Group study. J Clin Oncol 1985;3:1240.

Omura GA, Major FJ, Blessing JA, et al. A randomized trial of Adriamycin with and without dimethyl triazenoimidazole carboxamide in advanced uterine sarcomas. Cancer 1983;52:626.

Onsrud M, Kolstad P, Normann T. Postoperative external pelvic irradiation in carcinoma of the corpus stage I: a controlled clinical trial. Gynecol Oncol 1976;4:222.

Ozasa H, Noda Y, Mori T. A dynamic test of hormonal sensitivity of gynecologic malignancy by used of an antiestrogen, tamoxifen. Am J Obstet Gynecol 1988;158:1120.

Padwick MB, Endacott J, Whitehead MB. Efficacy, acceptability, and metabolic effects of transdermal estradiol in the management of postmenopausal women. Am J Obstet Gynecol 1985;152:1085.

Park RC, Patow WE, Petty WE, et al. Treatment of adenocarcinoma of the endometrium. Gynecol Oncol 1974;2:60.

Patsner B, Mann WJ, Cohen H, Loesch M. Predictive value of preoperative serum CA 125 levels in clinically localized and advanced carcinoma. Am J Obstet Gynecol 1988;158:399.

Peters WA 3d, Riokis SE, Smith MR, Tesh DE. Cisplatin and Adriamycin combination chemotherapy for uterine stromal sarcomas and mixed mesadermal tumors. Gynecol Oncol 1989;34:323.

Peters WA, Andersen WA, Tharton NJ, Morley GW. The selective use of vaginal hysterectomy in the management of adenocarcinoma of the endometrium. Am J Obstet Gynecol 1983;146:285.

Peterson EP. Endometrial carcinoma in young women: a clinical profile. Obstet Gynecol 1968;31:702.

Photopulos GJ, Zwaag RV, Simmons J. Lack of pelvic peritoneal closure and pelvic drain use correlated to operative morbidity in radical hysterectomy. Personal communication, 1991.

Podczaski ES, Woomert CA, Stevens CW, et al. Management of malignant, mixed mesodermal tumors of the uterus. Gynecol Oncol 1989;32:240.

Pollow K, Lubbert H, Boquol E, et al. Characterization and comparison of receptors for 17$_\beta$-estradiol and progesterone in human proliferative endometrium and endometrial carcinoma. Endocrinology 1975;96:319.

Quinn MA, Campbell JJ. Tamoxifen therapy in advanced/recurrent endometrial carcinoma. Gynecol Oncol 1989;32:1.

Reagan JW, Ng ABP. The cells of uterine adenocarcinoma. Baltimore: Williams & Wilkins, 1965.

Reid GC, Morley GW, Schmidt RW, Hopkins MP. The role of pelvic exenteration for sarcomatous malignancies. Obstet Gynecol 1989;74:80.

Reifenstein ECJ. The treatment of advanced endometrial cancer with hydroxyprogesterone caproate. Gynecol Oncol 1974;2:377.

Rosenwaks Z, Weitz AC, Jones GS, et al. Endometrial pathology and estrogens. Obstet Gynecol 1979;53:403.

Rutledge F. Role of radical hysterectomy in adenocarcinoma of the endometrium. Gynecol Oncol 1974;2:331.

Salazar OM, Bonfiglio TA, Pattern SF, et al. Uterine sarcomas. Natural history, treatment and prognosis. Cancer 1978;42:1152.

Salazar OM, DePapp EW, Bonfiglio TA, et al. Adenosquamous carcinoma of the endometrium. Cancer 1977;40:119.

Schroeder R. Nordwestdeutsche Gesellschaft fur Gynakolgie. Zbl Gynak 1922;46:193.

Segreti EM, Novotny DB, Soper JT, et al. Endometrial cancer: histologic correlates of immunohistochemical localization of progesterone receptor and estrogen receptor. Obstet Gynecol 1989;73:780.

Seski JC, Edwards CL, Herson J, et al. Cisplatin chemotherapy for disseminated endometrial cancer. Obstet Gynecol 1982;59:225.

Shimizu H, Inoue M, Tanizawa O. Adaptive cellular immunotherapy to the endometrial carcinoma cell line xenografts in nude mice. Gynecol Oncol 1989;34:195.

Siiteri PK, Schwarz BE, MacDonald PC. Estrogen receptors and the estrone hypothesis in relation to endometrial and breast cancer. Gynecol Oncol 1974;2:228.

Silverberg E, Boring CC, Squire TS. Cancer statistics, 1990. CA 1990;40:9.

Silverberg SG, Makowski EL. Endometrial carcinoma in young women taking oral contraceptives. Obstet Gynecol 1975;46:503.

Soper JT, Creasman WT, Clarke-Pearson DL, et al. Intraperitoneal chronic phosphate P-32 suspension therapy of malignant peritoneal cytology in endometrial carcinoma. Am J Obstet Gynecol 1985;153:191.

Sorbe B, Frankendal B, Risberg B. Intracavitary irradiation of endometrial carcinoma stage I by a high dose-rate afterloading technique. Gynecol Oncol 1989;33:135.

Spanos WJ Jr, Wharton JT, Gomez L, et al. Malignant mixed müllerian tumors of the uterus. Cancer 1984;53:311.

Stratton JA, Mannel RS, Rettenmaier MA, et al. Treatment of advanced and recurrent endometrial carcinoma: correlation of patient response to hormonal and cytotoxic chemotherapy and the response predicted by the subrenal capsule chemosensitivity assay. Gynecol Oncol 1989;32:55.

Sutton G. Hormonal aspects of endometrial cancer. Current Opinions in Obstet Gynecol 1990;2:69.

Swenerton KD. Treatment of advanced endometrial adenocarcinoma with tamoxifen. Cancer Treat Rep 1980;64:805.

Taina E, Maenpaa J, Erkkola R, et al. Endometrial stromal sarcoma: a report of nine cases. Gynecol Oncol 1989;32:156.

Tak WK, Marchant DJ, Munzenrider JE, Anderson B. Preoperative irradiation for carcinoma of the endometrium: indications and results. Gynecol Oncol 1977;5:18.

Thigpen JT, Blessing JA, Homesley H, et al. Phase II trial of cisplatin as first-line chemotherapy in patients with advanced or recurrent endometrial carcinoma: a Gynecologic Oncology Group study. Gynecol Oncol 1989;33:68.

Thomas DB. Steroid hormones and medications that alter cancer risk. Cancer 1988;62:1755.

Tsukamoto N, Hirakawa T, Matsukuma K, et al. Carcinoma of the uterine cervix with variegated histological patterns and calcitonin production. Gynecol Oncol 1989;33:395.

Turner DA, Gershenson DM, Atkinson N, et al. The prognostic significance of peritoneal cytology for stage I endometrial cancer. Obstet Gynecol 1989;74:775.

Twiggs LB, DiSaia PJ, Morrow PC, et al. Gravlee jet irrigator: efficacy in diagnosis of endometrial neoplasia. JAMA 1976;235:2748.

Ulbright TM, Roth LM. Metastatic and independent cancers of the endometrium and ovary: a clinicopathologic study of 34 cases. Hum Pathol 1985;16:28.

Vardi J, Tadros GH, Simindokht Z, et al. Stage IV endometrial carcinoma in a 25-year-old woman: a case report and review of the literature. Gynecol Oncol 1989;34:244.

Varia V, Rosenman J, Halle J, et al. Primary radiation therapy for medically inoperable patients with endometrial carcinoma—stages I–II. Int J Radiat Oncol Biol Phys 1987;13:11.

Walker AM, Jick H. Declining rates of endometrial cancer. Obstet Gynecol 1980;56:733.

Wharam MD, Phillips TL. The role of radiation therapy in clinical stage I carcinoma of the endometrium. Int J Radiat Oncol Biol Phys 1976;1:1081.

Wynder EL, Escher GC, Mantel N. An epidemiological investigation of cancer of the endometrium. Cancer 1966;19:489.

Zaloudek CJ, Norris HJ. Adenofibroma and adenosarcoma of the uterus. Cancer 1981;48:354.

Ziel HK, Finkle WD. Increased risk of endometrial carcinoma among users of conjugated estrogens. N Engl J Med 1975;93:1167.

Zucker PK, Kasdon EJ, Feldstein ML. The validity of Pap smear parameters as predictors of endometrial pathology in menopausal women. Cancer 1985;56:2256.

Surgical Treatment of Ovarian Cancer

FELIX N. RUTLEDGE

Of the three treatments (surgery, irradiation, and chemotherapy) for cancer of the ovary, surgery is the most curative. Thus excision should be emphasized unless the patient's physical strength or associated illness makes the operation too dangerous. More frequently surgery and chemotherapy are used sequentially because the operation is incomplete owing to metastases that are unresectable or are not discovered. For these reasons treatment usually is a combination of therapeutic methods. (The current staging system for ovarian cancer is shown in Table 44-1).

Surgery combined with postoperative irradiation has the longest history, and is effective for many patients with early-stage disease. However, irradiation became less popular when chemotherapy was perfected for this role. More effective chemotherapy demands accurate monitoring when clinical signs of the cancer disappear. Thus the need for repeat laparotomy has increased.

Multiple operations often are needed during the treatment for cancer of the ovary. These cancers usually are advanced, and surgery is difficult and demands special skills. The surgeon should be technically able to resect large cancers within the pelvic area, as well as large metastases that involve organs in the upper abdomen. The surgeon must be trained to perform operations to correct complications of the therapy or of the cancer itself, notably intestinal obstruction. When the cancer is less advanced, the surgeon's knowledge of spread pattern and common sites for subclinical metastases improves the accuracy of staging by discovery of microscopic-size metastases. Cancers of the ovary are diseases of multiple histologic types with differing growth and spread behaviors, factors that are important to consider when choosing treatment.

The incidence of each type has an age-frequency relation, and special surgical considerations apply for young patients. The correct operation for youthful women may not be applicable for older patients and vice versa. Not only are the prognosis and histologic types different, but preservation of fertility is more valuable in younger women. Technical skills alone are not enough. The surgeon should be aware of these differences, for they may qualify the patient for conservative surgery.

The conventional surgical treatment for epithelial ovarian cancer is hysterectomy with bilateral salpingo-oophorectomy. An exception may occur for young patients when the contralateral ovary appears normal and the histologic grade is low. Fertility is valued; thus by accepting a small risk that the opposite ovary harbors subclinical metastases, or may develop another cancer years later, the ovary that appears normal can be saved. This deviation from standard treatment would be intended for preservation of fertility. Preservation for hormone production alone would not be justified, since hormonal replacement medication is highly effective.

The policy for treatment of some epithelial cancers of the ovary by unilateral oophorectomy has dissenters. This opposition is supported by the known high incidence of bilaterality of epithelial tumors. Unless both ovaries are removed, subclinical-size cancer will be missed. An opportunity to cure also is missed by the effort to maintain fertility. Such management may be labeled injudicious, for if an incipient recurrence should exist, it will not manifest itself clinically until it is advanced and probably not curable. The lack of consensus about conservation is a minor aspect of the surgical treatment of ovarian cancer as a whole because the subset of patients who might qualify (early-stage, low-grade, with epithelial histologic type in the young)

TABLE 44–1
Stage Grouping for Primary Carcinoma of the Ovary

Stage I. Growth limited to the ovaries
    Stage IA. Growth limited to one ovary; no ascites present containing malignant cells. No tumor on the external surface; capsule intact
    Stage IB. Growth limited to both ovaries; no ascites present containing malignant cells. No tumor on the external surfaces; capsules intact
    Stage 1C.* Tumor either stage IA or IB but with tumor on the surface of one or both ovaries; or with capsule ruptured; or with ascites present containing malignant cells or with positive peritoneal washings

Stage II. Growth involving one or both ovaries with pelvic extension
    Stage IIA. Extension and/or metastases to the uterus and/or tubes
    Stage IIB. Extension to other pelvic tissues
    Stage IIC.* Tumor either stage IIA or IIB but with tumor on the surface of one or both ovaries; or with capsule(s) ruptured; or with ascites present containing malignant cells or with positive peritoneal washings

Stage III. Tumor involving one or both ovaries with peritoneal implants outside the pelvis and/or positive retroperitoneal or inguinal nodes. Superficial liver metastasis equals stage III. Tumor is limited to the true pelvis but with histologically verified malignant extension to small bowel or omentum
    Stage IIIA. Tumor grossly limited to the true pelvis with negative nodes but with histologically confirmed microscopic seeding of abdominal peritoneal surfaces
    Stage IIIB. Tumor of one or both ovaries with histologically confirmed implants of abdominal peritoneal surfaces, none exceeding 2 cm in diameter. Nodes negative
    Stage IIIC. Abdominal implants >2 cm in diameter and/or positive retroperitoneal or inguinal nodes

Stage IV. Growth involving one or both ovaries with distant metastasis. If pleural effusion is present there must be positive cytologic test results to allot a case to stage IV. Parenchymal liver metastasis equals stage IV

---

*In order to evaluate the impact on prognosis of the different criteria for allotting cases to stage IC or IIC it would be of value to know if rupture of the capsule was (1) spontaneous or (2) caused by the surgeon and if the source of malignant cells detected was (1) peritoneal washings or (2) ascites.
(Am J Obstet Gynecol 1987;156:263, and Am J Obstet Gynecol 1990;162:611.)

---

is uncommon. Most patients with epithelial cancer are prone to have metastatic disease when first discovered and in the older group.

Bilateral salpingo-oophorectomy usually is necessary if the tumor is of epithelial type and a hysterectomy is added. Although the uterus may appear normal, reasons for removal are as follows:

1. The corpus may contain metastases of ovarian carcinoma.
2. The endometrium may later develop an endometrial carcinoma.
3. Hormonal replacement medication may be advisable and, if used, may cause uterine bleeding when the uterus has not been removed.

These advantages for hysterectomy do not warrant pursuing difficult surgical dissection if the cancer should invade the cul-de-sac, and by removing the cervix, ovarian cancer may invade the exposed apex of the vagina to cause vaginal bleeding or offensive discharge.

OMENTECTOMY

The omentum is a favored site of the earliest intra-abdominal metastases. Excision of a generous sample of the omentum for biopsy should be part of an operation for ovarian cancer, whether performed at initial laparotomy or at "second-look" operation. When the ovarian cancer seems confined, the histologic study of the omentum is essential to determine the stage. In more advanced cancer patients the omentum often harbors a heavy burden of cancer. For these patients the omentectomy may easily accomplish tumor bulk reduction. To ensure the accuracy of second-look laparotomy for determining completeness of regression induced by chemotherapy, a major portion of the omentum should be excised.

Opinions vary about the value of omentectomy for metastatic potential in stages I and II. Advocates who favor routine omentectomy do so to exclude subclinical disease and as prophylaxis against recurrence in the organ. Others disagree, and perform total omentectomy only if there is metastases. Complete excision requires a longer abdominal incision for extra exposure of the upper abdomen with the risk of hemorrhage. Removal of that portion near the hilum of the spleen risks both hemorrhage and injury to the spleen. The literature about routine omentectomy is vague. In 1940 Pemberton advocated adding omentectomy to the standard operation, although the omentum may appear normal. In 1957 Munnell and coworkers advised that a special effort be made to excise the omentum involved with metastases. Many authors since have reported their experiences. However, the benefits for survival of removing the clinically negative omentum have not been possible to determine from the literature, because these reports do not state whether the entire omentum is excised or just the major part. Removal of the omentum that contains large metastases to reduce the bulk of cancer is beneficial.

LYMPHADENECTOMY

Lymph node metastases are a frequent finding for both epithelial and germ cell tumors. Deposits of cancer can be demonstrated by several imaging techniques: lymphangiography, computed tomography (CT), and sonography. Lymphangiography is superior, for it visualizes the architecture of the interior of the node and demonstrates the size of the node and the patency of the surrounding lymph vessels. However, lymphangiography fails to show metastases if the diameter is less than 5 mm, and also fails if the node is filled with cancer. Such nodes do not opacify. Lymph nodes filled with cancer may be suspected if the lymph vessels usually seen coursing through the region are not visible. Lymphangiography is not expected to find all nodes at risk. CT studies are more comprehensive, and may serve to investigate those lymphatics for which lymphangiography is unreliable. Also, lymphangiography may not be safe for older patients with low pulmonary reserve.

Whether or not diagnostic studies show spread to nodes, the nodes should still be investigated during laparotomy. The extent of this search and the degree of effort to locate the nodes should increase when the prognostic factors are unfavorable. Poorly differentiated and advanced stage are compelling conditions. Preoperative testing may assist the surgeon in locating positive nodes. Although we expect little therapeutic success from lymphadenectomy alone, the excision of cancerous masses may improve the chemotherapy effect.

EXPLORATION OF THE ABDOMINAL CAVITY

Faulty staging seems responsible for the postoperative recurrence rates of 25% for stage I and 50% for stage II disease. In both situations all the visible and grossly evident tumor is removed. Some metastases must escape detection, but the location is obscure. Cancer in the retroperitoneal area, implants on the diaphragm, and perhaps metastases on other peritoneal surfaces are likely sites. Several causes are suggested for these mistakes: (1) incomplete inspection of the upper abdomen, especially the subdiaphragm; (2) failure to collect specimens from peritoneal surfaces notable for subclinical metastases; (3) the proper site is not chosen and for some the sample is unsatisfactory; and (4) inadequate staging results when the search is neglected because the surgeon does not understand the disease.

CYTOREDUCTIVE SURGERY FOR ADVANCED OVARIAN CANCER

Since the 1970s the prevalent philosophy regarding the role of debulking for advanced cancer has reversed. Formerly, partial resection was held to be worthless. Some considered such surgery potentially harmful because it might facilitate cancer spread, and because short-term relief of pain by reducing the masses was not worth the discomfort caused by the operation. Therefore, many patients simply had biopsy at laparotomy with no effort made to resect, if the dissection would prove lengthy and hemorrhage could be expected. This attitude still prevails among some surgeons, but it is no longer an acceptable stance.

Today's surgeons must be mentally and technically prepared to aggressively resect large pelvic masses and to move into the upper abdomen to remove metastases that may require organ resection and, consequently, a colostomy. Resection need not be complete as long as a significant reduction of tumor mass and total cancer cell burden is accomplished.

Too often patients with advanced cancer of the ovary are declared inoperable before resectability has been amply tested. Tenacious effort is necessary. Thus a reluctant surgeon may fail to complete the needed resection if cancer was not suspected in the preoperative diagnosis. If the physical evidence indicated less serious disease, such as myomata, endometriosis, or dysfunctional cyst of the ovary, the surgical team will not be prepared for the diagnosis. If the intestinal tract has not been prepared for resection and the patient's permission for colostomy was not obtained, cytoreductive surgery may be deferred. The surgeon may not be accustomed to operating on the upper abdominal organs and may not have made provision for consultation or assistance. If the incision was too restrictive, tumor in the upper abdomen cannot be adequately resected.

A repeat attempt at tumor resection after proper preparation may still be warranted. If a repeat laparotomy is being contemplated, several considerations will aid in reaching a decision. The findings observed at the initial laparotomy should be reviewed. If metastases are multiple or diffusely distributed, or coat much of the viscera, then resection is impossible or at least ineffective. The presence of large paraaortic nodes or parenchymal metastases within the liver also indicates that the metastases are unresectable. When the metastases infiltrate deeply into vital organs in multiple sites, they will not be resectable; therefore, a repeat effort at tumor bulk reduction will fail.

The potential benefit of radical surgery to the patient relies on the chemotherapy afterward to deal with the unresectable, residual tumor. Without chemotherapy or radiation therapy to follow up with a continued attack on the cancer, rapid regrowth will erase the initial accomplishments of surgery. One can reasonably question whether the value of such partial resection is justified. There are several benefits. The anticancer effects of either irradiation or chemotherapy are improved after removal of a major portion of the tumor. Resection of some of the tumor mass stimulates cancer cell mitotic activity. The dormant cells in the fraction of the tumor begin cycling, thus making them more sensitive to cancericidal drugs. The consumption of immunologic defense products and defender cells is lessened when the bulk of the cancer is reduced.

In the late stages of cancer of the ovary intestinal function often is significantly disturbed. The relief of intestinal obstruction by tumor resection improves nutrition, and thereby helps the patient to tolerate the toxicity of irradiation or chemotherapy. Removal of large tumor masses lessens pain; thus there is an immediate benefit from such operations. Bladder and rectal function may be improved by surgical removal of large pelvic cancer masses.

Two thirds of the patients suspected of having cancer of the ovary will already be advanced with metastases above the pelvis, and will need to be prepared for a long operation with a significant likelihood of entry into the intestinal tract. If feasible, the operation should be delayed until body chemistries are restored to optimum. The more information that can be obtained about the status of the abdomen, the better prepared the surgeon is for the laparotomy. Laparoscopy is of little value in assessing the intra-abdominal status and does not decide resectability. It is both technically difficult and hazardous when the cancer is extensive.

Many of the large metastases of ovarian cancer are attached to organs that are not vital. Multiple organs often are fused together, for example, the omentum with the transverse colon and the spleen, the right ovary and the ileocecum, and the left ovary and the sigmoid colon. Occasionally the single site of metastasis is the omentum, and the resection is simple. However, the surgeon must be prepared for a complex resection.

It is important for the surgeon to be aware of the abdominal cavity compartments, for these provide access to metastases and serve as an approach for resection (Fig. 44-1). When the normal anatomy of the abdominal cavity is distorted by large masses, these anatomic spaces become important to the surgeon, for they are the most avascular pathway for circumscribing the tumor and for removal.

Certain techniques can make the approach to advanced cancer more efficient and safer. The vertical incision, preferably midline, may be extended to the entire length of the abdomen if necessary. Entering the abdominal cavity above the umbilicus is advised because the intestines are then less vulnerable to accidental injury. Many of these patients have had a prior operation in the region, which makes the intestines adherent to the old incisional scar. Even without prior laparotomy, the anterior abdominal wall above the umbilicus is safer for entry because the omentum intervenes between the abdominal wall and the underlying intestine.

Multiple metastases usually are encountered in advanced ovarian cancer; thus the surgeon must decide in what order they are to be resected. The ovarian masses

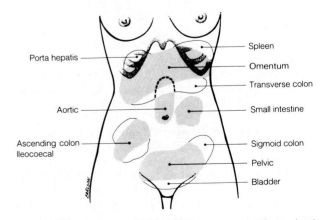

Figure 44-1. Sites within the abdomen commonly involved in metastases from ovarian cancer. Some of these metastases require resection of part of the organ harboring the cancer.

themselves have a high priority because they provide the most representative tissue for the pathologist to use in determining whether or not the cancer had its origin in the ovary. Effective chemotherapy depends on an accurate histologic diagnosis. Cancers that originate from other organs and grow on the ovaries may not be treated properly with agents used for primary carcinoma of the ovary.

When multiple masses at different sites must be resected, the largest and most troublesome usually are in the pelvic cavity. On initial assessment of the mass, resection may appear impossible. Yet persistent dissection often accomplishes removal. There are techniques that facilitate this dissection. Because ovarian cancer commonly involves the peritoneum along the pelvic wall, the bladder, and the sigmoid colon, there are advantages to approaching the resection through the retroperitoneal spaces (Fig. 44-2). Although the cancer may be adherent to the peritoneum, it seldom penetrates, and the best method for detaching the cancer is from outside the peritoneum. The blood supply to the cancer originates behind the peritoneum, and here blood vessels can be ligated for better control of hemorrhage. By using the retroperitoneal approach the pelvic peritoneum is removed, which may include microscopic-size implants. By this technique the ureters are exposed early and kept in view during the entire dissection, and risk of ureteral injury is lessened.

The retroperitoneal dissection begins at the pelvic brim, near the ovarian vessels where the ureter crosses the brim (Fig. 44-3). The ovarian vessels are safely ligated if the ureter is in view. Visual protection is maintained while the dissection progresses along the pelvic wall to the depth of the pelvic cavity. The peritoneum, with the attached cancer, is rolled medially as

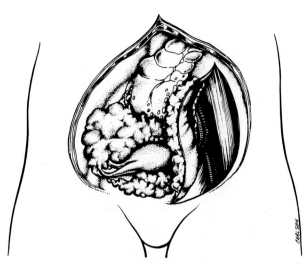

Figure 44–3. The retroperitoneal space is best entered along the pelvic brim, where the ovarian blood vessels can be ligated and the course of the ureter identified.

these tissues are freed (Fig. 44-4). The round ligament is then divided, the uterine and superior vesicle vessels are ligated, and the peritoneal covering of the bladder is removed if it is involved with the cancer.

The anterior and posterior cul-de-sac often are filled with cancer, and the conventional methods for separating the bladder from the uterus and the vagina from the rectum cannot be used. An alternative approach may be used if the bladder can be reflected downward, so that the vagina is exposed and amputated from the cervix (Fig. 44-5). Although the uterine vessels may not yet be secured, entry behind the cervix of the posterior cul-de-sac may be possible by dissecting in a retrograde manner through the posterior fornix. The uterine vessels are secured while dissecting up the cervix instead of down, the usual way. When the cancer cannot be separated from the rectosigmoid, segmental resection should be considered. Reanastomosis is desired, but if this is impossible, the lower end of the bowel may be closed as for a Hartmann's pouch with colostomy for the functional end.

For the total removal of the omentum, the gastroepiploic vessels and their branches can be exposed for a direct separation from the stomach. The branches to the greater curvature of the stomach should be ligated by suturing to the stomach wall to prevent displacement if the stomach becomes distended (Fig. 44-6). Gastric distention occurs after omentectomy, for some mysterious reason. If the metastases in the omentum are massive, the blood vessels may be concealed and not suited for a direct dissection. A safer approach begins the dissection beneath by separating the transverse colon. Access to the lesser omental sac mobilizes the mass

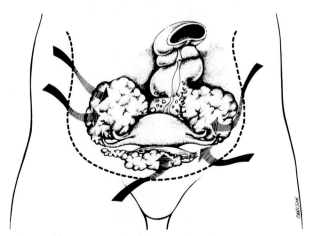

Figure 44–2. Arrows indicate the direction for the dissection to surround the cancerous masses within the pelvis. The retroperitoneal path is easier and safer.

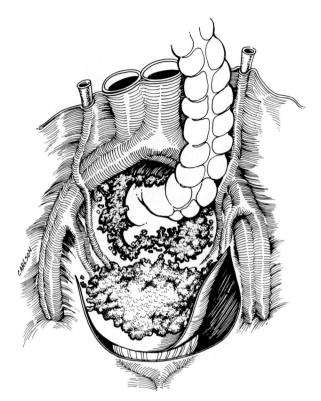

Figure 44–4. For some patients the peritoneal covering of the bladder is involved with implants of cancer and must be removed.

from the deeper structures, and the position of the blood supply becomes clearer. Exposure of this retrogastric space is helpful if splenectomy should be necessary.

PARAAORTIC EXPLORATION

The retroperitoneal nodes are important in the spread pattern of ovarian cancer. Total dissection of these nodes to reduce the cancer burden is not feasible; however, sampling of nodes in this area to search for metastases is essential for staging. We use one or more approaches to the paraaortic nodes. One approach is directly beneath the mesentery of the small intestine. In this region caution is needed to avoid dissecting too high and encountering the blood supply to the ileum or injuring the second portion of the duodenum. When this pathway to the aortic nodes is used the right ureter should be identified and protected. The thin vena cava is vulnerable to damage and may be the greatest potential source of hemorrhage. The surgeon also should be alert to the location of the superior and inferior mesenteric arteries. The latter is less valuable and can be sacrificed if needed.

Another approach to the aortic nodes is to free the right colon by dividing the peritoneum of the right paracolic gutter and rotating the bowel toward the midline. The proximal colon and terminal ileum can be rotated upward in a manner that is the reverse of its embryologic development (Fig. 44-7). Again, the right ureter can be deflected from the area of dissection. Essentially the same technique can be used on the left side with similar precautions (Fig. 44-8). The inferior mesenteric artery is more vulnerable from the left side dissection.

After the intra-abdominal operation has been completed, nonabsorbable sutures are used to approximate the abdominal wall. These are placed by the Smead-Jones method. This pulley-type stitch includes the fascia, muscles, and peritoneum about 2.5 cm away from the cut edge on both sides. This skin may be approximated by a variety of methods.

NONEPITHELIAL NEOPLASMS OF THE OVARY

Many of the same surgical procedures and therapeutic approaches applicable for epithelial cancer of the ovary apply to nonepithelial types. However, more of-

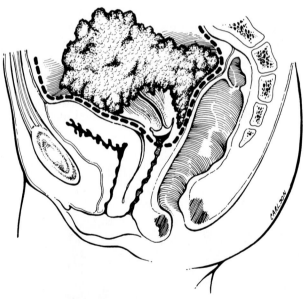

Figure 44–5. When ovarian cancer incorporates the uterus and a hysterectomy is needed, usually the tumor is freed from the sigmoid and lifted from the cul–de–sac before the upper vagina is transected to complete the hysterectomy. When this order of resection cannot be accomplished because of the cancerous mass, the reverse sequence may be attempted; access may be easier through the anterior cul–de–sac. The vagina can be divided, and the tumor in the posterior cul–de–sac can be freed by retrograde dissection.

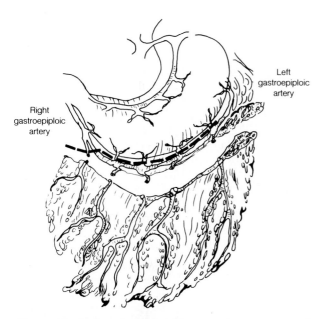

Figure 44–6. Site of excision of gastrocolic component of omentum in a total omentectomy. Partial omentectomy at the level of the transverse colon is safer and usually as effective as the higher level indicated by the broken line; however, a large part of the omentum between stomach, spleen, and splenic flexure of the colon will remain.

ten the contralateral ovary is normal and need not be removed.

Germ cell tumors are notable for development in children and teenagers and, in contrast with epithelial types, usually are unilateral. Preservation of the normal-appearing ovary does not compromise therapy in these patients. They are now being treated successfully with unilateral oophorectomy followed by chemotherapy, which preserves childbearing ability.

As a rule, ovarian tumors that occur in women under age 20 years are unilateral and, if stage Ia, only the involved ovary is removed. In more advanced cases, in which there are metastases, cytoreduction should be attempted. Tumor reductive resection may be less important for a cure for the nonepithelial varieties because the chemotherapy is more complete.

Management of the normal-appearing ovary in young patients with neoplasm in the opposite ovary has changed in recent years from bilateral to unilateral oophorectomy. For a while, during the development of this more conservative management, bisection of the ovary to be retained was common practice until the adverse effects on fertility were known. Today neither bisection nor biopsy is advised unless there is an abnormality.

The surgeon also should be aware that these tumors

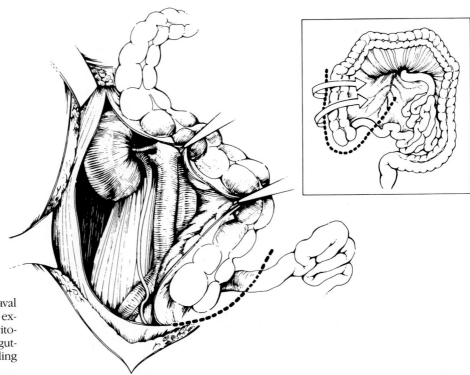

Figure 44–7. The precaval and paraaortic area can be exposed by dividing the peritoneum of the right paracolic gutter and rolling the ascending colon medially.

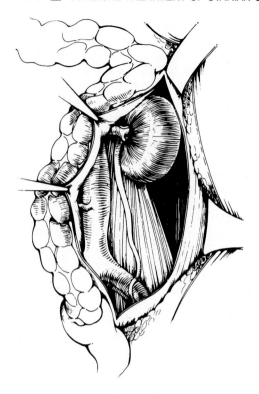

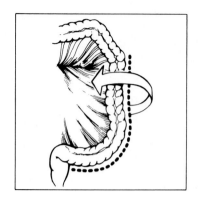

Figure 44–8. The descending colon can be retracted to expose the left paraaortic area. Because the inferior mesenteric vessel restricts exposure of this side when directed from the right, this left side approach is useful for the dissection of aortic nodes.

often produce markers that may help to monitor recurrences (ie, human chorionic gonadotropin, lactate dehydrogenase, alpha-fetoprotein, or carcinoembryonic antigen). Therefore, preoperative serum levels should be recorded. Because these tumors grow rapidly, they are prone to rupture spontaneously to produce intra-abdominal hemorrhage. The vascular pedicle may twist and occlude the vessels, causing necrosis and rupture. These events require emergency laparotomy.

As a group, the germ cell tumors (dysgerminomas, endodermal sinus tumors, and embryonal and immature teratomas) are rare. They constitute about 5% of all types of ovarian cancers that occur at any age.

Stromal tumors (eg, granulosa cell, Sertoli-Leydig, and theca) also are rare. They may appear in very young or older patients; thus the need for conservatism may arise when deciding what to remove. Stromal cell tumors in young patients usually are unilateral, but not so predictably as the germ cell tumors.

SECOND-LOOK LAPAROTOMY

The second-look laparotomy has a limited role in treating patients with epithelial carcinoma of the ovary. An accurate assessment of tumor regression when chemotherapy has been completed is important for judging and determining the effectiveness of the treatment.

Although ovarian cancer usually is sensitive to chemotherapy, in more than half the patients, the tumors either do not respond to treatment or develop regrowth after an initial response. To maintain control over this cancer, its behavior must be clinically watched with apprehension. Uncertainties may need surgical resolution.

Surveillance must be timely, continuous, and diligent. To learn the status of cancer in some patients requires reoperation, especially if no equally accurate alternative method is available. Near completion of a prescribed treatment regimen, the gynecologist must determine whether the cancer has been completely eradicated or whether regression has been only partial. The management plan for the future depends on the duration of the chemotherapy, the completeness of the regression, and especially whether total eradication of the cancer can be confirmed. Reexploration may be the only method for obtaining this information.

Since the 1970s gynecologists' common practice of performing second-look operations after chemotherapy has been supported on the premise that the antitumor action of cancer chemotherapy is an unstable and unreliable factor that frequently must be checked. Currently, however, regular use of the second-look laparotomy has been challenged to prove that survival increases as a result of the information learned from the operation. If residual cancer is found, further treatment is seldom successful, since there is no effective second-line chemotherapy. Thus the surgery has no therapeutic value. Nevertheless, patients who have microscopic-size residual cancer may benefit from additional chemotherapy (see Ch. 46).

The University of Texas M. D. Anderson Cancer Center Experience

The experience of the department of gynecology at the M. D. Anderson Cancer Center illustrates how information gained by second-look operation can be used to improve patient treatment. From 1971 to 1982, 246 patients with stage III or IV epithelial carcinoma of the ovary had a second-look laparotomy. The purpose was to determine with as much precision as possible the actual status of the cancer when a series of courses of chemotherapy has induced a complete clinical regression. We consider this information essential to avoid chronic toxicity from the drugs and to determine whether to end treatment.

Laparotomy identified evidence of gross residual cancer ("macroscopic positive") in 111 patients (45%). No cancer was found in 85 patients (35%). This was confirmed by samples collected at random from sites judged to be at high risk for residual disease. Also, cells from peritoneal spaces were benign. These patients were classified as "negative." In 50 patients (20%) no residual cancer was visible, yet biopsies or peritoneal cytology did identify cancer. These patients were classified as "microscopic positive" (Fig. 44-9).

Treatment was discontinued for patients in the negative category; however, those with macroscopic cancer were given more treatment. If cytoreductive surgery was feasible for patients with macroscopic cancer, the bulk of the cancer was resected and more chemotherapy administered, usually with drugs different from those previously used. The patients with microscopic residual disease received more of the same chemotherapy or, infrequently, radiation. For a time a third exploration was done after another year of chemotherapy. A "third-look," however, was found unnecessary, and this practice was discontinued.

At the time of the 1985 reports by Copeland and associates and Gershenson and colleagues 37 of 50 patients in the microscopic-positive category were surviving with no evidence of cancer. Eleven had died of cancer and two had died of other causes. These survivals support reinstituting chemotherapy. The patients in the negative category had been observed for a 3- to 5-year period and, generally, had done well, although 30% developed a recurrence. Among the 85 patients whose second-look was negative and who were observed for more than 4 years, 65 (76%) were alive with

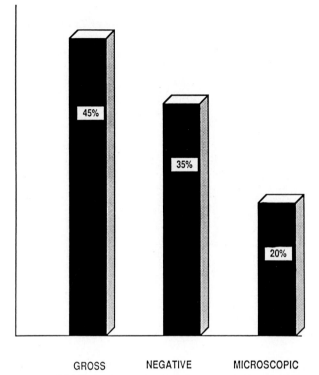

Figure 44–9. Findings of cancer in second–look laparotomy in 246 patients with stage III–IV disease. (Courtesy of M.D. Anderson Hospital Univ. of Texas Cancer Center, Dept. of Gynecology.)

no evidence of disease. Four were alive with recurrence and 16 had died of recurrence.

Experience with the second-look operation had produced valuable new understanding as to why patients' courses of disease are dissimilar. We now know that stage, histologic cell type, size of unresectable metastases, age of patient, and physical disabilities are prognostic factors. If they are all known at the start of treatment, an estimate of the clinical course can be made. Our experience observing the responses of patients with negative second-look laparotomies is summarized in Table 44-2.

About 75% of the patients with early-stage ovarian cancer obtain a complete clinical remission. In addition, about 50% of those with advanced-stage disease respond to chemotherapy, and about half of these patients are then candidates for repeat laparotomy. The second-look operation defines a complete clinical remission pathologically. A pathologic (surgical) complete remission currently is the best possible assessment of a negative cancer status.

There are other, less frequent reasons for reexploration. For example, the clinical examination of some

TABLE 44–2
M. D. Anderson Cancer Center Negative Second-Look Laparotomy Survival by Patient Characteristics

CHARACTERISTICS	NO. OF PATIENTS	ACTUARIAL SURVIVAL		
		5-year Survival (%)		P Value
Age				
≤40	15	100		0.03
>40	70	82		
Stage				
III	73	88		0.68
IV	12	73		
Grade				
1	11	100	1 versus 2	0.10
2	24	89	2 versus 3	0.47
3	50	80	1 versus 3	0.02
Residual disease at initial surgery				
0	17	100	i versus ii	0.09
≤2 cm	47	86	ii versus iii	0.37
>2 cm	21	69	i versus iii	0.03
All patients	85	85		

patients during chemotherapy may be confusing. The abdominal viscera may feel abnormal on palpation, but there is still uncertainty about interpreting this finding as cancer. Exploratory laparotomy may be needed to resolve the confusion.

Related Literature

Some cancer treatment centers use repeat laparotomy frequently. They incorporate it into the initial treatment scheme for all patients, provided response to chemotherapy is good. Other centers are more selective of which patients will receive a second look. Repeat laparotomy is especially helpful when new drugs are being tested.

Tables 44-3 and 44-4 summarize the frequency of negative second-look laparotomies and subsequent recurrence by stage of disease, as reported in the recent English literature. Because some authors have observed that laparotomies of patients with stage I or II frequently are negative, patients with early-stage disease are considered separately in Table 44-3. As expected, the percentage of patients free of cancer at second look is higher and the incidence of recurrence lower in that group than in patients with stage III or IV disease (Table 44-4). The variations in the recurrence percentages may be due to different follow-up intervals.

The low incidence of residual cancer after chemotherapy in patients with early-stage disease provides an option for individualized care, and repeat laparotomy may be omitted. Nevertheless, some patients with stage I or II cancer have residual disease; these patients will

TABLE 44–3
Negative Second-Look Laparotomy (Stages I and II)

AUTHOR	NUMBER EXPLORED	NEGATIVE	RECURRENCE
Barnhill et al. (1984)	41	30 (73%)	1 (3%)
Cain et al. (1986)	60	45 (75%)	4 (9%)
Podczaski et al. (1987)	28	24 (86%)	0 (0%)
Podratz et al. (1985)	57	47 (82%)	4 (9%)
Webb et al. (1982)	30	22 (73%)	3 (14%)
Total	216	168 (78%)	12 (7%)

TABLE 44–4
Negative Second-Look Laparotomy (Stages III–IV)

AUTHOR	NUMBER EXPLORED	NEGATIVE	RECURRENCE
Cain et al. (1986)	103	49 (48%)	13 (27%)
Gershenson et al. (1985)	246	85 (35%)	20 (24%)
Ho et al. (1987)	39	17 (44%)	9 (53%)
Podczaski et al. (1987)	66	25 (38%)	7 (28%)
Podratz et al. (1985)	77	29 (38%)	8 (27%)
Podratz et al. (1988)	134	50 (37%)	15 (30%)
Webb et al. (1982)	29	10 (34%)	1 (10%)
Total	694	265 (38%)	73 (28%)

respond better to additional treatment if they receive it promptly, while the cancer is minimal. If treatment is delayed until recurrence is large enough to be clinically evident, as may happen without laparotomy, optimal treatment conditions have passed.

Table 44-5 summarizes reports of positive second-look operations contained in the current literature. Six authors reported on a total of 579 patients explored, of whom 20% were classified as microscopic positive. This is the category wherein laparotomy may benefit future treatment.

Imaging techniques are rapidly improving, and there are roles for sonography, CT, and magnetic resonance imaging in evaluating residual disease. For some patients these noninvasive techniques have sufficed and have replaced the second-look laparotomy. However, they do not sufficiently demonstrate small metastases present in many patients; therefore, we still perform reexploration for these patients.

Surgical Techniques

The second-look operation must be more than a simple laparotomy. In addition to excising the ovaries, if they are still present, a major portion of the omentum must be removed. Samples of the pelvic wall nodes and lower paraaortic nodes must be collected, and multiple biopsies of the peritoneum also are recommended. The search should include samples of the peritoneal fluid, taken immediately after opening the abdomen, for cytologic examination.

Some basic surgical considerations should be observed to facilitate the search described above. The incision should give maximal access to all parts of the abdominal cavity. Because the diaphragm is most difficult to expose, the incision must extend as near to the rib margins as possible. Loops of the intestine can be expected to be adherent to the anterior abdominal wall, especially to an old incisional scar. Entry above the umbilicus is safer.

The frequency of second-look surgery recently has declined. There may be several explanations. Clinicians are more confident that patients with early-stage disease and no residual cancer will do well. They also are confident in their ability to manage chemotherapy toxicity, although there is still uncertainty about long-term effects. The generation of new knowledge by second-look operations has reached a plateau. Monitoring of the cancer under treatment has improved. Imaging and

TABLE 44–5
Positive Second-Look Laparotomy

AUTHOR	NUMBER EXPLORED	MACROSCOPIC POSITIVE	TOTAL POSITIVE*
Brenner et al. (1985)	52	25 (48%)	35 (67%)
Copeland et al. (1985)	246†	111 (45%)	161 (65%)
McCusker et al. (1987)	42	11 (26%)	22 (52%)
Miller et al. (1986)	88	32 (36%)	50 (57%)
Podczaski et al. (1987)	94	30 (32%)	45 (48%)
Stehman et al. (1988)	57	25 (44%)	34 (60%)
Total	579	234 (40%)	347 (60%)

*Macroscopic + microscopic positive.
† Stages III and IV.

tumor markers effectively signal tumor regression and recidivation but become blind when residual cancer masses are 1 cm or less in greatest diameter.

After cisplatin combinations, other chemotherapies have little success. A timely switch from a failing chemotherapy to different drugs, to sustain regression, is not possible with the current drugs. Information obtained by reexploration is superfluous if we are unable to treat patients whose disease remains.

There is consensus that stage and size of unresected cancer are strong prognostic factors. Experiences differ regarding grade, patient age, and drugs used. Prognostic factors are not wholly reliable. Nevertheless, perhaps some patients may be identified for whom a second-look operation has a low priority, for example, a young patient with well-differentiated and low-volume residual cancer. A second look at this patient will have an excellent chance of being negative, and even if biopsies and peritoneal cytology are positive, the prognosis will be marked by a slow progression of the disease. The benefits of additional chemotherapy would be minimal, and the risk of chronic toxicity from protracted chemotherapy would be high (see Ch. 46).

CONCLUSIONS

The management of patients with carcinoma of the ovary without surgery may be necessary in some instances, such as serious physical disability that makes laparotomy too hazardous. Unless severely contraindicated, primary laparotomy is necessary to establish the diagnosis, document the extent of spread, and eradicate the resectable cancer. For patients with advanced cancer maximum resection is important.

The duration of survival and cures improved by maximum, although often incomplete, resection is convincing, providing the separate unresectable tumor masses are small. This advantage usually is noted only when the residual inoperable cancer is 2 cm or less in diameter.

The prognosis can be influenced by the surgical team. It is axiomatic that a blend of knowledge and technical skills accomplishes the best surgical treatment. Perhaps the proper mental attitude toward the task accomplishes a small additional gain.

OVARIAN TUMORS COMPLICATING PREGNANCY

A. GATEWOOD DUDLEY

The coexistence of an ovarian tumor with pregnancy presents problems both to the clinician and the patient, with the most serious complication being that of

malignancy. This possibility must be discussed with the patient in obtaining informed consent prior to laparotomy. The therapeutic implications of possible hysterectomy and castration results in an emotionally charged environment because of the young age of the patient, the need to preserve the pregnancy (two patients), and the preservation of reproductive capacity as well as ovarian function.

Incidence

Fortunately, ovarian cancer is quite rare in pregnancy, ranking as the fifth most common cancer after cervix, breast, leukemia–lymphoma, and melanomas. The incidence of ovarian cancer is variously reported to be between 1/12,000 and 1/50,000 live births.

The incidence of benign ovarian tumors complicating pregnancy is more common. The exact incidence, however, depends on whether one considers simple cyst noted on ultrasound exam (1/50 live births) or pelvic exam (1/80 live births), or those that ultimately require laparotomy (1/1000 to 1/1500 live births). In our experience about 30% of ovarian masses complicating pregnancy are nonneoplastic ones, and only about 1% to 2% are malignant.

Koonings noted the incidence of ovarian tumors complicating cesarean section to be about 1/200 cesarean births, and Ballard observed ovarian tumors to complicate termination of pregnancy in 1/594 procedures. The incidence of ovarian tumor complicating abortion hysterectomy is about 1/77. Our recent review of the literature of ovarian tumors complicating pregnancy since 1939 reveals an approximate total of 825 benign and 330 malignant tumors requiring surgical exploration.

Diagnosis

The appropriate diagnosis of ovarian tumors complicating pregnancy depends upon the use of certain windows of opportunity, namely: (1) the initial pelvic examination in the first trimester, (2) the initial ultrasound, (3) careful evaluation at the time of operative intervention. This includes thorough pelvic examination at the time of termination of pregnancy and careful examination of the ovaries at the time of cesarean section or postpartum tubal ligation.

The increasing (nearly routine) use of ultrasound examination affords an excellent opportunity for the diagnosis of coexistent ovarian pathology, and it is for this reason that such an examination should always include the adnexa.

Resta and coworkers have reported that the upper

limits of normal size for the corpus luteum of pregnancy is 2 cm. Recent studies of ovarian cyst formation have therefore used this size in defining ovarian cyst formation. This is obviously smaller than those cysts noted on clinical pelvic examination. Therefore, there is a danger that many cysts which previously would have been unrecognized could be operated on unnecessarily during pregnancy. However, properly utilized high-quality ultrasound should reduce, not increase, the frequency of surgical intrusion on pregnant patients with simple ovarian cysts (Fig. 44-10). Grimes and coworkers have pointed out that most clinical cystic tumors will resolve by 16 weeks. Recent ultrasound evidence clearly documents this experience, although not all cystic corpus lutea resolve spontaneously. They may persist, become quite large, undergo torsion, and become symptomatic.

Lavery, in a review of 3918 ultrasound examinations at 20 weeks gestation, noted cyst formation greater than 2 cm in 2.4% of examinations. Only nine patients (0.23%) required surgical intervention. Hogston, in a review of 26,000 patients who received routine ultrasound, noted an incidence of cyst formation of 0.52%. All complex cysts and those greater than 6 cm were operated on primarily (10%). Eighty-five percent of the remaining patients who were followed conservatively showed a spontaneous resolution, with the exception of five patients (5%) who ultimately required laparotomy.

The first trimester is clearly the optimum time to diagnose the adnexal mass complicating pregnancy. Because tumors are rarely symptomatic during this period, the majority of such tumors are now being discovered by ultrasound examination (or later, as an incidental finding at cesarean section). With the increasing incidence of ultrasound evaluation and use of cesarean section, recent articles suggest that about 50% of ovarian tumors complicating pregnancy are asymptomatic. When symptomatic, the patient typically presents with abdominal pain, abdominal distention, and vague gastrointestinal complaints. All these symptoms may be directly attributable to pregnancy itself; therefore, it is not surprising that the most symptomatic ovarian tumors are not suspected.

Actually, ovarian tumors complicating pregnancy may be divided into three groups depending on the severity of presentation:

Those that are asymptomatic
Those with symptoms compatible with torsion
Those with catastrophic presentations consistent with shock, hemorrhage, and rupture.

Successful outcome for both mother and fetus depends upon a high index of suspicion with early diagnosis. One should consider an ovarian mass in any woman who experiences abdominal pain in pregnancy. Furthermore, torsion, rupture, infection, or hemorrhage of an ovarian tumor should be included in the differential diagnosis of any catastrophic abdominal obstetrical event. This is particularly true if occurring at times of rapid change in uterine size or position (such as 8 to 16 weeks), termination of pregnancy, labor and delivery, or during the immediate postpartum period.

The incidence of torsion complicating ovarian tumor in the nonpregnant state is about 2%. Torsion complicating ovarian tumor during pregnancy is clearly

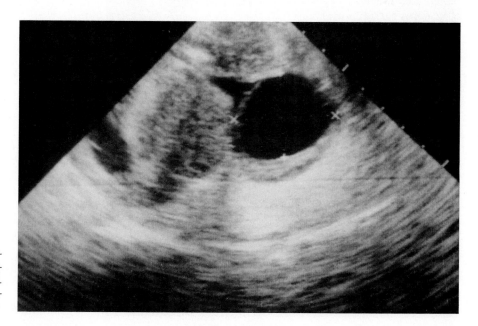

Figure 44–10. A simple ovarian cyst complicating early pregnancy was noted on ultrasound. Most such cysts resolve spontaneously.

higher, varying from 11% to 50%. As late as 1984, Young, in a review of 36 sex cord stromal tumors complicating pregnancy, reported an incidence of 28% torsion and rupture, and 21% dystocia. Other recent studies in which there is a high incidence of incidental asymptomatic tumors report much lower incidence of torsion, rupture, and dystocia. Nevertheless, it is clear that the unrecognized symptomatic ovarian tumor complicating pregnancy may become catastrophic accompanied by hemorrhage, shock, peritonitis, or death.

Pathology

Benign neoplasms complicating pregnancy include two tumorlike conditions with which every gynecologist should be familiar. Hyperreactio luteinalis (first described by Burger in 1938 as a grossly multicystic, usually bilateral, ovarian enlargement, often 15 to 20 cm in size) is a term used to describe multiple theca lutein cysts of the ovary complicating pregnancy (Fig. 44-11). Microscopically, one notes extensive luteinization of the theca and granulosa cell layers. Clinically, this condition is known to be associated with hydatidiform mole, multiple gestations, choreiocarcinoma, erythroblastosis fetalis, or other conditions associated with elevated levels of human chorionic gonadotrophins.

Hyperreactio luteinalis has also been associated with normal pregnancy.

Luteoma of pregnancy is a specific benign, usually unilateral, solid lutein cell tumor of the ovary found in late pregnancy, often noted at cesarean section (Fig. 44-12). First described by Sternberg in 1962, this tumor is grossly bosselated, soft, fleshy, yellow, or hemorrhagic. Microscopically, it exhibits an acidophilic granular cytoplasm with sparse lipid formation and a distinctive reticular pattern.

The important clinical implication with both of these lesions is that, if they are recognized or suspected, simple biopsy without further surgery is adequate therapy, as both will almost invariably resolve spontaneously.

The most common benign neoplasm of the ovary in pregnancy is the benign cystic teratoma, occurring in about 40% of such cases (Fig. 44-13). In our experience, the second most common group of ovarian tumors complicating pregnancy is that of functional tumors, such as corpus luteum or simple cysts (Fig. 44-14). These represent about 30% and may occur in late pregnancy. Tumors of epithelial origin represent about 20% to 30% of benign neoplasms complicating pregnancy with a relative increase in tumors of the mucinous type (Fig. 44-15). Endometrial (4%), paraovarian (6%), and other miscellaneous tumors constitute the remaining types of tumors.

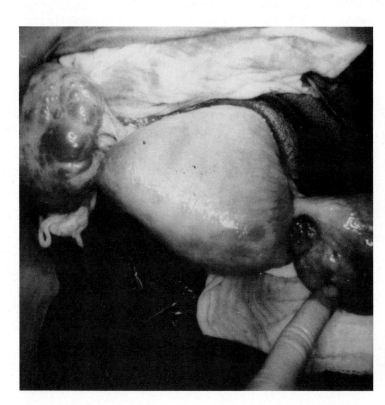

Figure 44–11. Hyperreactio luteinalis (multiple theca luteal cysts) is a tumor–like condition complicating pregnancy. Usually bilateral, it virtually always resolves spontaneously. (Photograph courtesy of David Barclay, Little Rock, Arkansas.)

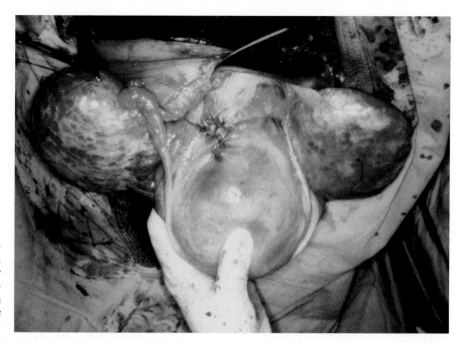

Figure 44–12. Luteoma of pregnancy. Typically occurring late in normal pregnancies, and usually unilateral and solid, this lesion resolves spontaneously. (Photograph courtesy of David Barclay, Little Rock, Arkansas.)

Malignant ovarian tumors constitute about 2% of all adnexal masses that complicate pregnancy and require surgical exploration. The single most common malignant ovarian tumor complicating pregnancy is probably the germ cell dysgerminoma (Fig. 44-16). Malignant tumors of epithelial origin as a group, however, are more common with a greater frequency of both mucinous types and tumors of borderline malignancy (Fig. 44-17). Sex cord stromal tumors are the third most common primary malignant ovarian neoplasm, representing about 8% to 14% (Fig. 44-18). Krukenberg and/ or other metastatic tumors represent about 15% of

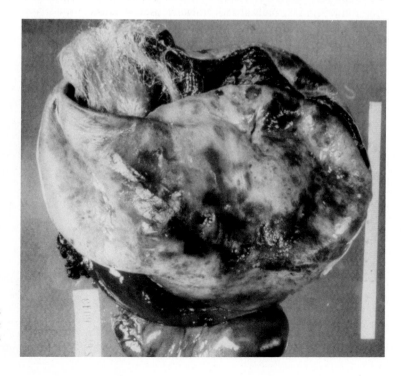

Figure 44–13. The benign cystic teratoma is the most common benign neoplasm of the ovary complicating pregnancy. This tumor has undergone torsion and infarction.

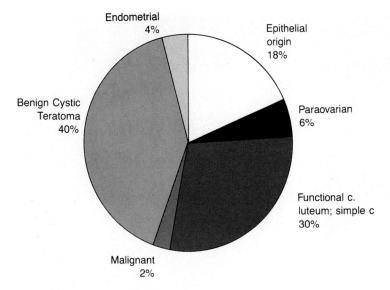

Figure 44–14. The relative frequency of ovarian tumors complicating pregnancy. Note that only 2% are malignant.

malignant ovarian neoplasms complicating pregnancy (Fig. 44-19).

Whether malignant or benign, the overwhelming majority of ovarian tumors complicating pregnancy are unilateral. Karlen reported 90% of dysgerminomas in pregnancy to be unilateral, and Young reported 35 of 36 sex cord stromal tumors to be unilateral when complicating pregnancy. Even malignant tumors of epithelial origin noted during pregnancy are unilateral in 90% of cases. The rarer germ cell tumors, such as endodermal sinus tumors, are virtually always unilateral as well. This

has important therapeutic implications. Viewed somewhat differently, it is also important to note that most bilateral tumors occurring in pregnancy are not malignant—for example, benign cystic teratoma, endometriosis, and hyperreactio luteinalis. The most common bilateral malignant ovarian tumors are the metastatic and Krukenberg type. Somewhat less commonly noted are primary malignant tumors of epithelial origin.

Virilization secondary to an ovarian tumor sometimes complicates pregnancy (Fig. 44-20). Historically, the classic painting entitled *Magdalena Ventura with*

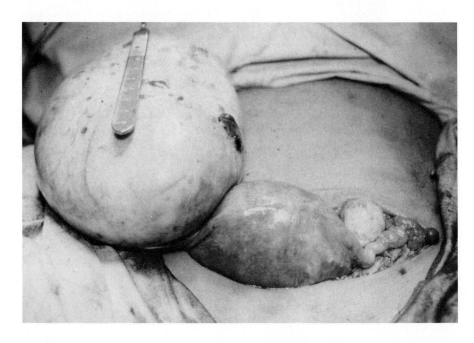

Figure 44–15. A mucinous cystadenoma complicating pregnancy. Tumors of epithelial origin are the second most common benign neoplasms of the ovary complicating pregnancy. Tumors of mucinous type are relatively more common in pregnancy.

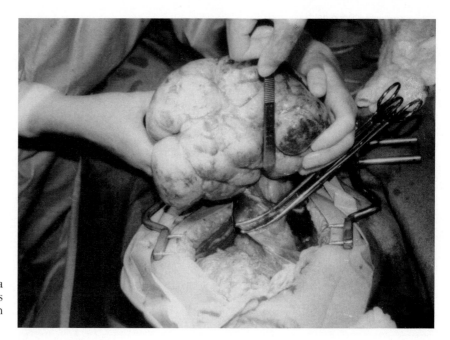

Figure 44–16. A dysgerminoma that has undergone torsion. This tumor is relatively more common when complicating pregnancy.

Husband and Son done in 1631 by Ribera documents such a problem (Fig. 44-21). Magdalena, after having several children, became virilized at age 37 with apparent infertility thereafter. However, when she was 52 a son was born. One would speculate that she probably had an ovarian Sertoli-Leydig cell tumor. Young, how-

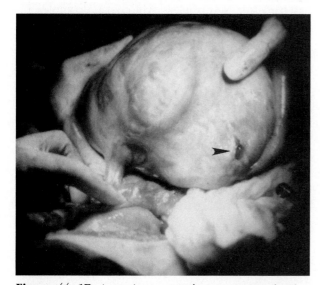

Figure 44–17. A mucinous cystadenocarcinoma that has undergone rupture (*arrow*). Failure to diagnose ovarian tumors may result in an increased incidence of rupture in later pregnancy. (Photograph courtesy of James Nelson, Valhalla, New York.)

ever, has pointed out that while about 50% of Sertoli-Leydig cell tumors in the nonpregnant state are functional, only about 15% of those complicating pregnancy result in maternal virilization. He proposed two possible explanations for this apparent decrease in virilization. The first is that the most active of such tumors result in anovulation, and therefore are selected out. The second is that the placenta may aromatize the tumor-produced androgens into estrogens.

In any event, Sertoli-Leydig cell tumors are not the most common tumors in pregnancy associated with virilization. This distinction falls to those tumors associated with a functioning ovarian stroma. Such tumors may be nonneoplastic, neoplastic, benign, or malignant (either primary or secondary). The most common virilizing ovarian tumor that complicates pregnancy is the luteoma, representing about one third of such cases. The second most common is the Krukenberg group, followed closely by tumors of the epithelial group, which are almost always mucinous in type (Table 44-6).

The clinical implications of virilizing tumors complicating pregnancy are somewhat different from those of such tumors in the nonpregnant state. Virilization usually occurs late in pregnancy, is of short duration, and is usually reversible. About one third of such cases, as previously mentioned, are secondary to luteoma and therefore resolve spontaneously. Fifty percent of such cases are associated with malignancy. If tumors of sex cord stroma or epithelial type are present, the ultimate outcome remains quite good. However, patients with Krukenberg lesions have a poor outcome.

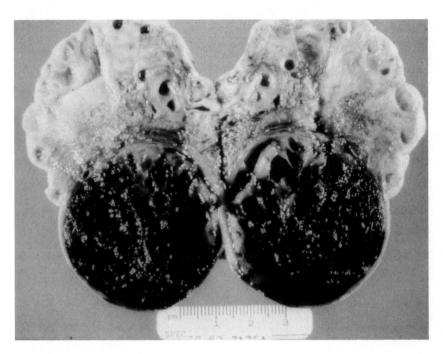

Figure 44–18. A sex cord stromal tumor complicating pregnancy, with considerable area of hemorrhage. Torsion, rupture, and hemorrhage occur frequently with this tumor in pregnancy. (Photograph courtesy of Robert Young, Boston, Massachusetts.)

Therapy

Surgery

The first successful oophorectomy for an ovarian tumor complicating pregnancy was performed in 1846 by Bund. Although the woman survived, the fetus aborted at 12 weeks gestation. At about the same time, J. Marion Sims performed the first successful removal of an ovarian tumor in which both the woman and the fetus survived. As late as 1906 McKerran reported a 21% maternal mortality and a 50% fetal mortality, with surgi-

cal management, when pregnancy and ovarian tumors coexist.

In general, one should avoid elective surgery in the first trimester, as many lesions represent the cystic corpus luteum of pregnancy and will resolve spontaneously. Buttery and others have also noted an abortion rate of about 30% in those patients operated on in the first trimester. Nevertheless, symptomatic, complex, bilateral, or solid tumors should be operated on immediately (Fig. 44-22). Preoperative evaluation should be limited to careful clinical evaluation and pelvic ultra-

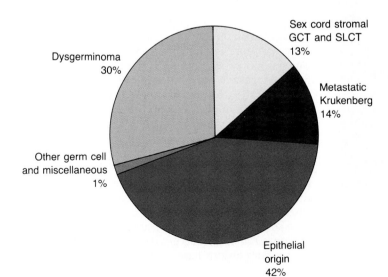

Figure 44–19. The approximate relative frequency of the most common malignant ovarian tumors.

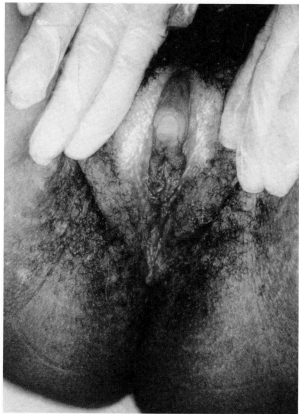

Figure 44–20. Virilization occurring in late pregnancy secondary to a pregnancy luteoma. Note clitoral hypertrophy and hirsutism. (Photograph courtesy David Barclay, Little Rock, Arkansas.)

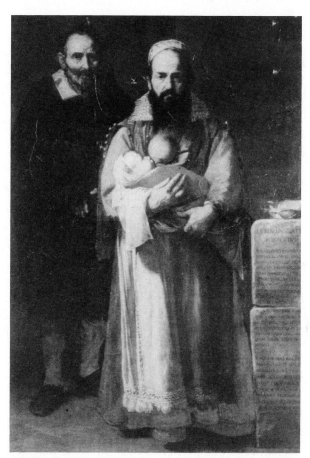

Figure 44–21. The painting by Ribera entitled *Magdalena Ventura With Husband and Son.* The most common virilizing tumors of the ovary complicating pregnancy are those with functioning stroma. (Reprinted with permission.)

TABLE 44–6
Published Cases of Virilzing Ovarian Tumors Associated with Pregnancy*

TUMOR TYPE	TOTAL NUMBER
Luteoma	33
Hyperthecosis	3
Hyperreactio luteinalis	1
Krukenberg	14
Sex cord stromal	11
Sertoli-Leydig	8
Granulosa cell	3
Epithelial origin	12
Mucinous	9
Benner	3
Serous	0
Oher	
Dermoid	3
Leydig	1
Lipoid	1
Total	102

*The luteoma of pregnancy is responsible for approximately one third of such cases.

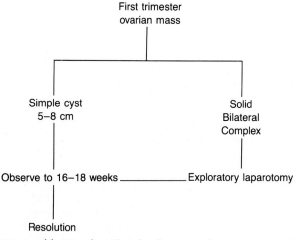

Figure 44–22. Algorithm for the surgical management of ovarian tumors complicating pregnancy in the first trimester. Symptomatic, solid, bilateral, and complex lesions should be operated on when discovered.

sound examination. Excretory urography, barium enema, computed tomography, and other such studies are best avoided.

The optimum time for surgical intervention is 16 to 18 weeks. In patients in whom the asymptomatic mass is noted at or near term, vaginal delivery should be avoided because torsion, rupture, and hemorrhage may occur during or immediately following labor. Delivery by cesarean section with careful surgical evaluation of the adnexa is more appropriate.

General anesthesia is the anesthesia of choice. One should remember that delayed gastric emptying and esophageal reflux may occur in pregnancy; therefore, appropriate precautions are necessary. One should also be aware of and prevent vena caval and aortic compression.

A vertical or paramedian incision is preferred, since after 16 weeks gestation the ovary is an abdominal rather than a pelvic structure. The incision should therefore be placed higher than usual.

At laparotomy, one should carefully assess the limits of disease. Thorough gross examination of the lesion, with frozen section, as well as evaluation of the upper abdomen, omentum, and paraaortic nodes should be performed, along with pelvic washings. The involved ovary should be sent for frozen section to establish a preliminary diagnosis. The contralateral ovary should be carefully inspected. However, biopsy or wedge resection of the contralateral ovary should be avoided if there is no gross evidence of involvement. One possible exception might be made if the primary is a dysgerminoma, because these tumors reportedly may involve the contralateral ovary in a clinically undetectable, microscopic manner.

One should avoid pelvic or paraaortic node sampling if the size of the uterus limits exposure or poses the risk of excessive manipulation. The uterus should be handled gently in any case, and frequent irrigation should be used to prevent the tissue from drying. When ovarian cystectomy is required, a plastic closure using internal cautery with a 5-0 internal closure should be used; alternatively, there may be no closure. The traditional Buxton-type closure should be avoided.

Prior to a decision to perform oophorectomy, one must always consciously exclude hyperreactio luteinalis and luteoma of pregnancy. Furthermore, since most malignant ovarian tumors are unilateral, total abdominal hysterectomy and bilateral salpingectomy are rarely indicated (Fig. 44-23). Total hysterectomy and removal of ovaries should *never* be performed on the basis of a frozen section diagnosis of borderline or low-grade malignancy, unless the patient clearly is not interested in future childbearing or preservation of ovarian function.

When faced with a clearly malignant bilateral tumor, one will usually treat the patient as if nonpregnant, with total hysterectomy, bilateral salpingo-oophorectomy, pelvic and abdominal washings, omentectomy, and pelvic and paraaortic node biopsies. Even with bilateral malignant disease, one could consider omitting hysterectomy if the uterus is not grossly involved, thus allowing preservation of the existing pregnancy. Although other tumors are known to metastasize only rarely to either the placenta or fetus, primary ovarian tumors almost never do so.

The role of progesterone in the postoperative period is unclear. Most recent publications suggest that it is of unproven value and therefore not recommended. There are no reports in the literature dealing with tocolytic therapy for premature labor associated with ovarian tumors complicating pregnancy.

Treatment Outcome

Conservative surgical treatment outcome for benign disease should be excellent. Even with malignant disease, overall 5-year survival should be 75% to 80%. In the largest series of malignant ovarian tumors, Woodruff reported a 5-year survival of 75%. Karlen, in a review of 27 dysgerminomas, reported a tendency toward local recurrence with conservative treatment, but an overall 5-year survival of 90%. Young, in a review of 36 sex cord stromal tumors, noted a 5-year survival of 100%, although he cautioned that granulosa cell tumors are prone to late recurrence.

Fetal mortality should also be minimal with early diagnosis and appropriate surgical intervention. Although Karlen reported a fetal mortality of 25%, two of the five deaths appeared to be iatrogenic, secondary to hysterotomy. Young reported 3 fetal deaths in 36 cases, two of which were iatrogenic. Mahone at Grady Memorial Hospital reported only 1 antenatal death in 136 surgical interventions with ovarian tumors complicating pregnancy.

Adjunctive Cytotoxic Chemotherapy

At no time is the treatment of cancer during pregnancy more complicated than when adjunctive therapy is indicated. Can such therapy be given safely during pregnancy? Although the teratogenic effect of single agent or combination chemotherapy is clear in the first trimester, it is now equally apparent that cytotoxic chemotherapy may be safely employed in the second and third trimesters. Specifically with antimetabolite therapy, both aminopterin and methotrexate have been reported to be associated with an increased rate of congenital abnormalities. The aminopterin syndrome, which consists of cranial dysostosis, hypertelorism, anomalies of the external ear, micrognathia, and cleft palate, has occurred in the fetuses of about 20% of

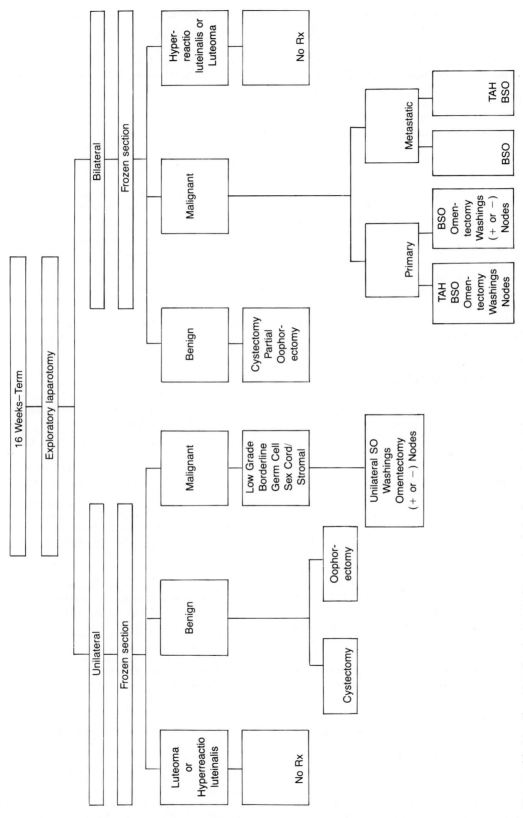

Figure 44–23. Algorithm for the surgical management of ovarian tumors occurring after 16 weeks gestation.

patients treated in the first trimester. However, no such anomalies have been noted with therapy in the second and third trimesters. The alkylating agent chlorambucil has been associated with congenital abnormalities, namely, renal aplasia, cleft palate, and skeletal anomalies. Again, no such relationship has been noted when therapy was initiated after the first trimester. Cisplatin has also been employed in a limited number of patients in the second and third trimesters without apparent problems.

There are, of course, other effects of cytotoxic chemotherapy, including hematopoietic depression and infection. For this reason, timing of chemotherapy in relationship to anticipated delivery must be assessed carefully so that delivery does not occur when the patient is pancytopenic.

There are now a number of individual case reports of apparent successful therapy of ovarian malignancies with adjunctive chemotherapy during pregnancy. These include tumors of epithelial origin, and at least four cases of endodermal sinus tumors treated during pregnancy, with the survival of three mothers (75%) and four infants (100%) (see Ch. 46).

CONCLUSIONS

The evaluation and management of ovarian tumors complicating pregnancy must be different from treatment of such tumors in the nonpregnant woman. Although many tumors are asymptomatic, torsion, rupture, and hemorrhage are more common during pregnancy and may adversely affect maternal and fetal outcome if not appropriately diagnosed.

However, the outlook for malignant ovarian tumors complicating pregnancy is much better than for those occurring in nonpregnant women. An increased incidence both of tumors of borderline malignancy and early stage epithelial tumors, as well as an increased incidence of germ cell tumors, allows more conservative therapy. Consequently, the pregnancy and future ovarian and reproductive function can be preserved. Furthermore, pregnancy does not preclude adjunctive cytotoxic chemotherapy, which may be initiated safely in the second and third trimesters.

In the final analysis, under optimum circumstances, achieving the therapeutic goal of both a healthy mother and a healthy child should be the rule rather than the exception when ovarian tumors complicate pregnancy.

Bibliography

Achari K, Prasad V. Ovarian tumours in pregnancy. J Obstet Gynaec Inda 1968;18:439.

Ahlvin RC, Bauer WC. Luteinized cysts in ovaries of infants born of diabetic mothers. AMA Am J Dis Child 1957;93:107.

Albukerk JN, Berlin M. Unilateral lutein cyst in pregnancy. NY State J Med 1976;76:259.

Amico JC. Pregnancy complicated by primary carcinoma of the ovary. Am J Obstet Gynecol 1957;74:920.

Andrews CJ, Nichoos AG. Bilateral ovarian dermoids complicating pregnancy treated by bilateral oophorectomy. Am J Obstet Gynecol 1940;39:453.

Ashkenazy M, Kessler I, Czernobilsky B, et al. Ovarian tumors in pregnancy. Int J Gynecol Obstet 1988;27:79.

Bailey H, Bragg HJ. Effects of irradiation on fetal development. Am J Obstet Gynecol 1923;5:461.

Ballard CJ. Ovarian tumors associated with pregnancy termination patients. Am J Obstet Gynecol 1984;149:384.

Barber HRK. Fetal and neonatal effects of cytotoxic agents. Obstet Gynecol 1981;58(suppl):41.

Barber HRK. Ovarian cancer complicating pregnancy. In: Ovarian carcinoma: etiology, diagnosis, and treatment. New York: Masson, 1982:167.

Barclay DL, Leverich EB, Kemmerly JR. Hyperreactio luteinalis: postpartum persistence. Am J Obstet Gynecol 1969;105:642.

Barkan A, Cassoria F, Loriaux DL, Marshall JC. Pregnancy in a patient with virilizing arrhenoblastoma. Am J Obstet Gynecol 1984;149:909.

Barnhill DR, Hoskins WJ, Heller PB, et al. The second-look surgical reassessment for epithelial ovarian carcinoma. Gynecol Oncol 1984;19:148.

Baxi Laxmi, Holub D, Hembree W. Bilateral luteomas of pregnancy in a patient with diabetes. Am J Obstet Gynecol 1988;159:455.

Beclere C. Accidents aigus de luteinisation ovarienne massive. Presse Med 1960;68:31.

Beischer NA, Buttery BW, Fortune DW, Macafee CAJ. Growth and malignancy of ovarian tumours in pregnancy. Aust NZ J Obstet Gynaecol 1971;11:208.

Bender S. Placental metastases in malignant disease complicated by pregnancy. Br Med J 1950;1:980.

Berek JS, Hacker NF, Lagasse LD, et al. Lower urinary tract resection as part of cytoreductive surgery for ovarian cancer. Gynecol Oncol 1982;13:87.

Berek JS, Hacker NF, Lagasse LD, et al. Survival of patients following secondary cytoreductive surgery in ovarian cancer. Obstet Gynecol 1983;61:189.

Berek JS, Hacker NF, Lagasse LD. Rectosigmoid colectomy and reanastomosis to facilitate resection of primary and recurrent gynecologic cancer. Obstet Gynecol 1984;64:715.

Bergman P. Bilateral multiple lutein cysts of the ovary complicating normal pregnancy. Obstet Gynecol 1983;21:28.

Betson, Jr. JR, Golden ML. Primary carcinoma of the ovary coexisting with pregnancy. Obstet Gynecol 1958;12:589.

Bianchi UA, Sartori E, Favall G, et al. New trends in treatment of ovarian dysgerminoma. Gynecol Oncol 1986;23:246.

Bloom M, Hendel D. Ovarian tumors in pregnancy. Harefuah 1975;88:63.

Bolli C. Premature delivery due to granulosa cell tumors of the ovary. Rupture of the tumor in the puerperium, hematoperitoneum, and death. Lav Inst Anat Unia, Perugia 1949;6:5. Abstracted by Narat JK. Int Abstr Surg 1950;90:492.

Bongiovanni AM, McFadden AJ. Steroids during pregnancy and possible fetal consequences. Fertil Steril 1960;11:191.

Booth RT. Ovarian tumors in pregnancy. Obstet Gynecol 1963;21:189.

Brenner DE, Shaff MI, Jones HW, et al. Abdominopelvic computed tomography: evaluation in patients undergoing second-look laparotomy for ovarian carcinoma. Obstet Gynecol 1985;65:715.

Brentnall CP. A case of arrhenoblastoma complicating pregnancy. J Obstet Gynaecol Br Commonw 1945;52:235.

Brill AB, Forgotson EH. Radiation and congenital malformations. Am J Obstet Gynecol 1964;90:1149.

Brock DR. Granulosa cell tumors of the ovary associated with pregnancy. Am J Obstet Gynecol 1962;83:109.

Brodsky JB, Cohen EN, Brown BW, et al. Surgery during pregnancy and fetal outcome. Am J Obstet Gynecol 1980;138:1165.

Brown EH. Identical twins with twisted benign cystic teratoma of the ovary. Am J Obstet Gynecol 1987;134:879.

Brune WH, Pulaski EJ, Shuey HE. Giant ovarian cyst. N Engl J Med 1957;257:876.

Buttery BW, Beischer NA, Fortune DW, Macafee CAJ. Ovarian tumors in pregnancy. Med J Aust 1973;1:345.

Cain JM, Saigo PE, Pierce VK, et al. A review of second-look laparotomy for ovarian cancer. Gynecol Oncol 1986;23:14.

Caspi E, Schreyer P, Bukovsky J. Ovarian lutein cysts in pregnancy. Obstet Gynecol 1973;42:388.

Caverly CE. Ovarian cyst complicating pregnancy. Am J Obstet Gynecol 1931;21:566.

Chai MS, Waltman R, Tricomi V. Abdominal pregnancy associated with ovarian carcinoma. Case report. NY State J Med Vol 1972;72:259.

Check JH, Rankin A, Teichman M. The risk of fetal anomalies as a result of progesterone therapy during pregnancy. Fertil Steril 1986; 45:575.

Chen SS, Bochner R. Assessment of morbidity and mortality in primary cytoreductive surgery for advanced ovarian carcinoma. Gynecol Oncol 1985;20:190.

Chez RZ. Proceedings of the symposium "Progesterone, progestins and fetal development." Fertil Steril 1978;30:16.

Chowdhury NNR. Ovarian tumors complicating pregnancy. Am J Obstet Gynecol 1962;83.

Christie RW. Lutein cysts of ovaries associated with erythroblastotic hydrops fetalis. Am J Clin Pathol 1961;36:518.

Clark DGC. The appropriate extent of bulk resection in advanced ovarian cancer. In: Ballon SC, ed. Gynecologic oncology: controversies in cancer treatment. Boston: GK Hall Medical Publishers, 1981:313.

Cohen CJ. Surgical considerations in ovarian cancer. Semin Oncol 1985;12(suppl 4):53.

Copeland LJ, Gershenson DM, Wharton JT, et al. Microscopic disease at second-look laparotomy in advanced ovarian cancer. Cancer 1985;55:472.

Copeland LJ, Wharton JT, Rutledge FN, et al. Role of "third-look" laparotomy in the guidance of ovarian cancer treatment. Gynecol Oncol 1983;15:145.

Croskloss HH, Nipe GM. Ovarian tumors in pregnancy. Obstet Gynecol 1953;2:513.

Cruikshank SH, McNeillis TM, Wise HD. Mucinous cystadenocarcinoma of the ovary associated with pregnancy. Case report and review. Mo Med 1982;79:695.

Csapo AL, Pulkkinen MO, Wiest WG. Effects of lutectomy progesterone replacement in early pregnant patients. Am J Obstet Gynecol 1973;115:759.

Cunningham JF, McGrath J. Dysgerminoma: A complete report of a case of bilateral dysgerminomata complicating pregnancy with malignant secondary deposits. J Obstet Gynecol Br Emp 1942; 49:36.

Daane TA, Lurie AO, Barton RK. Ovarian lutein cysts associated with an otherwise normal pregnancy. Obstet Gynecol 1969;34:655.

Darling MR, Hawkins DF. Sex homones in pregnancy. Clin Obstet Gynaecol 1981;8:2, 405.

Daro A, Carey CM, Zummo BP. Spontaneous rupture of a primary carcinoma of the ovary complicating pregnancy. Am J Obstet Gynecol 1949;57:1011.

Delant B, Fried A, van Nagell JR, et al. Ultrasonography in the diagnosis of tumors of the ovary. Surg Gynecol Obstet 1979;148:346.

Delclos L, Quinlan EJ. Malignant tumors of the ovary managed with postoperative megavoltage irradiation. Radiology 1969;93:659.

Delgado G, Oram DH, Petrilli ES. Stage III epithelial ovarian cancer: the role of maximal surgical reduction. Gynecol Oncol 1984;18:293.

Dembo AJ. Radiotherapeutic management of ovarian cancer. Semin Oncol 1984;11:238.

Diffle AW, O'Connor KA. Feminizing ovarian tumors and pregnancy. Am J Obstet Gynecol 1951;62:1071.

DiSaia PJ, Creasman WT. Clinical gynecologic oncology, 2nd ed. St. Louis: CV Mosby, 1984.

Dische FE, Ritichie JM. Luteoma of pregnancy. J Pathol 1970;100:77.

Donegan WI. Cancer and pregnancy. CA 1983;33:194-214.

Dougherty CM, Lund CJ. Solid ovarian tumors complicating pregnancy. Am J Obstet Gynecol 1950;60:261.

Downing GC. Bilateral multiple ovarian lutein cysts in pregnancy. Obstet Gynecol 1961;18:770.

Durie BHG, Biles HR. Successful treatment of acute leukemia during pregnancy. Arch Intern Med 1977;137:90.

Eckstein K, Marx GF. Aortocaval compression and uterine displacement. Anesthesiology 1974;40:92.

Editorial. Synthetic sex hormones and infant. Br Med J 1974;4:485.

Faulk HC, Bumkin IA. The management of ovarian tumors complicating pregnancy. Am J Obstet Gynecol 1947;54:82.

Fayad MM, Hussein MA, El-Ghar MA, et al. Unusual presentations of ovarian tumours during pregnancy. J Egypt Med Assoc 1978; 61:243.

Floyd WS. Theca-lutein cysts of the ovary in a multiple pregnancy. Obstet Gynecol 1960;15:743.

Forest MG, Orgiazzi J, Tranchant D, et al. Approach to the mechanism of androgen overproduction in a case of Krukenberg tumor responsible for virilization during pregnancy. J Clin Endocrinol Metab 1978;47:428.

Forney JP. Pregnancy following removal and chemotherapy of ovarian endodermal sinus tumors. Obstet Gynecol 1978;52:360.

Fuks Z, Rizel S, Anteby SO, et al. The multimodal approach to the treatment of stage III ovarian carcinoma. Int J Radiat Oncol Biol Phys 1982;8:903.

Galle PC, McCool JA, Elsner CW. Arrhenoblastoma during pregnancy. Obstet Gynecol 1978;51:359.

Garcia-Bunuel RG, Berek JS, Woodruff JD. Luteomas of Pregnancy. Obstet Gynecol 1975;45:407.

George PA, Fortner JG, Pack GT. Melanoma with pregnancy. Cancer 1960;13:854.

Gershenson DM, Copeland LJ, Wharton JT, et al. Prognosis of surgically determined complete responders in advanced ovarian cancer. Cancer 1985;55:1129.

Gillibrand PN. Granulosa-theca cell tumors of the ovary associated with pregnancy. Am J Obstet Gynecol 1966;94:1108.

Gillibrand CH, McCollough RH. Sudden and rapid virilization during pregnancy. Am J Obstet Gynecol 1972;113:XX.

Girouard DP, Barclay DL, Collins CG. Hypperreactio luteinalis: review of the literature and report of 2 cases. Obstet Gynecol 1964;23:513.

Gray LA. Ovarian cysts and myomas of uterus in pregnancy. South Med J 1961;54:632.

Greene GG, Smith AE, McClelland T. A malignant granulosa cell tumor associated with pregnancy. Am J Obstet Gynecol 1956; 60:686.

Griffiths CT. Surgical resection of tumor bulk in the primary treatment of ovarian carcinoma. Natl Cancer Inst Monogr 1975; 42:101.

Griffiths CT. Surgical treatment of ovarian carcinoma. Recent Adv Clin Oncol 1982;1:145.

Griffiths CT, Parker LM, Fuller AF Jr. Role of cytoreductive surgical treatment in the management of advanced ovarian cancer. Cancer Treat Rep 1979;63:235.

Grimes WH Jr, Bartholomew MD, Colvin ED, et al. Ovarian cyst complicating pregnancy. Am J Obstet Gynecol 1954;68:594.

Gustafson GW, Gardiner SH, Stout FE. Ovarian tumors complicating pregnancy. Am J Obstet Gynecol 1954;67:1210.

Haas JF. Pregnancy in association with a newly diagnosed cancer: a population based epidemiologic assessment. Int J Cancer 1984; 34:229.

Hacker NF, Berek JS, Lagasse LD, et al. Primary cytoreductive surgery for ovarian cancer. Obstet Gynecol 1983;61:413.

Halmo SD, Nisker JHA, Allen HH. Primary ovarian tumors in pregnancy. In: Allen HH, Nisker JA (eds): Cancer in pregnancy. Mt. Kisco, NY:Futura Publishing, 1986:269.

Heintz APM, Hacker NF, Berek JS, et al. Cytoreductive surgery in ovarian carcinoma: feasibility and morbidity. Obstet Gynecol 1986;67:783.

Hensleigh PA. Luteoma of pregnancy. Am J Obstet Gynecol 1975; 123:1053.

Hess LW, Peaceman A, O'Brien WF, et al. Adnexal mass occurring with itrauterine pregnancy: report of fifty-four patients requiring laparotomy for definitive mangement. Am J Obstet Gynecol 1988;158:1029.

Hess RL. Pregnancy and adnexal cysts. Two malignant cases. Am J Obst Gynec 1949;58:283.

Hill LM, Johnson CE, Lee RA. Ovarian surgery in pregnancy. Am J Obstet Gynecol 1974;122:565.

Ho AG, Beller U, Speyer JL, et al. A reassessment of the role of second-look laparotomy in advanced ovarian cancer. J Clin Oncol 1987;5:1316.

Hofmeister FJ, Miller JP. Bilateral dermoid cysts complicating pregnancy. Obstet Gynecol 1956;7:684.

Hogston P, Lifford RJ. Ultrasound study of ovarian cysts in pregnancy: prevalence and significance. Br J Obstet Gynaecol 1986;93:625.

Homesley HD. The appropriate extent of bulk resection in advanced ovarian cancer. In: Ballon SC, ed. Gynecologic oncology: controversies in cancer treatment. Boston: GK Hall Medical Publishers, 1981:321.

Horner EN. Placental metastases. Case report: maternal death from ovarian cancer. Obstet Gynecol 1960;15:566.

Horner H, Young JJ. Hyperreactio luteinalis. Obstet Gynecol 1955; 6:285.

Hurwitz A, Yagel S, Zion I, et al. The management of persistent clear pelvic cysts diagnosed by ultrasonography. Obstet Gynecol 1988;72:320.

Inoue M, Meda G, Yamaski M, et al. A follicullar adenoma arising from the thyroid tissue of a benign cystic teratoma during pregnancy: lithmicroscopical, ultrastructural and endocrinological studies. Acta Obstet Gynaecol Jpn 1980;32(7):953.

Ito M, Tohya T, Yoshimura T, et al. Theca lutein cysts with maternal viralization and elevated serum testosterone in pregnancy. Acta Obstet Gynecol Scand 1987;66:565.

Jolles CJ. Ovarian cancer: diagnosis, staging, grading, and epidemiology. Clin Obstet Gynecol 1985;28:L787.

Jolles CJ. Gynecologic cancer associated with pregnancy. Semin Oncol 1989;16(5):417.

Jones RT, Weinerman BH. MOPP (nitrogen mustard, vincristine, procarbazine and prednisone) given during pregnancy. Obstet Gynecl 1979;54:477.

Jones WJ, Huston JW. Bilateral theca lutein cysts associated with an apparently normal pregnancy. Am J Obstet Gynecol 1961; 81:1033.

Joshi SN, Limb DG. Ovarian cysts complicating pregnancy. J Obstet Gynecol 1985;5:143.

Joyeux H, Szawlowski AW, Saint-Aubert B, et al. Aggressive regional surgery for advanced ovarian carcinoma. Cancer 1986; 57:142.

Jubb ED. Primary ovarian carcinoma in pregnancy. Am J Obstet Gynecol 1963;85:345.

Karlen JR, Akbari A, Cook WA. Dysgerminoma associated with pregnancy. Obstet Gynecol 1979;53:330.

Katz Z, Lancet M, Skornik J, et al. Teratogenicity of progestogens given during the first trimester of pregnancy. Obstet Gynecol 1985; 65:775.

Kifle G. Case report. Ovarian cystic teratoma as a cause of obstructed labour. Ethiop Med J 1987;25:177.

Klein J. Pregnancy complicated by teratoma of the ovary. Obstet Gynecol 1954;3:93.

Koonings PP, Platt LD, Wallace R. Incidental adnexal neoplasms at cesarean section. Obstet Gynecol 1988;72:767.

Krepart GV, Lotocki RH. Chemotherapy during pregnancy. In Allen HH, Nisker JA (eds): Cancer in pregnancy. Mt. Kisco, NY: Futura Publishing, 1986:69.

Kristensen GB, Baunsgaard P, Hesseldahl H. Androblastoma associated with pregnancy in two sisters. Case report. Br J Obstet Gynaecol 1984;91:592.

Krueger JA, Davies RB, Felal C. Multiple drug chemotherapy in the management of acute lymphocytic leukemia during pregnancy. Obstet Gynecol 1976;48:324.

Lavery JP, Koontz WL, Layman L, et al. Sonographic evaluation of the adnexa during early pregnancy. Surg Gynecol Obstet 1986; 163:319.

Lee KH, Yeung KK. Rupture of a dermoid cyst during pregnancy. Aust NZ J Obstet Gynaecol 1971;11:58.

Lermer A, Villanueva C, Tannhauser S. Bilateral theca lutein cysts of the ovary in a case of erythroblastosis. Am J Obstet Gynecol 1958;75:203.

Levine W, Diamond B. Surgical procedures during pregnancy. Am J Obstet Gynecol 1961;81:1046.

Ling FW, Stovall TG, Welden SW. Intraperitoneal rupture of benign cystic teratoma after midtrimester pregnancy termination: a case report. J Reprod Med 1988;33:397.

Lowenthal RM, Funnell CF, Hope DM, et al. Normal infant after combination chemotherapy including teniposide for Burkitt's lymphoma in pregnancy. Med Pediatr Oncol 1982;10:165.

Luesley DH, Weaver JB, Rushton DI. A retrospective study of ovarian cysts in pregnancy. J Obstet Gynaecol 1984;4:161.

Lutz MH, Underwood PB, Rozier JC, et al. Genital malignancy in pregnancy. Am J Obstet Gynecol 1977;129:536.

Lynch MJG, Kyle PR, Raphael SS, Bruce-Lockhart P. Unusual ovarian changes (hyperthecosis) in pregnancy. Am J Obstet Gynecol 1959;77:335.

Matsuoka R, Kaneda S, Teshima H, et al. Delivery following removal and chemotherapy of ovarian endodermal sinus tumor. Asia-Oceania J Obstet Gynaecol 1987;13(2):137.

McCusker MC, Hoffman JS, Curry SL, et al. The role of second-look laparotomy in treatment of epithelial ovarian cancer. Gynecol Oncol 1987;28:83.

McGowan L. Cancer and pregnancy. Obstet Gynecol Surv 1964; 19:285.

Miller DS, Ballon SC, Teng NNH, et al. A critical reassessment of second-look laparotomy in epithelial ovarian carcinoma. Cancer 1986;57:530.

Milunsky A, Graef JW, Gaynor MF. Methotrexate-induced congenital malformation. J Pediatr 1968;72:790.

Moore GE. Debunking debulking. Surg Gynecol Obstet 1980;150:395.

Morton DL. Changing concepts of cancer surgery: surgery as immunotherapy. Am J Surg 1978;135:367.

Munnell EW. Primary ovarian cancer associated with pregnancy. Clin Obstet Gynecol 1949;6:983.

Munnell EW, Jacox HW, Taylor HC Jr. Treatment and prognosis in cancer of the ovary: with a review of a new series of 143 cases treated in the years 1944-1951. Am J Obstet Gynecol 1957; 74:1187.

Neijt JP, Aartsen EJ, Bouma J, et al. Cytoreductive surgery with or without preceding chemotherapy in ovarian cancer. Prog Clin Biol Res 1985;201:217.

Novak DJ, Lauchian SC, McCawley JC, Fairman C. Virilization during pregnancy. Am J Med 1970;49:281.

Novak ER, Lambrose CD, Woodruff JD. Ovarian tumors in pregnancy. Obstet Gynecol 1975;46:401.

Onarir R, Kazancigh A. Granulosa cell tumor of the ovary associated with pregnancy. Int J Gynaecol Obstet 1971;9:217.

Orr JW Jr, Shingleton HM. Cancer in pregnancy. Curr Probl Cancer 1983;8:1.

Ortega J. Multiple agent chemotherapy including bleomycin for non-Hodgkin's lymphoma during pregnancy. Cancer 1977; 40:2829.

Paoletti M, Pridjian G, Okagaki T, Talerman A. A stromal Leydig cell tumor of the ovary occurring in a pregnant 15-year girl. Cancer 1987;60:2806.

Pascal RR, Grecco LA. Mucinous cystadenoma of the ovary with stromal luteinization and hilar cell hyperplasia during pregnancy. Hum Pathol 1988;19:179.

Pemberton FA. Carcinoma of the ovary. Am J Obstet Gynecol 1940;40:751.

Podczaski ES, Stevebs CW Jr, Manetta A, et al. Use of second-look laparotomy in the management of patients with ovarian epithelial malignancies. Gynecol Oncol 1987;28:205.

Podratz KC, Malkasian GD Jr, Hilton JF, et al. Second-look laparotomy in ovarian cancer: evaluation of pathologic variables. Am J Obstet Gynecol 1985;152:230.

Podratz KC, Malkasian GD Jr, Wieand HS, et al. Recurrent disease after negative second-look laparotomy in stages III and IV ovarian carcinoma. Gynecol Oncol 1988;29:274.

Polansky S, DePapp EW, Ogden EB. Virilization associated with bilateral luteomas of pregnancy. Obstet Gynecol 1975;45:516.

Post WD, Steele HD, Gorwill RH. Mucinous cystadenoma and viralization during pregnancy. Can Med Assoc J 1978;118:948.

Pride GL, Pollock WJ, Norgard MJ. Metastatic Sertoli-Leydig cell tumor of the ovary during pregnancy treated by BV-CAP chemotherapy. Am J Obstet Gynecol 1982;143:231.

Quagliarello J, Blaustein A. Maternal virilization in pregnancy due to an unclassified sex-cord stromal neoplasm. Am J Obstet Gynecol 1985;152:570.

Quehl E. Pregnancy complicated by malignant ovarian mass. J Obstet Gynaecol Brit Emp 1950;57:253.

Resta P, Nardelli GB, Ambrosini A, et al. Limits of echography in the evaluation of ovarian tumors. Clin Exp Obstet Gynecol 1982; 9:165.

Rice BF, Barclay DL, Sternberg WH. Luteoma of pregnancy: steroidogenic and morphologic considerations. Am J Obstet Gynecol 1969;104:871.

Rice BF, Woody HB, Barclay DL, Sternberg WH. Virilizing luteoma of pregnancy: specific sterol and steroid hormone content. J Steroid Biochem 1971;2:183.

Rivera-Alsina ME, DeSanctis VM, Schmidt WA. Bilateral ovarian thecosis and virilization in pregnancy: a case report. J Reprod Med 1987;32:873.

Roberts JA. Management of gynecologic tumors during pregnancy. Clin Perinatol 1983;10:369.

Roberts RB, Shirley MA. Reducing the risk of acid aspiration during cesarean section. Anesth Analg 1979;53:859.

Rosenshein NB, Grumbine FC, Woodruff JD, Ettinger DS. Case report. Pregnancy following chemotherapy for an ovarian immature embryonal teratoma. Gynecol Oncol 1979;8:234.

Rouchy R, LeDall R. Le syndrome d'hyperluteinisation massive de l'ovaire par administration de gonadotrophines. Rev Fr Gynec Obstet 1959;54:135.

Rudolph AI, Barnett RV. Bilateral multiple lutein cysts of the ovary complicating a normal pregnancy. Obstet Gynecol 1956;8:293.

Saito J, Ueda G, Yamasaki M, et al. Pregnancy following removal and chemotherapy for a malignant mixed germ cell tumor of the ovary. Acta Obstet Gynecol Jpn 1985;37:1042.

Sarram M. Severe intra-abdominal hemorrhage from bilateral lutein cysts in Rh-isoimmunized pregnancy. Obstet Gynecol 1961; 17:366.

Schapira DV, Chudley AE: Successful pregnancy following continuous treatment with combination chemotherapy before conception and throughout pregnancy. Cancer 1984;54:800.

Schwatz PE. Combination chemotherapy in the management of ovarian germ cell malignancies. Obstet Gynecol 1984;64:564.

Shettles LB. Recurrent theca lutein cysts. Obstet Gynecol 1983;21:339.

Shuster E, Leake FM. Luteoma of pregnancy. Obstet Gynecol 1968; 32:637.

Sieber SM, Adamson RH. Toxicity of antineoplastic agents in man: chromosomal aberrations, antifertility effects, congenital malformations and carcinogenic potential. Adv Cancer Res 1975; 22:57.

Silva PD, Porto M, Moyer DL, Lobo RA. Clinical and ultrastructural findings of an androgenizing Krukenberg tumor in pregnancy. Obstet Gynecol 1988;71:432.

Simmer H, Hillemans HG. Arrhenoblastoma und Schwangerschatt. Arch Gynaekol 1962;196:541.

Sokal JE, Lessmann EM. Effects of cancer chemotherapeutic agents on the human fetus. JAMA 1960;172:151.

Spaun E, Toft B. Case report. Epithelial atypia in ovarian mucinous cystadenoma during the puerperium. Acta Obstet Gynecol Scand 1986;65:505.

Stehman FB, Calkins AR, Wass JL, et al. A comparison of findings at second-look laparotomy with preoperative computed tomography in patients with ovarian cancer. Gynecol Oncol 1988;29:37.

Steiner-Salz D, Yahalom J, Sanuelov A, et al: Non-Hodgkin's lymphoma associated with pregnancy. A report of six cases, with a review of the literature. Cancer 1985;56:2087.

Sternberg WH, Barclay DL. Luteoma of pregnancy. Am J Obstet Gynec 1966;95:165.

Struyk APHB, Treffers PE. Ovarian tumors in pregnancy. Acta Obstet Gynecol Scand 1984;63:421.

Sweet DL, Kinzie J. Consequences of radiotherapy and antineoplastic therapy for the fetus. J Reprod Med 1976;1976;17:241.

Taleman A. Theca cell tumors associated with pregnancy: report of a case. Obstet Gynecol 1968;31:45.

Taleman A, Scholte E, Daamen CBF, Grantama S. Granulosa-theca cell tumor associated with pregnancy. Int J Gynaecol Obstet 1975;13:113.

Tawan K, Baker TH. Ovarian tumors in pregnancy. Journal of the International College of Surgeons 41:60, 1964.

Thomas E, Mestman J, Henneman C, et al. Bilateral luteomas of pregnancy with virilization. Obstet Gynecol 1972;39:XXX.

Thornton JF, Wells M. Ovarian cysts in pregnancy: does ultrasound make traditional management inappropriate? Obstet Gynecol 1987;69:717.

Traut HF, Kuder A. Pelvic tumors complicating pregnancy. Internat Clin 1940;3:285.

Ulstein M, Rana G, Yangzom K, Gurung R. Case report. Prolapse of an ovarian tumor during labor. Acta Obstet Gynecol Scand 1987; 66:721.

Verhoeven ATM, Mastboom JL, Van Leusden HAIM, Van Der Velden WHM. Virilization in pregnancy coexisting with an (ovarian) mucinous cystadenoma: a case report and review of virilizing ovarian tumors in pregnancy. Obstet Gynecol Surv 1973;28:XXX.

Vicens E, Martinez-Mora J, Potau N, et al. Masculinization of a female fetus by Krukenberg tumor during pregnancy. J Pediatr Surg 1980;15(2):XXX.

Vrettos AS, Papaevangelow PI, Michalas SP. Int Surg 1969;52:41.

Wade M, Janovski NA, Bysshe SM. Pseudomucinous cystadenocarcinoma associated with pregnancy. Am J Obstet Gynecol, in press.

Warkany J. Aminopterin and methotrexate: folic acid deficiency. Teratology 1978;17:353.

Watson RM, Demick PE. Normal twin pregnancy and bilateral theca lutein cysts. Obstet Gynecol 1959;14:120.

Webb MJ, Snyder JA, Williams TJ, et al. Second-look laparotomy in ovarian cancer. Gynecol Oncol 1982;14:285.

Weinreb JC, Brown CE, Lowe TW, et al. Pelvic masses in pregnant patients: MR and US imaging. Radiology 1986;159:717.

White KC. Ovarian tumors in pregnancy: a private hospital ten year survey. Am J Obstet Gynecol 1973;116:544.

Wilson JG, Brent RI. Are female sex hormones teratogenic? Am J Obstet Gynecol 1981;141:567.

Wolfe E, Glasser M, Gordon GG, et al. Virilizing luteoma of pregnancy. Report of a case with measurements of testosterone and testosterone binding in plasma. Am J Med 1973;54:XXX.

Yemini M, Borenstein R, Dreazen E, et al. Prevention of premature labor by 17 a-hydroxprogesterone caproate. Am J Obstet Gynecol 1985;151:574.

Young RH, Dudley AG, Scully RE. Granulosa cell, Sertoli-Leydig cell, and unclassified sex cord stromal tumors associated with pregnancy: a clinicopathological analysis of thirty-six cases. Gynecol Oncol 1984;18:181.

Pelvic Exenteration

GEORGE W. MORLEY
MICHAEL P. HOPKINS

It has now been more than 40 years since Brunschwig introduced surgical evisceration as a significant step toward the control of cancers that involve the pelvic organs, especially those of gynecologic origin. In the beginning significant morbidity and mortality in the range of 50% to 70% was encountered, but over time these have decreased dramatically, thus providing an increased survival for those afflicted. The results of ultraradical pelvic surgery have been improved by a number of advances. Improved surgical techniques and training have decreased operative time and blood loss. Progress has been made through the control of infection, blood component therapy, improved anesthetic techniques, parenteral nutrition, and intensive care facilities provided by the entire medical team assigned to the service. It is well recognized that pelvic exenteration is indeed a formidable procedure, but now that there is a greater than 50% 5-year survival and a marked decrease in mortality, this procedure has gained wide acceptance in the minds of both patients and referring physicians (Table 45-1). Simply stated, pelvic exenteration has become the treatment of choice in certain types of advanced or recurrent tumors of the pelvis, and it has provided another chance at survival.

At the onset the attending physicians must focus on the careful selection of patients by a thorough and detailed preoperative assessment, so that control of disease can be contemplated. Strict guidelines regarding indications and contraindications must be met. The adaptation principle provided to those patients who survive is dramatic; however, most of those who succumb to their disease despite these somewhat heroic efforts do not die of uremia secondary to ureteral obstruction. Because the ureters have been diverted, in most instances, from the bed of neoplasm, these patients often die with intractable pain from intestinal obstruction or pulmonary, bone, or liver metastases.

Many modifications of the Brunschwig procedure have been instituted since its introduction in 1948. The most significant modification was introduced in 1950, when Bricker reported his classic ileal loop technique. This technique served as an isolated conduit for urinary diversion and was a substitute for the traditional "wet colostomies" or ureterosigmoidostomies of the past. Although the ileal loop is not the most common diversion used today, the principle of isolated urinary diversion persists and is always used if the bladder is removed. Although this has the disadvantage of requiring two stomas with appliances attached, it has markedly decreased the complications seen previously when the urinary and fecal systems were not separated. Other advances, such as the two-team approach, pelvic floor reconstruction, vaginal reconstruction, and the use of the stapling device for the gastrointestinal portion of the procedure, also have been significant and have improved the overall results and rehabilitation of these patients.

Total pelvic exenteration includes removal of the genital organs (vagina, uterus, tubes, and ovaries) as well as bladder and rectum. In current practice an isolated segment of bowel provides for a urinary reservoir, whether it be a segment of small or large bowel. Modifications of the total pelvic exenterative procedure include either an anterior or posterior exenteration or a total exenteration with a low rectal reanastomosis. In the anterior exenteration the bladder and genital organs are removed and the gastrointestinal system remains intact. In this situation a "bladder conduit" is developed from an isolated loop of bowel into which the ureters are anastomosed. The posterior exenteration, which involves the removal of the genital organs and rectum, allows for preservation of the urinary system. In selected patients who undergo a total pelvic exenteration a low rectal anastomosis can be accom-

TABLE 45–1
Surgical Mortality and 5-Year Survival Rates After Pelvic Exenteration

STUDY (YR)	NO. OF PATIENTS	SURGICAL MORTALITY (%)	5-YEAR SURVIVAL (%)
Parsons (1964)	112	14.2	21.4
Brunschwig (1965)	535	16.0	20.1
Rutledge and Burns (1965)	108	16.6	28.7
Kiselow et al. (1967)	207* (54)†	7.8 (1.8)†	35.0
Symmonds et al. (1968)	118	12.0	26.0
Ketcham et al. (1970)	162‡	7.4	38.0
Brunschwig et al. (1970)	225	8.0	19.3
Symmonds et al. (1975)	198 (102)§	8.1 (3.0)§	33.0
Rutledge et al. (1977)	296	13.3	48.3
Averette et al. (1984)	92	24.0	37.0
Morley et al. (1989)	100	2.0	61.0

* 1950–1965.
† 1960–1965.
‡ Includes 65 cases treated by primary exenteration.
§ 1963–1971.

plished if the lower 6 to 10 cm of rectum is preserved. A stapling device designed for this purpose is used to reconstruct the rectum low in the pelvis. This usually requires a protective colostomy, since the anastomosis usually is performed in an irradiated field. The colostomy can then be reversed at a later date, allowing the patient to eventually have only one ostomy.

INDICATIONS AND CONTRAINDICATIONS

The decision-making process begins when the physician first sees the patient and takes her history. The appropriate diagnostic steps are then taken. If the patient appears to be a candidate for a pelvic exenterative procedure, she is referred to a gynecologic oncologist who is experienced in the evaluation and treatment of these patients. The best results from pelvic exenterative surgery are achieved in patients who have a recurrent squamous cell carcinoma of the cervix or vagina. This therapy may be appropriate for advanced vulvar cancer when prior therapy has failed. Patients with carcinoma of the vulva initially may require a pelvic exenteration as primary treatment because of geographic spread of the disease to involve adjacent organs. Infrequently a recurrent adenocarcinoma of the cervix or endometrium or a sarcoma in the pelvis may respond satisfactorily to this therapy. Carcinoma of the ovary is almost an absolute contraindication, and this operation has a limited place in the treatment of this disease.

The primary indication for pelvic exenteration is re-

current or persistent squamous cell carcinoma of the cervix. This is not only because of its comparative frequency, but also because squamous cell lesions notably spread by continuity and contiguity along tissue planes, thus staying localized for longer periods of time before metastasizing to more remote areas. The adjacent tissues, such as the bladder, urethra, and bowel, however, often are involved, thus requiring their removal for control of the carcinoma. In addition, total pelvic exenteration is the most common type of exenteration performed in most reported series, since it is mandatory that we not only be well around the palpable disease, but also encompass that which is not palpable. Macroscopic disease can be seen or palpated; such is not the case in the presence of microscopic involvement. Therefore, the philosophy of instituting the widest margin of surgery at the earliest possible moment must prevail if we expect to eradicate the disease. The lesser forms of radical pelvic surgery, such as radical hysterectomy, not only have a high incidence of recurrence, but also an unacceptably high incidence of urinary or bowel fistulization, since these tissues have already been compromised by previous radiotherapy. Anterior or posterior exenteration in the irradiated pelvis also carries with it a high fistula rate.

Before the introduction of new diagnostic technologies, the clinical assessment of the patient along with intravenous pyelography were the only modalities available to assess whether or not the disease could be controlled by radical surgery. The often referred to "triad of trouble" used in this assessment consists of (1) an abnormal intravenous pyelogram demonstrating ureteral obstruction; (2) sciatic nerve distribution of pain, suggesting neural sheath involvement at or near the lateral pelvic wall; and (3) lower-extremity edema, implying venous or lymphatic compromise of the iliac vessels, again, in the lateral pelvis. In using this approach, if none or one of these features is present, the patient should be explored; if two or more of these abnormalities are present, the patient should not be explored. If there is doubt as to the resectability of the lesion, the patient should be explored, since the "court of last resort" is the operating room—not the conference room.

A number of significant diagnostic techniques can now help immeasurably in the assessment of these patients as to the feasibility of exploration with a reasonable chance of performing a curative procedure. A preoperative study that can demonstrate the presence of nonresectable disease helps to avoid exploratory laparotomy and its high preoperative false hope. The patient experiences a tremendous psychological dip when she is prepared preoperatively for the exenterative procedure only to be told postoperatively that she had an inoperable lesion and that the operation could not be performed.

The transvaginal Tru-Cut needle biopsy technique used to evaluate a large pelvic mass at the lateral pelvic wall can be helpful. This aids in the differentiation between the presence of recurrent neoplasm and post-irradiation fibrosis when thickened tissue is encountered throughout the pelvis. Fine needle aspiration of suspicious regional lymph nodes on lymphangiography can be helpful in the preoperative decision-making process. McDonald and coworkers reported an 85% accuracy rate in identifying positive nodes when this technique is used. Because the 5-year survival ranges from 0% to 14% if the pelvic lymph nodes are positive, pelvic exenteration is unrewarding, and these patients are not explored (Table 45-2). Finally, computed to-

mography (CT) can be most beneficial in assessing the presence or absence of lateral pelvic wall tissue invasion and unsuspected liver metastases as well as in a further evaluation of the retroperitoneal lymph nodal tissue.

The final diagnostic decision concerning the operability and curability of the existing disease must await the examination under anesthesia and the evaluation at the time of the exploratory laparotomy. Fixation in the pelvis caused by recurrent disease extending to the pelvic sidewall, penetration of the tumor into the peritoneal cavity with dissemination of cells intra-abdominally, and extrapelvic involvement of regional lymph nodes, omentum, liver, and other structures are all contraindications to the performance of pelvic exenteration. The physician performing the exploration must remember the philosophy of *primum non nocere*. These areas must be completely assessed through thorough palpation, visualization, and multiple frozen section biopsies, when indicated, before committing the patient to the more radical procedure with transection of the ureters or the bowel. The use of the avascular paravesical and pararectal spaces can be most helpful in evaluating the extent of the disease under these circumstances.

During a recent 20-year period 100 pelvic exenterations were performed on the gynecologic oncology service at the University of Michigan Medical Center. About 5000 patients were evaluated at the Gynecology Tumor Conference during this same period, with about 80% of them having a primary neoplasm and 20%, a recurrent lesion. Of the approximate 1000 patients with recurrent disease, 80% were not candidates for pelvic exenteration because of extensive local disease or regional or distant metastases, or because the primary nature of the disease was of an unacceptable type. Of the remaining 200 or so patients, 100 underwent some form of pelvic exenteration, indicating that essentially

TABLE 45–2
Effect of Pelvic Lymph Node Metastasis on Survival After Pelvic Exenteration

	NEGATIVE NODES		POSITIVE NODES	
STUDY (YR)	No. of Patients	5-Year Survival %	No. of Patients	5-Year Survival %
Barber and Jones (1971)	166	17.4	97	5.1
Creasman and Rutledge (1974)	29	27.0	14	14.0
Symmonds et al. (1975)	139	39.0	59	13.0
Averette et al. (1984)	92	—	6	0.0
Morley et al. (1989)	87	70.0	13	0.0

one out of every two patients who undergo exploratory laparotomy will actually have an exenteration performed. This ratio varies from institution to institution. Seventy percent of our patients were treated with total pelvic exenteration, and the stage of the primary lesion did not alter the chance of survival after the exenteration. In this series there was an approximate 60% 5-year survival rate.

Pelvic exenteration is not considered a treatment of choice for primary disease except in a limited number of patients with carcinoma of the vulva and in selected patients with nongynecologic lesions that involve the bladder or colon. In the past, stage IVa carcinoma of the cervix involving the bladder or rectum had been treated in this manner; however, the results were not considered superior to those achieved by full-course pelvic radiotherapy. Therefore, exenteration, as primary therapy for this lesion, has been universally abandoned, since Rutledge and Burns treated stage IV lesions with radiation therapy and showed an acceptable 28% survival. The same concept exists in regard to primary carcinoma of the vagina, for which radiation therapy is the preferred initial treatment.

From a prognostic point of view, even though it is not beneficial in the decision-making process, it is interesting to review the comparative survival rates as they relate to the disease-free interval. This is a measure of time from the initiation of primary therapy to the time the recurrence is detected. In all patients there is a direct relation of time from primary treatment to time of recurrence, since a greater than 90% 5-year survival has been reported at the University of Michigan when the disease-free interval is greater than 10 years, compared with less than 50% survival if this interval is 1 year or less.

Pelvic exenteration should only rarely be used to treat severely damaged irradiated tissue in the pelvis. Many patients with radiation necrosis experience intractable pain, copious foul-smelling discharge, and loss of excretory contents. These patients often can be relieved of their symptoms with specific diversionary therapy; but in the selected patient pelvic exenteration may be more appropriate.

Pelvic exenteration should not be used as a palliative procedure for cancer except under unusual circumstances. The morbidity, mortality, and complication rates are too high to justify this approach, especially when other palliative alternatives are available. The anticipated long-term hospitalization after this procedure precludes the patient from spending more of her remaining time at home with her friends and relatives. Parenthetically, it must be stated that even palliative urinary diversion in the presence of ureteral obstruction is contraindicated if the disease process cannot be controlled.

The presence of recurrent or persistent adenocarcinomatous lesions of the female pelvic organs is a relative contraindication to pelvic exenterative therapy. These lesions not only disseminate rapidly through the hematologic or lymphatic routes, but also often skip the more traditional, more orderly mode of spread. About 20% of patients with adenocarcinoma of the endocervix treated in this manner survive for 5 years; however, most, if not all, patients with recurrent adenocarcinoma of the endometrium die of disease before 5 years.

A sarcomatous carcinoma of the female pelvic organs, although rare, may respond satisfactorily to pelvic exenteration. In a small series from the University of Michigan reported by Reid and associates, five of nine patients, or 55%, were alive and well at 5 and 10 years. Patients with mixed müllerian tumors did not respond well to this form of therapy.

Age, religious orientation, obesity, and medical and psychological alterations must be considered as risk factors or as possible contraindications. Life expectancy beyond 70 years steadily diminishes; however, this factor alone is not an absolute deterrent to this procedure. A number of patients over age 70 have been treated successfully and without significant complications. Religious orientation is seldom a contraindication; however, the inevitability of blood replacement requires that the patient be willing to accept blood or blood products.

Although obesity is not an absolute contraindication to surgery, it should be noted that most patients with recurrent cancer of the cervix are not overweight; thus this deterrent is not frequently encountered. Obese patients should be operated on in an expedient manner, since time is of the essence. Massively obese patients present still further problems, and must be approached on an individual basis. Stomal construction can be extremely difficult in these patients, and this in itself may contraindicate the operation. Operating time is prolonged in these patients, and pulmonary function may be compromised in the postoperative period.

Medical complications and psychological incapacities are important factors in deciding whether or not to operate on some of these specific patients. All the surgical risks must be seriously weighed against the benefits of the procedure. In contemplating this operation there usually is no favorable alternative, and this must be shared with the patient and her relatives. Unlike other radical surgery, for which mortality figures usually are below 1 percent, the mortality for this ultraradical procedure can be 10% to 15%.

The medical and anesthetic assessments of the cardiopulmonary, renal, and nutritional status of the patient must be thorough, and consultants in these areas must be readily available during the intraoperative and postoperative periods. All patients, and especially high-risk patients, need this close surveillance. These patients also must be psychologically prepared for the significant alterations in their excretory systems and their sexual function. These patients often benefit immeasurably from being counseled by a sex therapist, psychologist, or psychiatrist, since these alterations are permanent and must be adapted to psychologically. This coverage may be more important than the surgery itself, and an informal exchange with a patient who has satisfactorily adjusted to the exigencies related to this procedure frequently is most beneficial and should not be overlooked.

Finally, the surgeon who undertakes pelvic exenterative therapy has an important responsibility, not only for the fact of life, but also for the quality of life remaining for the patient after the operation. The surgeon must be responsible for the long-term rehabilitation if she survives or for the long-term terminal care if she succumbs to her disease.

Preoperative Preparation

The initial planning for pelvic exenteration begins in the outpatient office setting. A full discussion is undertaken with the patient before planning definitive surgery. The complete operation, including the removal of the bladder, vagina, and rectum and the necessity of two ostomies, is fully outlined. Some patients elect to go no further and psychologically cannot adjust to the operation, thus refusing any further evaluation. However, this is rarely the case. For the patient who can psychologically accept the removal of all her pelvic viscera, a further discussion is undertaken, including her desire for reconstruction of the vagina. Whenever possible, the patient's husband or significant other should be included in these discussions.

Patients are admitted preoperatively about 2 days before surgery for a full bowel preparation as well as markings by the stomal therapist for stomal placement. Specimens for arterial blood gas analysis are routinely obtained; for patients with adequate screening blood gases, pulmonary function testing is not routinely performed. A central venous pressure line can be placed before surgery; however, there is the risk of pneumothorax when this is performed. It is possible to wait for the intraoperative decision as to whether or not to proceed with the exenteration before establishing this line. If the procedure is to be performed, the anesthesiologist can place the central line intraoperatively through an internal jugular approach. Preoperative hyperalimentation is not routinely used unless the patient has a nutritional deficit. The patient takes a shower with antiseptic soap the night before surgery. Antibiotics and heparin are given on call to the operating room, and the patient is shaved in the operating room.

The patient is prepared for surgery, using the "ski position" or spreader boards, which constitutes a modified ski position. This position allows simultaneous access to the abdominal and perineal areas not only for bimanual assessment of the lesion intraoperatively, but also for the "double team" approach to operating transabdominally and transvaginally at the same time, if desired.

Intraoperative Exploration

The abdomen is opened by either a true transverse incision or a vertical midline incision. The transverse incision allows greater pelvic exposure and facilitates the lateral pelvic wall assessment, but it can, on occasion, limit the upper abdominal evaluation. The transverse incision is an ideal incision for the obese patient and can allow for an easier performance of the pelvic portion of the operation (Fig. 45-1). On entry into the abdomen, careful palpation of all organs as well as the lymph node–bearing areas is undertaken. Particular attention is focused on the liver for evidence of metastatic disease. Cytologic washings and ascitic fluid, if present, are recovered and sent for immediate cytology analysis. Additional attention is paid to any areas that appeared abnormal on the preoperative diagnostic studies. If any look suspicious, biopsies are taken for frozen section analysis. Abnormal nodal findings are similarly analyzed with a specific focus on the pelvic, high common iliac, and paraaortic lymph nodes. The paraaortic lymph node dissection, if indicated, is performed by initially incising the peritoneum over the lower aorta (Fig. 45-2). The peritoneum is retracted with stay sutures of 3-0 silk, and the area is carefully evaluated by visual and tactile examination. The lymph node dissection is then begun at the bifurcation of the aorta, working cephalad. The fat pad is carefully freed from the aorta, using hemoclips to ligate the small perforating vessels. Using gentle upward traction and sharp dissection, the fat pad can be isolated to about the level of the inferior mesenteric artery. The uppermost pedicle is tied with 3-0 silk or ligated with an appropriate hemoclip. The fat pad over the inferior vena cava should then be isolated in a similar manner. Great care must be used over the inferior vena cava to avoid injury to this thin-walled great vessel. It is not necessary to completely mobilize the aorta or the inferior vena cava to obtain lymph nodes that are lateral to or behind the great vessels. Squamous cell carcinoma of the cervix spreads in a stepwise manner, and for this reason an extensive paraaortic node dissection to the level of the renal artery is not necessary. In the vast majority of instances, if the lower paraaortic tissue is negative for metastatic disease, none will be found at a higher level. The high common iliac and pelvic lymph nodes are similarly evaluated (Fig. 45-3).

When this evaluation is completed and there are no

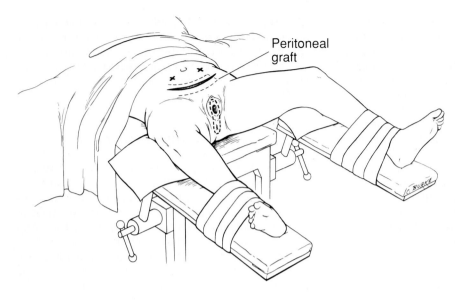

Peritoneal
graft

Figure 45–1. The patient is prepared on spreader boards and a true transverse incision is made to enter the abdomen. Sites for stoma placement have been marked with an X. The dotted peritoneal incision line demonstrates the incision for the peritoneal patch. The dotted perineal incision line demonstrates the approach for the perineal phase.

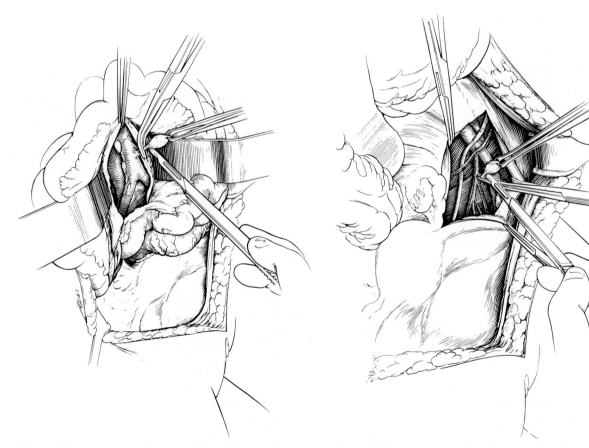

Figure 45–2. Paraaortic lymph node sampling is performed by first incising the peritoneum overlying the aorta. Small vessels are ligated with hemoclips as the fat pad is elevated from the aorta.

Figure 45–3. Suspicious lymph nodes have been sampled from the common iliac and pelvic region. The ureter and ovarian vessels are identified as they cross the pelvic brim near the bifurcation of the common iliac artery.

contraindications to proceeding, the round ligaments are divided and the pararectal and paravesical spaces are then opened. The paravesical space is exposed by bluntly sweeping the bladder away from the pubic symphysis in the space of Retzius and then continuing the dissection down until the fibrovascular pedicle is encountered at the 4 and 8 o'clock positions. These fibrovascular pedicles contain the uterine artery and vein, ureter, base of the broad ligament extending from the upper vagina and cervix to the pelvic sidewall, and the superior hemorrhoidal vessels. The evaluation of one pelvic sidewall at a time is appropriate. The peritoneum is then incised over the iliopsoas muscle. This exposes the pararectal space, which is developed by bluntly freeing the medial leaf of the broad ligament with the attached ureter from its areolar attachment to the pelvic sidewall structures. When the pararectal space is fully developed, the fibrovascular pedicle can then be palpated between the operator's thumb and index finger, allowing for evaluation of the pelvic sidewall. Any nodular or suspicious area in this region is biopsied and frozen section is obtained (Fig. 45-4). At this early stage in the operation the mass of neoplasm should be movable. Free spaces should be present between the neoplasm and the pelvic sidewalls in both the paravesical and pararectal spaces. If the mass is not freely movable, this suggests that a more extensive process is present, and it must be pursued.

To this point, the patient has not been committed to an exenteration, since neither the bowel nor the ureter has been transected. Once the decision to perform an exenteration is made, then the specific type—total, posterior, or anterior—must be decided. When deciding on the type of exenteration, the exact extent of the disease, with its questionable involvement of the bladder or bowel or both, must be estimated. Preoperative studies that have shown involvement of the bladder or rectum would mandate their removal. Again, the principle that microscopic disease cannot be seen by the naked eye or palpated with the examining fingers must be remembered. It is absolutely mandatory to encompass the entire neoplasm with the procedure selected. Absolute contraindications to pelvic exenteration include intra-abdominal metastases, malignant cells in the peritoneal washings or ascitic fluid, metastatic disease to regional lymph nodes, breakthrough of the tumor through the peritoneal surfaces, and presence of malignant disease at or beyond a surgically resected margin. When all frozen section reports have been returned, and if they are negative, then the decision is made to perform the exenteration.

Removal of Specimen

An en bloc dissection of the pelvic neoplasm is undertaken by successively clamping and dividing the fibrovascular pedicle of tissue along the pelvic sidewalls. Large pedicle clamps are used to doubly clamp the tissue and to control the bleeding from this area.

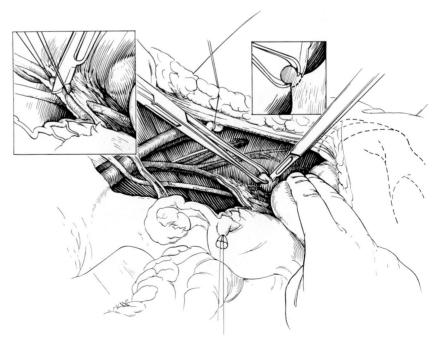

Figure 45-4. The pararectal and paravesical spaces have been developed. Thickened or suspicious areas of tumor extension to the sidewalls are sampled for frozen section analysis. The uterine artery is divided as it crosses over the ureter and tied with no. 2-0 silk.

The tissue is then divided and suture ligated using either nonabsorbable or absorbable suture or large hemostatic clamps. The uterine artery can be individually clamped, divided, and ligated lateral to the ureter, and the dissection is then continued along the pelvic sidewall. The ureters are freed from the medial leaf of the peritoneum with sharp dissection, doubly ligated with silk sutures, and transected. This ligation allows the proximal ureters to distend during the remainder of the case, facilitating the anastomosis into the urinary conduit. The sigmoid colon is then divided using the gastrointestinal anastomotic (GIA) stapler (Fig. 45-5). Before division, small epiploic vessels are divided and tied with 3-0 silk. A free space is then developed in the bowel mesentery just beneath the bowel wall. This allows introduction of either a bowel clamp or the GIA stapler. The peritoneum overlying the mesentery is incised, exposing the vessels to the sigmoid colon. These are then cross-clamped and tied with 3-0 silk. Transillumination of the vascular arcade leading to the bowel allows for preservation of the major blood supply. The major blood supply to the sigmoid colon and rectum consists of the sigmoidal and superior hemorrhoidal arteries arising from the inferior mesenteric artery, the middle hemorrhoidal arteries coming bilaterally from the hypogastric vessels, and the inferior hemorrhoidal vessels from the pudendal arteries. The sigmoidal artery usually is preserved, while the superior hemorrhoidal is ligated as a major blood supply to the specimen. When the sigmoid colon is divided and the superior hemorrhoidal vessel has been clamped

and divided, the sigmoid will then be freed from the sacrum and a free space becomes apparent. Using blunt dissection, the colon can be freed posteriorly to the levator ani muscles constituting the pelvic diaphragm. Care must be taken not to damage the sacral veins when bluntly dissecting the colon free in this area. If these sacral veins are torn, the resulting hemorrhage often is difficult to control. Clamping and ligating the vessels is uniformly unsuccessful, and tends only to aggravate the situation. The use of absorable hemostatic substances may be most beneficial in these instances. Sterile thumbtacks placed directly into the sacrum can be used to control this bleeding. This is an avascular plane, and the dissection should be directed toward the colon and away from the sacrum. Clamping of the middle hemorrhoidal vessels is then performed, further freeing the pelvic specimen. These pedicles entering from the 4 and 8 o'clock positions are suture ligated in a preferential manner (Fig. 45-6).

As the pelvic diaphragm is approached, the second team begins the perineal phase of the operation. The incision around the urethra, vagina, and rectum is outlined, and the dissection proceeds cephalad toward the pelvic diaphragm from below. These muscles are then transected circumferentially, and the specimen is removed in toto through the pelvis. The perineum is then reconstructed by approximating the levator muscles with absorbable sutures. A sufficient vault and adequate introitus are maintained, so that a split-thickness skin graft vaginoplasty can be performed at a later date. If a bilateral myocutaneous graft is to be used for vaginal

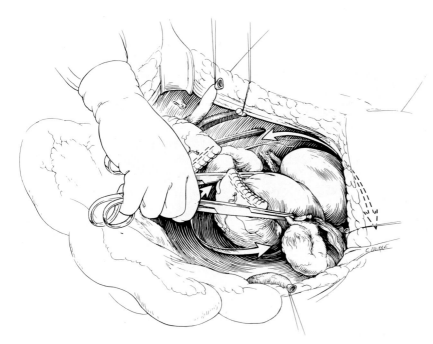

Figure 45–5. Ureters have been tied with silk and divided. The colon has been isolated and divided with the GIA stapler. The superior hemorrhoidal vessels have been clamped and divided previously. The colon is now swept free by gentle blunt dissection from the sacrum. Similarly, the bladder is swept free from the symphasis pubis (*arrows*).

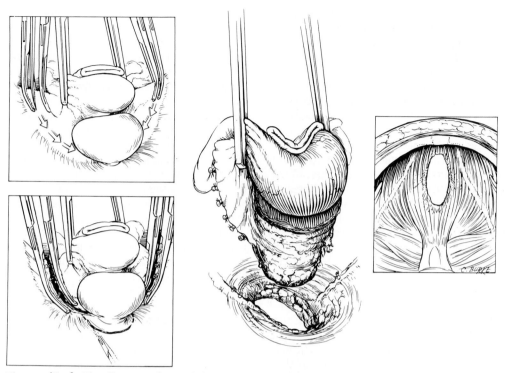

Figure 45–6. The fibrovascular pedicle is progressively clamped and divided down to the pelvic floor. The perineal dissection is simultaneously performed with isolation and removal of the pelvic mass in toto.

reconstruction, the second team at this point begins harvesting the grafts while the team operating in the abdomen begins construction of the urinary conduit.

Conduit Formation

We prefer the sigmoid conduit unless the colon has been heavily irradiated. About 15 cm of bowel is selected as the urinary conduit, and it is divided with the GIA stapler. The length of the conduit is important. If the conduit is too short, stomal retraction will occur with stenosis. An excessively long conduit can lead to stone formation or hyperchloremic metabolic complications. In the overweight to obese patient this requires measurement in the preoperative planning phase of the operation. In general, the conduit length should be 15 cm plus the difference between the anteroposterior diameter of the patient's abdomen in the lying and standing positions to account for the patient's panniculus. If the sigmoidal artery has been preserved, the blood supply to this portion of the bowel usually is excellent. The left colon can be mobilized by incising the peritoneal reflection to facilitate division of the colon. The ureters are further freed along their routes using blunt and sharp dissection. Care should be taken

to select an area of the ureter for anastomosis that is relatively free of radiation damage. When using the sigmoid conduit the left ureter does not need to be tunneled through the bowel mesentery, since it comes freely across the sacrum where the sigmoid colon has been removed. The ureters are then anastomosed to the bowel by first selecting an appropriate site for the anastomosis. This usually is 2 to 3 cm from the proximal end of the conduit. A No. 8 French Silastic pediatric feeding tube is placed through the lumen of the bowel and then directed through the selected anastomotic site. The site is opened sharply for about 1 cm. The stent is sutured to the colon with fine absorbable suture passing through the bowel wall and the feeding tube. Some surgeons choose not to use stents. The ureter is anchored with long-acting absorbable suture to the underside of the conduit, about 2 cm from the anastomosis. The ureter is then spatulated to a distance of about 4 to 5 mm. A mucosa-to-mucosa anastomosis of the ureter to the antimesenteric border of the isolated segment of bowel is then performed using fine (3 or 4-0) absorbable suture. Interrupted sutures or a continuous running suture may be used for the anastomosis. Absorbable sutures should be used to avoid stone formation at the ureterosigmoid anastomosis. The proximal end of the conduit is oversewn with a continuous absorbable suture in front of the staples, if they have been used to divide the colon. This will prevent stone formation from the metal staple line. When the conduit is completed it is sutured to the peritoneum for stability, and the distal end is brought through the preselected site on the abdominal wall (Fig. 45-7). A rosebud-type stoma is then fashioned to allow for ease of care and application of appliance. The new distal end of the sigmoid colon is then brought up through an appropriate site as a permanent diverting colostomy. It is not matured until the abdominal incision is closed, to avoid further contamination of the intra-abdominal contents. The colon is sutured to the lateral peritoneum with interrupted 3-0 silk to avoid an internal hernia.

Attention is then directed to the pelvic floor. The peritoneal graft has provided excellent results at the University of Michigan. A 10 × 12-cm peritoneal patch is isolated from the anterior parietal peritoneum, irrespective of the type of incision used to open the abdomen. It is placed in the lower portion of the pelvis to cover the pelvic aperture and sutured with nonabsorbable interrupted sutures to the ends of the transected levator ani muscles (Fig. 45-8). Care must be taken not to place the patch too high in the pelvis, as this will lead to a greater chance of postoperative bowel obstruction secondary to disruption of the *high* peritoneal patch. The omentum has been used as a pelvic floor with satisfactory results. If the omentum is chosen for this

purpose, it is isolated from the greater curvature of the stomach. When removing the omentum from the greater curvature hemostasis must be meticulous. The short gastric vessels should be isolated, clamped, and tied with silk ties. The operator must preserve the blood supply from the left gastroepiploic artery as the major blood supply to the omentum. This can then be laid into the pelvic basin as a carpet and sutured in place with absorbable interrupted sutures. Another option for the pelvic floor is to use absorbable synthetic mesh. When bilateral myocutaneous gracilis grafts are used, they fill the pelvic basin and can provide an adequate floor by themselves. Some type of pelvic floor should be used. Without such a floor there is the possibility of vaginal evisceration, which requires reoperation for replacement of the bowel contents. The perineal defect is then packed and, after closing the abdominal incision and maturing the colostomy, the patient is transferred to the surgical intensive care unit.

Stoma Construction

The sites for urinary and fecal stomas, which were selected preoperatively by the stomal therapist, are marked on the abdomen with sterile methylene blue before the patient is draped. The urinary conduit is brought through the abdominal wall in the right lower

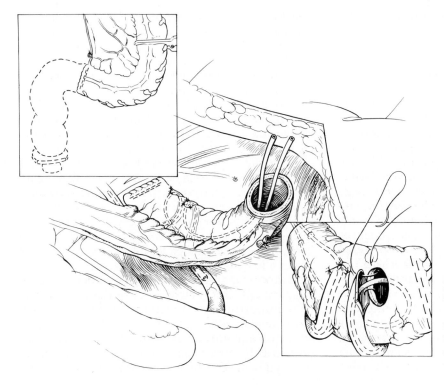

Figure 45–7. The sigmoid colon conduit is constructed from the distal 15 cm of the sigmoid colon. The ureters have been spatulated and sewn to the colon with absorbable suture. The conduit is anchored to the underlying tissue with interrupted sutures.

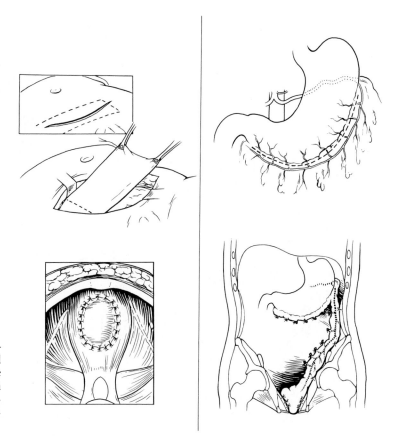

Figure 45–8. The pelvic floor is reconstructed using the free 10 × 12-cm peritoneal graft that was previously harvested from the anterior peritoneum of the abdominal wall. An omental pedicle isolated from the greater curvature of the stomach also is used as an alternative approach.

quadrant, midway between the umbilicus and the anterior superior iliac spines, where a flat skin surface is available for attachment of the prosthesis. If the transverse colon is used for the urinary conduit, it can be mobilized and located in the right lower quadrant. The sigmoid colostomy site is located in the left paraumbilical area. Ideally, the fecal stoma should be at a lower level than the urinary stoma. This helps to prevent contamination of the urinary stoma with fecal contents.

The abdominal wall aperture is prepared by removing an oval segment, 2 to 3 cm in diameter, through its entire thickness. Skin, subcutaneous fat, and external oblique fascia must all be excised, so that the flow of urine from the conduit will not be obstructed. The urinary conduit is brought through the abdominal wall, and the serosa of the bowel is sutured to the fascia of the abdominal wall. The bowel mucosa is everted, creating a raised, "rosebud" stoma, which projects at least 1 cm from the abdominal wall. The stoma is fashioned with interrupted sutures of No. 3-0 delayed absorbable suture, which passes initially through the skin edge, then anchors the serosa and musculature of the adjacent bowel wall, and finally passes through the free margin of the bowel mucosa. When the sutures are tied the mucosa is everted over the serosa of the bowel to

produce a raised stoma that directs the urine away from the skin surface, greatly reducing the chance for stricture of the ostium. Application of the urinary stoma bag also is facilitated by the raised opening.

The fecal stream is diverted through the left abdominal wall in a similar manner. The free end of the sigmoid colon is brought through the abdominal wall to the skin through the previously marked site. If anatomically feasible, the colostomy bud should be placed below the beltline, for cosmetic purposes (Fig. 45-9).

The serosa of both the urinary conduit and the sigmoid colostomy should be sutured to the lateral parietal peritoneum to avoid leaving peritoneal pockets for possible herniation and obstruction of the small bowel.

Anterior Exenteration

Anterior exenteration is a modification of total exenteration. After the ureters have been isolated and divided the rectum must be taken down from the posterior vagina. This is done by incising the peritoneum along the rectovaginal peritoneal reflection. When this free space has been entered the rectum can then be bluntly dissected from the posterior vagina. It is then

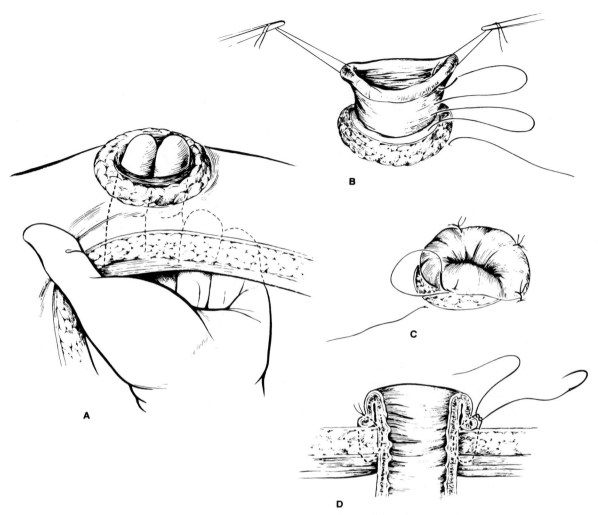

Figure 45–9. Technique for creating a bowel stoma that is elevated from the skin surface. This "rosebud" stoma is developed by (*A*) excising a wide segment of abdominal wall, (*B*) anchoring the skin margin with the adjacent wall of the exteriorized bowel, and (*C*) approximating the mucosal edge of the bowel to the skin. *D*, The cross-sectional view demonstrates how the bowel wall is anchored to the skin margin to prevent retraction.

freed laterally from the uterosacral ligament. The uterosacral ligaments are then clamped, divided, and suture ligated as close to the sacrum as possible. The procedure is then carried down the pelvic sidewalls, similar to a total exenteration. Great care is taken to ensure that the rectum is not damaged. When the perineal phase is performed the vagina is freed up from the rectum by dissecting the plane between the rectum and the vagina. The sigmoid conduit is not used when the colon remains intact. An ileal conduit is fashioned if the patient has not received previous radiation therapy. If the patient has received previous radiation, a transverse colon conduit or segment of ileum outside the irradiated field is the preferred segment of bowel to use.

Posterior Exenteration

Posterior exenteration is most often used for vulvar cancer, and is a modification of total exenteration. In this procedure the uterovesical peritoneum is incised and the bladder is freed from the cervix and vagina, using sharp and blunt dissection. After the uterine artery has been ligated the ureter must be dissected free down to the bladder. This is performed in a manner similar to that used for a radical hysterectomy. This allows for visualization of the ureter and frees it from the vagina, which is to be removed. The fibrovascular pedicle can then be divided in a manner similar to that used for a total exenteration. The ureter and bladder are preserved under direct visualization of these structures. The perineal phase separates the anterior vagina from the base of the bladder in the lowermost portion of the pelvis.

Total Exenteration with Rectal Reconstruction

In selected patients undergoing total pelvic exenteration the lower 6 to 10 cm of rectum may be preserved. This depends on the location of the recurrent tumor, and is an individual decision to be made at the time of surgery. When this lower portion of the rectum is preserved the sigmoid colon can be brought down and anastomosed to the rectal stump. This is greatly facilitated by use of the end-to-end anastomosis (EEA) device. A running suture of a 2-0 nylon starting on the outside is placed on the open end of the sigmoid colon and the rectal stump. The ends are not tied until the EEA has been introduced. The EEA is introduced through the rectum and positioned. The running purse-string sutures are then tied. When both ends of the bowel are aligned the device is slowly closed and fixed. When the device is removed a "doughnut" of tissue from each end of the bowel should be present in the removed EEA device. The anastomosis is then reinforced with interrupted 4-0 silk sutures. A diverting colostomy usually is necessary if the patient has been previously irradiated

or if there is undue tension on the anastomosis in the nonirradiated bowel.

POSTOPERATIVE CARE

Preoperative planning should include routine admission to the intensive care unit on completion of pelvic exenteration (Fig. 45-10). The continued oozing from the operative site with sequestration of fluids in the extravascular spaces causes significant fluid shifts; therefore, central venous pressure monitoring is essential. When left heart function and pulmonary function are adequate a Swan-Ganz catheter is not routinely used. When ureteral stents are used there is little chance for conduit obstruction from mucous plugging, and the urine output should accurately reflect kidney function. During the initial 24 hours volume usually is replaced with albumin and blood products, as indicated. Electrolytes and coagulation studies must be closely monitored as well as calcium and magnesium levels. By the 2nd to 4th day the patient usually is ready to leave the intensive care unit. Hyperalimentation, which is started on the 1st postoperative day, is continued until the patient begins to have spontaneous bowel function. Intravenous antibiotics are continued for about 5 days, and the perineal packing is changed daily after being left in place for about 3 days.

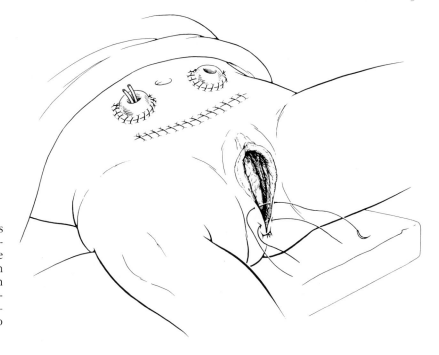

Figure 45–10. The perineal defect is partially closed with interrupted absorbable suture and a pack is placed in the lower pelvic cavity. A split-thickness skin graft vaginoplasty will be carried out in about 10 days. The operation is completed and the stomas have been matured. The patient is ready for transfer to the intensive care unit.

VAGINAL RECONSTRUCTION

Split-Thickness Skin Graft Vaginoplasty

After an adequate granulation bed has been established in the pelvic vault and the patient's bowel function has returned to normal, the decision is then made to perform the vaginoplasty. The patient usually is ready to have this performed 2 to 3 weeks after the primary surgery. The skin graft is taken from the buttocks or the posterior thigh as a split-thickness graft 10 to 15 cm in length at about .015 to .017 of an inch, using the air-powered dermatome. A vaginal stent is then fashioned around either an anoscope, a glass obturator, or a cotton ball mass and the visible end is sutured to the introitus (Fig. 45-11). The patient is then confined to bed with "logrolling" privileges for 3 days and ambulated on the 4th to 5th day. The vaginal packing is removed on the 6th to 7th day, after which an obturator of foam rubber is prepared as a vaginal obturator and the patient is instructed on its use. The patient leaves the obturator in continuously for 8 months to avoid stricture of the split-thickness skin graft. The condom covering the obturator is changed one to two times per week. In our experience this has provided an excellent result for vaginal reconstruction. Beemer and coworkers reported that 90% of patients achieved satisfactory coitus.

Myocutaneous Gracilis Graft

The myocutaneous gracilis graft can be used with favorable results. Construction at the time of initial exenteration surgery is required. This approach has the disadvantage of requiring additional operating time, additional incisions, and a full-thickness graft with a somewhat tenuous blood supply. If necrosis should occur, the patient may require multiple surgical debridements to remove the necrotic tissue. The advantages include immediate reconstruction of the vagina, and the tissue mass itself helps to fill the pelvic basin. An obturator is not required to maintain patency. When this approach is chosen it is best to have a second operating team "harvest" the grafts while the primary surgical team is completing the urinary diversion. The team approach minimizes the operating time required.

Myocutaneous grafts are constructed by obtaining bilateral full-thickness muscle, adipose, and skin grafts. The initial incision is made in an elliptical manner along an imaginary line extending from the superior aspect of the symphysis pubis to the medial condyle of the knee. The overlying skin to be taken should measure 10 to 15 cm in length by 6 to 8 cm in width. The underlying gracilis muscle is identified separate from the adductor group and is then divided, using the cautery at the lower portion of the graft. This is then mobilized toward the symphysis. Care must be taken not to damage the blood supply; if this occurs, the graft will be lost. The perforating vessels to the underside of the muscle are about 10 cm from the symphysis. When the muscle and overlying skin are fully mobilized they are brought through a tunnel into the introitus. This necessitates folding the gracilis on itself, which is done without undue tension. The posterior edge of the grafts from both sides are then sutured with absorbable interrupted sutures followed by a similar approximation of

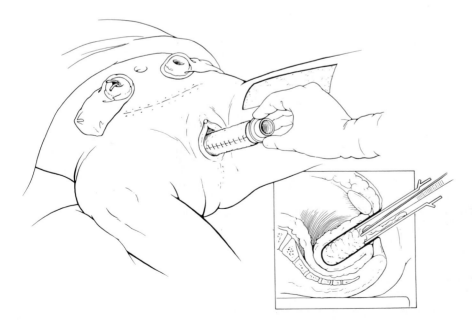

Figure 45–11. The split-thickness skin graft, .015-inch thick, has been harvested and fashioned around a hollow obturator. It is placed in the pelvic cavity and sutured to the introitus. The obturator is removed as the area is gently packed. The pack acts as an immobilizing stent.

the anterior edge. This graft is then introduced (or inserted) into the pelvic cavity and sutured to the sacral periosteum with long-acting absorbable or permanent 3-0 silk sutures. The opening to the new vaginal tube is then sutured to the introitus with interrupted absorbable sutures (Fig. 45-12).

COMPLICATIONS

As might be expected, the incidence of postoperative complications after pelvic exenteration is significant; complications occur in from 25% to 50% of patients undergoing this procedure. The most common major complications after this operation primarily involve the urinary or gastrointestinal tract. Other significant complications include bleeding, infection, thromboembolism, and, some time later, stoma problems such as stenosis, prolapse, and hernia.

The complications related to the urinary system are alleviated by the decreased use of posterior pelvic ex-

enteration. Its indication is limited, and the procedure frequently is complicated by a vesicovaginal fistula. Ureteral stricture and urinary leakage at the ureterointestinal anastomotic site still plague the pelvic surgeon; however, the occurrence of these problems has significantly decreased with improved techniques. Ureteral stricture, especially if ureteral obstruction coexists, must be surgically corrected without delay; most anastomotic leaks clear spontaneously without requiring repair. Transient anuria immediately after the exenteration secondary to localized edema has been reported, but this, too, clears spontaneously. Renal calculus formation does occur on occasion.

Intestinal obstruction occurs both as an early and a late complication and continues to be a serious problem. This has been alleviated by the institution of the peritoneal graft or the omental sac to cover the pelvic aperture at the level of the pelvic diaphragm. Most paralytic ileus problems seen in the postoperative period can be treated conservatively with traditional decompression. In our series two enteroperineal fistulae

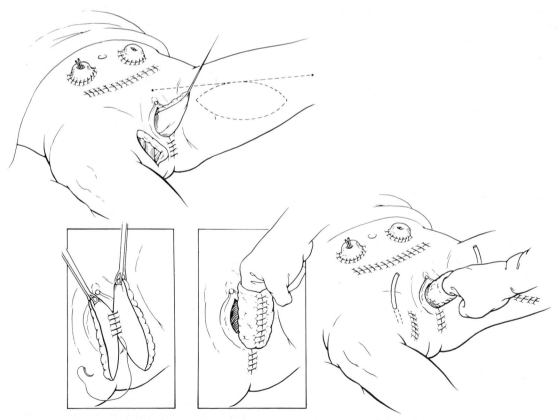

Figure 45–12. Full-thickness gracilis grafts are harvested from the medial thigh. These are about 10 × 6 cm in dimension. They are tunneled through the thigh and then sutured on themselves and positioned in the pelvic cavity. An alternative to a delayed split-thickness skin graft vaginoplasty is the myocutaneous vaginoplasty constructed at the time of the pelvic exenteration.

occurred, one as late as 7 years. They both occurred in patients who had not undergone reconstructive vaginal surgery. Bowel fistulae and intestinal obstructions occur in about 10% to 20% of patients reported. Five patients in our series experienced vaginal dehiscence, but all of these occurred during the time when only vaginal packing was used to fill the pelvis and before the use of the peritoneal graft.

Septicemia, which often is related to urinary tract infection, usually responds satisfactorily to intensive antibiotic therapy. Thromboembolic disease has become a less frequent postoperative complication now that low-dose heparin is used, even in the presence of a large denuded pelvic vault. We originally compartmentalized the inferior vena cava with staples, using the Codman stapler technique, but this prophylactic method has been replaced by prophylactic anticoagulant therapy. Wound and pelvic abscesses, although they occur infrequently, must be treated with multiagent antibiotic therapy and drainage. CT-guided drainage is preferred to laparotomy.

The operative mortality related to pelvic exenterative surgery has dramatically improved since the 1970s. Reports from the literature show a mortality rate ranging from 7% to 17% when other clinics are compared. In a 20-year report from the University of Michigan on 100 patients who had been operated on 5 or more years earlier there was a 2% mortality rate (see Table 45-1).

SUMMARY

During the past 40 years dramatic changes have taken place in our approach to patients whose lives have been significantly altered by the existence of persistent or recurrent gynecologic cancer that is localized to the pelvis and that has been resistant to prior therapeutic measures. By means of advances in preoperative diagnostic aids, improved surgical techniques, and sophisticated postoperative intensive care facilities, we can now offer these patients a second chance at survival through pelvic exenterative therapy. This approach does require the expertise of those who are well trained in ultraradical surgery and the constant vigilance of a tertiary care team during the immediate postoperative period. This coverage is necessary until the patient is physiologically and metabolically stabilized. Long-term supportive care, encouragement, and motivation after the surgery are equally important in bringing about a successful rehabilitation. No one person should be given the credit for these successes, since never before in the care of patients with gynecologic cancer has a team effort been so important.

In our opinion, the diagnosing physician plays a vital role in the initial detection of the problem; it must be remembered that there still may be something that can be done for this patient. Someone once said that to consider a situation hopeless often is to render it so. It therefore becomes incumbent on all of us to exhaust all possibilities in the evaluation and care of these patients until such time that the situation becomes irreversible. When the irreversibility is encountered, however, the physician must not persist in an effort to complete an ill-advised procedure.

The ultimate diagnostic step in evaluating a patient with persistent or recurrent pelvic cancer is the intraoperative evaluation using multiple frozen section biopsies at the time of the exploratory laparotomy. This final step in diagnosis as a determinant of the extent of disease should be taken when doubt as to resectability exists.

There is no place in our armamentarium for this operation as a palliative procedure. However, when it is performed with therapeutic control of the disease as the goal, the acceptance by the patient is excellent, and she usually adjusts to the exigencies in a mature manner. Certainly, the complications are major and the body alterations are significant, but if the patients are well informed about this reality of life and their chance for survival, they are understanding. No one wants this to occur unless it is the only chance one has for survival; therefore, we must continue our search for easier, better, and less radical ways of obtaining equal, or preferably better, survival in the future.

The selection of the appropriate patient on whom to perform this operation is of paramount importance if we are to improve our results in the future. A less than 5% operative mortality and a greater than 50% 5-year survival through proper selection should be our goal in caring for these patients.

Bibliography

Averette HE, Lichtinger M, Seven BU, et al. Pelvic exenteration: a 15-year experience in a general metropolitan hospital. Am J Obstet Gynecol 1984;150:179.

Barber HRK, Jones W. Lymphadenectomy in pelvic exenteration for recurrent cervix cancer. JAMA 1971;215:1945.

Beemer W, Hopkins MP, Morley GW. Vaginal reconstruction in gynecologic oncology. Obstet Gynecol 1988;72:911.

Bricker EM. Bladder substitution for pelvic evisceration. Surg Clin North Am 1950;30:1511.

Brunschwig A. Complete excision of the pelvic viscera for advanced carcinoma. Cancer 1948;1:177.

Brunschwig A. Surgical treatment of recurrent endometrial cancer. Obstet Gynecol 1961;18:272.

Brunschwig A. What are the indications and results of pelvic exenteration? JAMA 1965;194:274.

Brunschwig A. Some reflections on pelvic exenterations after twenty years experience. In: Sturgis SH, Taymor ML, eds. Progress in gynecology. Vol. 5. New York: Grune & Stratton, 1970:416.

Brunschwig A, Brockunier A Jr. Surgical treatment of squamous cell carcinoma of the vulva. Obstet Gynecol 1967;29:362.

Buchsbaum HJ, White AJ. Omental sling for management of pelvis floor following exenteration. Am J Obstet Gynecol 1973;117:407.

Cavanagh D, Shepherd JH. The place of pelvic exenteration in the primary management of advanced carcinoma of the vulva. Gynecol Oncol 1982;12:318.

Creasman WT, Rutledge F. Is positive pelvic lymphadenectomy a contraindication to radical surgery in recurrent cervical cancer? Gynecol Oncol 1974;2:482.

Green TH, Ulfelder H, Meigs JV. Epidermoid carcinoma of the vulva. analysis of 238 cases. Pt II. Therapy and end results. Am J Obstet Gynecol 1958;75:848.

Ketcham AS, Deckers PJ, Sugarbaker EV, et al. Pelvic exenteration for carcinoma of the uterine cervix: a fifteen year experience. Cancer 1970;26:513.

Kiselow M, Butcher HR Jr, Bricker EM. Results of the radical surgical treatment of advanced pelvic cancer: a 15-year survey. Ann Surg 1967;166:428.

McDonald TW, Morley GW, Choo YC, et al. Fine needle aspiration of para-aortic and pelvic lymph nodes showing lymphangiographic abnormalities. Obstet Gynecol 1983;61:383.

Morley GW. Cancer of the vulva: a review. Cancer 1981;48:597.

Morley GW, Hopkins MP, Lindenauer SM, Roberts JA. Pelvic exenteration: University of Michigan 100 patients at five years. Obstet Gynecol 1989;34:258.

Morley GW, Lindenauer SM. Peritoneal graft in total pelvic exenteration. Am J Obstet Gynecol 1971;110:696.

Parsons L. Pelvic exenteration. Clin Obstet Gynecol 1959;2:1151.

Parsons L, Friedell GH. Radical surgical treatment of cancer of cervix. Proc Natl Cancer Conf 1964;5:241.

Reid GC, Morley GW, Schmidt RW, Hopkins MP. The role of pelvic exenteration for sarcomatous malignancies. Obstet Gynecol 1989;74:80.

Rutledge FN, Burns BC Jr. Pelvic exenteration. Am J Obstet Gynecol 1965;91:691.

Rutledge FN, Smith JP, Wharton JT, O'Quinn AG. Pelvic exenteration: analysis of 296 patients. Am J Obstet Gynecol 1977;129:881.

Symmonds RE, Pratt JH, Webb MJ. Exenterative operations: experience with 198 patients. Am J Obstet Gynecol 1975;121:907.

Symmonds RE, Pratt JH, Welch JS. Exenterative operations. Am J Obstet Gynecol 1968;101:66.

Thornton WN, Flanagan WC. Pelvic exenteration in the treatment of advanced malignancy of the vulva. Am J Obstet Gynecol 1973;117:774.

Valle G, Ferraris G. Use of the omentum to contain the intestines in pelvic exenteration. Obstet Gynecol 1969;33:772.

Way S. The use of the "sac" technique in pelvic exenteration. Gynecol Oncol 1974;2:476.

Webb MJ, Symmonds RE. Management of the pelvic floor after pelvic exenteration. Obstet Gynecol 1977;50:166.

Chemotherapy of Gynecologic Malignancies

CARMEL J. COHEN

Patients with cancer have historically presented the discipline of gynecology a therapeutic challenge, which has been well met. From the time of Ephraim McDowell's brave performance on Christmas day of 1809 through the historic contributions of Victorian surgical adventurers and the latter-day contributions of pelvic surgeons in many countries, cancer of the female genital tract has been surgically diagnosed and excised, and the ravages of malignancies have been repaired and ameliorated. However, tumor cells too often defeat the most gifted and innovative surgeon.

Cancer cells, unlike normal host cells, fail to differentiate, retain embryonic characteristics, generate substances permitting direct invasion and distant metastasis, fail to respond to the normally programmed mortality schedule, and form masses that are ultimately physically diagnosable.

Although, it was tumor formation that historically attracted the surgeon's attention, his or her ability to excise the tumor was often only the initial therapeutic effort. Oncologists have long sought other means of dealing with malignancies. Stimulated by observations of the cytotoxic power of radium, radiation therapy was developed and enlisted in the treatment of gynecologic cancers.

The application of cytotoxic chemotherapy, a relatively new treatment, evolved from the observation during World War I that exposure to mustard gas in the trenches of Europe atrophied lymph nodes of the victims. However, it was not until 1942 that nitrogen mustard was administered therapeutically and found to produce objective tumor regréssion in patients with lymphoma (Gilman and Philips). An active search for cytotoxic activity in other compounds eventually identified antifolate drugs for the treatment of childhood leukemia (Farber and co-workers). Following this lead, Hertz demonstrated that the antifolate compound methotrexate inhibited the growth of fetal tissue by depriving it of the folic acid required for replication (Li and colleagues). When this discovery was clinically applied in 1956, complete remission was obtained for patients with choriocarcinoma, producing the first cure of a universally lethal cancer by cytotoxic chemoapy. Since that time, thousands of compounds have been screened for cytotoxic activity, hundreds have been developed as drugs for cancer treatment, and more than two dozen drugs have been employed, either singly or in combination, for the therapy of patients with gynecologic cancers. In April of 1990, there were 51 new medications in development for treating patients with cancers of the breast or gynecologic tract (American Cancer Society; Pharmaceutical Manufacturers Association). These ranged in their state of preparation from animal testing to completion of clinical trials and expectant approval by the Federal Drug Administration.

All approaches to cancer therapy are based on assumptions about cell replication and the ability to inhibit it. Fortunately, techniques are available for measuring cell division and cell viability, permitting the synthesis of hypotheses based on reproducible observations. Investigators are no longer limited to counting the number of metaphase figures in microscopic fields as an index of cell duplication. Instead, the tritiated thymidine labeling index measures the nuclear uptake of a radioactive DNA precursor during the synthetic phase (S) of the cell cycle, and this can be quantitatively assessed by autoradiography. Sophisticated techniques employing the uptake of monoclonal antibodies directed against specific proteins that are expressed during cell growth also offer a dynamic measurement of cell division without altering cell viability. Flow cytometry, although rapid and quantitative, often does not differentiate between cancer cells and other replicating cells in the aliquot of tissue being studied; however, with appropriate controls and careful management, the procedure can be used effectively to study cell biology. Fluorescence-activated cell sorting, by determining the proportion of dye-labeled DNA and RNA in a suspension of cells, can be programmed to reveal cell size, labeled targets within the cell, and other cell characteristics. These techniques can be focused on certain phases of the cell cycle, accurately assessing the percentage of cells in a given tumor population that are multiplying, resting, or not viable.

The most commonly employed measurement of cell kinetics is the DNA content of each cell, allowing identification of the S phase fraction (SPF). The replicating cells of the SPF are important because they are generally more susceptible to cytotoxic agents.

We can summarize the cell cycle by observing that a mammalian cell starts with a diploid (2n) number of chromosomes and diploid DNA content. In this beginning phase, it is classified as G_1 (Gap 1), and it spends a variable period in this presynthetic phase. However, some of these cells never replicate, never engage in DNA synthesis, and are classified by inference as G_0 (resting). After the G_1 cell becomes active in DNA synthesis, it is reclassified as an S phase cell. In mammalian cell populations, this synthetic phase lasts between 12 and 24 hours, during which the DNA content increases from 2n to 4n. The cell then enters the G_2 phase, during which some cells rest but most go on to the M phase, in which mitosis occurs. The M phase includes the formation of the mitotic plate, separation of chromosomes, and preparation for final division. This phase is the most consistent in mammals and usually occurs over 1 hour. Although there is great variation in the length of the mammalian cell cycle, range of means varies from 48 to 96 hours.

After division, the new cell can reprogram division and again become a G_1 candidate. If the cell remains active in replication, it is considered to be a part of the proliferative or *growth fraction* of the cell population, and when cells in this fraction continuously produce daughters that select G_1 status, they are called stem cells. Stem cells are basic progenitors for much of the subsequent population. Further differentiation of this progeny results in the specialized functions of tissues. However, cells can complete the M phase and enter a G_0 phase, during which they rest and comprise the *quiescent fraction* of the cell population. The final alternative for cells completing the M phase is death, and these cells comprise the *cell loss fraction*. The rate of tumor

expansion is directly proportional to the ratio of cells in these three categories, but there are paradoxical performances in different cell populations. For example, a tumor that seems not to be expanding may erroneously be inferred to be composed of slowly dividing cells. In fact, the tumor may have rapidly dividing cells that have a high cell loss fraction. Yet by virtue of the high number of mitoses, the statistical probability of a change in ploidy or random acquisition of drug resistance may be very high. An understanding of the biology of cell replication is mandatory for formulating rational therapy.

CELL KINETICS

Skipper established the "log-kill hypothesis," suggesting that a fixed dose of cytotoxic drug destroys a constant fraction of tumor cells, independent of the absolute number of cells present. Thus, the ultimate destruction of the cell population is a function of the dose of drug administered and frequency of treatment. Many studies support this notion. Figure 46-1 is from the work of Salmon and Apple, and it displays the natural history of a tumor transplanted into an animal host. The dotted line represents the cancer growth from time zero until the death of the host. The numbers in parentheses indicate the percentage of the cancer cells replicating at any given time. Most of the life of this cancer is spent in a subclinical mode, during which the total number of cancer cells is less than 10^9. One billion cells equate to a tumor mass of approximately a cubic centimeter or 1 g. There is a short period between clinical diagnosability and the onset of symptoms in the animal host, and there is also a relatively brief period between the onset of symptoms and the death of the host. If cytotoxic drugs are administered, as illustrated by the upper row of arrows, the growth of the tumor colony can be inhibited, but it will ultimately resume, requiring another cytotoxic effort. If these treatments are separated by long intervals, the tumor can repair sufficiently to overcome the cytotoxic effects, and the host dies, albeit at a later time than without therapy.

If, however, the cytotoxic treatments are pulsed rapidly, repeatedly killing a fixed percentage of surviving cells before the tumor can adequately replace them, then the absolute number of tumor cells is reduced to nearly zero or to a number that can be contained by the host surveillance and immunologic mechanisms.

The response to therapy depicted in the illustration assumes that the tumor is homogeneous, that all cells are replicating reasonably synchronously, and that all cells are sensitive to the cytotoxic therapy employed. In actuality, the model of Goldie and Coldman describes the development of cell resistance from spontaneous mutation every 10^5 to 10^6 divisions. The gene alterations produce differences in coatings for target proteins or other changes in regulation, resulting in cell heterogeneity. If administration of the cytotoxic drugs is not sufficiently frequent, then by spontaneous mutation cells resistant to the therapeutic agents will develop in sufficient numbers to render the treatment regimen ineffective. Norton and Simon suggested that the percentage of cells in replication may actually decrease as tumors respond to chemotherapy, making small terminal deposits of tumor more resistant to cytotoxic therapy than the larger, untreated cancers. This argues for dose intensification to achieve late consolidation and prevent small deposits of resistant clones from defeating the therapy.

Using cell cycle kinetics to reinspect Figure 46-1, it is clear that the most efficient cytotoxic technique for a clinically diagnosable cancer (10^9 cells) is surgical cytoreduction. This reduces the log number of cells, and it is likely to remove cells that have a low growth fraction and those that are indolent, necrotic, or hypoxic. Surgical intercession has been observed to synchronize the cell cycle of homogeneous cells. After maximal cytoreduction, a cytotoxic regimen of chemotherapy can be introduced before the cells replicate to their previous number, and by repeatedly and rapidly pulsing this cytotoxic treatment, the tumor can be controlled. To overcome the possibility of acquired resistance, the most intense dose tolerable should be administered as often as the patient can accept it. A combination of cytotoxic drugs, employed simultaneously or sequentially, can achieve a synergistic effect in cell kill, and if properly selected, can be administered without intolerable adverse effects.

There are two major classes of activity among drugs. Some drugs act only in a specific phase of the cell cycle and are only active when cells are not resting. Other drugs act at any phase of the cell cycle or when cells are resting. Because most cells, including cancer cells, spend most of the cell cycle in a resting or nonreplicating phase, the administration of a single cytotoxic agent that acts by only one mechanism is usually unsuccessful. The utility of combination chemotherapy was actually suggested and demonstrated by Greenspan when he found that treatment of breast cancer by a combination of thiotepa and methotrexate, drugs from different classes that acted through different mechanisms, produced a higher clinical response rate than single-drug treatment. Since that time, the notion of multidrug chemotherapy has been established in many tumor systems (DeVita and colleagues), and the concept of dose intensification has been confirmed empirically (Tormey) and by meta-analysis (Levin and Hryniuk).

CREATION OF DRUG REGIMENS

Cytotoxic drugs are selected from naturally occurring compounds, which have been observed to have cytotoxic properties, or they are designed prospectively by therapeutic pharmacologists. A new drug is screened for cytotoxic activity against panels of cancer cell cultures and then tested in animal studies. If it is active, it is introduced in a phase I trial for human application to determine optimal dose and schedule. If an effective schedule is identified, the drug is administered to a larger number of patients in a phase II trial to observe clinical response and adverse effects. After the drug is studied in these trials, it is compared in a phase III trial in randomized fashion with a drug already proven to be effective in the treatment of the disease being studied. If the new agent is equal to or superior to the standard therapeutic agent, it is accepted in phase IV trials for therapy. Each of the phases of investigation requires careful observation, close clinical monitoring, precision in biomathematical design and interpreta-

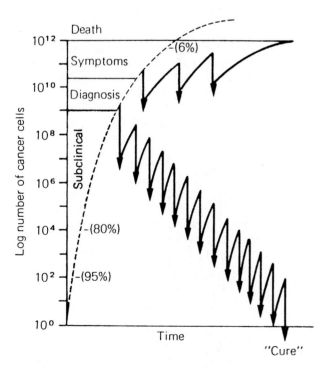

Figure 46–1. Tumor cell number compared with time of diagnosis, symptoms, treatment, and survival. (Salmon SE, Apple M. Cancer chemotherapy. In: Meyers FH, Jawetz E, Goldfien A, eds. Review of Medical Pharmacology. 5th ed. Los Altos, Calif.: Lange Medical Publications, 1976:470.)

tion, and usually a significant investment in funding and personnel.

DESIGNING A THERAPEUTIC PROGRAM

Cytotoxic chemotherapy should be administered only after the therapeutic goal has been well defined. The therapist and the patient should be unambiguous about whether they seek a cure of the disease, palliation of symptoms, short-term extension of life unrelated to quality, or investigation of drug behavior and host response. The distinction should further be drawn between adjunctive therapy (which is applied after initial therapy has reduced disease but has not been curative), and adjuvant therapy (which is applied after cure has possibly been achieved, but the rate of recurrence without further therapy is usually high). Only by establishing the direction of therapy can an informed consent be obtained and an appropriate regimen be selected.

Although curing a patient of her disease is the obvious goal of treatment, specific interval end points should be included in the construction of a therapeutic regimen. These options are disappearance of all disease (ie, complete clinical response) detectable by noninvasive surveillance, diminution but not disappearance of clinically detectable disease (ie, partial clinical response), biopsy-proven absence of disease (ie, complete pathologic response), and the progression-free interval measured from the time of completion of therapy.

If the patient is to be treated as part of an investigational effort, a formal, written protocol must be available. The protocol defines the background and rationale of the study, the rules of conduct for the study, the bounds of tolerance, reasons for stopping, forms for precise data collection, provision for detecting and repairing adverse effects, informed consent, and delineation of appropriate statistical tools, assuring a priori that the study can achieve its purpose because of good design and the probability of achieving adequate enrollment.

ANTINEOPLASTIC AGENTS

Antineoplastic agents can be assigned to one of seven categories based on similar mechanisms of action. These include the alkylating agents, antimetabolites, mitotic inhibitors, antineoplastic antibiotics, miscellaneous agents, hormones, and biologic response modifiers. Within each category are drugs that are commonly used in treating gynecologic cancers, and although they are frequently used in combination, it is

useful to understand their individual behaviors and distinguishing features. Typical treatment schedules with agents frequently employed in treatment of gynecologic cancers are listed in Table 46-1.

Alkylating Agents

Alkylating agents were the first chemotherapeutic drugs employed against human cancers. They were discovered to be inducers of lymphoid hypoplasia in those exposed to mustard gas during World War I. Because nitrogen mustard was an unstable vesicant, other analogues with chloroethylating function were derived. Melphalan (L-phenylalanine mustard), cyclophosphamide, and chlorambucil are three of the most commonly employed of these agents in treating gynecologic cancers. Dacarbazine (DTIC) has no chloroethylating components, but it still acts through the alkylating mechanism: it transfers its alkyl group to recipient cell constituents, whose functions are then impaired. This transfer occurs between the electrophilic functional groups provided by the alkylating agent to the nucleophilic targets, such as a guanine site in DNA. The alkylating agent may be polyfunctional and react with two or more targets, cross-linking different nucleic acid chains, two sites on the same chain, or an open site and other cellular complexes. Cross linkage prevents formation of a proper RNA template, disrupting cell replication. Despite the similarity in mechanism of action, acquired resistance to one alkylating agent need not result in resistance to all others, and substitution of alkylating agents may be appropriate therapy in some clinical circumstances.

Chlorambucil, a bifunctional chloroethyl alkylator was one of the earliest chemotherapeutic agents employed in the treatment of ovarian cancer. The medication was attractive because it could be administered orally and chronically. Although occasional nausea occurred, alopecia was uncommon, and the major adverse effect was myelosuppression.

Melphalan or L-phenylalanine mustard replaced chlorambucil in wide application and was accepted by patients because of the ease of administration and few discomforting adverse effects. The dose of 0.2 mg/kg/day for 5 days each month was widely employed in the treatment of ovarian cancer. Hematologic toxicity was the most important adverse effect until the reports of acute leukemia after treatment with alkylating agents, especially melphalan (Reimer and colleagues; Sotrel and co-workers). Although oral administration is usual, parenteral administration is possible. Doses of more than 150 mg m^2 of melphalan are being employed intravenously in autologous marrow transplant programs, and intraperitoneal application is being investigated.

Cyclophosphamide is a widely employed bifunctional alkylating agent, which can be administered orally or intravenously. It requires activation in the liver to achieve cytotoxicity, and it releases acrolein, an aldehyde that probably causes many of the drug's adverse effects. Gynecologic use of cyclophosphamide is primarily in combination with other drugs for the treatment of ovarian and endometrial cancers and some sarcomas. Because this drug has important immunosuppressive properties, it can be employed before transplantation of bone marrow. Like most alkylators, the drug is myelosuppressive, but its unique adverse effect is damage to the bladder epithelium with resultant hemorrhagic cystitis. Interstitial fibrosis of the lung has been reported, and it usually requires discontinuation of the drug.

Ifosfamide was synthesized as an analogue of cyclophosphamide. Initially, it seemed to have a wide spectrum of activity in many different tumor systems, but, its metabolite acrolein produced dose-limiting bladder urothelial toxic effects, and its use declined. Recently, certain thiol complexes, such as mesna, have been shown to protect the urothelium, allowing resumption of the clinical investigation of this drug. The Gynecologic Oncology Group tested doses of 1.2 to 1.5 g/m²/ day for 5 days with mesna administered every 4 hours for three doses after ifosfamide at a dose of 20% of the daily ifosfamide dose. Significant activity was demonstrated in patients who had previously failed treatment for ovarian or cervical cancer and especially for those treated unsuccessfully for mixed müllarian tumors of the uterus. Although renal, hematologic, and neurologic toxic effects were significant, the 30.7% response rate among patients with mixed müllarian tumors suggests a role for this agent in wider applications (Sutton and co-workers).

DTIC was originally designed as an antimetabolite, but its behavior is that of an alkylator. Like cyclophosphamide, this drug requires activation in the liver, and it then methylates nucleophilic sites. In gynecology, it has been employed in combination with other agents in the treatment of uterine sarcoma and is employed as a single agent in the treatment of malignant melanoma. Myelosuppression is not usually profound, but nausea and vomiting can be intense, and the drug is extremely irritating at injection sites, producing necrosis after extravasation.

Thiotepa is a trifunctional alkylating agent, which is administered parenterally, has few toxic effects other than hematologic, and has a wide spectrum of antitumor activity. It offers no particular advantage over the other alkylating agents, but provides a useful option in the treatment of ovarian cancer if other agents cannot be employed.

There are four nitrosoureas that are chemically related. They are different from the other alkylating agents in that they have a glucosamine structure and alkylate uniquely. They all cause severe nausea and vomiting, and their hematologic toxicity may be profound. These drugs, carmustine (BCNU), lomustine, semustine, and streptozotocin, are useful primarily in patients with brain metastases. Streptozotocin has activity against carcinoid, but it is toxic to pancreatic beta cells and can produce a variety of renal tubular disorders, resulting in chronic renal failure.

Antimetabolites

Although antimetabolites have different structures, the drugs include chemicals that are similar to normal metabolites. They act by substituting for the normal metabolite or by competing with a normal metabolite that acts at a regulatory site. Because most of these drugs are cycle-phase specific, they are rarely used as single agents.

Methotrexate, famous for producing the first chemotherapy cures for patients with trophoblastic disease, is an analogue of folic acid and binds to the site of the enzyme dihydrofolate reductase. This is a uniquely competitive inhibition process by which the reduction of dihydrofolate to tetrahydrofolate is inhibited, preventing the synthesis of purine precursors. Because the drug is S-phase specific, its success demands a high growth fraction in the tumor. Although the drug has a wide spectrum of activity, its primary use in gynecology is in the treatment of trophoblastic disease. It may be administered orally, parenterally, or intraperitoneally. Occasionally, intra-arterial and intrathecal administration have been useful. Because its transport is active, there is rationale for a high-dose regimen, and folinic acid or leucovorin can be administered after the methotrexate to "rescue" the normal cells after the cytotoxic action of methotrexate is accomplished. If the patient has renal insufficiency, the dose of methotrexate should be diminished, and rapid urine flow is essential to prevent deposition of methotrexate crystals in the renal tubules. Because the drug can be sequestered in body fluid pools, the dose should be diminished if there are effusions, or the effusions must be drained before treatment. If the drug leaks from its fluid storage sites and reenters the circulation over an extended period, it can cause serious adverse effects by creating a relative overdose. Myelosuppression is usual, but destruction of the mucous membranes in the orodigestive tract can be profound.

TABLE 46–1.

Chemotherapeutic Agents Frequently Employed in Treatment of Gynecologic Cancers

DRUG	ROUTE OF ADMINISTRATION	TYPICAL TREATMENT SCHEDULE	FREQUENT TOXICITIES
Alkylating agents			
Ifosfamide	IV	1.2–1.5 g/m² QD×5 MESNA 240 mg/m² q 4 h × 3 after ifosfamide dose	Hematologic, renal, urothelial, neurologic
Cyclophosphamide (Cytoxan)	PO, IV	PO: 100–250 mg/m² qd × 7–14 days IV: 400–1000 mg/m² q3 wk	Myelosuppression, hemorrhagic cystitis, bladder fibrosis, alopecia, hepatitis, amenorrhea, azoospermia
Hexamethylmelamine (Hexalen)	PO	150–250 mg/m² qd × 14 days q 4 wk	Myelosuppression, thrombocytopenia, neuropathy
Chlorambucil (Leukeran)	PO	0.03–0.10 mg/kg/day	Myelosuppression, hepatotoxicity, skin changes
Melphalan (Alkeran; L-PAM)	PO	0.2 mg/kg/day × 5 days q 4–6 wk	Myelosuppression, thrombocytopenia
Dacarbazine (DTIC)	IV	80–200 mg/m²/day × 5–10 days	Myelosuppression, nausea and vomiting, hepatotoxicity, asthenia
Thiotepa	IM, IV	8–10 mg/m² IV × 4 days; then q 1 wk	Myelosuppression, thrombocytopenia
Platinum analogues			
Cisplatinum (cisdiammino-dichloro) (Platinol)	IV	15–40 mg/m² IV qd × 5 q 3–4 wk 50–100 mg/m² IV q 3 wk 50–250 mg/m² IP q 3 wk	Nephrotoxicity, hearing loss, nausea and vomiting, thrombocytopenia, peripheral neuropathy, mineral loss
Carboplatin (Paraplatin)	IV	300 mg/m²/day × 1–3 days q 3–4 wk dose adjusted by Egorin or Calvert formulas	Thrombocytopenia, anemia, myelosuppression, nausea and vomiting, milder nephrotoxicity
Antitumor antibiotics			
Actinomycin D (dactinomycin; Cosmegen)	IV	0.3–0.5 mg/m² IV qd × 5	Nausea and vomiting, skin necrosis, mucosal ulceration, myelosuppression, hepatotoxicity, alopecia
Bleomycin (Blenoxane)	IV or IM	2.5 mg/m²/IV weekly 10 mg/m² IV or IM: q 1 wk For effusion: 60–120 units intracavitary	Fever, dermatologic reactions, alopecia, anaphylactic reactions, myelosuppression, bone pain, rigors, chills, pneumonitis, and pulmonary fibrosis at cumulative doses over 400 units
Mitomycin C (Mutamycin)	IV	10–20 mg/m² IV q 6–8 wk 2 mg/m² IV qd × 3 q 3 wk	Myelosuppression, nausea and vomiting, mucosal ulcerations, nephrotoxicity, hypercalcemia, tissue destruction at contact
Adriamycin	IV	50 mg/m² IV q 3 wk Daily escalating doses × 3 day q 3 wk	Alopecia, nausea and vomiting, mucositis, cardiotoxicity

Drug	Route	Dose	Side effects
Mitoxatrone	IV	12–14 mg/m² q 3 wk	Leukopenia, cardiac toxicity, discoloration of sclera, fingernails and urine, thrombocytopenia
Plant products			
Vincristine (Oncovin)	IV	1.4 mg/m²/weekly (maximum 2 mg)	Alopecia, neuropathy myelosuppression, muscular weakness, ileus areflexia
Vinblastine (Velban)	IV	3–4 mg/m² q 1–3 wk	Myelosuppression, alopecia, nausea and vomiting, neurotoxicity,
Etoposide (VP-16; VePesid)	IV / PO	50–150 mg/m²/day × 5 q 3 wk / 100–150 mg/m² qd × 5	Nausea and vomiting, alopecia, myelosuppression, hypotension, allergic reactions
Taxol	IV	175–250 mg/m² 24 hr IV infusion q 4 wk	Myelosuppression, nausea, vomiting mucositis, peripheral neuropathy, acute cardiopulmonary hypersensitivity reactions
Antimetabolites			
5-Fluorouracil (5-FU)	IV	500 mg/m²/day q 1 wk or qd × 5 1000 mg/m² continuous 24-h infusion q 3 wk	Stomatitis, diarrhea, myelosuppression, nausea and vomiting, anorexia
Methotrexate (MTX; amthopterin)	PO, IV	PO: 10–100 mg/m² qd × 1–5 d q 4 wk IM/IV:25–50 mg b.i.w. IM: 200 mg–10 g with leucovorin rescue q 3 wk Intrathecal: 12–15 mg q 1–3 wk	Mucosal ulceration, myelosuppression, hepatotoxicity
Hydroxyurea (Hydrea)	PO, IV	PO: 1–2 g/m²/day variously IV: 1–2 g/m²/day q d × 5	Myelosuppression, nausea and vomiting, anorexia
Cytarabine (ara-c)	IV, IP	100–200 mg/m²/day IV × 5 by continuous infusion IP 15–50 mg/m² q 2–4 d	Nausea, vomiting, bone marrow depression, megaloblastosis, leukopenia, thrombocytopenia
Hormones			
Medroxyprogesterone acetate (DepoProvera)	IM, PO	200–600 mg IM q 1–2 wk, 30–50 mg PO qd	Weight gain, personality change, edema
Megestrol acetate (Megace)	PO	20–40 mg PO q.i.d.	
Tamoxifen	PO	2–12 mg PO b.i.d.	Gastrointestinal discomfort, hot flashes, flare reaction, endomertial proliferation
Leuprolide	SC	1 mg q d × 12 wk	Acute menopausal symptoms

Hydroxyurea inhibits the enzymes necessary for production of DNA precursors. It also is S-phase specific and is taken orally. It is useful in some leukemias, and its activity in gynecologic tumors is mainly as a synchronizer of the cell cycle and as a radiosensitizer during radiation treatment of patients with squamous cell carcinoma of the cervix.

5-Fluorouracil (5-FU), a pyrimidine that inhibits thymidine synthetase, can incorporate into RNA and interfere with macromolecular synthesis. The drug is widely used in combination or alone for carcinoma of the colon, stomach, pancreas, and breast, and it has been employed intravenously and intraperitoneally against ovarian carcinoma, often in combination with other drugs. It has activity against endometrial cancer in combination with other agents and has been employed topically in treating preinvasive cancers of the lower genital tract. While myelosuppression is common, nausea, vomiting, and mucositis are often more profound. Photosensitivity and dermatologic adverse effects are common.

Floxuridine (FUDR) is the deoxyribose form of 5-FU and is immediately converted to 5-FU after intravenous administration. It should be employed only for regional use, such as arterial infusion. Its toxic effects are similar to those of 5-FU.

Cytarabine (cytosine arabinoside), an analogue of cytidine, is used primarily in the treatment of acute nonlymphocytic leukemia. Because there is a significant pharmacokinetic advantage when this drug is administered intraperitoneally, it has been used extensively in combination with other drugs in the treatment of ovarian cancer. Its adverse effects include those of the other antimetabolites, and mucositis may be severe and extensive.

Other antimetabolite preparations are not employed in the treatment of gynecologic cancers.

Mitotic Inhibitors

Mitotic inhibitors are plant-derived substances that include vincristine (Oncovin), vinblastine (Velban) produced from the periwinkle plant, and the epipodophyllotoxin derivatives etoposide VP-16 and teniposide VM-26, produced from the mandrake plant. All of these drugs are phase specific in their activity; require hepatic, biliary, and renal metabolism for elimination; and act by two different mechanisms. Vincristine and vinblastine act principally by arresting mitosis in metaphase, and they have acquired the description of "spindle-cell poisons." Etoposide and teniposide additionally react with topoisomerase II, an enzyme that is essential in DNA arrangement, replication, and transcription.

Vincristine is administered intravenously, is employed in combination with other drugs, and is active against sarcomas. Alopecia is prominent, but the major adverse effects are neurologic, including paresthesias, diminished neuromuscular activity, and paralytic ileus. Extravasation is painful and can produce necrosis. Because there is little myelosuppression, the drug is suitable for combination therapy.

Vinblastine is very similar in structure to vincristine, but its spectrum of activity is different. It is an extremely active drug against germ cell tumors and some sarcomas. Its neurotoxic effects are not as severe as those associated with vincristine. Myelosuppression is often the dose-limiting effect, and nausea, vomiting, and mucositis can be severe.

Etoposide is the most widely tested of the epipodophyllotoxin drugs. It can be administered intravenously or orally. It interrupts mitosis in metaphase, but the mechanism differs sufficiently from that of the vinca alkaloids to escape cross-resistance with those drugs. Myelosuppression is one of the dose-limiting toxicities, but occasional hypotension and bronchospasm are caused by rapid infusion. The oral route of administration produces a higher rate of gastrointestinal symptoms. The drug is useful in combination with several other agents employed against gynecologic cancers, and there is pharmacologic evidence of synergisms with platinum compounds.

Teniposide is similar to etoposide in its mechanism of action and structure and has shown activity against ovarian carcinoma. Its potential and range of adverse effects have not been completely defined.

Antitumor Antibiotics

There are six commercially available antitumor antibiotics, all of which are derived from *Streptomyces* species. All have been employed in the treatment of gynecologic cancers, but the most frequently used are doxorubicin (Adriamycin), dactinomycin (actinomycin D), and bleomycin (Blenoxane). The primary mechanism of action of this class of drugs is the disruption of DNA functions and RNA synthesis. The action of these agents depends on cell proliferation, but there is variability in the site of action and the specific phase during which cells are vulnerable. All of these agents have unsaturated ring structures, resulting in free radical production. Each agent has other functional moieties that can produce the effects of alkylating agents or act as inhibitors of enzyme activity.

Doxorubicin is the most widely used antitumor antibiotic. Its pharmacokinetics, structure, and mechanism of action have been widely studied, and it is believed to act by inhibiting DNA-directed RNA polymerase. The availability of free radicals creates havoc among the binding sites for the enzyme. The drug has a wide range of targets, including sarcomas, many adenocarcinomas, tumors of the urogenital ridge, and leukemias. It can be effective as a single agent in escalating doses, but it is more frequently employed in combination with other drugs. The drug is administered primarily intravenously but intracavitary instillation, although extremely caustic, has been effective in certain regimens. Excretion is hepatic and renal, and dose adjustments are essential if these functions are impaired.

Adverse effects of doxorubicin include marrow suppression, nausea and vomiting, orodigestive mucositis, reversible alopecia, and recall dermatitis in skin areas that have previously been radiated. Extravasation produces painful and serious necrosis and sluffing, occasionally requiring reconstructive surgery. The major adverse effect is cardiomyopathy, which can be fatal. Cardiomyopathy is dose related and can be avoided by careful measurement of ventricular efficiency before and during the course of doxorubicin therapy by any of several techniques. Discontinuation of the drug at the earliest sign of ventricular inefficiency usually prevents clinical manifestations and the cardiac reserve is sufficiently great to preserve performance status despite the measured impairment. Below a dose of 350 mg/m^2, the risk of congestive heart failure is insignificant. At a dose of 550 mg/m^2, the risk of clinical cardiotoxicity ranges from 1% to 10%. After the syndrome is discovered, supportive measures are useful, but there appears to be no reversibility of the myocardial damage. Careful monitoring and discontinuation of the drug, if there is an alternate regimen available, are the best strategies for avoiding this serious complication.

A spectrum of cardiac arrhythmias can develop idiosyncratically, sometimes progressing to pericarditis or myocarditis with secondary major cardiac dysfunction. This syndrome appears not to be dose related and occurs rarely.

Because of the potential for cardiotoxicity, doxorubicin has been replaced in many treatment programs by other drugs, including epirubicin, which was constructed to avoid cardiac toxicity. While the spectrum of activity of this agent is similar to that of doxorubicin, it has not provided an improved alternative.

Daunorubicin is an anthracycline derivative that is structurally similar to doxorubicin but has a narrower spectrum of activity, offers no advantage over doxorubicin, and is not employed in the treatment of gynecologic cancer.

Mitoxantrone, another of the drugs produced as alternatives to doxorubicin, comes from the same class of drugs, has diminished cardiac toxicity, but has a much narrower spectrum of activity. Because of its pharmacokinetic advantage when administered intraperitoneally, the drug appears to be ideal for treatment of ovarian cancers. Investigations are being conducted, but the efficacy and advantage of this compound have not yet been defined.

With careful monitoring, the anthracyclines can provide effective, safe, and versatile antitumor activity in the treatment of uterine sarcomas, germ cell tumors of the ovary, epithelial cancers of the ovary, and endometrial carcinoma.

Dactinomycin was the earliest antitumor antibiotic. It is cell-cycle specific, interferes with DNA and RNA synthesis, is administered intravenously, and requires hepatic and renal integrity for excretion. Myelosuppression is the dose-limiting adverse effect, but nausea, vomiting, mucositis, radiation recall, and alopecia can all be prominent. The drug is extremely useful in the treatment of trophoblastic disease and has wide activity against endodermal sinus tumor of the ovary, immature ovarian teratoma, mixed müllerian tumor of the ovary, ovarian germ cell tumors, and some uterine sarcomas.

Bleomycin is a mixture of peptide antibiotics from which a single clinical preparation, bleomycin A_2, has been prepared. The drug is cell-cycle specific and is very active in the M phase. It disrupts DNA synthesis, probably through the release of free radicals, not unlike the activity of doxorubicin. The drug can be administered by parenteral or intracavitary routes, and because of little cross-toxicity and some degree of marrow sparing, it is employed in combination therapy. Because the drug is inactivated by aminopeptidases, one of which, bleomycin hydrolase, is found universally except in lung and skin, the drug is quite toxic to both these sites. Pulmonary fibrosis, usually dose related and usually occurring at a cumulative dose of 450 mg, can be fatal. Although pretreatment testing of lung capacity and function are essential, they are poor predictors of pulmonary fibrosis, and careful monitoring during treatment is essential. Delayed adverse effects may occur after cessation of therapy. Other toxic effects, including febrile reactions, bone pain, hyperpigmentation of skin, inflammatory reaction of skin and joints, and stomatitis, can be dose limiting.

The commercially available antibiotic mitomycin C differs from the others by being metabolically converted to an alkylating agent and acting through mechanisms identical to traditional alkylators. The drug fell into disuse after investigators in the United States were unable to duplicate the findings of investigators in other countries and after reports of adverse effects, including universal nausea, vomiting, anorexia, and severe and often fatal marrow hypoplasia. However, recent inclusion of this drug in combination regimens for treatment of cervical cancer and its utility in intracavitary treatment in the peritoneal cavity and in the bladder have provoked its inclusion in the field of gynecologic oncology.

Miscellaneous Drugs

Many platinum compounds have been investigated as chemotherapeutic agents, and although some oncologists would classify them as alkylating agents, there are sufficiently prominent additional mechanisms of action to require a separate description of these compounds.

The earliest of this series and the first of the coordination complexes of heavy metals to demonstrate utility as a cytotoxic agent is cisplatin. The drug has ideal cytotoxic properties. It has activity against a wide variety of animal tumors and has produced clinical remission in drug-sensitive tumor systems. It is not species or strain specific in animal or culture systems, and it is active against tumors that are transplanted or induced by viral or chemical stimuli. The drug acts against primary and metastatic cancers, acts through more than one mechanism, and is synergistic with other drugs. Its use is modified by some of the platinum-related toxicities, which include universal nausea and vomiting, some myelosuppression, ototoxicity, peripheral neuropathy, and renal damage with mineral wasting.

Because of the wide use of cisplatin in different tumor systems, it has been extensively tested and found to be effective against virtually every gynecologic cancer, with the possible exception of trophoblastic disease. Despite its adverse effects, it is useful in combinations and is very effective as salvage therapy in patients who previously have not been treated with the drug. Experienced oncologists can prevent serious complications by hydrating patients before treatment, establishing osmotic diuresis, suppressing nausea and vomiting with vigorous antiemetic regimens, supplementing with calcium and magnesium substitutes, and carefully monitoring renal performance with creatinine determinations and neurologic performance by frequent interviews and examinations.

Other platinum analogues, such as carboplatin, are now commercially available. Carboplatin avoids the neuropathy and the nephropathy of cisplatin. In a trial comparing carboplatin plus cyclophosphamide and cisplatin plus cyclophosphamide for patients with previously untreated stage 3 or 4 epithelial ovarian carcinoma, the Southwest Oncology Group demonstrated no difference in response to the carboplatin or cisplatin regimens (Albert and associates). After patients with ovarian carcinoma are successfully treated with cisplatin and later fail, treatment with carboplatin produces a 30% response rate (Canetta and colleagues), suggesting that retreatment of initial platinum responders with any platinum compound is effective, or that carboplatin and cisplatin do not have identical spectra of activity. Other platinum analogues are being investigated, but none are as acceptable as carboplatin and cisplatin.

Taxol, a new plant derivative extracted from the bark of the western yew tree, acts by enhancing tubulin polymerization and microtubule stability in the cell cycle. This imposed stability resists the reorganization of microtubules essential to cell division in the mitotic process (Rowinsky and co-workers). Taxol was employed in a phase II study at the Johns Hopkins University and an objective response rate of 30% was observed in the treatment of patients who had previously failed other treatments for ovarian cancer. Six responses were observed among 25 patients whose disease progressed while receiving cisplatin (McGuire and colleagues). The Gynecologic Oncology Group independently confirmed these findings and established that the drug is not cross-resistant with platinum compounds (Thigpen and co-workers). Myelosuppression and a variety of hypersensitivity reactions, including cardiopulmonary and mucous membrane toxicities, require special monitoring, but this drug has great promise in the treatment of patients with ovarian cancer.

Hexamethylmelamine (Hexalen) is structured like most alkylating agents, but it acts as an antimetabolite. The drug is well tolerated orally and has demonstrated activity against ovarian cancer in patients who have received prior therapy with cisplatin (Manetta and co-workers) and in combination therapy for patients with previously untreated ovarian cancer (Bruckner and colleagues). Myelosuppression is usually easily managed, and dose-limiting toxicities are most frequently gastrointestinal and neurologic.

Hormones

Hormones have been employed longer than cytotoxic agents in the treatment of cancer. Hormone therapy is based on the assumption that target tissue requires hormones for growth and that depriving the target of its hormone or supplying exogenous competing hormone or antihormone inhibits the growth of target tissues. All indigenous steroid hormones are derived from cholesterol, and most tissues in the body synthesize this precursor.

There are five classes of steroid hormones, but only androgens, estogens, and progestins have therapeutic roles in gynecologic cancer. Hormones usually circulate bound to plasma proteins; but free hormone enters target cells more frequently by diffusion than by active transport and there binds to hormone-specific receptors. By saturating the receptor with a competing moiety or by producing an imbalance of a counteracting hormone, the normal cell metabolism can be changed.

The first hormonal modulation for patients with gynecologic cancer was oophorectomy for women with advanced or recurrent breast carcinoma. Paradoxically, estrogen was administered to other patients with breast cancer if they were menopausal or if oophorectomy failed.

The role of estrogen in the physiology of endometrial cancer had been suspected since Cullen's classic publication in 1900 describing the full spectrum of preinvasive and invasive endometrial neoplasia, but it remained for Gusberg in 1947 to suggest that patients with "unopposed" exposure to estrogen might develop the precursor to endometrial carcinoma and ultimately the disease itself. This rationalized the application by Kelly and Baker of progestational agents in the treatment of advanced or recurrent endometrial cancer; 30% of the patients so treated had objective responses. These investigators originally employed hydroxyprogesterone caproate (Delalutin) at a dose of 1 g 3 times weekly by intramuscular injection.

Although more powerful progestational agents have been synthesized requiring less volume of drug to be administered over longer intervals and although there are now oral compounds for daily use, the response rates among patients with advanced endometrial cancer have not changed.

The mechanism through which progestins control endometrial cancer is uncertain. It is possible that these agents have a direct cytotoxic effect on tumor cells. However, progestins also suppress gonadotropin, cortosol, and estridiol, but the significance of these observations for patients with endometrial cancer is unclear. It is known that progestins can decrease estrogen receptors, thereby diminishing the stimulation of cell replication and growth factors resulting from estrogen binding in the cell nucleus (Swain and Lippman).

In clinical application, progestin therapy is rarely successful against more than 30% of tumors; it may require 12 weeks to demonstrate clinical response and, in at least 67% of the patients, the progestins are never active. The best predictors of response seem to be differentiation of tumor, presence of progesterone receptors, and flow cytometric parameters suggesting diploidy. Unfortunately, these are the prognostic features of tumors that are unlikely to recur after conventional initial therapy, obviating their candidacy for progestin therapy.

The adverse effects of progestins are not life threatening, but weight gain, phlebothrombosis, fluid retention, and personality change can be unpleasant for many patients.

The most widely employed agents include medroxyprogesterone (Provera), which can be administered through long-acting injections of 200 to 600 mg weekly or orally at a dose of 30 to 200 mg daily. The other popular progestin is megestrol acetate (Megace), which is given in daily doses of 120 to 320 mg.

Although the steroids prednisone and dexamethazone are not generally employed in gynecologic oncology as cytotoxic agents, there are regimens in which they are administered as part of a supportive effort, usually to suppress noxious symptoms.

Androgens are not directly employed in treating gynecologic cancers. However, testosterone derivatives are highly active as anabolic compounds; they can stimulate appetite and support erythropoiesis.

Tamoxifen is generally regarded as an antiestrogen and, based on data derived from its effect on breast cancer cell lines, it was administered to patients with breast cancer. Its success in cancer control has led to increasing use. Tamoxifen's mechanism of action is complex: it binds to the estrogen receptor, and the complex binds with DNA, but there is then a paradoxical failure to express estrogen-related genes (Swain and Lippman). It changes the receptor itself, increases overall cell cycle transit time, is directly cytotoxic for some cells, and stimulates the production of certain growth inhibitors. Attempts were made to employ tamoxifen against endometrial cancer cell lines based on the observation that this agent elaborated progesterone receptors in endometrial tumors (Carlson and colleagues). No advantage was observed in employing tamoxifen over a conventional progestin.

Moreover, after breast cancers and endometrial cancers were transplanted into different sites of the same nude mouse and tamoxifen was administered, the breast cancer was inhibited and the endometrial cancer proliferated (Gottardis and co-workers).

A recent clinical trial employing adjuvant tamoxifen in patients after surgery for breast cancer randomized the patients between tamoxifen at a dose of 20 mg twice daily and no adjuvant endocrine therapy. The patients receiving tamoxifen experienced a significant increase in endometrial cancer (Forhander and colleagues). There are now more than 50 patients described in the literature who received tamoxifen at a dose of 10 mg twice daily who developed endometrial neoplasia (Dottino and co-workers). There are currently prospective screening studies in progress to detect the frequency of endometrial cancer in patients receiving tamoxifen therapy, but for the present, gynecologists should be alert to the increased risk and should immediately sample the endometrium of any patient who experiences bleeding while taking tamoxifen.

Because more than 50% of patients with ovarian epithelial carcinoma have estrogen or progesterone receptors or both (Schwartz and colleagues), there have been several attempts at secondary salvage with hormones in patients who failed primary cytotoxic chemotherapy regimens. Sikic and colleagues treated 47 patients, most of whom had previously failed platinum-containing combination therapy, with orally administered megesterol at 800 mg daily for 1 month, followed by 400 mg daily until progression. There were one complete and three partial responses. Geisler observed a 45% response rate in 22 similar patients, but this group had been treated primarily with non-platinum-containing regimens initially. The Gynecologic Oncology Group treated 105 patients who failed cisplatin regimens with tamoxifen daily and observed ten complete responses and seven partial responses. There was no correlation between clinical response and the presence, absence or level of estrogen or progesterone receptors (Beecham and associates).

Luteinizing hormone-releasing hormone (LHRH) agonists and antagonists have been synthesized in very large numbers. Gonadotropin-releasing hormone (GnRH) controls release of follicle-stimulating hormone and luteinizing hormone from the pituitary gland, and its release is modulated by a sensitive network of neurotransmitters and histamines, with negative feedback stimulated by estrogen and testosterone. GnRH agonists, represented by leuprolide, are commercially available, and although designated by the FDA specifically for treatment of prostatic cancer, there are several independent investigations testing the efficacy of these agents alone and in combination with progestins in patients with ovarian and endometrial cancers.

Biologic Response Modifiers

Biologic response modifiers are agents that modulate the immune system. Some are endogenously produced, others have been cloned from their naturally occurring forms and duplicated in volume commercially, and others are known immunostimulants, often exogenous bacteria or other biologic preparations. The naturally occurring biologic response modifiers include the cytokines: interleukins 1 through 6, interferons alpha, beta, and gamma, lymphotoxins, several colony-stimulating factors, tumor necrosis factor, and a series of growth factors, including transforming growth factor beta (TGF-β). Many of these agents have direct antitumor activity. Others, such as the interferons, are potent stimulators of natural cytotoxicity cells and modulate tumor destruction through other effectors. Most agents have multiple functions, and some behave paradoxically against the immunologic interest of the patient in resisting tumor cells.

A detailed discussion of the biotherapy of gynecologic cancer is beyond the scope of this chapter, and the reader is referred to the excellent review by Berek, Martinez-Maza, and Montz. However, salient observations about the use of biologic response modifiers in the field of gynecologic oncology can be summarized.

The initial enthusiasm for employing nonspecific immunostimulants, such as *Corynebacterium parvum (C. parvum)* or bacille Calmette-Guérin (BCG), with cytotoxic chemotherapy in the treatment of ovarian cancer has faded. Early pilot studies suggesting that the addition of these immunostimulants improved response rates and progression-free intervals, compared with the same chemotherapeutic regimen without the immunostimulants, have not been supported by groupwide studies in the Gynecologic Oncology Group (Alberts and colleagues; Gynecologic Oncology Group).

Berek described 19 patients with recurrent ovarian carcinoma who were treated by the administration of intraperitoneal *C. parvum,* with objective responses in six patients. In 14 patients with persistent ovarian cancer, intraperitoneal treatment with recombinant alpha interferon was administered weekly for 16 weeks. Of the 11 patients who had surgical reexploration, four had complete pathologic responses and one had a partial response. Most of the responders were patients who had lesions smaller than 5 mm before treatment. This signal experience suggests that the intraperitoneal application of biologic response modifiers in patients with minimal residual ovarian cancer can be effective.

Recombinant technology has made available a panoply of antibodies that can be labeled with radioisotopes for diagnosis, conjugated with radionuclides for delivery of focused radiation to antigenic tumor sites, or conjugated with toxins, such as ricin, abrin, diphtheria, or pseudomonas. Monoclonal antibodies can also be conjugated to many of the drugs routinely employed in intraperitoneal therapy, including methotrexate, vinblastine, and melphalan.

Colony-stimulating factors are glycoprotein hormones that regulate the production and function of blood cells. Molecular cloning has been accomplished for granulocytemacrophage colony-stimulating factor, granulocyte colony-stimulating factor, macrophage colony-stimulating factor, and interleukin-3. These factors are now produced in sufficient quantity to allow clinical trials, including the use of these agents in cytotoxic chemotherapy regimens. The colony-stimulating factors can restore hematopoiesis, stimulate functionally primed effector cells, which can contribute to host defense, and recruit cells into the S phase, allowing them to be better targets for cytotoxicity (Gabrilove).

Biologic therapy is new, but because of an intense focus on its vast potential, its use in gynecologic oncology should soon be better defined.

DRUG RESISTANCE

Cellular resistance to chemotherapeutic agents is related to several independent factors: altered transmembrane transport of the agent, altered cellular distribution, increased inactivation at the cell interface, random alterations in the target cell, increased target inactivating enzymes, and a diminished growth fraction, resulting in restricted cell exposure to cell-cycle-specific chemotherapeutic agents. Accommodations can be made for each of these variables by changing clinical approaches if the obstacles are identified. For example, aggressive surgical cytoreduction before chemotherapy and early dose intensification can avoid many of these obstacles. If the patient is unable to tolerate dose intensification, then autologous bone marrow transplantation is an alternative. The procedure has demonstrated utility in the treatment of patients with leukemias and breast cancer and is now being introduced for patients with refractory ovarian cancer. By this technique, the patient's marrow is extracted and stored, very high doses of chemotherapeutic agents are administered, the marrow is reinfused, and the patient is kept in isolation during the period of immunosuppression and potential susceptibility to infection. Although early experience with this modality resulted in significant mortality rates, the safety of this procedure has improved in experienced centers.

There is intriguing information derived from observations in Chinese hamster ovarian cells suggesting a genetic cause for multidrug resistance (MDR) (Riordan and Ling). Some cells concentrated cytotoxic agents less than others, and this rejection included many structurally unrelated agents. This functional resistance was associated with the expression of a membrane glycoprotein, and after cloning, it was established that the P-glycoprotein gene was amplified in drug-resistant cells (Riordan and colleagues). The structure of human P-glycoprotein has been described by Chen and has been identified in a variety of normal human tissues. The gene has also been overexpressed in samples of drug-resistant ovarian cancers (Bell and co-workers). Because membrane-active agents have reversed experimental drug resistance (Tsuro and associates), trials employing agents such as calcium channel blockers may overcome drug resistance after the product of the gene is detected.

Ozols described cross-resistance between alkylating agents, cisplatin, and irradiation associated with elevations in cellular glutathione levels. He further demonstrated in the mouse model that lowering glutathione levels by the administration of buthionine sulfoximine potentiated the cytotoxic effects of melphalan and improved survival by 72% in animals with ovarian cancer.

Chemosensitivity Testing

Because the penalty of retrospectively discovered drug resistance is so high for patients treated with chemotherapeutic agents, there has long been a search for techniques of predicting drug sensitivity in vitro before selection for clinical application. The work of Hamburger and Salmon and colleagues in describing the human tumor stem cell assay for anticancer drugs led to widespread application of this system in clinical investigation. Modification of the original assay were introduced to make the system more efficient and improve its accuracy (Ajani and associates). Other techniques, such as serial biopsy or tumors during therapy and placement of tumor samples in the subrenal capsule of small animals for in vitro assessment of drug effect, have also been widely employed. Some systems have achieved a range of 95% success in predicting resistance and 75% success in predicting sensitivity. With new technology and improved efficiency, there is commercial availability of this testing capacity outside of research centers. However, in gynecologic oncology, these systems are seldom employed outside of investigational programs, and it may be that the practical identification of the multidrug resistance gene, flow cytometric data predicting prognosis, and measurement of biologic parameters on very small samples will prove even more successful in predicting chemosensitivity.

ROUTES OF ADMINISTRATION AND ACCESS

The most convenient route for administering chemotherapy is usually oral. Drugs like hexamethylmelamine can only be given orally, but others, including cyclophosphamide, alkeran, methotrexate, and VP-16, can be administered orally or parenterally. Despite ease of administration, if a patient is anorexic, has impaired gastrointestinal absorption, or is otherwise unreliable, oral administration is ineffective, and potentially dangerous, and a parenteral route should be selected.

Intravenous administration is the route most widely employed, and techniques of temporary access are often preferable. To spare the veins, weekly blood tests should be performed though finger punctures, and even patients who are managed on an ambulatory basis and attend laboratories in their neighborhoods are able to be served in this way. Because of dilution factors, venous run-off, first-pass hepatic conversion of circulating drug, and protein binding in the vascular system, there is a maximum serum concentration achievable for each drug in a given patient when intravenous administration is performed. This maximum is not related to host tolerance, the adverse effects on marrow and other target tissues, or the cytotoxic effect of the drug.

If there are cancers in the peritoneal cavity, direct intraperitoneal installation is attractive. By selecting this route, the pharmacologic advantage of drug at the interface with tumor exceeds by a significant factor the concentration resulting from intravenous administration. Further, if the drug concentration in the peritoneal cavity fluid after intraperitoneal installation is compared with the plasma concentration after intravenous administration, there is an even larger advantage of the intraperitoneal route for cisplatin, cytosine arabisondide, 5-FU, and other drugs. Unfortunately, the pharmacologic advantage alone does not confer response advantage in all patients. Our experience and that of McVie and colleagues and Ozols suggest that approximately 30% of patients with small residual disease (< 5 mm) have tumor eradicated by intraperitoneal administration of cytotoxic agents.

After large doses of cytotoxic agents are introduced into the peritoneal cavity, the serum levels of those agents identified subsequently are often much higher than the levels attainable by intravenous administration. These high levels result from the multiple exit sites from the peritoneal compartment into the systemic circulation. If this reabsorbed drug is still cytotoxic after its transport into the systemic circulation, an added advantage accrues to the patient from intraperitoneal treatment. Unfortunately, cytotoxicity has not been established for each of the reabsorbed chemotherapeutic agents.

After peripheral venous access has been exhausted, the placement of semipermanent catheters in a large central neck vein might be necessary. The Broviac catheter with single or multiple entry ports is placed under the skin on the anterior chest wall and tunnelled into one of the veins of the jugular or subclavian systems. The entry ports remain external and require aseptic care and periodic injection of heparin to maintain patency. Other catheter systems, such as the Portacath, can be internalized with the reservoir placed subcutaneously and superficial to the ribs in a location convenient for percutaneous needle access. The disadvantage of the latter system is inability to use the port routinely for blood sampling.

Access to the peritoneal cavity can be by single percutaneous puncture with placement of a drum catheter for individual use, by placement of the traditional Tenckhoff dialysis type catheter with exterior ports, or by an internalized system, such as the Portacath, which is placed similarly to the system for the subcutaneously located reservoir in the venous access system.

Exterior catheters generally have a higher rate of infection in the venous and peritoneal systems. This complication can be overcome by administration of antimicrobials directly into the catheters, but it is a frequent cause of removal. Other complications in peritoneal access include hemorrhage, bowel obstruction, clot formation, and erosion of the catheter into a viscus.

Our experience with single-use catheters placed "blindly" produced only one adverse effect in 105 punctures. This was the placement of the catheter into the bladder in a patient who had not emptied her bladder and who had a short hypogastrium; the catheter was removed without sequelae. Further refinements of the single-use catheter have been made by insertion under sonographic control at the bedside. The advantage is the elimination of adverse effects caused by an indwelling foreign body during the six or eight cycles of intraperitoneal treatment.

The location of a tumor mass or the metabolic pathways for a cytotoxic agent may be better served by arterial administration of the drug. For patients with gynecologic cancer, this usually means catheterization of the iliac or hypogastric vessels. We favor having the interventional radiologists place the catheter through the left axillary artery to the appropriate side in the pelvis. After 24 or 48 hours of infusion, the catheter can be repositioned to the contralateral side or removed. We have repeated these cycles every 2 to 3 weeks, employing the same artery as the entry site without adverse effect.

CLINICAL TOXICITY

It is impossible to administer cytotoxic chemotherapy intensely without incurring a variety of adverse effects. Although therapists tend to worry most about life-threatening or permanent adverse effects, such as cardiac or renal impairment or marrow hypoplasia, these effects may be imperceptible to the patient. Of greater concern to her may be the noxious adverse effects of alopecia, nausea and vomiting, change in skin or nail pigments, mucositis with secondary dyspareunia and the inability to enjoy food, and general asthenia, especially during times of anemia or myelosuppression. Each of these effects must be addressed with sensitivity, patience, efficiency, and aggression to ensure that the patient continues a therapeutic program that is vital for her. Intimate consultation concerning cosmetics, hair prostheses, and general conduct are essential for chemotherapy patients. Also required are careful nutritional guidance, including the administration of androgens for marrow support and appetite stimulus, replacement of mineral wasting by appropriate oral and parenteral supplements, relief of mucositis by topical applications of analgesics and fungicides, and constant availability of supportive medical, social, and administrative services.

For purposes of regimen selection, the performance status of the patient can be essential. Table 46-2 depicts one scheme that measures performance, and this type of classification is frequently employed in the stratifica-

TABLE 46–2.
Gynecologic Oncology Group Criteria for Adverse Effects

SYSTEM	0	1 = MILD	2 = MODERATE	3 = SEVERE	4 = LIFE-THREATENING
*Hematologic**					
Hgb (g/dL)	>11.0	9.5–10.9	8.0–9.4	6.5–7.9	<6.5
WBC (/μL)	>4000	3000–3999	2000–2999	1000–1999	<1000
Granulocytes (/μL)	>1999	1500–1999	1000–1499	500–999	<500
Platelets (/μL)	>150,000	100,000–149,999	50,000–99,999	25,000–49,999	<25,000
Gastrointestinal					
Nausea and vomiting	None	Nausea only	Vomiting controlled by antiemetics	Vomiting 6 ×/day despite antiemetics	Life-threatening dehydration or bleeding

*Hgb = hemoglobin. Values are given in grams per deciliter. WBC = white blood cells. Values are given in number per microliter.

tion of patients for drug trials. Adverse effects often require dose reduction, and for purposes of comparing treatments, it is necessary to standardize the intensity of adverse effects and to build into each protocol standard drug reductions related to the level of toxicity. Each collaborative group has standard tables of adverse effects for most body functions. Table 46-3 depicts the hematologic adverse effects and a gastrointestinal toxicity rating system employed by the Gynecologic Oncology Group.

Effects on Gonadal Function

One of the adverse effects of chemotherapy most feared by patients in the reproductive age group is gonadal failure and infertility. Averette, Boike, and Jarrell summarized reports on the effects of chemotherapy on reproduction in men and women. In men and boys, the cytotoxic effects of chemotherapy on gonadal function have been studied by semen analysis, hormonal assessment, testicular biopsy, and observation of secondary sexual development. A cumulative dose of 18 g of cyclophosphamide produces consistent

TABLE 46–3.
Performance Scale

GRADE	CHARACTERISTICS
0	Asymptomatic
1	Symptomatic; full activity
2	Symptomatic; spends less than 50% of time in bed
3	Symptomatic; spends more than 50% of time in bed
4	Bedridden

permanent azoospermia. Nitrogen mustard and cyclophosphamide cause sterility in males treated by lymphoma. Methotrexate therapy does not appear to affect spermatogenesis. The MOPP regimen (ie, nitrogen mustard, vincristine, procarbazine, prednisone) causes sterility in patients being treated for Hodgkin's disease. Platinum-containing regimens appear to be less toxic to the gonads than other drug combinations. After male patients are treated with platinum, velban, and bleomycin, with or without doxorubicin, half retain normal sperm counts at the end of therapy, and recovery of spermatogenesis by the third year after therapy occurs in most patients. Although there are suggestions that some prepubertal boys are affected by chemotherapy, infertility is more common with age.

Ovarian failure is common among women who are treated after the age of 40 or those who have received a cumulative dose of chlorambucil of 1 g or 5.2 to 9.3 g of cyclophosphamide. Although the MOPP regimen produces amenorrhea in most female patients, treatment of patients with ovarian germ cell tumors by the combination of vincristine, dactinomycin, and cyclophosphamide produced amenorrhea in only 30%. Eleven of 16 patients who attempted pregnancy after therapy ended were able to deliver healthy children. Prepubertal girls treated with the same cytotoxic agents that cause amenorrhea in adulthood manifest no adverse effects. The children of women who were treated with cytotoxic chemotherapy do not appear to have an anomaly rate higher than the general population. Although there are reports of the efficacy of oral contraceptives in protecting ovaries during the administration cytotoxic chemotherapy (Chapman and Sutcliffe), other reports (Whithead and colleagues) are not as sanguine.

With the availability of in vitro fertilization and cryopreservation of embryos, it is incumbent upon the team treating a young woman to counsel her about the possibility of temporary amenorrhea, possible permanent ovarian failure, and irreversible infertility. A full discussion of the ethical and legal implications of cryopreservation should be conducted, and the patient's wishes should be carried out if at all possible.

Effects on the Fetus

There are three gross measurements of adverse effects on pregnancy: the rate of fetal wastage, the rate of congenital anomaly, and the ultimate performance of a child born to a mother who received chemotherapy during pregnancy. Fetal wastage is most easily measured. The incidence of fetal anomalies, although somewhat more difficult to assess immediately, can be quantified. Assessing the long-term effects on individuals gestated during chemotherapy presents a problem in follow-up and in examination. The example of the diethylstilbestrol-exposed population demonstrates how difficult evaluation of ultimate outcome can be.

Although some chemotherapeutic agents are more prominently teratogens than others, it is safest to consider all chemotherapeutic agents teratogenic, because they are designed to interrupt metabolic pathways in rapidly replicating tissues. However, it is remarkable that most of the congenital malformations observed at birth occurred in the offspring of patients who received cytotoxic chemotherapy during the first trimester of pregnancy. Patients who received chemotherapy during the first 4 weeks after the last menstrual period almost invariably abort. The period of greatest teratogenic risk is between the fifth and eleventh weeks of pregnancy. The risk is lowest in the second and third trimesters, despite exposure to the worst teratogens (ie, the antifolic chemotherapeutic agents and the alkylating agents).

In Sokal and Lessman's classic study, 50 different reports of women who received cytotoxic therapy during pregnancy were analyzed. None of the eight fetal abnormalities and 16 spontaneous abortions occurred in patients who received chemotherapy as single treatment in the second or third trimesters of pregnancy.

Cytotoxic chemotherapy should not be given during the first 4 weeks of pregnancy if fetal wastage is to be avoided. If it must be given, dose intensification should not be applied and further treatment should be avoided until the second trimester of pregnancy. Antifolates during pregnancy should be avoided if possible, and nursing should be discouraged. Patients must be counseled, and if they have been treated inadvertently during the critical portion of the first trimester, their risk of carrying a fetus with congenital anomalies requires elaboration.

CLINICAL SUMMARY

The role of cytotoxic chemotherapy in the treatment of patients with gynecologic cancers has expanded dramatically since the 1960s. Gestational trophoblastic disease can be cured by the administration of methotrexate or dactinomycin; patients with recurrent disease or patients who are at high risk can be treated with multidrug combinations that include methotrexate, dactinomycin, and chlorambucil; or that include etoposide, dactinomycin, methotrexate, folinic acid, vincristine, and cyclophosphamide.

Patients with epithelial ovarian cancers profit from cytotoxic chemotherapy or the administration of hormone or biologic therapy, except for those with low-grade, small stage I ovarian cancers. After aggressive cytoreductive surgery in patients with advanced cancer, therapy with platinum-containing regimens should produce a complete clinical response in at least 50% of the treated patients. Of those patients with optimal cytoreduction, 35% should enjoy complete pathologic responses, and in those in whom bulky disease remained, at least 15% are pathologically free of disease after chemotherapy. Patients with small residual disease can be retreated with platinum analogues other than those originally employed, or can be treated with ifosfamide, etoposide, or intraperitoneal biologic response modifiers with or without cytotoxic chemotherapy. Patients with germ cell cancers of the ovary can be treated with great success by a combination of vincristine, dactinomycin, and cyclophosphamide or by the combination of bleomycin, etoposide, and cisplatin. These tumors, once highly lethal, are now highly curable, and if confined to one ovary, reproductive function may be spared.

Endometrial carcinoma considered unsuitable for cytotoxic therapy just two decades ago is now treated with doxorubicin or cisplatin, with or without hormonal treatment, and a 30% response rate for patients with advanced or recurrent cancer can be anticipated.

Uterine sarcomas are sensitive to doxorubicin, ifosfamide, and cisplatin, and studies are underway to establish the possible superiority of combination therapy over single-agent treatment in these tumors.

Carcinoma of the fallopian tube is now understood to be treatable with regimens in common with epithelial ovarian cancers, and therapists should expect 40% to 45% of the patients to be disease free after 4 years.

Squamous cell carcinomas of the lower genital tract have not been treated with cytotoxic therapy until recently, but cisplatin and ifosfamide have been identified as active chemotherapeutic agents against these cancers and have been administered to patients with recurrent disease and employed as induction agents before combination treatment with radiation therapy or surgery.

With a better understanding of multidrug resistance, with better-defined roles for biologic response modifiers, and with improved techniques for managing adverse effects, the treatment of patients with cytotoxic chemotherapy will continue to be made more rational and more effective.

Bibliography

Ajani JA, Baker FL, Spitzer G, et al. Comparison between clinical response and in vitro drug sensitivity of primary human tumors in the adhesive tumor cell culture system. J Clin Oncol 1987; 5:1912.

Albert D, Green S, Hannigan E, et al. Improved efficacy of carboplatin/cyclophosphamide vs. cisplatin/cyclophosphamide: preliminary report of a phase III randomized trial in stages III–IV suboptimal ovarian cancer. [Abstract] Proc Am Soc Clin Oncol 1989; 8:588.

Alberts DS, Salmon SE, Moon TE, et al. Chemoimmunotherapy for advanced ovarian cancer with Adriamycin-cyclophosphamide ± BCG: early report of a Southwestern Oncology Group study. Recent Results Cancer Res 1978; 68:160.

American Cancer Society, New York, New York, data released 26 April 1990; and Pharmaceutical Manufacturers Association, data released 4 May 1990.

Averette HE, Boike GM, Jarrell MA. Effects of cancer chemotherapy on gonadal function and reproductive capacity. CA 1990; 40:199.

Beecham J, Blessing J, Creasman W, Hatch K. Tamoxifen is effective as second line therapy for certain patients with chemoresistant epithelial ovarian cancer: a Gynecologic Oncology Group study of 105 patients. [Abstract] Proc Am Soc Clin Oncol 1988; 7:135.

Bell DR, Gerlach JH, Kartner N. Detection of P-glycoprotein in ovarian cancer: a molecular marker associated with drug resistance. J Clin Oncol 1985; 3:311.

Berek JS, Martinez-Maza O, Montz FJ. Biologic response modifiers and monoclonal antibodies. In: Coppleson M, ed. Gynecologic Oncology. New York: MacMillan, 1990.

Bruckner HW, Cohen CJ, Feuer E, Holland JF. Modulation and intensification of a cyclophosphamide, hexamethylmelamine, doxorubicin and cis-platin ovarian cancer regimen. Obstet Gyncol 1988; 73:349.

Canetta R, Bragman K, Smaldone L, Rosenweig M. Carboplatin: current status and future prospects. Cancer Treat Rev 1988; 15:17.

Carlson JA Jr, Allegra JC, Day TG Jr, Wittliff JL. Tamoxifen and endometrial carcinoma: alterations in estrogen and progesterone receptors in untreated patients and combination hormone therapy in advanced neoplasia. Am J Obstet Gyncol 1984; 149:149.

Chapman RW, Sutcliffe SB. Protection of ovarian function by oral contraceptive in women receiving chemotherapy for Hodgkin's disease. Blood 1981; 58:849.

Chen CJ, Chin JE, Ueda K. Internal duplication and homology with bacterial transport proteins in the $mudr_1$ (P-glycoprotein) gene from multi-drug resistant human cells. Cell 1986; 47:381.

Cohen CJ. Therapeutic staging. In: Bruckner H, Cohen CJ, eds. Ovarian Cancer: New Approaches with Curative Intent. Morristown, NJ: Sieber and McIntyre, 1984: 37.

Creasman WT, Omura GA, Mark F, et al: A randomized trial of cyclophosphamide, doxorubicin, cis-platin with or without bacillus calmette-guerin in patients with sub-optimal stage III and IV ovarian cancer: a Gynecologic Oncology Group study. Gynecol Oncol 1990; 39:239.

Cullen TS. Cancer of the uterus, its pathology, symptomatology, diagnosis and treatment. Philadelphia: WB Saunders, 1900.

DeVita VT, Simon RM, Hubbard SM, et al. Curability of advanced Hodgkin's disease with chemotherapy. Ann Intern Med 1980; 92:587.

Dottino PD, Cohen CJ, Heller D, Bello G, Deligdisch L. Tamoxifen and endometrial neoplasia. Obstet Gynecol (Submitted for publication)

Farber S, Diamond LK, Mercer RD, Sylvester RF, Wolff JA. Temporary remissions in acute leukemia in children produced by folic acid antagonist, 4-aminopterol-glutamic acid (aminoperin). N Engl J Med 1948; 238:787.

Fornander T, Rutqvist LE, Cedermark B, et al. Adjuvant tamoxifen in early breast cancer: occurrences of new primary cancers. Lancet 1989; 1:117.

Gabrilove JL. Introduction and overview of hematopoietic growth factors. Semin Oncol 1989; 26(suppl 2):1.

Geisler EH. The use of high dose megesterol acetate in the treatment of ovarian adenocarcinoma. Semin Oncol 1985; 12(suppl 1):20.

Gilman A, Philips, FS. The biological actions and therapeutic applications of the β-chloroethyl amines and sulfides. Science 1946; 103:409.

Goldie JH, Coldman AJ. A mathematics model for relating the drug sensitivity of tumors to their spontaneous mutation role. Cancer Treat Rep 1979; 63:1727.

Gottardis MM, Robinson SP, Satyswaroop PG, Jordan VC. Contrasting actions of tamoxifen on endometrial and breast tumor growth in the athymic mouse. Cancer Res 1989; 49:2362.

Greenspan EM. Combination cytotoxic chemotherapy in advanced disseminated breast carcinoma. Mount Sinai J Med 1966; 33:1.

Gusberg SB. Precursors of corpus carcinoma: estrogen and adenomatous hyperplasia. Am J Obstet Gynecol 1947; 54:905.

Hamburger AW, Salmon SE. Primary bioassay of human tumor stem cells. Science 1977; 197:461.

Kelly RM, Baker WH. Progestational agents in the treatment of carcinoma of the endometrium. N Engl J Med 1961; 264:216.

Levin L, Hryniuk W. Dose intensity analysis of chemotherapy regimens in ovarian carcinoma. J Clin Oncol 1987; 5:756.

Li M, Hertz R, Spencer DB. Effects of methotrexate therapy upon choriocarcinoma and chioradenoma. Proc Soc Exp Biol Med 1956; 93:361.

Manetta A, MacNeill C, Lyter JA, et al. Hexamethylmelamine as a single second-line agent in ovarian cancer. Gynecol Oncol 1990; 36:93.

McGuire WP, Rowinsky EK, Rosenshein NG, et al. Taxol: a unique antineoplastic agent with significant activity in advanced ovarian epithelial neoplasms. Ann Intern Med 1989; 11:273.

McVie JG, Ten Bokkel Huinink WW, Aartsen E, et al. Intraperitoneal chemotherapy in minimal residual ovarian cancer with cis-platin and IV sodium thiosulfate protection. Proc Am Soc Clin Oncol 1985; 4:125.

Norton L, Simon R. Tumor size, sensitivity to therapy, and design of treatment schedules. Cancer Treat Rep 1977; 61:1307.

Ozols RF. Intraperitoneal chemotherapy in the management of ovarian cancer. Semin Oncol 1985; 12:1.

Ozols RF, Louie KG, Plowman J. Enhanced melphalan cytotoxicity in human ovarian cancer in vitro and in tumor-bearing nude mice by buthionine sulfoximine depletion of glutathione. Biochem Pharmacol 1987; 36:147.

Reimer PR, Hoover R, Fraumeni JF Jr. Acute leukemia after aklylating agent therapy of ovarian cancer. N Engl J Med 1977; 297:177.

Riordan JR, Deuchars K, Kartner N. Amplification of P-glycoprotein genes in multidrug resistant mammalian cell lines. Nature 1985; 316:817.

Riordan JR, Ling V. Genetic and biochemical characterization of multidrug resistance. Pharmacol Ther 1985; 28:51.

Rowinsky EK, Donehower RC, Jones RJ, Tucker RW. Microtubule changes and cytotoxicity in leukemia cell lines treated with taxol. Cancer Res 1988; 48:4093.

Salmon SE, Apple M. Cancer chemotherapy. Review of medical pharmacology. 5th ed. In: Meyers FH, Jawetz E, Goldfien A, eds. Los Altos, Calif: Lange Medical Publications, 1976: 470.

Salmon SE, Hamburger AW, Soehnlen B, et al. Quantitation of differential sensitivity of human-tumor stem cells to anti-cancer drugs. N Engl J Med 1978; 298:1321.

Schwartz PA, Merino MJ, Livolsi VA, et al. Histopathologic correlations of estrogen and progestin receptor protein in epithelial ovarian carcinomas. Obstet Gynecol 1985; 66:428.

Sikic BI, Scudder SA, Ballon SC, et al. High dose megesterol acetate therapy of ovarian carcinomas: a phase II study by the Northern California Oncology Group. Semin Oncol 1986; 13:26.

Skipper HE, Schabel FM Jr, Wilcox WS. Experimental evaluation of anticancer agents XII on the criteria and kinetics associated with "curability" of experimental tumors. Cancer Chemother Rep 1964; 35:1.

Sokal JE and Lessman EM. The effects of cancer chemotherapeutic agents on the human fetus. JAMA 1960; 172:1765.

Sotrel G, Jafari K, Lash AF. Acute leukemia in advanced ovarian carcinoma after treatment with alkylating agents. Obstet Gynecol 1976; 47:67S.

Sutton GP, Blessing JA, Photopulos G, Berman ML, Holmesley H. Gynecologic Oncology Group, experience with ifosfamide. Semin Oncol 17(suppl 4):6.

Swain SM, Lippman ME: Endocrine therapies of cancer. In: Chabner BA, Colllins JM, eds. Cancer Chemotherapy. Principles & Practice. Philadelphia: JB Lippincott, 1990:59.

Thigpen T, Blessing J, Ball H, et al. Phase II trial of Taxol as second line therapy for ovarian carcinoma; a Gynecologic Oncology Group study. Proc Am Soc Clin Oncol 1990; 9:156.

Tormey DC. On the Convergence of treatment and prevention in breast cancer. Chemotherapy Foundation Symposium IX, innovative chemotherapy for tomorrow. Cancer Invest 1990; 9(3):22.

Tsuro T, Lida H, Nojiri M. Circumvention of vincristine and adriamycin resistance in vitro and in vivo by calcium influx blockers. Cancer Res 1983; 43:2905.

Whitehead E, Shalet SM, Blackledge G, et al. The effect of combination chemotherapy on ovarian function in women treated for Hodgkin's disease. Cancer 1983, 52:988.

Index

Page numbers followed by *f* indicate figures; those followed by *t* indicate tabular material.

Emge, Ludwig, 849
Emmett, Thomas Addis, 5–6, 785
Emmett vaginal repair, 5–6
Emotional response to surgery,
14–19. *See also* Psychological
factors
anxiety as, 15
direct and indirect sexual disorders and, 17–18
grief as, 15–16
insecurity as, 14–15
offering help and, 21–22
regression and dependency as, 15
sexual dysfunction and, 17, 17t
surgeon's influence on, 18–19
touching and, 19
symbolic value of uterus and,
16–17
Emphysema
mediastinal, laparoscopy and, 380
of omentum, laparoscopy and, 380
problems associated with, 75
Endocervical curettage (ECC), in cervical intraepithelial neoplasia,
1152, 1155
Endocervical scraping, in endometrial cancer, 1262–1263
Endolymphatic stromal myosis, 1297,
1297f
Endometrial ablation
in dysfunctional uterine bleeding,
303
hysteroscopy and, 403–405
technique for, 404–405, 405f,
406f
laser, 520
Endometrial cancer, 494, 1253–1299
advanced, treatment of, 1282–1284
in clinical stage II, 1282–1283
in clinical stage III, 1283
in clinical stage IV, 1283–1284
chemotherapy in, 1289–1290
concomitant independent ovarian
cancer and, 1285
diagnosis of, 1262–1264
evaluation of symptomatic
women and, 1262–1263,
1263t
precursors of endometrial cancer and, 1264
screening and, 1262
exogenous estrogens and, 1257–
1262
oral contraceptives and, 1261
progesterone production and,
1260–1261
role of, 1258t, 1258–1260, 1259t
virulence of estrogen-induced
cancer and, 1261–1262
follow-up of, 1286–1288, 1288t

imaging techniques and, 283–284,
286f, 287f
incidence of, 1253–1255, 1254f,
1255f
postoperative treatment of, 1278t,
1279f, 1279–1282
irradiation therapy in, 1279t,
1279–1282, 1280f
prognosis for, 1286, 1286t, 1287f
prognostic factors for, 1271t,
1271–1278
age as, 1277
depth of myometrial invasion
as, 1274–1275, 1275t
histologic grade as, 1271f, 1271–
1272, 1272f, 1272t, 1273t
histologic type as, 1272–1274,
1273t
lymph node metastasis as,
1275–1277, 1276f
peritoneal cytology as, 1278
steroid receptors as, 1277–1278
tumor invasion as, 1278
radical (Clark-Wertheim) hysterectomy in, 1284
recurrence of, 1286–1288, 1288t
systemic treatment of, 1288t,
1288–1290
results of treatment of, 1286,
1286t, 1287f
risk factors associated with, 1255–
1257
diabetes mellitus as, 1256
hypertension as, 1256
obesity as, 1255–1256
syndromes of increased endogenous estrogen stimulation
as, 1256–1257
simultaneous cancers in other organs and, 1285–1286
staging of, 1264–1270
clinical, 1264, 1265t
preoperative studies and, 1265–
1267, 1266t
surgical, 1267–1270, 1270t
unsuspected, 1285
vaginal hysterectomy in, 1284–
1285
variable-level invasion limited to
adenomyosis and, 1285
Endometrial hyperplasia, 1264
adenomatous, as indication for
hysterectomy, 673
management of, 304
postmenopausal bleeding and, 304
Endometrial lavage, in endometrial
cancer, 1263
Endometrioma, imaging techniques
and, 290, 294f

Endometriosis, 463–494
adnexal masses and, 529
affecting gastrointestinal tract,
1026–1042
closed anastomosis in, 1026,
1030–1031f
colostomy in, 1035–1042, 1040–
1042f
enterostomy in, 1035, 1039f
open end-to-end anastomosis in,
1026, 1027–1029f
side-to-side anastomosis in,
1026, 1032–1033f
stapled anastomosis in, 1034–
1035, 1034–1038f
surgery of anus and rectum in,
1042
appendicitis associated with, 1003
of bladder
gross pathology of, 473
laparoscopic procedures for,
376–377
bladder injury and, 791
of bowel, laparoscopic procedures
for, 376–377
conservative surgery in, 488–491,
489f, 490f
definitive surgery in, 491–493
diagnosis of, 483–484, 484f
distribution and gross pathology
of, 468–475, 469f, 470t
evolving aspects of, 745–746. 746t
gross pathology of, 469, 471, 471f
histogenesis of, 477–479, 478f,
480–482f
histology of, 475, 476f
historical background of, 9
hormonal therapy in, 486–487,
488t
hysterectomy in, 491–492
imaging techniques and, 290
of incisional scars, gross pathology
of, 473–474
internal. *See* Adenomyosis
of intestine, gross pathology of,
472–473, 473f
irradiation in, 493
of kidney, gross pathology of, 473
laparoscopic procedures for, 376–
377
endometriosis of bladder,
bowel, and ureter and, 376–
377
ovarian endometriosis and, 376,
377f
resection and fulguration/vapor-
ization and, 376
laser surgery in, 512
fulguration or excision and, 517,
518t
laparoscopic, 513

ISBN 0-397-50835-2

9 780397 508358

90000